PRIMARY CARE OF THE

CHILD *with a* CHRONIC CONDITION

FIFTH EDITION

Patricia Jackson Allen, RN, MS, PNP, FAAN
Professor and Director
Pediatric Nurse Practitioner Specialty
Yale University School of Nursing
New Haven, Connecticut;
Professor Emerita
University of California, San Francisco
San Francisco, California

Judith A. Vessey, RN, PhD, MBA, DPNP, FAAN
Leila Holden Carroll Professor of Nursing
William F. Connell School of Nursing
Boston College
Chestnut Hill, Massachusetts

Naomi A. Schapiro, RN, PhD(c), CPNP
Associate Clinical Professor
Specialty Coordinator, Advanced Practice Pediatric Nursing Program
Department of Family Health Care Nursing
University of California, San Francisco
San Francisco, California

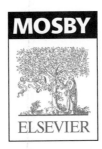

MOSBY

ELSEVIER

11830 Westline Industrial Drive
St. Louis, Missouri 63146

PRIMARY CARE OF THE CHILD WITH A CHRONIC CONDITION, Fifth Edition
Copyright © 2010, 2004, 2000, 1996, 1992 by Mosby, Inc., an affiliate of Elsevier Inc.

ISBN: 978-0-323-05877-3

Notice

Knowledge and best practice in this field are constantly changing. As new research and experience broaden our knowledge, changes in practice, treatment, and drug therapy may become necessary or appropriate. Readers are advised to check the most current information provided (i) on procedures featured or (ii) by the manufacturer of each product to be administered, to verify the recommended dose or formula, the method and duration of administration, and contraindications. It is the responsibility of the practitioner, relying on their own experience and knowledge of the patient, to make diagnoses, to determine dosages and the best treatment for each individual patient, and to take all appropriate safety precautions. To the fullest extent of the law, neither the Publisher nor the Authors assumes any liability for any injury and/or damage to persons or property arising out of or related to any use of the material contained in this book.

The Publisher

Previous editions copyrighted 1992, 1996, 2000, 2004

Library of Congress Control Number 978-0-323-05877-3

Senior Acquisitions Editor: Sandra E. Clark
Senior Developmental Editor: Cindi Crismon
Publishing Services Manager: Jeffrey Patterson
Project Manager: Mary G. Stueck
Design Direction: Paula Catalano

Printed in the United States of America

Last digit is the print number: 9 8 7 6 5 4 3 2 1

To my husband, Rick, who has become my soul mate and partner on life's journey,
To our children and their families, a continued source of pride and joy, and
To you, the health care provider, for assisting children and their families
to successfully meet the challenges of living with a chronic health condition.
Patricia Jackson Allen

To Diane and Harry, Eileen and Bill—
good friends who never cease to nourish my spirit.
Judith A. Vessey

To Kimi, whose love and support make everything possible,
and to our fabulous young adult daughters, Dannielle and Erica,
who have always managed to remind me what I didn't yet know about pediatrics.
Naomi A. Schapiro

Contributors

Patricia Jackson Allen, RN, MS, PNP, FAAN
Professor and Director
Pediatric Nurse Practitioner Specialty
Yale University School of Nursing
New Haven, Connecticut;
Professor Emerita
University of California, San Francisco
San Francisco, California
*Chapter 1.   The Primary Care Provider and Children
                       with Chronic Conditions*

Christina Baggott, APRN, BC, PhD(c), PNP, CPON
Doctoral Student
Department of Physiological Nursing
University of California, San Francisco
    School of Nursing
San Francisco, California
Chapter 16.   Cancer

Vanessa Battista, RN, MS, CPNP, CCRC
Pediatric Nurse Practitioner
Columbia University
Pediatric Neuromuscular Center/Spinal Muscular Atrophy
    Clinical Research Center
New York, New York
Chapter 34.   Muscular Dystrophy, Duchenne

Joan L. Blair, MSN, RN, PNP-BC
Pediatric Nurse Practitioner
Alfred I. duPont Hospital for Children
Division of Neurology
Wilmington, Delaware
Chapter 26.   Epilepsy

Anne Boekelheide, RN, MHSL, MSN, PNP
Nurse Coordinator for the Center for Craniofacial Anomalies
University of California, San Francisco Children's Hospital
San Francisco, California
Chapter 19.   Cleft Lip and Palate

Margaret A. Brady, PhD, RN, CPNP
Professor
Department of Nursing
California State University, Long Beach
Long Beach, California;
Adjunct Professor
School of Nursing
Azusa Pacific Universtiy
Azusa, California
Chapter 36.   Obesity

Stacy Suzanne Brown, BA
Vecinos Sanos/Healthy Neighbors Foundation
Santa Rosa, New Mexico
*Chapter 8.   Financing Health Care for Children
                     with Chronic Conditions*

Elizabeth Callard, RN, MS, PNP
Certified Pediatric Nurse Practitioner
Bone and Marrow Transplantation Program
Children's Hospital and Research Center
Oakland, California
Chapter 15.   Bone Marrow Transplantation

Julia Caschera, MSN, CPNP
Pediatric Nurse Practitioner
Annapolis Pediatrics
Annapolis, Maryland
Chapter 10.   Allergies

Angelique M. Champeau, MSN, CPNP
Pediatric Nurse Practitioner
University of California, San Francisco Children's Hospital
San Francisco, California
Chapter 20.   Congenital Adrenal Hyperplasia

Alana L. Clements, MSN, CPNP
Previously
Yale University School of Medicine, Department of Genetics
Yale–New Haven Hospital
New Haven, Connecticut
Chapter 38.   Phenylketonuria

Elizabeth H. Cook, RN, MS, PNP
Assistant Professor
Samuel Merritt University
Oakland, California
Chapter 21.   Congenital Heart Disease

Ann W. Cox, RN, PhD
Scientist and Site Coordinator
National Professional Development Center on ASD
Frank Porter Graham Child Development Institute
University of North Carolina at Chapel Hill
Chapel Hill, North Carolina
Chapter 4.   Transition to Adulthood

Donna L. Cullinan, MS, FNP-BC
Assistant Clinical Professor
William F. Connell School of Nursing
Boston College
Chestnut Hill, Massachusetts;
Family Nurse Practitioner
Milton Hospital
Milton, Massachusetts
Chapter 25.   Eating Disorders

Ginny Curtin, MS, RNC, PNP
Pediatric Otolaryngology, Head and Neck Surgery
Lucile Packard Children's Hospital at Stanford
Palo Alto, California
Chapter 19. Cleft Lip and Palate

Elizabeth A. Doyle, MSN, APRN, PNP-BC
Pediatric Nurse Practitioner
Pediatric Endocrine and Diabetes Specialists
Norwalk, Connecticut
Chapter 23. Diabetes Mellitus (Types 1 and 2)

Karen G. Duderstadt, PhD, RN, CPNP
Clinical Professor
Department of Family Health Care Nursing
University of California, San Francisco;
Pediatric Nurse Practitioner
San Francisco General Hospital
    Children's Health Center
San Francisco, California
Chapter 36. Obesity

Lisa V. Duffy, PhD(c), CPNP, CNRN
Pediatric Nurse Practitioner
Department of Neuroscience
Children's Hospital Boston
Boston, Massachusetts
Chapter 29. Hydrocephalus

Rita Fahrner, RN, MS, PNP
Clinical Nurse Specialist/Nurse Practitioner
San Francisco General Hospital
San Francisco, California
Chapter 28. HIV Infection and AIDS

Donna A. Gaffney, DNSc, PMHCNS-BC, FAAN
International Trauma Studies Program
New York, New York
Chapter 7. Ethics and the Child with a Chronic Condition

Bonnie Gance-Cleveland, PhD, RNC, PNP, FAAN
Director
Center for Improving Health Outcomes in Children, Teens,
    and Families
Arizona State University College of Nursing and Healthcare
    Innovation
Phoenix, Arizona
Chapter 36. Obesity

Mary Margaret Gottesman, PhD, RN, CPNP, FAAN
Professor, Clinical Director, Doctor of Nursing
    Practice Program
Director, Pediatric Nurse Practitioner Specialty
The Ohio State University College of Nursing
Columbus, Ohio
Chapter 36. Obesity

Margaret Grey, DrPH, RN, FAAN
Dean and Annie Goodrich Professor
Yale University School of Nursing
New Haven, Connecticut
Chapter 23. Diabetes Mellitus (Types 1 and 2)

Betsy Haas-Beckert, RN, MSN, CPNP
Adjunct Clinical Assistant Professor
University of California, San Francisco School of Nursing;
Clinical Nurse V, Pediatric Nurse Practitioner
University of California, San Francisco
San Francisco, California
Chapter 30. Inflammatory Bowel Disease

Randi Hagerman, MD
Professor of Pediatrics and Endowed Chair in Fragile X
    Research
Medical Director of the MIND Institute
University of California at Davis Medical Center
Sacramento, California
Chapter 27. Fragile X Syndrome

Leslie A. Hazle, MS, RN, CPN
Director of Patient Resources
Cystic Fibrosis Foundation
Bethesda, Maryland
Chapter 22. Cystic Fibrosis

Melvin B. Heyman, MD, MPH
Anita Ow Wing Endowed Chair
Professor of Pediatrics
Chief, Division of Gastroenterology, Hepatology,
    and Nutrition
Training Director, Pediatric GI/Nutrition
University of California, San Francisco
San Francisco, California
Chapter 30. Inflammatory Bowel Disease

Gloria C. Higgins, PhD, MD, FAAP, FACR
Associate Professor of Clinical Pediatrics
The Ohio State University
Nationwide Children's Hospital
Columbus, Ohio
Chapter 31. Juvenile Rheumatoid Arthritis

Sarah S. Higgins, PhD, RN, FAAN
Professor Emerita
University of San Francisco
San Francisco, California
Chapter 21. Congenital Heart Disease

June Andrews Horowitz, PhD, RN, PMHCNS-BC, FAAN
Professor
William F. Connell School of Nursing
Boston College
Chestnut Hill, Massachusetts
Chapter 33. Mood Disorders

Karla B. Jones, BS, MS, CPNP
Pediatric Nurse Practitioner
Nationwide Children's Hospital
Columbus, Ohio
Chapter 31. Juvenile Rheumatoid Arthritis

Susan Karp, RN, MS
Nurse Coordinator, Hemophilia Program
University of California, San Francisco
San Francisco, California
Chapter 14. Bleeding Disorders

Michelle M. Kelly, MSN, CRNP
Adjunct Clinical Faculty
Villanova University
Villanova, Pennsylvania;
Pediatric/Neonatal Nurse Practitioner
Alfred I. duPont Hospital for Children at Main Line Health
Bryn Mawr, Pennsylvania
Chapter 39. Prematurity

Gail M. Kieckhefer, PhD, PNP-BC, ARNP
Professor
The Joanne Montgomery Endowed Professor in Nursing
University of Washington;
Affiliate, Center on Human Development and Disability
and MCHB Pediatric Pulmonary Center
Seattle, Washington
Chapter 11. Asthma

Melanie S. Klein, RN, MSN, CNP
Nurse Practitioner
University Hospitals of Cleveland
Rainbow Babies and Children's Hospital
Cleveland, Ohio
Chapter 32. Kidney Disease, Chronic
Chapter 37. Organ Transplantation

Kathleen A. Knafl, PhD, FAAN
Associate Dean for Research
Francis Hill Fox Distinguished Professor
School of Nursing
University of North Carolina at Chapel Hill
Chapel Hill, North Carolina
Chapter 5. Chronic Conditions and the Family

Karen Marie Kristovich, RN, MSN, CPNP
Pediatric Stem Cell Transplant Nurse Practitioner
Lucile Packard Children's Hospital at Stanford
Palo Alto, California
Chapter 15. Bone Marrow Transplantation

Cynthia Colen Lazzaretti, RN
Clinical Coordinator
Spina Bifida, Pediatric Rehabilitation Programs
University of California, San Francisco Children's Hospital
San Francisco, California
Chapter 35. Myelodysplasia

Linda L. Lindeke, PhD, RN, CPNP
Associate Professor
School of Nursing
University of Minnesota;
Pediatric Nurse Practitioner
University of Minnesota Children's Hospital, Fairview
Minneapolis, Minnesota
Chapter 9. Systems of Care for Children with Chronic Conditions

Wendy Sue Looman, PhD, RN, CPNP
Assistant Professor
School of Nursing;
Pediatric Nurse Practitioner
Cleft Plate and Craniofacial Clinics
School of Dentistry
University of Minnesota
Minneapolis, Minnesota
Chapter 9. Systems of Care for Children with Chronic Conditions

Carol Anne Marchetti, PhD(c), RN, PMHCNS-BC, SANE
Doctoral Candidate/Clinical Nurse Specialist
William F. Connell School of Nursing
Boston College
Chestnut Hill, Massachusetts;
Behavioral Health Fellow
Harvard Vanguard Medical Associates;
Sexual Assault Nurse Examiner
Massachusetts Department of Public Health
Boston, Masachusetts
Chapter 33. Mood Disorders

Kathy Martin, MN, NP-Paeds.
Nurse Practitioner
Heart Transplant Program
The Hospital for Sick Children
Toronto, Ontario
Canada
Chapter 37. Organ Transplantation

Stephanie G. Metzger, DNP, RN, CPNP
Advanced Practice Nurse
Chester Pediatrics
Chester, Virginia;
RN Clinical Nurse IV
VCU Health System
Richmond, Virginia
Chapter 4. Transition to Adulthood

Ann Milanese, MD
Associate Professor of Pediatrics
University of Connecticut School of Medicine
Farmington, Connecticut;
Medical Director
Education and Rehabilitation Services
Connecticut Children's Medical Center
Hartford, Connecticut
Chapter 42. Traumatic Brain Injury

Wendy M. Nehring, RN, PhD, FAAN, FAAIDD
Dean and Professor
East Tennessee State University
Johnson City, Tennessee
Chapter 18.   Cerebral Palsy
Chapter 24.   Down Syndrome

Kaylie K. Nguyen, RN, MS, CPNP, CNS
Pediatric Nurse Practitioner
Department of Gastroenterology, Nutrition
    and Hepatology
Lucile Packard Children's Hospital at Stanford
Palo Alto, California
Chapter 17.   Celiac Disease

Caroline Pearson, RN, MS, CPNP
Department of Neurosurgery
University of California, San Francisco
San Francisco, California
Chapter 35.   Myelodysplasia

Robin H. Pitts, RN, MN, C-FNP
Sickle Cell Nurse Practitioner
Children's Healthcare of Atlanta;
Aflac Cancer Center
Atlanta, Georgia
Chapter 40.   Sickle Cell Disease

Marijo M. Ratcliffe, MN, ARNP
Nursing Faculty
Pediatric Pulmonary Center Training Grant
Department of Pediatrics;
Lecturer
School of Nursing
University of Washington;
Pediatric Nurse Practitioner, Pulmonary
Seattle Children's Hospital
Seattle, Washington
Chapter 11.   Asthma

Elizabeth O. Record, MSN, CPNP, DNP
Pediatric Nurse Practitioner
Children's Healthcare of Atlanta
Atlanta, Georgia
Chapter 40.   Sickle Cell Disease

Roberta S. Rehm, PhD, RN
Associate Professor
Department of Family Health Care Nursing
University of California, San Francisco
San Francisco, California
Chapter 6.   Family Culture and Chronic
    Conditions

James P. Riddel, Jr., RN, MS, CPNP
Assistant Clinical Professor/Doctoral Student
University of California, San Francisco
San Francisco, California;
Pediatric Nurse Practitioner
Hemostasis and Thrombosis Treatment Center
Children's Hospital and Research Center, Oakland
Oakland, California
Chapter 14.   Bleeding Disorders

Ann M. Riley, RN, MSN
Care Coordinator
The Special Kids Support Center
Connecticut Children's Medical Center
Hartford, Connecticut
Chapter 42.   Traumatic Brain Injury

Sostena Romano, APRN, MSN, MBA
Director and Clinical Coordinator
Global PMTCT Initiative
William J. Clinton Foundation HIV/AIDS Initiative
New York, New York
Chapter 28.   HIV Infection and AIDS

Kari Runge, RN, MS, CNS, CPNP
Pediatric Nurse Practitioner
Pediatric Gastroenterology, Hepatology, and Nutriton
Lucile Packard Children's Hospital at Stanford
Palo Alto, California
Chapter 17.   Celiac Disease

Sheila Judge Santacroce, PhD, APRN, CPNP
Associate Professor and Carol A. Beerstecher-Blackwell Chair
University of North Carolina at Chapel Hill
    School of Nursing
Advanced Practice Nurse
Chapel Hill, North Carolina
Chapter 5.   Chronic Conditions and the Family

Kathleen J. Sawin, DNS, CPNP-PC, FAAN
Professor and Research Chair in the Nursing of Children
University of Wisconsin–Milwaukee
Milwaukee, Wisconsin
Chapter 4.   Transition to Adulthood

Naomi A. Schapiro, RN, PhD(c), MS, CPNP
Associate Clinical Professor
Specialty Coordinator, Advanced Practice Pediatric Nursing
    Program
Department of Family Health Care Nursing
University of California, San Francisco
San Francisco, California
Chapter 41.   Tourette Syndrome and Obsessive-Compulsive
    Disorder

Janice Selekman, DNSc, RN, NCSN
Professor
School of Nursing
University of Delaware
Newark, Delaware
Chapter 3.   School and the Child with a Chronic Condition
Chapter 12.   Attention-Deficit Hyperactivity Disorder

Maureen Sheehan, RN, MS, CPNP
Assistant Clinical Professor
University of California, San Francisco
San Francisco, California;
Nurse Practitioner, Pediatric Neurology
Lucile Packard Children's Hospital at Stanford
Palo Alto, California
Chapter 13.   Autism Spectrum Disorder

Elizabeth Sloand, PhD, CRNP
Assistant Professor
Johns Hopkins University School of Nursing
Baltimore, Maryland
Chapter 10.   Allergies

Adrian T. Smith, BA
Research Coordinator
William F. Connell School of Nursing
Boston College
Chestnut Hill, Massachusetts
Chapter 25.   Eating Disorders

Brittney J. Sullivan, BSN
William F. Connell School of Nursing
Boston College
Chestnut Hill, Masachusetts
Chapter 2.   Chronic Conditions and Child Development

Judith A. Vessey, PhD, RN, DPNP, FAAN
Leila Holden Carroll Professor of Nursing
William F. Connell School of Nursing
Boston College
Chestnut Hill, Massachusetts
Chapter 2.   Chronic Conditions and Child Development
Chapter 3.   School and the Child with a Chronic Condition
Chapter 8.   Financing Health Care for Children with Chronic Conditions

Barbara E. Wolfe, PhD, APRN, FAAN
Associate Dean for Research and Professor
William F. Connell School of Nursing
Boston College
Chestnut Hill, Massachusetts
Chapter 25.   Eating Disorders

Reviewer

Marilyn Krajicek, RN, MS, EdD
Professor
Primary Care of Children Nursing Leadership, Pediatric
  Special Needs
University of Colorado at Denver and Health Sciences Center
  School of Nursing
Denver, Colorado

Preface

Among the greatest rewards and challenges of parenting are nourishing hopes and dreams for the child's future, and yet not knowing how or if these hopes and dreams will be realized. For parents of children who have chronic health conditions, their hopes and dreams may be more uncertain due to the unknowns associated with their child's health. Parents of children with chronic health conditions hope for the greatest quality of life and longevity for their children, with wide-ranging possibilities for an independent and fulfilling adulthood. And as pediatric primary care providers, we are committed to helping our families achieve their visions for their children's future.

Although some children with serious health conditions will die in infancy and others in childhood, most children with chronic and even life-threatening conditions now survive to adulthood. Their health care is often complex and costly, requiring multiple treatment modalities and specialists. In addition, medical responsibilities for this care have shifted from the hospital to community providers, as family members now provide treatments in the home that previously would have been the sole responsibility of professionals in acute care settings. Community-based providers, professional and lay, are shouldering this increasingly complex responsibility in the context of shrinking reimbursements and uncertainty about health care systems.

Over the past century the focus of pediatric primary care has shifted from disease management to a focus on health, including disease and injury prevention, growth and development counseling, and promoting healthy lifestyles for all children, regardless of health status. At the same time, because of the complexity of medical and surgical treatment for many chronic health conditions, primary care visits for children with chronic conditions now focus on the disease process instead of on holistic care for the child. With multiple specialties involved for some children, families and health care providers alike can overlook preventive services. Developing, implementing, and monitoring a care plan that ensures comprehensive, culturally sensitive, and family-centered care of the child, not the disease or condition, is critical in improving the quality of care for the child—and the family.

Faced with these imperatives, diverse professional and governmental agencies have launched initiatives to improve the quality of care coordination and preventive services for children with special health care needs, broadly known as a community-based medical home, or health care home (AAP, 2002; Maternal Child Health Bureau, n.d.; Perrin et al., 2007). Several models of a multidisciplinary medical home exist and are currently undergoing outcomes testing, including the participation of advanced practice nursing (Homer et al., 2008). Although the ultimate configuration of the medical home has yet to be determined, we can predict that community-based and primary health care providers will play a continuing and increasing role as the anchor of care for children living with chronic conditions.

As we go to press, we have witnessed an historic U.S. presidential election, are in the throes of a serious worldwide economic crisis, and are engaging in public dialogue that juxtaposes hope and uncertainty in new and creative ways. Families raising children, whether they are in excellent or compromised health, are coping during uncertain times with common childhood illnesses; educational challenges; uneven access to quality, affordable health care; and developmental, behavioral, and environmental health risks. For children growing up with a chronic condition, these challenges are inherently more difficult. The stresses of both the condition and its treatments may compromise their growth and development, increase their susceptibility to and severity of childhood illnesses, increase their risk of injury, and contribute to their behavioral dysfunction. Poor children have higher rates of chronic conditions, and related medical and caregiving expenses may impoverish additional families, jeopardizing their access to ongoing preventive care and illness treatment. The combined emotional, physical, and financial strains of raising a child with special health care needs can have unpredictable psychosocial effects on all family members and on overall family function.

This book provides pediatric health care professionals with the knowledge necessary to provide comprehensive primary preventive care to children with special health care needs. Part I addresses the major issues common to care of all children with chronic conditions: the role of the primary care provider, effect of a chronic condition on a child's development, school issues, family and cultural influences, transition to adulthood, ethical and cultural concerns, the financial resources—or lack thereof—available and necessary to support the care of a child with a chronic condition, and systems of care needed to coordinate primary care and specialty care for children with chronic health conditions. This knowledge is not condition specific but forms a nexus of core concepts upon which to base the delivery of care to all children with chronic conditions.

Part II identifies 33 chronic conditions found in children that necessitate alterations in standard primary care practices. Each condition-specific chapter was written by health care professionals with extensive experience in caring for the complex needs of children with the condition. Each chapter discusses the etiology, incidence, and prevalence of the condition; diagnostic criteria; clinical manifestations of the chronic condition; treatment, including complementary therapies; anticipated advances in diagnosis and treatment; and current prognosis. This information is then integrated into a primary care plan that addresses the health care maintenance, common illness management, and developmental issues needed by these children. This section stresses the importance of primary health care for children with chronic health conditions and the primary care needs are summarized at the end of each chapter for quick reference.

Decisions about which chronic conditions were included in this text were based on two criteria. First, the prevalence of the condition needed to be at least 1 in 10,000 or would likely reach this level if underreporting were not a problem. For a few other conditions, the decision of inclusion was based on how rapidly the incidence was increasing. The second criterion for inclusion was that the condition requires significant adaptations in primary care. To reflect the ever-changing landscape of chronic conditions seen in childhood, several changes have been made in the fifth edition of this text. First, in recognizing not just the many levels of care coordination, but also programs and state and federal organizations that may be involved in the care of the child with a chronic condition, the chapter on Care Coordination has been reconceptualized and renamed Systems of Care. We have also included four new condition-specific chapters in this fifth edition of *Primary Care of the Child with a Chronic Condition:* "Celiac Disease, Eating Disorders, Muscular Dystrophy, Duchenne," and "Obesity." Information on broncho-pulmonary dysplasia has been incorporated into the chapter on prematurity. Recognizing the increasing importance of addressing behavioral and mental health issues in primary care, the chapters on "Attention-Deficit/Hyperactivity Disorder" and "Mood Disorders" have had significant updates and revisions, including a discussion of the "Black box warnings" from the Food and Drug Administration about psychiatric and antiseizure medications and their implications. Last, the chapter "Head Injury" has been renamed "Traumatic Brain Injury" and "Renal Failure, Chronic" is now titled "Kidney Disease, Chronic," reflecting specialty-specific changes in nomenclature. Several changes in the headings and sub-headings for each condition-specific chapter also have been made. A section on Diagnostic Criteria has been added. Because of the rapid advancements in our understanding of the pervasive genetic basis of disease, genetic content has been incorporated into the section on etiology, and in most chapters the subheading Known Genetic Etiology has been eliminated.

Whenever possible, inclusive language regarding health care providers has been used throughout the text. We have extended this terminology to include nurse practitioners, physicians, and other health care providers because individuals with a variety of professional preparations provide primary care to children with chronic conditions. Readers will also note that the terms *patient* and *chronic illness* are rarely used and, whenever possible, we have used the wording "the child with (condition name)" rather than the "(condition name) child." Although we recognize that this sometimes makes for awkward grammar, it reflects our philosophy that children are children first instead of being defined by their condition and that wellness and illness are relative.

It would be presumptuous to edit such a text without acknowledging its scope and limitations. First, we assume that readers have a basic knowledge of growth and development and of common pediatric conditions and their management. Second, we believe there are many excellent texts available that review the diagnostic process required to determine a chronic condition in a child, so this content is covered in brief. Our intent is to provide the health care provider with a review of the condition's etiology, prevalence and incidence, clinical manifestations, and associated problems, treatment, and prognosis as a foundation for establishing a plan for primary health care. Finally, it is impossible to provide detailed information on treatment options for all secondary problems that may occur in conjunction with those highlighted. Wherever possible, readers are referred to another chapter of the text. If referral was not feasible, readers should consult the general pediatric literature for management protocols and review the extensive reference list accompanying each chapter.

The preparation of this text has been a professionally challenging and personally rewarding endeavor for us. As with any text, its successful completion depended on the help of numerous others. We wish to extend our gratitude to the contributors for their excellent, careful, and timely work and to all past contributors whose work and early development of each chapter has been so important in the evolution of this text. The contributions of the Yale University School of Nursing, the Boston College William F. Connell School of Nursing, and the University of California, San Francisco, Department of Family Health Care Nursing are recognized and sincerely appreciated. The assistance and support of the Elsevier staff editors, Sandra Clark, Cindi Crismon, and Mary Stueck are also warmly acknowledged. Their patience, humor, painstaking dedication to excellence, and commitment to the editorial process have been outstanding.

Just as parents cannot predict the futures that lie in store for their own children, we cannot predict the future of health care or even of our own professions. Yet, as the editors of this book, we can aspire to provide a solid foundation for primary health providers of many disciplines. We hope the information provided in this book will help ensure that children with chronic conditions receive more holistic family-centered primary care that will help them stay healthy, promote their growth and development, maximize their potential in all areas, and live successfully with their condition. This care can only be accomplished if health care professionals are willing to assume the challenge of providing comprehensive care to these children so they can reach their biological, intellectual, and social potential—and beyond.

Patricia Jackson Allen
Judith A. Vessey
Naomi A. Schapiro

American Academy of Pediatrics & Medical Home Initiatives for Children with Special Needs Project Advisory Committee. (2002). The medical home. *Pediatrics, 110,* 184-186.

Homer, C. J., Klatka, K., Romm, D., et al. (2008). A review of the evidence for the medical home for children with special health care needs. *Pediatrics, 122,* e922-937.

Maternal and Child Health Bureau. (n.d.) Achieving and Measuring Success: A National Agenda for Children with Special Health Care Needs. Available at http://mchb.hrsa.gov/programs/specialneeds/measuresuccess.htm. Retrieved February 22, 2009.

Perrin, J., Romm, D., Bloom, S., et al. (2007). A family-centered, community-based system of services for children and youth with special health care needs. *Arch Pediatr Adolesc Med.* 161, 933-936.

Table of Contents

PART ONE

Concepts in Pediatric Primary Care

1

The Primary Care Provider and Children with Chronic Conditions

Patricia Jackson Allen

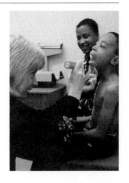

The Health of America's Children

Medical advances over the past 50 years have dramatically improved the health of children. Childhood infections have been greatly reduced through better public health, immunizations, and the development of effective antibiotic and antiviral medications. Safety standards and regulations, such as the use of infant car seats, safety caps on medications, and the removal of lead from paint, have greatly reduced the number of children with unintentional injuries. Advanced pediatric medical knowledge, surgical techniques, diagnostic procedures for infants and children, pediatric intensive care centers, and trauma centers have all improved the health outcomes of children requiring these services. Children with complex health conditions or disabilities, who previously would have died early in life, now survive; they require ongoing care and their medical needs are often complex, necessitating multiple providers to maximize the child's function and quality of life. Care, once only available in acute care hospitals, is now routinely provided by parents or community health care providers in the home, school, and community.

Child health is determined by a complex interplay of biologic, environmental, and societal factors. Children are cared for within the family unit, however defined (see Chapter 5), influenced by family culture (see Chapter 6), the family environment, socioeconomic status, and educational level, and the current health care systems in place to meet their medical or health promotion needs (see Chapter 9). A review of current child health statistics is necessary to establish the context for primary care of children with chronic conditions and their families.

Health Statistics for Children

Nationwide the number of children under 18 years of age grew 15% between 1990 and 2006 (from 63.6 million to 73.7 million) with minority children accounting for the majority of growth (Martin, Kung, Mathews, et al., 2008). In 2006, 58% of children were non-Hispanic white, 20% were Hispanic, 15% were black, 4% were Asian, and 4% were listed as other (Federal Interagency Forum on Child and Family Statistics, 2007). Children identified as Hispanic are the fastest growing racial or ethnic group, increasing from 9% of the population in 1980 to the current 20%, with a quarter of the registered births in the United States in 2005 being to Hispanic women (Hamilton, Minino, Martin, et al., 2007). It is estimated that by 2025, half of the children in America will be from a "racial minority." About one fourth of the children in the United States are immigrants, with 20% of children speaking a language other than English at home (Federal Interagency Forum on Child and

Family Statistics, 2007). Twenty-eight percent of families with foreign-born parents live below the Federal Poverty Level (FPL) (Table 1-1) and have parents with less than a high school degree (42%), both factors contributing to increased health risks in children (Federal Interagency Forum on Child and Family Statistics, 2007). Noncitizen foreign-born persons, legally or illegally residing in the United States, were estimated to number over 21 million people in 2004, or approximately 7.3% of the total population (National Center for Health Statistics [NCHS], 2007). They are disproportionately uninsured; not eligible for publicly funded supports for food, housing, or health care; and have difficulty with accessing services because of language skills (NCHS, 2007).

During the past decade only a few indicators of child health and well-being in the United States have improved, moving slowly closer to the goals and objectives of *Healthy People 2010* (Park, Brindis, Chang, et al., 2008; U.S. Department of Health and Human Services [DHHS], 2000, 2007). Child mortality rate has declined 5% from 2000 to 2005 in part because of improved medical and surgical care for children with cancer, heart disease, birth defects, and infectious disease and improved trauma services for children with unintentional and intentional injuries. Overall the pattern of mortality causes in children has not changed significantly from 2000; unintentional injuries remain the leading cause of death (42.4%) and assaults are the second leading cause of death (10.9%) in all age-groups except for children under 1 year of age (Martin et al., 2008) (Table 1-2). Although the incidence of birth defects does not vary significantly across racial groups, chronic health conditions and the incidence of injuries, with their subsequent health problems or disabilities, are more prevalent in children of racial minority groups. Gender discrepancies are now also being tracked for mortality and indicate a higher mortality rate for males in all age-groups and racial groups (U.S. DHHS, Centers for Disease Control and Prevention [CDC], NCHS, 2007) (Table 1-3).

Infant mortality rates declined slightly from 6.95 deaths per 1000 live births in 2002 to 6.89 per 1000 live births in 2005, but the infant mortality rate for non-Hispanic black infants (13.6 per 1000 live births) is over twice the rate for non-Hispanic white and Hispanic infants (5.7 per 1000 live births) and three times the rate for infants of mothers from Asia/Pacific Islands (4.5 per 1000 live births) (Hamilton et al., 2007; Martin et al., 2008). Preterm births, a major contributor to infant morbidity and mortality, have risen from 11.6% in 1998 to 12.7% in 2005 (U.S. DHHS, 2007; Martin et al., 2008). There continues to be a racial disparity for characteristics of mothers known to be associated with poor outcomes for newborns; overall, minority mothers are younger, have lower levels of education, more frequently are unmarried, are more likely

TABLE 1-1		

Poverty Guidelines for the 48 Contiguous States and the District of Columbia

Size of Family Unit	Poverty Guidelines	125% Poverty
1	$10,830	$13,538
2	$14,570	$18,213
3	$18,310	$22,888
4	$22,050	$27,563
5	$25,790	$32,238
6	$29,530	$36,913
7	$33,270	$41,588
8	$37,010	$46,263

From U.S. Department of State (n.d.). *2009 HHS poverty guidelines.* Available at http://aspe.hhs.gov/poverty/09poverty.shtml. Retrieved May 11, 2009.

to be poor, and have delayed or limited health care utilization (Hamilton et al., 2007). These social risk factors have been found to have a cumulative effect in increasing the odds that children will have poor health, increased social or emotional problems, poor dentition, and obesity (Larson, Russ, Crall, et al., 2008). Multiple factors (biologic, environmental, and societal) affect health, and there is growing recognition that situations affecting fetal and early childhood health have continued health implications into adulthood (Forrest & Riley, 2004; Mokdad, Marks, Stroup, et al., 2004).

Inequalities in Child Health

Disparities Based on Race/Ethnicity. The Institute of Medicine (IOM) released an extensive report titled *Unequal Treatment: Confronting Racial and Ethnic Disparities in Health Care* (2003). This report compiled evidence of broad-based health care disparities and individual racial discrimination in health care and health care systems that resulted in discrimination and poor quality of care provided to minority people. Although the majority of this report focused on disparities in health care for adults, the report does include discussion and analysis of research showing discrepancy in parents' reports of pediatric care under managed care by race/ethnicity (Morales, Spritzer, Elliott, et al., 2001), variable access to kidney transplant by race/ethnicity (Furth, Garg, Neu, et al., 2000), use of psychotropic medications (Zito, Safer, Riddle, et al., 1998), and use of prescription medications (Hahn, 1995). More recent reports support the disparity in health outcomes for children based on race/ethnicity and language (Andrulis, 2005; Blendon, Buhr, Cassidy, et al., 2008). For example, Hispanics who are not comfortable speaking English are less likely to have regular health care, go to an emergency department, have their prescription filled, or have health insurance (Agency for Healthcare Research and Quality [AHRQ], 2008), all factors that may result in significant consequences for children with chronic conditions.

Race, family structure (single parent vs. two parent), parent education, poverty, and culture/language are closely linked in the United States; many professionals question whether disparities in health care are more related to poverty, social class, family structure, or parent education rather than race/ethnicity (Bauman, Silver, & Stein, 2006; Committee on Pediatric Research, 2000; Shi & Stevens, 2005; Wise, 2004). In addition, disparities in access, quality, costs, health promotion, and early child development services have recently been found to have wide variation by state with strong regional patterns in quality of child health care performance; New England and the north-central states perform well on

indicators of health care access, quality, and equity for children, whereas many western and southern states did not have positive indicators of child health system performance (Shea, Davis, & Schor, 2008). Children with chronic conditions residing in regions with poorer access to health care and quality health services may not receive preventive care or early treatment of complications necessary to maintain optimal health and prevent complications from their chronic condition.

Health Insurance Coverage. There has been a gradual increase in the percentage of children with health insurance coverage over the past decade. The rise in health care coverage has been the result of increased public insurance coverage. In 2007, almost a third of children were covered by public insurance (Medicaid and State Children's Health Insurance Program [SCHIP]), and greater than 60% were covered by private insurance; 87.3% of children under 18 years of age were covered by health insurance for at least part of the year as compared with 76.6% of working-age adults, their parents (Cohen & Martinez, 2007). Unemployment and economic recessions often increase the number of children and families without private health insurance. Health care coverage for children varies dramatically by state; for example, 95% of children living in Michigan have coverage compared with only 80% of children in Texas (Shea et al., 2008). A sluggish economy and continued rise in health care costs increase the likelihood of even working families being without health care coverage for periods of time (see Chapter 8).

Disparities in coverage based on family income occur with 11.6% of poor children (less than 100% FPL) and 17.4% of near-poor children (income greater than 100% FPL but less than 200% FPL) not covered by health insurance (Cohen & Martinez, 2007). Even when coverage is available, costs of deductibles, co-pays, uncovered medical supplies or treatments, and medications can severely limit access to care and is a greater share of out-of-pocket expense in lower-income families compared to those families with higher incomes (Banthin, Cunningham, & Bernard, 2008; DeVoe, Baez, Angier, et al., 2007). The cost of health care can force families into poverty. Disparities in coverage are also present based on race; 40% (3.4 million children) of all uninsured children in the United States are Hispanic/Latino (Children's Defense Fund, 2007b) with greater than 70% of immigrant Hispanic children reported to be uninsured (Aiken, Freed, & Davis, 2004). One in eight non-Hispanic black children is uninsured (Children's Defense Fund, 2007a). Although insurance coverage is strongly correlated with access to care and utilization of health care, there is limited evidence of correlation of health insurance and health outcomes (Jeffrey & Newacheck, 2006). Multiple factors, such as poverty, education, and health behaviors, affect health. A study comparing morbidity and mortality statistics for children with public or no insurance compared to children with private insurance found that children with public insurance had significantly higher rates of hospital admissions, asthma, diabetes, vaccine-preventable diseases, psychiatric conditions, and ruptured appendix, with higher rates among nonwhite or Hispanic children than children with private insurance (Todd, Armon, Griggs, et al., 2006). Clearly, availability of insurance was not the only factor affecting health.

Inconsistent or disrupted insurance coverage is a significant barrier to health care access and utilization, especially among low-income families (Aiken et al., 2004; DeVoe et al., 2007). Children with inconsistent insurance or transitions in insurance were found

TABLE 1-2

Deaths and Death Rates for the Five Leading Causes of Death in Childhood by Age-Group, 2000 and 2005

Cause of Death by Age-Group	Rank	2005/n	2005/%	2005/Rate	2000/n	2000/%	2000/Rate
TOTAL 1-19 YEARS							
All causes		25,018	100.0	32.2	25,955	100.0	33.9
Accidents/unintentional injuries	1	10,619	42.4	13.7	11,560	45.0	15.1
Assault/homicide	2	2730	10.9	3.5	2641	10.0	3.4
Malignant neoplasm	3	2098	8.4	2.7	2179	8.0	2.8
Intentional self-harm	4	1857	7.4	2.4	1928	7.0	2.5
Congenital malformation/chromosomal abnormalities	5	1140	4.6	1.5	1119	4.0	1.5
Diseases of heart	6	756	3.0	1.0	855	3.0	1.1
Influenza/pneumonia	7	266	1.1	0.3	255	1.0	0.3
Cerebrovascular disease	8	229	0.9	0.3	190	0.7	0.2
Septicemia	9	223	0.9	0.3	202	1.0	0.3
Chronic lower respiratory disease	10	210	0.8	0.3	276	1.0	0.4
1-4 YEARS							
All causes		4749	100.0	29.3	4979	100.0	32.0
Accidents/unintentional injuries	1	1643	34.6	10.1	1826	36.7	12.0
Congenital malformations/chromosomal abnormalities	2	515	10.8	3.2	495	909	3.0
Malignant neoplasms	3	378	8.0	2.3	420	8.4	3.0
Assault/homicide	4	353	7.4	2.2	356	7.2	2.0
Disases of heart	5	147	3.1	0.9	181	3.6	1.0
5-9 YEARS							
All causes		2836	100.0	14.5	3253	100.0	15.8
Accident/unitnentional injuries	1	1070	37.7	5.5	1391	42.8	6.8
Malignant neoplasms	2	480	16.9	2.3	489	15.0	2.4
Congenita malformation/chromosomal abnormalities	3	193	6.8	1.0	198	6.1	1.0
Assault/homicide	4	120	4.2	0.6	140	4.3	0.7
Diseases of heart	5	100	3.5	0.5	106	3.3	0.5
10-14 YEARS							
All causes		3756	100.0	18.0	4160	100.0	20.3
Accidents/unintentional injuries	1	1340	35.7	6.4	1588	38.2	7.7
Malignant neoplasms	2	509	13.6	2.4	525	12.6	2.6
Intentional self-harm	3	268	7.1	1.3	300	7.2	1.5
Assault/homicide	4	215	5.7	1.0	231	5.6	1.1
Congenital malformations/chromosomal abnormalities	5	192	5.1	0.9	201	4.8	1.0
15-19 YEARS							
All causes		13,677	100.0	65.0	13,563	100.0	67.0
Accidents/unintentional injuries	1	6566	48.0	31.2	6755	49.8	33.0
Assault/homicide	2	2042	14.9	9.7	1914	14.1	9.0
Intentional self-harm	3	1587	11.6	7.5	1621	12.0	8.0
Malignant neoplasms	4	731	5.3	3.5	745	5.5	4.0
Diseases of heart	5	374	2.7	1.8	403	3.0	2.0

Data from Leading causes of death and numbers of deaths by age: United States, 1980 and 2005. (2008). In National Center for Health Statistics. *Health, United States, 2007.* Available at www.cdc.gov/nchs/data/hus/hus07. pdf#listtables.

to postpone medical care, postpone filling prescriptions (Aiken et al., 2004), have less routine care, have unmet medical needs, and have lower immunization rates (Federico, Steiner, Beaty, et al., 2007; Zhao, Mokdad, & Barker, 2004). Satchell and Pati (2005) found that preschool-age children had more frequent gaps in coverage leading to interference with routine primary health care and concerns about missed opportunities to identify health conditions early, when intervention services are most effective. They also found that children with chronic conditions were just as likely to be uninsured or have gaps in insurance as other children. When a child has an acute or a chronic health condition, postponing care or medications may have profound health consequences.

Poverty. Poverty has an overwhelming effect on family well-being in the domains of health, productivity, physical environment, emotional well-being, and family interaction (Currie & Lin, 2007; Jhanjee, Saxeena, Arora, et al., 2004; Park, Turnbull, & Turnbull, 2002). In 2006, the U.S. Census Bureau reported that there were 36.5 million people (12.3%) living in poverty (DeNavas-Walt, Proctor, & Smith, 2007). The Federal Interagency Forum on Child and Family Statistics (2007) report titled *American's Children: Key National Indicators of Well-Being, 2007* indicates over 13 million (18%) children under 18 years of age were poor (family income less than 100% of FPL), a higher rate than any other age-group, including people 65 years and older. The poverty rates were highest for black children (34%), followed by Hispanic children (28%) and white children (14%) (Table 1-4) (U.S. DHHS, CDC, NCHS, 2007). Forty-three percent of children living in single-parent female-headed households were living in poverty. The rising

TABLE 1-3

Death Rates for All Causes, by Sex, Race, Hispanic Origin, and Age: United States, Selected Years 2000, 2005

Sex, Race, Hispanic Origin, and Age	Deaths per 100,000 Resident Population		Sex, Race, Hispanic Origin, and Age	Deaths per 100,000 Resident Population	
	2000	2005		2000	2005
ALL PERSONS			**WHITE, NON-HISPANIC/LATINO MALE**		
Under 1 year	736.7	692.5	Under 1 year	658.7	625.7
1-4 years	32.4	29.4	1-4 years	32.4	29.9
5-14 years	18.0	16.3	5-14 years	20.0	17.4
15-24 years	79.9	81.4	15-24 years	103.5	105.8
MALE			**WHITE FEMALE**		
Under 1 year	806.5	762.3	Under 1 year	550.5	515.3
1-4 years	35.9	33.4	1-4 years	25.5	22.9
5-14 years	20.9	18.6	5-14 years	14.1	12.8
15-24 years	114.9	117.8	15-24 years	41.1	41.5
FEMALE			**BLACK OR AFRICAN AMERICAN FEMALE**		
Under 1 year	663.4	619.4	Under 1 year	1279.8	1179.7
1-4 years	28.7	25.1	1-4 years	45.3	36.7
5-14 years	15.0	13.9	5-14 years	20.0	19.4
15-24 years	43.1	42.7	15-24 years	58.3	51.2
WHITE MALE			**HISPANIC/LATINA FEMALE**		
Under 1 year	631.6	640.0	Under 1 year	553.6	555.4
1-4 years	29.4	30.9	1-4 years	27.5	24.5
5-14 years	17.9	17.1	5-14 years	13.4	12.0
15-24 years	108.3	110.4	15-24 years	31.7	36.6
BLACK OR AFRICAN AMERICAN MALE			**WHITE, NON-HISPANIC/LATINA FEMALE**		
Under 1 year	1,567.6	1,437.2	Under 1 year	530.9	496.5
1-4 years	54.5	46.7	1-4 years	24.4	22.2
5-14 years	28.2	27.0	5-14 years	13.9	12.9
15-24 years	181.4	172.1	15-24 years	42.6	42.2
HISPANIC OR LATINO MALE					
Under 1 year	637.1	670.2			
1-4 years	31.5	33.2			
5-14 years	17.9	15.3			
15-24 years	107.7	120.4			

From U.S. Department of Health and Human Services, Centers for Disease Control and Prevention, National Center for Health Statistics. (2007). *Health, United States, 2007.* Hyattsville, MD: National Center for Health Statistics.

price of oil and the related increased cost of gasoline, heating fuel, and food will increase the number of families facing difficulty meeting monthly household expenses (Krauss, 2008).

Lower family income is associated with poorer health in children with a cumulative effect; the longer the child experiences poverty, the greater the health problems the child will have (Chen, Martin, & Matthews, 2007; Malat, Oh, & Hamilton, 2005). Poverty is associated with higher odds for activity limitations, school problems, behavior problems, asthma, exposure to environmental pollutants, exposure to regular in-home smoking, obesity, substantiated child abuse, untreated dental caries, and high blood lead levels (Chen et al., 2007; Federal Interagency Forum on Child and Family Statistics, 2007). Parents living at or below the poverty level were more than twice as likely to report that their children were in good, fair, or poor health versus excellent or very good health as compared with parents' report of children living above the poverty level (34.9% vs. 15.5%). Additionally, children living at or below the FPL had higher rates of chronic conditions (18.1%

vs. 13.9%) and greater frequency of activity limitations (9.3% vs. 7.3%) (Bauman et al., 2006).

Food Insecurity. Poverty is often associated with food insecurity, the ability of the family to have access at all times to enough food for all members to support an active, healthy life (Federal Interagency Forum on Child and Family Statistics, 2007). The food security status of a household is determined by parental report of difficulty in obtaining enough food for each member, reduced food intake or food quality caused by inability to secure food, or concerns about being able to provide sufficient food for all family members. In 2005, 17% of children (12 million) resided in households classified as food insecure, but over 42% of children living in households at or below the poverty level were reported to have food insecurity (Federal Interagency Forum on Child and Family Statistics, 2007). Of particular concern is food insecurity in households with infants and young children when adequate nutrition is critical for brain growth and early development (Rose-Jacobs, Black, Casey, et al., 2008). One in eight households

TABLE 1-4

Persons and Families below Poverty Level, by Selected Characteristics, Race, and Hispanic Origin: United States, Selected Years 2000, 2005

All Persons/ Selected Characteristics	Percent Below Poverty	
	2000	**2005**
All races	11.3	12.6
White only	9.5	10.6
Black or African American only	22.5	24.9
Asian only	9.9	11.1
Hispanic or Latino only	21.5	21.8
White only/non-Hispanic	7.4	8.3
RELATED CHILDREN UNDER 18 YEARS OF AGE IN FAMILIES		
All races	15.6	17.1
White only	12.4	13.9
Black or African American only	30.9	34.2
Asian only	12.5	11.0
Hispanic or Latino only	27.6	27.7
White only/non-Hispanic	8.5	9.5
RELATED CHILDREN UNDER 18 YEARS OF AGE IN FAMILIES WITH FEMALE HOUSEHOLDER AND NO SPOUSE PRESENT		
All races	40.1	42.8
White only	33.9	38.8
Black or African American only	49.3	50.2
Asian only	38.0	25.6
Hispanic or Latino only	49.8	50.2
White only/non-Hispanic	28.0	33.1

From U.S. Department of Health and Human Services, Centers for Disease Control and Prevention, National Center for Health Statistics. (2007). *Health, United States, 2007.* Hyattsville, MD: National Center for Health Statistics.

(12.6%) with an infant is reported to be food insecure with this rising to one in six (16.1%) in immigrant households and greater than one in four (29%) in households living at or below the FPL (Bronte-Tinkew, Zaslow, Capps, et al., 2007).

Research has indicated potential long-term risks of food insecurity such as poorer quality-of-life indicators (Casey, Szeto, Robbins, et al., 2005; Vozoris & Tarasuk, 2003), early childhood obesity (Bronte-Tinkew et al., Center on Hunger and Poverty, 2002), maternal depression, less positive parenting, and behavior problems in children (Whitaker, Phillips, & Orzol, 2006). Family food insecurity has not been found to adversely affect diet as compared with children in families without food insecurity. This finding reportedly reflected the overall poor quality of nutrition in children in the United States as measured by the Healthy Eating Index (HEI), Centers for Disease Control and Prevention, National Health and Nutrition Survey (Federal Interagency Forum on Child and Family Statistics, 2007). Children in families with incomes below the poverty level had equal levels of diets that were poor (9%) or needing improvement (65%) as children whose families had incomes above the poverty level.

Chronic and Disabling Conditions in Children

There are basic differences in the type and profile of chronic conditions in children and adults. Children are affected by a wide spectrum of rare conditions and genetic or prenatal conditions, whereas adults are affected by a relatively small number of common conditions (e.g., heart disease, emphysema, hypertension, diabetes) that increase in morbidity with age. Children with chronic conditions have unique health and social needs. Chronic conditions in children are often not stable but subject to acute exacerbations and remissions that are superimposed on the child's growth and development. Children also depend on adults for care. Parent/family health, ethnicity, culture, socioeconomic status, education, and source of health care insurance all affect the child's access to services, use of services, and adherence to management plans.

Chronic Conditions in Children. The number of children who have a chronic condition and the relative severity of the conditions are unknown. Estimates of children with chronic conditions depend on the definition and method used to identify them (van der Lee, Mokkink, Grootenhuis, et al., 2007). Stein and Silver (1999) defined chronic conditions in children as conditions that at the time of diagnosis or during their expected course would produce one or more of the following current or future long-term sequelae: limitation of functions appropriate for age and development, disfigurement, dependency on medication or special diet for normal functioning or control of condition, dependency on medical technology for functioning, need for more medical care or related services than usual for the child's age, or special ongoing treatments at home or in school. Perrin (2002, p. 303) defined chronic conditions in children as simply "health conditions that at the time of diagnosis are predicted to last longer than 3 months." The prevalence of children with chronic health conditions varied depending on the definition used; Stein and Silver (1999) estimated that 14.8% of children had chronic health conditions whereas Perrin estimated that up to 31% of children under 18 years of age had chronic health conditions.

The incidence of many chronic conditions has not changed over the past decade (CDC, 2008) (see Chapters 22, 34, 38, and 40), but the prevalence of children affected has increased as a result of improved treatments increasing survival (see Chapters 14, 16, 21, and 37) and enhanced recognition (see Chapters 13, 17, 25, 33, and 41). The incidence of some chronic health conditions has increased (see Chapters 11, 12, 23, and 36) because of a variety of social, environmental, dietary, perinatal, and genetic conditions, all with long-term consequences for child and adult health (Perrin, Bloom, & Gortmaker, 2007) and with considerable implications for future health care utilization and costs (van der Lee et al., 2007).

Children with Special Health Care Needs (CSHCN). In 1995, the federal Maternal and Child Health Bureau's Division of Services for Children with Special Health Care Needs (DSCSHCN) established a group of professionals to develop a definition of children with special health care needs (McPherson, Arango, Fox, et al., 1998). Health, education, and social policy changes, as well as changes in child health and disability patterns, warranted a definition that was easily understood and used by federal and state programs for planning and developing comprehensive community-based, family-centered services for children with special health care needs. While this new definition was being created, eligibility criteria for existing state and federal Title V programs, special education, and Supplemental Security Income (SSI) programs were reviewed. The following definition was developed:

"Children with special health care needs are those who have or are at risk for a chronic physical, developmental, behavioral, or emotional condition and who also require health and related services of a type or amount beyond that required by children generally" (McPherson et al., 1998, p. 138).

This definition of children with special health care focuses on the criterion of need for additional services instead of an identified medical condition or functional impairment, recognizing the variability in condition severity, degree of impairment, and service needs among children with the same or differing diagnosis. This definition also recognizes that children at risk for developing chronic hysical, developmental, behavioral, or emotional conditions because of biologic or environmental characteristics also require health and related services beyond those generally required by children (McPherson et al., 1998; Newacheck, Rising, & Kim, 2006).

In 1998 the Child and Adolescent Health Measurement Initiative (CAHMI), a national collaborative coordinated by the Foundation for Accountability, brought together a task force of federal and state policymakers, pediatric health care providers, researchers, and consumer groups to develop a method to identify children with special health care needs based on the new definition. The Children with Special Health Care needs (CSHCN) Screener was developed by this task force (Box 1-1) (Bethell, Read, Stein, et al., 2002; van Dyck, McPherson, Strickland, et al., 2002). This short, five-question parent report screening tool identifies children based not on diagnosis but on functional limitation or service use needs that are the direct result of an ongoing physical, emotional, behavioral, developmental, or other health condition and should determine more accurately the prevalence of children with special health care needs in studied populations (Bethell, Read, Blumberg, et al., 2008).

The CSHCN Screener has been used in several large-scale population-based surveys to estimate prevalence of CSHCN (Bethell et al., 2008). The 2001 National Survey of Children with Special Health Care Needs (NS-CSHCN), the 2003 National Survey of Children's Health (NSCH), and the 2001–2004 Medical Expenditures Panel Survey (MEPS) used the questions from the CSHCN Screener to estimate prevalence and characteristics of CSHCN. Bethell and colleagues (2008) found that the prevalence estimates for CSHCN varied significantly by study ranging from the 2004 MEPS estimate of 18.8%, the 2003 NSCH estimate of 17.6%, and the 2001 NS-CSHCN finding of 12.8%. Across studies the most common criterion for identification of a special health care need was the need for prescription medications and the least common was the need for specialized therapies. The 2004 MEPS, the NS-CSHCN, and the NSCH datasets all indicated that an adjusted odds for special needs in children was greater for children living in poverty. Bethell and colleagues (2008) concluded that methodologic differences largely accounted for the variance in findings and that prevalence estimates would be best expressed as a range from 13% to 20% for CSHCN. Unfortunately, the CSHCN Screener does not identify children at risk because of genetic, social, and environmental factors or the notion of susceptibility and resilience (Newacheck et al., 2006).

The State and Local Integrated Telephone Survey (SLAITS) of Children with Special Health Care Needs (CSHCN), 2005–2006. In 2000 the Maternal and Child Health Bureau (MCHB) partnering with the National Center for Health Statistics (NCHS) created the State and Local Integrated Telephone Survey (SLAITS) to determine the prevalence and impact of special health care needs among children, using the definition of children with special health care needs (van Dyck et al., 2002). The initial SLAITS of CSHCN was collected in 12 languages between October 2000 and March 2002 and provided baseline data for *Healthy People 2010*. The survey was repeated again in 2005–2006 with many of the survey questions revised and indicators

redefined to improve the study design, making direct comparisons with the 2001 survey not possible in all areas (U.S. DHHS, Health Resources and Service Administration [HRSA], MCHB, 2007).

The 2005–2006 SLAITS of CSHCN found that a national prevalence of 13.9% of children from 0 to 17 years, 10.2 million children, met the definition of "children with special health care needs," and 21.8% of households with children had at least one child with special health care needs, both increases from 2001 (12.8% and 20%, respectively). These increases may indicate a true increase in prevalence or increased recognition by parents or providers of special health care needs. Significant variations were found with parents of Hispanic and Asian children reporting fewer children with special health care needs than parents of either non-Hispanic white or non-Hispanic black children (Figure 1-1). The reasons for this finding are unknown but may be associated with non-English fluency, because Hispanic parents who spoke English as their primary language reported a 13% prevalence for having a child with special health care needs, consistent with other racial groups, whereas parents who spoke Spanish only indicated a 4.6% prevalence. Prevalence of children with special health care needs was found to increase with age (Figure 1-2). This generally mirrors other studies on child health, reflecting the increased identification of children with chronic conditions limiting school participation or requiring related special services (see Chapter 3) and conditions not diagnosed until later in childhood.

Conditions and functional limitations were tabulated from parent reports. Table 1-5 identifies a list of selected conditions reported by parents in the 2005–2006 survey as present in 91% of their CSHCN; parents indicated that one third of their children with special health care needs had two or more of the conditions and a quarter of the children had three or more of the listed conditions (U.S. DHHS, HRSA, MCHB, 2007). When asked about functional difficulties, 57% of parents of CSHCN indicated that their child had difficulty with at least one bodily function, such as eating, dressing, or bathing; 50% said their child had difficulty with participation in some activity, such as walking or running; and 42% indicated emotional or behavioral difficulties in function. Fifteen percent of CSHCN were reported as not having any functional limitations, with 90% indicating that this lack of functional limitation was due to adequate treatment of their chronic condition. CSHCN had a combination of functional limitations as depicted in Figure 1-3, and the percent of CSHCN with functional difficulty was significantly higher in children living at or below the FPL (Figure 1-4). The impact of the child's condition on daily activities was also significantly greater in poor families (Figure 1-5). The type of chronic condition and functional involvement affects health care service needs. Table 1-6 lists the percentage of CSHCN needing specific health services, and Figure 1-6 identifies the variation in health services needed by the child's level of functional ability.

Insurance coverage for the previous 12 months for CSHCN increased from 88% to 91% between the 2001 and 2005–2006 SLAITS for CSHCN as a result of increased public insurance coverage. Fourteen percent of families living below 200% FPL were uninsured for some period of time in the past 12 months as compared with less than 3% of children in families living at 400% of FPL. Hispanic children were twice as likely as non-Hispanic white children to have been uninsured (15.1% vs. 7.1%). Overall, one third of parents with insurance for their child reported that the insurance was inadequate because it did not allow them to see necessary providers (9.3%), the benefits did not meet the perceived

BOX 1-1

Children with Special Health Care Needs (CSHCN) Screening Tool (Mail or Telephone)

1. Does your child currently need or use *medicine prescribed by a doctor* (other than vitamins)?
   Yes → Go to Question 1a
   No → Go to Question 2
   1a. Is this because of ANY medical, behavioral, or other health condition?
      Yes → Go to Question 1b
      No → Go to Question 2
   1b. Is this a condition that has lasted or is expected to last for *at least* 12 months?
      Yes
      No

2. Does your child need or use more *medical care, mental health,* or *educational services* than are usual for most children of the same age?
   Yes → Go to Question 2a
   No → Go to Question 3
   2a. Is this because of ANY medical, behavioral, or other health condition?
      Yes → Go to Question 2b
      No → Go to Question 3
   2b. Is this a condition that has lasted or is expected to last for *at least* 12 months?
      Yes
      No

3. Is your child *limited* or *prevented* in any way in his or her ability to do the things most children of the same age can do?
   Yes → Go to Question 3a
   No → Go to Question 4
   3a . Is this because of ANY medical, behavioral, or other health condition?
      Yes → Go to Question 3b
      No → Go to Question 4
   3b. Is this a condition that has lasted or is expected to last for *at least* 12 months?
      Yes
      No

4. Does your child need or get *special therapy,* such as physical, occupational, or speech therapy?
   Yes → Go to Question 4a
   No → Go to Question 5
   4a. Is this because of ANY medical, behavioral, or other health condition?
      Yes → Go to Question 4b
      No → Go to Question 5

4b. Is this a condition that has lasted or is expected to last for *at least* 12 months?
   Yes
   No

5. Does your child have any kind of emotional, developmental, or behavioral problem for which he or she needs or gets *treatment* or *counseling*?
   Yes → Go to Question 5a
   No
   5a. Has this problem lasted or is it expected to last for *at least* 12 months?
      Yes
      No

SCORING THE CHILDREN WITH SPECIAL HEALTH CARE NEEDS (CSHCN) SCREENING TOOL

Conceptual Background

The CSHCN screener uses consequences-based criteria to screen for children with chronic or special health needs. To qualify as having chronic or special health needs, the following set of conditions must be met:
   1. The child currently experiences a specific consequence.
   2. The consequence is due to a medical or other health condition.
   3. The duration or expected duration of the condition is 12 months or longer.
The first part of each screener question asks whether a child experiences one of five different health consequences:
   1. Use or need of prescription medication
   2. Above average use or need of medical, mental health, or educational services
   3. Functional limitations compared with others of same age
   4. Use or need of specialized therapies (occupational, physical, speech, etc.)
   5. Treatment or counseling for emotional or developmental problems
The second and third parts* of each screener question ask those responding "yes" to the first part of the question whether the consequence is due to any kind of health condition and if so, whether that condition has lasted or is expected to last for at least 12 months.
All three parts* of at least one screener question (or in the case of question 5, the two parts) must be answered "yes" for a child to meet CSHCN screener criteria for having a chronic condition or special health care need.
The CSHCN screener has three "definitional domains":
   1. Dependency on prescription medications
   2. Service use above that considered usual or routine
   3. Functional limitations

The definitional domains are not mutually exclusive categories. A child meeting the CSHCN screener criteria for having a chronic condition may qualify for one or more definitional domains (see diagram below).

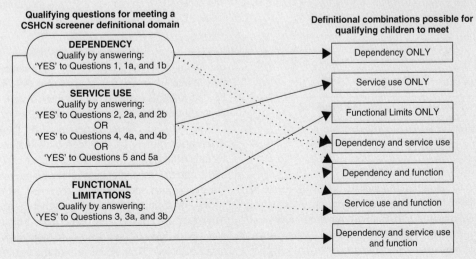

From FACCT: Foundation for Accountability CAMHI project/Chronic condition screener, January 2000. Reprinted with permission.
*Note: CSHCN screener question 5 is a two-part question. Both parts must be answered "yes" to qualify.

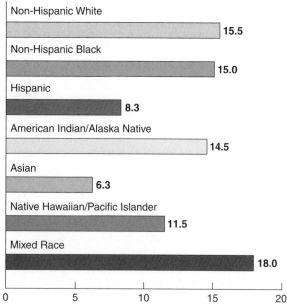

FIGURE 1-1 Prevalence of CSHCN: Race/ethnicity. (From U.S. Department of Health and Human Services, Health Resources and Services Administration. [n.d.]. *National survey of children with special health care needs chartbook 2005-2006.* Available at http://mchb.hrsa.gov/cshcn05/MI/intro.htm. Retrieved June 10, 2008.)

TABLE 1-5
Percent of CSHCN with Selected Conditions

Condition	Percentage (%)
Allergies	53.0
Asthma	38.8
Attention-deficit disorder; attention-deficit/hyperactivity disorder	29.8
Depression, anxiety, or other emotional problems	21.1
Migraine or frequent headaches	15.1
Mental retardation	11.4
Autism or autism spectrum disorder	5.4
Joint problems	4.3
Seizure disorder	3.5
Heart problems	3.5
Blood problems	2.3
Cerebral palsy	1.9
Diabetes	1.6
Down syndrome	1.0
Muscular dystrophy	0.3
Cystic fibrosis	0.3

Data from U.S. Department of Health and Human Services, Health Resources and Services Administration. (n.d.). *National survey of children with special health care needs chartbook 2005-2006.* Available at http://mchb.hrsa.gov/cshcn05/MI/intro.htm. Retrieved June 10, 2008.

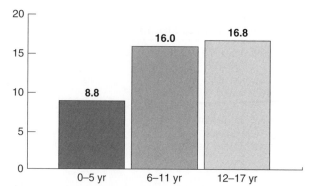

FIGURE 1-2 Prevalences of CSHCN: Age. (From U.S. Department of Health and Human Services, Health Resources and Services Administration. [n.d.]. *National survey of children with special health care needs chartbook 2005-2006.* Available at http://mchb.hrsa.gov/cshcn05/MI/intro.htm. Retrieved June 10, 2008.)

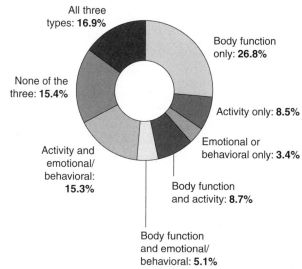

FIGURE 1-3 Distribution of functional difficulties among CSHCN. (From U.S. Department of Health and Human Services, Health Resources and Services Administration. [n.d.]. *National survey of children with special health care needs chartbook 2005-2006.* Available at http://mchb.hrsa.gov/cshcn05/MI/intro.htm. Retrieved June 10, 2008.)

uninsured children. Children who were uninsured had the greatest percentage of unmet health services (44.7%), problems getting needed referrals (39.2%), and highest overall out-of-pocket annual expenditures for health care needs for their CSHCN (see Chapter 8).

The *financial burden* experienced by families with CSHCN is determined largely by the degree of functional ability of the affected child, time required by parents or caretakers to care for the child, and the impact this has on the employment of the caretakers, family income, and insurance coverage. Almost 34% of families caring for children whose daily activities was affected "usually," "always," or "a great deal" experienced financial burden as compared with 7.5% of families where the child's daily activities were never affected. Time spent providing, arranging, or coordinating health care for CSHCN varied significantly, with 47% of families spending less than 1 hour per week in these activities, 34% spending

needs of the child (12.7%), and 28% indicated that the costs of health care needs covered by the insurance were not reasonable. Figure 1-7 shows the percent of CSHCN with reported health services needed but not received. Interestingly, families with private insurance and higher incomes were more likely to have higher out-of-pocket health expenses for their CSHCN than low-income families covered by Medicaid and SCHIP but not as high as for

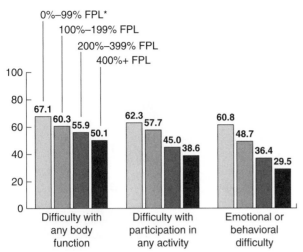

FIGURE 1-4 Percent of CSHCN with each type of functional difficulty: Family income. (From U.S. Department of Health and Human Services, Health Resources and Services Administration. [n.d.]. *National survey of children with special health care needs chartbook 2005-2006.* Available at http://mchb.hrsa. gov/cshcn05/MI/intro.htm. Retrieved June 10, 2008.)
*Federal Poverty Level, In 2005, the HHS poverty guidelines defined 100% of poverty as $19,350 for a family of four.

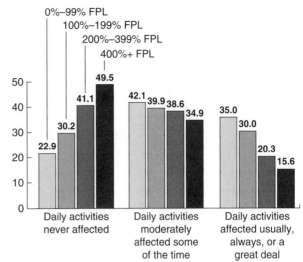

FIGURE 1-5 Impact of child's condition: Family income. (From U.S. Department of Health and Human Services, Health Resources and Services Administration. [n.d.]. *National survey of children with special health care needs chartbook 2005-2006.* Available at http://mchb.hrsa.gov/cshcn05/MI/intro.htm. Retrieved June 10, 2008.)

TABLE 1-6

Percent of CSHCN Needing Specific Health Services

Health Service	Percentage (%)
Prescription drugs	86.4
Preventive dental care	81.1
Routine preventive care	77.9
Specialty care	51.8
Eyeglasses/vision care	33.3
Mental health care	25.0
Other dental care	24.2
Physical, occupational, or speech therapy	22.8
Disposable medical supplies	18.6
Durable medical equipment	11.4
Hearing aids/hearing care	4.7
Home health care	4.5
Mobility aids/devices	4.4
Substance abuse treatment	2.8
Communication aids/devices	2.2

Data from U.S. Department of Health and Human Services, Health Resources and Services Administration. (n.d.). *National survey of children with special health care needs chartbook 2005-2006.* Available at http://mchb.hrsa.gov/cshcn05/MI/intro.htm. Retrieved June 10, 2008.

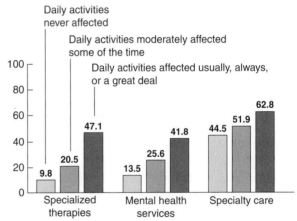

FIGURE 1-6 Percent of CSHCN needing specific health services: Impact of child's condition on functional ability. (From U.S. Department of Health and Human Services, Health Resources and Services Administration. [n.d.]. *National survey of children with special health care needs chartbook 2005-2006.* Available at http://mchb.hrsa.gov/cshcn05/MI/intro.htm. Retrieved June 10, 2008.)

1 to 4 hours per week, almost 9% spending 5 to 10 hours per week, and almost 10% spending over 11 hours per week. Time burden was greater on low-income families, with nearly 19% of poor families spending at least 11 hours per week providing needed care as compared with only 4.3% of families living at or above 400% FPL. Families with children whose activities were affected "usually," "always," or "a great deal" were also more likely (23.5%) to spend greater than 11 hours per week in care of their children, and 47%

reported having to cut back on work or stop altogether, affecting family income and sometimes insurance coverage. Only 3.2% of parents of children without limitations in daily activities reported spending more than 10 hours per week in time providing, arranging, or coordinating health care for their child and only 9% reported cutting back on work to care for the child. Families of uninsured children reported the highest financial burden (42%) as compared with those with public insurance (19.5%) and private insurance

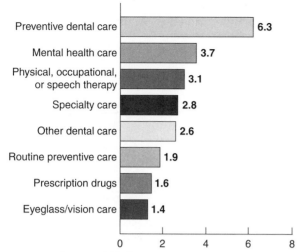

FIGURE 1-7 Percent of CSHCN with reported health services needed but not received. (From U.S. Department of Health and Human Services, Health Resources and Services Administration. [n.d.]. *National survey of children with special health care needs chartbook 2005-2006.* Available at http://mchb.hrsa. gov/cshcn05/MI/intro.htm. Retrieved June 10, 2008.)

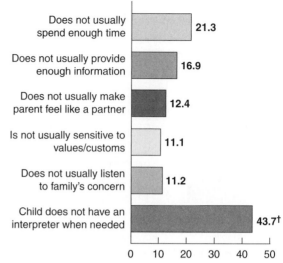

FIGURE 1-8 Percent of CSHCN who did not receive family-centered care: Individual component.* (From U.S. Department of Health and Human Services, Health Resources and Services Administration. [n.d.]. *National survey of children with special health care needs chartbook 2005-2006.* Available at http://mchb. hrsa.gov/cshcn05/MI/intro.htm. Retrieved June 10, 2008.)
*Parents reported that care did not "usually or always" meet this criterion.
[†]Among children who needed interpreter services.

(15%); the financial burden is higher on families of children with public insurance even though out-of-pocket expenses are lower because family income is lower, so costs are proportionally higher than for higher-income families.

Source of health care and availability of care consistent with the philosophy of a "medical home" for the CSHCN were also tabulated from parental response to questions in the 2005–2006 survey. Overall, 94% of CSHCN had at least one personal health care provider, nurse or doctor, overseeing their care and a usual source of care, with the vast majority (74%) receiving care in a private health care office. When parents were asked if they usually received help with coordinating services when needed and were satisfied with the communication between providers involved with the care of their child, components of coordinated care and the "medical home" initiative, only 46% of parents responded that they were satisfied with both components. Lack of communication between providers was the major concern; over half of the parents reported that they did not need assistance with coordinating services because they only saw one provider or the parents coordinated the care themselves.

The 2005–2006 survey asked several questions to determine if families were receiving family-centered care. Figure 1-8 identifies the percent of families reporting that they did not "usually" or "always" receive components of family-centered care, with 35% of families reporting that their care lacked one or more of the defining characteristics of family-centered care. Lack of satisfactory family-centered care was more common in families with incomes at or below the FPL (50%), and in children who were uninsured (55.4%) as compared with children with public insurance (44%) or private insurance (28.4%). As the level of functional difficulties increased from daily activities "never affected" to daily activities "usually" or "always" affected, the frequency of family-centered care not being reported by parents increased also (26% to 44%). In addition, family-centered care recognizes that families are the ultimate decision makers for their children until

the child matures and assumes this responsibility, and therefore optimal care is provided when health care providers partner with families to provide care and make informed health care decisions (Council on Children with Disabilities, 2007). Fifty-seven percent of parents of CSHCN reported that they usually or always felt like a partner and were very satisfied with the child's care. Families below 100% FPL reported feeling like partners in care and satisfied with care only 50% of the time as compared with 65% of families with incomes greater than 400% FPL. Seventy percent of families whose children's daily activities were "never affected" reported satisfaction as compared with 42% of families whose children's daily activities were affected "usually" or "always."

Disabilities in Children. Definitions of disability have also been changing in an attempt to standardize data collection to determine prevalence estimates and characteristics of children with disabilities. Common components of most definitions of disabilities are as follows: having a particular need for services (i.e., daily medication, respiratory therapy, routine catheterization); having a diagnosis of a physical or mental condition commonly associated with being disabled (i.e., mental retardation, hearing loss, cystic fibrosis); or exhibiting specific functional deficits that alter a person's ability to perform activities of daily living or require some means of accommodation (i.e., needing a wheelchair for mobility, needing gavage feedings, being blind) (NCHS, 2007; Westbrook, Silver, & Stein, 1998). Children with severe disabilities or functional limitations often have greater needs for services, including specialized educational services, care coordination, and referrals to specialists, and greater unmet needs than CSHCN without functional limitations (Nageswaran, Silver, & Stein, 2008). These complex care needs often result in parents feeling that the care provided their children is insufficient and that providers do not spend enough time in care of their child, do not provide enough information to parents, do not listen carefully, or do not make families partners in care of their child (Nageswaran et al., 2008).

The World Health Organization (WHO) has tried to standardize the definition and screening method for determining disabilities in people (Mbogoni & Me, 2002). Cultural variations in expected functions and recognition of the stigma often associated with disability impeding full inclusion of the individual in his or her environment have resulted in an International Classification of Functioning, Health, and Disability (ICF) (Clancy & Andersen, 2002). The definition of *disability* used by the WHO is "a person who is limited in the kind or amount of activities that he or she can do because of ongoing difficulties due to a long-term physical condition, mental conditions or health problems" (United Nations, 1998). The classic functions used to determine disability in adults (the ability to work, to perform household chores, and to care for oneself independently) are not appropriate in determining ability in children. Limitations in activities associated with play, the ability to attend and succeed in school, and the ability to develop self-care activities are more appropriate indicators of ability or limitations in children. In 2007, the WHO published the *International Classification of Functioning, Disability and Health: Children and Youth Version* (ICF-CY). The ICF-CY attempts to provide a common and universal language to facilitate the documentation and measurement of health and disability in children and youth so measurements can be used across disciplines, governments, and national boundaries. The documentation of disabilities in children is in support of the 1989 United Nations (UN) Convention on the Rights of the Child and the 2006 UN Convention on the Rights of Persons with Disabilities. ICF-CY describes children and youth with disabilities in two parts, each with two components (Box 1-2). A coding system has been developed to identify abilities or impairments in each of these areas as they apply to the normal activities and development during childhood. It is unclear at this time if this form of documentation will be adopted in the United States.

Barriers to Quality Comprehensive Care for Children with Special Health Care Needs

Lack of awareness or knowledge regarding health care needs may contribute to health care needs not being met. A health care need may go unrecognized by child, family, or primary care provider because of inconsistent care, inability to access a specialist, lack of knowledge regarding the benefit of specific care, or language or cultural differences. Family/social complexities (i.e., poverty, mental health problems, competing family demands) or chronic condition complexities may overshadow the perceived need for certain treatments or routine health care, such as immunizations or vision and hearing screening. Transportation to appropriate health facilities may be difficult or expensive or access to specialists may be restricted by lack of availability in a geographic region.

Availability of insurance and the adequacy of insurance positively affect access to care and utilization of care (Jeffrey & Newacheck, 2006). Some low-income families with CSHCN without insurance may be eligible for Medicaid or SCHIP but unaware of their eligibility or believe that the application process is too complicated to complete (Haley & Kenney, 2007). Some children

---

> **BOX 1-2**
>
> ## World Health Organization (WHO) International Classification of Functioning, Disability, and Health: Children and Youth Version, 2007
>
> Part 1. Functioning and disability
>   a. *Body functions and structures:* Identifies physiologic functions of body systems or anatomic parts of the body
>   b. *Activities and participation:* Identifies the ability of the child to execute a task or action or participate in activities of daily living
> Part 2. Contextual factors
>   a. *Environmental factors:* The physical, social, and attitudinal environment that supports or impedes the function of the child
>   b. *Personal factors:* Attributes such as race, gender, education, habits, coping styles; past and current experiences that foster ability or disability

Adapted from World Health Organization (WHO). (2007). *International Classification of Functioning, Disability and Health: Children and Youth Version.* Geneva, Switzerland: WHO Press.

---

with insurance, either public or private, are termed "underinsured" if their insurance coverage does not provide necessary health care services, their insurance coverage does not allow the child to see needed health care providers, or reasonable costs are not covered. Approximately one third of children with chronic health conditions whose family were low income (less than 200% FPL) were classified as underinsured and reported unmet health needs, difficulty obtaining specialty referrals, and financial problems as a result of health care costs (Davidoff, 2004b; Kogan, Newacheck, Honberg, et al., 2005). Hispanic children, children living in poverty, and children having more functional limitations or disabilities were more likely to be underinsured than their nonaffected peers (Kogan et al., 2005) (see Chapter 8).

Fragmentation of care may interfere with comprehensive care. Many children with chronic conditions receive the majority of their medical care in specialty clinics that do not provide routine health care management. When children are shuffled from specialist to specialist, they often miss the screenings, developmental assessments, anticipatory guidance, and immunizations that healthy children of the same age receive. The development of medical specialization has improved the disease control and life expectancy of children with special health care needs, but has also resulted in fragmentation of health care delivery and increased medical costs. The families of CSHCN have to interact with multiple institutions and systems providing some aspect of care for their child (e.g., early intervention programs; equipment vendors; social services; special education programs; federal, state, or private financial providers of care) (see Chapter 9). In addition, there are often medical subspecialists whose expectations may or may not be realistic for the family or child. Demands are sometimes conflicting, uncoordinated, and incomprehensible to the family. Subspecialists rarely address primary health care needs, developmental concerns, or common illness management. Primary care providers, on the other hand, frequently cite lack of specialty knowledge, lack of adequate time with children and families, lack of adequate reimbursement for care of children with complex medical or behavioral conditions, and unavailability of subspecialists to collaborate with in their community as barriers to their provision of comprehensive care to children with chronic conditions (Barclay, 2003).

Mental and behavioral health care needs should be part of comprehensive health care. It is estimated that 7% to 18% of children in primary care settings have identifiable psychosocial problems (Kelleher, McInerny, Gardner, et al., 2000). The 2005–2006 SLAITS CSHCN report found that 25% of CSHCN had emotional, developmental, or behavioral problems; adolescents were almost four times as likely to have reported mental health problems as preschool-age children (U.S. DHHS, HRSA, MCHB, 2007). An in-depth analysis of the National Survey of Children with Special Health Care Needs 2002 by Ganz and Tendulkar (2006) found that 25.7% of CSHCN reported needs for mental health services and 13.3% of other family members had some need for mental health care; severity of the child's condition and instability of the condition were associated with increased mental health care needs. The authors reported that 18.4% of the children and 21.3% of the family members had unmet mental health needs. Poverty, lack of insurance, lack of usual source of care, condition severity, family member unmet mental health care need, and being black were most strongly associated with unmet mental heath care needs in children. Parental depression has an adverse affect on children's health care utilization that can negatively affect chronic condition management (Sills, Shetterly, Xu, et al., 2007). Child maltreatment and neglect have been reported to be significantly higher in CSHCN possibly because the chronic condition places higher emotional, physical, economic, and social demands on the families (Hibbard, Desch, Committee on Child Abuse and Neglect, & Council on Children with Disabilities, 2007). Having a special health care need has also been found to increase the incidence of being bullied in school, especially if the child has a functional limitation or behavioral, emotional, or developmental problems (Van Cleave & Davis, 2006). The stress and psychological burden caretakers and family members experience caring for a child with special needs, while trying to balance personal and family needs, can be significant. The cumulative social disadvantages of poverty and mental health problems in parents should not be underestimated (Bauman et al., 2006; Ganz & Tendulkar, 2006; Sen & Yurtserver, 2007).

Oral health care needs are commonly identified (Federal Interagency Forum on Child and Family Statistics, 2007). Although rates of preventive dental care have risen from only 38% of U.S. children in 1996 to 72% in 2003–2004 due largely to increased coverage of pediatric dental care under SCHIP, low-income, foreign-born, and black or multiracial children were significantly less likely to have received dental care (Lewis, Johnston, Linsenmeyar, et al., 2007). Children with chronic conditions often have special diets or eating patterns that can affect oral health. Medications may affect tooth or gum development, and dental hygiene may be very difficult in children with severe disabilities or oral aversion. Dentists skilled in the care of children with complex conditions are often difficult to find but important in helping to maintain oral health and long-term adequate nutrition.

Comprehensive Care for Children with Special Health Care Needs

Concern over the access and importance of comprehensive health care benefits for children has resulted in the release of policy statements on access to health care for infants, children, adolescents, and pregnant women (Committee on Child Health Financing, 1998) and the scope of health care benefits needed

---

BOX 1-3

Specialized Services for Children with Special Health Care Needs

- Care coordination in a pediatric medical home
- Comprehensive case management
- Intermediate or skilled nursing care in residential and rehabilitation settings
- Availability of physical, occupational, speech, and respiratory therapy for rehabilitation and habilitation
- Home health services, including therapies, nursing, and home health aids
- Nutritional evaluation and counseling for eating disorders and nutritional deficiencies
- Special diets, formulas, and feeding devices for nutritional support
- Rental or purchase and maintenance of durable medical equipment
- Disposable medical equipment
- Palliative and hospice care for children with terminal illness

Adapted from Committee on Child Health Financing. (2006). Scope of health care benefits from birth through age 21. *Pediatrics, 117*(3), 979-982.

---

for children from birth to 21 years of age (Committee on Child Health Financing, 2006) by the American Academy of Pediatrics. The American Academy of Pediatrics advocates universal access to comprehensive evidenced-based health care, reflecting changes in treatment modalities and new technologies. This care should include preventive care services; acute, critical, and chronic care services; pediatric surgical care; emergency care services; behavioral health services; and all necessary services that (1) are appropriate for the child's age and health status; (2) will prevent or ameliorate the effects of a condition, illness, injury, behavior, or disorder; (3) will aid in the overall physical and mental development of the individual; or (4) will assist in achieving or maintaining functional capacity (Committee on Child Health Financing, 1998, 2006). Specialized services recommended for children with special health care needs by the American Academy of Pediatrics Committee on Child Health Financing (2006) are summarized in Box 1-3.

All Aboard the 2010 Express: A 10-Year Action Plan to Achieve Community-Based Service Systems for Children and Youth with Special Health Care Needs and Their Families. To address the complexity of care provision needed by children with special health care needs and health care system deficiencies, the American Academy of Pediatrics, the Maternal and Child Health Bureau, and Family Voices developed the goals of a community-based system of care for CSHCN in the document *All Aboard the 2010 Express: A 10-Year Action Plan to Achieve Community-Based Service Systems for Children and Youth with Special Health Care Needs and Their Families* (Maternal and Child Health Bureau, Health Resources and Services Administration, 2001) (Box 1-4). A major component of this action plan was the creation of the "medical home" initiative of care for CSHCN (American Academy of Pediatrics, Medical Home Initiative for Children with Special Needs Project Advisory Committee, 2002). A "medical home" (the term "health care home" is preferable because it implies the importance of health maintenance and health promotion) is the term used to connote an ideal health care practice in the child's community that offers a source of ongoing, comprehensive, family-centered care for children with special health care needs. A health care home

BOX 1-4

Goals Identified to Achieve Community-Based Service Systems for Children with Special Health Care Needs to Meet *Healthy People 2010* Goals

- *Goal 1:* Families of children with special health care needs will partner in decision making at all levels and will be satisfied with the services they receive.
- *Goal 2:* All children with special health care needs will receive coordinated, ongoing, comprehensive care within a medical home.
- *Goal 3:* All families of children with special health care needs will have adequate private and/or public insurance to pay for the services they need.
- *Goal 4:* All children will be screened early and continuously for special health care needs.
- *Goal 5:* Community-based services systems will be organized so families can use them easily.
- *Goal 6:* All youths with special health care needs will receive the services necessary to make transitions to all aspects of adult life, including adult health care, work, and independence.

From U.S. Department of Health and Human Services, Maternal and Child Health Bureau. (2001). All aboard the 2010 express: A 10-year action plan to achieve community-based service systems for children and youth with special health care needs and their families. *Pediatr Nurs, 27*(4), 429, 432.

offers the child and family preventive primary care services, as well as management of chronic and acute conditions, 24 hours per day, 7 days per week. Care coordination and collaboration among primary care providers, specialists, and community resources, in partnership with the child and family, are fundamental components of a health care home. Family-centered continuity care with an identified health care provider, nurse or doctor, who knows well the child, family, health condition, and community resources, has been identified as a major component of the medical home and source of parent satisfaction with care (Council on Children with Disabilities, 2007; American Academy of Pediatrics, Medical Home Initiative for Children with Special Needs Project Advisory Committee, 2002). Children who do not have a personal health care provider but receive care in community clinics or emergency/urgent care settings are more likely to have poor identification of chronic health conditions, complications of chronic conditions, inconsistency in management, lack of appropriate referrals, and lack of appropriate health care maintenance.

The results of the 2005–2006 SLAITS CSHCN (U.S. DHHS, HRSA, MCHB, 2007) report indicate that many families with CSHCN do not believe the *All Aboard the 2010 Express* goals have been met by the current health care system. Goal 1, receipt of family-centered care, was only reported in 50% to 75% of families depending on family income level, race/ethnicity, and functional ability of the child. Racial disparities in satisfaction with care and ease of using services has been identified by other authors (Ngui & Flores, 2006). Goal 2 addresses the need for coordinated and comprehensive care ideally in a "medical home." The 2005–2006 SLAITS CSHCN report indicated that 94% of CSHCN had a usual place for sick care and a personal nurse or doctor as a health care provider, but less than 50% of families reported receiving coordinated care and only 65% reported consistently receiving family-centered care. Goal 3 is for all CSHCN to have adequate insurance, but this has also not been met. CSHCN continue to be uninsured (9% to 15%) or underinsured (30%), affecting access to health care and resulting in poorer health outcomes (Kogan et al., 2005; Oswald, Bodurtha, Willis, et al., 2007). Statistics for goals

4 and 5 were not presented in the SLAITS CSHCNS Chartbook, 2005–2006 (U.S. DHHS, HRSA, MCHB, 2007). Transitioning of youth with special health care needs to appropriate adult services, Goal 6, is discussed at length in Chapter 4. Studies have found that overall only 50% of youths with special needs had discussed the need to transitions services with their provider (Lotstein, McPherson, Strickland, et al., 2005), with over 50% of youth with special health care needs reporting gaps in insurance coverage with a mean of 15 months not insured in the previous 36 months (Callahan & Cooper, 2007).

Role of the Primary Care Provider in Caring for Children with Chronic Conditions

Few professionals would argue that the pediatric subspecialists with advanced training and skills gained from caring for many children with similar conditions are the best professionals to deal with the medical complexities of many chronic conditions. If the broader needs of the child and family (i.e., education on well care and safety, health promotion, support, advocacy, referral to community resources)—needs that families have regardless of the specific chronic condition—are seen as the major focus of care, there is an obvious role for a primary care provider.

The primary care provider should be an integral part—if not the leading force—in the care of children with chronic conditions for the following reasons:

1. Holistic health care of children requires that they be viewed first and primarily as children, with the health care and developmental needs of any child.
2. The family must be seen as an integral part of the child's growth and development and recognized for its individual strengths and weaknesses. The development of partnership with families in the care of their children is a fundamental tenet of pediatric primary care.
3. Health promotion, disease prevention, and anticipatory guidance have even greater significance when children already have a condition putting them at increased risk. Subspecialists are experts in their area of disease management but often have limited knowledge of normal growth and development and standard health care practices for health maintenance.
4. Primary care providers most likely know a family's community resources better than subspecialists, who may have practices many miles from the family's home. This knowledge of community resources is extremely important in helping families receive optimal care and support for their children. Care coordination in partnership with families is essential, especially when the condition is complex or unstable, or the child has functional limitations.
5. Primary providers are best positioned to advocate for families' health care needs and to interact with the health care system. They can ensure that all families that are eligible for insurance, particularly Medicaid or SCHIP, are successful in obtaining insurance so access to care is enhanced. They can intercede with insurance companies to attempt to obtain coverage for uninsured services or items of medical necessity.
6. Primary care providers can evaluate the compounding effects of cumulative social disadvantages—poverty, food insecurity, language barriers, racial or cultural barriers, mental health problems, domestic or community violence—and how these

social issues affect health care of the child. Working with other health professionals or agencies in the family's community, such as social workers, mental health counselors, early parenting projects, and government and private agencies that assist the impoverished, immigrants, or people with a particular chronic condition, the primary care provider can help reduce the stress on families caring for a child with special needs. Although no primary care provider can resolve all social disadvantages, seemingly small changes (e.g., having a special formula donated to a family by the formula company, electricity bills covered by the utility company, finding a dentist willing and able to provide services to the child, or a mental health worker to meet with a depressed parent) can help parents of CSHCN feel supported by their health care team.

Levels of Primary Care Intervention for Children with Chronic or Disabling Conditions

Caring for children with chronic conditions is a challenging, often complex and time-consuming, but rewarding proposition. It requires a commitment to service beyond that required for routine ambulatory pediatric care, as well as increased knowledge about children, chronic conditions, community resources, systems of health care, insurance, interpersonal communication, and organizational skills necessary to provide optimal child and family care.

Levels of intervention in the primary care of children, as well as the knowledge base and skills primary care providers need at each level of intervention, are outlined in Box 1-5. These levels of intervention are cumulative (i.e., level 3 intervention cannot be attained until the knowledge base and skills of levels 1 and 2 are mastered). As the levels increase, so do the commitment of the provider and the comprehensiveness of care for the child and family. This model of care was inspired by work done in the area of family-centered care by Doherty and Baird (1987) and in child health leadership by the Maternal and Child Health Leadership Competencies Workgroup (2007), and further developed by the editors of this text.

Level 1 care is the provision of routine health care maintenance and common illness management to healthy children and their families. Some health care providers may elect not to care for children with chronic conditions because of practice restrictions, a knowledge base limited to the care of children without complex chronic conditions, or a lack of skills necessary to adequately manage more complex medical and psychosocial problems. Optimal care can be provided at level 1 but only to children and families without complex chronic health care needs.

Level 2 care is task-oriented care requiring minimal interaction with the child or family and no commitment to continuity care. Level 2 care is not primary care but may be used to supplement primary care when a certain task must be accomplished. The knowledge base and skill level needed for task-oriented care are limited to those necessary to complete the task efficiently, effectively, and safely. Examples of this level of care include the primary care provider administering immunizations, ordering laboratory tests, or performing a prehospitalization and camp physical examination on a child with special health care needs at the request of the managing subspecialist.

Level 3 care is provided when health care professionals offer routine primary care to children with chronic conditions, recognizing

the unique health care needs of the child and family. Providers are able to assess the child's chronic condition but refer this care to other individuals or agencies. Because of the complexity of some conditions, the provider's personal interest or knowledge, or practice restriction, primary care providers may elect to manage some children with chronic conditions at this level, for example, children with inflammatory bowel disease, while managing children with other conditions, for example, asthma, at a higher level.

Level 4 care is comprehensive primary health care that incorporates the unique complexities of the chronic condition, the child, and the family. At this level the practitioner assumes the primary health care responsibilities of the child and family and uses consultations or referrals for complex situations. This is the level of care often expected of primary care providers serving as gatekeepers in managed care systems. Practitioners do not abdicate care to subspecialists but work with them and the family to provide optimal care. As the health professional with the greatest knowledge of the family, the child, the health care system, and the community, the primary care provider assumes a leadership role in providing comprehensive continuity care.

Level 5 care takes the role of the primary provider one step further to that of care coordinator. A care coordinator assesses, plans, facilitates, implements, coordinates, monitors, and evaluates the education and service needs of a child and family (Antonelli, Stille, & Antonelli, 2008; Committee on Children with Disabilities, American Academy of Pediatrics, 1999; Lindeke, Leonard, Presler, et al., 2002). The care coordinator must know the available resources and how to access them, provide linkage between services, integrate services so they are not duplicative, and be able to set measurable goals to determine effectiveness of individual interventions. As systems of care for children with special health care needs become more complex, multiple interdisciplinary professionals may act as care coordinators, each assuming responsibility for their component of the child's care; that is, the primary care provider may assume the coordination of the health care system, the school nurse the coordination of the services delivered in the school setting, and the social worker the coordination of social services (Committee on Children with Disabilities, American Academy of Pediatrics, 1999). Care coordination of children with complex health care needs is critical if efficient, cost-effective, team-based approaches to care are expected.

Primary care providers may assume the role of care coordinator for the child's health services (Antonelli et al., 2008). This role is not defined with specific tasks but is dynamic and determined by the needs of the child and family (see Chapter 9). Barriers to the provision of care coordination by primary care providers include lack of knowledge about the specific condition and available community resources, lack of communication between health care professionals and organizations, and the time required to perform care coordination, which is usually not reimbursable by private and public insurance plans (Committee on Children with Disabilities, American Academy of Pediatrics, 1999). Subspecialty providers or treatment teams may also assume this role in children with complex conditions, such as organ transplantation. The need for care coordination has been recognized as critical to ensure quality continuity care. The Institute of Medicine identified care coordination for people with chronic conditions as one of the 20 priority areas to improve health care quality and delivery (Adams & Corrigan, 2002).

BOX 1-5

Hierarchic Intervention Framework for Practitioners Caring for Children with Chronic Conditions

LEVEL 1
Ongoing health care and illness management for children without chronic conditions

Knowledge Base Needed
- Routine health care maintenance and common condition management for children and youths without chronic conditions and their families
- Biologic, environmental, economic, racial, cultural, and societal factors affecting health and access to care for children
- Health insurance coverage of children and families receiving care

Skills Needed
- The ability to collect and record subjective and objective data related to child health maintenance and common pediatric conditions
- The ability to elicit relevant data related to family structure, socioeconomic environment, medical history, and current health problems and concerns
- The ability to listen effectively
- The ability to assess and critically evaluate objective and subjective information obtained to formulate a differential diagnosis
- The ability to assess and critically evaluate growth and development of children from birth to young adulthood
- The ability to identify and implement a treatment plan consistent with scientific evidence for children without chronic conditions and families
- The ability to effectively communicate treatment plans to children and families and obtain their assent to the plan
- The ability to monitor children's and families' response to treatment plans and make modifications as needed
- The ability to identify children with more complex needs requiring additional services
- The ability to provide culturally sensitive care to children and families
- The ability to provide care in an ethical and professional manner at all times

LEVEL 2
Task-oriented care for children with chronic conditions; primary care needs and specialty care needs managed by other professionals

Additional Knowledge Base Needed
- Task-related knowledge

Additional Skill Needed
- Performance of task in efficient, correct manner, consistent with evidence-based practice

LEVEL 3
Management of routine health care needs for children with chronic conditions; collaboration or referral for care related to the chronic condition

Additional Knowledge Base Needed
- Pathophysiology of chronic conditions
- Common associated problems of chronic conditions
- Biologic, environmental, economic, racial, cultural, and societal factors affecting health and access to care for children with chronic conditions and their families
- Noncategorical effect of chronic conditions and treatment on child development
- Role functions of interdisciplinary team members and how to access their services
- Community subspecialists, health care and social agencies, school systems, and tertiary care centers for children and youths with special health care needs
- Common health services needed by CSHCN and means of accessing these services

Additional Skills Needed
- The ability to teach/coach children and families regarding health care maintenance needs, management plans, and accessing chronic care services
- The ability to partner with families in their efforts to manage children's chronic condition, growth and development
- The ability to monitor and critically assess children with chronic conditions, identifying changes requiring consultation or referral to a specialist
- The ability to identify family strengths and incorporate them into the plan of care and make effective referrals for families having difficulty managing children's health care needs or coping with the demands of care
- The ability to communicate physical or psychosocial changes in children or families to the appropriate professional
- The ability to access community and educational services for children with special needs
- The ability to provide culturally sensitive care to children and families experiencing chronic health conditions

LEVEL 4
Comprehensive primary care of children with chronic conditions and their families

Additional Knowledge Base Needed
- In-depth pathophysiology of chronic conditions
- Unique primary care needs of children with chronic conditions
- Effective management of common associated problems found in chronic conditions
- Differential diagnosis for common pediatric illnesses occurring in children with chronic conditions
- Specific stressors for children and families with chronic conditions
- Effects of specific chronic conditions on children's growth, development, and activities of daily living
- Community resources, including educational resources, available to assist children and families and means of accessing these services
- Components of family-centered care in a "medical home"
- Insurance coverage for special services, equipment, or treatments for children and families
- Cost and scientific evidence of effectiveness of services provided to families

Additional Skills Needed
- The ability to systematically assess the medical condition and health care needs of children with chronic conditions
- The ability to plan and implement primary health care, including common illness management, that is individualized for the child, the family, and the chronic condition
- The ability to identify complications of the chronic conditions requiring more complex care and to make appropriate referrals
- The ability to educate/counsel families on the special health care needs of children with chronic conditions, management plans, and accessing of services
- The ability to access services within the health care system and community, including educational system, to meet the child's health care needs
- The ability to work with families to plan short- and long-term care consistent with medical needs and family function
- The ability to assist parents and children in problem solving both medical and family issues
- The ability to help families recognize the needs of individual members and balance these needs
- The ability to assist families in planning services and activities to reduce stress
- The ability to make interdisciplinary referrals communicating children and family needs and expectations
- The ability to provide consistent, available, long-term care in partnership with families

Continued

BOX 1-5

Hierarchic Intervention Framework for Practitioners Caring for Children with Chronic Conditions—cont'd

LEVEL 5
Care coordination of families and children with chronic conditions

Additional Knowledge Base Needed
- Service networks involved with children with special health care needs
- Information systems available to collect and communicate health information
- Cost of resources
- Quality outcome measures
- Service planning and systems coordination
- Team building and coordination
- Eligibility requirements, referral process, and utilization measures for agencies or services that might benefit families and children

Additional Skills Needed
- The ability to identify outcome measures of quality care for children with chronic conditions
- The ability to develop an alliance with families and children to work in partnership to plan and provide optimum care
- The ability to make a comprehensive needs assessment for children and families
- The ability to plan and initiate appropriate and successful referrals for services within the health care system and community
- The ability to work effectively in teams with other interdisciplinary professionals
- The ability to analyze cost/benefit ratio for services provided
- The ability to coordinate services and personnel working with the families and children
- The ability to use information systems to collect and evaluate outcome data and communicate health information
- The ability to measure and monitor progress in attaining identified goals in children and families
- The ability to make changes in management and service plans as necessary

- The ability to communicate findings from multiple interdisciplinary sources to families, children, and others involved in addressing the needs of children and families
- The willingness to function as child and family advocate

LEVEL 6
Leadership in systems advocacy for children with chronic conditions and their families

Additional Knowledge Base Needed
- Institutional structures governing care of children
- Health care systems and health economics
- Current rules, regulations, and laws at the institutional, local, state, and national levels regarding health care for children and families
- Legislative and regulatory process at the local, state, and national levels
- Community, state, and national policymakers
- Research on evidence-based practice and quality outcome indicators for children with chronic conditions and their families

Additional Skills Needed
- The ability to identify and articulate important children's health issues that are measurable and achievable
- The ability to communicate a vision of quality comprehensive family-centered services for children with special health care needs and their families
- The ability to influence decision making with available data
- The ability to build coalitions of individuals/professionals around children's health issues
- The ability to negotiate, compromise, and formulate alternative proposals
- The ability to work within the political and legislative systems and with politicians

---

In many instances parents become the central care coordinator, becoming the "coordinator of the coordinators." Parents who are knowledgeable about their child's condition and the health care systems involved can become empowered to perform this role but should always feel that they are partnered with concerned professionals. They should be assured that during times of high-intensity care coordination needs, such as during hospital discharge, a new diagnosis or complications, entrance into school, or transition to adulthood, additional care coordination will be available from the appropriate health professional. Respectful partnerships between professional care coordinators and families are necessary. "At all times, care coordinators must remember that the families are the continuous influence in children's lives and respect the parents' roles, needs, and culture" (Lindeke et al., 2002, p. 294).

As the complexity of medical management increases with knowledge and technology and the health care financial system becomes overtaxed with health care costs, service efficiency and cost-effectiveness will be central concerns. In the past, practitioners have been more likely to emphasize the quality of services and intensive care needs of clients, whereas administrators and funding sources often viewed service efficiency and cost-effectiveness as more important. The term "case management" has assumed the connotation of "cost containment" whereas care coordination assumes a broader role for systems organization. Primary care providers functioning as care coordinators must learn to assess, monitor, and document the effectiveness of the treatment programs used

by their clients to support the continuation of these programs in this era of shrinking health care dollars and rising incidences of chronic conditions in children.

Level 6 care goes beyond direct health care services and management of services to the macrosystems level of policies and political activism for child advocacy. Provision of quality health care services to individual children with special health care needs is critical and requires knowledgeable and skilled providers willing to take on the additional care requirements of these children. The barriers to optimal health for children with chronic conditions will not be altered, however, without significant changes in health care delivery systems, community awareness and acceptance of the special needs of such children, and legislative mandates for improved health care for all children.

Pediatric primary care providers must become leaders in child advocacy at the institutional, community, state, and federal levels—especially during periods of financial competition for service priorities. The barriers to optimal health care identified earlier (i.e., poverty, lack of insurance, minority/immigrant status, fragmentation of care) will not be reduced without fundamental changes in society's awareness and recognition of the health care needs of children and families. Pediatric health care providers can become effective child advocates by working with interdisciplinary colleagues to change the governing structure of health care organizations to ensure that the needs of children and families are addressed; by conducting or participating in evidenced-based research to determine outcome measures of quality care; by educating community service organizations and professional and community leaders on the need for comprehensive, culturally appropriate, and sensitive health care for all children and the common barriers to quality care; by being involved in the legislative process, negotiations, and conflict resolution to enable changes in laws or regulations affecting children's health care; and by becoming pediatric health care experts in development of policies governing pediatric health care (Maternal and Child Health Leadership Competencies Workgroup, 2007).

Primary care providers working with children with complex needs must identify their role and the roles of other health care professionals working with the child and family and communicate this role to all concerned, including the family. If primary care providers plan to only intervene at levels 1 to 3, the family must be informed of this decision and an appropriate professional identified to provide level 4 and level 5 care. Leaders in the care of children with special health care needs should aspire to level 6 care in order to have the greatest effect on health care systems and the quality of care provided to CSHCN.

If the chronic condition is medically complicated, uses complex technology, or requires prolonged use of resources housed in a tertiary care center, the subspecialty team (i.e., often more than one subspecialist or professional is working with a child) may assume the leadership role in total health care management of the child. In this situation the subspecialist should consult with or refer to a pediatric primary practitioner for normal health care maintenance appropriate for the child. Many specialty clinics are now using advanced nurse practitioners knowledgeable in both the specialty area and primary care to help facilitate communication and care among the specialty clinic, the primary provider, and the family.

Most chronic conditions of childhood are not so complex that the primary care practitioner with additional knowledge about the chronic condition and its implications for primary care, as well as a commitment to effective communication, cannot assume a leadership role in health care management. In many managed care plans, this is a requirement of the primary care provider as a gatekeeper to additional services. Providers of pediatric health care have long embraced the philosophy that it encompasses much more than disease management. The primary care provider must play a key role in establishing, organizing, monitoring and participating in health care systems if they are to provide the holistic, family-centered, health care promotion and maintenance needed to ensure the maximum health and potential of each child. Care—rather than cure—assumes greater meaning when working with children with chronic conditions, but there is much care in common with that needed by all children and their families.

The goal of health care maintenance for these children is to promote normal growth and development; to maximize the child's potential in all areas; to prevent or diminish the behavioral, social, and family dysfunction frequently accompanying a chronic condition; and to confine or minimize the biologic disorder and its sequelae (Committee on Children with Disabilities, 1993, 1998). The primary care provider who knows the child and family well, knows the resources of the community, and specializes in health care maintenance/promotion is most often the appropriate health care professional to assume leadership in the often complex care, care coordination, and systems management for children with special health care needs.

REFERENCES

Adams, K., & Corrigan, J.M.(Eds.) (2002). *Priority Areas for National Action. Transforming Health Care Quality*, Washington, DC: The National Academies Press.

Agency for healthcare Research and Quality (AHRQ). 2008. Demographics and health care access of limited-English-proficient and English-proficient Hispanics. *MEPS Research Findings #28.* Available at www.meps.ahrq.gov/mepsweb. Retrieved October 28, 2008.

Aiken, K.D., Freed, G.L., & Davis, M.M. (2004). When insurance status is not static: Insurance transitions of low-income children and implications for health and health care. *Ambul Pediatr, 4*(3), 237-243.

American Academy of Pediatrics,Medical Home Initiatives for Children with Special Needs Project Advisory Committee. (2002). The medical home. *Pediatrics, 110*, 184-186.

Andrulis, D.P. (2005). Moving beyond the status quo in reducing racial and ethnic disparities in children's health. *Public Health Rep, 120*(4), 370-377.

Antonelli, R.C., Stille, C.J., & Antonelli, D.M. (2008). Care coordination for children and youth with special health care needs: A descriptive, multisite study of activities, personnel costs, and outcomes. *Pediatrics, 122*(1), e209-e216.

Banthin, J.S., Cunningham, P., & Bernard, D.M. (2008). Financial burden of health care, 2001-2004. *Health Aff, 27*(1), 188-195.

Barclay, L. (2003), February 4. Limited time for pediatric visits compromises care: A newsmaker interview with Peter Holbrook, MD. *Medscape: Medical News* [online]. Available at www.medscape.com/viewarticle/448898. Retrieved March 4, 2003.

Bauman, L.J., Silver, E.J., Stein, R.E. (2006). Cumulative social disadvantage and child health. *Pediatrics, 117*(4), 1321-1328.

Bethell, C.D., Read, D., Blumberg, S.J., et al. (2008). What is the prevalence of children with special health care needs? Toward an understanding of variations in findings and methods across three national surveys. *Matern Child Health J, 12*, 1-14.

Bethell, C., Read, D., Stein, R.E.K., et al. (2002). Identifying children with special health care needs: Development and evaluation of a short screening instrument. *Ambul Pediatr, 2*(1), 38-48.

Blendon, R.J., Buhr, T., Cassidy, E.F., et al. (2008). Disparities in physician care: Experiences and perceptions of a multi-ethnic America. *Health Aff, 27*(2), 507-517.

Bronte-Tinkew, J., Zaslow, M. Capps, R., et al. (2007) Food insecurity and overweight among infants and toddlers: New insights into a troubling linkage. *Child Trends Research Brief, #2007-20,* Washington, DC.

Callahan, S.T., & Cooper, W.O. (2007). Continuity of health insurance coverage among young adults with disabilities. *Pediatrics, 119*(6), 1175-1180.

Casey, P.H., Szeto, K.L., Robbins, J.M., et al. (2005). Child health-related quality of life and household food security. *Arch Pediatr Adolesc Med, 159*, 51-56.

Center on Hunger and Poverty (2002). *The Consequences of Hunger and Food Insecurity for Children: Evidence from Recent Scientific Studies.* Waltham, MA: Author.

Centers for Disease Control and Prevention (CDC) (2008). Update on overall prevalence of major birth defects—Atlanta, Georgia, 1978-2005. *MMWR Morb Mortal Wkly Rep, 57*(01), 1-5.

Centers for Disease Control and Prevention (CDC), National Center for Health Statistics (NCHS). (September 12, 2002). *HHS issues report showing dramatic improvements in America's health over past 50 years* [online]. Available at www.cdc.gov/nchs/releases/02news/hus02.htm. Retrieved October 28, 2008.

Centers for Disease Control and Prevention (CDC), National Center for Health Statistics (NCHS), & Health Resources and Services Administration, Maternal and Child Health Bureau. (n.d.). *State and Local Area Integrated Telephone Survey (SLAITS) Survey of Children with Special Health Care Needs (CSHCN)* [online]. Available at http://ftp.cdc.gov/pub/Health_Statistics/NCHS/slaits/other%20info/factsheet_cshcn.pdf. Retrieved October 28, 2008.

Chen, E., Martin, A.D., & Matthews, K.A. (2007). Trajectories of socioeconomic status across children's lifetime predict health. *Pediatrics, 120*(2), e297-e303.

Children's Defense Fund. (2007a). *Black child health fact sheet.* Available at www.childrensdefense.org/site/PageServer?pagename=policy_ch_blackfactsheet. Retrieved May 20, 2008.

Children's Defense Fund. (2007b). *Latino child health fact sheet.* Available at www.childrensdefense.org/site/PageServer?pagename=policy_ch_latinofactsheet. Retrieved May 20, 2008.

Clancy, C.M., & Andersen, E.M. (2002). Meeting the health care needs of persons with disabilities. *Milbank Q, 80*(2), 381-391.

Cohen, R.A., & Martinez, M.E. (2007). *Health insurance coverage: Early release of estimates from the National Health Survey,* January-June 2007.

Committee on Child Health Financing (2006). Scope of health care benefits from birth through age 21. *Pediatrics, 117*(3), 979-982.

Committee on Child Health Financing, American Academy of Pediatrics (1998). Principles of child health care financing. *Pediatrics, 102*(4), 994-995.

Committee on Children with Disabilities, American Academy of Pediatrics. (1999). Care coordination: Integrating health and related systems of care for children with special health care needs. *Pediatrics, 104*(4), 978-981.

Committee on Children with Disabilities, American Academy of Pediatrics (1998). Managed care and children with special health care needs: A subject review,. *Pediatrics, 102*(3), 657-659.

Committee on Children with Disabilities & Committee on Psychosocial Aspects of Child and Family Health, American Academy of Pediatrics (1993). Psychosocial risks of chronic health conditions in childhood and adolescence (RE9338). *Pediatrics, 92*(6), 876-878.

Committee on Pediatric Research, American Academy of Pediatrics (2000). Race/ethnicity, gender, socioeconomic status—Research exploring their effects on child health: A subject review (RE9848). *Pediatrics, 105*(6), 1349-1351.

Council on Children with Disabilities (2007). The role of the medical home in family-centered early intervention services. *Pediatrics, 120*(5), 1153-1158.

Currie, J., & Lin, W. (2007). Chipping away at health: More on the relationship between income and child health. *Health Aff, 26*(2), 331-344.

Davidoff, A.J. (2004a). Identifying children with special health care needs in the National Health Interview Survey: A new resource for policy analysis. *Health Serv Res, 39,* 53-71

Davidoff, A.J. (2004b). Insurance for children with special health care needs: Patterns of coverage and burden on families to provide adequate insurance. *Pediatrics, 114*(2), 394-403.

DeNavas-Walt, C., Proctor, B.D., Smith, J., U.S. Census Bureau. (2007). *Income, Poverty, and Health Insurance Coverage in the United States: 2006. Current Population Reports, P60-233,* Washington, DC: U.S. Government Printing Office.

DeVoe, J.E., Baez, A., Angier, H., et al. (2007). Insurance + access ≠ health care: Typology of barriers to health care access for low-income families. *Ann Fam Med, 5*(6), 511-518.

Doherty, W., & Baird, M.A. (1987). *Family Centered Medical Care: A Clinical Casework.* New York: Guilford Press.

Federal Interagency Forum on Child and Family Statistics (2007). *America's Children: Key National Indicators of Well-Being, 2007. Federal Interagency Forum on Child and Family Statistics,* Washington, DC: U.S. Government Printing Office.

Federico, S.G., Steiner, J.F., Beaty, B., et al. (2007). Disruptions in insurance coverage: Patterns and relationship to health care, access, unmet needs, and utilization before enrollment in the State Children's Health Insurance Program. *Pediatrics, 120*(4), e1009-e1016.

Forrest, C.B., & Riley, A.W. (2004). Childhood origins of adult health: A basis for life-course health policy. *Health Aff, 23*(5), 155-164.

Furth, S.L., Garg, P.P., Neu, A.M., et al. (2000). Racial differences in access to the kidney transplant waiting list for children and adolescents with end-stage renal disease. *Pediatrics, 106*(4), 756-761.

Ganz, M.L., & Tendulkar, S.A. (2006). Mental health care services for children with special health care needs and their family members: Prevalence and correlates of unmet needs. *Pediatrics, 117*(6), 2138-2148.

Hahn, B.A. (1995). Children's health: Racial and ethnic differences in the use of prescription medications. *Pediatrics, 95*(5), 727-732.

Haley, J., & Kenney, G. (2007). Low-income uninsured children with special health care needs: Why aren't they enrolled in public health insurance programs? *Pediatrics, 119*(1), 60-68.

Hamilton, B.E., Minino, A.M., Martin, J.A., et al. (2007). Annual summary of vital statistics: 2005. *Pediatrics, 119*(2), 345-360.

Hibbard, R.A., Desch, L.W, Committee on Child Abuse and Neglect, & Council on Children with Disabilities. (2007). Maltreatment of children with disabilities. *Pediatrics, 119*(5), 1018-1025.

Institute of Medicine (2003). *Unequal Treatment: Confronting Racial and Ethnic Disparities in Health Care.* Washington, DC: National Academies Press.

Jeffrey, A.E., & Newacheck, P.W. (2006). Role of insurance for children with special health care needs: A synthesis of the evidence. *Pediatrics, 118*(4), e1027-e1038.

Jhanjee, I., Saxeena, D., Arora, J., et al. (2004). Parents' health and demographic characteristic predict noncompliance with well-child visits. *J Am Board Fam Pract, 17,* 324-331.

Kelleher, K.J., McInerny, T.K., Gardner, W.B., et al. (2000). Increasing identification of psychosocial problems: 1979-1996. *Pediatrics, 105,* 1313-1321.

Kogan, M.D., Newacheck, P.W., Honberg, L., et al. (2005). Association between underinsurance and access to care among children with special health care needs in the United States. *Pediatrics, 116*(5), 1162-1169.

Krauss, C. (June 9, 2008). Rural U.S. takes worst hit as gas tops $4 average. [Electronic version]. *New York Times.*

Larson, K., Russ, S.A., Crall, J.J., et al. (2008). Influence of multiple social risks on children's health. *Pediatrics, 121*(2), 337-344.

Lewis, C.W., Johnston, B.D., Linsenmeyer, K.A., et al. (2007). Preventive dental care for children in the United States: A national perspective. *Pediatrics, 119*(3), 544-553.

Lindeke, L.L., Leonard, B.J., Presler, B., et al. (2002). Family-centered care coordination for children with special needs across multiple settings. *J Pediatr Health Care, 16*(6), 290-297.

Lotstein, D.S., McPherson, M., Strickland, B., et al. (2005). Transition planning for youth with special health care needs: Results from the National Survey of Children with Special Heal Care Needs. *Pediatrics, 115*(6), 1562-1568.

Malat, J., Oh, H.J., & Hamilton, M.A. (2005). Poverty experience, race, and child health. *Public Health Rep, 120*(4), 442-447.

Martin, J.A., Kung, H.C., Mathews, T.J., et al. (2008). Annual summary of vital statistics: 2006. *Pediatrics, 121*(4), 788-801.

Maternal and Child Health Leadership Competencies Workgroup (Eds.). (2007). *Maternal and Child Health Leadership Competencies,* Version 2.0, Washington, DC: Maternal and Child Health Bureau.

Maternal and Child Health Bureau, Health Resources and Services Administration. (2001). *All aboard the 2010 express: A 10-year action plan to achieve community-based service systems for children and youth with special health care needs and their families* [online]. Rockville, MD: Author. Available at www.mchb.hrsa.gov/12010express/CHD-brochure.htm. Retrieved October 28, 2008.

Mbogoni, M., & Me, A. (2002, February 18-20) *Revising the United Nations census recommendations on disability.* Paper prepared for the first meeting of the Washington Group on Disability Statistics, Washington, DC [online]. Available at www.cdc.gov/nchs/about/otheract/citygroup/products/me_mbogoni1.thm. Retrieved October 28, 2008.

McPherson, M., Arango, P., Fox, H., et al. (1998). A new definition of children with special health care needs. *Pediatrics, 102*(1), 137-140.

Mokdad, A.H., Marks, J.S., Stroup, D.F., et al. (2004). Actual causes of death in the United States, 2000. *J Am Med Assoc, 291*(10), 1238-1245.

Morales, L.S., Spritzer, K., & Elliott, M., et al. (2001). Racial and ethnic differences in parents' assessments of pediatric care in Medicaid managed care. *Health Serv Res, 36*(3), 575-594.

Nageswaran, S., Silver, E.J., & Stein, R.E. (2008). Association of functional limitation with health care needs and experiences of children with special health care needs. *Pediatrics, 121*(5), 994-1001.

National Center for Health Statistics (2007). *Health, United States, 2007, with Chartbook on Trends in the Health of Americans.* Hyattsville, MD: Author.

National Center for Health Statistics. (n.d.) *Technical appendix: vital statistics of the United States: mortality.* Available at www.cdc.gov/nchs/datawh/statab/pubd/ta.htm. Retrieved June 24, 2008.

Newacheck, P.W., Rising, J.P., & Kim, S.E. (2006). Children at risk for special health care needs. *Pediatrics, 118*(1), 334-342.

Newacheck, P.W., Stoddard, J.J., Hughes, D.C., et al. (1997). Children's access to health care: The role of social and economic factors. In R. Stein (Ed.): Health care for children: *What's Right, What's Wrong, What's Next.* New York: United Hospital Fund.

Ngui, E.M., & Flores, G. (2006). Satisfaction with care and ease of using health care services among parents of children with special health care needs: The roles of race/ethnicity, insurance, language, and adequacy of family-centered care. *Pediatrics, 117*(4), 1184-1196.

Oswald, D.P., Bodurtha, J.N., Willis, J.H., et al. (2007). Underinsurance and key health outcomes for children with special health care needs. *Pediatrics, 119*(2), e341-e347.

Park, J., Turnbull, A.P., & Turnbull, H.R. (2002). Impacts of poverty on quality of life in families of children with disabilities. *Except Child, 68*(2), 151-170.

Park, M.J., Brindis, C.D., Chang, F., et al. (2008). A midcourse review of the Healthy People 2010: 21 critical health objectives for adolescents and young adults. *J Adolesc Health, 42*(2), 329-334.

Perrin, J.M. (2002). Health services research for children with disabilities. *Milbank Q, 80*(2), 303-324.

Perrin, J.M., Bloom, S.R., & Gortmaker, S.L. (2007). The increase of childhood chronic conditions in the United States. *J Am Med Assoc, 297*(24), 2755-2759.

Rose-Jacobs, R., Black, M.M., Casey, P.H., et al. (2008). House hold food inse-curity: Associations with at-risk infant and toddler development. *Pediatrics*, *121*(1), 65-72.

Satchell, M., & Pati, S. (2005). Insurance gaps among vulnerable children in the United States, 1999-2001. *Pediatrics*, *116*(5), 1155-1161.

Sen, E., & Yurtserver, S. (2007). Difficulties experienced by families with disa-bled children. *J Spec Pediatr Nurs*, *22*(4), 238-252.

Shea, K.K., Davis, K., & Schor, E. (2008). *U.S. variation in child health system performance: A state scorecard.* [online]. Available at www.commonwealthfund.org/publications/publications_show.htm?doc_id=687113. Retrieved June 25, 2008.

Shi, L., & Stevens, G.D. (2005). Disparities in access to care and satisfaction among U.S. children: The roles of race/ethnicity and poverty status. *Public Health Rep*, *120*(4), 431-441.

Sills, M.R., Shetterly, S., Xu, S., et al. (2007). Association between parental depression and children's health care use. *Pediatrics*, *119*(4), e829-e836.

Stein, R.E., & Silver, E.J. (1999). Operationalizing a conceptually based non-categorical definition: A first look at US children with chronic conditions. *Arch Pediatr Adolesc Med*, *153*, 68-74.

Todd, J., Armon, C., Griggs, A., et al. (2006). Increased rates of morbidity, mortality, and charges for hospitalized children with public or no health insurance as compared with children with private insurance in Colorado and the United States. *Pediatrics*, *118*(2), 577-584.

United Nations. (1998). *Principles and recommendations for population and housing censuses, Revision 1.* United Nations Publication, Sales No. E.98.XVII.8.

U.S. Department of Health and Human Services. (2007). *Progress review: Maternal, infant, and child health.* Available at www.healthypeople.gov/data/2010prog/focus16. Retrieved May 21, 2008.

U.S. Department of Health and Human Services (2000). *Healthy People 2010: Tracking Healthy People.* Washington, DC: U.S. Government Printing Office.

U.S. Department of Health and Human Services, Centers for Disease Control and Prevention, National Center for Health Statistics. (2007). *Health, United States, 2007.* Hyattsville, MD: National Center for Health Statistics.

U.S. Department of Health and Human Services, Health Resources and Service Administration, Maternal and Child Health Bureau (2007). *The National Survey of Children with Special Health Care Needs Chartbook 2005-2006.* Rockville, MD: U.S. Department of Health and Human Services.

U.S. Department of State. (n.d) *2008 poverty guidelines.* Available at http://travel.state.gov/visa/immigrants/info_1327.html. Retrieved June 25, 2008.

Van Cleave, J., & Davis, M.M. (2006). Bullying and peer victimization among children with special health care needs. *Pediatrics*, *118*(4), e1212-e1219.

Van der Lee, J.H., Mokkink, L.B., Grootenhuis, M.A., et al. (2007). Definitions and measurement of chronic health conditions in childhood. *J Am Med Assoc*, *297*(24), 2741-2751.

van Dyck, P.C., McPherson, M., Strickland, B.B., et al. (2002). The national sur-vey of children with special health care needs. *Ambul Pediatr*, *2*(1), 29-37.

Vozoris, N.T., & Tarasuk, V.S. (2003). Household food insufficiency is associ-ated with poor health. *J Nutr*, *133*, 120-126.

Westbrook, L.E., Silver, E.J., & Stein, R.E. (1998). Implications for estimates of disability in children: A comparison of definitional components. *Pediatrics*, *101*(6), 1025-1030.

Whitaker, R.C., Phillips, S.M., & Orzol, S.M. (2006). Food insecurity and the risks of depression and anxiety in mothers and behavior problems in their preschool-aged children. *Pediatrics*, *118*(3), 859-868.

Wise, P.H. (2004). The transformation of child health in the United States. *Health Aff*, *23*(5), 9-25.

World Health Organization (WHO) (2007). *International Classification of Functioning, Disability and Health: Children and Youth Version.* Geneva, Switzerland: WHO Press.

Zhao, Z., Mokdad, A.H., & Barker, L. (2004). Impact of health insurance status on vaccination coverage in children 19-35 months old, United States, 1993-1996. *Public Health Rep*, *119*(2), 156-162.

Zito, J.M., Safer, D.J., Riddle, M.A., et al. (1998). Prevalence variations in psy-chotropic treatment of children. *J Child Adolesc Psychopharmacol*, *8*(2), 99-105.

2 Chronic Conditions and Child Development

Judith A. Vessey and Brittney J. Sullivan

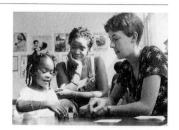

DEVELOPMENT does not exist in a vacuum; children's developmental domains are significantly influenced by their physiologic state, psychological competence, family and friends, and greater external environment. The presence of a chronic condition adds developmental and behavioral risks and can complicate children's attainment of developmental tasks (Council on Children with Disabilities, 2006). Because children with chronic conditions are more similar than different in respect to developmental challenges (Nehring, 2007; Sawyer, Drew, Yeo, et al., 2007), a noncategorical approach focusing on the commonalties of these children rather than just on the disease process will serve as the foundation for this chapter.

Children with chronic conditions may experience developmental lags in acquiring cognitive, communicative, motor, adaptive, and social skills compared with their unaffected peers. These maturational alterations may range from minor to all-encompassing and from transient to permanent. The presence of a chronic condition, however, does not necessarily connote the presence of a developmental disturbance or permanent disability. The development of many children with chronic conditions progresses without interruption.

The maturational alterations that accompany chronic conditions may be manifested within a single area of development (e.g., motor difficulty in a child with juvenile rheumatoid arthritis) or globally, affecting all developmental domains (e.g., those seen in a child with Down syndrome). Children whose developmental trajectories are delayed may advance through the normal sequence of milestones but at a rate slower than that of their peers of the same chronologic age. Such is the case of a child with a partially corrected congenital heart defect. Discrepancies in development across domains result from unevenly developed or damaged neurologic processes and result in disruptions in selected developmental sequences (e.g., a child with autism) (Reeve, 2001). The greater the severity of a condition, the more likely that the child will experience global delays, with some domains being more affected than others.

Development is ongoing and the maturation of structures and functions interdependent. For example, an integrated nervous system is modeled through repeated use, such as is seen with the development of normal 20/20 vision or, in the absence of repeated use, amblyopia (Reeve, 2001). Numerous physiologic and psychological variables can contribute to the occurrence and severity of maturational alterations associated with chronic conditions. For example, infants and mothers may have difficulty forming long-term emotional bonds with each other if they are physically, cognitively (e.g., brain damage), or emotionally (e.g., postpartum depression) separated from each other.

Developmental deviations in a child with a chronic condition are not directly related to a specific diagnosis. Rather, the type, intensity, and duration of developmental changes evolve from reciprocal interaction of condition-specific characteristics and child-specific attributes (Meijer, Sinnema, Bijstra, et al., 2002). These are more fully described in the next section. Because a child is still maturing, many potential and actual problems may be overcome if condition management programs proactively address these concerns. Specifically, clinical management requires capitalizing on the child's strengths so that development may be optimized. Improved developmental and clinical outcomes are realized by the child when families and providers engage in active partnerships when designing and implementing treatment regimens (Denboba, McPherson, Kenney, et al., 2006).

Characteristics of the Condition

The pathophysiology, severity, persistence, visibility, and prognosis of the condition, as well as any iatrogenic insults that may have occurred, influence a child's developmental outcome.

Pathophysiology, Severity, and Persistence

The pathophysiologic mechanisms of a condition (e.g., chronic hypoxemia, aberrant serum glucose levels, or malabsorption) and its related severity, persistence, and prognosis can alter development. The correlation between physiologic severity/persistence and developmental attainment is neither causal nor highly robust, and is moderated by a nexus of individual traits, available social support, and quality of symptom management. Children in the least and most disabled groups are at greater risk than those at intermediate severity.

Conditions associated with multisystem involvement, neurologic impairment, and unpleasant symptomatology place children at greater global developmental risk because their condition physically, mentally, or psychologically limits or prohibits them from completing developmental tasks. The interaction of pathophysiologic changes, availability for learning, and contact with the environment further compromises developmental attainment.

The pathophysiologic changes that children with mild conditions experience lack sufficient severity or are ameliorated by treatment so they readily adapt to them, and thus the potential for developmental insult is minimized. When conditions are marked by only occasional exacerbations, have limited visibility, or appear to cause only marginal problems, they may be ignored or denied by children and their families (Joachim & Acorn, 2000). This denial is often motivated by an effort to normalize the child's condition; yet when mild conditions are not recognized by others but do affect a child's performance, the child may be held to unrealistic expectations, such as is frequently seen in children with attention-deficit/hyperactivity disorder (ADHD). Unfortunately, children may have poorer developmental outcomes when denial interferes with symptom recognition, ongoing management regimens, and appropriate expectations of behavior.

Knowledge about untoward developmental sequelae secondary to prolonged disease states is also emerging. As research continues to advance health care technology, the mortality rate previously associated with many chronic conditions has been reduced. Usually, reductions in mortality rates initially result in escalating morbidity. The morbidity associated with survival of very low birth weight infants is an example (Petrini, Damus, Russell, et al., 2002) (see Chapter 39).

Other developmental limitations are secondarily imposed by the condition's pathophysiology and management. Conditions that are painful, embarrassing, or energy depleting place a child at greater developmental risk. Tremendous exertion may be necessary to cope with intensive treatment protocols or the time-consuming activities of daily life. For example, children with cystic fibrosis may spend more than 3 hours each day receiving pulmonary care. Additional energy is also required in adjusting to new or exacerbated symptoms (e.g., persistent pain, malaise, or fatigue). The activities of children who depend on technology are limited by physical constraints and the time needed to care for equipment such as ventilators and infusion pumps. Such expenditures of time and energy may limit children's opportunities to engage in recreational activities or predispose them to significant fatigue because participation requires too much effort. Moreover, in families where caregiving needs become the primary focus of daily living, parent-child interactions and other social activities are restricted.

Visibility

The visibility of a chronic condition may place the child at risk for stigmatization and can trigger self-consciousness (Immelt, 2006). Stigmatization is an act or process in which an individual is negatively labeled or characterized because of certain attributes or behaviors he or she possesses. Jones (as cited in Joachim & Acorn, 2000) lists six dimensions of stigma that can affect children's psychosocial development (Box 2-1). Visible conditions (e.g., Down syndrome, myelodysplasia [see Chapters 24 and 35]) place a child at risk for immediate stigmatization, and individuals may discredit the child's capabilities. However, children with visible disabilities who can effectively address their differences with others may fare better than their peers or children with hidden problems (Lawrence, Rosenberg, & Fauerbach, 2007; Lifshitz, Hen, & Weisse, 2007). For conditions that are invisible, such as inflammatory bowel disease (see Chapter 30), children may try to hide their condition and "pass" as normal, creating stress for fear of discovery. "Passing" may also require ignoring aspects of condition management, such as adolescents with diabetes or phenylketonuria (PKU) (see Chapters 23 and 38) who ignore dietary recommendations, thus impairing their health status. Choosing to disclose one's condition may promote stigmatization, as frequently occurs in children with epilepsy (see Chapter 26) (deBoer, Mula, & Sander, 2008). For children with deteriorating conditions, accidental disclosure is always a fear.

BOX 2-1

Dimensions of Stigma

Concealability: The degree to which the condition is hidden or visible.
Course of the condition: The extent to which a condition changes over time.
Strain: The effect of the condition's visibility and qualities on interpersonal relationships.
Aesthetic qualities: The extent to which a condition affects a child's appearance.
Cause of stigma: Whether the condition is congenital or acquired.
Peril: Dangers associated with being affiliated with a stigmatized child.

From Joachim, G., & Acorn, S. (2000). Stigma of visible and invisible chronic conditions. *J Adv Nurs, 32,* 243–248. Reprinted with permission.

Prognosis

Maturational progression is superimposed on the natural course of the condition. In conditions associated with ongoing pathophysiologic deterioration, children may initially achieve milestones but lose them as the condition worsens. This is always noted when there is progressive degeneration of the neurologic system (e.g., muscular dystrophy; see Chapter 34), but this is also a problem with any seriously compromised physiologic state. Even in nonprogressive conditions, developmental lags become noticeable as children mature and developmental expectations are higher. In part, the ability to sustain development depends on effectively managing the effects of the disease and promoting the child's functional status and psychosocial adjustment (Nageswaran, Silver, & Stein, 2008).

The uncertainty associated with a condition's trajectory that parents and children face is a major stressor and may influence a child's developmental outcomes (Burke, Kauffmann, LaSalle, et al., 2000; Garwick, Patterson, Meschke, et al., 2002; Stewart & Mishel, 2000). Children who have limited or uncertain futures or whose significant others (i.e., family, teachers) consider them to have a poor prognosis for reaching adulthood may be deprived of a past-present-future perspective of learning about one's cultural heritage or forming goals and personal aspirations. This longitudinal perspective plays an integral role in shaping cognitive processes. If individuals are misguided into thinking that such information is not worth transmitting or would be unduly upsetting, especially for children who recognize their potentially diminished longevity, this lack of information limits children's ability to learn. Children may also be held to differing behavioral expectations than their peers by sympathetic but misguided adults. Differing expectations can create anxiety in the child and resentment in siblings and peers.

Predicting prognoses is a risky business in light of rapid advances in medical science; nearly 90% of children with chronic conditions live into adulthood (Newacheck & Halfon, 1998). The life expectancies for children with cystic fibrosis, organ transplantation, cancer, human immunodeficiency virus (HIV), and numerous other conditions continue to increase at dramatic rates. If a poor medical prognosis is communicated to the family without a broader perspective of the child's future, it may become a self-fulfilling prophecy, resulting in poorer psychological outcomes as well.

Iatrogenic Insults

Selected treatment protocols impose their own risks. Developmental iatrogeny refers to health care interventions that hinder children from progressing through their normal developmental milestones.

Therapeutic interventions commonly associated with developmental iatrogeny are the associations between aminoglycosides and hearing loss (Turnidge, 2003); cancer therapies, transplantation, and late effects (Schwartz, Hobbie, Constine, et al., 2005); and oxygen and steroid administration and retinopathy of prematurity (Smolkin, Steinberg, Sujov, et al., 2008). Numerous other interventions, however, directly or indirectly influence development. Many classes of drugs (e.g., anticonvulsants, steroids) have been shown to alter cognition, perceptual abilities, or behavior and make children less available for learning (Graef, Wolfsdorf, & Greenes, 2008).

Characteristics of the Child

Each age-group gives rise to different sets of challenges for children with chronic conditions. The child's age at onset of a condition, however, affects adaptation and progression from one stage of development to the next. Achieving a developmental task that has never been acquired is very different from regaining a skill mastered and then lost. Overall, children with congenital conditions have greater developmental plasticity and more readily adjust to condition-imposed limitations because greater adaptive mechanisms come into play (Dennis, 2000); yet evidence suggests that the risk of behavioral difficulty associated with chronic conditions is inversely correlated with age (Frank, Thayer, Hagglund, et al. 1998; Sawyer et al., 2007), with younger children being at higher risk.

Infancy

The major developmental tasks of infancy include establishing trust and learning about the environment through sensorimotor exploration (Berk, 2006). For infants with congenital chronic conditions, these tasks may be difficult to accomplish. Parents who are mourning the loss of their perfect child may have little energy to care for their infants whose needs may be complex and demanding. If parents find little gratification in trying to meet their child's basic needs despite their best efforts, they may begin to view their child as vulnerable because of the extensive care required, and this attitude can affect future development. A poor prognosis may lead some parents to emotionally divorce themselves from their infants in an effort to insulate themselves from further emotional hurt. Infants subjected to prolonged or frequent hospitalizations may encounter repeated separations, the unpredictability associated with numerous caregivers, potentially unreliable or inadequate care, and painful experiences. All of these factors can inhibit attachment and the subsequent development of a trusting relationship (Vessey, 2003). For infants whose conditions are physically limiting or painful, exploration of and interaction with their environment are limited, further curtailing development.

Toddlerhood

The major developmental tasks of toddlerhood include acquiring a sense of autonomy, developing self-control, and forming symbolic representation through the acquisition of language (Berk, 2006). If a child's chronic condition requires careful limit setting and control of activities of daily living, independence in tasks such as toileting, feeding, or acquiring larger social networks may not be encouraged. For example, toddlers who are immunosuppressed need to be restricted in their social contacts and play arenas, and children with bleeding disorders (see Chapter 14) need more restrictions on exploring their environments. Mandatory prolonged dependency

can make separation difficult and contribute to a fragile self-image. Developmental tasks that have just been mastered are often easily lost in toddlers experiencing acute exacerbations of disease—with or without hospitalization (Vessey, 2003). This behavioral regression is a means of social and emotional adaptation whereby children revert to earlier, previously abandoned stages when they do not have the necessary psychic energy to maintain functioning at developmental levels already achieved (Freud, 1966). Behavioral regression is exacerbated by psychic and physiologic stress associated with fear, separation, pain, and other symptomatology. Depending on the severity and duration of a condition's exacerbation and the child's resilience and support, behavioral regression may deteriorate into frank psychopathology. Although regression can happen at any point along the developmental continuum, it is most commonly noted in this age-group.

Preschool Children

The primary developmental task for preschoolers is acquiring a sense of initiative to successfully meet the challenges of their ever-expanding world (Berk, 2006). Preschoolers with chronic conditions may not have the physical energy or motivation to design and perform such activities; therefore opportunities for learning about the environment, developing social relationships, and cultivating self-confidence and a sense of purpose are diminished. They may have difficulty forming a healthy self-concept, body image, and sexual identity, particularly if most of their body awareness is associated with disability and discomfort. The egocentricity and naive reasoning processes of preschoolers influence their understanding and interpretation of their condition. Although their understanding of illness and its relationship to morality is less enmeshed than previously thought, preschoolers still may think that their thoughts or behaviors cause their symptoms. Regardless, developing self-esteem and motivation to undertake new tasks may be compromised by their condition.

School-age Children

For school-age children, increasing independence and mastery over their environment are important developmental landmarks (Berk, 2006). Such activities contribute to gaining social skills, developing a sense of accomplishment, learning to effectively cope with stress, and acquiring the skills that result in self-sufficiency. Functional limitations in self-care, communication, mobility, stamina, and learning hinder children with chronic conditions from successfully participating in school and extracurricular activities that help develop independence and mastery (Msall, Avery, Tremont, et al., 2003; Tork, Lohrmann, & Dassen, 2007) and result in a poorer overall quality of life (Grootenhuis, Koopman, Verrips, et al., 2007).

Parental and child perceptions of the impact of their condition affect a child's developing sense of self-worth and psychological adjustment (Immelt, 2006). Enforced dependency—whether required by the treatment regimen or instituted by overprotective parents—creates additional social and emotional barriers between these children and their unaffected peers.

Children with a condition that is not highly visible may try to hide its existence until forced by circumstances to admit otherwise when they recognize that it distinguishes them from their peers, placing them at risk for stigmatization, ostracism, and bullying (Horowitz, Vessey, Carlson, et al., 2004; Joachim & Acorn, 2000;

Marin, 2005). When provided with the necessary skills to be socially competent, including communicating condition-specific information to their peers, these youths will be able to build and sustain friendships and thwart bullying attempts. Failure to do so frequently results in withdrawal, anxiety and depression, and other risks to their psychosocial well-being (LaGreca, Bearman, & Moore, 2002).

Adolescence

Adolescence is the transitional period from childhood to adulthood in which the primary developmental tasks are to (Betz, 2007)

1. Develop personal moral and ethical codes for behavior
2. Assume greater responsibility for academic endeavors and career planning
3. Master social rules
4. Avoid high-risk behaviors that threaten the adolescent's well-being

All of these tasks require that adolescents become increasingly independent of their parents. Because these tasks are complicated by the demands of a chronic condition, adolescents are at greater risk for chronic dependency and related psychological difficulties (Telfair, Alleman-Velez, Dickens, et al., 2005).

Adolescents need to begin to make decisions about future career and personal goals. For adolescents with chronic conditions, this requires expanding their networks for social support and assistance beyond their immediate family and friends to include help from an array of interdisciplinary services and professionals (Betz & Redcay, 2002). Adolescents are prone to two dangers in planning for the future: they may (1) overemphasize the potential barriers that accompany their condition and succumb to a sense of futility or despair or (2) deny realistic limitations and set themselves up for failure by holding unrealistic expectations. Chapter 4 more fully discusses these issues.

Adolescence is the time for assuming responsibility for care of their condition, but adolescents' relative inexperience and the complexity of care needs may preclude this from happening (Betz, 2007). Christian, D'Auria, and Fox (1999) identify three themes in the process of gaining self-responsibility. *Making it fit* refers to youths learning how to integrate condition management into their daily lives. *Ready and willing* reflects adolescents' acceptance of self-responsibility. *Having a safety net of friends* underscores the importance of supportive peers in condition management and assistance in case difficulties (e.g., insulin reaction) are encountered. When realistic expectations and meaningful social support are available, adolescents can learn from their choices and the natural consequences they experience (Reeve, 2001). For an adolescent who requires complex care or has a limited life expectancy, the developmental task of transitioning from parental care to self-care is more difficult to achieve and may go unmet.

Puberty is a time of rapid change and uncertainty for adolescents and may be more difficult for teens with chronic conditions. Delayed puberty accompanies many conditions, emphasizing the differences between affected and unaffected youths. Integrating limitations into a changing body image and self-concept amplifies these differences. Because this is a particularly difficult time to be viewed as different by one's peers, some adolescents may withdraw from social activities and relationships that promote

healthy psychosexual development (Cheng & Udry, 2002). Others may choose to engage in risky behaviors (e.g., smoking, unprotected sex), although it is unclear whether their rates are higher or lower compared to youths without chronic conditions (Sawyer et al., 2007; Telfair et al., 2005). Adolescents with chronic conditions, however, are particularly vulnerable to sexual exploitation as a way of seemingly being accepted by their peers. The exposure of youths with chronic conditions to sex education is generally consistent, but often insufficient, as it rarely addresses condition-specific issues. Although pubertal development may be slower and social isolation more common, youths with disabilities are as interested in pursuing intimate sexual relationships and are as sexually experienced as their counterparts (Cheng & Udry, 2002).

Individual Characteristics

Despite great odds, many children have intrapsychic and interpersonal resources that allow them to conquer virtually any disability and excel in life. A child's individual characteristics, or those relatively stable behavioral attributes that underlie a child's behavior (i.e., temperament, motivation, resilience, locus of control, intellect, attitudinal qualities, interpersonal skills), influence developmental attainment and adaptation to the child's condition (Cantrell, 2007; Meijer et al., 2002; Vessey, 2006).

Children with chronic conditions display the same scope of individual differences and developmental assets as children without chronic conditions. Some behavioral traits, such as temperament, are inborn, and others, such as self-concept, develop over time. The refinement of modifiable traits is influenced by social and environmental factors. A child's self-esteem is linked to fully mastering a variety of physical, intellectual, social, and emotional tasks during the appropriate developmental period. Failing such tasks does not bode well for physical or psychosocial health. Although children with chronic conditions are at a somewhat higher risk for developing behavioral problems, many are remarkably resilient and approach life's challenges with aplomb. Many learn to rapidly identify threats to their integrity, respond with justifiable anger to those who are prejudiced against them, and reject biased individuals as inferior. These children often work to simultaneously educate those around them, dispelling myths and inaccuracies that might interfere with their own developmental competence.

Children often live with multiple chronic conditions. Two or more conditions can occur within the same domain—chronic illnesses, developmental disabilities, or mental health problems—or across domains (Figure 2-1) (Vessey, 1999). Children with multiple chronic conditions are especially at increased risk for psychosocial problems, although condition severity alone does not affect a child's psychological outcome. Factors known to place children at greater risk for coexisting psychiatric conditions include (1) poor self-esteem, (2) inappropriate or underdeveloped coping mechanisms, (3) family dysfunction, (4) familial or geographic isolation, and (5) poverty (Chen, Martin, & Matthews, 2007; Farmer, Clark, Sherman, et al., 2005; Malat, Oh, & Hamilton, 2005; Meijer et al., 2002; Melnyk, Moldenhauer, Veenema, et al., 2001; Newacheck, Rising, & Kim, 2006; Parish & Cloud, 2006; Sawyer et al., 2007; Stewart, 2003). Gender differences are not well delineated. Boys experiencing behavioral problems tend toward externalizing disorders (e.g., conduct or oppositional disorders) that are more readily detected than disorders of girls, who tend toward internalizing disorders (e.g., depression).

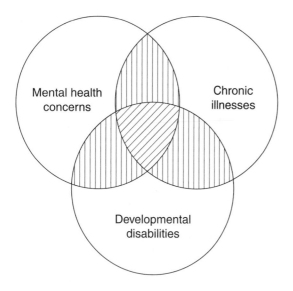

FIGURE 2-1 Co-occurring conditions.

The interrelationships of a child's positive self-esteem, perceived autonomy, easy temperament, internal locus of control, at least normal intelligence, adequate perceptual and communication skills, accurate cognitive appraisal of the condition, and coping skills in conjunction with environmental and family support all predict better adaptation (Meijer et al., 2002). When children are provided with the protective factors needed to balance out risk exposure, improved resilience and developmental attainment will result (Rink & Tricker, 2003; Vessey, 2006).

Role of Family and Social Networks

Healthy development depends on repeated, varied positive interactions between the growing child and the environment. Such reciprocity results in a spiral of mutually effective interactions. A child's family, and particularly parents, are important influences on a child's development and strong predictor of emotional well-being during early childhood (Immelt, 2006). Although maternal and paternal responses and roles differ, most parents are tremendously resilient despite the demands of the child's condition and effectively balance their role in normative parenting with meeting specific demands of the condition (Coffey, 2006; Knafl & Gillis, 2002; Pelchat, Lefebvre, & Levert, 2007). The converse is also true. Parental guilt, despair, or unfinished grief over the loss of the fantasized child may negatively affect a child's development. Other factors include parental depression, "nerves," poor self-esteem, and a chronically stressful environment. Children with disabilities are at higher risk for child abuse and neglect (Spencer, Devereux, Wallace, et al., 2005). Well-functioning families enhance their child's development, whereas those with discordant functioning curtail it (Coffey, 2006; Knafl & Gillis, 2002). Differing cultural orientation, language, social class, religiosity, and economic status of the family further influence development in children with chronic conditions (Nehring, 2007). As these orientations vary, so does the symbolic significance and semantic significance of the events, perceived origins, potential for stigma, and potential consequences. Differences between children and families who successfully adapt are related to their coping abilities, social support, and access to needed resources (see Chapter 5).

As children mature, their environments and social networks naturally expand, and extended family members, teachers, friends, and acquaintances influence their developmental attainment. Individuals who offer practical, tangible support, provide intellectual stimulation, plan activities that help the child excel, and take pride in the child's accomplishments truly serve as the child's advocates. Unfortunately, the benefits of informal social support are mixed because some individuals have had few experiences with children with special needs and may overcompensate for or reject a child's limitations (Pal, Das, Chaudhury, et al., 2005). For children whose conditions are associated with disfigurement, their development may be unwittingly at risk because of the reactions of others. Many uninformed individuals automatically assume that a physical handicap is associated with cognitive impairment. Children may be spoken of as if they are not present, or questions may be addressed to nearby family members or peers. The damage that can be done to a child's sense of self-worth is inestimable. The family can be helped to educate significant others about the child's strengths and limitations, mainstream their child into community activities, and use effective methods for working with insensitive individuals.

Developmental Perspectives of the Body, Illness, Medical Procedures, and Death

Children's perspectives about their bodies, illness, medical procedures, and death differ depending on age, cognitive abilities, and experience. Children with chronic conditions may develop expertise about selected topics within the range of their experiences and beyond that expected at their cognitive levels, but their understandings may be inconsistent, ranging from being extremely knowledgeable on content specific to their condition while holding less sophisticated views about general concepts of anatomy, physiology, illness, procedures, and treatments. Children may use advanced terminology that could confuse others into thinking that their comprehension exceeds what is normally expected. For example, a 4-year-old stated that he was receiving "methotrexate intravenously" but thought his blood filled an empty body cavity because blood vessels were an unknown entity. Children's self-concepts, interpersonal abilities, and adherence to treatment regimens are related to the beliefs they hold and influence their functional status, school performance, and psychosocial competence.

Understanding of the Body

Toddlers can point to various external body parts, but by the preschool period, children have well-defined concepts of their external bodies and the relationships of its parts. Their understanding of internal anatomy and physiology, however, is primitive in keeping with experience, cognitive level, and perceptual abilities. By preschool, children can name several internal body parts, with the heart, brain, bones, and blood being the most common. Children's descriptions of the parts and how they function tend to be global, undifferentiated, and laced with fantasy (e.g., hearts look like valentines) although there is a great deal of variation among children about their specific ideas. Knowledge of the interrelationships of the parts and their functions is equally hazy. Physiologic processes are seen as a series of static states, with each organ having a singular, autonomous function. By late elementary school, when children's causal reasoning and ability to differentiate mature, they begin to understand the complexities of anatomy and physiology.

Levels of the body's organization are differentiated and hierarchically integrated with each other. Progressively more complex information about body functions, much of it from school science classes, is incorporated throughout adolescence. Children with chronic conditions hold a slightly different—although not necessarily more sophisticated—view of their internal bodies than that of their unaffected peers. They may focus on the affected part of the body but do not identify fewer organs or organ systems (Schmidt, 2001; Vessey & O'Sullivan, 2000).

Understanding of Illness, Medical Procedures, and Treatments

Children's understanding of illness, medical procedures, and treatments is intrinsically linked to their knowledge about their body. For example, if children are considered by their parents to be sick, their developing views and personalization of illness and treatment regimens will negatively influence how they interpret their conditions. As children mature and their views of their body and disease processes evolve, primary care practitioners and significant others can assist them in developing positive images of their condition.

Infants do not have any mental representation of illness or understanding of procedures, which are interpreted only in light of how they intrude on personal comfort. When infants experience pain or other unpleasant symptomatology, or are subjected to hospitalization where they encounter repeated separation and unpredictable routines, behavioral responses such as agitation or withdrawal are common. All of these factors can inhibit attachment and curtail development.

By toddlerhood, children begin to understand the concept of illness. For children with chronic conditions, this is usually interpreted by how the condition interferes with desired activities. Many condition-specific treatments and procedures (e.g., injections of insulin, wearing a seizure helmet) are particularly onerous for this age-group.

As children mature, they begin to form ideas and articulate their feelings about illness. Because preschoolers are egocentric and engage in magical thinking, they often ascribe the causes of illness and associate treatments to their own thoughts or behaviors, especially as related to other temporally occurring events. The purpose of a procedure is viewed as independent of a child's health status, and little discrimination about its diagnostic or therapeutic purpose is made except by children who have undergone repetitive procedures. All procedures are designed to make them "better" or "sicker." Many associate treatment with punishment (Kato, Lyon, & Rasco, 1998); and because preschoolers' understanding of body boundaries is not well developed, virtually all invasive procedures are perceived as threats to their body integrity.

By school age, children's views of illness begin to reflect their evolving causal reasoning. Illness is initially perceived as occurring from contamination of, or physical contact with, the causal agent. Over time their understanding matures, and children begin to believe that illnesses are caused by external events (e.g., germs that enter the body). School-age children often are intrigued with medical procedures and are usually pleased when asked to participate in their own care. Multistep procedures and their purposes can be understood by school-age children, who can classify and order variables. Information may be interpreted quite literally, however, and misunderstandings can occur if the teaching explanations are not validated. School-age children respect health care personnel

and their hierarchic position. Although they sometimes express affection for their caregivers, children are often ambivalent about their relationships with health care providers.

With the development of formal operations, adolescents know progressively more about illness and pathophysiology. Illness causation is recognized as a complex, multifaceted process. Initial biologic and physiologic explanations that form the basis for explanations of illness later evolve into psychophysiologic descriptions with the relationship of behavior and emotion to illness being acknowledged.

Adolescents can understand the efficacy of specific medical procedures and the relationships between procedures and their health status, although their sense of invincibility and desire for experimentation affect their decision making. Informed decisions about alternative treatments are possible. Adolescents view the health care provider's authority as extending only as far as their willingness to adhere to their therapeutic regimens. Although the need for therapeutic adherence is understood, treatments are not automatically affectively and behaviorally assimilated into an adolescent's daily activities.

Understanding of Death

Death is the ultimate experience of separation and loss for children and their families. Children's understanding of death is formed along a developmental progression and reflects their cognitive maturation and experience (Karns, 2002; Slaughter & Griffiths, 2007). Infants do not comprehend death per se but react to phenomena (e.g., pain, separation) associated with death. By late toddlerhood and preschool age, children may talk freely about death but may describe its occurrence and attributes with magical thinking and an egocentric viewpoint. They may perceive their impending death as punishment, yet do not view death as permanent but rather as "sleep" or departure from the family. The permanence of death is not realized until the early grade school–age period, when the concepts of reversibility and irreversibility are learned. Children in this age-group often personify death as the bogeyman or some kind of monster. For children who are dying, this newly found knowledge enhances their fears of the unknown. Adolescents, with their new metacognitive abilities, conceptualize death as a process of the life cycle, readily comprehending the emotional, social, and financial implications of the loss occurring from death for themselves and their families. Of all age-groups, adolescents have the most difficulty in dealing with death.

Children with chronic conditions are often subjected to many intrusive and painful experiences and may have experienced the death of friends in the hospital. These experiences can exacerbate their anxieties about death. Depending on individual experience, a child's understanding of death may not follow the projected trajectory. Although information about how affected children's views of death differ from their nonaffected peers is limited, it appears that the fears associated with death are remarkably similar to the fears of hospitalization and intrusive procedures. Even preschool-age children may express fear of separation, despite the fact that death may not yet be conceptualized as irreversible.

For the dying child, how issues such as separation, mutilation, and loss of control are handled plays an important role in their personal conceptualization of death. Care must be taken to prevent unnecessary separation and help these children maintain their autonomy, sense of mastery, and other developmental skills whenever possible.

Primary Care Provider's Role in Promoting Development

Because "cure" is not possible for many chronic conditions, practitioners' condition management plans must focus on care. The goal of care is to minimize the manifestations of the disease and maximize the child's physical, cognitive, and psychosocial potential. Realization of this goal is facilitated by appreciating the family's ecology and adopting a family-centered approach. Family-centered care recognizes that the family is the constant in the child's life and as such is vital to children successfully meeting their potential. Practicing family-centered care requires professionals to do the following: (1) recognize and respect a family's strengths and individuality, (2) promote a family's confidence and competence in caring for the child, and (3) empower a family to advocate for their child when working with the health care system. Families repeatedly identify the need for clear, ongoing communication across the nexus of their child's primary care and specialty providers and providers' appreciation for the family's role as caregivers (Nageswaran et al., 2008; Stille, Primack, McLaughlin, et al., 2007). Lengthening the amount of time, increasing the number of visits, praising success, and being empathetic regarding challenges in a spirit of collaboration promotes families' satisfaction and adherence with treatment plans (Hart, Drotar, Gori, et al., 2006). Providing written educational materials and taping conversations further improves satisfaction and information recall. Telehealth and other Internet technologies can promote communication, but care must be taken not to allow technology to subsume direct clinical care and to ensure that privacy and confidentiality are maintained (Drotar, Greenley, Hoff, et al., 2006).

A noncategorical approach, incorporated with specific strategies for disease management and mitigating functional limitations, provides a nexus on which to base assessments and develop holistic management plans. A good maxim to follow is to generalize developmental information across diagnostic groups and then individualize it for each child and family.

Assessment and Management

Maturational alterations are rarely immutable and should not be thought of as such. Children with chronic conditions require comprehensive care including developmental surveillance to achieve their optimal level of functioning. Developmental lags or behavioral problems should be identified as soon as possible and vigorous intervention should ensue, followed by careful observation for progress with modifications in the treatment plan as necessary. Interventions are most effective when initiated in the preclinical period, that time when slight indications of developmental impairment may be detected but gross manifestations are not yet evident. A "wait and see" attitude is never warranted. Early intervention may prevent or ameliorate many secondary problems or those resulting from neglect or mistreatment of the original condition. For example, although a child may experience hearing loss from aminoglycosides, subsequent language and cognitive delays may be prevented with aggressive intervention.

Like all children, developmental surveillance should be incorporated into every primary care visit for children with chronic conditions as the primary care provider serves as the child's medical home, providing continuous and comprehensive care. Developmental surveillance is "a flexible, longitudinal, continuous, and cumulative process whereby knowledgeable health care professionals identify children who may have developmental problems"

(Council on Children with Disabilities, 2006, p. 407). It incorporates the following components: (1) identification and follow-up of parental concerns, (2) maintaining a documented developmental history, (3) careful observation of the child and parents, (4) identification of risk and protective factors, and (5) general and condition-specific screening using standardized screening instruments (Council on Children with Disabilities, 2006). The American Academy of Pediatrics' algorithm for developmental surveillance of all children (Council on Children with Disabilities, 2006, pp. 405-420) serves as a beginning template for developmental surveillance of children with chronic conditions.

For children with mild conditions, the standard surveillance schedule is probably sufficient. Providers must normalize developmental surveillance and parents must be counseled that ongoing surveillance is the standard of care for all children and not because their child has a chronic condition. This will help allay fears that their child is unduly vulnerable and creating self-fulfilling prophecies. Additional and ongoing assessment throughout a child's lifetime, however, is warranted for those children at risk for specific delays. Attention to expressed parental concerns is critical because these are highly correlated with developmental differences in their children (Glascoe, 1999).

Standardized assessment instruments are useful, necessary adjuncts to a complete history and physical examination for a comprehensive developmental evaluation. When used at regular intervals, these instruments provide objective data so that small developmental changes can be detected. Considering the ever-growing number of children with special needs being cared for in the community, primary care practitioners need to have a compendium of readily administered standardized instruments from which to draw (Table 2-1). They also should not rely only on broad-band developmental screening instruments that are designed to identify global delay rather than provide in-depth information on the type and severity of developmental problems. Focused instruments provide specific information that is useful as part of an in-depth evaluation.

Instruments should be carefully chosen and results thoroughly interpreted because most of these are norm referenced instead of criterion referenced. Other instruments and results are invalid if they measure one developmental construct based on performance in a different arena of development (e.g., the cognitive development of a child with a tracheostomy should not be assessed by an instrument requiring verbal responses). Timed tests may also bias results, particularly if a child has a motor or learning deficit. If a child tires easily, it is best to perform developmental assessments in short intervals so as not to obscure the child's true capabilities. Last, instruments must be culturally relevant to be valid (Nehring, 2007).

When untoward developmental manifestations are detected, the pediatric primary care provider can either provide treatment or, more likely, refer the child to subspecialists with expertise in the area of concern. Referrals should ideally be made to individuals who are parts of the specialty team or within the child's school setting, but additional local referrals may be necessary if the specialty team is far away or school services are inadequate. Adding another layer of care providers requires exquisite coordination of services if the child is to receive appropriate care without overlaps, gaps, or too many demands to cause fatigue (see Chapter 9). Coordination by the primary care provider helps ensure that care is seamless and integrated across the disciplines, especially in today's climate of cost constraint and restrictive insurance coverage (see Chapter 8).

Text continued on p.35

TABLE 2-1

Instruments Used in Developmental Assessment

Test/Score	Age Level	Method	Comments	Time; Examiner Qualifications Required
GENERAL DEVELOPMENT				
AAMR Adaptive Behavior Scale, 2nd ed. Authors: N. Lambert, K. Nihira, H. Leland Source: Pro-ed Website: www.proedinc.com	3–19 yr	Observation Performance tasks	Used as a screening tool and for instructional parent report. Can be an indicator in assessing children whose adaptive behavior indicates possible mental retardation, learning difficulties, or emotional disturbances; provides 16 domain scores. Software for scoring available (previously named AAMD Adaptive Behavior Scale).	15–30 min per domain, 1–2 hr in full
Ages and Stages Questionnaires (ASQ) Authors: J. Squires, L. Potter, D. Bricker Source: Brookes Publishing Co. Website: www.brookespublishing.com	4 mo–5 yr	Parent-completed questionnaire	Series of 79 age-specific questions. Screens communication, gross motor, fine motor, problem solving, and personal adaptive skills. Pass/fail scoring for domains.	10–15 min
Alberta Infant Motor Scale Authors: M. Piper, J. Darrah, L. Pinnell, T. Maguire, P. Byrne Source: Saunders, published Feb 1994 Website: www.elsevier.com; www.umanitoba.ca/	Birth–18 mo	Observation Performance-based, norm-referenced, observational tool.	58 items to measure gross motor developmental milestones. Assesses postural control in supine, prone, and sitting positions. Assesses delays or atypical motor performance and evaluates motor development over time.	20–30 min Rehabilitation therapists; health care professionals with knowledge of motor development in infants
Battelle Developmental Inventory (BDI-2) (2005) Authors: J. Newborg, J. Stock, L. Wnek, J. Guidubaldi, J. Syinicki Source: Riverside Publishing Co. Website: http://riverpub.com	Birth–8 yr	Structured test format Parent and teacher interview Observation	Includes a screening test that can be used to identify areas of development in need of a complete comprehensive BDI. Full BDI consists of 341 test items in five domains: personal-social, adaptive, motor, communication, and cognitive.	Screening test consists of 96 items taking 10–30 min to administer, 1–1½ hr to complete Low examiner qualifications
Bayley Infant Neurodevelopmental Screen (BINS) Author: G.P. Aylward Source: Psychological Corp. Website: www.harcourtassessment.com	3–24 mo	Observation	Series of 6-item sets screening basic neurologic functions; receptive functions (visual, auditory, and tactile input); expressive functions (oral, fine, and gross motor skills); and cognitive processes; results in risk category (low, moderate, or high risk).	10 min
Bayley Scales, 2nd ed. (1993) Author: N. Bayley Source: Psychological Corporation Website: http://harcourtassessment.com	1–42 mo	Observation Demonstration	Evaluates motor, mental, and social behavior of infants and toddlers. Diagnoses normal vs. delayed development. New scoring procedures allow examiners to determine a child's developmental age equivalent for each ability domain.	25–35 min for <15 mo, 60 min for >15 mo Qualified practitioner to examine and evaluate an infant
Bender Visual Motor Gestalt Test II Author: L. Bender Source: American Orthopsychiatric Association, Inc. Website: www.pearsonassessments.com	≥3 yr	Demonstration Visual-motor	A drawing test for evaluating developmental problems, learning disabilities, retardation, psychosis, organic brain disorders in children.	10–20 min Trained psychologist or psychiatrist
Brazelton Neonatal Behavioral Assessment Scale Author: T.B. Brazelton Source: The Brazelton Institute Website: www.brazelton-institute.com/intro.html	3 day–4 wk		Used as a predictive tool in clinical practice and research for behavioral and neurologic assessment. Tests 28 behavioral, 18 reflexive items in the areas of habituation, orientation, motor maturity, variation, self-quieting, and social.	20–30 min Administer by trained examiner
Child Behavior Checklist Author: T.M. Achenbach Source: ASEBA Website: www.aseba.org	1½–18 yr (two forms: 1½–5 yr, 6–18 yr)	Observation/interview	Provides an overview of the child's behavior. Parent and teacher forms available. Self-report form for adolescents.	Administrative form: 15 min Scoring: 3 min via computer, 20 min by hand
Child Development Inventory (CDI) Author: H. Ireton Source: Behavior Science Systems Website: www.childdevrev.com	1½–6 yr	Parent-completed questionnaire	Measures social, self-help, motor, language, and general developmental quotients and age equivalents for different developmental domains. Appropriate for more in-depth evaluation.	30–50 min

Continued

TABLE 2-1

Instruments Used in Developmental Assessment—cont'd

Test/Score	Age Level	Method	Comments	Time; Examiner Qualifications Required
Child Development Review-Parent Questionnaire (CDR-PQ) Author: H. Ireton Source: Behavior Science Systems Website: www.childdevrev.com	1½–5 yr	Parent-completed questionnaire	Professional-completed child development chart measures social, self-help, motor, and language skills.	10–20 min
Denver-II Developmental Screening Test Authors: W.K. Frankenburg, B.W. Camp, P.A. Van Natta Source: Denver Developmental Materials Website: www.denverii.com	Birth–6 yr	Directly administered tool	Screens for expressive and receptive language, gross and fine motor, and personal-social skills. Results in risk category (normal, questionable, abnormal).	10–20 min Administer by professional or trained paraprofessional
Developmental Indicators for Assessment of Learning (DIAL-3) (1998) Authors: C. Mardell-Czudnowski, D.S. Goldenberg Source: Pearson Assessments Website: www.pearsonassessments.com	3–7 yr	Observational	Screens five early childhood areas: motor, language, concepts, self-help, and social development.	20–30 min Scored by a trained professional or paraprofessional
The Early Screening Inventory (revised 1997) Authors: S. Meisels, D. Marsden, M. Wiske, L. Henderson Source: Pearson Learning Group Website: www.pearsonlearning.com	3–6 yr	Observation	Two separate tests: one for age 3–4 ½ yr, one for 4½–6 yr. Assesses visual-motor/adaptive skills, language cognition, and gross motor skills. Includes a parent checklist.	15–20 min Must be a trained professional
Hawaii Early Learning Profile (HELP, 1988) Authors: S.F. Furuno, K.A. O'Reilly, C.M. Kosaka, T.T. Inatsuka, T.L. Allman, B. Zeislott, S. Parks Source: Vort Corporation Website: www.vort.com	Birth–36 mo	Observation and parent interview	685 developmental tasks used to assess six domains: cognition, language, gross motor, fine motor, social-emotional, and self-help. Criterion referenced, curriculum based.	Each domain takes 15–30 min to administer Domains may be selected for individual use
Infant Development Inventory Authors: D.E. Creighton, R.S. Sauve Source: Behavior Science Systems, Inc. Website: www.childdevrev.com	Birth–1½ yr	Parent-completed questionnaire	4 open-ended questions followed by 87 items crossing 5 domains: social, self-help, gross motor, fine motor, and language skills.	10–20 min
Minnesota Infant Development Inventory (1988) Minnesota Early Child Development Inventory Minnesota Preschool Development Inventory Minnesota Childhood Development Inventory Authors: H. Ireton, E. Thwing Source: Behavior Science Systems, Inc. Website: www.childdevrev.com	Birth–15 mo 1–3 yr 3–6 yr	Observation/interview Parent report True/false	A first-level screening tool. Measures infant's development in five domains: gross motor, fine motor, language, comprehension, and personal-social. Provides a profile of the child's strengths and weaknesses. 60–80 items on each inventory.	10–30 min
Parents' Evaluation of Developmental Status (PEDS) Authors: F.P. Glascoe Source: Ellsworth & Vandermeer Press, LLC Website: www.pedstest.com	Birth–8 yr	Parent interview form	Screens for developmental and behavioral problems needing further evaluation. Single response form used for all ages. May be useful as a surveillance tool.	2–10 min
Peabody Individual Achievement Test: Revised (PIAT-R) 1989 Authors: L.M. Dumm, F.C. Markwardt, Jr. Source: Pearson Assessments Website: www.ags.pearsonassessments.com	6–18 yr	Interview Written test	Content areas: general information, reading recognition and comprehension, math, spelling, written expression. Used to screen for areas of weakness requiring more detailed diagnostic testing in scholastic achievement.	50–70 min Must be administered by a psychologist
Pediatric Symptom Checklist Authors: M. Murphy, M. Jellinek Source: Massachusetts General Hospital Website: http://psc.partners.org/	6–18 yr (2–5 yr-old version also)	Checklist completed by parent	Used to screen for areas of weakness requiring more detailed diagnostic testing in scholastic achievement. Parent-completed form or child self-report.	5 min

Test / Author / Source / Website	Age	Method	Description	Time / Comments
Riley Preschool Development Screening Inventory (RPDSI) Author: G.D. Riley Source: Western Psychological Services Website: www.wpspublish.com	3–5 yr	Observation	For children who have academic problems. Used to screen for emotional, learning, and behavioral issues.	Time varies To be administered by qualified clinician
Vineland Adaptive Behavior Scales, 2nd ed. Authors: S.S. Sparrow, D.A. Balla, D.V. Cicchetti Source: Pearson Assessments Website: www.ags.pearsonassessments.com	Birth–19 yr	Semi-structured interview with caregiver and observation	Assesses adaptive behavior in four sectors: communication, daily living skills, socialization, and motor skills. Can be used with mentally retarded and disabled individuals.	Interview edition: 20–40 min Expanded edition: 60–90 min
Wide Range Achievement Test (WRAT), 3rd ed. Authors: Jastak & Wilkinson Source: Wide Range Inc. and Psychological Assessment Resources Inc. Website: www3.parinc.com	5–75 yr	Paper-pencil subtests	Used for educational placement, vocational assessment, and job placement training. Measures skills needed to learn reading, spelling, and math. Large-print edition available.	15–30 min
TEMPERAMENT				
Carey Temperament Scales Early Infancy scale Revised Infant scale Toddler scale Behavioral Style questionnaire Middle Childhood questionnaire Authors: S.C. McDevitt, W.B. Carey Source: Pearson Assessments Website: http://pearsonassess.com	1–4 mo 4–11 mo 1–3 yr 3–7 yr 8–12 yr	Interview	Provides an objective measure of the child's temperament profile. Fosters more effective interaction between parent and child. 95 items, 6-point frequency scale.	Time varies. Counselors, educators, health practitioners, social workers, and psychologists may administer.
VISION				
Allen Picture Card Test of Visual Acuity Author: H.F. Allen Source: Western Ophthalmics Corporation Website: www.west-op.com	2½–6 yr	Observation	Preschooler screening test for visual acuity. No pretraining needed for preschool children.	Time varies
Denver Eye Screening Test (DEST) 1973 Authors: W.K. Frankenberg, A.D. Goldstein, J. Barker Source: Denver Developmental Materials, Inc. Website: www.denverii.com/DEST.html	6 mo–6 yr	Observation	Includes three different tests according to age. Identifies children with acuity problems. 6 mo–2½ yr (preschool-age children unable to respond to the Snellen Illiterate E Test): do a picture card test; takes 5 min. 3–6 year: Snellen Illiterate E Test.	6 mo–3 yr: 5 min, 3–6 yr: 10 min For use by health professionals, Headstart, daycare, and social services personnel.
HOTV (matching symbol test) Author: O. Lippmann Source: Veatch Instruments Website: www.veatchinstruments.com	≥2½ yr, or able to identify shapes	Flashcards	Good for young children or those who do not like to verbalize. Children name the four letters, H, O, T, V, on a chart for testing at 10–20 ft and match them to a demonstration card. Avoids the problem with image reversal and eye-hand coordination that can occur with the letter "E."	Time varies
Preschool (Allen) Acuity Test Card Author: H.F. Allen Source: Western Ophthalmics Website: www.west-op.com	≥2½ yr	Interview (i.e., "name the picture")	Identifies children with acuity problems.	10 min
Snellen Illiterate E Test Author: H. Snellen Source: American Academy of Ophthalmology; American Association of Ophthalmology Website: www.paao.org	≥3 yr	Observation using two persons as a team in screening	Intended as a screening measure for central acuity of preschool-age children and other children who have not learned to read	Time varies

Continued

TABLE 2-1

Instruments Used in Developmental Assessment—cont'd

Test/Score	Age Level	Method	Comments	Time; Examiner Qualifications Required
LANGUAGE/COGNITIVE				
The Bzoch-League Receptive Expressive Emergent Language Scale (REEL), 3rd ed. Authors: K.R. Bzoch, R. League. Source: Pearson Assessments. Website: www.pearsonassessments.com	Birth–3 yr	Paper-and-pencil inventory. Parent interview	To identify young children who have language impairments or other disabilities that interfere with language development.	20 min
Capute Scales (Cognitive Adaptive Test/Clinical Linguistic Auditory Milestone Scale [CAT/CLAMS]) Authors: R.G. Voigt, F.R. Brown, J.K. Fraley. Source: Paul H. Brookes Publishing Co. Website: www.pbrookes.com	3 mo–3 yr	Directly administered tool	Measures visual-motor/problem solving (CAT) and expressive and receptive language (CLAMS). Results in developmental quotient and age equivalent.	15–20 min
Communication and Symbolic Behavior Scales- Developmental Profile (CSBS-DP); Infant Toddler Checklist Authors: A.M. Wetherby, B.M. Prizant. Source: Paul H. Brookes Publishing Co. Website: www.pbrookes.com	6–24 mo	Parent-completed checklist	Screens for communication and symbolic abilities up to the 24-month age level. One-page parent-completed screening tool.	5–10 min
Denver Articulation Screening Exam (DASE) (1973) Authors: A.F. Drumwright, W.K. Frankenberg. Source: Denver Developmental Materials, Inc. Website: www.denverii.com/DASE.html	2½–7 yr	Observation	Designed to identify significant developmental delay in the acquisition of speech sounds. Good for screening children who may be economically disadvantaged and have a potential speech problem with articulation or pronunciation.	5–15 min To be administered by a qualified professional or a nonprofessional with special training
Early Language Milestone Scale (ELMS), 2nd ed. Author: J. Coplan. Source: PRO-ED Inc. Website: www.proedinc.com	Birth–36 mo	Interview. Observation	Screening instrument for auditory expressive, receptive, and visual components of language. 43 items arranged in 3 domains: expressive, receptive, and visual components of language.	1–10 min
Kaufman Brief Intelligence Test (K-BIT-2), 2nd ed. Authors: A.S. Kaufman, N.L. Kaufman. Source: Pearson Assessments. Website: www.ags.pearsonassessments.com	4–90+ yr	Structured test format	Quick measure of verbal and nonverbal intelligence. May not be substituted for comprehensive measure of intelligence. Assesses expressive vocabulary, definitions, and matrices.	15–30 min
McCarthur-Bates Communicative Development Inventory Authors: L. Fenson, P.S. Dale, D. Thal, E. Bates, J.P. Harding, S. Pethick, J.S. Relly. Source: CDI Advisory Board. Website: www.sci.sdsu.edu/cdi/cdi3_e.htm	8–30 mo and older developmentally delayed children	Parent report measuring vocabulary development	Measures vocabulary development (words and sentences) in children with and without developmental delays. Includes an extensive vocabulary checklist containing words that children typically produce in the second and third years; parents are asked to review and check all words that their child can spontaneously produce.	Time varies Administered by a speech therapist or pathologist, physician, or nurse
Peabody Picture Vocabulary Test, 4th ed. Author: L.M. Dunn. Source: Pearson Assessments. Website: http://ags.pearsonassessments.com	2–6 yr through 90+	Individual "point to" response test	More up-to-date/realistic pictures, balanced sex and race/ethnicities. IQ used to assess receptive vocabulary; not a measure of speech and language skills. Measures hearing vocabulary for standard American English. Used with non-English-speaking students to screen for mental retardation or giftedness.	10–20 min Administer by a qualified clinician
Riley Articulation and Language Test, Revised (RALT-R) Author: G.D. Riley. Source: Western Psychological Services. Website: www.wpspublish.com	≥4–8 yr	Performance tasks by the child	Screening test that identifies children in need of speech therapy. Uses three subjects: language proficiency and intelligibility, articulation function, and language function. Provides a quantified system for observing and measuring neurologic signs leading to problems in speech, language, and behavior.	3 min Administer by a qualified clinician

HEARING

Test	Age	Method	Description	Time/Notes
Noise Stik II Author: L.H. Eckstein Website: www.hearingreview.com/issues/articles/HPR_2002-03_99.asp	Infants, toddlers, and older persons	Behavioral response to auditory stimulation	2-sec tone which can be increased up to 5 sec. Hand-held free-field screener for early detection of infant hearing loss.	Time varies

MOTOR

Test	Age	Method	Description	Time/Notes
Early Motor Pattern Profile (EMPP) Authors: A.M. Morgan, J.C. Aldag Source: Early identification of cerebral palsy using a profile of abnormal motor patterns. *Pediatrics*, 98(4 P+1), 692-697. Website: None	6–12 mo	Physician-administered examination	Standard examination of movement, tone, and reflex development. Simple 3-point scoring system.	5–10 min Administer by physician
Motor Quotient (MQ) Authors: A.J. Capute, B.K. Shapiro Source: The motor quotient: A method for the early detection of motor delay. *Am J Dis Child*, 139(9), 940-942. Website: None	8–18 mo	Ratio quotients	Uses simple ration quotient with gross motor milestones for detecting delayed motor development. 11 total milestones; 1 per visit.	1–3 min
Peabody Developmental Motor Scales, 2nd ed. Authors: M. Folio, R. Fewell Source: Psychological Assessment Resources, Inc. Website: www3.parinc.com	Birth–5 yr	Observation	Assesses reflexes, stationary, locomotion, object manipulation, grasping, and visual-motor integration skills.	20 min Must be trained professional
Riley Motor Problems Inventory (RMPI) Author: G.D. Riley Source: Western Psychological Services Website: www.wpspublish.com	≥4 yr	Performance tasks by the child	Provides a quantified system for observation and measurement of neurologic signs that lead to problems in speech, language, learning, and behavior.	Time varies Must be qualified practitioner

PSYCHOSOCIAL DEVELOPMENT

Test	Age	Method	Description	Time/Notes
Brief Infant-Toddler Social and Emotional Assessment (BITSEA) Authors: M. Briggs-Gowan, A. Carter Source: Pearson Assessments Website: www.pearsonassess.com	1–3 yr	Parent form	Ideal for monitoring progress over time. 42-item parent form. Focuses on four domains: externalizing, internalizing, dysregulation, and competence.	5–15 min
Children's Depression Inventory (CDI) Author: M. Kovacs Source: Pearson Assessments Website: www.pearsonassessments.com	6–17 yr	Paper-and-pencil self-report	Assesses cognitive, affective, and behavioral signs of depression. Contains 27 items and is designed for schools, child guidance clinics, pediatric practices, and child psychiatric settings. First-grade reading level.	5–10 min
Piers-Harris Children's Self-Concept Scale, 2nd ed. Authors: E.V. Piers, D.B. Harris Source: Western Psychological Services Website: http://portal.wpspublish.com	7–18 yr	Self-report Descriptive statements used by groups or individuals	80 questions requiring yes/no answers. Assesses a raw self-concept score plus cluster scores for 60 items in six domains: behavioral adjustment, freedom from anxiety, intellectual and school status, happiness and satisfaction, physical appearance and attributes, and popularity. Test title is "The Way I Feel about Myself."	10–15 min

Continued

TABLE 2-1

Instruments Used in Developmental Assessment—cont'd

Test/Score	Age Level	Method	Comments	Time; Examiner Qualifications Required
STRESS AND ANXIETY				
Revised Children's Manifest Anxiety Scale Authors: C.R. Reynolds, B.O. Richmond Source: Western Psychological Services Website: www.wpspublish.com	6–19 yr	Self-report	Designed to assess the level and nature of anxiety in children and adolescents. For children over 9 it can be administered in a group. Based on 28 items and 9 items making up the "Lie Scale."	10–15 min
State-Trait Anxiety Inventory for Children (STAIC) (1997) Authors: C.D. Spielberg, C.D. Edwards, R.E. Lushene, J Montuori, D. Platzek Source: Mind Garden Website: www.mindgarden.com	Upper elementary and junior high school students	Self-administered in groups or individually	Measures anxiety in elementary school children. Test title is "How I Feel Questionnaire."	20 min
State-Trait Anxiety Inventory for Children (STAIC) (1984) Authors: C.D. Spielberger, C.D. Edwards, J. Montuori, R. Lushene Source: Mind Garden Website: www.mindgarden.com	Sixth-grade reading level	Group administration	Two 20-item scales. Designed to assess anxiety as an emotional state (S-Anxiety) and individual differences in anxiety proneness as a personality trait (T-Anxiety).	10–20 min
FAMILY FUNCTION				
Feetham Family Functioning Survey (FFFS) (1982) Authors: S. Feetham, S. Humenick Source: Springer Website: www.springerpub.com	Family	Self-reporting	25 questions evaluating 6 areas of functioning: household tasks, child care, sexual and moral relations, interaction with family and friends, community involvement, and sources of support. Used for identifying specific areas of dysfunction in a stressed family.	10 min
Home Observation for Measurement of the Environment (HOME) (1984) Authors: R. Bradley, B. Caldwell Source: Home Inventory LLC, University of Arkansas, Little Rock Website: www.ualr.edu/crtldept/home4.htm	Birth–3 yr; 3–6 years; middle childhood (6–10 yr); and early adolescence (10–15 yr)	Interview Direct observation of the interaction between the caretaker and the child	Two instruments designed to assess the quantity and quality of social, emotional, and cognitive support available to a child within the home. Inventory for birth–3 yr contains 45 items; 3–6 yr contains 55 items; 6–10 yr contains 59 items; and 10–15 yr contains 40 items	Each inventory takes approximately 1 hr

Obtaining services may require that the child's condition and associated problems be diagnostically labeled, although federal legislation has made this less common. Providing a label may help validate the concerns of children and families and direct future interventions and activities but must be done judiciously. Labeling often sets children apart from their peers and may result in different treatment by family members, teachers, and significant others. Diagnostic labels assigned in childhood follow children into adulthood and might prevent them from pursuing selected careers, joining the military, or being eligible for insurance. Although it is usually feasible to label specific disease entities, labeling associated with developmental manifestations should be done carefully. The ultimate long-term goal of care is for a child to reach and sustain optimal levels of functioning. Developing precise, measurable, short-term goals helps ensure that optimal functioning is obtained.

Fostering Psychosocial Health

Effective therapeutic interventions can strengthen a child's resiliency and improve general well-being and quality of life while preventing or mitigating coexisting psychological problems. Effective coping strategies, including seeking social support, managing condition-related stressors, and developing good social skills, help children with chronic conditions reduce the likelihood of developing behavioral problems (Meijer et al., 2002). Fostering a good parent-child relationship is the gateway to promoting childhood resilience (Letourneau, Drummond, Flemming, et al., 2001). Other strategies are listed in Box 2-2.

Children with and without chronic conditions enjoy participating in the same activities (Heah, Case, McGuire, et al., 2007). The role of schools should not be undervalued because they provide a measure of independence and opportunities for self-mastery and self-esteem building that are not readily achieved at home (see Chapter 3). Specialty camps help youths cope with their conditions, improve self-care skills, and foster healthy self-esteem (Plante, Lobato, & Engel, 2001; Thomas & Gaslin, 2001). Other extracurricular activities including a wide range of sports that showcase children's skills and encourage peer interaction are equally useful but must be selected in light of condition-specific limitations (Box 2-3) (Rice & Council on Sports Medicine & Fitness, 2008). Companion

---

BOX 2-2

Fostering Resilience

- Identify the child's and family's assets; help them develop assertiveness and self-advocacy skills.
- Nurture positive self-esteem and self-efficacy in all family members.
- Help youths see that their chronic condition is not an insurmountable problem.
- Help all family members develop flexible coping skills.
- Teach needed communication and problem-solving skills.
- Encourage academic attainment in youth.
- Encourage children to make social connections in school and through participation in extracurricular activities.
- Promote volunteerism in the community and other contributions to others.
- Help families develop healthy habits and youths develop appropriate self-care skills.
- Support youths in developing values, beliefs, and goals for their life.
- Encourage parents to role model appropriate behavior.
- Assist parents to set realistic but high expectations.

BOX 2-3

Categorization of Sports by Physical Contact Potential

HIGH-CONTACT SPORTS
- Basketball
- Boxing
- Cheerleading
- Diving
- Dodge ball
- Football
- Gymnastics
- Hockey
- Judo
- Kick boxing
- Lacrosse
- Mountaineering
- Parachuting
- Rugby
- Skiing/snowboarding
- Soccer
- Trampolining
- Water polo
- Wrestling

RESTRICTED-CONTACT SPORTS
- Baseball
- Cycling
- Fencing
- Football, touch
- Horseback riding
- Racquetball
- Rafting/sea kayaking
- Skating
- Skiing, cross-country and water
- Softball
- Surfing
- Squash
- Tae Kwon Do
- Track-and-field events
- Volleyball

NONCONTACT SPORTS
- Archery
- Badminton
- Bowling
- Canoeing/kayaking
- Crew/rowing
- Dance
- Fishing
- Golf
- Hiking
- Pilates
- Rope jumping
- Running
- Sailing
- Scuba diving
- Snowshoeing
- Swimming
- Tennis
- Track
- Yoga

Note: Depending on intensity of activity and of participants, amount of contact can change. Adapted from Rice, S.G., & Council on Sports Medicine and Fitness. (2008). Medical conditions affecting sports participation. *Pediatrics, 121,* 841–848.

animals also help children adapt to their chronic condition (Spence & Kaiser, 2002). Children who have shared their condition to close friends have found disclosure helpful (LaGreca et al., 2002). Suggestions for school reentry (see Chapter 3) can be adapted for returning to extracurricular activities as well.

Anticipatory Guidance and Education

Children with chronic conditions require the same anticipatory guidance as do their unaffected peers, although this needs to be adapted to their developmental (rather than chronologic) age and condition-specific limitations (Houtrow, Kim, Chen, et al., 2007). Primary care providers need to help prepare children in self-care behaviors and development of self-advocacy skills for dealing with the health care community. This is important for children and adolescents with chronic conditions because they are likely to use the health care system often throughout their lives. The transition between pediatric and adult care is a complex endeavor that is exacerbated by provider and system obstacles (Betz & Redcay, 2002) (see Chapter 4). Educating children and adolescents about their condition helps empower them to negotiate with the health care system effectively.

To accomplish the objectives of primary care, children must develop age-appropriate knowledge of anatomy, physiology, associated pathophysiology, and intricacies of the health care system. It is often incorrectly assumed that children are well versed about these topics because they know the jargon, appear comfortable with the health care environment, and have been diagnosed "for years." Accurate, developmentally appropriate information needs to be incorporated into the primary care of all children with chronic conditions because learning is more likely to occur in a nonthreatening environment where children are in a comparatively good state of health rather than when they are sick or hospitalized. A comprehensive plan managed by the primary care provider in conjunction with parents, subspecialty providers, and the school support services (see Chapter 3) will help ensure that this learning occurs. Teaching methods must be altered to fit the child's developmental age. Children will learn best when the material presented to them remains within one level of their current cognitive functioning. Information also needs to be reiterated with greater complexity as the child matures.

A multisensory approach (i.e., one that brings all of the child's senses to bear on the learning task at hand) is more likely to be effective with preschool- and school-age children than more traditional lecture methods. Materials need to be selected according to their age appropriateness, cultural relevance, and accuracy of information. For example, anatomically correct rag dolls or models, doll hospitals, and play equipment are highly effective teaching aids to use with younger children. For older youths, an ever-expanding array of professionally developed audiovisual media (e.g., books, videos, interactive computer programs, websites) are available and are useful adjuncts to individualized teaching plans. Practitioners should examine all materials in advance to determine if the information presented will correspond to the child's experiences and treatment plan. There is little sense in providing cute but inaccurate information to a child, because these myths will just need to be dispelled when the child matures. This is of particular significance for younger children who have not developed causal reasoning, engage in fantasy, and tend to interpret their environment from a singular perspective.

Therapeutic Adherence

Promoting therapeutic adherence is a critical role of the primary care provider, especially in light of current health care trends that shift the onus of treatment responsibilities to the family. Condition-management programs must be tailored to the child to maximize the likelihood of therapeutic adherence. A meta-analysis of interventions designed to promote adherence to pediatric treatment regimens for chronic conditions demonstrated that condition-specific education is necessary but insufficient in promoting adherence (Kahana, Drotar, & Frazier, 2008). Interventions with greater efficacy include those that use behavioral, cognitive-behavioral, self-regulatory skill training, or combined approaches (Haynes, Yackloo, Sahota, et al., 2008; Kahana et al., 2008). Therapeutic adherence is further enhanced when youths actively participate in health care decisions; feel supported by parents, peers, and practitioners; have the energy, motivation, and willpower to manage their treatment regimen; and the interventions are culturally appropriate (Kyngas & Rissanen, 2001; LaGreca et al., 2002; Nehring, 2007).

Revisiting adherence strategies needs to be an ongoing component of clinical management because adherence tends to diminish over time (Janse, Sinnema, Uiterwaal, et al., 2005a, 2005b; Kahana et al., 2008). Older children and adolescents should begin to take responsibility for more of the care regimens. Useful steps in this process include reeducating the youths about their conditions, helping parents and teens negotiate care responsibilities, and assisting parents to shift from close supervision so that by early adulthood, youths assume responsibility for all or most of their care whenever possible (Modi, Marciel, Slater, et al., 2008). Peers should be involved because they are an increasingly important part of a youth's social support system and, along with parental involvement, have a profound impact on youths' successful transition to self-care (Kef, 2002).

Assistive aids may help promote independence and therapeutic adherence. For example, beepers and watches with alarms help youths remember to take medications and personal digital assistants (PDAs) can be used in dietary decision making. For youths with physical or emotional disabilities, companion animals help create independence (Spence & Kaiser, 2002). Therapeutic adherence can be encouraged through open discussion and adoption of activities such as those listed in Box 2-4.

BOX 2-4

Promoting Therapeutic Adherence

Teach children in a developmentally appropriate manner about the following:
- Anatomy and physiology
- The pathophysiology of their condition
- Medication and treatment uses and effectiveness
- How to tell friends, teachers, and others about the condition

Explore the thoughts and feelings of children and parents about the treatment plan:
- Revisit as children mature
- Incorporate culturally relevant information

Adjust the treatment plan to fit within the child's and family's lifestyle.

Suggest the use of "props" to serve as reminders:
- Use beepers or watch or cell phone alarms for medication reminders
- Coordinate medications with mealtimes
- Adjust medications to the minimal number of pills and doses necessary
- Incorporate a reward system; use sticker charts or tokens with younger children

In evaluating therapeutic adherence, the clinician should seek information from both the child and parents and, when appropriate, other sources (e.g., schools) as well. Besides inquiring about the prescribed treatment plan, information regarding the use of complementary and alternative therapies needs to be sought (Committee on Children with Disabilities, 2001), because families and youths frequently use these as adjunct or replacement measures. Evidence indicates that neither parents nor children are necessarily accurate in their reports, particularly as children begin to move in social spheres exclusive of their parents (Burkhart, Dunbar-Jacob, & Rohay, 2001). Although nonadherence is an issue, determining the reason is critical before instituting any action. Nonadherence is usually not deliberate or consistent but due to misunderstanding the instructions, poor time management, forgetfulness, or other related behaviors. Some families with consistent but not deliberate nonadherence may be too disorganized to maintain a management plan. Smaller groups of children (and their parents) deliberately do not adhere to a treatment regimen because they believe it is inefficacious, fear side effects, find it too costly, or have similar reasons. Other families choose certain treatments as priorities and adhere to them while not adhering to others that they feel are of little value. Still others remain in denial as to the severity or ramifications of the condition. Interventions must specifically address the reason for nonadherence, and a referral for mental health counseling may be appropriate.

Advocacy

Many professionals are called on to care for the complex needs of children with chronic conditions. Although all have the same goal—to help the child reach maximum potential—conflicts may arise over the best approach for realizing it. Primary care providers are in the unique position to advocate for a child by identifying the range of treatment options and their implications, informing the child and family of available resources, and helping coordinate these interdisciplinary services (see Chapter 9). Advocacy extends to helping families acquire and maintain health insurance needed for receiving necessary services. This is especially critical in light of the changing service delivery and reimbursement patterns for chronic conditions (see Chapter 8).

Emergency Care. Children with chronic conditions are at higher risk for severe acute illnesses, often potentially preventable and tangential to the condition (Dosa, Boeing, & Kanter, 2001). They are also at higher risk for neglect or abuse from family members and others (Committee on Child Abuse and Neglect and Committee on Children with Disabilities, 2001). Clinicians can advocate for children's physiologic and psychological safety by helping ensure ongoing assessments and instituting appropriate interventions. Providers should also help families prepare for emergency care of their child should it be necessary. Because children with chronic conditions may require different and complex services not usually needed by the typical child, encouraging the family to ensure that the child wears a medical alert bracelet and providing a completed emergency information form to daycare, school, camp, and extracurricular activity personnel will help ensure that the child receives prompt care should this be necessary. For children on ventilators or who are disabled, a care plan should be filed with the local fire department and utility services in case of fire, flood, or power outage. A general emergency information form (in both English and Spanish), selected condition-specific forms, and disaster preparedness information are available from the American Academy of Pediatrics at www.medicalhomeinfo. org/tools/emer_med.html.

Counseling. Careful attention must be paid to the mental and emotional health of children with chronic conditions. Growing up is difficult, and the incidence of violence, substance abuse, depression, suicide, and other risks continues to climb among all children. Children with chronic conditions—especially those with diminished self-esteem—may be particularly vulnerable to mental health problems (Bethell, Read, Blumberg, et al., 2008; LaGreca et al., 2002; Telfair et al., 2005). Proactive efforts to prevent mental health problems from occurring include the following: (1) encouraging normal life experiences, (2) improving coping and adaptive abilities, (3) helping children empower themselves, (4) expanding social support networks, (5) addressing parental identified needs, and (6) coordinating care (Committee on Children with Disabilities and Committee on Psychosocial Aspects of Child and Family Health, 1993; Perrin, Lewkowicz, & Young, 2000).

Despite the prevalence of mental health concerns among children, many do not receive specialty mental health services; children from black, Hispanic, and poor families are disproportionately underserved (Inkelas, Ragahavan, Larson, et al., 2007; Ngui & Flores, 2007). The burden of identifying psychosocial problems falls on primary care providers. The longitudinal relationship that such individuals have with children and families is critical in helping to recognize that mental health problems might develop or may already exist. Unfortunately, the mental health problems of many children are overshadowed by the symptoms associated with their chronic condition and may go unrecognized and undiagnosed.

The first step for all pediatric providers is to recognize and appreciate the potential for psychological impairment in children with chronic conditions. Mental health problems may manifest as global behavioral or achievement problems or aberrant behaviors (e.g., psychosomatic complaints, extreme apprehension, deliberate therapeutic nonadherence, or dysfunctional communication) to family members and others. Adopting a healthy suspicion, conducting a careful health history, and providing an atmosphere for discussion will help identify children at risk. Mental health concerns are often missed if only the parents or only the child is interviewed, and less than half of parents will initiate discussions about psychosocial concerns. It is important to explore this possibility in discussions with all family members, stressing that information will be kept confidential unless the child is at risk (Telfair et al., 2005). Because standardized behavioral screening instruments have low sensitivity with populations of children with chronic conditions (Canning & Kelleher, 1994), careful observation and in-depth interviewing are important.

If no problems are apparent, the focus is on primary prevention where measures can be undertaken to avoid onset of emotional disturbance or enhance mental health. Programs may be based on counseling, skills training, health education, discussion groups, or combinations of these and are designed to develop resilience and coping skills. Most of these approaches have been shown to be effective. Referral to a mental health professional may be appropriate to help a child adapt to a new diagnosis or a deteriorating prognosis; deal with school, family, and peer group issues; or clarify interpersonal and career goals, which are usually very private concerns for older children and adolescents.

Secondary prevention seeks to treat symptoms of emotional distress early to prevent long-term sequelae of mental illness. When problems exist, an accurate diagnosis in accordance with the *Diagnostic and Statistical Manual of Mental Disorders IV-TR* (American Psychiatric Association, 2000) is important. After the diagnosis is made, appropriate interventions must be promptly initiated and may include individual or group counseling, judicious use of psychotropic medications, or referral to a mental health provider.

Unfortunately, the current insurance and health care delivery infrastructure accompanied by family resistance to mental health intervention is a significant barrier to the referral process. Moreover, seeking help while maintaining privacy may be difficult for children and families if their mobility around the community is limited. Primary care providers can facilitate such help.

Hospitalization. Hospitalization is not uncommon with this population of children, and care is usually transferred to the subspecialty team during this time. Pediatric primary care providers can assist in a smooth transition. In addition to giving information about the child's physical condition, parents must be encouraged to inform the subspecialty team about developmental enrichment programs or school services that the child is receiving. If the hospitalization is planned, every effort should be made for hospital-based educators or tutors to confer with school officials before the child's admission so that schooling is not interrupted. Properly preparing the child and family—especially for new situations—also smoothes the adjustment to hospitalization. Preparation must include procedural information about situations the child and family will encounter, definitions of medical jargon specific to the condition, and opportunities to process (i.e., through play, role playing, or discussion) new situations they may experience. For families who are nonassertive or overly aggressive, primary care providers can help to appropriately empower the child and family members for self-advocacy by working through these tasks.

Monitoring the child's adjustment to hospitalization and how it affects the child's future development is also an important part of advocacy. A child's personality and the severity of the condition affect adaptation to hospitalization (Vessey, 2003). Hospitalization is an intrusion into the lives of many children with chronic conditions, but other children have positive memories of previous hospitalizations and may see the hospital as a safe environment. These children may perceive the staff as friends and are often relieved to have a temporary respite from the stress of school, the harassment of other children, or the demands of daily activities. Primary care providers need to recognize that some children will occasionally try to become hospitalized to remove themselves from home or school situations that are particularly onerous, although this is uncommon.

Palliative Care. Palliative care is designed to relieve, rather than cure, symptoms caused by a child's condition. Palliative care helps children live more comfortably and improve their quality of life. It is not limited to dying children, but is appropriate for all children with severe chronic conditions for which there is no cure. It is estimated that palliative care would be appropriate for approximately 1.5 to 2 million children in the United States (Carroll, Torkildson, & Winsness, 2007), but these services are vastly underused. Families often confuse palliative care with hospice care and fear that the health care team has given up hope for their child. Primary care providers need to understand the differences between palliative care and hospice care and communicate these to the families.

Palliative care should be integrated into the care of children diagnosed with severe or profound disabilities or life-threatening or terminal conditions, regardless of outcome. Palliative care measures can be instituted even when restorative treatments are still being tried (Klick & Ballantine, 2007). The emphasis should be on symptom management, including pain, gastrointestinal problems (e.g., nausea, vomiting, constipation, diarrhea), and psychosocial distress (e.g., anger, anxiety, depression, suicide ideation) (Friedrichsdorf & Kang, 2007; Kersun & Shemesh, 2007; Santucci & Mack, 2007). Primary care providers need to be comfortable providing palliative care, whether directly or in tandem with a palliative care team.

Dying and Hospice Care. Despite everyone's best efforts, some children will die. For children with a downward clinical course, early discussions of hospice care before all curative options are exhausted are appropriate (Committee on Bioethics and Committee on Hospital Care, 2000). Hospitalization and home care both have advantages and disadvantages, and the decision of which to pursue must be made in concert with the child's wishes and the family's capabilities. Although some parents and children may feel more secure being in the hospital and surrounded by professionals they trust, increasingly families are choosing for children to die at home, where they are in familiar surroundings, separation is minimized, care is individualized, and they are in greater control of their situation. Primary care providers can be instrumental in facilitating either option.

For families who choose for their child to die at home, primary care providers, as members of the larger interdisciplinary team, help in planning for a seamless transition from hospital to home and providing hospice care during this difficult time. The need to identify child-appropriate services is critical when arranging hospice home care services for dying children and their families. Home hospice agencies that provide pediatric services need not only to provide appropriate end-of-life care for children of various ages, but also bereavement counseling to other family members, including siblings.

When selecting an agency, Carroll and colleagues (2007) identify the following steps providers should pursue:

1. Meet with the family to identify their goals and wishes for their child's care, exploring the limitations of treatment (i.e., antibiotics, oxygen, hydration, resuscitation, and other treatment modalities).
2. Verify insurance coverage.
3. Identify a qualified provider network and home hospice agency with pediatric specialty services.
4. Review the care plan with the insurance company to ensure that services are authorized and reimbursable.
5. Complete the referral to the selected home hospice agency.

Many hospice agencies are less comfortable with managing the care of dying children, and pediatric hospice care is not always available. Therefore the primary care practitioner needs to remain involved in the child's care, regularly communicating with hospice staff and family members while supporting hospice caregivers in managing symptoms and prescribing medications (Carroll et al., 2007). Throughout, the primary care provider needs to be sensitive to the family's culture and spiritual belief system and rituals.

Children should participate in decision making to the fullest extent possible (Committee on Bioethics and Committee on Hospital

Care, 2000). Primary care providers need to acknowledge that children frequently are aware of their impending death and help them communicate their wishes to their families and others. Some adolescents with chronic, life-threatening conditions may seek to discontinue treatment, and providers must balance the youth's and parents' desires and help mediate these conversations with the help of a hospital's ethics committee or palliative care/hospice personnel (Mercurio, 2007).

The psychosocial and emotional needs and fears of dying children need to be addressed from their cognitive level of development (Kane, Barber, Jordan, et al., 2000). Children often become anxious or depressed (Kersun & Shemesh, 2007). They must be reassured that they are not responsible for their illness and encouraged to talk about their feelings or express them through art or music therapy. Pharmacologic interventions may be considered. Primary care providers can help family members with this by modeling ways to communicate these sensitive issues and offering insights on how children's developmental levels affect their ability to conceptualize death. Children's questions are often upsetting to parents, such as when a 6-year-old requests detailed information about death rituals or a preschooler asks, "Who will read me stories after I die?" Many children are deeply spiritual, and their faith should not be left unexplored or unattended (Kane et al., 2000; McSherry & Smith, 2007). Helping family members and other significant individuals communicate effectively with the child and each other makes death easier to bear. The child's death does not conclude the primary care provider's responsibility because parents and siblings benefit from additional empathetic support in the following months.

Summary

Children with chronic conditions are at a higher risk for negative developmental sequelae than their nonaffected peers. The severity and persistence of the condition, the child's individual traits, family functioning, and the available network of social supports all influence the child's developmental outcomes. Comprehensive prospective care often can eliminate or significantly ameliorate negative outcomes. Careful assessment using an interdisciplinary, integrated approach helps identify potential or emerging problems associated with the child's disease progression, functional status, social interactions, or global development. Individualized intervention strategies—including therapeutic management, education, counseling, and advocacy—can then be designed and implemented to help children with chronic conditions reach their developmental potential. Partnering with families is essential to ensure optimal outcomes (Denboba et al., 2006).

Resources

Bright Futures
A national health promotion and disease prevention initiative that addresses children's health needs in the context of family and community. Diverse resources are available to help improve and maintain the health of all children and adolescents.
Website: www.brightfutures.aap.org

Children's Hospice and Palliative Care Coalition
A social movement led by children's hospitals, hospices, home health, and grassroots agencies to improve care for children with life-threatening conditions and their families.

65 Nielson St. #108
Watsonville, CA 95076
(831) 763-3070
Website: www.childrenshospice.org

Family Voices
A national grassroots network that advocates for health care services and provides information for families with children and youths with special health care needs.
3411 Candelaria NE, Suite M
Albuquerque, NM 87107
(888) 835-5669
Website: www.familyvoices.org

Starlight Starbright Children's Foundation
Improves the quality of life for children with serious medical conditions by providing entertainment, education, and family activities that help them cope with the pain, fear, and isolation of prolonged illness.
5757 Wilshire Blvd., Suite M100
Los Angeles, CA 90036
(310) 479-1212
Website: www.starlight.org

REFERENCES

American Psychiatric Association (2000). *Diagnostic and Statistical Manual of Mental Disorders. DSM-IV-TR.* (4th ed., Text Revision). Washington, DC: Author.

Berk, L.E. (2006). *Development Through the Lifespan.* Upper Saddle River, NJ: Allyn & Bacon.

Bethell, C.D., Read, D., Blumberg, S.J., et al. (2008). What is the prevalence of children with special health care needs? Toward an understanding of variations in findings and methods across three national surveys. *Maternal Child Health J, 12,* 1-14.

Betz, C.L. (2007). Facilitating the transition of adolescents with developmental disabilities: Nursing practice issues and care. *J Pediatr Nurs, 22,* 103-115.

Betz, C.L., & Redcay, G. (2002). Lessons learned from providing transition services to adolescents with special health care needs. *Iss Compr Pediatr Nurs, 25,* 129-149.

Burke, S.O., Kauffmann, E., LaSalle, J., et al. (2000). Parents' perceptions of chronic illness trajectories. *Can J Nurs Res, 32,* 19-36.

Burkhart, P.V., Dunbar-Jacob, J.M., & Rohay, J.M., et al. (2001). Accuracy of children's self-reported adherence to treatment. *J Nurs Scholarsh, 33,* 27-32.

Canning, E.H., & Kelleher, K. (1994). Performance of screening tools for mental health problems in chronically ill children. *Arch Pediatr Adolesc Med, 148,* 272-278.

Cantrell, M.A. (2007). Health-related quality of life in childhood cancer: State of the science. *Oncol Nurs Forum, 34,* 103-111.

Carroll, J.M., Torkildson, C., & Winsness, J.S. (2007). Issues related to providing quality pediatric palliative care in the community. *Pediatr Clin North Am, 54,* 813-827.

Chen, E., Martin, A.D., & Matthews, K.A. (2007). Trajectories of socioeconomic status across children's lifetime predict health. *Pediatrics, 120,* e297-e303.

Cheng, M.M., & Udry, J.R. (2002). Sexual behaviors of physically disabled adolescents in the United States. *J Adolesc Health, 31,* 48-58.

Christian, B., D'Auria, J.P., & Fox, L.C. (1999). Gaining freedom: Self-responsibility in adolescents with diabetes. *Pediatrics, 25,* 255-260, 266.

Coffey, J.S. (2006). Parenting a child with chronic illness: A metasynthesis. *Pediatr Nurs, 32,* 51-59.

Committee on Bioethics and Committee on Hospital Care (2000). Palliative care for children. *Pediatrics, 106,* 351-172.

Committee on Child Abuse and Neglect and Committee on Children with Disabilities (2001). Assessment of maltreatment of children with disabilities. *Pediatrics, 108,* 508-512.

Committee on Children with Disabilities (2001). Counseling families who choose complementary and alternative medicine for their child with chronic illness or disability. *Pediatrics, 107,* 598-601.

Committee on Children with Disabilities and Committee on Psychosocial Aspects of Child and Family Health (1993). Psychosocial risks of chronic health conditions in childhood and adolescence. *Pediatrics, 92,* 876-877.

Council on Children with Disabilities (2006). Identifying infants and young children with developmental disorders in the medical home: An algorithm for developmental surveillance and screening. *Pediatrics, 118,* 405-420.

deBoer, H.M., Mula, M., & Sander, J.W. (2008). The global burden and stigma of epilepsy. *Epilepsy Behav, 12,* 540-546.

Denboba, D., McPherson, M.G., Kenney, M.K., et al. (2006). Achieving family and provider partnerships for children with special health care needs. *Pediatrics, 118*(4), 1607-1615.

Dennis, M. (2000). Developmental plasticity in children: The role of biological risk, development, time, and reserve. *J Commun Disord, 33,* 321-331.

Dosa, N.P., Boeing, N.M., & Kanter, R.K. (2001). Excess risk of severe acute illness in children with chronic health conditions. *Pediatrics, 107,* 499-504.

Drotar, D., Greenley, R., Hoff, A., et al. (2006). Summary of issues and challenges in the use of new technologies in clinical care and with children and adolescents with chronic illness. *Children's Health Care, 35*(1), 91-102.

Farmer, J.E., Clark, M.J., Sherman, A., et al. (2005). Comprehensive primary care for children with special health care needs in rural areas. *Pediatrics, 116,* 649-656.

Frank, R.G., Thayer, J.F., Hagglund, K.J., et al. (1998). Trajectories of adaptation in pediatric chronic illness: The importance of the individual. *J Consult Clin Psychol, 66,* 521-532.

Freud, A. (1966). *The Ego Mechanism of Defense.* New York: International Universities Press.

Friedrichsdorf, S.J., & Kang, T.I. (2007). The management of pain in children with life-limiting illnesses. *Pediatr Clin North Am, 54,* 645-672.

Garwick, A.W., Patterson, J.M., Meschke, L.L., et al. (2002). The uncertainty of preadolescents' chronic health conditions and family distress. *J Child Fam Nurs, 8,* 11-31.

Glascoe, F.P. (1999). Using parents' concerns to detect and address developmental and behavioral problems. *J Soc Pediatr Nurs, 4,* 24-35.

Graef, J.W., Wolfsdorf, J.I., & Greenes, D.S., et al. (2008). *Manual of Pediatric Therapeutics.* (7th ed.). Philadelphia: Lippincott Williams & Wilkins.

Grootenhuis, M.A., Koopman, H.M., Verrips, E.G., et al. (2007). Health-related quality of life problems of children ages 8–11 years with a chronic disease. *Dev Neurorehabil, 10,* 27-33.

Hart, C.N., Drotar, D., Gori, A., et al. (2006). Enhancing parent-provider communication in ambulatory pediatric practice. *Pat Educ Counsel, 63,* 38-46. 2006.

Haynes, R.B., Ackloo, E., Sahota, N., et al. (2008). Interventions for enhancing medication adherence. *Cochrane Database Syst Rev* Issue 2. Art No: CD00011. DOI: 10.1002/1451858. CD0011. pub3.

Heah, T., Case, T., McGuire, B., et al. (2007). Successful participation: The lived experience among children with disabilities. *Can J Occup Ther, 74,* 38-47.

Horowitz, J.A., Vessey, J.A., Carlson, K.L., et al. (2004). Teasing and bullying experiences of middle school students. *J Am Psychiatr Nurs Assoc, 10,* 165-172.

Houtrow, A.J., Kim, S.E., Chen, A.Y., et al. (2007). Preventive health care for children with and without special health care needs. *Pediatrics, 119,* e821-828.

Immelt, S. (2006). Psychological adjustment in young children with chronic medical conditions. *J Pediatr Nurs, 21,* 362-377.

Inkelas, M., Ragahavan, R., Larson, K., et al. (2007). Unmet mental health need and access to services for children with special health care needs and their families. *Ambulat Pediatr, 7,* 431-438.

Janse, A.J., Sinnema, G., Uiterwaal, C.S.P., et al. (2005a). Quality of life in chronic illness: Perceptions of parents and pediatricians. *Arch Dis Child, 90,* 486-491.

Janse, A.J., Sinnema, G., Uiterwaal, C.S.P., et al. (2005b). A difference in perception of quality of life in chronically ill children was found between parents and pediatricians. *J Clin Epidemiol, 58,* 496-502.

Joachim, G., & Acorn, S. (2000). Stigma of visible and invisible chronic conditions. *J Adv Nurs, 32,* 243-248.

Kahana, S., Drotar, D., & Frazier, T., (2008). Meta-analysis of psychological interventions to promote adherence to treatment in pediatric chronic health conditions. *J Pediatr Psychol, 33*(6), 590-611.

Kane, J.R., Barber, R.G., Jordan, M., et al. (2000). Supportive/palliative care of children suffering from life-threatening and terminal illness. *Am J Hospice Palliat Care, 17,* 165-172.

Karns, J.T. (2002). Children's understanding of death. *J Clin Activ Assign Handouts Psychother Pract, 2,* 43-50.

Kato, P.M., Lyon, T.D., & Rasco, C. (1998). Reasoning about moral aspects of illness and treatment by preschoolers who are healthy or who have a chronic illness. *J Develop Behav Pediatr, 19,* 68-76.

Kef, S. (2002). Psychosocial adjustment and the meaning of social support for visually impaired adolescents. *J Vis Impair Blind, 96,* 22-37.

Kersun, L.S., & Shemesh, E. (2007). Depression and anxiety in children at the end of life. *Pediatr Clin North Am, 54,* 691-708.

Klick, J.C., & Ballantine, A. (2007). Providing care in chronic disease: The ever-changing balance of integrating palliative and restorative medicine. *Pediatr Clin North Am, 54,* 799-812.

Knafl, K.A., & Gillis, C.L. (2002). Families and chronic illness: A synthesis of current research. *J Fam Nurs, 8,* 178-198.

Kyngas, H., & Rissanen, M. (2001). Support as a crucial predictor of good compliance of adolescents with a chronic disease. *J Clin Nurs, 10*(6), 767-774.

LaGreca, A.M., Bearman, K.J., & Moore, H. (2002). Peer relations of youth with pediatric conditions and health risks: Promoting social support and healthy lifestyles. *J Develop Behav Pediatr, 24,* 271-281.

Lawrence, J.W., Rosenberg, L.E., & Fauerbach, J.A. (2007). Comparing the body esteem of pediatric survivors of burn injury with the body esteem of an age-matched comparison group without burns. *Rehabil Psychol, 52,* 370-379.

Letourneau, N., Drummond, J.U., Flemming, D., et al. (2001). Supporting parents: Can intervention improve parent-child relationships? Two pilot studies. *J Child Fam Nurs, 7,* 159-187.

Lifshitz, H., Hen, I., & Weisse, I. (2007). Self-concept, adjustment to blindness and quality of friendship among adolescents with visual impairments. *J Vis Impair Blind, 101,* 96-107.

Malat, J., Oh, H.J., & Hamilton, M.A. (2005). Poverty experience, race, and child health. *Pub Health Rep, 120*(4), 442-447.

Marin, S. (2005). The impact of epilepsy on the adolescent. *Mat Child Nurs, 30,* 321-326.

McSherry, W., & Smith, J. (2007). How do children express their spiritual needs? *Paediatr Nurs, 19*(3), 17-20.

Meijer, S.A., Sinnema, G., Bijstra, J.O., et al. (2002). Coping styles and locus of control as predictors for psychological adjustment of adolescents with a chronic illness. *Soc Sci Med, 54,* 1453-1461.

Melnyk, B.M., Moldenhauer, Z., Veenema, T., et al. (2001). The KySS (Keep your children/yourself Safe and Secure) Campaign: A national effort to reduce psychosocial morbidities in children and adolescents. *J Pediatr Health Care, 15,* 31A-34A.

Mercurio, M.R. (2007). An adolescent's refusal of medical treatment: Implications of the Abraham Cheerix case. *Pediatrics, 120,* 1357-1358.

Modi, A.C., Marciel, K.K., Slater, S.K., et al. (2008). The influence of parental supervision on medical adherence in adolescents with cystic fibrosis: Developmental shifts from pre to late adolescence. *Child Health Care, 37,* 78-92.

Msall, M.E., Avery, R.C., Tremont, M.R., et al. (2003). Functional disability and school activity limitations in 41,300 school-age children: Relationship to medical impairments. *Pediatrics, 111,* 548-553.

Nageswaran, S., Silver, E.J., & Stein, R.E., et al. (2008). Association of functional limitation with health care needs and experiences of children with special health care needs. *Pediatrics, 121,* 994-1001.

Nehring, W.M. (2007). Cultural considerations for children with intellectual and developmental disabilities. *J Pediatr Nurs, 22*(2), 93-102.

Newacheck, P.W., & Halfon, N. (1998). Prevalence and impact of disabling chronic conditions in childhood. *Am J Pub Health, 88,* 610-617.

Newacheck, P.W., Rising, J.P., & Kim, S.E. (2006). Children at risk for special health care needs. *Pediatrics, 118,* 334-342.

Ngui, E.M., & Flores, G. (2007). Unmet needs for specialty, dental, mental, and allied health care among children with special health care needs: Are there racial/ethnic disparities? *J Health Care Poor Underserved, 18,* 931-949.

Pal, D.K., Das, T., Chaudhury, G., et al. (2005). Is social support sometimes a mixed blessing?. *Child Care Health Dev, 31,* 261-263.

Parish, S.L., & Cloud, J.M. (2006). Financial well-being of young children with disabilities and their families. *Social Work, 51,* 223-232.

Pelchat, D., Lefebvre, H., & Levert, M. (2007). Gender differences and similarities in the experience of parenting a child with a health problem: Current state of knowledge. *J Child Health Care, 11,* 112-131.

Perrin, E.C., Lewkowicz, C., & Young, M.H. (2000). Shared vision: Concordance among fathers, mothers, and pediatricians about unmet needs. *Pediatrics, 105,* 277-285.

Petrini, J., Damus, K., Russell, R., et al. (2002). Contribution of birth defects to infant mortality in the United States. *Teratology, 66*(9(Suppl 1)), S3-S6.

Plante, W.A., Lobato, D., & Engel, R. (2001). Review of group interventions for pediatric chronic conditions. *J Pediatr Psychol, 26*(7), 435-453.

Reeve, A. (2001). Understanding the adolescent with developmental disabilities. *Pediatr Ann, 30*, 104-108.

Rice, S.G., & Council on Sports Medicine and Fitness. (2008). Medical conditions affecting sports participation. *Pediatrics, 121*, 841-848.

Rink, E., & Tricker, R. (2003). Resiliency-based research and adolescent health behaviors. *The Prevention Researcher, 10*(1), 1-4.

Santucci, G., & Mack, J.W. (2007). Common gastrointestinal symptoms in pediatric palliative care: Nausea, vomiting, constipation, anorexia, cachexia. *Pediatr Clin North Am, 54*, 673-689.

Sawyer, S.M., Drew, S., Yeo, M.S., et al. (2007). Adolescents with a chronic condition: Challenges living, challenges treating. *Lancet, 369*(9571), 1481-1489.

Schmidt, C.K. (2001). Development of children's body knowledge, using knowledge of the lungs as an exemplar. *Iss Compr Pediatr Nurs, 24*, 177-191.

Schwartz, C.L., Hobbie, W.L., Constine, L.S., et al. (2005). *Survivors of Childhood and Adolescent Cancer: A Multidisciplinary Approach.* New York: Springer.

Slaughter, V., & Griffiths, M. (2007). Death understanding and fear of death in young children. *Clin Child Psychol Psychiatry, 12*, 525-535.

Smolkin, T., Steinberg, M., Sujov, P., et al. (2008). Late postnatal systemic steroids predispose to retinopathy of prematurity in very low birth weight infants: A comparative study. *Acta Pediatr, 97*, 322-326.

Spence, L.J., & Kaiser, L. (2002). Companion animals and adaptation in chronically ill children. *West J Nurs Res, 24*, 639-656.

Spencer, N., Devereux, E., Wallace, A., et al. (2005). Disabling conditions and registration for child abuse and neglect: A population-based study. *Pediatrics, 116*, 609-613.

Stewart, J.L. (2003). Children living with chronic illness: An examination of their stressors, coping responses, and health outcomes. *Ann Rev Nurs Res, 21*, 203-243.

Stewart, J.L., & Mishel, M.H. (2000). Uncertainty in childhood illness: A synthesis of the parent and child literature. *Schol Inq Nurs Pract, 14*, 299-319.

Stille, C.J., Primack, W.A., McLaughlin, T.J., et al. (2007). Parents as information intermediaries between primary care and specialty physicians. *Pediatrics, 120*, 1238-1246.

Telfair, J., Alleman-Velez, P.L., Dickens, P., et al. (2005). Quality health care for adolescents with special health-care needs: Issues and clinical implications. *J Pediatr Nurs, 20*(1), 15-24.

Thomas, D., & Gaslin, T.C. (2001). "Camping up" self-esteem in children with hemophilia. *Iss Comprehen Pediatr Nurs, 24*, 253-263.

Tork, H., Lohrmann, C., & Dassen, T. (2007). Care dependency among school-aged children: Literature review. *Nurs Health Sci, 9*, 142-149.

Turnidge, J. (2003). Pharmacodynamics and dosing of aminoglycosides. *Infect Dis Clin North Am, 17*, 503-528.

Vessey, J.A. (1999). Psychologic comorbidity and chronic conditions. *Pediatr Nurs, 25*, 211-214.

Vessey, J.A. (2003). Children's psychological responses to hospitalization. *Ann Rev Nurs Res, 21*, 173-203.

Vessey, J.A. (2006). Health and behavior risk assessment. In M. Craft-Rosenberg & M. Krajicek (Eds.), *Nursing Excellence for Children and Families.* New York: Springer.

Vessey, J.A., & O'Sullivan, P. (2000). A study of children's concepts of their internal bodies: a comparison of children with and without congenital heart disease. *J Pediatr Nurs, 15*, 292-298.

3

School and the Child with a Chronic Condition

Janice Selekman and Judith A. Vessey

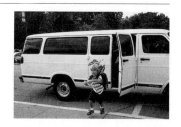

Role of School in a Child's Life

Receiving an education is an essential component in the life of a child. Every state constitution contains provisions related to the education of children and the minimum curriculum and educational requirements that are to be provided (Centers for Disease Control and Prevention [CDC], 2008). Almost 90% of American school-age children receive their education in a school setting (Riley-Lawless, 2006). School participation is especially important for children with chronic conditions, because it represents a component of their lives that is "normal" and age-appropriate. It is a time during each day when they can be and act like every other child.

The role of school should not be underestimated. It represents the second most influential environment in a child's life (Council on School Health, 2008). School provides opportunities for social, emotional, and cognitive development. In addition to the family, school is the major context in which children develop their sense of self and understanding of their place in relation to peers. Most children genuinely enjoy school, despite their protestations. This enjoyment of school may be particularly true for children with chronic conditions because they may have fewer opportunities to socialize outside the school setting. Another positive benefit of including children with chronic conditions in school activities is that nondisabled children can develop attitudes of acceptance and respect for their peers with special needs.

The United Nations Convention on the Rights of Persons with Disabilities stated that "Parties shall take all necessary measures to ensure the full enjoyment by children with disabilities of all human rights and fundamental freedoms on an equal basis with other children" and "In all actions concerning children with disabilities, the best interest of the child shall be a primary consideration" (National Council on Disability, 2008, p. 52). This chapter will examine the legislative mandates regarding the education of children with disabilities or chronic conditions that alter their ability to fully participate in the standard educational experience and then explore ways primary care providers can facilitate a child's school experience.

Children with Chronic Conditions in the School Setting

Before 1965, children with many chronic conditions were prevented from attending public schools because of the inability or unwillingness of schools to provide services and accommodations; many children with special needs were institutionalized or kept separate from their peers. The civil rights movement was the impetus to ensure that all children were eligible to receive an education.

Integrating children with chronic needs into the school setting, however, is not without problems. These children and their families experienced (and in many cases continue to experience) resistance and resentment from both within the community and within the school. Moreover, many schools have inadequate resources to educate children with special needs, despite the fact that educational services are mandated by law. There are two groups of children that must be considered in this discussion. One group includes all children with chronic conditions. The second group is a subset of this larger group, in that these are children whose chronic condition interferes with their ability to learn.

Laws on Education of Children with Chronic Conditions

With very few exceptions, laws specific to education and health are the prerogative of the states. Many of these legal exceptions are laws that protect the educational rights of children with chronic conditions. Legislative and judicial rulings over the past 45 years have dramatically changed the role of public educational institutions in providing services to children with chronic conditions. The change in public policy actually started with the civil rights movement when the landmark decision of *Brown v. Board of Education* (1954) banned segregated schools and affirmed education as a right of all U.S. citizens. The principle of "separate is not equal" was used almost 20 years later in *Pennsylvania Association for Retarded Citizens v. Pennsylvania* (1972) to challenge the state's right to exclude children with mental retardation from public education (National Council on Disability, 2000). That same year the Supreme Court ruled that a free and public education (known as FAPE) must be provided to all school-age children regardless of disability or degree of impairment (*Mills v. Board of Education of the District of Columbia*, 1972). This landmark Supreme Court decision paved the way for the federal government to enact legislation supporting public education for all children regardless of their health or ability.

Just as civil rights legislation of the 1960s was intended to prevent discrimination based on race, ethnic origin, and gender, the Vocational Rehabilitation Act of 1973 was enacted to prohibit discrimination of qualified persons on the basis of one's disability. This act was limited to programs and activities that received federal assistance, which includes the vast majority of educational settings. This was the first time people with disabilities were seen as a class—a minority group deserving basic civil rights protection in employment, education, housing, and access to society (Golden, Kilb, & Mayerson, 1993). The Americans with Disabilities Act

(ADA) of 1990 was also an antidiscrimination act, as it extended the prohibition against discrimination to all state and local government services, programs, or activities, regardless of whether they receive any federal funding (Office of Civil Rights, 2005). One of ADA's prime areas of focus was to eliminate barriers for individuals with disabilities into buildings, onto transportation, and with communication.

In 1965, the Elementary and Secondary Education Act Amendment was approved as an early attempt at special education for children with disabilities. It was amended a number of times and ultimately developed into the Education for All Handicapped Children Act (Public Law 94-142), passed by Congress in 1975 as an educational bill of rights for children 5 to 18 years of age. Public Law 94-142 entitled children, regardless of their handicap, to a "free and appropriate public education" (FAPE) including "special education and related services provided at public expense, under public supervision and direction, without charge, which meet the standards of the state educational agency, and are provided in uniformity with the Individualized Educational Program (IEP)" (Education for All Handicapped Children Act, 1975). This law affected every school that received federal funds and also mandated that "related services" necessary for the child to learn be included.

Public Law 94-142 was amended to include parents' rights, and in 1986 Public Law 99-457 was passed, which included the Handicapped Infants and Toddlers Program, Part H (Infant and Toddler Program, 1986). Public Law 99-457 extended services to children from birth to 21 years of age and required interagency and interdisciplinary collaboration, development of a child identification system, a care manager designated for the family, and the implementation of an individualized family service plan (IFSP) for children from birth through 2 years, analogous to the individualized educational program (IEP) required under PL 94-142 for older children (The Handicapped Infant and Toddler Program, 1986). This amendment dramatically increased the school systems' role in providing early intervention services to infants and toddlers who were at high risk for developing handicapping conditions, as well as preschool programs for children 3 to 5 years with developmental delays. In 1990 and 1991, these laws were merged and further amended under the Individuals with Disabilities Education Act (IDEA), Public Law 101-476. IDEA was also revised many times, with FAPE being required to be in the least restrictive environment (LRE). Parents' rights were further elaborated, transition services were mandated, and "person first" language was stressed. The latest amendment was in 2004 and was called the Individuals with Disabilities Education Improvement Act (IDEA) (PL 108-446).

Under IDEA, schools are accountable to identify students who have a disability that interferes with learning and to plan, implement, and evaluate the success of an IEP for the student. "However, nothing in IDEA holds schools accountable for the progress and academic performance of children with disabilities" (Cortiella, 2006, p. 9). The No Child Left Behind Act (NCLB) (2001) built on the early education laws from 1965 to improve the academic achievement of students. Although initially designed to assist children who were poor and disadvantaged, the intent of NCLB is to improve the achievement of all students and to ensure that all children have a fair, equal, and significant opportunity to receive a high-quality education and achieve at or above state standards. NCLB holds schools accountable for student achievement; this includes all students, including those with disabilities and chronic conditions. Therefore, whereas IDEA addresses the needs of individual students, NCLB focuses on the performance of schools (Cortiella, 2006).

Rehabilitation Act of 1973: Section 504

According to the Vocational Rehabilitation Act (1973), more commonly referred to as the Rehabilitation Act, a person with a disability is defined as someone who (1) has a mental or physical impairment that substantially limits one or more major life activities; (2) has a record of such impairment; or (3) is regarded as having such impairment. Physical or mental impairment includes "(A) any physiological disorder, cosmetic disfigurement or anatomical loss affecting one or more of the following systems: respiratory, including speech; cardiovascular; reproductive; digestive; genitourinary; hematologic and lymphatic; skin; and endocrine or (B) any mental or psychological disorder such as mental retardation, organic brain syndrome, emotional or mental illness and specific learning disabilities" (34 Code of Federal Regulations Part 104.3). The phrase "major life activities" means functions such as caring for oneself, performing manual tasks, walking, seeing, hearing, speaking, breathing, learning, and working. The Office of Civil Rights considers learning to be a major life activity.

Section 504 of the Rehabilitation Act of 1973 (PL 93-112) is one small component of a larger act that was primarily aimed at providing job opportunities and training to adults with disabilities. However, it is now interpreted as conferring the same rights and expectations to schools in the education of children with disabilities. The total section 504 states:

> No otherwise qualified individual with a disability in the United States, as defined in section 706(8) of this title, shall, solely by reason of her or his handicap, be excluded from participation in, be denied the benefits of, or be subjected to discrimination under any program or activity receiving Federal financial assistance or under any program or activity conducted by any Executive agency or by the United States Postal Service. [29 U.S.C. §794(a) (1973)]

The Rehabilitation Act covers *all* students with disabilities and chronic conditions. All students whose chronic conditions meet one of the aforementioned criteria are eligible for the services provided by Section 504. As applied to the schools, the language broadly prohibits the denial of public education participation or participation in school-related activities because of a child's disability. It requires that the educational needs of the disabled child must be met and strategies for classroom adaptation be implemented so that he or she can be educated as adequately as the nondisabled child in the least restrictive environment. The key words in implementing this law are "reasonable accommodations." Schools are to develop an "accommodation plan" for the student; this is also called a 504 plan. The goal should be to assist children to receive services, including related services and assistive technologic devices that enable them to participate more fully in the public school program so that the "student's disability will not limit her ability to benefit from educational programs" (CDC, 2008, p. 81).

Funds to support accommodations in education under Section 504 must come from the general education funds, not the funds earmarked for IDEA. Section 504 requires parental notice regarding identification, evaluation, and placement, but approval is not required. Periodic reevaluations are required, but Section 504 does not specify any timelines. The Federal Office of Civil Rights in the U.S. Department of Education has jurisdiction over implementation of Section 504, and conflicts between parents and school districts are mediated through this office.

The 504/Accommodation Plan. Anyone working with the student, including the students themselves or their families, can request an evaluation for school accommodations. A specially designated school team that can best determine the student's eligibility for necessary accommodations will meet with the parent, observe the child in the classroom, obtain input from the teachers and school nurse, and review the medical records (Moses, Gilchrist, & Schwab, 2005). Accommodations can be as simple as allowing children with inflammatory bowel disease to use the bathroom in the nurse's office and having a signal to the teacher when they have to quickly leave the classroom, to allowing children with diabetes to keep their glucose testing supplies on them and to test in the classroom. Children with hematologic or respiratory conditions may need accommodations in physical education that allow them to rest more often or avoid contact sports. Children with peanut or latex allergies may need more extensive plans that include cafeteria personnel, art teachers, and those responsible for purchasing materials for the classroom, as well as notifying all of the parents in the class. Other accommodations may include extended time for testing, organizational assistance, using behavioral management techniques, having exceptions made in the school's uniform policy, having an additional set of books at home, or alternative testing or homework/class assignments to demonstrate knowledge.

Individuals with Disabilities Education Improvement Act (IDEA): 2004 (PL 108-446)

The purpose of IDEA is to ensure that children with disabilities receive assistance with the educational needs that result from their disability so that they can be involved in and progress in the general curriculum in an educational setting. The goal of IDEA is to identify students who qualify for and would benefit from special education. IDEA is a complex statute divided into four parts: Part A contains general provisions, the purpose, goals, and definitions; Part B, "Assistance for Education of All Children with Disabilities," describes how the federal government provides assistance to states for the education of children with disabilities from ages 3 to 21 years, how state agencies must supervise and monitor the statute, and the basic rights and responsibilities of children with disabilities and their parents or guardians; Part C, "Infants and Toddlers with Disabilities," describes the program for children from birth to age 3 years; and Part D, "National Activities to Improve Education of Children with Disabilities," authorizes programs to improve teacher preparation and credentialing in the education of children with disabilities (U.S. Department of Education, 2008a). The final regulations were published in 2006.

IDEA reaffirmed the language regarding the importance of providing a free appropriate public education (FAPE) to all eligible children with disabilities and educating them in the least restrictive environment (LRE), including an emphasis on participation in the curriculum of general education; the rights of parents to be involved in educational decisions affecting their children, including eligibility and placement; the importance of functional behavioral assessments and strategies to promote positive behavior;

and the requirement that states develop annual performance goals and outcome measurements for children with disabilities as part of school and district-wide assessments. This legislation clarified that states are required to identify, locate, and evaluate all children with disabilities residing in the state, including children in private schools. This directive is referred to as "child find."

IDEA also expanded covered related services. The term "related services" was initially part of the 1975 Education for All Handicapped Children Act and includes transportation and developmental, corrective, and supportive services, including early identification and assessment of disabilities in children, speech-language pathology and audiology services, orientation and mobility services, parent counseling and training, psychological and counseling services, physical and occupational therapy, recreation, rehabilitation counseling services, social work services, interpreting services, transition services, and medical services. The term also includes school health services, including the services of the school nurse, and supplemental aids and supports needed to enable children with disabilities to be educated with nondisabled children to the most appropriate extent (IDEA, 2004).

Children with disabilities whose parents place them in nonpublic schools are referred to as "parentally placed private school children" (U.S. Department of Education, 2008b). These children are also eligible to receive the benefits and services under the law. It is the responsibility of local education agencies (LEAs) and state education agencies (SEAs) to ensure that children with disabilities participate equitably within the state's implementation of IDEA. "Parentally placed children with disabilities do not have an individual entitlement to services they would receive if they were enrolled in a public school. Instead, the LEA is required to spend a proportionate amount of IDEA federal funds to provide equitable services to this group of children" (U.S. Department of Education, 2008b, p. 1). Therefore the services provided, if any, may be different from those provided in a public school.

Eligibility for Special Education Services under IDEA. Although all students who qualify for services under IDEA also qualify under Section 504 of the Rehabilitation Act, not all children with chronic health conditions are eligible for special education services under IDEA (Lee & Janik, 2006). Only certain health conditions have been designated as making a child eligible for special education and related services. Not only do students need to have one of the conditions listed, they must also, by reason thereof, need special education and related services. The list of conditions is in Box 3-1. Those students who do not qualify under IDEA may be able to have their needs met through a 504 Plan. "For children ages 3 through 9, states have discretion to cover children with other impairments, such as developmental delay, who need special education and related services as a result of those impairments" (National Council on Disability, 2008, p. 92). Table 3-1 denotes the number of children ages 6 to 21 years served by IDEA in fall 2007, and Table 3-2 indicates the percent of children with each disability who receive services.

In 2006 and 2007, IDEA served over 6 million children, ages 3 to 21, almost 14% of the school-age children in the United States, and up to another million children from birth through age 5. The $10.6 million spent by the government for IDEA, less than $2 per child served, was distributed among the states to assist with the cost of providing special education services (Cortiella, 2006, 2007; IDEA Data, 2007). Federal enforcement of IDEA is through the Office of Special

BOX 3-1

Conditions Identified as Disabilities in Children under the Individuals with Disabilities Education Act (2004)

DISABILITIES AS DEFINED FOR CHILDREN 3 TO 21 YEARS OF AGE

Autism: A developmental disability significantly affecting verbal and nonverbal communication and social interaction.

Deaf-blindness: Children with both deafness and blindness; communication with others is severely impaired.

Deafness: Children with a hearing deficiency that impairs processing of linguistic information through hearing with or without amplification.

Hearing impairment: Permanent or fluctuating hearing loss that adversely affects the child's educational process.

Mental retardation: Significant subaverage general intelligence existing with deficits in adaptive behavior.

Multiple disabilities: Concomitant impairments other than deaf-blindness resulting in severe educational problems that cannot be addressed in a special education program solely for one impairment.

Orthopedic impairments: Severe orthopedic impairments that adversely affect the child's educational performance.

Other health impairments: Limited strength, vitality, or alertness, including a heightened alertness to environmental stimuli, that results in limited alertness with respect to the educational environment, resulting from chronic or acute health problems, such as asthma, a heart condition, lead poisoning, tuberculosis, rheumatic fever, nephritis, sickle cell anemia, hemophilia, epilepsy, leukemia, diabetes, attention-deficit/hyperactivity disorder (ADHD), or Tourette syndrome, and that adversely affects a child's educational performance.

Serious emotional disturbance: A child who exhibits over a prolonged period of time one or more of the following characteristics: an inability to learn that cannot be explained by intellectual, sensory, or health factors; an inability to build or maintain satisfactory interpersonal relationships; inappropriate behavior or feelings; depression or unhappiness; and a tendency to develop physical symptoms or fears associated with personal or school problems.

Specific learning disability: A disorder in one or more of the psychological processes involved in understanding or using spoken or written language; term does not apply to children who have learning problems primarily caused by other disabilities listed here or environmental, cultural, or economic disadvantages.

Speech or language impairment: A communication disorder caused by impaired articulation, problems with language development, or voice impairment that adversely affects a child's educational performance.

Traumatic brain injury: Acquired injury to the brain resulting in total or partial functional and/or psychosocial impairment.

Visual impairments (including blindness): Visual impairments, including ones that can be corrected, that adversely affect a child's educational performance.

DISABILITIES AS DEFINED FOR CHILDREN 3 TO 9 YEARS OF AGE

Children experiencing developmental delays, as defined by the state, in one or more of the following developmental areas: physical, cognitive, communication, social, emotional, or adaptive development.

Children meeting these requirements are eligible for services from their school district at age 3 years.

DISABILITIES AS DEFINED FOR INFANTS AND TODDLERS

Infants and toddlers from birth to age 2 years who (1) experience delay in cognitive, physical, communicative, social/emotional, or adaptive development; (2) are diagnosed with a physical or mental condition that has a high probability of resulting in developmental delay; or (3) are at risk of having developmental delays if early intervention services are not provided.

Adapted from U.S. Department of Education, Office of Special Education Programs, Data Analysis System (DANS), OMB #18200-043: "Children with Disabilities Receiving Special Education Under Part B of the Individuals with Disabilities Education Act," 2007. Data updated as of July 15, 2008.

TABLE 3-1

Number of Children Ages 6 to 21 Years Served in the U.S. under IDEA, Part B, by Disability, during Fall 2007

Disability	No. of Children
Specific learning disabilities	2,620,240
Speech or language impairment	1,154,165
Mental retardation	498,159
Emotional disturbance	440,202
Multiple disabilities	131,347
Hearing impairment	71,332
Orthopedic impairment	60,010
Other health impairments	625,187
Visual impairments	26,423
Autism	258,305
Deaf-blindness	1,380
Traumatic brain injury	23,864
Developmental delay	88,629
All disabilities	5,912,586

Data form U.S. Department of Education, Office of Special Education Programs, Data Analysis System (DANS), OMB #18200-043: "Children with Disabilities Receiving Special Education Under Part B of the Individuals with Disabilities Education Act," 2007. Data updated as of July 15, 2008.

TABLE 3-2

Percent of Children Ages 6 to 21 Years Served in the U.S. under IDEA, Part B, by Disability, Fall 2007

Disability	%
Specific learning disability	43.36
Speech or language impairment	19.25
Mental retardation	8.25
Emotional disturbance	7.42
Multiple disabilities	2.22
Hearing impairment	1.21
Orthopedic impairment	1.01
Other health impairments	10.57
Visual impairment	0.44
Autism	4.34
Deaf-blindness	.02
Traumatic brain injury	0.40
Developmental delay	1.5

Data form U.S. Department of Education, Office of Special Education Programs, Data Analysis System (DANS), OMB #18200-043: "Children with Disablities Receiving Special Education Under Part B of the Individuals with Disabilities Education Act," 2007. Data updated as of July 15, 2008. IDEA, Part B Child Count, in Cortiella, C. (2007). *Rewards and Roadblocks.* New York: National Center for Learning Disabilities.

Education and Rehabilitation Services in the U.S. Department of Education through each state's office. The federal government does not require reporting for Section 504, but one survey of public school principals estimated that only 1.2% of students received accommodation services through a 504 plan (Holler & Zirkel, 2008).

To receive special education services a pre-placement evaluation must be conducted to determine eligibility. This individual initial evaluation can be requested by the parent or guardian or by a public agency (school, preschool center, residential placement agency, etc.) with written approval of the parent or guardian. In order for a child to be eligible for special education services, including an IEP, the child must have a condition that is covered under one of the mandated categories (see Box 3-1) or test at and/or below a designated level of performance (i.e., often 1.5 to 2.0 standard deviations below the norm in specific or multiple areas of function) as a

BOX 3-2

Individualized Educational Program (IEP) Team as Required under the Individuals with Disabilities Education Act, Reauthorization of 2004

- The parents of the child
- At least one regular teacher of the child
- At least one special education teacher or provider of the child
- A representative of the school district who is:
  - Qualified to provide or supervise the provision of special education
  - Knowledgeable about the general curriculum
  - Knowledgeable about the availability of the district's resources
- An individual who can interpret the instructional implications of the evaluation results
- At the discretion of the parent or the school district, others who have knowledge or special expertise regarding the child, such as a health care provider
- When appropriate, the child or youth with the disability

Adapted from U.S. Department of Education, Office of Special Education Programs, Data Analysis System (DANS), OMB #18200-043: "Children with Disabilties Receiving Special Education Under Part B of the Individuals with Disabilities Education Act," 2007. Data updated as of July 15, 2008.

result of his or her disability. This latter component of inconsistent and below-level performance is being debated, especially related to specific learning disabilities; the newer requirement is to measure "response to intervention" (see later discussion).

The team that determines eligibility and develops the IEP goes by many names, including the IEP team, the special education team, or the multidisciplinary team. It must include the parents of the child, at least one regular education teacher of the child, at least one special education teacher of the child, a representative of the public agency, and someone who can interpret the instructional implications. Whenever it is appropriate, the child should also be included. Box 3-2 lists the people required by law to be part of the IEP team. This team is also responsible for evaluating the child's progress toward the goals, for determining if the plan is effective, and for making changes as needed. A complete reevaluation is required at least every 3 years; if it is done more frequently, by law, it does not have to be done more than once a year.

The law requires that testing evaluations be free and the child be evaluated in all areas related to his or her suspected disability, that is, health, vision, hearing, social and emotional status, general intelligence, academic performance, communication ability, and motor abilities. Input from the parents or guardians, teachers, and other professionals with knowledge of the child's condition is included in the evaluation process. Previously performed evaluations as part of the child's health care can also be submitted for review during this pre-placement phase and are often helpful in documenting the child's abilities and disabilities. This pre-placement evaluation must be sufficiently comprehensive to determine eligibility and what, if any, related services will be needed by the child. The findings from this evaluation process serve as the foundation for the child's IEP. This is also where input from primary care and specialty health care providers would be most helpful. When the pre-placement evaluation is initiated, by law, the parents or guardians must be given information about IDEA, special education services, related services, their rights as parents, and the appeal process. IDEA requires that procedural safeguards be established to protect the rights of parents or guardians and the child. Once initiated, the school system has 60 workdays to complete the pre-placement evaluation process.

Legal Principles Basic to IDEA. The following are the basic legal principles and mandated components of IDEA:

1. *Zero reject.* A student cannot be excluded from a local school district because of the nature of his or her disability. Therefore even children with the most severe disabilities and those with significant health and medical needs must be included in the educational process.
2. *Child find.* It is the responsibility of the school district to identify and locate children with disabilities from birth to age 21 and then to inform the parents of the available special education services. The identified children are to be evaluated at no cost to the families, and then the school must provide appropriate educational programs to these students.
3. *Nondiscriminatory testing.* Materials used for testing must be racially and culturally appropriate, "comprehensive and validated for the purpose for which they are being used, and be administered by trained personnel" in a nondiscriminatory manner, and in the native language of the child (CDC, 2008, p. 81). Parents may seek one independent evaluation at public expense if they disagree with the district's evaluation.
4. *Free and appropriate public education (FAPE).* This applies to all children with disabilities in the state where the family resides. This includes the opportunity to participate in physical education, including specially designed activities, if physical education is provided to nondisabled students.
5. *Least restrictive environment (LRE).* This speaks to the placement of the child, with the regular classroom being the preferred site. Children with disabilities should be educated with their nondisabled peers. "Special classes, separate schooling or other removal of children with disabilities from the regular education environment occurs only when the nature of the severity of the disability is such that education in regular classes with the use of supplementary aids and services cannot be achieved satisfactorily" (National Council on Disability, 2008, p. 91). Getting children with disabilities into regular classrooms was referred to as "mainstreaming" and "inclusion." The premise of this principle is that all students, no matter how severe their disability, have some aspects of their development that are typical (See the options for special education listed later.)
6. *Development of an individualized educational program (IEP).* This is described in the following section and includes both the process for development of the educational program and the specific IEP.
7. *Procedural due process.* Due process is to be explained to the families, and followed for mediation and for resolving conflicts among parents, school personnel, and educational professionals. It includes the evaluation process, protection of parental participation rights, and prevention of expelling a student or changing a student's educational placement without following due process.
8. *Parental participation.* Parents are to be involved in the process of developing an IEP. They must provide consent for the initial evaluation, as well as for follow-up evaluations, and their participation in the decisions made about placement and accommodations should be supported. Parents should be encouraged and supported in speaking up for the needs of their children. They should have access to all

records on their child and should receive the reports of all evaluations.

9. *Transition services.* This refers to a coordinated set of activities that focuses on facilitating "the child's movement from school to post-school activities, including post secondary education, vocational education, integrated employment (including supported employment); continuing and adult education, adult services, independent living, or community participation" (IDEA, 2004). These transition services should be based on the child's needs, but also take into consideration the child's strengths, preferences, and interests. The objectives and initiation of the transition plan should begin for the IEP that will be in effect on the child's sixteenth birthday, potentially as early as age 14. The child must be invited to the IEP team meeting for his or her input and approval; representatives from participating agencies likely to be part of the child's future plans should also be present (see Chapter 4).

Individualized Educational Program. The key component of IDEA is the development of the individualized educational program (IEP); it is mandated for every student who qualifies under IDEA. This document should outline the accommodations and instructional approaches necessary to allow the child to participate in the learning environment and to progress in the same curriculum as his or her peers. The desired academic content standards should be those set by the state under the No Child Left Behind Act.

The IEP must include the present level of the child's academic and functional performance, including how the disability or chronic condition affects the child's ability to learn or participate in the learning environment; measurable academic and functional annual goals for all students and short-term objectives for children with significant cognitive disabilities; a description of how and when the child's progress will be measured and reported; the specific interventions that will be provided, including the amount of special education and related services that will be provided, the supplementary aids and accommodations that are needed, and the extent to which the child will not participate with his or her nondisabled peers in regular class or school activities; dates and places where services will be provided; and, by age 16, transition planning for postsecondary goals (Rief, 2005) (Box 3-3).

Part of the IEP for each child in special education should address the child's need for assistive technology devices, defined as any item, piece of equipment, or product system that is used to increase, maintain, or improve the functional capabilities of a child with disability. Assistive technology devices can be simple items commercially available off the shelf, such as a magnifying glass, or complex communication devices, such as a laser-operated computer to establish communication with a severely physically disabled but cognitively intact child. Assistive technology devices have become more widely available, and the possibilities for augmenting a child's learning experience with computers, the Internet, and virtual reality seem endless. The financial cost of many of these devices limits their current use and places a severe financial strain on already underfunded school systems.

Special Education. *Special education* is defined by IDEA as specially designed instruction that meets the unique needs of a student with a disability through adaptation of the content, methodology, or delivery of instruction. Special education services can be provided

---

BOX 3-3

Content Included in an IEP Document

- *Present level of child's academic achievement and functional performance.*
- *Annual goals* that are measurable, including academic and functional goals that meet the child's needs that result from the disability to enable the child to be involved in and make progress in the general education curriculum and meet each of the child's other educational needs that result from the child's disability.
- *Special education and related services to be provided* including assistive technology devices, based on peer-reviewed research to the extent possible: All services required to meet the educational goals including supplemental aids (e.g., communication devices) must be identified.
- *Participation with nondisabled children:* Any time the child is not included in regular education programs with nondisabled children must be identified and explained.
- *Participation in state and district-wide assessments:* Modification needed for accomplishing state and district general education testing need to be listed. If the child cannot participate in these standard tests, alternative assessments aligned to alternative achievement standards, including short-term objectives, must be described, including how and when the child's progress toward meeting annual goals will be measured.
- *Dates and location of services:* When, how often, where, and for how long services will be provided must be stated.
- *Transition services needed:* Beginning not later than the child's sixteenth birthday, the IEP must list measurable postsecondary goals based on age-appropriate transition assessments related to training, education, employment, and, where appropriate, independent living skills and the transition services needed to assist the child in reaching these goals.
- *Transfer of rights:* Beginning not later than 1 year before the child reaches the age of majority under state law, the IEP must include a statement that the child has been informed of his or her rights under Part B, if any, that will transfer to the child on reaching the age of majority.

U.S. Department of Education (2008).

---

in a regular classroom, special classroom or facility, home, private nonprofit preschool, private school, college, hospital, and even state prison. Placement falls under the principle of least restrictive environment (LRE). Children eligible for services who attend private schools are still eligible through the public school system, but parents will need to bring them to public schools for services.

Although 53% of students who qualify under IDEA spend more than 80% of their school day in the regular education classroom, the rest of the students spend less time in the regular education classroom and more time in resource rooms or alternative settings receiving more individualized attention and the related services approved in their IEP (Cortiella, 2007). Table 3-3 denotes the percent of students ages 6 to 21 years covered under IDEA, Part B, by their educational environment. "Inclusion" is the term used when a child receiving special education services is in a regular daycare, preschool, or school program. This environment is seen as the least restrictive, providing children the fullest educational potential. They receive special education services (e.g., speech, physical, or occupational therapy) in the classroom or are removed briefly for services and then return to the classroom when the intervention is completed.

Children with severe disabilities or who are medically fragile will require services in special classrooms often found within regular school settings; in special schools, institutions, or hospitals; or at home (if the individual is unable to attend other facilities). Even profoundly handicapped children are required by law to receive educational services for a designated period of time each week. Depending on the size of the school district and the population

TABLE 3-3

Percent of Children Ages 6 to 21 Years Who Received Special Education Services by Their Educational Environment, Fall 2007

Educational Environment	%
80% in regular classroom	56.84
40%-70% in regular classroom	22.40
<40% in regular classroom	15.39
Separate school	3.00
Residential facility	0.41
Parentally placed in private schools	1.13
Correctional facility	0.39
Home or hospital environment	0.42

Data from U.S. Department of Education, Office of Special Education Programs, Data Analysis System (DANS), OMB #18200-043: "Children with Disablities Receiving Special Education Under Part B of the Individuals with Disabillties Education Act," 2007. Data updated as of July 15, 2008.

served, these special classes may be available in the child's school district or in adjoining school districts that contract out services. In some situations, school districts contract special education services to private institutions or programs.

Some children with disabilities have behaviors that interfere with the educational process and require disciplinary action. Although IDEA mandates that the IEP address behavior problems proactively through the use of functional behavior assessments and positive behavior strategies, interventions, and supports, IDEiA also established a process for school suspensions for children in special education consistent with suspension policies for nondisabled students. These regulations are summarized in Box 3-4. The 2004 regulations allow school personnel to consider unique circumstances on a case-by-case basis when the code of conduct for the school has been violated (IDEA, 2004).

Challenges to the Supreme Court. The Rowley decision in 1982 helped to define "related services" (Board of Education, 1982). In this case, an 8-year-old deaf child was doing well in school and the parents' request for an interpreter was denied; the ruling limited "related services" to those interventions necessary for the student to learn.

The Tatro case (Irving Independent School District, 1984) focused on a child with spina bifida and clarified that medical services, such as catheterization, must be provided if it will assist the student to benefit from special education and the service does not have to be performed by a physician. In 1999 in *Cedar Rapids Community School District v. Garret F.* (1999), the Supreme Court reaffirmed the requirement of schools to provide special education and related services to all children with disabilities, even if this required one-on-one, full-time registered nursing services for a child with complex medical needs.

Problems with Implementation of IDEA

Lack of adequate funding. The intent of IDEA is honorable, and it is an improvement over previous inequities and lack of services for children with disabilities. Problems exist, however, with funding, eligibility, responsibility for services, and the actual provision of services to the targeted child. Lack of adequate funding to support public education and services for children with special needs is the basis for most controversies. Federal programs mandate services but do not adequately provide the financial resources to supply these services to all children who would benefit from

BOX 3-4

Major Discipline Provisions of the 2004 IDEA Regulations

1. School personnel may remove a child with disability to an alternative educational setting for not more than 45 school days without regard to whether the behavior is determined to be a manifestation of the child's disability, if the child carries a weapon to or possesses a weapon at school, on school premises, or to or at a school function under the jurisdiction of a state educational agency (SEA) or a local educational agency (LEA); knowingly possesses or uses illegal drugs, or sells or solicits the sale of a controlled substance, while at school, on school premises, or to or at a school function under the jurisdiction of the state education agency or a local education agency; or has inflicted serious bodily injury on another person while at school, on school premises, or at a school function under the jurisdiction of an SEA or an LEA.
2. School personnel may remove a child with a disability who violates a code of student conduct from his or her current placement to an appropriate interim alternative educational setting, another setting, or suspension, for not more than 10 consecutive school days (to the extent those alternatives are applied to children without disabilities), and for additional removals of not more than 10 consecutive school days in the same school year for separate incidents of misconduct (as long as those removals do not constitute a change in placement under IDEA).
3. If the disciplinary charge is not related to the disability, the same disciplinary procedures may be used as those for nondisabled students, except as dictated in the IEP.
4. Within 10 school days of any decision to change the placement of a child with a disability because of a violation of a code of student conduct, the LEA, the parent, and relevant members of the child's IEP team must review all relevant information in the student's file, including the child's IEP, any teacher observations, and any relevant information provided by the parents to determine if the conduct in question was caused by, or had a direct and substantial relationship to, the child's disability or if the conduct was the direct result of the LEA's failure to implement the IEP.
5. If the behavior was determined to be a manifestation of the child's disability, the IEP team must either conduct a functional behavioral assessment, unless one had been conducted before the behavior that resulted in the change of placement occurred, and implement a behavioral intervention plan for the child or, if a behavioral intervention plan already has been developed, review the behavioral intervention plan, and modify it, as necessary, to address the behavior; and return the child to the placement from which the child was removed, unless the parent and the LEA agree to a change in placement as part of the modification of the behavioral intervention plan.

Modified from U.S. Department of Education, Office of Special Programs' IDEA Website (2008).

them. Funding to support special education services is given to the states "based on the number of children in the state receiving special education services multiplied by the average per-pupil cost of public education in the United States" (National Council on Disability, 2008, p. 90). However, Congress does not allocate enough funds to cover the 40% portion that is the federal government's responsibility, leaving states to absorb the costs. This results in poor communities having fewer financial resources to commit to special education services even though there may be more children needing services because of the risks associated with poverty.

Change in the eligibility criteria for learning disabilities. Children with learning disabilities (LDs) make up the largest group of students using special education services. LDs were federally designated as a "handicapping condition" in 1968 (Fletcher, Lyon, Fuchs, et al. 2007). Until the 2004 amendments, LDs were diagnosed by a significant discrepancy between achievement and ability, as measured on IQ tests. "The evidence base for its validity as a central feature of LD classification is weak to nonexistent" (Fletcher et al., 2007, p. 20). IDEA (2004) took the unprecedented step to redefine "learning disabilities" and eliminate the criteria for a discrepancy in performance and ability. The new criteria state that "when determining whether a child has a specific learning disability as defined in section 602, a local education agency shall not be required to take into consideration whether a child has a severe discrepancy between achievement and intellectual ability in oral expression, listening, comprehension, written expression, basic reading skill, reading comprehension, mathematical calculation, or mathematical reasoning." It goes on to state, "In determining whether a child has a specific learning disability, a local education agency may use a process that determines if the child responds to scientific, research-based intervention as part of the evaluation procedures" (U.S. Department of Education, 2006).

The practices are referred to as response to intervention (RTI) and, if implemented, require schools to use evidence-based targeted instructions as soon as the student demonstrates learning problems and to note the student's responses to those interventions (Kamphaus, Quirk, & Kroncke, 2006). There must be evidence that appropriate instruction is provided and that there is data-based documentation at repeated intervals (Fletcher et al., 2007). This format raises as many questions as did the criteria of significant discrepancy.

1. There is some concern that this process delays a diagnosis of LD and therefore accessing services under IDEA
2. There is no description of what is "typically achieving"
3. Implementation of RTI is not required
4. There is no professional assessment to differentiate LD from attention deficit hyperactivity disorder (ADHD) or LD from intellectual disability until classroom measures are tried first
5. There is no list of evidence-based classroom measures from which a teacher can choose

The law does allow funds that are intended for special education to be used to provide services to students in the classroom without them having qualified under IDEA (Cortiella, 2007).

Response to intervention puts the onus of responsibility on the teacher. However, if insufficient funds are distributed at this point, it is questionable if resources will be deflected to general education students who are struggling. Cortiella (2007) cites a 2001 report by Finn, Rotherham, and Hokanson that predicts that the number of children diagnosed as having an LD will decrease up to 70%. Interventions are scientific research–based programs used in addition to the core curriculum. The process involves providing many opportunities for preteaching, reteaching, review, and supervised practice. Because the law does not provide guidance for practitioners, the diagnosis of LD is thought to be just as subjective as it was when "significant discrepancy" was used (Flanagan, Ortiz, Alfonso, et al., 2006).

Schools' responsibility for medical services. Because educational systems are responsible for "related services," which include medical services and therapies needed by a child during the school day (e.g., tracheostomy suctioning, gavage feedings, intermittent catheterization, and medication administration), the educational systems have become the overseers and deliverers of medical care, often independent of the primary or specialty care providers. All services that can be provided by someone with less training than a physician are the responsibility of the school district.

A qualified school nurse is the most appropriate person to provide school health services (Selekman, 2006). As children with chronic conditions live longer and medical technology enables them to participate in school, concern has surfaced about the qualifications of school personnel to provide services to children with special needs. Many schools are without the services of a full-time school nurse, and have aides, secretaries, and even teachers performing skills for which they are ill prepared and limited. Although the *Healthy People 2010* objectives are to have one school nurse to every 750 students (U.S. Department of Health and Human Services, 2000), the goal is to have at least one nurse in every school building in America. In addition, the National Association of School Nurses recommends a school nurse caseload of 1:225 in the student populations that may require daily professional nursing services or interventions and 1:125 in student populations with complex health care needs (National Association of School Nurses, 2006). As more children enter the schools with chronic conditions, it is the school nurse who has the breadth of knowledge to provide optimum care in the school setting.

A significant number of public schools have established school-based clinics (referred to as wellness centers or health centers) to provide care to the school's children and staff. Often under the management of nurse practitioners, they provide a variety of services, most commonly primary and acute care (Luehr & Selekman, 2006). This may include these same services to children with chronic conditions.

School districts that identify therapeutic interventions for children with special needs in the IEP process are generally required to pay for these services, although Medicaid fee-for-service or other public funding can often be billed if the child is eligible. For children covered by Medicaid managed care or SCHIP, coverage varies substantially among plans. Private insurance will not usually cover services provided in the school setting. School systems are also financially responsible for providing the necessary equipment to support the child's educational program but can attempt to obtain reimbursement or funding from other sources, such as U.S. Maternal-Child Health Bureau Title V Services, Medicaid, the state children's insurance plans (SCHIPs), or other private health insurance plans (see Chapter 8).

Additional problems. A number of additional concerns exist in the implementation of IDEA:

1. IDEA states that personnel who teach and provide related services must meet state-approved, state-recognized licensure, registration, or other comparable requirements. No waivers are allowed, and LEAs must take measureable steps to recruit, hire, and retain qualified individuals. This requires a considerable amount of retraining for individuals practicing in the field who may need remediation on the current state of evidence-based practices.
2. Although there are regulations about the transition plan for adolescents, less attention is paid to transition from Part C to Part B of IDEA. There are reports of agencies that delay assessments on toddlers so that school districts will have to assume the expense and personnel once the child reaches his or her third birthday.
3. Some school administrators and educators have taken it on themselves to diagnose children with learning and behavioral problems and have even recommended or mandated

Family Educational Rights and Privacy Act

1. Protects the release of personally identifiable student information to others
2. Gives parents rights to access their child's educational records
3. Any information on a student within the school is considered an educational record
   a. Includes health records maintained by school employees who provide school health services, especially those that support the student's participation and progress in school
   b. Includes health screenings, immunization status, health room visits, individualized health plans (IHPs), and medication administration
4. Access to files is limited to those with a legitimate educational interest and may be released without parental permission to current school officials, other schools to which a student is transferring, specified officials for audits or accreditation, appropriate parties for financial aid to a student, state and local authorities within a juvenile justice system (regulated by state law) or in response to a subpoena, appropriate officials in cases of health and safety emergencies

Data from Kelly (2006) and U.S. Department of Education. Available at: www.ed.gov/policy/gen/guid/fpco/ferpa/index.html.

treatments to families. Such diagnoses and recommendations are outside the scope of their expertise. Under IDEiA (2004), school officials are explicitly prohibited from requiring parents to medicate children as a condition for attending school.

4. Concerns about the Health Insurance Portability and Accountability Act (HIPAA) have sometimes interfered with the continuity of care. HIPAA was intended to protect identifiable health data and prevent disclosure of protected health information without consent. This act applies to covered entities, including health care providers. It was never intended to interrupt necessary communication between health care providers, such as between primary care providers, school nurses, practitioners, and physicians. Protected health information can be shared for the purposes of treatment. "Therefore, healthcare providers should not feel restricted to share necessary information with the school nurse regarding specific treatments including medications or other interventions when a question arises about a specific student" (Kelly, 2006, p. 297). HIPAA privacy rules allow consultation with another health care provider about a patient for that provider's treatment of the individual (U.S. Department of Health and Human Services, 2008). This includes the primary care provider and the school nurse. In addition, nurse practice acts in each state require nurses to obtain authorization and clarification for treatments provided. Once information is shared with school nurses and advanced practice nurses (APNs), disclosure within the school system is regulated by the Family Educational Rights and Privacy Act (FERPA, 1974) (Box 3-5).

Americans with Disabilities Act of 1990

The Americans with Disabilities Act (ADA) (PL 101-336, 1990) prohibits discrimination against an individual with a disability in employment in government facilities and services and public accommodations operated by private entities, including public schools, public accommodations, telecommunications, and transportation. The ADA was based on the 1964 Civil Rights Act, which prohibited employment and accommodation discrimination by the

Americans with Disabilities Act (ADA) 1990 Definition of Disability

An individual with a disability is a person who
1. Has a physical or mental impairment that substantially limits one or more of the major life activities of the individual
2. Has a record of being impaired
3. Is regarded as having such an impairment

private sector against women and racial and ethnic minorities. Before the ADA, no federal law prohibited discrimination against people with disabilities in the private sector. Public schools must adhere to the ADA by ensuring reasonable accommodations so that students with disabilities can participate in school activities and access school services (CDC, 2008). Although this law has minimal effect on school programs, it has been extremely helpful in facilitating the transition of youths with disabilities into employment positions and independent housing, as well as ensuring accessibility for parents and staff with disabilities. ADA defined disability broadly using definition constructs first used under Section 504 (Box 3-6). Supreme Court decisions have indicated that the disability must not only be present but also be limiting the person's major life activities for the individual to be protected under the ADA. If a person's disability (i.e., severe myopia or severe hypertension) can be mitigated by corrective lenses or medication, that individual is no longer protected under ADA (*Sutton v. United Airlines, Inc*, 119 S. Ct 2139, 1999; *Murphy v. United Parcel Service, Inc*, 119 S. Ct. 2133, 1999) (see Mayerson & Mayer, 2000).

Role of Health Professionals in Determining Special Education Services

Primary Care Provider

The primary care provider's role starts with early identification and assessment of children with disabilities, as well as "children at risk" for disabilities as part of the mandated "child find" regulations of IDEA. If the primary care provider identifies a child at risk, the family should be referred to the school district's special education office to determine the appropriate public agency to evaluate the child. Children in the birth to 3 year age range may be evaluated through a variety of agencies depending on the state's implementation strategy for Part C of IDEA. Multiple services and assistive technology devices are available to infants and toddlers with disabilities through this program.

To initiate the IEP process, the parents or caretakers must request a special education assessment in writing. The primary care provider can provide the parents with a sample letter to initiate this process and inform them of their rights and their child's rights under IDEA (Box 3-7). A written letter by the primary care provider describing the child's diagnosis, known limitations, available test results, need for medical treatments, and so on can be critical because it provides medical documentation to support the request and can guide the comprehensiveness of the evaluation. The IEP assessment plan is determined by this initial request, so it is important to identify all areas of delay or potential risk.

The primary care provider can be part of the comprehensive multidisciplinary assessment process by providing health records and physical findings, with parental consent, to the IEP team. The

Sample Letter to Begin Special Education Assessment Process

Date: _____

To: Principal of Child's School or Director of Special Education Services School Address

Re: Student Name, Current Grade, School, and Teacher

I am writing to formally request my child be evaluated through the special education process because of his or her difficulty with _____.

I have discussed my concerns with his or her teacher. I request that the initial plan for assessment for eligibility be sent to me within 10 days so that I may review and approve if appropriate. I understand the school district has 80 days to complete the assessment process. Please keep me informed of scheduled assessments or evaluation of my child once I have approved the plan. Please send me information on the special education programs, eligibility, parental rights and due process, and the IEP process.

Thank you very much for assisting in this evaluation of my child. I look forward to working with you and your staff.

Sincerely,

Signature

Parent or guardian name

Relationship to child

Address

Phone numbers

E-mail address

From Siegel, L.M. (2001). *The complete IEP guide: How to advocate for your special ed child.* Berkeley, CA: Consolidated Printers, Inc; Nolo.com, Inc. Modified with permission.

primary care provider may participate in additional assessments or referrals to other specialists. Although the IEP team is responsible for explaining the assessment findings to the parents and child, the primary care provider may be able to offer additional insight or interpretation.

The primary care provider can be very helpful in making recommendations for interventions and for reviewing the plan with the family to determine its appropriateness for the child. If the provider and family think that the plan is not sufficient to meet the child's developmental and cognitive needs, it can be rejected and additional recommendations made to the IEP team. Recommendations supported by assessment findings or relevant literature are more likely to be accepted and incorporated into the plan. The primary care provider should act as an advocate for the parents and child when there is evidence of inappropriate or incomplete planning by the IEP team.

Although the aforementioned information speaks to the primary care provider's role in accessing and ensuring appropriate special education for children, the primary care provider should also be an advocate for students who need 504 accommodation plans. Children and families should be assisted to identify those accommodations that would facilitate learning in the school environment and then be supported in asserting for those rights in the school. The primary care provider can request specific accommodations to be included in the 504 plan. Although 504 plans are less comprehensive than IEPs, the process is also less formal, and often a simple letter from the primary care provider, or even a note on a prescription pad with the diagnosis and recommended accommodations, will provide sufficient documentation for the family and school.

Ongoing involvement of the primary care provider will facilitate a child's adjustment to school. Although the school district is the lead agency for services provided in the school setting, school personnel often welcome input from the child's primary care provider in coordinating health care information and services among specialty clinics, the school, and the child and family. If the school district has a nurse assigned to oversee health care services for children with chronic conditions, the primary care provider should establish a link with that individual.

The AAP Council on School Health recommends that "pediatricians should establish a working relationship with the school nurses who care for their patients with chronic conditions to ensure that individual patients' health plans are executed effectively within the school. In addition, pediatricians' communications with school nurses concerning their patients should be sufficiently clear and detailed to guide school nurses in overseeing the care of individual children" (Council on School Health, 2008, p. 1054).

Taras and Brennan (2008) conducted a study on the nature of the support of physicians who serve as consultants to schools for students with chronic diseases. They found that physician consultation interventions in the school fell into six primary categories:

1. Direct communication between the school physican consultant and the child's own physician
2. Recommending an appropriate level of school health services where there is a discrepancy of opinion
3. Providing medical input into the development of the individualized health care plan by the school nurse
4. Educating school staff on particular health conditions
5. Establishing ongoing communication between school personnel and the child's physician
6. Assisting the family with navigating the health system

These roles could also be those of an APN.

Before initiating any discussion with the school that could involve the release of medical information about the child, it is important for primary care providers to seek the permission of the child and the family and adhere to HIPAA regulations (see Chapter 8). The primary care provider should be aware that school district personnel, including nurses and APNs who are school district employees, are bound by FERPA guidelines that are not as restrictive as HIPAA. Although this will not be a problem for most families, establishing open communication and the limits of confidentiality with the school district may need to be explored (see Box 3-5 for a description of FERPA). Students may be hesitant to disclose information because they view their condition as a privacy issue (Betz and Redcay, 2002). If a condition is mild and not visible, families may not want information about the condition conveyed to school personnel to prevent their child from being labeled as "different." In other cases, parents or students genuinely fear ostracism or reprisal from the school community. Regardless, some students find dealing with the assumptions others hold about their condition more bothersome than the condition itself (Thies, 1999).

The family's wishes should be respected if at all possible. When withholding information about a child places that child at risk, however, the family must be counseled about the risks and benefits of disclosure, and appropriate legal action must be taken. For example, withholding information about an adolescent with uncontrolled epilepsy who is enrolling in driver's education is both dangerous and illegal. Parents' fears, guilt, and values need to be carefully assessed because these play critical roles in their children's school success.

BOX 3-8

Questions to Ask When Evaluating the Appropriateness of an IEP

1. What does the child know about the condition? How much of the care is the child responsible for? What help will he or she require?
2. Is the child's general health stable, improving, or worsening? Is the child terminally ill?
3. Are any classes or school activities contraindicated by the child's condition? Is the child placed in the least restrictive environment?
4. Is preferential seating in the classroom recommended? Are assistive devices required?
5. What modifications in diet exist? Does the child require any assistance in feeding?
6. What physical restrictions and exercise limitations exist? How are they best managed at school? Can the child access all school services? Is fatigue a problem?
7. What medications or treatments does the child receive during the school day? Can dosage times or treatments be modified around school hours?
8. Does the child require counseling, special therapies (e.g., occupational, physical, speech), adaptive equipment, protective devices, or transportation?
9. Does the child need assistance with any activities of daily living (i.e., toileting)?
10. What precautions, first aid interventions, and emergency procedures should school personnel be able to implement? Does the child wear a medical alert bracelet?

Box 3-8 lists multiple questions the primary care provider can ask to determine the appropriateness of the interventions identified on the IEP. When the child is approaching the age for transition services, the primary care provider can assist the child and family by providing instruction for the transition plan; ensuring that the child (or parent if the child is unable) has the necessary skills for self-care; and ensuring that the child (or parent if the child is unable) knows or has a list of his or her history and the accommodations needed to be successful.

School Nurses/Advanced Practice Nurses

The school nurse has an important leadership role in the provision of school health services for children with chronic conditions (Council on School Health, 2008; Selekman, 2006). The school nurse must assess the student's health, identify health problems needing to be addressed at school to enable the student to fully participate in the educational process, and develop a plan to address these issues. When children with chronic conditions require medical interventions in school, an individualized health plan (IHP), analogous to the IEP for educational services, must be written and approved by the parents and school officials. The school nurse obtains information from the parents, from the student, and, with parent/student permission, from other health care providers responsible for the child's medical care and establishes goals and objectives for medical care and therapies in the school setting. The contents of the IHP may be incorporated directly into the IEP.

The nurse functions as the coordinator/case manager of care and is responsible for ensuring continuity. One of the minimum health services identified by the American Academy of Pediatrics that should be offered by school nurses is that of "identification and management of students' chronic health care needs that affect educational achievement" (Council on School Health, 2008, p. 1054). Other roles of the school nurse include providing or supervising the acute, chronic, episodic, and emergency health care of all students in the assigned school; liaison among the family, health care professionals, the school, and the community; advocate for the child and family; and coordinating the school health services team.

An optimum potential for collaboration occurs when a school nurse and an advanced practice nurse (APN) are both in the same facility. When school-based health/wellness centers are present in a school, the opportunity exists for coordination of care and continuity of care. Either of these individuals could be the team leader for the IEP team for children with health-related conditions if the APN is an employee of the school. If school nurses are not on school grounds most of the time but a school health center is, it then becomes the responsibility of the APN to take the lead in the care of children with chronic conditions or to communicate with the responsible person within the school about the child. It should be noted, however, that most school-based health centers are freestanding entities that are not under the direction or employment of the school or school district.

The school nurse is in an ideal position to coordinate care with the primary care provider, specialists, and local public health and social services agencies. He or she "is the constant in the student's school experience over the years. It is the nurse who can see the whole picture of what is happening with a student over time" (Selekman & Gamel-McCormick, 2006).The nurse has the opportunity to see the child on a daily basis and can identify changes in health status, the effectiveness of newly prescribed interventions or medications, and the effectiveness of the IEP-related services and assistive technologic devices in meeting the educational goals for the child. Potential problems and strategies can be proactively identified and implemented, or changes in the child's condition can be easily communicated.

Facilitating the School Experience

An important developmental task of children at least 5 years old is to move beyond the family sphere into the school community, where regular attendance, academic achievement, and social competence are major goals; many children begin working on these goals through preschool education beginning at age 3. Condition severity and perceived limitations interfere with normal school activities for 6.5% of students; about 1.5% are unable to regularly attend school (Council on Children with Disabilities, 2005; Kaffenberger, 2006). Information regarding a student's academic performance, social skills, support networks, capabilities in performing daily living skills, health care needs, and stamina for handling the demands of the school day needs to be assessed and acted on to best help children cope with the limitations that may be encountered in school while helping them maintain independence.

The primary care provider must work in conjunction with the child, family, and school personnel (and ideally a school nurse), as well as auxiliary personnel (e.g., school bus drivers, coaches) to ensure a successful school experience. Decisions around whether, what, and to whom to disclose information about a student's condition need to balance the child's need to be treated normally with the need to ensure an optimal learning environment and safe supervision (Clay, 2004). For many children with chronic conditions, school nurses and counselors are critical partners for primary care providers because they can provide regular observations regarding students' health, their ability to engage in self-care, and the effectiveness of treatment protocols, including availability of needed medications and supplies (Erickson, Splett, Mullet, et al., 2006).

Because schools vary widely in their resources and commitment to students with chronic conditions, student needs must be addressed on a case-by-case basis. For underresourced schools, the primary care provider can assume a lead role in helping staff access accurate condition-specific information and receive necessary training. Students' school experiences will be enriched when school personnel are educated not only about specific conditions, but also as to the implications of this information for academic success (Cunningham & Wodrich, 2006). By understanding common expressions of chronic health problems in the classroom, teachers will be more likely to appropriately attribute learning and behavioral issues to a condition's pathology (Wodrich & Cunningham, 2008).

Factors Affecting Academic Performance

A successful school life is, in part, a function of academic performance. Youths with chronic conditions feel less affiliated with school and experience more academic difficulty than their peers (Telfair, Alleman-Velez, Dickens, et al., 2005). Disease severity is not directly correlated with academic performance. A nexus of factors facilitates or limits academic success, including school attendance, condition manifestations and management, a child's sense of self, teacher and family expectations, school connectedness, a child's perceived sense of safety both in school and traveling to and from school, components of the school's physical environment, and factors at home, including support for the school experience, as well as ensuring adequate nutrition, sleep, and care (Madan-Swain, Katz, & LaGory, 2004; Shaw & McCabe, 2008; Wodrich & Cunningham, 2008).

School Attendance and Absenteeism. The relationships among disease and chronicity, absenteeism, and school performance are complex. Illness alone is rarely a suitable excuse for academic difficulty and school failure. However, academic achievement is associated with attendance, and absenteeism is significantly higher among children with chronic conditions (Shaw & McCabe, 2008). School refusal is five-fold higher and absenteeism averages 16 days per year among students with chronic conditions compared with 3 days per year for nonaffected youth (McDougall, King, deWit, et al., 2004; Shiu, 2001).

The pattern of absences is more predictive of poor academic performance than the number of days missed, with frequent short-term interruptions more disruptive than a single, longer absence. Exacerbations in the child's condition, treatment side effects, fatigue, health care appointments, and family dysfunction are the primary reasons for absenteeism. Repeated absenteeism not only affects academic performance but can create a downward spiral in a child's self-concept, peer relations, and school connectedness (Kearney & Bensaheb, 2006), especially in this era of "high-stakes" testing. Parental guilt and anxiety can further contribute to absenteeism by fostering school resistance or school phobia. These consequences are difficult to reverse.

Families and professionals need to work together to reduce absenteeism. Parents must clearly communicate their expectations about school to their children and facilitate their attendance. Whenever possible, health care visits should be scheduled around school hours. If this is impossible, several appointments should be scheduled on one day so that the child does not have to miss several half days of class. Partnering with school-based clinics for routine monitoring also reduces students' absenteeism from class.

If a prolonged absence is anticipated, primary care providers can help parents arrange for home instruction. School policies vary, and delays as a result of child ineligibility, poor coordination of services, or unavailable teachers may be encountered before homebound education is initiated. If schools are not approached before the requisite length of absenteeism (i.e., usually 2 to 4 weeks) is met, additional delays are likely to be encountered before services are arranged. Most schools are willing to work with families in maintaining their child's education by providing homework assignments, communicating with hospital-based teachers, helping parents become informal tutors, and arranging for tutorial services or even dial-up participation from home to the classroom to begin as soon as the child is eligible. If hospitalizations are frequent or prolonged absences are anticipated, a specific objective should be included in the child's IEP or IHP to ensure uninterrupted schooling. This is an example of how case management and care coordination can benefit the child and family.

Condition Management Issues. Disease processes (e.g., poor oxygen diffusion, repeated hypoglycemia), side effects from various interventions (e.g., chemotherapies, long-term steroid use, cranial radiation), and associated fatigue all may affect academic motivation and learning (e.g., concentration, memory, information processing) (Shaw & McCabe, 2008). The coexistence of psychosocial problems such as anxiety, depression, or family difficulties further exacerbates the student's potential for poor academic performance. Of students with chronic illnesses, 45% report falling behind in their school work and 35% of high school students report failing grades (Thies, 1999). Clinicians need to identify and optimally manage symptomatology that impairs students' motivation and academic performance.

Mobility Concerns. Mobility is affected by physical impairments, diminished strength, and fatigue. Regardless of the cause, limited mobility can affect students' ability to achieve and compete. Physical changes can limit some children from participating fully in physical education, recess, sports, and afternoon activities. In the worst case scenario, limited mobility will hinder children from participating in critical learning activities.

If mobility is a problem, appropriate adaptations must be addressed in the student's IEP meetings. Two major approaches are used to facilitate a child's mobility: structuring the environment and improving mobility. School districts have eliminated many physical obstacles in compliance with the Americans with Disabilities Act, but individual schools may be more difficult to navigate than others. When choosing a school is an option, its physical layout (e.g., number of floors, width of hallways, presence of elevators, and location of bathrooms) needs to be considered. Providing the child with two sets of books, one for the classroom and one for home, eliminates the problem of transporting them. Scheduling classes in rooms close to one another and scheduling a study hall or lunch after physical education class gives the student more time to change and prevent tardiness. "Buddies" from the class can be assigned to assist a student to get from class to class.

The student's mobility will be improved and normalization promoted if appropriate assistive devices are used. For example, an adolescent in a large high school may prefer to use a wheelchair when traveling long distances between classes rather than limiting the class schedule to classes that are near each other. Adaptive aids can help children write, reach books on library shelves, or respond to questions in the classroom. Backpacks on rollers may assist the student in dragging rather than lifting books and supplies. For students who drive, access to handicapped parking needs to be ensured.

Fatigue. Fatigue is an integral part of many chronic conditions that affect children's overall quality of life, including school success and participation in scholastic activities (Eddy & Cruz, 2007). Fatigue may be a symptom of the disease (e.g., in heart disease or sickle cell disease), a physiologic side effect of treatment (e.g., chemotherapy, radiation), associated with time-consuming therapies (e.g., chest physiotherapy for cystic fibrosis), or a side effect of medications (e.g., those given for epilepsy). Severity of fatigue is further mediated by stress and mood (Schanberg, Gil, Anthony et al., 2005).

Strategies for reducing fatigue focus on structuring a child's educational experience in a way that is not physically taxing while promoting academic success and peer acceptance. For example, the child could be encouraged to use an MP3 recorder for note taking, serve as scorekeeper rather than participating in vigorous activity during physical education, or be assigned easy classroom chores such as sharpening pencils with an electric sharpener. Choosing classes in close proximity is particularly important in large schools or those with several buildings. Scheduling a study hall period immediately after lunch gives the child an opportunity to nap (ideally in a different setting) without missing instructional time. Another strategy is arranging the student's schedule so that the most important classes are either in the morning or in the afternoon; that way, if only half-day sessions are possible, the student can still learn the important content. The homework demands of various courses should also be taken into account when planning a child's schedule. It is better to defer one class than to have children take on a rigorous schedule that portends failure. Selected courses may be taken during summer school to lighten a child's academic load. Prospective academic planning is important, as schools have limited summer offerings. Students and families must be helped in setting reasonable expectations around participation in school activities.

Medications and Treatments. If medications are required during the school day, the general guidelines and criteria of each state and school district must be followed:

1. A legal prescriber must authorize the medication.
2. Parents must give written permission for medication to be given.
3. The medication should be properly labeled in its original container.
4. The medication must be stored in a locked area.
5. The school must document that the medication was administered.

Schools are responsible for having written policies regarding student confidentiality and medication storage and, in the absence of a school nurse if the state nurse practice act allows, designate an individual trained in medication administration (Committee on School Health, 2003).

To ensure smooth coordination among providers, the school, and the family, orders for any over-the-counter medications also need to be given. When it is desired that children carry their own

medications, such as with an asthma inhaler or Epi-pen, these must be cleared with the school district because policies vary across jurisdictions. If it is likely that a student will need to take medications ordered on an as-needed basis or on school field trips, clearly defined protocols should be made for their administration (Reutzel & Patel, 2001).

Medications that can interfere with learning need to be prescribed judiciously. Steroids, a mainstay with many chronic conditions, can lead to dysthymia, anxiety, sleep disturbances, weight gain, and other distressing symptoms that may interfere with academic performance and social acceptance (Thies, 1999). Other medications, including some analgesics, anticonvulsants, antidepressants, and antipsychotics, also affect academic performance. When monitoring a drug's efficacy in managing a specific condition, its side effects on learning must be assessed.

Whenever possible, clinicians should alter treatment protocols to occur around school schedules for several pragmatic reasons. The child with a chronic condition wants to be considered normal. Requiring the child to go to the nurse for medications may be met with resistance, particularly in this era of "safe and drug-free schools." Schools that have such programs unwittingly place the student with a chronic condition at risk for nonadherence. School nurses can adopt unobtrusive methods, such as instant messaging or vibrating beepers, to remind students about coming to take their medications. There are some cases, however, when the treatment provided by the school nurse is the best way of guaranteeing that the medication or treatment was given, usually because of an unstable home enviroment; therefore some primary care providers set up the schedule so that the child is guaranteed to have the treatment at least 5 days per week in the school setting.

Even in the best of circumstances, there may not be adequate time or qualified personnel within the school to administer medications or oversee treatments. As children enter adolescence, it is often appropriate to explore ways to help them develop self-care behaviors (e.g., self-medication, intermittent clean catheterizations, testing blood glucose levels). Such activities will help children become more autonomous, an important developmental goal.

Social and Emotional Needs

Students with chronic conditions have an array of social and emotional needs that have an impact on motivation, learning, and school success. Common internal (e.g., anxiety, depression, suicide ideation) and externalizing (e.g., impulsivity, anger) psychosocial problems are associated with school stress (Shaw & McCabe, 2008). Associated peer rejection, increased high-risk behaviors (including substance abuse), increasing somatization, and deteriorating self-esteem peak in adolescence (Erickson, Patterson, Wall, et al., 2005; Shiu, 2001).

Effective coping strategies and a healthy self-concept are paramount if children with chronic conditions are to become resilient in handling the demands of their condition and school pressures (Hampel, Rudolph, Stachow, et al., 2005). Many normative school activities (e.g., instruction in nutrition or sexuality) teach children health-promoting behaviors that can help build healthy self-concepts. Helping these children develop wholesome relationships and share their talents with other children is also beneficial; children who excel in a specific academic area or participate in sports and other extracurricular activities are more likely to be successful.

Participating in these activities not only helps build self-esteem but also enhances other spheres of development.

Developing healthy self-esteem in students with chronic conditions is not without difficulty. These children face unique stressors associated with their conditions that are further exacerbated by insensitive policies or a lack of privacy when taking medications or performing management tasks. They are more likely to be teased; many may experience bullying or even ostracism (Vessey & Horowitz, in press).

Helping youths with chronic conditions develop a social support network will positively influence their psychosocial adjustment and self-esteem (Kef, 2002). Opportunities must be created for these youth to interact with nonaffected peers in nonacademic settings, including sports teams, clubs, and other extracurricular activities. They benefit from interventions to strengthen their coping abilities, helping them deal constructively with peer rejection, loneliness, or isolation. Incorporating social skills training into the child's educational plan is one way to help the child and family become more confident in their interactions with others and their use of effective behaviors when dealing with discrimination. School personnel can assist by dealing with inappropriate behavior of other students and developing an awareness of what it is like to have a chronic condition.

Students' self-concepts are enhanced when they can successfully communicate information about their condition and its management to their friends and school personnel, thus creating a supportive environment and enhancing their own safety and security. This is especially important for adolescents who are increasingly independent of their parents. The primary care provider can role play situations with students, such as determining what friends they may trust and how to communicate selected information.

Parents, teachers, and school professionals often are challenged with how to best help foster emotional development and school connectedness in children with chronic conditions. Teachers and parents may be overprotective, be anxious that care needs will be addressed, have lowered academic expectations, or impose less discipline (Clay, 2004). They may need help to acknowledge that children with chronic conditions experience the same developmental stressors as their peers and therefore need to be treated similarly and taught the same coping skills. Using a variety of techniques to help these children normalize their school experience will be beneficial to developing their self-concept.

For a variety of reasons, the process of ensuring appropriate educational placement and accommodations for children with special health care needs can be contentious and stressful for families: inadequate school funding for special education, lack of a funding stream for 504 accommodations, and differing perspectives and lack of trust between parents and educators. From the school's perspective, parents may deny the presence of a chronic condition, refuse testing, or dispute the IEP team's finding that their child has special needs. From the parents' perspective, schools may delay or deny educational assessments, deny recommended therapies or educational aides, fail to provide adequate education in separate classes, or fail to enforce plans that are in place. Primary care providers are sometimes put in the middle of this process, and at other times may be unaware that encouraging the parent to "ask for an IEP" does not necessarily lead to a speedy and mutually satisfactory result. As a trustworthy third party, the primary care provider can effectively reinforce the benefits of adequate evaluation when communicating with the parents and the need for specific interventions when communicating with educational professionals.

Ensuring Safety

School systems are responsible for ensuring that students with chronic conditions are in a safe environment. Schools should have policies and procedures in place to handle emergency situations, including (1) the identification of qualified individuals to manage emergencies, (2) appropriate staff safety education, (3) an emergency kit and manual, and (4) parental notification procedures (Committee on School Health, 2001). Primary care providers can assist families in ensuring that these policies and procedures contain sufficient information to handle common emergencies associated with their child's condition.

Because many chronic conditions or their treatments place children at greater risk for infection, illness, or injury, each student's risks must be assessed individually. For example, students with asthma may have numerous classroom triggers (Sharma, Hansel, Matsui, et al., 2007). Impaired sensory function (e.g., cataracts, diminished vision) and lowered immunity may result from long-term use of steroids. The school's policy on notifying parents of possible exposure to communicable diseases must be clarified. Depending on the child's chronic condition, specific areas of concern may include "strep" throat, measles, varicella, meningitis, hepatitis A and B, salmonella, or shigella infections. Latex allergy is another potential threat for students with chronic conditions. Although students with myelodysplasia are the most likely to be affected (see Chapter 35), any child with repeated exposure to latex is at greater risk.

For children on life-sustaining equipment such as ventilators, electrical adaptive equipment must be periodically inspected with a reserve generator made available. Provisions for transporting a student with a physical disability during emergencies such as fires and earthquakes need to be determined and disseminated to all school personnel. Faculty and staff need to rehearse plans to retrieve students with mobility or cognitive deficits from classrooms, especially those not on the first floor.

Many students with chronic conditions participate in intramural and varsity athletics. Athletic trainers and coaches need to be informed and prepared to handle condition-specific emergencies such as hypoglycemia, seizures, or asthma attacks (Committee on School Health, 2001). Because such emergencies occur rarely, providing individualized procedure cards to be included in field emergency kits is useful, particularly if the team travels. Other students' conditions may prohibit them from participating on regular school teams. Special Olympics programs (www.specialolympics.org) may be an alternative. For younger children, adaptations in playground equipment may be necessary and should be individualized. Regardless of level of play, appropriate safety equipment must be used under adult supervision. Strengthening exercises also help prevent injury.

Under IDEA (2004), school buses may transport children with chronic conditions as young as 3 years of age for related services. Children with disabilities need individualized evaluation to determine the appropriate restraint system for their age, size, and disability. School buses need to be equipped with appropriate safety devices (i.e., communication system, fire extinguisher, first aid kit) that meet federal motor vehicle safety standards (FMVSS). Buses need to be equipped with height- and weight-appropriate, forward-facing seats with dynamically tested three-point restraints and/or four-point tie-down devices for wheelchairs that allow the passenger to face forward that meet FMVSS if transporting disabled children. Certified transit wheelchairs should be used whenever possible; lap boards should be removed and stored separately. Strollers are not permitted. Students under 50 pounds should be restrained with safety vests. Oxygen, suctioning equipment, or other specialized equipment needs to be stored appropriately and labeled. An aide or nurse should accompany selected medically fragile children. The school nurse will develop emergency action plans that direct lay personnel in the emergency measures to take for a particular child's condition until medical assistance arrives. Written emergency evacuation plans should be in place with drills held yearly (Committee on Injury, Violence, and Poison Prevention, 2007).

Transition between Hospital and School

Primary care providers should actively participate in school reintegration programs for youth who have had prolonged absences or dropped out (Betz & Redcay, 2002). Those returning to school with developmental changes or new disfigurements are especially at risk. A positive experience of reentry can provide children with a sense of accomplishment and social acceptance, strengthen faltering self-esteem, and lessen maladaptive emotional responses to their condition (Thies & McAllister, 2001).

Primary care providers can help promote a smooth transition for such children by proactively engaging the child, family members, and school personnel in determining strategies to facilitate school reentry. For children who are returning to school after a prolonged hospitalization, a three-phase approach is used. In phase 1, families are helped to identify school and community supports. In phase 2, communication occurs between hospitals and health care providers and school personnel (i.e., principal, school nurse, counselor) to help make the transition a positive experience for the child. An appropriate IEP or IHP (or both) should be initiated that addresses individualized educational strategies for the child and peer and teacher education. Last, in phase 3, follow-up to ensure that the transition has been successful is undertaken (Kliebenstein & Broome, 2000; Madan-Swain et al., 2004).

Most children with chronic conditions, however, no longer experience long hospitalizations but rather shorter hospital stays, and longer home recuperation with more outpatient services. These children have less access to hospital teachers, and parents may assume increasing health care and educational responsibilities. This makes transition planning more complex. Schools should tailor a student's educational program to allow for flexible attendance, offer differentiated instruction, and provide mechanisms for social support (Shaw & McCabe, 2008).

When a prolonged absence is anticipated, parents must arrange for home instruction. School policies vary, and delays as a result of child ineligibility or poor coordination of services may be encountered before homebound education or other alternatives are initiated. If schools are not approached before the requisite length of absenteeism (i.e., usually 2 to 4 weeks) is met, additional delays are likely to be encountered before services are arranged. Most schools are willing to work with families in maintaining their child's education by providing homework assignments, communicating with hospital-based teachers, helping parents become informal tutors, and arranging for tutorial services to begin as soon as the child is eligible. If hospitalizations are frequent or prolonged absences are

anticipated, a specific objective should be included a priori in the child's IEP to plan for uninterrupted schooling.

The two primary goals are to help the child and family anticipate situations they may encounter and to prepare teachers and classmates for the child's return. One helpful approach to preparing the child for reentry is role playing, wherein the primary care provider plays the role of a classmate and children play themselves. The purpose is to act out a variety of scenarios that may occur during the first day back at school so that the child can develop answers to potentially embarrassing questions or situations that may arise. Another useful strategy is to ask close friends to accompany the child and serve as a buffer on the return to school. Parents may also bring the child for several drop-in visits or sponsor a welcome back class party designed to promote peer acceptance.

A variety of approaches can be used to help teachers and classmates adjust. Two-way video conferencing while the child is still in the hospital or homebound is becoming more available. A child may be encouraged to write a letter or record a videotape for classmates about the experience of being in the hospital or undergoing treatment, which is then shared with teachers or classmates several days before the child's return. Providing visual images of a child—either on videotape or in photographs—allows time for "sanctioned staring" or for classmates to ask questions or express their concerns without fear of recrimination. This is particularly important if the child has undergone major physical changes (e.g., alopecia secondary to chemotherapy, scarring from burns). Role playing, science projects, literature assignments, and video presentations can be used by teachers to promote understanding and acceptance within the child's peer group. Careful advance planning will improve the likelihood of a successful return to school for the child.

The decision to repeat a grade must be made with great care. This setback can cause feelings of shame, inadequacy, and inferiority; but the decision to remain in the same grade may also enhance feelings of success because the work requirements may be easier. New classmates provide a second chance to form friendships.

School and the Student with a Terminal Condition

School is an appropriate activity for many children who are terminally ill because it provides a sense of normality, opportunities for socialization, and personal achievement. For children to have a successful school experience, the following must be considered:

1. A priori discussions on how and when information regarding the child's condition will be shared with the child, peers, school personnel, and other parents.
2. Academic programming is flexible and tailored to the specific child so that school remains relevant as the child's condition deteriorates. For example, an adolescent enrolled in a college preparatory curriculum needs to be helped to develop achievable objectives rather than giving up all hope for the future.
3. Efforts are made to help the child maintain a positive self-concept and body image, important albeit difficult when a child begins to manifest physical and mental changes. Children who are dying often need to exhibit more control over their lives and environments. Whenever possible, efforts must be made to help children reach the goals that they have set for themselves.

It is not enough to focus attention only on the dying child and the family because many students and school personnel have had little experience with a terminally ill peer or pupil. Development and experience moderate children's understanding of death. The attitudes of school personnel toward illness and death, as well as their ability to individualize instruction, their concern or need to protect the dying child, and their fear of an emergency arising in the classroom, can influence their effectiveness. Working with the school's nurse and school counselors, in consultation with palliative care or hospice programs, will help provide guidance throughout this difficult time. After a child's death, developmentally appropriate bereavement counseling for students and staff is imperative.

Do Not Resuscitate Orders

Comprehensive planning for end-of-life care for a child with a terminal condition may include promulgating the family's wishes that the child not be resuscitated if a cardiac arrest occurs. A comprehensive approach to responding to do not resuscitate (DNR) orders in the school requires school personnel to develop a protocol to follow when a child with a DNR order attends school. It should be noted that some facilities use the term allow natural death (AND) rather than DNR.

The National Education Association (NEA) has issued guidelines for DNR orders in school provided that a school district and state honor DNR orders in school (NEA, 2000). The NEA has suggested the following minimum conditions if a school board is to honor DNR:

1. The request should be submitted in writing and be accompanied by a written order signed by the student's physician.
2. The school should establish a team to consider the request and all available alternatives and, if no other alternative exists, to develop a medical emergency plan.
3. Staff should receive training.
4. Staff and students should receive counseling.

In its statement, the NEA delineated the following elements of the medical emergency plan:

1. The student's teacher specifies his or her actions if the student experiences a cardiac arrest or other life-threatening emergency.
2. Other school employees who supervise the student receive briefing sessions.
3. The student wears an identification bracelet indicating the DNR order.
4. The parents execute a contract with the local emergency medical service and send a copy to the superintendent.
5. The team reviews the plan annually.

In 2000 the Committee on School Health and Committee on Bioethics (2000) of the American Academy of Pediatrics released a joint policy statement on DNR orders in schools. This document is similar to that of the NEA, but goes further in recommending that pediatricians review the plan with the board of education and its legal counsel and update the plan every 6 months rather than yearly.

Individual states have highly varied DNR policies and laws that govern the actions of emergency medical personnel actions when treating students (Costante, 2001). Practitioners are encouraged to determine specific regulations for their state. Schools should develop protocols for responding to DNR orders in accordance with NEA guidelines, AAP policy, and state regulations and in a spirit of collaboration, respect, and sensitivity. Parents, educators, support personnel, and members of the health care team must be committed to a process that is flexible and responsive to the changing needs of the child. In some cases, it is appropriate for the child to be actively involved with planning. Essential to this process are ongoing forums where parents and educators can discuss their concerns, share their values and preferences about how certain situations should be handled, and define or revise plans. Within these discussions, it is crucial to define the range of possible scenarios that are likely to occur for the child and to build contingency plans for how they should be handled. Hospice personnel may be helpful in guiding these discussions.

Summary

Primary care providers must not lose sight of the fact that schools provide opportunities for social, emotional, and cognitive development. A team approach based on the principles of family-centered schools helps guarantee that students' educational and health care needs are met (Thies & McAllister, 2001). School success for the child with a chronic condition is predicated on successful communication and information dissemination across respective parties (Esperat, Moss, Roberts, et al., 1999). Primary care providers may assume the role of coordinator by bringing together the child, parents, peers, and school personnel and fostering open communication. Providing in-service training to school personnel and using a "referral pad" that lists contact information for the provider's office, federal and state agencies, organizations, mentor programs, and support groups are ways to foster communication (Betz & Redcay, 2002). Innovative school health programs based on delivering primary care in the school and linking it to the school program should be encouraged.

Resources

Centers for Disease Control and Prevention
Division of Adolescent and School Health
Provides information on the coordination of school health programs and important long-term studies on children, youth, and school health.
Website: www.cdc.gov/HealthyYouth/index.htm

Consortium for Citizens with Disabilities
1331 H St. NW
Suite 300
Washington, DC 20005
(202) 783-2229
Website: www.c-c-d.org

Council for Exceptional Children
1110 North Glebe Rd., Suite 300
Arlington, VA 22201
Voice phone: (703) 620-3660
TTY: (866) 915-5000
Fax: (703) 264-9494
E-mail: service@cec.sped.org
Website: www.cec.sped.org

Disability Rights Education and Defense Fund (DREDF)
2212 6th St.
Berkeley, CA 94710
(510) 644-2555
Website: www.dredf.org

Federation for Children with Special Needs Parents Training and Information Centers (PTI)
Each state has a PTI office.
Federation for Children with Special Needs (central office)
95 Berkeley St., Suite 104
Boston, MA 02116
(617) 482-2915
Website: www.fcsn.org

IDEA Practices: updates in IDEA from the Council for Exceptional Children
Website: http://205.241.44.100/law_res/doc/

National Association of School Nurses
Provides information on policy statements, local chapters, and a link to the *Journal of School Nursing.*
Website: www.nasn.org

National Association of State Boards of Education
State-level policy guides, publications, and annotated links to general school and health websites.
Website: www.nasbe.org

National Information Center for Children and Youth with Disabilities
PO Box 1492
Washington, DC 20013
(800) 695-0285, (202) 884-8200
E-mail: nichcy@aed.org
Website: www.nichcy.org

Office of Civil Rights
330 C St., SW
Washington, DC 20202
(202) 205-5413
Website: www.ed.gov/about/offices/list/ocr/index.html

U.S. Department of Education
Building the Legacy: IDEA 2004
Website: http://idea.ed.gov

U.S. Department of Education
Office of Special Education and Rehabilitation Services
330 C St., SW
Washington, DC 20202
(202) 205-5507
Website: www.ed.gov/about/offices/list/osers/index.html

REFERENCES

Americans with Disabilities Act (1990). Public Law 101-336, 42 USC 12101 et seq. Washington, DC: U.S. Government Printing Office.

Betz, C.L., & Redcay, G. (2002). Lessons learned from providing transition services to adolescents with special health care needs. *Issues Compr Pediatr Nurs, 25*, 129-149.

Board of Education of the Hendrick Hudson Central School District, Westchester County et al., Petitioners v. Amy Rowley, by her parents, Rowley et al. Respondent (1982). 80-1002 U.S.Supreme Court.

Brown v. Board of Education. (1954). U.S. Supreme Court 347, US, 483.

Cedar Rapids Community School District v. Garret F. 119 S. Ct. 992, 29 IDELR 966 (U.S. 199). Available at http://supct.law.cornell.edu/supct/html/96-1793.ZS.html. Retrieved August 2008.

Centers for Disease Control and Prevention (2008). A CDC review of school laws and policies concerning child and adolescent health. *J School Health, 78*(2), 69-128.

Clay, D.L. (2004). *Helping Schoolchildren with Chronic Health Conditions.* New York: Guilford Press.

Committee on Injury, Violence, and Poison Prevention (2007). School transportation safety. *Pediatrics, 120*, 213-220.

Committee on School Health (2001). Guidelines for emergency medical care in school. *Pediatrics, 107*, 336-435.

Committee on School Health (2003). Guidelines for the administration of medication in school. *Pediatrics, 112*, 697-699.

Committee on School Health & Committee on Bioethics (2000). Do not resuscitate orders in schools (RE9842). *Pediatrics, 105*, 878-879.

Cortiella, C. (2006). *NCLB and IDEA: What Parents of Students with Disabilities Need to Know and Do.* Minneapolis, MN: University of Minnesota, National Center on Educational Outcomes.

Cortiella, C. (2007). *Rewards and Roadblocks: How Special Education Students Are Faring Under No Child Left Behind.* New York: National Center for Learning Disabilities.

Costante, C. (2001). Do not resuscitate in the school setting: Determining the policy and procedures. In N. Schwab, & M. Gerlman, (Eds.), *Legal Issues in School Health Services: A Resource for School Administrators, School Attorneys, and School Nurses,* North Branch, MN: Sunrise River Press.

Council on Children with Disabilities. (2005). Care coordination in the medical home: Integrating health and related systems of care for children with special health care needs. *Pediatrics, 116*, 1238-1244.

Council on School Health. (2008). Role of the school nurse in providing school health services. *Pediatrics, 121*(5), 1052-1056.

Cunningham, M.M., & Wodrich, D.L. (2006). The effect of sharing health information on teachers' production of classroom accommodations. *Psychol Schools, 43*, 553-564.

Eddy, L., & Cruz, M. (2007). The relationship between fatigue and quality of life in children with chronic health problems: A systematic review. *J Spec Pediatr Nurs, 12*, 105-114.

Education for All Handicapped Children Act. (1975). Public Law 94-142, 20 USC. Washington, DC: U.S. Government Printing Office.

Erickson, C.D., Splett, P.L., Mullet, S.S., et al. (2006). The healthy learner model for student chronic condition management—I. *J School Nurs, 22*, 310-318.

Erickson, J.D., Patterson, J.M., Wall, M., et al. (2005). Risk behaviors and emotional well-being in youth with chronic health conditions. *Children's Health Care, 34*, 181-192.

Esperat, M., Moss, P., Roberts, K., et al. (1999). Special needs children in the public schools: Perceptions of school nurses and school teachers. *Issues Compr Pediatr Nurs, 22*, 167-182.

Family Educational Rights and Privacy Act. (1974). 20, U.S.C.A. 1232g, regulations at 34 C.F.R.

Flanagan, D., Ortiz, S., Alfonso, V., et al. (2006). *The Achievement Test Desk Reference: A Guide to Learning Disability Identification.* Hoboken, NJ: Wiley & Sons.

Fletcher, J., Lyon, G.R., & Fuchs, L., et al. (2007). *Learning Disabilities: From Identification to Intervention.* New York: Guilford Press.

Golden, M., Kilb, L., & Mayerson, A. (1993). *Americans with Disabilities Act: An Implementation Guide.* Berkeley, CA: Disability Rights Education and Defense Fund, Inc (DREDF).

Hampel, P., Rudolph, H., and Stachow, R., et al. (2005). Coping among children and adolescents with chronic illness. *Anxiety, Stress, and Coping, 18*, 145-155.

Holler, R., & Zirkel, P. (2008). Section 504 and public schools: A national survey concerning "section-504-only" students. *National Association of Secondary School Principals, 92*(1), 19-43.

Individuals with Disabilities Education Act. (1991). 20 U.S.C. 1400 et seq. Public Law 101-119. Washington, DC: U.S. Government Printing Office.

Individuals with Disabilities Education Improvement Act. (2004). Public Law 108-446. Washington, DC: U.S. Government Printing Office.

Individuals with Disabilities Education Act Data. (2007). Data tables for OSEP state reported data. Available at https://www.ideadata.org. Retrieved November 4, 2008.

Infant, and Toddler Program, Part H. et al. (1986). Public Law 99-457. Washington, DC: U.S. Government Printing Office.

Irving Independent School District v. Tatro Et Ux., Individually and as Next Friends of Tatro, a Minor Certiorari (1984). United States Court of Appeals for the Fifth Circuit No. 83-558.

Kaffenberger, C. (2006). School re-entry for students with chronic illness: A role for professional counselors. *Prof School Counsel, 9*, 223-230.

Kamphaus, R., Quirk, M., & Kroncke, A. (2006). Learning disabilities. In R. Kamphaus & J.Campbell (Eds.), *Psychodiagnostic Assessment of Children*, Hoboken, NJ : John Wiley & Sons.

Kearney, C.A., & Bensaheb, A. (2006). School absenteeism and school refusal behavior: A review and suggestions for school-based health professionals. *J School Health, 76*, 3-7.

Kef, S. (2002). Psychosocial adjustment and the meaning of social support for visually impaired adolescents. *J Vis Impair Blind, 96*, 222-237.

Kelly, L. (2006). Legislation affecting school nurses. In J. Selekman, (Ed.), *School Nursing: A Comprehensive Text*. Philadelphia: F.A. Davis.

Kliebenstein, M.A., & Broome, M.E. (2000). School re-entry for the child with chronic illness: Parent and school personnel perceptions. *Pediatr Nurs, 26*, 579-583.

Lee, S., & Janik, M. (2006). Provision of psychoeducational services in the schools: IDEA, Section 504, and NCLB. In L.Phelps, (Ed.), *Chronic Health-Related Disorders in Children*, Washington, DC: American Psychological Association.

Luehr, R.E., & Selekman, J. (2006). Collaboration with the community. In J.Selekman (Ed.), *School Nursing: A Comprehensive Text*. Philadelphia: F.A. Davis.

Madan-Swain, A., Katz, E.R., & LaGory, J., (2004). School and social reintegration after a serious illness or injury. In R.T. Brown, (Ed.) *Handbook of Pediatric Psychology in School Settings*, Mahwah, NJ: Erlbaum.

Mayerson, A.B., & Mayer, K.S. (2000). *Defining disability in the aftermath of Sutton:* Where do we go from here? Berkeley, CA: Disability Rights Education and Defense Fund (DREDF) [online]. Available at http://64.143.22.161/articles/mayerson.html.

McDougall, J., King, G., deWit, D.J., et al. (2004). Chronic physical health conditions and disability among Canadian school-aged children: A national profile. *Disabil Rehabil, 26*, 35-45.

Mills, v. Board of Education of the District of Columbia. (1972). U.S. Court of Appeals 348F, Supp. 866.

Moses, M., Gilchrest, C., & Schwab, N. (2005). Section 504 of the Rehabilitation Act: Determining eligibility and implications for school districts. *J Sch Nurs, 21*(1), 48-58.

National Association of School Nurses. (2006). *Position statement: Caseload assignments*. Available at www.nasn.org. Retrieved August 1, 2008.

National Council on Disability. (2000). *Back to school on civil rights,* January 25, 2000. Available at www.ncd.gov/newsroom/publications/backto-school_1.html.

National Council on Disability (2008). *Finding the Gaps: A Comparative Analysis of Disability Laws in the United States to the United Nations Convention on the Rights of Persons with Disabilities*. Washington, DC: Author.

National Education Association. (2000). *Providing safe health care: The role of educational support personnel*. Available at www.nea.org/esphome/images/safecare.pdf.

No Child Left Behind Act. (2001). Public Law 107-110. Washington, DC: U.S. Government Printing Office.

Office of Civil Rights, U.S. Department of Education. (2005). *Protecting students with disabilities*. Available at www.ed.gov/about/offices/list/ocr/504faq.html. Retrieved July 29, 2008.

Pennsylvania Association for Retarded Citizens v. Pennsylvania. (1972). U.S. Court of Appeals, 343 F.

Reutzel, T.J., & Patel, R. (2001). Medication management problems reported by subscribers to a school nurse Listserv. *J Sch Nurs, 17*, 131-139.

Rief, S. (2005). *How to Reach and Teach Children with ADD/ADHD*. San Francisco, CA: Jossey-Bass.

Riley-Lawless, K. (2006). The demographics of children and adolescents. In J. Selekman, (Ed.) *School Nursing: A Comprehensive Text*. Philadelphia: F.A. Davis.

Schanberg, L.E., Gil, K.M., Anthony, K.K., et al. (2005). Pain, stiffness, and fatigue in juvenile polyarticular arthritis: Contemporaneous stressful events and mood as predictors. *Arthritis Rheum, 52*, 1196-1204.

Selekman, J. (Ed.). (2006). *School Nursing: A Comprehensive Text*. Philadelphia: F.A. Davis.

Selekman, J., & Gamel-McCormick, M. (2006). Children with chronic conditions. In J. Selekman, (Ed.), *School Nursing: A Comprehensive Text*. Philadelphia: F.A. Davis.

Sharma, S.R., Hansel, N.N., and Matsui, E. et al. (2007). Indoor environmental influences on children's asthma. *Pediatr Clin North Am, 54*, 103-120.

Shaw, S.R., & McCabe, P.C. (2008). Hospital-to-school transition for children with chronic illness: Meeting the new challenges of an evolving health care system. *Psychol Schools, 45*, 74-87.

Shiu, S. (2001). Issues in the education of students with chronic illness. *Int J Disabil, Dev Educat, 48*, 269-281.

Siegel, L.M. (2001). *The Complete IEP Guide: How to Advocate for Your Special Ed Child.* (2nd ed.) Berkeley, CA: Consolidated Printers.

Taras, H., & Brennan, J. (2008). Students with chronic diseases: Nature of school physician support. *J Sch Health, 78*(7), 389-396.

Telfair, J., Alleman-Velez, P.L., and Dickens, P., et al. (2005). Quality health care for adolescents with special health-care needs: Issues and clinical implications. *J Pediatr Nurs, 20*, 15-24.

Thies, K.M. (1999). Identifying the educational implications of chronic illness in school children. *J Sch Health, 69*, 392-397.

Thies, K.M., & McAllister, J.W. (2001). The Health and Education Leadership Project: A school initiative for children and adolescents with chronic health conditions. *J Sch Health, 71*, 167-172.

U.S. Department of Education (2006). 34 CFR, Parts 300 & 301: Assistance to states for the education of children with disabilities and preschool grants for children with disabilities. Final rules. *Federal Register, 71*, 46540-46845.

U.S. Department of Education. (2008a). *Office of Special Programs' IDEA* website. Available at http://idea.ed.gov/explore/view/p/%2Croot%2Cstatute%2CI%2C. Retrieved July 29, 2008.

U.S. Department of Education (2008). *The Individuals with Disabilities Education Act (IDEA): Provisions Related to Children with Disabilities Enrolled by Their Parents in Private School*. Washington, DC: Author.

U.S. Department of Health and Human Services. (2000). *Healthy People 2010: National Health Promotion and Disease Prevention Objectives*. Washington, DC: U.S. Department of Health and Human Services, Public Health Service.

U.S. Department of Health and Human Services. (2008). *HIPAA—frequent questions*. Available at www.hhs.gov/hipaafaq/index.html. Retrieved August 1, 2008.

Vessey, J.A., & Horowitz, J. (in press). A conceptual framework for understanding teasing and bullying. *J Pediatr Nurs.*

Vocational Rehabilitation Act (1973). Public Law 93-112, 29 USC, Section 504, 45CFR Washington, DC: U.S. Government Printing Office.

Wodrich, D.L., & Cunningham, M.M. (2008). School-based tertiary and targeted interventions for students with chronic medical conditions: Examples from type 1 diabetes mellitus and epilepsy. *Psychol Schools, 45*, 52-62.

4 Transition to Adulthood

Kathleen J. Sawin, Ann W. Cox, and Stephanie G. Metzger

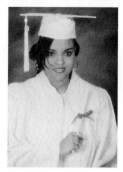

TRANSITION planning for adolescents with chronic conditions is a much more pressing issue for primary care providers than it has been in the past (American Academy of Pediatrics [AAP], 2002a). Although there have been substantial philosophic developments (AAP, 2002a, 2002b; Betz, 2000) and an expansion of resources (see Resources at the end of this chapter) for adolescents, their families, and primary health care providers, the challenges remain essentially unchanged. The life expectancy for youths with chronic conditions has dramatically increased in the last 20 years. Most data suggest that 90% of all children with chronic health conditions (CHCs) now live beyond age 20 years. Today more than 2 million young people between 10 and 18 years of age (i.e., 3.8% of our population) have some functional limitation caused by chronic and disabling conditions, which is a 100% increase since 1960 (Betz, 2000). Therefore, by the year 2000, more than 1 million young Americans with CHCs had transitioned to young adulthood.

An expanded civil rights movement has demanded equal life options for individuals with CHCs (Table 4-1). The most influential event in this movement has been the adoption of the Americans with Disabilities Act (ADA) of 1990. This act was designed to ensure that persons with disabilities have the same rights as those without disabilities: specifically, the right to a free public education and the right to have access to public transportation, clinics, restaurants, stores, and recreational facilities. The rights to live in the community and hold a job are hallmarks of the ADA. The thrust of the legislation was to "normalize" life for persons with a disability. Discrimination against those with disabilities from chronic conditions in school, health care, or community living is prohibited. These changes have made the concept of purposeful planned transition a priority for primary care providers.

Outcome data suggest that youths with CHCs are not making the transition to a full adult life in the areas of education, employment, development of meaningful relationships, and independent community living (Beresford, 2004; Lotstein, McPherson, Strickland, et al., 2005; National Council on Disability [NCD], 2008; Reid, Irvine, McCrindle, et al., 2004). More than 1 of 5 people with a CHC failed to complete high school (22%), compared with less than 1 of 10 people without a CHC (9%)—a gap of 13% (National Organization on Disability [NOD], 2000). Of those with CHCs who finished high school, the college graduation rates are less than one half. The number of students with CHCs who graduated from high school has increased since 1995 (Table 4-2), whereas the number who dropped out has decreased. However, data differ greatly by condition. Only 15% of those with visual impairments drop out whereas 30% of those with other health impairments and 55% of those with emotional disturbances dropped out. Conversely, 35% with emotional disturbances, 49% with other health impairments, and 69% with visual impairments graduated with a regular diploma. Those who did not graduate or drop out either aged out or received a certificate of completion. Clearly, progress has been made for some with CHCs more than others (U.S. Department of Education & Office of Special Education Programs, 2007).

Of all working-age people with CHCs (18 to 64 years), only approximately 3 out of 10 (32%) have full-time or part-time employment, compared with approximately 8 in 10 working-age people without CHCs (81%)—a gap of 49%. However, among those who are able to work despite their condition or health problem, 56% of people with CHCs are working, and the gap decreases to 25%. Native American youths with chronic conditions have an even more difficult time, with fewer than 30% employed or living independently. Of those unemployed with chronic conditions, 72% indicate that they would prefer to work. In addition, 40% of adults with CHCs have household incomes of $15,000 or less compared with only 16% of those without CHCs (NOD, 2000), and many young adults with CHCs do not live independently after high school. However, recent data suggest that progress has been made, especially for women, youths from higher socioeconomic settings, and those who had prevocational training and work experience (Ross & Nehring, 2007).

Youths with CHCs are also at greater risk for other compromising behavioral morbidities. For instance, there is a higher than average prevalence of depression and attempted suicide among this population, reflecting the social isolation experienced by many youths with CHCs (Keith, 2001). Substance abuse rates among these youths may be twice as high as those for the general population (Wolkstein, 2002), again with a disproportionate rate in minority communities. In addition, segregation, dependency, and nonproductivity occur for many of these young adults (Hollar, Weber, & Moore, 2002). These comorbidity outcomes make it more difficult to obtain an independent and fulfilling adult life.

Unsuccessful transition to adult life has become a concern to health professionals, educators, and community activists, and barriers to optimal transition have been identified. The ultimate goal of transition planning is to provide comprehensive health, education, and vocational services that are seamless, coordinated, developmentally appropriate, and psychosocially sound. Educators and health care providers, directed by the 1997 revision to the Individuals with Disabilities Education Act (IDEA), have begun to initiate transitional planning for youths with chronic conditions during middle school. Whether formal or informal, assessment and counseling interactions must focus on developing skills in adolescents that enhance competency, autonomy, and responsibility, which are all necessary to make transition successful (Blum, 2002). As with the concept of "discharge planning begins with admission," transition planning must begin early in childhood. Attainment of competency requires time for maturation and training and therefore must begin early and build over time. The primary care provider has a significant role to play in the purposeful endeavor of transition.

TABLE 4-1

Legislation Affecting the Transition to Adulthood for Youths with Chronic Conditions

Americans with Disabilities Act of 1990	Prohibits discrimination against persons with disability in employment, public accommodations, and public services
Rehabilitation Act—1992 and 1998, amendments of the 1973 Act	Strengthens the focus on employment for youths with disabilities, expanded eligibility criteria, and expanded customer choice
Section 504 of Rehabilitation Act	Prohibits discrimination for those with disabilities by any program or agency receiving federal funds; mandates equal opportunity to participate in or receive services from programs or activities and requires accommodations necessary to participate
Individuals with Disabilities Education Improvement Act (IDEA) amendments of 2004 (PL 108-446)	Redefined "transition services" to include a results-based process to address academic and functional achievement to facilitate movement to postschool activities.
School to Work Opportunities Act of 1994 with 1998 amendments (PL 103-239)	Support to build high school learning systems to prepare students for further education and careers
Title XIX of the Social Security Act, Medicaid amendments, Home- and Community-Based Services Waiver (PL 97-35), 1990	Provides funds to support community services that enhance community living options
Community Supported Living Arrangements (CSLA) (PL 101-508), 1990	Promotes development of statewide systems of individual supported living
Independence Plus Waiver (2002)	Allows greater control by persons with disabilities to manage personal assistant services
"Money Follows the Person" Rebalancing Initiative Deficit Reduction Act of 2005 (DRA)	Allows services to move with the person from institutional to community-based services
Real Choice Systems Change Grants for Community Living (an initiative of the Centers for Medicare and Medicaid)	State grants to revamp Medicaid state system to realign funding to support community living for people with disabilities
Supplemental Security Income (SSI) and Social Security Disability Insurance (SSDI)	Provides income benefits for youths (over 18 years of age) with substantial disabilities and low income; parental income is not considered; usually provides Medicaid benefits
Health Insurance Portability and Accountability Act (HIPAA) of 1996	Allows health care eligibility coverage to be portable from a previous plan to a new plan
Ticket to Work and Work Incentives Improvement Act of 1999	Provides incentives to states for workers with disabilities to purchase Medicaid to maintain employment
New Freedom Initiative 2001	Proposes to reduce barriers to full community integration for people with disabilities

TABLE 4-2

Numbers of Students with Disabilities Ages 14 to 21 Years Exiting School by Graduation with High School Diploma or Dropping Out 1995–2003

	1995–1996	1996–1997	1997–1998	1998–1999	1999–2000	2000–2001	2001–2002	2002–2003
High school diploma (regular)	42%	43%	46%	47%	47%	49%	51%	52%
Dropped out	47%	47%	44%	43%	42%	40%	37%	35%

Data from U.S. Department of Education & Office of Special Education Programs. (2007). 27th annual report to Congress on the implementation of the Individuals with Disabilities Education Act for year 2005, vol 1. Washington, DC: Author.

An emerging issue in primary care during transition and indeed throughout childhood for children and youths with chronic conditions (called "children with special health care needs" [CSHCN] by several federal initiatives) is the medical home initiative, "Every Child Deserves a Medical Home" (Kelly, Kratz, Bielski, et al., 2002) (see Chapter 9). The AAP (2002b) has issued a policy statement regarding medical homes, asserting that children with special health care needs should have accessible, continuous, comprehensive, family-centered, coordinated, compassionate, and culturally effective medical care delivered through a primary provider. Recent data would suggest that children with these services are more likely to have plans for transition and have discussed transition with their provider (Lotstein et al., 2005).

Adolescence and Emerging Adulthood: A Universal Time of Change

The central developmental task during adolescence is achieving a sense of personal identity based on adaptation to a new physical, cognitive, and social self. Youths with chronic conditions confront obstacles similar to those experienced by all adolescents living and growing up in our complex and pluralistic society, but they encounter additional challenges associated with the demands and restrictions of their conditions. Primary health care providers must be aware of both the typical and condition-based challenges encountered by youths with a CHC in order to effectively support their need for autonomy as they transition into adulthood.

All adolescents, including youths with CHCs, must meet the same fundamental requirements if they are to grow up to be healthy, constructive adults. In a seminal report, the Carnegie Council on Adolescent Development (1995, pp. 10-11) summarized these competencies as follows:

- Finding a valued place in a constructive group
- Learning how to form close, durable human relationships
- Feeling a sense of worth as a person
- Achieving a reliable basis for making informed choices
- Knowing how to use the available support systems
- Expressing constructive curiosity and exploratory behavior
- Finding ways of being useful to others
- Believing in a promising future with real opportunities

While striving toward these outcomes, youths experience an array of interconnected challenges that are related to the following:

1. The biologic changes of puberty that result in reproductive capacity and new social roles
2. The movement toward psychological and physical independence from parents
3. The search for friendship and belonging among peers

Today's youths are growing up in a climate marked by dramatic changes in American families; less time spent with adults; changing work expectations; earlier reproductive capacity but later marriage and financial independence; dominance of electronic media; and a more diverse, pluralistic society. The result is that a series of new morbidities plague adolescents: higher rates of suicide, depression, and reported abuse (Keith, 2001); earlier experimentation with drugs; earlier sexual activity (Alan Guttmacher Institute, 2002); inadequate learning (Wirt, Choy, Gerald, et al., 2002); and more health-damaging behaviors (Kann, Kinchen, Williams, et al., 2000). Today, younger adolescents exhibit many of the risky behaviors that were once associated with middle and late adolescence.

Youths with chronic conditions find that the integration of their chronic condition with their self-identity only reinforces a sense of being different at a time when sameness is desired. Further, the physiologic changes of maturation may influence the actual management of a chronic condition (e.g., diabetes, asthma), and social role expectations may be inconsistent with cognitive ability (e.g., with mental retardation). The challenges of puberty, autonomy, personal identity, sexuality, education, and vocational choices may all be influenced by physical or mental abilities, pain, medical setbacks, forced dependence, and perceived prognosis. Arnett (2004) proposes that the ages 18 to 25 years are actually an extended time of emerging adulthood. Evidence suggests that emerging adulthood is a distinct period with a focus on love and work. This period is characterized by identity explorations but is also called the age of instability; the self-focused age; or the age of feeling "in-between." Interviews indicate youths as hopeful even though uncertain, very optimistic even if their current situation is unsettled. During this time the individual accepts responsibility for himself or herself, makes independent decisions, and becomes financially independent. In addition, most live independently and many expand their education.

Several authors propose that adolescents with chronic conditions may lag behind their peers in these transition activities by several years. It is important to assess continued progress, even if, for some with chronic conditions, the transition is on a slightly different timetable than is typical for those without chronic conditions (Buran, Sawin, Brei, et al., 2004; Davis, Shurtleff, & Walker, 2006).

Key developmental parameters of early and mid-to-late adolescence and those of early or emerging adulthood are provided in Table 4-3, along with the associated implications of CHCs. These implications are generic in nature because specificities of conditions are addressed in subsequent chapters. The heterogeneity of youths with CHCs implies that primary providers must take the time to know the individual's and family's uniqueness.

Understanding Transition

Transition is a process—not an event (Meleis, Sawyer, Im, et al., 2000). Bridges (1994, p. 5) defines it as "the psychological process people go through to come to terms with the new situation. Change is external, transition is internal." For life changes to be described as transitional, they must involve both an internal shift (i.e., how people understand and feel about themselves and the world) and an external visibility of this change reflected in a reorganization of personal competence and roles or relationships with significant others.

Transitions can be classified as (1) developmental; (2) situational; (3) health or illness; and (4) organizational. The process and outcome of transition are powerful determinants of an enhanced sense of subjective well-being, role mastery, and the well-being of relationships, which enables the individual to function with increased confidence and skill in future challenges. Characteristics of transition identified were awareness (perception, knowledge, and recognition of the transition), engagement in the process, change, and difference (dealing with feelings of difference), happening over a time span, and often having critical points or events (i.e., moving out of the home) (Meleis et al., 2000).

Lenz (2001) discusses the use of this theory in adolescent transition, including the role of anticipatory guidance and planning in facilitating transition and the negative impact of ignoring the transition. Lenz also discussed the contribution of counseling and developmental frameworks in this specific transition. Developmental theory delineates the issues in adolescent transition, especially the questions about who adolescents will become, including family, employment, and careers. Counseling theory supports the role of the environment, the characteristics of the individual, the role change undertaken, the degree of stress involved in transition, and the need for all of these components to be addressed in counseling.

Adolescents with chronic conditions enter into developmental, health or illness, and potentially situational transitions. Primary care providers are in an excellent position to assess the factors associated with the quality of the transition experience and the factors that inhibit or facilitate transition and intervene with adolescents and families to optimize outcomes. To do this effectively, primary care providers need to understand the family and individual factors that can moderate the transitional process.

Family Factors Moderating Transition

The family is a constant factor in all transition endeavors working to prepare youths to consider options, set goals, develop the skills to work with service agencies and bureaucracies, find and use community support services, and solve problems to shape their lives and environments. Primary care providers have an opportunity to facilitate parent practices to facilitate independence in youths and reduce stress in the family.

The adolescent transitional years are stressful for all parents—but especially for those whose dependents have severe CHCs. Families with adolescents with CHCs indicate continued protectiveness and worry (Sawin, Brei, Buran, et al., 2002b). Parents of preadolescents whose life expectancies are uncertain or those who have intermittently unpredictable symptoms report greater family/social disruption, emotional strain, and financial burden than parents whose preadolescents with a chronic condition have a more certain future (Garwick, Patterson, Meschke, et al., 2002).

The transition to independent living may be delayed by several years for youths with severe CHCs or other special needs. In such situations, families must advocate for their adolescents to achieve supported living arrangements. Families with youths who have severe physical or intelligence limitations and who plan to remain

TABLE 4-3

Key Developmental Parameters and Associated Implications of Chronic Conditions

Typical Developmental Parameters	Chronic Condition/Disability Implications
EARLY ADOLESCENCE (GENERALLY AGE 11-14 YR)	
Rapid physical growth: Particularly sensitive to their changing bodies	Certain developmental and disease conditions can alter rate of physical growth. Primary providers need to address these with youths and their families. In some conditions sexual maturation is accelerated by several years.
Sexual maturation: Initiation of the biologic changes of puberty; new social roles reinforced	Anticipate interaction of sex hormones with other medication, and counsel accordingly. Education regarding emerging sexuality and consequences of resultant choices is essential.
Relationships: Shift from family to peer groups as a source of security and status; intense need to belong to a group, usually of the same gender	Social isolation is a critical issue. Encourage peer group activities at and away from home.
Cognitive: Generally remain in concrete operational thought	Teens are eager for information about their development and need accurate information about chronic conditions or disabilities, especially implications for sexuality and fertility.
Self-concept/self-esteem: Described in terms of physical features and likes; less tolerant of deviations from the "norm"	Respectfully deal with their many questions and concerns.
Health issues: Nutrition, acne, smoking, alcohol consumption; homicide from firearms has more than doubled in this age-group; increase in reported victims of child abuse and neglect	At risk for some health consequences. Reported to have higher risk for victimization because of the desire to "fit in."
Career awareness: Typically begin thinking about the future	Career awareness activities are often overlooked by youths with disabilities. Have high and realistic expectations, and communicate these.
MIDDLE AND LATE ADOLESCENCE AND EMERGING ADULTHOOD (AGE 15-25 YR)	
Physical growth: Continued physical growth but at a slower rate; strength and endurance increase	Physical activity may be limited by certain conditions or disabilities; alternative means of physical activity must be provided
Sexuality: Sexual maturation and/or experimentation heightened; sexual development typically completed by 16 yr of age; intimate sexual relationships develop	Information on risks associated with sexual activity is needed. Contraception is explored, and implications of interactions with other medications are provided. If sexual maturation is delayed, this must be addressed with adolescent.
Relationships: Achieving psychological independence from parents becomes particularly important; peer relationships become central; although family relationships are changing, they remain important	In many settings, because of age or physical development, appropriate social skills are expected. Even individuals who are developmentally or cognitively disabled must be taught appropriate public behavior.
Cognitive skills: Rapid growth and increasingly comprehend abstractions; movement into formal operation and abstract thinking	Youths vary in their ability to assume independent activities because of skills, cognition, or the complexity of the condition, but every effort should be made to foster choice in decisions related to health condition.
Self-concept/self-esteem: Increasing individuation with some diminishing or peer influence; self is defined by including interpersonal traits and abstract categories	Address strengths, and encourage positive self-concept.
Health issues: Experimentation with alcohol, cigarettes, and illicit drugs increases; unintentional injury, homicide, and suicide are leading causes of morbidity and mortality; exposure to or participation in violence may arise; females report higher incidence of depression than males	There are some particularly dangerous interactions between prescribed medications and other drugs and substances. Additional nutritional education is particularly relevant because youths with limited mobility can be overweight and experience resultant complications. Abuse and victimization are higher among youths with disabilities than nondisabled peers.
Career: Planning emphasizes examination of own interests, aptitude qualities, and occupational aptitudes	Emphasis should be on developing self-sufficiency skills, vocational and career decisions, and future planning. Active transition planning in health care, employment, and independent living must begin.

in the family home face increasing responsibility as school eligibility terminates and family members' daily care responsibilities increase. Often resources to employ other caregivers are limited in the community. These families need support and resource information to connect them with independent living centers and other community programs that offer alternative options and respite care. Families of youths who need continual supervision also must consider developing plans for custody and financial arrangements to ensure ongoing supervision when parents die or are unable to provide care. Medicaid-financed homes and daycare programs for adults with disabilities are scarce, so many parents must continue to care for their adult children at home. Advocates for people with intellectual disabilities have filed class action suits to require states to provide housing and daycare services to these families.

Extensive studies of parents and adolescents without CHCs confirm that authoritative parenting produces adolescents who achieve in school, have positive mental health, are more self-reliant, have higher self-esteem, and are less likely to participate in antisocial behavior, including delinquency and drugs. Authoritative parents are warm and involved and offer strong support to their

adolescents, but at the same time they are firm and consistent in establishing and enforcing guidelines, limits, and developmentally appropriate expectations. During adolescence they encourage and permit the adolescents to develop their own opinions and beliefs (Steinberg, 2000). Data support similar family characteristics supportive of youths with chronic conditions with family cohesion, warmth, satisfaction, and family activity related positively to outcome (Sawin, Buran, Brei, et al., 2002c). In addition, more positive parent-provider relationships are related to fuller discussion of transition issues in families (Scal & Ireland, 2005).

One difference in families of adolescents with CHCs may be the issue of overprotection. In a qualitative study exploring the experience of parenting an adolescent with spina bifida, parents of adolescents who had normal intelligence simultaneously reported an interest in supporting independence and a need to protect their adolescents (Sawin, Brei, Buran, et al., 2002b). Similarly, paradoxical findings support the crucial function of families in developing transition skills. Although some adolescents experience social isolation and their family essentially becomes their peer group, data also support the modeling of families. Adolescents who participate in more activities with their families are also more likely to participate in more activities with their friends and participate fully in society (Sawin, Buran, Brei, et al., 2003).

Participants in a study of "successful" young adults with CHCs reported several family themes associated with effective transitions. Families (1) treated them as typical children and adolescents; (2) expected them to participate fully in family responsibilities; (3) gave them no preferential treatment; (4) facilitated their participation in leisure activities; (5) focused on their strengths; (6) discussed their CHC with them; and (7) assisted them in accommodating challenges. These young adults valued family experiences and discussions that allowed them to develop skills, participate in risk taking, and cope with social rejection. These youths perceived that their family was a safe and nurturing environment where competence was developed.

Providers need to assess family knowledge and family behaviors that facilitate the development of competence. Primary care providers working with families of youths with chronic conditions should begin to talk to parents about strategies that foster effective transition into adulthood when the affected child is still young. Many parents of children with chronic or disabling conditions have difficulty letting go and encouraging independence and may see their children as vulnerable. Early discussions on the importance of fostering autonomous decision-making skills and independence in the activities of daily living may help parents realize the importance of assisting their child to build the necessary skills for a successful transition into adulthood.

Factors Moderating Individual Transition

Cognitive ability, personal philosophy of self-competence, ability to solve problems, degree of autonomy, and peer relationships are all factors that influence an adolescent's ease and success in the transition to adulthood.

Cognitive Ability. Cognition plays a major role in transition planning. Self-sufficiency assumes the intellectual abilities necessary to carry out the education, employment, and management of health care and community living. An adolescent's developmental abilities and age need to be considered in individual planning. If intellectual ability is moderately or significantly impaired, families or advocates must increase their participation in the planning and implementation of the transition plan. Many people with significant intellectual disabilities, however, can be competent, self-determined individuals. Achieving this goal may require individual skill building, alteration of the environment and interaction patterns, and use of available supports (Betz, 2007). Youths with intellectual disabilities must be afforded the basic rights that accompany the belief that all people are worthy of respect and dignity. Supportive employment has been shown to facilitate skill building and social outcomes in adolescents and young adults with CHCs (Betz, 2007).

At age 18 years all youths obtain the legal right to make decisions about life activities. When cognition is impaired, legal guardianship of a young adult should be considered and pursued by family members. Once the age of majority is reached, medical, school, and financial information, as well as consent to treatment, is not accessible to others without the youth's or guardian's permission. It is important to be clear about access to information and consent of the individual, family, school, primary care provider, and other agencies involved. Youths can determine access to

information unless a court finds otherwise. Issues of information sharing should be openly discussed with youths and their families; a plan should be created as youths near age 18 years.

Self-Competence. All transition programs are constructed on the assumption that youths are being educated to develop self-competence. Self-competence is thought to be a function of two domains: (1) skills or efficacy and (2) a sense of well-being (Ellison, Matuszewski, Phillips, et al., 2001) and comprises self-determination, self-advocacy, assertiveness, coping, and self-esteem. Activities, experiences, and programs should be designed to develop self-competence and each of its components (Betz, 2000).

Problem Solving and Autonomy. Studies of youths with chronic conditions have identified that problem solving and autonomy skills are related to positive health outcomes (Holmbeck, Johnson, Wills, et al., 2002; Sawin et al., 2002c). Interestingly, many youths with CHCs have limited experience making basic life decisions, much less decisions about health care (Buran et al., 2004; Sawin et al., 2002c). Knowledge about health care, knowledge of the specific chronic condition, and experience in making decisions are prerequisites for making decisions about health (see Chapter 2). By practicing decision making in other areas (e.g., what clothes to purchase, how to wear your hair, what to do with friends, how to budget money), youths will gain confidence through experience. Without these basic decision-making skills, choices related to health care are not possible. Because all problem solving is context based, experience is essential to solving potential health care dilemmas. Simple choices (e.g., whether to take medication with applesauce or gelatin) should be given as early as developmentally possible so that there is a gradual movement to making all choices about health care management.

Specific interventions to enhance autonomy through skill development have been developed over the last decade. Evaluations indicated that significant gains in knowledge and autonomy were achieved with these interactive approaches. One exemplar program is designed to systematically promote self-determination and functional competence by reducing learned helplessness and promoting motivation and self-efficacy expectations. This comprehensive program has components of skill development, the role of mentors, and peer and parental support. Qualitative and quantitative evaluations support the effectiveness of this program to promote self-efficacy, self-determination, and social adjustment (Ellison et al., 2001).

Additional data on the effectiveness of adolescent interventions can be expected in the near future from the Healthy and Ready to Work (HRTW) programs (see Resources at the end of this chapter). Another interesting program is Oregon's empowerment program (see Resources). In addition, a program funded by the National Institutes on Disability and Rehabilitation Research (NIDRR) at the University of Florida offers to provide new insights into the transition experience for those who traverse it. This program has both a research and a program arm (see Resources).

Attitudes, Beliefs, Perceptions, and Peer Relationships. An adolescent's attitudes, beliefs, and perceptions, such as hope, communication, self-efficacy, coping, and future expectations, can have a major impact on outcomes. Although problem solving and autonomy are critical skills necessary to develop self-management and independence, attitudes and beliefs have been found to be the strongest predictors of mental health measures, such as depression, behavior problems, and health-related quality of life. Indeed, in a study of adolescents with spina bifida, attitude was the strongest predictor of developmental competence and quality of life (r = .56 to .62) but was not a significant predictor of functional status or self-management outcomes. In contrast, decision-making skill and household responsibility had strong relationships (r = .42 to .61) with functional status and self-management but not with developmental competence and quality of life (Sawin, Bellin, Roux, et al., 2002a).

Establishing meaningful friendships with others is the hallmark of successful social interaction. Friendships are the basis for the social, emotional, and practical support needed to become truly integrated into society and are one measure of success in community integration. The social skills necessary for successful peer relationships are the ability to read both verbal and nonverbal cues from others, make judgments about those cues, and respond in a socially appropriate manner. Mastering these social skills can be hard for many individuals with learning disabilities or neurodevelopmental deficits. Social expectation for displays of affection, caring, anger, and frustration must be learned in adolescence if not acquired during childhood. Social immaturity, social isolation, restricted social lives, and lack of social skills may all be present in youths with chronic conditions (Murphy & Young, 2005). Transition plans must aggressively identify mechanisms for integrating youths with chronic conditions with their peers in educational, recreational, sports, and social activities. Adults who have made successful transitions report that peer and inclusion activities are fundamental to achieving independence.

Sexuality. Sexuality is a basic component of a full, adult life. Developing an identity as a sexual being is a universal developmental task of adolescents and young adults and should not be confused with sexual activity. Youths with chronic conditions are sexual beings with desires and interests similar to those of their unaffected peers, yet society often views and treats them as asexual. This can have disastrous consequences for youths (i.e., from being uneducated about sex and vulnerable to exploitation to feeling they have to prove their sexuality through risky behaviors) (Murphy & Young, 2005). Adolescents report having limited sources of sexuality information and wanting more sexuality information, both general information and condition-specific information (Sawin, Buran, Brei, et al., 2008). Like their peers, adolescent women with CHCs who experience pregnancy may be at increased risk to drop out of school because of pregnancy or childbearing issues.

For a successful transition, sexuality education should start with a focus on the physical changes of puberty integrated with alterations caused by the youth's condition (Murphy & Young, 2005; Sawin et al., 2008). Discussions over time should include abuse and pregnancy prevention, access to reproductive health care, and responsible sexual decision making. Youths, particularly females in this population, are at high risk for sexual and substance abuse (American Academy of Pediatrics, 2001; Nosek, Hughes, Taylor, et al., 2006). Early sexuality education is important for youths with chronic conditions because of their high risk for sexual abuse (Sawin & Horton, in press). Unfortunately, issues of sexuality for children and youths with chronic conditions are not routinely addressed by school programs, families, health care providers, or other transition team members (Murphy & Young, 2005; Sawin et al., 2008). Thus issues of sexuality can pose major threats to the transition plan if overlooked (Murphy & Young, 2005).

Condition-specific information is critical. For example, it is important for youths with spina bifida, who have a very high incidence of latex allergy, to avoid latex condoms. Likewise, women with spinal cord injuries may not be good candidates for oral contraceptives because of their high risk for deep vein thrombosis. Young women with epilepsy treated with select anticonvulsants have an increased risk of fetal anomalies if the type and dose of the medications are not altered before conception. It is also important to realize that seizure medication can interact with some oral contraceptives, decreasing their effectiveness (American Academy of Neurology, 1998). All young women of childbearing age should be taking a multivitamin with 0.4 mg of folic acid. Because women with spina bifida, epilepsy, and diabetes have an increased risk of bearing an infant with neural tube deficits, it is especially important for these women to take a multivitamin and have preconception counseling. However, in one survey 20% of adolescents in the highest risk category were unaware of this need (Sawin et al., 2002c).

Neurologic deficits (e.g., those from spinal cord injury, spina bifida, or muscular dystrophy and musculoskeletal limitations, such as those associated with severe juvenile rheumatoid arthritis or a high degree of spasticity) may limit some sexual positions or practices (Metzger, 2004). Alternative strategies for sexual gratification must be openly discussed.

Transition Planning for Health Care
Condition Self-Management

To begin the transition to adult health care, adolescents must have a basic understanding and awareness of their CHC. Each contact with the adolescent is an opportunity to assess self-care knowledge and to provide further education (AAP, American Academy of Family Practice [AAFP], & American College of Physicians–American Society of Internal Medicine [ACP-ASIM], 2002). The primary care provider must assist adolescents in developing age-appropriate self-care skills for health promotion and condition management, such as knowing their condition, medications, and management in detail and knowing how to use the health care system to address their needs (see Chapter 2). A wide range of educational materials in multiple formats and openness to exploring new ways to acquire the knowledge necessary to build self-management skills are essential. The Internet is a powerful source of information that can be used to encourage knowledge acquisition, as are condition-specific chat lines. Web TV is being used to provide health-related information on a variety of subjects. Adolescents and their parents must be cautioned about privacy and accuracy of information from the Internet and encouraged to discuss what they learn with health care providers. Agencies or organizations with a broad focus (e.g., the March of Dimes) can often be a source of program support for other educational materials. Condition-specific resources such as those found in endocrine, oncology, and transplantation literature are being developed as survival into adulthood is becoming normative (Ginsberg, Hobbie, Carlson, et al., 2006; Hanna, DiMeglio, & Fosretnberry, 2007; Stabile, Rosser, Porterfield, et al., 2005). Additional avenues for education include conferences sponsored by condition-specific agencies, camps, and mentoring by an adult with a similar CHC.

Developing self-care skills to manage CHCs must begin as early as developmentally feasible and be emphasized as the child approaches adolescence. Self-care skills include all activities of daily living, use of medical prostheses or equipment, administration of medication,

TABLE 4-4

Developmentally Based Skills Checklist

Health Promotion and Condition Management	Medications, Supplies, and Other Equipment	Health Care System
EARLY ADOLESCENCE (11-14 YR)		
Knows simple anatomy, physiology, and pathology	Knows names of medication taken, dose, reason, expected response	Knows the difference in kinds of health care providers (e.g., obstetrician vs. optometrist)
Able to tell health care provider what is wrong	Is aware of amount of regularly taken medication remaining in container and alerts parents or caregiver when low	Knows date of and reason for next health appointment
Discusses diagnosis and management plans with parents and providers	Understands the difference between illicit drugs and medications	Knows where primary care providers and specialists are located and how to contact them
Knows name(s), dates, and significance of any chronic illness and significant injuries	Takes medications for chronic condition correctly	
Can perform appropriate first aid	Knows use and care of equipment and supplies and can notify parents when problems occur	
Knows CPR		
Knows any allergies and can outline avoidance and emergency treatment actions		
Takes responsibility to monitor chronic condition and quickly notify parents of any new developments		
Manages aspects of chronic condition in predictable or common situations, accessing consultation for family or other resource people in unfamiliar situations		
If assistance with ADLs needed, can identify needs and preferences and knows the tasks to be carried out by others		
Has opportunity to develop decision making and has responsibilities at home		
Knows about basic money management (e.g., function of checking and saving accounts) and manages small personal resources		
MIDDLE ADOLESCENCE (15-17 YR)		
Knows date of last menstrual period (girls) and keeps record on personal or family calendar (i.e., may be early task for females with early-onset menses)	Calls pharmacy to reorder own medications or calls own provider about need for refill	Makes own health care appointments
Knows the basics of own health history, including family history	Knows the difference between generic and proprietary medication	Knows basic facts of own health insurance; knows limitations and issues for insurance in ordering supplies or medications and other equipment
Knows year of last tetanus shot	Selects own medications for minor illnesses (e.g., URI, headaches)	
Knows about TSE and BSE; performs regularly	Orders new supplies or equipment with supervision; can reorder these materials independently	
Manages chronic conditions in less predictable situations; seeks consultation when needed; requires minimal day-to-day supervision	Arranges for transportation to get medication supplies or for appointments	
Can plan ahead to anticipate problem areas and generate options		
If assistance with ADLs needed, knows care well enough to direct others in what he or she is unable to do		
Has increasing responsibility in family		
Has a savings or checking account and manages it with supervision from parents if needed		
LATE ADOLESCENCE AND EMERGING ADULTHOOD (18-25 YR)		
Manages stable chronic condition independently; uses parents or professionals to get advice regarding complex situations but makes management decisions	Independently manages medication, manages assessment and repair of any equipment, and pays for or arranges payment for medications and supplies	Understands the complexities of own health insurance plan
Participates in discussions regarding adult health care options		Understands effect of change in employment or school status on insurance options
Understands the connection among mind, body, and spirit in health and illness		Keeps updated file of own health records
Engages in healthy lifestyle activities; chooses healthful foods; exercises regularly; avoids caffeine, tobacco, illicit substances; gets adequate amount of sleep		Takes responsibility to initiate contact with providers when transition to new living or educational environment occurs
If assistance for ADLs needed, participates in the hiring, supervision, and termination of attendant caregiver		

Key: *ADLs*, activities of daily living; *BSE*, breast self-examination; *CPR*, cardiopulmonary resuscitation; *TSE*, testicular self-examination; *URI*, upper respiratory infection.

health promotion activities, prevention of secondary conditions, and how to access health care services. Table 4-4 provides a developmental checklist for acquisition of needed self-care skills.

In addition to the tables presented in this chapter, four other resources may be useful for transition:

1. The California Healthy and Ready to Work Project (Betz, 2000) has created the Developmental Guidelines for Teaching

Health Care Self-Care Skills to Children. These guidelines address self-care skill development by age category (infant, toddler, school-age child) and by participant (parent, child). The guidelines delineate for the health care provider competencies in three areas: knowledge of health condition and management, preventive health behaviors, and emergency measures.

2. The CHOICES project (AAP, 2002a; Betz, 2000) has also developed Transition Guidelines by age and focus area. The

guidelines identify expected outcomes and useful interventions in five areas: health promotion and disease prevention, health problem management, development and self-care, coping and stress, and family and community support.

3. The autonomy checklist (http://depts.washington.edu/healthtr/Checklists/home.htm) can be a useful tool for adolescent, family, and provider to evaluate the presence of important autonomy skills.
4. An outcome tool, the Adolescent Self-Management and Independence Scale (AMIS II) (Sawin et al., 2008) may be used by providers to evaluate outcomes of their intervention programs. This instrument measures outcomes in the area of self-management (i.e., condition knowledge, prevention activities, medication management) and independent living skills (i.e., ordering supplies, making appointments, household skills, arranging for community transportation, managing finances).

Close evaluation of the development of self-management skills is critical (Betz & Ayres, 2007). Familiarity with language and procedures may make young and middle adolescents with chronic conditions appear to be more knowledgeable or sophisticated than they really are. The gradual transfer of responsibility for complex self-care is optimal but can be overwhelming for young adolescents striving to assume total responsibility for managing their condition. Moreover, it can lead to poor condition outcomes. The driver's license model is a useful analogy for establishing self-care responsibility. That is, youths drive under supervision for a prolonged period and many parents often restrict them to familiar routes and provide them with a way of obtaining help in unexpected or complex situations. If youths are driving long distances or to unfamiliar territory, parents intervene by providing discussions on how to manage unforeseen occurrences. Even when an adolescent with a chronic condition masters a skill, occasional help or a holiday from selected responsibilities helps maintain the commitment necessary for care of a chronic condition. Stewart (2006) appraised five review articles related to transition and concluded that skill development, environmental support, and an individualized approach contribute to best practices for transition.

Adolescents unable to care for themselves need to develop the ability to supervise others caring for them. There is little in the literature, however, on how to teach adolescents or families to recruit, train, evaluate, and hold attendants or personal care providers accountable—critical skills for youths in transition who need assistance in activities of daily life. In addition, service animals may be a reasonable resource for youths who are not functionally independent. Several states currently have or are developing Medicaid waiver programs that will give adolescents and their families more control over issues such as attendant care (see Chapter 8). Such resources and an array of technologic resources must be explored when considering transition planning for adolescents who are not independent in activities of daily living (Nehring, 2007).

Health Care Maintenance

The development of a condition-specific health care maintenance plan for adults is an important part of transition planning. Open communication regarding key roles and responsibilities is essential (Geenen, Powers, & McVey, 2003). Key issues include nutrition, exercise, dental care, safety, injury prevention, substance abuse, and mental health. Although the goals are the same for all adolescents making the transition into adulthood, adaptations and accommodations must be made for individuals with intellectual impairments, impaired mobility, and altered physiologic states. For example, planning for the transition to an adult dental care provider needs to include discussions about issues of spasticity, latex allergy, and decreased cognition or behavioral difficulties if such exist.

Youths with chronic conditions are generally at greater risk for substance abuse and mental health issues, but a chronic condition is not a cause of psychiatric illness in either individuals or families. However, youths with chronic conditions and their families do have psychosocial and adaptive issues that can be severe. A person with a CHC has a higher risk of abusing alcohol and other drugs than a person without a CHC. Rates of abuse in persons with CHCs range from 15% to 30%, which is well above the national average (SARDI, 2002; Wolkstein, 2002). Most youths with CHCs take two or more prescription medications. The dangers of prescription drug abuse, selling prescription drugs, and mixing prescriptions with alcohol or other street drugs are often overlooked by the adolescent, parents, professionals, and friends. Even when adolescents ask about the possible interaction of their prescribed medication with recreational drugs, the answers are often not readily available. Initiating a no-nonsense discussion of the potential interactions of street and prescription drugs, as well as the legal consequences of illicit drug use, is often useful to adolescents. When referral is necessary, it must be made to a professional with training and compassion for the struggles and transition needs of youths with chronic or disabling conditions. The "dual diagnosis" must be addressed in any counseling program (Wolkstein, 2002).

Prevention of Secondary Disabilities

The prevention of secondary disabilities must be a major theme of each health care transition plan. This prevention is accomplished by the following: (1) aggressively addressing health maintenance and condition-specific primary prevention issues; (2) aggressively addressing condition-specific management issues; (3) facilitating the development of a philosophy of self-competence in the adolescent; and (4) identifying condition-specific, high-risk issues and developing a plan for early recognition of the need for treatment and specific management plans.

The Centers for Disease Control and Prevention (CDC) now sponsors the National Center for Chronic Disease Prevention and Health Promotion. The purpose of this center is to influence both the prevention of disability and the quality of life of those living with a CHC. The center, partnering with state health and education agencies, voluntary associations, private organizations, and other federal agencies, will be undertaking a number of initiatives to better understand the causes of these diseases, support programs to promote healthy behaviors, and monitor the health of the nation.

Access to Health Care as an Adult

The majority of adolescents with chronic conditions receive their health care in the pediatric primary care setting. It is the responsibility of the pediatric primary care provider to facilitate the transition from child-centered to adult-centered health care. This responsibility is identified and supported by both the AAP (1996, 2002a, 2002b) and the Society of Adolescent Medicine (Blum, Garell, Hodgman et al., 1993); and jointly by AAP, AAFP, and ACP-ASIM

(2002). The primary care provider often initiates and facilitates the transition for youths with chronic conditions by helping the adolescent and family to develop competency in condition self-management (i.e., including knowledge and self-care skills, health care maintenance, and prevention of secondary or associated conditions). Studies have demonstrated a host of barriers to effective transition to adult care (Reiss & Gibson, 2002; Reiss, Gibson, & Walker, 2005; Scal, 2002; Telfair, Alexander, Loosier, et al., 2004), including the following:

- Lack of adult care providers
- Different focus: the adult provider focuses on the medical condition of the adolescent rather than the broader social, developmental, and family focus of the pediatric providers
- Differing transition expectations and perception of program needs
- Limited experience of adult providers with managing conditions previously only thought to be chronic conditions of children
- Protectiveness of pediatric providers
- Bond between pediatric providers and families
- Not beginning early
- Focus of the teen on the here and now
- Structural issues (e.g., age limits to Title V programs; licensing and practice limitations; mission of facilities and charities, such as children's hospitals)
- Organizing, financing, and delivery of care

Health care providers need to initiate and coordinate referral to an adult-focused health care system. The AAP and other experts (National Association of Pediatric Nurse Practitioners, 2008; Reiss & Gibson, 2002) recommend that in "some cases" health care providers with skills in the health care needed by certain youths may provide care into adulthood. One of the barriers to an effective transition to adult care is the perception among many pediatric primary care providers that there is a lack of knowledgeable, sensitive providers in the adult health care system to care for adult survivors of congenitally acquired conditions (AAP, 2002a, 2002b; Scal, 2002). The focus must be on consulting adult specialists to enable them to address the needs of young adults with chronic conditions—not on keeping these individuals in the pediatric health care system (AAP, AAFP, & ACP-ASIM, 2002). Further, research is critically needed that evaluates both specific services/service models and long-term outcomes of young people as they move into adulthood (Beresford, 2004).

Health Insurance Issues

The quality and amount of health care available to transitioning adolescents may be adversely affected by insurance limitations and a lack of coordinated case management. Insurance coverage becomes an issue as youths transition into adulthood and are no longer covered by their parents' insurance or federal and state programs established for care of children. Youths with CHCs over age 18 or 19 often lose health insurance (White, 2002). Once a young adult leaves school, parental insurance is usually terminated. The cutoff age for students still in school varies by policy, but almost no coverage exceeds age 25 years. Youths in college can access the student health center for primary care but may need to have

another source of inpatient coverage. Most medical plans for college students, however, have a preexisting condition clause that may eliminate eligibility.

Youths can opt to continue parental insurance through the Consolidated Omnibus Budget Reconciliation Act of 1986 (COBRA insurance program). This program allows youths to retain parental insurance with the same coverage for 18 months, but the cost is high and extended benefits must be applied for within 60 days of loss of group coverage. The Health Insurance Portability and Accountability Act of 1996 (HIPAA) provisions allow eligibility coverage to be portable from a previous plan to a new plan, thus avoiding the preexisting conditions clause. Youths in some states can join a high-risk insurance plan supplemented by the state, but this option is also costly and usually has no sliding scale for income. Options for individuals to buy into a Medicaid plan on a sliding-fee scale have received federal approval and are now state options (AAP, 2002a). The Ticket to Work and Work Incentives Improvement Act of 1999 includes incentives to states to allow workers with CHCs to purchase Medicaid to maintain employment, as well as an option to workers to maintain Medicare coverage. Families and health care providers must advocate for innovative state insurance options that would support optimal transition outcomes and ensure continued health care.

Further complicating the loss of personal insurance is the termination at a specific age of supplemental benefits available in most states through block grant programs (e.g., Title V programs) for children with special health care needs. Federal block grants give states financial resources to provide specialty clinical services, care coordination, and supplemental fiscal support for families with children with special health care needs (see Chapters 1, 8, and 9). These programs were created as a health care safety net for at-risk children and families and cease at age 21. Eligible youths may apply for Supplemental Security Income (SSI) or Social Security Disability Insurance (SSDI), which come with automatic Medicaid benefits in many states. Employment, however, may result in loss of eligibility and termination of financial and medical benefits (see Chapter 8). Youths with CHCs will automatically lose SSI benefits when they turn 18 years old unless they are redetermined to be eligible under the adult SSI criteria. This must occur during the month preceding their eighteenth birthday. Thus youths in transition may lose the medical support available from the state and not be able to access any other type of insurance. If insurance is available to youths in transition, the benefits may be severely restricted, especially for therapies important to youths with mobility, communicative, or psychological challenges. If services are provided, they are often limited in amount and duration, which is a problem that may be accentuated if an individual's coverage includes only limited resources and restricted referral options. If these youths are to become independent members of society, new policies and solutions for health insurance need to be developed to address these important insurance issues for youths with CHCs (White, 2002).

Transition Planning in the School System

Although the focus of transition planning in the health care system is accessing adult health care services, the focus in the school system is preparing individuals for life in the community and meaningful employment (see Chapter 3). The Individuals with Disabilities Education Improvement Act (IDEA) is the only federal legislation that requires a planning process to enable students with CHC to achieve a smooth, gradual, and planned transition to community life. Transition provisions were first set forth in the 1990 reauthorization of IDEA that required schools to develop individualized transition plans (ITPs) for students with CHCs who are 16 years old. IDEA (2004) (1) simplified the rules for transition services by requiring that transition services and planning begin at age 16; and (2) strengthened the involvement of the vocational rehabilitation system with students while still in secondary school. The 2004 legislation and subsequent regulations of 2006 define *transition services* as

> *a coordinated set of activities for a child with a disability that (a) is designed to be within a results oriented process, that is focused on improving the academic and functional achievement of the child with a disability to facilitate the child's movement from school to post-school activities, including postsecondary education, vocational education, integrated employment (including supported employment), continuing and adult education, adult services, independent living, or community participation; (b) is based on the individual child's needs, taking into account the child's strengths, preferences, and interests; and (c) includes instruction, related services, community experiences, development of employment and other post-school adult living objectives, and if appropriate, acquisition of daily living skills and provisions of a functional vocational evaluation. (34 CFR 300.43[a]) (20 U.S.C. 1401[34])*

This expanded definition redefines transition services to focus not on just the academic achievement of a student but also the youth's functional development. Further, it facilitates transition to postsecondary activities by focusing exit evaluations on recommendations to assist youths in meeting postsecondary goals, and providing students with a summary of their academic achievement to present to employers or postsecondary schools.

The National Secondary Transition Technical Assistance Center (NSTTAC) is a center funded by the U.S. Department of Education's Office of Special Education Programs through 2010. Among other purposes, this center is identifying research-based transition practices to enhance states' capacity to improve transition outcomes for students with disabilities.

Students with chronic or disabling conditions who are not eligible for special education and therefore do not have an individualized education plan (IEP) can and should receive transition services under Section 504 of the Rehabilitation Act. Students with CHCs (e.g., diabetes, asthma) often have transition services addressed in their individual health service programs (IHPs). Neither 504 plans nor IHPs have legal mandates for transition planning, even though it is a recommended practice (U.S. Department of Health and Human Services, 2000). Primary care providers may need to advocate for appropriate school-based services for youths who do not have a legal mandate for transition planning in the school.

School nurses and other related service providers in schools have unique opportunities to support high school students through an impending developmental transition and address quality-of-life issues, as well as disease management issues (Lenz, 2001), yet these professionals may not be participating in transition services to their fullest potential (Kardos & White, 2005) or may be underusing them. Primary care providers often find that requesting the

involvement of the school nurse in all IEP, IHP, or 504 processes facilitates communication among the family, school, and primary care practice (Betz & Nehring, 2007). Primary care providers, especially those who have embraced the medical home initiative for children with special health care needs, often participate in the IEP, especially if attendance can be by phone or held in the provider's office (AAP, 2002a). Educational transition teams often overlook the health care issues that must be addressed for successful planning. If health care issues are not adequately addressed, a successful transition into postsecondary education or full-time employment, community living, and self-sufficiency will be jeopardized.

Postsecondary Education

The statistical profile of college students with CHCs and disabilities reveals that in the 2003–2004 school year, 11.3% of undergraduate students attending postsecondary educational institutions self-reported disabilities (U.S. Department of Education, National Center for Education Statistics, 2006). More than half of all undergraduates with self-reported disabilities are students with hidden disabilities (i.e., learning, mental health, etc.). Many are significantly concerned about financing their college education, often receiving financial aid from vocational rehabilitation funds. Many used special support programs offered at colleges and reported having been influenced by a role model or mentor to go to college.

Plans for a transition from high school to college should be reflected in an IEP, IHP, or 504 accommodation plan. Certain collegiate schools around the United States are especially noted as having strong support programs for those with chronic conditions. Youths—especially those with severe physical CHCs—may find the extensive educational, health, recreational, and social support services of these universities helpful. Almost all colleges and universities have an office of disabled student services. Contacting this office before applying to determine available services is often useful. Some students are unwilling to identify themselves as having a CHC because of the stigma associated with differences in our society. Students should be encouraged to use all services available to them to enhance their potential for success.

As with other college students, financial considerations are important. Early consultation in high school with the Division of Vocational Rehabilitation Services can determine if a student is eligible for any educational or support services. Services vary across states, and early consultation is important because staff in all agencies have a heavy caseload. Youths and their parents must be clear about what services are available and then vigorously pursue them.

A major source of information about postsecondary education is the HEATH Resource Center (see Resources) located at George Washington University. HEATH is the national clearinghouse on postsecondary education for individuals with disabilities. Support from the U.S. Department of Education enables the center to serve as a resource for exchange of information about educational support services, policies, procedures, adaptations, and opportunities at American campuses, vocational-technical schools, and other postsecondary training entities. In operation since 1984, HEATH offers a multitude of resource papers, monographs, guides, and directories focusing on a broad range of disability-related topics, such as accessibility, career development, classroom and

---

BOX 4-1

Useful Questions in Assessing a Postsecondary Education Environment

WHAT ARE THE MEDICAL AND HEALTH NEEDS OF THIS YOUNG ADULT?
- Will a plan for health care transition need to be developed?
- What factors would be included in the health component of the transition plan?
- When should the health transition process be initiated?

HOW WILL THE CHRONIC HEALTH CONDITION AFFECT THIS INDIVIDUAL?
- How does the chronic health condition affect this youth's educational process?
- How does the chronic health condition affect this individual's living environment?
- How does the chronic health condition affect activities of daily living?

DISCLOSURE
- Should the individual disclose the chronic health condition when applying to colleges or other postsecondary training institutions? To whom? When?
- What laws are in place to protect the rights of people with disabilities? How do they relate to young adults with chronic illness?

ACCOMMODATIONS
- What educational or environmental accommodations or modifications will need to be in place to increase independence?
- What accommodations are postsecondary educational institutions required by law to provide?
- If this individual needs additional accommodations or modifications, who will pay for them?
- How can this individual assess the ability of the postsecondary institution and the surrounding community in meeting his or her needs?

LOCATING RESOURCES
- When should financial, medical, and support service resources begin?
- Who can assist at the postsecondary site?
- Whose responsibility is it?

From Edelman, A. (1995). Maximizing success: Transition planning for education after high school for young adults with chronic illness. Information from *HEATH 15*(1), 3. Reprinted with permission.

laboratory adaptations, financial aid, independent living, transition resources, training and postsecondary education, vocational education, and rehabilitation. Providers should encourage youths and their families to access this information via the public library or Internet early in the planning process. At a minimum, youths and families need to ask basic questions about a school. Box 4-1 outlines useful questions proposed by HEATH.

Some universities have preenrollment programs for students with severe CHCs, especially those who will need attendant care. The focus of the health providers in these situations is evaluation of the attendant care needs of the student, as well as—and more importantly—the student's independent ability to teach others to provide the necessary care. Each student must determine if health care should be transferred from his or her home community to either the college health care center or a local specialty provider or if the community provider should be maintained. Access to emergency health care must always be evaluated, and youths should have a copy of all critical health care records with them if they are far from their usual sources of health care.

Vocational Training and the Transition to Work

The 1992 and 1998 Amendments to the Rehabilitation Act of 1973 (PL 102-569) strengthened the role of vocational rehabilitation to work collaboratively with special education in preparing youths for transition into adult life while they are in school. Having already initiated the independent living movement with the 1986 amendments, the Rehabilitation Act of 1992 addressed the needs of youths and young adults for personal assistant services, supported employment opportunities, and a broad range of assistive technology. The 1998 amendments reinforce that employment is the intended outcome of vocational rehabilitation services. Two of the characteristics identified as important in the transition process were preparation and knowledge (Meleis et al., 2000). Most high school students identified as having a disability intend to enter the workforce on leaving school but face many employment barriers. Youths who were in special education from low-income households had poorer postschool outcomes. Those who had sensory or motor disabilities benefited the most from special education, and concentrated vocational education (i.e., several courses focusing on a specific area)—as opposed to one course from a variety of concentrations—yielded higher employment and income rates. Even with vocational courses, however, outcomes for employment were still low compared with those of youths not in special education.

The major resource for youths making the transition to work is the vocational rehabilitation service in their state. The changes in the Rehabilitation Act in 1992 and 1998 strengthened the focus on employment and changed the criteria for service. The only criterion is that the adolescent would benefit from employment, and the definition of employment has been broadened to include supported employment. The act also provides technologic resources and personal assistance services if necessary to provide assistance in activities of daily living on or off the job. Even with these resources, however, the transition to work is often problematic, which is due, in part, to numerous work disincentives (National Council on Disability [NCD], 2008). Early referral to vocational support services and conveying the expectation that work, in some form, is an expected outcome must be the focuses of the home, school, and health care communities. The NCD (2008) recommends that the Federal Partners Workgroup expand its role and develop plans for bringing the resources of each member agency to bear more effectively in addressing and solving the problems that hinder seamless transition from school to work or to adult services for youths with CHCs.

A supportive workplace is a critical factor for transition-age youths. Butterworth, Hagner, Helm, and colleagues (2000) found that multiple-context relationships, specific social supports, a personal and team-building management style, and interdependent job designs individually and collectively made for a supportive workplace. Providers may need to guide youths and their families to successful first-workplace experiences. However, this time of change may also result in vulnerability and risks that affect health.

Transitioning from Home to Community Living

The transition to independent living is difficult for many youths and young adults with cognitive, physical, and emotional disabilities to achieve because necessary support systems are not readily available. Youths with chronic unstable health conditions find this transition particularly difficult if they have not developed the skills necessary to manage their conditions and solve problems associated with their condition and limited functional capacity.

Several legislative initiatives have given communities the impetus to develop supports for young adults who want to study, work, and live as independently as possible in the community. These initiatives include the Americans with Disabilities Act (ADA) of 1990 (PL 101-336), the 1992 and 1998 Amendments to the Rehabilitation Act of 1973 (PL 102-569), the New Freedom Initiative launched in February 2001, and the Individuals with Disabilities Education Improvement Act (IDEA) of 2004. The latter was created to reduce barriers to full community integration for people with CHCs. These programs are often underfunded, however, and there are often insufficient resources available in the community to meet the needs of youths and adults with CHCs who seek independence.

Several amendments to the Medicaid program have provided funding mechanisms to support community living for young adults with CHCs (see Chapter 8). The Home and Community Based Services (HCBS) waiver, which was first enacted in 1982, has gained momentum and is rapidly replacing Title XX as the major source of federal funding for community services (White, 2002). Although originally intended to support the movement of individuals from institutional care to residential care, this program now finances case management, homemakers, home health aides, personal care, residential habilitation, day habilitation, respite care, transportation, supported employment, adapted equipment, and home modification. The Community Supported Living Arrangements (CSLA) amendment of 1990 promotes the development of statewide systems of individualized supported living. This program provides person-centered planning processes and provides individuals with the support needed to enable them to live in their own homes, apartments, or family homes. The Ticket to Work and Work Incentives Improvement Act of 1999 allows states to create Medicaid buy-in programs to ensure health coverage for the working disabled. The Independence Plus Waiver of 2002 encourages greater control by persons with disabilities to manage personal assistant services. And, finally, the "Money follows the Person" Rebalancing Initiative allows funding for services to move with the person from institutions to communities. The support services available through these programs are critical for many youths and young adults with disabling conditions making a transition to the community.

If young adults with CHCs are to be successful living independently, they must have the social skills—including the skills necessary to make appropriate decisions about their health and activities of daily living—as well as the technical skills or assistance to actually meet their daily needs for physical care, communication, and transportation. Most youths with chronic conditions and those with mild degrees of disability negotiate the road to community living much like youths without disabilities. Youths with moderate to severe degrees of functional disability will have more difficulty.

Learning to be as independent as possible with activities of daily living does not mean doing things without help or modification. On the contrary, distinguishing between when and how much assistance is needed is indicative of mature decision making for many young persons with CHCs. Ideally, the development of self-help skills that began at home and continued throughout school was geared toward the ultimate goal of independent living. These skills include personal hygiene; domestic skills; transportation; safety; financial management, including banking, purchasing, and spending; and seeking and developing meaningful leisure activities.

Coordination of Transition Planning

Families report not only frustrations with obtaining a coordinated transition plan but also confusion about where to turn for assistance. Care coordination across all the systems, family, education, employment, community, and health care, is complex, and communication among providers, transition team members, and the family is essential for transition into adulthood (see Chapter 9). Families are often the leaders in the transition process, but the primary care provider may facilitate both the process and communication across systems. When an individual's health problems are significant, the primary care provider may need to assume a leadership role in the transition process. To facilitate the plan, the primary care provider must know the needs of the adolescent and family; the agencies and team members involved; and the family, school, community, and health care resources available. The AAP (2001, 2002a, 2002b) has developed several position statements addressing youths with special health care needs and transition issues.

When the family is articulate and knowledgeable and can access resources, the primary care provider may only need to coordinate health information and referrals to community health agencies. Primary care providers may provide health information on a regular basis for school transition team conferences, as well as for community experiences such as "camperships" and athletic teams, and also serve as consultants. If there is a significant health component to the transition plan, the primary care provider may actually be the case manager or can be the team leader while a specialty provider is the case manager. To achieve a smooth transition to adult health care, all transition team members need to have similar goals.

As adulthood approaches, primary care providers must encourage youths and their families to address future planning for education, health care, employment, and community living options with referrals to appropriate resources. In preparation for adulthood, the primary health care provider has an obligation to do the following: (1) educate and inform adolescents of their conditions, including future expectations and preventive health care; (2) encourage parents to adopt parenting styles that support the transition to independent adulthood; (3) recognize and plan for opportunities to support young adults' autonomous decision making regarding health care, building on the strengths of the individual; (4) convey a positive attitude about the potential of young adults and provide information to agencies or people who can help them reach their full potential; (5) be knowledgeable about the evolving community system of supports and legal mandates for services; (6) help individuals access appropriate health care services and function as a consultant to adult providers when necessary; (7) advocate at the legislative level for insurance coverage and community services to enable individuals to live as full and healthy adult lives as possible; (8) advocate for appropriate and comprehensive transition services that integrate systems of care and educational, health, community, and family resources; and (9) provide genetic and family planning information and resources.

Resources

DisabilityInfo.gov.
The *New Freedom Initiative's* online resource for Americans with disabilities.
Website: www.disabilityinfo.gov/digov-public/public/Display-Page.do?parentFolderId=500

Organizations

ABLEDATA
A database of products.
Website: www.abledata.com

Adolescent Health Transition Project
Provides checklists for ongoing assessment of independence skills.
Website: http://depts.washington.edu/healthtr/

Alliance for Technology Access
Provides access to technology for people with disabilities.
Website: www.ataccess.org

HEATH Resource Center of The George Washington University, Graduate School of Education and Human Development
An online clearinghouse on postsecondary education for individuals with disabilities.
Website: www.heath.gwu.edu

Maternal Child Health Bureau (MCHB) Healthy and Ready to Work Program
Policy briefs, national demonstration projects, and useful tools. A variety of activities by state.
Website: www.hrtw.org

National Center for Chronic Disease Prevention and Health Promotion
Promotes preventions and quality of life for children with special health care needs.
Website: www.cdc.gov/nccdphp

National Center on Secondary Education and Transition (NCSET)
Website: www.ncset.org

National Council on Disability
Website: www.ncd.gov

National Information Center for Children and Youth with Disabilities (NICHCY)
Provides information in English and Spanish.
Website: www.nichcy.org

National Organization on DisABILITY
Website: www.nod.org

National Organization for Rare Diseases
Websites: www.rarediseases.org; www.ucp.org

National Secondary Transition Technical Assistance Center (NSTTAC)
Website: www.nsttac.org

Parent Training and Information Centers (PTI), Technical Assistance to Parents Program (TAPP)
Includes Parenting Educational Advocacy Training Center. Provides links to almost every disability organization.
Website: www.peatc.org

SARDI (Substance Abuse Resources and Disability Issues)
Website: www.med.wright.edu/citar/sardi

TASH
An international advocacy association.
Website: www.tash.org

The Transition Center: A resource for family members.
Website: www.thetransitioncenter.org/flash/index.htm

University Centers for Excellence in Developmental Disabilities Education, Research, and Service (UCEDD)
Located at major universities and teaching hospitals
Website: www.aucd.org

Youth Empowerment Program –University of Oregon
Website: www.omhrc.gov/templates/content.aspx?ID=4879

Lay Resources for Teens and Families

Kaufman, M. (1995). *Easy for You to Say: Questions and Answers for Teens Living with Chronic Illness or Disability.* Toronto: Key Porter Books.

Kriegsman, K.H., Zaslow, E.L., & D'Zmura-Rechsteiner, M.A. (1992). *Taking Charge: Teenagers Talk about Life and Physical Disability.* Bethesda, MD: Woodbine House.

REFERENCES

Alan Guttmacher Institute (2002). *Sexuality Education.* New York: Author.

American Academy of Neurology (1998). Practice parameter: Management issues for women with epilepsy. *Neurology, 51,* 944-948.

American Academy of Pediatrics (2001). Sexuality education for children and adolescents. *Pediatrics, 108,* 498-502.

American Academy of Pediatrics (2002a). *Every Child Deserves a Medical Home: Component Five—Transitioning Children and Youth to Adulthood.* Elk Grove Village, IL: Author.

American Academy of Pediatrics (2002b). The medical home. *Pediatrics, 110*(1), 184-186.

American Academy of Pediatrics, American Academy of Family Practice, & American College of Physicians–American Society of Internal Medicine. (2002). A consensus statement on health care transitions for young adults with special health care needs. *Pediatrics, 100*(Suppl 6), 1304-1306.

American Academy of Pediatrics, Committee on Children with Disabilities and Committee on Adolescence (1996). Transition of care provided for adolescents with special health care needs. *Pediatrics, 98*(6), 1203-1206.

Arnett, J.J. (2004). *Emerging Adulthood: The Winding Road from the Late Teens Through the Twenties.* New York: Oxford University Press.

Beresford, B. (2004). On the road to nowhere? Young disabled people and transition. *Child Care Health Dev, 30*(6), 581-587.

Betz, C.L. (2000). California healthy and ready to work transition health care guide. *Issues Compr Pediatr Nurs, 23,* 203-244.

Betz, C.L. (2007). Facilitating the transition of adolescents with developmental disabilities: Nursing practice issues and care. *J Pediatr Nurs, 22*(2), 103-115.

Betz, C.L., & Ayres, L. (2007). Promoting health care self-care and long-term disability management. C.L. Betz & W.M. Nehring (Eds.), *Promoting Health Care Transitions for Adolescents with Special Health Care Needs and Disabilities.* Baltimore: Paul H. Brookes.

Betz, C.L., & Nehring, W.M. (2007). Integrating health-related needs into individualized education programs and 504 plans.In C.L. Betz & W.M. Nehring (Eds.), *Promoting Health Care Transitions for Adolescents with Special Health Care Needs and Disabilities,* Baltimore: Paul H. Brookes.

Blum, R.W. (Ed.). (2002). Improving transition for adolescents with special health care needs from pediatric to adult-centered health care. *Pediatrics, 100*(Suppl 3), 1301-1335.

Blum, R.W., Garell, D., Hodgman, C.H., Jorissen, T.W., Okinow, N.A., et al. (1993). Transitions from child-centered to adult-care systems for adolescents with chronic conditions: A position paper of the Society of Adolescent Medicine. *J Adolesc Health, 14*(7), 570-576.

Bridges, W. (1994). *Transitions—Making Sense of Life's Changes.* Reading, MA: Addison-Wesley.

Buran, C.F., Sawin, K.J., Brei, T.J., et al. (2004). Adolescents with myelomeningocele: Their activities, beliefs, expectations, and perceptions. *Dev Med Child Neurol, 46,* 244-252.

Butterworth, J., Hagner, D., Helm, D., et al. (2000). Workplace culture, social interactions, and supports for transition-age young adults. *Ment Retard, 38*(4), 342-353.

Carnegie Council on Adolescent Development. (1995). *Great Transitions: Preparing Adolescents for a New Century.* New York: Carnegie Council of New York.

Davis, B.E., Shurtleff, D.B., & Walker, W.O. (2006). Acquisition of autonomy skills in adolescents with myelomeningocele. *Dev Med Child Neurol, 48*(4), 253-258.

Edelman, A. (1995). Maximizing success: Transition planning for education after high school for young adults with chronic illnesses. *HEATH, 15*(1), 3.

Ellison, R., Matuszewski, J., Phillips, A., et al. (2001). A multi-component intervention to promote adolescent self-determination (Take Charge Field Test). *J Rehabil, 67*(4), 13-19.

Garwick, A.W., Patterson, J.M., Meschke, L.L., et al. (2002). The uncertainty of preadolescents' chronic health conditions and family distress. *J Fam Nurs, 8*(1), 11-31.

Geenen, S., Powers, L., & McVey, C.W. (2003). Understanding the role of health care providers during the transition of adolescents with disabilities and special health care needs. *J Adolesc Health, 32*(3), 225-233.

Ginsberg, J.P., Hobbie, W.L., Carlson, C.A., et al. (2006). Delivering long-term follow-up care to pediatric cancer survivors: Transitional care issues. *Pediatr Blood Cancer, 46*(2), 169-173.

Hanna, K.M., DiMeglio, L.A., & Fosretnberry, J.D. (2007). Brief report: Initial testing of scales measuring parent and adolescent perceptions of adolescents' assumption of diabetes management. *J Pediatr Psychol, 32*(3), 245-249.

Hollar, D., Weber, J., & Moore, D. (2002). Educational and employment outcomes for youth with disabilities who use alcohol and drugs: Analysis of NELS:88 longitudinal data. *Drug Alcohol Depend, 66*, S81.

Holmbeck, G.N., Johnson, S.Z., Wills, K.E., et al. (2002). Observed and perceived parental overprotection in relation to psychosocial adjustment in preadolescents with a physical disability: The mediational role of behavioral autonomy. *J Consult Clin Psychol, 70*(1), 96-110.

Individuals with Disabilities Education Improvement Act of 2004, PL 108-446, *20* U.S.C. §§1400 et seq Washington, DC: US. Government printing office.

Kann, L., Kinchen, S.A., Williams, B.I., et al. (2000). Youth risk behavior surveillance—United States, 1999. MMWR. CDC surveillance summaries. *MMWR Morb Mortal Wkly Rep. CDC Surveillance Summaries, 49*(5), 1-2.

Kardos, M., & White, B.P. (2005). The role of the school-based occupational therapist in secondary education transition planning: A pilot survey study. *Am J Occup Ther, 59*(2), 173-180.

Keith, C. (2001). Suicide in teenagers: Assessment, management and prevention. *J Am Med Assoc, 286*, 3120-3125.

Kelly, A.M., Kratz, B., Bielski, M., et al. (2002). Implementing transitions for youth with complex chronic conditions using the medical home model. *Pediatrics, 110*(6, Suppl), 1322-1327.

Lenz, B. (2001). The transition from adolescence to young adulthood: A theoretical perspective. *J School Nurs, 17*(6), 300-306.

Lotstein, D.S., McPherson, M., Strickland, B., et al. (2005). Transition planning for youth with special health care needs: Results from the National Survey of Children with Special Health Care Needs. *Pediatrics, 115*(6), 1562-1568.

Meleis, A., Sawyer, L., Im, E., et al. (2000). Experiencing transitions: An emerging middle-range theory. *ANS Adv Nurs Sci, 23*(1), 12-28.

Metzger, S.G. (2004). Individual with disabilities. In E. Youngkin et al. (Eds.), *Pharmacotherapeutics: A Primary Care Clinical Guide* (2nd ed.). Upper Saddle River, NJ: Pearson/Prentice Hall.

Murphy, N., & Young, P.C. (2005). Sexuality in children and adolescents with disabilities. *Dev Med Child Neurol, 47*(9), 640-644.

National Association of Pediatric Nurse Practitioners (2008). Position statement on age parameters for pediatric nurse practitioner practice. *J Pediatr Healthcare, 22*, e1-e2.

National Council on Disability. (2008). *National disability policy: A progress report.* Available at www.ncd.gov/newsroom/publications/2008/National DisabilityPolicy:AProgressReport.html. Retrieved January 17, 2008.

National Organization on Disability. (2000). *The 2000 N.O.D./Harris Survey of Americans with Disabilities.* Washington, DC: Author. Available at www. NOD.org.

Nehring, W.M. (2007). Accommodations for school and work. In C.L. Betz & W.M. Nehring (Eds.), *Promoting Health Care Transitions for Adolescents with Special Health Care Needs and Disabilities.* Baltimore: Paul H. Brookes.

Nosek, M.A., Hughes, R.B., Taylor, H.B., et al. (2006). Disability, psychosocial, and demographic characteristics of abused women with physical disabilities. *Violence Against Women, 12*(9), 838-850.

Reid, G.J., Irvine, M.J., McCrindle, B.W., et al. (2004). Prevalence and correlates of successful transfer from pediatric to adult health care among a cohort of young adults with complex congenital heart defects. *Pediatrics, 113*(3 pt 1), e197-e205.

Reiss, J., & Gibson, R. (2002). Health care transition: Destinations unknown. *Pediatrics, 111*(Suppl 6), 1307-1314.

Reiss, J.G., Gibson, R.W., & Walker, L.R. (2005). Health care transition: Youth, family, and provider perspectives. *Pediatrics, 115*(1), 112-120.

Ross, R., & Nehring, W.E. (2007). Working with job developers and employers. In. C.L. Betz & W.E. Nehring (Eds.), *Promoting Health Care Transitions for Adolescents with Special Health Care Needs and Disabilities.* Baltimore: Paul H. Brookes.

SARDI: (2002, October/November). Substance abuse and students with a disability *HEATH,* 5-6.

Sawin, K.J., Bellin, M., Roux, G., et al. (2002a). *The experience of parenting an adolescent with spina bifida: Trying to decide where to cut the umbilical cord and how much.* Unpublished manuscript. Virginia Commonwealth University.

Sawin, K.J., Brei, T.J., Buran, C.F., et al. (2002b). Factors associated with quality of life in adolescents with spina bifida. *J Holistic Nurs, 20*(9), 279-304.

Sawin, K.J., Buran, C.F., Brei, T., et al. (2002c). Sexuality issues in adolescents with a chronic neurological condition. *J Perinat Educ, 11*(1), 22-34.

Sawin, K.J., Buran, C.F., Brei, T.J., et al. (2003). Correlates of functional status, self management, and developmental competence in adolescents with spina bifida. *SCI Nurs, 20*(2), 72-86.

Sawin, K.J., Buran, C.F., Brei, T.J., et al. (2008). *The Development of the Adolescent Self-Management and Independence Scale. AMIS II manual.* University of Wisconsin–Milwaukee.

Sawin, K.J. & Horton, J. (in press). ACCESS for women with disabilities. In C.I. Fogel & N.F. Woods (Eds.), *Women's Health Care* (2nd ed.). Thousand Oaks, CA: Sage Publishers.

Scal, P. (2002). Transition for youth with chronic conditions: Primary care physicians' approaches. *Pediatrics, 110*(Suppl 6), 1315-1321.

Scal, P., & Ireland, M. (2005). Addressing transition to adult health care for adolescents with special health care needs. *Pediatrics, 115*(6), 1607-1612.

Stabile, L., Rosser, L., Porterfield, K.M., et al. (2005). Transfer versus transition: Success in pediatric transplantation brings the welcome challenge of transition. *Progression in Transplantation, 15*(4), 363-370.

Steinberg, L. (2000). Family at adolescence: Transition and transformation. *J Adolesc Health, 27*, 170-178.

Stewart, D. (2006). Evidence to support a positive transition into adulthood for youth with disabilities. *Phys Occup Ther Pediatr, 26*(4), 1-4.

Telfair, J., Alexander, L.R., Loosier, P.S., et al. (2004). Providers' perspectives and beliefs regarding transition to adult care for adolescents with sickle cell disease. *J Health Care Poor Underserved, 15*(3), 443-461.

U.S. Department of Education, National Center for Education Statistics (2006). *Profile of Undergraduates in U.S. Postsecondary Education Institutions: 2003-04.* Washington, DC: Author.

U.S. Department of Education & Office of Special Education Programs. (2007). *27th annual report to Congress on the implementation of the Individuals with Disabilities Education Act for year 2005,* vol 1. Washington, DC: Author. Available at www.eric.ed.gov/ERICDocs/data/ericdocs2sql/content_storage_01/0000019b/80/37/0f/f0.pdf.

U.S. Department of Health and Human Services. (2000). *Healthy People 2010.* (2nd ed.) Washington, DC: Author.

White, P.H. (2002). Access to health care: Health insurance considerations for young adults with special health care needs/disabilities. *Pediatrics, 110*(Suppl 6), 1328-1335.

Wirt, J., Choy, S., Gerald, D., et al. (2002). *The Condition of Education.* Washington, DC: National Center for Education Statistics.

Wolkstein, D. (2002). *Second Annual Conference on Substance Abuse and Co-existing Disabilities. Baltimore RTTC in Drugs and Disability.* Dayton, OH: Wright State University.

5 Chronic Conditions and the Family

Kathleen A. Knafl and Sheila Judge Santacroce

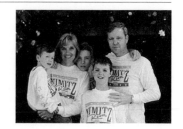

BETWEEN 13% and 20% of children in the United States are estimated to have a chronic condition, and for most it is experienced in the context of the family (Bethell, Read, Blumberg, et al., 2008; van Dyck, Kogan, McPherson, et al., 2004). Approximately one third of these children have moderate to severe conditions that limit their activity (Barlow & Ellard, 2006). Childresn who have a chronic condition often require additional health and social services for themselves and for their families (Davidoff, 2004). For example, Williams and colleagues reported that "children with special health needs experience 5 times as many admissions and 10 times as many days in hospitals compared with children without special needs." (2004, p. 384)

There is considerable evidence in the literature for the existence of a strong reciprocal relationship between illness and child and family functioning (McClellan & Cohen, 2007; Preechawong, Zauszniewski, Heinzer, et al., 2007). The importance of this relationship is especially salient in the context of a childhood chronic condition. Giammona and Malek (2002) observed that in children diagnosed with cancer "the ability of the child and [the child's] family to adapt to this new reality and all of its life-altering changes has a tremendous effect on the course of treatment" (p. 1063). Attention to this reciprocal relationship is predicated on a view of the family as a system interacting with other systems. Children with a chronic condition, along with their families, face multiple challenges that are of concern to both the families and the health care providers with whom they interact. Typically parents are expected to master new, often sophisticated, medical information and complex regimens, and children are expected to cooperate with and adhere to treatments and the lifestyle changes that may ensue.

The literature indicates that families respond in varying ways to a child's chronic condition. Although many families report that they are able to lead normal, satisfying lives despite the challenges of their child's condition, others describe their lives as an ongoing struggle that takes its toll on both individual and family well-being (Knafl & Deatrick, 2003; Knafl & Gilliss, 2002). Giammona and Malek (2002) noted that the "response of the family varies throughout the process of the diagnosis and treatment of the illness, and is affected by the coping styles chosen by individual members of the family as well as by the family system itself at different stages of the process" (p. 1076). A unique array of strengths and limitations shapes each family's condition management and the difficulties they experience; some families struggle to master a child's treatment regimen whereas others who have mastered the regimen remain stymied in their efforts to make condition management a less intrusive or less conflict-laden aspect of family life. This diversity of family responses necessitates individualized interventions if optimal child and family functioning is to be supported.

To understand the varying ways in which families and children respond to the challenges of a child's chronic condition, it is useful to understand the broader social context of the contemporary American family, current research on family response to childhood chronic conditions, and key family concepts and conceptual frameworks that can guide the primary care of children with chronic conditions. Knowledge in these three areas provides the evidence base for practice and contributes to the practitioner's ability to develop individualized interventions. Ideally, interventions address the unique needs of individual children and families and contribute to the family's ability to manage childhood chronic conditions in ways that result in both disease control and well-adjusted child and family functioning.

The Contemporary American Family

Families and nurses interact in the social context of contemporary American society. Changes over the past 40 years in marital roles, prevailing family structures, and the cohesiveness of the family unit touch all families, including those experiencing a child's chronic condition. These changes in concert with the sociocultural diversity of the American family mean that practitioners are more likely than ever to encounter a varied array of family types and circumstances. Both the popular and professional literatures are replete with statistics meant to convey important information about the current state of children and family life in America such as those listed in Box 5-1, which summarizes data from the Federal Interagency Forum on Child and Family Statistics (2007). Typically, statistics such as these are linked to concerns about the current well-being of children and the ability of the family to provide a safe environment that supports healthy child development. As such, the statistics provide useful information for shaping policies and programs.

Knowing that growing numbers of children are in need of child care and that single parents are more likely to express considerable difficulty with their parental role suggests a need for certain kinds of services and support systems. The statistics inform us about current trends, high-risk groups, and broad social needs. However, they are less useful in guiding direct practice and the kinds of interactions that take place between practitioners, children, and family members. Knowing that single parents statistically are more likely to live in poverty tells the practitioner only that the single parents they encounter fall into a high-risk group. The statistics can alert the practitioner to key areas for assessment, but they reveal nothing about the unique needs of individual children and families and never replace the need for careful assessment.

Although the statistics raise concerns about the ability of the American family to provide a safe and healthy environment for

BOX 5-1

Characteristics of Families in the United States

- In 2006, 67% of American children lived with two parents, down from 69% in 2000 and 77% in 1980.
- In 2006, 76% of white, non-Hispanic children lived with two parents, compared with 35% of black children and 66% of children of Hispanic origin.
- In 2005, 37% of all births were to unmarried women, compared with 33% in 1999. Single mothers are disproportionately more likely to be poor, and poverty has been associated with multiple negative outcomes for children.
- In 2005, 60.8% of all prekindergarten children ages 0-6 years received some form of child care on a regular basis from persons other than their parents, compared with 60.1% in 1995.
- In 2005, 11% of all American children lacked health insurance, compared with 14% in 1999.

Data from the Federal Interagency Forum on Child and Family Statistics. (2007). *America's children: Key national indicators of wellbeing 2007. Federal Interagency Forum on Child and Family Statistics.* Washington, DC: U.S. Government Printing Office.

children, another considerable body of literature indicates that family members are highly involved in the care of ill members and health care providers increasingly encourage them to be so. As Campbell (2000) noted, "families, not health care providers, are the primary caretakers of patients with chronic illness" (p. 166). Such involvement is seen as both cost effective and in the family member's best interest, and families typically prefer high levels of involvement in managing their members' health care needs. Providers and health insurance carriers typically encourage, and increasingly require, that families take considerable responsibility for managing the health care requirements of children with chronic conditions.

Statistics also are used to highlight the ethnic and cultural diversity of the American family. An early national census conducted in 1860 included only three ethnic categories—black, white, and "quadroon," or persons of mixed racial heritage. In contrast, the most recent 2000 census listed 30 ethnic categories, including 11 subcategories under "Hispanic." This striking change in census reporting reflects the growing recognition of ethnicity as a key aspect of identity, one that often is linked to beliefs about family, child rearing, illness behavior, and health care. The 2000 census reported that as a nation, we are approximately 71% white, 12% black, 12% Hispanic, 4% Asian/Pacific Islander, and less than 1% American Indian, Eskimo, and Aleut Islander. However, as with the statistics on characteristics of families, these figures provide an overview of national trends, but are of little direct use in guiding practice. They point to the likelihood that practitioners will need to take into account ethnically based beliefs about health and illness when delivering family-centered care for children with a chronic condition and their families, but provide minimal, if any, guidance on how to address ethnically based health care beliefs. The array of ethnic groups in the United States today, including recently arrived immigrants, presents a considerable challenge to practitioners who are committed to providing culturally sensitive care. How do we meet the needs of diverse families confronting diverse chronic conditions? How do we integrate our clinical and academic expertise of families and chronic conditions in order to help families meet condition-specific demands while sustaining a satisfying family life? The diversity of families speaks against the likelihood of coming up with definitive guidelines for helping certain kinds of

families facing certain kinds of health care challenges. The individuality of each family precludes the development of specific guidelines for assessment and intervention. On the other hand, there are a number of useful concepts and conceptual models available that contribute to understanding how families experience chronic conditions and that suggest important topics and issues to take into account when interacting, assessing, and developing interventions that support family management of chronic conditions.

In the remainder of this chapter, an overview of current research and conceptual models that have proven useful in guiding practice with families of children with chronic conditions will be presented. The conceptual models provide insights into what is important with regard to the nature of the challenges families face when a child member has a chronic condition. At the same time, the concepts and frameworks discussed accommodate family diversity because they do not prescribe or judge observations; as such, they are meant to guide efforts to encourage families to share their experiences and work collaboratively with practitioners to develop effective interventions.

Families and Chronic Conditions: The Evidence Base for Practice

Transition to Living with the Diagnosis of a Pediatric Chronic Health Condition

Almost all of what is known about the transition to living with the diagnosis of a pediatric chronic health condition and initial responses to such diagnoses has to do with parents. The related literature about children addresses their responses to specific illness-related events and circumstances, such as painful procedures and hospitalization, rather than to the diagnosis. The focus on parental responses is justified because parents play a critical role in delivering medical treatments to the child with a chronic health condition, mediating condition-related distress for the affected child and healthy siblings, promoting the child's psychological and social adaptation to a chronic condition, and managing day-to-day family life. Optimal care for children with chronic health conditions and their families requires an understanding of usual parental responses to the diagnosis of a pediatric chronic condition and the development of supports for parents.

The transition to living with the diagnosis of a pediatric chronic health condition does not occur at the point in time when a clinician meets with the parents to formally pronounce the child's medical diagnosis, give population-based estimates for the child's prognosis and long-term survival, and make recommendations for the child's medical treatment. More accurately, this transition is a process that begins when parents become aware of changes in their child and is completed when family members absorb the implications of the condition for the child and the family. Davis (1963) first described the process that families experience as it applied to families of children with poliomyelitis (Box 5-2). Cohen (1993a, 1995a) found support for Davis's depiction and extended his work through family interviews and review of the autobiographical literature about families of children with a broad array of chronic health conditions. Clarke-Steffen (1993a) has developed a model of the process as it occurred for families of children with cancer. Research about children with type 1 diabetes (Grey, Cameron, Lipman, et al., 1995; Hatton, Canam, Thorne, et al., 1995) and children diagnosed at birth with a chronic health condition (Sharkey,

Transition to Living with the Diagnosis of a Chronic Condition

1. Prediagnostic stage
   a. Parents aware of changes in the child
   b. Parents and PCP define symptoms as normal and attempt to manage
   c. Parents and PCP redefine symptoms as serious and seek subspecialty evaluation
2. Diagnostic stage
   a. Subspecialty evaluation is initiated
   b. Formal pronouncement of the diagnosis and treatment recommendations
   c. Initiation of treatment
3. Living with the diagnosis
   a. Parents responsible for administering treatment
   b. Parental awareness of the implications of the diagnosis for child and family

Key: *PCP,* Primary care provider.

1995) shows that the transition process is realized when the family undertakes implementation of the child's medical regimen and develops an accurate sense of the implications of the health condition for the affected child and family life.

According to Cohen (1995a), the onset of the transition to living with the diagnosis of a pediatric chronic health condition, which she referred to as the prediagnostic period, comprises three stages. The onset of the transition begins with a parent's awareness that something is going on with his or her child and continues until the formal diagnostic announcement. Before the first or lay-explanatory stage, the child's symptoms, for example, bone aches or irritability, are so ordinary as not to be noticed. The lay-explanatory stage begins when the child's symptoms enter the parent's awareness and become a focus of attention. Parents, especially those with little experience with serious pediatric health conditions, commonly apply a normal developmental explanation such as growing pains or a desire for attention, or a benign medical explanation such as the flu, to account for the symptoms; primary care providers may do the same thing. When the child's symptoms are defined as evidence of a nonmedical problem, parents use interactional strategies such as ignoring, nagging, punishing, or paying extra attention to the child to manage the child's symptoms. When the symptoms are defined as evidence of a medical problem, parents use medical strategies such as rest and over-the-counter medications for symptom management (Cohen, 1995a).

After symptom management strategies are initiated, parents wait to see improvement in the child's symptoms. If the problem gets worse or does not resolve within a reasonable amount of time, parents question the plausibility of the lay explanation and start to legitimate the need for medical intervention. The second, or legitimizing, stage of the acute phase of the transition to living with the diagnosis of a pediatric chronic health condition commences when the parent redefines the child's symptoms as worrisome and originates a strategic plan in anticipation of a parent-provider interaction. Parents devote considerable effort to developing a strategic plan to guide their interactions with professionals. Parents do this because they fear being made to feel like an alarmist; fear that the child's symptoms will be dismissed by health care providers, just as the parents had previously dismissed the symptoms; and, particularly in the current health care climate, to quickly gain the referral that many insurers require from a primary care provider before setting an appointment for evaluation by a specialist. Parents use a broad range of strategies to enact the strategic plan for interactions with providers, including raising their concerns during a routine health care visit, acquiring knowledge to counter a provider's appraisal of the child's symptoms as normal, paying out-of-pocket costs for nonauthorized referral to obtain the care they believe is indicated, and embellishing the nature or severity of the child's symptoms (Cohen, 1995a). Adverse consequences of the prolonged lay-explanatory or legitimizing phases are loss of parents' confidence in their ability to perform the parental role as it applies to monitoring the child's physical health, distinguishing normal variations from symptoms of illness, and inappropriate disciplining of the child. This loss of confidence applies not only to parenting affected children but also their healthy siblings (Cohen & Martinson, 1988).

The third, or medical diagnostic, stage of the transition to diagnosis begins when the parent makes an appointment for the child to be seen by a physician or other specialist and ends when the diagnosis is confirmed and formally announced to the family. The duration of this stage is determined by the extent to which there are unambiguous physical findings in the child, the degree to which the provider acknowledges parental concerns, and the degree to which a provider allows the relative frequency of a disease to influence diagnostic testing. For example, the relatively low incidence of childhood leukemia versus viral illness may cause a health care provider to attribute the general symptoms of fever, bone pain, and pallor to viral illness and delay blood tests for leukemia. When the medical diagnosis phase is protracted, the long wait for diagnostic certainty becomes unbearable, causing existential agony and extreme psychosocial stress for parents (Clarke-Steffen, 1993b). Adverse consequences of a prolonged medical diagnosis phase consist of parental anger with providers, institutions, and systems of care; lack of parental confidence in the provider's ability to assess and treat the child; and hypersensitivity to provider statements and behaviors (Clarke-Steffen, 1993b; Davis, 1963) that can be so extreme as to resemble paranoia. When the medical diagnostic phase has been prolonged, parents have reported extreme relief in response to the diagnoses of even potentially fatal pediatric health conditions (Cohen, 1995b; Santacroce, 2000). Parental relief is supported by provider statements reflecting the expectation that the condition can be managed by available treatment, specific treatment recommendations, the health care team's expertise with delivering treatment and supportive care, and a plan for initiating treatment (Santacroce, 2000).

Parents have likened the diagnosis of a chronic health condition in their child to a "physical assault by a powerful force" (Cohen, 1995a, p. 47). In 1994, the American Psychological Association (APA, 1994) recognized the diagnosis of a life-threatening condition in a child as a traumatic event for parents, and this continues to be the case (APA, 2000). The diagnosis may be particularly traumatic in the contemporary sociomedical context owing to cognitive dissonance between what is expected and what is experienced. In the past, families expected to experience childhood death from disease. There were few available means to prevent or treat infectious diseases. Available technologies did not allow for early diagnosis of life-threatening disease and there were few available means to manage late-stage disease or the side effects of crude treatments. Preparation for the child's certain and usually imminent death often followed the diagnostic announcement. Given medical and technologic developments over the past five decades, today's parents expect healthy children who will outlive them. Modern Western beliefs include personal responsibility for health, healthy living as a way to ensure personal and family health, and the availability of definitive "cures" for disease and other health conditions through widespread access to state-of-the-science medicine and supportive care technologies (Comaroff & Maguire, 1981).

With the diagnosis of a pediatric chronic health condition that has no definitive cure, or when the application of available "curative" treatments generates a distinct set of problems, the previously held assumptions come apart and parents' beliefs about themselves, science, and the world, and sometimes God, are shattered. Uncertainty about the nature of the problem that existed during the prediagnostic phase changes to uncertainty that permeates every aspect of daily family life. Parents experience intense helplessness with being unable to prevent the child's health condition and protect the child from harm, guilt at their real or imagined role in causing or failing to recognize the condition, horror at witnessing the child's suffering and thoughts that the child may die, and fear about what the child and the family will have to endure in the future (Clarke-Steffen, 1997; Cohen, 1993a). These parental reactions may be heightened when there is a genetic component to the chronic condition. Grandparents may also respond to the child's diagnosis with helplessness, guilt, horror, and fear. Overcome by their intense, distressing emotions, they may not be as emotionally or physically available to mediate parental or child distress as parents or children may need or desire.

Four to six weeks after the diagnosis of cancer in their child, parents have reported symptoms similar to those seen in persons with an extreme response to traumatic stressors such as combat, natural disaster, or sexual assault: posttraumatic stress disorder (PTSD) (Santacroce, 2002). Symptoms of PSTD include insomnia, irritability, difficulty concentrating and remembering, recurrent intrusive daytime thoughts or nightmares about the traumatic event, detachment and inability to experience loving or pleasurable feelings, amnesia for important aspects of the trauma, careful avoidance of cues that recall the trauma, intense reactivity with exposure to these cues, a sense of a foreshortened future, and separation of cognition and emotion (APA, 2000). Such symptoms imply full-blown PTSD when symptoms in each of three clusters, that is, reexperiencing, avoidance/numbing, and heightened arousal, are present for 1 month or more with significant psychological or social impairment as a result of the symptoms (APA, 2000). Wijnberg-Williams, Kamps, Klip, and colleagues (2006) found that in parents of children diagnosed with cancer, "levels of reported distress, psychoneurotic symptoms and state anxiety significantly decreased across time" (p. 1), falling to normal levels at 12 months after diagnosis, but observed that a significant number of parents still experienced clinical distress after 5 years. Some parents may be more vulnerable than others to developing full-blown PTSD or long-term PTSD-associated symptoms following the diagnosis of a childhood chronic condition. Risk factors for developing full-blown PTSD include female gender, acute emotional distress, depression and lack of social support after the trauma, and a history of exposure to interpersonal trauma (Bisson, 2002; Kessler, 2000). Mothers may be at greater risk for the development of PTSD than fathers by virtue of their gender and because, generally, mothers assume responsibility for the day-to-day care of their children and

are thus more likely to experience cyclic retraumatization during treatments, procedures, and health care visits. Across a range of traumatic events, children are more likely to develop full-blown PTSD or its symptoms when their parents have the full-blown disorder or its symptoms (Santacroce, 2003). For parents of long-term survivors of childhood cancer, higher trait anxiety, smaller social network, and greater perceived intensity of treatment and threat to the child's life predicted PTSD-associated symptoms (Kazak, Stuber, Barakat, et al., 1998).

In the immediate period following diagnosis, especially when there is an acute threat to the child's life, PTSD-associated symptoms are normative and protective in that they restrict parental awareness of upsetting events, dampen potentially overwhelming distressing emotions, and allow parents to make treatment decisions and take other steps to preserve child and family life. Conversely, PTSD-associated symptoms can impede parental ability to comprehend and remember detailed information about their child's condition and its treatment, learn critical condition-management skills, mediate their child's emotional distress, utilize social support, and plan for the future (Santacroce, 2002). Over time, as immediate threats to the child's life are eliminated, protective "symptoms" generally abate, allowing more comprehensive cognitive awareness of condition-related events. It is also when the child's condition is stabilized that parents usually assume responsibility for managing the child's medical regimen. Hatton and colleagues (1995) found that when parents of children with type 1 diabetes assumed responsibility for managing the child's medical regimen at home, they developed a more complete absorption of the diagnosis, including an understanding of the widespread implications and pervasive influence of the condition on each member of the family. In children with type 1 diabetes, Grey and colleagues (1995) found increased levels of depressive symptoms and reduced levels of self-efficacy over the second year following the diagnosis. The researchers attributed the increased levels of depression and reduced self-efficacy to experience with managing the medical regimen and the development of an understanding of the meaning of the diagnosis and its implications; that is, that diabetes (and diabetes self-management) is forever.

In a study about families of children with conditions requiring home care, Sharkey (1995) found that the child's discharge home was associated with heightened awareness of the physical work and family environmental and lifestyle changes required to accommodate the child's health condition while maintaining some sense of normal family life. Taken together, these findings indicate that the transition to living with the diagnosis of a pediatric chronic health condition is not complete when the diagnosis is announced; instead, the transition is complete when responsibility for managing the child's condition-related and usual daily care is assumed by family members and the child and family develop genuine awareness of the implications of the diagnosis and the medical treatment regimen for individual and family life over the longer term. Clinical experience suggests that this idea is applicable beyond families of children with diabetes or children requiring home care.

The transition to living with the diagnosis of a pediatric health condition is a process that begins when the child's symptoms enter the parent's awareness and is complete when parental understanding of the meaning of the diagnosis for child and family life develops with experience managing the child's care. There may be parallel critical points in the child's transition to living with the diagnosis of a chronic health condition. That is, the child's transition may be advanced during late school age with the experience of beginning responsibility for self-management and completed during late adolescence or young adulthood with cognitive awareness of both the immediate and future implications of the condition and its treatment.

Living with a Chronic Condition

Research on the interplay between childhood chronic conditions and child and family functioning has focused on the family's contribution to the child's functioning, the quality of family functioning in the context of childhood illness, and the patterns of family response to the child's chronic condition. Studies in these areas have generated considerable knowledge with regard to child and family functioning and provide the practitioner with an understanding of the range of child and family responses one is likely to encounter in practice. These studies also highlight family and child characteristics that may lead to adjustment difficulties as well as concepts that are likely to help primary care providers understand the family context of childhood chronic conditions and support families' efforts to care for their child's condition in a way that contributes to healthy child development and family functioning.

Impact of a Chronic Condition on Child and Family Functioning

Impact of a Chronic Condition on Child Functioning. The relationship between family and child functioning when a child has a chronic condition typically is discussed in terms of the family's impact on the child's psychosocial adjustment, condition control, and treatment adherence. A large body of research has focused on children's psychosocial adjustment to a chronic condition. Studies carried out over the past 50 years have shown that children with chronic physical problems are at increased risk for emotional and behavioral problems, suggesting that primary care providers need to be alert for the special needs of this particular group of children. For example, an early meta-analysis of 87 studies that compared the psychological adjustment of children with chronic conditions to that of either study controls or normative data found a mean difference in overall psychological adjustment of approximately half of a standard deviation (Lavigne & Faier-Routman, 1992), indicating that having a chronic condition puts children at significant risk for psychosocial problems. Similarly, Wallendar and Varni (1998) concluded that prior research, including major epidemiologic surveys, has established the risk status of children with chronic conditions. At the same time, they, along with other investigators, are quick to point out that "although the prevalence of maladjustment is higher, only a minority of children with chronic disorders appeared maladjusted" (Wallender & Varni, 1998, p. 31). More recently, Barlow and Ellard (2006) reported the results of prior syntheses and meta-analyses of research on the psychosocial well-being of children with chronic conditions, concluding as well that these children "are at slightly elevated risk for psychological distress, although the number of children who fall within clinical parameters is relatively small" (p. 29).

Family functioning is an important predictor of adjustment in children with chronic conditions (Friedman, Holmbeck, Jandasek, et al., 2004; Graf, Landolt, Capone, et al., 2006; Knafl & Gilliss, 2002; Mitchell, Lemanek, Palermo, et al., 2007; Rodenburg, Meijer, Dekovic, et al., 2005; Salewski, 2003; Sawyer, Antoniou, Rice, et al., 2000; Sawyer, Spurrier, Kennedy, et al., 2001; Sawyer, Spurrier, Whaites, et al., 2000; Thompson, Armstrong, Link, et al., 2003; Wood, Lim, Miller, et al., 2007). For example, Sawyer, Spurrier, and colleagues (2000) found that in children with chronic asthma, there was a significant relationship between the mental health of children and family functioning despite the lack of a significant relationship between their physical health and family functioning. In a separate study, Sawyer and colleagues (2001) demonstrated that "independent of their frequency, the extent to which asthma symptoms upset and bother children varies depending on the level of the functioning of the children's families" (p. 279). Although different studies have linked varying characteristics of the family to child adjustment, the variables of family cohesion and absence of conflict consistently have been associated with better adjustment in children. As a group, these studies indicate that providers should expect the majority of children with chronic conditions in their practice to be well adjusted. On the other hand, they also point to the importance of including family variables in any assessment of adjustment difficulties a child may be experiencing. Moreover, there is a growing body of literature that demonstrates the benefits of normalization as a coping strategy that helps both the child and the family adjust to the chronic condition (Deatrick, Knafl, & Murphy-Moore, 1999; Knafl, Deatrick, & Kirby, 2001). As discussed later in this chapter, health care professionals can play a key role in helping parents create normal lives for children with chronic conditions and their families.

Impact of a Chronic Condition on Family Functioning. Investigators have addressed how childhood chronic conditions affect family life, as well as the quality of family functioning in the context of chronic conditions (Knafl & Gilliss, 2002; McClellan & Cohen, 2007). Studies address various aspects of family functioning including problem solving, communication, and coping. The coping function of families, or their ability to maintain stability in the face of change, has been a particular concern of researchers interested in family. The results of these studies, which typically used standardized measures to assess family functioning, present a mixed picture of the impact of a chronic condition on family life. Some authors found evidence that families continue to function well when a member has a chronic condition (Gerhardt, Vannatta, McKellop, et al., 2003; Rodrigues & Patterson, 2007; Thanarattanakorn, Louthrenoo, Sittipreechacharn, et al., 2003). For example, Gerhardt and colleagues (2003) studied 64 parents of children with juvenile rheumatoid arthritis and found family functioning levels similar to those of comparison families. Similarly, Rodrigues and Patterson (2007), in a study of 262 two-parent families of infants and children with varied conditions, found that families functioned as well as or better than families in a normative comparison group. Overall, the investigators in these studies found that families expressed satisfaction with family life and did not perceive the chronic condition to be the dominant focus of their life.

In contrast, other studies documented negative outcomes for family functioning when a child had a chronic condition (Holmbeck, Greenley, Coakley, et al., 2006; Rodenburg et al., 2005; Spieth, Stark, Mitchell, et al., 2001). These studies suggest that families who are facing multiple stressors or have a child who has a condition characterized by an uncertain disease course are more likely to experience impaired family functioning. For example, based on a review of 35 studies of functioning in families with children with epilepsy, Rodenburg and colleagues (2005) concluded that "families with a child with epilepsy generally fare worse on a whole range of family factors, indicating lower parent-child relationship quality, more depression in mothers, and problems with family functioning" (p. 488). Other authors have reported varying quality of family functioning over time as changes in the condition or the family's situation make adapting to the challenges of managing the condition more or less difficult (Knafl & Deatrick, 2002; Mussatto, 2006).

Descriptive studies have provided insights into the cognitive and behavioral strategies that support optimal family functioning over the course of a child's chronic condition. As such, they serve to guide the assessment of key aspects of family life. These studies provide evidence that adaptation is a process that often occurs in a series of stages (Gilliss & Knafl, 1999; Knafl & Deatrick, 2003; Knafl & Gilliss, 2002). For example, Horner (1998), in a qualitative study of 12 families in which a school-age child had asthma, identified three phases of adaptation: learning the ropes, dealing with asthma, and coming to terms with the asthma. She described how, over time, families mastered the treatment regimen and were able to balance asthma care with other aspects of family life. Other investigators have noted the importance of developing a routine for carrying out the treatment regimen that minimizes its intrusiveness on family life. These authors also noted that families typically were able to develop such a routine, but often struggled to do so during the first few months following the diagnosis and during subsequent developmental transitions as the child's responsibility for self-care increased.

Helping families to master the treatment regimen and develop a management routine that accommodates other family activities and responsibilities is an important goal for health care providers. Burke, Kauffmann, Harrison, and colleagues (1999) have developed a useful tool for helping families manage a child's condition. The "Burke Assessment Guide to Stressors and Tasks in Families with a Child with a Chronic Condition" was based on a series of interviews with over 300 parents of children with a chronic condition and is meant to support the comprehensive assessment of critical issues for families and to focus ongoing nursing interventions. Box 5-3 lists the 11 major areas of stressors and tasks included in the assessment (see Burke et al., 1999, for a more detailed description).

Underlying Dimensions of Chronic Conditions. Much of the research on family response to chronic conditions addresses the challenges that specific conditions present to children and families. However, both researchers and clinicians have noted the limitations of focusing exclusively on condition categories when the primary interest is the psychosocial as opposed to the physiologic consequences of chronic conditions (Rolland, 1994; Stein & Jessop, 1982; Wallender & Varni, 1998). Noncategorical frameworks are particularly useful because they direct the clinician's attention away from an exclusive focus on the condition to the experience of living with the condition. As early as 1975, Pless and Pinkerton discussed the benefits of taking a noncategorical approach to the care and study of children with chronic conditions and their families. They argued that it is neither possible nor particularly useful to try to chronicle the distinct challenges posed by each chronic condition. Since their seminal work, clinicians and researchers have identified underlying dimensions of chronic conditions that cut across disease entities and play an important role in shaping individual and family response. In their review of the effects of chronic physical illness on children and their families, Wallender and Varni (1998) noted that an approach that "focuses on commonalities in the class of chronic physical disorders could enhance the understanding of the impact on the psychosocial adjustment of children and their families and could improve care" (p. 29). Several frameworks have been devised that highlight generic dimensions of the chronic condition experience (Jessop & Stein, 1985; LoBato, Faust, & Spirito, 1988; Rolland, 1994; Stein & Jessop, 1982). Although varied, these frameworks reveal some common themes and important psychosocial dimensions of a chronic condition that increase family stress (Box 5-4).

The condition onset dimension is related to the abruptness with which the condition occurs. Conditions such as diabetes and spinal cord injury have a sudden onset allowing little time for family adaptation and requiring immediate changes in family life. On the other hand, conditions such as arthritis, muscular dystrophy, and attention-deficit/hyperactivity disorder permit more gradual adjustments in family life, although the uncertainty surrounding the diagnostic period may be the source of considerable stress. The course of the chronic condition addresses the relative stability and predictability of the condition. In general, conditions such as lupus and epilepsy that are unstable or unpredictable impose greater psychosocial demands on the family. The degree and nature of functional limitation associated with the condition also have implications for the quality of child and family adaptation. Rolland (1984) goes so far as to say that it is the presence or absence of any major incapacitation rather than the exact nature of the incapacitation that is the salient functional dimension of a chronic condition. Visibility also has been identified as an important dimension of the chronic condition experience, although the nature of its influence is somewhat unclear with some authors linking visibility with better and some with poorer adaptation (Wallender & Varni, 1998).

BOX 5-3

Major Stressors and Tasks Included in the Burke Assessment Guide

1. Gaining and interpreting knowledge, skills, and experience to manage the child's problem
2. Acquiring and managing physical resources and services to manage the child's health problem
3. Acquiring and managing financial resources to care for the child's health problem
4. Establishing and maintaining effective social supports
5. Rearing a child with a chronic condition
6. Developing beliefs, values, and a philosophy of life
7. Managing the care of the child
8. Identifying and managing sibling issues
9. Managing spousal, parental, and nuclear family relationships
10. Maintaining health of other family members
11. Maintaining effective relationships with the health care system and other sources of care

---

BOX 5-4

Characteristics of Chronic Conditions Resulting in Increased Family Stress

- Sudden onset
- Instability in course of condition
- Functional limitations
- Visibility of condition

Underlying Dimensions of Genetic Conditions

Recent advances in genomic research have contributed to the growing recognition of the unique challenges of genetic conditions for families (Van Riper & Gallo, 2006). Rolland and Williams (2005, 2006) have developed a model of common psychosocial challenges of genetic conditions that builds on Rolland's earlier work on the noncategorical dimensions of chronic illness (1994). Rolland and Williams' Family Systems Genetic Illness (FSGI) model groups different genetic conditions based on the pattern of psychosocial demands they present to the family and identifies key time phases in living with a genetic condition. The model, which is applicable to a broad spectrum of genetic conditions, identifies four components of psychosocial demand that cut across multiple genetic conditions: likelihood of developing a condition, clinical severity, timing of clinical onset, and prevention and treatment. Each of these four components varies across genetic conditions, and the FSGI model includes a typology of 36 different types of genetic conditions based on the distinct psychosocial challenges they are likely to present. For example, in families with a history of sickle cell disease, the likelihood of having a child who will have or be a carrier of the condition is known, the clinical severity is high, the diagnosis is made prenatally or at birth, and there are multiple treatment options. On the other hand, for families in which there is a history of Duchenne muscular dystrophy, there is a similar pattern of known likelihood, childhood onset, and high severity, but there are limited effective treatment options. This key difference between sickle cell disease and Duchenne muscular dystrophy is likely to contribute to a very different experience and set of psychosocial challenges for families. The FSGI model also describes four illness phases: awareness, pretesting, testing and posttesting, and long-term adaptation. These phases include the time span before the onset of symptoms and highlight a unique challenge of genetic conditions: families often have to adapt to the possibility of having the condition before they have to adapt to living with the actual condition. For clinicians, the FSGI model is a useful framework for identifying the kinds of challenges varying types of genetic conditions present to families over time. Rolland and Williams (2005, 2006) also have identified likely challenges at different illness phases, and readers with an interest in genetics are encouraged to review this model more fully.

Key Concepts for Understanding Family Response to Illness

Health care providers have a number of concepts to draw on to help them understand how families experience and respond to childhood chronic conditions. Uncertainty, stigma, normalization, and survivorship are concepts that capture important aspects of many families' experiences (Box 5-5).

Uncertainty. Uncertainty has been identified as the single greatest source of psychosocial stress for people affected by chronic health conditions (Koocher, 1985). For parents, uncertainty pervades the experience of a child's illness, from the time around diagnosis through long-term survivorship or bereavement (Santacroce, 2001). Over the course of pediatric chronic health conditions, parents experience uncertainty as an unbearable urge to know what is not knowable about the child's future: what the child will be asked to endure, whether or not the child will ultimately survive, and, if the child survives, the child's quality of life and level of function (Clarke-Steffen, 1993b; Cohen & Martinson, 1988).

BOX 5-5

Key Concepts in Family Responses to Pediatric Chronic Conditions

1. *Uncertainty* about the nature of the child's problem spreads to every aspect of family life at diagnosis
2. *Stigma* can interfere with accessing available social supports and health care utilization
3. *Normalization* includes integrating condition with usual life to maximize medical outcomes and promote family function
4. *Survivorship* applies to affected individual as well as family members

---

Parental uncertainty has been defined as a parent's or other family caregiver's ability to determine meaning relative to illness events in a family member, specifically a child (Mishel, 1983; Santacroce, 2001). In adults, uncertainty has been shown to have four dimensions: ambiguity about the illness state; lack of information about the illness, its treatment and side effects, and their management; complexity in what information is known, the health care system, and relationships with health care providers; and unpredictability of the future (Mishel, 1981, 1997). Parental uncertainty in child chronic health conditions has been shown to share these features (Mishel, 1983; Santacroce, 2001).

Uncertainty is intrinsically neutral, but can be appraised as dangerous or beneficial (Mishel, 1988). It seems to be a robust predictor of parental psychological adaptation in the setting of chronic childhood conditions (Carpentier, Mullins, Chaney, et al., 2006). Adults initially tend to appraise uncertainty as dangerous. When they appraise uncertainty as dangerous, people next evaluate if they have the skills and resources to reduce uncertainty. When their skills and resources seem sufficient, adults act to resolve uncertainty. In the perceived absence of skills and resources, or when distressing emotions and negative beliefs impede action, people manage uncertainty by restricting their awareness of what produces uncertainty (Mishel, 1988). Uncertainty has been consistently associated with higher levels of emotional distress, reduced quality of life and poorer psychosocial adjustment (Mast, 1995; Mishel, 1997). Higher levels of distress have predicted less functional coping (Mishel, 1997).

With the explosion of information about the role of genetic mutations in the development of childhood and adult health conditions, uncertainty now includes preclinical phases. Before genetic testing, the core uncertainty may be whether or not an individual child has a specific genetic mutation. When a genetic mutation with high penetrance, that is, the likelihood of developing clinical disease, is clearly present, parents may experience ongoing uncertainty about the nature and severity of the child's disease course. For genetic mutations with low penetrance, ongoing parental uncertainty can also include whether or not the child will actually develop clinical disease. Knowing for certain the results, affirmative or negative, of genetic testing for highly penetrant mutations that underlie chronic conditions with relatively predictable courses and outcomes can be more psychologically manageable than chronic uncertainty; the parent can have some sense of what lies ahead and the corresponding plans that need to be made (Rolland & Williams, 2006). Box 5-6 identifies some key triggers of uncertainty.

BOX 5-6
Triggers of Uncertainty

- Anniversaries, birthdays, holidays
- Changes in the treatment regimen, treatment completion
- Communications with health care practitioners
- Genetic testing
- Waiting for the results of regular tests and procedures
- Nighttime
- Onset of symptoms present at diagnosis of cancer
- Questions from family and friends
- Routine medical appointments
- Stories in the media
- Usual life transitions
- Variations in mood or behavior or physical condition

For the most part, parents cope with uncertainty by managing information (Stewart & Mishel, 2000). Information management typically takes two forms: intensive pursuit of information concerning the child's condition with hypervigilance to cues regarding the state of the child's health and potential threats in the environment, and careful avoidance of social encounters or cues that call to mind the child's condition and draw attention to negative aspects of uncertainty (Clarke-Steffen, 1993b; Cohen, 1993b, 1995b; Cohen & Martinson, 1988; Davis, 1963; Hinds, Birenbaum, Clarke-Steffen, et al., 1996; Santacroce, Deatrick, & Ledlie, 2002). Intense pursuit of information and hypervigilance to the child's condition can exhaust parents and impede child development through over-restriction of child and family activities beyond what is medically indicated. Avoidance of social encounters and other reminders of the child's condition can lead to lack of adherence to treatment regimens, social isolation, and diminished family communication.

The four domains of adult uncertainty also have been shown to be salient and distressing aspects of the experience for adolescents and young adults with chronic health conditions, including cancer (Haase & Rostad, 1994; Neville, 1998), asthma (Carpentier, Mullins, & Van Pelt, 2007; Van Pelt, Mullins, Carpentier, et al., 2006), and type 1 diabetes (Mullin, Wolfe-Christensen, Pai, et al., 2007). For adolescents with cancer, the level of uncertainty was found to be fairly consistent by disease phase but there were phase-specific areas of concern (Decker, Haase, & Bell, 2007). Throughout the cancer experience, adolescents have been shown to manage uncertainty through the use of the specific avoidance strategies of selective attention and distraction (Weekes & Kagan, 1994). In long-term survival, adult survivors of childhood cancer report coping with chronic uncertainty about the future by living for today, putting their worries aside, and accepting what seems out of their ability to control (Parry, 2003). Although avoidance strategies may be effective means to control intense emotional distress, their use may impede health care use, information seeking, and the development of daily self-management behaviors that can minimize risk for developing chronic health problems secondary to treatment (Santacroce & Lee, 2006).

Child uncertainty during the diagnosis and treatment of childhood cancer has been shown to have four domains that are similar to the dimensions of adult uncertainty: not understanding (complexity), not knowing (lack of information), not being able to predict (unpredictability), and not being sure what things mean (ambiguity) (Stewart, 2003). The main consequence of child uncertainty is the worry or fear that is experienced most intensely

during diagnosis and treatment but which can be triggered at any time by body sensations that recall the initial symptoms of cancer. Children say they cope with illness uncertainty by learning from their experiences, by focusing on the routine versus the unpredictable in their everyday lives, and by viewing the unpredictable as normal and expected (Stewart, 2003).

Similarly, adults can adopt a view that normalizes uncertainty and considers its beneficial features (Mishel, 1990). For example, uncertainty about the ultimate prognosis for a particular child can come to be a source of family hope that their child will survive long-term. Change in appraisal of uncertainty from danger to normal and even beneficial can be encumbered by social isolation and sizeable family responsibilities (Mishel, 1990, 1999). Parents of children with chronic health conditions are often socially isolated and carry considerable responsibility for the care of the child who is ill. Families may need assistance with the development of a broader range of functional strategies for managing uncertainty that is appraised as dangerous and support for acknowledging the positive features of uncertainty in childhood chronic conditions.

Stigma. Children with chronic health conditions can have characteristics that differ from norms and set the child and family apart in undesirable ways from peers and also life before the onset of the condition. These characteristics can potentially stigmatize, or disgrace, people with chronic health conditions, their families, and their caregivers, and thus interfere with the communication of important information, utilization of available social supports, formation of trusting relationships with health care providers, and maximal management of the underlying condition.

In ancient Greece, *stigma* referred to bodily signs designed and inflicted to warn the larger community about the inferior moral state of an individual (Goffman, 1963). Stigma has come to refer to social and personal intolerance of characteristics that are viewed as either undesirable or not typical and thus discrediting of a person's social identity (Goffman, 1963). The assumption that people with potentially stigmatizing characteristics have internalized the larger society's negative views about these traits is inherent in the idea of stigma.

Goffman (1963) proposed a typology of stigma that can be applied to understanding family responses to childhood chronic conditions: discredited and discreditable. Discrediting stigma are those that are readily evident. Among pediatric chronic conditions, discrediting conditions are those with obvious physical or developmental differences, medications and equipment requirements, or diet or activity restrictions. A discreditable stigma is one that is not easily perceivable or readily apparent. Stigma can also be inferred through records such as a person's medical record that includes a history of engagement in risky behaviors or the results of genetic testing, transmitted through a lineage to all members of the line, and extended to the family and close associates. People with discreditable stigma and their families tend to expend great effort to obscure traces of the potentially stigmatizing characteristic through the use of strategies that include information management, impression management, and "passing" (Goffman, 1963). Santacroce, Deatrick, and Ledlie (2002) found that mothers of children with perinatally acquired human immunodeficiency virus (HIV) infection delayed medical treatment for their children when they believed that multidrug regimens would make a nonapparent condition readily obvious to family, friends, and educators, that is, shift the stigma from the discreditable to discredited type. Thus stigma has the potential to compromise both psychosocial and medical outcomes when health care use is compromised because of negative expectations about stigma.

Child obesity (see Chapter 36) provides a contemporary example of an obvious and potentially manageable chronic health condition in which providers can unwittingly engage in stigmatizing behaviors. Parents of children who are overweight report feeling blamed and held responsible by providers for their child's weight status (Edmunds, 2005). Women who are overweight have been found to be more likely than other adults to avoid health care because they do not want to be lectured about weight (Wee, McCarthy, Davis, et al., 2004). Similarly, mothers may avoid pediatric care for a child or adolescent who is obese to avoid comments that they perceive as being critical and the feelings that can result (O'Dea, 2005), resulting in fewer opportunities for health education and interventions that aim to improve child health. Practitioners should examine their attitudes and beliefs about potentially stigmatizing health conditions, and attempt to promote health care use and limit unhelpful interactions with children and parents by adopting a holistic focus on health and health improvement via healthy lifestyle rather than highlighting potentially stigmatizing characteristics such as weight.

Normalization. As noted in the prior discussion of the family's transition to having a child with a chronic condition, the events surrounding the diagnostic process and the family's initial period of adjustment can be a difficult stressful time. However, over time many families are able to incorporate the treatment regimen into their ongoing family routine and life resumes a "taken for granted" quality. Robinson (1993) noted that "the preferred or dominant story for many individuals and families managing a chronic condition is one of normalization, that is, essentially normal persons leading normal lives" (p. 7). The concept of normalization has received considerable attention in the literature and can help guide practitioners' efforts to help families balance condition-related demands with the responsibilities of ongoing family life.

Based on a comprehensive review of research related to normalization of family life in the context of childhood chronic conditions, Deatrick and colleagues (1999) identified five defining attributes of the concept (Box 5-7). The literature indicates that for many families of children with a chronic condition normalization is a valued goal and the five defining attributes can guide the practitioner's assessment of the family's normalization status. These attributes also can help to pinpoint areas where the family is experiencing normalization difficulties (Knafl & Deatrick, 2002). For example, are difficulties the result of the failure of other systems, such as the school or health care, to support the family's normalization efforts? Or are difficulties based on problems with carrying out the treatment regimen or a change in the child's health status? When establishing interventions to support the family's ability to normalize their situation, it is important to remember that the five attributes are based on the assumption that views of normalcy are highly subjective, are likely to vary considerably across families, and may differ from those of the practitioner.

Families who normalize their life recognize the seriousness of their child's condition and the importance of the treatment regimen. However, these families also believe that the chronic condition is only one aspect of their family and child. They see themselves as essentially normal with a particular problem that has to be managed. Moreover, they often are quick to point out that although not

---

BOX 5-7
Attributes of Normalization

1. Acknowledge the condition and its potential to threaten lifestyle.
2. Adopt a "normalcy lens" for defining the child and the family.
3. Engage in parenting behaviors and a family routine that are consistent with a normalcy lens.
4. Develop a treatment regimen that is consistent with a normalcy lens.
5. Interact with others based on a view of their child and family as normal.

---

all families have a child with a chronic condition, all families do, in fact, have problems that must be managed. Families who normalize the chronic condition are likely to develop a flexible approach to adhering to the treatment regimen. In their article on the "tricks of the trade" parents develop for managing the treatment regimen, Gallo and Knafl (1998) noted that parents not only modified the treatment plan to make life more livable, but relied on the advice and support of health care providers to do so. As indicated by the fifth attribute listed in Box 5-7, families who normalize life in the context of a childhood chronic condition also expect others, both individuals and systems, to treat them and their child as normal; that is, health care providers are expected to help in the modification of treatment regimens so the child can participate in usual childhood activities, and school systems are expected to minimize restrictions placed on the child as a result of the condition.

Although there is a considerable body of literature indicating that many families achieve normalization, there also is evidence of families who view normalization as an impossible or inappropriate goal (Knafl & Deatrick, 2002). In these families, the child may be viewed as different from peers in multiple, important ways or the work of managing the treatment regimen may become the focus of family life. Normalizing families experience a chronic condition as one of many concerns of family life, compared with families who are unable to normalize family life who experience the condition as the pervasive focus of family life. However, Rehm and Bradley's (2005) research on families in which there is a medically fragile/technology-dependent child found that even in families where normalization was not possible because of the complexity and severity of the child's condition, parents believed their family had a good life, though not one that was normal by usual standards. This key finding points to the importance of recognizing that even in the absence of normalization, families can function and lead a satisfying life.

Health care professionals are likely to work with families whose primary need is for support for the normalized routine they have developed, as well as with families who are struggling to achieve or sustain a normalized family life. Parents who indicate that they have been successful in incorporating the condition into everyday family life appreciate being commended for their efforts. Moreover, they need to know that health care providers understand their desire for flexibility in the treatment regimen and are willing to work with the family to develop a routine that supports optimal condition control without making the condition the sole focus of family life. On the other hand, families who see normalization as an unattainable goal may need help in recognizing the many normal aspects of their child and the various family strengths they have to draw on to make life, in the context of the chronic condition, more livable. The Nursing Intervention Classification (Dochterman & Bulechek, 2004) described 24 different activities that nurses can do to promote normalization. Examples of these activities include deemphasizing the uniqueness of the child's condition; identifying adaptations needed to accommodate the child's limitations so the child can participate in normal activities; and encouraging the family to maintain usual family habits, rituals, and routines.

It also is important to bear in mind that normalization may not always be an appropriate goal and that there are times when it is necessary to focus on the condition because of an exacerbation or a change in the usual treatment routine. However, a temporary focus on the condition need not signal the end of a normalized family life (Knafl & Deatrick, 2002).

Survivorship. The Centers for Disease Control and Prevention and the Lance Armstrong Foundation define *cancer survivorship* as the experience of living with, through, and beyond a cancer diagnosis. People with cancer are considered survivors from the point of diagnosis and for the balance of life as are their family and friends, because they too are greatly affected by the diagnosis (Centers for Disease Control and Prevention, 2004). This definition of survivorship and its application are germane not only to childhood cancer, a chronic condition, but to the entire set of chronic health conditions that can affect families. Survivorship has been conceptualized as having three phases: (1) acute, which occurs around the time of diagnosis and initial treatment; (2) extended, which appears when the disease has been controlled or the intensive treatment phase has been completed; and (3) permanent, which is a time of periodic monitoring and possibly intermittent treatment (Mullan, 1985).

In clinical pediatric oncology, survivorship denotes the phase in which the young person has successfully completed primary therapy plus a period of intensive monitoring for recurrence, and is considered "cured." Entry to the survivorship phase does not mean that the risk for disease recurrence has become zero, nor does it mean that toxic side effects have been resolved or are even fully known. Mounting evidence shows that effective treatment regimens can place long-term survivors at high risk relative to non-ill siblings for developing multiple chronic health conditions, referred to as "late effects," that require lifelong self-management and medical follow-up (Oeffinger, Mertens, Sklar, et al., 2006). Based on these findings, childhood cancer survivors are among the most vulnerable populations seen by health care providers (Oeffinger & Hudson, 2004). Specific late effects have been associated with specific treatment exposures and, overall, can occur in any body organ and in the psychosocial realm (Children's Oncology Group, 2006). These associations can be used to guide risk-based clinical assessment and laboratory monitoring, as well as health education, for survivors.

Although, for the most part, late effects apply to the individual who has been treated for cancer, psychosocial late effects such as posttraumatic stress (PTS) symptoms can arise in family members who have secondarily experienced diagnosis and treatment. In one study, the majority of families had at least one parent with a moderate to severe level of PTS symptoms (Alderfer, Cnaan, Annunziato, et al., 2005). In another, most (81%) siblings of childhood cancer survivors had elevated PTS symptoms, with 39% having a moderate level (Alderfer, Labay, & Kazak, 2003). Given these findings, primary care practitioners should apply a family-centered care approach to survivorship by screening siblings and parents of children with chronic health conditions for psychosocial late effects, including symptoms of depression, anxiety, and PTS.

Although monitoring for late effects in survivorship has focused almost exclusively on undesired sequelae, advantageous outcomes

have also been evidenced in adolescent survivors of childhood cancer and their mothers and fathers (Barakat, Alderfer, & Kazak, 2005). As a whole, these types of changes are referred to as posttraumatic growth (PTG) and seem to result from positive interpretations and finding meaning in the illness experience. The five domains of PTG have been shown to include personal strength, new possibilities, relating to others, appreciation of life, and spiritual changes (Calhoun & Tedeschi, 2006). Posttraumatic growth and symptoms of PTS are not mutually exclusive; both can be present, and levels can shift with time. Providers can help families by understanding that the experience of a chronic childhood health condition can have outcomes that are beneficial and also harmful, offering anticipatory guidance about them to families, and acknowledging and supporting family members' expression of both types of outcomes.

The idea of survivorship has become increasingly relevant with the development of intensive and time-limited "curative" therapies such as surgical cardiac repairs or solid organ transplantation for conditions that can nonetheless relapse, or when the therapies may bear their own possibilities for adverse health outcomes. As a result, more and more children with chronic health conditions will survive well into adulthood, for some yet unknown amount of time, and experience the implications of their condition and its treatment for themselves, their families, and their future offspring. In response, programs have been developed that provide comprehensive long-term follow-up. Development of these programs rests on the view that long-term survivors, including the family, have unique needs that deserve attention from educated and trained providers. To maximize quality of life in survivorship, childhood cancer survivors, and possibly survivors of other chronic childhood health conditions, need care that includes the following: risk-based medical and psychosocial monitoring, reproductive and sexuality counseling, genetic counseling for individuals with hereditary conditions, interventions as clinically indicated, ongoing support, education about the risks to which they are susceptible, and preventive approaches that have been effective for the general population (Hewitt, Weiner, & Simone, 2006). Given its nature, the care should be multidisciplinary and guided by knowledge of the individual's condition, treatment, and the evidence about the persistent and late-onset complications that have been associated with them. Access to research that aims to describe and identify effective ways to manage survivorship issues is another essential feature of the necessary care (Aziz, Oeffinger, Brooks, et al., 2006; Friedman, Freyer & Levitt, 2006).

In childhood cancer, the treatment center usually assumes responsibility for long-term follow-up care that may be offered in a distinct survivorship clinic where practitioners with a particular interest and expertise in survivorship apply a holistic and wellness-oriented approach to care. When the treating practitioner also gives long-term follow-up care, the approach tends to be more disease focused. Among other advantages, the use of the survivorship clinic model can allow the identification of patterns in late effects, which, in turn, can compel fine-tuning efficacious treatment regimens to maintain the survival advantage while reducing late effects in future affected individuals. However, the needs of adult survivors are not best addressed in pediatric settings. It is conceivable for long-term follow-up to be delivered in primary care settings during routine health visits. Although this approach could better foster a sense of return to normalcy, some community providers may lack knowledge about potential late effects, as well as time to sufficiently address them. In each model communication between specialty and primary care providers is essential (Friedman et al., 2006; Hewitt et al., 2006).

The Children's Oncology Group's "Long-Term Follow-Up Guidelines for Survivors of Childhood, Adolescent, and Young Adult Cancers" version 2 (Children's Oncology Group, 2006) provides an excellent example of the evidence-derived recommendations for risk-based monitoring and health education that can be developed for populations of survivors. Ideally, pediatric specialty and primary care providers will facilitate the reduction of potential late effects such as secondary cancers by initiating health education, including avoidance of tobacco smoke, use of sunscreen, and protection against genital human papillomavirus infection. Promoting these behaviors will help families to maintain or adopt targeted risk-reduction healthy lifestyle behaviors and to enhance family hope and sense of control over possible late effects (Greving & Santacroce, 2005; Pagano-Therrien & Santacroce, 2005).

Conceptual Frameworks for Understanding Families and Guiding Practice

Nursing has a long-standing interest in working with families in which a child has a chronic condition. A number of well-established models exist to help the nurse understand important dimensions of the family experience of a childhood chronic condition and develop interventions that support healthy child and family functioning. Stress and coping models address family functioning in the context of a childhood chronic condition. In contrast, the family management model focuses more narrowly on the treatment regimen and how the family incorporates the illness into daily family life. The Calgary Assessment and Intervention Models provide a framework for intervening to help families cope with the challenges of a childhood chronic condition (Wright & Leahey, 2005).

Stress and Coping Models

As generally applied to the study of human responses to illness, stress and coping models use an information processing perspective to explain how individuals cognitively process illness events to create meaning and adapt. Stress and coping models assume that stress is not inherent in illness but depends on the individual's cognitive appraisal of stress, that is, an appraisal that an illness event is dangerous and its demands exceed available resources. Variation in what individuals appraise as stress has been largely attributed to personal differences in internal and external characteristics and resources for coping.

The Family Resilience Framework (FRF) (Coleman & Ganong, 2002) represents a research-based and clinical practice–informed derivative of stress and coping models for use with families experiencing events that are generally recognized as extreme stressors: natural disasters, interpersonal violence (including war), and serious illness or a chronic condition. When employed in the study of family responses to chronic conditions, FRF addresses how the family as a unit responds and adapts. The feature that distinguishes FRF from other stress and coping models is its emphasis on strengths and protective factors and functional coping strategies, such as resilience and problem-solving communication patterns, rather than on pathology (Coleman & Ganong, 2002). The overarching goal for assessments and interventions derived from the

FRF is the identification and development of existing and potential strengths and competencies to enhance family function and well-being.

Resilience, the central construct in FRF, had previously been viewed as an impervious characteristic possessed by extraordinary individuals. Within this perspective, studies of resilient individuals highlighted the role of extrafamilial caring adults in helping resilient individuals rise above their hopelessly dysfunctional families (Walsh, 2002). Gradually, informed by research, resilience came to be seen as more ordinary, arising from normative adaptive functions by individuals, families, and communities (Masten, 2001).

Resilience is most currently conceptualized as the dynamic process of adaptation in the context of significant stress. Resiliency is the constructive behavioral patterns and functional competencies that families demonstrate under difficult circumstances. These patterns and competencies support a family's ability to ensure the well-being of its members and maintain the integrity of the family as a whole (McCubbin, Thompson, & McCubbin, 1996). The current view incorporates both ecological and developmental perspectives, seeing the family as an open system that is influenced by the broader sociocultural context with the potential for change and growth over time. Stress emerges from interactions among individual and family vulnerabilities, life experiences, and the sociocultural context. Family distress arises from unsuccessful attempts to cope with stress. The pile-up of internal and external stressors can overwhelm the family and heighten risk for future problems (McCubbin & Patterson, 1983).

According to the FRS, assessment is a multisystem process and should attend to concurrent and multiple family stressors over time, multigenerational influences, family processes for coping with adversity, and family functioning in the context of both normative and unpredictable stressful events. Interventions can be focused at the level of the individual, couple, family, multiple family groups, or the larger system, for example, school and health care systems, depending on the relevance of the system level to resolution of the problem. In the present view, parents rather than extrafamilial adults are the key mediators of individual and family stress and a focus of interventions to enhance family resilience. The current perspective recognizes growth as a potential outcome of "struggling well" (Rolland & Walsh, 2006) with stress or adversity, and emphasizes preventive efforts and interventions that enhance families' abilities to not only overcome specific current challenges but also to broadly apply their skills and resources to handle future situations more effectively (Walsh, 2002).

The stressors associated with serious pediatric chronic conditions pose a significant challenge to families and require considerable amounts of resilience and other resources for functional coping, adaptation, and growth. The FRF is a suitable framework for studying family responses to chronic childhood conditions and designing strength-based interventions to promote functional family coping in the context of a serious childhood chronic condition. There is evidence of the utility of the FRF in studying the predictors of functional family coping with the stressors and demands associated with the diagnosis and active treatment phases of childhood cancer (McCubbin, Balling, Possin, et al., 2002). Six resiliency factors for families of children with cancer have been identified: rapid mobilization and reorganization; support from the health care team in the form of availability, information, and respect; support from extended family in the form of respite care, transportation, and emotional support; support from the community in the form of financial assistance, home maintenance, and emotional assistance; support from the workplace in the form of flexible scheduling, time off, and job assurance; and personal and family beliefs that allow a focus on the positive. The factors indicate areas for assessment of resilience in families of children with serious health conditions, as well as targets for interventions to promote resilience.

Family Management Models

In recent years there has been a growing interest in uncovering patterns of family response to childhood chronic conditions and developing typologies of response that can be used to guide individualized interventions. Because they are based on multiple aspects of family life, typologies have the advantage of preserving and conveying how the family as a unit responds to a chronic condition.

Over the past 40 years, a number of investigators have identified patterns or typologies of response to childhood chronic conditions. For example, in two early studies of family response to a childhood chronic condition, Davis (1963) reported two overarching patterns of response (normalization and disassociation) and Darling (1979) identified four patterns of response (normalization, altruism, crusadership, and resignation). Both of these typologies support the observation made in the previous section on normalization that some, but not all, families report being able to lead a normal family life despite their child's condition.

Building on earlier efforts to identify typologies of family response to chronic conditions, Knafl and Deatrick (1990) formulated the Family Management Style Framework (FMSF) to guide research efforts directed toward further typology development and clinical assessment of families in which there is a child with a chronic condition. The most current version of the framework (Knafl & Deatrick, 2003) conceptualizes family management style (FMS) as the pattern formed by individual family members' definitions of the situation, management behaviors, and perceived illness consequences. The FMSF directs the researcher or clinician to focus on how family members are actively engaged in the management of the illness and how their subjective views of their situation and the impact of the chronic condition on family life shape their management efforts. The framework takes into account the definitions of the situation, management behaviors, and perceived consequences of all or a subset of family members. The actual management style is the pattern formed across family members. Family members' subjective perceptions of sociocultural factors also shape their FMS, which, in turn, influences individual and family functioning.

The FMSF is composed of three conceptual dimensions: definition of the situation, management behaviors, and perceived consequences. Definition of the situation is the subjective meaning family members attribute to their situation. Management behaviors are the discrete behavioral accommodations that family members use to manage the condition on a daily basis. These include efforts directed to caring for the condition, as well as those aimed at incorporating condition management into everyday family life. Perceived consequences are family members' perceptions of the impact of condition management on family life. The framework conceptualizes sociocultural context as family members' subjective perceptions of factors influencing their approach to

TABLE 5-1	
Major Components and Conceptual Themes of the Family Management Model	
Conceptual Component	**Conceptual Themes**
Definition of the situation	*Child identity:* Parents' views of the child and the extent to which those views focus on illness or normalcy and capabilities or vulnerabilities
	Illness view: Parents' beliefs about the cause, seriousness, predictability, and course of the illness
	Management mindset: Parents' views of the ease or difficulty of carrying out the treatment regimen and their ability to manage effectively
	Parental mutuality: Parents' beliefs about the extent to which they have shared or discrepant views of the child, the illness, their parenting philosophy, and their approach to illness management
Management behaviors	*Parenting philosophy:* Parents' goals, priorities, and values that guide the overall approach and specific strategies for illness management
	Management approach: Parents' assessment of the extent to which they have developed a routine and related strategies for managing the illness and incorporating it into family life
Perceived consequences	*Family focus:* Parents' assessment of the balance between illness management and other aspects of family life
	Future expectation: Parents' assessment of the implications of the illness for their child's and family's future

illness management. At any point, family members may identify sociocultural influences such as past experiences with health care providers, culturally based beliefs about illness, or family rules and boundaries as exerting an influence on how they define and manage their child's chronic condition and how they perceive its consequences.

Research across a broad range of chronic conditions has contributed to the further specification of themes that comprise the three major components of the framework. These themes are summarized in Table 5-1. By questioning families about the defining themes, the clinician develops a comprehensive understanding of the family's beliefs about the child, the condition, and their ability to work as a family unit to manage the condition. The management behavior themes provide insights into the extent to which condition management is guided by a particular set of goals and values and has been integrated into everyday family routines. Questions addressing the perceived consequences themes provide information on whether or not the condition is viewed as foreground or background in family life and if family members see the condition as shaping their child's and their family's future. An understanding of how these themes are manifested in individual families contributes to the practitioner's understanding of both family strengths and areas of difficulty with regard to condition management. For example, assessment may reveal that parents have shared views of the child, the illness, and their management goals, but are finding it difficult to develop a routine that accommodates the treatment regimen and other family life responsibilities. Based on this assessment, the practitioner may direct interventions toward developing a flexible illness management routine that lessens the family's focus on condition management. Most recently the developers of the FMSF have developed a standardized measure for assessing family management, the Family Management Measure (FaMM) (Knafl, Deatrick, Gallo, et al., 2007). The measure, as well as detailed information on its development and use, is available at www.ohsu.edu/son/famm.

Assessment and Intervention Models

Before closing at the end of 2007, the faculty associated with the Family Nursing Unit (FNU) of the University of Calgary nursing program had provided direct care for over 25 years to families experiencing a member's chronic condition. The FNU also served as a training ground for practitioners worldwide who were interested in applying the Calgary Assessment and Intervention Models. The models have been described in major publications (Wright & Leahey, 2005; Wright, Watson, & Bell, 1996), and additional training is available through videotapes. Directed toward practitioners in a variety of primary care settings (community, pediatric, maternity, mental health), the Calgary Models are intended to be practical guidelines for practitioners committed to providing family-centered care. The Calgary Models are predicated on the assumption that both practitioners and families have important areas of expertise related to the family's illness experiences, that there is no single, correct solution to any problem, and that practitioners and family members work together to create solutions to condition-related problems (Leahey & Harper-Jaques, 1996) .

The intent of the Calgary Family Assessment Model (CFAM) is to provide a "map of the family . . . so that family strengths and problems can be identified" (Wright & Leahey, 2005, p. 12). Assessment occurs across three major aspects of family life—structural, developmental, and functional. Wright and Leahey (2005) specify categories of data that might be relevant in each area and provide examples of questions that could be used to elicit data. For example, structural family data includes information on the internal family (e.g., composition, subsystems), the external family (e.g., extended family, other systems) and the family's social context (e.g., ethnicity, spirituality). Developmental assessment directs the practitioner's attention to the tasks associated with different stages of the family's life cycle. Functional assessment focuses on routine aspects of daily living such as meal preparation and treatment regimen management, as well as the roles and interactions associated with carrying out usual family activities. CFAM offers a comprehensive "menu of possibilities" for assessment, and the practitioner is advised to be selective in determining the ones that are relevant and appropriate areas for assessment in a given family. For example, the assessment of developmental issues may be especially relevant in the family of a child with diabetes who is making the transition to adolescence. On the other hand, functional assessment targeting the family's usual routine may be more appropriate in families who are having difficulty carrying out a prescribed treatment regimen. Wright and Leahey (2005) advocate the use of three-generation family genograms and ecomaps as useful strategies for engaging families in the assessment process and eliciting considerable information about key aspects of family life. The ecomap is a diagram of each family member's ties to persons and systems outside of the family. Taken together, the genogram and ecomap efficiently summarize considerable information about the family's internal and external structure.

The Calgary Family Intervention Model (CFIM) is a problem- and solution-focused approach for promoting or sustaining family functioning in the context of a condition-related challenge. CFIM is not a long-term therapy approach, and its focus on solving current problems makes it a useful tool for the primary care practitioner. CFIM assumes that families have the ability to solve their own problems related to living with a chronic condition and that the role of the provider is to offer, rather than prescribe, possibly helpful solutions. According to this model, interventions take place across three domains of family life—cognitive, affective, and behavioral. Cognitive interventions target family beliefs that make living with the condition more difficult. For example, the practitioner might note parents' firmly held beliefs about the fatal nature of cancer and provide information on survivorship programs in order to change beliefs about the condition and lessen fears about the future. Wright and Leahey (2005) note that commendations that identify family strengths are especially powerful cognitive interventions that help family members form a more positive view of themselves and their ability to address health-related problems.

In contrast to cognitive interventions, which focus on family beliefs, affective interventions focus on decreasing emotional response to the condition as a way to set the stage for effective problem solving; acknowledging the normalcy of an intense emotional response can help family members consider when such responses are appropriate and when they impede problem solving. The third category of interventions, behavioral, invites family members to do certain things such as become more directly involved in condition care or take a respite from caregiving, both of which can contribute to a parent's sense of competence as caregivers.

For primary care practitioners interacting with families in which a child has a chronic condition, the Calgary Assessment and Interventions Model can provide a practical, comprehensive guide that promotes both problem solving and a positive working relationship between the practitioner and the family.

The Family and Primary Care Practitioners

The challenges presented by chronic conditions for primary care practitioners are clearly different from those facing the family. For the practitioner, the challenge is identifying interventions that contribute to optimal child and family adaptation. Family-practitioner communications that are characterized by courtesy, respect for the family as unique and also knowledgeable, and mutual engagement in arriving at decisions that balance quality of life and medical goals are critical to beneficial health care encounters and optimal health outcomes (Thorne, Harris, Mahoney, et al., 2004). When chronic condition outcomes depend on adherence to medications and other aspects of self-management, acknowledging that the family is doing its best given the complexities of life and using a nonjudgmental approach to problem solving are particularly important (Thorne et al., 2004).

The challenges for primary care practitioners include not only communications with the family but also with the team of specialty practitioners with whom they collaborate to provide care for children with chronic health conditions. Primary care practitioners usually recognize the need for diagnostic evaluation, help children and families with decision making and communication, and facilitate specialty referrals. After the diagnostic process is completed, primary care practitioners require information from specialists about diagnosis and management, implications for other family members, and available supportive services even when the condition is asymptomatic or specialists assume prime responsibilities for coordinating medical care (McDaniel, Peters, & Acheson, 2006). During treatment phase(s), primary care practitioners hold responsibility for routine health maintenance and management of coexisting conditions that are not under specialty care. Care may be transferred back to primary care practitioners when the child's condition is stable or some years after intensive treatment has been completed, with referral back to specialists for periodic evaluation and when problems arise. Collaborative care relies on information sharing, the frequency of which is determined by risk for disease progression/recurrence and secondary health problems. Electronic medical records are a means of creating records that summarize the child's medical history, treatment, and actual and potential problems. Web-based electronic records can be accessed and updated by authorized providers to improve practitioner communications (Oeffinger & McCabe, 2006). Equipped with information, primary care providers are well positioned to make important contributions to the family's ability to adapt to the challenges of a child's chronic condition in ways that maximize child health and child and family quality of life.

REFERENCES

Alderfer. M., Cnaan, A., & Annunziato, R., et al. (2005). Patterns of posttraumatic stress symptoms in parents of childhood cancer survivors. *J Fam Psychol, 19,* 430-440.

Alderfer, M., Labay, L., & Kazak, A. (2003). Brief report: Does post-traumatic stress apply to siblings of childhood cancer survivors? *J Pediatr Psychol, 28,* 282-286.

American Psychological Association. (1994). *Diagnostic and Statistical Manual of Mental Disorders: DSM IV* (4th ed.). Washington, DC: Author.

American Psychological Association. (2000). *Diagnostic and Statistical Manual of Mental Disorders: DSM IV-TR* (5th ed.). Washington, DC: Author.

Aziz, N., Oeffinger, K., & Brooks, S., et al. (2006). Comprehensive long-term follow-up programs for pediatric cancer survivors. *Cancer, 107,* 841-848.

Barakat, L., Alderfer, M., & Kazak, A. (2005). Posttraumatic growth in adolescent survivors of cancer and their mothers and fathers. *J Pediatr Psychol, 31,* 413-419.

Barlow, J., & Ellard, D. (2006). The psychosocial well-being of children with chronic disease, their parents and siblings: An overview of the research evidence base. *Child Care, Health Dev, 32,* 19-31.

Bethell, C., Read, D., & Blumberg, S., et al. (2008). What is the prevalence of children with special health care needs? Toward an understanding of vitiations in findings and methods across three national surveys. *Mat Child Health J, 12,* 1-14.

Bisson, J. (2002). Post-traumatic stress disorder. In S.Barton (Ed.), *Clinical Evidence* (7th ed., pp.177-178). London: BMJ Publishing Group.

Burke, S., Kauffmann, E., & Harrison, M., et al. (1999). Assessment of stressors in families with a child who has a chronic condition. *Am J Mat Child Nurs, 24,* 98-106.

Calhoun, L., & Tedeschi, R. (Eds.). (2006). *Handbook of Posttraumatic Growth Research and Practice.* Mahwah, NJ: Lawrence Erlbaum Associates.

Campbell, T. (2000). Physical illness: Challenges to families. In S. Price, (Ed.), *Families and Change: Coping with Stressful Events and Transitions,* Thousand Oaks, CA: Sage.

Carpentier, M., Mullins, L., Chaney, J., et al. (2006). The relationship of illness uncertainty and attributional style to tong-term psychological distress in parents of children with type 1 diabetes mellitus. *Children's Health Care, 35,* 141-154.

Carpentier, M., Mullins, L., Van Pelt, J. (2007). Psychological, academic, and work functioning in college students with childhood-onset asthma. *J Asthma, 44,* 119-124.

Centers for Disease Control and Prevention. (2004). *A national action plan for cancer survivorship: Advancing public health policy.* Available at www.cdc.gov/cancer/survivorship/survivorpdf/plan. Retrieved January 21, 2008.

Children's Oncology Group (2006). *Long-term follow-up guidelines for survivors of childhood, adolescent, and young adult cancers V.2.* Available at from www.survivorshipguidelines.org/pdf/LTFUGuidelines.pdf. Retrieved November 3, 2008.

Clarke-Steffen, L. (1993a). A model of the family transition to living with childhood cancer. *Cancer Pract, 1,* 285-292.

Clarke-Steffen, L. (1993b). Waiting and not knowing: The diagnosis of cancer in a child. *J Pediatr Oncol Nurs, 10,* 146-153.

Clarke-Steffen, L. (1997). Reconstructing reality: Family strategies for managing childhood cancer. *J Pediatr Nurs, 12,* 278-287.

Cohen, M. (1993a). Diagnostic closure and the spread of uncertainty. *Issues Compr Pediatr Nurs, 16,* 135-146.

Cohen, M. (1993b). The unknown and the unknowable—managing sustained uncertainty. *West J Nurs Res, 15*(1), 77-96.

Cohen, M. (1995a). The stages of the prediagnostic period in chronic, life-threatening childhood illness: A process analysis. *Res Nurs Health, 18,* 39-48.

Cohen, M. (1995b). The triggers of heightened parental uncertainty in chronic, life-threatening childhood illness. *Qual Health Res, 5,* 63-77.

Cohen, M., & Martinson, I. (1988). Chronic uncertainty: Its effects on parental appraisal of a child's health. *J Pediatr Nurs, 3*(2), 89-96.

Coleman, M., & Ganong, L. (2002). Resilience and families. *Family Relations, 51,* 101-102.

Comaroff, J., & Maguire, P. (1981). Ambiguity and the search for meaning: Childhood leukemia in the modern clinical context. *Soc Sci Med, 15B,* 115-123.

Darling, R. (1979). *Families Against Society: A Study of Reactions to Children with Birth Defects.* Beverly Hills, CA: Sage.

Davidoff, A.J. (2004). Identifying children with special health care needs in the national health interview survey: A new resource for policy analysis. *Health Serv Res, 39,* 53-71.

Davis, F. (1963). *Passage Through Crisis: Polio Victims and Their Families.* Minneapolis: Bobbs-Merrill.

Deatrick, J., Knafl, K., & Murphy-Moore, C. (1999). Clarifying the concept of normalization. *Image: J Nurs Sch, 31,* 209-214.

Decker, C., Haase, J., & Bell, C. (2007). Uncertainty in adolescents and young adults with cancer. *Oncol Nurs Forum, 34,* 681-688.

Dochterman, J., & Bulechek, G. (2004). *Nursing Interventions Classification (NIC)* (4th ed.). St. Louis: Mosby.

Edmunds, L. (2005). Parents' perceptions of health professionals' responses when seeking help for their overweight children. *J Fam Pract, 22,* 287-292.

Federal Interagency Forum on Child and Family Statistics (2007). *America's Children: Key National Indicators of Wellbeing 2007. Federal Interagency Forum on Child and Family Statistics.* Washington, DC: U.S. Government Printing Office.

Freidman, D., Freyer, D., & Levitt, G. (2006). Models of care for survivors of childhood cancer. *Pediatr Blood Cancer, 46,* 159-168.

Friedman, D., Holmbeck, G.N., Jandasek, B. et al (2004). Parent functioning in families of preadolescents with spina bifida: Longitudinal implications for child adjustment. *J Fam Psychol, 18,* 609-619.

Gallo, A.M., & Knafl, K. (1998). Parents' reports of "tricks of the trade" for managing childhood chronic illness. *J Soc Pediatr Nurs, 3,* 93-100.

Gerhardt, C.A., Vannatta, K., McKellop, J.M., et al. (2003). Comparing parental distress, family functioning, and the role of social support for caregivers with and without a child with juvenile rheumatoid arthritis. *J Pediatr Psychol, 28,* 5-15.

Giammona, A.J., & Malek, D.M. (2002). The psychological effect of childhood cancer on families. *Pediatr Clin North Am, 49,* 1063-1081.

Gilliss, C., & Knafl, K. (1999). Nursing care of families in non-normative transitions: The state of the science and practice. In A. Hinshaw, S. Feetham, & J. Shaver (Eds.), *Handbook for Clinical Nursing Research,* Newbury Park, CA: Sage.

Goffman, E. (1963). *Stigma: Notes on the Management of Spoiled Identity.* Englewood Cliffs, NJ: Lawrence Erlbaum Associates.

Graf, A., Landolt, M.A., Capone Mori, A., et al. (2006). Quality of life and psychosocial adjustment in children and adolescents with neurofibromatosis type 1. *J Pediatr, 149,* 348-353.

Greving, D., & Santacroce, S.J. (2005). Cardiovascular late effects. *J Pediatr Oncol Nurs, 2,* 38-47.

Grey, M., Cameron, M., Lipman, T., et al. (1995). Psychosocial status of children with diabetes over the first two years. *Diabetes Care, 18,* 1330-1336.

Haase, J., & Rostad, M. (1994). Experiences of completing cancer therapy: Children's perspectives. *Oncol Nurs Forum, 21,* 1483-1492.

Hatton, D., Canam, C., Thorne, S., et al. (1995). Parents' perceptions of caring for an infant or toddler with diabetes. *J Adv Nurs, 22,* 569-577.

Hewitt, M., Weiner, S., & Simone, J. (2006). *Childhood Cancer Survivorship: Improving Care and Quality of Life.* Washington, DC: National Academies Press.

Hinds, P., Birenbaum, L., Clarke-Steffen, L., et al. (1996). Coming to terms: Parents' response to a first cancer recurrence in their child. *Nurs Res, 45,* 148-153.

Holmbeck, G.N., Greenley, R.N., Coakley, R.M., et al. (2006). Family functioning in children and adolescents with spina bifida: An evidence-based review of research and interventions. *J Dev Behav Pediatr, 27,* 249-277.

Horner, S. (1998). Catching the asthma: Family care for school-aged children with asthma. *J Pediatr Nurs, 13,* 356-366.

Jessop, D.J., & Stein, R.E. (1985). Uncertainty and its relation to the psychological and social correlates of chronic illness in children. *Soc Sci Med, 20*(10), 993-999.

Kazak, A., Stuber, M., Barakat, L., et al. (1998). Predicting posttraumatic stress disorders in mothers and fathers of survivors of childhood cancers. *J Am Acad Child Adolesc Psychiatry, 37,* 823-831.

Kessler, R. (2000). Posttraumatic stress disorder: The burden to an individual and society. *J Clin Psychiatry, 61*(S5), 4-12.

Knafl, K., & Deatrick, J. (1990). Family management style: Concept analysis and development. *J Pediatr Nurs, 5,* 4-14.

Knafl, K., & Deatrick, J. (2002). The challenge of normalization for families of children with chronic conditions. *J Pediatr Nurs, 28,* 49-53.

Knafl, K., & Deatrick, J. (2003). Further refinement of the family management style framework. *J Fam Nurs, 9,* 232-256.

Knafl, K., Deatrick, J., Gallo, A., et al. (2007). The analysis and interpretation of cognitive interview for instrument development. *Res Nurs Health, 30,* 224-234.

Knafl, K., Deatrick, J., & Kirby, A. (2001). Normalization promotion. In M. Craft-Rosenberg, & J. Denehy, (Eds.). *Nursing Interventions for Infants, Children, and Families.* Thousand Oaks, CA: Sage.

Knafl, K., & Gilliss, C. (2002). Families and chronic illness: A synthesis of the literature. *J Fam Nurs, 8,* 178-198.

Koocher, G.P. (1985). Psychosocial care of the child cured of cancer. *Pediatr Nurs, 11*(2), 91-93.

Lavigne, J.V., & Faier-Routman, J. (1992). Psychological adjustment to pediatric physical disorders: A meta-analytic review. *J Pediatr Psychol, 17,* 133-157.

Leahey, M., & Harper-Jaques, S. (1996). Family-nurse relationships: Core assumptions and clinical implications. *J Fam Nurs, 2,* 133-151.

LoBato, D., Faust, D., & Spirito, A. (1988). Examining the effects f chronic disease and disability on children's sibling relationships. *J Pediatr Psychol, 13,* 389-407.

Mast, M. (1995). Adult uncertainty in illness: A critical review of research (including commentary by Mishel, M.). *Sch Inq Nurs Pract, 9,* 3-29.

Masten, A. (2001). Ordinary magic: Resilience processes in development. *Am Psychol, 56,* 227-238.

McClellan, C., & Cohen, L. (2007). Family functioning in children with chronic illness compared to healthy controls: A critical review. *J Pediatr, 150,* 221-223.

McCubbin, M., Balling, K., Possin, P., et al. (2002). Family resiliency in childhood cancer. *Family Relations, 51,* 103-111.

McCubbin, M., & Patterson, J. (1983). The family stress process: The double helix ABCDX model of adjustment and adaptation. In H. McCubbin, M. Sussman, & J. Patterson, (Eds.), *Social Stress and the Family: Advances in Family Stress Theory and Research,* New York: Haworth.

McCubbin, H., Thompson, A., & McCubbin, M. (1996). *Family Assessment: Resiliency, Coping, and Adaptation.* Madison, WI: University of Wisconsin.

McDaniel, S., Peters,., J., & Acheson, L. (2006). Professional collaboration to assess and care for genetic disorders. In S. Miller, S. McDaniel, J. Rolland, et al. (Eds.), *Individuals, Families, and the New Era of Genetics: Biopsychosocial Perspectives,* New York: W.W. Norton.

Mishel, M.H. (1981). The measurement of uncertainty in illness. *Nurs Res, 30,* 258-263.

Mishel, M.H. (1983). Parents' perception of uncertainty concerning their hospitalized child. *Nurs Res, 32,* 324-330.

Mishel, M.H. (1988). Uncertainty in illness. *Image J Nurs Sch, 20,* 225-232.

Mishel, M.H. (1990). Reconceptualization of uncertainty in illness theory. *Image J Nurs Sch, 22,* 256-262.

Mishel, M.H. (1997). *Uncertainty in Illness Scale Manual.* Chapel Hill, NC: University of North Carolina.

Mishel, M.H. (1999). Uncertainty in chronic illness. *Ann Rev Nurs Res, 17,* 269-294.

Mitchell, M.J., Lemanek, K., Palermo, T.M., et al. (2007). Parent perspectives on pain management, coping, and family functioning in pediatric sickle cell disease. *Clin Pediatr (Phil), 46,* 311-319.

Mullan, F. (1985). Seasons of survival: Reflections of a physician with cancer. *N Engl J Med, 313,* 270-273.

Mullin, L., Wolfe-Christensen, C., Pai, A., et al. (2007). The relationship of parental overprotection, perceived child vulnerability and parenting stress to uncertainty in youth with chronic illness. *J Pediatr Psychol, 32,* 973-982.

Mussatto, K. (2006). Adaptation of the child and family to life with a chronic illness. *Cardiol Young, 16*(Suppl 3), 110-116.

Neville, K. (1998). The relationship among uncertainty, social support, and psychological distress in adolescents recently diagnosed with cancer. *J Pediatr Oncol Nurs, 15,* 37-46.

O'Dea, J. (2005). Prevention of child obesity: "First do no harm." *Health Educ Res, 20,* 259-265.

Oeffinger, K., & Hudson, M. (2004). Long-term complications following child and adolescent cancer: Foundations for providing risk-based health care for survivors. *CA Cancer J Clin, 54,* 208-236.

Oeffinger, K., & McCabe, M. (2006). Models for delivering survivorship care. *J Clin Oncol, 24,* 5117-5124.

Oeffinger, K., Mertens, A., Sklar, C., et al., for the Childhood Cancer Survivor Study. (2006). Chronic health conditions in adult survivors of childhood cancer. *N Engl J Med, 355,* 1572-1582.

Pagano-Therrien, J., & Santacroce, S.J. (2005). Bone mineral density decrements and children diagnosed with cancer. *J Pediatr Oncol Nurs, 22,* 328-338.

Parry, C. (2003). Embracing uncertainty: An exploration of the experiences of childhood cancer survivors. *Qual Health Res, 13,* 227-246.

Pless, I., & Pinkerton, P. (1975). *Chronic Childhood Disorder: Promoting Patterns of Adjustment.* Chicago: Year Book Medical Publishers.

Preechawong, S., Zauszniewski, J.A., Heinzer, M.M., et al. (2007). Relationships of family functioning, self-esteem, and resourceful coping of Thai adolescents with asthma. *Issues Ment Health Nurs, 28,* 21-36.

Rehm, R.S., & Bradley, J.F. (2005). Normalization in families raising a child who is medically fragile/technology dependent and developmentally delayed. *Qual Health Res, 15,* 807-820.

Robinson, C.A. (1993). Managing life with a chronic condition: The story of normalization. *Qual Health Res, 3,* 6-28.

Rodenburg, R., Meijer, A.M., Dekovic, M., et al. (2005). Family factors and psychopathology in children with epilepsy: A literature review. *Epilepsy Behav, 6,* 488-503.

Rodrigues, N., & Patterson, J. (2007). Impact of severity of a child's chronic condition on the functioning of two-parent families. *J Pediatr Psychol, 32*(4), 417-426.

Rolland, J. (1984). Toward a psychosocial typology of chronic and life threatening illness. *Fam Syst Med, 2,* 245-262.

Rolland, J. (1994). *Families, Illness, and Disability. An Integrative Treatment Model.* New York: Basic Books.

Rolland, J., & Walsh, F. (2006). Facilitating family resilience with childhood illness and disability. *Curr Opin Pediatr, 18,* 527-538.

Rolland, J., & Williams, J. (2005). Toward a biopsychosocial model for 21st century genetics. *Fam Process, 44,* 3-4.

Rolland, J., & Williams, J. (2006). Toward a psychosocial model for the new era of genetics. In S. Miller, S. McDanile, J. Rolland, (Eds.), *Individuals, Families, and the New Era of Genetics: Biopsychosocial Perspectives,* New York: W.W. Norton.

Salewski, C. (2003). Illness representations in families with a chronically ill adolescent: Differences between family members and impact on patients' outcome variables. *J Health Psychol, 8,* 587-598.

Santacroce, S.J. (2000). Support from health care providers and parental uncertainty during the diagnosis of perinatally-acquired HIV infection. *J Assoc Nurs AIDS Care, 22,* 63-75.

Santacroce, S.J. (2001). Measuring parental uncertainty during the diagnosis phase of serious illness in a child. *J Pediatr Nurs, 16,* 3-12.

Santacroce, S.J. (2002). Uncertainty, anxiety, and symptoms of posttraumatic stress in parents of children recently diagnosed with cancer. *J Pediatr Oncol Nurs, 19,* 104-111.

Santacroce, S.J. (2003). Parental uncertainty and symptoms of posttraumatic stress in serious childhood illness. *J Nurs Sch, 35,* 45-51.

Santacroce, S.J., Deatrick, J., & Ledlie, S. (2002). Redefining treatment: How biological mothers manage their child's treatment of perinatally acquired HIV. *AIDS Care, 14,* 247-260.

Santacroce, S.J., & Lee, Y.-L. (2006). Uncertainty, posttraumatic stress and health behaviors in young adult childhood cancer survivors. *Nurs Res, 55,* 259-266.

Sawyer, M., Antoniou, G., Rice, M., et al. (2000). Childhood cancer: A 4-year prospective study of the psychological adjustment of children and parents. *J Pediatr Hematol Oncol, 22,* 214-220.

Sawyer, M., Spurrier, N., Kennedy, D., et al. (2001). The relationship between the quality of life of children with asthma and family functioning. *J Asthma, 38,* 279-284.

Sawyer, M., Spurrier, N., & Whaites, L., et al. (2000). The relationship between asthma severity, family functioning and the health-related quality of life of children with asthma. *Qual Life Res, 9,* 1105-1115.

Sharkey, T. (1995). The effects of uncertainty in families with children who are chronically ill. *Home Health Nurse, 134,* 37-42.

Spieth, L., Stark, L., & Mitchell, M., et al. (2001). Observational assessment of family functioning at mealtime in preschool children with cystic fibrosis. *J Pediatr Psychol, 26,* 215-224.

Stein, R.E., & Jessop, D. (1982). A non-categorical approach to chronic childhood illness. *Public Health Rep, 97,* 354-362.

Stewart, J. (2003). Getting used to it: Children finding the ordinary and routine in the uncertain context of cancer. *Qual Health Res, 13,* 394-407.

Stewart, J., & Mishel, M. (2000). Uncertainty in childhood illness: A synthesis of the parent and child literature (including commentary by Hayes, V.). *Sch Inq Nurs Pract, 14,* 299-319, 321-326.

Thanarattanakorn, P., Louthrenoo, O., Sittipreechacharn, S., et al. (2003). Family functioning in children with thalassemia. *Clin Pediatr, 42,* 79-82.

Thompson, R., Armstrong, D., Link, C., et al. (2003). A prospective study of the relationship over time of behavior problems, intellectual functioning, and family functioning in children with sickle cell disease: A report from the Cooperative Study of Sickle Cell Disease. *J Pediatr Psychol, 28,* 59-65.

Thorne, S., Harris, S., Mahoney, K., et al. (2004). The context of health communication in chronic illness. *Pat Educ Counsel, 54,* 299-306.

van Dyck, P., Kogan, M., McPherson, M., et al. (2004). Prevalence and characteristics of children with special health care needs. *Arch Pediatr Adolesc Med, 158,* 884-890.

Van Pelt, J., Mullins, L., Carpentier, M., et al. (2006). Illness uncertainty and dispositional self-focus in adolescents and young adults with childhood-onset asthma. *J Pediatr Psychol, 31,* 840-845.

Van Riper, M., & Gallo, A. (2006). Families, health, and genomics. In D. Crane & E. Marshall, (Eds.). *Handbook of Families and Health.* Thousand Oaks, CA: Sage.

Wallender, J., & Varni, J. (1998). Effects of pediatric chronic physical disorders on child and family adjustment. *J Child Psychol Psychiatry, 39,* 29-46.

Walsh, F. (2002). A family resilience framework: Innovative practice applications. *Fam Relations, 51,* 130-137.

Wee, C., McCarthy, E., Davis, R., et al. (2004). Obesity and breast cancer screening. *J Gen Int Med, 26,* 233-246.

Weekes, D., & Kagan, S. (1994). Adolescents completing cancer therapy: Meaning, perception and coping. *Oncol Nurs Forum, 21,* 663-670.

Wijnberg-Williams, B.J., Kamps, W.A., & Klip, E.C., et al. (2006). Psychological adjustment of parents of pediatric cancer patients revisited: Five years later. *Psycho-Oncol, 15,* 1-8.

Williams, T.V., Schone, E.M., & Archibald, N.D., et al. (2004). A national assessment of children with special health care needs: Prevalence of special needs and use of health care services among children in the military health system. *Pediatrics, 114,* 384-393.

Wood, B.L., Lim, J., Miller, B.D., et al. (2007). Family emotional climate, depression, emotional triggering of asthma, and disease severity in pediatric asthma: Examination of pathways of effect. *J Pediatr Psychol, 32,* 542-551.

Wright, L., & Leahey, M. (2005). *Nurses and Families: A Guide to Family Assessment and Intervention* (4th ed.). Philadelphia: F.A. Davis.

Wright, L., Watson, W., & Bell, J. (1996). *Beliefs: The Heart of Healing in Families and Illness.* New York: Basic Books.

6

Family Culture and Chronic Conditions

Roberta S. Rehm

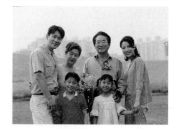

Historical Roots of Diversity

Because America has a long and complex multicultural heritage, it is important for health care providers to understand the roles that culture plays in modern American society in order to provide sensitive and appropriate care for children and families from diverse cultural backgrounds. The components of cultural identity are complex and vary even among people of the same ethnic, racial, or religious group. This chapter explores the interaction of culture and health care and discusses the cultural implications for providing care to children with chronic conditions and their families.

North American Multicultural Heritage

The early seventeenth century English Pilgrims are the best known of the early permanent immigrants to the United States, but explorers, refugees, and immigrants seeking a better life began arriving on North American lands long before the Pilgrims. Scientists believe that humans began migrating to North America from Asia across the Bering land bridge perhaps 12,000 years ago and may be ancestors of some of the peoples now called Native Americans or American Indians (O'Neill, 2005). Although the exact history of the earliest settlers varies according to each tribe's origination myths, it is certain that migration has always been an important factor in U.S. history. Spanish conquistadors began exploring what would become the American Southwest in the early sixteenth century. They led the first permanent colonial era settlers, who arrived in New Mexico in 1598. This group of 800 colonists consisted mostly of natives of Spain or Portugal but also included Mexican Indians and Africans who were servants to the soldiers and settlers (Lavash, 2006).

The foreign-born portion of the U.S. population reached its peak at 14.7% in 1910. In 2003, foreign-born U.S. residents constituted 11.7% of the total population, or 33.5 million people (Larson, 2004). Europeans made up the largest percentage of immigrants to the United States from 1820 (when formal immigration records began) until 1970. Since then the proportion of Hispanic and Asian immigrants has grown significantly. In 2003, 13.7% of immigrants came from Europe, 25% from Asia, and 53.3% from Latin America. Of the Latin American immigrants, 36.9% came from Mexico and Central America, 10.1% from the Caribbean, and 6.3% from South America. Besides these legal entrants, the U.S. government estimates that a million immigrants illegally entered the United States in 2003 or 2004, and over 11 million undocumented immigrants reside in the United States (U.S. Office of Immigrant Statistics, 2006). In the past decade, the number of children in immigrant families has grown seven times faster than the number in families born in the United States; moreover, immigrant children are less likely to have a regular source of health care and less likely to have health insurance than native-born children (Huang, Yu, & Ledsky, 2006).

Dynamic Nature of Culture

These trends in immigration reflect the changing face of our society and the dynamic nature of American culture. It was once presumed that most immigrants would give up traditional values, languages, and ways of life to join the "melting pot" of U.S. society, but scholars now recognize that the melting pot is an American myth. Esmer (2006) found, however, that despite widespread globalization in many areas of economic and political life, over a 20-year period there was little evidence of convergence of values in 20 countries. There are many—not one—American cultures, and no one set of values and practices clearly defines the United States. Increasing migration around the world in the last decade has contributed to the heterogeneity of many nations.

Culture can be characterized in terms of customs and behaviors and meanings exhibited in people's everyday lives, or it can be defined in complex terms that account for tradition, history, recurrent patterns, and common values (Baumeister, 2005; Giger & Davidhizar, 2003). Important definitions of cultural terms are found in Table 6-1. Definitions of culture must be fluid enough to recognize that although all cultural groups have commonalties, there is a great deal of intracultural variation.

Cultural identity can influence health and lifestyles affecting health. Airhihenbuwa, Kumanyika, TenHave, and colleagues (2000) found that people with a strong identity as black or bicultural were likely to make positive health choices such as lower-fat diets and not smoking. Racial identity and ethnic identity form strong components of culture, but many people may personally identify more with cultural subgroups based on less obvious factors than ethnic or racial identity (Schwartz, Zamvoanga, & Weisskirch, 2008). Among the shared understandings that constitute cultural subgroups are those based on factors such as religious beliefs or affiliation (e.g., fundamentalist Christian, Sunni Muslim), physical ability (e.g., mobility impairment, athletic nature), sexual preference or identity (e.g., heterosexual, lesbian), occupation (e.g., plumber, accountant), educational attainment (e.g., illiterate, college student), socioeconomic status (e.g., inherited wealth, homeless), and women's issues (e.g., feminism, maternal status) (Betancourt, Green, Carillo, et al., 2005).

TABLE 6-1
Definitions of Cultural Terms

Culture	A dynamic and negotiated social construction arising from interaction and resulting in shared understandings among people in contact with one another
Discrimination	Different treatment, including restricted opportunities or choices, of people because of factors such as race, class, or physical ability
Ethnicity	A socially, culturally, and/or politically constructed group of individuals that holds a set of characteristics in common; often based on language, national origin, and/or religion
Ethnocentrism	The belief that one's own ways are the best or preferred way to think, believe, or behave
Institutional racism	Intentional or unintentional manipulation or tolerance of institutional policies that unfairly restrict the opportunities of particular groups
Prejudice	Preconceived ideas or opinions about an individual or group based solely on factors such as race, gender, or physical ability
Race	Originally, it was human biologic variation, but racial mixing has given the term little biologic significance; race retains social and political significance and may reflect individual or group identity factors
Racism	An oppressive system of racial relations justified by an ideology in which one racial group benefits from dominating another and defines itself and others through this domination

Religious and Spiritual Influences

Religious and spiritual beliefs are among the most powerful forces that shape human experience. Health care providers for children can incorporate exploration of families' spiritual beliefs into health maintenance visits as part of family-centered pediatric primary care (American Academy of Pediatrics, 2003), although it must be recognized that many families are not overtly religious and may not characterize themselves as religious or spiritual at all. Specific belief systems vary widely and are even sometimes directly contradictory, yet religious faith and spiritual beliefs often provide a sense of comfort, strength, and direction for families coping with concerns about health, illness, life, and death (Coyle, 2002; Robinson, Thiel, Backus, et al., 2006). A concept analysis of holistic nursing in pediatric settings described spirituality as an important component of holistic nursing care. The authors claimed that spirituality is an ever-present force pervading all human experience (Tjale & Bruce, 2007). Spirituality includes practices and beliefs that give meaning to life and help an individual to cultivate inner strength to meet the challenges of daily life. Spirituality may be expressed in an organized religious setting with formal rituals of prayer and worship or more independently with individual practices. Both organized religious belief systems and spirituality that arises from life experiences may provide a set of values by which life can be lived (Sessanna, Finnell, & Jezewski, 2007).

Chronic conditions of childhood may present particular challenges for families, especially in the face of children's suffering, the need for ongoing care, and the possibility of disability or death. Many families seek an explanation for these difficulties in religious beliefs; others use their beliefs to find solace or strength to face the future. One study found that Mexican American parents recognized

three key influences in determining the outcome of their child's chronic condition: God, family, and health care providers (Rehm, 1999). Although these parents gave the ultimate authority to God, they felt that it was important to take excellent care of the child themselves and to seek the best possible professional care to ensure the greatest chance for survival and healing.

In rare instances, families' religious tenets bring them into conflict with health care providers (e.g., when beliefs preclude certain forms of medical care, such as blood transfusion, or lead to preferences for prayer or other healing rituals over biomedical treatment). In such cases, an open dialogue must be maintained with families, and legal and ethical concerns must be formally balanced. When negotiation does not reach a solution acceptable to both the family and the health care provider, the courts may be consulted. Because the dominant value in the United States usually includes preservation of a child's life, families are sometimes forced to accept care that is against their wishes and belief systems (Wilson, 2005). Health care providers must recognize the profound effect of such a situation and work to preserve respectful relationships with the family to ensure ongoing care for the child and to try to avoid future legal conflicts if possible.

Socioeconomic Status and Health

Around the world, economic inequalities and the gap between rich countries and poor countries are growing, facts reflected in continuing disparities in health status (Lewis, 2008; Martens & Rotmans, 2005). Children in the United States are also profoundly affected by poverty. The number of children living in poverty in the United States is growing and included nearly 13 million children in 2005; moreover, poor children are also more likely to lack health insurance coverage (Children's Defense Fund, 2006). Socioeconomic status exerts a profound influence—sometimes even more than ethnic or racial characteristics—on health and well-being. Children from economically secure homes are healthier, do better in school, are more likely to graduate from high school and less likely to commit criminal acts, and earn more money as adults than those from poverty-stricken homes (Zedlewski, 2002). There is a well-established link between poverty and the risk for childhood disability.

Welfare reform legislation, which changed eligibility for income support for children and families, and a generally robust U.S. economy in the 1990s encouraged many mothers and children to leave welfare programs in recent years. More recent downturns in the national economy have focused attention on the still-marginal economic status of many families with one or more employed adults. Families with low-wage jobs often do not receive benefits, such as health insurance, and may not earn enough income to leave poverty behind (Zedlewski, 2002).

Although the majority of poor Americans are white, people of color are disproportionately burdened by poverty and health problems. Black, Latino, and Native American children are more likely than white and Asian children to be uninsured, and less likely to have a usual source of health care (Flores & Tomany-Korman, 2008).

Cultural Power Struggles and the Impact of Globalization

Perhaps because of the nation's long association with European immigrants and their descendants, political and decision-making power has traditionally been held by white European Americans.

Although this group continues to command the greatest degree of political clout, some changes have occurred at both the local and national level, with blacks, Asians, and Latinos playing a larger role in municipal and legislative activities. The 2008 election of Barack Obama as the first African American president of the United States is a particularly striking example. Of foreign-born U.S. residents, 32% have become naturalized U.S. citizens—a percentage that tends to increase with length of residence (Passel, 2005). Over time, most residents of the United States adopt English for official and public transactions, although many people continue to speak other languages in their homes and communities.

There is growing recognition that people around the world are interdependent and that issues related to health, environmental, and economic well-being readily cross national borders. Crigger (2008) examined notions of social justice and nursing ethics in an era of globalization to facilitate discussion of transnational and cross-cultural issues that arise as nurses seek to reduce health disparities for all people. She identified technology and global businesses as particular factors that present dilemmas for fairness and justice that may affect nursing around the world. Within the United States, ethics may assume great importance to practitioners if they find themselves caught between the imperative to provide care for children with special needs and regulations affecting access to care, particularly eligibility for reimbursement of medical expenses. This ethical quandary may be particularly acute when caring for undocumented immigrants, when the requirement to enforce official rules and policies is pitted against personal or professional values to provide care to all in need (Rehm, 2003a; Young, Flores, & Berman, 2004).

Ethnocentrism and Racism

Ethnocentrism and racism (see definitions in Table 6-1) arise when those in privileged or powerful positions fail to recognize nondominant viewpoints as legitimate or are prejudiced against those from other racial and ethnic groups. These forms of discrimination can be enacted by individuals or become institutionalized and reflective of wider societal attitudes. Health care providers are sometimes ethnocentric in expecting children and families to accept advice or treatment based on their own values instead of those of the family. For example, children and parents are sometimes given diagnostic information and asked to make critical decisions without being able to first consult members of the extended family. This is an untenable position for families from cultures in which decision making is not necessarily centered in the nuclear family.

Technologic advances can also create ethical dilemmas, including who will have access to new, expensive forms of treatment and how decisions should be made about when to use these therapies. This is especially difficult for nurses when treatment appears to be futile or families make choices that differ from those of providers (Montagnino & Ethier, 2007). Advances in knowledge about genetic conditions pose challenges for families and providers in genetic testing and counseling. There is a great need for culturally sensitive genetic counseling, but Wang (2001) points out that it is not enough to rely on culture-specific group norms to ensure that the counseling needs of all families are met. Providers need to incorporate multicultural competencies into education, research, and practice. Such competencies include "clarifying one's own racial and cultural identities, developing self-acceptance, and having the ability to respectfully relate and function with people from all racial-cultural groups" (Wang, 2001, p. 212).

In a classic article, Barbee (1993) described three forms of racism that are common among health care providers in the United States: denial, color-blind perspectives, and aversive racism. Barbee posits that denial arises from attributes of the health professions (i.e., a preference for homogeneity and a need to avoid conflict), as well as an idealistic mission to serve all persons, which has allowed providers to avoid acknowledging and examining racism within the profession. Idealism may also lead to a color-blind perspective, which occurs when providers assert that they treat all people the same regardless of race or ethnicity and can lead to a lack of recognition and respect for cultural differences, which may then be labeled as deviance. Aversive racism occurs when clinicians do not acknowledge the conflict between an egalitarian value system and negative feelings and beliefs toward other cultural groups. Because aversive racists may believe they are not prejudiced, discrimination becomes subtle and providers experience great ambivalence. Health care professionals can and must learn to recognize ethnocentrism and racism and enhance their sensitivity to all clients by working to establish personal and institutional cultural competence.

Intracultural Variation and Diversity

Although it is helpful to learn about the common history, values, and practices of particular cultural groups, it can never be presumed that any particular individual or family is fully represented by these descriptions. Written descriptions of broad cultural groups are offered by authors in order to facilitate the acquisition of knowledge of other cultures; however, these depictions often present the most conservative cultural viewpoint, which stands in greatest contrast to that presumed to be "typically" American. These general descriptions rarely account for the dynamic nature of culture, in which traditional values and ways of life are incorporated into modern circumstances and familial needs (Culley, 2006). There is great diversity within particular ethnic, racial, and religious populations, and many people belong to several subcultures while identifying themselves with one major cultural group. Schwartz, Zamvoanga, & Weisskirch (2008) studied cultural identity in a diverse group of young adults and found that there were three dimensions of cultural identity: American-culture identity, heritage-culture identity, and biculturalism. These factors crossed white, black, and Latino cultural groups and were influenced to varying degrees by family socialization, perceived discrimination, and acculturation.

Acculturation and Biculturalism

Acculturation is the process whereby one group of people adapts to living with another, which often includes learning the dominant group's language, as well as adopting certain behaviors and practices (Birman, Trickett, & Buchanan, 2005). Acculturation can be bidirectional (i.e., both groups influence each other), although the most established culture is likely to remain dominant and to wield greater influence than less-powerful subgroups (e.g., ethnic foods, rituals, and holidays have become popular and are widely enjoyed in the United States without changing the political dominance of powerful groups in most locales).

In individuals exposed to two cultures or languages over long periods, it is common to see biculturalism and bilingualism enabling them to function well in both cultures. For example, Devos

(2006) studied Mexican American and Asian American college students and found that they identified strongly and equally with both American culture and their culture of origin. Wald and Knutson (2000) found that deaf adolescents who had received cochlear implants had very similar identity beliefs to deaf children who had not received the implants. Although both groups expressed approval of bicultural identity statements, children receiving implants were more likely to say that emulating the hearing majority was a desirable goal. Biculturalism can be helpful to children and families, allowing them to meet the demands of the dominant culture while retaining aspects of their cultural heritage (e.g., language, rituals, family relationships). Biculturalism may cause strain, however, when family members have different levels of acculturation and varying expectations about family roles and obligations.

Potential Differences in the Values of Health Care Providers and Families

Throughout the world, the family is the basic unit of society; however, different societies use family members in various ways to fulfill their basic functions of protecting, nurturing, and educating children. Parenting stress related to children's chronic conditions has been recognized internationally. For example, findings from one study of 206 mothers of 5- to 18-year-old children with intellectual disabilities, conducted in Ireland, Jordan, and Taiwan, indicated that mothers experienced increased levels of child-related stress and poor mental health and family functioning in each of these diverse nations (McConkey, Truesdale-Kennedy, Chang, et al., 2008). In the United States—unlike many parts of the world—it is common for the nuclear family (i.e., parents and their children) to live apart from other family members; therefore presumptions of nuclear family autonomy are widespread among health care providers. Nevertheless, Schwartz (2007) found that familism, a concept of family centeredness, collectivism, and interdependence, was similar across Hispanic, non-Hispanic white, and non-Hispanic black young adults, implying that diverse ethnic groups may share notions about the importance of both nuclear and extended family relationships. Hospital policies may fail to recognize the wide variety of existing family constellations and the interdependence of extended family members that are common throughout the world, as well as in many subcultures in the United States. Many health care providers are harried and distressed when large family groups arrive to visit in small hospital rooms or when family members besides parents seek information about hospitalized children.

When extended family interdependence is customary, decisions about a child's health and well-being often reach far beyond the parents. Parents may wish to consult with, or even rely on, a variety of important people (e.g., grandparents, family or community elders, religious leaders or counselors, native healers) when making critical decisions. When possible, parents should be given time and opportunities for these important consultations; and when the situation is critical or immediate decisions are crucial, families should be encouraged to keep vigil with important members present or nearby.

Although there is no one "American" value system in the multicultural United States, there are many values held widely among particular groups of people, including health care providers, who often share many common traits (e.g., most are white, middle class, and relatively well educated). Some values commonly held by providers (e.g., gender equality) may contrast with those of certain families. When providing care for people who live by contrasting values professionals may find themselves in conflict with those they seek to serve (Gillette, 2006). In analyzing situations when health care providers need to collaborate with individuals and families to make important decisions around health, Pellegrino (2006) points out that values and behaviors of both the provider and the family being cared for are important, but unlikely to always be in sync in today's pluralistic environment. He poses three important questions for consideration during health care: What is wrong? What can be done? What ought to be done? The answer to the last question must be determined with a full consideration of the life context of the child and family and must allow both the provider and the family to retain their fundamental moral values. Pellegrino suggests that the fundamental ethical power must rest in the notion of a compassionate relationship between provider, child, and family that may involve sharing power, information, and whatever common moral ground exists. Underlying the principles of cultural competence is the goal of achieving a level of cultural respect that allows care to be congruent with a family's cultural beliefs, viewpoints, and decisions. Nevertheless, Pellegrino remarks that clinicians are not required to abandon their own principles. Rather, they have an obligation to talk with families, to try to understand their viewpoints and prejudices, and to critically examine their own biases. In such a dialogue, neither the caregiver nor the family may change stances, but each may understand the other better. Where good communication and constructive relationships continue, change may eventually result.

Cultural Competence

Culturally competent health care is sensitive to the needs, backgrounds, and wishes of children with chronic conditions and their families. To be truly culturally competent requires health care providers to acquire knowledge about themselves and others; to adopt attitudes of tolerance, curiosity, patience, and appreciation of difference; and to practice interpersonal skills that foster good communication and trust. The persistence of disparities in health and access to health care is associated with a lack of cultural competence among providers and in health care systems (Betancourt et al., 2005).

Hallmarks of culturally competent caregiving and caregiving systems are described in Boxes 6-1 and 6-2. The information given there reiterates that culturally competent care is only achieved when caregivers and institutions form individual relationships with families. In a classic study of black, Hispanic, and white families interviewed about improving services for children with chronic conditions, the authors stated, "Surprisingly, there were no distinctive differences in families' recommendations based on ethnicity alone. Participants stressed the importance of individualizing care rather than providing culturally specific care for particular ethnic groups" (Garwick, Kohrman, Wolman, et al., 1998, p. 446). Nevertheless, recent research indicates that there are disparities in parents' satisfaction with care for children with special health care needs. In a large, nationally representative study, black and Hispanic parents were significantly more likely than white parents to be dissatisfied with care (Ngui & Flores, 2006). These differences were largely attributed to parental language and the presence of family-centered care measures, providing targets for intervention to improve the cultural competence of pediatric care.

BOX 6-1

Hallmarks of Culturally Sensitive Caregiving

- An asset model based on recognizing cultural differences in child rearing, family strengths, and culturally based coping methods should be used:
  - Information gathering: health records, cultural reading, family interviews
  - Family strengths serve as the basis for planning care for the child
- Families are directly involved in the family treatment and service plan:
  - Family decision makers are consulted
  - Family helps prioritize goals of care
  - Family's orientation to care providers as authority figures or joint decision makers is determined before care is planned
- Family goals permit intracultural variation on a case-by-case basis:
  - Standard care plans are altered as needed or desired
  - Alternative modes of care are incorporated as possible
- Self-sufficiency of the family is encouraged by promotion of self-esteem, cultural identification, and skill building to negotiate complicated medical systems:
  - Importance of family decision makers and caregivers is acknowledged
  - Family strengths are recognized and praised
  - Community resources are used
- Individual family/cultural values are respected:
  - Parent-child interaction patterns are taught in a culturally appropriate manner
  - Differences between family and caregiver goals are negotiated with goodwill, patience, and willingness to compromise

Data from Adams, E.V. (1990). *Policy-planning for culturally comprehensive special services: Bureau of Maternal and Child Health.* Washington, DC: U.S. Department of Health and Human Services; Bernstein, H.K., & Stettner-Eaton, B. (1994). Cultural inclusion in part H: System development. *Infant-Toddler Intervention, 4*(1), 43-50; Betancourt, J.R., et al. (2002). *Cultural competence in health care: Emerging frameworks and practical approaches (field report).* New York: The Commonwealth Fund; Dunn, A.M. (2002). Cultural competence and the primary care provider. *J Pediatr Health Care, 16,* 105-111.

BOX 6-2

Hallmarks of Culturally Sensitive Caregiving Systems

- Primary care providers and caregiving systems seek community participation in all stages of program design, development, implementation, and evaluation, including outreach, policy making, and problem solving.
  - Formal and informal community leaders (e.g., church leaders, traditional healers, elders) are involved in defining culturally appropriate care.
  - Community outreach to families is ongoing and culturally appropriate, involving bilingual providers, bicultural providers, and community members when possible.
- Intake systems are sensitive to family and cultural values:
  - Family privacy and previous experiences leading to mistrust must be respected.
- Team members must have ongoing, culturally appropriate training.
- Educational materials, media, evaluation, and monitoring instruments are field-tested for cultural appropriateness and congruency in language, content and emotional meaning.
- Programs are continuously evaluated to ensure cultural appropriateness and program effectiveness:
  - The child's progress is monitored by the family, the program, and external evaluators.
  - Family perceptions of interventions are sought and used in program revisions.

Data from Adams, E.V. (1990). *Policy-planning for culturally comprehensive special services: Bureau of Maternal and Child Health.* Washington, DC: U.S. Department of Health and Human Services; Bernstein, H.K., & Stettner-Eaton, B. (1994). Cultural inclusion in part H: System development. *Infant-Toddler Intervention, 4*(1), 43-50; Betancourt, J.R., et al. (2002). *Cultural competence in health care: Emerging frameworks and practical approaches (field report).* New York: The Commonwealth Fund; Dunn, A.M. (2002). Cultural competence and the primary care provider. *J Pediatr Health Care, 16,* 105-111.

Providers seeking cultural competence must explore their own contribution to enhancing or impeding cross-cultural interactions (i.e., their own values, beliefs, and communication patterns). Unconscious prejudices or ethnocentrism may be reflected in strained cross-cultural interactions and require thoughtful self-reflection to identify and rectify. The cross-cultural context of encounters among individuals, providers, and the health care system includes both societal factors (e.g., economic, political, and policy influences) and the immediate environment of the clinical setting (e.g., language congruency, privacy, and the acuity of the individual's health needs) (Dunn, 2002).

Cultural competence is a complex phenomenon that requires knowledge of self and others; an open-minded and tolerant attitude toward human differences; and skills in critical thinking, communication, and assessment of the outcomes of cross-cultural interactions. An ongoing effort is generally required to develop cultural competence over time. A recent field report recommended that organizations could better achieve cultural competence by encouraging a more diverse workforce, by involvement of community members in planning and quality improvement programs, and by promotion of underrepresented minorities into positions of leadership (Betancourt et al., 2005). The same report urged health care systems to remove barriers to care, such as a lack of interpreters and culturally or linguistically inappropriate educational materials. The authors urged education for clinical personnel on topics such as racial/ethnic disparities in health, assessment of community members' health beliefs and behaviors, and methods to help diverse individuals develop self-advocacy skills while negotiating complex care systems.

Cultural Variations in the Impact of Childhood Chronic Conditions

A variety of chronic conditions have been reported to occur more frequently in certain ethnic or racial groups. Recent immigrants, including children adopted from outside the United States, must be assessed for conditions that are prevalent in their region of origin, and all children with chronic conditions need comprehensive family and developmental assessment, as well as well-child care, in addition to care for their chronic condition (Grogg & Grogg, 2007). Children from immigrant families now constitute more than 20% of all children in the United States, and are less likely to have health insurance and access to health care than native-born poor children (Ku, 2007). It is important to recognize that definitions of chronic conditions may vary and some cultures may consider minor differences in health or ability as acceptable variants of normal.

In recent national surveys, children who have or are at increased risk for chronic physical, developmental, behavioral, or emotional conditions, and also require health and related services beyond those generally required for children, have been estimated to make up approximately 13% to 19% of all U.S. children less than 18 years of age (Bethell, Read, Blumberg, et al., 2008). An epidemiologic profile of these children found that 14% of white children, 13% of black children, 8.5% of Hispanic children, and 11% of children from other racial and ethnic groups were classified as having special health care needs (van Dyck, Kogan, McPherson, et al., 2004). Boys were about one third more likely to have a special health need than girls, and children whose family incomes were at or below the federal poverty level were also about one third more likely to have special needs than those with higher income levels. Children from single-parent families are about 40% more likely to have special health care needs than those from two-parent families.

The implementation of the State Children's Health Insurance Program (SCHIP) has decreased disparities in health care access for black and Hispanic children as compared with white children, including improving access to a usual source of care, and improving continuity and quality of care for all three groups (Shone, Dick, Klein, et al., 2005). Despite these improvements in disparities between ethnic/racial groups, 19% of all children in each of the three groups continued to have unmet health care needs.

Communications

At the heart of all successful relationships, including parent-nurse relationships within family-centered care environments, is good communication. Cultural factors (e.g., respect for authority, differences in social class) among families and providers may influence a family's attitude about accepting advice from health care providers or willingness to share reservations or objections to treatment plans. Some families may consider care providers to be partners or consultants whose advice can be considered and either accepted or discarded, but others may consider caregivers to be authority figures whose advice—accepted or not—should never be openly questioned. Therefore follow-ups and ongoing dialogue are necessary to ensure that mutually acceptable care and outcomes are established (Corlett & Twycross, 2006).

Besides words, communication is established through body language, touch, eye contact, and other nonverbal indicators. To convey respect and establish comfort, health care providers must be good observers and responsive to cues from children and families. Many care providers use direct, to-the-point communication; full eye contact; and firm handshakes, which are common courtesies for many people but may be aggressive or rude gestures to individuals used to indirect approaches and a lack of physical contact among strangers (Giger & Davidhizar, 2003).

The subtleties of effective communication are particularly complicated when interpreters are necessary. Children or friends of the family should not be used as interpreters because their presence may inhibit parents from a frank discussion of sensitive issues. Family members who can usually communicate adequately in English may find themselves tongue-tied or unable to understand complex medical concepts and vocabulary during times of crisis or stress (Rehm, 2003b). Moreover, parents may desire interpretation to their native language to fully understand explanations related to a child's chronic condition. It is important that interpreters be highly skilled communicators in both languages and cultures and that they convey more than simple, word-for-word translations of dialogue in clinical settings so that the actual meaning of the message is accurately portrayed (Nailon, 2006). When an interpreter is used, it is important to speak in short units of speech; to use simple, nontechnical language; to speak to family members directly—not just to the interpreter; and to listen to the individual and family and check their understanding often by asking them to restate the message in their own words.

Variations in Perceptions of Causality and Meaning of Chronic Conditions

Perceptions about the cause and meaning of disability and chronic conditions of childhood vary widely among families. Some of these variations are associated with cultural or religious beliefs or may be related to parental educational levels and past experiences. Nurse researchers examined parental illness representations of asthma, juxtaposed them to those of providers, and evaluated the impact of parental representations on the adequacy of the medication plan for the child (Yoos, Kitman, Henderson, et al., 2007). They found that parent and professional descriptions of asthma differed markedly, and that parent models of the illness were negatively affected by low education levels, inaccurate symptom evaluation, and a poor parent–health care provider relationship. Families with belief systems that consider social factors and spiritual influences, as well as pathophysiologic associations, may attribute a child's condition to multiple factors, including environmental, interpersonal, and genetic influences. Chronic conditions may be stigmatizing if thought to result from unacceptable behavior, inherent weaknesses, or external threats that could endanger the rest of the family or community (e.g., hexes, spirit possession, bad karma) (Burnard, Naiyapatana, & Lloyd, 2006). Children with such conditions may be kept at home and out of view to protect either the family from shame or the child from potentially disapproving or threatening community restrictions.

In many communities, however, families caring for children with chronic conditions are admired and offered ongoing support. Belief in causative factors beyond those generally recognized by biomedicine does not often interfere with acceptance and use of modern medical diagnosis and treatment. For example, Rao (2006) examined the hierarchy of choices for treatment regimens by Asian Indian migrants to the United States and found that people used folk remedies and ayurvedic, homeopathic, and allopathic treatments. They were more likely to choose home remedies and traditional Indian alternatives for minor ailments and Western medicines for serious or chronic conditions. A family's current practices must be determined, and planned treatments besides those proposed by primary care providers must be recognized. It may be important to determine the effects of herbs or other pharmacologic agents to assess drug interactions and safety, but folk healers are often willing to cooperate with health care providers; a blending of rituals and healing techniques can be both medically effective and helpful to the family. Prayer and other religious/spiritual rituals are among the most commonly reported alternative therapies (Yoon & Black, 2006). Pediatric care providers may facilitate joint practices when, for example, blessing ceremonies are conducted before an invasive procedure (e.g., Mormons) or amulets are worn by children for protection (e.g., some American Indians).

Expectations for the survival of infants and children influence the kinds of familial and community resources that parents seek and provide for their children with chronic conditions. Residents or recent immigrants from parts of the world that are less technologically oriented than the U.S. medical system may be unaware of recent advances in medical care that facilitate survival for many children who would ordinarily die or be profoundly disabled without the surgical, pharmacologic, and mechanical supports routinely available here. Expectations for children with chronic conditions vary widely and require ongoing education in the face of changing life circumstances, available support services, and official policies.

Family- and community-sanctioned roles for children and adults with chronic conditions help determine the kinds of educational, health, and other resources that are expended on such individuals. The official U.S. policy (i.e., in the form of laws such as the Americans with Disabilities Act [ADA] and the Individuals with Disabilities Education Improvement Act [IDEA]) explicitly entitles children and adults with disabling conditions to the same educational, occupational, and social opportunities as those without such conditions (see Chapter 3). These laws reflect the widely held American beliefs that most people should be independent and self-supporting and therefore are entitled to education and opportunities to ensure such measures of success. These expectations are often modified depending on individual circumstances, and the belief that each person should strive for the highest possible level of independence may need to be modified in light of individual or family preference, or the need for ongoing support, for example, in the widespread practice of group-home living for individuals who cannot live alone. Researchers and clinicians have noted the presence of a "disability paradox" in which adults or youths with serious illnesses or disabilities report a high quality of life, and a level of adaptation to their individual abilities and needs that allows them to pursue valued factors such as relationships and individual interests (Jorgensen, 2005; Saigal & Rosenbaum, 2007).

Cultural Assessment

Cultural competence requires that children with chronic conditions and their families are assessed to determine their cultural identities and any particular beliefs or needs that should be incorporated into care plans. There are many excellent, in-depth cultural assessment tools (Andrews & Boyle, 2007; Giger & Davidhizar, 2003). Cross-cultural assessment of a family with a child with a chronic condition is described in Table 6-2. These tools are particularly helpful when health care providers see families repeatedly over time because the many questions can be incorporated into several interviews. Many times, however, care providers are uncertain if they will see families repeatedly or the nature of the contact is time limited and problem focused. In such cases, it is helpful to distill a few key questions from these larger tools and focus attention on the aspects of assessment that are most relevant to the current encounter.

Key Questions for Brief Encounters in the Primary Care Setting

In the primary care setting, it is helpful to supplement the general child and family history with key questions, such as the following:

1. Would you be more comfortable with a translator present?
2. Who are your child's primary caregivers at home?
3. Is there anyone else who needs to know the treatment plan and have the opportunity to ask questions?
4. What kinds of home remedies have you been using for your child, and what others might you use for this situation?
5. Are you satisfied with the care plan made at this visit, and is there anything that you anticipate might interfere with your ability to carry it out?

In an acute situation or when it is necessary to make major decisions or changes in the care plan, it is important to add the following questions about the family's decision-making procedures:

1. Who are the appropriate people to make this decision for your child?
2. Do you want/need to bring in other family members or authority figures to receive information to help you make this decision?

It may be useful to get to know the family with these key questions and incorporate the answers into a larger assessment that can be left in the chart and completed over time. Primary care providers can bring in additional questions relating to the reason for the visit (e.g., questions about medication acceptability and use, dietary preferences and restrictions, or developmental goals). Many questions asked by clinicians as part of the routine history and physical clearly have cultural relevance, and once practitioners are sensitive to that fact, cultural assessment can be incorporated into all encounters and does not have to take up large blocks of time. A clinician's respect, nonjudgmental attitude, and sincere interest and curiosity about the child and family are likely to foster trust and open communication. It is important to assure families that their input is valuable and to verify that the plan of care is acceptable to them.

Research and Culture

Along with the increasing diversity of the American population has come an explosion in research including diverse samples, both in the United States and globally. Investigators have extensively described the effect of chronic conditions on children and their family members in both qualitative and quantitative studies (see Chapters 2, 3, 5, and 7). Nevertheless, despite this extensive research foundation, it is often difficult to find data-based information on the experiences or outcomes of particular cultural groups with specific chronic conditions. Agencies that fund research often require samples that reflect the local community, including studies about children with chronic conditions and their families. However, the definitions of racial/ethnic categories are often ambiguous or unspecified and the numbers of participants from any particular cultural group or subpopulation are often small, so the information related to them is subsumed into the findings of the larger study (Hunt & Megyesi, 2008). Moreover, people of color and cultural subgroups are often not studied within the context of their own culture.

Despite current regulations that require the inclusion of across–the–life span and ethnically diverse samples in government-funded studies, children, women, and nondominant ethnic groups continue to be underrepresented in many forms of research studies, particularly clinical trials. Although these regulations help ensure that all U.S. residents are represented in research, few studies focusing on particular cultural groups, which could help overcome oft-repeated stereotypes, are conducted. Perhaps these studies are rare because there is an assumption that such research is best conducted by members of a particular culture. If this assumption is accepted, important questions about particular cultural groups may not be answered because cultural minority groups are vastly underrepresented among the ranks of scholars. Currently, there are innovative programs being implemented to try to increase the numbers of doctorally prepared nurses with mentoring and intensive training in the conduct of research (Wallen, Rivera-Goba, Hantings, et al., 2005). One innovative program, funded by the National Institute of Nursing Research, creates partnerships between a majority dominant research intensive institution and a historically minority serving university in order to facilitate culturally competent research and examine how culture, race, and ethnicity influence health disparities and health outcomes (Hutchinson, Davis, Jemmont, et al., 2007).

TABLE 6-2

Cross-Cultural Assessment of a Family with a Child with a Chronic Condition

Family Demographics	Who lives in your family (i.e., members, ages, genders)?
	What kind of work do members of the household do?
	What is your family's socioeconomic status?
	What kind of health insurance coverage do you have?
	Which family members are covered?
	Which child are you seeking care for today?
	What chronic conditions or symptoms does the child have?
	How would you describe the problems that have brought you here today?
	Who is the primary caretaker in your family?
Orientation	Where were the members of the family born?
	What is the ethnic background of the family members?
	How many years have family members lived in the United States? (Note: Only ask if appropriate.)
	In your family is it important to be on time for an appointment or to get to an appointment based on everyone's schedule for that day?
	Why do you think your child has the chronic condition (e.g., punishment for a parent's past behavior such as conceiving a child out of wedlock, the result of a genetic problem, or a gift given because of the family's patience and love)?
Communication	What language(s) and dialect(s) are spoken at home?
	Who reads English in the family? If no one reads English, in what language would you prefer printed materials?
	Do parents and children make eye contact when spoken to, or do they look down?
	To whom should questions be addressed?
	What can be asked of the child directly? (Note: Avoid using the child as a translator because of the strain this imposes.)
Family Relationships	Besides the immediate household, who else makes up the members of this family?
	Who makes the decisions in this family (e.g., mother-in-law, father, both partners, other family or friends, group decision)?
	Who cares for the child and the child's medical needs?
	What are the housing arrangements (e.g., space, number of rooms, members living in the home)?
	What is the child's or family's usual daily routine like?
	To whom do you turn when you need help with or have questions about your child?
Beliefs about Health	What is the present health status of family members?
	What illnesses or conditions are present in the current family members?
	What illnesses or conditions were present in deceased family members?
	How often and for what reasons have family members used Western medicine in the past?
	What complementary therapies are used by your family routinely and specifically for the child (e.g., acupuncture, healers, prayer, massage)?
	What do you do when your child is in pain?
	Who takes care of the child if the child is hospitalized?
	Is it important to keep the child at home or to use institutional placement?
	What do you think will help clear up the problem?
	Are there things that help your child get better that the physicians should know?
	What problems has your child's illness caused your family?
Education	How much schooling have members of the family completed?
	What ways are the best for you to learn about your child's condition (e.g., pamphlets, videos, direct child teaching, home visits, return demonstrations)?
	From whom are you most comfortable learning about your child's condition (e.g., physician, nurse, social worker, home health aide, other family members)?
Religion	What religion(s) are practiced in your family?
	What religious things do you do to help your child (e.g., pray, meditate, attend a support group, practice the laying on of hands)?
	What things does your religion say you should *not* do for this child (e.g., have blood transfusions, allow strangers or dangerous circumstances to affect child)?
Nutrition	When are usual mealtimes for your family?
	With whom does the child eat?
	What foods does the child usually eat?
	What special foods does the child eat when the child is sick?
	What foods do you *not* give the child and when?

From Andrews, M.M., & Boyle, J.S. (2007). *Transcultural concepts in nursing care* (3rd ed.). Philadelphia: Saunders; Davis, B., & Voegtle, K. (1994). *Culturally competent health care for adolescents.* Chicago: American Medical Association. Modified with permission.

Studies of disadvantaged cultural populations must recognize the effects of racial, class, and other forms of discrimination, as well as seek solutions to health problems through interventions beyond those aimed at individuals who do not conform to generally accepted healthy behaviors. Researchers have demonstrated the effects of poverty and social class on health (Zedlewski, 2002) but seldom acknowledge other societal factors, such as repeated discrimination, exposure to high levels of pollutants and violence, and lack of opportunity for educational or occupational advancement. Interventions that address these factors, as well as those most commonly aimed at individual behavior changes, are necessary.

Victimization of and prejudice against children with chronic conditions have received relatively little attention from researchers. However, studies offer preliminary evidence that children's psychologic adjustment and mental health can be adversely affected by negative peer interactions, suggesting that much more work is needed in this area (Immelt, 2006; Shtayermman, 2007). The potential for discrimination against people with genetic conditions has been recognized by clinicians and researchers managing information gleaned from the Human Genome Project, and protection of privacy is an emerging area of interest and concern (Quick, 2005). Federal lawmakers are considering legislation to protect against genetic discrimination, which will have implications for children with special health care needs and their families.

Summary

As the United States becomes more culturally diverse, health care providers must develop cultural competence to ensure that sensitive and effective care is delivered. Cultural competence will help prevent racism and ethnocentrism in practice and research by helping providers to assess their own cultural viewpoints and biases while learning about the issues and needs of children and their families. Care should be congruent with the cultural beliefs and practices of individuals whenever possible, and increasing cultural competence will enhance effective communication and facilitate respect and appreciation for the range of human diversity. Researchers must investigate culturally relevant questions and test interventions in a wide variety of populations in order to develop the baseline knowledge that will provide clinicians with a sound foundation on which to develop primary care practices that are culturally aware and responsive.

REFERENCES

Airhihenbuwa, C.O., Kumanyika, S.K., & TenHave, T.R., et al. (2000). Cultural identity and health lifestyles among African Americans: A new direction for health intervention research. *Ethn Dis, 10,* 148-164.

American Academy of Pediatrics. (2003). Family pediatrics: Report of the task force on the family. *Pediatrics, 111,* 1541-1571.

Andrews, M.M., & Boyle, J.S. (2007). *Transcultural Concepts in Nursing Care.* (5th ed.). Philadelphia: Lippincott Williams & Wilkins.

Barbee, E.L. (1993). Racism in U.S. nursing. *Med Anthropol Q, 7,* 346-362.

Baumeister, R.F. (2005). *The Cultural Animal: Human Nature, Meaning, and Social Life.* New York: Oxford University Press.

Betancourt, J.R., Green, A.R., Carillo, E., et al. (2005). Cultural competence and health care disparities: Key perspectives and trends. *Health Aff, 24,* 499-505.

Bethell, C.D., Read, D., Blumberg, S.J., et al. (2008). What is the prevalence of children with special health care needs? Toward an understanding of variations in findings and methods across three national surveys. *Matern Child Health J, 12,* 1-14.

Birman, D., Trickett, E.J., & Buchanan, R.M. (2005). A tale of two cities: Replication of a study on the acculturation and adaptation of immigrant adolescents from the former Soviet Union in a different community context. *Am J Commun Psychol, 35,* 83-101.

Burnard, P., Naiyapatana, W., & Lloyd, G. (2006). Views of mental illness and mental health care in Thailand: A report of an ethnographic study. *J Psychiatr Ment Health Nurs, 13,* 742-749.

Children's Defense Fund. (2006). *New Census Data Shows 1.3 million children have fallen into poverty since 2000.* Available at www.childrensdefense.org/site/News2?page=NewsArticle&id=7887. Retrieved May 10, 2008.

Corlett, J., & Twycross, A. (2006). Negotiation of parental roles within family-centered care: A review of the research. *J Clin Nurs, 15,* 1308-1316.

Coyle, J. (2002). Spirituality and health: Towards a framework for exploring the relationship between spirituality and health. *J Adv Nurs, 37,* 589-597.

Crigger, N.J. (2008). Towards a viable and just global nursing ethics. *Nurs Ethics, 15,* 17-27.

Culley, L. (2006). Transcending transculturalism? Race, ethnicity and health care. *Nurs Inq, 13,* 144-153.

Devos, T. (2006). Implicit bicultural identity among Mexican Americans and Asian American college students. *Cultur Divers Ethnic Minor Psychol, 12,* 381-402.

Dunn, A.M. (2002). Culture competence and the primary care provider. *J Pediatr Health Care, 16*(3), 105-111.

Esmer, Y. (2006). Globalization, "McDonaldization" and values: Quo vadis? *Comp Sociol, 5*(2-3), 183-202.

Flores, G., & Tomany-Korman, S.C. (2008). Racial and ethnic disparities in medical and dental health, access to care, and use of services in US children. *Pediatrics, 121,* e286-e298.

Garwick, A.W., Kohrman, C., Wolman, C., et al. (1998). Families' recommendations for improving services for children with chronic conditions. *Arch Pediatr Adolesc Med, 152,* 440-448.

Giger, J.N., & Davidhizar, R.E. (2003). *Transcultural Nursing: Assessment and Intervention.* (4th ed.). St. Louis: Mosby.

Gillete, G. (2006). Medical science, culture, and truth. *Philosophy, Ethics, and Humanities in Medicine* (online). Available at www.pubmedcentral.nih.gov/picrender.fcgi?artid=1769504&blobtype=pdf. Retrieved May 10, 2008:

Grogg, S.E., & Grogg, B.C. (2007). Intercountry adoptions: Medical aspects for the whole family. *J Am Osteopath Assoc, 107,* 481-489.

Huang, Z.J., Yu, A.M., & Ledsky, R. (2006). Health status and health service access and use among children in US immigrant families. *Am J Pub Health, 96,* 634-640.

Hunt, L.M., & Megyesi, M.S. (2008). The ambiguous meanings of the racial/ethnic categories routinely used in human genetic research. *Soc Sci Med, 66,* 349-361.

Hutchinson, M.K., Davis, B., Jemmont, L.S., et al. (2007). Promoting research partnerships to reduce health disparities among vulnerable populations: Sharing expertise between majority institutions and historically black universities. *Ann Rev Nurs Res, 25,* 119-159.

Immelt, S. (2006). Psychological adjustment in young children with chronic medical conditions. *J Pediatr Nurs, 21,* 362-377.

Jorgensen, M. (2005). A disability paradox. *Can Fam Physician, 51,* 1474-1476.

Ku, L. (2007). Improving health insurance and access to care for children in immigrant families. *Ambul Pediatr, 7,* 412-420.

Larson, L.J. (2004). The foreign born population in the United States: March 2003. *Current Population Reports, P20-551.* Washington, DC: U.S. Census Bureau.

Lavash, D.P. (2006). *A Journey Through New Mexico History.* Santa Fe, NM: Sunstone Press.

Lewis, D. (2008). *200 Million Children World Wide Lack Basic Health Care.* Available at www.tennessean.com/apps/pbcs.dll/article?AID=/20080508/COLUMNIST0107/805080390/1008/OPINION01. Retrieved May 1, 2008.

Martens, P., & Rotmans, J. (2005). Transitions in a globalizing world. *Futures, 37,* 1133-1144.

McConkey, R., Truesdale-Kennedy, M., Chang, M., et al. (2008). The impact on mothers of bringing up a child with intellectual disabilities: A cross-cultural study. *Int J Nurs Studies, 45,* 65-74.

Montagnino, B.A., & Ethier, A.M. (2007). The experiences of pediatric nurses caring for children in a persistent vegetative state. *Pediatr Crit Care Med, 8,* 440-446.

Nailon, R.E. (2006). Nurses' concerns and practices with using interpreters in the care of Latino patients in the emergency department. *J Transcult Nurs, 17,* 119-128.

Ngui, E.M., & Flores, G. (2006). Satisfaction with care and ease of using health care services among parents of children with special health care needs: The roles of race/ethnicity, insurance, language, and adequacy of family-centered care. *Pediatrics, 117,* 1184-1196.

O'Neill, D. (2005). *The Last Giant of Beringia: The Mystery of the Bering Land Bridge.* Boulder, CO: Westview Press.

Passel, J.S. (2005). Unauthorized migrants: Numbers and characteristics. *Pew Hispanic Center* (online). Available at: www.migrantclinician.org/_resources/pew_hispanic_center.pdf. Retrieved May 5, 2008.

Pellegrino, E.D. (2006). Toward a reconstruction of medical morality. *Am J Bioethics, 6,* 65-71.

Quick, J.J. (2005). Genetic discrimination and the need for federal legislation. *J Biolaw Bus, 8,* 22-26.

Rao, D. (2006). Choice of medicine and hierarchy of resort to different health alternatives, among Asian Indian migrants in a metropolitan city in the USA. *Ethn Health, 11,* 153-167.

Rehm, R.S. (1999). Religious faith in Mexican American families living with chronic childhood illness. *Image J Nurs Sch, 31,* 33-38.

Rehm, R.S. (2003a). Legal, financial and ethical ambiguities for Mexican American families caring for children with chronic conditions. *Qual Health Res, 13*, 789-802.

Rehm, R.S. (2003b). Cultural intersections in the care of Mexican American children with chronic conditions. *Pediatr Nurs, 29*, 434-439.

Robinson, M.R., Thiel, M.M., Backus, M.M., et al. (2006). Matters of spirituality at the end of life in the pediatric intensive care unit. *Pediatrics, 118*, e719-e729.

Saigal, S., & Rosenbaum, P. (2007). What matters in the long term? Reflections on the context of adult outcomes versus detailed measures in childhood. *Semin Fetal Neonat Med, 12*, 415-422.

Schwartz, S.J. (2007). The applicability of familism to diverse ethnic groups: A preliminary study. *J Soc Psychol, 147*, 101-118.

Schwartz, S.J., Zamvoanga, B.L., & Weisskirch, R.S. (2008). Broadening the study of the self: Integrating the study of personal identity and cultural identity. *Soc Personal Psychol Compass, 2*, 635-651.

Sessanna, L., Finnell, D., & Jezewski, M.A. (2007). Spirituality in nursing and health-related literature. *J Holistic Nurs, 25*, 252-262.

Shone, L.P., Dick, A.W., Klein, J.D., et al. (2005). Reduction in racial and ethnic disparities after enrollment in the State Children's Health Insurance Program. *Pediatrics, 115*, e697-e705.

Shtayermman, O. (2007). Peer victimization in adolescents and young adults diagnosed with Asperger's syndrome: A link to depressive symptomatology, anxiety symptomatology and suicidal ideation. *Issues Compr Pediatr Nurs, 30*, 87-107.

Tjale, A.A., & Bruce, J. (2007). A concept analysis of holistic nursing care in paediatric nursing. *Curationis, 30*(4), 45-52.

U.S. Office of Immigration Statistics, Policy Directorate (2006). *Estimates of the Unauthorized Immigrant Population Residing in the United States: January 2005.* Washington, DC: Population Estimates: Homeland Security.

van Dyck, P., Kogan, M.D., McPherson, M.G., et al. (2004). Prevalence and characteristics of children with special health care needs. *Arch Pediatr Adolesc Med, 158*, 884-890.

Wald, R.L., & Knutson, J.F. (2000). Deaf cultural identity of adolescents with and without cochlear implants. *Ann Otol Rhinol Laryngol, 185*(Suppl), 87-89.

Wallen, G.R., Rivera-Goba, M.V., Hantings, C., et al. (2005). Developing the research pipeline: Increasing minority nursing research opportunities. *Nurs Educ Perspect, 26*, 29-33.

Wang, V.O. (2001). Multicultural genetic counseling: Then, now and in the 21st century. *Am J Med Genet, 106*, 208-215.

Wilson, P. (2005). Jehovah's Witness children: When religion and the law collide. *Paediatr Nurs, 17*, 34-37.

Yoon, S.L., & Black, S. (2006). Comprehensive, integrative management of pain for patients with sickle-cell disease. *J Altern Complement Med, 12*, 995-1001.

Yoos, L.H., Kitman, H., Henderson, H., et al. (2007). The impact of the parental illness representation on disease management in childhood asthma. *Nurs Res, 56*, 167-174.

Young, J., Flores, G., & Berman, S. (2004). Providing life-saving health care to undocumented children: Controversies and ethical issues. *Pediatrics, 114*, 1316-1320.

Zedlewski, S.R. (2002). Family economic resources in the post-reform era. *Future Child, 12*(1), 120-145.

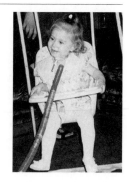

7 Ethics and the Child with a Chronic Condition

Donna A. Gaffney

Decision Making along the Course of Chronic Conditions

The course of a chronic condition is likely to include diagnosis and treatment; periods of recovery, exacerbations, stability, or instability; and, in some cases, deterioration and death. These phases are often punctuated by recurring ethical issues, including the following:

1. Defining what constitutes a life worth living
2. Recognizing the threshold for certainty in diagnosis and treatment
3. Choosing a decision maker to decide about treatment or nontreatment
4. Determining the role of minors in making treatment decisions
5. Deciding whether to pursue experimental or innovative therapies
6. Knowing how to resolve conflicts

The range of chronic conditions in childhood and adolescence is paralleled by the range of values held by people with chronic conditions or caregivers of those with chronic conditions. Competing ethical obligations can create a set of problematic situations for children, families, and health care providers.

The Ethical Domain

A moral or ethical course of action is based on guiding principles of doing what is right (i.e., ethics is concerned with "what ought to be" and how individuals think about and discuss "what ought to be"). Ethics is concerned with the behavior, choices, and character of individuals and groups. Ethical questions arise alongside—but differ from—fundamental social, legal, political, professional, and scientific questions. For example, public policies and laws (e.g., the death penalty) set boundaries for human behavior but do not necessarily correspond to an individual's sense of "what ought to be." It is within this context that ethical discourse occurs.

There are many ways of discerning the ethical dimensions of an issue or quandary. The process of discernment is complex and influenced by emotions, scientific facts, values, interpersonal relationships, culture, religion, the essence of who we are, and myriad situational factors—all of which converge to shape the way ethical questions are framed.

Ethical questions arise because an individual is unsure of the right thing to do or the proper outcome to pursue. For example, primary care providers may be concerned about whether to offer an experimental treatment protocol to a family when the likelihood of altering the natural course of the child's condition is remote and pursuing such treatment will require the family to pay out-of-pocket costs. Ethical questions may also arise because there are genuine value conflicts about the right thing to do or the proper outcomes to pursue. For example, primary care providers and families may disagree about whether it is justified to continue aggressive treatment for a child with end-stage cystic fibrosis. The providers may reason that continued treatment is burdensome and will prolong death; in contrast, the parents may believe that extending life is the appropriate goal to be pursued—despite the burden endured by the child. In both instances, careful consideration of the judgments and the justifications that are used to defend one's position and behavior is warranted.

Ethical deliberation involves the process of discerning, analyzing, and articulating ethically defensible positions and then acting on them. Ethical thinking provides a reasoned account of an ethical position and helps one move beyond intuition or emotions. The goal of ethical deliberation is not to achieve absolute certainty about what is right but to achieve reliability and coherence in behavior, choices, character, process, and outcomes.

Ethical theories and principles provide a foundation for ethical analysis and deliberation (Box 7-1), as well as a guide for organizing and understanding ethically relevant information in a dilemma or conflict situation. These theories and principles also suggest directions and avenues for resolving competing claims and supply reasons that justify moral action. Ethical principles are universal in nature but are not absolute. Each case involves particular principles and values integral to the decision-making process. One must balance the claims generated from competing principles relevant to a particular case. Moreover, factors such as family dynamics, the nature of relationships, contextual features, integrity, and faithfulness to commitments are also morally relevant to the decision-making process. Even when one chooses a morally justifiable course of action, there are always unmet obligations when resolving ethical dilemmas (i.e., a "moral remainder").

Ethical theories and principles must be applied systematically within the decision-making process. Ethical analysis is enhanced when a framework that provides a systematic process of decision making is used and mistakes are avoided by using only logic and reason (Box 7-2). In addition, because some decisions (e.g., those

The author gratefully acknowledges the contribution of Teresa A. Savage, PhD, RN, and Cynda Hylton Rushton, DNSc, RN, FAAN, the authors of this chapter in the previous edition.

Normative Ethical Theories and Principles

ETHICAL THEORIES
- *Teleologic theories:* Determine an action to be right or wrong based on the consequences the action produces. For example, in utilitarianism the principle of utility (i.e., maximizing the good or minimizing harm) is the central criterion for action.
- *Deontologic theories:* Focus on doing one's duty. The intrinsic quality of the act itself or its conformity to a rule—not its consequences—determines whether an act is right or wrong.

SELECTED ETHICAL PRINCIPLES
- *Beneficence:* The duty to do good; to promote the welfare of the individual.
- *Nonmaleficence:* The duty not to harm or burden.
  - Medical harm
  - Pain
  - New therapies
  - Maltreatment
- *Autonomy:* Self-determination.
- *Respect for persons:* Recognizing another person as sharing a common human destiny.
  - Informed consent
- *Justice:* Fairness. Distributive justice refers to the equitable distribution of benefits and burdens under conditions of scarcity and competition.
  - Macroallocation
  - Microallocation
  - Beneficence and justice

DERIVATIVE PRINCIPLES
- *Veracity:* The duty to tell the truth.
- *Fidelity:* The duty to keep one's promise or word.

Modified from Beauchamp, T.L., & Childress, J.F. (2001). *Principles of Biomedical Ethics* (5th ed.). New York: Oxford University Press. Modified with permission.

Process to Facilitate Ethical Decision Making

1. Identify the ethical problem(s); distinguish from clinical, administrative or legal problems.
2. Identify the key players (including the family members and what their roles are); identify your role.
3. Identify the ethical issue(s); describe/define them in terms of principles, values of key players, and potential conflicts.
4. Identify the preferences of the key players regarding the decision to be made.
5. Identify the decision maker(s).
6. Identify options, the range of permissible actions for this situation, and the ethical ramifications of each action.
7. Make decision/facilitate decision/abide by decision.
8. Evaluate the decision-making process and your role in the process.
9. Consider what you would do differently in the future and why.

A Moral Framework for Decision Making

- Beneficence
  - Balancing benefit and burden
- Respect for persons
  - Informed consent
- Justice
  - Macroallocation and microallocation of resources
  - Individual vs. society needs
- An ethic of care

to withhold or withdraw certain therapies) help determine the timing and consequences of death, other important social, ethical, and religious values come into play.

A Moral Framework for Decision Making

A specific framework provides a mechanism for individuals, families, and providers dealing with the ethical dimensions of difficult situations. For adults, a morally defensible framework for decision making is relatively straightforward and widely accepted (President's Commission for the Study of Ethical Problems in Medicine and Biomedical and Behavioral Research, 1983) (Box 7-3). Consistent with the Western view of autonomy, treatment options should promote the well-being of the individual according to that individual's understanding of well-being. When individuals lack the capacity to make choices for themselves, someone else must represent their particular values and preferences. Ethical decision making is a process with multiple contributors; it is a combination of the health provider's expertise on the available choices and the individual's or surrogate's expertise on which choices best promote that individual's life goals and values. This decision-making process is also influenced by the family system, culture, religious and spiritual affiliations, and personal values and preferences (Blustein, 1998; Jonsen, Siegler, & Winslade, 1998).

For children, ethical decision making is more complex because most lack the capacity to make informed, independent decisions.

Children have not formulated the life goals and values on which to base such decisions. The capacity to be involved in decision making varies according to a child's level of maturity, and as a result it is generally assumed that children need surrogate decision makers (Committee on Bioethics, 1994). However, more recent findings suggest that child decision making is based on more factors than stages of cognitive development (Alderson, Suttcliffe, & Curtis, 2006). In fact, a growing body of research supports the involvement of children in their health care decisions (Beidler & Dickey, 2001; Martenson & Fagerskiold, 2007). Decisions made on behalf of children lack a key feature of the moral framework for adults: an individual's unique assessment of his or her own well-being. Despite this, minors can be involved in meaningful ways in decisions about their own health care (see the section later in this chapter on respect for persons). The moral principles involved in adult decision making do, however, provide a valuable framework for making decisions on behalf of children (Ross, 1997; Savage, 1997). It is often useful to use ethical principles as an organizational framework for addressing ethical issues in decision making for children.

Beneficence

The primary principles involved in decision making are beneficence (i.e., doing good) and its corollary, nonmaleficence (i.e., avoiding or minimizing harm). Treatment options should include those that benefit the infant or child and clearly outweigh the associated burdens and harms. This "best interest" standard is often used as a hallmark when making decisions for children; it establishes a presumption in favor of life because existence is usually required for other interests to be advanced. Generally, life should be saved when possible. When life cannot be saved or the chance of survival is minimal, however, burdensome treatment should not be provided and palliative care should be considered (Hynson & Sawyer, 2001). Burdens for children with chronic conditions include repeated pain and suffering associated with invasive procedures, symptoms, or disability, as well as emotional distress caused by fear, immobilization, prolonged hospitalization, or isolation from family and friends. Decisions about a child whose chances of dying are great might reasonably focus on the comfort associated with dying instead of on therapies to prolong life.

An additional standard, the "relational potential" standard, has also been suggested as an adjunct to the "best interest" standard when balancing the benefits and burdens of various courses of action (McCormick, 1974). This standard focuses on the child's cognitive and intellectual capacities, the degree of neurologic impairment, the prognosis of reversing the neurologic condition, and whether the outcome of the condition can be altered through treatment or therapy. For example, infants or children who are permanently unconscious have no capacity to feel either pleasure or pain, so their "interests" are limited to prolonging biologic life. Because such children cannot be burdened in the usual sense and most of the reasons for treatment (e.g., better function, fewer symptoms, the opportunity for human relationships or greater opportunity to achieve life's goals) are gone, many would argue that treatment is not obligatory (Fost, 1999). The Baby Doe regulations (Public Law 98-457, 1984), for example, regard permanent unconsciousness as a condition that does not require life-sustaining treatment; yet there are a wide range of views on the degree of neurologic impairment that justifies limiting or forgoing treatment. In addition, Saigal and colleagues (Saigal & Doyle, 2008; Saigal & Tyson, 2008) have attempted to learn the perspectives of former "preemies" (now adults) on their present quality of life. Their insights debunk conventional thinking about the relationship of function with perceived quality of life.

The challenge for children, parents, and health care providers is to understand the unique meaning of the concepts of health, sickness, disability, suffering, care, and death for a child in a particular situation. The meaning that these concepts give to an individual's life is influenced by that individual's values, interests, aims, rights, and duties. A holistic understanding of a child's life, a recognition of important values that give direction to treatment decisions, and the tenor of the professional–family-child relationship evolve and change over time; therefore discovering the threshold for balancing benefits and burdens in a certain case may change as the child's condition changes. For example, the initial goals for a newborn with multiple congenital anomalies resulting in neurologic impairment and severe physical disability may be to understand the extent of the child's condition and to preserve life. In this instance, parents and professionals may agree to tolerate a high degree of burden to the child in order to diminish the uncertainty surrounding diagnosis and prognosis. However, 2 years later, after the diagnosis and prognosis have been clarified, parents and professionals may have a different view of how much burden the child must tolerate to sustain life, especially when continued treatment will not alter the prognosis and may impose significant burdens.

Beneficence is promoted by helping the child and family construct a meaningful life by balancing the burdens of the condition with the positive dimensions of living. Beneficence is expressed by identifying individualized care outcomes that enhance the child's well-being (e.g., adequately managing symptoms, accommodating to limitations imposed by the chronic condition, maximizing functional capacities). Therefore treatment interventions must be designed to contribute to the individualized goals that enhance quality of life and promote the child's sense of integrity despite the limitations related to the condition.

Parents and professionals must openly discuss the uncertainty in diagnosis and prognosis and explore the extent of certainty necessary for both parental and professional decision making. At times, the need for greater certainty of either parents or professionals may result in burdensome diagnostic evaluations that do not contribute to the child's well-being or outcome. Alternatively, parents may accept uncertainty when professionals are compelled to seek further evidence to support their recommendations. The dynamic nature of the condition's course may create special challenges for caregivers and parents. Ideally, a shared vision and a common understanding of the balance of benefit and burden that is acceptable for a certain child are created.

Nonmaleficence

Health care providers have a duty to prevent or remove harms, yet the interventions they pursue to benefit a child sometimes cause harm. Certain medical interventions are painful and uncomfortable and can cause permanent injury or disability. These unintended harms may be justified if they are proportional to the overall benefit that the child will derive from the treatment. Unintended harms can occur with or without negligence. For instance, interacting with the health care system puts children at risk of iatrogenic harm, failure to adequately assess and treat pain can lead to increased suffering, or certain complementary and alternative medical therapies intended to help may pose the risk of harm when their side effects are unknown. In extreme cases children with chronic conditions may receive intentional injuries because of maltreatment. Each of these categories of potential harm will be discussed further.

Medical Harms. Health care providers strive to prevent harm. With technologic interventions that support and improve health, there are often trade-offs in terms of comfort, side effects, restrictions of mobility, and, unfortunately, iatrogenicity. In the decision to accept treatment, parents and children (when developmentally appropriate) weigh the potential benefits against the known or potential harms that can occur with treatment. Chemotherapy usually causes side effects of temporary immunosuppression, gastrointestinal disturbances, hair loss, and fatigue and more permanent complications of peripheral neuropathy or sensorineural hearing loss. Even with careful symptom management, some children cannot escape the side effects. However, for many families, the potential benefit of cure (beneficence) over the burdens of treatment justifies the harm.

Other harms can befall children with chronic conditions who interact with health care professionals. Infiltrations of intravenous fluids, nosocomial infections, and skin breakdown are among the complications that can occur in an inpatient setting. The most common harm that occurs in pediatrics is medication error (Kaushal, Bates, Landrigan, et al., 2001; Kaushal, Jaggi, Walsh, et al., 2004). Children have less physiologic ability to sustain a medication error, yet there are often more opportunities for error. More calculations and steps are required in ordering, dispensing, and administering medication to children than adults, increasing the likelihood of error at each juncture. Progress has been made in computerizing orders and altering how medications are administered, but the safety of children depends on the vigilance of the care providers (Ferranti, Horvath, Cozart, et al., 2008; Wang, Herzog, Kaushal, et al., 2007).

Pain Assessment and Management. It is unequivocally substantiated that children have pain associated with disease and treatments. In 2001, standards for assessing and managing pain were required by the Joint Commission on Accreditation of Healthcare Organizations (2001) under the category of "Rights, Responsibilities, and Ethics." The standard requires systematic assessment and monitoring of the child's response to treatment. Unless the pain provides a therapeutic, necessary use (aid in diagnosis or progression of symptoms), it should be treated, and then it should be reduced to the lowest possible level. When a child's pain is not treated adequately, the child experiences unjustified harms. Concern about oversedation, difficulty with assessment, or the dismissal of the child's self-report contributes to the undertreating of pain in children. Nonverbal children, very young children, or children with significant disabilities are especially vulnerable, and the health care providers must depend on the parents' interpretation of the child's behavior to assess pain and pain relief (Carter, McArthur, & Cunliffe, 2002). Health care providers have a duty to stay abreast of assessment techniques, interventions, and professional guidelines (www.guidelines.gov) for relieving pain in children (American Academy of Pediatrics & American Pain Society, 2001).

New Therapies. The introduction of new therapies for children with chronic conditions often raises ethical concerns. There are two categories of new therapies—complementary and alternative therapies and experimental therapies. Complementary and alternative medicine (CAM) has become increasingly popular. Micozzi (2001, pp. xxiii-xxv) identifies three major areas: alternative medical therapies, such as homeopathy and naturopathy; complementary medicine, such as psychoneuroimmunology, mind-body interventions, humor, or expressive and creative arts therapies; and traditional medical systems, such as yoga, Chinese medicine, and curanderismo. Davis and Darden (2003) cite that 10% to 15% of all children use these therapies, with their usage higher in children with chronic conditions, so it behooves practitioners to be familiar with them. Numerous ethical issues revolve around their use, with the safety of the therapies being paramount (Vohra & Cohen, 2007). For parents to make an informed decision about the use of CAM, they need information. Health care providers can assist the parents in finding reliable information on CAM, although there is limited research evidence. As with all decisions that parents make, the health care providers strive to ensure that parents have as much available information as possible to make their decision. The parents' choice of CAM may reflect their values stemming from their culture. Unless providers believe that the use of CAM represents a real danger to the health of the child, parents are given wide latitude in their use of CAM. The health care provider and the parents together can evaluate the available data, analyze the possible risks and benefits, and come to a decision in the best interests of the child.

Another view of "new" therapies is the use of experimental treatments or procedures in children. In addition, the National Institutes of Health (NIH) mandates that children be included in all federally funded research unless it is inappropriate, but the investigator must justify excluding children (NIH, 1998). Although research on children can be extremely crucial in discovering efficacious treatments,

the NIH mandate is controversial. The Food and Drug Administration issued a Pediatric Rule requiring pharmaceutical companies to conduct clinical trials in children, but this rule was overturned by a federal court in late 2002 (Albert, 2002). Researchers must be aware of the different approaches that are necessary when conducting research in children (Punch, 2002).

Before children are included in clinical research, investigators must get approval from their institutional review board (IRB) to conduct their study in a particular institution. The IRB follows federal regulations for children, which stipulate four conditions under which a child may be included in a study. Briefly, those conditions are when the research (1) poses minimal risk to the child; (2) poses greater than minimal risk but there is the possibility of direct benefit to the child; (3) poses greater than minimal risk, there is no direct benefit, but the research should generate generalizable knowledge about the disorder or condition; and (4) would not otherwise be approved but "presents an opportunity to prevent, or alleviate a serious problem affecting the health or welfare of children" (U.S. Department of Health and Human Services, 1991, 2008). Many, if not all, oncology treatments for children are through enrollment of the child in a national clinical trial. Parents must understand the nature of the research, risks, benefits, and alternatives. Again, the ethical imperative is to foster a complete and thorough understanding of the information for parents to make an informed decision. For children developmentally capable of giving assent, obtaining the child's assent is required, unless the study offers the prospect of a direct benefit.

It is important for health care providers to be aware of the "therapeutic misconception" that parents may have. Although they are told that the child will be randomized into the standard therapy or the experimental therapy, parents may believe that the inclusion of the child in a study is for the child's good. Although it is hoped that the child will benefit from inclusion, clinical equipoise exists; that is, it is not known which treatment, the standard therapy or the experimental therapy, is better. It is ethical therefore to randomize the child into one of the two groups. However, the purpose of the study is to determine the better treatment, thereby helping children in the future, but not guaranteeing the children in the study will be helped.

Primary care providers, children, and families must consider the balance of benefit and burden of both CAM and experimental therapies. To address these challenging situations, parents and caregivers should engage in ongoing, open discussions about poorly tested therapies or experimental treatments. For example, when an innovative surgical procedure is considered for a young child with an orthopedic deformity, the health care provider must disclose the uncertainty surrounding its effectiveness.

Maltreatment. Horner-Johnson and Drum (2006) found that maltreatment of individuals with disabilities ranges between 11.5% and 28%, compared with a rate of 1.24% for children without disabilities (based on data from U.S. Department of Health and Human Services, Administration on Children, Youth and Families, 2005). Many of the same factors that contribute to maltreatment of children without chronic conditions are also present in families of children with chronic conditions, such as dysfunctional families, high levels of stress in the parents, low socioeconomic status (SES), and lower educational level of parents (Goldson, 2001). However, maltreatment of children crosses all SES and educational levels; it is likely that poor, uneducated parents are reported for suspected or actual abuse and neglect more often than parents of higher SES and educational levels. It is also likely that fatalities caused by maltreatment are under-recognized (Crume, DiGuiseppi, Byers, et al., 2002). Primary care providers should be aware of the increased risk and assess families for parenting stress. Recognition and early intervention may reduce the incidence of maltreatment (Committee on Child Abuse and Neglect and Committee on Children with Disabilities, 2001). Advocacy in the political arena for improved services for families of children with disabilities or chronic conditions may also aid in reducing the parental stresses contributing to maltreatment.

Autonomy

A child's autonomy, or self-determination, develops as the child matures. Before the child becomes an independent decision maker, parents make decisions for their children. Underlying the principle of autonomy is respect for persons.

Respect for Persons

A fourth principle involved in decision making is respect for persons. Respect for persons means respecting another person as sharing a common human destiny. Adult decisions focus on the unique life goals and values of the individual out of respect for that individual and the integrity of each life. The uniquely human freedom of each person to create a meaningful life is highly valued. Even though children are neither autonomous nor self-determining, respect is still required because their lives also have unique meaning. To treat individuals with respect is to acknowledge and value who they are outside of a medical context, rather than to only treat them in accordance with how professional goals and values are advanced. Most children live in families that provide nurturance and care. The relationships that arise within families are inherently valuable to the well-being of children. To respect a child is to acknowledge the importance of the child's world and the relationships that are central to it. Unilateral decision making by health care professionals based solely on "medical indications" denies a child fullness of life and relationships that are also benefiting and sustaining.

A central problem associated with parental or other surrogate decisions is the inherent difficulty of judging the quality of a child's life and the benefits and burdens that are experienced. The child, family members, and health care providers may attach different meanings to the child's life. Although life is regarded as valuable, professionals and surrogate decision makers cannot consider the prolongation of life exclusively. Decisions need to benefit and respect the child as an individual but recognize that the child relies on the family for nurturance and physical care. The values that parents place on their parenting roles may make it difficult for them to separate the benefits and burdens of parenting a child with special needs from the benefits and burdens that the child experiences. These decisions are even more complex for primary care providers as they attempt to discern what is best for the child in the context of the family. The choice of interventions can positively or negatively affect the comfort or ease with which a child lives.

Respect for others is enhanced and evidenced by nonjudgmental attitudes and behaviors. It is important to stress that being nonjudgmental does not mean relinquishing values or being blind or indifferent to personal principles. Instead, the goal is openness to different ways of viewing and acting on personal commitments and life circumstances. An essential dimension of nonjudgmental behavior is not imposing personal judgments on others.

Informed Consent.   The standard of informed consent is derived from the principle of respect for persons. Autonomy (i.e., self-determination) is the central moral value expressed through the process of informed consent. Legally, informed consent requires disclosure, comprehension, and voluntary agreement or consent by the competent individual or surrogate. To every possible extent, relevant information about diagnosis and treatment—including a description of the nature and purpose of the treatment or procedure, the benefits and risks, the problems related to recovery, the likelihood of success, and alternative treatments—must be discussed with the surrogate and the child (Claassen, 2000; Savage, 1997). The person giving consent (i.e., usually a parent) must be able to understand relevant information, to reason and deliberate according to his or her values and preferences and the perceived values and preferences of the child, and to communicate the choices to others. Finally, consent must be given voluntarily without coercion. The informed consent process must be evaluated as the child matures and altered as necessary to include the child's expressed decisions or concerns.

Veracity and Fidelity

As part of respect for persons, the health care provider has a duty to be truthful and faithful. In caring for children, the health care provider may feel a conflict in loyalties; sometimes the provider feels a conflict between being truthful with the child and following the request of the parents. For example, a conflict may arise when total parental nutrition (TPN) is being recommended for a 12-year-old girl with Crohn's disease. Her parents have requested that she not be told her diagnosis or the length of time she is expected to need TPN. The health care team expresses their desire to engage the child in decisions affecting her care, but the parents are steadfast in demanding she not be told. In another example, a child who has sustained a spinal cord injury is told by his parents that his paralysis is not permanent. Despite his direct questions, his parents tell him that his condition is temporary and he will walk again "soon." Although the relationships between providers and parents can become tense, open, honest communication and transparency in decision making can facilitate decisions in the child's best interests. If a mutually acceptable approach to veracity cannot be reached, health care providers have the option of negotiating a smooth transfer of care to another appropriate health care provider when they believe they cannot, in good conscience, participate in a child's care. However, the transfer is not always feasible or desirable.

Justice

Justice pertains to fair and equal treatment of others. Therefore justice also refers to an individual's access to an adequate level of health care and the distribution of available health care resources. Caregivers promote the principle of justice by being fair in providing care and attending to children and their families. For example, the *Code of Ethics for Nurses* focuses on delivery of care with respect for human dignity, which is not to be defined in terms of personal attributes, socioeconomic status, or the nature of an illness (American Nurses Association, 2001). This provision requires that a criterion (e.g., age, gender, wealth, religious beliefs, social unacceptability) should not be a factor in deciding between individuals competing for the same treatment. This provision strives for genuine impartiality, equal respect for all persons, and refusal to create a hierarchy of individual worth. Prejudicial treatment on the basis of personal or other attributes is a violation of a moral norm and ideal precious to the health care professions for generations.

Consistent with the ethical obligations of justice, children with chronic conditions are legally protected from discriminatory treatment by state and federal laws. Section 504 of the Rehabilitation Act of 1973 (Public Law 93-112, 1973) grants protection from discrimination based on disability, whereas the Individuals with Disabilities Education Improvement Act (IDEA) (Public Law 101-476, 2004) guarantees access for children with disabilities to education by establishing a federal grant program to help states provide a free and appropriate public education to all children in need of special education (see Chapter 3). The Americans with Disabilities Act (ADA) (1990) gives civil rights protection to individuals with disabilities by guaranteeing equal opportunity to public accommodations, employment, transportation, state and local government services, and telecommunications. Such laws create important obligations for both parents and health care providers and must be considered within the ethical analysis of troubling cases.

Macroallocations of Justice.   Health policies for children with chronic conditions address some of the concerns encompassed in the principle of justice. These policies include strategies to avoid discrimination, stigmatization, and the exploitation of dependence. Strategies to support health insurance reform, delivery of family-centered service, access to employment, and educational opportunities, as well as the community's role in supporting children and their families, are consistent with a justice perspective.

Issues involving the just distribution of health care resources arise at two levels. The macroallocation level refers to the share of societal resources allocated to specific societal goods, such as health care. Resources allocated to support the health, development, and education of children with chronic conditions reflect society's values and willingness to recognize and address the unique circumstances and needs of these children. Unfortunately, health care coverage for children rarely includes habilitation-rehabilitation services, and access to long-term care and other services (e.g., home nursing, some durable and nondurable equipment, or services for children without clear diagnoses) is usually limited. Eligibility is often restricted and based on income or physical, mental, or emotional disabilities. In addition, by not establishing uniform eligibility requirements for Medicaid or the State Children's Health Insurance Programs (SCHIPs) from state to state, children who depend on either of these insurance plans for support services and care in one state may not be able to obtain the same services if they move to another state (see Chapter 8). These issues reflect some of the challenges of devising a national health policy that supports the interests of children with chronic conditions.

Within health care, macroallocation refers to division of a resource (e.g., money) among various services (e.g., transplantation programs, critical care, outpatient services) (Beauchamp & Childress, 2008). This issue is particularly relevant at the institutional level, where costs and priorities for allocating scarce resources are determined. In an era of cost containment and downsizing, institutions and programs providing specialized services to children with chronic conditions are particularly vulnerable. For example, providers may reason that the expenditures for specialized services for children with organ transplants consume a disproportionate share of the overall budget for pediatric care. They may conclude that more children can be helped if money is spent on preventive services. Such reasoning focuses on the consequences of actions by evaluating their utility based on how they can maximize the benefits and outcomes for the greatest number of children. Focusing on a single criterion, such as utility, may not account for other important moral values (e.g., protection of vulnerable populations, existing obligations toward those in the greatest need of services).

Microallocation of Justice.   The term "microallocation" is applied at the individual level; these decisions involve determining the distribution of a specific resource. In general, the professional's main concern is for the individual, but the needs of others may impinge on an individual's care—especially during periods of shortages of human and material resources. Health care providers participate in microallocation decisions when determining which child needs the greatest amount of care, thereby limiting care to others perceived as less needy. Microallocation issues arise when resources are limited and there is not enough of a resource to provide for all who need it.

Beneficence and Justice.   The ethical principles of beneficence and justice are central to issues of resource allocation and rationing. The principle of beneficence requires health care providers to help others and promote good. This principle is evident on two levels: the societal level and the individual level (Beauchamp & Childress, 2008). Each level includes different considerations about allocating limited resources. To realize beneficence at the societal level, resources are allocated based on the needs of society. From a utilitarian perspective, the greatest good for the entire community is considered. The focus shifts from crisis care and doing good for the individual to preventive care and actions that benefit society. This shift is particularly important for children with chronic conditions because greater emphasis on prevention may diminish the specialized services designed to meet their needs. As resources become scarce, difficult decisions must be made to balance the needs of individuals—especially those with chronic conditions—with the needs of society.

On the individual level, health care providers fulfill the duty of beneficence by allocating resources based on individual needs. Scarce resources are distributed to those with immediate needs without regard for the needs of other potential clients or the community at large. For example, when an infant is born with spina bifida, a cadre of medical, developmental, educational, and social resources is mobilized regardless of socioeconomic status, cultural or religious heritage, or ability to pay. This initial commitment to provide equitable and fair services for all families may not be sustained. Cost constraints, lack of available resources, and accessibility of resources may limit services for some children as they mature.

An Ethic of Care

Traditional ethical reasoning requires providers to ascertain the rights of the individual and weigh the ethical principles in order to resolve conflicting obligations. Applying ethical principles alone cannot resolve the clinical quandaries that arise during the care of a child with a chronic condition. The language and method used to analyze a particular case can either clarify or confound the situation. When the rights of children are held in opposition to the rights of their parents, for example, an adversarial tension can be established that may polarize discussion. In contrast, if it is recognized that most parents are motivated to promote their child's interests, such polarity may be avoided. Considering other aspects of the moral life (e.g., virtue, individual experience) may reduce adversarial tensions between the rights of children and their parents and allow for a more comprehensive appreciation of the attitudes, values, and moral commitments of decision makers within the context of family relationships. This perspective is often referred to as an ethic of care.

From the care perspective, the resolution of ethical quandaries is focused on the child's needs in the context of the family's and the provider's corresponding responsibilities within the provider–family–child relationship. Primary care providers can focus on the special circumstances and context of the specific situation in which moral action occurs instead of merely considering the individual's interests and preferences in isolation. Becker and Grunwald (2000) identify contextual dynamics of ethical decision making in the neonatal intensive care unit, but their sociologic observations resonate with other health care settings that care for children with chronic conditions. Such a model supports efforts to help children and their families find unique meaning or purpose in living or dying and realize goals that promote a meaningful life or death.

From this vantage point, the values and expectations involved in certain roles and relationships are primary. Therefore being an advocate for a child with a chronic condition involves appreciating the relationships significant to the child and understanding how those relationships affect care. Children with chronic conditions develop an intricate web of relationships that support and sustain them throughout their lives. In keeping with a family-centered philosophy of care, families are viewed as essential partners in the treatment and care of a child. Professionals must recognize and respect these interconnections as central to the well-being of a child. A care perspective also emphasizes the interrelationships of the members of the health care team. Therefore it recognizes that nurses, physicians, and other caregivers work collaboratively to advance the interests and goals of children with chronic conditions.

Ethical principles (e.g., beneficence, nonmaleficence, autonomy, respect for persons, veracity, fidelity, justice) and an ethic of care provide a framework for approaching ethical questions that occur in clinical practice. It must also be acknowledged that although these are the most common, they may not be the only principles that are relevant to a particular case. The challenge for primary care providers is to discern how these and other principles can help illuminate the ethical issues and guide the resolution of competing obligations.

The Process of Decision Making
Shared Decision Making
Traditionally, a model of shared decision making is based on the assumption that decisions are shared among children (if capable), parents, and professionals (Box 7-4). Treatment decisions must represent a combination of the individuals' expertise in order to select choices that best promote the life goals and values of the child. Parents do not have the expertise to act as surrogate health care professionals, and health care professionals cannot replace the expertise of parents. Shared decision making means that parents and professionals should agree about general treatment goals, but professionals may provide more input into decisions about which treatment modalities are necessary to advance the agreed-on goals.

> **BOX 7-4**
> ## Shared Decision Making
>
> - Role of parents
> - Limits of parental authority
> - Role of minors
>   - Legal issues in role of minors
> - Reality of shared decision making

Endorsement of a model of shared decision making ideally means that parents and children (if capable) engage fully in the process by understanding the range of treatment possibilities and the consequences of each and sharing their goals, values, and aspirations in a meaningful way. Such a model goes beyond the legal requirements for disclosure, comprehension, and voluntary consent (Bauchner, 2001). Although professionals theoretically embrace the ideal of shared decision making as the desired model of parent-professional decision making, accomplishing it remains difficult (Ladd & Mercurio, 2003; Perrin, Lewkowicz, & Young, 2000).

Role of Parents in Treatment Decision Making
Based on the moral framework of shared decision making described here, someone must represent the interests of the child. There is a strong presumption that parents should make judgments about the best interest of the child (Perrin et al., 2000). Parents are appropriate surrogates because their strong bonds of affection and commitment are likely to yield the greatest concern for the well-being of their children. Parents are expected to protect their children from harm and to do as much good for them as possible.

There is a direct connection between the well-being of parents and children; the identities of each are inextricably linked. For example, a woman who defines herself as a mother regards her own welfare partly in terms of the welfare of her child. Harm to the child constitutes personal harm to the mother. Such relationships are valuable to both parents and children, and society needs to limit its interference in this private realm (Caplan & Cohen, 1987; Cardol, De Jong, & Ward, 2002). Further, parents are identified as primary decision makers because of the importance of the family institution. Families play an essential role in maintaining the integrity of society. Children learn values of cooperation and commitment within the family context that can then be generalized to other members of society.

Parents must be involved in treatment decisions for their infants and children because there are lifelong consequences of these decisions. Parents will be responsible for the ongoing physical, emotional, medical, and financial care of the infant or child who survives with serious disabilities and will also live with the consequences of those decisions. Long after health care professionals have forgotten a case, the family will remember and have incorporated such momentous decisions into the fabric of their lives.

Limits of Parental Authority
In addition to being members of their immediate families, children are also members of a broader community. A moral community shares an interest in the life and well-being of each member. There are certain community standards of best interest (e.g., preservation of life) that may override a family's interpretation of a child's best interest. Although there are compelling reasons to support the

decision-making authority of parents, such authority is not absolute. The interests of the parents and the family must take a high priority but should not override the fundamental respect for the best interest of the infant or child. Ideally, the family and providers engage in a partnership to include the child in decision making as appropriate (Cavet & Sloper, 2004).

Even when parents and professionals presume shared responsibility to promote the well-being of a child, there are times when parents should be disqualified as primary decision makers. This disqualification may be the result of incapacity or choosing a course of action that is clearly against the child's best interest (President's Commission for the Study of Ethical Problems in Medicine and Biomedical and Behavioral Research, 1983). If a parent has a known psychiatric condition and is behaving irrationally or has a documented history of child abuse or neglect, the primary care provider may question parental capacity to advocate on behalf of the child. If there is a dispute about parental intentions or capacity to function as decision makers, it is incumbent that those who substitute another decision maker provide convincing evidence why the parents should be disqualified. For example, even though respect for religious beliefs is an important community value, so is the value of life. Although adults who are Jehovah's Witnesses can choose to forgo a lifesaving blood transfusion for themselves, they are often not permitted to make a similar decision for their children. Moreover, children are entitled to grow up and make independent assessments of their own religious beliefs.

In such circumstances health care providers must advocate for children and uphold the community standard of best interest. There will always be cases in which such assumptions are challenged; but these are likely to be few. Those who challenge parental motives and commitments must prove that parents should be disqualified as decision makers instead of having parents prove that their motives and commitments are authentic. Safeguards to protect the interests of children, families, and professionals will continue to be necessary and prudent. Assessing when community standards should outweigh a family determination is extremely difficult.

Whether the disqualification of parents always requires court intervention is the source of much debate (President's Commission, 1983; Ridgeway, 2004). When parents are disqualified, a surrogate decision maker should know all relevant facts and be able to perceive and represent the feelings and interests of those involved. Surrogate decision makers should also be free of serious conflicts of interest that may bias a decision. A court-appointed guardian ad litem often serves as a surrogate decision maker. In special circumstances, such as obtaining permission for withholding resuscitation for a child with significant disabilities who is a ward of the state, it is difficult to identify a single surrogate. The personnel in the child welfare agency may not know the child well, the foster parents may not know the child well, and the natural parents may not have any contact with the child. In these instances, an ethics consultation may aid in identifying key people and designing a process for arriving at a decision in the best interests of the child (Savage & Michalik, 2002).

Role of Minors in Treatment Decision Making

Professionals who care for children and adolescents with chronic conditions are increasingly concerned about the role minors play in making decisions about their health care. Many adolescents experience catastrophic physical and mental health problems associated with severe disabilities, malignancies, or cardiac, pulmonary, and hepatic organ disease without having the legal right to decide about their treatments.

As client advocates, primary care providers must be concerned with how to promote the interests of adolescents in decisions regarding their health care. The concerns of adolescents escalate when parents and primary care providers seem to disregard the adolescent's previously expressed preferences or embark on a course of treatment that is inconsistent with the adolescent's life goals and values. Many health professionals are questioning the adequacy of current decision-making models and searching for creative solutions, perhaps through the advent of advance directives for minors.

From a moral viewpoint, minors with decision-making capacities have a legitimate claim to be involved in decisions about their health care. This claim is based on a respect for persons that recognizes that adolescents and young adults can be self-determining and therefore should have a voice in their care and the extent of medical interventions provided. Such respect for them as individuals and members of families and society compels primary care providers to take their preferences seriously when treatment decisions are made. Moreover, adolescents' interpretations of the benefits and burdens of treatment should be considered.

The standards for determining the decision-making capacity of minors are the same as those for adults (American Academy of Pediatrics Committee on Bioethics, 1994):

1. The ability to comprehend essential information about their diagnosis and prognosis
2. The ability to reason about their choices in accordance with their values and life goals
3. The ability to make a voluntary informed decision, which includes being able to recognize the consequences of various courses of action

Based on our knowledge of conceptual development, most children do not reach this level of maturity until they are 11 or 12 years of age (White, 1994), although there is wide variation and controversy concerning theories and stages of cognitive development (Alderson et al., 2006). These standards are straightforward, but applying them in clinical practice requires clinicians to be skilled in systematically assessing and documenting the decision-making capacity of minors.

Despite the importance of self-determination and well-being in justifying the participation of minors in treatment decisions, there is another competing value at stake: the interests of parents in making decisions for their minor children. It has traditionally been assumed that minors require surrogates to make decisions for them. Parents are generally identified as the appropriate surrogates for their children and have been afforded considerable discretion in making treatment decisions.

Currently, treatment decisions for adolescents are made through a joint determination by the physician or health care team and the parent or guardian for the child. Joint decisions to withhold or withdraw therapeutic interventions are difficult for both parents and health care providers to formulate. Parents may seek any possible intervention to prolong their child's life, regardless of the burden to be endured. Alternatively, they may wish to relieve their child's suffering by forgoing certain life-sustaining treatments. The physician or health care team and the parent or guardian may have different agendas for either continuing or initiating certain therapeutic interventions or, instead, forgoing certain interventions; yet both groups may interpret their decisions as being in the best interest of the child. Despite their assessments, neither group may truly understand the adolescent's perspective. In many cases, the adolescent may already understand the pain and consequences of the treatment options, including the finality of death. Unfortunately, parents and health care providers may hesitate to consider adolescents as legitimate decision makers about medical treatment.

As the model of decision making enlarges to include a definitive role for minors with decision-making capacity, health care providers must recognize that such a departure will also challenge the traditional process of decision making and may create conflicts between minors and their parents. The potential for such moral and legal conflicts will necessitate the determination of a mechanism for resolving disputes. Researchers combined information from three studies on decision making in pediatric oncology, published literature, and professional associations' positions to posit evidence-based practice guidelines for end-of-life decision making by adolescents, their parents, and health care providers (Hinds, Oakes, Furman, et al., 2001). These guidelines may be useful outside the oncology setting as well.

Legal Viewpoint on the Role of Minors in Decision Making. The legal system has determined that adolescents in certain circumstances have specific rights and responsibilities associated with their decision-making capabilities for health care. Emancipated minors are children under 18 years of age who are in the armed forces or are financially self-supporting and live away from home (Dickens & Cook, 2005). Most states have legislation recognizing the rights and responsibilities of emancipated minors. Emancipation is rarely determined by the courts and is generally implied through factors such as marital status, pregnancy or parenthood, and financial self-sufficiency. Emancipated minors do not need parental consent for medical treatment and have rights similar to adults in refusing medical treatment (Dickens & Cook, 2005; Traugott & Alpers, 1997).

The courts have also classified some adolescents as mature minors in relation to their decision-making capacity for seeking and accepting health care interventions. Mature minors are at least 15 years of age and thought to have the capacity to understand the nature and risk of medical interventions. Adolescents classified as mature minors may consent to treatment that benefits them and does not involve any substantial risk. Derish and Vanden Heuvel (2000) present the various arguments, pro and con, for the mature minor's right to refuse life-sustaining treatment.

State statutes generally support a minor's (i.e., a 14- to 17-year-old's) rights to consent to ordinary medical care. For example, some state statutes support the right of minors to consent to specific medical treatment (e.g., contraceptive therapies) without parental notification and consent; the right to consent to abortion, however, is complex and varied. The Omnibus Reconciliation Act of 1990, which is also called the Patient Self-Determination Act (PSDA) of 1990, supports the right of adults (i.e., at least 18 years old) admitted to health care facilities to accept or refuse medical treatment. This age limit is based on the belief that only adults have the capacity and the right to determine what should be done to their bodies—even if executing this right means implementing

their right to die. It is crucial, however, that health care providers do not ignore the plight of thousands of adolescents (i.e., 12- to 17-year-olds) who face similar catastrophic and terminal conditions but are not given this legal right.

Although the PSDA was created for adults, the spirit of the PSDA provides an opportunity to examine the potential role of minors in their treatment decisions and ultimately their right to determine the circumstances of their death. It is likely that many young children and adolescents have the capacity to help make their own treatment decisions and determine what is in their best interest. There has been minimal guidance from the courts or from legislation on a minor's right to refuse lifesaving medical care. In the few decisions that have been rendered, the application of the mature minor status was used to support the minor's decision-making capacity to refuse treatment and understand the consequences of this decision. Unfortunately, because there are minimal and vague legal guidelines available to support a minor's rights to refuse treatment, health care providers are reluctant to intervene and support the minor's decision to withhold treatment—especially if this opposes the parents' wishes.

Involving minors in decision making about treatment requires families and professionals to create a system that supports the participation of minors. Such a system must include comprehensive guidelines for assessment, intervention, and ongoing revision (Hallstrom & Elander, 2005; McCabe, Rushton, Glover, et al., 1996).

Making Shared Decisions a Reality

Regardless of the child's age, the family's composition and dynamics, or professionals' involvement, resolution of ethical concerns is supported by an authentic model of shared decision making that accommodates the diverse ways children and families choose to participate. To resolve ethical concerns, it is necessary to move beyond a procedural model of informed consent to an authentic partnership in which parents, the child, and professionals create an alliance that promotes the child's interests. The foundation for this alliance is a mutual understanding of each other's aspirations and goals, perspectives on what makes life meaningful for the child, and concepts of benefit and burden. In addition, parents need to share their goals, values, and definition of being good parents, and professionals must share their uncertainties and boundaries of their professional responsibility.

Shared decision making requires a vision that results from collaboration and open, effective communication using language without technical terminology and jargon. One reason achieving shared decision making fails is that professionals may focus primarily on the decision itself, instead of on the process. Parents also may have difficulty separating emotions from facts. A revised model of shared decision making would focus more on the context of the situation—especially the relational dimensions, the parents' unique concept of good parenting, and the factors that mediate decision making—rather than on the decision itself.

Professionals must begin to appreciate the parents' perspective in decision making and not try to force them into a traditional, rational, stepwise model that is incongruent with their perspective. Therefore the goals of the parent-professional relationship, the outcomes of the process, and the process itself must be closely scrutinized. For example, if the goal of the relationship with families is to get them to see the world in the same way as the professional, dissenting views cannot be articulated or respected. Parents should be engaged early in a variety of choices about their child's care so that their involvement is not reserved for required consents for treatment or decisions about life-sustaining treatment. Parents need and want professionals to be partners in the care of their child—regardless of the outcome—and want professionals to help them be good parents in the process. Therefore sharing in decision making must begin early in the management of the condition.

Authentic shared decision making does not mean that differences will not exist or that everyone will come to the same conclusion about when and how to advance the child's interests. Nor does it mean that all participants will have the same skills, abilities, or preferences. Shared decision making is a process in which differences are discussed, differing opinions are valued, and the quality of care ultimately provided to the child and family is enhanced.

Transition to Adulthood

In most states, people 18 years of age and older are legally responsible for giving or refusing consent for medical treatment. People with chronic conditions often continue to be treated by pediatric subspecialists into their twenties and thirties because children with these disorders (e.g., spina bifida) in the past did not survive into adulthood. Unfortunately, some pediatric health care providers operate under a child-focused model of decision making and do not transition to an adult model when young adults are legally able and willing to serve as primary decision makers. Many transition programs are in place or being developed, but these are not without ethical problems (see Chapter 4). Ideally, the adolescent or young adult would have increasingly participated in decision making as developmentally appropriate. However, in some families, children with chronic conditions are prevented from participation because their parents see them as too immature and unable to make rational decisions. The child's lack of experience makes the parents' impression a self-fulfilling prophecy. Lacking the experience, the child is unable to participate or fears participating in decision making. The health care team can educate parents to identify and foster the capabilities for decision making in their child: understanding information, manipulating information, appreciating the impact of the decision on one's own situation, and making a choice (Grisso & Appelbaum, 1998).

Many older adolescents and young adults demonstrate a sophisticated level of understanding of their conditions and treatment. Members of the health care team can honor the autonomy of older adolescents and young adults by preparing them to participate in decisions and acting on their choices after the informed consent process (Dickens & Cook, 2005). There are other older adolescents or young adults who—because of cognitive comorbidity or immaturity—do not have the capacity to make decisions. Although they may be legally competent because they have not been declared incompetent by the courts, their ability to reason may be legitimately questioned. An assessment of their decision-making capacity, specific to the decision, should be undertaken and documented. Traditionally, parents or guardians have retained decision-making authority in such circumstances. Clinicians must work to foster decision making within the family context. To avoid confusion, parents should be counseled to seek legal guardianship for adult sons or daughters who lack decision-making capacity. Unfortunately, the cost of doing so is prohibitive for some families. Persons who lack the capacity to make decisions (e.g., those with

severe developmental disabilities) should be respectfully allowed to participate in the decision-making process. As with young children, every child should be afforded the opportunity to be prepared for medical interventions, to receive developmentally appropriate explanations, and to express preferences. The more important the decision in the life of the person, the greater the care in assessing that person's decision-making capacity pertinent to what the specific decision should be. Health care providers must be familiar with their institution's policies on surrogate decision making for adults who lack decisional capacity.

The Olmstead decision (*Olmstead v. L.C.*, No. 98-536, U.S. Supreme Court, June 22, 1999) bolstered the move toward independent and assisted living. Young adults who previously would have remained at home or been placed in residential facilities may choose the most integrated setting possible versus the most restrictive. The public entity, such as a state-supported institution, must facilitate placement in the most integrated setting appropriate to the needs of qualified individuals with disabilities. In the transition program, the health care provider who is knowledgeable about the Olmstead decision can assist in removing barriers so often faced by young adults with chronic disabling conditions.

Strategies for Ethical Decision Making
Increased Knowledge of Ethics, Laws, and Policies

Professionals can enhance their effectiveness in resolving ethical conflicts by seeking opportunities to enhance their knowledge of and skills in ethical analysis, as well as by identifying resources to assist them in resolving dilemmas. Further, knowledge of legal, public, and professional policies is advantageous. In particular, primary care providers who care for children with chronic conditions should be aware of pertinent state statutes and case laws that may affect their health care. Primary care providers must be particularly aware of institutional policies on discontinuing life-sustaining treatment, if such policies exist, and participate in developing them if they do not. Institutional policies that permit information to be withheld from parents or effectively deny parental access to divergent medical opinions should also be examined and challenged.

Proactive Dialogue, Assessment, and Planning

Children with chronic conditions and their families often have a high level of personal interaction with primary care providers. Because many chronic conditions persist over a lifetime, there are many natural opportunities to examine, revise, or abandon various goals or dimensions of the treatment plan. With proactive planning, it is also possible and desirable to anticipate the ethical conflicts that accompany the treatment plan. Ongoing dialogue about the treatment plan is essential for optimal planning and must not be reserved for crisis situations associated with acute episodes or illness, deteriorating conditions, or death.

Many children with chronic conditions and their families and providers will confront difficult decisions about treatment that will create significant moral tension. Questions about parental acceptance of psychoactive medications to treat children with attention-deficit/hyperactivity disorder or to try an experimental protocol for treating cancer may arise. Such morally difficult decisions are best made when there is adequate time for education, discussion, and reflection. Therefore ethical issues should be anticipated and discussions begun early.

Genetic Testing: Privacy and Confidentiality

Ethical questions regarding the use of genetic testing and new or experimental techniques for treating genetic disorders are arising. Genetic testing has long been accepted in newborn testing for the purposes of early identification for treatment. Technology has advanced to be able to identify many genetic disorders. Parents may be offered the opportunity to have genetic testing for themselves and their child in an attempt to diagnose their child's condition. When signs and symptoms indicate that a child may have a genetic disorder, even if a cure is not available, the family may benefit by knowing the diagnosis, planning for the child's future needs, and learning the probability of future children being affected. Although parents may have an intense desire to discover their child's diagnosis, they may fear that their child will be stigmatized and discriminated against by insurance companies, schools, and eventually employers. The Health Insurance Portability and Accountability Act of 1996 (HIPAA) (2002) contained no special provisions protecting genetic information. However, newer federal legislation, the Genetic Information Nondiscrimination Act (GINA), passed in 2008, is designed to protect Americans against discrimination based on their genetic information when it comes to health insurance and employment. Additionally, there is extensive relevant state legislation (see www.genome. gov/PolicyEthics/LegDatabase/pubsearch.cfm for a list of all legislation).

Although the technique of obtaining a blood test or a buccal smear or performing a skin biopsy in the office may seem rather benign, the ramifications of the findings can have profound consequences on the child's and family's future. Primary care providers can guard the privacy and confidentiality of a child's medical information by developing and implementing institutional policies on informed consent for genetic testing, special disposition of test results, and special procedures for releasing medical records containing test results (i.e., to schools, insurers, and others) National Task Force on Confidential Student Health Information. (2000). Many institutions currently have special procedures for tests (e.g., human immunodeficiency virus [HIV]) that protect individuals from unwarranted disclosure of information.

Presymptomatic genetic testing for adult-onset conditions (e.g., Huntington's disease, breast cancer) generally is not recommended for children (American Academy of Pediatrics, 2005; American Academy of Pediatrics Committee on Bioethics, 2001; Ross & Moon, 2000), but decisions should always be made in the best interest of the child (Twomey, 2006). Predictive testing may be done according to the "rule of earliest onset" for selected conditions (Kodish, 1999) and at the discretion of the parents for late childhood–onset disorders, with the child's input where appropriate. However, government-sponsored predictive screenings "do not fulfill public health screening criteria" (Ross, 2002, p. 225).

Testing one member of the family can yield information about other members. Families need to be aware of the ramifications of testing. Genetic counselors are skilled in assisting families in making decisions to share or withhold information about a tested relative. Sometimes it is necessary to test relatives. Again, genetic counselors assist families in understanding the extent to which other family members need to be involved to yield useful information

(Hodge, 2004). Guidelines in protecting privacy of family members for genetics research may also prove useful for protecting privacy for nonresearch testing. Doukas and Berg (2001) propose a family covenant model in working with families who have genetic testing. The family covenant recognizes the family as a unit and its members in the context of the family. With genetic knowledge increasing exponentially, professionals working with children with chronic conditions and their families should stay abreast of genetic advances and applicable laws. Programs such as the Ethical, Legal, and Social Implications (ELSI) branch of the National Human Genome Research Institute provide leadership in this area and post emerging news and information in this dynamic field (www. genome.gov). Professional organizations may also provide information and advocacy on advances in genetics.

Enormous advances in gene therapy and stem cell research are being realized. Hundreds of gene transfer protocols are underway or will be underway for conditions such as cystic fibrosis, hemophilia, muscular dystrophy, Fanconi anemia, Gaucher disease, and Canavan disease. As with any clinical trial, parents need as much information as possible to make an informed decision, and the child, if capable, should be included in the discussions. Additional ethical issues surrounding genetic advances, such as their availability and limitations, will need to be addressed in the future.

Strategies for Dealing with Conflict

Even when communication among children, parents, and professionals is optimal, conflicts arise. In fact, good communication may illuminate points of real ethical dispute. Participants often prioritize values differently and employ different processes to reach morally defensible conclusions. Therefore activities that promote multidisciplinary sharing, analysis, and decision making in an atmosphere of openness, objectivity, and diversity can lead to more tolerance of others' views.

When moral disagreements occur, strategies for resolution include the following:

1. Obtaining the most current factual information on points of controversy
2. Reaching a consensus about the language used for concepts or definitions
3. Agreeing on a framework of moral principles to guide discussions
4. Engaging in a balanced discussion of the positive and negative aspects of a viewpoint

Institutions can review difficult or disputed cases through institutional ethics committees and other means of efficiently accessing legal, governmental, and consultative services. An internal review process can serve several purposes, including

1. Verifying the facts of the case
2. Confirming the propriety of decisions
3. Resolving disputes
4. Making referrals to public agencies when appropriate

Institutional ethics committees are often consultants to staff and families experiencing ethical conflict. Multidisciplinary membership (i.e., including a parent) provides a broad representation of different viewpoints. In general, these committees are primarily consultative without any binding authority. The opportunity for uninvolved parties to assist in reviewing difficult cases, however, can provide constructive recommendations for resolution. Ethics committees or the use of ethics consultants is increasing in home health agencies, nursing homes, and community health facilities.

Mechanisms to resolve conflicts between minors and their parents must be developed as the process of involving minors in treatment decisions unfolds. Based on a model of family-centered care, mechanisms supporting individual self-determination within the context of the family system are necessary. Strategies will also be needed to support families as they allow their minor children to be more involved in decision making. Mechanisms for examining the decision-making patterns of families and the roles of children and parents in other types of decisions within the family are also necessary. Finally, strategies to prepare minors to participate in decisions about health care through community or school educational programs and as part of routine health care encounters are important prerequisites (Cavet & Sloper, 2005).

Summary

The resolution of ethical conflicts requires that health care professionals recognize there is a moral problem, use a systematic process of moral reasoning, and take action. As a prerequisite to such analysis, primary care providers who care for children with chronic conditions and their families must examine their own values about the content and structure of treatment decisions. Such clarification is necessary to ensure that the ideal of authentic shared decision making becomes a reality.

Resources

Alliance of Genetic Support Groups, Inc.
Website: www.geneticalliance.org
American Nurses Association
Website: www.nursingworld.org
American Society for Bioethics and Humanities
Website: www.asbh.org
Academic Bioethics Centers
Website: http://bioethics.od.nih.gov/academic.html
Center for Bioethics
University of Pennsylvania Medical Center
Website: www.bioethics.upenn.edu
Center for Clinical Ethics and Humanities in Health Care
University of Buffalo
Website: www.wings.buffalo.edu/faculty/research/bioethics
Council for Responsible Genetics
Website: www.gene-watch.org
Eubios Ethics Institute
Website: www.eubios.info
International Society of Nurses in Genetics (ISONG)
Website: www.isong.org
Kennedy Institute of Genetics
Georgetown University
Website: http://bioethics.georgetown.edu
MacLean Center for Clinical Ethics at University of Chicago
Website: http://medicine.uchicago.edu/centers/ccme/index.htm

National Bioethics Advisory Commission
Website: www.bioethics.gov
National Human Genome Research Institute
Website: www.genome.gov
National Library of Medicine
Website: www.nlm.nih.gov
National Reference Center for Bioethics Literature
Website: http://bioethics.georgetown.edu/nrc/visitNRCBL.htm

REFERENCES

Albert, T. (2002). *Federal court overturns FDA pediatric drug testing rule.* Available at www.ama-assn.org/amednews/2002/11/18/gvsc1118.htm. Retrieved November 19, 2008.

Alderson, P., Sutcliffe, K., & Curtis, K. (2006). Children's competence to consent to medical treatment. *Hastings Cent Rep, 36*(6), 25-34.

American Academy of Pediatrics. (2005). AAP publications retired and reaffirmed. *Pediatrics, 115*, 1438.

American Academy of Pediatrics Committee on Bioethics (1994). Guidelines on forgoing life sustaining medical treatment. *Pediatrics, 3*, 533-535.

American Academy of Pediatrics Committee on Bioethics. (2001). Ethical issues with genetic testing in pediatrics. *Pediatrics, 107*(6), 1451-1455.

American Academy of Pediatrics & American Pain Society. (2001). The assessment and management of acute pain in infants, children and adolescents. *Pediatrics, 108*(3), 793-797.

American Nurses Association. (2001). *Code of Ethics for Nurses with Interpretive Statements.* Washington, DC: Author.

Americans with Disabilities Act of 1990. (1990). Available at www.ada.gov/pubs/ada.htm. Retrieved November 12, 2008.

Bauchner, H. (2001). Shared decision making in pediatrics. *Arch Dis Child, 84*, 246.

Beauchamp, T.L., & Childress, J.F. (2008). *Principles of Biomedical Ethics* (6th ed.). New York: Oxford University Press.

Becker, P.T., & Grunwald, P.C. (2000). Contextual dynamics of ethical decision making in the NICU. *J Perinat Neonat Nurs, 14*(2), 58-72.

Beidler, S.M., & Dickey, S.B. (2001). Children's competence to participate in healthcare decisions. *JONA's Healthc Law Ethics Regulation, 3*, 80-87.

Blustein, J. (1998). The family in medical decision making. In J.F. Monagle & D.C. Thomasma (Eds.), *Health Care Ethics: Critical Issues for the 21st Century.* Gaithersburg, MD: Aspen Systems.

Caplan, A., & Cohen, C. (1987). *Ethics and the Care of Imperiled Newborns: A Report by the Hastings Center's Research Project on Ethics and the Care of Imperiled Newborns.* New York: Hastings Center.

Cardol, M., De Jong, B.A., & Ward, C.D. (2002). On autonomy and participation in rehabilitation. *Disabil Rehabil, 24*(18), 970-974.

Carter, B., McArthur, E., & Cunliffe, M. (2002). Dealing with uncertainty: Parental assessment of pain in their children with profound special needs. *J Adv Nurs, 38*, 449-457.

Cavet, J., & Sloper, P. (2004). Participation of disabled children in individual decisions about their lives and in public decisions about service development. *Children & Society, 18*(4), 278-290.

Child Abuse Amendments of 1984. (1984). 42 U.S. Code 10401 et seq: Interpretive Guidelines. (45 CFR Part 1 1340:15 et eq.) Washington, DC: U.S. Government Printing Office.

Claassen, M. (2000). A handful of questions: Supporting parental decision making. *Clin Nurse Spec, 14*(4), 189-195.

Committee on Bioethics. (1994). Guidelines for forgoing life-sustaining medical treatment. *Pediatrics, 93*(3), 532-536.

Committee on Child Abuse and Neglect and Committee on Children with Disabilities. (2001). Assessment of maltreatment of children with disabilities. *Pediatrics, 108*, 508-512.

Crume, T.L., DiGuiseppi, C., Byers, T., et al. (2002). Underascertainment of child maltreatment fatalities by death certificates, 1990-1998. *Pediatrics, 110*, e18.

Davis, M.P., & Darden, P.M. (2003). Use of complementary and alternative medicine by children in the United States. *Arch Pediatr Adolesc Med, 157*, 393-396.

Derish, M.T., & Vanden Heuvel, K. (2000). Mature minors should have the right to refuse life-sustaining medical treatment. *J Law Med Ethics, 28*, 109-124.

Dickens, B.M., & Cook, R.J. (2005). Adolescents and consent to treatment. *Int J Gynecol Obstet, 89*(2), 179B-184B.

Doukas, D.J., & Berg, J.W. (2001). The family covenant and genetic testing. *Am J Bioethics, 1*(3), 2-10.

Ferranti, J., Horvath, M.M., Cozart, H., et al. (2008). Reevaluating the safety profile of pediatrics: A comparison of computerized adverse drug event surveillance and voluntary reporting in the pediatric environment. *Pediatrics, 121,* e1201-e1207.

Fost, N. (1999). Decisions regarding treatment of seriously ill newborns. *J Am Med Assoc, 281*(21), 2041-2043.

Geron Ethics Advisory Board (1999). Research with human embryonic stem cells: Ethical considerations. *Hastings Cent Rep, 29*(2), 31-36.

Goldson, E. (2001). Maltreatment among children with disabilities. *Infants and Young Children, 13*(4), 44-54.

Grisso, T., & Appelbaum, P.S. (1998). *Assessing Competence to Consent to Treatment.* New York: Oxford University Press.

Hall, M.A., & Rich, S.S. (2000). Genetic privacy laws and patients' fear of discrimination by health insurers: The view from genetic counselors. *J Law Med Ethics, 28,* 245-257.

Hallström, I., & Elander, G. (2005). Decision making in paediatric care: An overview with reference to nursing care. *Nursing Ethics, 12*(3), 223-238.

Health Information Portability and Accountability Act (HIPAA). (2002). Available at www.hhs.gov/ocr/hipaa. Retrieved May 25, 2008.

Hinds, P.S., Oakes, L., & Furman, W., et al. (2001). End-of-life decision making by adolescents, parents, and healthcare providers in pediatric oncology: Research to evidence-based practice guidelines. *Cancer Nurs, 24*(2), 122-134.

Hodge, J.G. (2004). Ethical issues concerning genetic testing and screening in public health. *Am J Med Genet Part C, 125*(1), 66-70.

Horner-Johnson, W., & Drum, C.E. (2006). Prevalence of maltreatment of people with intellectual disabilities: A review of the recently published research. *Ment Retard Dev Disabil, 12,* 57-69.

Hynson, J.L., & Sawyer, S.M. (2001). Paediatric palliative care: Distinctive needs and emerging issues. *J Paediatr Child Health, 37*(4), 323-325.

Individuals with Disabilities Education Amendments of 1997. (1997). Public Law 105-17. Washington, DC: U.S. Government Printing Office.

Individuals with Disabilities Education Improvement Act of 2004. (2004). Public Law 108-446. Washington, DC: U.S. Government Printing Office.

Joint Commission on Accreditation of Healthcare Organizations (2001). *Comprehensive Accreditation Manual for Hospitals: The Official Handbook.* Oakbrook Terrace, IL.: Author.

Jonsen, A.R., Siegler, M., & Winslade, W.J. (1998). *Clinical Ethics.* (4th ed.). New York: McGraw-Hill.

Kaji, E.H., & Leiden, J.M. (2001). Gene and stem cell therapies. *J Am Med Assoc, 285,* 545-550.

Kaushal, R., Bates, D.W., & Landrigan, C., et al. (2001). Medication errors and adverse drug events in pediatric inpatients. *J Am Med Assoc, 285*(16), 2114-2120.

Kaushal, T., Jaggi, K., Walsh, E.B., et al. (2004). Pediatric medication errors: What do we know? What gaps remain? *Ambul Pediatr, 4*(1), 73-81.

Kodish, E. (1999). Testing children for cancer genes: The rule of earliest onset. *J Pediatr, 135*(3), 390-395.

Ladd, R.E., & Mercurio, M.R. (2003). Deciding for neonates: Whose authority, whose interests? *Semin Perinatol, 27,* 488-494.

Martenson, E.K., & Fagerskiold, A.M. (2007). A review of children's decision-making competence in health care. *J Clin Nurs, Sep, 19*(7), 40-43.

McCabe, M.A., Rushton, C.H., Glover, J., et al. (1996). Implications of the Patient Self-Determination Act: Guidelines for involving adolescents in medical decision-making. *J Adolesc Health, 19*(5), 319-324.

McCormick, R. (1974). To save or let die: The dilemma of modern medicine. *J Am Med Assoc, 229*(2), 172-176.

Micozzi, M.S. (2001). *Fundamentals of Complementary and Alternative Medicine* (2nd ed.). New York: Churchill Livingstone.

National Institutes of Health. (1998). *Policy and guidelines on the inclusion of children as participants in research involving human subjects.* Available at http://grants1.nih.gov/grants/guide/notice-files/not98-024.html. Retrieved November 12, 2008.

Olmstead v. L.C. (98-536) U.S. Supreme Court, decided June 22, 1999. Available at http://supct.law.cornell.edu/supct/html/98-536.ZO.html. Retrieved November 19, 2008.

Omnibus Reconciliation Act (Patient Self-Determination Act [PSDA]), Title IV. Section 4206, h12456-h12457, *Congressional Record,* October 26, 1990.

Perrin, E.C., Lewkowicz, C., & Young, M.H. (2000) Shared vision: Concordance among fathers, mothers, and pediatricians about unmet needs of children with chronic health conditions. *Pediatrics, 105*(Suppl 1), 277-285.

President's Commission for the Study of Ethical Problems in Medicine and Biomedical and Behavioral Research. (1983). *Deciding to Forgo Life-Sustaining Treatment.* Washington, DC: U.S. Government Printing Office.

Punch, S. (2002). Research with children the same or different from research with adults?. *Childhood, 9*(3), 321-341.

Ridgeway, D. (2004). Court-mediated disputes between physicians and families over the medical care of children. *Arch Pediatr Adolesc Med, 158,* 891-896.

Ross, L.F. (1997). Health care decision making by children: Is it in their best interest? *Hastings Cent Rep, 27*(6), 41-45.

Ross, L.F. (2002). Predictive genetic testing for conditions that present in childhood. *Kennedy Inst Ethics J, 12*(3), 225-244.

Ross, L.F., & Moon, M.R. (2000). Ethical issues in genetic testing of children. *Arch Pediatr Adolesc Med, 154*(9), 873-879.

Saigal, S., & Doyle, L.W. (2008). An overview of mortality and sequelae of preterm birth from infancy to adulthood. *Lancet, 371*(9608), 261-269.

Saigal, S., & Tyson, J. (2008). Measurement of quality of life of survivors of neonatal intensive care: Critique and implications. *Semin Perinatol, 32,* 59-66.

Savage, T.A. (1997). Ethical decision-making for children. *Crit Care Nurs Clin North Am, 9*(1), 97-105.

Savage, T.A., & Michalik, D.R. (2002). Finding agreement to limit life-sustaining treatment for children who are in state custody. *Curr Pract Pediatr Nurs, 27,* 594-597.

Section 504 of the Rehabilitation Act of 1973. (1973). Public Law 93-112. Washington DC: U.S. Government Printing Office.

Traugott, I, & Alpers, A. (1997). In their own hands: Adolescents' refusals of medical treatment. *Arch Pediatr Adolesc Med, 151*(9), 922-927.

Twomey, J.G. (2006). Issues in genetic testing of children. *MCN Am J Matern Child Nurs, 31,* 156-163.

U.S. Department of Health and Human Services. (1991). Office for Human Research Protections. *45 CFR 46 Subpart B. 46.* 404-407.

U.S. Department of Health and Human Services. (2008, January 3). Office for Human Research Protections (OHRP). OHRP 45 CFR part 46. *Frequently asked questions.* Available at www.hhs.gov/ohrp/45CFRpt46faq.html. Retrieved on Novmeber 12, 2008.

U.S. Department of Health and Human Services, Administration on Children, Youth and Families. (2005). *Child maltreatment 2003.* Washington, DC: U.S. Government Printing Office.

Vohra, S., & Cohen, M.H. (2007). Ethics of complementary and alternative medicine use in children. *Pediatr Clin North Am, 54,* 875-884.

Wang, J.K., Herzog, N.S., & Kaushal, R., et al. (2007). Prevention of pediatric medication errors by hospital pharmacists and the potential benefit of computerized physician order entry. *Pediatrics, 119,* e77-e85.

White, B.C. (1994). *Competence to Consent.* Washington, DC: Georgetown University Press.

8

Financing Health Care for Children with Chronic Conditions

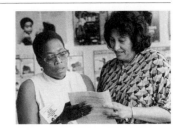

Judith A. Vessey and Stacy Suzanne Brown

USING the Maternal and Child Health Bureau's definition, it is estimated that 13.9% of children have special health care needs (referred to as *children with special health care needs,* or CSHCN)* These children require access to a wide range of health care and supportive services, many of which are quite costly. Although access to health insurance positively influences utilization of services and health outcomes of children with chronic conditions (Jeffrey & Newacheck, 2006), financing their health care remains an issue. With few exceptions, there is no universal health care entitlement for these children (Szilagyi, 2003). The *National Survey of Children with Special Health Care Needs Chartbook 2005–2006* indicates that 91% of CSHCN had continuous insurance coverage for the study year, but 9% of this cohort was uninsured for at least a part of the year; many others are underinsured (U.S. Department of Health and Human Services [U.S. DHHS], Health Resources and Services Administration [HRSA], Maternal and Child Health Bureau [MCHB], 2008a).

CSHCN are more likely to be insured than children without special health care needs, but there are disparities. Over 14% of uninsured CSHCN come from families below the federal poverty level compared with 2.9% of CSHCN from families at or above 400% of the federal poverty level. For fiscal year (FY) 2009 and a family of four, this translates to $22,050 and $88,200, respectively (see http://aspe.hhs.gov/poverty/09poverty.shtml). Racial/ethnic disparities in insurance coverage also are in evidence. Approximately 15% of CSHCN who lack health insurance are Hispanic and 11.0% are black, non-Hispanic as compared with 7.1% of white, non-Hispanic CSHCN (U.S. DHHS, HRSA, MCHB, 2008a).

Although some improvements in coverage for CSHCN have been noted since 2001, insurance coverage remains a burden (Liu, Zaslavsky, Ganz, et al., 2005). Barriers to enrollment continue to restrict a number of eligible children with chronic conditions from enrolling in public programs such as Medicaid or the State Children's Health Insurance Program (SCHIP) (Haley & Kenney, 2007). For children with health insurance, whether private or public, all coverage is not equal and approximately one third of CSHCN remain underinsured for the severity of their conditions. Underinsurance was more likely for children with complex needs, who lived in poverty, or who come from Hispanic backgrounds (Kogan, Newacheck, Honberg, et al., 2005). Many parents report that their child's coverage is inadequate in terms of access, quality, and cost. Nine percent of parents stated that their child could not see needed providers, 13% thought their plan did not meet their child's needs, and 28% thought the charges were unreasonable (U.S. DHHS, 2008). Limited access to subspecialists, long waiting times for appointments, and poor coordination of services between providers and insurance companies were further identified by families as problematic (Sobo, Seid, & Gelhard, 2006). "Wraparound" insurance coverage that provides financial protection for prescription medications, therapies, dental care, and additional ambulatory care is desperately needed by these families but frequently is unattainable (Newacheck & Kim, 2005). Perceived quality of insurance coverage is moderated by condition severity, with 26% of parents of mildly affected children reporting dissatisfaction compared with 41% of parents of CSHCN with complex problems (U.S. DHHS, 2008).

Decreased utilization of services is seen in the one third of CSCHN who are underinsured or have unstable coverage (Satchell & Pati, 2005). They are less likely to report a regular source of care and more likely to have an unmet health need (Haley & Kenney, 2007; Newacheck, McManus, Fox, et al., 2000). The number of specialty care visits is over twice as high (26% vs. 10.2%) for children with chronic conditions in general than those without, regardless of type of insurance, gender, family status, or geographic locale. Yet, for those without any health insurance, only 16.9% of children with chronic conditions sought specialty care, significantly below those that have insurance (Kuhlthau, Nyman, Ferris, et al., 2004). Failure to access needed services can result in profound negative health outcomes for children with chronic conditions.

Financing health care is essential but expensive for children with chronic conditions (Parish & Cloud, 2006). Overall, CHCSN have roughly three times the health care expenditures as other children (Newacheck & Kim, 2005). But for those with severe or catastrophic conditions, costs escalate dramatically. A snapshot of these differences can be seen in the analyses of a large health system's cost by Neff, Sharp, Muldoon, and colleagues (2004). They reported that in calendar year (CY) 1999 for the 82% of children classified as healthy, their mean and median annual health care costs were $485 and $191, respectively. But for 9.2% of children with one or more chronic conditions, these costs escalated dramatically. Mean and median costs ranged from $2,303 to $76,143 and from $1,151 to $19,456 depending on group health status and condition severity. Patterns of service usage also varied. Collectively, children with chronic conditions accounted for 31.8% of all physician, 41.8% of outpatient, 47.7% of pharmaceutical, 60.7% of inpatient, and 75.5% of other (e.g., home health, durable medical equipment, etc.) charges (Neff et al., 2004). These costs continue to escalate annually.

---

* *Children with special health care needs* (CSHCN) are defined as "those who have or are at increased risk for a chronic physical, developmental, behavioral, or emotional condition and who also require health and related services of a type or amount beyond that required by children generally." See Chapter 1 for more details.

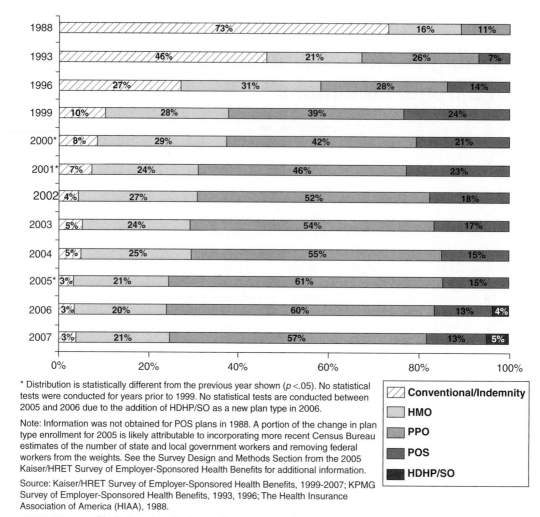

* Distribution is statistically different from the previous year shown (*p* <.05). No statistical tests were conducted for years prior to 1999. No statistical tests are conducted between 2005 and 2006 due to the addition of HDHP/SO as a new plan type in 2006.

Note: Information was not obtained for POS plans in 1988. A portion of the change in plan type enrollment for 2005 is likely attributable to incorporating more recent Census Bureau estimates of the number of state and local government workers and removing federal workers from the weights. See the Survey Design and Methods Section from the 2005 Kaiser/HRET Survey of Employer-Sponsored Health Benefits for additional information.

Source: Kaiser/HRET Survey of Employer-Sponsored Health Benefits, 1999-2007; KPMG Survey of Employer-Sponsored Health Benefits, 1993, 1996; The Health Insurance Association of America (HIAA), 1988.

FIGURE 8-1 Distribution of health plan enrollment for covered workers, by plan type, 1988–2007. Data from Kaiser/ HRET Survey of Employer-Sponsored Health Benefits, 1999–2007; KPMG Survey of Employer-Sponsored Health Benefits, 1993, 1996; The Health Insurance Association of America (HIAA), 1988.

Sources of Funding

Today in the United States, care for children with chronic conditions is financed by complex methods that are generally categorized as follows:

1. Private, employer-sponsored or employer-subsidized health insurance
2. Private, personal policies
3. Public health insurance programs (e.g., Medicaid, SCHIP, and other federal and state categorical programs)
4. Federal supplemental security insurance
5. Local educational systems
6. Private, philanthropic sources
7. The family's own funds

A child's health care costs may be supported by one or a combination of these methods. Indeed, as financing strategies and care needs become more complex, the number of CSHCN that are funded by multiple sources is expanding rapidly. The sources of financial coverage depend on a number of factors, including the type of health condition, the family's socioeconomic status, the state

and county of residence, the existence of a voluntary organization for the specific condition, and the availability of health care and legal personnel to advocate for the child's rights for specific sources of financial assistance.

Methods for financing health care are dynamic; as costs continue to soar and greater disparities in access are seen, both the private and public sectors are constantly modifying standard insurance schemes and testing new and creative new financing mechanisms (Figure 8-1). The goal is to control costs of care while improving both access to and quality of care. These changes, which are driven by population-based health care needs, have had mixed results. Moreover, they are often insensitive to the needs of special populations, including children with chronic conditions.

Major Financing Structures of Insurance
Traditional Indemnity, Fee-for-Service Plans

Historically, private and government insurance was *fee-for-service, indemnity* coverage (Box 8-1 gives definitions of italicized terms). Fee-for-service, indemnity coverage is an insurance scheme that separates payments from care-delivery systems and is determined

Glossary of Italicized Terms

Adverse selection: When a larger proportion of individuals with poorer health status enroll in specific plans or select specific options. Plans with a subpopulation of higher-than-average costs are adversely selected.

Capitation: A method of payment wherein a fixed amount per enrollee per month is paid to the provider to cover a specified set of services regardless of the actual services rendered.

Case management: A system of improving the quality of care while managing costs by monitoring and coordinating the delivery of health services to individuals with complex health problems.

Co-insurance: A method of cost sharing in which the insurer and insured party share payment for an approved charge of covered services according to a predetermined specified ratio after payment of the deductible.

Co-payment: A method of cost sharing in which the insured party pays part of the amount due on receiving services and the insurer pays the remaining portion.

Deductible: A method of cost sharing in which the insured party pays a predetermined amount with the insurance covering the balance.

ERISA: The Employee Retirement Income Security Act, which exempts self-insured health plans from state laws governing health insurance.

Exclusions: Populations or services that are not covered by an insurance plan.

Fee-for-service: Plans in which the payer (i.e., either patients or insurers) agrees to pay the fee set by the provider after the service is provided.

Gatekeeper: An MCO employee who authorizes patient referrals for specialty care.

Health maintenance organization (HMO): A managed care plan that integrates financing and delivery of a comprehensive set of health services to an enrolled population.

    Group model HMO: An HMO that pays a medical group a negotiated, per capita rate that the group distributes among its providers, often as salary.

    Independent practice association (IPA): An HMO that contracts with individual providers to provide services to enrollees as a negotiated per capita or fee-for-service rate. Providers may see other patients besides those enrolled in the HMO plan.

    Network model HMO: An HMO that contracts with several medical groups, often at a capitated rate.

    Staff model HMO: An HMO where providers practice solely as employees and provide services exclusively to HMO plan enrollees.

Healthcare Effectiveness Data and Information Set (HEDIS): A standardized set of measures used in evaluating health plan performance.

High deductible health plan (HDSP): A health insurance plan that provides traditional coverage but has a high minimum deductible, which does not cover the initial costs or all of the costs of medical expenses; usually associated with a *savings option* account.

Integrated service networks (ISNs): Organizations that are accountable for the costs and outcomes associated with delivering a full continuum of health care services to a defined population. All necessary health services are provided for a fixed payment.

Outliers: Cases with extremely long lengths of stay or extraordinarily high costs.

Out-of-pocket expense: Payments made by an individual for medical services, which may include direct payments to providers, deductibles, co-insurance, and for services not covered by the plan and/or charges in excess of the plan's limits.

Pay-for-performance: Providers are rewarded for the quality of health care services they provide.

Point-of-service (POS) plan: A managed care plan that combines features of both prepaid and fee-for-service insurance. Enrollees decide whether to use network or nonnetwork providers, generally with sizable co-payments for selecting the latter.

Population carve-outs: A population carve-out provides health care to a designated population that is targeted or defined by a specific health condition.

Preexisting condition exclusion: A practice of some health insurers to deny coverage to individuals for a certain period for health conditions that already exist when coverage is initiated.

Preferred provider organizations (PPOs): A health plan with a network of providers whose services are available to enrollees at lower cost than services of nonnetwork providers.

Prospective payment: A method of paying health care providers in which rates are established in advance. Providers are paid these rates regardless of the costs they actually incur.

Savings options account: A tax-advantage medical savings account for individuals enrolled in a high deductible health care plan. Also known as health savings accounts (HSAs), medical savings accounts (MSAs), and health reimbursement accounts (HRAs).

Service carve-outs: A set of specific services provided outside a mainstream plan.

Stop-loss provision: The amount that the enrollee must pay out-of-pocket in a calendar year before the plan pays 100% of further covered charges.

by a variety of market forces, including custom, altruism, profit, and administrative costs. These plans charge premiums and pay the bills; the relationship between the client and the provider remains distinct. Neither the provider nor the client is concerned about the cost of care provided. The plan pays fees for services without significant oversight of the providers or health care arena. The more services that are provided, the greater the fee paid.

Benefits that are likely to be covered by fee-for-service plans generally include hospital room costs, miscellaneous hospital expenses, surgery, physicians' nonsurgical services rendered in a hospital, and related outpatient diagnostic radiographic examinations and laboratory expenses. Room and board in an extended care facility may be included when there is proof that continued medical—as opposed to custodial—care is required. Other benefits may be included, but are highly variable across plans. Fee-for service plans are generally desirable by families and providers because of the perceived advantages of unlimited access and, by extension, higher-quality care. But because they do not employ any techniques designed to constrain care charges, pure fee-for-service

plans are costly and rare. Discounted indemnity plans are a variant on traditional indemnity insurance. These plans have adopted some cost containment measures (e.g., discounted, negotiated rates) to stay competitive.

Managed Care Plans

Managed care plans were initiated in the 1920s and 1930s but remained relatively unknown until 1973, with the passage of the HMO Act (Kongstvedt, 2007), which required companies of more than 25 individuals to offer such a plan as an alternative to indemnity insurance should they be approached by a health maintenance organization (HMO) agent. HMOs and other managed care entities became a major market force in the 1990s when the gross domestic product (GDP) for health care goods and services began to approach 14%, up from 5.1% in 1960 and 8.9% in 1980, with double-digit increases projected. Managed care was seen as a viable alternative for curtailing spiraling costs. Today, the majority of health plans are rooted in managed care principles (Kongstvedt, 2007).

Managed care is an integrated system of health insurance, financing, and service delivery functions that attempts to control and coordinate its enrolled members' use of health services in order to contain health expenditures, eliminate inappropriate care, and improve quality. In the classic managed care arrangement, the insured individual and dependents had access to selected providers who had agreed to furnish a defined set of health care services at a fee lower than what was considered "usual and customary" by indemnity plans. This typically was done through *prospective payment* and *capitation,* although these have fallen from favor and are being replaced with new schemes such as *pay-for-performance* and discounted reimbursement for delivered services. There are many types of managed care plans, including HMOs, *preferred provider organizations (PPOs),* and *point-of-service (POS)* plans. There also are different models of HMOs, such as (1) the *staff model,* (2) the *group model,* (3) the *network model,* and (4) the *independent practice association (IPA),* to name but a few.

These terms are still widely used by health plans, although their structures, restrictions, and services provided vary greatly within and across plan types, creating numerous hybrids. These hybrid plans have been fueled by initial consumer and provider dissatisfaction regarding restrictions imposed by traditional managed care plans (Lesser & Ginsburg, 2000). Consumers were concerned that under the first and more restrictive forms of managed care, providers would put their financial considerations and practice obligations ahead of client well-being, while providers reacted negatively to a variety of cost-containment measures. Managed care plans responded by offering broader provider networks; curtailing preauthorization, concurrent utilization management controls, and limited formularies; and reducing reliance on capitation, *gatekeeping,* and other measures designed to improve cost containment (Reed & Trude, 2002). Numerous state consumer (patient) protection legislation also mandates some of these changes, although no federal patient's bill of rights has been enacted.

Regardless of their title, managed care organizations (MCOs) provide similar services to those traditionally provided by fee-for-service plans with the addition of preventive health services as a covered benefit because they have a strong financial incentive to keep their enrollees healthy. Managed care plans operate by providing the insured with a list of providers enrolled with their plan. The insured chooses a primary care provider for all routine care and has little or no *out-of-pocket expenses.* To go outside the plan for care, the insured must pay a significantly higher share of the costs. MCOs may restrict access to specialty health care in the interest of controlling overall health plan costs. For example, access to pediatric specialty care may be restricted by limiting referrals to selected specialty providers, requiring the family to bear a higher share of the total cost of out-of-plan services, or penalizing the primary care provider for referrals to out-of-plan specialists or subspecialists. This may result in children not having ready access to specialists and subspecialists, health care facilities, and ancillary health care services (e.g., physical therapy, in-home care) that can improve their health outcomes and enhance the family's quality of life.

Managed care plans may use *service carve-outs* as a way of providing care to an historically difficult and expensive group of beneficiaries who are often referred to as *outliers.* Care for children with selected conditions, primarily prematurity and those that are behavioral in nature, are handled under a separate managed health care contract that is often held by a different agency. Carve-outs provide specialty care to populations formerly denied access to managed care (e.g., population carve-outs).

As managed care options have matured and competition among plans has expanded beyond cost to include access and quality issues, care available to children with chronic conditions has improved. Sophisticated health plans use a definition of medical necessity that is sensitive to the needs of children with chronic conditions, have a larger number of pediatric providers and pediatric subspecialists on the plan's roster, adapt utilization review standards for special populations, use risk-adjusted capitation and other financial incentives to help achieve quality of care standards, and coordinate case management activities with their service carve-out affiliates (Kastner & Committee on Children with Disabilities, 2004; Shenkman, Tian, Nackashi, et al. 2005). Although data on the quality of care are incomplete, preliminary findings indicate that relative to fee-for-service arrangements, children with chronic conditions receive fewer services and less specialty care but with no deterioration in access or perceived unmet needs; this is particularly true with capitated service carve-out programs (Davidoff, Hill, Courtot, et al., 2007; Garrett, Davidoff, & Yemane, 2003; Kuhlthau et al., 2004). These findings suggest that managed care may be offering better care coordination, including preventive services, for children with chronic conditions because it is in the MCO's best interest to do.

High Deductible Health Plans with Savings Options (HDHPs/SOs)

Consumer-driven health care, a more recent development in health insurance, has resulted in the creation of *high deductible health plans* (HDHPs) with *savings options* (SOs); either a health savings account (HSA) (also referred to as a medical savings account [MSA]) or a health reimbursement account (HRA) (also called a health reimbursement arrangement [HRA]). HDHPs/SOs were established by the Medicare Prescription Drug Improvement and Modernization Act of 2003 (Public Law 108-173) and are a variation on traditional fee-for-service plans. They are designed to curtail inappropriate usage and overusage of health care. HDHPs/SOs remove the majority of financial risk from insurers and generally cost less for employers. Individuals and/or their employers purchase major medical policies (i.e., HDHPs) that have low monthly premiums and high annual *deductibles.* There is no coverage for health care expenditures until the individual exceeds an annual predetermined maximum amount, often $2,000 to $4,000 per year. In conjunction with the HDHP, a separate SO is created for each enrollee. These SOs function by having insured individuals place tax-exempt money in personal savings accounts reserved for health care expenditures. Monies individuals and/or their employers saved from higher premiums are deposited into the insured SOs, where it accrues and earns interest until needed. The major medical policy applies if a certain amount equal to the high annual deductible is expended or if the account is depleted. HDHPs are permitted but not required to cover preventive care before meeting the deductible. Of employers offering HDHPs/SOs, only 30% included the "safe harbor for preventive benefits" option (Committee on Child Health Financing, 2007). HDHPs/SOs are popular with many employers, but when given insurance plan options, are selected less frequently by employees.

Selecting a Plan

Parents of children with chronic conditions must carefully consider their health insurance options to choose the best coverage for their particular needs. Families must consider a plan's structural characteristics (e.g., providers, adequacy of benefits, funding mechanisms), process indicators (level of coordination), and outcome measures (health outcomes, family satisfaction) (Szilagyi, 2003). Table 8-1 on p. 118 provides a guide for families to use in evaluating plans. When choosing a plan, it must be remembered that children with chronic conditions differ from adults with similar conditions. The changing dynamics of children's development combined with the situational stressors of serious illness or disability can significantly, and irreversibly, affect a child's developmental attainment. Moreover, the epidemiology of chronic conditions in pediatric populations is quite different from that in adult populations. Children with chronic conditions are best served by plans that allow for a medical home and contract with knowledgeable pediatric clinicians, including access to pediatric specialists and subspecialists (Kastner & Committee on Children with Disabilities, 2004).

Unfortunately, insurance options are becoming increasingly curtailed for families who use employer-based insurance. To reduce their costs, companies are offering fewer types of plans from which employees can select and often these plans have fewer benefits and more restrictions, such as only offering an HDHP/SO plan. HDHPs/SOs are not well suited for children with chronic conditions because they are primarily consumer-driven plans. They have no intermediaries (e.g., human resources offices, managed care contracts) to negotiate discounted fees but rely on competition in the marketplace to reduce expenditures, ultimately resulting in significant out-of-pocket costs for the insured. Visits to specialists and associated tests and therapies do not fall under the "safe harbor" provision should a family's plan offer this option. Instead, payments come from the insured's HSA/HRA, or, if depleted, out-of-pocket, becoming quite costly for families. Failure to have a medical home, increased use of episodic care, and delays in seeking necessary care are likely to occur (Committee on Child Health Financing, 2007).

Regardless of whether the insurance coverage is private or public, attention must be given to ensuring that parents and providers file claims accurately and promptly, work with a claims agent and care coordinator who understand the family's problems, and follow up rejected claims with convincing evidence of the treatment or medical equipment's importance to the child's well-being. The primary care provider can help parents better advocate for their children by encouraging them to keep records of all their child's health encounters and supporting documentation. These can be useful in contesting payment denials or seeking additional services, such as Supplemental Security Income (see p. 123). Although somewhat controversial because of potential security lapses, online repositories (e.g., Google Health) exist to help families with this task. Parents also need to be encouraged to begin planning well in advance for ensuring that their child has continuous insurance coverage after they "age out" of plans in which they were covered as dependents. Gaps in coverage are common in this population (see Chapter 4) (Callahan & Cooper, 2007).

Private Health Insurance

Private insurance remains the major method of financing health care in the United States, although small decreases in the percent of expenditures, as well as in the number of people covered, have been realized during the last decade. For CSHCN, the percent covered by private health insurance has decreased from 65% from 59% over a 5-year period (U.S. DHHS, 2008). Still, the role of private health insurance in paying the costs of care for children with chronic conditions remains substantial. The heterogeneity in the types of coverage, scope of covered services, and level of coverage make it difficult to comprehend trends or draw generalizations regarding coverage for CSHCN. However, parents whose CSHCN only had private insurance report greater dissatisfaction with their coverage than those whose children have public or a combination of private and public coverage (U.S. DHHS, 2008).

Private coverage is dependent on the parent's employment. The type, amount, and cost of coverage vary dramatically depending on the type, size, and altruism of the employer, the employee's position, state laws, and the general economy. Where small firms are subjected to underwriting if permitted by state regulation, the likelihood that affordable coverage is available for employees or dependents with chronic conditions may be reduced or nonexistent (Davidoff, 2004). One state, Massachusetts, requires all employers with ten or more employees to contribute to their employee's health insurance; other states are studying this program. Where both parents are eligible for dependent private insurance, increased coverage for the CSHCN may be realized but is offset by additional employee contributions to premium expenses and the need to coordinate provider payments (Davidoff, 2004). Private, nongroup coverage is very difficult and expensive to obtain for anyone with a major disability or complex condition.

Private health insurance is generally categorized by the method of reimbursement. Historically, most of these plans were indemnity, fee-for-service plans, but managed care is now the dominant organizational form (Kongstvedt, 2007).

Indemnity, Fee-for-Service Plans

Despite the decreased availability of private indemnity and discounted indemnity arrangements, families of children with chronic conditions may prefer this type of coverage. Ferris, Perrin, Manganello, and colleagues (2001) demonstrated that despite virtually identical coverage but higher costs, families strongly preferred indemnity plans over managed care plans with gatekeeping because they perceived fewer restrictions on choice of providers and care facilities.

In fee-for-service arrangements, the insured person usually pays an annual fee or deductible, usually $250 for the insured or $500 to $1000 per family, before insurance benefits are realized. The insured individual may also pay *co-insurance*, which is approximately 20% of physician, hospital, and other related fees. There is usually also a *stop-loss provision*, as well as a maximum lifetime benefit. Providers are reimbursed for services rendered based on schedules of usual and customary charges (Association of Health Insurance Plans [AHIP] & Agency for Healthcare Quality, 2007). In general, coverage is good for medical supplies and equipment. Most plans have only minimal coverage for preventive services or therapies (e.g., speech, occupational, and physical therapy; nutrition support; and home care). Mental health services also may be covered with limitations on the number of visits and the type of provider.

The problems faced by families who depend on employer-sponsored fee-for-service private health insurance to finance care for a child with a chronic condition are evident by looking at the exclusions and limitations of these health care policies. The insurer

TABLE 8-1

Plan Features to Evaluate

Pediatric Services Covered	Extent of Coverage	In-Plan Cost Sharing	Out-of-Plan Cost Sharing
PEDIATRIC PREVENTIVE CARE SERVICES			
Well-child and adolescent visits, including developmental screening			
Immunizations			
Vision and hearing			
Dental care			
Health education			
PEDIATRIC PRIMARY AND OTHER SERVICES			
Physician services			
Hospital services			
Emergency services			
Surgical care			
Prescription medications			
Laboratory and radiographic services			
PEDIATRIC CHRONIC CARE SERVICES			
Medical subspecialists and surgical specialty services			
Occupational, physical, speech, and respiratory therapy services			
Mental health and chemical dependency services			
Durable medical equipment, supplies, and assistive technology devices			
Home health care			
Nutrition services and products			
Care coordination services			
Other			
COST-SHARING PROVISIONS AND CATASTROPHIC PROTECTIONS	Amount		
Annual premium			
Annual deductible			
Annual out-of-pocket cost limit			
Lifetime out-of-pocket cost limit			
PEDIATRIC PROVIDER NETWORK CAPACITY		Yes	No
Are pediatricians included as primary care clinicians?			
Does the plan recruit physicians and other health professionals with expertise in the care of children with chronic conditions?			
Does the plan make exceptions to allow specialists to serve as primary care clinicians for certain children with complex conditions?			
Does the plan allow for shared management of children with chronic conditions between primary care physicians and subspecialists?			
If the primary or specialty care provider of a child with a chronic condition is not in the plan's network, are exceptions made to reimburse the physician to ensure continuity of care?			
Does the plan rely on pediatric (not adult) subspecialists to care for children with chronic conditions?			
Does the plan have an up-to-date inventory that lists and describes pediatric professionals within the plan who are experts in the care of children with chronic conditions?			
Does the plan include or contract with the following primary care pediatricians, pediatric medical subspecialists, and pediatric surgical specialists in the following areas? (If not, what alternative arrangements are used to ensure access to these pediatric subspecialists?)			
		Yes	No
Adolescent medicine			
Allergy/immunology			
Anesthesiology			
Cardiology			
Child and adolescent psychiatry			
Critical care			
Dermatology			
Development/behavioral medicine			
Emergency medicine			
Endocrinology			
Gastroenterology			
Genetics			
Hematology/oncology			
Infectious disease			

TABLE 8-1

Plan Features to Evaluate—cont'd

Pediatric Services Covered	Extent of Coverage	In-Plan Cost Sharing	Out-of-Plan Cost Sharing
Neonatology/perinatology			
Nephrology			
Neurosurgery			
Ophthalmology			
Oral surgery			
Orthopedics			
Otolaryngology			
Pediatric surgery			
Plastic surgery			
Pulmonology			
Radiology			
Rheumatology			
Urology			
Does the plan include or contract with the following other pediatric specialty health professionals and facilities? (If not, what alternative arrangements are used to ensure access to these other pediatric specialty providers?)			
Nurses with pediatric expertise			
Child and adolescent psychologists			
Social workers with pediatric expertise			
Physical therapists with pediatric expertise			
Occupational therapists with pediatric expertise			
Speech therapists with pediatric expertise			
Respiratory therapists with pediatric expertise			
Home health providers with pediatric expertise			
Nutritionists with pediatric expertise			
Genetic screening and counseling services			
Care managers with pediatric expertise			
Dentists or orthodontists with pediatric expertise			
Hospitals or medical centers specializing in the care of children			
Does the plan encourage coordination and integration of physical and mental health services for children with chronic conditions?			
Does the plan include state-designated pediatric centers of care (e.g., perinatal, hemophilia, trauma, transplant care)?			
Are multidisciplinary teams available for the care of children with chronic conditions through the following:			
Contracts with hospital outpatient departments that specialize in the care of children?			
Contracts with specialty pediatric clinics?			
Contracts with developmental centers?			
Other arrangements?			
Do durable medical equipment vendors have the capacity to individualize and customize equipment for children?			
Are the plan's utilization review and appeals processes performed by appropriate pediatric specialists and subspecialists?			

From Institute for Child Health Policy, Gainesville, FL. Available at www.ichp.edu/managed/materials/purchaser/pedserv.html. Reprinted with permission.

usually does not pay for *preexisting conditions*. Thus if a family was not adequately covered before their child acquired the chronic condition, a fee-for-service plan will not often cover the medical expenses related to the chronic condition. Other common exclusions are payments for preventive health care, rehabilitation services and equipment, and expenses associated with the birth of an infant up to the first 30 days of life. Coverage for health needs defined as nonmedical (e.g., special education, transportation to health care facilities, home renovations needed to care for a child with a chronic condition) are rarely included in fee-for-service plans.

Separate from general health insurance policies are major medical expense policies (e.g., catastrophic coverage) that provide additional protection. They cover a broad range of catastrophic medical expenses above a designated and generally very high deductible. These policies generally have a maximum lifetime limit of $1 million to $3 million, usually enough to cover the costs of most catastrophic illnesses. The cost of major medical insurance is controlled by sizable deductible fees and co-insurance fees for medical expenses that exceed the deductible. They are generally most helpful in catastrophic situations when a person's basic coverage is either a hospital-surgical policy or a major medical policy with a lower-than-adequate lifetime limit (AHIP & Agency for Healthcare Quality, 2007). Major medical plans are not necessarily advantageous for children with chronic conditions because their health care needs do not fit into the designated structure of catastrophic coverage.

Managed Care Plans

It is hard to evaluate the effectiveness of private managed care plans in providing care for children with chronic conditions because of their structural diversity and rapid evolution. The majority of MCOs, however, avoid *adverse selection* and do not actively enroll children with special needs or develop programs for them;

population and service carve-outs are common. Most plans do not actively restrict the enrollment of such children, but there is little incentive for them to do so. Many primary care providers also may be reluctant to care for children with special health care needs if capitation and other contractual arrangements with the MCO provide financial disincentives (Smucker, 2001).

Of the various types of private managed care plans, traditional HMOs have the potential to provide more comprehensive services to children with chronic conditions because they may include (1) comprehensive outpatient services, including basic mental health care; (2) coverage for ancillary therapies; (3) home health services; (4) coverage for durable medical equipment, supplies, and prescription drugs; and (5) access to pediatricians and pediatric subspecialists, pediatric nurse practitioners, psychologists, nutritionists, and social service workers with expertise in various problems of living with a chronic condition (Fox, Wicks, & Newacheck, 1993). Other advantages are that preexisting conditions are generally not excluded, *co-payment*s are small, and there may be no deductible or co-insurance provision.

Conversely, gatekeeper activities that restrict access to the best providers for a child's condition can be a serious limitation of HMO plans (Smucker, 2001). Moreover, a large number of services are excluded when a child goes out-of-plan, which may be very costly to the family. Out-of-pocket expenses can become a substantial burden. Although care coordination or *case management* services are included, they may be ineffective in providing higher-quality care but vary depending on the sophistication of the managed care organization.

Self-Insured Plans

Self-insured plans, whether they are fee-for-service or managed care, are not governed by the same laws as other private health insurance plans. They may offer even fewer benefits to children than other private insurance plans that are subject to the statutory and common-law doctrines regulating insurance. Self-insured plans are governed by the Employee Retirement Income Security Act of 1974 (ERISA), which makes them exempt from state and federal insurance regulations and allows employers to establish, modify, and cancel employee medical benefits without state or federal interference (Kongstvedt, 2007). The children of employees on self-insured plans can be left without coverage for costly conditions, and their families have little legal recourse. ERISA protections are currently being challenged in a number of legal proceedings. Many individuals do not realize that their health plan is a self-insured plan and subject to ERISA as many companies contract with private insurance carriers to manage their plans.

Paul Wellstone and Pete Domenici Mental Health Parity and Addiction Equity Act of 2008

This amendment to ERISA requires health plans to provide the same coverage for mental health conditions as they do for other medical conditions. Specific health plan mental health service restrictions such as the number of allowable outpatient visits and inpatient days or higher co-payments and deductibles of health plans are now eliminated. The new law will make is easier for children to receive care for conditions such as depression, autism, and eating disorders. The terms of the new law apply to businesses that employ 50 or more people. It goes into effect in 2010 so the full extent of law for families of children with chronic conditions is unknown (www.ncsl.org/programs/health/Federal_Parity08.htm).

Health Insurance Portability and Accountability Act

The Health Insurance Portability and Accountability Act, more commonly known as HIPAA, was passed in 1996 to provide additional protections for families with private health insurance. Of specific note for children with chronic conditions and their families, HIPAA limits group health plans from discriminating against potential subscribers for previous poor health and limits the use of preexisting condition exclusions. It also guarantees selected small employers and individuals who have lost their job-related coverage the right to purchase health insurance and the ability to renew the coverage, regardless of any health conditions covered by the policy (U.S. DHHS, Centers for Medicare and Medicaid Services [CMS], 2005d, December 14). These are important protections for families with children with chronic conditions. HIPAA is limited, however, in that it does not require selected benefits to be covered in group health plans or control the amount an insurer may charge for coverage. Health plans may seek to opt out of selected HIPAA requirements if they increase the plan cost above 1% and they meet other federal requirements.

HIPAA has improved group coverage protections, but access to individual coverage has not improved. It also has changed the way health plans are regulated by states and the federal government. Further legal interpretations of this law will determine its eventual impact on the private insurance market and consumer protections.

Government Health Care Programs

There are public health care financing programs for individuals and families who do not have access to employer-based health insurance, cannot afford to purchase private insurance, or are federal employees or are categorically protected groups. These programs may be entirely supported by federal money or may be jointly administered and funded by the federal government and the states. States also may have revenue-sharing agreements with counties or other local health jurisdictions to provide financial coverage for health care through public revenue (Wysen, Pernice, & Riley, 2003).

The likelihood of a child being covered by health insurance rises with parental income. Approximately 11.7% of all children, but 19.3% of poor children, are without coverage (U.S. Bureau of Commerce, U.S. Census Bureau, 2007). Several federal programs—Medicaid and SCHIP—help fill this gap. Other federal programs such as Supplemental Security Income and services offered under the aegis of the Maternal and Child Health Bureau are specifically directed toward improving the quality of lives for categorically eligible children. Finally, the federal government insures special populations including military personnel and Native Americans. These publicly sponsored programs vary widely in their breadth and depth of services offered, eligibility requirements, and quality.

Medicaid

Medicaid (Title XIX of the Social Security Act) is a federal-state matching entitlement program that pays for medical assistance for selected needy populations. As the largest public health care program in the United States, it is administered by the Centers for Medicare and Medicaid Services (CMS) within the U.S. Department of Health and Human Services (U.S. DHHS). It was established in 1965 and soon surpassed any other federally funded public health care program serving children. Medicaid guarantees eligible children a comprehensive package of health insurance benefits, which is generally more extensive than those of private insurance plans.

Medicaid programs vary among states. Within broad federal statutes and policies, each state (1) establishes its own eligibility standards; (2) determines the scope of services; (3) sets payment rates; and (4) administers its own program. The complexity of Medicaid regulations accompanied by the state's latitude in designing programs has resulted in disparity among state plans.

Eligibility. States have some discretion in determining which groups to cover under their Medicaid programs. Eligibility for federal funds also requires states to provide Medicaid coverage for selected "categorically needy" groups, which include the following (U.S. DHHS, CMS, 2005a, 2005h):

1. Low-income families with children who meet certain eligibility requirements of their state's Aid for Dependent Children (AFDC) program that was in effect on July 16, 1996
2. Children under 6 years of age and pregnant women whose family income is at or below 133% of the federal poverty level (FPL)
3. Supplemental Security Income recipients (in most states)
4. Infants born to Medicaid-eligible women
5. Recipients of adoption assistance and foster care under Title IV-E of the Social Security Act
6. Selected Medicare recipients
7. Special protected groups (i.e., typically individuals who lose their cash assistance because of increased work earnings or increased Social Security) for a limited period of time

States have the option of providing Medicaid coverage to "categorically related" groups including but not limited to the following (U.S. DHHS, CMS, 2008b):

1. Infants up to age 1 year and pregnant women whose family income is no more than 185% of the FPL
2. Optional targeted low-income children
3. Children under age 21 who meet income and resources eligibility requirements of their state's AFDC program but who are otherwise ineligible for AFDC
4. Institutionalized individuals with limited income and resources
5. Children who are receiving care under home- and community-based waivers
6. Recipients of state supplementary payments

An additional Medicaid option is the "medically needy program," which gives states the opportunity to extend Medicaid eligibility to persons who would be eligible for Medicaid under other criteria except that their income and/or resources are too high. "Medically needy" eligibility requirements are not as extensive as those for "categorically needy" eligibility. Individuals may qualify immediately or may "spend down" by incurring medical expenses that reduce their income to state-designated levels (U.S. DHHS, CMS, 2005f). Just over 50% of states offer a "medically needy" program (U.S. DHHS, CMS, 2005b). If states choose to have a medically needy program, they must include services for medically needy children under age 18 years and pregnant women (U.S. DHHS, CMS, 2005f).

Legal residents, including children, who are not citizens and entered the United States after August 22, 1996, are generally restricted from receiving Medicaid and SCHIP for 5 years; refugees, persons seeking asylum, Cuban and Haitian entrants, and several other finite groups are exempt (U.S. DHHS, CMS, 2008a, March 5). The eligibility of other groups of legal resident noncitizens is an option left up to individual states.

It is very important that families of children with chronic conditions and their primary care providers are informed of the Medicaid service rights and entitlement programs of the state where the child resides. All states that receive funds from the Developmentally Disabled Assistance and Bill of Rights Act of 1978, the Protection and Advocacy for Mentally Ill Individuals Act of 1986, the Protection and Advocacy of Individual Rights Act of 1992, and the Technology-Related Assistance for Individuals with Disabilities Act of 1988 are required to have a protection and advocacy organization to inform persons with disabilities of their rights to payment for health care through Medicaid. Information on how to contact these advocacy groups may be gotten from the local Medicaid office. In most states, eligibility for Medicaid for individuals and families is determined by the Department of Social Services in each county. Social workers in hospitals, public health, child welfare, and other human services agencies can help families with children with chronic conditions to determine if they are eligible for Medicaid coverage.

Basic Service Provisions. A full range of preventive-related and illness-related services are covered by Medicaid. These include inpatient, outpatient, rural health clinic, and federally qualified health center services; prenatal care; vaccines for children; physician, nurse practitioner, and midwife services; family planning services and supplies; laboratory and radiographic services; skilled nursing services or home health care; and the Early Periodic Screening Diagnosis and Treatment Program (EPSDT) for those eligible (U.S. DHHS, CMS, 2005e, December 14).

EPSDT is of particular importance to children with chronic conditions. This preventive health program was added to Medicaid in 1972 and amended in the 1989 Omnibus Budget Reconciliation Act, Public Law 101-329 (1989). The 1989 revisions require states to establish standards for medical, vision, hearing, and dental screenings. Section 1905(r)(5) of the Social Security Act further require states to offer additional screening and services, including a comprehensive health and developmental history, a comprehensive physical examination, appropriate immunizations, needed laboratory tests (including lead toxicity screens), and health education. Additional services needed to treat a suspected illness or condition found in the EPSDT screen are to be furnished at other than the mandated scheduled intervals. States must offer these services whether or not such services are otherwise covered by the state plan (U.S. DHHS, CMS, 2005e, December 14).

Children enrolled in Medicaid are entitled to case management. As defined by the federal government, case management consists of services that help Medicaid beneficiaries "gain access to needed medical, social, education, and other services" and are targeted toward groups such as those with developmental disabilities or chronic mental illness (U.S. DHHS, CMS, 2008, April 21). Widespread misuse resulted in a redefinition of these services as part of section 6052 of the Deficit Reduction Act of 2005. Current case management services must be targeted to an individual and provide comprehensive and coordinated services that result in a specific care plan, service referral, and monitoring activities (U.S. DHHS, CMS, 2005h, December 14; U.S. DHHS, CMS, 2008, April 21).

Traditional Medicaid. Medicaid was originally fashioned along the same lines as private fee-for-service insurance and designed as a program of inclusion. That is, eligible families were able to seek care from any provider, and then Medicaid reimbursed willing providers at set rates for services. There were nominal participation requirements, and each state oversaw the statutes and regulations of provider participation (Stein, 1997). During its first 25 years, Medicaid liberalized its eligibility criteria several times, allowing increased enrollment for children, but especially for those who were medically needy.

Major problems faced by traditional Medicaid programs in the early 1990s were spiraling costs and low provider reimbursement rates, often significantly lower than the prevailing rates in the community. Although children had access to services, they frequently were not available because of low provider participation. These issues were addressed by the U.S. government by applying managed care principles to Medicaid.

Medicaid Managed Care. The majority of states have adopted a variety of managed care strategies in their Medicaid programs to improve access and quality while conserving funds. It is estimated that by 2004, 60% of Medicaid enrollees were receiving benefits through managed care arrangements (U.S. DHHS, CMS 2008, February 27). By 2008, all states with the exception of Alaska, New Hampshire, and Wyoming were using managed care arrangements to cover all or a portion of their Medicaid population (U.S. DHHS, CMS 2008, February 27). The majority of these programs have been designed and implemented under several Medicaid waivers authorized by the U.S. Department of Health and Human Services under the Social Security Act.

Comprehensive health care reform waiver research and demonstration projects. The majority of Medicaid managed care programs fall under section 1115 waivers (U.S. DHHS, CMS, 2005g, December 14). This waiver program was designed by CMS' precursor, the Health Care Financing Administration (HCFA), to allow states to develop innovative solutions to health and welfare problems and expand coverage to additional populations provided while remaining "budget neutral," that is, the proposed program does not increase the proportion of federal spending (U.S. DHHS, CMS, 2005g, December 14).

1915(b): Freedom of Choice Waivers 1915(c): Home and Community Based Waivers. 1915(b): Freedom of Choice Waivers allow states to mandate Medicaid beneficiaries to enroll in a Medicaid managed care program. States may use the savings realized to expand services to other Medicaid populations. These waivers are limited to current Medicaid beneficiaries and cannot be used to expand coverage to other populations. States have the option of using any savings realized to provide additional services not covered under the state plan to Medicaid beneficiaries (U.S. DHHS, CMS, 2008, March 11). States can use 1915(c): Home and Community Based Waivers in their Medicaid packages to provide home- and community-based alternatives to institutional care for children with complex medical needs. Populations of individuals with severe physical disabilities, developmental disabilities, mental retardation, and mental illness may be covered. They offer a wide range of individual supports, including up to 24-hour live-in care and respite care (U.S. DHHS, CMS, 2008, June 3). States may simultaneously use the authorities of the 1915(b) and 1915(c) waiver programs to provide long-term services in a managed care environment for special populations provided that the federal regulations of both waiver programs are met (U.S. DHHS, CMS, 2005c, December 14).

Plan Type. Medicaid managed care plans are similar to the plans described earlier for private insurance. State Medicaid agencies sign service agreements with MCOs to provide Medicaid services. Like private insurance, states use a variety of managed care products, including contracting with commercial HMOs and PPOs, establishing Medicaid-only MCOs, operating prepaid health plans, and providing primary case management MCOs. (U.S. DHHS, CMS, 2005g, December 14). Although providers participating in Medicaid must accept Medicaid reimbursement as payment in full, states may impose nominal deductibles, co-insurance, or co-payments for selected groups of beneficiaries or services. All Medicaid managed care programs must operate against the backdrop of Medicaid regulations and other relevant state and federal laws.

If the state plan is well constructed, joining a managed care plan could benefit children with special health care needs because a more comprehensive range of preventive health services and other therapies may be available and better coordinated than under the traditional Medicaid fee-for-service plan (Mitchell & Gaskin, 2007; Schuster, Mitchell, & Gaskin, 2007). Better coordination also can result in fewer unnecessary visits and subsequent cost savings (Davidoff et al., 2007).

When a state plan is not well constructed or adequately funded, numerous problems can result. Some plans' contract constraints limit access and services for children with chronic conditions. Plans may be underfunded by states; the proportion of physicians who care for Medicaid beneficiaries, now at 85.4%, has decreased annually since 1997 (Cunningham, 2002). When MCOs are underfunded, the capitation rate may be too low to refer a child to pediatric specialty providers outside the plan, and pediatric specialty providers and services may not be available within the plan. Benefit packages offered by HMOs contracted with Medicaid may be less comprehensive than those under Medicaid fee-for-service plans because many optional services are eliminated (Fox, McManus, Almeida, et al.,1997). As with private MCOs, Medicaid-contracted MCOs have little incentive to establish a link with community agencies unless mandated in state contracts. Another problematic area is the relationship between Medicaid-contracted MCOs and the responsibility for, and payment of health services provided to, children with special needs by school districts under Public Law 101-476: IDEA (see Chapter 3). Many MCOs also have little experience providing selected Medicaid-required services (e.g., transportation). Last, disparate federal policy directives from 2006 to 2008 focus on reducing costs by reducing eligibility for enrollment and limiting access to services (Rosenbaum, 2008). Medicaid may prove to be the major funding source for children with chronic conditions, and especially CSHCN, because of its generous benefits package (Mele & Flowers, 2000).

Enrollment in Medicaid can be a tremendous help for families of children with chronic conditions. Unlike other types of insurance, there is no waiting period, no restrictions on preexisting conditions, and no exclusions for the types of conditions covered once eligibility criteria are met (Rosenbaum, 2008). Providers who are familiar with Medicaid regulations can advocate for families who may be denied services to which they are entitled. The provider should know the local protection and advocacy staff and parent advocacy groups who stay abreast of issues regarding the various laws affecting both private and public health insurance plans and are able to protect the civil, legal, and service rights of children with chronic conditions. Social workers can help primary care providers to remain informed of Medicaid's ever-changing services, eligibility requirements, and linkages with SCHIP. Receiving Medicaid coverage for health care does not preclude receiving assistance from other federal programs for services and equipment not covered by Medicaid.

Children's Health Insurance Program

The Children's Health Insurance Program Reauthorization Act (CHIPRA) was one of the first pieces of legislation passed in early 2009 under the Obama administration. It extends and expands the State Children's Health Insurance Program (SCHIP) (Public Law 105-100: Title XXI of the Social Security Act) that enabled states to expand insurance coverage to uninsured, low-income children through a program of matching funds. Initially, SCHIP was included in the Balanced Budget Act of 1997 in response to the growing percentage of children without health insurance, due in part to legislative reforms in the 1990s (Public Law 105-33, 1997). These reforms included replacing Aid to Families with Dependent Children (AFDC) with Temporary Assistance to Needy Families (TANF), which unlinked Medicaid eligibility with cash welfare payments, as well as more restricted eligibility requirements for Medicaid and Supplemental Security Income (SSI). SCHIP has been remarkably successful in reaching its goal—that states provide health care coverage for all uninsured children in families with incomes below 200% of the FPL or 50% above their Medicaid eligibility level, or whichever was higher. Since its enactment, all states have expanded their children's health insurance programs using Title XXI funds; most have met the federal goal of expanding coverage to children in families at 200% of the FPL, with 19 states exceeding the 200% threshold (U.S. DHHS, CMS, 2006; Committee on Child Health Financing, 2007).

Rates of childhood uninsurance were reduced from 23% in 1997 to 14.4% in 2004, access to care has improved, and fewer children have unmet health needs (Committee on Child Health Financing, 2007). Under CHIPRA, an additional 6.5 million children could be covered by 2013. About two thirds of these would be otherwise uninsured. It is estimated that approximately 5.5% of all CSHCN are covered by SCHIP because of improved outreach efforts, better case finding, and simplified enrollment procedures (U.S. DHHS, CMS, 2006). This percentage should increase under CHIPRA through a number of fiscal incentives to states to increase enrollments.

Indicators specific to the CSHCN cohort indicate that SCHIP enrollees are a heterogeneous group. Although the percent enrollment appears to mirror that of children without special needs, there may be some adverse selection and poorer retention because CSHCN are expensive to care for and a disincentive for aggressive enrollment marketing (Stein, Shenkman, Wegner, et al., 2003; Szilagyi, Shenkman, Brach, et al., 2003).

SCHIP programs vary widely in structure and coverage because the federal government gave states considerable latitude in designing their programs in accordance with their political and fiscal climates (U.S. Public Law 105-100, 1997). These will not change considerably under CHIPRA. The following broad mechanisms have been used: (1) establishing or expanding a separate child health insurance program (18 states); (2) expanding the state's Medicaid program (11 states); and (3) combining the former two options (21 states). Medicaid expansion programs must meet federal Medicaid

program guidelines and benefits packages (see discussion earlier in this chapter). The federal government has established benchmarks for non–Medicaid-based programs that mirror those of health plans offered to state and/or federal employees (Public Law 105-100, 1997). Across these three mechanisms, three payment systems—fee-for-service, managed care, or blended models—are used.

Within this program design and payment structure nexus, four highly variable approaches are used by SCHIP programs to provide care to CSHCN. These are (1) standard approaches used by all SCHIP-eligible children; (2) wraparound approaches that offer supplementary coverage and benefits that mirror Medicaid benefits; (3) service carve-outs; and (4) specialized systems of care (Szilagyi, 2003). For states with separate SCHIP plans and major CSHCN initiatives, benefits can be more generous than what is found in a standard Medicaid package. States offering generous packages often include services such as nutrition support, transportation, respite care, or behavioral health care. For states offering restricted benefits, services for therapies (e.g., physical therapy, occupational therapy), durable medical equipment, and mental health are likely to be curtailed. Care coordination efforts are highly variable across state plans. Unfortunately, states with plans to expand only Medicaid generally do not offer special service provisions for CSHCN. Moreover, Medicaid entitlements do not universally apply to SCHIP programs (U.S. DHHS, CMS, 2005b). CHIPRA specifically addresses some of SCHIP's limitations, now requiring dental care and mental health parity, both important services for CSHCN.

Regardless of how generous the plan, CSHCN often require services beyond what are offered. The benchmarks of the benefits set by federal legislation provide limited coverage for the many specialized services required by CSHCN. State plans include a wide variety of cost-sharing requirements, such as premiums, deductibles, co-payments, and co-insurance, although the level of cost sharing is restricted in accordance with the family's income level. Because of the child's increased care needs, however, the level of cost sharing required by families of children with chronic conditions is likely to be higher than the cost sharing required by other families. To better meet the needs of CSHCN, some states have made adjustments for this in their cost-sharing requirements for populations with special needs. Better quality performance measurement monitoring is needed to develop policies and funding mechanisms that provide more consistent, comprehensive care to CSHCN across states (Brach, Lewit, VanLandeghem, et al., 2003). As with Medicaid, recent federal policy directives are limiting children's access to the full range of available services (e.g., in schools, rehabilitation) (Rosenbaum, 2008).

But despite the discrepancies among state plans for addressing the needs of CSHCN, SCHIP was considered a success by families, providers, and policymakers alike. CHIPRA will capitalize on these successes through increased enrollment and expanded services.

Supplemental Security Income

The Supplemental Security Income (SSI) program, which is Title XVI of the Social Security Act, was established by Congress in 1972 for aged, blind, and disabled adults and in 1976 for children less than 16 years of age with disabilities. This program is based on the assumption that those with substantial disabilities and little income have increased costs for health care and daily living. Income support is provided to help recipients become as self-sufficient as possible within the limits of their disability. SSI does not pay directly for the health care costs of a child with a chronic condition, but its recipients are generally categorically eligible to receive health care services through Medicaid, although 11 states have Medicaid eligibility requirements that are more restrictive than those of SSI (U.S. Social Security Administration, 2008). With the exception of California, SSI recipients also are eligible for food stamps.

Eligible children are those who are U.S. citizens, permanent residents, or selected classes of documented noncitizen residents (e.g., refugees, asylees, special immigrant groups), have significant disabilities, and live in low-income households. Until 1990, children with disabilities were less likely than adults with disabilities to be eligible for SSI because children's impairments had to meet or equal those on a specified list of conditions designed for adults. This definition of disability for children seeking SSI was contested in the courts. On February 20, 1990, the Supreme Court upheld a lower court ruling that the policy for determining SSI eligibility for children was unfair and inconsistent with the statutory standards of comparable severity, and the regulations were changed. The definition of disability for children was again revisited in the 1996 Personal Responsibility and Work Opportunity Reconciliation Act (Public Law 104-193). The current definition requires that a child have a physical or mental condition that can be medically proven and results in marked and severe functional limitations *and* that the medically proven physical or mental condition(s) must last or be expected to last at least 12 months or expected to result in death (U.S. Social Security Administration, 2008). If a child has 1 of 15 specific impairments he or she may be found to be "presumptively eligible," allowing payments to begin quickly (Committee on Children with Disabilities, 2001). Examples of these impairments are Down syndrome, total deafness or blindness, terminal cancer with hospice care, leg amputations, acquired immunodeficiency syndrome (AIDS), and birth weight of less than 1200 g and under 6 months of age.

The SSI program has expanded dramatically—from 297,000 enrollees in 1989 to 7.0 million enrollees in 2007; with 421,000 (18.6%) being disabled youths under age 18 years (U.S. Social Security Administration, 2008). Despite the initial expansion of the program in 1990, selected children have lost their eligibility because of the new definition of disability adopted in 1996. Since then, enrollment has remained steady. Today, the program limits its support to those children with severe developmental and behavioral problems. Children with chronic conditions who do not meet the current SSI eligibility requirements may, however, still be eligible for Medicaid or SCHIP depending on their state's eligibility requirements.

The financial requirements for SSI eligibility are complex. The first step is to document that the applicant must be beneath the maximum income level. The amount of SSI paid to an individual and the administration of the program vary by state because states have the option of supplementing the payments. SSI rules allow eligible children from families up to 200% of the FPL to enroll (U.S. Social Security Administration, 2008). Many states administer their own supplementary payments, and the recipients receive this payment separately from that of the federal program. Other states elect to have the federal SSA issue the federal payment and the state supplement in one check; four states (Arkansas, Kansas, Tennessee, and West Virginia) offer no supplementation. Applications for SSI payments are made at Social Security Administration district field offices or through Social Security Administration teleservice centers, where supporting documentation on age, income, and assets is examined (U.S. Social Security Administration, 2008).

The second step in determining financial eligibility is to know the cash value of the applicant's resources, which for children involves determining the portions of the parents' income that are available to the child. This process is referred to as "deeming." The regulations must be carefully studied to understand how the amount of available income is calculated. Countable income, which is the amount of parental income determined to be available to the child or any income earned by the child, reduces this amount, and state supplements increase it. Providers can advocate for children and families by encouraging them to keep accurate records, learning the rules for eligibility, and seeking professional or legal advice if necessary.

SSI eligibility is evaluated periodically. Nonmedical eligibility is generally evaluated every 1 to 6 years. Medical reviews are required (1) within 12 months after birth where low birth weight is a contributing factor to the disability; (2) at least every 3 years for recipients under age 18 whose conditions are likely to improve; and (3) within 1 year of turning age 18 for those receiving benefits under the disabled child eligibility criteria (U.S. Social Security Administration, 2008).

Medicare

Medicare is authorized under Title XVIII of the Social Security Act. Children are generally not entitled to any health care benefits under Medicare because it provides health insurance protection for persons over 65 years of age and persons under 65 years of age who are collecting Social Security or Railroad Retirement Benefits. Children with end-stage renal disease, however, may be eligible to receive health care benefits to cover the costs of peritoneal dialysis or hemodialysis and related services in the hospital or home. This program is subject to change as the Center for Medicare and Medicaid Services attempts to streamline services between the agencies and as Medicare continues to adopt a managed care structure.

TRICARE: The Department of Defense Insurance Program

Approximately 9.2 million active duty and retired military personnel and their dependents are eligible for health care benefits. This includes 2 million children, an estimated 24.5% of whom are designated as CSHCN, higher than national rates (Williams, Schone, Archibald, et al., 2004).

Historically, the Department of Defense provided health insurance to military personnel, their dependents, and other eligible individuals through the Civilian Health and Medical Program of the Uniformed Services (CHAMPUS), an indemnity-style insurance plan. TRICARE, a series of managed care alternatives, replaced CHAMPUS and is the current health plan offered by the Department of Defense (U.S. Department of Defense, 2008). TRICARE brings together military health care resources and supplements them with networks of civilian care. TRICARE operations are divided into three regions, the south, north, and west, each of which contracts with a single managed care plan for benefits administration. TRICARE offers a variety of health, dental, and special program options. The scope and structure of these options vary as widely as their costs.

The first option is TRICARE Prime, an HMO-style arrangement. It offers the most affordable and comprehensive coverage.

The majority of care comes from a military treatment facility and is augmented by the TRICARE contractor's preferred provider network. Although there is no enrollment fee for active duty personnel and their families, other eligible persons pay an annual fee. A primary care manager supervises and coordinates care, and serves as the gatekeeper for specialty referrals. Priority access to military health care is provided. There also is a point of service (POS) option available for all enrollees except active duty personnel for an additional fee. A small fee per visit to civilian providers is assessed if the claimant is not from an active duty family. One major disadvantage is that standard TRICARE Prime is not universally available and enrollees must live in a Prime Service Area (PSA) (U.S. Department of Defense, 2008). Active duty personnel stationed in the United States but outside of a PSA are eligible for TRICARE Prime Remote, where the majority of care is received through an assigned network or, if not available, a TRICARE-authorized provider. TRICARE Prime Overseas is a managed care option for active duty personnel and their families at selected worldwide locations. Approximately 60% of eligible children are enrolled in TRICARE Prime. Roughly 23% of CSHCN from military families are enrolled in this plan (Williams et al., 2004).

TRICARE Standard is a fee-for-service option that is the same as the traditional CHAMPUS plan. This plan is widely available and allows an unrestricted choice among TRICARE-authorized providers. TRICARE Extra is essentially a preferred provider organization arrangement; it differs from TRICARE Standard in that participating individuals choose a TRICARE-authorized provider from within the TRICARE network. Out-of-pocket expenses are reduced with TRICARE Extra. There is no enrollment fee or primary care manager. Significant cost sharing is imposed through deductibles, co-payments, and balances for nonparticipating provider charges that exceed the insurance cap. Participants only may receive care at a military treatment facility on a space-available basis. TRICARE Reserve Select is available to qualified National Guard and Reserve members. It offers coverage similar to TRICARE Standard and Extra.

Services for CSHCN vary according to plan and are similar to those offered by indemnity and managed care plans in the private sector. Additional special services for CSHCN are available to active duty personnel through the TRICARE Extended Care Health Option (ECHO), initiated in 2005. To qualify, a family member must have "(1) moderate to severe mental retardation, (2) a serious physical disability, or (3) extraordinary physical or psychological conditions of such complexity that the beneficiary is homebound." TRICARE ECHO provides extended services such as rehabilitation, durable equipment, assistive devices, special education, in-home services, and respite care. All TRICARE enrollees must pay a sliding scale monthly cost share based on military rank (Shin, Rosenbaum, & Mauery, 2005). Public services (e.g., special education) must be sought before service authorization.

Early results indicate that health service usage for military dependent CSHCN approximates that of civilian CSHCN populations (Williams et al., 2004). CSHCN had a greater proportion of primary care visits than specialty care and no greater rates of hospitalizations, suggesting that the military health care system is managing these children's care satisfactorily. The military views Medicaid, SCHIP, Title V services, and SSI as important supplements to TRICARE coverage, and concerted efforts are made to link eligible CSHCN dependents to these programs (Shin et al., 2005). Military

organizations provide families of children with chronic conditions with information, financial assistance, and health care within the military community or through local community, state, and federal agencies. Health benefits advisors located on military bases facilitate access to both military and public programs in coordination with the multidisciplinary medical and social service support from the Army's Exceptional Family Member Program, the Air Force's Children's Programs, and the Navy's Family Support Program. Eligible families with children with chronic conditions must choose the plan that best fits their needs after considering the issues of access to care, quality of care, overall out-of-pocket costs, other nonmilitary insurance coverage, and the need for other services, such as home care, durable medical equipment, drugs and supplies, or physical, occupational, or speech therapy.

Indian Health Service

The Indian Health Service (IHS) is an organization within the Public Health Service of the U.S. DHHS that is the principal health care provider to more than 1.5 million American Indians and Alaska Natives (AIs/ANs) who belong to 557 federally recognized tribes in 35 states. In conjunction with maximal tribal involvement, IHS seeks is to provide a comprehensive health care delivery system by offering an array of services including primary and tertiary care, rehabilitation services, health education, school-based services, mental health services, and other community and environmental health programs (U.S. DHHS, IHS, n.d.). The IHS integrates health services delivered directly through IHS facilities with purchased contract health services (CHSs) from the private sector. CHSs help pay for care when other sources (e.g., private insurance, SCHIP) are not available. Referrals for CHS funds are based on medical priorities and are not available in all instances.

Although data for AI/AN CSHCN are not available, all major health indicators, including infant morbidity and mortality rates and conditions (e.g., alcoholism, mental health problems) known to contribute to child vulnerability, are worse than population norms. Cultural barriers, geographic isolation, low income, and inadequate insurance coverage are contributing factors. Data for 2005 indicate that only 45% of AIs/ANs had private health insurance coverage, 21.3% relied on Medicaid coverage, and 30% of AIs/ANs had no health insurance coverage (U.S. DHHS, Office of Minority Health, 2008).

The extent to which children with chronic conditions are well served in this system depends on the staff at the local IHS unit's skill in determining the family's eligibility for third-party payment for health services, making appropriate referrals, and providing culturally sensitive counseling and education. The IHS interacts with other federal and state agencies and public and private institutions to develop ways to deliver health services, stimulate consumer participation, and apply resources. These resources include tribal-operated hospitals and health centers and rural and urban health programs that receive both state and federal funding and are subject to regulations of Medicaid, SCHIP, and private health plans. In 2007 and 2008, legislative attempts to amend the Indian Health Care Improvement Act sought to revise requirements for health care programs and services for Indians, Indian tribes, tribal organizations, and urban Indian organizations. Proposed amendments that would benefit CSHCN included the following: (1) expanded coverage for qualified Indians in SCHIP and Medicaid; (2) increase related payments to Indian Health Programs and Urban

Indian Organizations; and (3) consolidation of existing programs into a new program of comprehensive behavioral health, prevention, treatment, and aftercare for Indian tribes. These amendments also would reauthorize the Indian Health Care Improvement Act through FY 2017. At the time of this writing, this legislation is currently pending.

Information on eligibility and the location and health care programs of the local IHS unit may be obtained from the IHS headquarters in Washington, D.C., from the western headquarters in Albuquerque, through one of the IHS area service offices, or at www.ihs.gov.

Maternal and Child Health Bureau

The Maternal and Child Health Bureau (MCHB) is a division of the Health Resources Services Administration (HRSA) of the U.S. DHHS. MCHB administers seven major programs, which, in FY 2007, had a total budget of $838.2 million (U.S. DHHS, HRSA, MCHB, n.d., a). These programs include the following:

- The Maternal and Child Health Services Block Grant (Title V, Social Security Act), $693 million
- The Healthy Start Program (Public Health Service Act), $101.5 million
- Emergency Medical Services for Children Program (Public Health Service Act), $19.8 million
- Traumatic Brain Injury (Public Health Service Act), $8.9 million
- Universal Newborn Hearing Screening (Public Health Service Act), $9.8 million
- Sickle Cell Service Demonstration (American Jobs Creation Act of 2004), $2.2 million
- Family to Family Health Information Centers (Title V, Social Security Act), $3 million

Activities sponsored under Title V legislation are the most salient regarding financing care for CSHCN.

Maternal and Child Health Services Block Grant. This grant is the largest of MCHB's programs and is a federal-state program established under Title V of the Social Security Act of 1935. The purpose of Title V is to improve the health of mothers and children and is the only federal program solely devoted to this population (U.S. DHHS, HRSA, MCHB, n.d.). Title V legislation grew out of increased recognition at the turn of the century that the federal government should bear some responsibility for the well-being of mothers and children and that federal assistance to state health departments would enable the states to provide needed services on the local level. MCHB's predecessor, the Children's Bureau, was established in 1912; the Maternal and Infancy (Sheppard-Towner) Act of 1920–1929 then set the precedents for federal assistance to states for services for pregnant women and for infants and children with disabilities or conditions that might lead to a disability. Although the Sheppard-Towner Act only survived briefly, states had the opportunity to establish a public health unit for mothers and children, improve birth registration, and increase public health nursing services. These positive experiences with federal support of state public health programs helped lessen resistance to federal intervention in health care on the part of private physicians and enabled passage of Title V (Kruger, 2001). Over time, expansion in the number and variety of categorical services was realized.

In 1981, with passage of the Omnibus Budget Reconciliation Act (Public Law 97-35), specific Title V programs were consolidated and continued as the MCH Services Block Grant. Control was returned to the states, and the federal government's role in organizing health services for mothers and children was diminished (Stein, 1997). The MCH Block Grant, as amended in 1989 (Public Law 101-329), continues the original purpose of the 1981 act, but efforts at consolidation and state control eroded as Congress began mandating categorical services as a requirement of funding. Provisions to strengthen connections between health services for mothers and children on Medicaid and its EPSDT program were included in these mandates. The 1989 MCH Block Grant legislation also specified connections between the infants' and children's immunization programs of the U.S. Public Health Service, the Centers for Disease Control and Prevention (CDC), and the supplemental feeding program for low-income women, infants, and children (WIC) in the Department of Agriculture. Today, Title V seeks to broaden its scope of services to mothers and children by embracing a "family health" perspective, recognizing that improving the lives of children and mothers is difficult to accomplish in isolation from the larger family unit (Whitehand & Kagan, 2001).

Working with a wide range of public and private sector partners, Title V provides both a framework and a focal point for MCH efforts at the national, state, and local levels. Through Title V, MCHB provides funds to all 50 states and territories to support a statewide MCH program, including a program for CSHCN. The largest portion of Title V goes to the states through a formula-based matching block grant process. Each state's share of the total allocation is based in part on the number of births and the percentage of the nation's low-income children residing in each state and prior grant experience. The states are required to match each $4 of federal funds with $3 in cash or in-kind services (U.S. DHHS, HRSA, MCHB, n.d., b). Collectively, this $5 billion federal/state partnership develops service systems designed to do the following (U.S. DHHS, HRSA, MCHB, n.d., a):

- Significantly reduce infant mortality rate and incidence of handicapping conditions
- Provide and ensure access to comprehensive care for women
- Promote the health of children by providing preventive and primary care services
- Increase the number of children who receive health assessments, diagnostic services, and treatment services
- Provide family-centered, community-based, coordinated care for children with special health care needs

To meet its diverse mandate, Title V is organized into five divisions, two of which are of particular interest to primary care providers for CSHCN: the Division of Services for Child, Adolescent, and Family Health and the Division of Services for Children with Special Needs. The central objective of the Division of Services for Child, Adolescent, and Family Health is to support the development, expansion, and enhancement of comprehensive, community-based, family-centered care. The central objective of the Division of Services for Children with Special Needs is to support development and implementation of comprehensive, culturally competent, coordinated systems of care for children who have or are at risk for chronic physical, developmental, behavioral, or emotional conditions and who require more health care services than generally required by children (U.S. DHHS, HRSA, MCHB, n.d., b). These objectives are met through providing direct health care services, enabling services (e.g., transportation, health education, family support services), and infrastructure services (e.g., evaluation, planning, policy, and standards development) (U.S. DHHS, HRSA, MCHB, n.d., b) (see Chapter 9).

In addition to financing direct care services, Title V sets aside 15% of block grant funds to be used for special projects of regional and national significance (SPRANS grants) and community-integrated service systems (CISS) projects. CISS projects may help with coordinating eligibility criteria among health and social programs, coordinating the financing of services, improving shared data and information systems, and coordinating services with the medical home (see Chapter 9). Selected SPRANS programs directly affect financing of care for children with chronic conditions, including the following:

- Genetic services
- Hemophilia diagnostic and treatment centers
- Maternal and child health improvement projects
- Traumatic brain injury demonstration projects (U.S. DHHS, HRSA, MCHB, n.d., a)

States have some authority to prioritize how they will meet the goals of the program but are required to allocate at least 30% of Title V funds for pediatric primary care services (e.g., service utilization, benchmarking, benefits package design, etc.) and 30% for CSHCN. No more than 10% of the state allocation may be spent on administrative costs (U.S. DHHS, HRSA, MCHB, n.d., b).

Today, services for CSHCN are primarily coordinated by the Division of Services for Children with Special Health Needs. Their primary mission is to improve the infrastructure for service delivery, including projects supporting the medical home (see Chapter 9), rather than providing direct care services. This is a significant change from earlier Title V activities and reduces overlap with services financed by Medicaid and SCHIP. Numerous legislative mandates have been enacted to promote coordination and reduce overlaps between Title V and Title XIX (Medicaid). Efforts to date include a variety of Title V research and demonstration projects (e.g., service utilization tracking, benchmarking, benefits package design, etc.) that directly benefit Medicaid recipients (U.S. DHHS, HRSA, MCHB, 2008b).

Ryan White HIV/AIDS Program

In 1990, the Ryan White Comprehensive AIDS Resources Emergency (CARE) Act was enacted to improve the availability and quality of care for uninsured and underinsured individuals with human immunodeficiency virus (HIV)/acquired immunodeficiency syndrome (AIDS). It is administered by HRSA and was most recently amended and reauthorized in 2006. The CARE Act primarily funds local and state primary care and support services to uninsured individuals with HIV/AIDS. The most recent amendment increases direct care funding, requiring grantees to spend 75% of selected funding on core medical services. The CARE Act also funds the development and operations of community-based primary health care and social service systems, health care provider training, technical assistance to programs, and demonstration projects (U.S. DHHS, HRSA, n.d.).

Individuals with Disabilities Education Improvement Act. The Education for All Handicapped Children Act (Public Law 94-142,

1975) resulted from legal decisions establishing that children with disabilities had a constitutional right to a publicly funded education in the least restrictive environment. This law and its amendments covered children ages 3 to 21 years. The Education for the Handicapped Amendments of 1986, Public Law 99-457, Part H, extended the benefits of Public Law 94-142 to handicapped children from birth to 2 years of age. This act designated funds for the development of a statewide comprehensive, coordinated, multidisciplinary interagency system to provide early intervention services. The Individuals with Disabilities Education Act (IDEA: Public Law 101-476, 1990) and its 1997 and 2004 reauthorizations and amendments (Public Law 105-17, 1997; Public Law 108-446, 2004 [Individuals with Disabilities Education Improvement Act]) further expanded and clarified the educational mandate for children with chronic conditions. An expanded description of this legislation and its ramifications for health care may be found in Chapter 3. Under IDEA, health services deemed necessary to the educational program must be provided. These services may include speech and hearing therapy, psychologic services, physical and occupational therapy, recreation, counseling, social work, and nursing and medical services. School districts may bill Medicaid or SCHIP for these services if allowable by state law and according to regulations set forth by the Centers for Medicare and Medicaid Services (CMS).

Future Trends in Financing Health Care for Children with Chronic Conditions

Improving health outcomes for children with chronic conditions requires (1) expanding access to high-quality health care services; (2) understanding the unique stressors that families face; (3) providing training for health care professionals, families, and community members about chronic conditions and their management; and (4) fostering collaboration among interested parties and coordination of services (Liptak, Orlando, Yingling, et al., 2006). All of these recommendations are predicated on adequate financing, availability of quality services, and universality of care.

Unfortunately, health care financing and delivery in the United States remains highly fragmented, especially for those with complex conditions. The presence or absence of health insurance is a powerful indicator of children's access to care. Analyses suggest that significant disparities to health care access between uninsured and insured children remain (Kuhlthau et al., 2004), despite reform efforts targeting health care's organization, financing, and delivery.

New federal, state, and private initiatives are being implemented to help eliminate barriers to care, provide efficacious care more efficiently, and curtail unnecessary expenditures (see Chapter 9). Because CSHCN use such a disproportionate amount of health care and health care dollars, these initiatives will directly affect this population. The ratio of disproportionate use of services continues to expand as more sophisticated—and more expensive—therapies are developed and increasing morbidities replace declining mortality rates.

All health insurance programs, both public and private, are becoming increasingly complex as efforts are made to balance the quality and cost of care with access to services. Variations on traditional managed care models as well as new insurance schemes are being tested with mixed success. Often these new iterations fail to foster high-quality care for those with chronic conditions because they fail to address the underlying issues of reimbursement and fragmented delivery (Tynan & Draper, 2008). Access to quality, private insurance is becoming more difficult and only is favorable for those who are steadily employed in large, family-friendly corporations or members of strong labor unions that can negotiate comprehensive benefit packages in a strong economy. With these changes, CSHCN are at risk for losing needed coverage and access to services. If this were to happen, significant decreases in CSHCN's functional abilities and condition management would result (Stein & Silver, 2005).

The issues faced by families of CSHCN and other high-user groups have served as a catalyst for discussions for broad-based reforms, not only for CSHCN but for other at-risk groups as well. Increasingly, the public sector is being challenged by family advocacy groups and health care organizations to expand access to federal/state insurance coverage for CSHCN and to improve the range of services covered and the reimbursement rates. There is growing broad-based support by policymakers, health care professionals, and citizens to achieve universal coverage, although there is dissension as to how this should be accomplished. The dilemma faced by families, providers, and children's advocates is how to ensure high-quality pediatric care, especially for the most vulnerable children, in this volatile environment. Better case finding with presumptive eligibility clauses and streamlined enrollment also are needed.

Implications for Primary Care

Primary care providers must be informed about how families of children with chronic conditions in their caseloads are paying for care, help them realize the benefits for which they are eligible, and identify alternative sources of funding. Parents whose private coverage is inadequate need to be encouraged to apply for additional public coverage. Medicaid and SCHIP programs have the potential to provide coverage for virtually all CSHCN from underserved economic and ethnic cohorts. Yet, parents' insufficient knowledge, difficulty in completing application forms, and to a lesser extent, lack of interest, are all barriers to achieving adequate insurance coverage for their child (Haley & Kenney, 2007). Accessing federal-state public benefits requires dedication and persistence on the part of the family. The primary care provider is crucial to providing the necessary supports and referrals during this process. Professionals and families need to effectively advocate for CSHCN by joining together, becoming informed of their rights under the law, and using the legal system for access to care. Their collective voice can have a further impact on health care reforms, including the move toward universal health care.

Resources

Federal

HIPAA
Website: http://cms.hhs.gov/HIPAAGenInfo
HIV/AIDS Bureau
Website: www.hab.hrsa.gov
Indian Health Service
Website: www.ihs.gov
Maternal and Child Health Bureau
Website: www.mchb.hrsa.gov

Medicaid
Website: http://cms.hhs.gov/medicaid
SCHIP
Website: http://cms.hhs.gov/schip
State CSHCN data
Website: http://mchb.hrsa.gov/cshcn05/SD/dc.htm
Supplemental Security Income
Website: http://ssa.gov/ssi
TRICARE (military insurance)
Website: www.tricare.mil

Advocacy and Policy Organizations

Center for Studying Health Systems Change
600 Maryland Ave., SW, Suite 550
Washington, DC 20024-2512
(202) 484-5261
Website: www.hschange.org
Families USA
1334 G St., NW, 3rd floor
Washington, DC 20005
(202) 628-3030
Website: www.familiesusa.org
Kaiser Family Foundation
2400 Sand Hill Rd.
Menlo Park, CA 94025
(650) 854-9400
Website: www.kff.org
National Center for Children in Poverty
Mailman School of Public Health
Columbia University
215 W. 125th St., 3rd floor
New York, NY 10027
(696) 284-9600
Website: www.nccp.org

REFERENCES

Association of Health Insurance Plans & Agency for Healthcare Quality. (2007). *Questions and answers about health insurance. A consumer guide.* Available at www.ahip.org/content/default.aspx?bc=41|329|20888. Retrieved July 31, 2008.

Balanced Budget Act of 1997. (1997). Public Law 105-33. Subtitle J—State Children's Health Insurance Program; Establishment of Program, Section 4901.

Brach, C., Lewit, E.M., VanLandeghem, K., et al. (2003). Who's enrolled in the State Children's Health Insurance Program (SCHIP)? An overview of findings from the Child Health Insurance Research Initiative. *Pediatrics, 112,* e499-e507.

Callahan, S.T., & Cooper, W.O. (2007). Continuity of health insurance coverage among young adults with disabilities. *Pediatrics, 119,* 1175-1180.

Committee on Child Health Financing (2007). High-deductible health plans and the new risks of consumer-driven health insurance products. *Pediatrics, 119,* 622-626.

Committee on Children with Disabilities (2001). The continued importance of Supplemental Security Income (SSI) for children and adolescents with disabilities (RE0040). *Pediatrics, 107,* 790-793.

Cunningham, P.J. (2002). Mounting pressures: Physicians serving Medicaid patients and the uninsured, 1997-2001. *Tracking Report: Results from the Community Tracking Study* (Center for Studying Health System Change), no, 29, 2.

Davidoff, A. (2004). Insurance for children with special health care needs: Patterns of coverage and burden on families to provide adequate insurance. *Pediatrics, 114,* 394-403.

Davidoff, A., Hill, I., Courtot, B., et al. (2007). Effects of managed care on service use and access for publicly insured children with chronic health conditions. *Pediatrics, 119*, 956-964.

Education for All Handicapped Children Act. (1975). Public Law 94-142.

Education of the Handicapped Children Act. (1986). Public Law 99-457.

Ferris, T.G., Perrin, J.M., Manganello, J.A., et al. (2001). Switching to gate-keeping: Changes in expenditures and utilization for children. *Pediatrics, 108*, 283-290.

Fox, H.B., McManus, M.A., Almeida, R.A., et al. (1997). Medicaid managed care policies affecting children with disabilities: 1995 and 1996. *Health Care Financ Rev, 18*(4), 23-26.

Fox, H.B., Wicks, L.B., Newacheck, P.W. (1993). Health maintenance organizations and children with special needs. A suitable match? *Am J Child, 147*, 546-552.

Garrett, B., Davidoff, A.J., & Yemane, A. (2003). Effects of Medicaid managed care models. *Health Serv Res, 38*, 575-594.

Haley, J., & Kenney, M.A. (2007). Low-income uninsured children with special health care needs: Why aren't they enrolled in public health insurance program?. *Pediatrics, 119*, 60-68.

Individuals with Disabilities Education Act. (1990). Public Law 101-476.

Individuals with Disabilities Education Act Amendments of 1997. (1997). Public Law 105-17.

Individuals with Disabilities Education Improvement Act of 2004. (2004). Public Law 108-446.

Jeffrey, A.E., & Newacheck, P.W. (2006). Role of insurance for children with special health care needs: A synthesis of the evidence. *Pediatrics, 118*(4), e1027-e1038.

Kastner, T.A., & Committee on Children with Disabilities (2004). Managed care and children with special health care needs. *Pediatrics, 114*, 1693-1698.

Kaiser Commission on Medicaid and the Uninsured (2009, February).*Children's Health Insurance Program Reauthorization Act of 2009 (CHIPRA).* Available at http://kff.org/medicaid/upload/7863.pdf. Retrieved February 26, 2009.

Kogan, M.D., Newacheck, P.W., Honberg, L., et al. (2005). Association between underinsurance and access to care among children with special health care needs in the United States. *Pediatrics, 116*, 1162-1169.

Kongstvedt, P.R. (2007). *Essentials of Managed Health Care.* (5th ed.). Gaithersburg, MD: Aspen.

Kruger, B.J. (2001). Title V-CSHCN: A closer look at the shaping of the national agenda for children with special health care needs. *Policy, Politics, and Nursing Practice, 2*, 321-330.

Kuhlthau, K., Nyman, R.M., Ferris, T.G., et al. (2004). Correlates of use of specialty care. *Pediatrics, 113*, e249-e255. Available at www.pediatrics.org/cgi/content/full/113/3/e249. Retrieved November 13, 2008.

Lesser, C.S., & Ginsburg, P.B. (2000). Update on the nation's health care system: 1997-1999. *Health Aff, 19*, 206-216.

Liptak, G.S., Orlando, M., & Yingling, J.T., et al. (2006). Satisfaction with primary health care received by families of children with developmental disabilities. *J Pediatr Health Care, 20*, 245-252.

Liu, C., Zaslavsky, A.M., & Ganz, M.L., et al. (2005). Continuity of health insurance coverage for children with special health care needs. *Matern Child Health J, 9*, 363-375.

Medicare Prescription Drug Improvement and Modernization Act of 2003. (2003). Public Law 108-173.

Mele, N.C., & Flowers, J.S. (2000). Medicaid managed care and children with special health care needs: A case study analysis of demonstration waivers in three states. *J Pediatr Nurs, 15*, 63-72.

Mitchell, J.M., & Gaskin, D.J. (2007). Caregivers' ratings of access: Do children with special health care needs fare better under fee-for-service or partially capitated managed care? *Med Care, 45*, 146-153.

National Conference of State Legislators (2008). *Mental Health Parity and Addiction Equity Act of 2008 (HR 1424).* Available at www.ncsl.org/programs/health/Federal_Parity08.htm. Retrieved November 13, 2008.

Neff, J.M., Sharp, V.L., & Muldoon, J., et al. (2004). Profile of medical charges for children by health status group and severity level in a Washington state health plan. *Health Serv Res, 39*, 73-89.

Newacheck, P.W., & Kim, S.E. (2005). A national profile of health care utilization and expenditures for children with special health care needs. *Arch Pediatr Adolesc Med, 159*, 10-17.

Newacheck, P.W., McManus, M., & Fox, H.B., et al. (2000). Access to health care for children with special health care needs. *Pediatrics, 105*, 760-766.

Omnibus Budget Reconciliation Act of 1981, Section 2176. (1981). Public Law 97-35.

Omnibus Budget Reconciliation Act of 1989, Section 6403. (1989). Public Law 101-329.

Parish, S.L., & Cloud, J.M. (2006). Financial well-being of young children with disabilities and their families. *Social Work, 51*, 223-232.

Personal Responsibility and Work Opportunity Reconciliation Act of 1996. (1996). Public Law 104-193.

Reed, M.C., & Trude, S. (2002). Who do you trust? Americans' perspectives on health care, 1997-2000. *Center for Health System Change Tracking Report,* no. 3.

Rosenbaum, S. (2008). CMS' *Medicaid regulations: Implications for children with special health care needs.* Available at www.cbpp.org/2-13-08health. htm. Retrieved June 15, 2008.

Satchell, M., & Pati, S. (2005). Insurance gaps among vulnerable children in the United States, 1999-2001. *Pediatrics, 116*, 1155-1169.

Schuster, M.P.P., Mitchell, J.M., & Gaskin, D.J. (2007). Partially capitated managed care versus FFS for special needs children. *Health Care Financ Rev, 28*, 109-123.

Shenkman, E., Tian, L., & Nackashi, J., et al. (2005). Managed care organization characteristics and outpatient specialty care use among children with chronic illness. *Pediatrics, 115*, 1547-1554.

Shin, P., Rosenbaum, S., & Mauery, D.R. (2005). *Medicaid's role in treating children in military families.* Available at www.gwumc.edu/sphhs/departments/healthpolicy/chsrp/downloads/Medicaid_military_102405.pdf. Retrieved May 30, 2008.

Smucker, J.M. (2001). Managed care and children with special needs. *J Pediatr Health Care, 15*, 3-9.

Sobo, E.J., Seid, M., & Gelhard, L.R. (2006). Parent-identified barriers to pediatric health care: A process-oriented model. *HSR: Health Serv Res, 41*, 148-172.

State Children's Health Insurance Program, Section 4901, HCFA. (1997). Public Law 105-100.

Stein, R.E.K. (1997). *Health Care for Children: What's Right, What's Wrong, What's Next.* New York: United Hospital Fund.

Stein, R.E.K., Shenkman, E., & Wegener, D.H., et al. (2003). Health of children in Title XXI: Should we worry? *Pediatrics, 112*, e112-e118.

Stein, R.E.K., & Silver, E.J. (2005). Are rates of functional limitations associated with access to care? A state-level analysis of the National Survey of Children with Special Health Care Needs. *Matern Child Health J, 95*(Suppl), S33-S39.

Szilagyi, P.G. (2003). Care of children with special health care needs. *Future of Children, 13*, 137-151.

Szilagyi, P.G., Shenkman, E., & Brach, C., et al. (2003). Children with special health care needs enrolled in the State Children's Health Insurance Program (SCHIP): Patient characteristics and healthcare needs. *Pediatrics, 112*, 3508-3520.

Tynan, A., & Draper, D.A. (2008). *Getting What We Pay For: Innovations Lacking in Provider Payment Reform for Chronic Disease Care. Research Brief #6.* Washington, DC: Center for Studying Health System Change.

U.S. Bureau of Commerce, U.S. Census Bureau. (2007). *Income, poverty, and health insurance coverage in the United States, 2006.* Available at www.census.gov/prod/2007pubs/p60-233.pdf. Retrieved June 15, 2008.

U.S. Department of Defense. (2008). *TRICARE benefit information.* Available at www.tricare.mil. Retrieved July 28, 2008.

U.S. Department of Health and Human Services. (2008, January 23) (2008). poverty Guidelines. *Federal Register, 73*(15), 3917-3972.

U.S. Department of Health and Human Services, Centers for Medicare and Medicaid Services. (2005a, December 14). *Mandatory eligibility groups.* Available at www.cms.hhs.gov/MedicaidEligibility/03_MandatoryEligibilityGroups.asp. Retrieved July 27, 2008.

U.S. Department of Health and Human Services, Centers for Medicare and Medicaid Services. (2005b). *Medicaid at a glance 2005. A Medicaid information source.* Available at www.cms.hhs.gov/MedicaidEligibility/Downloads/MedicaidataGlance05.pdf. Retrieved July 27, 2008.

U.S. Department of Health and Human Services, Centers for Medicare and Medicaid Services. (2005c, December 14). *Combined 1915(b)/(c) waivers.* Available at www.cms.hhs.gov/MedicaidStWaivProgDemoPGI/06_Combined1915bc.asp. Retrieved July 27, 2008.

U.S. Department of Health and Human Services, Centers for Medicare and Medicaid Services. (2005d, December 14). *HIPAA general information.* Available at www.cms.hhs.gov/hipaaGenInfo. Retrieved June 15, 2008.

U.S. Department of Health and Human Services, Centers for Medicare and Medicaid Services. (2005e, December 14). *Medicaid early and periodic screening and diagnostic treatment benefit.* Available at www.cms.hhs.gov/MedicaidEarlyPeriodicScrn. Retrieved July 27, 2008.

U.S. Department of Health and Human Services, Centers for Medicare and Medicaid Services. (2005f, December 14). *Medically needy.* Available at www.cms.hhs.gov/MedicaidEligibility/06_Medically_Needy.asp. Retrieved July 27, 2008.

U.S. Department of Health and Human Services, Centers for Medicare and Medicaid Services. (2005g, December 14). *Research and demonstration projects.* Section 1115. Available at www.cms.hhs.gov/MedicaidSt-WaivProgDemoPGI/03_Research&;DemonstrationProjects-Section1115.asp. Retrieved July 27, 2008.

U.S. Department of Health and Human Services, Centers for Medicare and Medicaid Services. (2005h, December 14). *Technical summary.* Available at www.cms.hhs.gov/MedicaidGenInfo/03_TechnicalSummary.asp. Retrieved July 27, 2008.

U.S. Department of Health and Human Services, Centers for Medicare and Medicaid Services. (2006, November 6). *SCHIP state plan amendments.* Available at www.cms.hhs.gov/LowCostHealthInsFamChild/06_SCHIP-StatePlanAmmendments.asp. Retrieved June 15, 2008.

U.S. Department of Health and Human Services, Centers for Medicare and Medicaid Services. (2008, February 27). *Medicaid managed care. Overview.* Available at www.cms.hhs.gov/MedicaidManagCare. Retrieved July 27, 2008.

U.S. Department of Health and Human Services, Centers for Medicare and Medicaid Services. (2008a, March 5). *Immigrants.* Available at www.cms.hhs.gov/MedicaidEligibility/05a_Immigrants.asp. Retrieved July 27, 2008.

U.S. Department of Health and Human Services, Centers for Medicare and Medicaid Services. (2008b, March 5). *Optional eligibility groups.* Available at www.cms.hhs.gov/MedicaidEligibility/04_OptionalEligibility.asp. Retrieved July 27, 2008.

U.S. Department of Health and Human Services, Centers for Medicare and Medicaid Services. (2008, March 11). *Managed care/freedom of choice waivers.* Section 1915(b). Available at www.cms.hhs.gov/MedicaidStWaiv-ProgDemoPGI/04_MC_FC_1915b.asp. Retrieved July 27, 2008.

U.S. Department of Health and Human Services, Centers for Medicare and Medicaid Services. (2008, April 21). *Case management regulation.* Available at www.cms.hhs.gov/DeficitReductionAct/025_Case%20Management%20Regulation.asp. Retrieved July 27, 2008.

U.S. Department of Health and Human Services, Centers for Medicare and Medicaid Services. (2008, June 3). *HCBS Waivers.* Section (1915(c). Available at www.cms.hhs.gov/MedicaidStWaivProgDemoPGI/05_HCBSWaivers-Section1915(c).asp. Retrieved July 27, 2008.

U.S. Department of Health and Human Services, Health Resources and Services Administration. (n.d.). *The HIV/AIDS Program: Ryan White.* Parts A-F. Available at http://hab.hrsa.gov/aboutus.htm. Retrieved June 10, 2008.

U.S. Department of Health and Human Services, Health Resources and Services Administration, Maternal and Child Health Bureau. (n.d., a). *Maternal Child Health Bureau. Overview.* Available at http://mchb.hrsa.gov/about/overview.htm. Retrieved July 27, 2008.

U.S. Department of Health and Human Services, Health Resources and Services Administration, Maternal and Child Health Bureau. (n.d., b). *Understanding Title V of the Social Security Act.* Available at ftp://ftp.hrsa.gov/mchb/titlevtoday/UnderstandingTitleV.pdf; and http://mchb.hrsa.gov/about/overview.htm. Retrieved July 20, 2008.

U.S. Department of Health and Human Services, Health Resources and Services Administration, Maternal and Child Health Bureau. (2008a). *The National Survey of Children with Special Health Care Needs Chartbook 2005-06.* Rockville, MD: Author. Available at http://mchb.hrsa.gov/cshcn05. Retrieved June 10, 2008.

U.S. Department of Health and Human Services (2008). Health Resources and Services Administration, Maternal and Child Health Bureau. (2008b). *State MCH-Medicaid Coordination. A Review of Title V and Title XIX Interagency Agreements* (2nd ed.). Washington, DC: Author.

U.S. Department of Health and Human Services, Indian Health Service. (n.d.). *About the Indian Health Service.* Available at www.ihs.gov. Retrieved June 13, 2008.

U.S. Department of Health and Human Services, Office of Minority Health. (2008). *American Indian/Alaska Native profile.* Available at www.omhrc.gov/templates/browse.aspx?lvl=2&lvlID=52. Retrieved June 13, 2008.

U.S. Social Security Administration. (2008, April 10). *Supplemental Security Income.* Available at www.ssa.gov/ssi. Retrieved July 27, 2008.

Whitehand, L., & Kagan, J. (2001, September). *Family health: The next generation of MCH?* Available at www.amchp1.org/news/FHealthSurveyRpt.pdf. Retrieved June 10, 2008.

Williams, T.V., Schone, E.M., & Archibald, N.D., et al. (2004). A national assessment of children with special health care needs: Prevalence of special needs and use of health care services among children in the military health system. *Pediatrics, 114,* 284-293.

Wysen, K., Pernice, C., & Riley, T. (2003). How public health insurance programs for children work. *Future of Children, 12,* 171-183.

9

Systems of Care for Children with Chronic Conditions

Linda L. Lindeke and Wendy Sue Looman

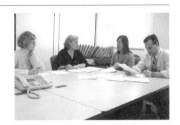

Background

Children with chronic conditions and their families need complex health, education, and related services across a wide range of systems and settings. Their needs both *are similar to* and *are different from* the needs of all developing children and families. Children with special health care needs (CSHCN) by definition require medications, need more medical care than children without special needs, require mental health care or special education services, have limitations on their activities, or require special therapy, counseling, or treatments (Bethell, Read, Stein, et al., 2002). A telephone survey of a representative sample of CSHCN conducted in all 50 states in 2005–2006 found that 86% of the children needed prescription medications, 52% needed specialist care, 25% needed mental health care, 23% needed specialized therapies, and 11% used durable medical equipment; among these same children, 85% had functional difficulties, 57% had difficulty with bodily functions, 49% had difficulty participating in activities, and 42% had emotional or behavioral difficulties (Child and Adolescent Health Measurement Initiative [CAHMI], 2007). Families with children with chronic conditions require accessible, coordinated, and comprehensive services. They usually do not have the medical knowledge, understanding of the multiple health care systems involved with their child's care, or the time and resources to fully advocate for their own needs. Thus health care professionals caring for CSHCN must develop the necessary knowledge and skills to help families obtain comprehensive coordinated services within complex health care systems. Leadership in advocacy and system change is required to meet the needs of CSHCN and their families.

Healthy People 2010

The nation's prevention agenda, known as *Healthy People 2010,* reinforces the need to build community-based systems of care for CSHCN (U.S. Department of Health and Human Services [U.S. DHHS], 2000). The two goals of *Healthy People 2010* are (1) to increase quality and years of healthy life and (2) to decrease health disparities. The Maternal and Child Health Bureau (MCHB) released a 10-year action plan to address *Healthy People 2010* goals and objectives for CSHCN (MCHB, n.d.). This plan identifies six core goals (Box 9-1) to guide the achievement of the *Healthy People 2010* objectives for CSHCN (McPherson & Honberg, 2002). Selected strategies derived from these six goals directly relate to coordination of care. These include developing models of coordination among primary care, specialty, and community providers; implementing medical homes; improving

pediatric-adult medical transitions for young adults; supporting telehealth initiatives; and developing financial models for reimbursement for care coordination (U.S. DHHS, 2001). Goal three clearly states that all children with special heath care needs will receive coordinated, ongoing, comprehensive care within a medical home, that is, at the community-based primary care level. To ensure that states are working on this goal the Maternal Child Health Block Grants require that all state Title V–CSHCN programs annually report the percent of CSHCN who receive coordinated care within a medical home. Collectively, the Title V legislative mandate, *Healthy People 2010* integration of CSHCN, and the MCHB action plan and accountability requirements are the driving forces to ensure that goals are met.

Recent studies have shown mixed results in achieving these goals over a 5-year period. Unchanged from 2001 through 2006 was the finding that only 57% of parents of CSHCN indicated that they were satisfied with their children's health care, and only 57% stated that professionals considered them partners in decision making for their children's care (CAHMI, 2007) (Table 9-1). There was a significant increase in the percentage of parents (from 73% in 2001 to 89% in 2006) who reported that community-based services were organized in ways that made them easier to use, although 38% of parents reported unmet health care needs because of inadequate private or public insurance coverage. Kogan, Newacheck, Honberg, and colleagues (2005) reviewed the health care of nearly 40,000 CSHCN to determine the prevalence of underinsurance as defined by four criteria:

1. Did insurance benefits cover the child's needs?
2. Were the costs not covered by insurance reasonable?
3. Did the health insurance plan allow the child to see the health care providers needed?
4. Was the child currently covered by health insurance and had the child been covered for the previous 12 months?

The authors found that 32% of the parents reported their coverage "never" or only "sometimes" met these criteria, 5.2% were uninsured at the time of the study, and an additional 6.4% had a period with no insurance in the past 12 months. Overall, 21% of families reported financial burdens as a result of their child's medical needs. Mangione-Smith, DeCrostofaro, Setodji, and colleagues (2007) reviewed medical records of 1536 children in a randomized, multistate study of ambulatory care in children and found that children received 67.6% of the acute care indicated, 53.4% of the chronic care indicated by their diagnosis, and only 40.7% of the recommended preventive care for their

BOX 9-1

Healthy People 2010 Action Plan for Children, Youths, and Families with Special Health Care Needs

Goal 1. Families of children with special health care needs will partner in decision making at all levels and will be satisfied with the services they receive.

Goal 2. All children with special health care needs will receive coordinated, ongoing, comprehensive care within a medical home.

Goal 3. All families of children with special health care needs will have adequate private and/or public insurance to pay for the services they need.

Goal 4. All children will be screened early and continuously for special health care needs.

Goal 5. Community-based service systems will be organized so families can use them easily.

Goal 6. All youths with special health care needs will receive the services necessary to make transitions to all aspects of adult life, including adult health care, work, and independence.

From U.S. Department of Health and Human Services (2001). *All Aboard the 2010 Express: A 10-Year Action Plan to Achieve Community-Based Service Systems for Children and Youth with Special Health Care Needs and Their Families.* Washington, DC: Author.

TABLE 9-1

Comparison of MCHB Core Outcomes, 2001 and 2005/2006

MCHB Core Outcome from *2010 Express* Goals	CSHCN Achieving Outcome (2001)	CSHCN Achieving Outcome (2005/2006)
1. CSHCN whose families are partners in decision making at all levels, and are satisfied with the services they receive	57.5%	57.4%
2. CSHCN who receive coordinated, ongoing, comprehensive care within a medical home	52.6%	47.1%
3. CSHCN whose families have adequate private and/or public insurance to pay for the services they need	59.6%	62%
4. CSHCN who are screened early and continuously for special health care needs	Not assessed in 2001	63.8%
5. CSHCN whose community-based services are organized in ways so families can use them easily	73.4%	89.1%
6. Youths with special health care needs who receive the services necessary to make appropriate transitions to adult health care, work, and independence	5.8%	41.2%

Adapted from the Child and Adolescent Health Measurement Initiative (CAHMI), 2007. Source: *Data Resource Center for Child and Adolescent Health,* www.childhealthdata.org.

age. Clearly there is a need for advocacy for comprehensive coordinated care for families and children with special health care needs.

Levels of Systems of Care for Children with Chronic Conditions: Microsystems, Mesosystems, and Macrosystems

Comprehensive coordinated systems of care for children with special health care needs and their families requires a holistic assessment of the systems of care involving the child and family. The

Model for Effective Chronic Illness Care (Figure 9-1), developed with the support of the Robert Wood Johnson Foundation, addresses the need to move beyond episodic provision of acute and chronic care by designing comprehensive systems for chronic condition care (Wagner, 1998). Improved outcomes for CSHCN and families require coordination between community resources and policies and health delivery systems. Productive interactions between informed empowered families and prepared proactive practice teams of health care providers will improve both functional and clinical outcomes for the child. Services and resources often sought by families of CSHCN are found in Table 9-2, and can include financial support, health/medical care, educational support, and family assistance.

The World Health Organization (WHO) has further developed this model as the basis of the WHO Innovative Care for Chronic Conditions (ICCC) Framework. This framework recognizes that optimal care for the child with a chronic health condition requires partnerships between families and health care providers, community agencies that provide resources needed for comprehensive care, and the broader system of health care organizations, funding sources, and government policies (see www.who.int/diabetesactiononline/about/ICCC/en/index.html).

To provide comprehensive and coordinated systems of care, the care must be provided and evaluated at three levels: the microsystem level, mesosystem level, and macrosystem level. Systems at the microsystem level include interactions at the level of child/family/health care team/community and include direct care, as well as care coordination or case management. The goal of the microsystem level of care is for families to receive needed services that are accessible, affordable, seamless, and coordinated through interagency collaborative relationships (Perrin, Romm, Bloom, et al., 2007). The mesosystem level of care includes health care organizations and community organizations, the services provided, information systems in place, and their effectiveness in delivering quality care and meeting the needs of populations served. The macrosystem level includes policies and financing of health care systems, insurance programs, eligibility requirements, government (federal, state, and local) agencies, and legal protections for families and children with chronic health conditions (Perrin et al., 2007). Entities involved at this level globally would include the WHO and the United Nations, and at the national level would include, but are not limited to, the Maternal and Child Health Bureau, the Social Security Administration, and Medicaid. The state level includes the State Children's Health Insurance Program (SCHIP), the public school systems, and the social services system. For care to be comprehensive, coordinated, and accessible to families, all three levels must be functioning in partnership.

Microsystem Level of Care for Children with Special Health Care Needs

Microsystem care refers to the direct interactions among children, families, and health care providers within complex care delivery systems, as well as the coordination of those services. A number of circumstances influence the development of models and financing mechanisms for care coordination for families of CSHCN within primary care settings. Some of the factors discussed in this chapter are the historic advocacy of federal and state maternal and child health services under Title V and *Healthy People 2010*, family access to a myriad of fragmented services, the shift in health care

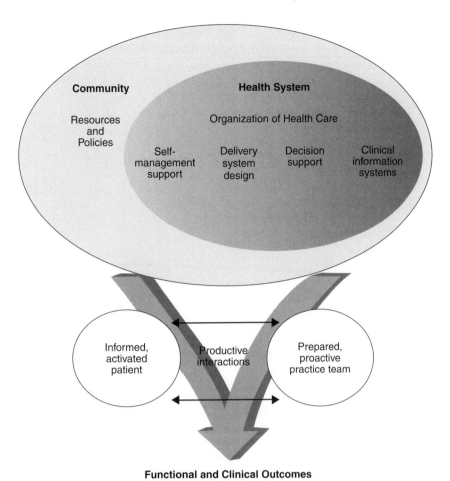

Functional and Clinical Outcomes

FIGURE 9-1 The model for effective chronic illness care. From Wagner, E.H., Davis, C., Schaefer, J., et al. (1999). A survey of leading chronic disease management programs: Are they consistent with the literature? *Managed Care Q, 7*(3), 56-66.

services delivery, and an emerging model of primary care delivery called the "medical home." Primary care providers are particularly well situated to collaborate with families and community partners to improve child and family outcomes by developing community-based coordinated systems of care and ensuring that families receive the individualized care needed to promote optimal well-being for their children with special needs (American Academy of Pediatrics [AAP] & Committee on Children with Disabilities, 1999a, 1999b).

Family-Centered Care Coordination for Children with Chronic Conditions. Care coordination occurs at the microsystem level. It is the process of arranging and integrating the delivery of health and related services over time, across providers and community agencies, for individual families and their CSHCN. A major component of care coordination is the "transfer of information about children's needs, their family context, and their prior experiences with and responses to health care" (Stille & Antonelli, 2004, p. 700). Care coordination for CSHCN has an historical basis in community health nursing and social work and has also been discussed as an essential role for pediatricians for many decades. The most commonly disseminated definitions or descriptions of care coordination specific to CSHCN are promoted by the Maternal and Child Health Bureau (MCHB) within the Department of Health and

Human Services and the American Academy of Pediatrics (AAP& Committee on Children with Disabilities, 1999b). They focus on the process of connecting both child and family to resources to achieve positive health outcomes. Care is considered "coordinated" when an individualized plan of care exists that includes all relevant information (both historical and current), with tracking of referrals and laboratory data, evaluation of outcomes, and retrievable documentation. The plan must be communicated to family, child, and providers. Care coordination is a *proactive process* that plans, implements, and evaluates the delivery of comprehensive services. School nurses report involvement with care coordination for this population (AAP & Committee on School Health, 2001; Erickson, Splett, Mullett, et al., 2006). Nurse practitioners are involved in coordinating care of children accessing hospital-based chronic condition or specialty programs (Horst, Werner, & Werner, 2000) and coordinating the overall health needs of CSHCN in community settings (Lindeke, Krajicek, & Patterson, 2001).

"Case management" is another term associated with service delivery for children with chronic conditions. Care coordination and case management can be described as separate end points on a continuum of services according to a multistate study of Medicaid managed care programs (Rosenbach & Young, 2000). In these programs, care coordination was based on a social service model whose

TABLE 9-2			
Services and Resources that May Be Sought by Families of CSHCN			
Financial Support	**Health/Medical Care**	**Educational Support**	**Family Assistance**
Health care costs	Primary care	Assistive technology	Home adaptations
Durable supplies costs	Dental care	Early intervention services	Automobile adaptations
Durable equipment costs	Specialty care	Employment support	Assisted living services
Food, housing, clothing	Hospital care	Disability advocacy	Child behavior counseling
Transportation costs	Rehabilitation care	Transition services	Child care services
Pharmacologic costs	Developmental services	Sheltered workshop	Family advocacy
SCHIP	Mental health services	Adult daycare	Group home services
Medicaid	Counseling	Special education services	Foster care/adoption
SSI	Skilled nursing services	Head Start programs	Marriage support
Title V-CSCHN programs	WIC nutritional services	Preschool services	Divorce/custody services
Waiver programs	School health services	Therapeutic arts	Parenting support
		Educational advocacy	Parent-to-parent groups
			Family resource centers
			Recreation
			Summer camps
			Respite care
			Sibling support
			Faith community support
			Legal aid

Adapted from State of New Hampshire. (2002). *Information and Referral Report, 1991-2001.* Concord, NH: Special Medical Services Bureau, Office of Health Planning and Medicaid.
Key: *SCHIP,* State Children's Health Insurance Program; *SSI,* Supplemental Security Income; *TANF,* Temporary Assistance for Needy Families; *Title V–CSCHN,* federally mandated state funding for children with special health care needs; *WIC,* Women, Infants, and Children nutrition program.

goal was to facilitate access to quality care across a broad range of programs in the community for vulnerable populations. Case management, in contrast, was focused on containing costs within a medical model of service delivery for high users of costly services. More significantly, "care coordination" is the term families of CSHCN prefer. Definitions of case management also exist from the American Nurses Association (Bower, 1992) and the international, interdisciplinary Case Management Society of America (2002) that include all populations. The commonalties among all these processes of care coordination and case management include the identification of short-term individual outcomes (meet planned health needs, ensure access to services), long-term individual outcomes (positive health status, self-management, empowerment), and system outcomes (improved quality and cost-effective use of resources).

"Family-centered care" is a term used to describe care in which families are fully integrated into all aspects of health care decisions; it implies that families are the experts in the care of their children and able to identify child and family needs. Family-centered care requires that all health care providers collaborate with families, share unbiased information, show respect, and approach families from an individualized strengths-based perspective (Shelton & Stepanek, 1994) versus the typical emphasis on childhood disease/disability and family problems/needs (Dunst & Trivette, 1994). Family strengths are defined as the characteristics and resources (cognitive, attitudinal, and behavioral) that enhance family functioning and well-being.

All families and children have strengths. For example, families have traditions that bring them unity and meaning; they show ingenuity in identifying resources and solving problems; and they often have supportive family members who share caregiving tasks and provide support (Looman, 2004). One model of family-centered care is the Presler (1998) Model of Care Coordination (Box 9-2) first developed for the nation's 21 Shriners Hospitals for Children as part of a 10-year project called "CHOICES (1990–1999)" and jointly funded by MCHB and Shriners Hospitals for Children.

Presler's care coordination model focuses on the importance of the child/youth and family as the key decision makers in every aspect of planning and implementing the plan of care. Care coordinators become partners with families and youths as they negotiate complex systems of care (primary and specialty health care, developmental/educational/vocational services, community support services, and public/private funding resources). Care coordination is a proactive, family-/youth-centered, collaborative, and outcome-focused process. Care coordinators anticipate child and family developmental stages and take measures to prepare children and families though anticipatory guidance. They function as consultants, advocates, brokers, expert clinicians, teachers, and learners. The overarching goal of care coordination at each developmental stage is to prepare children and youths to leave pediatric systems of care healthy and ready to live fully, inclusively, and as independently as possible. Care coordination continually focuses on enhancing child/youth and family well-being, preventing secondary disabilities, and supporting the best possible health, developmental, educational, and vocational outcomes while also improving quality of care and using resources as efficiently as possible. The step-wise Presler Model is systematic, but it is not linear, in that the various steps will be repeated over time and may sometimes occur simultaneously. For example, *Step 1, Identifying and engaging families,* may need to be renegotiated if health, services, or family circumstances change; *Step 3, Developing family-/child-/youth-centered interdisciplinary/interagency plan of care,* will need to be changed if a child is hospitalized and discharge will require new home care accessories, home schooling, or transportation services; and *Step 6, Disengaging active care coordination,* may occur during periods when the chronic condition and family situation are stable and services by a care coordinator are not needed because the family is able to coordinate their care needs. Care coordination services can be reengaged when needed and are greatly facilitated if comprehensive records have been maintained.

BOX 9-2

Components of the Presler Model of Care Coordination for Children, Youths, and Families

Step 1. Identifying and engaging families

Step 2. Assessing children, youths, and families related to
- Needs, concerns, priorities
- Strengths and resources
- Current health/functional status, including health records review
- Need for symptom management, services, or resources to improve quality of life
- Access to primary and specialty health services
- Access to health care insurance (public or private)
- Access to therapies, nursing services, durable medical equipment or supplies
- Technology or environmental supports or modifications currently used or needed
- Access to basic resources such as food, housing, transportation, respite care
- School placement and satisfaction
- Community inclusion and satisfaction
- Perceived need for care coordination services and desired role of the care coordinator

Step 3. Developing family-/child-/youth-centered interdisciplinary/interagency plan of care
- Identifying family's/youth's preference for their primary care coordinator
- Identifying current and future goals and priorities
- Developing comprehensive health services plan that includes
  - Medical/health care home
  - Specialty care referrals and integration
  - Home health care needs and services
  - School/daycare health services needs
  - Emergency services

Step 4. Implementing the plan of care
- Teaching the child/youth and family about the importance of health promotion, health condition management, and prevention of secondary disabilities
- Teaching the child/youth/family essential skills for self-advocacy, self-management, and care coordination
- Providing resource information
- Facilitating interdisciplinary and interagency referrals
- Arranging for and coordinating services
- Advocating for and with the child/youth/family as needed
- Working with third-party payers to ensure access and payment
- Promoting information exchange with community agencies, schools, and health system providers, including adult health care providers at age of transition
- Preparing for and facilitating transition to adult systems of care, roles, and responsibilities as developmentally appropriate at each encounter

Step 5. Monitoring and evaluating the plan of care
- Assessing child/youth/family outcomes
- Assessing systems-related outcomes
- Advocating for systems change to improve outcomes
- Providing resource information

Step 6. Disengaging active care coordination
- Determining child's/youth's/family's desire and ability to coordinate care
- Maintaining care coordination records
- Periodically assessing child's/youth's/family's desire or need for care coordination
- If care coordination services are needed, return to Step 2

Created with input from B. Presler, PhD, RN, CPNP, Shriners Hospitals, May 2008.

Nolan, Orlando, and Liptak (2007) used the Presler Model of Care Coordination to survey 83 families receiving care in a specialty practice for children with disabilities to determine parental perception and perceived value of specific care coordination services received through the clinic. Almost all of the parents in this study indicated that they were responsible for making their own medical appointments, sharing medical information, and accessing insurance and prescriptions. Most of the parents had no problem getting referrals to interdisciplinary specialists such as physical therapists or speech and language pathologists. The parents identified having access to care for both acute and nonacute services; being involved in decisions regarding their child's health care, communication among providers and between systems of care (i.e., between primary and specialty providers), and between providers and educational or community resource systems; and being informed about treatment options, alternatives and choices, programs, and services as the most important components of care coordination. Professional help was needed by 46% of the families to optimize their child's care needs in the educational system, and nearly 50% of families reported needing assistance in obtaining medical equipment for home use. Families stressed the importance of communication among all persons involved with their child's care. The authors noted that their study was done before the implementation of the Health Insurance Portability and Accountability Act (HIPAA) and these new regulations may pose a challenge to the sharing of information. Providers will need to discuss and obtain HIPAA release forms from parents to exchange information. On the other hand, care coordination communication built on the infrastructure of the Internet and electronic records could be greatly improved (Nolan et al., 2007).

An activity assessment tool was used to objectively measure the care coordination activities in six practices over 8 months (Antonelli, Stille, & Antonelli, 2008). The study demonstrated that office-based nurses provided extensive care coordination that avoided significantly higher costs and a large majority of emergency department visits. Care coordination costs ranged from about $4 to $12 per encounter (2003 data), with an overall mean of $7.78 per episode. This study demonstrated the cost-effectiveness and prevention focus of care coordination.

Multiple Systems of Care Coordination. Families of children with chronic conditions may simultaneously have several systems of care coordination (Lindeke, Leonard, Presler, et al., 2002). This may occur because care coordinators are embedded in different systems of care. For example, there may be health system coordinators (located in medical home/health care clinics, specialty clinics, hospitals), education system coordinators (school-based coordinators for the individualized family service plan or individualized educational program [see Chapter 3]), and payment system coordinators (Medicare/Medicaid coordinators, private insurance/managed care coordinators). At times, the various care coordinators may have disparate or even incongruent goals for children and families; families and professionals must be aware of potential conflicts of interest embedded in the overlapping care coordination processes, particularly related to cost containment and the quality and quantity of services provided (Lindeke et al., 2002). Families may be challenged to coordinate the efforts of these multiple systems of care coordination, and some parents report that their role often is to "coordinate the coordinators."

Ideally, there should be one lead care coordinator, based on family choice and the best match with family needs. Selecting the most appropriate lead coordinator may depend on the child's type of care needs, the family's knowledge and skill to manage caregiving, and the family's desire to coordinate care. The selected coordinator, often personnel from the child's medical/health care home, would assume responsibility for working with the family and all other key players, systems, and providers to implement the best possible and most inclusive plan of care. Over time, many families develop skills in navigating health care systems and advocating for their child's needs. A study of over 12,000 parents of hospitalized children found that parents of children with chronic conditions reported fewer care-related problems compared with parents of hospitalized children who did not have chronic conditions (Mack, Co, Goldmann, et al., 2007). The authors theorized that parents of children with chronic conditions had more experience advocating for their children's needs and knew the health care system better than parents of children who did not have chronic conditions. Effective communication and parent-physician partnerships were the factors most strongly related to perceived care quality in this study, and parents with CSHCN may have developed these critical skills and relationships over time because of the child's chronic health problems (Mack et al., 2007).

Some care coordination services focus on particular age-groups (e.g., birth to 3 years) or on specific functions (e.g., transition from hospital to home) and are therefore time-limited services. When services are terminated by one agency, families with continued service needs should be transitioned to other appropriate agencies and care coordinators. If care is being coordinated through hospital-to-home programs, transferring care coordination to community providers avoids disruption in support and services. Transitioning to adult health services from pediatric care is a critical need for adolescents with special needs (see Chapter 4). Other transitions may occur if parents change employment or move and have to select different health plans and care providers. Whether this occurs within the same town or across state lines, there should be communication between care settings to ensure continuity of care. State Title V programs, children's hospitals, and condition-specific organizations (e.g., Cystic Fibrosis Foundation, American Lung Association, etc.) are valuable sources for information for professionals acting as care coordinators and families who relocate or must change whole systems of care.

Varying Needs for Care Coordination Over Time. Families may not require the same intensity of care coordination over time, since needs fluctuate with changes in the child's conditions and developmental stage. Consequently, families enter and exit care coordination processes as needed, alternating between high- and low-intensity periods. Discharge or disengagement from care coordination is relatively common. The benefit of family-centered care coordination originating from a medical/health care home is that it can be available over time and is not condition specific (categorical eligibility). Some families assume the major care coordination responsibility; other families will request considerable assistance. Thus the amount and configuration of care coordination is a choice made by families if family-centered principles are truly followed.

Arranging referrals to professional and community services and following up after referrals are completed, whether done by families or professionals can consume a lot of time. Referrals to specialists or selected services must be authorized, tracked, and integrated into children's plans of care. Some health plan policies require that families obtain prior authorization permission from their health plans (the payers) before referrals take place. Other health plans have "open access" to subspecialists and do not require families to obtain prior authorizations. It can be empowering for families to be able to directly access specialty providers without involving primary care "gatekeepers." However, the results of referrals must be communicated to all care providers to integrate the new information and coordinate the care, a task that might be challenging for parents without the support of professional care coordinators.

Care coordination activities range from the trivial to the profound. At a minimum, care coordinators eliminate barriers to care through excellent communication, negotiation, and advocacy. Care coordinators assist families to schedule multiple appointments in a medical center on a single day to minimize travel time and loss of employment and school time. For families with transportation difficulties, care coordinators locate rides from local community services or teach families to negotiate with health care plans to access appropriate transportation. Coordinators may need to assist families to mobilize a system of supports, such as respite care, child care, recreation, and social support. Families not established in their communities or unable to rely on friends or family members require help obtaining these services. It can be frustrating when family support resources either do not exist or are in limited supply. Mobilizing respite services for families with children with special health care needs may mean piecing together providers from a variety of sources (extended family, neighbors, church volunteers, nursing students, and agencies) and educating them to provide appropriate care. Coordinators may work with young adults who are in the process of transitioning to adult services to obtain health coverage, identify adult providers, and help them develop self-advocacy skills. At the most profound level, care coordination leads to deep relationship-based care (Koloroutis, 2004) that assists the child and family to maximize their full potential and quality of life through ongoing therapeutic professional-family partnerships.

Coordinators may need to arrange and oversee in-home services and create an emergency medical services plan for a child's home care, transfer to the hospital in the event of a sudden change in health status, or evacuation to a special needs shelter in the event of a community disaster. These child- and family-focused emergency plans identify roles and responsibilities among family members, primary care providers, visiting nurses, hospitals, police/fire departments, and emergency medical services personnel. Emergency plans can become very complex. For example, if the family residence is remote, county commissioners may need to address road improvement. Connections must be made with agencies responsible for evacuation and placement of individuals with special needs. The experiences of disabled populations following Hurricane Katrina have emphasized this need. Typically, states, counties, and cities have emergency response plans that assign responsibilities to a combination of agencies for medical services, shelter placement, and special transportation to ensure that residents with special health care needs are identified and entered into a database for emergency plans.

The Importance of Comprehensive, Accessible Health Care Records. Care coordination can only be accomplished if the child's health care records are made available to the care coordinator. Families must sign release of information forms to facilitate requests for health and education records and telephone communications.

Primary care providers must collect the names and contact information for specialists, subspecialists, tertiary center services, habilitative/rehabilitative services, education (including early intervention and special education), dental services, community support (transportation, recreation, parent-support programs), and health insurance plans used by the child and family. A chronologic summary of health care interventions and community involvement in supporting care of the child will provide information about the progression of the child's condition. Comprehensive record-keeping is essential so the care coordinator can monitor care, uncover gaps and breaks in care continuity, evaluate services, and anticipate needs.

Monitoring is the periodic review and documentation of whether, when, and how well services were implemented and referrals completed. It is an important component of the health care record. Monitoring requires that care coordinators maintain and nurture their relationships with families and providers. Frequent contact with families creates opportunities to reassess family priorities, anticipate needs, and revise plans. A "tickler" or reminder system (manual or computer generated) should be implemented in records to ensure that care coordinators track completion of planned services. Monitoring systems should "catch" families when they do not return for scheduled office visits or complete referrals or when telephone contact is disrupted and mail is returned. Families who have not returned for visits and who send requests to transfer medical records to other facilities should be flagged and followed to ensure continuity of care and communication with the new providers. Follow-up should become customary practice through written reminders and telephone calls to home or work. School nurses and public health nurses should be enlisted to help locate families who have not returned for appointments. Follow-up should not be viewed as optional for families whose children have chronic conditions because interruption in care may significantly jeopardize children's health. Eventually, families lost to follow-up from one system of care will reappear somewhere in the health care system. Care coordinators must anticipate child and family needs and proactively guide families back to primary and specialty care rather than have them use episodic or emergency department care.

Mesosystem Level of Care for Children with Special Health Care Needs

Although changes at the microsystem level have improved care for the individual family and child with a chronic condition, reform at the mesosystem level is also essential. The mesosystem level looks at the systems of care affecting health care delivery to children. An excellent definition of the ideal pediatric "system of care" and care reform was originally articulated by Stroul and Friedman (1986) and further refined by Pires (1996). They defined a "system of care" as a comprehensive spectrum of services organized into a coordinated network to meet the multiple and changing needs of children and their families. Early identification and prompt intervention are also emphasized. The system of care concept has since been applied to all children with serious disorders by Pires (2002), who stated that a system of care

"incorporates a broad array of services and supports... organized into a coordinated network . . . [and] integrates care planning and management across multiple levels, is culturally and linguistically competent, and builds meaningful partnerships with families and youth[s] at service delivery and policy levels." [p. 3]

Effective system builders "recognize the strategic importance of connecting to related reform initiatives—to minimize duplication of efforts, maximize resources, and reduce service fragmentation for families" (Pires, 2002, p. 186). Services should be comprehensive, individualized, and coordinated, and they should involve families and youths as full partners (Bronheim & Tonnigest, 2004). Systems of care for children with chronic conditions and their families will be most successful when they move from provider-focused, deficit-based, crisis-oriented approaches to family-focused, strengths-based, and prevention-oriented approaches. Table 9-3 highlights focal points for systems reform.

The MCHB, AAP, March of Dimes, and Family Voices (a national parent-run advocacy and support organization) formed a coalition of organizations in 2000 and proposed a system of care for children with special health care needs; *All Aboard the 2010 Express: A 10-Year Action Plan to Achieve Community-Based Service Systems for Children and Youth with Special Health Care Needs and Their Families* proposed a change in the system of care for CSHCN to an integrated model of care delivery called a "medical home" (AAP & Medical Home Initiatives for Children with Special Needs Project Advisory Committee, 2002; McPherson & Honberg, 2002; U.S. DHHS, 2001).

Medical/Health Care Home Model of Care. Emerging from the *Healthy People 2010* goal-setting initiative was the health care system reform model under the umbrella term "medical home" (sometimes also referred to as "health care home"). The "medical/

TABLE 9-3

Characteristics of Systems of Care Reform

System Characteristics Needing Change	Ideal System Characteristics
Provider focused	Family focused
Categorical programs	Shared service arrangements
Tight central control	Increased local discretion, lateral control
Quality = process + rules compliance	Quality = outcomes for people
Paperwork-intensive processes	Electronic information intensive processes
Control by professionals	Partnerships with families
Only professional services	Partnership between natural and professional supports and services
Multiple case managers	Single point-of-service coordinator within a team
Fragmented service delivery	Coordinated service delivery
Categorical programs/funding	Multidisciplinary teams and blended resources
Reactive, crisis-oriented approach	Focus on prevention/early intervention
Centralized authority	Community-based ownership
Needs/deficit assessments	Strengths-based assessments
Families/youths as "problems"	Families/youths as "partners" and therapeutic allies
Cultural blindness	Cultural competence
Highly professionalized	Coordination with informal and natural supports
Child and family must "fit" services	Individualized/wraparound approach
Input-focused accountability	Outcomes-/results-oriented accountability
Funding tied to programs	Funding tied to populations
Office based	Home and neighborhood based

Adapted from Pires, S. (1996). *Characteristics of Systems Reform Initiatives.* Washington, DC: Human Service Collaborative.

health care home" is a community-based, family-centered, and family-directed care delivery model. This model of care attempts to overcome barriers of fragmented service delivery through care coordination and ongoing family-provider partnerships. Nurses and nurse practitioners must be embedded in medical/healthcare home models (Duderstadt, 2008).

The values and principles associated with the medical home model specify that care be accessible, continuous, comprehensive, family centered, coordinated, compassionate, and culturally effective. The medical home has become the main care model proposed for children and youths with special health care needs and their families in many states through Title V programs and nationally in various demonstration projects. Funders of medical/health care home demonstration projects have mandated that clinics receiving this designation must use electronic health records for children's care coordination.

Medical homes are also required to organize their office systems around the needs of children and families, and they must engage the help of parents to transform existing practices into medical homes. Parents are formally designated as consultants in designing medical home projects. Bridging the gap between family expectations and care delivery requires relationship building, continuing professional education, and significant system changes. Change processes focus on increasing provider knowledge about resources, finding practical ways to reduce care coordination time and financial constraints, and monitoring care quality. Medical/health care home care quality evaluation must be ongoing and integrated, which requires concerted effort to improve outcomes. Primary care providers, nurses, nurse practitioners, social workers, and trained parent advocates from a medical home clinic can be the lead persons to collaborate with families and agencies to improve child and family outcomes by developing community-based, coordinated systems of care.

Establishing medical homes is a challenging and time-consuming process within existing financial structures and systems. A demonstration project, the Pediatric Alliance for Coordinated Care (Palfry, Sofis, Davidson, et al., 2004) assessed the feasibility of medical homes for children with chronic conditions in six community-based pediatric practices, providing services to 150 families of diverse economic, cultural, and ethnic backgrounds. One pediatric nurse practitioner (PNP) in each practice spent 8 hours per week doing home visits for assessments and illness care, system development for ordering medical equipment and supplies, and making appointments for their cohort of children with special health care needs. In addition, the PNPs developed individualized health plans (IHPs) for each child that were maintained at the primary care site and contained relevant clinical information. These IHPs were faxed to subspecialists, emergency departments, hospitals, and schools for information sharing and referral coordination. Each pediatric practice site also hired a parent consultant for family peer support and resource development in the community. Evaluation data were collected before launching the program and after 2 years of implementation of the program. The results indicated that there was a clear correlation between the level of PNP involvement and positive outcomes; 87% of families reported easier access to care (i.e., getting an appointment) as a result of the system change, with families of children with more severe conditions reporting greater improvement in communication, including time until telephone

calls were returned, prescriptions filled, and referrals made. PNP involvement was also related to fewer missed work days for parents and fewer hospitalizations of children, ease of obtaining community resources and respite care, goal setting for the child, and understanding of medical conditions by families leading to improved communication and relationships between the pediatrician and families. This study demonstrated that it is feasible to develop medical homes for children with special health care needs with a modest financial investment (about $400 per child per year). The authors stated that formal relationships with a medical center, cultural/language expertise, and family "buy-in" to the model of care were keys to its success (Palfrey et al., 2004).

The article by Palfrey and colleagues (2004) demonstrated how a mesosystem-level initiative (the medical home) helped transform the microsystem level of care into a model that can be adapted to many sites. There are many practical tools to guide primary care practices in transforming systems into medical homes. The Center for Medical Home Improvement (http://medicalhomeimprovement.org) provides extensive resources including validated measurement tools to assess how well primary care settings provide care (measures of "medical homeness"). The domains measured reflect the needs of children and families and include organizational capacity, chronic condition management, care coordination, community outreach, data management, and quality improvement. Many state Title V offices have dedicated staff to work with primary care teams, parents, and community agencies to improve the quality of care for children and their families through medical/health care home programs. Medical/health care home models are part of the ideal comprehensive care system for chronic care improvement. A recent meta-analysis (Homer, Klatka, Romm, et al., 2008) of 30 studies of medical/healthcare home projects concluded that there is "moderate support for the hypothesis that medical homes provide improved health-related outcomes for children with special healthcare needs" (p. e992). Research including comparison groups is needed to test all aspects of the medical home model. Additionally, provider-inclusive language is necessary in policies and laws being developed to fund this type of care delivery to ensure that nurse practitioners are fully included (Duderstadt, 2008). Children and families will benefit when healthcare/medical homes are based on collaboration of families, nurses and physicians.

Macrosystem Level of Care for Children with Special Health Care Needs

The macrosystem level of health care involves policies and financing of health care systems; insurance programs; local, state, and federal governmental agencies; their rules, regulations, and processes; and legal protection for families and children with chronic health conditions. The main responsibilities of this level "relate to organization and financing services through coordinating eligibility determinations, enabling flexible funding streams and providing clear programmatic responsibility and accountability for service provision" (Perrin et al., 2007, p. 935). Major entities at this system level include the Social Security Administration, the Maternal and Child Health Bureau, federal and state insurance programs, the educational system, the juvenile justice system, and federal, state, and local social service systems. Perrin and colleagues (2007) indicate that developing services for CSHCN at the macrosystem level requires the following:

1. Standardized eligibility protocols
2. Legal and accounting mechanisms for flexible funding streams
3. Development of cost-sharing mechanisms to allocate costs fairly among all payers, including families
4. Measures to eliminate duplication of effort based on resource allocation
5. A flexible point of entry such that a family need only apply once to access all needed services

To accomplish these macrosystem-level services for CSHCN will require major changes in legislation, interagency agreements, funding sources, and political commitment to health services for all people in need (Perrin et al., 2007). Health care professionals must be knowledgeable regarding the importance of and restrictions created by the macrosystem-level of policies, regulations, and laws, and become involved at the local, state, and national levels to educate those in positions of power on needed changes to improve care for CSHCN.

Culturally Appropriate Services for Children with Chronic Conditions and their Families

Discussion of systems of care for children and families must include the cultural appropriateness of services. Critical to service design and delivery is the extent to which systems focus on family and community uniqueness, including the diversity of backgrounds of those seeking care within the systems (see Chapter 6). A much-cited model by Cross, Bazron, Dennis, and colleagues (1989) is a good starting place for systems design and evaluation related to inclusivity and diversity. Cross and colleagues (1989) include congruent behaviors, attitudes, and policies as key components of systems, agencies, and professional practice. Their work has been expanded to include measures of inclusivity related to race, ethnicity, class, religion, gender, geography, and income. Linguistic services are key to quality care but are not sufficient. Adapted from Cross and colleagues (1989) are the following five ideal organizational characteristics:

1. Valuing diversity
2. Carrying out cultural self-assessment
3. Promoting awareness of cultural interaction dynamics
4. Building the organization's knowledge base about culture
5. Adapting services according to cultural knowledge

Creating climates of tolerance and safety with processes for addressing conflict must be intentional and constantly monitored. Integrity, authenticity, and legal protections must be modeled throughout systems, organizations, and professions, with clear expectations and sanctions when goals are not met. Weaving inclusivity into the fabric of organizations that care for children and families is mandated by the MCHB. Practical resources and leadership support are available from groups such as the MCHB-funded National Center for Cultural Competence in the Georgetown University Center for Child and Human Development.

Leadership Development In Improving Systems of Care for Children with Special Health Care Needs

The Maternal and Child Health Bureau recently released the *Maternal and Child Health Leadership Competencies* (Maternal Child Health Leadership Competencies Workgroup, 2007). These interprofessional competencies were developed during a series of national meetings to address the need for maternal and child health leaders at the local, state, and national levels. The progression of leadership is viewed as starting with "self," then "others" (colleagues, co-workers), and then moving to the "wider community." Leadership in the professional's care of children starts with development of the individual provider's knowledge and skills in care of children and the process of leadership. As the individual's knowledge and skills increase, he or she extends this knowledge to co-workers, colleagues, and families, influencing them to support quality pediatric care. To influence and change health care policy at the community, state, or national level, leadership skills need to be developed to understand the change process, factors affecting change over time, and the role politics plays in health care policy. The Maternal and Child Health Bureau identified 12 leadership competencies (Box 9-3). A definition of each competency, knowledge areas needed, and basic and advanced skills for each competency are identified in *Maternal and Child Health Leadership Competencies* and are available on the Internet (www.leadership.mchtraining.net).

Doctor of Nursing Practice: An Educational Innovation for Improving Systems of Care

Despite decades of efforts to improve systems of care for children and families, many barriers exist, and health care costs are spiraling upward with predicted levels that far exceed the available funds. A new graduate degree has been developed for those seeking practice-based advanced nursing education at the doctoral level to address health care at all three system levels. This clinical doctorate, most commonly awarded as a doctor of nursing practice (DNP) degree, was first supported in 2004 when the American Association of Colleges of Nursing (AACN) passed a resolution to develop a doctoral degree to reflect achievement at the highest level of education for nursing practice (AACN, 2004). The DNP is an alternative to the doctor of philosophy (PhD) in nursing, considered

---

BOX 9-3

Maternal and Child Health Leadership Competencies

- Maternal child health knowledge base
- Self-reflection
- Ethics and professionalism
- Critical thinking
- Communication
- Negotiation and conflict resolution
- Cultural competency
- Family-centered care
- Developing others through teaching and mentoring
- Interdisciplinary team building
- Working with communities and systems
- Policy and advocacy

the highest degree for nursing knowledge discovery (Sperhac & Clinton, 2008). Since the 2004 vote at AACN, nearly 200 programs have launched DNP degrees and more than 80 universities and colleges have enrolled students in their newly created DNP programs (www.aacn.nche.edu/DNP/DNPProgramList.htm).

The competencies established by AACN for the graduates of the DNP programs address many of the systems-level challenges in providing coordinated, comprehensive, quality care to children with special health care needs and their families. The DNP competencies include the following areas:

1. Advanced nursing practice
2. Scientific underpinnings for practice
3. Organizational and systems leadership for quality improvement and systems thinking
4. Clinical scholarship and analytical methods for evidence-based practice
5. Information systems/technology and patient care technology for the improvement/transformation of health care
6. Health care policy for advocacy in health care
7. Interprofessional collaboration for improving individual and population health outcomes

The competencies of the DNP degree will prepare nurse leaders and care providers with in-depth scientific knowledge and skills in clinical practice who can provide quality, evidence-based care to children with complex health and social conditions; use information systems to communicate health needs across systems of care; understand health care organizations and how to effect change in these systems while working collaboratively with other professionals and community agencies to improve services for an individual child, and children in general, with chronic conditions; and work to influence health care policy at the institution, local, state, and federal levels to improve health care. The *Maternal and Child Health Leadership Competencies* (www.leadership.mchtraining. net) complement the DNP competencies, and are also interdisciplinary in their approach. The assumption is that DNP-prepared nurses will have strong systems leadership skills and will be key players in quality improvement initiatives. This bold professional initiative could address the complex health care issues and the gaps in health care coverage impeding quality comprehensive care delivery to CSHCN, thereby improving systems of care for children with special health care needs and their families.

Summary

Systems of care for children with special health care needs and their families must encompass many factors, including accessible community resources. Care providers, whether in community agencies, clinics, hospitals, or educational systems, must respect child and family autonomy through practice models of *family-directed* and *family-centered care*. Providers must communicate with each other and with families for joint problem solving and resource procurement. Providers must work together with families to identify gaps in service delivery and to advocate systems change at the microsystem, mesosystem, and macrosystem levels. Leadership, collaboration, and advocacy are essential if quality, cost-effective, community-based systems of care for families of CSHCN are to be realized.

Resources

CarePages
Family-focused information and support for those coping with illness.
Website: www.carepages.com

Center for Medical Home Improvement
Provides a medical home improvement kit, including medical home measurement tool and parent resources.
Website: www.medicalhomeimprovement.org

Champions, Inc.
Assists communities in developing inclusive environments for children with special needs and their families.
Website: www.championsinc.org

Doctor of Nursing Practice Competencies
Website: www.aacn.nche.edu/DNP/pdf/Essentials.pds

FamilyDoctor.org
Consumer health information from the American Academy of Family Physicians.
Website: http://familydoctor.org

Family Voices
A national family advocacy organization with links to state family coordinators and resources.
Website: www.familyvoices.org/

Foundation for Accountability
The children with special health care needs (CSHCN) screening tool.
Website: www.facct.org/facct/doclibFiles/documentFile_446.pdf

HealthFinder
A service of the U.S. Department of Health and Human Services.
Website: www.healthfinder.gov

HRTW National Resource Center
Resources for transitioning young adults from pediatric care to adult services, employment, and independence.
Website: www.hrtw.org

Improving Chronic Illness Care
Model of chronic care system.
Website: www.improvingchroniccare.org

KidsHealth
Site provides child-focused health information.
Website: http://kidshealth.org

Maternal and Child Health Bureau
National goals for improving the care of children with special health care needs and their families.
Website: http://mchb.hrsa.gov/programs/specialneeds/measure-success.htm

Medicalhomela.org
Resources for families, providers, and training materials, as well as a family notebook called "All About Me."
Website: www.medicalhomela.org

National Center of Medical Home Initiatives for Children with Special Needs
National center resources, screening tools, and technical assistance.
Website: www.medicalhomeinfo.org/index.html

National Center on Physical Activity and Disability(NCPAD)
Provides information about physical activity and disability.
Website: www.NCPAD.org

National Dissemination Center for Children with Disabilities
Provides state-by-state lists of organizations and agencies for children with disabilities and their families.
Website: www.nichcy.org/states.htm

National Initiative for Children's Health Care Quality
Website: www.nichq.org/NICHQ
National Survey of Children with Special Health Care Needs
Website: www.cshcndata.org
New Freedom Initiative
Governmental resources for inclusion of people with disabilities into full community participation.
Website: www.hhs.gov/newfreedom
World Health Organization
Site for chronic care models.
Website: www.who.int/diabetesactiononline/about/ICCC/en/index.html

REFERENCES

American Academy of Pediatrics & Committee on Children with Disabilities. (1999a). The pediatrician's role in development and implementation of an Individual Education Plan (IEP) and/or an Individual Family Service Plan (IFSP). *Pediatrics, 104,* 124-127.

American Academy of Pediatrics & Committee on Children with Disabilities. (1999b). Care coordination: Integrating health and related systems of care for children with special health care needs. *Pediatrics, 104,* 978-981.

American Academy of Pediatrics & Committee on School Health. (2001). The role of the school nurse in providing school health services. *Pediatrics, 108,* 1231-1232.

American Academy of Pediatrics & Medical Home Initiatives for Children with Special Needs Project Advisory Committee. (2002). The medical home. *Pediatrics, 110,* 184-186.

American Association of Colleges of Nursing (2004). *AACN Position Statement on the Practice Doctorate in Nursing.* Washington, DC: Author.

Antonelli, R., Stille, C., & Antonelli, D. (2008). Care coordination for children and youth with special health care needs: A descriptive, multisite study of activities, personnel costs and outcomes. *Pediatrics, 122,* e209-e216.

Bethell, C.D., Read, D., and Stein, R.E., et al. (2002). Identifying children with special health care needs: Development and evaluation of a short screening instrument. *Ambul Pediatr, 2,* 38-47.

Bower, K.A. (1992). *Case Management by Nurses.* Kansas City, MO: American Nurses Publishing.

Bronheim, B., & Tonnigest, T. (2004). *Strengthening the community system of care for children and youth with special health care needs and their families: Collaboration between health care and community service systems.* Georgetown University Center for Child and Human Development, Washington, DC. Available at www.medicalhomeinfo.org/tools/gen_med_materials/BSOFwkbkfinal.pdf. Retrieved February 25, 2008.

Case Management Society of America (2002). *CMSA Standards of Practice for Case Management.* 8201 Cantrell Road. Suite 230, Little Rock, AR: 72227.

Child and Adolescent Health Measurement Initiative. (2007). *National survey of children with special health care needs 2005-2006.* Data Resource Center for Child and Adolescent Health website. Available at http://cshcndata.org. Retrieved February 25, 2008.

Cross, T., Bazron, B., Dennis, K., et al. (1989). *Towards A Culturally Competent System of Care: A Monograph on Effective Services for Minority Children Who Are Severely Emotionally Disturbed.* (Vol. I). Washington, DC: Georgetown University Child Development Center.

Duderstadt, K. (2008). Medical home: Nurse practitioners' role in health care delivery to vulnerable populations. *J Pediatr Healthcare, 22,* 390-393.

Dunst, C.J., & Trivette, C.M. (1994). Empowering case management practices: A family-centered perspective. In C.J. Dunst, C.M. Trivette, & A.G.Deal (Eds.), *Supporting and Strengthening Families: Methods, Strategies and Practices.* (Vol. 1). Cambridge, MA: Brookline Books.

Erickson, C.D., Splett, P., Mullett, S.S., et al. (2006). The healthy learner model for student chronic condition management. Part I. *J School Nurs, 22,* 310-318.

Homer, C.J., Klatka, K., Romm, D., et al.: (2008). A review of the evidence for the medical home for children with special health care needs. *Pediatrics, 122,* 3922-e927.

Horst, L., Werner, R.R., & Werner, C.L. (2000). Case management for children and families. *J Child Fam Nurs, 3,* 5-14.

Kogan, M., Newacheck, P., Honberg, L., et al. (2005). Association between underinsurance and access to care among children with special health care needs in the United States. *Pediatrics, 115,* 1162-1169.

Koloroutis, M.(Ed.). (2004). *Relationship-Based Care: A Model for Transforming Practice.* Minneapolis, MN: Creative Health Care Management.

Lindeke, L., Leonard, B., Presler, B., et al. (2002). Family-centered care coordination for children with special needs across multiple settings. *J Pediatr Health Care, 16,* 290-297.

Lindeke, L.L., Krajicek, M., & Patterson, D.L. (2001). PNP roles and interventions with children with special needs and their families. *J Pediatr Health Care, 15,* 138-143.

Looman, W. (2004). Defining social capital for nursing: Experiences of family caregivers of children with chronic conditions. *J Fam Nurs, 10,* 412-428.

Mack, J., Co, J., and Goldmann, D., et al. (2007). Quality of health care for children. *Arch Pediatr Adolesc Med, 161,* 828-834.

Mangione-Smith, R., DeCrostofaro, A., Setodji, C., et al. (2007). The quality of ambulatory care delivered to children in the United States. *N Engl J Med, 357,* 1515-1523.

Maternal and Child Health Bureau. (n.d.) *Achieving and measuring success: A national agenda for children with special health care needs.* Available at http://mchb.hrsa.gov/programs/specialneeds/measuresuccess.htm.Retrieved February 25, 2008.

Maternal Child Health Leadership Competencies Workgroup. (Eds). (2007). *Maternal child health leadership competencies.* Available at http://leadership.mchtraining.net. Retrieved February 25, 2008.

McPherson, M., & Honberg, L. (2002). Identification of children with special health care needs: A cornerstone to achieving *Healthy People 2010. Ambul Pediatr, 2,* 22-23.

Nolan, K., Orlando, M., & Liptak, G. (2007). Care coordination services for families with special health care needs: Are we there yet? *Families, Systems and Health, 25,* 293-306.

Palfrey, J., Sofis, L., Davidson, E., et al. (2004). The Pediatric Alliance for Coordinated Care: Evaluation of a medical home model. *Pediatrics, 113,* 1507-1516.

Perrin, J., Romm, D., Bloom, S., et al. (2007). A family-centered, community-based system of services for children and youth with special health care needs. *Arch Pediatr Adolesc Med, 161,* 933-936.

Pires, S. (1996). *Characteristics of Systems Reform Initiatives.* Washington, DC: Human Service Collaborative.

Pires, S. (2002). *Building Systems of Care: A Primer.* Washington, DC: Georgetown University National Technical Assistance Center for Children's Mental Health.

Presler, B. (1998). Care coordination for children with special health care needs. *Orthop Nurs, 17,* 45-51.

Rosenbach, M., & Young, C. (2000). *Care Coordination and Medicaid Managed Care: Emerging Issues for States and Managed Care Organizations.* Princeton, NJ: Mathematica Policy Research Inc.

Shelton, T.L., & Stepanek, J.S. (1994). *Family-Centered Care for Children Needing Specialized Health and Developmental Services.* Association for the Care of Children's Health, 7910 Woodmont Avenue, Suite 300, Bethesda, MD 20814;(301) 654-6549.

Sperhac, A., & Clinton, P. (2008). Doctorate of nursing practice: Blueprint for excellence. *J Pediatr Health Care, 22,* 145-151.

Stille, C., & Antonelli, R. (2004). Coordination of care for children with special health care needs. *Curr Opin Pediatr, 16,* 700-704.

Stroul, B., & Friedman, R. (1986). *A System of Care for Severely Emotionally Disturbed Children and Youth.* Washington, DC: CASSP Technical Advisory Committee, Georgetown University Child Development Center.

U.S. Department of Health and Human Services. (2000). *Healthy People 2010.* Available at www.health.gov/healthypeople/document/html/volume2/16mich.htm. Retrieved February 28, 2008.

U.S. Department of Health and Human Services (2001). *All Aboard the 2010 Express: A 10-Year Action Plan to Achieve Community-Based Service Systems for Children and Youth with Special Health Care Needs and Their Families.* Washington, DC: Author.

Wagner, E.H. (1998). Chronic disease management: What will it take to improve care for chronic illness?. *Effective Clinical Practice, 1,* 2-4.

Chronic Conditions

10 Allergies

Elizabeth Sloand and Julia Caschera

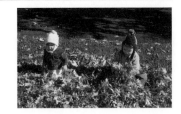

Etiology

Allergy is an unwanted response of the body to what is perceived as a "foreign" substance, or allergen. Allergens, or "foreign" substances, are not always harmful and can also trigger a positive response. A positive or beneficial response results in the development of immunity, whereas a negative or unwanted response results in the development of atopy, or an immunoglobulin E (IgE)–mediated condition. The term "atopy" is often used interchangeably with the term "allergy" and contributes to the confusion surrounding the condition. *Atopy* is defined as a personal or familial tendency to produce IgE antibodies in response to low-dose allergens, confirmed by a positive skin-prick test result (Greer, Sicherer, Burks, & Committee on Nutrition and Section on Allergy and Immunology, 2008). The IgE-related conditions that run in families and are encountered most often include allergic rhinitis, atopic dermatitis, allergic asthma, and gastrointestinal allergies; these are often referred to as atopic conditions (McGeady, 2004). Allergens are usually proteins, and numerous ones have been identified, including dust mites, animal dander, cockroaches, molds and spores, and pollen. Foods can also cause allergic symptoms, and include cow's milk, eggs, peanuts, soy, and others (Box 10-1). Although allergy is a broad topic, this chapter will specifically cover the common chronic conditions of allergic rhinoconjunctivitis and food allergies. Medication allergies, allergic reactions to insect bites and venom, and allergic dermatitis will not be comprehensively covered in this chapter.

Allergy is the result of an immunologically based acquired change in the body of an individual child. In most cases, the response to a foreign substance can be classified as either a Th-1 or a Th-2 response. This refers to the type of cytokine that is activated. A Th-1 response is linked to the development of immunity that protects against many infections, and a Th-2 response contributes to atopy and allergy symptoms (McGeady, 2004). Allergic reactions all involve the production of antigen-specific mediators and a complex cascade of reactions. Histamines or other mediators are released from a mast cell or basophil, which causes inflammation. The resulting respiratory, dermatologic, and eye symptoms vary with the individual's sensitivities and may include sneezing; itching of the nose, ears, and eyes; and rhinitis, wheezing, conjunctivitis, and rash. When the offending agent is a particular food, the child may experience abdominal pain, diarrhea, vomiting, and skin rashes, alone or in addition to respiratory symptoms. Food allergies that are specifically IgE-mediated reactions occur in infants and children. However, the term "food allergies" is also commonly used for less specific food reactions and intolerances that are a result of nonallergic causes, such as pharmacologic, toxic, or metabolic mechanisms, as well as gastrointestinal (GI) intolerances, such as lactose.

The strong role of genetic factors in the development of atopy has long been known. It has become increasingly clear, however, that atopic conditions are "complex" conditions in which multiple major and minor genes interact. Additionally, genes may themselves be modulated by nongenetic factors such as the level and frequency of allergen exposure (McGeady, 2004). Although some genes have been recognized as possible contributors to the development of allergies, no definitive candidates have been identified. There are two reasons for this: first, multiple genes in various combinations are responsible for a variety of allergy phenotypes; second, it is difficult to interpret and compare studies that use different definitions and phenotypes of allergies (Holloway, Cakebread, & Holgate, 2003).

Although no specific gene has been identified for allergies, there is clear indication of a hereditary factor leading to increased susceptibility to asthma, eczema, and allergies in affected families. There are two methods for identifying the genes responsible for allergies: (1) search for candidate genes, genes that are in regions known to be involved in the immunologic response to allergens; and (2) a genome-wide search for potentially involved genes (Holloway et al., 2003).

Atopy has been linked to some human leukocyte antigen (HLA) histocompatability types and various chromosome locations (Kliegman, Behrman, Jenson, et al., 2007). Researchers are exploring multiple factors that either affect the expression of particular genes or trigger their expression. Scientists are targeting various chromosomes and genes as potential contributors to atopy. The discovery of genes such as *ADAM33* and *SPINK5* that appear to be involved in the pathogenesis of bronchial hyperresponsiveness related to asthma and atopic dermatitis, respectively, show that genetic approaches can lead to identification of new biologic pathways involved in the pathogenesis of an allergic condition, the development of new therapeutic approaches, and the identification of at-risk individuals (Holloway et al., 2003). Many other genes are still under investigation. It is likely that multiple genes are responsible for various parts of the inflammatory pathway (including inhibitors, modifiers, and enhancers), and that different combinations of such genes are responsible within a particular individual or family.

Understanding allergies and their rising prevalence will depend not only on continued research in the field of genetics, but also on a greater understanding of the contributing environmental factors. Clearly, the dramatic rise in condition prevalence cannot be attributed to an equally significant change in the existing gene pool (de Groot, Brand, Fokkens, et al., 2007; Holloway et al., 2003; Troye-Blomberg, 2002).

BOX 10-1
Common Allergens
ENVIRONMENTAL ALLERGENS
• Dust mites
• Animal dander
• Cockroaches
• Molds and spores
• Pollen
FOOD ALLERGENS
• Cow's milk
• Eggs
• Peanuts, tree nuts
• Soy
• Wheat
• Fish and shellfish

One of the leading hypothesis to explain the increasing prevalence of atopy is the hygiene hypothesis. Encompassed in this hypothesis are several theories. One theory proposes a relationship between the increased use of antibiotics, the subsequent decrease in infection, and the increased prevalence of atopy. Many have suggested that decreased exposure to infection discourages the development of Th-1–type cytokine response and in turn increases the Th-2 response leading to atopy (Liu & Murphy, 2003; von Mutius, 2002). More recently, researchers have moved beyond the hygiene hypothesis and are exploring the role of timing of allergen exposure, gut flora maturation, and immunoregulation contributors to increased prevalence of atopic condition (Kligler, Hanaway, & Cohrssen, 2007). It seems reasonable to expect that a complex interplay of genetics and environmental conditions are responsible for allergy development.

A second theory involves family size and its inverse relationship to allergies. Researchers found that an increased number of siblings results in a decrease in atopy, particularly for the younger siblings (Westergaard, Rostgaard, Wohlfahrt, et al., 2005). Scientists theorize that an increased number of siblings directly correlates with increased exposure to infection and therefore a switch from a Th-2 default response to a Th-1 immunity response. Similarly, some research has shown that exposure to pets at birth or early in life influences immune development and thereby attenuates atopic conditions including allergic rhinitis, asthma, and eczema. It appears that early pet exposure may have a protective effect against the development of allergies, though those findings are controversial because they have not been duplicated in all studies (Bufford & Gern, 2005; Gern, Reardon, Hoffjan, et al., 2004; Naydenov, Popov, Mustakov, et al., 2008; Ownby, Johnson, & Peterson, 2002; Platts-Mills, 2002; Pohlabeln, Jacobs, & Bohmann, 2007; Weiss, 2002).

In a third hypothesis, researchers found that there is a lower prevalence of atopy and allergic rhinitis in children who have lived on farms (Perkin & Strachan, 2006). Floistrup, Swartz, Bergstrom, and colleagues (2006) report that an anthroposophic lifestyle is protective against atopy into adulthood. An anthroposophic lifestyle restricts the use of antibiotics, limits immunizations, and includes a diet that contains live lactobacilli because of the production and preservation of foods (Floistrup et al., 2006). Although it is yet to be determined which aspects of this lifestyle affect the decreased development of atopy, the possibilities include diet, decreased antibiotic use, having had measles, increased allergen exposure at a young age, and increased exposure to infection via a greater number of siblings (Floistrup et al., 2006; Westergaard et al., 2005).

Incidence and Prevalence

Up to 25% of the pediatric population worldwide is known to have some allergic condition (Bielory, Wilson, & Wagner, 2003; Singh & Kumar, 2003). Children from all countries, all ethnic groups, and all age-groups experience allergies and over 500 million people throughout the world experience allergies (Bousquet, van Cauwenberge, Khaled, et al., 2006). The incidence and prevalence of allergies are very low until age 2, but from age 2 and extending upward throughout childhood, there is a steady increase in the prevalence of allergies to 15% by age 7 (Liu, Martinez, & Taussig, 2003). Clinicians and epidemiologists report that the prevalence of allergic rhinitis, asthma, hay fever, and atopic dermatitis has increased worldwide over the past few decades (Huebner, Kim, Ewart, et al., 2008; von Mutius, 2002).

Rhinoconjunctivitis is very common. A recent study showed that 32% of children with allergies had an ocular condition as the single manifestation of their allergies (Bielory et al., 2003). Exact numbers are elusive because of varying definitions of the disorder, underdiagnosis, and the existence of comorbid conditions (Schoenwetter, 2000; Wang, Niti, Smith, et al., 2002).

Approximately 6% to 8% of children younger than 3 years experience allergic reactions to food (Huang, 2007). In contrast to other allergies, the prevalence of food allergies in infancy is higher, with approximately 2% to 8% affected by cow's milk or soy allergies, and decreases to less than 2% by adulthood (Spergel & Pawlowski, 2002). These numbers reflect those allergies confirmed by history and food challenges, and contrast with the number of people who believe they have a food allergy but are not formally diagnosed, which includes approximately 25% to 30% of Americans (Spergel & Pawlowski, 2002). Approximately 30,000 food-induced anaphylactic episodes occur in the United States each year, resulting in 2000 hospitalizations and 200 deaths; peanuts, tree nuts, fish, and shellfish account for most severe food anaphylactic reactions (Sampson, 2003).

Allergic rhinitis, which was virtually unknown 200 years ago in Europe and North America, now affects 35% to 40% of the population (Liu & Murphy, 2003; McGeady, 2004). Currently, allergic rhinitis is the most common atopic condition and one of the leading chronic conditions in children and adolescents (Gentile, Shaprio, & Skoner, 2003). Although the reasons for these changes are not fully known, they are most likely multifactorial and reflect environmental influences and genetic predisposition (Huebner et al., 2008). Recent changes such as the increased insulation of homes, the rising popularity of carpeting and upholstered furniture, and a change in lifestyle that results in children spending more time indoors may put children in increasing contact with rising levels of common indoor allergens, such as house dust mites and animal dander.

A worldwide study of atopic prevalence was recently done in a large number of centers around the world. The investigators found increases in atopic disorders in children, ages 6 to 14, with differing prevalence from one location to another and in different age-groups. They speculate that the differences are related to environmental factors, lifestyle, economic status, climate variation, dietary habits, microbial exposure, and management of symptoms

(Asher, Montefort, Bjorksten, et al., 2006). Other hypotheses to explain the rising prevalence of allergies and atopy include increased exposure to pollution (McGeady, 2004), increased early vitamin D exposure (Oren, Banerji & Camargo, 2008), and prenatal influences on immune system development (Troye-Blomberg, 2002).

Diagnostic Criteria

In primary care practices, allergies are most often diagnosed based on the clinical presentation and response to antihistamine therapy. Diagnostic tests, including in vivo skin testing and in vitro testing, may be indicated if the allergy symptoms are severe or persistent, to assess for the child's triggers (Cartwright & Dolen, 2006). Identifying particular allergens can encourage the family to avoid the offending agents such as dust mites, animals, and foods.

In Vivo Skin Testing

Skin testing, specifically IgE antibody testing, is usually done in the allergist's office. This process involves "pricking the skin" to expose the individual to a small amount of allergen. A positive test results in a reaction caused by IgE antibodies to the allergen, and should be followed by in vitro testing for confirmation (Allison, 2007). Before skin testing, children must be reminded to discontinue their H_1 antihistamines for 7 days and H_2 receptor antagonists for 48 hours to avoid masking a reaction (Nolte, 2007).

In the case of food allergies, negative skin tests rather that positive skin tests are more useful in identifying or ruling out a possible allergen. Positive results should be confirmed with double-blind placebo-controlled food challenges before a food is implicated (Bock, 2003; Nolte, 2007). This should not be done if anaphylaxis to a food is suspected. Often, food allergens are identified by the relief from symptoms following elimination of a food from the diet. This is a useful method if a particular food, such as shellfish, is strongly suspected and is easily eliminated from the diet.

In Vitro Testing

Blood testing for specific IgE immunoassay, commonly referred to as radioallergosorbent testing (RAST), is more expensive and less specific than skin testing, but can be useful if particular issues make skin testing impossible, such as overwhelming atopic dermatitis or behavioral concerns (Allison, 2007; Bock, 2003; deShazo & Kemp, 2007). It requires routine phlebotomy, and there is no medication interference and no risk of allergic reaction to the testing (Dowdee & Ossege, 2007).

Elevated total serum IgE is consistent with atopy but is not a specific indicator for allergies. Blood eosinophilia may be used as a screening test, but it has a low sensitivity. A nasal smear with eosinophils clearly indicates allergies, but does not implicate a specific allergen. For children with severe allergies, testing for egg and gelatin allergies may be done before immunization administration. There may also be some indication for period-specific allergy screening for new allergens.

In summary, no single screening test is recommended for identifying persons with allergies. When needed, skin testing is the standard diagnostic tool. The entire clinical picture, including a thorough family history, is the most valuable and practical diagnostic tool, used either in conjunction with diagnostic testing or alone.

Clinical Manifestations at Time of Diagnosis

Allergic Rhinitis ("Hay Fever")

Symptoms of allergic rhinitis (AR) include nasal itching, nasal congestion, rhinorrhea with clear nasal discharge, and bouts of sneezing. Clinical signs include pale, bluish, boggy nasal mucosa and turbinates, clear nasal discharge, and nasal obstruction. Specific signs of allergic rhinitis include a crease across the nose (referred to as an "allergic salute"), allergic shiners (dark circles under the eyes; Figure 10-1), Dennie sign (lines under the lower lid margin), throat clicking or clucking, and nose twitching and facial grimacing. Experts have made recent attempts to standardize the definition of allergic rhinitis to ultimately enhance the quality of life for those affected. The International Consensus Report defines allergic rhinitis as causing one or more of the classic symptoms, such as nasal itching, rhinorrhea, nasal obstruction, and sneezing, with the affected person exhibiting at least two of the symptoms on most days (Wang et al., 2002). Symptoms can be seasonal or year round. The World Health Organization (WHO) recommends using the terms "intermittent allergic rhinitis" and "persistent allergic rhinitis" instead of the older terms of "seasonal" and "perennial" (Box 10-2) (Bousquet et al., 2006).

Occasionally, a child may have epistaxis, especially in the winter, due to excessive dryness in the home. Some children exhibit a characteristic facial development. This adenoid-type facies (Figure 10-2) is a result of chronic nasal obstruction and subsequent mouth breathing that forces currents of breathed air through the mouth and changes the growth pattern of the soft bones of the face, resulting in an open gaping mouth, dental malocclusion, and high arched hard palate.

Allergic Conjunctivitis

Allergic conjunctivitis may occur in combination with allergic rhinitis, or it may occur alone. The hallmark symptom is significant itching of the eyes. The accompanying vasodilation appears superficial and pink rather than a deep red. The eye has a general glassy appearance and tarsal cobblestone-like papillae are also present on the palpebral conjunctiva (Ono & Abelson, 2005).

General Symptoms

In addition to rhinitis or conjunctivitis, other more general symptoms may be present. These can include dry sore throat; itching of ears, nose, and throat with accompanying grimacing, twitching, and picking; dry cough; ear popping and fullness; and headache (Kliegman & Behrman, 2007). Any of these symptoms may be intermittent or persistent. Symptoms may be present for weeks or months, and may look like "a cold that never quite goes away." There is typically no fever or adenopathy to accompany these symptoms.

Food Allergies

Food allergies may manifest with a wide variety of symptoms, affecting the skin, oral area, GI system, respiratory system, and cardiovascular system. Mild symptoms can include skin rash, stomachache, nausea, diarrhea, nasal congestion, and sneezing, but some children have much more severe symptoms, such as respiratory distress and anaphylaxis (Allison, 2007). Usually, severe symptoms appear immediately after ingestion of the causative food. Cow's milk allergy is the most common food allergy in infants, and symptoms include rash, vomiting, diarrhea, bloody stools, reflux, wheeze, rhinitis, and impaired growth (Skripak, Matsui, Mudd, et al., 2007).

Clinical Manifestations at Time of Diagnosis

ALLERGIC RHINITIS
Symptoms
- Nasal itching
- Nasal congestion
- Clear nasal discharge
- Sneezing

Clinical signs
- Blue or pale boggy nasal mucosa and turbinates
- Clear nasal discharge
- Nasal obstruction
- Allergic salute
- Allergic shiners and Dennie sign
- Throat clicking and facial grimacing

ALLERGIC CONJUNCTIVITIS
Symptoms
- Itching of eyes
- Tearing

Clinical signs
- Bilateral redness of conjunctiva
- Profuse watery discharge
- Cobblestone appearance of palpebral conjunctiva

General symptoms
- Dry sore throat
- Itchy throat or ears
- Dry cough
- Ear popping and fullness
- Headache

FOOD ALLERGIES
Symptoms
- Stomachache
- Nausea or diarrhea
- Sneezing
- Nasal congestion
- Feeding difficulties

Clinical signs
- Rash
- Impaired growth in infants

SKIN MANIFESTATIONS
Symptoms
- Pruritus varies in severity
- Rash may be very transient, with each lesion lasting less than 24 hours

Clinical signs
- Edematous plaques or wheals with pale centers
- Erythematous borders
- Rash may be confluent

BEHAVIORAL MANIFESTATIONS
Symptoms
- Irritability, sleep disorders
- Fearfulness, anxiety, fatigue

Clinical signs
- Decreased ability to concentrate

ANAPHYLAXIS
Symptoms
- Rash, pruritus
- Cough
- Difficulty breathing

Clinical signs
- Facial edema
- Lip, throat, and tongue swelling
- Urticaria
- Wheezing

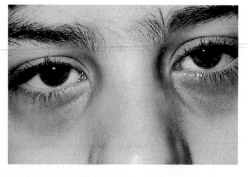

FIGURE 10-1 Allergic shiners, or dark circles beneath the eyes, in patient with allergic rhinitis. From Zitelli, B.J., & Davis, H.W. (2002). *Atlas of Pediatric Physical Diagnosis* (4th ed.). St. Louis: Mosby.

BOX 10-2

Classification of Allergic Rhinitis

1. "Intermittent" means that symptoms are present
   - Less than 4 days a week
   - Or for less than 4 weeks
2. "Persistent" means that symptoms are present
   - More than 4 days a week
   - And for more than 4 weeks
3. "Mild" means that none of the following items are present
   - Sleep disturbance
   - Impairment of daily activities, leisure and/or sport
   - Impairment of work or school
   - Troublesome symptoms
4. "Moderate-severe" means that one or more of the following items are present
   - Sleep disturbance
   - Impairment of daily activities, leisure and/or sport
   - Impairment of work or school
   - Troublesome symptoms

From ARIA Workshop Report. (2007). Allergic rhinitis and its impact on asthma. *J Allergies Clin Immunol, 108*(5), 1-205.

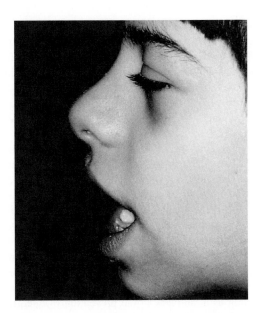

FIGURE 10-2 Characteristic adenoid-type facies in patient with long-standing allergic rhinitis. Note the open mouth and gaping habitus. From Zitelli, B.J., & Davis, H.W. (2002). *Atlas of Pediatric Physical Diagnosis* (4th ed.). St. Louis: Mosby.

Skin Manifestations

Urticaria (or hives) that is IgE mediated affects 20% of people at some point in their lifetimes. Most cases in children are secondary to IgE-mediated reactions or viral infections. Urticarial lesions appear as edematous plaques or wheals with pale centers and erythematous borders. The rash may be confluent, and lesions are transient, lasting for less than 24 hours, with new lesions continually appearing, giving the rash a sort of migratory nature. Pruritus is usually present and varies in severity. Food and drug reactions are common causes for urticaria. Foods that are most often responsible for urticaria include eggs, milk, wheat, peanuts, tree nuts, soy, shellfish, fish, and strawberries (Kliegman et al., 2007). The clinician should carefully elicit a complete history; however, the exact cause of the lesions is often not discovered.

Behavioral Manifestations

Some children with allergies show behavioral manifestations such as irritability, sleep disorders, and decreased ability to concentrate. Children may be so uncomfortable during allergy season that they misbehave at school or home. Allergies may lead to impaired daytime concentration, daytime sleepiness, and nighttime sleep disturbances. These impairments affect school and work performance. Clinicians must take care not to confuse these symptoms for those of attention-deficit/hyperactivity disorder or other behavioral disorders (see Chapter 12). Many believe that these behavioral signs may be due to a lack of sleep or to the use of over-the-counter medicines, many of which have sedating side effects. Finally, individuals with rhinitis find it socially embarrassing to be seen repeatedly sneezing, sniffling, or blowing their nose (Juniper, Stahl, Doty, et al., 2005).

Anaphylactic Reactions

Anaphylaxis is a systemic reaction to an allergen, rather than an organ- or system-limited response. Although rare, occurring in approximately 0.6% of children and up to 2% of the general population, it can be a life-threatening event (McIntyre, Sheetz, Carroll, et al., 2005). Among children, the most common cause of anaphylaxis is allergies to foods, stinging insects, and medications (Chiu & Kelly, 2005; McIntyre et al., 2005). The majority of fatal food anaphylaxis is caused by peanut and tree nut hypersensitivity (Kliegman et al., 2007). Of note, these foods also tend to induce persistent sensitivity in the vast majority of children, in contrast to other foods such as milk, soy, eggs, and wheat, that are frequently associated with milder allergic reactions and are usually outgrown (Powers, Bergren, & Finnegan, 2007). As children get older and develop other atopic symptoms, such as asthma, it is not uncommon for them to experience more severe anaphylaxis symptoms (Eghrari-Sabet, 2008; Sampson, 2003). Therefore those children with asthma who concurrently have food allergies should be identified as high risk for an anaphylactic reaction. Parents and caregivers should be educated on the potential signs and symptoms of anaphylaxis to ensure rapid recognition and treatment. The onset of symptoms, the sequence in which symptoms develop, and the severity of symptoms vary among individuals. The symptoms of anaphylaxis generally include the following systems: cutaneous, GI, respiratory, cardiovascular, and neurologic (Chiu & Kelly, 2005; Sampson, 2003; Young, 2003).

Treatment

The first line of defense against allergies is avoidance. In some cases, such as the child with dust mite allergy, that may be nearly impossible. Other potential components of the treatment plan include medications, education of child and parents about the condition and management plan, referral to an allergist, and immunotherapy ("allergy shots"). The treatment plan must be individualized for each child, and developed in partnership with the family and affected child.

Treatment

- Avoidance
- Medications/pharmacologic therapy
- Parent and child education
- Immunotherapy

Avoidance

Rhinitis and Conjunctivitis. The health care provider can assist the family in identifying the allergens for a particular child, and then endeavor to avoid, minimize, or control them. Families can try to avoid aerosol products as much as possible. Environmental

---

BOX 10-3

Avoidance of Allergens at Home

- Do not use aerosol products.
- Use dehumidifiers in damp places, such as in basements.
- Do not allow smoking in the family's home or car.
- Control dust with vacuuming, air filtration systems, wet mopping, and keeping "dust catchers," such as stuffed toys and open shelving, out of bedrooms.
- Keep windows closed or use air conditioning.
- Enclose pillows and mattresses in hypoallergenic covers.

tobacco smoke is a great offender for many children with respiratory allergies, and smoking should not be allowed in the family's home or car. Molds can be controlled using dehumidifiers, especially in the basement of the home.

Furry pets, unfortunately, are common allergens. The best clinical option is to keep all such pets out of the home. When this is not acceptable to the child or family, the pet should at least be confined to areas of the house where the child is least present; at the very minimum, the animal must be kept out of the bedroom. Frequent washing of a cat has been proposed and studied as a possible strategy. Significant reductions in airborne allergens were seen with a combination of air filtration and washing the cat, but later studies showed that the decrease lasted only a few days (Eggleston, 2005).

Dust mite is the most common indoor allergen, and frequent cleaning to control house dust can be helpful in decreasing symptoms. Vacuuming, air filtration systems, and wet mopping of non-carpeted floors are worthwhile strategies. Bedrooms, in particular, should be kept free of as many "dust catchers" as possible, including stuffed toys, carpets, curtains, large pillows, and open shelving filled with books and toys. In addition, mattresses and pillows can be encased in hypoallergenic covers, and only hypoallergenic pillows and bedding should be used. Some studies investigating measures to decrease dust mite exposure indicate that such efforts are not effective in improving asthma (de Vries, van den Bemt, Aretz, et al., 2007). Limited clinical trials show that measures to avoid dust mites as described previously may be somewhat effective in the reduction of allergic rhinitis symptoms, but more work needs to be done in this area to provide clear recommendations regarding the role of dust mite control in the management of symptoms (Sheikh & Hurwitz, 2003).

When a child has allergies to specific seasonal allergens, such as various pollens, it is wise to limit time outdoors during days with high pollen counts. Pollen counts can be found in local newspapers or on websites such as the Environmental Protection Agency (EPA) website (www.epa.gov). Keeping windows closed and using an air conditioner will also help control symptoms.

Food Allergies. Most children with food allergies must completely avoid all offending foods. Careful reading of food labels is essential (see Resources at the end of this chapter). The Food Allergen Labeling and Consumer Protection Act, in effect since 2006, has been a great help to parents of children with severe allergies. The act requires that manufacturers clearly label foods that contain any amount of milk, egg, fish, crustacean shellfish, tree nuts, peanuts, wheat, and soy (U.S. Food and Drug Administration Center for Food Safety and Applied Nutrition, 2008). These foods are responsible for over 90% of food allergens (Green, LaBelle, Steele, et al., 2007). Children must be taught to avoid particular foods as they grow more independent and spend more time away from home and parents. They must learn to avoid any sharing of foods in daycare, in school, or at the homes of friends. Effective education is necessary for parents, schools, daycare providers, and any other caregivers for the affected child, so that they are fully informed of significant food allergies (Jackson, 2002). Special care must be taken when eating in restaurants and reading labels, because the U.S. Food and Drug Administration reported an investigation of food companies in which 25% of the products contained undeclared allergic ingredients, often from cross-contamination (Mofidi & Sampson, 2008). Parents and caregivers must routinely ask about food components in restaurants to avoid serious or fatal food reactions. For those highly allergic, ingestion may not even be required for an allergic reaction, as reactions have been reported following superficial contact or merely being in the vicinity of the offending food. Currently, many manufacturers are adding warning labels to their packaging such as "may contain..." to alert consumers to potential cross-contamination (Mofidi & Sampson, 2008).

Infancy presents special challenges. Breastfeeding is best in almost all cases. Babies may have allergic reactions to infant formulas, and changing to a soy-based formula is sometimes necessary. If soy allergic, the infant must be switched to a protein hydrolysate formula. When babies who are at a high risk for an allergic condition due to a positive atopic family history are fed exclusively with breast milk or partial whey hydrolysate formula for at least 4 months, there is some evidence that they will have a lower incidence of atopy and food allergies (Greer et al., 2008; Sorensen & Niolet, 2007). The American Academy of Pediatrics considers breastfeeding as a hallmark in the prevention of allergies. However, although breastfeeding is clearly advantageous to the general health of the infant by decreasing some respiratory and GI infection rates, studies regarding its effect on the development of subsequent atopy may need to be interpreted taking into account the complex immunomodulatory role of early infections (Friedman & Zeiger, 2005). Even if, as some studies suggest, breastfeeding might sensitize some infants to more allergenic foods at an early age, other studies suggest it is protective. At the present time, there is lack of evidence that maternal dietary restrictions during pregnancy play a significant role in the prevention of atopy in infants. Similarly, antigen avoidance during lactation does not prevent atopy, with the possible exception of atopic eczema, although more data are needed to substantiate this conclusion (Greer et al., 2008). It would be unwise to suggest that a chance of sensitization would be a reason to forego the nutritional, psychological, and other immunologic benefits of breastfeeding (Friedman & Zeiger, 2005). In summary, a conservative approach of advocating breast milk or partial whey hydrolysate formula should be encouraged for the high-risk infant (de Jong, Scharp-Van Der Linden, Aalberse, et al., 2002; Friedman & Zeiger, 2005).

Food allergies may manifest as reactions to the foods the breast-feeding mother eats. The mother may need to eliminate certain offending foods from her diet. In extreme cases, the health care provider may recommend a hypoallergenic infant formula, such as Alimentum, Nutramigen, or Pregestimil (Friedman & Zeiger, 2005). Cow's milk allergy is particularly significant in infancy, when a child's nutritional need for milk is great. It must be carefully diagnosed, because elimination of cow's milk from the diet may have serious implications for growth and development.

Pharmacologic Therapy

Rhinitis and Conjunctivitis. Many over-the-counter and prescription medications can be employed in controlling allergy symptoms (Table 10-1). Antihistamine preparations are the mainstay of treatment, and are used to reduce itching, sneezing, and rhinorrhea within 1 hour, symptoms that result from histamine release in the allergic response (Figure 10-3) (deShazo & Kemp, 2007).

Most of the over-the-counter antihistamines are readily available, effective, and reasonable in price. They are prepared in both tablet and liquid form, and include diphenhydramine hydrochloride

TABLE 10-1

Medications Used in the Treatment of Allergic Rhinoconjunctivitis

	Route	Age	Dosing	Adverse Effects
SYSTEMIC ANTIHISTAMINES				
Allegra (fexofenadine HCl)	Oral	≥12 yr 2-11 yr	180 mg once daily or 60 mg twice daily 30 mg twice daily	Headache
Alavert OTC (loratadine)	Oral (quick-dissolving tablets)	≥6 yr	10 mg once daily	Nervousness, wheezing, dry mouth
Claritin OTC (loratadine)	Oral	≥6 yr 2-5 yr	10 mg once daily 5 mg once daily	≥12 yr: Headache, somnolence, fatigue, dry mouth <12 yr: Nervousness, wheezing, fatigue
Clarinex (desloratadine)	Oral	≥12 yr 6-11 yr 12 mo-5 yr 6-11 mo	5 mg once daily 2.5 mg once daily 1.25 mg 1.0 mg	Sore throat, dry mouth
Zyrtec (cetirizine HCl)	Oral	≥6 yr 2-5 yr 6-23 mo	5-10 mg once daily 2.5-5 mg once daily or 2.5 twice daily 2.5 mg once daily	≥12 yr: Somnolence, fatigue, dry mouth <12 yr: Headache, somnolence
Benadryl OTC (diphenhydramine HCl)	Oral	2-6 yr 6-11 yr >12 yr 6-11 yr	6.25 mg three or four times daily 12.5-25 mg three or four times daily 25-50 mg three or four times daily 5 mg/kg/day in 3 or 4 divided doses	Drowsiness, excitability
Chlor-Trimeton OTC (chlorpheniramine maleate)	Oral	>12 yr 6-12 yr 4-6 yr	4 mg q4-6hr 2 mg q4-6hr 1 mg q4-6hr	Drowsiness, excitability
Dimetapp OTC	Oral	6-12 yr	1 cap q4hr, max 4 doses/day	CNS stimulation, dizziness, blurred vision, palpitations, GI upset, anxiety, weakness, insomnia, excitability, drowsiness, anticholinergic effects
Tavist OTC (clemastine fumarate)	Oral	≥12 yr	1 tab (1.34 mg) twice daily	Drowsiness, excitability
TOPICAL ANTIHISTAMINES				
Astelin (azelastine HCl)	Nose	≥12 yr 5-11 yr	2 sprays/nostril twice daily 1 spray/nostril twice daily	Bitter taste, headache, somnolence
Emadine (emedastine)	Eyes	≥3 yr	1 drop up to four times daily	Transient burning, stinging, discomfort
Livostin (levocabastine HCl)	Eyes	>12 yr	1 drop per affected eye up to four times daily	Local irritation immediately after instillation
TOPICAL MAST CELL STABILIZERS				
Nasalcrom (cromolyn sodium)	Nose	≥2 yr	1 spray each nostril q4-6hr Prevention: Begin 1 wk before exposure to known allergen	Transient stinging, sneezing
Opticrom (cromolyn sodium)	Eyes	≥4 yr	1-2 drops/affected eye four to six times daily	Transient stinging or burning on instillation
Alomide (lodoxamide tromethamine)	Eyes	≥2 yr	1-2 drops four times daily for up to 4 mo	Burning, stinging, or discomfort
Zaditor (ketotifen fumarate)	Eyes	≥3 yr	1 drop per affected eye q8-12hr	Conjunctival infection, headache, rhinitis
Alocril	Eyes	≥3 yr	1-2 drops in affected eye twice daily	Headache, burning, irritation, stinging, unpleasant taste, nasal congestion

Data from Crisalida, T., Kaline, M.A., & Turkeltaub, M. (2002). *Allergies and asthma pocket guide.* New York: Adelphi Inc.; Boguniewicz, M. (2007). Allergic disorders. In W.W. Hay, M.J. Levin, J.M. Sondheimer, & R.R. Deterding (Eds.), *Current Pediatric Diagnosis and Treatment* (18th ed.). New York: Lange Medical Books/McGraw-Hill.
Key: *CNS,* central nervous system; *GI,* gastrointestinal.

TABLE 10-1

Medications Used in the Treatment of Allergic Rhinoconjunctivitis—cont'd

	Route	Age	Dosing	Adverse Effects
LEUKOTRIENE RECEPTOR ANTAGONIST				
Singulair (montelukast)	Oral	≥15 yr 6-14 yr 6 mo-5 yr	10 mg once daily 5 mg once daily 4 mg once daily (Note: Approved 6 mo and older for perennial allergic rhinitis only)	Fatigue, headache
TOPICAL STEROIDS				
Flonase (fluticasone propionate)	Nose	≥4 yr	1-2 sprays/nostril once daily	Epistaxis, headache, pharyngitis
Nasacort AQ (triamcinolone acetonide)	Nose	≥6 yr 2-5 yr	1-2 sprays/nostril once daily 1 spray/nostril once daily	Epistaxis, pharyngitis, increase in cough
Nasonex (mometasone furoate monohydrate) Rhinocort (budesonide)	Nose	≥12 yr 2-11 yr	2 sprays/nostril once daily 1 spray/nostril once daily	Epistaxis, headache, viral infection, pharyngitis
Nasal inhaler	Nose	≥6 yr	2 sprays/nostril twice daily (morning and evening) or 4 sprays/nostril once daily (morning)	Epistaxis, nasal irritation, pharyngitis, cough
Aqua nasal spray	Nose	≥6 yr	1 spray/nostril once daily	Epistaxis, pharyngitis, bronchospasm, cough, nasal irritation
Veramyst nose spray (fluticasone furoate)	Nose	>12 yr 2-11 yr	2 sprays/nostril per day 1 spray/nostril per day	Headache, epistaxis, pharyngitis, nasal ulceration
MAST CELL ANTIHISTAMINES				
Patanol (olopatadine HCl)	Eyes	≥3 yr	1 drop/affected eye twice daily	Headache, asthenia, blurred vision
Pataday (olopatadine HCl)	Eyes	≥3 yr	1 drop/affected eye once daily	Headache, asthenia, blurred vision
Patanase (olopatadine HCl)	Nose	>12 yr	2 sprays/nostril twice daily	Bitter taste, headache, epistaxis
NONSTEROIDAL ANTIINFLAMMATORY DRUGS (NSAIDs)				
Acular (ketorolac tromethamine)	Eyes	≥3 yr	1 drop/affected eye qid	Transient stinging and burning on instillation
ANAPHYLAXIS				
Epinephrine Auto-injector	IM, thigh only	>30 kg <30 kg	EpiPen 0.3 mg EpiPen Jr 0.15 mg	Palpitations, tachycardia, sweating, nausea and vomiting, respiratory difficulty, pallor, dizziness, weakness. tremor, headache, apprehension, nervousness, anxiety

(Benadryl), brompheniramine maleate (Dimetapp), clemastine fumarate (Tavist), and chlorpheniramine maleate (Chlor-Trimeton). These first-generation antihistamines may be reasonable choices for intermittent, mild symptoms or acute flares that do not require daily medications. The most common troublesome side effect of these medications is drowsiness (deShazo & Kemp, 2007; Juniper et al., 2005). Because of their sedative effect, bedtime dosing is often recommended to avoid daytime drowsiness and allow children to be awake and alert for school and activities. Current practice of using first-generation antihistamines is not well supported in the literature, and use of the second-generation antihistamines is encouraged whenever possible (deShazo & Kemp, 2007; Juniper et al., 2005).

Many second-generation antihistamines are available. They are not necessarily more effective, but most have minimal sedating side effects and a longer duration of action, making them better choices for children with more severe or persistent symptoms. Those that have been approved for use in young children include fexofenadine hydrochloride (Allegra), loratadine (Claritin), and cetirizine hydrochloride (Zyrtec).

Rhinitis. Topical nasal steroid sprays are the first-line treatment for persistent nasal symptoms, and can be used in children as young as 2 years old (de Groot et al., 2007; Lai, Casale, & Stokes, 2005; Seth, Secord, & Kamat, 2007). They include budesonide (Rhinocort Nasal or Rhinocort Aqua), fluticasone furoate (Veramyst), fluticasone propionate (Flonase), mometasone furoate monohydrate (Nasonex), and triamcinolone acetonide (Nasacort AQ); several are now available in long-acting preparations. Many studies have been done to investigate the impact of intranasal steroid use on children's growth and on the suppression of the hypothalamic-pituitary-adrenal axis, and little evidence has been found of adverse effects (Agertoft & Pedersen, 2000; *Fluticasone furoate [Veramyst] for allergic rhinitis,* 2007; Juniper et al., 2005; Skoner, Rachelefsky, Meltzer, et al., 2000). Although there is lingering concern about this issue, the use of nasal steroids should be time limited and be employed when symptoms are persistent and have a significant impact on daily functioning such that the benefits outweigh the potential risks. As with all steroids, the lowest possible dose should be employed to minimize side effects, and growth monitoring should be done regularly.

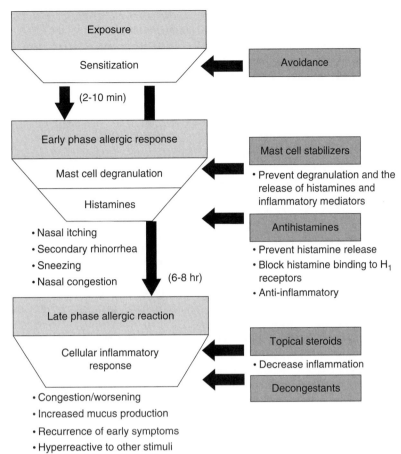

FIGURE 10-3 Etiology of allergic responses and the corresponding treatment.

There are a variety of topical nonsteroidal nasal sprays to choose from to manage the symptoms of rhinitis. Cromolyn sodium (NasalCrom) spray, a nonsteroidal antiinflammatory agent, is a mast cell stabilizer. It is a very safe medication; however, its utility is limited by the need for frequent dosing (deShazo & Kemp, 2007). For full effect it must be used four to six times per day during the allergy season or continually for perennial symptoms. Adherence to such a rigorous medication schedule is nearly impossible for children who spend most full days in daycare, school, or camp. Another option in the form of a nasal spray is azelastine hydrochloride (Astelin), which is a topical antihistamine and can be used in children 5 years of age and older.

Sneezing and nasal itching correlate best with histamine levels in allergic rhinitis. Nasal congestion correlates with leukotriene levels (deShazo & Kemp, 2007). Another class of medications that is approved to treat allergic rhinitis is the leukotriene modifier, montelukast (Singulair). When given alone, it seems to be less effective than topical steroids in treating allergic rhinitis; however, it also seems beneficial to use montelukast in combination with loratadine (deShazo & Kemp, 2007). Montelukast can be given to children age 6 months and older for year-round (indoor) allergies and to children age 2 years and older for seasonal (outdoor) allergies (Merck, 2008). If children experience epistaxis with nasal sprays despite proper technique, montelukast would be a good second choice (deShazo & Kemp, 2007).

Decongestants, both oral and topical, are available for use in children with significant nasal congestion. Use of over-the-counter oral antihistamines and decongestants, however, is not recommended for most children. The Food and Drug Administration (FDA) issued a public advisory notice that declared these products to be unsafe and ineffective for children under age 2 years (U.S. Food and Drug Administration & Center for Drug Evaluation and Research, 2008). Research continues to determine the safety and efficacy of these products in children ages 2 to 11 years. For infants and young children, nasal saline drops, the use of a bulb syringe to clear nasal secretions, and a cool mist humidifier are other safe treatments that are available. Decongestant nasal sprays are readily available over the counter in pharmacies and are very effective for fast relief of nasal symptoms. They can cause severe rebound congestion (rhinitis medicamentosa) when used for more than 3 days. Their use must be restricted to 1 or 2 days when optimum nasal clearing is absolutely essential. For example, the child who has a championship soccer game and another who is to perform in a vocal concert may be reasonable candidates for a few doses of a decongestant nasal spray. Providers must emphasize the significance of the rebound effect in these preparations to the child and parent, and their long-term or repeated use must be strongly discouraged.

Conjunctivitis. There are a wide variety of eye drops available to relieve symptoms of allergic conjunctivitis. The mast cell stabilizers are very effective and include cromolyn sodium (Opticrom), lodoxamide tromethamine (Alomide), nedocromil sodium (Alocril), and ketotifen fumarate (Zaditor). They vary in frequency of administration, which can be particularly important with a younger child who is fearful of or combative with eye drops. Some of the mast cell stabilizers are approved for children as young as 2 years old. Olopatadine hydrochloride (Patanol) is a mast cell stabilizer that also has antihistamine properties. Nonsteroidal antiinflammatory eye drops can also be employed, and include ketorolac tromethamine (Acular) and diclofenac (Voltaren). Another classification of eye drops is the antihistamines, such as emedastine difumarate (Emadadine) and lovocabastine (Livostin). Eye drops containing steroids are not recommended for children. In addition to pharmacotherapy, the child may gain some relief from ocular itching with the application of cool compresses, especially during a period of acute discomfort.

Food Allergies. Medications are used in two specific circumstances related to food allergies: to treat food-induced urticaria and to give immediate treatment for anaphylaxis. In the case of food-induced urticaria, a course of oral antihistamines, usually diphenhydramine, is useful to decrease itching and inflammation.

Anaphylaxis. The key to treating anaphylaxis is early recognition and rapid treatment with self-administered epinephrine. The recommended dose is epinephrine 1:1000 (aqueous), 0.01 mL/kg/dose, up to 0.5 mL, repeated every 10 to 20 minutes for up to three doses (Pickering & American Academy of Pediatrics Committee on Infectious Diseases, 2006). For best protection of children at risk for anaphylaxis, primary care providers should prescribe an epinephrine autoinjector (EpiPen, EpiPen Jr, Twinject) for use at home, in school, and wherever an allergic reaction may occur (Eghrari-Sabet, 2008; Hodges, Clack, & Hodges, 2007). Studies show that in many cases epinephrine is not readily available or used because of lack of prescribing by providers, poor instruction and lack of understanding on how to use the device, or not having the device on hand when an episode occurs, sometimes with fatal results (Chiu & Kelly, 2005; Eghrari-Sabet, 2008). It is critical that parents, teachers, caregivers, and the child with allergies know the signs of anaphylaxis, know the proper treatment, and are able to take prompt action when needed. A food allergy action plan that details the particular child's needs is advised; a template is available at www.foodallergy.org.

When there is any doubt about the severity of a reaction, epinephrine should be given. Whereas the potential side effects of an overdose of epinephrine are minimal, the potential consequence of withholding treatment is death. To facilitate proper administration, use of the epinephrine autoinjector device should be clearly taught and reinforced during routine visits (Figure 10-4). The most critical steps for proper use of the device include removing the gray cap, placing the black end flush against the thigh, applying pressure to the end opposite the black end until a click is heard, and holding the autoinjector in place for 10 seconds. After administration of epinephrine the child should be immediately transported to an emergency facility, even if symptoms subside. This safety measure is needed because a delayed or secondary reaction occurs in many children. At minimum, observation should continue for at least 4 hours after a mild episode of anaphylaxis, and 24 hours after a severe episode (Chiu & Kelly, 2005; Eghrari-Sabet, 2008; Pickering et al., 2006). Because of the potential for a biphasic reaction, some advocate prescribing two autoinjectors for each child so that a second one is available if needed (Eghrari-Sabet, 2008; Hodges et al., 2007).

Child and Parent Education

As with almost all chronic conditions, the education and involvement of the family are hallmarks of good care for allergies and will promote the optimum health of affected children. All family members and caregivers must have some understanding of the condition, its chronic nature, the offending agents (allergens), and the goals of treatment.

A clear understanding of any medications to be used and their proper administration is critical. For instance, some nasal sprays and eye drops are preventive in nature, such as steroid nasal sprays and mast cell stabilizer ophthalmic preparations. The family and child must understand that for optimum effectiveness, the medications should not be used only when symptoms are present, but must be used regularly throughout the allergy season.

Young children can be very fearful of eye drops, kicking and fighting to prevent administration. Clinicians can help teach caregivers the least traumatic ways to administer eye drops: first, the parent must hold down the child's lower lid, and then dispense the drop into the pocket created by the palpebral and bulbar conjunctiva, trying not to splash the eye drop into the center of the eye. Another effective method, useful in the younger child who has his or her eyes squeezed shut, is to simply dispense the eye drop on the closed eye, holding the child's head back. Eventually, the child will open his or her eyes, and the drop will roll into the eye.

Children and parents must be proficient in reading food labels when the child has food allergies. This is particularly important with prepared foods, which often have a long list of ingredients. Parents must also be able to identify hidden sources of foods in unfamiliar ingredients (see Resources at the end of this chapter). In addition, they must be assertive in talking with restaurant managers and food handlers at daycare, school, camp, and other such arenas. Clinicians can educate children and parents about these matters and practice needed skills.

There is a vast array of family education and support groups in many regions of the United States, as well as a growing list of reliable websites (see Resources at the end of this chapter). When working on environmental measures, the family may benefit from additional home-based intervention. For instance, clinicians can seek out the local chapter of an allergy support organization, local health department, university program, or home health agency with a fitting supportive or intervention program.

Immunotherapy

Immunotherapy is an effective treatment when used in carefully selected situations. Children who have severe allergies, and for whom avoidance and medications are not effective in relieving nasal symptoms or the cost of immunotherapy will be less than the cost of long-term medication, may benefit from immunotherapy (Huggins & Looney, 2004). In these cases, a pediatric allergist is consulted who will test the child for specific allergies and prepare an individualized serum. The serum is administered in a series of frequent injections that desensitize the child to the specific allergens. Approximately 75% of children respond well to immunotherapy, becoming desensitized to specific allergens. It can be used for pollen allergies, dust mite allergies, and stinging insect hypersensitivity (Matsui, 2008). Immunotherapy must be administered frequently and for several years, so it must be employed judiciously. Parents and providers can work together to help children and adolescents through the difficulties of immunotherapy. A developmental approach may help the child to understand the basic facts of immunotherapy and the reasons that parents and providers believe the treatments should be tried. Examples of developmentally based education include allowing a young child to inject a

EpiPen® DIRECTIONS FOR USE

1. Unscrew the yellow or green cap off of the EpiPen® or EpiPen® Jr carrying case (A) and remove the EpiPen® or EpiPen® Jr auto-injector from its storage case (B).

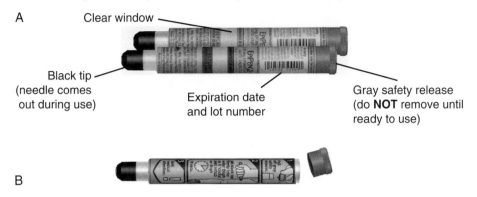

A   Clear window

Black tip
(needle comes
out during use)

Expiration date
and lot number

Gray safety release
(do **NOT** remove until
ready to use)

B

2. Grasp unit with the black tip pointing downward.

3. Form fist around the unit (black tip down).

4. With your other hand, pull off the gray safety release.

5. Hold black tip near outer thigh (C).

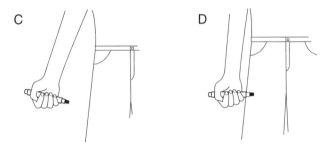

C   D

6. Swing and jab firmly into outer thigh until it clicks so that unit is perpendicular (at a 90-degree angle) to the thigh. (Auto-injector is designed to work through clothing.) (D)

7. Hold firmly against thigh for approximately 10 seconds. (The injection is now complete. Window on auto-injector will show red.)

8. Remove unit from thigh and massage injection area for 10 seconds.

9. Call 911 and seek immediate medical attention.

10. After use, carefully place the used auto-injector (without bending the needle), needle-end first, into the storage tube of the carrying case that provides built-in needle protection. Then screw the cap of the storage tube back on completely, and take it with you to the hospital emergency room.

Note: Most of the liquid (about 90%) stays in the auto-injector and cannot be reused. However, you have received the correct dose of the medication if the red flag appears in window.

FIGURE 10-4 How to treat anaphylaxis with self-administered epinephrine. **A** to **D,** Epi-Pen.

Twinject® DIRECTIONS FOR USE

First Dose Administration (E)

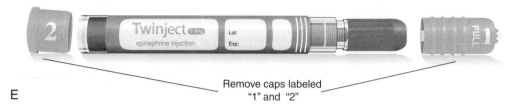

Remove caps labeled
"1" and "2"

E

1. Remove caps labeled "1" and "2."

2. Place rounded tip against the middle of the outer thigh. The needle may be injected through clothing. Press down hard until auto-injector fires. Hold in place while slowly counting to 10.

3. Immediately call 911.

Note: Never place thumbs, fingers, or hands over rounded tip.

Second Dose Administration (F)

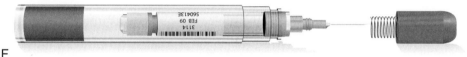

F

If symptoms have not improved within about 10 minutes after the first injection, a second dose is needed.

1. Unscrew rounded tip.

2. Pull syringe from barrel, and slide yellow collar off plunger.

3. Put needle into thigh. Push plunger down all the way.

FIGURE 10-4, cont'd E, Twinject first dose administration; **F,** Twinject second dose administration.

doll or teddy bear with a play syringe, use of a star chart that marks successful injection visits and is linked to a reward system, and recommending one of the child- or teen-focused allergy websites (see Web Resources at the end of this chapter). There is also a risk of serious reactions with immunotherapy, including anaphylaxis, especially in the early induction stage of therapy. Because of these risks, immunotherapy should only be given in a health care facility with skilled personnel and appropriate equipment to deal effectively with an anaphylactic reaction. Immunotherapy is not used for the treatment of ocular symptoms alone or food allergies.

Complementary and Alternative Therapies

Complementary and alternative medicine (CAM) practice in North America is increasing. Studies evaluating the use of CAM by children with chronic conditions found a user rate as high as 72% (Jean & Cyr, 2007). This can be correlated with the rising prevalence of allergies, but is also a result of parental and child frustration in not finding adequate relief for allergy symptoms with conventional therapies. The limited understanding of the etiology of allergies, the pervasive nature of offending allergens, nonadherence with prescribed therapies, the lack of a standardized classification system for the diagnosis and management of allergies, and the impact of symptoms on the daily lives of those affected all contribute to treatment failure.

Treatments that have been used by families seeking complementary and alternative therapies include herbal remedies, relaxation, supplementation, elimination diets, and rotation diets. Research is ongoing to evaluate the mechanisms and efficacy of various CAM treatments in the United States and internationally, but the

evidence to date is not convincingly supportive of these treatments (Goldsobel, 2007; Ko, Lee, Munoz-Furlong, et al., 2006; Passalacqua, Compalati, Schiappoli, et al., 2005; Schafer, 2004; Ziment & Tashkin, 2000). Providers should remember that there are some risks with CAM, particularly herbs that are not benign but can cause direct toxicity; decreased adherence with traditional therapies is another concern (Bielory, 2004; Heimall & Bielory, 2004). Studies specific to the pediatric population are scarce, though some work is being done with pregnant women and the effect of prenatal treatment on later infant inflammatory conditions (Blazek-O'Neill, 2005). Continued investigation remains to be done by researchers regarding the clinical effectiveness and usefulness of these modalities, particularly with children.

Probiotics, the use of live microbial food ingredients to treat many different kinds of allergies, is a therapy garnering some recent attention. The theory regarding the use of probiotics suggests that atopic individuals are lacking specific microbes in the commensal gut microflora, making them susceptible to the development of allergies (Kligler et al., 2007; Prescott & Bjorksten, 2007; Rautava, Kalliomaki, & Isolauri, 2005). Some studies report that *Lactobacillus rhamnosus* GG, a probiotic strain, is effective in the treatment of allergic inflammation of the gut (Prescott & Bjorksten, 2007; Rautava et al., 2005) Studies have suggested its usefulness in the prevention of atopic eczema when given to mothers during pregnancy and breastfeeding (Prescott & Bjorksten, 2007; Kalliomaki, Salminen, Arvilommi, et al., 2001). Other researchers have shown no benefit from *Lactobacillus rhamnosus* GG (Helin, Haahtela, & Haahtela, 2002). The positive findings regarding lactobacillus and its availability have contributed to its use outside of conventional therapies, particularly for food allergies where little other treatment is available.

Anticipated Advances in Diagnosis and Management

The latter part of the twentieth century saw large increases in the prevalence of allergic conditions, implicating changing environment and lifestyles as significant causes. It is difficult to determine the influence of the environment versus genetic variation of the immune system (Tovey & Kemp, 2005). Allergic conditions result from combinations of, and interactions among, mild defects rather than massive genetic disruptions. The fact that genetic variants occur at increasing numbers of positions along the complex pathway regulating IgE provides for an almost infinite variety of individual genotypes. Advances in genetic therapy for allergies include highlighting interleukin-13 (IL-13) as a critical effector of allergic inflammation. Future advances regarding allergies and atopy will not only depend on identifying the genes responsible but also the complex interaction between genes and the environment.

Some anticipated advances in treating children with food allergies include anti-IgE, probiotics, and food allergy vaccines. These advances may provide helpful therapy for children with food allergies and prevent development of food allergies in at-risk infants. These will have to be studied at great length for risk of toxicity and long-term effects of suppressing antibodies. These new approaches have the potential to bring real hope to people for whom no specific therapy is currently available (Nowak-Wegrzyn, 2003).

There are several anticipated advances with regard to immunotherapy. First, alternative routes of immunotherapy administration are being researched, including oral, sublingual, and intranasal delivery. Researchers have examined the efficacy of oral and sublingual swallow immunotherapy and demonstrated some improvement in asthma and allergic rhinitis symptoms (Matsui, 2008). Second, immunotherapy has traditionally been used as a therapeutic intervention rather than a preventive one. However, some evidence suggests that specific immunotherapy may have a future role in the secondary prevention of allergic conditions. The research evidence is preliminary, but there is a suggestion that immunologic intervention at an early stage of immune development may alter the natural progression of the allergic phenotype (Matsui, 2008; Moss, 2005). The cost-effectiveness of immunotherapy seems clear with respect to decreased use of medications and other treatments (Hankin, Cox, Lang, et al., 2008).

Associated Problems of Allergies and Treatment

Children with allergies often are brought to the clinician with one or more clinical manifestations because there is a strong association between sensitization and symptoms of allergy. Children with asthma, eczema, or rhinitis are more likely to be sensitized to one or more allergens than those without these conditions (Almqvist, Li, Britton, et al., 2007). The term "atopic march" refers to the sequential development of allergic conditions in childhood, beginning with atopic dermatitis and food allergies in infancy and early childhood, then proceeding to asthma and allergic rhinitis (Hahn & Bacharier, 2005). Besides asthma and atopic dermatitis (eczema), other associated problems include upper respiratory infections (sinusitis, pharyngitis, and acute otitis media), eustachian tube obstruction, sleep apnea, and dental malocclusion. A link between psychiatric comorbidities and allergies has been made in the adult population, particularly depression and allergic rhinitis, but this link has not been explored in children and adolescents (Slattery, 2005).

Associated Problems of Allergies and Treatment

- Asthma
- Atopic dermatitis (eczema)
- Respiratory infections (sinusitis, pharyngitis, acute otitis media)
- Eustachian tube obstruction
- Sleep apnea
- Dental malocclusion

Asthma

One of the most prominent associated conditions is asthma (see Chapter 11). Studies show that 88% of children with asthma were sensitized to at least one inhalant allergen (Lack, 2001; Liu & Murphy, 2003; Thomas, 2006). Asthma and allergies often coexist, and because of some shared symptomatology, the diagnosis of asthma often is confounded by the presence of allergic rhinitis. When a child is affected by both of these conditions, both must be aggressively treated. Fortunately, there is some evidence to suggest that treatment of children with allergic rhinitis improves the coexisting asthma, emphasizing the importance of vigilant treatment of allergic rhinitis (Bousquet et al., 2006; Lack, 2001; Thomas, 2006). In addition, when aggressive allergen avoidance is successful, both conditions may improve because they both have the common underlying cause of allergic sensitization.

Atopic Dermatitis (Eczema)

Atopic dermatitis (AD) is a chronic inflammatory rash, characterized by severe pruritus, overall dryness of the skin, and a pattern of exacerbation and remission. Recent evidence suggests that atopic dermatitis may be the first indication of the development of allergies later on in life (Sorensen & Niolet, 2007). Allergic rhinitis develops in approximately 30% of children with AD. Like asthma, the incidence and prevalence of AD are rising and the environmental risk factors are similar to those of allergic rhinitis and asthma (Leung & Boguniewicz, 2003; Williams, 2005). AD is one of the most common symptoms of food allergies, comprising the majority of allergic manifestations among infants (Dowdee & Ossege, 2007). Approximately one third of children who have AD also have at least one food allergy (Scurlock, Lee, & Burks, 2005). For infants older than 6 months of age, however, there are insufficient data to support a protective effect of any dietary intervention for the development of atopic conditions (Greer et al., 2008).

Upper Respiratory Infections

Sinusitis, pharyngitis, and acute otitis media sometimes complicate allergic rhinitis. Clinicians should be careful to follow the current treatment guidelines and avoid overuse of antibiotics. Children who have recurrent bouts of these related infections should be referred to a pediatric otolaryngologist for consultation. In cases of persistent cough or recurrent respiratory tract infections, a pediatric pulmonologist may be consulted.

Eustachian Tube Obstruction

Allergies often involve inflammation of the eustachian tubes, which may cause obstruction, accumulation of fluid in the inner ear, and infection. Hearing can be affected, and if the inflammation is chronic, speech problems can develop. This is of particular concern between ages 6 months and 3 years, a critical period for speech development.

Sleep Apnea

Children with allergic rhinitis may be more prone to obstructive sleep apnea because of upper airway edema and lymphoid hypertrophy. One study suggests that systemic and airway inflammation may contribute to daytime sleepiness associated with obstructive sleep apnea syndrome (OSAS) (Bender & Leung, 2005). Guidelines have been developed by the American Academy of Pediatrics regarding childhood OSAS recommending that *all* children be screened for snoring as a part of routine health maintenance visits (Section on Pediatric Pulmonology & Subcommittee on Obstructive Sleep Apnea Syndrome, 2002). Children with allergies who have habitual snoring or evidence of disturbed sleep should receive further workup for OSAS.

Once snoring is recognized in a child, a more focused history and examination is necessary to identify the child's potential for OSAS. Detailed information regarding the quality of the snoring and the subsequent pauses, snorts, or gasps is important in distinguishing OSAS from primary snoring. History and physical alone are not diagnostic, but are useful in determining which children need further testing and treatment, as well as to avoid unnecessary and expensive interventions (Section on Pediatric Pulmonology & Subcommittee on Obstructive Sleep Apnea Syndrome, 2002). Parents can audiotape their child sleeping to help in the diagnosis and treatment plan. The timely diagnosis and management of this disorder is important to avoid the complications associated with OSAS. A trial of allergy medications and environmental measures may help alleviate the problem. Referral to a pediatric otolaryngologist or pediatric sleep specialist may be indicated when symptoms persist.

Dental Malocclusion

Allergic rhinitis causes mouth breathing for many children. The result may be dental malocclusion, causing an overbite that could benefit from an orthodontia referral.

Prognosis

In the past, many have seen allergies, particularly allergic rhinitis and conjunctivitis, as an insignificant health issue. It has become increasingly clear, however, that it is a significant condition in many ways, including the number of persons affected, the economic burden, and the effect of the condition on quality of life and productivity. The direct medical cost of allergies in the United States has been estimated to be $5.9 billion annually, and children 12 years and younger account for 38% of this total (Bielory et al., 2003). Total economic burden is much greater when the impact on school performance, family function, and parental work productivity is considered.

Beyond the condition, with its cost, symptoms, and adverse effects of sedating medications, allergic rhinitis has a significant role in the development of life-threatening comorbidities such as asthma (ARIA, 2007; Bousquet, van Cauwenberge, & Khaltaev,

2001). Managing allergies more consistently and aggressively will lessen the burden associated with the condition and may also prevent the development of asthma or minimize its severity.

Allergic rhinitis and conjunctivitis are chronic conditions that may come and go over time. Approximately 10% to 20% of affected children with allergic rhinitis have a lessening or disappearance of symptoms in several years (deShazo & Kemp, 2007). Of those with symptoms that persist into adulthood, improvement generally occurs in the majority of people over the years, though skin test reactivity may not change. Exacerbations and remissions often occur throughout the lifetime as a result of environmental changes.

Milder food allergies often resolve over time, though some more severe allergies, such as allergies to peanuts, tree nuts, and fish, persist throughout life (Bender & Leung, 2005; Sampson, 2002; Zeiger, 2003).

PRIMARY CARE MANAGEMENT

Health Care Maintenance
Growth and Development

Allergies may result in inadequate food intake and consequently affect growth. Chronic congestion may cause a child to have a poor appetite or allergies to various common foods may severely limit a child's intake. Decreased rates of skeletal growth have been a concern with long-term steroid use, particularly large-dose oral administration. Research shows that intranasal corticosteroids delivered once daily do not inhibit children's growth (Gradman, Caldwell, & Wolthers, 2007; Murphy, Uryniak, Simpson, et al., 2006), though it appears that twice-daily delivery is associated with slight reductions in growth (Juniper et al., 2005). Providers should carefully monitor growth of children receiving long-term steroids.

Decreased ability to concentrate, disordered sleep, and sedative effects from allergy medications are associated with lower levels of performance on tests and can compromise a child's success in school (Bender & Leung, 2005). Allergic rhinitis may have a detrimental effect on adolescents' academic testing, alter their memory and affect decision-making ability (Walter, Khan-Wasti, Fletcher, et al., 2007; Fineman, 2002). Providers must be sure to consider allergies when developmental delay or poor school performance is the presenting problem.

The child with severe seasonal allergies may need to avoid being outdoors, even when fully medicated. When this is the case, providers, parents, and child can work together to identify other age-appropriate activities that would be enjoyable for the child and enhance development.

Diet

The child with allergies may have a poor appetite (Lack, 2001). Sore throats from persistent postnasal drip may also deter a child from eating. Ensuring adequate intake of a well-balanced variety of foods may take extra effort for the child with allergies.

The American Academy of Pediatrics advises avoidance of solids for 4 to 6 months for the prevention of allergic conditions (Kleinman & American Academy of Pediatrics, 2004). There is conflicting information about the relationship between early introduction of solids and the development of allergic conditions (Tarini, Carroll, Sox, et al., 2006). A recent study found no evidence to recommend a delayed introduction of solids beyond 4 to 6 months for the prevention of asthma, allergic rhinitis, and food or inhalant sensitization at age 6 years (Zutavern, Brockow, Schaaf, et al., 2008). In view of this, clinicians should caution parents with a family history of food allergies to wait until age 4 to 6 months before offering any solid foods, to help guard against allergy development (Zeiger, 2003). At 6 months, parents are encouraged to proceed slowly with the introduction of each new food. Parents may carefully introduce a small amount, approximately one teaspoon, of one food at a time. After 3 to 5 days, another food can then be introduced. This allows parents to more easily identify an offending food if any reactions occur. Avoid giving high-risk children certain foods that are more likely to cause symptoms; these include citrus fruits and juices, peanuts and peanut butter, eggs, and wheat. After 1 year of strict avoidance, some foods can be introduced successfully. Particular care should be taken with peanut allergies because of the greater risk of anaphylaxis. An open food challenge, supervised by an allergist, where parents and child are aware of the food being ingested, may be offered to parents of children with peanut allergies, because it would be a clear advantage for the family to know that the child is no longer allergic (Mofidi & Sampson, 2008).

Managing the diet of a child with food allergies can be particularly challenging. Because avoidance is the mainstay of treatment, parents must become experts in deciphering food labels, and be continually vigilant for hidden sources of the offending food. Several websites provide useful tips for identifying hidden foods on product labels (see Web Resources at the end of this chapter). Equally challenging is making sure the child with food allergies is getting all nutrients in adequate amounts. For example, a child who has an allergy to milk and milk products must consume other sources of calcium or take a supplement. Helping parents to find alternatives is an important aspect of the primary care provider's role in promoting good health. In situations of multiple food allergies, providers may refer the family to a nutritionist.

Safety

Children with allergies to foods must be assessed regarding the need for injectable epinephrine. Factors that contribute to a greater risk of anaphylactic reactions to foods include a past medical history for asthma, young age, and eczema (Sampson, 2003). The foods most commonly implicated in severe food anaphylaxis reactions include peanuts, tree nuts, seafood, and shellfish (Sampson, 2003). A toddler with peanut allergy, who reacted with minimal cutaneous and GI symptoms before developing asthma, may experience a more severe anaphylactic reaction after ingesting peanuts in later years. However, subsequent allergic reactions are highly variable and may manifest as milder, similar, or more severe reactions (Sampson, 2003). It is critical that health care providers be knowledgeable in prescribing and instructing families in using self-injectable epinephrine (EpiPen). An EpiPen can be a life-saving medication if available and used promptly and properly. Unfortunately, in many cases of anaphylaxis, either an EpiPen is not available or it is improperly used (McIntyre et al., 2005; Munoz-Furlong, 2007). Parents and providers all need to be better educated about the use of EpiPens, and, in turn, need to educate all others who may be caring for their children, including teachers, daycare providers, camp leaders, and others who may

be the first person to recognize early allergic reaction symptoms (McIntyre et al., 2005; Munoz-Furlong, 2007). The child should be instructed in self-injection techniques when developmentally appropriate. If the EpiPen 2-Pak or EpiPen Jr 2-Pak is prescribed, the pack includes a training device that can be used with parents and children to learn and practice administration. The condition of the emergency epinephrine must be monitored by parents and children, so that appropriate replacement can be made if the solution is discolored or if the medication expires. After using an EpiPen, the child must immediately be transported to the local hospital emergency department for follow-up care. Emergency plans should be developed and on file in schools and daycare centers to detail the plan of action in case of anaphylaxis, including a picture of the child when multiple caregivers or teachers are involved. A medical alert bracelet to identify the child's allergy is recommended.

Immunizations

Routine immunizations are recommended for most children with allergies. This includes yearly influenza vaccine, now recommended for all children ages 6 months to 18 years (Centers for Disease Control and Prevention, n.d.). Children younger than 5 years old and those with significant allergies should be a priority because they are at higher risk for more severe influenza complications compared with other children. Providers must be alert for the small number of children with allergies who have serious contraindications to immunizations. Those who are on long-term, high-dose oral steroid therapy should have live virus vaccines (measles-mumps-rubella [MMR], varicella, influenza) postponed until after steroid treatment is completed (Committee on Infectious Diseases, 2006; Verstraeten, Jumaan, Mullooly, et al., 2003). It is also imperative for providers to carefully screen all children who have a history of anaphylaxis. Those with anaphylaxis to eggs should not receive influenza vaccine; those with anaphylaxis to gelatin should not receive MMR or varicella (Committee on Infectious Diseases, 2006). If there is known anaphylaxis to gelatin before the first does of MMR, the vaccine should be given in a facility prepared to handle an anaphylactic reaction. If anaphylaxis is discovered after the first dose, titers should be checked to confirm immunity and the second dose should be deferred (Committee on Infectious Diseases, 2006).

Screening

Vision. Routine screening is recommended for all children. In addition, ocular symptoms or use of ocular medications may require closer evaluation of a child's eyes on physical examination.

Hearing. The child with allergies may require more frequent hearing screens to evaluate for hearing deficit that may be secondary to recurrent otitis media or transient and due to congestion.

Dental. Routine screening is recommended. Malocclusion may occur due to prolonged mouth breathing.

Blood Pressure. Routine screening is recommended.

Hematocrit. Routine screening is recommended.

Urinalysis. Routine screening is recommended.

Tuberculosis. Routine screening is recommended.

Condition-Specific Screening

No condition-specific screening is recommended other than screening tests for diagnosis (see Diagnostic Criteria).

Common Illness Management

Differential Diagnosis for Common Illnesses

Asthma. Asthma can be mistakenly diagnosed as allergies, and allergies as asthma. The most frequent reason for this is the existence of the shared symptom of cough, which constitutes an area of clinical overlap between rhinitis and asthma. In young children, cough is often the result of postnasal drip, but is sometimes diagnosed as asthma or cough-variant asthma. When this happens, the child may appear to have more severe asthma and therefore may be overtreated with asthma medications. This is particularly problematic when the medications include steroids.

Acute Viral Rhinitis. Acute viral rhinitis, or upper respiratory infection (URI), is the most frequent infection in all children, and is easily confused with allergic rhinitis. Both may cause cough, nasal congestion, and discharge. Usually, the nasal discharge in URI is time limited, lasting less than 2 weeks. However, this situation is more difficult to evaluate when the child has the more complicated history of recurrent bouts of URI, a common case in the school-age child or child in daycare.

The diagnosis of seasonal allergic rhinitis is usually straightforward. The clinician who is knowledgeable about local environmental pollens can correlate the clinical signs and symptoms with the seasonal time frame, recorded pollen counts, and personal and family health history, and make the diagnosis. The clinician can also differentiate URI from allergies by evaluating for erythematous nasal mucosa, fever, and purulent nasal discharge, all of which are commonly seen in URI.

Vasomotor Rhinitis. Vasomotor rhinitis is a poorly defined nasal condition that is manifested by some degree of nasal obstruction, profuse rhinorrhea, and congestion. Symptoms often occur with exposure to nonspecific factors, such as exercise, temperature changes, or air pollution, and generally appear and depart quite suddenly. There is usually a negative family history. The etiology is unclear, and the symptoms rarely improve with environmental controls or medications.

Acute Infectious Sinusitis, Pharyngitis, and Conjunctivitis. Acute sinusitis, pharyngitis, and conjunctivitis can be mistaken for allergies. The affected child may have nasal obstruction, sore throat, headache, red eyes, and fatigue. In these cases, the clinician must be alert for signs of infection, such as lymphadenopathy, fever, erythema, and purulent discharge. There is often a history of contagious contacts in the family, school, or daycare setting. Some of the hallmark signs of allergies, such as pruritus and clear discharge, are not present with infections. An atopic history may be absent. A rapid strep test or throat culture can help determine if antibiotics are needed. Infectious conjunctivitis can be differentiated

---

Differential Diagnosis

- Asthma
- Acute viral rhinitis
- Vasomotor rhinitis
- Acute infectious sinusitis, pharyngitis, and conjunctivitis
- Rhinitis medicamentosa
- Substance abuse
- Urticaria
- Gastroenteritis and other gastrointestinal problems

---

from allergic causes of red eye, primarily with history and physical evidence of infection such as purulent discharge, the presence of preauricular lymph nodes, and eye crusting.

The child with allergies can develop an infectious condition in addition to the allergic condition. The clinician must be alert for this episodic situation, and treat with antimicrobial agents as appropriate. Allergy medications should be continued. For the child who has recurrent pharyngitis, recurrent otitis media, or snoring, a referral to pediatric otolaryngology should be considered.

Rhinitis Medicamentosa. Rhinitis medicamentosa is severe rebound nasal congestion that occurs as a result of frequent prolonged use of proprietary nasal decongestant sprays. When the child stops using the spray, the rebound congestion is acute and intensely uncomfortable. When eliciting the health history, the provider must directly question the child and parent on the use of over-the-counter medications, specifically nasal sprays.

Substance Abuse. Adolescents who are snorting cocaine or abusing other medications may show symptoms that are highly suggestive of an allergic condition, including rhinorrhea, rhinitis, nasal polyps, epistaxis, conjunctivitis, and nasal congestion (Chrostowski & Pongracic, 2002; Williams & Storck, 2007). Chronic use can also cause perforation of the nasal septum. Clinicians should watch for these symptoms, especially when other components of the history or physical are suggestive of substance abuse. Behavioral and developmental indicators, such as school failure, deterioration of relationships with family or peers, mood alterations, or changes in sleep and eating patterns, may reinforce such diagnostic exploration. Another key to diagnosis is when adolescents do not improve with standard allergic rhinitis medical treatment, which may point to underlying substance abuse, not allergic condition. Physical examination may assist in the diagnosis, as the nasal mucosa in substance abuse may bleed easily and is often erythematous, instead of the pale and boggy mucosa that is typical of allergies.

Urticaria. Urticaria (hives) that are related to food allergies often present a confusing dilemma to the clinician. When an offending food cannot be identified, other diagnoses are entertained. Urticarial wheals may mimic many conditions, including insect bites, adverse medication reactions, contact dermatitis, and urticarial vasculitis. If a medication is suspected, future avoidance is paramount. Treatment of most urticaria with antihistamines is the same, regardless of cause. Although the exact cause of many cases of urticaria remains a mystery, the history, distribution, and progression of the rash often provide the clinician with important diagnostic clues.

Gastroenteritis and Other Gastrointestinal Problems. Stomach upset, diarrhea, and vomiting are common symptoms in children, with a myriad of causes other than food allergies, including lactose intolerance, acute gastroenteritis, parasitic infestations, and colic. Intolerance to a food is an inability of the body to digest the food, but it is not an allergy in that it is not an IgE-mediated response and is not likely to have the same long-term effects as allergy (Ewing & Allen, 2005). True food allergy, such as cow's milk allergy, may be a precursor for later development of other allergies, asthma, or eczema. Differentiating between actual allergies and intolerance is important but can be difficult based on clinical presentation alone. Typically, the child with allergies to a food will have skin and respiratory symptoms in addition to GI symptoms.

Acute gastroenteritis has an onset of less than 1 week, may or may not be accompanied by a fever, and is always time limited. With a bacterial cause, critical aspects of the history include presence of bloody diarrhea, fever, chills, and cramps. When caused by a virus, the diarrhea is typically watery. A wait-and-see approach is reasonable in the case of mild gastroenteritis, focusing more on adequate intake of fluids and maintaining hydration. Other helpful clues for discriminating between food allergies and gastroenteritis include the season at time of presentation (viral more likely in winter and summer) and contact with other sick individuals. The diagnosis of a parasitic infestation depends ultimately on stool cultures, but a history of recent travel or blood or mucus in the stool increases the likelihood of parasitic infection.

Colic is most commonly seen beginning in the second week of life, with a peak at 1 to 2 months and a decline by 3 to 4 months. Although some suggest that colic is secondary to GI upset, there is no clear evidence for this theory (Savino, 2007). Lactose intolerance can be either primary or secondary. In primary lactose intolerance, the infant has diarrhea following feedings, the infant may vomit, and the stool is typically frothy. More common is secondary or acquired intolerance. This is seen usually at about 3 to 5 years of age and more often in children of African American, Hispanic, Ashkenazi Jewish, American Indian, or Asian decent (Heyman, 2006). The presenting symptom is stomachache after drinking or eating milk or milk products.

Diagnosing food allergies is a long and arduous process. A definitive diagnosis is only made with a double-blind placebo-controlled food challenge.

Drug Interactions

There are many medications used to manage the symptoms associated with allergies (see Table 10-1). Many have limited potential for interaction with other drugs used in primary care because they are administered topically (intranasal or ophthalmic preparations). Systemic preparations used for allergy management frequently have potential for central nervous system stimulation and/or drowsiness and therefore, other medications with similar reactions, including alcohol, should be used with caution. Parents must be cautioned about the potential hazards of over-the-counter medications for coughs, colds, and allergies and educated to read medication labels to avoid the possibility of over-medicating their child. Parents should be instructed to contact the primary care provider if they believe the child needs additional medication to control allergy symptoms.

Developmental Issues

Sleep Patterns

Nasal obstruction and itching can disrupt the sleep of children with allergies. It can result in restlessness, shortened naps, and waking during the night. Additionally, the child with allergies may also have obstructive sleep apnea (see section on associated problems earlier in this chapter). The resulting sleep deprivation can cause irritability and an inability to concentrate, disturbing home and school activities. When this happens, providers should be careful not to mislabel a child with attention-deficit/hyperactivity disorder or a learning disability. In turn, daytime sleepiness may be attributed to the sedative effects of some antihistamines rather than a lack of sleep. The clinician must be alert for these more subtle signs of allergies, be certain that the child's treatment plan is appropriately aggressive, and be sure the plan is well understood by the child and family in order to promote adherence. In addition, clinicians must encourage a reasonable bedtime and consistent bedtime ritual.

Toileting

Food allergies with accompanying symptoms of diarrhea can cause additional challenges in the toddler who is toilet training. When this occurs, it is best to caution the parent to wait until the diarrhea subsides before proceeding with toilet training.

Discipline

Caregivers must be reminded that behavioral manifestations may be due to inadequately treated allergies. Itching of the eyes, nose, skin, and ears can be extremely uncomfortable. Children can feel totally miserable but be unable to fully verbalize the symptoms. This is especially true with young children, but can also apply to the older child or adolescent. Sometimes, children just feel bad, get irritable, and cry or act out in some other way. The whole family can be disrupted, and parents may feel compelled to employ stronger disciplining methods. However, if the true underlying cause of the misbehavior is allergies, caregivers should be encouraged to seek help in reevaluating the treatment plan with the provider, and adapt as necessary to achieve better control of allergy symptoms.

Child Care

Child care providers are usually very vigilant about contagious conditions, and it is not unusual for a child with red, teary eyes, a runny nose, cough, or sneezing to be sent home for fear that other children will be exposed to the illness. Parents of children with allergies can be quite frustrated when this happens repeatedly. If the red eyes or runny nose is exclusively allergy related, the clinician can work with the parents to reassure the daycare center that the child poses no threat to the other children. Usually, a statement from the clinician verifying that this is not a contagious condition is sufficient. It may also be helpful to send additional written information to reinforce the facts. There are excellent resources for parents and caregivers that can be used or the clinician can adapt (see Web Resources at the end of this chapter).

One important issue in daycare concerns the child who has a severe food allergy. Daycare providers must be informed of the allergy and provided with whatever additional information they need to fully understand the problem and how it should be handled. Ideally, a food allergy action plan should be in place, as described in the earlier section on anaphylaxis. In cases of severe food allergies, an EpiPen Jr and diphenhydramine hydrochloride (Benadryl) should be kept at the daycare center with explicit instructions. When there are multiple food allergies, a list of offending foods can be posted in both the daycare kitchen and classroom areas, especially if the daycare center employs multiple caregivers. Clear distinctions should be made between food intolerances, mild food allergies, and severe food allergies. Information should be distributed to all parents who may also bring food into the school or daycare setting to avoid accidental exposure to an offending food. Special event and craft foods are particularly problematic. A study of peanut and tree nut reactions in the school setting showed that 79% of the reactions that occurred in the classroom were from food brought in for class projects or celebrations (Munoz-Furlong, 2007).

Schooling

Up to 25% of individuals with allergic rhinitis miss time from school or work. Those who do manage to go to school or work are significantly less productive and less able to learn. These problems are due to the symptoms of the condition, particularly impaired restorative sleep, and also to the sedating effects of some of the medications used to treat allergic rhinitis (Bender, 2005; Fineman, 2002).

The school setting can be a source of many allergens. Common sources of allergic triggers in school include chalk dust, classroom pets, plants, upholstered furniture or pillows, and carpeting. School-age children should be seated as far away from the blackboard as possible if it is the chalk-type board. This will minimize exposure to chalk dust. Other, less obvious, sources of allergens include mold and industrial cleaning agents. If a child's allergies are much worse during school days, with improvement during the weekends or vacations, vigilant parents and clinicians will suspect that the school is the primary site of allergen exposure. For children with specific environmental allergies, school personnel can be instructed to close the windows when grass is being cut or leaves are being raked. Depending on particular school regulations, the school nurse or designated person may be able to administer medications as needed, such as antihistamines, to a child with acute symptoms.

Physical education, recess period activities, and after-school sports programs do not usually cause additional problems for the child with allergies, unless such activities take place outside during the high-pollen season. School personnel may have to alter the child's schedule to avoid being outside on high-pollen days. The family and the school nurse can collaborate to be aware of those days and make appropriate adjustments.

School nurses and teachers should be informed about a child with allergic rhinitis or allergic conjunctivitis. Even with appropriate treatment, the child may sometimes have inflamed eyes or a runny nose. Similar to daycare providers, school personnel will usually take any potential exposure to an infectious condition very seriously, so they must be reassured that the child is not contagious and is getting proper treatment. As in the daycare situation, clinicians and parents must provide the needed documentation to allay any fears of school personnel.

The school-age child who is treated with antihistamines may be drowsy during school, decreasing school performance. Researchers report a statistically significant difference in the learning capacity of schoolchildren with allergic rhinitis (Bender, 2005). Children usually do better if treated with a second-generation antihistamine versus no treatment, but perform worse if given diphenhydramine hydrochloride (a first-generation antihistamine) versus no treatment (Blaiss, 2004). Conversely, the school-age child who is taking a decongestant may be overactive and therefore have trouble focusing on schoolwork. For both of these reasons, providers must be careful to recommend the minimum medication with the least adverse side effects, while achieving optimum symptom control.

Anaphylactic reactions that occur outside the hospital are most commonly related to food allergies (McIntyre et al., 2005; Munoz-Furlong, 2007). Discussion with school administrators and thorough education of the school nurse, teachers, cafeteria workers, and other school personnel are imperative, because school policies are frequently inadequate (McIntyre et al., 2005; Munoz-Furlong, 2007). School nurses can play a key role in the safety and care of children with allergies by ensuring that each child has current information about allergies and treatment on file and that appropriate personnel are fully aware of the plan for care (Powers et al., 2007; Weiss, 2002; Weiss, Munoz-Furlong, Furlong, et al., 2004). An emergency health care plan, ideally the food and allergy action plan as described earlier, should be devised in conjunction with the clinician, parent, and school nurse. This plan includes specifics regarding the child's allergies, typical reactions, early symptoms of potential anaphylaxis, and a plan to administer epinephrine. Emergency epinephrine (EpiPen or EpiPen Jr) should be readily available in the classroom, nurse's office, or school office, and should accompany the child on all field trips and outings. In addition, the plan should include notifying an emergency medical team (EMT) and the parent. Last, the plan should explain typical effects of epinephrine and other care the child requires until the EMT arrives. It is essential that parents and guardians of affected children keep school emergency information up to date, with all phone numbers and other contact information kept current. The school emergency plan should be updated at least yearly. All school personnel who may be in a setting to respond to an anaphylactic emergency should have a copy of the plan. Attaching a photo of the child is useful for rapid identification.

Sexuality

Age-appropriate anticipatory guidance regarding sexuality should be provided for preadolescents and adolescents with allergies, similar to that given to their peers. If there is a known allergy to latex, information about avoidance of latex condoms and diaphragms should be discussed. In this case the child must also be aware of the risk for anaphylaxis, along with a plan of action including epinephrine (see section on associated problems earlier in this chapter).

Transition to Adulthood

The majority of children with allergies will progress to adulthood with some allergy symptoms. For this reason, children and adolescents must be encouraged to move gradually toward independence in their self-management care. As with most chronic conditions, such a transition must start early, with young children learning the basics of their condition and care. By adolescence, the parents can assume a supportive role, while the teenager practices self-care. Parents, however, must remain actively aware of their adolescent's moods, behaviors, and subtle allergies symptoms; with the often-chaotic haze of adolescence, this can be challenging for parents. Attention to alleviating allergy symptoms will often go a long way in improving adolescent mood and function.

Family Concerns

When managing the child with allergies it is important to recognize the strong familial link and the likelihood that several other family members may also have allergies. The provider should inquire about allergies in other family members to ascertain how they are managing their condition and discourage the sharing of medications.

Food allergies require the vigilance of the whole family. Avoiding foods often necessitates change on the part of the entire family. Using nutritionists specializing in food allergies can help the family to maintain a balanced diet while avoiding offending foods. Linking families to resources and support groups is a critical aspect of management. As with any chronic condition, dealing with food allergies is a disruption of normal daily life. The families of children with food allergies must live with constant uncertainties and fear (Mofidi & Sampson, 2008). For this reason, a careful and accurate diagnosis must be made, followed by education and emotional support.

In the case of allergic rhinitis and conjunctivitis, total avoidance is a challenging goal. Television and newspaper weather reports are good sources of daily information regarding the pollen count. In addition, there are websites that routinely report the pollen count for a given region on a daily basis (see Resources). This may be an integral part of the family's regular routine in high-pollen seasons. Altering the home environment by installing air conditioning, removing carpeting, or even getting rid of the family pet may be essential to controlling allergen exposure. Treating allergies, whether or not others in the family share the condition, will always include treating the family as a unit.

Resources

Web Resources

Air Now
AIRNow is a government-backed program. Through AIRNow, Environmental Protection Agency (EPA), National Oceanic and Atmospheric Administration (NOAA), National Park Service (NPS), news media, tribal, state, and local agencies work together to report conditions for ozone and particle pollution.
Website: www.airnow.gov

Allergic-Child
Good materials on "how to read a food label." Also provides links to many other useful sites.
Website: www.allergicchild.com

Allergies and Asthma Network, Mothers of Asthmatics
Excellent site with a wide variety of information from avoidance tips to developing anaphylaxis action plan. Includes information both on asthma and allergies, including food allergies.
Website: www.aanma.org

Allergies, Asthma and Sinus Relief, National Supply, Inc.
This site provides a resource for ordering supplies used to decrease allergens in the home including healthy bedding, HEPA vacuum cleaners, and more. There is also a toll-free number to ask for expert advice on which products would help.
Website: www.natlallergy.com
Phone: (800) 522-1448

American Academy of Allergies, Asthma, and Immunology
Resources for patients and providers. Provides local pollen count and maps with pollen seasons identified.
Website: www.aaaai.org

Anaphylaxis.com
Excellent resource for providers and patient about anaphylaxis and EpiPens from the company that manufactures them. Even includes an animated movie on how to use an EpiPen.
Website: www.anaphylaxis.com

Asthma and Allergies Foundation of America
This site is primarily focused on asthma; however, it also discusses allergies. It provides a link to connect with a local support group and a link to ask an allergist. The site also provides information devised for different age-groups and a map to identify the 100 most challenging places to live with allergies.
Website: www.aafa.org

Food Allergies and Anaphylaxis Network
Provides good information about food allergies and anaphylaxis. Provides information about unlabeled sources of common allergic foods. Provides downloadable tools for a food allergy action plan and excellent information on anaphylaxis. Special section for children and teens. Supported with references and reviewed by a medical advisory board.
Website: www.foodallergy.org

Food Allergies Initiative
A nonprofit organization providing information on eating in restaurants with food allergies and food labeling.
Website: www.foodallergyinitiative.com

Pollen Count
General allergy website with immediate information about local pollen counts, based on zip code.
Website: www.pollen.com

Other Resource

Jones, M.H. (2001). *The Allergies Self-Help Cookbook* New York: Rodale.
Provides excellent information on allergies, nutrition, and methods for preparing foods with atypical ingredients or substitutions.

Summary of Primary Care Needs for the Child with Allergies

HEALTH CARE MAINTENANCE

Growth and Development
- Chronic congestion and restrictions secondary to food allergies may adversely affect intake; offer a wide variety of healthful foods and monitor for impact on growth.
- Prolonged intranasal steroid may affect growth; monitor height.
- Allergy medications and disordered sleep secondary to allergies can impede a child's ability to learn and concentrate. The goal for treatment should be adequate control of symptoms with minimal side effects to enhance school performance.
- Age-appropriate alternatives for outdoor activities may be necessary to promote development during high-pollen days.

Diet
- Solid foods should not be introduced before 4 to 6 months. There is no evidence that delaying introduction beyond this period has a protective effect on the development of atopic conditions. Introduce one food every 3 to 5 days to monitor for adverse reactions to new foods.

- Avoid giving high-risk children citrus fruits and juices, peanuts and peanut butter, eggs, and wheat. After a year of strict avoidance some foods are often successfully tolerated.
- Parents of children with food allergies may need guidance in selecting appropriate substitutions or supplementations to ensure a balanced diet. A referral to a nutritionist may be necessary.
- Poor appetite secondary to congestion and sore throat secondary to postnasal drip may inhibit adequate intake of foods.

Safety
- Children with food allergies who are at high risk for anaphylaxis (past medical history for asthma, young age, eczema) need injectable epinephrine for home and school.
- Most common foods implicated in anaphylaxis include tree nuts, peanuts, and seafood.
- Providers, parents, and children need regular instruction regarding the use of epinephrine. It is safer to give epinephrine than to withhold treatment. The child should always be taken to the emergency department (ED) for follow-up care and evaluations.

Continued

Summary of Primary Care Needs for the Child with Allergies—cont'd

- Emergency plans are an important aspect for the care of children with food allergies attending daycare or school. A medical alert bracelet identifying the allergy and treatment is recommended.

Immunizations

- Routine immunizations are recommended.
- Children with a history of anaphylaxis to eggs or gelatin should be identified before administration of influenza, measles-mumps-rubella (MMR), or varicella vaccines. Immunizations may be given by an allergist.

Screening

- *Vision.* Routine screening. Ocular symptoms or use of ocular medications may require increased evaluation of a child's eyes on physical examination.
- *Hearing.* The child with allergies may require more frequent hearing screens to evaluate for hearing deficit that may be secondary to recurrent otitis media or transient and due to congestion.
- *Dental.* Routine screening recommended. Malocclusion may require orthodontic care.
- *Blood pressure.* Routine screening recommended.
- *Hematocrit.* Routine screening recommended.
- *Urinalysis.* Routine screening recommended.
- *Tuberculosis.* Routine screening recommended

Condition-Specific Screening

- Skin testing for IgE antibodies is usually done in the allergist's office; families must be reminded to discontinue antihistamines 2 to 7 days before testing.
- Administration of double-blind, placebo-controlled food challenges by an allergist is the best method for confirming suspected food allergies; use caution if anaphylaxis is suspected.
- Radioallergosorbent tests (RASTs) can be used when atopic dermatitis, failure to discontinue antihistamines, possible anaphylaxis, or child refusal makes skin testing impossible.

COMMON ILLNESS MANAGEMENT

Differential Diagnosis

- *Asthma.* Cough is a common symptom in both asthma and allergies. Distinguish between cough-variant asthma and cough secondary to postnasal drip to avoid inappropriately medicating.
- *Acute viral rhinitis.* Nasal discharge is purulent and time limited, lasting less than 2 weeks; fever and erythematous nasal mucosa are present.
- *Vasomotor rhinitis.* Nasal obstruction, profuse rhinorrhea, and mucoid or clear nasal discharge are secondary to exposure to nonspecific factors such as exercise, temperature changes, or air pollution and generally appear and depart suddenly.
- *Acute infections, sinusitis, pharyngitis, and conjunctivitis.* Signs of an infectious process include lymphadenopathy, fever, erythema, and purulent discharge in conjunction with a history of a sick contact.
- *Rhinitis medicamentosa.* Severe rebound nasal congestion secondary to overuse of decongestant nasal sprays. Their use should be strongly discouraged.
- *Substance abuse.* When allergy symptoms in an adolescent fail to improve with standard treatment, consider underlying substance abuse. Keys to diagnosis may be perforated nasal septum, erythematous nasal mucosa with a tendency to bleed, and behavioral changes.

- *Dermatitis and other skin manifestation.* Urticaria or hives may manifest secondary to food exposure.
- *Gastrointestinal problems.* Clues to distinguishing between acute gastroenteritis, parasitic infections, and food allergies are characteristics of diarrhea (bloody, mucus, frothy, watery), fever, length of symptoms, associated cramping and vomiting, age of child, past history of signs and symptoms, sick exposure, time of year, and travel history.
- *Other, less common, conditions.* Nasal foreign body, adenoidal hypertrophy, drug interactions, nasal polyps, nasopharyngeal tumors, congenital syphilis, and rhinorrhea of cerebrospinal fluid can all mimic the symptoms of allergies.

DEVELOPMENTAL ISSUES

Sleep Patterns

- Nasal obstruction, itching, and obstructive sleep apnea can disrupt sleep.
- A regular and reasonable bedtime routine is advisable.
- Daytime use of first-generation antihistamines may cause drowsiness.

Toileting

- Diarrhea secondary to food allergies may interfere with toilet training; training should be postponed until diarrhea subsides.

Discipline

- Behavioral manifestations of allergies may provoke unwarranted discipline; good control of allergy symptoms is necessary to avoid this.

Child Care

- Child-care providers may need documentation from the primary care provider of the diagnosis of allergies and not infection to continue attendance at daycare.
- Care providers of children with food allergies must be informed in writing of the child's allergies, typical reaction, signs of anaphylaxis, and plans for emergency action (including administration of epinephrine). Other children's parents must also be aware of a child's allergies to avoid accidental exposure from foods.

Schooling

- Allergic triggers, including chalk dust, classroom pets, plants, upholstered furniture or pillows, and carpeting: Measures should be taken to decrease the presence of these allergens for the child with allergies.
- Alternatives to physical education and school sports may be necessary on days when the pollen count is extremely high.
- School personnel should be informed of typical allergic symptoms so as not to confuse them with infectious condition symptoms. Medications for symptom relief may need to be given in school. Some medications may make the child drowsy.
- Schools must be prepared with an emergency plan for the child with food allergies at risk for anaphylaxis. Self-injectable epinephrine should be available at school and on field trips.

Sexuality

- Allergies to latex may be a concern for the sexually active adolescent; risk should be assessed and information provided.

Summary of Primary Care Needs for the Child with Allergies—cont'd

Transition to Adulthood

- Allergy symptoms may diminish or completely subside as adolescents enter their adult years.
- Children and adolescents should be encouraged to gradually assume responsibility in managing their allergy care as appropriate.

FAMILY CONCERNS

- It is important to recognize that several family members may also have allergies; medication sharing should be discouraged.

- Avoidance of food allergens requires vigilance of the entire family and may require a change in diet for the entire family; a referral to a dietitian may be useful.
- Avoidance of triggers for allergic rhinitis and conjunctivitis may also require changes that will affect the entire family, including installing air conditioning, removing carpeting, and getting rid of the family pet.

REFERENCES

Agertoft, L., & Pedersen, S. (2000). Effect of long-term treatment with inhaled budesonide on adult height in children with asthma. *N Engl J Med, 343,* 1064-1069.

Allison, B.A. (2007). Pediatric food allergy. *Am J Nurse Pract, 11,* 10-19.

Almqvist, C., Li, Q., Britton, W.J., et al. (2007). Early predictors for developing allergic disease and asthma: Examining separate steps in the "allergic march." *Clin Exp Allergy, 37,* 1296-1302.

ARIA. (2007). *ARIA at-a-glance pocket reference.* World Health Organization, GA2LEN, and AllerGen. Available at www.whiar.org/docs/ARIA_Glance_WM.pdf. Retrieved March 22, 2008.

Asher, M.I., Montefort, S., Bjorksten, B., et al. (2006). Worldwide time trends in the prevalence of symptoms of asthma, allergic rhinoconjunctivitis, and eczema in childhood: ISAAC Phases One and Three repeat multicountry cross-sectional surveys. *Lancet, 368,* 733-743.

Bender, B.G. (2005). Cognitive effects of allergic rhinitis and its treatment. *Immunol Allergy Clin North Am, 25,* 301-312.

Bender, B.G., & Leung, D.Y. (2005). Sleep disorders in patients with asthma, atopic dermatitis, and allergic rhinitis. *J Allergy Clin Immunol, 116,* 1200-1201.

Bielory, L. (2004). Complementary and alternative interventions in asthma, allergy, and immunology. *Ann Allergy Asthma Immunol, 93,* S45-S54.

Bielory, L. Wilson, T. & Wagner, R. (2003). Allergic and immunologic eye disease. In D. Leung, H. Sampson, R. Geha, & S.J. Szefler (Eds.), *Pediatric Allergy: Principles and Practice.* St. Louis: Mosby.

Blaiss, M.S. (2004). Allergic rhinitis and impairment issues in schoolchildren: A consensus report. *Curr Med Res Opin, 20,* 1937-1952.

Blazek-O'Neill, B. (2005). Complementary and alternative medicine in allergy, otitis media, and asthma. *Curr Allergy Asthma Rep, 5,* 313-318.

Bock, S.A. (2003). Diagnostic evaluation. *Pediatrics, 111,* 1638-1644.

Bousquet, J., van Cauwenberge, P., Khaled, N., et al. (2006). Pharmacologic and anti-IgE treatment of allergic rhinitis ARIA update. *Allergy, 61,* 1086-1096.

Bousquet, J., van Cauwenberge, P., & Khaltaev, N. (2001). Allergic rhinitis and its impact on asthma. *J Allergy Clin Immunol, 108,* S147-S334.

Bufford, J.D., & Gern, J.E. (2005). The hygiene hypothesis revisited. *Immunol Allergy Clin North Am, 25,* 247-262.

Cartwright, R.C., & Dolen, W.K. (2006). Consultation with the specialist: Who needs allergy testing and how to get it done. *Pediatr Rev, 27,* 140-146.

Centers for Disease Control and Prevention. (n.d.). *2008 immunization schedules.* Available at www.cdc.gov/vaccines/recs/schedules/default.htm. Retrieved May 13, 2008.

Chiu, A.M., & Kelly, K.J. (2005). Anaphylaxis: Drug allergy, insect stings, and latex. *Immunol Allergy Clin North Am, 25,* 389-405.

Chrostowski, D., & Pongracic, J. (2002). Control of chronic nasal symptoms. Directing treatment at the underlying cause. *Postgrad Med, 111,* 77-84, 87.

Committee on Infectious Diseases. (2006). *Red Book: Report of the Committee on Infectious Diseases.* Elk Grove Village, IL: American Academy of Pediatrics.

de Groot, H., Brand, P.L., Fokkens, W.F., et al. (2007). Allergic rhinoconjunctivitis in children. *Br Med J, 335,* 985-988.

de Jong, M.H., Scharp-Van Der Linden, V.T.M., Aalberse, R., et al. (2002). The effect of brief neonatal exposure to cows' milk on atopic symptoms up to age 5. *Arch Dis Child, 86,* 365-369.

deShazo, R.D., & Kemp, S.F. (2007). *Management of allergic rhinitis (rhinosinusitis).* Available at www.UpToDate.com/online. Retrieved April 28, 2008.

de Vries, M.P., van den Bemt, L., Aretz, K., et al. (2007). . House dust mite allergen avoidance and self-management in allergic patients with asthma: Randomised controlled trial. *Br J Gen Pract, 57,* 184-190.

Dowdee, A., & Ossege, J. (2007). Assessment of childhood allergy for the primary care practitioner. *J Am Acad Nurse Pract, 19,* 53-62.

Eggleston, P.A. (2005). Improving indoor environments: Reducing allergen exposures. *J Allergy Clin Immunol, 116,* 122-126.

Eghrari-Sabet, J. (2008). Preparing for anaphylactic reactions in severely allergic children. *School Nurse News, 25,* 14-17.

Ewing, W.M., & Allen, P.J. (2005). The diagnosis and management of cow milk protein intolerance in the primary care setting. *Pediatr Nurs, 31,* 486-493.

Fineman, S.M. (2002). The burden of allergic rhinitis: Beyond dollars and cents. *Ann Allergy Asthma Immunol, 88,* 2-7.

Floistrup, H., Swartz, J., Bergstrom, A., et al. (2006). Allergic disease and sensitization in Steiner school children. *J Allergy Clin Immunol, 117,* 59-66.

Fluticasone furoate (Veramyst) for allergic rhinitis. (2007). *Med Lett,* November 5, 2007, issue 1273.

Friedman, N.J., & Zeiger, R.S. (2005). The role of breast-feeding in the development of allergies and asthma. *J Allergy Clin Immunol, 115,* 1238-1248.

Gentile, D., Shapiro, G., & Skoner, D. (2003). Allergic rhinitis. In D. Leung, H. Sampson, R. Geha, & S.J. Szefler, (Eds.), *Pediatric Allergy: Principles and Practice,* St. Louis: Mosby.

Gern, J.E., Reardon, C.L., Hoffjan, S., et al. (2004). Effects of dog ownership and genotype on immune development and atopy in infancy. *J Allergy Clin Immunol, 113,* 307-314.

Goldsobel, A.B. (2007). Use of complementary and alternative medicine. *Pediatrics, 120*(Suppl), S119-S120.

Gradman, J, Caldwell, M.F., & Wolthers, O.D. (2007). A 2-week, crossover study to investigate the effect of fluticasone furoate nasal spray on short-term growth in children with allergic rhinitis. *Clin Ther, 29,* 1738-1747.

Green, T.D., LaBelle, V.S., Steele, P.H., et al. (2007). Clinical characteristics of peanut-allergic children: Recent changes. *Pediatrics, 120,* 1304-1310.

Greer, F.R., Sicherer, S.H., Burks, A.W., & Committee on Nutrition and Section on Allergy and Immunology. (2008). Effects of early nutritional interventions on the development of atopic disease in infants and children: The role of maternal dietary restriction, breastfeeding, timing of introduction of complementary foods, and hydrolyzed formulas. *Pediatrics, 121,* 183-191.

Hahn, E.L. & Bacharier, L.B. (2005). The atopic march: The pattern of allergic disease development in childhood. *Immunol Allergy Clin North Am, 25,* 231-246.

Hankin, C.S., Cox, L., Lang, D., et al. (2008). Allergy immunotherapy among Medicaid-enrolled children with allergic rhinitis: Patterns of care, resource use, and costs. *J Allergy Clin Immunol, 121,* 227-232.

Heimall, J., & Bielory, L. (2004). Defining complementary and alternative medicine in allergies and asthma: Benefits and risks. *Clin Rev Allergy Immunol, 27,* 93-103.

Helin, T., Haahtela, S., & Haahtela, T. (2002). No effect of oral treatment with an intestinal bacterial strain, *Lactobacillus rhamnosus* (ATCC 53103), on birch-pollen allergy: A placebo-controlled double-blind study. *Allergy, 57,* 243-246.

Heyman, M.B. (2006). Lactose intolerance in infants, children, and adolescents. *Pediatrics, 118,* 1279-1286.

Hodges, B., Clack, G., & Hodges, I.G. (2007). Severe allergy: An audit and service review. *Paediatr Nurs, 19,* 26-31.

Holloway, J., Cakebread, J., & Holgate, S. (2003). The genetics of allergic disease and asthma. In D. Leung, H. Sampson, R. Geha, & S.J. Szefler, (Eds.), *Pediatric Allergy: Principles and Practice,* St. Louis: Mosby.

Huang, S.W. (2007). Follow-up of children with rhinitis and cough associated with milk allergy. *Pediatr Allergy Immunol, 18*, 81-85.

Huebner, M., Kim, D.Y., Ewart, S., et al. (2008). Patterns of GATA3 and IL13 gene polymorphisms associated with childhood rhinitis and atopy in a birth cohort. *J Allergy Clin Immunol, 121*, 408-414.

Huggins, J.L., & Looney, R.J. (2004). Allergen immunotherapy. *Am Fam Physician, 70*, 689-696.

Jackson, P.L. (2002). Peanut allergy: An increasing health risk for children. *Pediatr Nurs, 28*, 496.

Jean, D., & Cyr, C. (2007). Use of complementary and alternative medicine in a general pediatric clinic. *Pediatrics, 120*, e138-e141.

Juniper, E.F., Stahl, E., Doty, R.L., et al. (2005). Clinical outcomes and adverse effect monitoring in allergic rhinitis. *J Allergy Clin Immunol, 115*, S390-S413.

Kalliomaki, M., Salminen, S., Arvilommi, H., et al. (2001). Probiotics in primary prevention of atopic disease: A randomised placebo-controlled trial. *Lancet, 357*, 1076-1079.

Kleinman, R.E., & American Academy of Pediatrics. (2004). *Pediatric Nutrition Handbook*. (5th ed). Elk Grove Village, IL: American Academy of Pediatrics.

Kliegman, R.M., Behrman, R.E., Jenson, H.B., et al. (2007). *Nelson Textbook of Pediatrics*. (18th ed.). Philadelphia: Elsevier Saunders.

Kligler, B., Hanaway, P., & Cohrssen, A. (2007). Probiotics in children. *Pediatr Clin North Am, 54*, 949-967.

Ko, J., Lee, J.I., Munoz-Furlong, A., et al. (2006). Use of complementary and alternative medicine by food-allergic patients. *Ann Allergy Asthma Immunol, 97*, 365-369.

Lack, G. (2001). Pediatric allergic rhinitis and comorbid disorders. *J Allergy Clin Immunol, 108*, S9-S15.

Lai, L., Casale, T.B., & Stokes, J. (2005). Pediatric allergic rhinitis: Treatment. *Immunol Allergy Clin North Am, 25*, 283-299.

Leung, D.Y., & Boguniewicz, M. (2003). Advances in allergic skin diseases. *J Allergy Clin Immunol, 111* (Suppl) S805-S812.

Liu, A., Martinez, F., & Taussig, L. (2003). Natural history of allergic diseases and asthma. In D. Leung, H. Sampson, R. Geha, S.J. Szefler, (Eds.), *Pediatric Allergy: Principles and Practice*, St. Louis: Mosby.

Liu, A.H., & Murphy, J.R. (2003). Hygiene hypothesis: Fact or fiction? *J Allergy Clin Immunol, 111*, 471-478.

Matsui, E. (2008). Immunology for allergic disease. In D. Leung, H. Sampson, R. Geha, S.J. Szefler (Eds.), *Pediatric Allergy: Principles and Practice*. St. Louis: Mosby.

McGeady, S.J. (2004). Immunocompetence and allergy. *Pediatrics, 113*, 1107-1113.

McIntyre, C.L., Sheetz, A.H., Carroll, C.R., et al. (2005). Administration of epinephrine for life-threatening allergic reactions in school settings. *Pediatrics, 116*, 1134-1140.

Merck. (2008). *I. Singulair prescribing information*. Available at www.singulair.com/montelukast_sodium/singulair/hcp/allergies/product_information/pi/index.jsp. Retrieved April 22, 2008.

Mofidi, S.M., & Sampson, H. (2008). Management of food allergy. In D. Leung, H. Sampson, R. Geha, S.J. Szefler (Eds.), *Pediatric Allergy: Principles and Practice*. St. Louis: Mosby.

Moss, M.H. (2005). Immunotherapy: First do no harm. *Immunol Allergy Clin North Am, 25*, 421-439.

Munoz-Furlong, A. (2007). *Food allergy in schools and camps*. Available at www.UpToDate.com/online. Retrieved March 20, 2008.

Murphy, K., Uryniak, T., Simpson, B., et al. (2006). Growth velocity in children with perennial allergic rhinitis treated with budesonide aqueous nasal spray. *Ann Allergy Asthma Immunol, 96*, 723-730.

Naydenov, K., Popov, T., Mustakov, T., et al. (2008, February). The association of pet keeping at home with symptoms in airways, nose and skin among Bulgarian children. *Pediatr Allergy Immunology*. Available at www3.interscience.wiley.com/cgi-bin/fulltext/120122826/PDFSTART. Retrieved November 18, 2008.

Nolte, H.K.K.D.L. (2007). *Overview of skin testing for allergic disease*. Available at www.UpToDate.com/online. Retrieved March 20, 2008.

Nowak-Wegrzyn, A. (2003). Future approaches to food allergy. *Pediatrics, 111*, 1672-1680.

Ono, S.J., & Abelson, M.B. (2005). Allergic conjunctivitis: Update on pathophysiology and prospects for future treatment. *J Allergy Clin Immunol, 115*, 118-122.

Oren, E., Banerji, A., & Camargo, C.A., Jr. (2008). Vitamin D and atopic disorders in an obese population screened for vitamin D deficiency. *J Allergy Clin Immunol, 121*, 533-534.

Ownby, D.R., Johnson, C.C., & Peterson, E.L. (2002). Exposure to dogs and cats in the first year of life and risk of allergic sensitization at 6 to 7 years of age. *J Am Med Assoc, 288*, 963-972.

Passalacqua, G., Compalati, E., Schiappoli, M., et al. (2005). Complementary and alternative medicine for the treatment and diagnosis of asthma and allergic diseases. *Monaldi Arch Chest Dis, 63*, 47-54.

Perkin, M.R., & Strachan, D.P. (2006). Which aspects of the farming lifestyle explain the inverse association with childhood allergy? *J Allergy Clin Immunol, 117*, 1374-1381.

Pickering, L.K., & American Academy of Pediatrics Committee on Infectious Diseases (2006). *Red Book: 2006 Report of the Committee on Infectious Diseases*. (27th ed.). Elk Grove Village, IL: American Academy of Pediatrics.

Platts-Mills, T.A. (2002). Paradoxical effect of domestic animals on asthma and allergic sensitization. *J Am Med Assoc, 288*, 1012-1014.

Pohlabeln, H., Jacobs, S., & Bohmann, J. (2007). Exposure to pets and the risk of allergic symptoms during the first 2 years of life. *J Investig Allergol Clin Immunol, 17*, 302-308.

Powers, J., Bergren, M.D., & Finnegan, L. (2007). Comparison of school food allergy emergency plans to the Food Allergy and Anaphylaxis Network's standard plan. *J Sch Nurs, 23*, 252-258.

Prescott, S.L., & Bjorksten, B. (2007). Probiotics for the prevention or treatment of allergic diseases. *J Allergy Clin Immunol, 120*, 255-262.

Rautava, S., Kalliomaki, M., & Isolauri, E. (2005). New therapeutic strategy for combating the increasing burden of allergic disease: Probiotics—A Nutrition, Allergy, Mucosal Immunology and Intestinal Microbiota (NAMI) Research Group report. *J Allergy Clin Immunol, 116*, 31-37.

Sampson, H.A. (2002). Clinical practice. Peanut allergy. *N Engl J Med, 346*, 1294-1299.

Sampson, H.A. (2003). Anaphylaxis and emergency treatment. *Pediatrics, 111*, 1601-1608.

Savino, F. (2007). Focus on infantile colic. *Acta Paediatr, 96*, 1259-1264.

Schafer, T. (2004). Epidemiology of complementary alternative medicine for asthma and allergy in Europe and Germany. *Ann Allergy Asthma Immunol, 93* (Suppl) S5-S10.

Schoenwetter, W.F. (2000). Allergic rhinitis: Epidemiology and natural history. *Allergy Asthma Proc, 21*, 1-6.

Scurlock, A.M., Lee, L.A., & Burks, A.W. (2005). Food allergy in children. *Immunol Allergy Clin North Am, 25*, 369-388.

Section on Pediatric Pulmonology & Subcommittee on Obstructive Sleep Apnea Syndrome. (2002). Clinical practice guideline: Diagnosis and management of childhood obstructive sleep apnea syndrome. *Pediatrics, 109*, 704-712.

Seth, D., Secord, E., & Kamat, D. (2007). Allergic rhinitis. *Clin Pediatr (Phila), 46*, 401-407.

Sheikh, A., & Hurwitz, B. (2003). House dust mite avoidance measures for perennial allergic rhinitis: A systematic review of efficacy. *Br J Gen Pract, 53*, 318-322.

Singh, A.B., & Kumar, P. (2003). Aeroallergens in clinical practice of allergy in India. An overview. *Ann Agric Environ Med, 10*, 131-136.

Skoner, D.P., Rachelefsky, G.S., Meltzer, E.O., et al. (2000). Detection of growth suppression in children during treatment with intranasal beclomethasone dipropionate. *Pediatrics, 105*, e23.

Skripak, J.M., Matsui, E.C., Mudd, K., et al. (2007). The natural history of IgE-mediated cow's milk allergy. *J Allergy Clin Immunol, 120*, 1172-1177.

Slattery, M.J. (2005). Psychiatric comorbidity associated with atopic disorders in children and adolescents. *Immunol Allergy Clin North Am, 25*, 407-420.

Sorensen, R., & Niolet, P. (2007, August 1). Eating away allergies. *Contemporary Pediatrics*. Available at www.modernmedicine.com/modernmedicine/Features/Eating-away-allergies/ArticleStandard/Article/detail/450928. Retrieved: November 17, 2008.

Spergel, J.M., & Pawlowski, N.A. (2002). Food allergy: Mechanisms, diagnosis, and management in children. *Pediatr Clin North Am, 49*(1), 73-96.

Tarini, B.A., Carroll, A.E., Sox, C.M., et al. (2006). Systematic review of the relationship between early introduction of solid foods to infants and the development of allergic disease. *Arch Pediatr Adolesc Med, 160*, 502-507.

Thomas, M. (2006). Allergic rhinitis: Evidence for impact on asthma. *BMC Pulm Med, 6*(Suppl 1), S4.

Tovey, E.R., & Kemp, A.S. (2005). Allergens and allergy prevention: Where to next? *J Allergy Clin Immunol, 116*, 119-121.

Troye-Blomberg, M. (2002). T-cell reactivity in neonates: Influence of environmental and genetic factors. *Allergy, 57*(2), 69-72.

U.S. Food and Drug Administration & Center for Drug Evaluation and Research. (2008). *Public health advisory nonprescription cough and cold medicine use in children*. Available at www.fda.gov/cder/drug/advisory/cough_cold_2008.htm. Retrieved April 22, 2008.

U.S. Food and Drug Administration Center for Food Safety and Applied Nutrition. (2008). *Questions and answers regarding Food Allergen Labeling and Consumer Protection Act of 2004.* Available at www.cfsan.fda.gov/%7Edms/alrguid4.html. Retrieved April 22, 2008.

Verstraeten, T., Jumaan, A.O., & Mullooly, J.P., et al. (2003). A retrospective cohort study of the association of varicella vaccine failure with asthma, steroid use, age at vaccination, and measles-mumps-rubella vaccination. *Pediatrics, 112,* e98-e103.

von Mutius, E. (2002). Environmental factors influencing the development and progression of pediatric asthma. *J Allergy Clin Immunol, 109* (Suppl) S525-S532.

Walter, S., Khan-Wasti, S., Fletcher, M., et al. (2007). Seasonal allergic rhinitis is associated with a detrimental effect on examination performance in United Kingdom teenagers: Case-control study. *J Allergy Clin Immunol, 120,* 381-387.

Wang, D.Y., Niti, M., Smith, J.D., et al. (2002). Rhinitis: Do diagnostic criteria affect the prevalence and treatment? *Allergy, 57,* 150-154.

Weiss, C., Munoz-Furlong, A., Furlong, T.J., et al. (2004). Impact of food allergies on school nursing practice. *J Sch Nurs, 20,* 268-278.

Weiss, S.T. (2002). Eat dirt: The hygiene hypothesis and allergic diseases. *N Engl J Med, 347,* 930-931.

Westergaard, T., Rostgaard, K., Wohlfahrt, J., et al. (2005). Sibship characteristics and risk of allergic rhinitis and asthma. *Am J Epidemiol, 162,* 125-132.

Williams, H.C. (2005). Clinical practice. Atopic dermatitis. *N Engl J Med, 352,* 2314-2324.

Williams, J.F., & Storck, M. (2007). Inhalant abuse. *Pediatrics, 119,* 1009-1017.

Young, M.C. (2003). General treatment of anaphylaxis. In D.Y. Leung, H.A. Sampson, R.S. Geha, & S.J. Szefler (Eds.), *Pediatric Allergy: Principles and Practice,* St. Louis: Mosby.

Zeiger, R.S. (2003). Food allergen avoidance in the prevention of food allergy in infants and children. *Pediatrics, 111,* 1662-1671.

Ziment, I., & Tashkin, D.P. (2000). Alternative medicine for allergy and asthma. *J Allergy Clin Immunol, 106,* 603-614.

Zutavern, A., Brockow, I., Schaaf, B., et al. (2008). Timing of solid food introduction in relation to eczema, asthma, allergic rhinitis, and food and inhalant sensitization at the age of 6 years: Results from the prospective birth cohort study LISA. *Pediatrics, 121*(1), e44-e52.

11 Asthma

Marijo M. Ratcliffe and Gail M. Kieckhefer

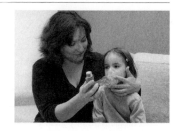

Etiology

Although asthma is difficult to define, the *Guidelines for the Diagnosis and Management of Asthma* describes asthma as follows (Expert Panel Report 3 [EPR-3], 2007, sec. 2):

"Asthma is a chronic inflammatory disorder of the airways in which many cells and cellular elements play a role: in particular mast cells, eosinophils, T lymphocytes, macrophages, neutrophils, and epithelial cells. In susceptible individuals, the inflammation causes recurrent episodes of wheezing, breathlessness, chest tightness and cough particularly at night and/or early morning. These episodes are usually associated with widespread but variable airflow obstruction that is often reversible either spontaneously or with treatment. The inflammation also causes an associated increase in the existing bronchial hyperresponsiveness to a variety of stimuli. Reversibility of airflow limitation may be incomplete in some patients with asthma." (p. 14)

Our current understanding of asthma continues to expand and includes the knowledge, based on research over the past 25 years, that asthma is a heterogeneous disorder with variable expression in different individuals, indicating phenotypic differences and genetic patterns that influence the response to treatments. Different phenotypes of asthma have been described as overlapping symptoms of a complex entity, with categories of common phenotypes depicted as allergic or nonallergic, exercise induced, occupational, aspirin induced, and those based on severity or response to treatment (EPR-3, 2007; Wenzel, 2006). Regardless of the descriptor, asthma symptoms are the result of exposure to an agent, often called a trigger, which leads to a cascade of physiologic changes creating the acute inflammatory episode that occurs on an often already chronically inflamed airway and leads to the usual symptoms of an asthma exacerbation: cough, wheeze, chest tightness, and shortness of breath. The manner in which any individual's asthma first manifests may be related to genetic factors and the environment interacting during development of the immune system (Eder, Ege, & von Mutius, 2006). Airway remodeling, resulting from permanent alterations in airway structure, along with bronchospasm and inflammation, is now included in the description of asthma because not all individuals continue to have reversible responses to treatment (Holgate & Polosa, 2006).

Although current research is aimed toward finding a strategy/treatment to prevent asthma, there is no specific prevention or cure at this time. Day-to-day efforts center on controlling asthma. There is much a health care provider, child, and family can do to reduce the number or minimize the severity of acute exacerbations. Continuing research is dedicated to improving chronic monitoring and treatment to prevent long-term morbidity (EPR-3, 2007; Hoffjan, Nicolae, Ostrovnaya, et al., 2005). An acute asthma episode is initiated by at least one of two types of offending triggers: (1) inflammatory triggers (e.g., allergens, chemical sensitizers, and viral infections); and/or (2) irritants (e.g., particulates in the air, smoke, cold air, exercise, etc.). Inflammatory triggers cause symptoms from an immunoglobulin E (IgE)–dependent release of mediators, increasing the frequency and severity of airway smooth muscle contraction and enhancing airway hyperresponsiveness through inflammatory mechanisms. Noninflammatory triggers and irritants cause a bronchospastic response that narrows the airways and may become more severe if there is already elevated responsiveness or chronic inflammation.

Early, late, and mixed responses can occur as a result of an asthma trigger (Bjermer, 2007). Initial exposure causes a response within 10 to 20 minutes. The allergen/antigen binds to the allergen-specific IgE surface, causing activation of resident airway mast cells and macrophages. Proinflammatory mediators such as histamine and leukotrienes are released. These provoke contraction of the airway's smooth muscles, increased secretion of mucus, and vasodilation. Consequently, microvascular leakage and exudation of plasma into the airway walls cause them to become thickened and edematous with subsequent airway lumen constriction. Additionally, plasma may pass through the epithelial layer to collect in the airway lumen itself, causing further problems in removal of mucus and increasing airflow obstruction. This early response is therapeutically addressed through bronchodilation with short-acting beta agonist (SABA) medications.

Subsequently, occurring up to a few hours later, the inflammatory response predominates. Recruitment, release into circulation, and activation of CD4+ T cells, eosinophils, neutrophils, basophils, prostaglandins, and other macrophages by the initial early phase stimulation mediator release causes further airway wall inflammation and bronchospasm. Treatment for this process involves not only smooth muscle relaxation through SABAs or long-acting beta-2 agonists (LABAs), but also requires acute and long-term control with routine antiinflammatory medication. An ongoing cycle of proinflammatory mediator release leads to further cell activation, recruitment, and, ultimately, a cycle of persistent inflamed airways and bronchial hyperreactivity (Cohn, Elias, & Chupp, 2004).

It appears that both genetic susceptibility and environmental influences determine the expression of asthma in a child (McLeish & Turner, 2007). Asthma is a multifactorial, polygenic condition with not one or two but rather multiple specific gene sites responsible for its pathology (Bierbaum & Heinzmann, 2007; Ober, 2005; Singh, Moore, Gern, et al., 2007). T lymphocytes are known to be one of the many cells types involved in the inflammation of airways characteristic of asthma. Genetic factors (at birth) may determine the direction of T lymphocytic cytokine production tendency toward one of two subtypes, Th-1 cytokine or Th-2 cytokine responses, both present and known to be circulating in an infant's body. Allergic sensitization results from a Th-2 cell response to produce proinflammatory cytokines that stimulate IgE production and tissue eosinophilia with airway hyperreactivity. If the infant's response can be directed toward a stronger balance of Th-1 response, the hope is that atopic asthma will be repressed (Xepapadaki & Papadopoulos, 2007).

In utero and in infancy, the existing physiologic tendency is to favor a Th-2 cytokine profile. Environmental factors early in life may lead to up-regulation of the Th-2 cytokine response because of respiratory infections, allergen exposure, and pollutants. Viral bronchiolitis, use of antibiotics, living in a relatively "clean" versus "dirty" environment, having few if any siblings, and receiving immunizations also seem to promote a stronger Th-2 response (Liu, 2007). Ostensibly, as a result, the child experiences the characteristic response of bronchospasm, inflammation, and production of mucus.

Conversely, attempting to repress the Th-2 response or increase the Th-1 response during this sensitive time of life is another approach being explored. There appears to be a protective influence against the development of asthma if a child has older siblings; attends day care; develops a bacterial infection, measles, or hepatitis A; or acquires an acute gastrointestinal infection (Ball, Castro-Rodriguez, Griffith, et al., 2000; Sabina, Von Mutius, Lau, et al., 2001). The prevention of asthma is the ideal long term strategy, and attempting to identify young children (younger than 2 years of age) at risk for persistent asthma through ascertaining their atopic status has been proposed in order to initiate timely appropriate care and early interventions (Sly, Boner, Björksten et al, 2008). Ongoing research continues to explore attempts to promote Th-1 expression in utero, as well as the use of medications, probiotics, and vaccinations to modify the neonatal tendency toward the Th-2 immune response (EPR-3, 2007; Furrie, 2005).

In the 1990s, bronchoscopy documented the predominant presence of T-helper 2 cell profiles with their corresponding cytokine mediators associated with inflammatory cells, such as eosinophils in the airway and IgE production. Although this is thought to be the main pathologic basis of most asthma, severe persistent asthma may be immunologically different because it has principally neutrophilic airway inflammation and may not respond as expected to traditional treatment (Diamant, Boot, & Virchow, 2007).

If the ongoing inflammatory cycle is not interrupted, a more chronic phase emerges with nonspecific bronchial hyperresponsiveness leading to airway wall remodeling. Remodeling causes submucosal damage with airway smooth muscle hypertrophy, mucous gland enlargement, vascularization, increased collagen and fibronectin in the airway wall, and abnormalities in elastin and collagen deposition in the connective tissue (Bjermer, 2007; Cohn et al., 2004). Although the bronchial epithelial layer may heal, the submucosal layer regenerates abnormally, ultimately causing irreversible reduced pulmonary function and growth, with an accelerated decline in forced expiratory volume in 1 second (FEV_1) beyond that of normal aging (Barbato, Turato, Baraldo, et al., 2003). Early intervention with inhaled corticosteroids (ICSs) to control the inflammation reduces morbidity and daily symptoms but does not change the natural course of asthma, with symptoms recurring when treatment is discontinued (Guilbert, Morgan, Zeiger, et al., 2006; Murray, Woodcock, Langley, et al., 2006).

The pathogenesis of exercise-induced bronchospasm (EIB), also known as exercise-induced asthma, is not yet well described. The most commonly accepted cause is that symptoms of cough, wheeze, and chest tightness with shortness of breath are the result of cooling and drying of airways caused by an increased ventilatory rate with mouth versus nasal breathing. This is hypothesized to lead to vasoconstriction and osmolarity changes in the airways, which activate mast and epithelial cells to release proinflammatory mediators. Rewarming of the airways and vascular bronchial congestion with edema follows the vasoconstriction, and, as a result, airways narrow (Miller, Weiler, Baker, et al., 2005; Weiler, Bonini, Coifman, et al., 2007). An additional inflammatory basis of EIB is postulated since mast cell mediators and inflammatory eicosanoids have been found in airways of exercising subjects 12 to 59 years of age (Hallstrand, Moody, Wurfel, et al., 2005). It may thus be logical to propose treatment with antiinflammatory leukotriene receptor antagonists (LTRAs) and antihistamines instead of bronchodilators in order to address or prevent the inflammation. In the general population, EIB is present in 5% to 20% of people; in those with asthma, up to 90% have EIB. Among elite athletes, 30% to 70% who are involved in cold air sports will have symptoms of EIB (O'Hallaren, 2002; Weiler et al., 2007). All providers must carefully evaluate whether any child with EIB symptoms also has untreated underlying asthma because treatment of underlying disease may help EIB.

Although genetic host factors predispose the individual to developing asthma, environmental factors contribute to the presence of clinically recognized asthma phenotypes, with the interaction of these two factors leading to the expression of asthma (Wenzel, 2006). The prenatal environment (maternal smoking) and infant environment (exposure or lack thereof to various immunologic stimuli such as viruses, endotoxins, and animal dander) are continuing to be investigated for their role in the rising prevalence of asthma in Western cultures during the 1980s and 1990s, as well as for a preventive role (Bierbaum & Heinzmann, 2007; Campo, Kalra, Levin, et al., 2006; Perkin & Strachan, 2006). Prenatal exposure to maternal periodontal microbes leads to an increase in maternal IgG antibodies and is associated with lower asthma prevalence (Arbes, Sever, Vaughn, et al., 2006). The question remains as to whether the overall microbial burden experienced versus any one isolated illness during infancy, or possibly in utero, primes the immunologic system for the child's later phenotypic expression of his or her genetic asthma predisposition.

Although wheeze is common in infancy and childhood, the persistence of wheeze and the development of atopy appear to come from a complex interaction among gender, age, environment, and genetics (EPR-3, 2007). Parental asthma and atopy may differentially influence the inheritance patterns for asthma and atopy in children. However, if both parents have asthma, the child's risk of developing asthma is enhanced, with parental atopy alone being a less important but still significant factor (Bjerg, Hedman, Perzanowski, et al., 2007). The ability to predict which early wheezing child will develop persistent asthma is fraught with inconsistencies, but factors indicating a greater possibility are identification of certain genetic variations, parental asthma, exposure to tobacco smoke, airway hyperresponsiveness, reduced lung function at a young age, and atopy (Bouzigon, Corda, Aschard et al, 2008, Illi, von Mutius, Lau, et al., 2006; Toelle, Xuan, Peat, et al., 2004).

Incidence and Prevalence

The National Center for Health Statistic's annual National Health Interview Survey (NHIS) from 2006 documented 6.8 million children (9%) younger than 18 years of age with asthma, with males' prevalence higher than that of females (11% versus 8%) (Bloom & Cohen, 2007). After puberty, asthma is more prevalent in women (Vonk & Boezen, 2006).

Ethnic and racial prevalence differences were noted, being greater for black (13%) than white (9%) and Hispanic (9%) children. Puerto Rican Hispanics had significantly higher prevalence (14.5%) than Mexican Hispanics (3.9%) (Bloom & Cohen, 2007). Between 2001 and 2003, families below the poverty level had increased asthma prevalence (10.3%) as compared with those at or above poverty (6.4% to 7.9%). Asthma is the third leading cause of hospitalization in children under 15 years and results in an estimated 14 million days of school lost per year. The highest hospitalization rate remains in children 4 years of age and younger (10.0 per 100 children). The number of children who died from asthma tripled between the years 1980 and 1996 at a time when asthma prevalence was growing at 4% per year. Risk factors for asthma-related deaths are listed in Box 11-1. Asthma prevalence has stabilized while both mortality rates and hospitalizations have decreased, which may indicate better treatment, monitoring, or condition management (Moorman, Rudd, Johnson, et al., 2007).

Diagnostic Criteria

The 2007 "Guidelines for the Diagnosis and Management of Asthma" (EPR-3, 2007) recommends the following criteria for the most accurate diagnosis of asthma:

- Medical history and physical examination to determine the presence of airflow obstruction, most often on a recurrent and episodic basis, but can also be daily.
  - Wheezing, heard most often on expiration
  - History of any of the following: cough (particularly worse at night), recurrent wheeze, chest tightness, and shortness of breath
  - Symptoms that occur or worsen with exercise, viral infections, allergens, irritants (smoke, airborne chemicals, odors), weather changes, strong emotions, stress, peri-menstrual period
  - Symptoms that occur frequently or worsen at night, disrupting sleep

- Spirometry in all children 5 years of age and older to determine the reversibility of the airway obstruction, which should be at least partially reversible. After albuterol administration, FEV_1 should increase by 10% to 12% to be considered significant, indicating reversibility. However, it is important to remember that data in very young children are difficult to interpret, do not correlate with adult-validated diagnostic criteria (Galant, Morphew, Amaro, et al., 2007) and must be incorporated along with clinical judgment.
- In infants and children younger than 4 years, asthma diagnosis is particularly difficult because of lack of objective parameters. The need for chronic treatment is recommended in the following instances:
  - Four or more episodes of wheezing in the past 12 months that lasted longer than 1 day and affected sleep *and* infant/child has positive asthma risk profile with one of following:
    - Parental history of asthma, health care provider diagnosis of atopic dermatitis, sensitization to aeroallergens, *or*
    - Two of following: sensitization to foods, 4% or greater blood eosinophilia, wheezing outside of *colds*
  - Require SABA more than 2 days per week for 4 weeks
  - Infant/child has experienced two exacerbations that required oral corticosteroids within 6 months
- Elimination of other possible diagnoses and causes of similar (asthma-like) symptoms (see Other Conditions Causing Cough and Wheeze, later in this chapter).
- Diagnosis of EIB can be attempted with an exercise challenge resulting in subsequent 15% decrease in FEV_1 before and after exercise at 5-minute intervals over 20 to 30 minutes of activity. Cold air challenge is also used to clarify this diagnosis and is generally conducted in a specialty center.

Clinical Manifestations at Time of Diagnosis
Acute Symptoms

Many children with asthma initially have an acute episode of cough, wheezing, or shortness of breath associated with exposure to an allergen or irritant or with an upper respiratory infection (URI). URI symptoms typically include a 2- to 3-day history of rhinorrhea and slight fever. The child may have tachypnea, use of accessory muscles and nasal flaring with difficulty walking and talking at the same time, or need to stop and breathe between words. Children with sternocleidomastoid muscle involvement and supraclavicular indrawing have significant airway obstruction and need rapid assessment of their cardiorespiratory status, including pulse oximetry, and immediate intervention. Preference for an upright body position, use of abdominal muscles to expel air, and alterations in mental status are concerning. Auscultation for adventitious sounds can elicit the following, which represent increasing airway obstruction: prolongation of the expiratory phase, expiratory wheeze, inspiratory and expiratory wheeze, and absence or distancing of breath sounds. This last is an ominous sign indicating little air exchange and possible impending respiratory arrest. The child's chest wall may have an increased anterior-posterior (AP) diameter, which can indicate longstanding pulmonary obstruction or acute disease in an infant. If an AP and lateral chest film is indicated because of rales, concerns for consolidation, or unequal/decreased breath sounds with a significant fever, one may note hyperinflation, as evidenced by flattened diaphragm and increased AP diameter. In severe obstructive disease, the liver may be palpated below the right costal margin. Even with severe asthma, however, clubbing of extremities in a child is rare.

Clinical Manifestations at Time of Diagnosis

ACUTE SYMPTOMS
- Prolongation of expiratory phase
- Wheezing and/or chest tightness/pain and cough
- Tachypnea, accessory muscle use, retractions, nasal flaring
- Agitation or altered mental status
- Evidence of hyperinflation, increased anterior-posterior diameter with or without x-ray findings

CHRONIC SYMPTOMS
- Chronic cough, especially at night
- Prolonged cough with colds and triggers
- Allergic symptoms and/or rhinitis
- With or without enlarged anterior-posterior diameter of chest wall
- Wheeze, though it may only be evident during acute episodes or with activity
- Atopic dermatitis
- Recurrent pneumonia and/or sinusitis
- Shortness of breath on exercise (EIB)
- Seasonal pattern
- Response to beta agonist therapy

Key: *EIB*, exercise-induced bronchospasm.

Chronic Symptoms

When examining a child who is not acutely ill, a different set of chronic findings may be present on history and physical examination. Chronic cough in the absence of a URI or audible wheezing and persistent nocturnal cough and wheeze are the most frequent symptoms. Cough may be the principal manifestation of asthma in very young children. Allergic symptoms are also common (see Chapter 10). Breath sounds are often clear except during an acute exacerbation; a soft wheeze might be heard on expiration or elicited during a forced expiration. It is important to discern if dry skin patches with evidence of eczema are present or if there is a family history of asthma or atopy because these conditions heighten the suspicion of allergies and asthma in all children. Other conditions that prompt consideration of asthma include history of recurrent pneumonia, recurrent croup with wheeze, frequent sinus infections, and posttussive emesis with chronic cough. In older children and teenagers, decreased ability to exercise with complaint of shortness of breath, chest pain or pressure, and a history of cough or wheeze about 10 or 15 minutes after starting or completing exercise is indicative of EIB.

Seasonal Pattern of Symptoms

A seasonal pattern to asthma symptoms is likely when airborne allergens trigger exacerbations, such as during the spring when grasses, weeds, and pollens are endemic and during fall when mold and ragweed can be prevalent outdoors. A return to school usually heralds further environmental exposures leading to exacerbations, especially since it coincides with the fall virus season. It is helpful to have return clinic visits scheduled just before the child's problematic seasons to allow adaptation of treatment regimens and updates of school forms and asthma management plans.

Other Conditions Causing Cough and Wheeze

Because children display a variety of common symptoms with asthma, other conditions must be considered and eliminated before initiating treatment.

A child with a history of premature birth and bronchopulmonary dysplasia resulting in relatively smaller, scarred airways may show subsequent asthma-like symptoms. Children who have a history of cough, wheeze, recurrent pneumonia, or sinusitis and otitis—even with no evidence of malabsorption—need a quantitative pilocarpine ionophoresis (i.e., sweat chloride test) for cystic fibrosis (see Chapter 22). In young children, monophonic wheezing or stridor may indicate foreign body aspiration in the trachea or esophagus. Similar symptoms may also be due to tracheal airway compression from an aberrant vessel, tracheal stenosis, tracheomalacia or bronchomalacia, pertussis, and primary ciliary dyskinesia. Gastroesophageal reflux with ascending aspiration or dysphagia leading to descending aspiration may also cause chronic congestion, coughing, stridor with laryngomalacia, and wheezing (Zoumalan, Maddalozzo, & Holinger, 2007). Environmental tobacco exposure can lead to increased coughing and secretions.

A child or infant should be referred to an asthma specialist if:

- Signs and symptoms are atypical, making diagnosis unclear and additional testing needed
- Comorbid conditions are contributing to poor response to treatment
- Determining the role of allergy in children with persistent asthma, need for immunotherapy, or need for immunomodulators is being considered
- A medium-strength ICS is needed in children younger than 12 years of age

---

Treatment

The current asthma treatment reflects the understanding that airway inflammation is predominant. Although therapy must be individualized to the particular child within a family, it is universally recognized that it is critical (with persistent asthma) to control underlying inflammation with long-term controllers. The hope of preventing

---

Treatment
- Education for shared management
- Treatment appropriate to level of severity
  - Intermittent
  - Mild persistent
  - Moderate persistent
  - Severe persistent
- Written action plan
- Medications/pharmacologic therapy
  - Short-acting beta-2 agonists (i.e., rescue medications)
  - Nonsteroidal antiinflammatory agents
  - Inhaled corticosteroids
  - Long-acting beta-2 agonists
  - Systemic corticosteroids
  - Leukotriene receptor agonists
  - Methylxanthines
- Treatment of exercise-induced bronchospasm
- Environmental manipulation

airway remodeling and preserving the child's pulmonary function by treating the airway hyperreactivity and inflammation through appropriate and timely antiinflammatory treatment drives the current controller treatment regimens (EPR-3, 2007). Bronchoconstriction, as the main cause of the early, acute symptoms, is still treated with a short-acting rescue medication.

As a chronic condition, asthma requires lifelong learning and family participation in shared management with the health care provider. Pharmacologic therapy, environmental control, the family's and the child's education (with accurate measures of asthma assessment), and careful monitoring will all be necessary to control asthma for most children (EPR-3, 2007). For treatment to be effective it will need to be comprehensive and multipronged.

National Heart, Lung, and Blood Institute Guidelines for the Diagnosis and Management of Asthma

The primary goal of treatment is to allow the child to live as normal a life as possible with as close to normal lung function as possible. The child should be able to participate in normal childhood activities, experience exercise tolerance similar to peers, and attend school to grow intellectually and develop socially. The current "Guidelines for the Diagnosis and Management of Asthma" articulates current best evidence-based practices and incorporates expert opinion in order to translate research findings into clinical practice (EPR-3, 2007). This document provides a framework to guide clinical decision making by the primary care provider and serves as the basis for recommendations advocated in this chapter. Because knowledge is rapidly expanding, providers must regularly review updated online reports on best practice; evidence-based management strategies from the National Heart, Lung, and Blood Institute (NHLBI) Information Center at www.nhlbi.nih.gov; and other relevant professional organizations such as the American Academy of Pediatrics (www.aap.org) and National Association of Pediatric Nurse Practitioners (www.napnap.org).

Summary of the Recommendations in the Treatment of Asthma in Children. See Tables 11-1 through 11-5, and Figure 11-1 on p. 175.

- Age-groups are divided into 0 to 4, 5 to 11, and 12 or greater years of age.
- Focus on asthma control in addition to asthma severity.
  - Asthma severity is initially determined *before* initiating therapy and is divided into intermittent, mild persistent, moderate persistent, and severe persistent levels with respect to frequency and timing of symptoms, interference with daily activities, objective parameters from pulmonary function testing, and need for short-acting relief medications. Asthma severity is classified based on the most severe level of symptoms or impairment. If already on asthma therapy, severity is ascertained or inferred by the type of medications needed to maintain control.
  - Once treatment has started, asthma control is evaluated based on the level of *impairment* and *risk* when on a daily treatment regimen.
  - The concept of impairment reflects the functional impact on the family's and child's daily life activities (i.e., sleep, school attendance, physical activity), frequency of use of SABAs, and current pulmonary function. Classifying risk entails judging the occurrence of further exacerbations that will require oral steroids, problematic medication side effects, and the decline

of lung function (low FEV_1 is a predictor of exacerbations) in order to determine treatment needs with greater precision.
- Asthma control requires an emphasis on daily monitoring and considers impairment and risk factors to define asthma that is well controlled, not well controlled, or poorly controlled for all three age-groups. Recommendations for ongoing treatments are linked to these assessments.
- Asthma medication treatment is divided into six steps across all three age-groups starting with lowest level of severity, intermittent asthma, followed by mild persistent, moderate persistent, and concluding with severe persistent asthma. Treatment is defined by medications, including those preferred and those labeled alternatives for long-term chronic management.
- Risk and impairment influence the foundation of assessment of severity and control of asthma for subsequent ongoing treatment.

A reduction in severe exacerbations has been noted when inhaled corticosteroid (ICS) treatment is started within 2 years of disease onset (Vonk & Boezen, 2006). Determining which children need daily treatment for persistent asthma can be difficult in the 0 to 4-year age-group because they may have minimal impairment but a high level of risk (see Diagnostic Criteria, earlier in this chapter, for recommendations for initiating treatment). Closely monitoring children in this age-group once treatment is started is emphasized because of limited outcome data, making a therapeutic trial often necessary. If there is no improvement with daily treatment after 4 to 6 weeks of therapy, other diagnoses should be considered (see Other Conditions Causing Cough and Wheeze and Differential Diagnosis).

Education for Shared Management. When the diagnosis of asthma is made during an acute exacerbation, the family first needs education on immediate care, signs of deterioration that require immediate contact with the provider, how to administer medications, and action and side effects of medications. Once the crisis has passed, the provider plans with the family for ongoing, comprehensive asthma education that includes asthma pathophysiology, monitoring, prevention, environmental assessments, and treatment options. Families have noted that it takes them up to a year to gain a sense of ease with the comprehensive asthma management. The components of an asthma education program have been logically sequenced and are summarized in Box 11-2 (EPR-3, 2007).

BOX 11-2

EPR-3 (2007) Asthma Education Program Components

- Basic facts about asthma
- Roles of medications
- Skills—inhaler/spacer/holding chamber/peak flow meter use
- Self-monitoring and management
- Written asthma management plan
- Agree on treatment goals and plan
- Environmental control measures and exposure to allergens
- When and how to take rescue actions
- When to call health care provider
- Lifelong learning with education at every interaction or point of care

Data from United States Department of Health and Human Services. National Institutes of Health. National Heart, Lung and Blood Institue. (2007) *National Heart, Lung, and Blood Institute National Asthma Education and Prevention Program Expert Panel Report 3: Guidelines for the Diagnosis and Management of Asthma. Full Report 2007.* NIH Publication No. 07-4051. Orginally Printed July 1997. Revised June 2002, August 2007.

TABLE 11-1

Classifying Asthma Severity and Initiating Therapy in Children

Components of Severity	Intermittent Ages 0-4	Intermittent Ages 5-11	Persistent — Mild Ages 0-4	Mild Ages 5-11	Moderate Ages 0-4	Moderate Ages 5-11	Severe Ages 0-4	Severe Ages 5-11
IMPAIRMENT								
Symptoms	≤2 days/wk	≤2 days/wk	>2 days/wk but not daily	>2 days/wk but not daily	Daily	Daily	Throughout the day	Throughout the day
Nighttime awakenings	0	≤2 times/mo	1-2 times/mo	3-4 times/mo	3-4 times/mo	>1 time/wk but not nightly	>1 time/wk	Often 7 times/wk
Short-acting beta-2 agonist use for symptom control	≤2 days/wk	≤2 days/wk	>2 days/wk but not daily	>2 days/wk but not daily	Daily	Daily	Several times/day	Several times/day
Interference with normal activity	None	None	Minor limitation	Minor limitation	Some limitation	Some limitation	Extremely limited	Extremely limited
Lung function FEV$_1$ (predicted) or peak flow (personal best)	N/A	Normal FEV$_1$ between exacerbations >80%	N/A	>80%	N/A	60%-80%	N/A	<60%
FEV$_1$/FVC		>85%		>80%		75%-80%		<75%
RISK								
Exacerbations requiring oral systemic corticosteroids (consider severity and interval since last exacerbation)	0-1/year (see Notes)	0-1/year (see Notes)	≥2 exacerbations in 6 mo requiring oral systemic corticosteroids, ≥4 wheezing episodes/1 yr lasting >1 day AND risk factors for persistent asthma	≥2 times/yr (see Notes) Relative annual risk may be related to FEV$_1$				
Recommended Step for Initiating Therapy	Step 1 (for both age-groups)	Step 1 (for both age-groups)	Step 2 (for both age-groups)	Step 2 (for both age-groups)	Step 3 and consider short course of oral systemic corticosteroids	Step 3: Medium-dose ICS option and consider short course of oral systemic corticosteroids	Step 3 and consider short course of oral systemic corticosteroids	Step 3: Medium-dose ICS option OR Step 4 and consider short course of oral systemic corticosteroids

In 2-6 wk, depending on severity, evaluate level of asthma control that is achieved.

Children 0-4 yr old: If no clear benefit is observed in 4-6 wk, stop treatment and consider alternative diagnoses or adjusting therapy.

Children 5-11 yr old: Adjust therapy accordingly.

From National Heart, Lung, and Blood Institute. (2007). *National Asthma Education and Prevention Program Expert Panel Report 3. Guidelines for the Diagnosis and Management of Asthma*, NIH Publication 08-5846, U.S. Department of Health and Human Services.

Key: *FEV$_1$*, forced expiratory volume in 1 sec; *FVC*, forced vital capacity; *ICS*, inhaled corticosteroid; *ICU*, intensive care unit; *N/A*, not applicable.

Notes

- Level of severity is determined by both impairment and risk. Assess impairment domain by caregiver's recall of previous 2-4 wk. Assign severity to the most severe category in which any feature occurs.
- Frequency and severity of exacerbations may fluctuate over time for children in any severity category. At present, there are inadequate data to correspond frequencies of exacerbations with different levels of asthma severity. In general, more frequent and severe exacerbations (e.g., requiring urgent, unscheduled care, hospitalization, or ICU admission) indicate greater underlying disease severity. For treatment purposes, children with two or more exacerbations described above may be considered the same as children who have persistent asthma, even in the absence of impairment levels consistent with persistent asthma.

TABLE 11-2

Assessing Asthma and Control and Adjusting Therapy in Children

Components of Control	Assessing Asthma Control and Adjusting Therapy in Children					
	Well Controlled		**Not Well Controlled**		**Very Poorly Controlled**	
	Ages 0-4	Ages 5-11	Ages 0-4	Ages 5-11	Ages 0-4	Ages 5-11
IMPAIRMENT						
Symptoms	≤2 days/wk, but not more than once on each day		>2 days/wk or multiple times on ≤2 days/wk		Throughout the day	
Nighttime awakenings	≤1 time/mo		>1 time/mo	≥2 times/mo	>1 time/wk	≥2 times/wk
Interference with normal activity	None		Some limitation		Extremely limited	
Short-acting beta-2 agonist use for symptom control (not prevention of EIB)	≤2 days/wk		>2 days/wk		Several times per day	
Lung function						
FEV$_1$ (predicted) or peak flow personal best	N/A	>80%	N/A	60%-80%	N/A	<60%
FEV$_1$/FVC		>80%		75%-80%		<75%
RISK						
Exacerbations requiring oral systemic corticosteroids	0-1 time/year		2-3 times/year	≥2 times/year	>3 times/year	≥2 times/year
Reduction in lung growth	N/A	Requires long-term follow-up	N/A		N/A	
Treatment-related adverse effects	Medication side effects can vary in intensity from none to very troublesome and worrisome. The level of intensity does not correlate to specific levels of control but should be considered in the overall assessment of risk.					

Recommended Action for Treatment		
(See "Stepwise Approach for Managing Asthma" for treatment steps.) **The stepwise approach is meant to assist, not replace, clinical decision making required to meet the individual child's needs.**	Maintain current step Regular follow-up every 1-6 mo Consider step down if well controlled for at least 3 mo	Step up one step Step up at least one step Before step up: • Review adherence to medication, inhaler technique, and environmental control • If alternative treatment was used, discontinue it and use preferred treatment for that step • Reevaluate the level of asthma control in 2-6 wk to achieve control; every 1-6 mo to maintain control • Children 0-4 yr old: If no clear benefit is observed in 4-6 wk, consider alternative diagnoses or adjusting therapy • Children 5-11 yr old: Adjust therapy accordingly • For side effects, consider alternative treatment options.	Consider short course of oral systemic corticosteroids Step up one or two steps

From National Heart, Lung, and Blood Institute. (2007). *National Asthma Education and Prevention Program Expert Panel Report 3. Guidelines for the Diagnosis and Management of Asthma,* NIH Publication 08-5846, U.S. Department of Health and Human Services.

Key: *EIB,* exercise-induced bronchospasm; *FEV*$_1$, forced expiratory volume in 1 sec; *FVC,* forced vital capacity; *ICU,* intensive care unit; *N/A,* not applicable.

Notes
- The level of control is based on the most severe impairment or risk category. Assess impairment domain by child's or caregiver's recall of previous 24 wk. Symptom assessment for longer periods should reflect a global assessment, such as whether the child's asthma is better or worse since the last visit.
- At present, there are inadequate data to correspond frequencies of exacerbations with different levels of asthma control. In general, more frequent and intense exacerbations (e.g., requiring urgent, unscheduled care, hospitalization, or ICU admission) indicate poorer disease control.

Educating the family and maturing child to become effective partners with the primary care provider in the day-to-day management of asthma remains a primary treatment goal. This requires age-appropriate sharing of responsibilities among family members and the primary care provider. The purpose of shared management education is to help prevent episodes of asthma exacerbation, minimize the severity of episodes that cannot be prevented, enhance the family's ability to understand and implement treatment strategies, improve their capabilities along with their sense of control, and provide healthy responses to life changes that may be necessitated by asthma (Wolf, Guevara, Grum, et al., 2003).

Family education in shared management promotes a sense of teamwork (Bonner, Zimmerman, Evans, et al., 2002; Holgate, Price, & Valovirta, 2006). The foundations should be laid early at diagnosis, with primary care providers drawing families into treatment decisions as their basic knowledge and skills increase. Community organizations recruiting families from a variety of providers have offered formal education programs and developed and extensively tested curricular guides for several programs, which are useful, relatively inexpensive, and easy to implement. Consistent with the EPR-3 (2007), the primary care provider should play a central role with the family in ensuring a comprehensive mix of ongoing

TABLE 11-3

Stepwise Approach for Long-Term Management of Asthma in Children 0 to 4 and 5 to 11 Years of Age

Step up if needed (first check inhaler technique, adherence, environmental control, and comorbid conditions) →

ASSESS CONTROL

← Step down if possible (and asthma is well controlled at least 3 mo)

Intermittent Asthma	Persistent Asthma: Daily Medication (Consult with asthma specialist if Step 3 care or higher is required. Consider consultation at Step 2.)				
Step 1	**Step 2**	**Step 3**	**Step 4**	**Step 5**	**Step 6**
CHILDREN 0-4 YR OF AGE					
Preferred					
SABA PRN	Low-dose ICS	Medium-dose ICS	Medium-dose ICS + LABA *or* montelukast	High-dose ICS + LABA *or* Montelukast	High-dose ICS + LABA *or* montelukast + Oral corticosteroids, ICS
Alternative	Cromolyn or montelukast				

EACH STEP: EDUCATION AND ENVIRONMENTAL CONTROL
Quick-Relief Medication: SABA as needed for symptoms. Intensity of treatment depends on severity of symptoms.
With Viral Respiratory Symptoms: SABA q4-6hr up to 24 hr (longer with physician consultation). Consider short course of oral systemic corticosteroids if exacerbation is severe or child has history of previous severe exacerbations.

Intermittent Asthma	Persistent Asthma: Daily Medication (Consult with asthma specialist if Step 4 care or higher is required. Consider consultation at Step 3.)				
CHILDREN 5-11 YR OF AGE					
Preferred					
SABA PRN	Low-dose ICS	Low-dose ICS + LABA *or* LTRA *or* theophylline	Medium-dose ICS + LABA	High-dose ICS + LABA	High-dose ICS + LABA + Oral corticosteroids
Alternative	Cromolyn, LTRA, nedocromil, or theophylline	Medium-dose ICS	Medium-dose ICS + LTRA *or* theophylline	High-dose ICS + LTRA *or* theophylline	High-dose ICS + LTRA *or* theophylline + Oral corticosteroids

EACH STEP: EDUCATION, ENVIRONMENTAL CONTROL, AND MANAGEMENT OF COMORBIDITIES
Steps 2-4: Consider subcutaneous allergen immunotherapy for children who have persistent, allergic asthma.
Quick-Relief Medication: SABA as needed for symptoms. Intensity of treatment depends on the severity of symptoms: up to three treatments at 20-min intervals as needed. Short course of oral systemic corticosteroids may be needed.
Caution: increasing use of SABA or use >2 days/wk for symptom relief (not prevention of EIB) generally indicates inadequate control and the need to step-up treatment.

From National Heart, Lung, and Blood Institute. (2007). *National Asthma Education and Prevention Program Expert Panel Report 3. Guidelines for the Diagnosis and Management of Asthma*, NIH Publication 08-5846, U.S. Department of Health and Human Services.
Key: *ICS,* inhaled corticosteroid; *LABA,* inhaled long-acting beta-2 agonist; *LTRA,* leukotriene receptor antagonist; *oral corticosteroids,* oral systemic corticosteroids; *SABA,* inhaled short-acting beta-2 agonist.

Notes for children 0-4 yr of age
- The stepwise approach is meant to assist, not replace, the clinical decision making required to meet the individual child's needs.
- If an alternative treatment is used and the response is inadequate, discontinue it and use the preferred treatment before stepping up.
- If clear benefit is not observed within 4-6 wk, and child's/family's medication technique and adherence are satisfactory, consider adjusting therapy or an alternative diagnosis.
- Studies on children 0-4 yr of age are limited. Step 2 preferred therapy is based on Evidence A. All other recommendations are based on expert opinion and extrapolation from studies in older children.
- Clinicians who administer immunotherapy should be prepared and equipped to identify and treat anaphylaxis that may occur.

Notes for children 5-11 yr of age
- The stepwise approach is meant to assist, not replace, the clinical decision making required to meet the individual child's needs.
- If an alternative treatment is used and the response is inadequate, discontinue it and use the preferred treatment before stepping up.
- Theophylline is a less desirable alternative due to the need to monitor serum concentration levels.
- Steps 1 and 2 are based on Evidence A. Step 3 ICS and ICS plus adjunctive therapy are based on Evidence B for efficacy of each treatment and extrapolation from comparator trials in older children and adults—comparator trials are not available for this age-group; Steps 4-6 are based on expert opinion and extrapolation from studies in older children and adults.
- Immunotherapy for Steps 2-4 is based on Evidence B for house-dust mites, animal danders, and pollens: evidence is weak or lacking for molds and cockroaches. Evidence is strongest for immunotherapy with single allergens. The role of allergy in asthma is greater in children than adults.
- Clinicians who administer immunotherapy should be prepared and equipped to identify and treat anaphylaxis that may occur.

TABLE 11-4

Classifying Asthma Severity and Initiating Therapy in Youths 12 Years of Age and Adults: Assessing Severity and Initiating Treatment for Individuals Who Are Not Currently Taking Long-Term Control Medications

Components of Severity	Classification of Asthma Severity ≥12 Yr of Age			
	Intermittent	**Persistent**		
		Mild	Moderate	Severe
IMPAIRMENT				
Symptoms	≤2 days/wk	>2 days/wk but not daily	Daily	Throughout the day
Nighttime awakenings	≤2 times/mo	3-4 times/mo	>1 time/wk but not nightly	Often 7 times/wk
Short-acting beta-2 agonist use for symptom control (not prevention of EIB)	≤2 days/wk	>2 days/wk but not daily, and not more than 1× on any day	Daily	Several times per day
Interference with normal activity	None	Minor limitation	Some limitation	Extremely limited
Lung function (normal = 85% for this age group)	Normal FEV_1 between exacerbations >80% FEV_1 >80% predicted FEV_1/FVC normal	FEV_1 >80% predicted FEV_1/FVC normal	FEV_1 >60%, but <80% predicted FEV_1/FVC reduced 5%	FEV_1 <60% predicted FEV_1/FVC reduced >5%
RISK				
Exacerbations requiring oral systemic corticosteroids	0-1/year (see Notes)	≥2/year (see Notes) ————————————————————————————————→		
	←———————— Consider severity and interval since last exacerbation. ————————→ Frequency and severity may fluctuate over time for patients in any severity category. Relative annual risk of exacerbations may be related to FEV_1.			

Recommended Step for Initiating Therapy			
Step 1	Step 2	Step 3	Step 4 or 5
(See "Stepwise Approach for Managing Asthma" for treatment steps)	In 2-6 wk, evaluate level of asthma control that is achieved and adjust therapy accordingly.		Consider short course of oral systemic corticosteroids.

From National Heart, Lung, and Blood Institute. (2007). *National Asthma Education and Prevention Program Expert Panel Report 3. Guidelines for the Diagnosis and Management of Asthma,* NIH Publication 08-5846, U.S. Department of Health and Human Services.
Key: *EIB,* exercise-induced bronchospasm; *FEV_1,* forced expiratory volume in 1 sec; *FVC,* forced vital capacity; *ICU,* intensive care unit.

Notes
- The stepwise approach is meant to assist, not replace, the clinical decision making required to meet individual patient needs.
- Level of severity is determined by both impairment and risk. Assess impairment domain by patient/caregiver's recall of previous 2-4 wk and spirometry. Assign severity to the most severe category in which any feature occurs.
- At present, there are inadequate data to correspond frequencies of exacerbations with different levels of asthma severity. In general, more frequent and intense exacerbations (e.g., requiring urgent, unscheduled care, hospitalization, or ICU admission) indicate greater underlying disease severity. For treatment purposes, patients who had ≥2 exacerbations requiring oral systemic corticosteroids in the past year may be considered the same as patients who have persistent asthma, even in the absence of impairment levels consistent with persistent asthma.

educational experiences. This requires knowledge of community programs and other available age-appropriate resources, ongoing documentation of what has been taught/learned, and the family's/child's response to the information. Online and comprehensive printed compilations of resources for asthma are available at www.nhlbi.nih.gov/guidelines/asthma/index.htm and www.lungusa.org.

Most asthma education programs contain information on the basic pathophysiology of asthma and control of triggers, knowledge of early warning signs that signal the onset of a problem, how to manage an exacerbation (including when to contact the primary care provider), knowledge of strategies for relaxation and controlled breathing and problem solving, medication names, actions and when to alter their use according to set guidelines, and proper use of equipment. Programs have shown effectiveness in reducing child and family anxiety, increasing asthma management behavior, improving school attendance, and reducing costly emergency department and hospital use (Clark, Brown, Joseph, et al., 2004; Walders, Kercsmar, Schluchter, et al., 2006). Before a child is referred to a program, the primary care provider should review the program to ensure that it is consistent with the provider's treatment philosophy; know whether it is an individualized or group approach; and identify the age, child, and type of family for whom the program has previously worked best. When the provider is knowledgeable

about the shared management program and can reinforce learning during routine health care visits with the family, a true child-parent-provider partnership is enhanced to ultimately improve the child's overall health status.

Education must be viewed in the context of lifelong learning. Changes in the child's and family's capabilities and in treatment modalities necessitate ongoing education. This ensures that the family gains depth in their knowledge and skills and keeps pace with current treatment guidelines. With the overarching goal of independence in mind, the family moves toward the child learning, understanding, and providing greater levels of his or her own care as the child moves through the teen years, unless significant developmental delays exist.

Treatment Appropriate to Level of Severity. Because asthma is a chronic condition with episodic symptoms, asthma management entails treatment based on the needs or severity of the child's underlying airway pathology, seasonal changes, as well as growth and development of the child. It requires the provider to "step up treatment" if asthma symptoms emerge and remain uncontrolled or "step down" treatment after control has been achieved. Step-down therapy is advocated if the child's asthma has been under control for at least 3 months, reducing ICS dose by 25% to 50% at a time to the lowest possible dose while maintaining control (EPR-3, 2007). Specific questions about day/nighttime symptoms versus global perceptions

TABLE 11-5

Assessing Asthma Control and Adjusting Therapy in Youths ≥12 Years of Age and Adults

Components of Control	Classification of Asthma Control (≥12 Years of Age)		
	Well Controlled	**Not Well Controlled**	**Very Poorly Controlled**
IMPAIRMENT			
Symptoms	≤2 days/wk	>2 days/wk	Throughout the day
Nighttime awakenings	≤2 times/mo	1-3 times/week	≥4 times/wk
Interference with normal activity	None	Some limitation	Extremely limited
Short-acting beta-2 agonist use for symptom control (not prevention of EIB)	≤2 days/wk	>2 days/wk	Several times per day
FEV$_1$ or peak flow	>80% predicted/personal best	60%-80% predicted/personal best	<60% predicted/personal best
Validated questionnaires			
ATAQ	0	1-2	3-4
ACQ	≤0.75	≥1.5	N/A
ACT	≥20	16-19	≤15
RISK			
Exacerbations requiring oral systemic corticosteroids	0-1/yr	≥2/yr (see Notes)	
	Consider severity and interval since last exacerbation		
Progressive loss of lung function	Evaluation requires long-term follow-up care		
Treatment-related adverse effects	Medication side effects can vary in intensity from none to very troublesome and worrisome. The level of intensity does not correlate to specific levels of control but should be considered in the overall assessment of risk.		

Recommended Action for Treatment			
(See "Stepwise Approach for Managing Asthma" for treatment steps.)	Maintain current step	Step up one step	Consider short course of oral systemic corticosteroids
	Regular follow-up every 1-6 mo to maintain control	Reevaluate in 2-6 wk	Step up one or two steps
	Consider step down if well controlled for at least 3 mo	For side effects, consider alternative treatment options	Reevaluate in 2 wk
			For side effects, consider alternative treatment options

From National Heart, Lung, and Blood Institute. (2007). *National Asthma Education and Prevention Program Expert Panel Report 3. Guidelines for the diagnosis and management of asthma,* NIH Publication 08-5846, U.S. Department of Health and Human Services.
Key: *EIB,* exercise-induced bronchospasm; *ICU,* intensive care unit.
*ACQ values of 0.76-1.4 are indeterminate regarding well-controlled asthma.

Notes
- The stepwise approach is meant to assist, not replace, the clinical decision making required to meet the individual's needs.
- The level of control is based on the most severe impairment or risk category. Assess impairment domain by individual's recall of previous 2-4 wk and by spirometry or peak flow measures. Symptom assessment for longer periods should reflect a global assessment, such as inquiring whether the patient's asthma is better or worse since the last visit.
- At present, there are inadequate data to correspond frequencies of exacerbations with different levels of asthma control. In general, more frequent and intense exacerbations (e.g., requiring urgent, unscheduled care, hospitalization, or ICU admission) indicate poorer disease control. For treatment purposes, patients who had two or more exacerbations requiring oral systemic corticosteroids in the past year may be considered the same as patients who have not-well-controlled asthma, even in the absence of impairment levels consistent with not-well-controlled asthma.
    ATAQ = Asthma Therapy Assessment Questionnaire
    ACQ = Asthma Control Questionnaire
    ACT = Asthma Control Test
    Minimal Important
    Difference: 1.0 for the ATAQ; 0.5 for the ACQ; not determined for the ACT.

Before step up in therapy
- Review adherence to medication, inhaler technique, environmental control, and comorbid conditions.
- If an alternative treatment option was used in a step, discontinue and use the preferred treatment for that step.

are needed to accurately assess asthma control, asking for both the parent and child's perceptions (Cabana, Slish, Nan, et al., 2005).

Timely treatment of an asthma exacerbation requires recognition of early warning signs in a child and rescue treatment appropriate to the level of severity. Early warning signs may be unique to a particular child (e.g., tickle in the throat, frequent yawning or sighing, fatigue) or fairly common (e.g., a cough especially at night, tightness in the throat with URI symptoms of a runny nose and congestion, and a decreased peak expiratory flow rate [PEFR]).

Written Action Plans. All children with asthma need a written action plan to be implemented in times of exacerbation and to describe chronic management of their disease. Children with even mild asthma may have a severe exacerbation that requires an emergency action plan in addition to a written daily management plan. The emergency action plan is meant to reduce the severity and length of the exacerbation and prevent the need for emergent medical care (EPR-3, 2007). The daily management plan provides a strategy to control underlying inflammation/daily symptoms and prevent exacerbations while allowing the child's caretakers or the child to plan for any contingency. For example, a written plan for everyday management may include morning and evening controller medications per metered-dose inhaler

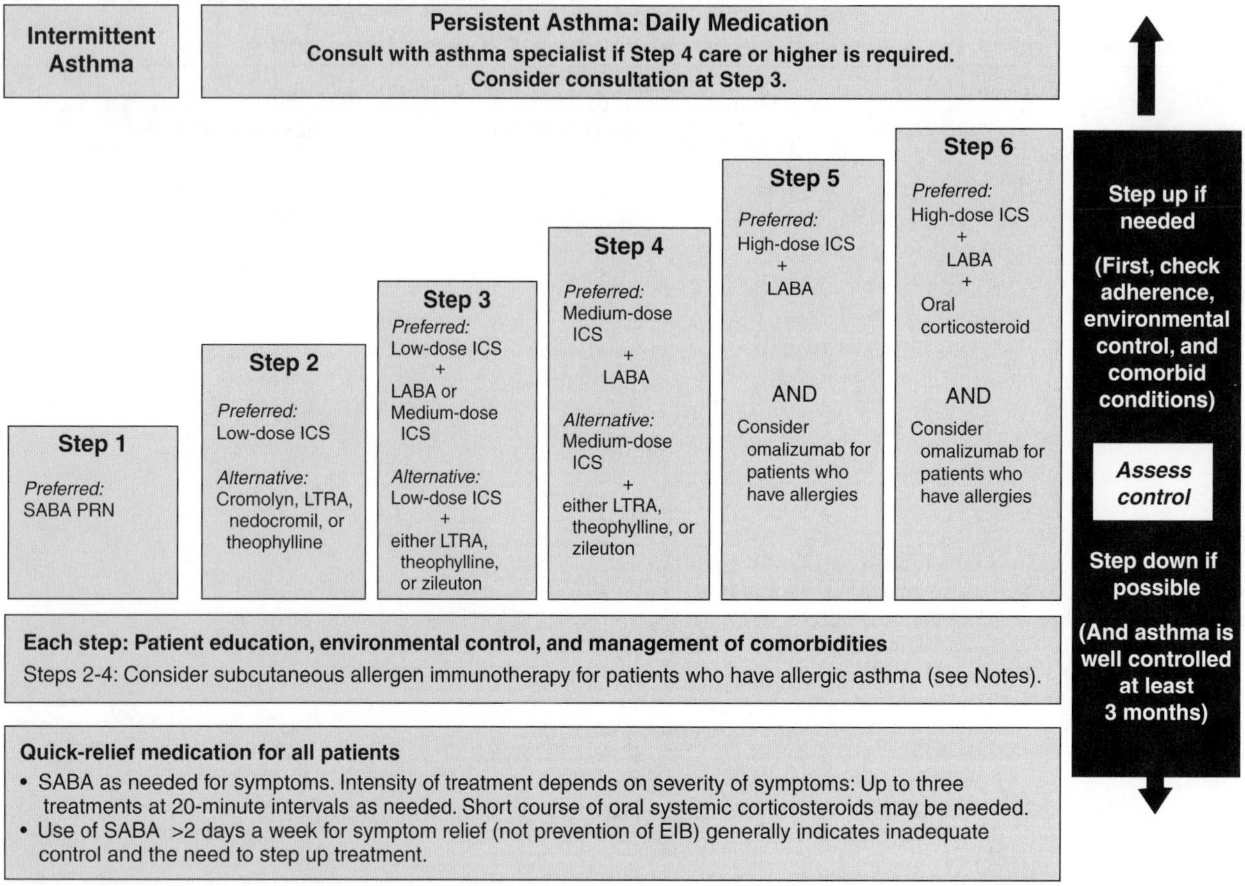

Intermittent Asthma	**Persistent Asthma: Daily Medication** Consult with asthma specialist if Step 4 care or higher is required. Consider consultation at Step 3.

Step 1

Preferred:
SABA PRN

Step 2

Preferred:
Low-dose ICS

Alternative:
Cromolyn, LTRA, nedocromil, or theophylline

Step 3

Preferred:
Low-dose ICS
+
LABA or
Medium-dose ICS

Alternative:
Low-dose ICS
+
either LTRA, theophylline, or zileuton

Step 4

Preferred:
Medium-dose ICS
+
LABA

Alternative:
Medium-dose ICS
+
either LTRA, theophylline, or zileuton

Step 5

Preferred:
High-dose ICS
+
LABA

AND

Consider omalizumab for patients who have allergies

Step 6

Preferred:
High-dose ICS
+
LABA
+
Oral corticosteroid

AND

Consider omalizumab for patients who have allergies

Step up if needed

(First, check adherence, environmental control, and comorbid conditions)

Assess control

Step down if possible

(And asthma is well controlled at least 3 months)

Each step: Patient education, environmental control, and management of comorbidities

Steps 2-4: Consider subcutaneous allergen immunotherapy for patients who have allergic asthma (see Notes).

Quick-relief medication for all patients

- SABA as needed for symptoms. Intensity of treatment depends on severity of symptoms: Up to three treatments at 20-minute intervals as needed. Short course of oral systemic corticosteroids may be needed.
- Use of SABA >2 days a week for symptom relief (not prevention of EIB) generally indicates inadequate control and the need to step up treatment.

Key: Alphabetical order is used when more than one treatment option is listed within either preferred or alternative therapy. *ICS*, inhaled corticosteroid; *LABA*, long-acting inhaled beta-2 agonist; *LTRA*, leukotriene receptor antagonist; *SABA*, inhaled short-acting beta-2 agonist.

Notes
- The stepwise approach is meant to assist—not replace—the clinical decision making required to meet individual patient needs.
- If alternative treatment is used and response is inadequate, discontinue it and use the preferred treatment before stepping up.
- Zileuton is a less desirable alternative due to limited studies as adjunctive therapy and the need to monitor liver function. Theophylline requires monitoring of serum concentration levels.
- In Step 6, before oral corticosteroids are introduced, a trial of high-dose ICS + LABA + either LTRA, theophylline, or zileuton may be considered, although this approach has not been studied in clinical trials.
- Steps 1, 2, and 3 preferred therapies are based on Evidence A; Step 3 alternative therapy is based on Evidence A for LTRA, Evidence B for theophylline, and Evidence D for zileuton. Step 4 preferred therapy is based on Evidence B, and alternative therapy is based on Evidence B for LTRA and theophylline and Evidence D for zileuton. Step 5 preferred therapy is based on Evidence B. Step 6 preferred therapy is based on EPR-2, 1997 and Evidence B for omalizumab.
- Immunotherapy for Steps 2-4 is based on Evidence B for house-dust mites, animal danders, and pollens; evidence is weak or lacking for molds and cockroaches. Evidence is strongest for immunotherapy with single allergens. The role of allergy in asthma is greater in children than in adults.
- Clinicians who administer immunotherapy or omalizumab should be prepared and equipped to identify and treat anaphylaxis that may occur.

FIGURE 11-1 Stepwise approach for managing asthma in youths 12 years of age and older and in adults. From National Heart, Lung, and Blood Institute. (2007). *National Asthma Education and Prevention Program Expert Panel Report 3. Guidelines for the diagnosis and management of asthma*, NIH Publication 08-5846, U.S. Department of Health and Human Services.

(MDI) with spacer. An action plan to implement during exacerbation might additionally include the following: (1) begin or increase rescue SABA medication up to every 4 hours at home; (2) start oral steroid "burst" at prescribed dose if symptoms are not improved or are getting worse after taking SABA; and (3) notify primary care provider within 24 hours if starting oral steroids. All of the child's caregivers, including schools, day care centers, babysitters, relatives, and so on, should have a copy of the asthma management plan and have it reviewed with a family member. Symptom-based action plans have resulted in less need for acute care visits (Bhogal, Zemek, & Ducharme, 2006). It is advantageous for an action plan to contain both symptoms and peak flow values to give families the maximum information.

If symptoms do not respond to home management, the child needs further evaluation and treatment in a primary care provider's office, if appropriate monitoring and treatment equipment are available, or in

BOX 11-3
Medications

QUICK-RELIEF MEDICATIONS
- *Short-acting beta agonists*: Therapy of choice for relief of acute symptoms and prevention of EIB
- *Anticholinergics*: Ipratropium bromide may provide some additive benefit to inhaled beta-2 agonists in severe exacerbations; may be an alternative bronchodilator for children who do not achieve optimal benefit from inhaled beta-2 agonists alone
- *Systemic corticosteroids*: Used for moderate-to-severe exacerbations to speed recovery and prevent hospitalization

Key: EIB, exercise-induced bronchospasm.

an emergency department or hospital setting. These settings offer the ability to monitor the child's breath sounds and air movement, work of breathing, oxygenation, and blood gases; administer oxygen as needed; perform spirometry; continuously monitor cardiac and respiratory status; and give medications frequently in a controlled environment.

Pharmacologic Therapy

Delineated treatment modalities for management of all the severity levels of asthma are available to facilitate decision making in any setting (see Tables 11-1 through 11-5 and Figure 11-1). These guideline tables include use of validated self-assessment tools that are not discussed in this chapter because of space limitations. Several types of medications are used in treatment. For quick relief, inhaled "rescue" medications or SABAs are used. In emergency department settings (Box 11-3), anticholinergics and systemic corticosteroids may be added. A wider array of long-term controller or maintenance medications includes inhaled or systemic corticosteroids, sometimes combined with LABAs, cromolyn sodium, nedocromil, and LTRAs. Table 11-6 provides a comparative listing of inhaled corticosteroids' strengths.

Quick Relief or "Rescue" Medications. For most children the first medication chosen for symptomatic treatment of an acute exacerbation is a quick-acting SABA, such as albuterol, which inhibits the early bronchospastic response. All beta agonists can cause tachycardia and may cause tremor of the hands; some parents of young children also note hyperactivity, irritability, and sleeplessness. An isomer of albuterol, levalbuterol (Xopenex), may have fewer side effects and is available for use for relief of bronchospasm in place of albuterol (Micromedex, 2008).

Using an air compressor with an updraft nebulizer and aerosol mask to deliver a beta-adrenergic medication is common; however, children and even infants can be treated with a metered-dose inhaler (MDI, or puffer) if a spacer with an attached facemask is used, with equally effective results (Cates, Bestall, & Adams, 2006). A spacer is a chamber that attaches to the MDI, allowing the medicine to be puffed into the chamber. The child then inhales from the spacer to receive the medication. This avoids having to coordinate compressing the MDI while slowly inhaling, an almost impossible feat for most young children. If a spacer is not used, much of the medication will impact on and deposit in the mouth or throat rather than the airways, leading to more side effects and less therapeutic effect. Dry powder inhalers (DPIs), which involve inhaling a powder form of the medication, do not require a coordinated effort like an MDI, are used to deliver a variety of medications, but usually require the inspiratory effort of a child 5 or 6 years of age or older. Delivery devices are being altered

to reduce environmental chlorofluorocarbons (CFCs) with hydrofluoroalkane (HFA) because they are safer for the environment and more ozone-friendly. Because of the wide variety of delivery devices available, each with unique steps to activate, maneuvers to inhale, and cleaning requirements, the provider must know and diligently review the directions for proper use and have office staff consistently teach and review proper techniques with the child and family.

Nebulized treatments with a facemask offer several advantages, including the following: (1) direct deposition of aerosolized medication in the respiratory tract; (2) fewer side effects than oral medication; (3) better delivery than an MDI when tidal volume is reduced during an acute episode; and (4) ability to mix beta-adrenergic medications with other medications (e.g., cromolyn sodium or ipratropium sulfate).

Oral syrups containing beta-adrenergic agents are also available, but onset of action takes 30 minutes, causes greater hyperactivity in many children, and is not recommended as preferred treatment. For convenience, some older children favor a pill rather than use an MDI, and therapeutic adherence may be improved if given this choice. However, any oral preparation will have a longer onset compared with an inhaled medication, which is less than ideal in a "rescue" medication.

Nonsteroidal Antiinflammatory Agents. Antiinflammatory agents are the first-choice daily preventive medication for children with persistent asthma because they block the late phase response to an allergen, reduce airway hyperreactivity, and inhibit inflammatory mediator migration and activation of inflammatory cells. Nedocromil and cromolyn sodium, nonsteroidal antiinflammatory mast cell stabilizers, are currently recommended as alternatives to ICSs for mild persistent asthma and as an alternative to a bronchodilator before exercise. They require three or four doses daily for effectiveness (EPR-3, 2007).

Inhaled Corticosteroids. Corticosteroids inhibit the late phase asthmatic response and are used to treat the inflammation and edema associated with asthma, thereby earning the title of "controller" or "maintenance" medications. Thus preferred treatment of children with more than intermittent asthma includes the long-term use of ICSs at the lowest effective dose. Even young children may be able to use an ICS via MDI with a spacer and mask or nebulizer and reduce their need for systemic treatment. Children using a spacer with an ICS should rinse their mouth and spit and then wipe the facial area that was covered by the mask after use to prevent development of thrush. Pulmicort Respules (a budesonide suspension) is available in nebulized form for treatment of children older than 1 year of age. The nebulized medication should be administered via mask, keeping the mist away from the eyes, to prevent a theoretic but potential complication of cataract formation.

Triamcinolone acetate (Azmacort) and beclomethasone (Beclovent, Vanceril, Qvar HFA) have long been used as ICSs. Mometasone (Asmanex) DPI is now available for daily controller medication (Berger, Milgrom, Chervinsky, et al., 2006), as is budesonide (Pulmicort), available in DPI and nebulized forms, and fluticasone (Flovent) in DPI and MDI formulations. All reduce resident inflammatory cells in the airways, migration and activation of circulating inflammatory cells, and obstruction. All are available in different concentrations and dosages.

Long-Acting Beta-2 Agonists. For the child with moderate or severe persistent asthma whose symptoms remain uncontrolled with an ICS, an LABA such as salmeterol (Serevent) or formoterol (Foradil) should be added to the regimen and its effects evaluated. In children 4 years of age or younger, the addition of LABA should be considered only after a medium-dose ICS has been attempted (treatment step 4). Current recommendations include considering a trial

TABLE 11-6

Estimated Comparative Daily Dosages for Inhaled Corticosteroids (EPR-3, 2007)

Drug	Low Daily Dose			Medium Daily Dose			High Daily Dose		
	Child 0-4 Years of Age	Child 5-11 Years of Age	Child ≥ 12 Years of Age and Adult	Child 0-4 Years of Age	Child 5-11 Years of Age	Child ≥ 12 Years of Age and Adult	Child 0-4 Years of Age	Child 5-11 Years of Age	Child ≥ 12 Years of Age and Adult
Beclomethasone HFA 40 or 80 mcg/puff	N/A	80-160 mcg	80-240 mcg	N/A	>160-320 mcg	>240-480 mcg	N/A	>320 mcg	>480 mcg
Budesonide DPI 90, 80, or 200 mcg/inhalation	N/A	180-400 mcg	180-600 mcg	N/A	>400-800 mcg	>600-1200 mcg	N/A	>800 mcg	>1200 mcg
Budesonide inhaled, Inhalation suspension for mobilization	0.25-0.5 mg	0.5 mg	N/A	>0.5-1.0 mg	1.0 mg	N/A	>1.0 mg	2.0 mg	N/A
Flunisolide 250 mcg/puff	N/A	500-750 mcg	500-1000 mcg	N/A	1000-1250 mcg	>1000-2000 mcg	N/A	>1250 mcg	>2000 mcg
Flunisolide HFA 80 mcg/puff	N/A	160 mcg	320 mcg	N/A	320 mcg	>320-640 mcg	N/A	≥ 640 mcg	>640 mcg
Fluticasone HFA/MDI 44, 110, or 220 mcg/puff	176 mcg	88-176 mcg	88-264 mcg	>176-352 mcg	>176-352 mcg	>264-440 mcg	>352 mcg	>352 mcg	>440 mcg
Fluticasone DPI: 50, 100, or 250 mcg/inhalation	N/A	100-200 mcg	100-300 mcg	N/A	>200-400 mcg	>300-500 mcg	N/A	>400 mcg	>500 mcg
Mometasone DPI 200 mcg/inhalation	N/A	N/A	200 mcg	N/A	N/A	400 mcg	N/A	N/A	>400 mcg
Triamcinolone acetonide 75 mcg/puff	N/A	300-600 mcg	300-750 mcg	N/A	>600-900 mcg	>750-1500 mcg	N/A	>900 mcg	>1500 mcg

From National Heart, Lung, and Blood Institute. (2007). *National Asthma Education and Prevention Program Expert Panel Report 3. Guidelines for the diagnosis and management of asthma,* NIH Publication 08-5846, U.S. Department of Health and Human Services.

Key: *DPI,* dry powder inhaler; *HFA,* hydrofluoroalkane; *MDI,* metered-dose inhaler; *N/A,* not available (either not approved, no data available, or safety and efficacy not established for this age-group).

Therapeutic issues

- The most important determinant of appropriate dosing is the clinician's judgment of the individual's response to therapy. The clinician must monitor the individual's response on several clinical parameters and adjust the dose accordingly. Once control of asthma is achieved, the dose should be carefully titrated to the minimum dose required to maintain control.
- Preparations are not interchangeable on a mcg or per puff basis. This table presents estimated comparable daily doses. See EPR-3 (2007) for full discussion.
- Some doses may be outside package labeling, especially in the high-dose range. Budesonide nebulizer suspension is the only inhaled corticosteroid (ICS) with FDA-approved labeling for children <4 yr of age.
- For children <4 yr of age: The safety and efficacy of ICSs in children <1 yr has not been established. Children <4 yr of age generally require delivery of ICS (budesonide and fluticasone HFA) through a facemask that should fit snugly over nose and mouth and avoid nebulizing in the eyes. Wash face after each treatment to prevent local corticosteroid side effects. For budesonide, the dose may be administered once to three times daily. Budesonide suspension is compatible with albuterol, ipratropium, and levalbuterol nebulizer solutions in the same nebulizer. Use only jet nebulizers, because ultrasonic nebulizers are ineffective for suspensions. For fluticasone HFA, the dose should be divided two times daily; the low dose for children <4 yr of age is higher than for children 5-11 yr of age because of lower dose delivered with facemask and data on efficacy in young children.

Potential adverse effects of inhaled corticosteroids

- Cough, dysphonia, oral thrush (candidiasis).
- Spacer of valved holding chamber with non–breath-actuated MDIs and mouthwashing and spitting after inhalation decrease local side effects.
- A number of the ICSs, including fluticasone, budesonide, and mometasone, are metabolized in the gastrointestinal tract and liver by CYP 3A4 isoenzymes. Potent inhibitors of CYP 3A4, such as ritonavir and ketoconazole, have the potential for increasing systematic concentrations of these ICSs by increasing oral availability and decreasing systemic clearance. Some cases of clinically significant Cushing syndrome and secondary adrenal insufficiency have been reported.
- In high doses, systemic effects may occur, although studies are not conclusive, and clinical significance of these effects has not been established (e.g., adrenal suppression, osteoporosis, skin thinning, and easy bruising). In low-to-medium doses, suppression of growth velocity has been observed in children, but this effect may be transient, and the clinical significance has not been established.

of the addition of an LABA to any child 5 years of age or older with moderate or severe persistent asthma who are already taking a low- or medium-dose ICS (treatment step 3 and greater) (see Table 11-3). However, a new recommendation regarding children 12 years of age and older is to also consider increasing from a low- to medium-dose ICS before the addition of LABA, because of safety concerns that led to a black box warning on all LABA preparations (Israel, Chinchilli, Ford, et al., 2004; Nelson, Weiss, Bleecker, et al., 2006).

A controversial treatment of asthma exacerbations is the use of combinations of ICS and LABA "as needed" during exacerbations, in addition to maintenance controller therapy. In a randomized, controlled, double-blind study, budesonide/formoterol combination (Symbicort) as a reliever therapy was compared with either an SABA or formoterol alone (Rabe, Atienza, Magyar, et al., 2006). Compared with the other two therapies, results indicate less frequent exacerbations and a longer period of time to a severe exacerbation with "as-needed" Symbicort administered when first symptomatic. An adjunct expectation is that combinations may obviate the need for oral corticosteroids. Further research is needed in this area before a recommendation is made.

Leukotriene Receptor Antagonists. Leukotriene receptor antagonists, also referred to as leukotriene modifiers by some, are another class of medications that intervene in the inflammatory cascade, predominantly through antieosinophilic action (Diamant et al., 2007). Montelukast decreases arachidonic acid metabolites that lead to potent inflammatory mediator release of cysteinyl leukotrienes, which activate neutrophils and eosinophils, cause microvascular leakage, produce mucus, and constrict airways. Montelukast (Singular), an LTRA, is approved for children older than 1 year of age and zafirlukast (Accolate) is approved for ages 7 and older. For children older than 12 years of age, zileuton (Zyflo) is available but requires liver function monitoring. Leukotriene receptor antagonists have been investigated as a possible first-line treatment in place of ICSs in children younger than 5 years of age and found to produce a modest improvement in lung function. In children younger than 2 years of age, asthma outcomes were improved on LTRA compared with placebo (Bisgaard, Zielen, Garcia-Garcia, et al., 2005; Ostrom, Decotiis, Lincourt, et al., 2005; Zeiger, Szefler, Phillips, et al., 2006). Leukotriene receptor antagonists are suggested as an adjunct to ICSs in children 12 years old and younger, but in older children, a trial of an LABA with an ICS is preferred first. When compared with low-dose ICSs, several different randomized controlled trials have noted that children receiving LTRAs were more likely to experience an exacerbation requiring systemic steroids (Ducharme, 2004). Secondary outcomes, including nocturnal awakenings, rescue medication use, quality of life, and improvement of FEV_1 and PEFR, were also more favorable for those taking an ICS compared with an LTRA alone. Leukotriene receptor antagonists were noted to be efficacious with exercise-induced asthma, although the first recommendation for EIB is still a beta-2 agonist.

Systemic Corticosteroids. Children who continue to have frequent symptoms or exacerbations even with combination therapy may require systemic corticosteroid treatment in either a short burst (3 to 10 days) or a longer period (EPR-3, 2007). In children who require prolonged or repeated short treatments, reevaluation is needed every 2 to 3 months. Evaluation includes review and documentation of treatment effects, appropriate use of medications and delivery devices, review of any comorbidities, environmental evaluation for new triggers/allergies, and family understanding of the treatment regimen. At each visit a thorough interval history is necessary to determine any adverse effects from corticosteroid therapy.

To prevent problems with growth suppression or, more seriously, suppression of the hypothalamic-pituitary-adrenal (HPA) axis, the total dose of oral, inhaled, and topical corticosteroids should be adjusted to the cumulative lowest level necessary to maintain symptom control. Awareness of potential HPA suppressive affects may include severe chickenpox, risk to bone density, insulin intolerance, systemic hypertension, and cataract development and ocular hypertension. Appropriate and timely assessment of adrenal function, depending on steroid exposure, is controversial (Zollner, 2007), but if concerned, consultation with an endocrinologist is advised. Table 11-6 provides comparative daily dosages for ICS to ensure appropriate selection (EPR-3, 2007). After reviewing the current evidence, national asthma guidelines continue to emphasize that the effectiveness of ICS in treatment of asthma, when used at appropriate doses, outweighs concerns regarding growth (EPR-3, 2007).

Concerns regarding the use of ICSs are not confined to growth. Effects on bone metabolism and adrenal function are being scrutinized. The appropriate dose, method of delivery, and type of ICS appears to influence whether these problems can be avoided. Small doses of ICS bring no significant risk of side effects. When larger doses are required, use of a spacer prevents extraneous deposition of drug on the oral mucosa, limiting steroid systemic circulation that is not therapeutic for asthma. Use of medications that allow first-pass inactivation in the liver, such as fluticasone and budesonide, may also help prevent HPA axis suppression (Allen, 2006). Fracture risk with oral corticosteroid use has been addressed in studies evaluating fracture outcomes in adults who had childhood asthma (Melton, Patel, Achenbach, et al., 2005) and children 4 to 17 years of age (Melton III, Patel, Achenbach, et al., 2005). Both studies reported concerns regarding skeletal development, identified lack of normative data in bone quality, and recommended further research on biomechanical bone competence over time, noting that "fractures do not represent a substantial problem for most children with asthma" (Melton III et al., 2005).

The Childhood Asthma Management Program (Kelly, Van Natta, Covar, et al., 2008) follow-up study evaluated the interaction of oral corticosteroid (OCS) bursts in addition to ICS, as recommended in current asthma guidelines, on bone mineral density in the lumbar spine. Over the 4.5 years that the children were progressing through puberty, a significant dose-dependent response was noted in boys receiving five or more OCS bursts while taking daily ICSs, resulting in a greater risk for osteopenia and reduced bone mineral accretion. This effect was not found in girls. Long-term ICS treatment without OCS bursts was deemed safer, revealed a lesser effect in boys, and, once again, no effect was noted in girls. Although fractures in these children remained minimal, it emphasized the need for controlling underlying inflammation with the lowest possible dose of ICS to prevent the (frequent) need for OCS bursts.

Anticholinergics. Anticholinergic agents (e.g., ipratropium bromide [Atrovent]) block cholinergic reflex bronchoconstriction by antagonizing the effect of acetylcholine at muscarinic receptors, and may be most useful in children with bronchitic symptoms of increased mucous secretion when used with beta agonists or antiinflammatory agents. These agents, however, are not particularly helpful against allergic challenges and do not block late phase response or inhibit mediators from mast cells. Ipratropium bromide is the only anticholinergic drug currently approved for treatment of airway disease (EPR-3, 2007). It is also used concomitantly with an SABA in moderate to severe exacerbations as an additive bronchodilator, usually in the emergency department. It may be of benefit to children who respond poorly or adversely to SABAs. Delivery of ipratropium is by MDI or nebulizer. It can be mixed with albuterol and cromolyn sodium for the convenience of providing three medications with one aerosol treatment. Side effects include dry mucous membranes, cutaneous flush, and fever (Micromedex, 2008).

Methylxanthines (Long-Acting Bronchodilators). Some children may benefit from the addition of theophylline if antiinflammatory and beta-adrenergic agents do not control their asthma symptoms. Methylxanthines in combination with beta-adrenergics work synergistically to produce bronchodilation and may improve control of nocturnal asthma symptoms in particular. A high level of provider and family monitoring is necessary. Metabolism and toxicity, with permanent central nervous system side effects, varies among individuals and age-groups. The dose must be individually adjusted by monitoring theophylline levels in the blood, especially when there are signs of toxicity or viral illness, or when the child experiences persistent or recurring asthma episodes on maintenance medications. Sustained-release theophylline is not a preferred treatment for mild persistent asthma with children, and its only role may be as an alternative/adjunct treatment with ICS (EPR-3, 2007).

Immunomodulators. A new group of medications, immunomodulators, is available for consideration as an adjunct to long-term controller therapy in a very specific population of children with severe persistent asthma by pulmonary or allergy specialists. Several agents are included in this group, such as methotrexate, new LTRAs, cyclosporin A, and intravenous immunoglobulin (IVIG). The most commonly used therapy is an anti-IgE humanized monoclonal antibody called Xolair. These medications are adjuncts to therapy used for their steroid-sparing strategy. Omalizumab (Xolair) is considered with children 12 years of age or older requiring step 5- or step 6-level therapy who have allergies and elevated total serum IgE levels with severe persistent asthma. As a recombinant deoxyribonucleic acid (DNA)-derived monoclonal antibody to IgE, it prevents the binding of IgE to receptors on mast cells and basophils, leading to a decrease in release of inflammatory mediators when exposed to allergens. Studies have shown a modest decrease in steroid dose, small improvement in pulmonary function, reduced exacerbations and emergency care requirements, and clinically significant improvement in quality-of-life scores (Buck, Hofer, & McCarthy, 2007; EPR-3, 2007). Xolair is expensive and cost-effectiveness must be considered. Xolair is administered subcutaneously, every 2 to 4 weeks depending on serum IgE level and the child's weight, in a setting that has the ability to observe the child and respond to postinjection anaphylaxis.

Immunotherapy. Allergen immunotherapy should be considered when a specific symptom-producing allergen is identified in the child's environment, one that cannot be eliminated and leads to increasing asthma therapy. Although not always lifelong, reduction in asthma symptoms and medications can be achieved when allergen and therapy are matched (Abramson, Puy, & Weiner, 2003). Success requires adherence with repeat appointments on the part of the child and family. As with Xolair, immunotherapy must be administered in a medical facility that allows observation for and treatment of anaphylaxis.

Food and Drug Administration-Approved Medications. Many of the recommendations for treatment of young children are extrapolated from studies in older children and adults. Currently, in young children, the following long-term control medications are Food and Drug Administration (FDA) approved:

- ICS budesonide nebulizer solution (1 to 8 years of age)
- ICS fluticasone DPI (older than 4 years of age)
- LABA salmeterol in combination with ICS (older than 4 years of age)
- ICS/LABA combination, Symbicort HFA MDI (12 years and older)
- LTRA montelukast, chewable tablets 2 to 6 years, granules 1 year and older

Treatment of Exercise-Induced Bronchospasm. Exercise-induced bronchospasm is a phenotype of asthma. When a child experiences EIB, a short-acting or beta-2 agonist or, occasionally, a nonsteroidal antiinflammatory agent (e.g., cromolyn) can be used to block the symptoms that inhibit the child's continued exercise. When taken to prevent EIB, these agents should be inhaled with a spacer if using MDI formulation, approximately 15 minutes before participation in scheduled exercise. Protection against symptoms of EIB lasts 3 to 4 hours with an SABA such as albuterol (Miller et al., 2005). As reflected in Table 11-3 and Figure 11-1, current recommended pediatric use of LABA is only when paired with ICS and never used as an independent agent for EIB or maintenence asthma therapy. Prescription of an SABA is still required for rescue from acute symptoms (EPR-3, 2007). Although an LTRA may reduce symptoms of EIB in those taking the medication as part of a daily regimen, they are not currently advised as monotherapy for EIB. Wearing a mask or scarf over the mouth if feasible or an extended warm-up session before activity (such as 10 to 15 minutes of fast walking, then slow jogging before running) may reduce EIB symptoms in conjunction with medication.

Environmental Manipulations

Avoidance of common environmental triggers can improve asthma control in children. Any type of environmental smoke is a trigger in children. Tobacco smoke should be avoided along with smoke from pipes, cigars, wood-burning stoves, and campfires. Using motivational interviewing with parents and guiding them to smoking cessation support services when they are ready to quit smoking can be helpful. Health care providers should discuss the damage smoking will do as the child moves into later childhood and throughout adolescence. Helping the youth develop risk-avoidance behaviors to smoking and avoidance of the smoke of peers through positioning is critical.

Dust mites and cockroaches are also common triggers for asthma problems, especially when these are found in the child's sleeping room. Biweekly damp mopping, pillow and mattress covers, and elimination of mold may reduce the number of asthma exacerbations. Outside air pollution, especially high levels of particulate matter, exacerbate asthma. Some families have found it useful to monitor these and pollen levels through the Asthma and Allergy Foundation of America website at www.aafa.org or their local American Lung Association chapter at www.lungusa.org and adapt the child's outdoor activity when levels are high.

Cats, dogs, rodents, and other furry pets can be a trigger for exacerbation in children with allergies. These pets should never be allowed into the child's sleeping room or on furniture where the child will recline. If pets are suspected triggers, allergy testing is indicated, and, if positive, pets should be removed from the home. It may take months for allergens to be eliminated and symptoms to be reduced, which means evaluation of the effects of such removal should be after an extended time period.

Complementary and Alternative Therapies

The use of complementary and alternative medication (CAM) therapy either alone or in concert with allopathic medicine for treatment is increasing, although there are few published studies among families with children, especially minority children. Seventy-nine percent of parents living in one inner city reported use of CAM in treating their child's asthma (Adams, Murdock, & McQuaid, 2007). Those with chronic persistent asthma, poorly controlled symptoms, frequent health care visits, and adverse reactions to bronchodilators, and those on corticosteroids, were most likely to use complementary therapies. Parental beliefs regarding CAM, asthma outcomes, and a desire for a more "holistic" approach to asthma care influence use.

The most common therapies used are breathing techniques, yoga, herbal remedies, acupuncture, diet, homeopathy, traditional medicines from the country of ethnic origin, and over-the-counter medications. Buteyko breathing, advocated to restore normal breathing patterns and reduce hyperventilation, has yielded a reduction in rescue medication (Shaw, Thompson, & Sharp, 2006) but not in corticosteroid use, hospitalization rate, or quality of life in one randomized clinical trial (Opat, Cohen, Bailey, et al., 2000). Yoga, with its stress management results, has shown reduced airway hyperresponsiveness. The National Asthma Council of Australia's website at www.NationalAsthma.org.au has summarized current evidence of CAM effects on asthma control. Therapies are graded 3+ (strong evidence for effectiveness) to -3 (strong evidence for lack of effectiveness), with 0 for insufficient evidence. Given the caveat that there is inadequate evidence-based information regarding many of the therapies, randomized clinical trials available found that only three therapies had a 2+ level (probably effective) on asthma symptoms: Buteyko breathing, a traditional Japanese medication, and an Ayurvedic medication. No research found 3+ level evidence of effectiveness, but several had insufficient or strong evidence for lack of effect.

Although some herbal remedies may be harmless, others, such as ephedra or Ma Huang, have been found to be dangerous. If herbal supplements are taken, they should be listed in the medication history so consideration of interaction or adverse effects can be made. Content, variability, and cost of herbal supplements should be discussed with the family.

Studies regarding dietary addition of omega-3 fatty acids, selenium, vitamins C and E, magnesium, *Lactobacillus acidophilus,* and salt were also reviewed and summarized by the National Asthma Council of Australia with none showing strong or probable effectiveness. Only magnesium and selenium supplements yielded possible effectiveness. Reliance on over-the-counter medications, if used as a substitute for medically supervised management, can be harmful, although some (antihistamines) may be helpful in managing allergic reactions. A provider's willingness to understand a family's rationale for using complementary therapies, as well as an openness to explore evidence of help/harm, is critical to successfully integrating complementary with allopathic treatments and the principles of family-centered care.

Anticipated Advances in Diagnosis and Management

- Since remodeling of the airways may take place in early childhood, more aggressive identification and treatment of asthma has been researched, with the hope of changing the natural course of the disease. Findings indicate that early and sustained treatment to reduce airway inflammation with ICSs brings significantly better clinical and lung function outcomes during treatment (Guilbert et al., 2006; Martinez, 2003, 2007).

- An increased appreciation of the role of bronchial hyperresponsivness is undergoing scrutiny. Hyperresponsivness is now thought to be a strong determinant of FEV_1 and FEV_1/FVC ratio, which may be a more accurate indicator of lung growth and lung function in children (Bacharier, Strunk, Mauger, et al., 2004). With or without the presence of the classic asthma symptoms of wheezing and cough, bronchial hyperresponsivness may be of greater importance and predict the future pattern of lung growth and airway performance, becoming the object of future research and therapies hoping to modify the natural course of asthma (Koh & Irving, 2007).

- Research over the past two decades reveals an increased risk of recurrent wheezing or asthma after respiratory syncytial virus (RSV) in infants up to 36 months of age, but this association decreases as the child increases in age (Perez-Yarza, Moreno, Lazaro, et al., 2007). Whether early infection with RSV has a causative role in asthma or merely heralds asthma in a genetically predisposed child is now being investigated. Evaluation of a new monoclonal antibody (MEDI-524) against RSV is being investigated. In animal models it has been more effective than palivizumab. Work is also continuing in development of vaccines against RSV (Panitch, 2007).

- There is a continuing need for noninvasive objective measures of pulmonary inflammation. Exhaled nitric oxide (E_{NO}), a measure of eosinophilic inflammation, and breath condensate, a measure of inflammatory markers, have been researched and may have a place in clinical management soon. Titration of inhaled steroids by tracking E_{NO} was evaluated with significant improvement in airway hyperresponsiveness and inflammation in the E_{NO}-tracked group compared with the symptom-tracked group, with no change in steroid dose by either group (Pijnenburg, Bakker, Hop, et al., 2005). E_{NO} may assist in evaluating compliance with ICS therapy and aid in diagnosis of asthma. Further research is continuing because there are still questions regarding the interpretation of results, that is, what other conditions may lead to increased (viral illness) or decreased (primary ciliary dyskinesia) E_{NO} and appropriate application to practice. Normal values have been researched in children (Buchvald, Baraldi, Carraro, et al., 2005). Any child able to perform spirometry can complete E_{NO} evaluation (i.e., at least 5 or 6 years of age).

- Infant pulmonary function testing is becoming more available in specialty or tertiary care centers. It requires administering sedation and supporting the recovery of the child when the test is complete. Therefore it is currently indicated and performed on specific populations of infants, such as those with bronchopulmonary dysplasia and cystic fibrosis (Beydon, Davis, Lombardi, et al., 2007).

- Further investigation into methods to evaluate airway obstruction in preschool children is needed. Measuring resistance by using an interruptor technique (Rint) involves tidal breathing through a mouthpiece-shutter-pneumotachograph system and requires limited cooperation. Standard procedures and values have yet to be established (Couriel & Child, 2004; Larsen, Kang, Guilbert, et al., 2005). The forced oscillation technique is both noninvasive and effort independent, suitable for the preschool age-group. Specific reference values for children, interpretation, and the appropriate place in therapy are under study (Frei, Jutla, Kramer, et al., 2005).
- Current research is addressing asthma phenotype-directed therapy. Severe asthma phenotype remains an enigma in terms of underlying etiology, as well as treatment. The role of subcutaneous etanercept, a soluble tumor necrosis factor-alpha (TNF-α) receptor that promotes the Th-1 response, is being investigated.
- New medications to treat chronic inflammation are a constant source of inquiry. Recently, a new generation of ICS, ciclesonide, has been investigated in Europe with adults for its antiinflammatory effect. Compared with budesonide, it has been found effective, well tolerated, and with reduced HPA axis suppression (Hansel, Benezet, Kafe, et al., 2006). Ongoing studies are being conducted in the United States.

Associated Problems of Asthma and Treatment

Allergies

All children who have allergies do not have asthma, but the majority of children with asthma have allergies. These allergies can also be expressed in the form of atopic dermatitis or allergic rhinitis (see Chapter 10). A strong history of allergic reactions associated with respiratory symptoms or unsuccessful escalation of therapy suggests consideration for skin-prick tests or radioallergosorbent test (RAST) allergy blood testing in conjunction with total IgE level, to determine specific problematic allergens. Antihistamines for treatment of allergic rhinitis may relieve the postnasal drip that accompanies sinusitis and triggers an asthma episode. It is vital to review possible allergens and triggers with the family, discussing avoidance or, at the minimum, modification of the child's environment to reduce exposures.

Associated Problems of Asthma and Treatment

- Additional allergies
- Medications (aspirin/NSAIDs) and other sensitivities
- Gastroesophageal reflux
- Swallowing disorders
- Allergic rhinitis

Key: *NSAIDs,* nonsteroidal antiinflammatory drugs.

Sensitivity to Aspirin and Nonsteroidal Antiinflammatory Drugs

Aspirin and nonsteroidal antiinflammatory drugs (NSAIDs) may precipitate an asthma episode in adults and possibly in children. Aspirin is rarely indicated in children, and parents should be taught to read over-the-counter drug labels because aspirin can be combined with other substances, especially cold remedies. Ibuprofen is commonly used in children and may have cross-sensitivity to aspirin and NSAIDs. In one study of 100 children between 6 and 18 years of age, approximately 2% had ibuprofen-sensitive asthma (Debley, Carter,

Gibson, et al., 2005). The authors excluded all children with severe asthma for ethical reasons, meaning their results are conservative estimates, but if there are approximately 6 million children with asthma in the United States, approximately 120,000 may be at risk for NSAID-induced bronchospasm. If NSAID sensitivity is suspected, referral to a specialist for confirmatory testing can be done.

Gastroesophageal Reflux

Gastroesophageal reflux (GER) is found in many children with chronic lung disease. Reflux of gastric secretions into the esophagus can initiate a reflex vagal response with increased production of airway secretions and cough. Cough itself can induce reflux episodes. Theophylline is known to increase gastric secretions and decrease lower esophageal pressure and thus may aggravate GER in some children. In a study of 44 children ages 8 to 15 years with moderate persistent asthma and GER, significant clinical improvement without any change in pulmonary function testing was noted when treated with a prokinetic pump inhibitor versus an H_2 blocker alone. The authors recommended a year of treatment for gastroesophageal reflux disease, but noted that some children may require longer treatment (Khoshoo & Haydel, 2007). Management of GER includes upright positioning following thickened feedings for infants, smaller feedings, and use of medications that reduce acidity or increase gastric motility.

Swallowing Disorders

Some infants and young children have dysphagia, or swallowing disorders, that may cause episodes of microaspiration, with or without obvious symptoms of cough. Aspiration of food or formula into the lungs will trigger a chronic inflammatory response that will exacerbate a child's asthma and require escalating therapy. If suspected, a video fluoroscopic swallowing study can document aspiration with resulting feeding adaptations required until, and if, the swallow is normally developed. Adaptations may include thickened feedings, positioning, or occupational therapy evaluation.

Allergic Rhinitis

Allergic rhinitis may contribute to lower airway inflammation, triggering asthma exacerbation, and predispose the child to chronic or recurrent sinusitis. Chronic infections of the sinuses with fever, pain, and thick postnasal secretions can irritate lower airways and trigger an asthma exacerbation. Treatment of allergic rhinitis and the infection is necessary to reduce this trigger and may involve routine nasal washes with antibiotic/saline solutions, intermittent nasal or oral steroids, and antibiotics. Treatment may be needed over a prolonged period, because chronic sinusitis is a notoriously difficult infection to eradicate.

Prognosis

Understanding the natural history of asthma continues to be an area of discussion and research. Longitudinal research studies have noted that wheezing is common in infants and young children (Ly, Gold, Weiss, et al., 2006; Martinez, Wright, Taussig, et al., 1995), yet wheezing does not always persist into childhood and adulthood. Forecasting which children will have ongoing symptoms, determining the appropriate treatment, and predicting which children may benefit from more aggressive treatment to prevent pulmonary functional decline drives much of the research.

Attempts to predict which young children will have asthma as an adult and which children will attain remission is still a puzzle. Increased asthma severity in childhood is predictive of reduced lung function in adulthood. Young children with episodic asthma and no severity markers (FEV₁% predicted >80%, no chronic use of ICS with minimal symptom scores) tend to have only intermittent asthma or complete remission 9 years later (Koh & Irving, 2007). Atopy is associated with persistence of asthma into adulthood, and, in those children who do have remission of symptoms, atopy is associated with greater rates of relapse later in life (Taylor, Cowan, Greene, et al., 2005). In one longitudinal study, children who were without symptoms by 16 years of life had an increased risk of relapse in midlife, often related to atopy and current smoking (Butland & Strachan, 2007). The main predictors of persistent wheezing into adulthood are a reduced level of lung function in childhood and significant bronchial hyperresponsiveness to histamine in the childhood years (Morgan, Stern, Sherrill, et al., 2005).

PRIMARY CARE MANAGEMENT

Health Care Maintenance
Growth and Development
Investigators continue to explore the degree to which asthma has a direct influence on growth. The practitioner should measure height and weight, calculate body mass index (BMI), and record these measurements on the child's growth charts at each acute care and monitoring visit. Major deviations from population norms (i.e., less than the 10th or above the 90th percentile) or departure (i.e., two or more zones) from the child's individualized curve should be noted and assessed in detail to determine if lack of asthma control or treatment may be influencing growth. Genetic, social, and nutritional factors, unassociated with asthma, must be considered when evaluating patterns in growth. Alterations may need to be monitored over time for their significance to be appreciated. During a series of acute exacerbations, a plateau or small drop in weight may take place; however, with improved health status, catch-up growth should occur. If it does not, the cause of the weight loss should be further explored.

The first year of ICS use may lead to a temporary decrease in growth velocity, but this should disappear in subsequent years (EPR-3, 2007; Guilbert et al., 2006). Primary care providers need to carefully monitor growth at least every 6 to 12 months after age 2 years to evaluate cost/benefit ratios of treatment protocols. Although the adolescent growth spurt may be slightly delayed, with optimal management of the disease, maximal height attainment is thought to be possible (Agertoft & Pedersen, 2000; Allen, 2004). Adjunctive long-term control therapy may reduce the need for high-dose inhaled or systemic steroids and thus minimize the dose-dependent undesirable effects of treatment (EPR-3, 2007).

Standard infant, child, and adolescent assessment tools are appropriate for assessing development at the typically recommended ages (Bright Futures, 2007; Drotar, Stancin, Dworkin, et al., 2008; Glascoe & Robertshaw, 2007). Delayed development is rarely documented in children with asthma. When found, the delay is not necessarily related to the physiologic severity of the asthma but to imposed limitations placed on a child's experiences. Limitations typically involve reductions in physical activity or social experiences, including childcare and school attendance. Therefore practitioners should encourage normalization of experiences whenever possible and provide treatment adequate to allow normative activities (Milton, Whitehead, Holland, et al., 2004).

If age-typical experiences must be discouraged to avoid specific asthma triggers, primary care providers should assist parents and children to identify alternative experiences that could provide similar developmental stimulation. For example, if the child cannot play competitive soccer because of grass allergy, poor response to medication/immunotherapy, or refusal to take preventive medication, the child and family should be helped to identify an alternative sport. Sports such as swimming or gymnastics allow the child to exercise and participate in a competitive team sport and provide the opportunity to engage in an age-appropriate social and skill-building activity without outdoor allergen exposure. Helping a child find an enjoyable sport/physical activity should be a significant goal to improve overall health (Welsh, Kemp, & Roberts, 2005). Without normalized experiences a child's self-image, self-esteem, perception of bodily control, and overall level of health are likely reduced and anxiety, fear, and dependent behavior increased (Ortega, Huertas, Canino, et al., 2002). During adolescence these problems have been found related to symptoms of exercise-induced bronchoconstriction (Hallstrand, Curtis, Aitken, et al., 2003). Consultation with or referral to a mental health practitioner should be considered if problems emerge, before they become deeply established and more difficult to improve (EPR-3, 2007).

Repeated brief school absences can impair academic achievement (Moonie, Sterling, Figgs, et al., 2006). Concerns have also been linked to some medications, but the demonstrated negative effect of asthma or medications on cognitive capabilities is not universal. Prevention and swift management of exacerbations reduces the number and length of school absences, limiting the factor contributing most to lower academic achievement (Guevara, Wolf, Grum, et al., 2003; Wolf et al., 2003).

Diet
Today's children and families eat many meals away from home, so dietary restrictions could affect family habits. Sulfites, used to enhance the appearance of fresh foods, have been implicated in severe asthma exacerbations in some children, and, once such sensitivity is identified, sulfites need to be avoided. Sulfite use has decreased and FDA has ruled that foods containing sulfites must be clearly labeled, but they are still found in processed potatoes, shrimp, dried fruits and vegetables, nonfrozen lemon and lime juice, and wine (U.S. Food and Drug Administration, 2008). Although parents and providers often feel that foods exacerbate asthma in children, the incidence of documented food allergy is low (Beausoleil, Fiedler, & Spergel, 2007). Restrictive diets without proven specific allergy are thus inappropriate (see Chapter 10).

Obesity. The association between asthma and obesity is complex (Hasan, Zureikat, Nolan, et al., 2006). However, if the BMI rises, especially if greater than the 85th percentile, the provider should discuss opportunities to increase the child's routine activity and provide appropriate pharmacologic support before focusing on diet. Reducing portion sizes and high-calorie/high-fat food intake can be discussed. Advocating changes by the entire family rather than focusing just on the child's habits is more effective in stabilizing the child's weight.

Although obesity can result from inactivity associated with asthma, more recent explorations examine the role obesity plays in the emergence of asthma (Beuther & Sutherland, 2007). Prospective research suggests that obesity precedes the development of asthma. Questions linking obesity to the underlying pathology of airway inflammation and hyperresponsiveness, presence of atopy, and mechanical changes in chest wall function are being explored. Early data suggest that weight loss may decrease asthma symptoms (Story, 2007) (see Chapter 36).

Safety

Electrical burns are possible when equipment (e.g., nebulizers, dehumidifiers) is run in the child's presence. Infants and young children should never be left alone where they can reach equipment, cords or open sockets. School-age children and adolescents should be properly instructed in the safe use of electrical equipment and demonstrate their use to parents or the provider before being encouraged to use the equipment independently.

Medications kept in the home must be safely stored in their original containers in a locked location that is inaccessible to infants and young children. Children will ultimately need to develop age-appropriate responsibility for medication administration, however, and families benefit from provider help to create an effective parent-child shared management plan. Practitioners can help parents identify their child's developmental capabilities and limits for safely assisting with medication by providing age-normative suggestions. For example, when a child is an infant or a toddler, the parents must speak about the medications as such—not as candy. With maturation, toddlers can be taught how to hold facemasks or take slow breaths to assist in therapy. Preschool-age children typically have the manual dexterity to take part in the medicinal therapy by helping parents assemble inhalers or count doses in the parent's presence. Young, school-age children may be asked to get the medication and take it in the presence of a parent. When older school-age children can tell time, they can assume greater responsibility to prompt the parent when medication is needed, get the medication, take the medication in the parent's presence, and return it to its proper storage place. School-age children should also become increasingly responsible for taking needed medication while at school. Parents can monitor and encourage safe and knowledgeable use by discussing or having a child count and record on a calendar the number of times medication was taken. Most states now have mandates that children can carry asthma rescue medication on their person if trained to do so and have parental and provider permission. During adolescence, more autonomy should be given for independently taking, and replenishing, both controller and rescue medication and ensuring that the medication is in all needed locations (e.g., home, school, sports bag). Parents need to be reminded that one consistent finding in successful adolescent adherence to prescribed regimens is, however, the continued support and age-appropriate assistance of their parents. This support is not shown by "doing for" or "nagging" but by demonstrating faith in the adolescent's capabilities and offering assistance when problems arise; parents can maintain an interested, interdependent attitude to best assist their adolescent. Greater details on how to promote shared management can be found elsewhere (Kieckhefer & Trahms, 2000).

Parents and children need help in learning how to monitor the number of doses remaining in the child's rescue or daily medication if a counter is not on the delivery device. Although new, DPIs show the number of remaining puffs or require a capsule for each dose; MDIs do not have this advantage. The typical MDI contains 200 actuations; therefore, with a two-puff dose, it will take 100 doses to empty the MDI. Historically, families were told to estimate how much medication remained in the MDI by observing its sinking (full)/floating (empty) in a water container. This is discouraged because this process would destroy DPI medication. Most pharmacies now recommend that families count the actual doses the child takes or keep an extra medication dispenser of, at least, the rescue medication on hand to ensure that they do not run out.

The child's skill in using the inhaler should be observed at each visit with the practitioner (EPR-3, 2007). Up to 50% of children can improve proper technique when this is done (Minai, Martin, & Cohn, 2004). Use of spacers with MDIs for all age-groups lessens problems and enhances widespread medication deposition in the lungs. New, breath-activated devices may also help in children old enough to inhale with adequate inspiratory effort. Usually children able to perform spirometry are able to appropriately inhale medication from these DPIs (e.g., 4 years).

With age and increasing time spent away from parents, children must independently recognize when their treatment is not effective and seek assistance. An episode that does not respond to treatment as expected may herald a particularly severe exacerbation requiring need for systemic corticosteroids. A written action plan containing the daily long-term control recommendations, as well as a plan to be implemented if an acute exacerbation begins or does not respond to initial treatment, is essential for every person with asthma. Written plans serve as a concrete means to communicate the treatment plan to the child, parent, childcare workers, teachers, and others who provide care to the child. Examples of these plans are provided in "Guidelines for the Diagnosis and Management of Asthma" (EPR-3, 2007).

Immunizations

The most recent recommendations of the Committee on Infectious Diseases are available online at http://aapredbook.aappublications. org should guide immunization decisions. Although the Committee on Infectious Diseases notes that vaccination with live-virus vaccines can lead to airway inflammation and therefore increased hyperresponsivity in children with asthma, the standard schedule of childhood immunizations is still recommended for most children, with additional considerations for the child's total corticosteroid load as noted in the following (American Academy of Pediatrics, 2008b):

- *Low-potency topical corticosteroids,* either on the skin, in the respiratory system by aerosol, or intraarticular, bursal, or tendon injection, usually do not result in immunosuppression that contraindicates administration of live-virus vaccines. If evidence of systemic immunosuppression results from prolonged application, live-virus vaccines should not be given until steroid therapy has been discontinued for at least 1 month.
- *Low/moderate doses of systemic corticosteroids given daily or on alternate days:* Children under 10 kg receiving less than 2 mg/kg/day of prednisone/equivalent can receive live-virus vaccines while on treatment.
- *High-dose systemic corticosteroids given daily or on alternative days for less than 14 days:* Children receiving 2 mg/kg/day or greater of prednisone/equivalent, or 20 mg or greater (more if they weigh greater than 10 kg), can receive live-virus vaccines immediately after discontinuation of treatment.
- *High doses of systemic corticosteroids given daily or on alternate days for 14 days or longer:* Children receiving 2 mg/kg/day or

greater of prednisone/equivalent, or 20 mg/day or greater if they weigh more than 10 kg, should not receive live-virus vaccines until steroid therapy has been discontinued for at least 1 month.

Although infants and children with asthma may have frequent signs of respiratory infection, these signs alone, in the absence of specific published contraindication, should not be the basis for deferring immunizations (American Academy of Pediatrics, 2008b). Inadequate immunization with subsequent risk of infection is of greater concern. Individualized assessment of the child with respiratory symptoms, including progressive signs of pulmonary dysfunction, should guide decisions about immunization in these cases.

Severe and even fatal varicella has been reported in otherwise healthy children receiving intermittent courses of high-dose corticosteroids (greater than 2 mg/kg of prednisone or equivalent) for treatment of asthma and other conditions. The risk is especially high when corticosteroids are given during the incubation period for chickenpox. Oral acyclovir should be considered for unvaccinated children exposed to and up to within the first 72 hours of rash who have been receiving even short intermittent aerosolized corticosteroids. Intravenous antiviral therapy is recommended for immunocompromised children being treated with chronic corticosteroids (American Academy of Pediatrics, 2008b).

Children with asthma may experience complications with influenza (e.g., increased wheezing, bronchitis, pneumonia, and increased school absences and medical care visits). Therefore, despite recent or current prednisone bursts, children with asthma should annually receive an influenza vaccine after age 6 months (American Academy of Pediatrics, 2008b). Inactivated influenza vaccines are licensed for children over 6 months. Live-attenuated influenza vaccine is licensed for those over 2 years and is being tested for those as young as 6 months. Prolonged corticosteroid doses of greater than 2 mg/kg/day may impair antibody response, but immunization should not be deferred if doing so will compromise the likelihood of immunization before the influenza season. Parents and siblings should also receive the influenza vaccine.

Routine pneumococcal immunization is recommended. Ongoing immunization of children after 24 months, who are on high-dose oral corticosteroids, with 23-valent vaccine is warranted because of their presumed high-risk status for serious infection (American Academy of Pediatrics, 2008b).

Screening

See Box 11-4.

Vision. Routine screening is recommended unless the child is taking daily high-dose corticosteroids because these drugs are known to cause inflammatory changes, cataracts, and glaucoma in adults. If abnormal findings are identified during routine monitoring examinations, the child should be referred to an ophthalmologist.

Hearing. Routine screening is recommended.

Dental. Routine screening is recommended. Inhaled medication may alter the pH of the oral cavity, increasing development of caries (Tootla, Toumba, & Duggal, 2004). Rinsing the mouth after inhaling all medications should be routinely taught.

Blood Pressure. Blood pressure should be evaluated at each visit because of possible elevation with sympathetic medications or corticosteroids. With a potential link between asthma and obesity and obesity and high blood pressure, monitoring is essential to identify early rises (Din-Dzietham, Liu, Bielo, et al., 2007).

BOX 11-4
Summary of Screening Activities

ROUTINE CHILDHOOD SCREENING
- Vision: See text
- Hearing: Routine
- Dental: Routine
- Blood pressure: See text
- Hematocrit
- Urinalysis: See text
- Tuberculosis: Routine

CONDITION-SPECIFIC SCREENING
- Lung function
  - Spirometry
  - Peak expiratory flow rate
- Theophylline levels
- Allergic triggers
- Bone density

Hematocrit. Routine screening is recommended.

Urinalysis. Routine screening is recommended unless the child is taking high-dose corticosteroids daily, which may cause glycosuria. If glycosuria is present, the child should be referred to a pulmonary specialist for evaluation and possible treatment alteration.

Tuberculosis. Routine screening is recommended.

Condition-Specific Screening

Lung Function. Ongoing monitoring in the office setting is essential to assess current function, lung growth, and effects of treatment. Spirometry, using American Thoracic Society–approved spirometers loaded with reference values appropriate to the population being tested, should be done at diagnosis and when the child is under good control to establish baseline lung function. Spirometry is also recommended following any step up or step down of treatment and annually when treatment is stable (EPR-3, 2007). Spirometry can assess severity of both small and larger airway obstruction. Child norms can be found in pediatric pulmonary publications (Wang, Dockery, Wypij, et al., 1993). Spirometry should always be evaluated in the context of the clinical history because, when used alone, it can underestimate disease severity and control (Cowen, Wakefield, & Cloutier, 2007).

Peak flow meters have been previously used in the primary care office to measure the greatest rate of airflow during a forced exhalation (PEFR) and guide treatment decisions. PEFR, however, is effort dependent, predominantly reflects large airway function, is highly dependent on using the same meter, and provides less information than spirometry. Thus the PEFR meter is no longer recommended for office use but instead as an aid for the child and family in their home to objectively screen for evaluating large airway status, especially when the child has poor perception of changing asthma symptoms (EPR-3, 2007). Asthma action plans given to the family to help them manage asthma outside the clinic may include both symptoms and PEFR readings to best guide family management decisions (EPR-3, 2007). PEFR meters are relatively inexpensive and easy to use. The objective data can help the child and family decide when to initiate early treatment and to evaluate the child's response to treatment. See www.mayoclinic.com/health/asthma/MM00399 (Mayo Clinic, 2008) for a video demonstrating proper use of a flow meter and EPR-3 (2007) for written directions on flow meter use. Table 11-7 depicts a common way PEFR values are used in action plans using a green/yellow/red zone approach.

Theophylline Levels. Theophylline remains an infrequently used alternative treatment adjunct because of the need for close monitoring of drug levels due to its narrow therapeutic index (EPR-3, 2007; Seddon, Bara, Ducharme, et al., 2006). Because theophylline preparations come in quick-release, sustained-release, or ultra-sustained-release forms, monitoring theophylline levels is determined by the preparation and following the manufacturer's guidelines is critical. Monitoring level should be drawn at the same time (e.g., always 4 hours after the dose of a sustained-release preparation) to ensure consistency. In the case of suspected theophylline toxicity, levels must be obtained immediately. See Table 11-8 for a summary of factors affecting serum theophylline levels.

Allergic Triggers. A biannual review of possible environmental allergens and irritants is helpful. If it appears that allergies are implicated in asthma exacerbations, this review can be done more frequently and consideration given for initial or repeat allergy testing. Results can aid in education for environmental alterations or immunotherapy (EPR-3, 2007). There is no age limit as to when allergy testing can be done. Referral to a specialist is recommended for children under 2 years because of difficulties in interpretation of results (Douglass & O'Hehir, 2006).

TABLE 11-7
Zone Action Plan

PEFR (Best or Predicted for Age)	Action
GREEN ZONE	
80% to 100%	All clear, continue regular management plan
YELLOW ZONE	
50% to 80%	Caution, implement action plan predetermined with primary care provider
RED ZONE	
50% or less	Medical alert, implement action plan predetermined with primary care provider; if PEFR does not return to yellow or green zone, call provider

Key: *PEFR*, Peak expiratory flow rate.

TABLE 11-8
Factors Affecting Serum Theophylline Levels

	Factors Increasing Serum Levels Because of Decreased Clearance	Factors Decreasing Serum Levels Because of Increased Clearance
Age	Infants	12 mo to 12 yr
Medications	Erythromycin—alone or in combination	Phenobarbital
	Azithromycin (Zithromax)	Phenytoin (Dilantin)
	Clarithromycin (Biaxin)	Rifampin (Rifadin)
	Cimetidine (Tagamet)	
	Oral contraceptives	
	Propranolol (Inderal)	
	Carbamazepine (Tegretol)	
	Zileuton (Zyflo)	
Illnesses	Liver or heart dysfunction	
	Acute viral illnesses	
Other	Obesity	Cigarette or marijuana smoking
	Fever for over 24 hr	

Bone Density. Currently, bone scans are encouraged for children over 12 years of age on systemic corticosteroids. Some researchers believe that all children on prolonged high-dose ICSs should also have bone scans, but norms are not well established for this younger age-group (Ducharme, Chabot, Polychronakos, et al., 2003).

Common Illness Management
Differential Diagnosis

Cough and Wheezing. See Other Conditions Causing Cough and Wheeze, earlier in this chapter.

Sinusitis. Sinusitis can cause nighttime cough and headache, and may be associated with complaints of purulent nasal drainage and foul breath odor. These symptoms will not respond to asthma medications. Because sinusitis can trigger an asthma episode, there may also be increased wheezing in the child with concurrent asthma. When diagnosed, sinusitis and allergic rhinitis should be treated early and aggressively to improve asthma control (Corren, Manning, Thompson, et al., 2004; Sandrini, Ferreira, Jardim, et al., 2003).

Differential Diagnosis

- *Cough and wheezing:* Foreign body aspiration, upper respiratory infection, other airway diseases, structural abnormalities, GER, neurologic/cardiac disease
- *Sinusitis:* Adequate treatment may reduce asthma exacerbations
- *Vocal cord dysfunction:* Wheezing caused by adduction of the vocal cords
- *Drug interactions:* To be evaluated on an individual basis

Key: *GER*, gastroesophageal reflux.

Vocal Cord Dysfunction. Vocal cord dysfunction, defined as adduction versus abduction of the vocal cords during the respiratory cycle, may mimic sounds much like an asthmatic wheeze (Noyes & Kemp, 2007). The "wheeze" does not respond to asthma medications, and the child has near-normal spirometry findings and oxygen saturations. Reduced voice quality may be noted or the inspiratory loop on the flow volume curve during spirometry may be flattened during times of breathlessness. This disorder may be clinically recognized but is definitively diagnosed via flexible laryngoscopy during an acute episode if the history, pulmonary function, and response to treatment are unclear. Speech therapy and relaxation techniques may be recommended for treatment (Weinberger & Abu-Hasan, 2007).

Drug Interactions. Drug interactions need to be evaluated on an individual basis. Some ICSs (e.g., fluticasone, budesonide, mometasone) are metabolized in the gastrointestinal tract and liver by CYP 3A4 isoenzymes. Inhibitors of these isoenzymes (e.g., ketoconazole) could lead to increased systemic concentration of the ICS (Johnson, Marion, Vrchoticky, et al., 2006; Samaras, Pett, Gowers, et al., 2005). Children with asthma are often atopic and receive topical in addition to inhaled steroids. The provider must be aware of the potential cumulative effects because it is the total body load of steroid that is related to side effects (EPR-3, 2007). Medications children most commonly take whose formulations at this time do not appear to have drug interactions with asthma medications include antibiotics, anti-gastric reflux medications, and antihistamines. Because new drugs are being continually developed and interactions discovered, checking for interaction using an online resource or pharmacist is always recommended when adding a new medication to the child's regimen.

Developmental Issues

Sleep Patterns

The sleep of young children is often disrupted during asthma exacerbations. Even when an exacerbation is not evident, a child may awaken and cough during the night or early morning and report low overall sleep quality (Chugh, Khanna, & Shah, 2006; Esnault, Fang, Kelly, et al., 2007; Kieckhefer & Lentz, 2006). Parental perception of nocturnal symptoms is as low as 40% (Cabral, Conceicao, Saldiva, et al., 2002). Parents and children may report different levels of symptoms, which necessitates asking both during the history (Kieckhefer & Lentz, 2006). The tendency for early morning problems probably represents both circadian- and sleep-driven changes in airway caliber and steroid production/responsiveness. Because nocturnal symptoms represent an exaggeration of existing bronchial hyperresponsivity, optimizing daytime control and reducing environmental irritants in the sleeping room often reduces symptoms.

Carpets, stuffed toys, curtains, or anything that retains dust should be removed from the sleeping room and the change in symptoms noted. Dust mite covers for the pillow and mattress can be tried with a cost of as little as $100 total. Pets should remain out of the sleeping room and windows should be kept closed, reducing pollen and grass allergens. Mold-producing agents such as houseplants should be removed. The regional American Lung Association may have a Home Environmentalist Program that can provide a comprehensive in-home assessment on family request.

Persistent sleep problems may necessitate an evening dosage of an LTRA or, infrequently, a short- or long-acting theophylline preparation. If improvements are not seen in several weeks, referral to a pulmonary clinic or sleep specialist is warranted.

Most young children find a nighttime ritual soothing. Primary care providers should help parents establish a bedtime ritual that is relaxing and can be easily implemented by the family. A consistent bedtime is helpful because frequent deviation may cause difficulty in settling a child, may delay sleep onset, and is associated with reduced daytime alertness and attentiveness (Sadeh, Gruber, & Raviv, 2003).

Toileting

Toileting needs are typically not altered by a child's asthma. Bowel and bladder training is achieved at the expected ages. Clinicians report that a small proportion of children experience problems with enuresis when taking theophylline preparations, possibly because of its diuretic action. The exact incidence, however, is undocumented. If standard behavioral interventions are not effective in eliminating enuresis, most primary care providers recommend an alternative medication regimen. Constipation could occur if the child becomes dehydrated during exacerbations.

Discipline

Parents may report that they find it difficult to deal with discipline for fear of upsetting the child and initiating an asthma exacerbation. Because children with asthma may experience some degree of bronchospasm with intense crying, parental concern is understandable. Crying cannot be entirely avoided, but parents should be reassured that most discipline can be implemented by rewarding desirable behaviors, if this is done routinely and begun early in a child's life.

Inconsistent limit setting for undesirable behavior only confuses children and makes it more difficult for them to learn and internalize the limits chosen by the parents. Well grounded popular parenting books used with children not having asthma can be recommended for the parent of a child having asthma (Faber & Mazlish, 2002).

Another parental concern is that the child's irritability, refusals, or acting-out behavior is caused by illness or medications. Medications and illness may influence the child's behavior, but consistency of parental expectations is of greater importance. Blaming the illness or medication does not remove the necessity to help a child develop behaviors desired by the family and social networks. A child will ultimately need to develop a strong sense of internal control to effectively participate in shared management of asthma. Early, consistent, positive expectations set by the parents will form the foundation for a child's later self-discipline and sense of mastery and control. Avoiding discipline early in a child's life will not make the ensuing years more pleasant for parents or help the child learn socially expected behaviors. Thus primary care providers should initiate discussion about positive discipline early during an infant's first year of life, assuring parents that with time this issue should become less burdensome as the child is able to verbally express emotion without excessive crying leading to bronchospasm.

Child Care

Most families find it desirable or necessary to use childcare services on either a regular or sporadic basis. Having a child with asthma should not prohibit this. Because upper respiratory infections trigger exacerbations of asthma in many children less than 5 years of age, a smaller site with less chance of exposure to these infections may reduce the number of asthma exacerbations. Parents should evaluate the childcare environment for any known triggers. Licensed childcare centers prohibit exposure to secondhand smoke and are evaluated for dust mite catchers (e.g., carpets, stuffed toys, or furniture), molds or mildew, and animals. If unlicensed, private, or in-home childcare arrangements do not need to meet state requirements, parents must take the initiative to evaluate for these known triggers. The local chapter of the American Lung Association or Asthma and Allergy Foundation may be of assistance in this regard along with the local health department. With proper communication and explanation, childcare can be safely accomplished with a responsible, interested caretaker. Whether childcare is at a center or is home based, provided by a relative, neighbor, or professional, information must be shared by parents to ensure success in asthma management.

Parents are responsible for providing all relevant information to the caretaker; that is, what triggers the child's asthma, early warning signs of an impending asthma episode, what the caretaker should do first and what should be done next if the action is not fully effective, how the parent and other responsible parties (i.e., including health care provider) can be reached, and what information must be passed on to emergency personnel if they are called. The recommended way to provide this information is in written format, using an asthma management plan created with the health care provider. Examples of these written plans can be found online at www.nhlbi.nih.gov (National Heart, Lung, and Blood Institute Health Information Center), www.aafa.org (Asthma and Allergy Foundation of America), or www.aanma.org (Allergy and Asthma Network: Mothers of Asthmatics) or in the *Guidelines for the Diagnosis and Management of Asthma* (EPR-3, 2007). Parents can be encouraged to share the action plan they receive or the provider can obtain parental permission to mail a copy directly to the childcare provider, whichever best ensures that the childcare site obtains the needed paperwork.

If the childcare provider is to give any treatments, the parent must demonstrate the procedures and observe the provider's repeat performance. In addition, center-based programs may require written prescriptions from the primary health care provider and written permission of the parent for the childcare provider to perform the treatment. Parents must maintain close contact with the childcare provider to learn about changing triggers or emerging early warning signs. Anyone in repeated contact with the child who observes responses to treatments should also relay that information to the parent. This information can then be integrated into the overall routine reevaluation of the treatment plan. Treatment modifications should be immediately related to the childcare provider so that a consistent approach is provided to the child regardless of setting. Frequent and open communication is the key to successful childcare arrangements. At times, direct communication between the childcare site and the health care provider, with parental consent, may be beneficial.

Schooling

Surveys consistently find that children with asthma have increased numbers of school absences when asthma is uncontrolled (Gustafsson, Watson, Davis, et al., 2006). Parents report that communicating with school personnel is essential but often difficult. Many fears and misconceptions about children with asthma still exist in the general public. Many teachers do not recognize a cough as a sign of poorly controlled asthma. They may believe the child has an infectious disease that should restrict school attendance. Teachers and administrators may attempt to limit the child more than the parents or primary care provider believes necessary, especially in regard to sports participation. With proper therapy and education, only those children with severe persistent asthma require regular limitations (EPR-3, 2007). With appropriate warm-up, pacing, hydration, and preventive pharmacologic therapy, almost all children with asthma will be able to participate in active school activities on a regular basis. Field trips also do not need limitations, although an SABA and a copy of the asthma management plan must accompany the child on each field trip.

Three online resources for the health care provider to support the parent in working with school personnel are www.cdc.gov/healthyyouth/healthtopics/asthma, Centers for Disease Control and Prevention; www.lungusa.org/site/pp.asp?c=dvLUK9O0E&b=22590, American Lung Association; and www.epa.gov/iaq/schools/asthma.html, U.S. Environmental Protection Agency.

Fitting in with school peers and maintaining positive peer relationships are essential to the child's full development. Parents can actively arrange peer gatherings, encourage the child to join clubs or organizations, and allow the child age-appropriate independence in visiting friends to ensure social experiences. Friends may question why the child is taking medications or has special equipment in the home. Simple explanations about the child's asthma should be given with the assurance that asthma is not contagious. This might also be done in school as a class presentation with the teacher's assistance because, with asthma one of the most common chronic conditions of childhood, several children in any classroom may have asthma. Parents are encouraged to discuss their child's asthma with parents of their child's peers so that all may have an honest understanding of the child's condition and abilities, as well as of any temporary limitations or needs for treatment. The American Lung Association's program, "Open Airways," for school-age children is available at www.lungusa.org/site/pp.asp?c=dvLUK9O 0E&;b=44142, and the "Asthma Care Training" program is available from the Asthma and Allergy Foundation of America at http://aafa.org/display.cfm?id=4&sub=79&cont=351.

Sexuality

As noted earlier, pubertal development may be delayed if asthma has not been adequately controlled to allow regular growth. Systemic corticosteroids historically have been associated with delay in development because of their effect on the adrenal glands and corticosteroid production. Current treatment regimens that rely on recently developed ICSs with limited systemic bioavailability and infrequent bursts of systemic corticosteroids appear to have reduced the adverse effects on general and pubertal growth patterns for most children, but more needs to be known about the subtle effects of these long-term approaches (Acun, Tomac, Ermis, et al., 2005; Ferguson, Van Bever, Teper, et al., 2007). If an adolescent becomes sexually active and wishes to use oral or depot contraceptives, drug interactions must be considered. It is known that these contraceptives may interfere with the breakdown of theophylline, thus increasing the likelihood of toxicity. As new asthma and contraceptive medications are developed, their interactions must be considered.

Transition to Adulthood

As youths with asthma enter adulthood, it is important that they continue to increase and periodically update their understanding of asthma and its management. Formal review and updating education might take place before a move to college or a switch in primary care providers. College students need to have access to their medications and an emergency care provider while away from home. If persons with a history of moderate to severe asthma are currently symptom free, they should be reminded to inform their adult provider of their asthma history because symptoms may return later in life. If the history is complex, a formal request for transfer of records to the adult health care provider should be made. Maintaining a smoke-free work environment is essential. Some vocations that involve inhaled irritants or allergens and overexposure to known triggers (e.g., work with laboratory animals, cleaning fluids, or painting products) may be best avoided.

Family Concerns

Family members may express guilt during the child's exacerbations because of the genetic nature of asthma. Parents should be reminded that there is little they could have done to prevent asthma in their child but much they can do to prevent exacerbations. Eliminating all exacerbations is an ideal but difficult goal to achieve (Gustafsson et al., 2006). Eliminating the number and extent of problems and learning something about prevention or management from each episode is achievable.

If family members have a history of asthma, they may retain outdated beliefs and habits regarding treatment. The primary care provider must respect the family's beliefs but also stress new knowledge and discuss the development of new therapies to encourage the family to take advantage of current information. Given the familial nature of asthma, cultural and ethnic considerations are important. In the United States, minority ethnicity and poverty continue to be linked to potential reduced access to care, lower quality of care, and reduced implementation of recommended care with subsequent higher risks of morbidity and mortality (Erickson, Iribarren, Tolstykh, et al., 2007; Greek, Kieckhefer, Kim, et al., 2006; National Institutes of Health, 2004a, 2004b). Providers must be child advocates for reducing environmental exposures that cause asthma and its exacerbation (e.g., prenatal tobacco smoke, preterm birth, housing with poor ventilation, mold and mildew, early URI). Providers can support policies and legislation that ensure comprehensive systems with the ability to meet the needs of children with asthma and universal access to health care, because both have been found to influence asthma outcomes (American Academy of Pediatrics, 2008a; Kieckhefer, Greek, Joesch, et al., 2005; National Association of Pediatric Nurse Practitioners, 2008). Exploring values, beliefs, and health practices of diverse families should enable the creative primary care provider to partner with families to individualize critical elements of practice guidelines. This individualization helps ensure the greatest acceptance and implementation of the recommended care by tailoring the management program to the cultural realities of the child and family. It is within the ongoing trusting relationship between the family and caregiver that further information regarding cultural beliefs and practices can be discussed (Mosnaim, Kohrman, Sharp, et al., 2006; Svavarsdottir, Rayens, & McCubbin, 2005).

Prenatal exposure to tobacco is linked to developing asthma, and smoking by a family member is also associated with increased asthma flare-ups (Alati, Al Mamun, O'Callaghan, et al., 2006; Pattenden, Antova, Neuberger, et al., 2006). Changing the smoking habits of family members is difficult for health care providers and family members alike. When the provider is recommending behavior changes, a motivational approach may increase the likelihood of success (Levensky, Forcehimes, O'Donohue, et al., 2007). When advising families to eliminate smoke from their child's environment, the practitioner should convey resources for smoking cessation or, at minimum, risk avoidance. If unable to stop smoking, parents must be reminded to only smoke outside (i.e., not in another room, near an open window, or in car) and wear a "smoking jacket" (i.e., an outer layer to prevent smoke retention on clothes). In-home smoking can lead to more frequent need for systemic steroids, can lead to hospitalizations with extended stays, and, in some extreme situations, may be considered child endangerment.

Many parents express ambivalence about long-term medication regimens, especially when the child has been taking medications for years (Kieckhefer & Ratcliffe, 2000). Although parents acknowledge the effectiveness of these regimens, many also hold the belief that long-term medication—especially steroids—can be harmful to their child. Helpful approaches for supporting parents include acknowledging and discussing these common feelings while presenting your belief that more detrimental effects of asthma come from poor control. It is also useful to reinforce that the long-term treatment program will continue to be tailored to their individual child, trying to decrease medication to the minimum amount needed for symptom control.

Asthma, like all chronic conditions, can disrupt the life of the child's family. This disruption is marked when the child is young but can be minimized by actively involving all family members in concrete, daily management tasks. Disruption comes not only from the disease but also from management activities. It is important to recognize the effort families exert and point out successes for them to reflect on, as well as continuing to implement the simplest, most effective treatment regimen.

Resources

Primary care providers should become familiar with the local offices of national organizations (see list that follows) to identify community-based services in the area that can complement their health care services. Many of these community-based services have programs that are useful to children and parents in managing the day-to-day effects of asthma. Programs typically offer education about asthma and training in shared management skills for the child and parents.

If the primary care provider's practice is large enough, educational programs for similar-age children may be effectively implemented. A well-stocked lending library of reading materials and videotapes on asthma helps parents and children learn how to manage asthma effectively. Practitioners can provide families with information on how to obtain these materials for their own use. Some of the most reputable are listed here. A comprehensive list is available in the *Guidelines for the Diagnosis and Management of Asthma* (EPR-3, 2007).

Asthma Education

Allergy and Asthma Network: Mothers of Asthmatics
2751 Prosperity Ave., Suite 150
Fairfax, VA 22030
Website: www.breatherville.org
(703) 641-9595; (800) 878-4403

American Academy of Allergy, Asthma, and Immunology
555 East Wells St., Suite 100
Milwaukee, WI 53202-3823
Website: www.aaaai.org
(414) 272-6071

American Association for Respiratory Care
9125 North MacArthur Blvd., Suite 100
Irving, TX 75063
Website: www.aarc.org
(972) 243-2272

American College of Allergy, Asthma, and Immunology
85 West Algonquin Rd.
Suite 550
Arlington Heights, IL 60005
Website: www.acaai.org
(847) 427-1200; (800) 842-7777

American Lung Association
61 Broadway
New York, NY 10006
Website: www.lungusa.org
(800) 586-4872

Association of Asthma Educators
1215 Anthony Ave.
Columbia, SC 29201
Website: www.asthmaeducators.org
(888) 988-7747

Asthma and Allergy Foundation of America
1233 20th St. NW., Suite 402
Washington, DC 20036
Website: www.aafa.org
(800) 727-8462

Centers for Disease Control and Prevention
1600 Clifton Rd.
Atlanta, GA 30333
Website: www.cdc.gov
(800) 311-3435

Food Allergy and Anaphylaxis Network
11781 Lee Jackson Hwy., Suite 160
Fairfax, VA 22033
Website: www.foodallergy.org
(800) 929-4040

National Heart, Lung, and Blood Institute
P.O. Box 30105
Bethesda, MD 20824-0105
Website: www.nhlbi.nih.gov
(301) 592-8573

National Jewish Medical and Research Center
1400 Jackson St.
Denver, CO 80206
Website: www.njc.org
(800) 222-LUNG

U.S. Environmental Protection Agency
P.O. Box 42419
Cincinnati, OH 45242-0419
Website: www.airnow.gov
(800) 490-9198

Summary of Primary Care Needs for the Child with Asthma

HEALTH CARE MAINTENANCE

Growth and Development

- It is important to measure and record height, weight, and body mass index. Variations from the expected norms must be investigated.
- Prolonged or systemic use of steroids, inhaled steroids may affect growth; must be monitored carefully.
- Delayed adolescent growth is associated with poor control with exacerbations or chronic oral corticosteroids.
- Delayed development is only noted when unnecessary limitations are imposed on the child.
- Impaired cognitive development is most clearly linked to repeated school absences.

Diet

- The role of obesity in asthma is unclear. Children who are overweight or obese should be encouraged to increase exercise and decrease excess calorie intake. A family approach to weight management is important.
- Children may have allergies to sulfites or foods.

Safety

- Electrical burns are possible from nebulizers or steamers.
- Medication safety varies with developmental age.
- Caution is needed on repeated use of quick-relief medications if improvement is not achieved.
- Adherence is an issue with adolescents.

Immunizations

- Routine immunizations are recommended.
- Caution is necessary with use of live-virus vaccines in children on systemic or long-term steroids.
- If a child has documented egg sensitivity, vaccines using other media must be considered.
- Influenza vaccine is recommended for children over 6 months of age. Pneumococcal immunization (Prevnar) is currently recommended in the schedule advocated for all children at 2, 4, 6, and 12 to 15 months of age. Pneumococcal polysaccharide vaccine, the 23-valent pneumococcal vaccine, is still recommended to expand serotype coverage to children 24 months of age and older deemed at high risk for invasive pneumococcal disease, including those children with significant chronic pulmonary disease.

Screening

- *Vision.* Routine screening is recommended unless daily high-dose corticosteroids are taken, which may result in cataracts or glaucoma, then referral to ophthalmologist is required for complete eye examination.
- *Hearing.* Routine screening is recommended.
- *Dental.* Routine screening is recommended.
- *Blood pressure.* Should be evaluated at each visit because of possible sympathetic stimulation from medications or corticosteroids.
- *Hematocrit.* Routine screening is recommended.
- *Urinalysis.* Routine screening is recommended unless daily doses of corticosteroids are taken, which may result in glycosuria. If glycosuria is present, refer to specialist for reevaluation of asthma management.
- *Tuberculosis.* Routine screening is recommended; should be screened for bone density after 12 years of age.

Condition-Specific Screening

- *Lung function tests.* Spirometry should be done at diagnosis, when major changes in treatment are contemplated, and routinely every 1 to 2 years in age-appropriate children, typically over 4 years.
  - PEFR testing in the home by the family should be advised for added assistance with decision making when poor symptom recognition exists or if the family/child finds the objective data helpful.
- *Theophylline levels.* Should be monitored with change in therapy, growth, and illness.
- *Allergic triggers.* Updated at each visit. Allergy testing may be indicated depending on history and therapy response.

Summary of Primary Care Needs for the Child with Asthma—cont'd

- *Bone density.* Children on high-dose ICSs or systemic corticosteroids should be screened for bone density after 12 years of age.

COMMON ILLNESS MANAGEMENT

- *Sinusitis.* May be confused with symptoms associated with asthma. May trigger asthma. Both sinusitis and allergic rhinitis should be treated.
- *Vocal cord dysfunction.* May mimic sound of wheeze but not associated with abnormal spirometry findings.
- *Drug interactions.* Total steroid use from topical, inhaled, and systemic steroids must be evaluated.

DEVELOPMENTAL ISSUES

Sleep Patterns

- Exacerbation may interfere with sleep.
- It is important to reduce environmental allergens in sleep area.
- If medications disturb sleep, an alternative regimen should be tried.

Toileting

- Toileting is routine.
- Few children experience enuresis while on theophylline.

Discipline

- Concern over discipline initiating asthma attack.
- Rewarding desirable behavior should be encouraged.
- The influence of medication and illness on behavior is often a concern of parents and needs discussion.
- Consistency of expectation is important.

Child Care

- Evaluate childcare environment for known or common triggers.
- Childcare workers must be provided with information on asthma triggers, early warning signs of asthma, a written action plan for treatment, emergency contacts, and medications used in day care.

Schooling

- Repeated school absences may interfere with academic performance.
- School personnel must be educated to evaluate child's symptoms and use of medications.
- School personnel need a written copy of the asthma action plan.
- Encourage participation in asthma education programs if available.
- Enhancing the child's strengths in all areas will support peer acceptance.
- Sports/activity participation should be encouraged.

Sexuality

- Sexual development may be delayed in severe cases or with prolonged corticosteroid use.
- Oral contraceptives may interfere with breakdown of theophylline.

Transition to Adulthood

- Begin plan for transitioning responsibilities of care throughout the child's life.
- Update knowledge and mature shared management roles.
- Inform new primary care provider.
- Discuss vocational issues.

FAMILY CONCERNS

- Familial nature of asthma may contribute to outdated beliefs of treatment.
- Parents may be ambivalent regarding long-term medication regimens.
- Smoking in home is detrimental to children with asthma. Parents who smoke need support and assistance in quitting.
- Ethnic minority and poverty have been linked with increased prevalence, morbidity, and mortality rates.
- System changes to improve access to care are necessary, especially for uninsured children.

Key: *GER,* gastroesophageal reflux; *ICS,* inhaled corticosteroid; *PEFR,* peak expiratory flow ate.

REFERENCES

Abramson, M.J., Puy, R.M., & Weiner, J.M. (2003). Allergen immunotherapy for asthma. *Cochrane Database Syst Rev* (4). CD001186.

Acun, C., Tomac, N., Ermis, B., et al. (2005). Effects of inhaled corticosteroids on growth in asthmatic children: A comparison of fluticasone propionate with budesonide. *Allergy Asthma Proc, 26*(3), 204-206.

Adams, S.K., Murdock, K.K., & McQuaid, E.L. (2007). Complementary and alternative medication (CAM) use and asthma outcomes in children: An urban perspective. *J Asthma, 44*(9), 775-782.

Agertoft, L., & Pedersen, S. (2000). Effects of long-term treatment with inhaled budesonide on adult height in children with asthma. *N Engl J Med, 343*(15), 1064-1069.

Alati, R., Al Mamun, A., O'Callaghan, M., et al. (2006). In utero and postnatal maternal smoking and asthma in adolescence. *Epidemiology, 17*(2), 138-144.

Allen, D.B. (2004). Systemic effects of inhaled corticosteroids in children. *Curr Opin Pediatr, 16*(4), 440-444.

Allen, D.B. (2006). Effects of inhaled steroids on growth, bone metabolism, and adrenal function. *Adv Pediatr, 53*, 101-110.

American Academy of Pediatrics. (2008a). *The National Center of Medical Home Initiatives for Children with Special Needs.* Available at www.medicalhomeinfo.org/tools/med_home.html. Retrieved April 21, 2008.

American Academy of Pediatrics. (2008b). *The red book.* Available at http://aapredbook.aappublications.org. Retrieved April 23, 2008.

Arbes, S.J., Jr., Sever, M.L., Vaughn, B., et al. (2006). Oral pathogens and allergic disease: Results from the Third National Health and Nutrition Examination Survey. *J Allergy Clin Immunol, 118*(5), 1169-1175.

Bacharier, L.B., Strunk, R.C., Mauger, D., et al. (2004). Classifying asthma severity in children: Mismatch between symptoms, medication use, and lung function. *Am J Respir Crit Care Med, 170*(4), 426-432.

Ball, T.M., Castro-Rodriguez, J.A., Griffith, K.A., et al. (2000). Siblings, day-care attendance, and the risk of asthma and wheezing during childhood. *N Engl J Med, 343*(8), 538-543.

Barbato, A., Turato, G., Baraldo, S., et al. (2003). Airway inflammation in childhood asthma. *Am J Respir Crit Care Med, 168*(7), 798-803.

Beausoleil, J., Fiedler, J., & Spergel, J. (2007). Food intolerance and childhood asthma: What is the link?. *Paediatr Drugs, 9*(3), 157-163.

Berger, W.E., Milgrom, H., Chervinsky, P., et al. (2006). Effects of treatment with mometasone furoate dry powder inhaler in children with persistent asthma. *Ann Allergy Asthma Immunol, 97*(5), 672-680.

Beuther, D.A., & Sutherland, E.R. (2007). Overweight, obesity, and incident asthma: A meta-analysis of prospective epidemiologic studies. *Am J Respir Crit Care Med, 175*(7), 661-666.

Beydon, N., Davis, S.D., Lombardi, E., et al. (2007). An official American Thoracic Society/European Respiratory Society statement: Pulmonary function testing in preschool children. *Am J Respir Crit Care Med, 175*(12), 1304-1345.

Bhogal, S., Zemek, R., & Ducharme, F. (2006). Written action plans for asthma in children. *Cochrane Database Syst Rev* (3), article number CD005306.

Bierbaum, S., & Heinzmann, A. (2007). The genetics of bronchial asthma in children. *Respir Med, 101*(7), 1369-1375.

Bisgaard, H., Zielen, S., Garcia-Garcia, M.L., et al. (2005). Montelukast reduces asthma exacerbations in 2- to 5-year-old children with intermittent asthma. *Am J Respir Crit Care Med, 171*(4), 315-322.

Bjerg, A., Hedman, L., Perzanowski, M.S., et al. (2007). Family history of asthma and atopy: In-depth analyses of the impact on asthma and wheeze in 7- to 8-year-old children. *Pediatrics, 120*(4), 741-748.

Bjermer, L. (2007). Time for a paradigm shift in asthma treatment: From relieving bronchospasm to controlling systemic inflammation. *J Allergy Clin Immunol, 120*(6), 1269-1275.

Bloom, B., & Cohen, R.A. (2007). Summary health statistics for U.S. children: National Health Interview Survey, 2006. *Vital Health Stat, 10*(234), 1-79.

Bonner, S., Zimmerman, B., Evans, D., et al. (2002). An individual intervention to improve asthma management among urban Latino and African-American families. *J Asthma, 39*(2), 167-179.

Bouzigon, E., Corda, E., Aschard, H., et al. (2008). Effect of 17q21 Variants and Smoking Exposure in Early-Onset Asthma. *N Engl J Med.* 2008 Oct 15. (Epub ahead of print.)

Bright Futures. (2007). *Bright Futures at Georgetown University.* Available at www.brightfutures.org/tools/index.html. Retrieved December 18, 2007.

Buchvald, F., Baraldi, E., Carraro, S., et al. (2005). Measurements of exhaled nitric oxide in healthy subjects age 4 to 17 years. *J Allergy Clin Immunol, 115*(6), 1130-1136.

Buck, M., Hofer, K., & McCarthy, M. (2007). Omalizumab for the management of refractory allergic asthma in children. *Pediatr Pharmocother, 13*(6).

Butland, B.K., & Strachan, D.P. (2007). Asthma onset and relapse in adult life: The British 1958 birth cohort study. *Ann Allergy Asthma Immunol, 98*(4), 337-343.

Cabana, M.D., Slish, K.K., Nan, B., et al. (2005). Asking the correct questions to assess asthma symptoms. *Clin Pediatr (Phila), 44*(4), 319-325.

Cabral, A.L., Conceicao, G.M., Saldiva, P.H., et al. (2002). Effect of asthma severity on symptom perception in childhood asthma. *Braz J Med Biol Res, 35*(3), 319-327.

Campo, P., Kalra, H.K., Levin, L., et al. (2006). Influence of dog ownership and high endotoxin on wheezing and atopy during infancy. *J Allergy Clin Immunol, 118*(6), 1271-1278.

Cates, C.J., Bestall, J., & Adams, N. (2006). Holding chambers versus nebulisers for inhaled steroids in chronic asthma. *Cochrane Database Syst Rev* (1), CD001491.

Chugh, I.M., Khanna, P., & Shah, A. (2006). Nocturnal symptoms and sleep disturbances in clinically stable asthmatic children. *Asian Pac J Allergy Immunol, 24*(2-3), 135-142.

Clark, N.M., Brown, R., Joseph, C.L., et al. (2004). Effects of a comprehensive school-based asthma program on symptoms, parent management, grades, and absenteeism. *Chest, 125*(5), 1674-1679.

Cohn, L., Elias, J.A., & Chupp, G.L. (2004). Asthma: Mechanisms of disease persistence and progression. *Ann Rev Immunol, 22*, 789-815.

Corren, J., Manning, B.E., Thompson, S.F., et al. (2004). Rhinitis therapy and the prevention of hospital care for asthma: A case-control study. *J Allergy Clin Immunol, 113*(3), 415-419.

Couriel, J., & Child, F. (2004). Applied physiology: Lung function testing in children. *Curr Paediatr, 14*(5), 444-451.

Cowen, M.K., Wakefield, D.B., & Cloutier, M.M. (2007). Classifying asthma severity: Objective versus subjective measures. *J Asthma, 44*(9), 711-715.

Debley, J.S., Carter, E.R., Gibson, R.L., et al. (2005). The prevalence of ibuprofen-sensitive asthma in children: A randomized controlled bronchoprovocation challenge study. *J Pediatr, 147*(2), 233-238.

Diamant, Z., Boot, J.D., & Virchow, J.C. (2007). Summing up 100 years of asthma. *Respir Med, 101*(3), 378-388.

Din-Dzietham, R., Liu, Y., Bielo, M., et al. (2007). High blood pressure trends in children and adolescents in national surveys, 1963 to 2002. *Circulation, 116*(13), 1488-1496.

Douglass, J.A., & O'Hehir, R.E. (2006). 1. Diagnosis, treatment and prevention of allergic disease: The basics. *Med J Aust, 185*(4), 228-233.

Drotar, D., Stancin, T., Dworkin, P.H., et al. (2008). Selecting developmental surveillance and screening tools. *Pediatr Rev, 29*(10), e52-e58.

Ducharme, F.M. (2004). Inhaled corticosteroids versus leukotriene antagonists as first-line therapy for asthma: A systematic review of current evidence. *Treat Respir Med, 3*(6), 399-405.

Ducharme, F.M., Chabot, G., Polychronakos, C., et al. (2003). Safety profile of frequent short courses of oral glucocorticoids in acute pediatric asthma: Impact on bone metabolism, bone density, and adrenal function. *Pediatrics, 111*(2), 376-383.

Eder, W., Ege, M.J., & von Mutius, E. (2006). The asthma epidemic. *N Engl J Med, 355*(21), 2226-2235.

Erickson, S.E., Iribarren, C., Tolstykh, I.V., et al. (2007). Effect of race on asthma management and outcomes in a large, integrated managed care organization. *Arch Intern Med, 167*(17), 1846-1852.

Esnault, S., Fang, Y., Kelly, E., et al. (2007). Circadian changes in granulocyte-macrophage colony-stimulating factor message in circulating eosinophils. *Ann Allergy Asthma Immunol, 98*(1), 75-82.

Expert Panel Report 3 (EPR-3). (2007). EPR-3: Guidelines for the diagnosis and management of asthma—summary report 2007. *J Allergy Clin Immunol, 120*(5 Suppl), S94-S138.

Faber, A., & Mazlish, E. (2002). *How To Talk So Kids Will Listen and Listen So Kids Will Talk.* New York: Quill Publishing.

Ferguson, A., Van Bever, H., Teper, A., et al. (2007). A comparison of the relative growth velocities with budesonide and fluticasone propionate in children with asthma. *Respir Med, 101*(1), 118-129.

Frei, J., Jutla, J., Kramer, G., et al. (2005). Impulse oscillometry: Reference values in children 100 to 150 cm in height and 3 to 10 years of age. *Chest, 128*(3), 1266-1273.

Furrie, E. (2005). Probiotics and allergy. *Proc Nutr Soc, 64*(4), 465-469.

Galant, S.P., Morphew, T., Amaro, S., et al. (2007). Value of the bronchodilator response in assessing controller naive asthmatic children. *J Pediatr, 151*(5), 457-462.

Glascoe, F., & Robertshaw, N. (2007). New AAP policy on detecting and addressing developmental and behavioral problems. *J Pediatr Health Care, 21*(6), 407-412.

Greek, A.A., Kieckhefer, G.M., Kim, H., et al. (2006). Family perceptions of the usual source of care among children with asthma by race/ethnicity, language, and family income. *J Asthma, 43*(1), 61-69.

Guevara, J.P., Wolf, F.M., Grum, C.M., et al. (2003). Effects of educational interventions for self management of asthma in children and adolescents: Systematic review and meta-analysis. *Br Med J, 326*(7402), 1308-1309.

Guilbert, T.W., Morgan, W.J., Zeiger, R.S., et al. (2006). Long-term inhaled corticosteroids in preschool children at high risk for asthma. *N Engl J Med, 354*(19). 1985-1997.

Gustafsson, P.M., Watson, L., Davis, K.J., et al. (2006). Poor asthma control in children: Evidence from epidemiological surveys and implications for clinical practice. *Int J Clin Pract, 60*(3), 321-334.

Hallstrand, T., Curtis, J., Aitken, M., et al. (2003). Quality of life in adolescents with mild asthma. *Pediatr Pulmonol, 36*(6), 536-543.

Hallstrand, T.S., Moody, M.W., Wurfel, M.M., et al. (2005). Inflammatory basis of exercise-induced bronchoconstriction. *Am J Respir Crit Care Med, 172*(6), 679-686.

Hansel, T.T., Benezet, O., Kafe, H., et al. (2006). A multinational, 12-week, randomized study comparing the efficacy and tolerability of ciclesonide and budesonide in patients with asthma. *Clin Ther, 28*(6), 906-920.

Hasan, R.A., Zureikat, G.Y., Nolan, B.M., et al. (2006). The relationship between asthma and overweight in urban minority children. *J Natl Med Assoc, 98*(2), 138-42.

Hoffjan, S., Nicolae, D., Ostrovnaya, I., et al. (2005). Gene-environment interaction effects on the development of immune responses in the 1st year of life. *Am J Hum Genet, 76*(4), 696-704.

Holgate, S.T., & Polosa, R. (2006). The mechanisms, diagnosis, and management of severe asthma in adults. *Lancet, 368*(9537), 780-793.

Holgate, S.T., Price, D., & Valovirta, E. (2006). Asthma out of control? A structured review of recent patient surveys. *BMC Pulm Med, 6*(Suppl 1), S2.

Illi, S., von Mutius, E., Lau, S., et al. (2006). Perennial allergen sensitisation early in life and chronic asthma in children: A birth cohort study. *Lancet, 368*(9537), 763-770.

Israel, E., Chinchilli, V.M., Ford, J.G., et al. (2004). Use of regularly scheduled albuterol treatment in asthma: Genotype-stratified, randomised, placebo-controlled cross-over trial. *Lancet, 364*(9444), 1505-1512.

Johnson, S.R., Marion, A.A., Vrchoticky, T., et al. (2006). Cushing syndrome with secondary adrenal insufficiency from concomitant therapy with ritonavir and fluticasone. *J Pediatr, 148*(3), 386-388.

Kelly, H.W., Van Natta, M.L., Covar, R.A., et al. CAMP Strunk Research Group. (2008). Effect of long-term corticosteroid use on bone mineral density in children: A prospective longitudinal assessment in the Childhood Asthma Management Program (CAMP) study. *Pediatrics, 122*(1), e53-e61.

Khoshoo, V., & Haydel, R., Jr. (2007). Effect of antireflux treatment on asthma exacerbations in nonatopic children. *J Pediatr Gastroenterol Nutr, 44*(3), 331-335.

Kieckhefer, G.M., Greek, A.A., Joesch, J.M., et al. (2005). Presence and characteristics of medical home and health services utilization among children with asthma. *J Pediatr Health Care, 19*(5), 285-292.

Kieckhefer, G., & Lentz, M. (2006). Nocturnal asthma in children. *Nurse Pract, 14*(1), 53-56.

Kieckhefer, G.M., & Ratcliffe, M. (2000). What parents of children with asthma tell us. *J Pediatr Health Care, 14*(3), 122-126.

Kieckhefer, G.M., & Trahms, C.M. (2000). Supporting development of children with chronic conditions: From compliance toward shared management. *Pediatr Nurs, 26*(4), 354-363.

Koh, M.S., & Irving, L.B. (2007). The natural history of asthma from childhood to adulthood. *Int J Clin Pract, 61*(8), 1371-1374.

Larsen, G.L., Kang, J.K., Guilbert, T., et al. (2005). Assessing respiratory function in young children: Developmental considerations. *J Allergy Clin Immunol, 115*(4), 657-666; quiz 667.

Levensky, E.R., Forcehimes, A., O'Donohue, W.T., et al. (2007). Motivational interviewing: An evidence-based approach to counseling helps patients follow treatment recommendations. *Am J Nurs, 107*(10), 50-58; quiz 58-59.

Liu, A.H. (2007). Hygiene theory and allergy and asthma prevention. *Paediatr Perinat Epidemiol, 21*(Suppl 3), 2-7.

Ly, N.P., Gold, D.R., Weiss, S.T., et al. (2006). Recurrent wheeze in early childhood and asthma among children at risk for atopy. *Pediatrics, 117*(6), e1132-e1138.

Martinez, F.D. (2003). Toward asthma prevention—Does all that really matters happen before we learn to read? *N Engl J Med, 349*(15), 1473-1475.

Martinez, F.D. (2007). Asthma treatment and asthma prevention: A tale of 2 parallel pathways. *J Allergy Clin Immunol, 119*(1), 30-33.

Martinez, F.D., Wright, A.L., Taussig, L.M., et al. (1995). Asthma and wheezing in the first six years of life. The Group Health Medical Associates. *N Engl J Med, 332*(3), 133-138.

Mayo Clinic. (2008). Tools for healthier lives. Available at www.mayoclinic.com/health/asthma/MM00399. Retrieved April 21, 2008.

McLeish, S., & Turner, S.W. (2007). Gene-environment interactions in asthma. *Arch Dis Child, 92*(11), 1032-1035.

Melton, L.J., III, Patel, A., Achenbach, S.J., et al. (2005). Long-term fracture risk among children with asthma: A population-based study. *J Bone Miner Res, 20*(4), 564-570.

Micromedex. (2008). Available at www.micromedex.com. Retrieved April 23, 2008.

Miller, M.G., Weiler, J.M., Baker, R., et al. (2005). National Athletic Trainers' Association position statement: Management of asthma in athletes. *J Athl Train, 40*(3), 224-245.

Milton, B., Whitehead, M., Holland, P., et al. (2004). The social and economic consequences of childhood asthma across the lifecourse: A systematic review. *Child Care Health Dev, 30*(6), 711-728.

Minai, B., Martin, J., & Cohn, R. (2004). Results of a physician and respiratory therapist collaborative effort to improve long-term metered-dose inhaler technique in a pediatric asthma clinic. *Respir Care, 49*(6), 600-605.

Moonie, S.A., Sterling, D.A., Figgs, L., et al. (2006). Asthma status and severity affects missed school days. *J Sch Health, 76*(1), 18-24.

Moorman, J.E., Rudd, R.A., Johnson, C.A., et al. (2007). National surveillance for asthma—United States, 1980-2004. *MMWR Surveill Summ, 56*(8), 1-54.

Morgan, W.J., Stern, D.A., Sherrill, D.L., et al. (2005). Outcome of asthma and wheezing in the first 6 years of life: Follow-up through adolescence. *Am J Respir Crit Care Med, 172*(10), 1253-1258.

Mosnaim, G., Kohrman, C., Sharp, L.K., et al. (2006). Coping with asthma in immigrant Hispanic families: A focus group study. *Ann Allergy Asthma Immunol, 97*(4), 477-483.

Murray, C.S., Woodcock, A., Langley, S.J., et al. (2006). Secondary prevention of asthma by the use of Inhaled Fluticasone propionate in Wheezy INfants (IFWIN): Double-blind, randomised, controlled study. *Lancet, 368*(9537), 754-762.

National Association of Pediatric Nurse Practitioners. (2008). NAPNAP position statement on access to care. Available at http://download.journals.elsevierhealth.com/pdfs/journals/0891-5245/PIIS0891524506006936.pdf. Retrieved April 21, 2008.

National Institutes of Health. (2004a). *Strategic plan and budget to reduce and ultimately eliminate health disparities.* Vol. 1: Fiscal years 2002-2006 (NIH 2004). Available at www.nih.gov. Retrieved October 30, 2008.

Nelson, H.S., Weiss, S.T., Bleecker, E.R., et al. (2006). The Salmeterol Multicenter Asthma Research Trial: A comparison of usual pharmacotherapy for asthma or usual pharmacotherapy plus salmeterol. *Chest, 129*(1), 15-26.

Noyes, B.E., & Kemp, J.S. (2007). Vocal cord dysfunction in children. *Paediatr Respir Rev, 8*(2), 155-163.

O'Hallaren, M. (2002). Exercise induced asthma. In. R. Slavin & R. Reisman (Eds.), *Asthma.* Philadelphia: American College of Physicians.

Ober, C. (2005). Perspectives on the past decade of asthma genetics. *J Allergy Clin Immunol, 116*(2), 274-278.

Opat, A., Cohen, M., Bailey, M., et al. (2000). A clinical trial of the Buteyko breathing technique in asthma as taught by video. *J Asthma, 37*(7), 557-564.

Ortega, A.N., Huertas, S.E., Canino, G., et al. (2002). Childhood asthma, chronic illness, and psychiatric disorders. *J Nerv Ment Dis, 190*(5), 275-281.

Ostrom, N.K., Decotiis, B.A., Lincourt, W.R., et al. (2005). Comparative efficacy and safety of low-dose fluticasone propionate and montelukast in children with persistent asthma. *J Pediatr, 147*(2), 213-220.

Panitch, H.B. (2007). The relationship between early respiratory viral infections and subsequent wheezing and asthma. *Clin Pediatr (Phila), 46*(5), 392-400.

Pattenden, S., Antova, T., Neuberger, M., et al. (2006). Parental smoking and children's respiratory health: Independent effects of prenatal and postnatal exposure. *Tob Control, 15*(4), 294-301.

Perez-Yarza, E.G., Moreno, A., Lazaro, P., et al. (2007). The association between respiratory syncytial virus infection and the development of childhood asthma: A systematic review of the literature. *Pediatr Infect Dis J, 26*(8), 733-739.

Perkin, M.R., & Strachan, D.P. (2006). Which aspects of the farming lifestyle explain the inverse association with childhood allergy? *J Allergy Clin Immunol, 117*(6), 1374-1381.

Pijnenburg, M.W., Bakker, E.M., Hop, W.C., et al. (2005). Titrating steroids on exhaled nitric oxide in children with asthma: A randomized controlled trial. *Am J Respir Crit Care Med, 172*(7), 831-836.

Rabe, K.F., Atienza, T., Magyar, P., et al. (2006). Effect of budesonide in combination with formoterol for reliever therapy in asthma exacerbations: A randomised controlled, double-blind study. *Lancet, 368*(9537), 744-753.

Sabina, I., Von Mutius, E., Lau, S., et al. (2001). Early childhood infectious diseases and the development of asthma up to school age: A birth cohort study. *Br Med J, 322*, 390-395.

Sadeh, A., Gruber, R., & Raviv, A. (2003). The effects of sleep restriction and extension on school-age children: What a difference an hour makes. *Child Dev, 74*(2), 444-455.

Samaras, K., Pett, S., Gowers, A., et al. (2005). Iatrogenic Cushing's syndrome with osteoporosis and secondary adrenal failure in human immunodeficiency virus-infected patients receiving inhaled corticosteroids and ritonavir-boosted protease inhibitors: Six cases. *J Clin Endocrinol Metab, 90*(7), 4394-4398.

Sandrini, A., Ferreira, I.M., Jardim, J.R., et al. (2003). Effect of nasal triamcinolone acetonide on lower airway inflammatory markers in patients with allergic rhinitis. *J Allergy Clin Immunol, 111*(2), 313-320.

Seddon, P., Bara, A., Ducharme, F., et al. (2006). Oral xanthines as maintenance treatment for asthma in children. *Cochrane Database Syst Rev* (1), CD002885.

Shaw, A., Thompson, E., & Sharp, D. (2006). Complementary therapy use by patients and parents of children with asthma and the implications for NHS care: A qualitative study. *BMC Health Serv Res, 6*, 76.

Singh, A.M., Moore, P.E., & Gern, J.E., et al. (2007). Bronchiolitis to asthma: A review and call for studies of gene-virus interactions in asthma causation. *Am J Respir Crit Care Med, 175*(2), 108-119.

Sly, P.D., Boner, A.L., Björksten, B., et al. (2008). Early identification of atopy in the prediction of persistent asthma in children. *Lancet, 372*(9643), 1100-1106.

Story, R.E. (2007). Asthma and obesity in children. *Curr Opin Pediatr, 19*(6), 680-684.

Svavarsdottir, E.K., Rayens, M.K., & McCubbin, M. (2005). Predictors of adaptation in Icelandic and American families of young children with chronic asthma. *Fam Community Health, 28*(4), 338-350.

Taylor, D.R., Cowan, J.O., Greene, J.M., et al. (2005). Asthma in remission: Can relapse in early adulthood be predicted at 18 years of age?. *Chest, 127*(3), 845-850.

Toelle, B.G., Xuan, W., Peat, J.K., et al. (2004). Childhood factors that predict asthma in young adulthood. *Eur Respir J, 23*(1), 66-70.

Tootla, R., Toumba, K.J., & Duggal, M.S. (2004). An evaluation of the acidogenic potential of asthma inhalers. *Arch Oral Biol, 49*(4), 275-283.

U.S. Food and Drug Administration. (2008). *Protecting and promoting your health.* Available at www.fda.gov. Retrieved April 21, 2008.

Vonk, J.M., & Boezen, H.M. (2006). Predicting adult asthma in childhood. *Curr Opin Pulm Med, 12*(1), 42-47.

Walders, N., Kercsmar, C., Schluchter, M., et al. (2006). An interdisciplinary intervention for undertreated pediatric asthma. *Chest, 129*(2), 292-299.

Wang, X., Dockery, D.W., Wypij, D., et al. (1993). Pulmonary function between 6 and 18 years of age. *Pediatr Pulmonol, 15*(2), 75-88.

Weiler, J.M., Bonini, S., Coifman, R., et al. (2007). American Academy of Allergy, Asthma and Immunology Work Group report: Exercise-induced asthma. *J Allergy Clin Immunol, 119*(6), 1349-1358.

Weinberger, M., & Abu-Hasan, M. (2007). Pseudo-asthma: When cough, wheezing, and dyspnea are not asthma. *Pediatrics, 120*(4), 855-864.

Welsh, L., Kemp, J.G., & Roberts, R.G. (2005). Effects of physical conditioning on children and adolescents with asthma. *Sports Med, 35*(2), 127-141.

Wenzel, S.E. (2006). Asthma: Defining of the persistent adult phenotypes. *Lancet, 368*(9537), 804-813.

Wolf, F.M., Guevara, J.P., Grum, C.M., et al. (2003). Educational interventions for asthma in children. *Cochrane Database Syst Rev* (1), CD000326.

Xepapadaki, P., & Papadopoulos, N.G. (2007). Viral infections and allergies. *Immunobiology, 212*(6), 453-459.

Zeiger, R.S., Szefler, S.J., Phillips, B.R., et al. (2006). Response profiles to fluticasone and montelukast in mild-to-moderate persistent childhood asthma. *J Allergy Clin Immunol, 117*(1), 45-52.

Zollner, E.W. (2007). Hypothalamic-pituitary-adrenal axis suppression in asthmatic children on inhaled corticosteroids (part 2)—The risk as determined by gold standard adrenal function tests: A systematic review. *Pediatr Allergy Immunol, 18*(6), 469-474.

Zoumalan, R., Maddalozzo, J., & Holinger, L.D. (2007). Etiology of stridor in infants. *Ann Otol Rhinol Laryngol, 116*(5), 329-334.

12 Attention-Deficit/Hyperactivity Disorder

Janice Selekman

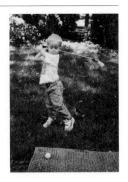

Etiology

Attention-deficit/hyperactivity disorder (ADHD) was identified as a condition in 1902, although it was described in a German nursery rhyme, "Fidgety Phil," in 1865 (Barkley, 2006). The current diagnosis of ADHD has been preceded by many other labels, including brain damaged, minimal brain dysfunction, hyperactive child syndrome, hyperkinetic disorder of childhood, and attention-deficit disorder with and without hyperactivity.

The definition of ADHD also continues to evolve; it is currently defined by the *Diagnostic and Statistical Manual of Mental Disorders IV–Text Revised (DSM-IV-TR)* as a "persistent pattern of inattention and/or hyperactivity-impulsivity that is more frequent and severe than is typically observed in individuals at a comparable level of development" (American Psychiatric Association [APA], 2000, p. 85).

This disorder is intrinsic to an individual and presumed to be the result of central nervous system (CNS) dysfunction. Even though ADHD can occur with other disabling conditions (e.g., sensory impairment, intellectual disability, serious psychosocial and emotional disturbances) or extrinsic influences (e.g., insufficient or inappropriate instruction or parenting), it is not the direct result of those conditions or influences. ADHD is a nonprogressive, highly heterogeneous, neurologic condition.

The causes and the exact mechanisms involved remain unknown, although multiple areas are under investigation. The primary contributors to ADHD appear to be neurologic and genetic. The proposed neurologic causes being explored are neurobiologic and neuroanatomic. The neurobiologic hypothesis focuses on the imbalance and dysregulation of neurotransmitters—especially catecholamines (dopamine, norepinephrine, and possibly serotonin) (Kieling, Goncalves, Tannock, et al., 2008). It is believed that there is a deficit in catecholaminergic neurotransmission resulting in not enough catecholamine being available to hold onto a task, such as attention (Solanto, 2001). Because most of the medications with proven efficacy for ADHD stimulate receptors to increase dopamine release and inhibit reuptake of neurotransmitters, deficits in this system seem to be supported as one of the primary causes of ADHD.

The neuroanatomic research attempts to identify structural anomalies of, or damage to, the brains of children with ADHD. The prefrontal cortex is rich in dopamine receptors and is therefore the subject of much exploration. In some studies using neurologic scanning techniques, it appears that the right prefrontal cortex and parts of the cerebellum are about 5% smaller, on average, in children with ADHD, with decreased blood flow to, and decreased electrical activity in, the area compared with those without the disorder (Barkley, 2006; Kieling et al., 2008; Nigg, 2006). The blood flow deficits appear to be reversed following administration of stimulant medication (Anastopoulos & Shelton, 2001). The right prefrontal cortex is involved in inhibiting behavior and sustaining attention; it is also the site where the coordination of complex planned behavior occurs, as well as emotional control, social judgment, and the ability to override inappropriate responses (Nigg, 2006). The identified areas of the cerebellum are responsible for allowing the cortex time to process stimuli and coordinate input among the regions of the cortex. The research findings, although potentially helpful from an etiologic aspect, are not useful tools for diagnosis in individuals at this time.

It is recognized that there are specific conditions that can result in the symptoms of ADHD. Brain damage can occur as a result of brain infections, hypoxic or anoxic episodes, or trauma; approximately 20% of this population, especially those with damage to the prefrontal cortex, develops impulsivity and inattention (Jensen, 2000). In the history of ADHD, the first cases were described following cases of encephalitis. Premature birth is another risk factor for the symptoms of ADHD, especially for infants weighing less than 2.2 lb (1 kg) at birth, who are at a greater risk of developing impulsivity and have trouble with concentration and with social interactions (Kieling et al., 2008). Children who underwent cardiac surgery as newborns for cardiac anomalies have a higher risk of ADHD during the school-age years (Shillingford, Glanzman, Ittenbach, et al., 2008). Maternal alcohol and tobacco use during pregnancy, as well as fetal exposure to other substances of abuse, especially crack cocaine, has also been correlated with the development of alterations in behavior and attention. Nicotinic acetylcholine plays a major role in brain development and nicotine binds to those receptors. This results in a "twofold increase in the risk for ADHD diagnosis in those individuals whose mothers smoked during pregnancy" (Kieling et al., 2008, p. 288) and a 2.5 times increase if the mothers drank alcohol during their pregnancy. Exposure to high levels of lead in young children can also result in the development of hyperactivity and inattention (Kieling et al., 2008). Questions have been raised as to whether these conditions actually *cause* ADHD or are merely associated with it. There is no evidence that the various child-rearing practices cause ADHD (Pliszka & American Academy of Child and Adolescent Psychiatry [AACAP] Work Group on Quality Issues, 2007).

Barkley (2006) has proposed that ADHD is not a disorder of attention but rather a defect or delay in response inhibition that results in difficulty "self-regulating" one's impulsive motor behavior.

Consequently, one becomes hyperresponsive to stimuli, and hyperactivity results. This neurologic defect in inhibition and self-control leads to alterations in an individual's ability to carry out executive functions (e.g., deflecting distractions, recalling goals by using hindsight and using problem solving to reach them by using forethought). It also includes changes in the ability to follow rules, control emotions and behaviors, and exhibit flexibility. This lack of self-regulation interferes with one's ability to inhibit a response that has not yet started, stop one in progress, and prevent interference by extraneous stimuli (Solanto, 2001).

ADHD is considered to be "among the most heritable of psychiatric disorders" (Mick & Faraone, 2008, p. 262), with a heritability estimate of 76% and a range of 60% to 91% (Kieling et al., 2008). The idea of genetic predisposition is supported for ADHD in a significant number of cases. Genetic studies with twins have suggested that the condition is polygenic, with eight different genes implicated (Pliszka & AACAP Work Group on Quality Issues, 2007). There is an 81% concordance rate for monozygotic twins and a 29% concordance rate for dizygotic twins (Barkley, 2006). Siblings of a child with ADHD have up to a 32% chance of also having ADHD. In the twin studies, the effect of a "shared environment" does not help explain the differences seen among children in the same family (Barkley, 2006).

Because of the belief that the symptoms of ADHD are due to pathophysiology of the neurotransmitters and their receptors, investigators are studying the genes that encode for these transmitters and their receptors, as well as the neurocircuitry of the frontal lobe. Research on the dopamine receptor gene on chromosome 11 *(DRD4)* demonstrated a number of sections that repeat themselves, leading to an increased association with the incidence of ADHD (Mick & Faraone, 2008). It is hypothesized that the increased number of repeats may result in a rapid turnover of dopamine at the synapse, leading to a greater increase in the hyperactive-impulsive type of ADHD (Solanto, 2001). Other genes being investigated are the dopamine receptor genes *(DRD2, DRD5),* the dopamine transporter gene on chromosome 5 *(DAT1),* and the genes that regulate the dopamine pathways that direct neural activity in the frontal basal ganglia (Mick & Faraone, 2008; Pliszka & AACAP Work Group on Quality Issues, 2007). "DAT1 is important in reuptake of dopamine at the synapse, which in turn is important for regulating dopamine neural transmission" (Nigg, 2006, p. 205). The D4 receptor is prevalent in the frontal lobe, which is the part of the brain implicated in ADHD (Mick & Faraone, 2008). It is unlikely that any one gene is responsible for the majority of cases of ADHD. The bottom line is that ADHD probably is caused by multiple genes interacting with factors in the environment, especially during pregnancy and shortly after delivery (Kieling et al., 2008).

Incidence and Prevalence

ADHD is one of the most common psychiatric disorders seen in childhood (Mick & Faraone, 2008). As the diagnostic criteria have changed over time, so have the prevalence rates. Estimates of the number of children with ADHD range from 2% to 26%, with the international prevalence rate ranging from 5.23% to 12% (Mick & Faraone, 2008; Polanczyk & Jensen, 2008). According to the Centers for Disease Control and Prevention, "the rate of lifetime childhood diagnosis of ADHD was 7.8%, whereas 4.3% (or only 55% of those with ADHD) had ever been treated with medication for

the disorder" (Pliszka & AACAP Work Group on Quality Issues, 2007, p. 895). Froehlich, Lanphear, Epstein, and colleagues (2007) surveyed over 3000 children between ages 8 and 15 and found the prevalence to be 8.7%, and the National Adolescent Health Information Center indicates that 8.9% of 12- to 17-year-olds have ADHD (Knopf, Park, & Mulye, 2008). Because of the differences in the *DSM-IV-TR* and the World Health Organization's International Classification of Diseases, 10th edition (ICD-10) diagnostic criteria, those using *DSM-IV-TR* criteria generally have higher prevalence rates than those using ICD-10. When functional impairment is required for the diagnosis, the prevalence rates are lower (Polanczyk & Jensen, 2008).

Two percent to 6% of preschool-age children meet the criteria for ADHD (Greenhill, Posner, Vaughan, et al., 2008). In 2000, it was estimated that 3% to 5% of the school-age population had ADHD; that number is now thought to be between 6% and 12% of those between 5 and 13 years of age. From 60% to 85% of children with ADHD will continue to meet the criteria for ADHD during their adolescence (Pliszka & AACAP Work Group on Quality Issues, 2007). This means that 4.5 million children in the United States between ages 3 and 17 have ADHD (U.S. Department of Health and Human Services, 2007).

The prevalence of ADHD appears to peak around age 9 and then decreases somewhat over time (Kieling et al., 2008), perhaps because of symptomatology that is less well defined for the teenager. The rate of ADHD appears to decline in adulthood, with the prevalence of ADHD in adults estimated to be 4.4% (Pliszka & AACAP Work Group on Quality Issues, 2007). This decline may be tied to the reduction in available diagnostic and treatment services.

More boys than girls have been diagnosed with ADHD. This is thought to be due to the fact that more males have noticeable signs of hyperactivity and more females exhibit symptoms consistent with the inattentive type of ADHD, leading to a delayed or missed diagnosis. Although the ratios differ by the setting, the general ratio of males to females with this condition is approximately 2.4:1, with an average of 11.3% of males having ADHD compared with 5.4% of females (Polanczyk & Jensen, 2008). Approximately 4.4% of children meet the criteria for the inattentive type of ADHD; 2% meet the criteria for the hyperactive-impulsive type of ADHD; and 2.2% meet the criteria for the combined type (Froehlich et al., 2007).

Diagnostic Criteria

The current subtypes of ADHD are the predominantly inattentive type (ADHD-I), the predominantly hyperactive-impulsive type (ADHD-H/I), and the combined type (inattentive, hyperactive, and impulsive) (ADHD-C) (APA, 2000). According to the *DSM-IV-TR,* for an individual to be labeled ADHD predominantly inattentive, at least six of the nine symptoms must have persisted for at least 6 months (Box 12-1). For ADHD predominantly hyperactive-impulsive, at least six of the nine characteristics in that category must have persisted for at least 6 months. A diagnosis of the combined type requires at least six symptoms from each of the sets of categories. Regardless of the type of ADHD, some symptoms must have been present before age 7 years (APA, 2000). The criteria have been found to be valid for children as young as 3 years (Kieling et al., 2008). In a practical sense, any child who is experiencing significant dysfunction across settings should be evaluated further.

BOX 12-1

Diagnostic Criteria for Attention-Deficit/Hyperactivity Disorder

A. Either (1) OR (2):

(1) Six (or more) of the following symptoms of inattention have persisted for at least 6 mo to a degree that is maladaptive and inconsistent with developmental level

Inattention:

a. Often fails to give close attention to details or makes careless mistakes in school work, work, or other activities

b. Often has difficulty sustaining attention in tasks or play activities

c. Often does not seem to listen when spoken to directly

d. Often does not follow through on instructions and fails to finish school work, chores, or duties in the workplace (not because of oppositional behavior or failure to understand instructions)

e. Often has difficulty organizing tasks and activities

f. Often avoids, dislikes, or is reluctant to engage in tasks that require sustained mental effort (e.g., school work or homework)

g. Often loses things necessary for tasks or activities (e.g., toys, school assignments, pencils, books, tools)

h. Is often easily distracted by extraneous stimuli

i. Is often forgetful in daily activities

(2) Six (or more) of the following symptoms of hyperactivity-impulsivity have persisted for at least 6 mo to a degree that is maladaptive and inconsistent with developmental level

Hyperactivity:

a. Often fidgets with hands or feet or squirms in seat

b. Often leaves seat in classroom or in other situations in which remaining seated is expected

c. Often runs about or climbs excessively in situations in which it is inappropriate (in adolescents or adults, may be limited to subjective feelings of restlessness)

d. Often has difficulty playing or engaging in leisure activities quietly

e. Is often "on the go" or often acts "as if driven by a motor"

f. Often talks excessively

Impulsivity:

g. Often blurts out answers before questions have been completed

h. Often has difficulty awaiting turn

i. Often interrupts or intrudes on others (e.g., butts into conversations or games)

B. Some hyperactive-impulsive or inattentive symptoms that caused impairment present before age 7 yr

C. Some impairment from the symptoms present in two or more settings (e.g., at school or work and at home)

D. Clear evidence of clinically significant impairment in social, academic, or occupational functioning

E. Symptoms do not occur exclusively during the course of a pervasive developmental disorder, schizophrenia, or other psychotic disorder and are not better accounted for by another mental disorder (e.g., mood disorder, anxiety disorder, dissociative disorder, personality disorder)

From American Psychiatric Association. (2000). *Diagnostic and Statistical Manual of Mental Disorders* (4th ed., Text Revision). Washington; DC: Author. Reprinted with permission.

The *DSM-IV-TR* (APA, 2000) changed the wording of the symptomatology to better address symptoms experienced or observed in preschoolers as well as in adolescents or adults with ADHD. Some controversy has been raised regarding the DSM-IV-TR age-of-onset criterion of 7 years for ADHD, particularly in light of the increasing interest in diagnosis of adolescents and adults with ADHD. Diagnostic issues include the following: (1) the validity of historical recollection and self-report of symptoms; (2) the later awareness of impairment, especially with the predominantly inattentive subtype of ADHD; (3) the problem of separating out symptoms of frequent comorbid disorders in adolescents and adults with ADHD; and (4) the fact that an onset before age 7 years was selected without empiric field trials. The individual who cannot document symptoms of ADHD before age 7 years but who does meet the criteria at the time of diagnosis is usually labeled *ADHD—Not Otherwise Specified* (APA, 2000). It is important to note that all children under age 7 years are likely to manifest some of the behaviors associated with ADHD at times as part of the normal developmental process.

Diagnostic Measures

The American Academy of Child and Adolescent Psychiatry (AACAP) recommends that screening for ADHD should be part of every child's mental health assessment (Pliszka & AACAP Work Group on Quality Issues, 2007). Because no gold standard exists, no one test or tool can diagnose a child as having ADHD. Therefore a diagnosis of ADHD must be viewed with caution. The primary care provider (PCP) needs to know which criteria were used to make the diagnosis and which differential diagnoses were ruled out. Multiple data sources collected over time should have been used to make the diagnosis. These sources include the following: (1) family history; (2) perinatal history; (3) developmental history with current developmental assessment; (4) assessment of past and current temperament of the child; (5) health history; (6) assessment of academic performance; (7) any history of physical or psychological trauma the child may have experienced; (8) current stressors; (9) comprehensive age-appropriate psychological and intelligence testing, and (10) comprehensive physical assessment with an emphasis on neurologic and motor abilities. According to expert opinion, there is no need for laboratory or neurologic testing if the child's health history is unremarkable (Pliszka & AACAP Work Group on Quality Issues, 2007).

Evidence must be directly obtained from parents or caregivers and the children themselves regarding the symptoms displayed in various settings, the age of onset, and the duration and frequency of the symptoms. It is important to distinguish the presence of symptoms from the presence of impairment (Pliszka & AACAP Work Group on Quality Issues, 2007). Evidence should also be provided by the classroom teacher or other school personnel. Although it is helpful for a clinician to observe a child's performance and behavior in structured and unstructured activities, it is usually not realistic. Whereas these criteria are used for diagnostic purposes, the same criteria are also used to monitor the child's response to treatment regimens. Therefore it is important for the PCP to be familiar with them.

A variety of behavior rating scales (Table 12-1) can be used by parents and teachers for providing supplemental, standardized data when screening for ADHD and assessing treatment efficacy (Garcia-Barrera & Kamphaus, 2006; Pliszka & AACAP Work Group on Quality Issues, 2007). Comparing a teacher's objective evaluation of a child's behavior with that of his or her same-age peers or using a symptom frequency count with the parent's assessment can be especially valuable. Although hyperactivity can be rated as a physical measurement, inattention cannot be measured directly; it must be "inferred" by the rater. These same rating scales can be used intermittently throughout the year by teachers and parents to monitor the child's response to treatments.

TABLE 12-1

Selected Behavior Rating Scales for Screening and Assessing Treatment Efficacy in ADHD

Scales	Age Range	Responders	Comments
Achenbach's Child Behavior Checklist	6-18	Parent Teacher	Adaptive and maladaptive functioning
Attention Deficit Disorder Evaluation Scale (ADDES-3)	4-18	Parent Teacher	Subtypes of ADHD
ADD-H Comprehensive Teacher's Rating Scale (ACTeRS)	6-14	Parent Teacher	Hyperactivity, attention, social skills, oppositional behavior
ADHD Rating Scale–IV (ADHD-IV)	5-17	Parent Teacher Clinician	Subtypes of ADHD
Conners Parent and Teacher Rating Scale	3-17	Parent Teacher Student	Subtypes of ADHD plus cognitive problems, oppositional, anxiety, and social problems
SNAP-IV Rating Scale–Revised (SNAP-IV-R)	6-18	Parent Teacher	Subtypes of ADHD plus other DSM diagnoses
Vanderbilt ADHD Diagnostic Parent and Teacher Rating Scales	6-12	Parent Teacher	Subtypes of ADHD plus comorbid conditions and performance

Data from Garcia-Barrera, M., & Kamphaus, R. (2006). Diagnosis of attention-deficit/hyperactivity disorder and its subtypes. In R. Kamphaus & J. Campbell (Eds.), *Psychodiagnostic Assessment of Children: Dimensional and Categorical Approaches*. Hoboken, NJ: John Wiley & Sons; Pliszka, S., & AACAP Work Group on Quality Issues. (2007). Practice parameter for the assessment and treatment of children and adolescents with attention-deficit/hyperactivity disorder. *J Am Acad Child Adolesc Psychiatry, 46*(7), 894-921.

More recently, there has been an emphasis on the need for the presence of functional impairments in addition to meeting diagnostic criteria to receive the diagnosis of ADHD. Children who exhibit all the behavioral characteristics in *DSM-IV-TR* but do not exhibit "functional impairments" in social or academic activities do not fit the criteria for ADHD (Leach & Brewer, 2005). This concept is based on the implication that there are only subjective measures to determine when a child's behavior is inappropriate, atypical, or dysfunctional. Adaptive functioning measures the child's degree of self-sufficiency in the activities and demands of daily living, such as self-care skills, respect for property, accomplishing developmental tasks, communication skills, and awareness of self (Barkley, 2006). Children with ADHD have diminished overall adaptive functioning relative to nondisabled children. They have a discrepancy between what they know (their ability) and what they do (Barkley, 2006).

Many conditions may mimic symptoms seen in ADHD; a complete assessment will rule out these conditions. Box 12-2 contains a list of common conditions that should be considered as possible alternative causes for the symptomology. Allergy-based signs and symptoms can result in a child being tired, irritable, or restless. Symptoms such as difficulty breathing or pruritus can interrupt a child's attention. Obstructive sleep disorders such as apnea or upper airway resistance syndrome can result in fatigue and inattention (Chervin, Archbold, Dillon, et al., 2002). Even hypoglycemia from skipped breakfasts can result in irritability and inattention. These conditions can easily be identified and treated. In addition, many psychiatric conditions, especially conduct disorder and oppositional defiant disorder, may mimic the signs and symptoms of ADHD and must be identified, if present.

Trials of stimulant medications to determine their effect on the child without a complete assessment are both inappropriate and unethical; this practice has no place in the diagnostic process. As with any chronic condition, the diagnostic period may be especially difficult for the parents, and guidance and support by the knowledgeable PCP are especially helpful.

BOX 12.2

Conditions that Mimic ADHD

- Abuse
- Allergies
- Anemia
- Asthma
- Bipolar disorder
- Brain injury or brain infection
- Brain tumor
- Conduct disorder
- Congenital adrenal hyperplasia (rare)
- Family disruptions or dysfunctional family
- Fetal alcohol syndrome
- Generalized anxiety disorder
- Hearing and vision problems
- Hypoglycemia
- Lead toxicity
- Learning disabilities
- Major depressive disorder
- Neurologic trauma

- Nutritional deficiency, especially iron deficiency anemia
- Obstructive sleep problems
- Oppositional defiant disorder (ODD)
- Other psychiatric conditions, such as anxiety disorders, Asperger syndrome, autism, depression, conduct disorder (CD), posttraumatic stress disorder (PTSD), or Tourette syndrome
- Seizure disorders, especially absence seizures, which may be misinterpreted as inattentive ADHD
- Sleep apnea
- Thyroid abnormalities
- Use of over-the-counter or prescribed medications where the side effects may be overactivity or sluggishness

Data from Galanter, C., & Leibenluft, E. (2008). Frontiers between attention deficit hyperactivity disorder and bipolar disorder. *Child Adolesc Psychiatr Clin North Am, 17*(2), 325-346; Heilbroner, P., & Castaneda, G. (2007). *Pediatric Neurology: Essentials for General Practice*. Philadelphia: Lippincott Williams & Wilkins.

Clinical Manifestations at Time of Diagnosis

The past emphasis on hyperactivity as the primary component of ADHD has changed; impulsivity, inattention, and hyperactivity are now recognized as equally important. These manifestations occur in all facets of a child's life and often become worse in situations requiring sustained attention. Therefore the school setting is frequently where these features result in a referral for evaluation. Although symptoms are often identified in early childhood, they

Clinical Manifestations at Time of Diagnosis

POSSIBLE BEHAVIORAL MANIFESTATIONS
- Suspensions from daycare or preschool
- Hyperactivity—inability to sit still; fidgeting, toe-tapping
- Impulsivity—blurting out answers, difficulty taking turns
- Difficulties with attention, specifically related to persistent effort
- Sluggish cognitive tempo—increase in daydreaming
- Disorganization at school, home, or work
- Executive function difficulties
- Difficulties with social interaction
- Older adolescents—possible criminal behavior, drug or alcohol use disorders

may not be identified until after a child enters a structured school environment. Even then, children (most often girls) with the inattentive type are less likely than other children with ADHD to be referred for evaluation. Children with the inattentive form of ADHD are less likely to exhibit the level of behavior difficulty observed in those with the combined or hyperactive-impulsive types (APA, 2000). The average age for diagnosis of ADHD-I is 7 to 10 (Greenhill et al., 2008), although symptoms were obvious to most parents and teachers 3 to 5 years earlier.

Children with the inattentive subtype "have their greatest difficulties with aspects of attention related to persistence of effort, or sustaining their attention (responding) to tasks; this is sometimes called 'vigilance' and is believed to be mediated through frontal brain attention circuits" (Barkley, 2006, p. 78). They spend more time off task than on, as they are highly distractible and have difficulty with persistence. It has been suggested that some of those who have the inattentive subtype have a "sluggish cognitive tempo," as they appear passive, hypoactive, and daydreaming, as if they are "in a fog" (Barkley, 2006, p. 78).

ADHD in Preschool Children

More preschoolers are diagnosed with the hyperactive-impulsive subtype of ADHD rather than the inattentive form, the latter of which may not be as impairing or as obvious in this young age-group. "However, a proportion of children diagnosed as preschoolers changed to another ADHD subtype over the next 8 years, questioning the stability and validity of ADHD subtyping in this population" (Greenhill et al., 2008, p. 349). Studies have demonstrated that preschool children diagnosed with ADHD have a significant increase in suspensions from their daycare/preschool, often due to disruptive behavior, compared with their non-ADHD peers; they also have more difficulty with their academic tasks (Greenhill et al., 2008).

Young children diagnosed with ADHD are at increased risk for developmental delay, especially language disorder (Greenhill et al., 2008). Greenhill and colleagues (2008) warn that early diagnosis of preschoolers with ADHD may result in overidentification of children with this disorder and subsequent treatment in children who ultimately will be found not to have ADHD. For those who do have preschool-onset symptoms, fewer than one in five receive appropriate services.

ADHD in Older Adolescents and Adults

Although most researchers have acknowledged that most children with ADHD have the disorder into adolescence (60% to 85%) and adulthood (40%), it has been implied that there are many older adolescents and adults with ADHD who were never identified as having the disorder as children. Older adolescents and adults suspected of having ADHD exhibit symptoms slightly different from those in the *DSM-IV-TR,* because these criteria were designed for school-age children. Two percent to 8% of adults have the full syndrome (meeting six of the nine criteria), yet many more adults are significantly impaired when meeting less than six of the criteria (Pliszka & AACAP Work Group on Quality Issues, 2007). These symptoms include poor social interaction with possible antisocial and criminal behavior, substance and/or alcohol use disorders, high levels of school failure, anxiety disorders, poor work histories, marital difficulties, and low self-esteem. Other symptoms include heightened motor activity, such as fingers tapping and knees going up and down fairly continuously, restlessness, distractibility, failure to stay on task, disorganization with schedules, and executive function difficulties. These symptoms may reflect sequelae of undiagnosed and consequently unmanaged ADHD. These adults are often undereducated and assume lower occupational levels.

Treatment

ADHD is a chronic condition that generally causes significant functional impairment across several domains at home, at school, and in the community. Because of this, effective treatment must necessarily address behavioral, educational, and health care needs. This comprehensive multimodal approach typically requires involvement of the family and primary care clinician and a number of other professionals, such as teachers, administrators, school psychologists, social workers, psychiatrists, psychologists, and the school nurse.

Children diagnosed with ADHD are more frequent users of medical and mental health services than their nonaffected peers (Greenhill et al., 2008). Many primary care clinicians are likely to see individuals who have already been diagnosed and are currently under treatment. In such cases, the effectiveness of the current management needs to be evaluated and maintained or adjusted as necessary, based on parent, teacher, and child feedback and/or consultation with the treating clinician.

Multimodal Treatment

Multimodal treatment addresses the core symptoms of ADHD. The premier studies that systematically evaluated the efficacy of various approaches to treatment were the National Institute of Mental Health MTA (Multimodal Treatment Study of Children with ADHD) and the Multimodal Psychosocial Treatment Study of Children with ADHD (Pliszka & AACAP Work Group on Quality Issues, 2007). The results of these landmark studies suggested that pharmacologic management involving close follow-up and feedback from school personnel or a combination of pharmacologic management and behavioral intervention were more effective than intensive behavioral treatment alone.

Treatment
- Multimodal treatment
- Behavioral intervention
- Pharmacologic therapy
  - Stimulant medication
  - Nonstimulant medication
  - Second-line medications

Every few years, "state-of-the-science" practice parameters are released to guide specialists and primary care providers in the care of children with ADHD. In 2007, the American Academy of Child and Adolescent Psychiatry released an official statement to guide the assessment and treatment of children and adolescents with ADHD. The "Practice Parameter for the Assessment and Treatment of Children and Adolescents with Attention-Deficit/Hyperactivity Disorder" (Pliszka & AACAP Work Group on Quality Issues, 2007) recommends that a comprehensive and well-thought-out treatment plan be developed for each child.

Behavioral Intervention

Behavioral interventions comprise a wide array of strategies that may be recommended by specialists in mental health (psychiatrists, psychologists, counselors, social workers) or primary care clinicians (Box 12-3). Recommended interventions and strategies are likely to be most effective if they are implemented relatively consistently across settings by parents, caregivers, and teachers. This is one of the aspects of ADHD management that makes it a very complex undertaking. Psychosocial intervention strategies, especially behavioral parent training, appear to be most effective for younger children. Maternal coping strategies are especially important. "Negative, inconsistent parental behavior and high levels of family adversity are associated with early-onset behavioral problems and are predictors of their persistence. Mothers of at-risk preschoolers exhibited more negative behavior and less encouragement with heightened situational demands" (Greenhill et al., 2008, p. 357).

Components of parent training programs include understanding the facts and correcting the myths about ADHD, understanding the causes of disruptive child behavior and the principles of behavior management, improving positive attending skills, and knowing how and when to praise and discipline (Barkley, 2006). Educating parents about ADHD and the treatments, providing anticipatory guidance related to developmental challenges the child may face, and advocating for resources in ensuring that the child is able to benefit from a quality academic education are all part of the role of the primary care provider.

Behavior management skills are generally based on behavioral principles, such as positive reinforcement, withdrawal of privileges (response-cost intervention), and token economies, or a combination of these. Response to these interventions can be highly variable, even in the same individual. Examples of functional disparities in the child with ADHD may include difficulties engaging in and completing schoolwork, homework, and chores; consistently negative interactions with siblings; lack of compliance with directions from parents, teachers, or other authority figures; disorganization and forgetting; and impaired social skills. In general, most activities that require sustained mental effort (except those that are highly stimulating and of the child's choosing, such as video or computer games) will present problems to the child with ADHD. Tangible reinforcers, such as tokens and stickers for school-age children, are more effective in improving behavior and academic performance than are social reinforcers such as increased attention (Anastopoulos & Shelton, 2001).

Because ADHD manifests itself primarily through excessive activity, inattention, and academic or behavioral problems, parents (particularly mothers) are frequently targeted as ineffective and responsible for their child's difficulties. Parents frequently feel as though they must be doing something wrong, particularly if the affected child is their first. Clinicians can help to dispel the myth of poor parenting as a cause of ADHD. These children may not respond to conventional parenting wisdom and discipline strategies, leaving parents with few effective options for managing misbehavior. The core symptoms of ADHD frequently preclude the child from responding to cues, learning from past disciplinary actions, or generalizing a set of rules to a different setting.

Clinicians can be most helpful by recognizing and validating the inherent difficulties of parenting a child with ADHD and facilitating healthy coping through information and knowledge of community resources. Referral for instruction in behavioral management techniques specific to the child with ADHD may be beneficial.

Behavior rating scales, such as the Connors Parent and Teacher Rating Scales, are useful in assessing baseline status and as an evaluation tool for selected interventions and for periodic assessments of the effectiveness of intervention modalities. In general, the more structured and predictable the environment (both home and school), the better the child with ADHD is likely to function. Daily routines should be as consistent as possible, allowing extra time for the child to overcome his or her frequently limited organizational skills. For the younger child, picture charts or written reminder lists can be helpful in getting mornings off to a productive start. If medications are administered, it may be helpful to give the morning dose before the child gets out of bed so that some absorption and effect have occurred at the beginning of the day, facilitating a smoother morning routine.

Children affected by ADHD may benefit from involvement in recreational or competitive sports activities. Summer camps or experiential education activities can offer opportunities for social and emotional growth and enhanced self-esteem. Some children can manage in regular camp situations; others may benefit from camps or programs specific to the child affected with ADHD. It is helpful for the clinician to support and encourage these opportunities where available.

BOX 12-3

Behavior Management Strategies

STRATEGY: POSITIVE REINFORCEMENT

- *Description:* Immediate reward given for desired behavior; tangible reinforcers, such as small treats, stickers, or inexpensive toys, are the most effective. Other reinforcers include special privileges or activities.
- *Example:* Child performs targeted behavior and receives previously agreed on reinforcer. Child completes task, receives praise and small treat.

STRATEGY: WITHDRAWAL OF PRIVILEGES (COST-RESPONSE INTERVENTION)

- *Description:* Undesirable behavior results in loss of desired privilege.
- *Example:* Access to computer time or favorite TV show is withdrawn if targeted misbehavior occurs. Alternatively, time-out removes child temporarily from setting where misbehavior occurred.

STRATEGY: TOKEN ECONOMIES

- *Description:* Tokens are awarded for each appropriate behavior, which can be accumulated and used to acquire a desired activity or object. Alternatively, the child starts with a given number of tokens, and each incidence of targeted misbehavior results in loss of a token. A certain number of tokens must be acquired or retained by child to access special privileges or items.
- *Example:* Desired behavior occurs; token is awarded. Alternatively, undesirable behavior occurs; token is withdrawn. Different numbers of tokens can be traded for small toys, games, or special privileges at the end of a specified time period.

Although pharmacotherapy can significantly improve the behavior of the child with ADHD, the results are inconsistent regarding their impact on peer relationships, family dysfunction, and academic achievement (Antshel & Barkley, 2008). Academic and social adjustments are most difficult for these children because of deficient behavioral and executive function skills. Behavioral interventions are helpful adjuncts to pharmacotherapy, and this combination can offer synergistic and cost-effective benefits. Health care professionals, educators, and parents must help these children set appropriate goals and then guide them to organize and prioritize strategies to obtain them. The support of professionals for child-parent training and for teacher training is important in helping a family and child effectively cope with a chronic, difficult situation.

Pharmacologic Therapy

Strong evidence supports the use of stimulant medications in the treatment of the core symptoms of ADHD; 65% to 75% of children with ADHD respond favorably to stimulants (Pliszka & AACAP Work Group on Quality Issues, 2007). It is the first line of treatment for ADHD without comorbid conditions. Stimulant medications are among the most studied of all the pharmacologic interventions for ADHD, with hundreds of controlled studies in school-age children. They have excellent effectiveness and safety profiles and are the mainstay of therapeutic medications for ADHD symptoms. It should be noted, however, that improvement in ADHD symptoms usually only occurs while the medication is being used. Many parents, however, are reticent to give them.

The goal of treatment is to maximize the desired effect and minimize any adverse effect. The stimulant medications used for ADHD are sympathomimetic drugs similar to endogenous catecholamines and one of their actions is to block the dopamine transporter (Mick & Faraone, 2008). The widely held belief that stimulants have a paradoxical calming effect on children with ADHD is erroneous; they are thought to work by affecting certain neurotransmitters, such as serotonin, dopamine, and norepinephrine, which have to do with selectivity, focus, and attention. Indeed, ADHD itself can be conceptualized as paying attention to every stimulus at once, instead of selectively focusing on the most important one.

Stimulant Medication

Prescribing principles. Stimulant dosing is not usually weight dependent, but "using weight as a rough guideline for determining a starting dose continues to be recommended" (Connor, 2006a, p. 632). Recommended acceptable ranges for each medication are listed in Table 12-2. Methylphenidate preparations range from 0.3 to 0.5 mg/kg/dose to 0.9 to 1.2 mg/kg/dose. Amphetamine preparations range from 0.2 to 0.6 mg/kg/dose (Connor, 2006a). In general,

---

TABLE 12-2

Psychostimulants Used for ADHD

Drug	Dosage (Individualized)	Range	Approximate Duration
METHYLPHENIDATE			
Ritalin	5, 10, 20 mg tablets	5-60 mg/day in divided doses	4 hr
Methylin	5, 10, 20 mg tablets	5-60 mg/day in divided doses	4 hr
Focalin	2.5, 5, 10 mg tablets	2.5-30 mg/day in divided doses	4 hr
Ritalin SR	20 mg tablets	10-60 mg	Up to 8 hr
Metadate ER	10, 20 mg cap	10-60 mg	Up to 8 hr
Methylin ER	10, 20 mg cap	10-60 mg	4-6 hr
Ritalin LA*	20, 30, 40 mg	20-60 mg	Up to 8 hr
Concerta†	18, 27, 36, 54 mg cap	18-72 mg	10 hr
Metadate CD*	10, 20, 30, 40, 50, 60 mg	20-60 mg	Up to 12 hr
Daytrana patch‡	10, 15, 20, 30 mg	10-30 mg	12 hr
Focalin XR	5, 10, 15, 20 mg	5-30 mg	10 hr
DEXTROAMPHETAMINE			
Dexedrine	5 mg tablet	2.5 mg for children 3-5 yr	4-5 hr
Dextrostat	5, 10 mg tablets	5-10 mg	4-5 hr
Dexedrine spansule	5, 10, 15 mg cap	5-40 mg	8-12 hr
Lisdexamfetamine (Vyvanse)	30, 50, 70 mg cap	30-70 mg	12 hr
MIXED SALTS OF DEXTRO- AND LEVO-AMPHETAMINE			
Adderall	5, 7.5, 10, 12.5, 15, 20, 30 mg	5-40 mg/day in divided doses	6 hr
Adderall XR*	5, 10, 15, 20, 25, 30 mg cap	10-30 mg	12 hr
SELECTIVE NOREPINEPHRINE REUPTAKE INHIBITOR			
Atomoxetine (Strattera)	10, 18, 25, 40, 60, 80, 100 mg cap	<70 kg; 0.5 mg/kg/day for 4 days; then 1 mg/kg/day for 4 days; then 1.2 mg/kg/day	

Data from Biederman, J., & Spencer, T. (2008). Psychopharmacological interventions. *Child Adolesc Psychiatr Clin North Am, 17*(2), 439-458; Heilbroner, P., & Castaneda, G. (2007). *Pediatric Neurology: Essentials for General Practice.* Philadelphia: Lippincott Williams & Wilkins; Pliszka, S., & AACAP Work Group on Quality Issues. (2007). Practice parameter for the assessment and treatment of children and adolescents with attention-deficit/hyperactivity disorder. *J Am Acad Child Adolesc Psychiatry, 46*(7), 894-921.
*Capsules can be opened and sprinkled on soft food.
†Nonabsorbable tablet shell may be seen in stool.
‡Wear for 9 hours and remove; works for another 3 hours.

"there is a linear relationship between dose and clinical response" (Pliszka & AACAP Work Group on Quality Issues, 2007, p. 904).

There are increasing numbers of studies of stimulant medication use in preschool populations. The weight-determined dosage for preschoolers should be less than that for older children, with a maximum of 0.7 (±0.4) mg/kg/day of methylphenidate (Pliszka & AACAP Work Group on Quality Issues, 2007). At higher dosages, preschool children may exhibit social withdrawal, irritability, and uncontrolled crying. It appears that clearance of methylphenidate in preschoolers, which is moderately effective for this age-group, takes longer than the same dose given to older children (Greenhill et al., 2008).

The stimulant dose-response curve is highly variable in its effect among individuals and with respect to specific behaviors and learning. The recommended strategy for initiating stimulant medication is to begin with a low dose and slowly titrate upward at weekly intervals, with feedback from parents, teachers, and the child himself or herself to assess for an optimal clinical response or any adverse effects (Connor, 2006a). The effectiveness of stimulants is measured by behavioral changes (e.g., decreased motor activity, increased attention span and concentration). Behavioral changes can be identified within 30 to 90 minutes of ingestion. It is recommended that new doses of stimulant medications be started on Saturday mornings so that parents can observe the child for the first 2 days and so that teachers would have 3 days to evaluate if any changes in the child are noted. The health care provider can then be informed by Thursday or Friday so that dosage adjustments can be recommended for the following week's cycle. It is recommended that children are initially followed monthly to assess for efficacy and side effects.

The most commonly used stimulant medications include methylphenidate products (Ritalin, Methylin, Concerta, Metadate, Focalin) and amphetamines and their derivatives (Dexedrine, Dextrostat, Adderall, Adderall-XR). The two groups are equally efficacious in the treatment of ADHD for 41% of affected individuals; another 44% respond better to one class over another. If a child does not respond to one stimulant, others should be tried before moving on to second-line agents, because efficacy may occur with one stimulant but not another (Pliszka & AACAP Work Group on Quality Issues, 2007).

Creative delivery systems have resulted in varied dosing recommendations. Short-acting, intermediate-acting, and long-acting preparations are available and are equally efficacious. Children who weigh less than 16 kg often are started on short-acting preparations until the proper dosage can be determined for the symptoms; children who only have difficulty during school hours, when concentration and attention are required, may also benefit from short-acting stimulants (Connor, 2006a). Because of the short half-life of the short-acting stimulants, it is possible for behavior to deteriorate as the medication is wearing off. This behavioral rebound may be decreased with the use of either a long-acting preparation or administering a short-acting product 1 hour before rebound symptoms occur (Connor, 2006a).

Long-acting preparations decrease the need for children to receive medication during school hours and increase compliance. Using long-acting agents to initiate stimulant therapy is now the accepted standard of care (Connor, 2006a). First choice is usually either a methylphenidate or an amphetamine preparation. Some medications in capsule form can be opened and sprinkled on applesauce to aid in administration for children who are unable to swallow tablets whole; however, the granules cannot be chewed. The long-acting methylphenidate medications may sometimes need to be augmented in the afternoon with a short-acting one if symptoms are not well controlled during evening homework time.

Methylphenidate is now available through a transdermal delivery system (Daytrana). This patch is applied once daily and delivers a consistent amount of methylphenidate while the patch is on. The patch is worn for 9 hours; once removed, the medication continues to work for another 3 hours, making it effective for 12 hours. "The drug does not go through first-pass metabolism in the liver, thereby allowing more methylphenidate to be bioavailable" (Biederman & Spencer, 2008, p. 445). Mild erythema and pruritus may occur at the application site, but these do not constitute a significant reaction.

Prodrugs bind D-amphetamine to an amino acid rendering the amphetamine therapeutically inactive. Lisdexamfetamine dimesylate (Vyvanse) converts to active D-amphetamine after enzymatic hydrolysis in a rate-limited manner at or following absorption. "The saturable rate-limited hydrolysis releases active amphetamine slowly, creating a predictable long-acting delivery of active drug" (Biederman & Spencer, 2008, pp. 445-446). The most common adverse events with Vyvanse were decreased appetite, insomnia, upper abdominal pain, headache, irritability, vomiting, weight loss, and nausea (Biederman, Krishnan, Zhang, et al., 2007).

Treatment with stimulants has resulted in demonstrated improvement in school productivity and improved performance in academic testing (Biederman & Spencer, 2008). Reasons to stop increasing the dosage of a particular stimulant are (1) if the maximum dose for the stimulant is reached; (2) if the symptoms of ADHD remit; or (3) if side effects make it uncomfortable or unsafe to continue (Pliszka & AACAP Work Group on Quality Issues, 2007). If the stimulant does not appear to have an effect on the symptoms, the health care provider should carefully review the diagnosis and consider an alternative treatment plan. The stimulants are not a cure; their use is frequently compared with the use of insulin for the child with diabetes or glasses for the child who has visual difficulties.

Contraindications to the use of stimulant medications include symptomatic cardiovascular disease or children with structural cardiac defects, moderate to severe hypertension, marked anxiety or agitation, narrow-angle glaucoma, or a history of drug abuse. The use of stimulants in children with tic disorders is controversial because some children experience worsening of tic problems with stimulant use (Connor, 2006a). Children with both ADHD and tic disorders often demonstrate a decrease in their tics when treated with a stimulant (Pliszka & AACAP Work Group on Quality Issues, 2007). It should also not be given to those with psychotic conditions, because it may exacerbate symptoms.

A 3-year follow-up of the MTA study demonstrated that the strong advantage and effectiveness of stimulant medication over other modalities peaked at 1 to 2 years and then decreased by 3 years. This change was possibly related to "age-related decline in ADHD symptoms, changes in medication management intensity, starting or stopping medications altogether, or other factors not yet evaluated" (Jensen, Arnold, Swanson, et al., 2007, p. 989).

The AACAP practice parameters suggest that diagnosed individuals be assessed periodically to determine if the need for continued treatment still exists and if symptoms have remitted or changed (Pliszka & AACAP Work Group on Quality Issues, 2007). This is especially true for adolescents. If they are growing well, have not needed a dose adjustment during the past year, and have not deteriorated when a dose is missed, decreasing the medication should be considered (Pliszka & AACAP Work Group on Quality Issues, 2007).

Nonstimulant Medication. Atomoxetine (Strattera) is an active metabolite of bupropion (Wellbutrin) that appears to be safe and effective in school-age children with ADHD, with less risk of seizure than bupropion. It is a specific norepinephrine reuptake inhibitor with an effect similar to methylphenidate. The dosing for atomoxetine starts at 0.5 mg/kg/day for 2 weeks and then increases to 1.2 to 1.8 mg/kg/day (Biederman & Spencer, 2008; Spencer, 2006). Identified adverse effects include appetite suppression, gastrointestinal discomfort (pain and vomiting), sedation, and mood and sleep disorders (Vitiello, 2008). It may result in weight loss and a decrease in height of 2.7 cm less than would be expected (Vitiello, 2008). Acute liver failure is a rare possibility, with two cases reported with 2 million doses administered; however, the drug should be immediately discontinued in anyone experiencing jaundice or other signs that indicate liver involvement (Biederman & Spencer, 2008). Drug holidays are not an option with atomoxetine because the therapeutic effect requires continuous dosing. Cardiovascular effects can also be seen with atomoxetine similar to those seen with the stimulants; from 2002 to 2005, there were seven cases of sudden death among children using this medication (Vitiello, 2008).

Management of Adverse Effects. Side effects of the medications are seen in up to 22% of children (Connor, 2006a). The most common side effects of the stimulant classes of medications, as well as atomoxetine, are appetite suppression and sleep disturbances, especially delay of sleep onset. These effects are variable for any given preparation. Other common side effects are rebound behavioral difficulties when the drug is wearing off, irritability, stomachache, nausea, headache, dizziness, and growth delay (Taketomo, Hodding, & Kraus, 2005). Mood disturbances, ranging from tearfulness and nervousness to depression, have been known to occur. As a result, black box warnings have been proposed to both stimulant and nonstimulant drugs used to treat ADHD that warn of possible psychiatric events, such as severe depression and suicidal ideation during the first few months of treatment, as well as possible cardiovascular events, such as increased blood pressure and sudden death (Pliszka & AACAP Work Group on Quality Issues, 2007).

Suggested solutions to some of these effects include taking medication just before or with meals for appetite suppression, nausea, or abdominal pain; using nutritional supplements such as Ensure as needed to add necessary calories, and eating high-calorie snacks at bedtime when stimulant effects are wearing off; dosing earlier in the day or using short-acting stimulants to avoid sleep problems and considering administering low doses of clonidine or melatonin; reducing the stimulant dose or switching to a long-acting preparation if dizziness occurs, while also monitoring blood pressure; using long-acting stimulants to avoid rebound and irritability; and evaluating the child for mood disorders or medication side effects (Connor, 2006a).

Stimulant drugs are thought to decrease growth acceleration in children. Although weight loss is seen during the first few months of treatment, the effect on height takes over a year to become detectable (approximately 1 cm per year for the first 1 to 3 years) (Vitiello, 2008). Some believe that the weight loss that occurs because of the anorexia may be the cause of the growth delay whereas others believe it may be intrinsic to the condition itself. Regardless of the cause, final adult health is not thought to be affected (Biederman & Spencer, 2008; Vitiello, 2008). Some

believe that drug holidays should be used to allow the child to provide growth "catch-up." However, consideration of a drug holiday for children taking stimulants for ADHD needs to be evaluated on the basis of the child's academic performance and behavior without medication and the impact these have on the child and family. School vacations and weekends are the best times for trials off medication, when there is generally less pressure on the child. However, if there is an expectation that homework or projects are to be accomplished on weekends or over holidays, it is likely to put the school-age child at a serious disadvantage if medication is withdrawn during these times.

The impact of stimulants on the cardiovascular system has resulted in concerns and additional cautions regarding these medications. Stimulants are sympathomimetic drugs and therefore result in mild increases in pulse and blood pressure, although the clinical significance is unknown; it can certainly become a problem if an overdose of the stimulant is taken. The increase averages 2 to 6 beats per minute for heart rate, 2 to 4 mm Hg for systolic blood pressure, and 1 to 3 mm Hg for diastolic blood pressure compared with those taking placebo (Vitiello, 2008). Because of 28 sudden cardiac deaths in children under age 19 who were taking the various stimulants over a 13-year period, children with a family history of early cardiac arrhythmias or cardiac death or a personal history of cardiac structural abnormalities, chest pain, palpitations, or syncope of unclear origin either before or while using stimulants warrant further evaluation before these medications are prescribed (Biederman & Spencer, 2008). Other contraindications would be those with "serious structural cardiac abnormalities, cardiomyopathy, or serious heart rhythm abnormalities" (Vitiello, 2008, p. 468). Twelve of the children who died were found to have structural cardiovascular abnormalities (Vitiello, 2008). In light of this information, it is important to note that the risk of sudden death in teen athletes not on stimulants is higher than for the general population of those children with ADHD taking stimulants (Wilens, Prince, Spencer, et al., 2006).

If some side effects, such as headaches, mood swings, or stomachaches, do not resolve after a few weeks on the medication, perhaps changing to another product within the same category of drugs should be tried. If the child appears "spacey," has a flat affect, or has exaggerated hyperactivity or motor or vocal tics, the dosage may need to be decreased (Heilbroner & Castenada, 2007).

One of the greatest concerns of parents is that stimulant use will lead to an addiction. This is not the case. The stimulants are not addictive when taken in the doses prescribed and for the conditions for which they are needed, and children with ADHD do not get high from the stimulants they take (Biederman & Spencer, 2008). Studies have consistently demonstrated that children treated with stimulant medication for their ADHD were at decreased risk of substance abuse during adolescence compared with their non-ADHD peers and with those with ADHD who were not medicated. In young adulthood however, individuals with ADHD treated with medication were more likely than those who were not to report use of cocaine (Looby, 2008). Stimulant medication may actually serve as a protective effect against substance abuse during adolescence. The long-acting preparations are less able to be abused because of their delivery system and the new prodrugs that are being developed alter the rate of conversion to the active drug, thus providing "a barrier to euphoric abuse" (Biederman & Spencer, 2008, p. 443). However, the risk of substance abuse should not be a reason to avoid the use of pharmacotherapy for children with ADHD. Of greater concern is the increased use of stimulant abuse by those without a diagnosis of ADHD. Individuals who do not have ADHD, especially college students, attempt to access stimulant drugs to "help them study." Studies indicate that up to 8% have used/misused stimulant drugs, including amphetamines and methylphenidate (Szobot & Bukstein, 2008). Lisdexamfetamine is a prodrug. Its unique properties provide a "barrier to euphoric abuse" (Biederman & Spencer, 2008, p. 443).

Second-Line Medications. When stimulant drugs (or atomoxetine) are not effective, when the side effects cannot be tolerated, or when comorbid conditions exist, second-line medications may be prescribed (Table 12-3). Nonstimulant medications, such as tricyclic antidepressants (TCAs), selective serotonin reuptake inhibitors (SSRIs), and alpha-adrenergic agonists, are sometimes used. Use of these agents seems to be increasing, but they are still not approved by the Food and Drug Administration (FDA) for use in children with ADHD. Although most studies of nonstimulant medications for ADHD have involved administration of TCAs or other atypical antidepressants, such as bupropion, SSRIs have a better safety profile with little risk of cardiotoxicity and have largely replaced TCAs in the management of ADHD with comorbid mood disorders. However, the usefulness of SSRIs "in the treatment of core ADHD symptoms is not supported by clinical experience" (Spencer, 2006, p. 651). Full therapeutic effects may not be achieved until 3 to 6 weeks after therapy has been initiated.

TCAs have a half-life of approximately 12 hours, so only once-a-day dosing is required (Spencer, 2006). Nortriptyline (Pamelor) or imipramine (Tofranil) is favored over desipramine (Norpramin) because of four unexplained deaths that occurred in children with ADHD treated with desipramine (Spencer, 2006). TCAs are used when ADHD co-occurs with depression, anxiety, and tic disorders. They are effective and generally well tolerated but have fallen out of favor because of the concerns over their potential cardiac

effects. "TCAs more consistently improve behavioral symptoms . . . than they improve cognitive function" (Spencer, 2006, p. 650). In addition to their positive effect on mood, they also decrease sleep and tic problems. However, they can cause dry mouth, anorexia, and significant cardiac problems. A baseline electrocardiogram (ECG) needs to be obtained before treatment is initiated and then rechecked at regular intervals while the child is taking TCAs, because they may prolong the conduction of electrical activity of the heart (Vitiello, 2008) and increase the heart rate. After the maintenance dose is reached, ECGs can be done twice yearly.

Bupropion (Wellbutrin), a heterocyclic antidepressant, has been shown to be an effective second-line drug for treating ADHD (Spencer, 2006). Several well-conducted studies have found bupropion to be similar in efficacy to methylphenidate (Biederman & Spencer, 2008). It is also considered to have a decreased risk of being misused and abused (Szobot & Bukstein, 2008). Adverse effects with this agent include agitation, exacerbation of tic disorders, and a slightly increased risk of seizures (Spencer, 2006).

Clonidine (Catapres) and guanfacine are presynaptic alpha-adrenergic agonists that have been widely used in the treatment of ADHD, especially in individuals with a comorbid tic disorder, insomnia related to stimulant therapy, and aggression to minimal environmental provocation. "Alpha-adrenergic antagonists do not improve attention span as dramatically as stimulants, but may be helpful in decreasing the over-arousal that contributes to behavior problems in these children" (Connor, 2006a, p. 636). It has not been demonstrated to be effective with the inattentive type of ADHD (Connor, 2006b).

The availability of transdermal patches (applied every 5 days) is an advantage for clonidine, and clonidine can be useful in improving a child's ability to fall asleep. Although not approved by the FDA for these indications, clonidine has been prescribed both alone and in combination with stimulants, especially for those with sleep disturbances (because side effects include drowsiness, dizziness, and sedation) and those whose excessive hyperactivity is not controlled with stimulants alone (Connor, 2006b). Because clonidine (as well as guanfacine) is an antihypertensive, it can decrease the pulse and blood pressure and result in orthostatic hypotension, dizziness, palpitations, and tachycardia or bradycardia (Vitiello, 2008). Gradual tapering is recommended, because an abrupt discontinuation of the medication can result in rebound hypertension (Connor, 2006a).

A baseline ECG should be obtained before considering clonidine, and pulse and blood pressure should be monitored weekly during the first 2 months of treatment, especially observing for hypotension and bradycardia. Starting doses range from 0.025 mg in small children to 0.05 mg in older children, with very small increases in titration every 4 to 5 days given in divided doses. It takes 2 to 5 weeks to reach a full dose, and treatment effects are not seen for 1 month after that point (Connor, 2006b). If the patch is used, it should be placed on a hairless area. It is not affected by showering/bathing or perspiration, but may need to be replaced after swimming (Connor, 2006b). Contact dermatitis is possible, requiring changing sites and possibly using a topical steroid cream. Guanfacine (Tenex), a longer-acting, less-sedating, more receptor-specific alpha-adrenergic agonist than clonidine, has also been reported to be effective in ADHD treatment (Biederman & Spencer, 2008). In general, a child with ADHD whose condition seems to require more than one medication should be referred for specialty consultation

---

TABLE 12-3
Nonstimulant Medications for Treating ADHD

Drug	Dosage	Maximum
TRICYCLIC ANTIDEPRESSANTS		
Imipramine (Tofranil)	Start 10-25 mg/day (child) (1.5-5.0 mg/kg/day)	2-4 mg/kg/day (child)
Nortriptyline (Pamelor)	10-25 mg/day	2 mg/kg/day
ATYPICAL ANTIDEPRESSANT		
Bupropion (Wellbutrin)	3 mg/kg in divided doses	6 mg/kg/day or 300 mg/day
ALPHA-ADRENERGIC AGONISTS		
Clonidine (Catapres)	<45 kg: 0.05 mg q hs	0.2 mg
	>45 kg: 0.1 mg q hs	0.4 mg
Clonidine transdermal patches	5-day application	
Guanfacine (Tenex)	<45 kg: 0.5 mg q hs	2-3 mg
	>45 kg: 1 mg q hs	4 mg

Data from Biederman, J., & Spencer, T. (2008). Psychopharmacological interventions. *Child Adolesc Psychiatr Clin North Am, 17*(2), 439-458; Pliszka, S., & AACAP Work Group on Quality Issues. (2007). Practice parameter for the assessment and treatment of children and adolescents with attention-deficit/hyperactivity disorder. *J Am Acad Child Adolesc Psychiatry, 46*(7), 894-921.
Key: *q hs*, at bedtime.

with a mental health professional after a comprehensive physical examination by the PCP.

Complementary and Alternative Therapies

Many parents elect to explore alternative therapies for their children with ADHD because of concerns regarding initiating psychopharmacologic agents. Alternatives to traditional therapies include dietary regimens, vitamin and mineral supplements, herbal preparations, supplements, and homeopathic remedies. Dietary supplements and herbal preparations are not regulated for safety, efficacy, or standardized contents, and there is no evidence to support dietary modification in the management of ADHD (Pliszka & AACAP Work Group on Quality Issues, 2007). There is no empiric support for dietary chemicals, such as sucrose or aspartame, as causes for ADHD. Although it is proposed that a very small percentage of children with ADHD may demonstrate a high degree of sensitivity to certain food additives, withdrawal of the suspected substances should eliminate the symptoms and no further treatment would be needed. These children do not exhibit hyperactivity but may demonstrate decreased attention and behavior problems and are not considered to have ADHD. However, if dietary changes have been initiated by the family, it is essential that the health care provider ensure that the diet is nutritionally balanced for carbohydrates, proteins, fats, and vitamins and minerals.

Use of herbals in the treatment of ADHD has not been systematically evaluated, in part because such studies are not required before marketing herbals or supplements. Labeling is not regulated and may not reflect actual ingredients, and parents should be so advised. Nonetheless, herbals and supplements are likely to continue to be sought by parents who prefer a "natural" approach to symptom management. Thus it is helpful for the clinician to be aware of those substances. Megavitamin treatments may be dangerous and pose a risk of hepatotoxicity and peripheral neuropathy (National Resource Center on AD/HD, 2003). Sedative herbs that may be used to promote sleep and that are recognized by the FDA include chamomile, valerian, and melatonin. Safety has not been established for children, nor have any of these products been demonstrated to have an impact on the core symptoms of ADHD. Melatonin, a hormone produced in the pineal gland, was tested on children with neuropsychiatric conditions and demonstrated to have reduced time to fall asleep, but had no effect on the behaviors of ADHD (National Institutes of Health [NIH], 2008). The NIH only recommends melatonin for short-term use, because it may lower the seizure threshold, increase blood sugar, lower blood pressure, and result in mood changes and mild gastrointestinal discomfort. Primary care clinicians need to actively inquire about usage of alternative regimens and be knowledgeable about potential interactions, toxicology, and relative effectiveness of the various intervention strategies.

Other myths related to the causes of ADHD that have no validity include fluorescent lighting, tar and pitch, soaps and detergents, disinfectants, yeast, insect repellants, vitamin deficiencies, stress, television viewing (Stevens & Mulsow, 2006), and social adversity in the family. Although poor child-rearing and teaching styles have been ruled out as causes of ADHD, certain styles can exacerbate or lessen symptomatology (Barkley, 2006). Other proposed therapies where the efficacy has never been established or has been demonstrated to not be effective for children and adolescents with ADHD include cognitive-behavioral therapy, electroencephalogram (EEG)

and electromyogram (EMG) biofeedback, sensory integration training, social skills training, interactive metronome training, cerebellar training, vestibular stimulation, and visual training (Barkley, 2004; National Resource Center on AD/HD, 2003). At one time, optometric training, sensory integration therapy, and applied kinesiology were suggested for ADHD, but these were primarily for those with learning disabilities and other sensorimotor problems and not for ADHD. Although some children with ADHD also have coordination difficulties, coordination training does not improve the learning difficulties experienced by the child with ADHD. Biofeedback is based on programs that change the electrical activity of the brain, yet no deficit in the EEG has been identified for ADHD. This lengthy, time-consuming, costly program does not have scientific evidence supporting its efficacy (Antshel & Barkley, 2008; Pliszka & AACAP Work Group on Quality Issues, 2007).

Anticipated Advances in Diagnosis and Management

A number of areas are being investigated but have not yet resulted in clinical application. Multiple candidate gene studies are underway, because ADHD is suspected of being mediated by multiple genes (Mick & Faraone, 2008). Additional work is exploring the prefrontal cortex to better understand its influence on cognitive and affective processes. Functional imaging studies are attempting to identify an objective tool to diagnose ADHD (Bush, 2008). New medication mechanisms of action continue to be developed in an attempt to decrease the adverse effects of the current therapies; the prodrugs are one example. Finally, there is a great deal of discussion about changing the diagnostic criteria for ADHD when the DSM-V is published.

Associated Problems of ADHD and Treatment

An International Consensus Statement on ADHD (2002) noted that "ADHD leads to impairments in major life activities, including social relations, education, family functioning, occupational functioning, self-sufficiency, and adherence to social rules, norms, and laws" (p. 90). Up to one third of those with ADHD drop out of school; 30% may repeat a grade in school; and only 5% to 10% complete college. Over half have few or no friends and slightly less than half engage in antisocial activities. They are more likely to experience teen pregnancy (40%), contract sexually transmitted

---

Associated Problems of ADHD and Treatment

- Learning disabilities
- Conduct disorder (CD), oppositional defiant disorder (ODD), and other mental health disorders
- Co-existing psychiatric conditions
  - Anxiety disorders
  - Mood disorders
  - Tourette syndrome and tic disorders
- Drug and alcohol abuse/tobacco use
- Psychosocial sequelae: Low self-esteem, inadequate social skills, academic difficulties, multiple failures, family conflict, exercising of poor judgment, altered peer relationships, antisocial behavior (especially with ADHD and CD), psychosomatic complaints, failure to reach potential, labeling

diseases (16%), speed excessively and have multiple car accidents, and underperform at work (Barkley, 2006).

It is estimated that 44% of children with ADHD also have at least one other psychiatric condition; 32% have two (Barkley, 2006). This overlap is even more prevalent in preschoolers, where 64% to 74% have at least one coexisting psychiatric condition (Greenhill et al., 2008). The increased recognition of significant co-occurring psychiatric conditions with ADHD has complicated the diagnosis of ADHD and both the pharmacologic and nonpharmacologic management strategies. The presence of coexisting conditions may decrease the individual's response to stimulant medication and may result in more or different side effects than those seen in children with ADHD alone. Most guidelines are designed for the child with ADHD alone. The priority for treatment should be on the condition that is causing the greatest impairment in the child's life (Pliszka & AACAP Work Group on Quality Issues, 2007). The most common conditions seen with ADHD include learning disabilities (LDs), oppositional defiant disorder (ODD), and conduct disorder (CD).

Academic difficulties are commonly associated with ADHD. Whether the student has a coexisting LD or whether "many months or years of not listening in class, not mastering material in an organized fashion, and not practicing academic skills (not doing homework, etc.) [has led] to a decline in achievement relative to the patient's intellectual ability" must be determined (Pliszka & AACAP Work Group on Quality Issues, 2007, p. 901). Psychological testing is not required to make a diagnosis of ADHD, but is required for an LD. If a child does have both conditions, it is recommended that the child's ADHD be optimally treated before testing for the LD.

Learning Disabilities

An estimate of the prevalence of LDs is 8% to 9.2%, or 4.7 million children between ages 3 and 17 (Knopf et al., 2008; U.S. Department of Health and Human Services, 2007). This breaks down to 8.5% of boys 5 to 11, 11% of boys 12 to 17, 4.4% of girls 5 to 11, and 7.4% of girls 12 to 17 (Knopf et al., 2008). Approximately 25% to 35% of children with ADHD have an LD (Pliszka & AACAP Work Group on Quality Issues, 2007). LDs are very different from ADHD; LDs affect the brain's *ability* to learn in a particular way, whereas ADHD interferes with the individual's *availability* for learning (Selekman, 2006). Learning disabilities are deficits in academic skills whereas ADHD is a deficit in academic performance; children with ADHD have the skill, but they do not demonstrate their knowledge in the classroom on a consistent basis (DuPaul & Stoner, 2003). Neurotransmitters are not implicated in the cause of LDs. Although many of the environmental and behavioral interventions are similar for the two conditions, no medications are appropriate in the treatment of LDs.

The diagnosis of LD requires that one must have at least a normal intelligence quotient (IQ), whereas ADHD can be found across all intelligence levels (Anastopoulos & Shelton, 2001). Although some children with ADHD are gifted or average in academic abilities, in general, "children with ADHD display lower levels of intellectual performance [by about 9 points] than either nondisabled children or their own siblings do" (Barkley, 2006, p. 122), perhaps because intelligence is related to executive function. LDs can be diagnosed by psychological testing on multiple parameters, with the evaluators looking for discrepancies among and between the components and response to interventions. Whereas symptoms of ADHD should be present before age 7 years, there is no age requirement for LD.

Conduct Disorder (CD), Oppositional Defiant Disorder (ODD), and Other Mental Health Disorders

Between 30% and 84% of children with ADHD also have CD and/or ODD (Kieling et al., 2008; Pliszka & AACAP Work Group on Quality Issues, 2007). The combination of ADHD with CD or ODD significantly increases the risk of later delinquency, substance abuse, and antisocial behaviors. Individuals with these comorbidities have high levels of aggression, increased anxiety, decreased self-esteem, and increased rates of psychopathology among family members (Barkley, 2006). They have less education, are less likely to graduate from college, and are more likely to be in prison.

Other Coexisting Psychiatric Conditions

Rates of coexisting psychiatric conditions are much higher in clinical populations than in community samples. Other conditions that are often found in conjunction with ADHD include mood disorders (in 15% to 75%), anxiety disorders (in 10% to 35%), obsessive-compulsive disorder, and Tourette syndrome (see Chapter 41). (Barkley, 2006; Pliszka & AACAP Work Group on Quality Issues, 2007). Psychological conditions such as chronic anxiety, fear of failure, and those that develop from family stress (i.e., divorce, illness, and death in the family; teen pregnancy; poverty; malnutrition) may result in difficulty attending to academic tasks but should not be confused with a worsening of the disability. Adolescents who are found to have LDs or depression may have their diagnosis of ADHD delayed because the learning and behavior problems displayed may be classified as secondary to the depression.

The PCP needs to ensure that referrals are made for children who have coexisting psychiatric conditions. The manic phase of bipolar disorder (BD) may be similar to hyperactivity in both activity and speech with the corresponding disordered attention; however, BD is considered to be an episodic condition, whereas ADHD is ongoing. "Youth[s] who have ADHD are not at elevated risk for BD, but youth[s] who have BD are at elevated risk for ADHD. . . . Of those who had ADHD, 3.8% had BD. Of those who had BD, 11.1% had ADHD" (Galanter & Leibenluft, 2008, p. 327). Verbal and motor tics occur in 4% to 18% of the general pediatric population; however, they occur in 34% of those with ADHD. Tourette syndrome is found in only 0.1% to 0.5% of the general population. When looking at that small population with Tourette syndrome, however, between 25% and 85% also have ADHD (Barkley, 2006).

Drug and Alcohol Abuse/Tobacco Use

Between 15% and 19% of those with ADHD use tobacco or illicit drugs (Pliszka & AACAP Work Group on Quality Issues, 2007). "Youth[s] who have ADHD are at increased risk for cigarette smoking and substance abuse during adolescence and tend to show a longer course of addiction compared with non-ADHD peers" (Kieling et al., 2008, p. 299) and poorer results in cessation intervention programs (Szobot & Bukstein, 2008). A study from 1996 reported that "behavioral undercontrol at age 3 years (impulsivity, impersistence, and difficulty sitting still) predicted alcohol dependence at age 21 years" (Caspi et al., as reported by Szobot & Bukstein, 2008, p. 310). The connection made between substance abuse and ADHD relates to the fact that dopamine is implicated in both (Szobot & Bukstein, 2008). For example, cocaine increases dopamine and has a similar effect to that provided by the stimulant medications for ADHD (Szobot & Bukstein, 2008). There is also speculation that youths with ADHD may overestimate their competence, have difficulty in evaluating the negative consequences of substance abuse, or have difficulty with the decision-making process of how to refuse or avoid use of these products (Szobot & Bukstein, 2008). As mentioned earlier in this chapter, taking stimulants does not predispose the child with ADHD to substance abuse of other drugs later in life.

Psychosocial Sequelae

Children who are not diagnosed in grade school or not treated effectively may experience many years of academic difficulties that may lead to frustration and failure. The psychological sequelae of multiple failures can result in poor self-esteem. Chronic school pressures and failure can result in frustration, anxiety, depression, an inner sense of restlessness, psychosomatic complaints, and school absenteeism or resignation. Teachers may misinterpret their behaviors and label these children as lazy or insensitive or dismiss them from the classroom. They are at increased risk of failing and being suspended or expelled (Barkley, 2006). One important point for health care providers is to remember that increased emotional lability or "spacey" behavior may be a result of the side effects of the psychotropic medication being taken.

A number of children with ADHD have difficulty with peer relationships, as well as interpersonal relationships with adults (Rief, 2005; Shattell, Bartlett, & Rowe, 2008). Their poor self-control, poor problem-solving skills, difficulty in inhibiting their behavior, and overreactivity result in them being easily provoked into angry outbursts and making poor choices. They also may misread the verbal and nonverbal cues of others that signal the need to modify their behaviors when interactions with others are not going well (Rief, 2005). Shattell and colleagues (2008) found that college students with ADHD described their childhood and adolescence as feeling lonely, being isolated, and feeling different. Family relationships are also affected.

Although most of the research has been done on those with the hyperactive-impulsive and combined subtypes, those with inattentive ADHD may be "unsure, anxious, initially withdrawn in social situations, and reluctant to take social risks . . . and may lack the language skills to keep up verbally—remaining quiet or making inappropriate or out-of-context comments" (Rief, 2005, p. 55).

One problem in identifying children as having ADHD is the effect of labeling. The label allows the child to receive necessary services to compensate for deficits and adjust to the consequences but may also result in a self-fulfilling prophecy if only the negative aspects of the label are emphasized. The title of texts such as *Making ADHD a Gift: Teaching Superman How to Fly* (Cimera, 2002) and *The Gift of ADHD: How to Transform Your Child's Problems into Strengths* (Honos-Webb, 2005) put ADHD in a more positive light. These books, however, should not negate or make light of the significant difficulties children with ADHD and their families face throughout life.

Prognosis

There is a consistent decline in the childhood symptoms of ADHD over time; however, many adults who grew up with the disorder have continued impairment as adults. Approximately 15% continue to meet the full diagnostic criteria for ADHD as adults; 40% to 65% have partial resolution of symptoms (Kieling et al., 2008; Polanczyk & Jensen, 2008), meaning that most will continue to manifest some of the symptoms of ADHD as adolescents and over half will meet some of the diagnostic criteria as adults. This decrease in symptomatology is more prevalent among those with hyperactivity-impulsivity than with the inattentive type (Kieling et al., 2008). A study of the prevalence rates of Americans 18 to 44 years of age determined that 4.4% had ADHD (Polanczyk & Jensen, 2008).

Although many individuals with ADHD grow up to become successful adults, the "developmental trajectory does not result in normalization necessarily. The persistence of ADHD is associated with a range of educational and social adjustment outcomes, including less formal schooling and lower-ranking occupational positions" (Kieling et al., 2008, p. 298). Of those with ADHD, 18% to 53% "will be academic underachievers, performing significantly below their level of intelligence" (Anastopoulos & Shelton, 2001, p. 49). Studies of long-term outcomes in ADHD demonstrate considerable variation in results. Adults report increased interpersonal problems resulting in having fewer friends, increased job terminations (especially in jobs requiring adult problem solving, prioritizing, task completion, and self-control), and restlessness.

PRIMARY CARE MANAGEMENT

Health Care Maintenance
Growth and Development

Careful attention must be given to routinely (i.e., about every 6 months) measuring weight and physical growth parameters if a child is taking stimulant medication for symptom management (Connor, 2006a; Pliszka & AACAP Work Group on Quality Issues, 2007). The effect of stimulant medication on growth appears to be temporary and minimal, with no significant differences seen by the end of adolescence (Biederman & Spencer, 2008). The growth rate may be slowed approximately 1 centimeter per year for 1 to 3 years, but then it approaches normal with no long-term effects on health (Vitiello, 2008). It should be noted, however, that one large study did not support the theory of a growth rebound (Swanson, Elliott, Greenhill, et al., 2007). Weight loss may be seen during the early months of treatment with stimulant drugs and with atomoxetine (Vitiello, 2008). If the height and weight, as plotted on growth charts, decreases and crosses two percentile lines, a drug holiday is suggested (Pliszka & AACAP Work Group on Quality Issues, 2007). The possibility of drug holidays is discussed earlier in this chapter under managing adverse medication side effects (see page 202).

Children with ADHD should demonstrate the normal progression of attaining developmental milestones, especially in the early years. As the child reaches the preschool years, some delay in the development of a longer attention span, as well as the increased activity level of the child, may signal a need for a referral for psychoeducational evaluation.

ADHD is not routinely diagnosed until a child begins school. The Individuals with Disabilities Education Improvement Act (2004) requires that children at risk for developing ADHD be assessed in the first 3 years of life if signs and symptoms are evident (see Chapter 3). This places more responsibility on health care providers to develop and use tools that can identify the components of

ADHD at an earlier age. Because children may learn to compensate for their disabilities, and in some cases the nature of their disabilities changes as they grow and develop, it is important to reevaluate a child's cognitive, motor, and psychosocial level of development at each well-child visit. Whichever screening tools were used in the initial assessment of ADHD can be used periodically to monitor the child's progress with the treatment interventions.

Diet

There are no dietary restrictions, and no empiric evidence suggests that diets that restrict sugars, refined carbohydrates, food additives, or food colors result in any improvement in the symptomatology, nor do they cause ADHD (Barkley, 2006).

Children taking stimulant medication may have a decreased appetite, and their increased activity level may warrant an increased caloric intake. These children may be easily distracted from the meal and leave the table before they are finished eating. They may also experience a stomachache as a side effect of the medications; if this is the case, medication should be taken on a full stomach. Meals and snacks that are high in protein and calories and easy to eat should be encouraged to enhance nutritional status; because of the timing of medications, it may be easier to promote a healthy intake for breakfast and at bedtime, before and after the action of the stimulants has peaked. Nutritional supplements may also be encouraged. Establishing a mealtime routine may also be beneficial. Parents and caregivers should look for windows of opportunities to provide nutritious foods, such as after school and at bedtime.

Safety

There are a number of safety issues for children and adolescents with ADHD. Children with ADHD have an increased risk for accidents and unintentional injuries and are much more likely than non-ADHD children to be seen in emergency departments. This is especially true of toddlers and preschoolers who are hyperactive, even when treated with psychostimulants (Greenhill et al., 2008; International Consensus Statement on ADHD, 2002). Behaviors that resulted in accidents included leaning out of windows, running into the street, accidental poisonings, and stretching over burners. They have a decreased ability to tolerate delays or to think before acting; they often act without considering potential outcomes. Because of this impulsive behavior and altered judgment, they are at higher risk for engaging in unsafe activities.

A significant number of adolescents with ADHD have decreased judgment of speed, space, and distance. These deficits, plus a decreased ability to pay attention to things such as conditions of the road and driving speed, result in an increase in motor vehicle accidents in this population (Barkley, 2006). This trend continues for adults with ADHD. Driving is an activity that requires multiple tasks and decision making simultaneously. Adolescents who have difficulty in these areas are advised to delay driving for a few years.

Abuse of prescription drugs by those for whom they were not prescribed, including stimulant medications, has become a significant problem among those in high school and college. It is the second most common form of illicit drug abuse, next to marijuana, among college students (Greydanus, 2006). Almost one quarter of high school students legally taking stimulant drugs and 29% of college students with ADHD were solicited to sell or give their stimulant medications to others (Greydanus, 2006). Medication

safety should always be a consideration in teaching and in storing medication. Using containers that mark the pills for each day of the week may be helpful for children who are self-administering their medications. Standard precautions for keeping medications safely secured should be followed not only for the child with ADHD but also for siblings and classmates because many of the medications can be easily sold on the street. There are multiple reports of stimulants being stolen from the offices or desks of school personnel designated to administer stimulants who were not following guidelines to secure the drugs. The use of extended-release and longer-acting stimulant medications and use of the methylphenidate patch have lowered the potential for abuse.

Immunizations

No changes in the routine schedule of immunizations are needed.

Screening

Vision. Comprehensive vision testing should be performed during the diagnostic period; poor vision could also be a reason why a child might appear inattentive in the classroom. Routine screening at recommended intervals should then occur.

Hearing. Comprehensive audiometric testing should also be performed during the diagnostic period; poor hearing might be a reason a child appears to be inattentive and in his or her own world. Routine screening at recommended intervals should then occur.

Dental. Routine screening is recommended.

Blood Pressure. Blood pressure alterations may occur as a result of receiving stimulants, tricyclics, clonidine, or guanfacine; thus blood pressure should be monitored every few months (Barkley, 2006). Children not taking medication for ADHD should have routine blood pressure screening.

Hematocrit. Routine screening is recommended.

Urinalysis. Routine screening is recommended.

Tuberculosis. Routine screening is recommended.

Condition-Specific Screening

Learning Issues. Because of the increased academic problems experienced by those with ADHD and because of the association of learning disabilities with ADHD, it is essential to monitor children for them. Differentiation must be made between the child's ability to learn and the child's not being "available" for learning to occur. This may also include ongoing speech and language assessment, especially for those demonstrating receptive or expressive language disorders.

Psychological Screening. Because of the high incidence of comorbidity of ADHD with other psychiatric conditions and because of the complications of some of the psychotropic medications, the child's mental health should evaluated at each visit. Change in mood may suggest anxiety or depression. Self esteem should also be assessed continuously.

Cardiac Function. Because of the potential cardiac events associated with children taking stimulants, atomoxetine, TCAs, and clonidine, those being considered for treatment with these medications will need a more thorough cardiac assessment. Children born with structural heart anomalies, those with any cardiac symptomatology, and those with a family history of heart problems or stroke should have a baseline ECG, which can be repeated with dose increments (Biederman & Spencer, 2008; Vitiello, 2008). If tachycardia and chest pain "are severe or recurrent, the stimulant medication should be discontinued" and the child should be seen by a cardiologist (Heilbroner & Castaneda, 2007, p. 99). Mild increases in pulse rate as a result of stimulant medication usually disappear within 1 month.

Common Illness Management

Differential Diagnosis

Children with ADHD are three times more likely to have fair or poor health status compared with children without ADHD (19% vs. 7%) (U.S. Department of Health and Human Services, 2007). The diagnostic and recovery phases of illness may sometimes be compromised by the symptoms or treatments for ADHD. It is important to differentiate the clinical manifestations of ADHD, such as irritability and inability to attend to a task, with those same symptoms seen when a child is ill or experiencing emotional trauma.

Side effects of stimulant medications or the characteristics of the conditions themselves (e.g., anorexia, weight loss, stomachache, headache, insomnia) may mask the symptoms of other physical and psychological illnesses. The lack of appetite, insomnia, and difficulty resting the body may interfere with the healing process, as well as with taking in the fluids and nutrients needed in recovery. In general, children with ADHD require no modification in diagnosis or treatment of common childhood illnesses, keeping in mind the potential medication interactions.

Drug Interactions

Medications used to treat ADHD have a number of interactive effects when given with other drugs. When stimulant drugs are administered simultaneously with sympathomimetic medications used for cold and allergy symptoms (i.e., pseudoephedrine), a heightened stimulant effect can result (Heilbroner & Castaneda, 2007), resulting in hypertension and arrhythmias. Some individuals who take both beta-agonists for asthma and stimulant drugs for ADHD report feeling "jittery."

Stimulants should not be prescribed concurrently or within 14 days of having taken monoamine oxidase inhibitors (MAOIs) because MAOIs retard the metabolism of psychostimulants, which can lead to toxic effects, especially a potentially lethal hypertensive crisis (Connor, 2006a).

Dextroamphetamines can impair the hypotensive effects of guanethidine (Ismelin), possibly resulting in arrhythmias. Clearance of amphetamines is enhanced by urinary acidifiers, resulting in lower levels of the amphetamine; alkalinizers result in impaired renal tubular clearance. Dextroamphetamine may increase the risk of cardiovascular effects with beta-blockers, and phenothiazines may decrease the effect of dextroamphetamine (Dexedrine) (Bindler & Howry, 2005).

Methylphenidate may elevate levels of tricyclic antidepressants (TCAs) and warfarin. TCAs can decrease the effects of clonidine. The effects of the TCAs are increased by phenothiazine, cimetidine, and oral contraceptives. The effects of TCAs are decreased by barbiturates and smoking. Increased CNS depression is noted with concurrent use of clonidine or guanfacine with TCAs, and the antihypertensive effect of clonidine may be antagonized with TCA use. Clonidine decreases the effects of beta-adrenergic blockers, which heightens the rebound hypertension that can occur when it is discontinued (Hodgson & Kizior, 2008). Those

taking clonidine concurrently with stimulants will need periodic ECG monitoring because of the cardiac arrhythmias associated with this combination (Heilbroner & Castaneda, 2007). "Because atomoxetine is metabolized by the hepatic 2D6 enzymatic system, care should be taken with coadministration of medications that inhibit 2D6 (e.g., floxetine, paroxetine)" (Biederman & Spencer, 2008, p. 449).

When working with adolescents who may be engaging in high-risk behaviors, counseling on drug use is essential. "The combination of cocaine and a stimulant is exceptionally dangerous and could be life threatening due to the additive sympathomimetic effect of these substances" (Heilbroner & Castaneda, 2007, p. 100).

Developmental Issues

Sleep Patterns

Sleep issues (especially the amount of time it takes to fall asleep) are identified by parents as a chronic problem in children with ADHD. Some parents may come to the primary health care provider with complaints of the child's sleep problems; they may describe their child's difficulty falling asleep, waking frequently, or rising early in the morning. These problems may not always be related to use of stimulant medications but do result in fewer total sleep hours.

In children with ADHD, medication timing or inability to settle down may affect falling asleep. The drug administration schedule should be assessed. If insomnia does not resolve, however, decreasing the doses, scheduling administration earlier in the day, and changing between long- and short-acting preparations may help. Some recommendations include exercising regularly, but not in the evening; changing the type of bedding or the amount and type of noise and light in the room; keeping a regular sleep schedule, with presleep rituals; and going to bed only when tired (Cimera, 2002). Some clinicians recommend a second medication to assist with the onset of sleep; however, as a general rule, it is best not to treat one medication's side effect with another medication. Practitioners should be alerted to the fact that extreme sleepiness may be a sign of overmedication.

Toileting

Enuresis and encopresis may occur in the child with ADHD because of inattention to body cues. This may result in a lengthened time for toilet training. Routine toilet breaks should be a part of the daily schedule. Elementary schools should also be sensitive to this need and incorporate toileting into daily activities.

Discipline

All children act out and misbehave at various intervals in the developmental process. As with other children, discipline should fit the seriousness of the misbehavior. Children with ADHD, however, do not learn well from past experiences and may not be able to control their behavior. Even after these children have done something wrong, they may not relate their activity to the discipline and will need frequent clarification from adults. Frequent feedback related to progress is important.

Behavior modification techniques over a prolonged period may help a child develop self-control. Time-outs should be used only for serious offenses; if time-outs are used, children must be told when the period of restriction has ended. They need to be reminded of the reasons for the punishment and consistently helped to differentiate between "the act being wrong or bad" and "the child being bad." Although behavior modification helps to improve targeted behaviors and skills, it does not reduce inattention, hyperactivity, or impulsivity.

Rewards for good behavior are effective, especially if given immediately after the behavior is identified or the short-term task completed. Punishment should be used sparingly; give the child alternatives and remove positive reinforcers. Barkley (2006) recommends a reward-oriented home token system as an external motivation to complete parent-requested activities. Teach adaptive behaviors to replace the problems. Identify the target behavior and the antecedents to and consequences of it.

For hyperactive children, parents need help determining to what degree their child's normal behavior requires discipline. Parenting classes may help them to make this differentiation and provide clear instructions with positive reinforcement. Parents must be sensitive to the child with ADHD's inability to self-regulate behavior and make necessary modifications in their own discipline techniques while balancing sibling needs and discipline issues as well.

Discipline should be part of the daily routine and must be consistent. Limit setting is an important component of the day. Structuring the daily routine of the home environment helps these children establish acceptable patterns of behavior. Parents should be reminded to also teach the recommended behavioral approaches to a child's significant others (e.g., grandparents, caregivers). It is also important for the teachers and other school personnel to differentiate the behaviors caused by the ADHD from defiant behavior that is counter to the rules of the school when discipline is being determined. Parents are encouraged to have a contingency plan of action if behavior becomes a problem in a public setting.

PCPs may need to help families and older children develop plans to structure their environment and their activities. Breaking down activities into component parts and using checklists may help children be more aware of their behavior. Parents should be advised that normal activities may take more time, and they should keep the child's schedule simple to prevent it from becoming overloaded. Identifying the antecedents to the behavior can also help families focus on decreasing some of the problem issues.

Child Care

Child care that has a small class or group size, a structured and safe environment, constant adult supervision, and an opportunity to engage in gross motor play outdoors should be selected. Predictability of schedule and personnel is reassuring to children with ADHD because they often do not handle surprises or changes well. It is important to talk with personnel about ADHD and to listen to them when they express concern about the child in their care.

Schooling

ADHD has a major effect on the education of children and adolescents; problems in both the academic and behavioral arenas are common in the school setting. Children should be evaluated for school readiness before kindergarten. Teachers need to understand that ADHD is "a problem of sustaining attention, effort, and motivation and inhibiting behavior in a consistent manner over time, especially when consequences are delayed, weak, or absent. This is a disorder of performing what one knows, not of knowing what to do" (Pfiffner, Barkley, & DuPaul, 2006, p. 549).

Children who are not yet diagnosed when they enter school may experience a series of barriers. Teachers are not permitted to identify a child as hyperactive, lest they be making a diagnosis. Neither teachers nor principals may mandate that children be placed on medication before being able to return to school; those are medical decisions. Some districts discourage staff from recommending testing to parents because it is then the district's responsibility to pay for the testing. Practitioners should be familiar with the internal policies of the school districts in which they practice and support parents in their requests for testing and evaluation through special education if a child's history and physical findings are consistent with ADHD. There is no benefit in waiting to see if a child "outgrows" the condition if school failure is already occurring.

Any child experiencing school difficulties should be evaluated for learning and behavioral disorders, and this evaluation can be provided through the public school district at no expense to the parents. It is on the basis of this evaluation (if diagnosed with ADHD) that the school is required by law to implement an accommodation plan under Section 504 of the Rehabilitation Act, if one is appropriate. These accommodations apply to both the classroom and disciplinary policies. Federal and state laws requiring schools to provide accommodations for children with ADHD do not ensure that this help is readily available in any given school system or that there are quality services (see Chapter 3).

Some of the behaviors that most interfere with learning include the following: failure to complete work, failure to write down or bring home homework assignments, unwillingness to begin work at the designated time, lack of persistence, and carelessness in the work.

Children with ADHD are more likely to display disruptive classroom behavior and to underperform based on their IQ and ability (Barkley, 2006). They need accommodations, as well as more positive and negative consequences. Children with ADHD benefit from small, structured classes. They may be educated in regular classrooms, use the resource room, attend special education classes, be tutored, or use a combination thereof. The goal is inclusion into normal classrooms, but special education classrooms and resource rooms are also acceptable therapies. In resource rooms (supplementary help) and special education (self-contained) classrooms, teachers can limit the number of students in the classroom, decrease the amount of distraction, and provide specific interventions based on a child's needs. Many of these interventions can also be implemented by the classroom teacher (Box 12-4). Parents, with support from the PCP, can work with school personnel to help plan the child's school day. Information on when would be the best times of the day for the child to learn, where the child should sit, how to break content into short segments, and how frequently breaks are needed would be important and helpful for the teachers.

Children who continue to have academic difficulty resulting in failure need counseling support and assistance in dealing with the related stress. By high school, the inattention of ADHD may be manifested as chronic academic underachievement and motivation problems. Children with ADHD need to understand that even though they failed a course (or examination), they are not failures. It is not appropriate to tell children to "try harder." A child's decreased performance is not often because of a lack of effort or anyone's fault. These children need to be reassured that they are not stupid and that requests for repetition of directions and clarification of content are not a nuisance.

BOX 12-4

Behavioral, Educational, and Environmental Strategies for the Child with ADHD

- Identify the child's strengths, and build on them; catch the child "being good."
- Provide immediate and specific positive reinforcement for effort and achievement; only reinforce the positive.
- Make a hierarchy of rules; implement rules and consequences consistently.
- Provide parent coaching and child coaching.
- Provide learning activities when medication is at its peak.
- Get the child's attention first; put the child's head or shoulders gently in your hands; ask the child what he or she was just told (speak in a neutral tone).
- Give verbal *and* written instructions; list the steps on a 3 × 5 card; have the child repeat the request on instructions.
- Remind the child of critical behavior before an activity.
- Help the child distinguish between feelings and actions.
- Help the child understand labels and teasing.
- Use physical activities (e.g., role playing) for instruction.
- Use a notebook for daily homework assignments.
- Institute classroom rule that no laughing is allowed when someone makes a mistake.
- Help the child to develop a relationship with an adult (e.g., college student, Big Brother) to promote social interaction and supervised learning experiences.
- Decrease the length of tasks, plan frequent breaks, divide large projects into smaller components.
- Keep a second set of books at home.
- Post a daily schedule, and make to-do lists (use pictures if necessary).
- Pace the child; do not let the child get overloaded.
- Allow extra time for the child to overcome limited organizational skills.
- Use a kitchen timer to keep the child on task.
- Anticipate change, and frequently tell the child what is going to happen.
- Build the child's self-esteem and self-confidence at every opportunity.
- Use calm reminders (e.g., "What should you be doing now?")
- Model behaviors, respectful language, and tone of voice.
- Assist the child to feel "connected" with the school and his or her peers.

LEARNING ENVIRONMENT
- Use muted wall colors.
- Decrease clutter (desks, worksheets, classroom).
- Seat the child in the front of the room, away from doors, windows, and distractions.
- Seat the child near an on-task peer.
- Structured environment is preferred over open, unstructured environment.
- Have a place for everything with a picture on it.
- Provide consistency; keep daily routines.
- Use calendars, assignment books, structured schedule, untimed, and oral testing and/or testing in separate quiet room.
- Give extra time to answer questions.
- Use technologic assistive devices (e.g., tape recorders, word processors).

A significant part of the educational plan is to help children learn to compensate for their particular disability. Children need to understand which accommodations work best for them. It may be more helpful to present material in writing, pictorially, or with hands-on demonstration. Short lists of directions, calendars, or check-off sheets also help with organization. Peer coaches, buddies, behavior aides, or mentors may also be helpful.

Constant feedback to ensure their understanding of subject matter is essential. These children should be given extra time to answer questions; timed or competitive testing may be extremely stressful. It may be helpful to highlight texts to help them find the important information. A second set of textbooks that can be kept at home can minimize the effect of forgetting to bring them home.

Administration of medication during school hours has presented some problems for children. Some children forget to get their lunchtime dose because they often have to leave their friends to go to the school nurse or office, are involved in group activities, or may feel guilty or self-conscious about having to take pills—especially if "drug-free schools" information is being promoted. In addition, state and local policies on administration of medication in schools must be considered when prescribing medicines. Many of these issues have been resolved with the use of long-acting preparations that allow children to skip a lunchtime dose.

Most important in the success of the child in the school is significant collaboration and communication among the school, the health care provider, and the child's parents. Daily behavior report cards and homework lists are often helpful. It is often very helpful for the parent to observe their child in the classroom at least twice a year; this provides an excellent opportunity for parents who want to "blame it all on the teacher" to see their child's behaviors compared with the child's peers.

Sexuality

Providing sex education for children and adolescents is an important role for the PCP. Sex education must be individualized to the child and be repetitive and developmentally appropriate. Role playing can be helpful because problem solving may be difficult. Using a calendar for girls to predict oncoming menses may be helpful. Because of impulsivity and the lack of attention to planning ahead, parents need to constantly reinforce to adolescents with ADHD that they do not have to engage in high-risk activities for peer approval. Opportunities for open dialogue regarding puberty and sexuality must be made available by parents, counselors, or clinicians. Adolescents need to be made aware of community resources that offer information and services related to their developing sexuality.

Transition to Adulthood

The transition of older adolescents into adulthood is a critical point for families of children with ADHD. The underlying condition and its associated risks do not go away, so adolescents working on the developmental tasks of separation from parents and family, establishing a sense of identity, and formulating personal and occupational goals often require professional help. Youths with ADHD often have unresolved issues from earlier developmental phases, less developed executive functioning skills and problem-solving skills, and less confidence and may have limited awareness of the ramifications of their disability.

As children enter adolescence, they should begin to be responsible for taking their medication. However, parents must maintain control of the medications, because many are controlled substances. Keeping records of how many pills are in the vial, getting confirmation that the school nurse has received the number of pills sent to the school, and keeping the medications stored in a secure site away from other children in the family are essential for assisting the adolescent in transitioning to full responsibility for his or her own health.

Successful transitions are aided by empowering youths with ADHD to understand the condition they have, understand how it manifests (so that they can identify when behaviors have changed), identify the accommodations they will need as they enter college or obtain a job, and be responsible for continuing with their treatment plan (Selekman, 2006). It is the health care provider's responsibility to assist these young people in transitioning to adult health care services to a provider who understands ADHD and the treatments needed by young adults.

Family Concerns

Unlike many children's chronic health problems, ADHD is not likely to generate a sympathetic response from school administrators, teachers, other family members, and the health care system itself. Parents must frequently be tireless advocates to accomplish any type of effective intervention. Rewards are few, and the barriers to success are many.

Parents of children with ADHD experience greater parenting stress (Barkley, 2006). Discipline is a more complex process, the relationship between parent and child is strained as there is less child compliance, and parents may feel less competent as parents. Family conflicts can especially be expected when comorbid conditions exist. Many parents benefit from the step-by-step information available through support groups, such as Children and Adults with Attention-Deficit/Hyperactivity Disorder (CHADD), local parent information centers, and books about the special education process. These may especially be helpful for those parents who themselves have ADHD but who never received assistance during their formative years. An advocate of the parent's choosing (frequently a mental health professional) may accompany the parents to school accommodation or Individualized Educational Program (IEP) planning meetings. Attention should also be paid to siblings of children with ADHD.

The costs associated with the long-term management of children with ADHD are considered comparable to those of a child with asthma (Greenhill et al., 2008). The continuous contact with health care providers recommended in the multimodal approach can rapidly become cost prohibitive if families are underinsured or uninsured. Mental health insurance coverage typically has its own set of restrictions and may not allow sufficient coverage for the long-term treatment of ADHD and its associated behavioral problems.

Parents and siblings of a child with ADHD must learn strategies to facilitate their abilities. There are a number of programs that guide parents in behavior management strategies for their children. Children with ADHD and their families will need to readjust to the child's condition at every new developmental stage. The psychological effect of ADHD results in specific psychosocial needs. Building a child's self-esteem and self-confidence, as well as an accurate self-perception, becomes even more important when the child is experiencing chronic academic difficulty.

Environmental control in the home is similar to that discussed for the classroom. Decreasing clutter, developing routines, scheduling ample time for activities, and providing clear directions in the format that best meets the child's needs may be beneficial. Parents typically give more commands, directions, and supervision to these children than to a "normal" child. Parents are concerned about the child's potential for schooling and vocational choices, as well as the child's ability to assume an independent lifestyle. This concern may result in increased parental stress, depression, and marital discord. Parents, as well as their children, need coping strategies and consistent support.

Resources

Books on ADHD for Parents and Teachers

Barkley, R.A. (2000). *Taking Charge of ADHD: The Complete Authoritative Guide for Parents.* New York: Guilford Press.

CHADD Educator's Manual. (2006). Landover, MD: Children and Adults with Attention Deficit/Hyperactivity Disorder.

Cimera, R. (2002). *Making ADHD a Gift: Teaching Superman How to Fly.* Lanham, MD: Scarecrow Education.

Honos-Webb, L. (2005). *The Gift of ADHD: How to Transform Your Child's Problems Into Strengths.* Oakland, CA: New Harbinger Publications.

Levine, M. (2002). *A Mind at a Time.* New York: Simon & Schuster.

Rief, S. (2005). *How to Reach and Teach Children with ADD/ADHD: Practical Techniques, Strategies, and Interventions.* San Francisco: Jossey-Bass.

Books on ADHD for Children

Gantos, J. (2000). *Joey Pigza Loses Control.* New York: Farrar, Strauss, & Giroux.

Gordon, M. (1991). *Jumpin' Johnny: Get Back to Work: A Child's Guide to ADHD/Hyperactivity.* DeWitt, NY: GSI Publications.

Levine, M. (1992). *All Kinds of Minds: A Young Student's Book About Learning Abilities and Learning Disorders.* Cambridge, MA: Educators Publishing Service, Inc.

Mosa, D. (1989). *Shelly, the Hyperactive Turtle.* Bethesda, MD: Woodbine House.

Quinn, P., & Stern, J. (1991). *Putting on the Brakes: Young People's Guide to Understanding Attention Deficit Hyperactivity Disorder.* New York: Magination Press.

Organizations

ADD Warehouse
300 Northwest 70th Ave., Suite 102
Plantation, FL 33317
(800) 233-9273
Website: www.addwarehouse.com

American Academy of Child and Adolescent Psychiatry
3615 Wisconsin Ave., N.W.
Washington, DC 20016-3007
(202) 966-7300

American Academy of Pediatrics
141 Northwest Point Blvd.
Elk Grove Village, IL 60007-1098
(847) 434-4000
Website: www.aap.org

American Association of Child and Adolescent Psychiatry
Website: www.aacap.org

Attention Deficit Disorder Association (ADDA)
15000 Commerce Pkwy., Suite C
Mt. Laurel, NJ 08054
(856) 439-9099
Website: www.add.org

Children and Adults with Attention-Deficit/Hyperactivity Disorder (CHADD)
8181 Professional Pl., Suite 201
Landover, MD 20785
(800) 233-4050
Website: www.chadd.org

Health Resource Center (National Clearinghouse for Postsecondary Education for People with Disabilities)
1 DuPont Circle N.W., Suite 800
Washington, DC 20036-1193
Website: www.acenet.edu/Programs/heath/home.html

Learning Disabilities Association of America
4156 Library Rd.
Pittsburgh, PA 15234
(412) 341-1515
Website: www.ldanatl.org

National Center for Learning Disabilities (NCLD)
381 Park Ave. S, Suite 1401
New York, NY 10016
(212) 545-7510
Website: www.ncld.org

National Information Center for Children and Youth with Disabilities (NICHCY)
PO Box 1492
Washington, DC 20013-1492
(800) 695-0285
Website: www.nichcy.org

National Initiative for Children's Healthcare Quality (NICHQ)
Website: www.nichq.org

National Institute of Mental Health
Office of Communications and Public Liaison
Information Resources and Inquiries Branch
6001 Executive Blvd., Room 8184, MSC 9663
Bethesda, MD 20892-9663
(301) 443-4513
Website: www.nimh.nih.gov

National Resource Center on AD/HD
Website: Help4adhd.org

Summary of Primary Care Needs for the Child with Attention-Deficit/Hyperactivity Disorder

HEALTH CARE MAINTENANCE

Growth and Development
- Medications for hyperactivity cause appetite suppression; assess height and weight every 6 months.
- Early identification of problems related to behaviors that do not fall within normal ranges will promote early interventions and decrease morbidity.

Diet
- Children may be poor eaters. Decreased appetite may occur if they are taking stimulant medication. A nutritious diet with adequate protein and calories for growth is important.
- Stomachache may be a side effect of stimulant medication and atomoxetine. Give medication on a full stomach.

Safety
- There is a risk of injury because of impulsive behaviors and altered judgment. Teenagers of driving age may need to delay getting their license.
- Children with ADHD have increased incidence of injuries.
- Use of long-acting stimulants has decreased the risk of having drugs sold or stolen by those who do not have ADHD.
- Medication should be kept safely out of reach of young children.

Immunizations
- Routine schedule is recommended.

Screening
- *Vision.* Comprehensive visual testing is done initially as part of differential diagnosis.
- *Hearing.* Comprehensive audiometric testing is done initially as part of differential diagnosis. Children may have difficulty with audiometric testing because of attention needed.
- *Dental.* Routine screening is recommended.
- *Blood pressure.* Routine screening is recommended. If a child is taking medication for ADHD, screening must be done more often because of possible hypotension or hypertension.

- *Hematocrit.* Routine screening is recommended.
- *Urinalysis.* Routine screening is recommended.
- *Tuberculosis.* Routine screening is recommended.

Condition-Specific Screening
- *Learning issues.* Testing may need to differentiate altered ability to learn from altered availability to learn. This may include speech and language screening.
- *Psychological.* Comprehensive assessment of the child's mental health is required for children taking stimulant medications or atomoxetine; they may develop severe depression and suicidal ideation in the first few months of treatment. Change in mood may suggest referral for anxiety or depression. Assess self-esteem.
- *Cardiac function.* ECG is necessary for children taking stimulants, atomoxetine, tricyclic antidepressants, and clonidine.

COMMON ILLNESS MANAGEMENT

Differential Diagnosis
- Irritability, anorexia, weight loss, and insomnia are side effects of stimulants.
- Increased inattention or somnolence may indicate that the dosage needs to be decreased.

Drug Interactions
- Stimulants should not be given with MAOIs.
- There may be some negative interaction when combining dextroamphetamine with beta-adrenergic blockers, phenothiazines, and guanethidine.
- TCAs and warfarin are affected by methylphenidate.
- TCAs decrease the effect of clonidine.

DEVELOPMENTAL ISSUES

Sleep Patterns
- Children with ADHD taking stimulant medication may have insomnia if it is given late in the day or in large doses.

Continued

Summary of Primary Care Needs for the Child with Attention-Deficit/Hyperactivity Disorder—cont'd

Toileting

- Enuresis or encopresis may be present as a result of inattention to body cues.

Discipline

- Children may have difficulty responding to directions and may not understand discipline or learn from past experiences. Consistency in expectations is important.
- Behavior modification may be effective. A bad behavior must be differentiated from a bad child.

Child Care

- Children perform better in a small, structured, safe environment with constant adult supervision.

Schooling

- Education strategies to decrease distraction in a regular classroom, in addition to creative teaching modalities appropriate to the specific learning needs of the child, should be implemented. Building a child's self-esteem and confidence is essential. Children should be helped to learn to compensate for their disability. Development of the Individualized Education Program (IEP) or accommodation plan is a team effort.

Sexuality

- Learning techniques individualized for particular adolescents must be used when teaching sexuality and birth control material.

Transition to Adulthood

- Professional help may be necessary to facilitate the transition to more autonomous living and work situations; peer coaching may be helpful.
- The child needs to be empowered to understand his or her condition, how it manifests, what accommodations are needed, and what treatments are used.
- Career development counseling may be helpful in identifying an appropriate vocation based on a child's strengths and weaknesses.

FAMILY CONCERNS

- The child and the family need to readjust to this disability at every new developmental stage. Family counseling can provide information and emotional support.

REFERENCES

American Psychiatric Association (2000). *Diagnostic and Statistical Manual of Mental Disorders: Text Revision* (4th ed.). Washington, DC: Author.

Anastopoulos, A., & Shelton, T. (2001). *Assessing Attention-Deficit/Hyperactivity Disorder*. New York: Kluwer Academic/Plenum Publishers.

Antshel, K. & Barkley, R. (2008). Psychosocial interventions in attention deficit hyperactivity disorder. *Child Adolesc Clin North Am, 17*(2), 421-437.

Barkley, R. (2004). Adolescents with attention-deficit/hyperactivity disorder: An overview of empirically based treatments. *J Psychiatr Pract, 10*(1), 39-56

Barkley, R.(Ed.). (2006). *Attention-Deficit Hyperactivity Disorder: A Handbook for Diagnosis and Treatment*. New York: Guilford Press.

Biederman, J., Krishnan, S., Zhang, Y., et al. (2007). Efficacy and tolerability of lisdexamfetamine dimesylate (NRP-104) in children with attention-deficit/hyperactivity disorder: A phase III, multicenter, randomized, double-blind, forced-dose, parallel-group study. *Clin Ther, 29*(3), 450-463.

Biederman, J., & Spencer, T. (2008). Psychopharmacological interventions. *Child Adolesc Clin North Am, 17*(2), 439-458.

Bindler, R., & Howry, L. (2005). *Pediatric Drug Guide*. Upper Saddle River, NJ: Prentice Hall.

Bush, G. (2008). Neuroimaging of attention deficit hyperactivity disorder: Can new imaging findings be integrated in clinical practice? *Child Adolesc Clin North Am, 17*(2), 385-404.

Chervin, R., Archbold, K., Dillon, J., et al. (2002). Inattention, hyperactivity and symptoms of sleep-disordered breathing. *Pediatrics, 109*(3), 449-456.

Cimera, R. (2002). *Making ADHD a Gift: Teaching Superman How to Fly*. Lanham, MD: Scarecrow Education.

Connor, D. (2006a). Stimulants. In R. Barkley, (Ed.), *Attention-Deficit Hyperactivity Disorder: A Handbook for Diagnosis and Treatment*, New York: Guilford Press.

Connor, D. (2006b). Other medications. In R. Barkley, (Ed.), *Attention-Deficit Hyperactivity Disorder: A Handbook for Diagnosis and Treatment*. New York: Guilford Press.

DuPaul, G., & Stoner, G. (2003). *ADHD in the Schools: Assessment and Intervention Strategies*. New York: Guilford Press.

Froehlich, T., Lanphear, B., Epstein, J., et al. (2007). Prevalence, recognition, and treatment of attention-deficit/hyperactivity disorder in a national sample of U.S. children. *Arch Pediatr Adolesc Med, 161*(9), 857-864.

Galanter, C., & Leibenluft, E. (2008). Frontiers between attention deficit hyperactivity disorder and bipolar disorder. *Child Adolesc Psychiatr Clin North Am, 17*(2), 325-346.

Garcia-Barrera, M., & Kamphaus, R. (2006). Diagnosis of attention-deficit/hyperactivity disorder and its subtypes. In R. Kamphaus, J. Campbell (Eds.), *Psychodiagnostic Assessment of Children: Dimensional and Categorical Approaches*. Hoboken, NJ: John Wiley & Sons.

Greenhill, L., Posner, K., Vaughan, B., et al. (2008). Attention deficit hyperactivity disorder in preschool children. *Child Adolesc Psychiatr Clin North Am, 17*(2), 347-366.

Greydanus, D. (2006). Stimulant misuse: Strategies to manage a growing problem. *In Use and Misuse of Stimulants: A Guide for School Health Professionals*. Englishtown, NJ: American College Health Association.

Heilbroner, P., & Castaneda, G. (2007). *Pediatric Neurology: Essentials for General Practice*. Philadelphia: Lippincott Williams & Wilkins.

Hodgson, B., & Kizior, R. (2008). *Nursing Drug Handbook 2008*. St. Louis: Saunders/Elsevier.

Honos-Webb, L. (2005). *The Gift of ADHD: How to Transform Your Child's Problems Into Strengths*. Oakland, CA: New Harbinger Publications.

International Consensus Statement on ADHD (2002). *Clin Child Fam Psychology Rev, 5*(2), 89-111.

Jensen, P. (2000). ADHD: Current concepts on etiology, pathophysiology and neurobiology. *J Am Acad Child Adolesc Psychiatry, 9*(3), 557-572.

Jensen, P., Arnold, L.E., Swanson, J., et al. (2007). 3-Year follow-up of the NIMH MTA study. *J Am Acad Child Adolesc Psychiatry, 46*(8), 989-1002.

Kieling, C., Goncalves, R., Tannock, R., et al. (2008). Neurobiology of attention deficit hyperactivity disorder. *Child Adolesc Psychiatr Clin North Am, 17*(2), 285-307.

Knopf, D., Park, M.J., & Mulye, T. (2008). *The Mental Health of Adolescents: A National Profile*. San Francisco: National Adolescent Health Information Center.

Leach, D., & Brewer, D. (2005). The assessment and diagnosis of attention deficit hyperactivity disorder (ADHD) in children. In R, Waugh, (Ed.), *Frontiers in Educational Psychology*. New York: Nova Science Publishers.

Looby, A. (2008). Childhood attention deficit hyperactivity disorder and the development of substance use disorders: Valid concern or exaggeration? *Addict Behav, 33*(3), 451-563.

Mick, E., & Faraone, S. (2008). Genetics of attention deficit hyperactivity disorder. *Child Adolesc Psychiatr Clin North Am, 17*(2), 261-284.

National Institutes of Health. (2008). *Drugs and supplements: All herbs and supplements.* Available at www.nlm.nih.gov/medlineplus/druginformation. html. Retrieved May 2008.

National Resource Center on AD/HD. (2003). *Complementary and alternative treatments for AD/HD. Children and adults with attention deficit disorder (CHADD).* Available at www.help4adhd.org. Retrieved May 2008.

Nigg, J. (2006). *What Causes ADHD?* New York: Guilford Press.

Pfiffner, L., Barkley, R., & DuPaul, G. (2006). Treatment of ADHD in school settings. In R. Barkley (Ed.), *Attention-Deficit Hyperactivity Disorder.* New York: Guilford Press.

Pliszka, S., AACAP Work Group on Quality Issues. (2007). Practice parameter for the assessment and treatment of children and adolescents with attention-deficit/hyperactivity disorder. *J Am Acad Child Adolesc Psychiatry, 46*(7), 894-921.

Polanczyk, G., & Jensen, P. (2008). Epidemiologic considerations in attention deficit hyperactivity disorder: A review and update. *Child Adolesc Psychiatr Clin North Am, 17*(2), 245-260.

Rief, S. (2005). *How to Reach and Teach Children with ADD/ADHD: Practical Techniques, Strategies, and Interventions.* San Francisco: Jossey-Bass.

Selekman, J. (2006). *School Nursing: A Comprehensive Text.* Philadelphia: F.A. Davis.

Shattell, M., Bartlett, R., & Rowe, T. (2008). "I have always felt different": The experience of attention-deficit/hyperactivity disorder in childhood. *J Pediatr Nurs, 23*(1), 49-57.

Shillingford, A., Glanzman, M., Ittenbach, R., et al. (2008). Inattention, hyperactivity, and school performance in a population of school-age children with complex heart disease. *Pediatrics, 121*(4), e759-e767.

Solanto, M. (2001). Attention-deficit/hyperactivity disorder: Clinical features. In M. Solanto, A. Arnsten, & F.X. Castellanos (Eds.), *Stimulant Drugs and ADHD: Basic and Clinical Neuroscience.* New York: Oxford University Press.

Spencer, T. (2006). Antidepressant and specific norepinephrine reuptake inhibitor treatments. In R. Barkley (Ed.), *Attention-Deficit Hyperactivity Disorder: A Handbook for Diagnosis and Treatment,* New York: Guilford Press.

Stevens, T., & Mulsow, M. (2006). There is no meaningful relationship between television exposure and symptoms of attention-deficit/hyperactivity disorder. *Pediatrics, 117*(3), 665-672.

Swanson, J., Elliott, G., Greenhill, L., et al. (2007). Effects of stimulant medication on growth rates across 3 years in the MTA follow-up. *J Am Acad Child Adolesc Psychiatry, 46*(8), 1015-1027.

Szobot, C., & Bukstein, O. (2008). Attention deficit hyperactivity disorder and substance use disorders. *Child Adolesc Psychiatr Clin North Am, 17*(2), 309-323.

Taketomo, C., Hodding, J., & Kraus, D. (2005). *Pediatric Dosage Handbook.* Hudson, OH: LexiComp.

U.S. Department of Health and Human Services (2007, September). *Summary health statistics for U.S. children: National Health Interview Survey, 2006.* Series 10(234). Atlanta: Centers for Disease Control and Prevention.

Vitiello, B. (2008). Understanding the risk of using medications for attention deficit hyperactivity disorder with respect to physical growth and cardiovascular function. *Child Adolesc Clin North Am, 17*(2), 459-474.

Wilens, T., Prince, J., Spencer, T., et al. (2006). Stimulants and sudden death: What is a physician to do? *Pediatrics, 118*(3), 1215-1219.

13 Autism Spectrum Disorder

Maureen Sheehan

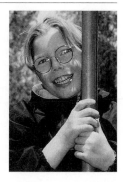

Etiology

Autism and autism spectrum disorders (ASDs) are gaining increasing prominence among neurodevelopmental disorders. Parents and medical and educational professionals are increasingly aware of the signs and symptoms of autism and the need for early evaluation, identification, and treatment of children with autism. Despite this increasing awareness, however, less than 10% of primary care providers (PCPs) routinely screen for ASDs (Dosreis, Weiner, Johnson, et al., 2006).

Autism was first described by Leo Kanner in 1943, who thought that children with autism were of normal intelligence and the product of cold and distant parenting. His description of the 11 children he studied focused on their social impairment and, to a lesser extent, their insistence on "sameness" (Kanner, 1943). Autism is now known to be a neurodevelopmental disorder recognized as one of a spectrum of pervasive developmental disorders (PDDs) (American Psychiatric Association, 2000). Children with autism have impaired communication skills and social interactions and one or more repetitive and stereotyped behaviors. Autism becomes apparent in a child by age 3 years, although delays in diagnosis can and frequently do occur. Many children with autism also have mental retardation.

The exact etiology of autism is unknown. What is known is that autism and the ASDs are heritable and that the etiology involves primarily genetic factors. The variation in the clinical manifestations of autism among all children with autism, monozygotic twins and siblings with autism, and other family members with ASDs has led to research into environmental factors that might interact with genetic susceptibility for autism or cause autism. In addition, although most children with autism do not experience normal social and language development, some children with autism do (Davidovitch, Glick, Holtzman, et al. 2000). Many potential environmental causes of this regression have been proposed and are being studied.

In 1998, Wakefield, Murch, Anthony, and colleagues proposed a link among the measles-mumps-rubella (MMR) vaccine, colitis, and the development of PDD in 12 children. By 2004, though, 10 of the 13 authors retracted their interpretation of these findings (Murch, Anthony, Casson, et al., 2004). Epidemiologic studies in Japan, Canada, the United States, and Denmark have been unable to find any evidence to support the idea that the MMR vaccine induces autism (DeStefano, 2007). The Danish study, which included more than 500,000 children, almost 100,000 of whom had not received the MMR, found no difference in rates of autism in the two groups (Madsen, Hviid, Vestegaard, et al., 2002). Fombonne, Zakarian, Bennett, and colleagues (2006) found a significant increase in the prevalence of PDDs in Montreal from 1987 to 1998 at the same time MMR vaccination rates showed a significant decrease. In children born in California between 1980 and 1994 and enrolled in California kindergartens, there was a 373% increase in the diagnosis of autism whereas MMR vaccine coverage increased only 14% (Dales, Hammer, & Smith, 2001). The Institute of Medicine (IOM) Immunization Safety Review Committee has concluded that sufficient evidence exists to refute a causal relationship between autism and the MMR vaccine (Levenson, 2004).

Thimerosal exposure through vaccinations is thought by a number of parents of children with autism to play a causative role in their child's disorder. A prospective cohort study of over 14,000 children in the United Kingdom unexpectedly suggested that thimerosal exposure may have a beneficial effect (Heron, Golding, & ALSPAC Study Team, 2004). These findings were replicated in a cohort study of over 1000 children ages 7 to 10 in the United States that also found no causal association between thimerosal-containing vaccines (TCVs) and neuropsychological deficits (Thompson, Price, Goodson, et al., 2007). The IOM Immunization Safety Review Committee has determined that scientific evidence does not support a causal association between TCVs and autism (Parker, Schwartz, Todd, et al. 2004).

Numerous studies have identified prenatal, perinatal, and neonatal complications that have occurred in children with autism. The problems observed (e.g., threatened abortion, labor induction, epidural anesthesia, precipitous labor, fetal distress, breech presentation, low Apgar score, low birth weight, prematurity, and cerebral hemorrhage) have not been consistently seen, are not specific to autism, and cannot be used to predict autism (Glasson, Bower, Petterson, et al., 2004; Larsson, Eaton, Madsen, et al., 2005; Limperopoulos, Bassan, Gauvreau, et al., 2007; Maimburg & Vaeth, 2006). Although there does seem to be a consistent association between complications during pregnancy, labor and delivery, and the neonatal period and the later development of autism, recent findings suggest that these are not independent risk factors but rather the result of a compromised fetal genotype, which contributes to a compromised fetal environment (Glasson et al., 2004; Larsson et al., 2005; Limperopoulos et al., 2007; Maimburg & Vaeth, 2006).

Maternal and paternal risk factors for autism that have been identified include advanced maternal and/or paternal age and parental psychiatric history, including psychosis, affective disorders, and substance abuse (Croen, Najjar, Fireman, et al., 2007; Larsson et al., 2005; Reichenberg, Gross, Weiser, et al., 2006). Advanced paternal age as a risk factor may be explained by the age-associated increase in de novo mutations in male germ cells.

Both neuroimaging and neuropathologic studies show that there are differences in brain growth and organization arising in the prenatal period that extend into adulthood (Johnson, Myers, & Council on Children with Disabilities, 2007). Neuropathologic studies of brain tissue from people with autism have found abnormalities in the hippocampus, amygdala, limbic system, Purkinje cells, and cerebellum—structures important to processing social and environmental information (DiCicco-Bloom, Lord, Zwaigenbaum, et al., 2006; Moldin, Rubenstein, & Hyman, 2006). Magnetic resonance imaging (MRI) studies have found thinning of the corpus callosum and increased cortical thickness (Hardan, Muddasani, Vemulapalli, et al., 2006; Hughes, 2007). The largest MRI study showed excessive brain growth early in life that then slowed to below normal growth during the school-age years (Courchesne, Karns, Davis, et al., 2001). This pattern was observed in both the gray and white matter, a finding that may help explain why the deficits of autism are pervasive and lifelong (Courchesne et al., 2001). Functional magnetic resonance imaging (fMRI) done primarily with children and adults with ASDs indicates abnormalities in information processing such as face recognition and executive functioning (Johnson et al., 2007). Evidence from neuroimaging and neuropathologic studies supports new theories of cortical underconnectivity and dysfunction in the recently discovered mirror neuron system (Just, Cherkassky, Keller, et al., 2007; Minshew & Williams, 2007).

Neurochemical abnormalities found in animal models of ASDs and people with autism include dysregulation of human growth factor, the neuroprotein reelin, neurotrophins, and neurotransmitters, particularly serotonin (Pardo & Eberhart, 2007). The relationship of these findings to the pathology of autism is unclear.

Idiopathic autism (without an identified cause) is a heritable disorder (Muhle, Trentacoste, & Rapin, 2004). Family members of children with ASDs report a higher rate of both psychiatric and developmental disorders than in the population as a whole (Brimacombe, Ming, & Parikh, 2007). The recurrence rate among siblings, which may be artificially low due to "stoppage" (parents forgoing having more children after having one with autism), is 2% to 8%, significantly larger than the general population (Muhle et al., 2004). Three epidemiologically based twin studies report an average concordance rate of greater than 60% among monozygotic twins and a 0% concordance rate among dizygotic twins (Folstein & Rosen-Sheidley, 2001). There are several theories to explain this discrepancy. Autism may be a heterogenetic disorder, environmental factors may influence gene expression, an epigenetic mechanism (heritable changes in gene expression not caused by deoxyribonucleic acid [DNA] sequence changes) could be at work, or de novo mutations in parental germ lines affect critical gene loci (Johnson et al., 2007; Muhle et al., 2004; Zhao, Leotta, Ksutanovich, et al., 2007).

Although there is a strong genetic component to autism, no specific genes for autism have yet been found. One or more autism-linked abnormalities have been found on virtually every chromosome, with some chromosomes (X, 2, 3, 7, 15, 17, and 22) being implicated more frequently (Johnson et al., 2007; Muhle et al., 2004). Identification of suspect genes is only the first step toward the understanding of how they contribute to the development of autism. The manifestations of autism vary widely among individuals, and delineating how genetic abnormalities affect these manifestations will be an arduous task.

Incidence and Prevalence

Autism is found in all ethnic and socioeconomic groups. It is generally more common in boys than in girls, by a ratio of 3.4:1 to 6.5:1, although the ratio between boys and girls approaches 1:1 as severity of coexisting mental retardation increases (Centers for Disease Control and Prevention [CDC], 2007; Croen, Grether, Hoogstrate, et al., 2002). Autism is now recognized as a common disorder of childhood, more common in the pediatric population than cancer, diabetes, spina bifida, and Down syndrome (Filipek, Accardo, Baranek, et al., 1999).

Studies over the past 20 years have shown an increase in the incidence and prevalence of autism. Prevalence of ASDs is now estimated to be approximately 6 per 1000 children (Nicholas, Charles, Carpenter, et al., 2008). Studies performed since the millennium generally include children with Asperger syndrome (AS) and PDD, whereas studies done in the last quarter of the twentieth century evaluated the prevalence of autistic disorder (AD) (Johnson et al., 2007). A few current studies have focused on the prevalence of AD and have found the prevalence rate for autism to be 2.2 to 2.7 per 1000 (Fombonne et al., 2006; Honda, Shimizu, Imai, et al., 2005).

Several factors might explain this increase in the rate of autism. As specific behavioral criteria for a diagnosis of autism have been delineated by the American Psychiatric Association *(Diagnostic and Statistical Manual of Mental Disorders, Fourth Edition, Text Revision [DSM-IV-TR])* (2000), a wider spectrum of children and adults with autism has been identified. A population-based study of eight successive California birth cohorts from 1987 to 1994 found that the incidence of autism increased by 9.1 cases per 10,000; at the same time, the incidence of mental retardation of unknown etiology decreased by 9.3 cases per 10,000 (Croen et al., 2002). Shattuck (2006) examined special education data which showed that whereas prevalence of autism among school-age children increased from 0.6 to 3.1 per 1000 from 1994 to 2003, prevalence of mental retardation (MR) and learning disabilities (LDs) declined by 2.8 and 8.3, respectively, per 1000. In British Columbia, Coo, Ouellette-Kuntz, Lloyd, and colleagues (2008) found that 30% to 50% of the increase in the prevalence of autism was caused by children changing special education classification to autism from MR and LDs. These studies support the theory of "diagnostic substitution." This suggests that changes in the diagnosis of autism and reclassification of diagnosis for some children from MR to autism account for much of the reported increase in the prevalence of autism.

Other factors responsible for the increasing prevalence of autism include heightened public and parental awareness of autism, entry of children into schools as state hospitals closed, and children with genetic disorders such as Down syndrome now also being diagnosed with ASD (Johnson et al., 2007). As intensive treatments for children with autism became the standard of care in many areas, children previously diagnosed as having an ASD may have been reclassified as having autism so that they might qualify for services, such as year-round schooling, not generally available to children without the diagnosis of autism (Croen et al., 2002; Johnson et al., 2007). Some parents prefer the diagnosis of autism to one of mental retardation, viewing it as more hopeful and less stigmatizing. For example, data from Texas showed that greater increases in prevalence of autism were found in school districts with higher revenues and fewer poor children (Shattuck, 2006). There are now financial incentives for many parents for a diagnosis of autism. In Maryland, a child with autism can receive a Medicaid waiver if the family does not qualify financially for Medicaid; however, children with mental retardation cannot receive this waiver. Private insurances also may cover services such as speech therapy for children with autism that are not covered for other diagnoses (Grinker, 2007). Clinicians may base their diagnosis of a child on what they perceive the child's treatment and educational needs are rather than adhering to the diagnostic criteria of the *DSM-IV-TR* (Grinker, 2007).

Finally, it is possible that the actual incidence of autism has increased over the past two decades. Studies with consistent and rigorously defined diagnostic criteria conducted with defined populations over a period of years have not been done. Incidence studies would help more precisely define the prevalence of autism. Changes in diagnostic criteria over time, however, preclude a definitive answer to the question of whether the incidence and prevalence of autism have actually increased.

Diagnostic Criteria

The symptoms of autism required for diagnosis fall into three categories: impaired communication skills (both verbal and nonverbal); impaired social interactions; and restricted and rigid play, activities, and interests (American Psychiatric Association, 2000). To be diagnosed with autism, a child *must* meet the criteria for autistic disorder of the American Psychiatric Association in the *DSM-IV-TR* (Box 13-1).

Clinical Manifestations at Time of Diagnosis

Although all children with autism will exhibit the triad of symptoms listed in the preceding paragraph, the severity of these symptoms varies among children, which can lead to a delay in diagnosis (Wiggins, Baio, & Rice, (2006). Most parents notice abnormalities by 18 months of age (Chawarska, Klin, Paul, et al., 2007). Parents typically initially report language delays although earlier prespeech deficits are present (Johnson et al., 2007) (Box 13-2). There are a number of parental reports in the lay literature that diagnosis is often delayed until age 3 years or later for two reasons: parents are offered false reassurance by PCPs who may be unfamiliar with autism and unsure of what to recommend to parents, and parents do not raise their concerns about a possible diagnosis of autism by reassuring themselves that if a problem exists the PCP will raise the issue (Grinker, 2007; Koegle & LaZebnik, 2004). Although autism may manifest in infancy as a lack of attention to faces, people, or the environment; interest in objects instead of faces; and inability to point or wave bye-bye, most children with autism are diagnosed as toddlers (i.e., between their second and third birthdays) when their delayed language is quite apparent.

Social deficits are the most specific symptom of autism, occurring earlier than communication deficits and restricted behaviors. Social deficits are often subtle and less likely to be reported by parents than delays in communication (Johnson et al., 2007). In 72% to 100% of 1- to 2-year-olds, nine red flags identified children with an ASD from those with developmental delay or typical development (Wetherby, Woods, Allen, et al., 2004). These red

---

BOX 13-1

Diagnostic Criteria for Autistic Disorder

A total of six (or more) items from (1), (2), and (3), with at least two from (1) and one each from (2) and (3).

(1) Qualitative impairment in social interaction, as manifested by at least two of the following:
- Marked impairment in the use of multiple nonverbal behaviors, such as eye-to-eye gaze, facial expression, body postures, and gestures to regulate social interaction
- Failure to develop peer relationships appropriate to developmental level
- Lack of spontaneous seeking to share enjoyment, interests, or achievements with other people (e.g., by a lack of showing, bringing, or pointing out objects of interest)
- Lack of social or emotional reciprocity

(2) Qualitative impairments in communication as manifested by at least one of the following:
- Delay in, or total lack of, the development of spoken language (not accompanied by an attempt to compensate through alternative modes of communication, such as gesture or mime)
- In individuals with adequate speech, marked impairment in the ability to initiate or sustain a conversation with others
- Stereotyped and repetitive use of language or idiosyncratic language
- Lack of varied, spontaneous make-believe play or social imitative play appropriate to developmental level

(3) Restricted repetitive and stereotyped patterns of behavior, interests, and activities, as manifested by at least one of the following:
- Encompassing preoccupation with one or more stereotyped and restricted patterns of interest that is abnormal either in intensity or focus
- Apparently inflexible adherence to specific, nonfunctional routines or rituals
- Stereotyped and repetitive motor mannerisms (e.g., hand or finger flapping or twisting, complex whole-body movements)
- Persistent preoccupation with parts of objects

Delays or abnormal function in at least one of the following areas, with onset before age 3 years: (a) social interaction, (b) language as used in social communication, or (c) symbolic or imaginative play.

The disturbance is not better accounted for by Rett disorder or childhood disintegrative disorder.

From American Psychiatric Association. (2000). *Diagnostic and Statistical Manual of Mental Disorders: Text Revision* (4th ed.). Washington, DC: American Psychiatric Publishing. Reprinted with permission.

---

flags included gaze abnormalities, lack of shared attention and pointing, and repetitive movements of body parts and/or objects. Further questioning by the provider may uncover impairment in play, including the absence or impoverishment of imaginative play and an inflexible adherence to routine (National Institute of Neurological Disorders and Stroke, 2007). Providers and parents should be particularly aware of the development of joint attention (JA). JA starts with a baby's smiling in response to his or her parent and progresses to following a point with looking back at the parent, protoimperative pointing, and then protodeclarative pointing (Johnson et al., 2007). Normally JA begins in the first few months of life and evolves throughout the first 18 months of a child's life. Functional language development appears to require the development of JA (Johnson et al., 2007).

Parents of children ages 13 to 15 months later diagnosed with autism reported more social deficits such as poor eye contact, failure to attend to name, and lack of joint attention than parents of children the same age with delayed development but not autism (Werner, Dawson, Munson, et al., 2005). Testing with the Mullen

Clinical Manifestations at Time of Diagnosis

DELAYED OR ABSENT COMMUNICATION
- Expressive language delay: lack of reciprocal babbling (6-9 months), lack of expressions such as "oh oh"
- Receptive language delay: unable to follow one-step command (12-14 months)

IMPAIRMENT OF SOCIAL INTERACTION
- Deficits in joint attention: not looking when parents point or not looking back to parent after parent points
- Failure to make eye contact
- Lack of response to parent saying child's name
- Lack of protoimperative pointing: pointing to request an object (12-14 months)
- Lack of protodeclarative pointing: pointing to share an object/event (14-16 months)
- Fascination with objects rather than people

RESTRICTIVE AND REPETITIVE BEHAVIOR, INTERESTS, AND ACTIVITIES
- Organizes toys, rather than manipulates them
- Throws tantrums when repetitive behaviors are interrupted
- Hand flapping, twirling, toe walking

RESISTANCE TO CHANGES IN SCHEDULE OR ENVIRONMENT
- Narrow food preferences
- Auditory hypersensitivity

BOX 13-2

Parental Concerns that are Red Flags for Autism

COMMUNICATION CONCERNS
- Does not respond to his or her name
- Cannot tell parent what he or she wants
- Language delayed
- Does not follow directions
- Appears to be deaf at times
- Seems to hear sometimes but not others
- Does not point or wave bye-bye
- Used to say a few words but does not now

SOCIAL CONCERNS
- Does not smile socially
- Seems to prefer to play alone
- Gets things for himself or herself
- Is very independent
- Does things "early"
- Has poor eye contact
- In his or her own world
- Tunes parents out
- Is not interested in other children

BEHAVIORAL CONCERNS
- Tantrums
- Is hyperactive, uncooperative, or oppositional
- Does not know how to play with toys
- Rigid about routines
- Has unusual attachments to toys (e.g., always is holding a certain object)
- Lines things up
- Is oversensitive to certain textures or sounds
- Has odd movement patterns

ABSOLUTE INDICATIONS FOR IMMEDIATE FURTHER EVALUATION
- No babbling by 12 months
- No gesturing (pointing, waving bye-bye, etc.) by 12 months
- No single words by 16 months
- No two-word spontaneous (not just echolalic) phrases by 24 months
- *Any* loss of *any* language or social skills at *any* age

From Filipek, P.A., et al. (1999). The screening and diagnosis of autistic spectrum disorders. *J Autism Dev Disord, 29*(6). Reprinted with permission.

Scales of Early Learning (MSEL) prospectively showed no significant differences among 6-month-olds but a significant decrease in development during the second year of life; at 24 months of age the ASD group was significantly worse in all areas of development (Landa & Garrett-Mayer, 2006). In a group of 75 children examined prospectively, all toddlers whose parents had concerns about autism at or after age 18 months were diagnosed with autism by age 4 years (Chawarska et al., 2007).

Although social deficits are more specific for autism, parents are more likely to raise language delay as a concern. Toddlers with ASD may babble and have some words at their first birthday but fail to move on to complex babbling, rapid acquisition of words, and development of two-word phrases by their second birthday (Filipek et al., 1999; Werner et al., 2005). Those who do attain some language, usually those with milder symptoms of autism, will often have language that is not functional. These children can recite entire television commercials, may clearly repeat things said to them (echolalia), and say the alphabet or count but cannot use these "skills" to communicate their needs or wants.

The restricted, repetitive, and stereotypic behaviors that are part of the triad of autistic symptoms are not specific to young children with autism because these behaviors can also be observed in typically developing toddlers and those with mental retardation (Johnson et al., 2007). Lower-level repetitive behaviors such as hand and finger mannerisms and persistent use of certain objects are not associated specifically with autism, though higher-level repetitive behaviors that generally do not appear until after age 3 are associated specifically with autism (Mooney, Gray, & Tonge, 2006). These behaviors include resistance to change, circumscribed interests, and abnormal preoccupations and attachments to objects (Mooney et al., 2006).

Developmental regression resulting in the appearance of the symptoms of autism is reported in a small group of children. The majority of these children did not have normal development before their regression (Richler, Luyster, Risi, et al., 2006). There are no perceptible developmental differences between toddlers with reported regression and those without at 24 months old (Werner & Dawson, 2005). Chawarska and colleagues (2007) theorized that regression in toddlers with autism may be similar to that seen in deaf toddlers; that is, language skills are lost when the connections necessary for continued progress are missing.

Screening and Diagnosis

In 2007 the American Academy of Pediatrics published a clinical report on the identification and evaluation of ASDs (Johnson et al., 2007). This report's goal is to assist in the identification of children with ASD before age 4 by providing a surveillance and screening algorithm (Figure 13-1). It recommends a dual process for the identification of children with autism: surveillance for ASD for all children and then screening of children identified to be at risk.

Surveillance begins with the identification of risk factors. Chief among these is having a sibling with ASD. Landa, Holman, and

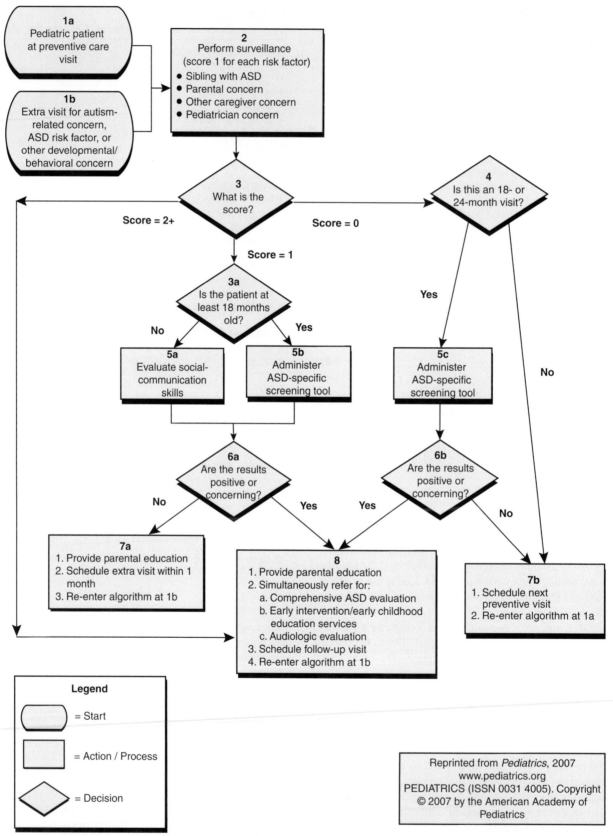

FIGURE 13-1 Surveillance and screening algorithm: Autism spectrum disorders (ASDs). From Johnson, C.P., Myers, S., & Council on Children with Disabilities. (2007). Identification and evaluation of children with autism spectrum disorders. *Pediatrics, 120,* 5.

1a
Pediatric patient at preventive care visit

1a: Developmental concerns, including those about social skill deficits, should be included as one of several health topics addressed at each pediatric preventive care visit through the first 5 years of life. *(Go to step 2)*

1b
Extra visit for autism-related concern, ASD risk factor, or other developmental behavioral concern

1b: At the parents' request, or when a concern is identified in a previous visit, a child may be scheduled for a "problem-targeted" clinic visit because of concerns about ASD. Parent concerns may be based on observed behaviors, social or language deficits, issues raised by other caregivers, or heightened anxiety produced by ASD coverage in the media. *(Go to step 2)*

2
Peform surveillance (score 1 for each risk factor)
• Sibling with ASD
• Parental concern
• Other caregiver concern
• Pediatrician concern

2: Developmental surveillance is a flexible, longitudinal, continuous, and cumulative process whereby health care professionals identify children who may have developmental problems. There are five components of developmental surveillance: eliciting and attending to the parents' concerns about their child's development, documenting and maintaining a developmental history, making accurate observations of the child, identifying the risk and protective factors, and maintaining an accurate record and documenting the process and findings. The concerns of parents, other caregivers, and pediatricians all should be included in determining whether surveillance suggests that the child may be at risk of an ASD. In addition, younger siblings of children with an ASD should also be considered at risk, because they are ten times more likely to develop symptoms of an ASD than children without a sibling with an ASD. Scoring risk factors will help determine the next steps. *(Go to step 3)*

For more information on developmental surveillance, see "Identifying Infants and Young Children with Developmental Disorders in the Medical Home: An Algorithm for "Developmental Surveillance and Screening" (*Pediatrics* 2006; 118:405-420).

3
What is the score?

3: Scoring risk factors:
• If the child does not have a sibling with an ASD and there are no concerns from the parents, other caregivers, or pediatrician: Score = 0 *(Go to step 4)*
• If the child has only one risk factor, either a sibling with ASD or the concern of a parent, caregiver, or pediatrician: Score = 1 *(Go to step 3a)*
• If the child has two or more risk factors: Score = 2+ *(Go to step 8)*

3a
Is the patient at least 18 months old?

3a:
• If the child's age is <18 months, *go to step 5a.*
• If the child's age is ?18 months, *go to step 5b.*

4
Is this an 18- or 24-month visit?

4: In the absence of established risk factors and parental/provider concerns (Score = 0), a level-1 ASD-specific tool should be administered at the 18- and 24-month visits. *(Go to step 5c)* If this is not an 18- or 24-month visit, *go to step 7b.*

Note : In the AAP policy, "Identifying Infants and Young children with Developmental Disorders in the Medical Home: An Algorithm for Developmental Surveillance and Screening," a general developmental screen is recommended at the 9-, 18-, and 24- or 30-month visits and an ASD screening is recommended at the 18-month visit. This clincal report also recommends an ASD screening at the 24-month visit to identify children who may regress after 18 months of age.

5a
Evaluate social-communication skills

5a: If the child's age is <18 months, the pediatrician should use a tool that specifically addresses the clinical characteristics of ASDs, such as those that target social-communication skills. *(Go to step 6a)*

5b
Administer ASD-specific screening tool

5b: If the child's age is ?18 months, the pediatrician should use an ASD-specific screening tool. *(Go to step 6a)*

5c
Administer ASD-specific screening tool

5c: For all children ages 18 to 24 months (regardless of risk factors), the pediatrician should use an ASD-specific screening tool. *(Go to step 6b)*

AAP-recommended strategies for using ASD screening tools: *"Autism: Caring for Children with Autism Spectrum Disorders: A Resource Toolkit for Clinicians" (in press)**

6a
Are the results positive or concerning?

6a: When the result of the screening is *negative, go to step 7a.*

When the result of the screening is *positive, go to step 8.*

6b
Are the results positive or concerning?

6b: When the result of the ASD screening (at 18- and 24-month visits) is *negative, go to step 7b.*

When the result of the ASD screening (at 18- and 24-month visits) is *positive, go to step 8.*

7a
1. Provide parental education
2. Schedule extra visit within 1 month
3. Re-enter alogorithm at 1b

7a: If the child demonstrates risk but has a negative screening result, information about ASDs should be provided to parents. The pediatrician should schedule an extra visit within 1 month to address any residual ASD concerns or additional developmental/ behavioral concerns after a negative screening result. The child will then re-enter the algorithm at 1b. A "wait-and-see" approach is discouraged. If the only risk factor is a sibling with an ASD, the pediatrician should maintain a higher index of suspicion and address ASD symptoms at each preventive care visit, but an early follow-up within 1 month is not necessary unless a parental concern subsequently arises.

7b
1. Schedule next preventive visit
2. Re-enter algorithm at 1a

7b: If this is not an 18- or 24-month visit, or when the result of the ASD screening is *negative,* the pediatrician can inform the parents and schedule the next routine preventive visit. The child will then re-enter the algorithm at 1a.

8
1. Provide parental education
2. Simultaneously refer for:
   a. Comprehensive ASD evaluation
   b. Early intervention early childhood education services
   c. Audiologic evaluation
3. Schedule follow-up visit
4. Re-enter algorithm at 1b

8: If the screening result is *positive* for possible ASD in step 6a or 6b, the pediatrician should provide peer-reviewed and/or consensus-developed ASD materials. Because a positive screening result does not determine a diagnosis of ASD, the child should be referred for a comprehensive ASD evaluation to early intervention/early childhood education services (depending on child's age), and an audiologic evaluation. A categorical diagnosis is not needed to access intervention services. These programs often provide evaluations and other services even before a medical evaluation is complete. A referral to intervention services or school also is indicated when other developmental/behavioral concerns exist, even though the ASD screening result is negative. The child should be scheduled for a follow-up visit and will then re-enter the algorithm at 1b. All communication between the referral sources and the pediatrician should be coordinated.

AAP information for parents about ASDs includes: *"Is Your One-Year-Old Communicating with you?"** and *"Understanding Autism Spectrum Disorders."**

*Available at www.aap.org

FIGURE 13-1, cont'd Surveillance and screening algorithm: Autism spectrum disorders (ASDs). From Johnson, C.P., Myers, S., & Council on Children with Disabilities. (2007). Identification and evaluation of children with autism spectrum disorders. *Pediatrics, 120,* 5.

Garrett-Mayer (2007) found that more than one third of the siblings of children with ASD in their prospective study of development were diagnosed with ASD themselves by age 3 years. Parents who enrolled their toddlers in this study may have already had concerns, another risk factor for ASD, but it does emphasize the necessity of close developmental surveillance for siblings of children with ASD. This surveillance should include careful attention to gesture production (eye contact, joint attention, pointing) before age 18 months, a time when verbal measures of development are less reliable (Mitchell, Brian, Zwaigenbaum, et al., 2006). Surveillance must also include asking parents about and observing for the "red flags" included in the American Academy of Neurology and Child Neurology Society practice parameter on screening and diagnosis of autism: no babbling or pointing or other gestures by 12 months, no single words by 16 months, no spontaneous two-word phrases by 24 months, and *any* loss of language or social skills at *any* age (Filipek, Accardo, Ashwal, et al., 2000).

When surveillance indicates a child with two or more risk factors for ASD (sibling with ASD, parent, other caregiver or PCP concerns) or any of the "red flags" and the child is 18 months old, the child should be screened with an ASD-specific screening tool (Johnson et al., 2007). The Modified Checklist for Autism in Toddlers (M-CHAT) is a 23-item simple questionnaire that can be completed by parents of children 18 months or older while they are at their child's PCP visit (Carr & LeBlanc, 2007). Five items on the M-CHAT have the strongest predictive value for autism: lack of pointing, not following a parent's pointing, not bringing things to show parents, little or no interest in other children or in imitation, and the child's inability to respond to his or her name (Robins, Fein, Barton, et al., 2001). The M-CHAT is freely available (see Resources section at the end of this chapter).

Evaluation of a child for autism includes an audiology examination to rule out hearing impairment as the reason for the child's speech delay. The audiology examination often requires brainstem auditory evoked response (BAER) testing, often with sedation, because of the challenging behavior of children with autism. If the audiology examination and a lead screen are normal and the results of the screening are in any way concerning, the child and family should be referred for formal diagnostic testing by clinicians experienced with autism and to the local school district or early intervention program (Filipek et al., 2000). Referral does *not* require a diagnosis of autism, only the suspicion of an ASD. In North Carolina referrals for evaluation for ASD of 2-year-olds by their PCPs resulted in the diagnosis of ASD for 75% of them, almost all of whom still had this diagnosis at 9 years old, indicating the competency of PCPs in identifying children at risk of ASD (Lord, Risi, DiLavore, et al., 2006). The worst that can result from false-positive referrals is that parents will be reassured by expert testing and opinion that their child does not have an ASD (Miller, 2007). The lay literature documents the dissatisfaction of parents with premature reassurance and dismissal of their concerns by the PCP with advice that their child "will grow out of it" (Grinker, 2007; Miller, 2007). The American Academy of Pediatrics and National Research Council recommend early intervention as soon as the diagnosis of ASD is suspected by parents or providers (Johnson et al., 2007).

After a child has been diagnosed with autism, the PCP can help the child and parents by coordinating additional assessments aimed at identifying an etiology. Because of the low yield of diagnostic testing, about 10%, a thorough history and physical should be the guide for all evaluation of a child with autism (Battaglia & Carey, 2006). A positive yield is correlated with coexisting mental retardation, dysmorphic features, or both. Referral to an academic genetics clinic is reasonable for any child with autism and these conditions.

The workup includes a skin examination, preferably with a Wood's lamp, looking for the hypopigmented macules of tuberous sclerosis, and high-resolution chromosome and DNA testing for fragile X syndrome (see Chapter 27) (Johnson et al., 2007). Routine electroencephalogram (EEG) studies are necessary only if the child has seizures or a clinically significant loss of language, particularly after age 3 years (Tuchman, 2006). Likewise, brain MRI, which will usually require sedation or anesthesia, and metabolic testing are indicated only when there are specific clinical findings (Battaglia & Carey, 2006). There is inadequate evidence to recommend positron emission tomography (PET) scanning; routine hair or stool analysis; allergy, immunology, micronutrient, or urinary peptide testing; or mitochondrial disorder and thyroid function tests (Filipek et al., 1999; Hyman, Rodier, & Davidson, 2001).

Treatment

Treatment will not "cure" autism because most children with ASD will continue to have ASD as adults. Treatment outcomes vary widely. Children with mental retardation or very impaired social skills are less likely to improve (Ben-Itzchak & Zachor, 2007; Magiati, Charman, & Howlin, 2007). Thus treatment should begin with a baseline assessment of the deficits of autism done with standardized tools by an autism center.

As the genetic and neurobiologic basis for the deficits of autism has become more apparent, approaches to treatment focus on the specific symptoms of autism. A comprehensive treatment plan for a child with autism must include both education and behavior management and often pharmacologic treatment. Treatment goals include maximizing functioning and quality of life for both the child and family and minimizing the deficits of autism (Myers, Johnson, & Council on Children with Disabilities, 2007). The plan should define language, social, and educational goals, define and prioritize target behavioral symptoms for intervention, and provide for periodic assessment of the child's functioning at home and school (Volkmar, Cook, Jr., Pomeroy, et al., 1999). Reassessment is especially important for children diagnosed before age 3 years and those with relatively mild symptoms because they are most likely to change diagnostic classification with either apparent improvement or decline (Turner & Stone, 2007).

Treatment

- Early intervention and education
  - One-on-one teaching
  - Therapeutic preschools
  - Social skills and speech therapy
- Behavioral management
- Pharmacologic therapy
  - Risperidone
  - Stimulants
  - Selective serotonin reuptake inhibitors (SSRIs)
  - Other pharmacologic treatments
    - Atypical antipsychotics
  - Complementary and alternative therapies

Early Intervention and Education

Early intervention and intensive education should begin when the diagnosis of ASD is suspected. There are three principal methods based on behavioral, developmental/relationship, or structured teaching principles. What all three methods share are education provided by specialists, parent inclusion, involvement of the child for 25 to 40 hours per week year round, low student-to-teacher ratio, and a focus on addressing the core deficits of autism. For toddlers and preschoolers a focus on the gestural aspects of communication, imitation, and social skills is important because these skills can be taught and are necessary for the future development of language (Landa et al., 2007). Ongoing assessment is essential to modify the child's treatment program in response to gains and plateaus in development.

Intensive early intervention (i.e., between birth and 4 years old) with an applied behavioral analysis (ABA) program has been shown to improve children's level of development as measured by intelligence quotient (IQ) and Autism Diagnostic Observation Schedule (ADOS) scores (Ben-Itzchak & Zachor, 2007). Also referred to as early and intensive behavioral intervention (EIBI), ABA is a skills-based intensive behavioral treatment based on operant conditioning principles as developed by Lovaas (1987). It is the only early intervention method that has been shown in controlled studies to produce gains in some children in IQ, language, and some social skills (Myers et al., 2007). Most ABA programs are home based and use one-to-one teaching. Clearly, not all families have the financial resources and community support necessary to carry out 25 to 40 hours per week of one-to-one teaching. Parents are increasingly turning to their school districts for help with one-to-one early intervention and often meeting with resistance, resulting in litigation (Grinker, 2007).

Other early educational approaches include therapeutic preschools employing Greenspan's developmental/relationship approach, which is based on learning through "floor time" sessions and other techniques to encourage social interactions with the child's parent/caregiver (Wieder & Greenspan, 2005). Evidence of the success of this approach is limited and based on measurement using nonstandardized tools (Mahoney & Perales, 2005). The Treatment and Education of Autistic and Related Communication-Handicapped Children (TEACCH) program is a structured teaching approach relying primarily on group instruction and extensive teaching through visual means to compensate for the verbal deficits of children with autism (Probst & Leppert, 2008). It is widely available in the United States and has had positive evaluation data, though no controlled studies have been conducted (Carr & LeBlanc, 2007).

Speech therapy is an essential part of any early intervention program for children with autism. Functional spoken language by age 6 years is an important predictor of future outcome (Volkmar et al., 1999). Speech therapy also includes the development of imitation and gestural joint attention, both necessary precursors for the ability to "learn to learn." Sign language and the Picture Exchange Communication System (PECS) are important alternatives to spoken language that some children with autism can master, thus allowing them to communicate with family members and at school and reducing the frustration of unmet needs that can lead to behavioral outbursts (Elder, 2002). They may enhance learning spoken language by teaching children with autism how symbolic communication works (Myers et al., 2007). Regardless of the specific communication therapy taken, intensive therapy done in conjunction with the child's school and family is essential, because low-intensity pull-out group sessions are unlikely to be effective (American Speech-Language-Hearing Association, 2006).

Behavioral Management

Behavioral management is an essential part of the treatment plan for a child with autism and should begin as soon after diagnosis as possible, before problematic behaviors are deeply entrenched. Parents may be reluctant to set the firm limits that even a very young child with autism requires to prevent the establishment of inappropriate behaviors. Parents can be reminded that removing a screaming 3-year-old from a store is embarrassing, but removing a screaming 13-year-old may be impossible.

Behavior management begins with a functional assessment of the child's inappropriate behaviors and their antecedents and what the child gains from the behaviors. Interventions are then tailored to modify the events provoking inappropriate behavior and teach the child new, appropriate responses. Early intensive behavioral treatment carries over into a child's language, academic, and social skills (Myers et al., 2007). Behavior specialists work in homes and schools. Trained behavior analysts and specialists can be found through the Behavior Analyst Certification Board (www.bacb.com), schools, autism centers, and state and local programs for children with developmental disabilities. Most children with autism will require behavioral management at home and school throughout their lives.

Pharmacologic Therapy

Medication is not a substitute for appropriate education and behavioral management but may be a useful adjunct to these therapies and enable a child to make full use of them. Medications are generally used to treat targeted, specific symptoms of autism. A medication trial should be considered when disruptive behaviors impair a child's functioning and learning, negatively affect the child and family's quality of life, or present a risk of harm to the child and his or her environment. Behavioral symptoms that may be targets of pharmacologic intervention include self-injurious and aggressive behaviors, compulsions, obsessions and perseveration, anxiety, labile moods, and poor attention and hyperactivity (Myers et al., 2007). Although many parents are reluctant to treat their child with psychotropic medications, surveys show that about half of individuals with ASDs receive some type of psychotropic medication (Myers et al., 2007). The PCP can reassure parents that no medication intervention is irrevocable.

A trial of any medication should include concrete, objective behavioral goals that are measurable and a predetermined time period for the use of the medication, during which its performance will be objectively evaluated. If improvement is shown at the end of this period, the parents and provider may decide to slowly withdraw the medication and monitor for return of the targeted behaviors. A return of the targeted behaviors indicates that the medication is effective. Medications that are not working should be gradually stopped. One of the most common confounding factors in pharmacologic intervention is the addition of one treatment after another without stopping previous medications that do not appear to be helping.

The primary care provider may want to consult a child psychiatrist, a pediatric neurologist, or personnel from autism clinics for

TABLE 13-1

TABLE 13-1

Medications with Demonstrated Efficacy in Autism by Randomized Controlled Studies

Drug Name	Symptom Improvement
Clomipramine	Aggression, Irritability, repetitive behavior
Clonidine	Aggression, hyperactivity, irritability
Fluoxetine	Anxiety, repetitive behavior
Fluvoxamine	Aggression, repetitive behavior
Methylphenidate	Aggression, hyperactivity
Naltrexone	Hyperactivity
Risperidone	Aggression, self-injurious behavior, repetitve behavior, irritability

From Posey, D.J., & McDougle, C.J. (2001). Pharmacotherapeutic management of autism. *Expert Opin Pharmacother, 2*(4), 587-600; Chavez, B., Chavez-Brown, M., Sopko Jr, M.A., & Rey, J. (2007). Atypical antipsychotics in children with pervasive development disorders. *Pediatr Drugs, 9,* 249-266; Kolevzon, A., Mathewson, K.A., & Hollander, E. (2006). Selective serotonin reuptake inhibitors in autism: A review of efficacy and tolerability. *J Clin Psychiatry, 67,* 407-414; Leskoves, T., Rowles, B., & Findling, R. (2008). Pharmacological treatment options for autism spectrum disorders in children and adolescents. *Harv Rev Psychiatry, 16,*97-112; Parikh, M.S., Kolevzon,A., & Hollander, E. (2008) Psychopharmacology of aggerssion in children and adolescents with autism: A critical review of efficacy and tolerability. *J Child Adol Psychopharm, 18,*157-178.

TABLE 13-2

Target Symptoms of Autism and Medications with Possible Efficacy

Symptom	Medication
Aggression/self-injurious behavior	Alpha$_2$-adrenergic agonists
	Atypical antipsychotics
	Anticonvulsants
	Clomipramine
	SSRIs
Anxiety/agitation/irritability	Alpha$_2$-adrenergic agonists
	Antipsychotics
	Buspirone
	Clomipramine
	SSRIs
Inattention/hyperactivity/impulsivity	Stimulants
	Atypical antipsychotics
Repetitive behaviors	Atypical antipsychotics
	Nonselective SRI (clomipramine)
	SSRIs
Sleep disturbance	Alpha$_2$-adrenergic agonists
	Atypical antipsychotics
	Clomipramine
	Clonidine
	Melatonin
	Mirtazapine

From Posey, DJ., & McDougle, C.J. (2001). Pharmacotherapeutic management of autism. *Expert Opin Pharmacother, 2*(4), 587-600; Chavez, B., Chavez-Brown, M., Sopko Jr, M.A., & Rey, J. (2007). Atypical antipsychotics in children with pervasive developmental disorders. *Pediatr Drugs, 9,* 249-266; Kolevzon, A., Mathewson, K.A., & Hollander, E. (2006). Selective serotonin reuptake inhibitors in autism: A review of efficacy and tolerability. *J Clin Psychiatry, 67,* 407-414; Leskoves, T., Rowles, B., & Findling, R. (2008). Pharmacological treatment options for autism spectrum disorders in children and adolescents. *Harv Rev Psychiatry, 16,*97-112; Parikh,M.S., Kolevzon,A., & Hollander, E. (2008) Psychopharmacology of aggerssion in children and adolescents with autism: A critical review of efficacy and tolerability. *J Child Adol Psychopharm, 18,*157-178.
Key: *SSRIs,* selective serotonin reuptake inhibitors.

their expertise about medications that may be useful in treating specific behaviors. Although many medications are prescribed for children with autism, risperidone is the only one approved by the U.S. Food and Drug Administration (FDA) for use in children with autism (U.S. FDA, 2006). Before any medication trial parents should be told both verbally and in writing of potential adverse side effects, how to report and manage them, and how to determine if the medication is helping their child. To minimize the possibility of adverse side effects, dosing should start low and go slow.

A growing number of studies have demonstrated the safety and efficacy of psychotropic medications in children but with small numbers of children and with some adverse side effects and reactions reported (Tables 13-1 and 13-2).

Risperidone. In 2006 the FDA approved risperidone for the treatment of aggressive behavior, including self-injury and tantrums, in children and adolescents with autism (Myers et al., 2007). In double-blind placebo-controlled studies, risperidone has ameliorated one of the symptom triad of autism: the repetitive, restricted, and stereotyped behaviors (McDougle, Scahill, Aman, et al., 2005). Unfortunately, risperidone does not improve the social and communication deficits (McDougle et al., 2005). Risperidone can also reduce aggressive and self-injurious behaviors and temper tantrums (Research Units on Pediatric Psychopharmacology Autism Network [RUPPAN], 2005). Positive effects are often achieved with a modest dose of 2 mg/day. The most common adverse side effects of risperidone are weight gain and sleepiness (Shea, Turgay, Carroll, et al., 2004). Sleepiness can be managed with adjustments in dose or dose schedule but usually spontaneously resolves (Shea et al., 2004). Parents must be informed of the real possibility of unwanted weight gain and advised to take a proactive approach by providing their child with a healthy diet and limiting intake of high-fat, high-calorie food and drink when treatment with risperidone begins. Risperidone has an extremely low incidence of extrapyramidal symptoms (EPS) and tardive dyskinesia (TD) in children, and the EPS and TD resolve when risperidone is discontinued (Correll & Kane, 2007; Dinca, Paul, & Spencer, 2005).

Stimulants. In a double-blind, placebo-controlled study, methylphenidate (Ritalin) decreased hyperactivity and impulsiveness and increased attention (RUPPAN, 2005). Children with autism do not respond to stimulant medication as often as children with isolated attention-deficit/hyperactivity disorder (ADHD) but can experience the same side effects such as decreased appetite, difficulty falling asleep, and irritability. In children with autism and epilepsy, stimulants can lower the child's seizure threshold and precipitate an increase in seizures. This may necessitate an adjustment in the child's antiepileptic regimen or discontinuation of the stimulant.

Selective Serotonin Reuptake Inhibitors. Because serotonin dysfunction has been documented in autism and repetitive symptoms such as those found in people with obsessive-compulsive disorder are also core symptoms in autism, treatment with selective serotonin reuptake inhibitors (SSRIs) may reduce these symptoms (Posey, Erikson, Stigler, et al., 2006). Placebo-controlled and open-label studies with fluoxetine (Prozac) and fluvoxamine (Luvox) have demonstrated a reduction in repetitive behaviors, anxiety, and aggression (Kolevzon, Mathewson, & Hollander, 2006; Posey et al., 2006). Agitation was the most significant adverse side effect reported. No SSRI has been shown to be more effective than any other (Moore, Eichner, & Jones, 2004). Like risperidone, SSRIs have not improved social and communication skills.

Other Pharmacologic Treatments. Carbamazapine (Tegretol, Carbatrol), divalproex sodium (Depakote), topiramate (Topamax), and lamotrigine (Lamictal) are anticonvulsants that may also be useful for decreasing self-injury and aggression (Hardan, Jou, & Keshavan, 2004; Myers et al., 2007). There are case reports and small clinical trials regarding a variety of other medications frequently used in children with neuropsychiatric disorders. Clonidine (Catapres), trazodone (Desyrel), steroids, and atypical antipsychotic medications (olanzapine, ziprasidone, quetiapine, aripiprazole) have all been reported to ameliorate the behavioral and social problems of some children with autism (Stachnik & Nunn-Thompson, 2007). None of the studies, either in support of these medications or suggesting caution in their use, have been conducted with large enough populations or in randomized clinical trials to definitively rule them in or out in the pharmacotherapy of autism.

Complementary and Alternative Therapies

Autism is a clinical, not laboratory-based, diagnosis. The deficits of autism are profound and to many parents seem to appear out of nowhere after their child has been developing typically. There are treatments for symptoms, although not always successful. It comes as no surprise that parents have sought out and tried every possible type of treatment. In fact, parent surveys indicate that the majority of children with autism have received at least one complementary and alternative therapy/medicine (CAM), often before they have been officially diagnosed with autism (Myers et al., 2007). PCPs need to ask parents about their use of CAM because parents will often not volunteer this information (Weber & Newmark, 2007).

A number of alternative treatments for autism are available. They fall into three broad categories: those that are unproven but relatively benign (e.g., low-dose vitamin supplements), those that pose a risk to the child and family in terms of time and money that are redirected from treatments with some proven efficacy to those that may disrupt ongoing education and management (e.g., hyperbaric oxygen therapy), and those that present an actual danger to the child (e.g., chelation therapy) (*Chelation therapy and autism,* 2006). The PCP is the ideal provider to help parents with a risk-benefit analysis of the many CAM treatments marketed to parents.

The gluten-free/casein-free diet is the most popular CAM with a website supporting at least 130 support groups (Christison & Ivany, 2006). There is insufficient evidence to recommend this treatment, but clinical trials are ongoing. Within trials individual children have shown improvement and there are numerous anecdotal reports of reduction in autistic symptoms (Elder, Shankar, Shuster, et al., 2006; Millward, Ferriter, Calver, et al., 2004). Megadose vitamin B_6 and magnesium have been tried to improve speech and behavior based on the idea that they can enhance neurotransmitter function. There is insufficient evidence to recommend their use (Nye & Brice, 2005). They can cause diarrhea and peripheral neuropathy, so if parents are administering them, their use should be monitored by a clinician. Dimethylglycine (DMG), a dietary supplement, was found to be no different in improving behavior from placebo in a double-blind, placebo-controlled study (Kern, Van Miller, Evans, et al., 2002).

Secretin, a gastrointestinal hormone, was proposed as a treatment for the social and communication deficits of autism after a report of a single child given a single injection of porcine secretin appeared to show dramatic improvement in these areas (Carey, Ratliff-Schaub, Funk, et al., 2002). There is no evidence that secretin reduces the symptoms of autism (Williams, Wray, & Wheeler, 2005). It is an invasive treatment and so should be recommended against.

The Committee on Children with Disabilities of the American Academy of Pediatrics and the Cochrane Collaboration have concluded that auditory integration training and facilitated communication are treatments warranted only as part of research protocols (Sinha, Silove, Wheeler, et al., 2004). The Cochrane Collaboration found that music therapy provided by a trained music therapist improved nonverbal and, to a lesser degree, verbal communication skills (Gold, Wigram, & Elefant, 2006).

Regardless of the CAM therapy the parents choose to use, the PCP should become familiar with it and approach its use as objectively and compassionately as possible (Committee on Children with Disabilities, 2001a). PCPs can help the family set objective, measurable goals regarding the symptoms to be treated and assist in defining a length of time the treatment will be used before its efficacy is evaluated. Parents should be cautioned to try only one new treatment at a time so that any changes observed can be ascribed to that treatment. The PCP must balance his or her role as an advocate and guardian for the child's well-being with a commitment to family-centered care (Committee on Children with Disabilities, 2001b).

Anticipated Advances in Diagnosis and Management

Research has established that the diagnosis of autism is stable in most children by age 2 years, and the average age of diagnosis is now 3 years (Mandell, Novak, & Zubritsky, 2005). The benefits of early intervention have also been demonstrated (Volkmar, Lord, Bailey, et al., 2004). Prospective studies with high-risk populations (e.g., siblings of children with autism) are being developed to identify reliable autistic symptoms as they emerge in infancy, to examine regression, and to track the long-term development of children diagnosed with autism. Prospective studies may make earlier diagnosis and intervention possible, leading to better outcomes.

In 2001 the National Institutes of Health (NIH) announced a research program aimed at some of the key questions regarding autism (National Institutes of Health [NIH], 2001). Areas that the government identified as needing further research include epidemiology, early diagnosis, genetics, brain mechanisms, communication skills, cognition, and behavioral and biologic interventions (NIH, 2001). These studies must be scientifically rigorous and multidisciplinary and must enroll sufficient numbers of children and adults with autism to arrive at significant conclusions. Research sites have been established throughout the United States and can be accessed at www.nih.gov.

The quest for autism susceptibility genes is complicated by the complex and extremely variable behavioral phenotype of autism and the now-established genetic heterogeneity of autism (Muhle et al., 2004). Identifying genes is a small first step. Research then must determine how abnormal genes are expressed in brain function. To integrate genetic research with clinical research into treatment methods and outcomes, more precise definitions of autistic symptoms, their development, and their outcomes are needed. Because of the wide continuum of behavioral phenotypes observed in autism, future research must include assessment of infants and children at risk for autism, with autism, and family members to delineate the boundaries of autism and the milder phenotypes (Volkmar, Chawarska, & Klin, 2005). Primary care providers can assist with this search by referring families to genetics clinics and the NIH for direction to studies in which they might participate.

Neuroimaging and neuropathologic studies have discovered abnormalities in the brains of both children and adults with autism. How these differences affect connectivity in the brain and resulting development of the child is the next frontier (Volkmar et al., 2004). Neuropathologic studies may be advanced if families of children with autism who die for any reason are encouraged by PCPs to consent to tissue donation (see Resources at the end of this chapter).

Advances in educational and behavioral treatment may focus more on the study of the learning processes of children with autism in more naturalistic settings than performance of isolated tasks. As with all research in autism, the challenge is devising studies with criteria specific enough to be replicated, with a large enough number of participants with homogenous symptoms, and long-term follow-up (McConachie & Diggle, 2007). Evaluation of parent training as a mode of delivering intervention is also on the horizon (McConachie & Diggle, 2007).

Psychopharmacology may be the answer to some of the most troubling behavioral manifestations of autism, although medications have not been shown to be effective in improving social and communication skills. There is a dearth of rigorously conducted, double-blind, placebo-controlled, large, long-term studies of both the efficacy and safety of the many neuropsychiatric medications being tried empirically in children. Future research in psychopharmacology using systematic, randomized clinical trials of medications is needed (Myers et al., 2007). There is also a need for standardization of outcome measures, which would make comparison of studies possible (Jesner, Aref-Adib, & Coren, 2007).

Associated Problems of Autism Spectrum Disorder and Treatment

Autism can be found coexisting with any medical or psychiatric conditions of childhood. Because autism-specific services improve the outcomes of many children with autism, all children, regardless of any preexisting condition, should be screened for autism. Symptoms of autism should not be overlooked and simply attributed to the child's preexisting condition. In a study published in 2008 one quarter of very low birth weight infants had positive scores on the M-CHAT, most of whom had normal MRIs of the brain (Limperopoulos, Bassan, Sullivan, et al., 2008). Congenital anomalies are found in approximately 10% of children with ASD (Wier, Yoshida, Odouli, et al., 2006). When chromosome and mitochondrial respiratory chain abnormalities discovered by systematic laboratory testing are included, the rate of physiologic comorbidities is 20% (Oliveira, Ataide, Marques, et al, 2007). Associated medical conditions increase in proportion with degree of mental retardation (Barton & Volkmar, 1998).

Associated Problems of Autism Spectrum Disorder and Treatment
- Mental retardation/intellectual disability
- Epilepsy
- Tuberous sclerosis
- Fragile X syndrome
- Tourette syndrome
- Psychiatric disorders
- Landau-Kleffner syndrome

Mental Retardation/Intellectual Disability

Children with autism may have IQs ranging from profound retardation to superior intelligence. Reported rates of intellectual disability range from 25% to 75% with children on the milder end of the autism spectrum less likely to have cognitive impairment (Johnson et al., 2007). The rate of mental retardation may be trending downward as testing of children with challenging behaviors improves and more children on the milder end of the spectrum are diagnosed with autism. Children with autism usually have higher nonverbal than verbal IQ scores, and testing must be done by an experienced psychologist who can work with the child's potential negativity, distractibility, and comprehension difficulties (Geiger, Smith, & Creaghead, 2002). Because a child's cognitive ability can help predict the child's future course and outcome, accurate assessment of a child's IQ provides the child's family with important information for treatment planning (Korkmaz, 2000).

When children with mental retardation are evaluated for ASDs, the prevalence ranges from 7% in Down syndrome (see Chapter 24) to almost 17% in nonspecific mental retardation (De Bildt, Sytema, Kraijer, et al., 2005; Dykens, 2007). Diagnosis is often delayed in children with Down syndrome until they reach school age (Dykens, 2007). This may be due to the common view of children with Down syndrome as happy and social and attribution of their autistic symptoms to their underlying mental retardation rather than co-occurring autism (Dykens, 2007).

Epilepsy

Up to one third of people with autism have been reported to develop epilepsy, a clinical diagnosis made when the child has recurrent unprovoked seizures (Danielsson, Gillberg, Billstedt, et al., 2005; Johnson et al., 2007). There is a bimodal peak onset of seizures during early childhood and again in adolescence (Filipek et al., 1999). The risk of developing epilepsy is higher in children with autism who also have severe mental retardation and in children with tuberous sclerosis and autism (Bolton, 2004; Tuchman & Rapin, 2002). Epilepsy is most likely a symptom of the same neurologic dysfunction that is responsible for the child's autism (Levisohn, 2007). Because of the high rate of epilepsy in children with autism, PCPs should obtain an EEG if parents report convulsions or staring episodes unresponsive to physical stimulation. Febrile seizures, rage attacks, and breath-holding spells are usually not epileptic seizures (Gabis, Pomeroy, & Andriola, 2005). Primary generalized, complex partial, atypical absence, and other types of seizures—alone or in combination—have all been reported (Tuchman & Rapin, 2002) (see Chapter 26).

Tuberous Sclerosis

Tuberous sclerosis, a neurocutaneous syndrome, is found in 1% to 4% of individuals with autism and in as many as 8% to 14% of individuals with autism and epilepsy (Wong, 2006). Epilepsy, particularly infantile spasms, and mental retardation are significant risk factors in the development of autism in tuberous sclerosis (Smalley, 2002). The PCP should thoroughly examine the skin of any child with autistic symptoms to look for the hypopigmented macules (i.e., ash-leaf spots) characteristic of tuberous sclerosis (Johnson et al., 2007). The presence of even one lesion indicates the need for a tuberous sclerosis workup including evaluation for autism.

Fragile X Syndrome

Fragile X syndrome, the most common genetic cause of mental retardation, also includes a number of social symptoms and repetitive behaviors similar to the deficits of autism (Belmonte & Bourgeron, 2006). The prevalence of autism in individuals with fragile X syndrome is thought to be 4% or less and found primarily in children with both autism and mental retardation (Zafeiriou, Ververi, & Vargiami, 2006). Testing for Fragile X syndrome is recommended for all children with autism and mental retardation (see Chapter 27).

Tourette Syndrome

Chronic motor tics can be distinguished from the usual stereotypes of autism in a number of ways. Tics are typically brief, interrupt the flow of behavior, are contextually inappropriate, and are seen more often in the face, shoulders, and arms than hands and fingers. Motor tics can be found in 11% of children with autism and Tourette syndrome (both motor and vocal tics) in up to 11% (Canitano & Vivanti, 2007). Like autism, Tourette syndrome is a genetic disorder but no specific genes have been identified. Medications to control tics can be considered when the tics interfere with the child's daily activities and quality of life (see Chapter 41).

Psychiatric Disorders

As with physiologic disorders, autism coexists with all psychiatric disorders of childhood. Symptoms of depression and ADHD are two to four times more prevalent in children with autism than children with typical development or mental retardation (Brereton, Tonge, & Einfeld, 2006; McCarthy, 2007). Although the *DSM-IV-TR* does not allow a diagnosis of ADHD if the child has ASD, up to 75% of children with ASD meet the DSM criteria for a diagnosis of ADHD (Lee & Ousley, 2006). A clinical diagnosis of ADHD can and should be made because the educational and pharmacologic treatments for isolated ADHD will also often be effective in children with both ASD and ADHD (Brereton et al., 2006) (see Chapter 12). Disruptive, repetitive, and anxious behaviors are also common in ASD (McCarthy, 2007). They can be difficult for both caregivers and teachers to manage and make out-of-home placement a necessity for the safety of the child and family. These symptoms are also frequently amenable to both behavioral and pharmacologic management.

Landau-Kleffner Syndrome

Landau-Kleffner syndrome is not an associated condition of autism but is discussed here because of the interest in the autism community in this syndrome and the belief by many parents of children with autism that Landau-Kleffner syndrome might be responsible for their child's developmental problems.

Landau-Kleffner syndrome (i.e., acquired aphasia with convulsive disorder in children) was originally described in 1957 by Drs. Landau and Kleffner. It was based on six children they studied who had had normal language and development and then, after age 3 years, had rapid onset of aphasia accompanied by seizures. Recovery occurred spontaneously in some children and after treatment with antiepileptic medications and speech therapy in others (Landau & Kleffner, 1998).

Landau-Kleffner syndrome has two necessary symptoms: acquired aphasia and a sleep-activated abnormal EEG (National Institute of Neurological Disorders and Stroke [NINDS], 2008).

The epilepsy of Landau-Kleffner syndrome, which occurs in about 70% of diagnosed individuals, is usually easily and well controlled (Tatum, Genton, Bureau, et al., 2001). Intelligence and social skills are preserved, and behavioral stereotypes are not seen. The onset of the aphasia is rapid, occurring over days, and with receptive aphasia usually preceding expressive (Tatum et al., 2001). Evaluation and diagnosis require EEG monitoring of deep sleep that can only be accomplished with an overnight EEG, either in the home or as an inpatient in an epilepsy monitoring unit. Treatment usually involves antiepileptic medication, corticosteroids, and speech therapy. Surgery may be an option for children who do not respond to medication. The prognosis for the recovery of speech varies but improves with early speech therapy and when onset is after age 6 years (NINDS, 2008).

Chromosome Disorders

Over 40 chromosome disorders have been reported in children with ASD. Chromosome disorders most likely to predispose a child to the development of autism include tuberous sclerosis, Angelman syndrome, Down syndrome, DiGeorge syndrome, and Smith-Lemli-Opitz syndrome with rates ranging from 15% to 75% (Bukelis, Porter, Zimmerman, et al., 2007; Fine, Weissman, Gerdes, et al., 2005; Zafeiriou et al., 2006).

Primary care providers must recognize that children with any medical condition might also have autism and that children with autism can also have another, possibly unrelated, condition. When possible, treatment of the comorbid condition can result in an improvement in the child's autistic symptoms. In addition, information about associated problems—even when a problem cannot be treated—can be important for genetic counseling and educating the family about their child's diagnosis and prognosis (Zafeiriou et al., 2006).

Prognosis

The outcome for children with autism, similar to the expression of the syndrome itself, varies. Almost all children diagnosed with autism will continue to meet the diagnostic criteria in adulthood (McGovern & Sigman, 2005). At one end of the spectrum are individuals with average or above-average cognitive abilities who have attended college, have careers, and can live independently. This group is a minority and they continue to have symptoms of autism, particularly social skill deficits and ritualistic behaviors (Howlin, Goode, Hutton, et al., 2004). Rarely is an adult with autism able to work at a job that requires social interaction or flexibility or be involved in intimate relationships. Even adults with average intelligence and academic achievement may have such serious social and judgment deficits that holding a job and living independently are impossible (Howlin et al., 2004). The one caveat to this rather grim picture is that these results are from adults not generally exposed to early, intensive, and continual therapeutic education and treatment. As research on autism continues and findings are put into clinical practice, more children may be able to function independently or semi-independently when they reach adulthood.

Performance and verbal IQs greater than 70 are an important prognostic factor (Coplan & Jawad, 2005). Children who have both autism and mental retardation will usually make developmental progress but more slowly than children with either of these disorders in isolation and will require a supportive living environment throughout their lives (Howlin et al., 2004). Young children who demonstrate joint attention behaviors (i.e., communication signals such as pointing to direct someone's attention to an experience they want to share) are more likely to develop better language skills (Chawarska, Paul, Klin, et al., 2006).

The natural course of autism varies over time. When the diagnosis of autism is made after age 30 months, it is very stable (Turner & Stone, 2007). Children diagnosed at age 2 years with autism who improve enough to no longer meet the criteria for diagnosis will virtually always continue to have developmental problems such as learning disabilities and ADHD (Turner & Stone, 2007). It is unclear if the improvement seen is the result of maturation, intensive intervention, early diagnosis, or some combination of these factors. Adults with ASD continue to exhibit greater impairment in social skills as compared with repetitive and maladaptive behaviors, which decrease in many individuals as they get older (Shattuck, Seltzer, Breenberg, et al., 2007). There is a small minority of children whose symptoms worsen with age. There is no research available that indicates how to predict accurately an individual child's outcome, although Coplan and Jawad (2005) have developed a statistical model that strongly suggests coexisting mental retardation is the most salient feature of children with autism who will require lifelong care.

Individuals with autism appear to have an increased mortality rate (Pickett & Paculdo, 2006). This increase is particularly associated with respiratory illness in people with more severe mental retardation and/or epilepsy and accidental causes such as drowning and suffocation (Shavelle, Strauss, & Pickett, 2001).

PRIMARY CARE MANAGEMENT

Health Care Maintenance
Growth and Development
Children with autism have the same basic health care maintenance needs as typically developing children (Myers et al., 2007). Perhaps the most challenging aspect of providing primary care to a child with autism is enlisting the child's cooperation. Before a child's visit, consultation with the parents regarding the child's behavioral symptoms, fears, and positive reinforcers can give the PCP information important for making the child's visit a success. With the parent's written permission, the PCP may also find it useful to talk with the child's teacher or behavioral therapist about the best ways to approach the child. Together, the PCP and parents can devise a plan for the examination that will help the PCP, the staff, and the child begin to form a working relationship and lead the PCP from the child's most to least favorite parts of the examination. A flexible and unhurried approach is best with time for talking before the PCP touches the child and for the child to handle objects such as the stethoscope. A reward at the completion of the examination can be planned, available, and referred to during the examination as necessary. Because many children with autism are highly distractible, time spent in the waiting room with other children and parents can leave them overstimulated and unable to fully cooperate. Appointments are best scheduled as the first appointment of the morning or afternoon. Children with autism often need more frequent clinic visits for both medical and psychiatric management

and longer appointments with plenty of time for both the examination and talking with the parents (Croen, Najjar, Ray, et al., 2006). Parents want to discuss their child's development, education, and use of complementary and alternative medicine with their PCP but feel they are imposing on the PCP unless the PCP is the one to initiate this conversation. PCPs may feel unable to provide a medical home for a child with autism because of time constraints, lack of training, and a lack of knowledge about resources available to both them and families (Brachlow, Ness, McPheeters, et al., 2007). Parents, though, report that their children with special needs have better health when the PCP provides a medical home for the child (Brachlow et al., 2007).

Children with autism may have their growth affected by disease symptomatology or pharmacologic therapies. Weight gain and height increases may falter as the result of decreased caloric intake secondary to restricted food preferences. The use of stimulant medication can decrease a child's appetite. Conversely, valproic acid and some atypical antipsychotic medications can result in unwanted weight gain because of their appetite-stimulating effects. Parents should be educated about the possible effects of medication on the child's growth and encouraged to monitor the child's growth and consult the PCP if there are concerns. Parents of children taking the atypical antipsychotics need nutritional guidance as their child begins taking them, including advice to limit portion sizes and restrict snacks to water and low-fat foods. Children with risk factors for altered growth should be measured every 6 months.

Neonatal head circumferences are usually normal for children with autism at birth but increased at a greater than normal rate from age 6 to 10 months for over half of babies in one study (Webb, Nalty, Munson, et al., 2007). Macrocephaly occurs in about 20% by age 3 years (Webb et al., 2007). These large head circumferences are nonpathologic and do not require further investigation with neuroimaging unless the child's neurologic examination reveals focal or cranial nerve abnormalities (Filipek et al., 2000). One hypothesis for the development of macrocephaly in autism is that there is a period of accelerated brain growth in the first year of life followed by deceleration (Courchesne & Pierce, 2005). Head circumferences should be measured at every well-child visit until age 5 years and annually thereafter if a child also has tuberous sclerosis.

Children with autism will have delayed development in their language and social skills. A majority will also have cognitive and motor skill delays (Provost, Lopez, & Heimerl, 2007). The extent of their delays will depend on the degree of their intellectual disability, interference with development from repetitive and self-stimulatory behaviors, and their response to educational and behavioral interventions, speech, physical, and occupational therapies, and medication when it is used. The success of a child's treatment for autism is measured empirically. Therefore the child will need to be annually reevaluated by a multidisciplinary team during the first few years of treatment and thereafter every few years. These evaluations will serve as the basis for treatment planning.

Primary care providers should continue to monitor motor, cognitive, language, and social-emotional development at all well-child care visits, using a standardized developmental questionnaire completed by the parent and/or an objective screening tool of the PCP's choice (Johnson et al., 2007) (see Chapter 2).

Diet

Throughout the lifetime of a child with autism, parents, teachers, therapists, and providers are faced with decisions about when and when not to accommodate the child's insistence on sameness. There is no one right answer for every child and family. Each family, with the help of their child's provider, should assess their own values, needs, and level of tolerance and make decisions accordingly.

Many children with autism have feeding and eating difficulties. Restricted food preferences are widely reported. Preferences appear to arise from sensitivities to texture, smell, color, and even the sound of the food being eaten. Adequacy of dietary intake should be evaluated at each well-child visit. An excessive adherence to routine and an abhorrence of changes in the environment may lead children with autism to reject their parents' efforts to provide them with a balanced diet. Children may have periods when they eat only one or a few foods. Families should be encouraged to follow their typical food preferences because these preferences have been shown to have more of an influence on the child's eating habits than their autistic symptoms (Schreck & Williams, 2006).

The feeding patterns of typically developing children have not been well studied, leaving uncertainty about just how abnormal the food rejection behaviors of some children with autism are (Ahearn, Castine, Nault, et al., 2001). Some of these difficulties may be ameliorated through the interventions of the child's behavioral therapist. If the child insists on using certain dishes and cups for eating, the PCP may advise the parents to have multiple sets of the preferred items. A daily multivitamin supplement is recommended to ensure adequate vitamin and mineral intake. Parents of children taking valproic acid and atypical antipsychotics should be encouraged to provide them with plenty of low-calorie, low-fat snacks and water instead of juice or soda, to prevent excessive weight gain.

The gluten-free, casein-free diet is extremely popular among the parents of children with autism (see previous section on CAM). Boys on a casein-free diet have been shown to have bone thickness 20% less than expected (Hediger, England, Molloy, et al. 2007). Parents using this diet with their children may benefit from a consultation with a dietitian and information regarding the potential risks of restricted diets during childhood.

Safety

The parents of children with autism are faced with a number of safety issues that arise from the cognitive and behavioral deficits of autism. Because of their poor judgment and lack of impulse control, children with autism must be supervised at all times. Their ability to recognize a potentially dangerous activity (e.g., tree climbing) is usually far below expectations for their chronologic age and gross motor capabilities. Children with autism have been known to swallow an entire bottle of medication in the time it takes a parent to turn away and answer the telephone.

Morbidity and mortality can be the result of momentary lapses in supervision. Deaths in children with autism during seizures, drowning, and suffocation were more than three times higher compared with the general population in one study (Shavelle et al., 2001). Children between 5 and 10 years old were particularly at risk for premature death, perhaps because teenagers with autism engage in fewer high-risk behaviors such as driving and recreational drug use than their typically developing peers (Shavelle et al., 2001).

Children with autism, especially those who also have epilepsy, must never be left alone in a bathtub or near a spa or any body of water. Providers will often find that parents need education regarding this precaution. They often do not realize that "never" includes those few seconds it may take to answer the phone or doorbell. Supervision during swimming means a specific adult being assigned to watch the child whenever the child is in or near the water. Drowning has occurred when a group of children is swimming with a group of adults nearby but no single adult is responsible for observing the child with autism.

Childproofing the home of a child with autism is essential. Medications must be out of reach and securely locked. Other dangerous objects (e.g., knives, matches) must be kept out of reach. Hot stoves and liquids present a constant danger to children with autism.

Personal safety is a concern for any child with autism. Wandering off is not uncommon. Children should wear an ID bracelet. Parents should prepare emergency forms that describe their child's condition and symptoms, a photo and description of identifying physical characteristics, and contact information for home, school, and the PCP. These forms should be kept in the family car, school office, and child's backpack and with all child-care providers.

Personal safety includes teaching all children about appropriate behavior toward strangers and how to both avoid and report potentially abusive situations. Visual aids and role playing can be used with children whose language is limited. When evaluating a sudden deterioration in behavior, the PCP must always consider the possibility of physical or sexual abuse. Behaviors correlated with physical and sexual abuse in children with autism include sexual acting-out behavior, self-injurious behavior, and running away (Mandell et al., 2005).

Children with autism may develop self-injurious behaviors such as head banging, hand biting, and scratching or picking at their skin. Some of these behaviors may be gentle and are probably self-stimulatory. Other self-injurious behavior, however, can cause significant body harm, and parents must stop this behavior even if the child becomes aggressive. Parents of children with self-injurious behavior must work with the child's PCP and autism treatment team to devise a plan for responding to this behavior. This plan may include pharmacotherapy and behavior modification techniques such as immediate removal from the situation and a firm "no." Self-injurious behaviors are extremely upsetting to parents, and they will need a great deal of support and assistance as they attempt to manage and prevent these behaviors.

The presence of self-injurious behaviors is complicated by an apparent decreased sensitivity to pain in many children with autism (Rapin, 1997). That is, they may fail to respond with tears or a painful outcry to painful stimuli (e.g., a hot stove, a laceration). They often fail to approach their parents for comfort when they have been injured or are ill. Because of their lack of communication and social skills, the only sign that a child with autism is in pain may be an exacerbation of their autistic symptomatology. Children with autism have died from gastrointestinal bleeding and bowel rupture that may not have been diagnosed rapidly enough because of the child's inability to communicate. The health care provider must pay attention to parental reports that their child's behavior is different for no apparent reason because this may be the only clue that the child has suffered an injury or is in pain.

Immunizations

Children with autism should be vaccinated following the schedule for all children recommended by the American Academy of Pediatrics, including receiving the MMR vaccine. The IOM Immunization Safety Review Committee has concluded that sufficient evidence exists to refute a causal relationship between autism and the MMR (DeStefano, 2007). Children with autism who also have epilepsy should be vaccinated following the guidelines of the American Academy of Pediatrics for children with epilepsy (see Chapter 26).

Because of their insensitivity to pain and inability to report discomfort, children with autism may be given acetaminophen or ibuprofen prophylactically 1 hour before and periodically for 24 hours following the administration of vaccinations.

Screening

Vision. A child with autism needs a thorough ophthalmologic examination at the time of diagnosis to look for the ocular signs of tuberous sclerosis: hypopigmented spots in the iris and choroid hamartomas. Following this initial screening, routine screening is recommended.

Hearing. Following an initial evaluation by an audiologist (which often requires BAER) to rule out hearing loss as a cause of speech delay, routine screening is recommended.

Dental. Routine screening is recommended. Children with autism who are also taking phenytoin for epilepsy are prone to develop gum hyperplasia and need to have their gums checked at least semiannually. Referral to a dentist familiar with treating children with developmental disabilities is essential because children with autism will often require sedation or general anesthesia for dental examinations and procedures. Indicators that a child with autism may be able to cooperate with dental examinations include being able to sit still for a haircut, brushing their own teeth, and having some receptive and expressive language (Marshall, Sheller, Williams, et al., 2007).

Blood Pressure. Routine screening is recommended. Blood pressure testing can be very upsetting to children with autism and may be deferred to the end of the examination when the child's cooperation is more important for other aspects of the visit. Children with autism may take clonidine either to treat a concomitant tic disorder or to decrease hyperactivity and improve attention. Clonidine can cause both hypotension and hypertension. Blood pressure should be monitored before initiation of therapy. Lowering the dose of clonidine or stopping it completely must be done very slowly with blood pressure monitoring after each dose change. A rapid decrease in the clonidine dose can precipitate potentially dangerous rebound hypertension (Posey & McDougle, 2001).

Hematocrit. Routine screening is recommended. Children with autism who are taking carbamazepine or valproic acid should have complete blood counts (CBCs) with platelets before initiation of therapy and several weeks after establishment of the maintenance dose. These tests should be repeated annually and should also be done if the child develops symptoms of thrombocytopenia or liver dysfunction, such as unusual bruising or petechiae, unusual bleeding, jaundice, vomiting, or hepatomegaly.

Urinalysis. Routine screening is recommended.

Tuberculosis. Routine screening is recommended.

Condition-Specific Screening

Liver Function Tests. Aspartate aminotran sferase (AST) and alanine aminotransferase (ALT) levels should be measured before a child begins taking either carbamazepine or valproic acid. Liver function tests and serum drug levels should be obtained several weeks after the maintenance dose is reached and annually after that. Slight elevations in liver functions are usually nonpathologic if asymptomatic and can be followed semiannually.

Common Illness Management
Differential Diagnosis

Because of their social, communication, and cognitive deficits, most children with autism cannot accurately report symptoms of illness to their parents or providers. Parents or caretakers of children with autism are the experts on their child's baseline behavior and level of functioning. Regression in a child's skills, a negative change in behavior, or self-injurious behaviors are often the first indication that a child with autism is ill (Oliver & Petty, 2002). Facial grimacing in a nonverbal child has been correlated with pain (Messmer, Nader, & Craig, 2007). Head banging or other self-injurious or aggressive behaviors may suddenly begin as a response to a painful illness, such as otitis media, urinary tract infection or obstruction, appendicitis, or a tooth abscess. It is important for PCPs to listen carefully to parental reports of children who are not behaving in their customary ways and schedule a clinic visit to look for physical causes of behavioral symptoms.

Injury. Children with autism are at higher risk for injuries of many types, including head and facial injuries, poisoning, cuts, and burns (Lee, Harrington, Chang, et al., 2007; McDermott, Zhou, & Mann, 2008). The frequency of accidental injury may obscure the occurrence of nonaccidental injury that can result from caretaker fatigue and the extremely trying and sometimes dangerous behavior of a child with autism. Self-injurious behaviors (e.g., hand biting, head banging) can also cause injuries that may require both treatment of the injury and behavioral and pharmacologic intervention to prevent further injury.

Seizures. Because of the high incidence of epilepsy in children with autism, the PCP should have a high degree of suspicion when a parent reports a seizure-like episode. Children with autism may have any one of the various types of seizures: simple or complex partial seizures, absence seizures, atonic, or generalized tonic or clonic seizures. Many of the self-stimulatory behaviors seen in children with autism can appear to be seizure activity. Nonepileptic events, such as self-stimulatory behaviors, tics, and staring and inattention, can be differentiated from epileptic events in several ways. Nonepileptic events are usually asymmetric and arrhythmic, they can be interrupted by firm physical stimulation from the

---

Differential Diagnosis

- Communication and cognitive deficits make assessment difficult
- Change in behavior may indicate underlying medical problem
- Injury vs. sequelae from self-injurious behavior vs. nonaccidental injury
- Seizures vs. repetitive or stereotypical behaviors of autism
- Gastrointestinal complaints and pica
- Medication side effects (e.g., gastrointestinal symptoms, ataxia, lethargy, tremulousness)

caregiver, and children remain responsive during them. Children who manifest signs of seizure activity (e.g., rhythmic jerking, stiffening, staring with unresponsiveness to physical stimulation, eye fluttering or deviation) should have an EEG at a diagnostic laboratory experienced in obtaining EEGs in children. Clinical seizures indicate the need for consultation with or referral to a pediatric neurologist.

When there is suspicion that the child has experienced language regression that may be Landau-Kleffner syndrome, an overnight EEG to obtain deep sleep is necessary for diagnosis. This can be obtained as a 24-hour ambulatory EEG in the child's home or with an overnight inpatient stay in an epilepsy monitoring unit.

Gastrointestinal Complaints. A significant minority of children with autism have gastrointestinal complaints, either chronic diarrhea or constipation (Myers et al., 2007). Milk consumption has been implicated in the development of constipation (Afzal, Murch, Thirrupathy, et al., 2003). Only about half of children with constipation and impaction will have fecal soiling (Afzal et al., 2003). As with other causes of discomfort in nonverbal children, deterioration in baseline behavior may be the first symptom. Workup and treatment should proceed as for any child with diarrhea or constipation.

Pica (the eating of nonfood substances) is not uncommon in children with autism and can result in gastrointestinal obstruction. Some of the more frequently ingested items are the small magnets now commonly found as part of toy trains and construction equipment. These magnets are especially dangerous because of their ability to be swallowed individually but then meet and stick to each other in the intestinal tract, creating a larger object than the child could be expected to eat. Symptoms of obstruction include appetite and weight loss, soiling, and disruptive behavior.

Medication Side Effects. Although there are no routinely prescribed medications for children with autism, many take medications for controlling seizures or behavioral disturbances. Parents are often reluctant to use medications in their children, particularly for symptoms that are defined clinically rather than by laboratory test. The PCP can guide parents in appropriate trials of medications to control seizures and behavioral disturbances by educating them about potential benefits and possible adverse side effects. The decision to medicate a child is not irrevocable; a medication can and should be stopped if it does not control the targeted symptom or has unacceptable side effects.

PCPs should know what medications a child is taking and the common and adverse side effects and signs of toxicity of each. When evaluating symptoms that may be adverse side effects, PCPs should consider whether the medication has been recently introduced because side effects are more common early in a medication trial. Although these medications will have been prescribed by the child's neurologist or psychiatrist, parents will call the PCP first if the child develops nausea and vomiting, ataxia, daytime sleepiness and lethargy, tremor, or other potential symptoms of toxic drug levels. It is up to PCPs to be aware of what medications, if any, a child is taking and their possible adverse side effects. Priapism is a potential adverse side effect of trazodone, so it should be used cautiously in postpubertal males (Kem, Posey, & McDougle, 2002).

Drug Interactions

The use of erythromycin in children taking carbamazepine should be avoided. Erythromycin increases carbamazepine blood levels, which can result in toxicity (see Chapter 26 for other antiepileptic drug interactions). There is a theoretical risk of lowering a child's seizure threshold with stimulants, even when the child is taking antiepileptic medications. If a stimulant is tried and seizures recur or become more frequent, the stimulant can be stopped and a return to the child's baseline seizure frequency can be expected.

Developmental Issues

Sleep Patterns

Sleep diaries kept by parents of children with autism and polysomnography show that their children take longer to fall asleep and wake more frequently than typically developing children (Malow, Marzec, McGrew, et al., 2006). Insomnia has been correlated with increased behavior problems during the day, including inattention and aggressiveness (Malow et al., 2006). Parents are affected also as they may train themselves to sleep lightly or get up frequently during the night. The reasons for the increased incidence of insomnia in autism are unknown. There is speculation that it may be caused by abnormal melatonin regulation, depression and anxiety, and behaviors seen more frequently in autism such as bruxism and nightmares (Malow, 2004). In addition, it is now known that children with typical development or chronic conditions other than autism are much more likely to have sleep disorders than previously thought (Mindell, Emslie, Blumer, et al., 2006). The PCP should refer the child, particularly one who snores, to a pediatric sleep disorder clinic for evaluation of structural causes of insomnia such as obstructive sleep apnea.

Prevention of insomnia should be discussed with parents as soon as a child is suspected of having autism and is having problems falling or staying asleep. Teaching the child to fall asleep in her or his own bed after a consistent bedtime ritual must be the focus, even if the child protests. If insomnia develops, sleep hygiene and behavioral interventions to improve sleep are the first steps in the treatment plan. Avoidance of caffeine, regular exercise, not allowing daytime sleeping, and highly structured bedtime rituals are essential (Malow et al., 2006). Initially, a child may need a parent at the bedside until the child falls asleep. Parents can gradually move themselves farther and farther from their child's bed until their presence is no longer needed. This is a process that may take weeks or even months (Wing, 2001). Because children with autism may awaken and get out of bed during the night, their rooms must be safe and free of objects with which the children could harm themselves. Some children with autism learn to play alone in their room, even in the dark. The door of the room must be secured, however, so that a child cannot wander about the house and engage in potentially dangerous behavior. A Dutch door is a useful alternative for some families. Parents will need reassurance that this aberrant sleep pattern is not unusual for some children, both with and without autism, and that it is all right for the child to be awake and playing at night.

When sleep hygiene measures do not cure insomnia, medication can be considered. Children who are already on medicines that may have sedative side effects, such as antiepileptics, atypical antipsychotics, clonidine, or benzodiazepines, may have improved sleep if their final dose of the day is given 30 to 60 minutes before bedtime (Malow, Marzec, & McGrew 2006). Diphenhydramine is effective in helping some children fall asleep, although it may have a paradoxical effect and is best tested on a night when the family can tolerate a child who may be awake and agitated for hours.

Although melatonin is not FDA approved because it is not considered a medication, there are many reports from parents about its usefulness in promoting sleep and one research study that supports its efficacy in autism (Andersen, Kaczmarska, McGrew, et al., 2008). It is a naturally occurring hormone with excessive sleepiness and enuresis reported as infrequent side effects (Andersen et al., 2008). Doses of 0.5 to 10 mg have been found to be effective in many children with autism (Andersen et al., 2008). When given as part of the bedtime ritual, trazodone or the newer hypnotic medications zolpidem and zaleplon may help the child both fall asleep and stay asleep (Owens, Rosen, & Mindell, 2003). There is no evidence, however, that any medication will help without a highly structured and consistent bedtime routine used simultaneously.

Toileting

Toilet training is a challenge for most children with autism. It is also one of the most important developmental milestones a child can attain. A toilet-trained child is much easier to care for at home, at school, and in the community. Toilet training saves families significant amounts of time and money. Although the goal of toilet training is the child's self-initiation of toileting, some children with the inability to communicate may be trained to stay dry between scheduled toileting times. For many children with autism and mental retardation, the goal will be the child requesting to be taken to the toilet rather than completely independent toileting.

Children with autism do not respond to many of the standard toilet-training strategies parents use (e.g., being encouraged to imitate the parent or wear "big kid underwear") but can often be toilet trained using a behavioral approach with food, a favorite toy, or a favorite activity as a reward. Toilet training can take weeks. It can proceed when a child is able to sit for 5 minutes, can stay dry for at least 1½ hours, and can cooperate with simple instructions (Cicero & Pfadt, 2002). Thus some children will need a behavioral training program to learn to sit before toilet training can start.

Research on toilet training both children with autism and typically developing children has indicated that the fastest and most successful training incorporates positive reinforcement, easy access to the toilet or potty chair, wearing underwear rather than diapers during training, and with the child sitting on the toilet or potty chair both on a schedule and as soon as the child starts to have a urination accident (Cicero & Pfadt, 2002). There are no negative consequences using this approach. Training is accomplished through proactive teaching using an intensive approach with toilet training the focus of the child's day. Extra fluids during training increase the opportunities for teaching but should be stopped once training is completed. Following successful training, prompts to use the toilet at scheduled times such as after meals and before bed may need to continue. Detailed information about toilet training children with autism using these principles is available in an excellent article by Cicero and Pfadt (2002).

Discipline

Discipline is an all-day, every-day, lifetime requirement for children with autism. As questions arise about appropriate behavior management, providers will want to consult the child's treatment team. Parents will need guidance about establishing and prioritizing behavioral goals and target symptoms for intervention (Matson & Nebel-Schwalm, 2007). Challenging behaviors that require intervention may include aggression, property destruction, repetitive

and perseverative behaviors, and tantrums. A functional analysis of the child's problematic behaviors can help with determining what factors might contribute to any single behavior (e.g., boredom, frustration, attention-getting attempts). Once the trigger for any specific behavior is identified, it is often easier to replace the challenging behavior with a more appropriate behavior rather than try simply to extinguish the challenging behavior. For example, if hand-flapping is found to occur when a child is bored, providing the child with a task or toy that requires use of the hands and praise for participating in the task may be more effective in stopping the hand-flapping than negative reinforcement when it occurs.

A highly structured and consistent approach is necessary for a child to learn socially appropriate behavior and refrain from dangerous behavior. Behavior modification techniques may be the most successful interventions for challenging behaviors. Many children will benefit from concurrent use of psychoactive medications that will temper the behaviors and the child's distress enough to make the successful use of positive and negative reinforcement possible. The use of positive reinforcers (e.g., play with favorite objects, food) is essential. Time-out for negative behaviors can also be employed if positive reinforcement is not totally successful. Negative reinforcement, such as a firm "no" and restraint or removal from the situation, may be necessary for potentially dangerous or self-injurious behaviors. Parents should be advised that children with autism do not readily generalize from one situation to another and often only attend to one very specific component of a situation, so teaching appropriate social and adaptive behaviors must be ongoing throughout the child's life (Koegel & LaZebnik, 2004). Koegel and LaZebnik's book *Overcoming Autism* (2004) is an excellent guide to strategies parents and professionals can use for reducing a child's autistic symptoms. Dr. Koegel is a psychologist at the Autism Research Center in Santa Barbara, California, and Mrs. LaZebnik is the mother of a child with autism.

In certain situations, parents may feel the need to discipline their child with autism even when they are not sure that the child will understand the discipline. For example, Harris (1994) relates the story of a mother who sent her daughter with autism for a time-out after she broke her brother's favorite toy. Although she knew her daughter might not learn from the time-out, she thought it was important for her son to see his sister receive appropriate consequences for her actions.

Child Care

Finding safe, reasonably priced, and developmentally appropriate child care is one of the more challenging tasks for parents of children with autism. Parents may have to balance their desire to have their child fully included in a child-care center for typically developing children with the child's need for intensive one-to-one social and behavioral training. Local and state laws regarding children with special needs and autism and their inclusion in child care vary. The state agency for people with developmental disabilities can advise parents about local laws and resources.

Three types of child care may be essential for the parents of children with autism: traditional child care during the hours the child's parents are working, respite care (i.e., care provided so that the child's parents may have time away from the constant responsibility of caring for their child with autism), and care for their unaffected children during the time the parents are taking the child with autism to clinic appointments and therapy sessions.

Children with autism are often easily overstimulated and can respond by withdrawing into self-stimulatory behaviors. They generally cannot interact with peers without teaching and supervision from adults. For these reasons, large-group child care is inadvisable unless a child has an accompanying aide to ensure that the child is appropriately occupied or the daycare provider has been taught specifically to care for children with autism. When both parents and daycare providers are educated and supported through lectures and on-site consultation, children with autism who attended child care with trained providers made significant gains in language as compared with children with autism whose parents and providers were not trained and supported. The daycare provider must be educated about the special behavior training and safety needs of the child with autism and willing to take on the challenge of integrating the child into activities with other children.

Therapeutic after-school programs are increasingly becoming available for school-age children with autism and may be covered under the related services clause of the Individuals with Disabilities Education Act (IDEA; see Chapter 3). These programs feature a low staff/child ratio and activities designed to teach social skills and appropriate public behavior. Although some children with autism can be fully included in regular after-school programs, many find these programs too unstructured and unpredictable.

Respite care is sometimes provided in the home by a trained respite care worker. Out-of-home respite care is provided by a licensed worker in the worker's home or in a group home or facility designed to provide short-term respite care. The PCP can be instrumental in referring the family to local respite services. Parents may be reluctant to use these services because they are fearful that their child will not be adequately cared for and that their need for respite services is a reflection on their parenting. The PCP can reassure parents that by taking care of themselves and the other children in the family, they will have more energy with which to meet the needs of their child with autism. Out-of-home respite care is also excellent practice for the transition to living away from home that many children with autism make in young adulthood.

Schooling

Public Law 101-426, the Individuals with Disabilities Education Improvement Act (IDEA), has made free and appropriate education the right of every child in America. For children with autism, however, what is "appropriate" is often debated by educators, clinicians, and parents. School services that are available to children with autism vary widely, but should always provide consistent structure and focus on developing functional communication and social skills and decreasing problematic behaviors.

The effectiveness of early intensive intervention with toddlers and preschoolers is now accepted (Myers et al., 2007). This includes year-round education 25 or more hours per week with at least some of the time devoted to one-to-one teaching (Myers et al., 2007). Objectives must be clearly identified and address all three deficits of autism: social, language, and play and behavior. Parent involvement and training is crucial to promote consistency between expectations at school and home. Academic skills may be included in an early intervention program but more important are functional skills such as toilet training, self-feeding, and independent dressing that will enable the child with autism to participate in activities with the child's typically developing peers.

There are three educational programs offered to school-age children with autism. A child's placement often depends on his or her cognitive ability and language skills, with the child's social deficits often not considered (White, Scahill, Klin, et al., 2007). Options range from full inclusion in a standard classroom, often with a paraprofessional aide, to a school day divided between time in a standard classroom and resource classes (e.g., speech therapy) to placement in a special day class solely for children who qualify for special education. A child's placement in first grade is generally an accurate predictor of the child's placement throughout his or her school career (White et al., 2007).

Full inclusion can be a successful strategy for educating children with ASD, but there are caveats. There must be flexibility in the curriculum to meet the individual's needs, cooperation between parents and teachers, and attention paid to the social environment for the child with autism who can easily be isolated. There are arguments both pro and con in the educational and developmental disability literature regarding full inclusion for children with autism versus self-contained special education classrooms. There are studies showing that both approaches have had positive results. Parents ultimately know their child best and will need to consider education options with their child's strengths and impairments in mind. When full inclusion is chosen it is imperative that the teacher and paraprofessional aide (if one is employed) have training in the unique deficits of children with autism and the particular needs of the child with whom they will be working.

Although increased opportunities for socialization seem to exist in a class with typically developing children, research has shown that children with autism find it impossible to interact with their peers without specific guidance from adults and peers who have been taught how to play and work with children with autism (Laushey & Heflin, 2000). Children as young as kindergarten age can be taught to use a "stay, play, and talk" approach with their peers with autism to improve their social skills (Laushey & Heflin, 2000). Regardless of the setting, education for children with autism needs to take place year-round in a structured and predictable environment that limits the opportunities for repetitive and ritualistic behaviors and consistently rewards appropriate behaviors (Myers et al., 2007).

Throughout a child's school years, parents need to participate in Individualized Educational Program (IEP) meetings. During these meetings the child's school placement is determined. Parents must carefully evaluate all alternatives for their child and choose the one that they and the treatment team agree is most appropriate. Parents should be prepared to present the reasons for their choice at the IEP meeting because federal law neither guarantees the best possible education for the child nor adequately funds programs to provide the highest standard of care (Siegel, 2003). Many parents will be helped by attending IEP training classes or bringing a friend or advocate with them to IEP meetings.

Parents should work closely with their child's speech therapist and consider adding augmentative communication methods (e.g., Picture Exchange Communication System [PECS], sign language, computers) to their child's program if the child does not begin to develop functional language spontaneously. There is no evidence that introducing augmentative communication methods delays or prevents the development of spoken language; in fact, the evidence is to the contrary (Millar, Light, & Schlosser, 2006).

Primary care providers should work with parents and the child's educational team to ensure that regular evaluation of the various domains of the child's functioning occurs. This includes addressing the child's behavioral adjustment, adaptive daily living skills, academic skills when appropriate, communication skills, and social interaction with family members and peers.

Sexuality

Children with autism must be taught appropriate behaviors regarding their sexuality that are tailored to their developmental level and educated to refrain from the inappropriate behaviors they may exhibit. Because of their communication and social deficits, children with autism will not necessarily independently learn behaviors such as refraining from masturbating or undressing in public and shutting the door when using the bathroom. This is significant because many adolescent and adult males and a significant minority of females with autism regularly masturbate. Many individuals engage in this and other sexual behaviors in community settings, although most are able to state that these activities should take place in their bedrooms (Stokes & Kaur, 2005). There was no significant difference in the frequency of these behaviors between individuals with autism who were verbal and high functioning and those without language who were low functioning. Specific rules about private behavior can be taught using repetition, redirection, positive reinforcement, and modeling.

Children and adolescents with ASD want to have friendships and romantic relationships. Their impaired social functioning causes them to pursue relationships indiscriminately with both individuals known to them and strangers (Stokes, Newton, & Kaur, 2007). They are often perseverative about relationships as they are about other interests, and their intrusiveness may rise to the level of stalking (Stokes et al., 2007). Children and adolescents with ASD need social skills education included in any sexual education program (Stokes et al., 2007).

PCPs can work with parents to identify problematic sexual behaviors and solicit help from the child's treatment team in developing a plan to ameliorate them. No research indicates that teaching children with autism about their sexuality encourages the development of aberrant behaviors, although many parents fear this. The PCP can reassure parents that many children with autism display inappropriate sexual behaviors but that these behaviors can be dealt with using behavior management techniques for nonsexual behaviors. To prevent the development of inappropriate behaviors, parents should be guided to teach their children very specific and concrete rules about acceptable and unacceptable sexual behavior throughout the child's life, not waiting until adolescence when such behavior may increase.

Transition to Adulthood

Children with autism grow up to be adults with autism. For most of these individuals autism will be a severely disabling condition (McGovern & Sigman, 2005). Adults who have cognitive deficits in addition to autism will require lifelong care, support, and supervision, including residential placement, sheltered workshop employment, continued education, and behavioral management. Adults with autism and normal intelligence will have continuing social deficits that will generally prevent them from employment commensurate with their intellectual capabilities. They have reported difficulties with relationships at work, understanding the

nuances of work and personal conversations, how to carry on a work-related or personal conversation, and how to interact with members of the opposite gender (Sperry & Mesibov, 2005).

The National Institute of Mental Health (NIMH) (2002) states that about one third of all adults with autism can live and work in the community with some degree of independence. The persistent social deficits of autism (e.g., poor judgment in social situations, limited conversation skills, impaired problem solving) preclude most adults with autism from completely independent employment and marriage. Work skills based on an individual's abilities, communication skills, and interests and that incorporate the adult's propensity for structure and repetition can be taught (NIMH, 2002). Most adults with autism will qualify for Supplemental Security Income (see Chapter 8). Parents may be directed to their local Social Security office by their child's school counselor, their case worker at the center for people with developmental disabilities, or their PCP.

The parents of children with autism must be encouraged and counseled by their child's PCP to plan for the child's future. Education is mandated for children with significant disabilities until they are 22 years of age (see Chapter 3). Those individuals able to attend college will still need a great deal of support and assistance with organization and planning. The end of mandated education may also be an appropriate time for a young adult to enter residential or community placement. Planning for this and locating a suitable home with an opening can take years. In early adolescence, the child's PCP should guide parents to begin exploring their options.

Finally, the PCP must help the parents find adult primary care for their child. As more children with developmental disabilities grow to adulthood and live and work in the community, family and adult providers will need to learn how to care for nonverbal individuals with continuing behavioral disturbances.

Family Concerns

Receiving a diagnosis of autism is intensely painful for most families. It may be months or even years from the time a toddler's delayed speech development is first recognized until the final diagnosis of autism is made. During this time, parents may have heard from several different providers in various specialties, including the child's PCP, that something is wrong with their child and it might be autism. The wait for the final diagnosis can be agonizing and delays implementation of appropriate interventions. The presentation of the diagnosis should be given in a setting that provides adequate time for discussion of test results and needs of the child and family. Because there is no biologic marker for autism, the diagnosis is made based on neuropsychological testing, careful history taking, and observation of the child's behavior. This relatively subjective way of diagnosing such a serious and lifelong condition is often difficult for parents to understand. This method of diagnosis, the apparently typical period of development of children with autism during the first year of life, unknown etiology of autism for most children, and the lack of a cure have contributed to a plethora of alternative diagnostic procedures and treatments that parents consider pursuing (Dale, Jahoda, & Knott, 2006). PCPs can play a crucial role in educating parents about the diagnosis, how it is determined, and the evidence-based treatments that are available.

Parents of children with autism have higher levels of stress and depression than parents of children with any other chronic condition or developmental disability (Lounds, Seltzer, Greenberg, et al., 2007). This stress stems from the difficulty of caring for their child, being bothered by and angry with their child's behavior, and sacrificing more of their life than expected to try and meet their child's needs (Schieve, Blumberg, Rice, et al., 2007). When a child is a toddler or preschooler this stress is heightened by the child's social disconnect from the parent (Davis & Carter, 2008). By the child's adolescence, mothers will have formed a relationship with their child; the mother's stress is then more likely to be caused by the child's behavior problems (Lounds et al., 2007). Parents do show resilience and the ability to adapt to their child's autism but need ongoing support throughout the child's life (Smith, Seltzer, Tager-Flusberg, et al., 2008). PCPs can point out examples of a family's resilience to the parents, including their ability to mobilize resources, change in perspective on life and its challenges, and development of patience and compassion (Bayat, 2007). Parent education, behavior management training, and counseling can improve both the physical and mental health of parents (Tonge, Brereton, Kiomall, et al., 2006). PCPs should ask parents about their sleep; levels of depression, anxiety, and stress; and physical complaints and refer them to the local family resource center for people with developmental disabilities and the websites listed at the end of this chapter (Meltzer, 2008; Montes & Halterman, 2007). Referral to a psychologist or psychiatrist for an evaluation for medication management can also reduce parental stress; parents of children taking psychotropic medications report a lessening of parental stress and anxiety (Lounds et al., 2007).

Many health insurance plans exclude autism and mental retardation as conditions for which they will pay for behavioral health services (Peele, Lave, & Kelleher, 2002). A growing number of states have enacted legislation requiring these conditions to be covered (Peele et al., 2002). Even when autism is a covered condition, many plans are reluctant to pay for the neuropsychological testing necessary for the diagnosis and follow-up of a child with autism. PCPs must advocate for the child and family in pursuing appropriate referrals and payment for them.

All parents of children with autism should receive counseling to inform them of the fifty-fold risk of having another child with autism (Myers et al., 2007). Referral to a genetics clinic is appropriate because knowledge about the genetics of autism increases constantly and there are a number of research studies involving families of children with autism of which family members should be made aware.

As families raise their child with autism, they will hear unkind remarks about their child's behavior and poor social skills and be given conflicting advice about how their child should be parented, treated, and educated. They will often have to struggle with school systems and after-school programs that are not designed to meet the special needs of a child with autism. Parents will need to educate all those who interact with their child about autism, their child's individual case, and the latest advances in the field of autism. In addition to educating parents, PCPs will need to be open to receiving information from parents about their child and the subject of autism in general.

Parenting a child with autism is a tremendous physical, emotional, and financial challenge. A family with a child with an ASD can expect to have about a 14% reduction in annual household income, perhaps due to the cost of educational and behavioral therapies and decreased earning secondary to the child's constant need for supervision (Montes & Halterman, 2008). A great deal of time and energy may be directed toward the child with autism and away from other relationships and family members—especially siblings. Siblings may be embarrassed by or afraid of the behavior of their sibling with autism and thus reluctant to bring friends home (Benderix & Sivberg, 2007). Siblings complain most about aggressive behavior in their sibling with autism (Ross & Cuskelly, 2006). They often cope with suppressing their anger at the situation, wishing that their sibling or home life was different, and withdrawing (Ross & Cuskelly, 2006). Siblings are at increased risk for depression and stress-related illness, secondary both to possible genetic predisposition related to their sibling's autism and lack of a positive relationship with their sibling resulting from their sibling's communication, social, and behavioral problems (Orsmond & Seltzer, 2007). Siblings are at increased risk for developmental problems, also adding to the parents' burden. Primary care providers can direct families to support groups, social services, and organizations that can address these issues.

Resources
Organizations
American Academy of Pediatrics
Website: www.aap.org
Autism Collaboration
Website: www.autism.org
Autism Research Institute
4182 Adams Ave.
San Diego, CA 92116
(866) 366-3361
Website: www.autism.com
Autism Society of America
7910 Woodmont Ave., Suite 300
Bethesda, MD 20814-3067
(301) 657-0881; (800) 3AUTISM
Website: www.autism-society.org
Autism Speaks
Park Ave, 11th Floor
New York, NY 10016
(212) 252-8584; Fax: (212) 252-8676
Website: www.autismspeaks.org
Centers for Disease Control and Prevention, National Center on Birth Defects and Developmental Disabilities
Website: www.cdc.gov/ncbddd

Information about Autism and Clinical Trials
National Institute of Neurological Disorders and Stroke, National Institutes of Health
Website: www.ninds.nih.gov

Free M-CHAT and Developmental Screening Tools
First Signs
Website: www.firstsigns.org

To Donate Brain Tissue for Research
Autism Tissue Program
(877) 333-0999
Website: www.brainbank.org

Summary of Primary Care Needs for the Child with Autism Spectrum Disorder

HEALTH CARE MAINTENANCE

Growth and Development

- Height and weight are usually within normal range but may be altered by medication side effects or restricted food preferences.
- Measure head circumference annually until age 5 years. If child also has tuberous sclerosis, annual measurement of head circumference should continue after age 5 years.
- Delayed language development is usually noticed between 18 and 30 months of age.
- Refer for diagnostic evaluation as soon as autism is suspected.

Diet

- Child's insistence on sameness may affect food intake.
- Well-balanced diet is encouraged.
- Multiple-vitamin supplements may be indicated.
- Valproic acid and atypical antipsychotics may cause increased hunger and excessive weight gain.

Safety

- Risk of injury is increased because of lack of impulse control, inability to generalize safety rules from one situation to another, and motor abilities more advanced than judgment. Constant supervision is required.
- Childproofing the environment is required.
- Self-injurious behavior can result in injury because of increased pain tolerance and inability to communicate injury.
- There is an increased risk of drowning. Children with autism and epilepsy must follow safety guidelines for children with epilepsy, including no unsupervised baths or swimming.
- Diagnosis of acute and chronic medical conditions can be delayed by child's inability to report symptoms.
- Sudden deterioration in behavior may indicate pain or abuse.

Immunizations

- Routine schedule is recommended, including MMR.
- Children with autism and epilepsy should follow the guidelines for children with epilepsy.

Screening

- *Vision.* Routine screening is recommended after initial ophthalmologic examination to look for signs of tuberous sclerosis.
- *Hearing.* Routine screening is recommended after initial audiology evaluation, which may include brainstem auditory evoked response testing to rule out hearing loss as a cause of communication delay.
- *Dental.* Routine dental care is recommended.
  - Children receiving phenytoin therapy require more frequent dental care for gum hyperplasia.
  - Sedation for dental care of the child with autism may be necessary.
- *Blood pressure.* Routine screening is recommended.
  - Children receiving clonidine therapy require blood pressure monitoring before initiation of therapy and with all dosage changes.
- *Hematocrit.* Routine screening is recommended.
  - Children receiving carbamazepine or valproate therapy should have a complete blood count (CBC) with platelets done before initiation of therapy, after establishment of maintenance dose, and annually thereafter.

- *Urinalysis.* Routine screening is recommended.
- *Tuberculosis.* Routine screening is recommended.

Condition-Specific Screening

- *Other laboratory tests.* Children receiving carbamazepine or valproate should have liver function testing (AST, ALT) before starting therapy, after establishment of maintenance dose, and annually thereafter.

COMMON ILLNESS MANAGEMENT

Differential Diagnosis

- Communication and cognitive deficits make assessment difficult.
- Change in behavior can indicate injury or illness.
- *Injury.* Cause of injury, accidental injury, self-injury, and nonaccidental injury must be determined and appropriate intervention identified.
- *Seizures.* Seizure activity must be differentiated from repetitive or stereotypical behaviors.
- Gastrointestinal complaints and pica.
- Medication side effects must be considered.

Drug Interactions

- Erythromycin can increase plasma levels of carbamazepine.

DEVELOPMENTAL ISSUES

Sleep Patterns

- Difficulty falling asleep and staying asleep is commonly reported by parents.
- Highly structured, consistent bedtime rituals are a necessity.
- Bedrooms must be thoroughly childproofed and secured so children cannot wander out alone or harm themselves at night.
- Pharmacologic management using melatonin or antihistamines or scheduling trazodone, atypical antipsychotics, or antidepressants for evening dosing may help with sleep.

Toileting

- Training is often delayed.
- Child must have performance IQ of 30 before training should be attempted.
- Structured, behavioral approach with reward system is usually needed.
- Mimicking parental behavior is usually not effective.

Discipline

- Highly structured and consistent approach is necessary.
- Continuous discipline is necessary because children with autism do not readily generalize from one situation to another.
- Concrete positive reinforcement (e.g., food) is essential.
- Negative reinforcement may be needed for dangerous behavior.

Child Care

- Family daycare or therapeutic child-care setting is recommended.
- After-school care may be covered under the related services clause of the Individuals with Disabilities Education Act (IDEA).
- Respite care can be important for primary caretaker and other family members.

Schooling

- Early, intense intervention, which may include 1:1 teaching, is often needed and most effective.

Summary of Primary Care Needs for the Child with Autism Spectrum Disorder—cont'd

- Families will need support during the individualized educational plan (IEP) process to advocate for their child.
- Year-round structured schooling is important.
- Parents must choose from a range of options from full inclusion to self-contained schools for children with autism.
- Augmentative communication methods are often helpful.

Sexuality

- Appropriate sexual behavior must be taught using behavior management techniques.
- Specific and concrete rules about sexuality are necessary.

Transition to Adulthood

- Most adults with autism require lifelong care, support, and supervision.
- Work that involves concrete and repetitive tasks and little social interaction may be most suitable.

- Most adults will qualify for Supplemental Security Income.
- Parents need to plan for child's future, including finding appropriate adult primary care.

FAMILY CONCERNS

- Diagnosis is based on neuropsychological testing and observation and appears relatively subjective; families may find it hard to comprehend.
- Genetic etiology of autism requires referral to genetics clinic after child is diagnosed with autism.
- Health insurance plans often exclude behavioral health services for autism.
- Lack of understanding of autism in the community contributes to lack of supportive services.
- Siblings and others may be afraid of or embarrassed by behavior of the child with autism.

REFERENCES

Afzal, N., Murch, S., Thirrupathy, K., et al. (2003). Constipation with acquired megarectum in children with autism. *Pediatrics, 112*, 939-942.

Ahearn, W.H., Castine, T., Nault, K., et al. (2001). An assessment of food acceptance in children with a pervasive developmental disorder—not otherwise specified. *J Autism Dev Disord, 31*(5), 505-511.

American Psychiatric Association. (2000). *Diagnostic and Statistical Manual of Mental Disorders: Text Revision* (4th ed.). Washington, DC: American Psychiatric Publishing.

American Speech-Language-Hearing Association. (2006). *Guidelines for speech-language pathologists in diagnosis, assessment, and treatment of autism spectrum disorders across the lifespan.* Available at www.asha.org. Retrieved May 15, 2008.

Andersen, I.M., Kaczmarska, J., McGrew, S.G., et al. (2008). Melatonin for insomnia in children with autism spectrum disorders. *J Child Neurol, 23*, 482-485.

Barton, M., & Volkmar, F. (1998). How commonly are known medical conditions associated with autism?. *J Autism Dev Disord, 28*, 273-278.

Battaglia, A., & Carey, J.C. (2006). Etiologic yield of autistic spectrum disorders: A prospective study. *Am J Med Genet C Semin Med Genet, 142*, 3-7.

Bayat, M. (2007). Evidence of resilience in families of children with autism. *J Intellect Disabil Res, 51*(pt 9), 702-714.

Belmonte, M.K., & Bourgeron, T. (2006). Fragile X syndrome and autism at the intersection of genetic and neural networks. *Nature Neurosci, 9*, 1221-1225.

Benderix, Y., & Sivberg, B. (2007). Siblings' experiences of having a brother or sister with autism and mental retardation: A case study of 14 siblings from five families. *J Pediatr Nurs, 22*, 410-418.

Ben-Itzchak, E., & Zachor, D.A. (2007). The effects of intellectual functioning and autism severity on outcome of early behavioral intervention for children with autism. *Res Dev Disabil, 28*, 287-303.

Bolton, P.F. (2004). Neuroepileptic correlates of autistic symptomatology in tuberous sclerosis. *Ment Retard Dev Disabil Rev Res, 10*, 126-131.

Brachlow, A.E., Ness, K.K., McPheeters, M.L., et al. (2007). Comparison of indicators for a primary care medical home between children with autism or asthma and other special health care needs. *Arch Pediatr Adolesc Med, 161*, 399-405.

Brereton, A.V., Tonge, B.J., & Einfeld, S.L. (2006). Psychopathology in children and adolescents with autism compared to young people with intellectual disability. *J Autism Dev Disord, 36*, 863-870.

Brimacombe, M., Ming, X., & Parikh, A. (2007). Familial risk factors in autism. *J Child Neurol, 22*, 593-597.

Bukelis, I., Porter, F.D., Zimmerman, A.W., et al. (2007). Smith-Lemli-Opitz syndrome and autism spectrum disorder. *Am J Psychiatry, 164*, 1655-1661.

Canitano, R., & Vivanti, G. (2007). Tics and Tourette syndrome in autism spectrum disorders. *Autism, 11*, 19-28.

Carey, T., Ratliff-Schaub, K., Funk, J., et al. (2002). Double-blind placebo-controlled trial of secretin: Effects on aberrant behavior in children with autism. *J Autism Dev Disord, 32*, 161-167.

Carr, J.E., & LeBlanc, L.A. (2007). Autism spectrum disorders in early childhood: An overview for practicing physicians. *Prim Care, 34*, 343-359.

Centers for Disease Control and Prevention. (2007). Prevalence of autism spectrum disorders—autism and developmental disabilities monitoring network, six sites, United States, 2000. Prevalence of autism spectrum disorders—autism and developmental disabilities monitoring network, 14 sites, United States, 2002. Evaluation of a methodology for a collaborative multiple source surveillance network of autism spectrum disorders—autism and developmental disabilities monitoring network, 14 sites, United States, 2002. *MMWR Morb Mortal Wkly Rep, 56*(SS-1), 1-40.

Chawarska, K., Klin, A., Paul, R., et al. (2007). Autism spectrum disorder in the second year: Stability and change in syndrome expression. *J Child Psychol Psychiatry, 48*, 128-138.

Chawarska, K., Paul, R., Klin, A., et al. (2006). Parental recognition of developmental problems in toddlers with autism spectrum disorders. *J Autism Dev Disord, 37*, 62-72.

Chelation therapy and autism (2006). *MMWR Morb Mrtl Wkly Rep, 55*, 204-207.

Christison, G.W., & Ivany, K. (2006). Elimination diets in autism spectrum disorders: Any wheat amidst the chaff? *J Dev Behav Pediatr, 27*, S162-S171.

Cicero, F.R., & Pfadt, A. (2002). Investigation of a reinforcement-based toilet training procedure for children with autism. *Res Dev Disabil, 23*, 319-323.

Committee on Children with Disabilities (2001a). Counseling families who choose complementary and alternative medicine for their child with chronic illness or disability. *Pediatrics, 107*(3), 598-601.

Committee on Children with Disabilities (2001b). The pediatrician's role in the diagnosis and management of autistic spectrum disorders in children. *Pediatrics, 107*(5), 1221-1226.

Coo, H., Ouellette-Kuntz, H., Lloyd, J.E.V., et al. (2008). Trends in autism prevalence: Diagnostic substitution revisited. *J Autism Dev Dis, 38*, 1036-1046.

Coplan, J., & Jawad, A.F. (2005). Modeling clinical outcome of children with autistic spectrum disorders. *Pediatrics, 116*, 117-122.

Correll, C., & Kane, J.M. (2007). One-year incidence rates of tardive dyskinesia in children and adolescents treated with second generation antipsychotics: A systemic review. *J Child Adolesc Psychopharm, 17*, 647-656.

Courchesne, E., Karns, C.M., Davis, H.R., et al. (2001). Unusual brain growth patterns in early life in patients with autistic disorder. *Neurology, 57*, 245-254.

Courchesne, E., & Pierce, K. (2005). Why the frontal cortex in autism might be talking only to itself: Local over-connectivity but long-distance disconnection. *Curr Opin Neurobiol, 15*, 225-230.

Croen, L.A., Grether, J.K., Hoogstrate, J., et al. (2002). The changing prevalence of autism in California. *J Autism Dev Disord, 32*, 207-215.

Croen, L.A., Najjar, D.V., Fireman, B., et al. (2007). Maternal and paternal age and risk of autism spectrum disorders. *Arch Pediatr Adolesc Med, 161*, 334-340.

Croen, L.A., Najjar, D.V., Ray, G.T., et al. (2006). A comparison of health care utilization and costs of children with and without autism spectrum disorders in a large group-model health plan. *Pediatrics, 118*, e1203-e1211. Available at www.pediatrics.org. Retrieved December 27, 2007.

Dale, E., Jahoda, A., & Knott, F. (2006). Mothers' attributions following their child's diagnosis of autistic spectrum disorder: Exploring links with maternal levels of stress, depression and expectations about their child's future. *Autism, 10*, 463-479.

Dales, L., Hammer, S.J., & Smith, N.J. (2001). Time trends in autism and in MMR immunization coverage in California. *J Am Med Assoc, 285*(22), 2852-2853.

Danielsson, S., Gillberg, I.C., Billstedt, E., et al. (2005). Epilepsy in young adults with autism: A prospective population-based follow-up study of 120 individuals diagnosed in childhood. *Epilepsia, 46*, 918-923.

Davidovitch, M., Glick, L., Holtzman, G., et al. (2000). Developmental regression in autism: Maternal perception. *J Autism Dev Disord, 30*(2), 113-119.

Davis, N.O., & Carter, A.S. (2008). Parenting stress in mothers and fathers of toddlers with autism spectrum disorders: Associations with child characteristics. *J Autism Dev Disord* (electronic publication). Available at www.springerlink.com. Retrieved May 16, 2008.

De Bildt, A., Sytema, S., Kraijer, D., et al. (2005). Prevalence of pervasive developmental disorders in children and adolescents with mental retardation. *J Child Psychol Psychiatry, 46*, 257-286.

DeStefano, F. (2007). Vaccines and autism: Evidence does not support a causal association. *Clin Pharmacol Ther, 82*, 257-286.

DiCicco-Bloom, E., Lord, C., Zwaigenbaum, L., et al. (2006). The developmental neurobiology of autism spectrum disorder. *J Neurosci, 26*, 6897-6906.

Dinca, O., Paul, M., & Spencer, N.J. (2005). Systematic review of randomized controlled trials of atypical antipsychotics and selective serotonin reuptake inhibitors for behavioural problems associated with pervasive developmental disorders. *J Psychopharmacol, 19*, 521-532.

Dosreis, S., Weiner, C.L., Johnson, L., et al. (2006). Autism spectrum disorder screening and management practices among general pediatric providers. *J Dev Behav Pediatr, 27*, S88-S94.

Dykens, E.M. (2007). Psychiatric and behavioral disorders in persons with Down syndrome. *Ment Retard Dev Disabil Res Rev, 13*, 272-278.

Elder, J.H. (2002). Current treatments in autism: Examining scientific evidence and clinical implications. *J Neurosci Nurs, 34*, 67-73.

Elder, J.H., Shankar, M., Shuster, J., et al. (2006). Prevalence of pervasive developmental disorders in children and adolescents with mental retardation. *J Autism Dev Disord, 36*, 413-420.

Filipek, P.A., Accardo, P.J., Ashwal, S., et al. (2000). Practice parameter: Screening and diagnosis of autism. *Neurology, 55*, 468-479.

Filipek, P.A., Accardo, P.J., Baranek, G.T., et al. (1999). The screening and diagnosis of autistic spectrum disorders. *J Autism Dev Disord, 29*, 439-484.

Fine, S.E., Weissman, A., Gerdes, M., et al. (2005). Autism spectrum disorders and symptoms in children with molecularly confirmed 22q11.2 deletion syndrome. *J Autism Dev Disord, 35*, 461-470.

Folstein, S.E., & Rosen-Sheidley, B. (2001). Genetics of autism: Complex aetiology for a heterogeneous disorder. *Nature Rev Genet, 2*, 943-955.

Fombonne, E., Zakarian, R., Bennett, A., et al. (2006). Pervasive developmental disorders in Montreal, Quebec, Canada: Prevalence and links with immunizations. *Pediatrics, 118*, e139-e150. Available at www.pediatrics.org. Retrieved March 30, 2008.

Gabis, L., Pomeroy, J., & Andriola, M.R. (2005). Autism and epilepsy: Cause, consequence, comorbidity, or coincidence? *J Epilepsy Behav, 7*, 652-656.

Geiger, D.M., Smith, D.T., & Creaghead, N.A. (2002). Parent and professional agreement on cognitive level of children with autism. *J Autism Dev Disord, 32*, 307-312.

Glasson, E.J., Bower, C., Petterson, B., et al. (2004). Perinatal factors and the development of autism. *Arch Gen Psychiatry, 61*, 618-627.

Gold, C., Wigram, T., & Elefant, C. (2006). Music therapy for autistic spectrum disorder. *Cochrane Database of Systematic Reviews,2, art.* no. CD 004381.

Grinker, R.R. (2007). *Unstrange Minds: Remapping the World of Autism.* Cambridge, MA: Basic Books.

Hardan, A., Jou, R., Keshavan, M., et al. (2004). Increased frontal cortical folding in autism: A preliminary MRI study. *Psychiatry Res, 131*, 263-268.

Hardan, A., Muddasani, S., Vemulapalli, M., et al. (2006). An MRI study of increased cortical thickness in autism. *Am J Psychiatry, 163*, 1290-1292.

Harris, S.L. (1994). *Siblings of Children with Autism.* Bethesda, MD: Woodbine House.

Hediger, M.L., England, L.J., Molloy, C.A., et al. (2007). Reduced bone cortical thickness in boys with autism or autism spectrum disorder. *J Autism Dev Disord* (electronic publication). Available at www.springerlink.com. Retrieved May 15, 2008.

Heron, J., Golding, J., ALSPAC Study Team (2004). Thimerosal exposure in infants and developmental disorders: A prospective cohort study in the United Kingdom does not support a causal association. *Pediatrics, 114*, 577-583.

Honda, H., Shimizu, Y., Imai, M., et al. (2005). Cumulative incidence of childhood autism: A total population study of better accuracy precision. *Dev Med Child Neurol, 47*, 10-18.

Howlin, P., Goode, S., Hutton, J., et al. (2004). Adult outcome for children with autism. *J Child Psychol Psychiatry, 45*, 212-229.

Hughes, J.R. (2007). Autism: The first firm finding = underconnectivity? *Epilepsy Behav, 11*, 20-24.

Hyman, S.L., Rodier, P.M., & Davidson, P. (2001). Pervasive developmental disorders in young children. *J Am Med Assoc, 285*, 3141-3142.

Jesner, O.S., Aref-Adib, M., & Coren, E. (2007). Risperidone for autism spectrum disorder. *Cochrane Database of Systematic Reviews, 1, art. no.* CD005040.

Johnson, C.P., & Myers, S.M. & Council on Children with Disabilities. (2007) Identification and evaluation of children with autism spectrum disorders. *Pediatrics, 120*, 1183-1215.

Just, M.A., Cherkassky, V.L., Keller, T.A., et al. (2007). Functional and anatomical cortical underconnectivity in autism: Evidence from an fMRI study of an executive function task and corpus callosum morphometry. *Cereb Cortex, 17*, 951-961.

Kanner, L. (1943). Autistic disturbances of affective contact. *Nervous Child, 2*, 217-250.

Kem, D.L., Posey, D.J., & McDougle, J. (2002). Priapism associated with trazodone in an adolescent with autism. *J Am Acad Child Adolesc Psychiatry, 41*, 758.

Kern, J.K., Van Miller, S., Evans, P.A., et al. (2002). Efficacy of porcine secretin in children with autism and pervasive developmental disorder. *J Autism Dev Disord, 32*, 153-160.

Koegel, L.K., & LaZebnik, C. (2004). *Overcoming Autism.* New York: Viking.

Kolevzon, A., Mathewson, K.A., & Hollander, E. (2006). Selective serotonin reuptake inhibitors in autism: A review of efficacy and tolerability. *J Clin Psychiatry, 67*, 407-414.

Korkmaz, B. (2000). Infantile autism: Adult outcome. *Semin Clin Neuropsychiatry, 5*(3), 164-170.

Landa, R., & Garrett-Mayer, E. (2006). Development in infants with autism spectrum disorders: A prospective study. *J Child Psychol Psychiatry, 47*, 629-638.

Landa, R.J., Holman, K.C., & Garrett-Mayer, E. (2007). Social and communication development in toddlers with early and later diagnosis of autism spectrum disorders. *Arch Gen Psychiatry, 64*, 853-864.

Landau, W.M., & Kleffner, F.R. (1998). Syndrome of acquired aphasia with convulsive disorder in children. *Neurology, 51*(5), 1241-1249.

Larsson, H.J., Eaton, W.W., Madsen, K.M., et al. (2005). Risk factors for autism: Perinatal factors, parental psychiatric history, and socioeconomic status. *Am J Epidemiol, 161*, 916-925.

Laushey, K.M., & Heflin, L.J. (2000). Enhancing social skills of kindergarten children with autism through the training of multiple peers as tutors. *J Autism Dev Disord, 30*, 183-193.

Lee, D.O., & Ousley, O.Y. (2006). Attention-deficit hyperactivity disorder symptoms in a clinic sample of children and adolescents with pervasive developmental disorders. *J Child Adolesc Psychol, 16*, 737-746.

Lee, L.C., Harrington, R.A., Chang, J.J., et al. (2007). Increased risk of injury in children with developmental disabilities. *Res Dev Disabil* (electronic publication). Available at www.sciencedirect.com. Retrieved May 19, 2008.

Levenson, D. (2004). Institute of Medicine rejects vaccine-autism link. *Rep Med Guidel Outcomes Res, 15*, 9-10, 12.

Levisohn, P.M. (2007). The autism-epilepsy connection. *Epilepsia, 48*, 33-35.

Limperopoulos, C., Bassan, H., Gauvreau, K., et al. (2007). Does cerebellar injury in premature infants contribute to the high prevalence of long-term cognitive, learning, and behavioral disability in survivors? *Pediatrics, 120*, 584-593.

Limperopoulos, C., Bassan, H., Sullivan, N.R.M.,, et al. (2008). Positive screening for autism in ex-preterm infants: Prevalence and risk factors. *Pediatrics,* *121,* 758-765.

Lord, C., Risi, S., DiLavore, P.S., et al. (2006). Autism from 2 to 9 years of age. *Arch Gen Psychiatry, 63,* 694-701.

Lounds, J., Seltzer, M.M., Greenberg, J.S., et al. (2007). Transition and change in adolescents and young adults with autism: Longitudinal effects on maternal well-being. *Am J Ment Retard, 112,* 401-417.

Lovaas, O. (1987). Behavioral treatment and normal educational and intellectual functioning in young autistic children. *J Consult Clin Psychol, 55*(1), 162-164.

Madsen, K.M., Hviid, A., Vestegaard, M., et al. (2002). A population-based study of measles, mumps, and rubella vaccination and autism. *N Engl J Med, 347,* 1477-1482.

Magiati, I., Charman, T., & Howlin, P. (2007). A two-year prospective follow-up study of community-based early intensive behavioural intervention and specialist nursery provision for children with autism spectrum disorders. *J Child Psychol Psychology, 48,* 803-812.

Mahoney, G., & Perales, F. (2005). Relationship-focused early intervention with children with pervasive developmental disorders and other disabilities: A comparative study. *J Dev Behav Pediatr, 26,* 77-85.

Maimburg, R.D., &Vaeth, M. (2006). Perinatal risk factors and infantile autism. *Acta Psychiatr Scand, 114,* 257-264.

Malow, B.A. (2004). Sleep disorders, epilepsy, and autism. *Ment Retard Dev Disabil Rev, 10,* 122-125.

Malow, B.A., Marzec, M., McGrew, S., et al. (2006). Characterizing sleep in children with autism spectrum disorders: A multidimensional approach. *Sleep, 29,* 1563-1571.

Mandell, D.S., Novak, M.M., & Zubritsky, C.D. (2005). Factors associated with age of diagnosis among children with autism spectrum disorders. *Pediatrics, 116,* 1480-1486.

Marshall, J., Sheller, B., Williams, B., et al. (2007). Cooperation predictors for dental patients with autism. *Pediatr Dent, 29,* 369-375.

Matson, J.L., & Nebel-Schwalm, M. (2007). Assessing challenging behaviors in children with autism spectrum disorders: A review. *Res Dev Disabil, 28,* 567-579.

McCarthy, J. (2007). Children with autism spectrum disorders and intellectual disability. *Curr Opin Psychiatry, 20,* 472-476.

McConachie, H., & Diggle, T. (2007). Parent implemented early intervention for young children with autism spectrum disorder: A systematic review. *J Eval Clin Pract, 13,* 120-129.

McDermott, S., Zhou, L., & Mann, J. (2008). Injury treatment among children with autism or pervasive developmental disorder. *J Autism Dev Disord, 38,* 626-633.

McDougle, C.J., Scahill, L., Aman, M.G., et al. (2005). Risperidone for the core symptom domains of autism: Results from the study by the Autism Network of the Research Units on Pediatric Psychopharmacology. *Am J Psychiatry, 162,* 1142-1148.

McGovern, C.W., & Sigman, M. (2005). Continuity and change from early childhood to adolescence in autism. *J Child Psychol Psychiatry, 46,* 401-408.

Meltzer, L.J. (2008). Brief report: Sleep in parents of children with autism spectrum disorders. *J Pediatr Psychol, 33,* 1-7.

Messmer, R.L., Nader, R., & Craig, K.D. (2007). Brief report: Judging pain intensity in children with autism undergoing venipuncture: The influence of facial activity. *J Autism Dev Disord.* Available at www.springerlink.com. Retrieved May 16, 2008.

Millar, D.C., Light, J.C., & Schlosser, R.W. (2006). The impact of augmentative and alternative communication intervention on the speech production of individuals with developmental disabilities: A research review. *J Speech Lang Hear Res, 49,* 248-264.

Miller, J. (2007). Screening children for developmental behavioral problems: Principles for the practitioner. *Prim Care, 34,* 177-201.

Millward, C., Ferriter, M., Calver, S., et al. (2004). Gluten- and casein-free diets for autistic spectrum disorder. *Cochrane Database of Systematic Reviews,* 2. art, no. CD003498.

Mindell, J.A., Emslie, G., Blumer, J., et al. (2006). Pharmacologic management of insomnia in children and adolescents: Consensus statement. *Pediatrics, 117,* e1223-e1232. Available at www.pediatrics.org. Retrieved January 28, 2008.

Minshew, N.J., & Williams, D.L. (2007). The new neurobiology of autism: Cortex, connectivity, and neuronal organization. *Arch Neurol, 64,* 945-950.

Mitchell, S., Brian, J., Zwaigenbaum, L., et al. (2006). Early language and communication development of infants later diagnosed with autism spectrum disorder. *J Dev Behav Pediatr, 27,* 69-78.

Moldin, S.O., Rubenstein, J.L., & Hyman, S.F. (2006). Can autism speak to neuroscience? *J Neurosci, 26,* 6893-6896.

Montes, G., & Halterman, J.S. (2007). Psychological functioning and coping among mothers of children with autism: A population-based study. *Pediatrics, 119,* e1040-e1046. Available at www.pediatrics.org. Retrieved February 8, 2008.

Montes, G., & Halterman, J.S. (2008). Association of childhood autism spectrum disorders and loss of family income. *Pediatrics, 121,* e821-e826.

Mooney, E.L., Gray, K.M., & Tonge, B.J. (2006). Early features of autism: Repetitive behaviours in young children. *Eur Child Adolesc Psychiatry, 15,* 12-18.

Moore, M.L., Eichner, S.F., & Jones, J.R. (2004). Treating functional impairment of autism with selective serotonin-reuptake inhibitors. *Ann Pharmacother, 38,* 1515-1519.

Muhle, R., Trentacoste, S.V., & Rapin, I. (2004). The genetics of autism. *Pediatrics, 113,* e472-e486. Available at www.pediatrics.org. Retrieved November 5, 2007.

Murch, S., Anthony, A., Casson, D., et al. (2004). Retraction of an interpretation. *Lancet, 363,* 750.

Myers, S.M., Johnson, C.P. Council on Children with Disabilities. (2007). Management of children with autism spectrum disorders. *Pediatrics, 120,* 1162-1182.

National Institute of Mental Health. (2002). *Autism.* Available at www.nim.nih.gov. Retrieved March 30, 2008.

National Institute of Neurological Disorders and Stroke. (2007). *Autism fact sheet.* Available at www.ninds.nih.gov/health. Retrieved February 18, 2008.

National Institute of Neurological Disorders and Stroke. (2008). *Landau-Kleffner syndrome information sheet.* Available at www.ninds.nih.gov. Retrieved February 18, 2008.

National Institutes of Health. (2001). *Program announcement number PA-01-051.* Available at http://grants.nih.gov/grants/guide. Retrieved March 30, 2008.

National Institutes of Health. (2002). *Research on autism and autism spectrum disorders.* Available at http://grants.nih.gov/grants/guide. Retrieved March 30, 2008.

Nicholas, J.S., Charles, J.M., Carpenter, L.A., et al. (2008). Prevalence and characteristics of children with autism-spectrum disorders. *Ann Epidemiol, 18,* 130-136.

Nye, C., & Brice, A. (2005). Combined vitamin B6-magnesium treatment in autism spectrum disorder. *Cochrane Database of Systematic Reviews, 4,* art. no. CD003497.

Oliveira, G., Ataide, A., Marques, C., et al. (2007). Epidemiology of autism spectrum disorder in Portugal: Prevalence, clinical characterization, and medical conditions. *Dev Med Child Neurol, 49,* 726-733.

Oliver, C., & Petty, J. (2002). Self-injurious behavior in people with intellectual disability. *Curr Opin Psychiatry, 15*(5), 477-481.

Orsmond, G.I., &Seltzer, M.M. (2007). Siblings of individuals with autism or Down syndrome: Effects on adult lives. *J Intellect Disabil Res, 51,* 682-696.

Owens, J.A., Rosen, C.L., & Mindell, J.A. (2003). Medication use in the treatment of pediatric insomnia: Results of a survey of community-based pediatricians. *Pediatrics, 111,* e628-e635.

Pardo, C.A., & Eberhart, C.G. (2007). The neurobiology of autism. *Brain Pathol, 17,* 434-447.

Parker, S.K., Schwartz, B., Todd, J., et al. (2004). Thimerosal-containing vaccines and autism spectrum disorder: A critical review of published original data. *Pediatrics, 114,* 793-804.

Peele, P.B., Lave, J.R., & Kelleher, K.J. (2002). Exclusions and limitations in children's behavioral health care coverage. *Psychiatr Serv, 53*(5), 591-594.

Pickett, J.A., & Paculdo, D.R. (2006). Letter to the editor: 1998–2002 update on "Causes of death in autism.". *J Autism Dev Disord, 36,* 287-288.

Posey, D.J., Erickson, C.A., Stigler, K.A., et al. (2006). The use of selective serotonin reuptake inhibitors in autism and related disorders. *J Child Adolesc Psychopharmacol, 14,* 181-186.

Posey, D.J., & McDougle, C.J. (2001). Pharmacotherapeutic management of autism. *Expert Opin Pharmacother, 2*(4), 587-600.

Probst, P., & Leppert, T. (2008). Brief report: Outcomes of a teacher training program for autism spectrum disorders. *J Autism Dev Disord.* Available at www.springerlink.com. Retrieved May 15, 2008.

Provost, B., Lopez, B.R., & Heimerl, S. (2007). A comparison of motor delays in young children: Autism spectrum disorder, developmental delay, and developmental concerns. *J Autism Dev Disord, 37,* 321-328.

Rapin, I. (1997). Autism. *N Engl J Med, 337*(2), 97-104.

Reichenberg, A., Gross, R., Weiser, M., et al. (2006). Advancing paternal age and autism. *Arch Gen Psychiatry, 63*, 1026-1032.

Research Units on Pediatric Psychopharmacology Autism Network (RUPPAN) (2005). Risperidone treatment of autistic disorder: Longer-term benefits and blinded discontinuation after 6 months. *Am J Psychiatry, 162*, 1361-1369.

Richler, J., Luyster, R., Risi, S., et al. (2006). Is there a 'regressive phenotype' of autism spectrum disorder associated with the measles-mumps-rubella vaccine? A CPEA study. *J Autism Dev Dis, 36*, 299-316.

Robins, D.L., Fein, D., Barton, M.L., et al. (2001). The Modified Checklist for Autism in Toddlers: An initial study investigating the early detection of autism and pervasive developmental disorders. *J Autism Dev Disord, 31*(2), 131-144.

Ross, P., & Cuskelly, M. (2006). Adjustment, sibling problems and coping strategies of brothers and sisters of children with autism spectrum disorder. *J Intellect Dev Disabil, 31*, 77-86.

Schieve, L.A., Blumberg, S.J., Rice, C., et al. (2007). The relationship between autism and parenting stress. *Pediatrics, 119*, S114-S121.

Schreck, K.A., & Williams, K. (2006). Food preferences and factors influencing food selectivity for children with autism spectrum disorders. *Rev Dev Disabil, 27*, 353-363.

Shattuck, P.T. (2006). The contribution of diagnostic substitution to the growing administrative prevalence of autism in US special education. *Pediatrics, 117*, 1028-1037.

Shattuck, P.T., Seltzer, M.M., Breenberg, J.S., et al. (2007). Change in autism symptoms and maladaptive behaviors in adolescents and adults with an autism spectrum disorder. *J Autism Dev Disord, 37*, 1735-1747.

Shavelle, R.M., Strauss, D.J., & Pickett, J. (2001). Causes of death in autism. *J Autism Dev Disord, 31*(6), 560-576.

Shea, S., Turgay, A., Carroll, A., et al. (2004). Risperidone in the treatment of disruptive behavioral symptoms in children with autistic and other pervasive developmental disorders. *Pediatrics, 114*, e634-41. Available at www.pediatrics.org. Retrieved January 23, 2008.

Siegel, B. (2003). *Helping Children with Autism Learn: Treatment Approaches for Parents. Oxford. England.* : Oxford University Press.

Sinha, Y., Silove, N., Wheeler, D., et al. (2004). Auditory integration training and other sound therapies for autism spectrum disorders. *Cochrane Database of Systematic Reviews, 1.* art. no. CD003681.

Smalley, S.L. (2002). Autism and tuberous sclerosis. *J Autism Dev Disord, 28*(5), 407-414.

Smith, L.E., Seltzer, M.M., Tager-Flusberg, H., et al. (2008). A comparative analysis of well-being and coping among mothers of toddlers and mothers of adolescents with ASD. *J Autism Dev Disord, 38*, 876-889.

Sperry, L.A., & Mesibov, G.B. (2005). Perceptions of social challenges of adults with autism spectrum disorder. *Autism, 9*, 362-376.

Stachnik, J.M., & Nunn-Thompson, C. (2007). Use of atypical antipsychotics in the treatment of autistic disorder. *Ann Pharmacother, 41*, 626-634.

Stokes, M., & Kaur, A. (2005). High-functioning autism and sexuality: A parental perspective. *Autism, 9*, 266-289.

Stokes, M., Newton, N., & Kaur, A. (2007). Stalking, and social and romantic functioning among adolescents and adults with autism spectrum disorder. *J Autism Dev Disord, 37*, 1969-1986.

Tatum, W., Genton, P., Bureau, M., et al. (2001). Less common epilepsy syndromes. In E.Wylie (Ed.), *The Treatment of Epilepsy: Principles and Practice*, (3rd ed.) Philadelphia: Lippincott Williams & Wilkins.

Thompson, W.W., Price, C., Goodson, B., et al. (2007). Early thimerosal exposure and neuropsychological outcomes at 7 to 10 years. *N Engl J Med, 357*, 1281-1292.

Tonge, B.J., Brereton, A., Kiomall, M., et al. (2006). Effects on parental mental health of an education and skills training program for parents of young children with autism: A randomized controlled trial. *J Am Acad Child Adolesc Psychiatry, 45*, 561-569.

Tuchman, R. (2006). Autism and epilepsy: What has regression got to do with it? *Epilepsy Currents, 6*, 107-111.

Tuchman, R.T., & Rapin, I. (2002). Epilepsy in autism. *Lancet Neurol, 1*, 352-358.

Turner, L., & Stone, W. (2007). Variability in outcome for children with an ASD diagnosis at age 2. *J Child Psychol Psychiatry, 48*, 793-802.

U.S. Food and Drug Administration. (2006). *FDA approves the first drug to treat irritability associated with autism, risperdal.* Available at www.fda.gov. Retrieved May 15, 2008.

Volkmar, F., Chawarska, K., & Klin, A. (2005). Autism in infancy and early childhood. *Ann Rev Psychol, 56*, 315-336.

Volkmar, F., Cook, E.H, Jr., Pomeroy, J., et al. (1999). Practice parameters for the assessment and treatment of children, adolescents, and adults with autism and other pervasive developmental disorders. *J Am Acad Child Adolesc Psychiatry, 38*, 32S-54S.

Volkmar, F., Lord, C., Bailey, A., et al. (2004). Autism and pervasive developmental disorders. *J Child Psychol Psychiatry, 45*, 135-170.

Wakefield, A.J., Murch, S.H., Anthony, A., et al. (1998). Ileal-lymphoid-nodular hyperplasia, non-specific colitis, and pervasive developmental disorder in children. *Lancet, 351*, 637-641.

Webb, S.J., Nalty, T., Munson, J., et al. (2007). Rate of head circumference growth as a function of autism diagnosis and history of autistic regression. *J Child Neurol, 22*, 1182-1190.

Weber, W., & Newmark, S. (2007). Complementary and alternative medical therapies for attention-deficit/hyperactivity disorder and autism. *Pediatr Clin North Am, 54*, 983-1006.

Werner, E., & Dawson, G. (2005). Validation of the phenomenon of autistic regression using home videotapes. *Arch Gen Psychiatry, 62*, 889-895.

Werner, E., Dawson, G., Munson, J., et al. (2005). Variation in early developmental course in autism and its relation with behavioral outcome at 3-4 years of age. *J Autism Dev Disord, 35*, 337-350.

Wetherby, A.M., Woods, J., Allen, L., et al. (2004). Early indicators of autism spectrum disorders in the second year of life. *J Autism Dev Disord, 34*, 473-493.

White, S.W., Scahill, L., Klin, A., et al. (2007). Educational placements and service use patterns of individuals with autism spectrum disorders. *J Autism Dev Disord, 37*, 1403-1412.

Wieder, S., & Greenspan, S.I. (2005). Climbing the symbolic ladder in the DIR model through floor time/interactive play. *Autism, 7*, 425-435.

Wier, M.L., Yoshida, C.K., Odouli, R., et al. (2006). Congenital anomalies associated with autism spectrum disorders. *Dev Med Child Neurol, 48*, 500-507.

Wiggins, L.D., Baio, J., & Rice, C. (2006). Examination of the time between first evaluation and first autism spectrum diagnosis in a population-based sample. *J Dev Behav Pediatr, 27*, S79-S87.

Williams, W.K.W., Wray, J.J, & Wheeler, D.M. (2005). Intravenous secretin for autism spectrum disorder. *Cochrane Database for Systematic Reviews, 3.* art. no. CD003495.

Wing, L. (2001). *The Autistic Spectrum.* Berkeley, CA: Ulysses Press.

Wong, V. (2006). Study of the relationship between tuberous sclerosis complex and autistic disorder. *J Child Neurol, 21*, 199-204.

Zafeiriou, D.I., Ververi, A., & Vargiami, E. (2006). Childhood autism and associated comorbidities. *Brain Dev, 29*, 257-272.

Zhao, X., Leotta, A., Ksutanovich, V., et al. (2007). A unified genetic theory for sporadic and inherited autism. *Proc Natl Acad Sci U S A, 104*, 12831-12836.

14 Bleeding Disorders

Susan Karp and James P. Riddel, Jr.

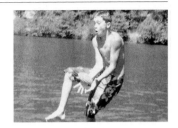

Etiology

Normal hemostasis occurs as a result of a set of regulated processes to accomplish two functions; first, it maintains blood in a fluid, clot-free state; and second, it induces a rapid and localized hemostatic plug at the site of vascular injury. "Hemostasis" is a dynamic process whereby blood coagulation is initiated and terminated in a rapid and tightly regulated fashion. Blood coagulation, also called hemostasis, is the cessation of blood loss from a damaged vessel and is the result of a complex interplay of various blood components. When a vessel is injured, platelets adhere to macromolecules in subendothelial tissues at the site of injury and then aggregate to form the primary hemostatic plug (Figure 14-1). Platelets stimulate the local activation of *plasma coagulation factors,* which leads to the generation of a fibrin clot that reinforces the platelet aggregate. Later, as wound healing occurs, the platelet aggregate and the fibrin clot are broken down and removed. Hemostasis is regulated by three basic components: namely, the vascular wall, platelets, and the activity coagulation factors. This chapter addresses three common hereditary bleeding disorders: hemophilia A (factor VIII deficiency), hemophilia B (factor IX deficiency), and von Willebrand disease (VWD), with the latter being the most common, albeit less symptomatic, disorder (Montgomery, Cox-Gill, & DiPaola, 2008; Riddel, Aouizerat, Miaskowski, et al., 2007).

Hemophilia

Hemophilia involves a defect in the intrinsic hemostatic mechanism. Factor VIII deficiency (e.g., classic hemophilia, hemophilia A) accounts for approximately 80% to 85% of hemophilia cases, whereas factor IX deficiency (e.g., Christmas disease, hemophilia B) accounts for 15% to 20% of such cases (Montgomery, Cox-Gill, & DiPaola, 2008; Smith & Smith, 2006). Less common factor deficiencies exist but are not specifically discussed in this chapter. Severity of hemophilia is defined by the percentage of activity of the deficient coagulation protein (Table 14-1) (Smith & Smith, 2006).

Hemophilia is inherited in an X-linked pattern (Figure 14-2). Most frequently, female carriers pass the disorder to their sons. The severity of hemophilia remains constant within families, although clinical symptoms may vary based on lifestyle and treatment regimens. Approximately one third of all people with hemophilia have a negative prior family history (Kulkarni, Ponder, James, et al., 2006). A woman is considered to be an obligate carrier if hemophilia has been diagnosed in her father, two of her sons, or one son and one other relative. Carriers of hemophilia A or B are expected to have, on average, factor VIII or IX levels that are approximately 50% of normal. Because of lyonization, however, some carriers have very low factor levels with resultant symptoms of excessive or unusual bleeding—particularly menorrhagia, which validates the need for determination of factor VIII/IX coagulant levels—even in obligate carriers (Lee, Chi, Pavord, et al., 2006).

The use of deoxyribonucleic acid (DNA) testing to detect carriers has an estimated accuracy of 95% to 99% (Peyvandi, Jayandharan, Chandy, et al., 2006). The factor VIII inversion is a genetic defect found in approximately 50% of people with severe hemophilia A and occurs when the distal end of the X chromosome containing part of the factor VIII gene flips over so that the factor VIII message is interrupted by irrelevant genetic material. If an affected male has this inversion, all female relatives who are carriers will also have it. This inversion test has an accuracy rate of 100%. Carrier testing for factor IX hemophilia using DNA analysis is also available (Peyvandi et al., 2006; Street, Ljung, & Lavery, 2008).

Prenatal diagnosis may be performed by amniocentesis as early as 13 to 16 weeks of gestation, by chorionic villus sampling at 10 to 13 weeks of gestation, or by fetal blood sampling (i.e., using percutaneous umbilical blood sampling) at 18 to 20 weeks of gestation. Male fetuses can be diagnosed as having hemophilia in utero by the use of DNA testing or the inversion test. If percutaneous umbilical blood sampling is performed, the hemophilia diagnosis is made by either DNA testing or a factor VIII or IX level (Chi, Lee, Shiltagh, et al., 2007; Kulkarni et al., 2006; Peyvandi et al., 2006).

von Willebrand Disease

von Willebrand disease (VWD) is caused by a deficiency or abnormality of von Willebrand factor (VWF) and is the most common inherited bleeding disorder in humans. VWF performs two major roles in hemostasis: first, it mediates the adhesion of platelets to sites of vascular injury, making it essential for platelet plug formation; second, it functions as a carrier protein that stabilizes coagulation factor VIII. Three main variants of the disorder exist: in type 1, the most common and generally the mildest variant, there is a partial quantitative deficiency of qualitatively normal VWF; in type 2 (which includes subtypes 2A, 2B, 2M, and 2N), there is a qualitative deficiency (or abnormal function) of VWF; and in type 3, there is a virtual absence of the VWF protein (Lillicrap, 2007).

von Willebrand disease is notable for considerable heterogeneity of its molecular basis. Although molecular studies have been successful in defining the genetic defects associated with type 2 and type 3 VWD, determining the genetic defects associated with type 1, the most common form of VWD, remains a challenge. Most types of VWD are inherited as an autosomal dominant trait, and thus there is often evidence of a family history of excessive bleeding.

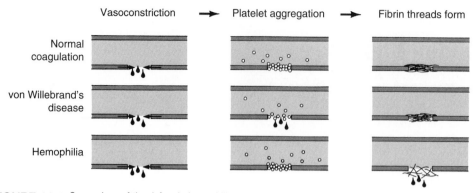

FIGURE 14-1 Comparison of the defect in hemophilia and von Willebrand disease with normal coagulation after a break in a vessel wall. Defect in von Willebrand disease is in platelet aggregation. Defect in hemophilia is in fibrin thread formation.

TABLE 14-1		
Severity of Hemophilia		
Severity	**Factor VIII and IX Coagulant Activity***	**Frequency and Type of Bleeding**
Severe	Less than 1%	By school age, several bleeding episodes that require treatment often occur each month. Bleeding may be spontaneous or the result of injury.
Moderate	1%-5%	Frequency of bleeding is variable. Spontaneous bleeding is less common.
Mild	5%-25%	Bleeding is generally only a result of trauma or surgery.

*Note that normal factor VIII and IX coagulant levels are generally 50% to 150% (0.50 to 1.5 U/dL).

Most forms of the condition show incomplete penetrance of the phenotype, and variable expressivity of bleeding symptoms within families. In contrast, the severe type 3 form of the condition or genetic defect shows a recessive pattern of inheritance with parents who do not usually manifest clinical symptoms. Finally, type 2N VWD, in which isolated low factor VIII levels occur, also shows a recessive pattern of inheritance, in which a family history may also be absent (James & Lillicrap, 2006; Kessler, 2007; Lillicrap, 2007).

Incidence and Prevalence

Hemophilia

Hemophilia A and B are uncommon, with an incidence of 1 in 5000 live male births for hemophilia A and 1 in 30,000 live male births for hemophilia B. The Centers for Disease Control and Prevention (CDC) estimates that there are approximately 18,000 people with hemophilia in the United States (Montgomery et al., 2008).

von Willebrand Disease

Although the true incidence of VWD is not known, it is thought to be the most common inherited bleeding disorder. It is estimated that VWD is present in more than 1% of the general population (Lillicrap, 2007).

Diagnostic Criteria

Approximately 30% of male infants with severe hemophilia have prolonged bleeding after a circumcision. In addition, 1% to 2% of neonates with hemophilia may experience an intracranial hemorrhage (Maclean, Fijnvandraat, Beijlevelt, et al., 2004; Montgomery et al., 2008). The majority of children with hemophilia are diagnosed at birth because of family history. It is recommended that male newborns of known carriers not diagnosed prenatally be tested for hemophilia by cord or peripheral blood sampling, especially prior to circumcision (Kulkarni & Lusher, 2001; Kulkarni et al., 2006; Street et al., 2008). In addition, neonates with no family history of hemophilia and unexplained subgaleal or intracranial hemorrhage should be screened for a hereditary bleeding disorder. Cesarean delivery is not routinely recommended in nontraumatic situations (Kulkarni & Lusher, 2001; Kulkarni et al., 2006; Street et al., 2008).

Although factor VIII levels generally rise above 50% during pregnancy, carriers whose baseline levels are below 50% may be at particular risk for postpartum hemorrhage. Factor VIII and IX levels should be checked several weeks before anticipated delivery to assess the possible need for hematologic intervention at delivery. Factor IX levels do not rise in pregnancy, and carriers with low levels of factor IX are more likely to need hematologic support with delivery (Kadir & Aledort, 2000; Kulkarni & Lusher, 2001; Peyvandi, 2005; Street et al., 2008).

Considerations in the Newborn Period

In the newborn period when there is a family history of hemophilia or other high level of suspicion, circumcision, heel sticks, and intramuscular immunizations and injections should ideally be delayed until a definitive diagnosis is made. Vitamin K may be given subcutaneously instead of intramuscularly to reduce the risk of hematoma development. It is best if phlebotomy is performed by a skilled technician in pediatrics, in order to avoid significant tissue hematoma.

As stated previously, in approximately one third of children, the occurrence of hemophilia represents a new (spontaneous) mutation. In these children, the diagnosis is often made when the child begins to crawl and walk. Common symptoms include easy bruising; oral bleeding, especially from a torn frenulum; hemarthroses (bleeding into joints); and intramuscular hemorrhages (bleeding into muscles) (Montgomery et al., 2008).

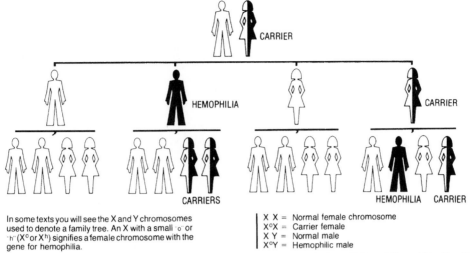

In some texts you will see the X and Y chromosomes used to denote a family tree. An X with a small "o" or "h" (X° or X^h) signifies a female chromosome with the gene for hemophilia.

X X = Normal female chromosome
X°X = Carrier female
X Y = Normal male
X°Y = Hemophilic male

FIGURE 14-2 Inheritance pattern for hemophilia. From Eckert, E.F. (1990). *Your Child and Hemophilia.* New York: National Hemophilia Foundation. Reprinted with permission.

When the diagnosis of hemophilia is suspected either on the basis of clinical finding or a positive family history, an initial diagnostic workup may include determination of prothrombin time (PT); partial thromboplastin time (PTT); a platelet function analysis (PFA) and fibrinogen or thrombin time; a platelet count; and studies to identify VWD, including a VWF antigen, von Willebrand ristocetin co-factor and factor VIII activity. If the PTT is prolonged, assays for factor VIII and factor IX should be done. The diagnosis of hemophilia is based on the absence or low levels of either the factor VIII or the factor IX protein. A severity level is then determined (see Table 14-1) (Montgomery et al., 2008; Smith & Smith, 2006).

In VWD, the diagnosis is made on the basis of the following clinical and laboratory components: a personal history of excessive mucocutaneous bleeding (i.e., nose bleeding, mouth bleeding, heavy menstrual bleeding), a family history of excessive bleeding, and a laboratory evaluation that is consistent with quantitative (factor VIII and VWF) or qualitative (ristocetin co-factor) defect in VWF (Lillicrap, 2004).

Clinical Manifestations at Time of Diagnosis

Clinical manifestations in infancy include intracranial hemorrhage, excessive bruising and hematomas, cephalohematoma, or bleeding following circumcision and venipuncture (Kulkarni & Lusher, 2001; Kulkarni et al., 2006; Maclean et al., 2004; Street et al., 2008). Bleeding from the umbilical cord stump may be indicative of factor XIII deficiency (Baur, 2008). Intracranial hemorrhage may be life threatening and occurs in approximately 1% to 5% of newborns with moderate to severe hemophilia; one half of these newborns develop neurologic deficits (Kulkarni & Lusher, 2001; Kulkarni et al., 2006; Maclean et al., 2004; Smith, Leonard, & Kurth, 2008; Street et al., 2008).

By 12 to 18 months of age, most children with severe hemophilia are diagnosed because of positive family history or unusual bleeding (see the Clinical Manifestations box) (Jones, 2002). Before diagnosis, parents may be questioned about child abuse because of excessive bruising. Children who first show signs of bleeding later in childhood or in adolescence more often have mild

Clinical Manifestations at Time of Diagnosis

HEMOPHILIA
- Bleeding following circumcision or heel stick
- Excessive bruising
- Hematomas after venipuncture or minimal injury
- Bleeding from the umbilical cord stump
- Intracranial bleeding
- Cephalohematoma
- Prolonged oral bleeding (i.e., after frenulum tear, dental extraction, tooth loss)
- Hemarthrosis (i.e., generally not the first symptom)

VON WILLEBRAND DISEASE
- Prolonged or repeated epistaxis
- Prolonged or excessive menstrual bleeding
- Gastrointestinal bleeding

to moderate hemophilia. A frequent misconception is that children with hemophilia can bleed to death from a typical childhood cut or scratch, but this does not happen. They may, however, demonstrate joint bleeding (i.e., hemarthrosis); muscle hematomas; excessive postoperative bleeding; or excessive or prolonged oral bleeding following frenulum tears, lost deciduous teeth, tooth eruption, and dental extractions (Jones, 2002).

von Willebrand disease is commonly manifested by bleeding from the mucous membranes. Although epistaxis is most frequently noted, excessive oral, gastrointestinal (GI), and menstrual bleeding also occurs (James & Lillicrap, 2006; Kessler, 2007; Lillicrap, 2007). Diagnostic testing is often requested when there is a positive family history of the disorder or when an increased PTT is obtained during routine preoperative screening. Because the levels of the von Willebrand protein and factor VIII may vary over time, coagulation testing may need to be repeated to establish a diagnosis (James & Lillicrap, 2006; Kessler, 2007; Lillicrap, 2007). Despite the relatively high incidence of this disorder, it is often not diagnosed because the common symptoms of epistaxis and heavy menstrual bleeding are often not brought to medical attention.

Treatment

Comprehensive Care in Hemophilia Treatment Centers

The standard of care for hemophilia is a collaborative interdisciplinary approach facilitated by local hemophilia treatment centers (HTCs). These centers, which are funded in part by the U.S. government, provide comprehensive management of inherited coagulation disorders. The core team consists of a pediatric hematologist, nurse coordinator, and social worker. A genetic counselor and physical therapist are other integral team members. A pediatric dentist and orthopedic surgeon provide consultative services. With the advent of human immunodeficiency virus (HIV), HTCs have also been mandated by the government to either provide or procure comprehensive management for individuals exposed to HIV. Individuals exposed to hepatitis C are often seen by a liver specialist as an adjunct to the HTC team. Services of the HTC include interdisciplinary comprehensive evaluations, counseling and support services, child and family education, carrier detection, access to new technology treatment products through clinical trials, and instruction on home infusion (Sharathkumar & Pipe, 2008; Soucie, Nuss, Evatt, et al., 2000).

All children and adolescents with hemophilia and VWD should receive regular comprehensive evaluations at the nearest HTC (Figure 14-3). The frequency of these evaluations should be every 3 to 12 months, depending on the severity of the child's bleeding disorder, use of prophylaxis (see section on prophylaxis), and other problems the child or family may be having. At these visits, children and their families are seen by the members of the interdisciplinary team. The family and primary care provider receive updated information on the status of a child's health and development, treatment options, new treatment products, and readiness

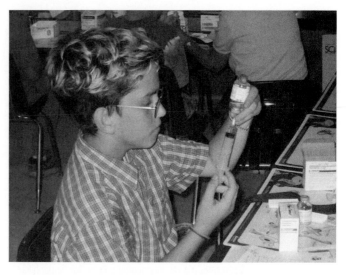

FIGURE 14-3 Adolescent learns the steps for self-injection. (Photo by Ken Hatfield.)

for home therapy is evaluated. HTCs work closely with primary care practitioners to provide comprehensive, coordinated, and accessible care for day-to-day management of pediatric health care. A federally funded study found that individuals receiving care at a hemophilia comprehensive care treatment center were 30% less likely to die than were those who did not receive hemophilia comprehensive care (Hoots, 2003; Soucie et al., 2000).

General Guidelines to Control Bleeding

The primary goal of treatment for a child who has hemophilia is the prevention of bleeding episodes. The second goal is early and aggressive treatment of bleeding episodes using a multidisciplinary team approach. Each bleeding episode should be treated on a case-by-case basis. When a bleeding episode is identified or suspected, therapy must be instituted promptly (Dunn & Abshire, 2004; Hoots, 2003; Rodriguez & Hoots, 2008; Sharathkumar & Pipe, 2008) (Table 14-2).

Prophylaxis

Prophylaxis is the regularly scheduled venous infusion of clotting factor concentrate with the goal of preventing most bleeding episodes. The use of home therapy and prophylactic therapy has revolutionized the care of children with hemophilia. In view of the demonstrated benefits of prophylaxis, the Medical and Scientific Advisory Council (MASAC) of the National Hemophilia Foundation recently issued recommendations that prophylaxis be considered optimal therapy for individuals with severe hemophilia A or B (Manco-Johnson, Abshire, Shapiro, et al., 2007; MASAC, 2006a).

Venous access is therefore critical to the treatment of hemophilia and one of the major barriers to treatment. Although peripheral venipuncture remains the first choice for venous access, it is often difficult and traumatic in young children. The use of implanted venous access devices (IVADs) has been helpful when prophylactic or frequent treatment is needed in children with poor venous access. However, these devices are not without complications, the most common being infection. Each child needs to be evaluated individually with a thorough discussion with the family and caregivers in making the choice to use an IVAD (Valentino & Kapoor, 2005).

Treatment

- Comprehensive care in hemophilia treatment centers
- General guidelines to control bleeding
- Prophylaxis
- Acute bleeding episodes
  - Major bleeding episodes: Head, muscle, joint, gastrointestinal, urinary, eye, throat, and neck
  - Minor bleeding episodes: Bruises, small cuts and scrapes, nosebleeds, and mouthbleeds
- Pharmacologic therapy for hemophilia (see Table 14-3)
  - Clotting factor concentrates
  - Recombinant factor VIII and factor IX
  - Dosing and cost of pharmacologic treatment
  - Plasma-derived factor VIII and IX concentrates
  - Desmopressin acetate (DDAVP)
- Pharmacologic therapy for von Willebrand disease
  - Use of synthetic and plasma-derived products (see Table 14-2)
  - Desmopressin acetate treatment choice for types 1 and 2A: intravenous or intranasal spray administration
- Hormonal therapy for women
- Oral antifibrinolytic agents
- Topical hemostatic agents
- Pain management
- Physical therapy
- Surgery

TABLE 14-2

Assessment and Treatment of Common Bleeding Episodes

Site of Bleeding	Signs and Symptoms	Treatment
Subcutaneous and/or soft tissue	*Mild:* Not interfering with ROM, not enlarging	Ice, Ace wrap
	Moderate: Occurring in wrist, volar surface of forearm, plantar surface of foot; interferes with ROM or is enlarging	Ice, splint/Ace wrap FVIII: 20-30 U/kg, or desmopressin* FIX: 30-50 U/kg†
	Severe: Pharyngeal; areas listed in "moderate" category accompanied by change in neurologic signs	Admit to hospital FVIII: 50 U/kg and follow-up doses FIX: 80-100 U/kg and follow-up doses†
Joint	*Earlier:* Moderate swelling, mild to moderate pain, warmth, stiffness, limited motion	Rest, splint/crutches FVIII: 20-30 U/kg, or desmopressin* FIX: 30-50 U/kg†
	Later: Tense swelling, moderate to severe pain, marked decrease in ROM; hip bleeding; limited abduction or adduction	Rest, splint/crutches PT plan May need repeat doses FVIII: 30-40 U/kg FIX: 40-50 U/kg† Ultrasound follow-up for hip bleed
Muscle	*Mild:* Swelling does not greatly affect ROM; mild discomfort	Rest, crutches, PT plan Ice, splint/Ace wrap FVIII: 20-30 U/kg or desmopressin* FIX: 30-40 U/kg†
	Severe: Swelling with neurologic changes; decreased ROM	Rest, splint/Ace wrap PT plan FVIII: 50 U/kg and follow-up doses FVIII: 80-100 U/kg†
	Iliopsoas: Abdominal, inguinal, or hip area pain; limited hip extension; numbness from nerve compression	Strict bed rest/ hospitalization Will need repeat doses FVIII: 50 U/kg FIX: 80-100 U/kg†
Nose	*Mild:* 10 min *Severe:* Prolonged or recurrent	Pressure to nares Collagen hemostat fibers and nasal pack VWD: Desmopressin, EACA FVIII: 20 U/kg, or desmopressin* FIX: 40 U/kg†
Oral areas	Dental extractions; frenulum, tongue, or lip bleeding	Topical hemostatic agent Epsilon-aminocaproic acid May need follow-up dose May need hospitalization if hard to control or severe anemia VWD: Desmopressin* FVIII: 30-40 U/kg, or desmopressin* FIX: 50-100 U/kg†
Gastrointestinal system	Abdominal pain; hypotension; blood in emesis; tarry or bloody stools; weakness	Hospitalization likely VWD: Desmopressin*/FVIII product with high level VWD FVIII: 50 U/kg and follow-up doses FIX: 100 U/kg and follow-up doses†
Central nervous system	Head, neck, or spinal injury; blurred vision; headaches; vomiting; unequal pupils; change in speech or behavior; drowsiness If no symptoms yet significant injury, treat and observe	Hospitalization and immediate consultation with hematologist depending on injury CT scan VWD: Desmopressin*/FVIII product with high level VWD factor FVIII: 50 U/kg two or three times/day FIX: 80-100 U/kg twice/day† May require follow-up prophylaxis if positive MRI or CT

Follow-up: By daily telephone contact or office visits through resolution of bleeding episode. If family is receiving home therapy, they should have telephone or office consultation if head, neck, or throat injury occurs; if more than two treatments are needed; or if bleeding occurs in hip, iliopsoas muscle, or urinary tract.

Data from Jones, P. (2002). *Living with Haemophilia* (5th ed.). Oxford, England: Oxford University Press; Hemophilia of Georgia. (2007). *The Hemophilia of Georgia Handbook* (4th ed.). Atlanta: Author; Kessler, C.R., & Lozier, J.N. (2000). Clinical aspects and therapy of hemophilia. In R. Hoffman et al. (Eds.), *Hematology: Basic Principles and Practice* (3rd ed.). New York: Churchill Livingstone.

NOTE: specific dosages may vary for individual patients; consult with the child's hematologist.

Key: *CT*, computed tomography; *EACA*, antifibrinolytic: epsilon-aminocaproic acid; *FIX*, factor IX hemophilia; *FVIII*, factor VIII hemophilia; *MRI*, magnetic resonance imaging; *PT*, physical therapy; *ROM*, range of motion; *U/kg*, units of factor VIII or IX per kilogram (factor concentrate vial contains a given number of FVIII or FIX activity units); VWD, von Willebrand disease.

*Desmopressin may be used if, after a test dose, the child with mild hemophilia has achieved a factor VIII coagulant level equal to the level that would be achieved after the recommended dose of factor VIII concentrate. Example: For a moderate soft tissue bleed in the calf, a dose of 20 to 30 U/kg should raise a child's factor VIII level to 40% to 60%. If after desmopressin the child reached a peak of only 25%, it is likely desmopressin would not be beneficial.

†Recombinate factor IX (BENEFIX) should be dosed at 20% higher.

Acute Bleeding Episodes

Bleeding episodes are usually categorized into two types, minor and major, and the type of bleed will dictate the *initial* treatment. The main treatment for hemophilia is replacement therapy (giving or replacing the clotting factor that is too low or missing) through a peripheral vein or central venous catheter.

The unit of measurement for products that replace the deficient factor protein is calculated in international units of factor VIII or IX activity. Choice of a particular dose is based on the type of hemophilia, the child's weight, the severity of the bleeding episode, the half-life of the chosen product, and the occurrence of bleeding in a chronically affected joint (see Table 14-3). Repeat doses may be necessary until clinical resolution is observed.

Major Bleeding Episodes: Head, Muscle, Joint, Gastrointestinal, Urinary, Eye, Throat, and Neck. Most episodes of major bleeding can be controlled with intermittent factor infusions; however, in the setting of life- or limb-threatening bleeding (e.g., iliopsoas muscle bleed) or surgical procedures during which constant factor levels are required, a continuous infusion of the factor replacement may need to be considered (see Table 14-3). For bleeding into a joint, treatment may begin when a child notes tingling in the joint. Many children have come to know this as the first indicator of oozing blood into the joint. For some children, symptoms of mild swelling, mild pain, or loss of range of motion of a joint may be the first recognizable indicators. In other children who have high pain tolerances or little self-awareness of body changes, the bleeding episode may not be recognized until there is severe swelling, major limitation of joint motion, and severe pain. Joint and bone radiographic examinations are generally not needed unless the child has a history of trauma and a broken bone is suspected. Treatment is usually given on demand as soon as the bleeding is identified but factor replacement may be given prophylactically to facilitate healing when bleeding is recurrent or severe or before high-risk or invasive procedures (e.g., surgery, dental extractions, physical therapy of a chronically affected joint) (Christie, 2002; Hemophilia of Georgia, 2007).

Minor Bleeding Episodes: Bruises, Small Cuts and Scrapes, Nosebleeds, and Mouthbleeds. In general, minor bleeding episodes can be treated with standard first aid measures. Bruises are common in children with hemophilia. Although these bruises may seem lumpy and slow to disappear, they are not usually a cause for alarm unless they are large or involve a joint or the head. Mild bruises rarely need treatment with factor replacement, and if a bump or hit to the skin is witnessed, an ice pack can be applied to slow the bleeding from the small blood vessels under the skin. Children do not usually need to take factor replacement for small cuts and scrapes because platelet adhesion is usually sufficient to control this type of bleed. If a cut or laceration appears to require sutures, factor replacement is necessary. Epistaxis, or nose bleeding, is a common manifestation in children with bleeding disorders; local measures such as pressure, tilting the head forward (this prevents blood from pooling in the posterior pharynx, thereby avoiding nausea and airway obstruction) (Kucik & Clenney, 2005), and applying ice to the bridge of the nose are usually sufficient. Bleeding from the gums around the teeth, the tongue, the lips, and the inside of the cheek often requires factor replacement for hemostasis. It is generally recommended that the child also start taking an oral antifibrinolytic to prevent clot lysis. This also holds true for episodes of epistaxis (Hemophilia of Georgia, 2007).

Pharmacologic Therapy for Hemophilia

The most exciting technologic advance in factor replacement therapy is the use of recombinant DNA to manufacture recombinant factor VIII and factor IX, rendering current therapies for hemophilia extremely safe and effective in preventing or treating bleeding (Table 14-3). The treatment product of choice should be determined by consulting with the child's hematologist. This information should be updated at least yearly to incorporate changes in manufacturing technologies. The current recommended treatment products are the recombinant factor VIII and factor IX products (MASAC, 2006a). These high-purity products, such as the recombinant VIII and IX concentrates, unfortunately are extremely costly. A school-age child with severe hemophilia who is receiving prophylactic therapy may use close to 180,000 units of factor VIII or IX per year at a cost of approximately $200,000. There have been reports by several HTCs in the United States and abroad of anaphylactic reactions occurring in children within the first 10 to 20 treatment episodes with factor IX, along with the development of an inhibitor factor. This has been reported particularly in children with factor IX deficiency with a specific gene deletion. Therefore, during the initial treatment of children with hemophilia B (factor IX deficiency), it is strongly recommended that the infusion occur in the medical setting where the child can be monitored and safety established (Warrier, 2005).

Vials of factor concentrate come in various sizes with varying numbers of factor units per vial. When a child is prescribed a specific dose of factor (i.e., expressed in factor VIII or IX units), this is considered a minimum dose and the child should be given the full number of vials that provide the desired dose without discarding any of the factor from an individual vial. This minimum dosing rule is due to the high cost of the medication and the lack of adverse sequelae from a dose slightly higher than that originally prescribed.

Desmopressin acetate (DDAVP) is also effective in raising the levels of factor VIII in many children with mild factor VIII deficiency and VWD and has relatively few major side effects (Franchini, 2007). DDAVP has been successfully used for children to prevent bleeding complications in connection with dental or surgical procedures and for acute bleeding such as joint, muscle, or mucosal bleeding. Not all children with mild hemophilia A respond adequately, and a "test of treatment" needs to be performed before any procedure or bleeding episode.

Pharmacologic Therapy for von Willebrand Disease

The standard treatment for VWD encompasses both synthetic and plasma-derived products. Primary care providers are urged to consult the child's hematologist, the local HTC, or the National Hemophilia Foundation for the most current treatment recommendations (MASAC, 2006b).

Desmopressin acetate (see Table 14-3), which is a synthetic analog of vasopressin, is the treatment of choice for persons with types 1 and 2A von Willebrand disease but not subtype 2B (Franchini, 2007). Although the mechanism of action is not completely understood, it is thought that desmopressin releases stores of factor VIII and the von Willebrand protein from the endothelial lining of the blood vessels. Stores may be depleted, however, if treatment is

TABLE 14-3

Products Available to Treat Individuals with Bleeding Disorders

Factor VIII Products Licensed in the United States — Recombinant Factor VIII Products

Product Name	Manufacturer	Method of Viral Depletion or Inactivation	Stabilizer	Human or Animal Protein Used in Culture Medium	Specific Activity of Final Product (IU Factor VIII/mg Total Protein)	Viral Safety Studies in Humans with This Product
Advate	Baxter	Immunoaffinity chromatography Solvent/detergent	Trehalose	None	4000-10,000	Yes
Helixate FS	Bayer (distributed by Aventis Behring)	Immunoaffinity chromatography	Sucrose	Human plasma protein fraction	4000*	Yes
Kogenate FS	Bayer	Immunoaffinity chromatography	Sucrose	Human plasma protein fraction	4000*	Yes
Recombinate	Baxter	Immunoaffinity chromatography	Human albumin	Bovine calf serum	1.65-19	Yes
ReFacto	Wyeth	Immunoaffinity chromatography Solvent/detergent (TNBP and Triton X-100)	Sucrose	Human serum albumin	11,200-15,500	Yes
Xyntha	Wyeth	1. Solvent/detergent(TNBP/ polysorbate80) 2. Nanofiltration	Sucrose	None	5500-9000	Yes

Immunoaffinity Purified Factor VIII Products Derived from Human Plasma

Product Name	Manufacturer	Method of Viral Inactivation	Specific Activity of Final Product (IU Factor VIII/mg Total Protein)	Hepatitis Safety Studies in Humans with This Product	Viral Safety Studies in Humans with Another Product but Similar Viral Inactivation Method
Hemofil M	Baxter	Immunoaffinity chromatography Solvent/detergent (TNBP and octoxynol 9)	2-15	Yes	No
Monarc-M	Manufactured by Baxter for American Red Cross (ARC) from ARC-collected plasma (distributed by ARC)	Immunoaffinity chromatography Solvent/detergent (TNBP and octoxynol 9)	2-15	No	Yes
Monoclate-P	Aventis Behring	Immunoaffinity chromatography Pasteurization (60°C, 10 hr)	5-10	Yes	Yes

Adapted from The Medical and Scientific Advisory Committee: The National Hemophilia Foundation. *MASAC Document #182*. Updated annually (www.hemophilia.org).
Key: *FDA*, U.S. Food and Drug Administration; *IV*, intravenous; *SQ*, subcutaneous; *TNBP*, tri(*N*-butyl)phosphate.
*Valid as long as product is kept under refrigeration as recommended by the manufacturer.

Continued

TABLE 14-3

Products Available to Treat Individuals with Bleeding Disorders—cont'd

Factor VIII Products Derived from Human Plasma that Contain von Willebrand Factor

Product Name	Manufacturer	Method of Viral Inactivation	Specific Activity of Final Product (IU Factor VIII/mg Total Protein)	Hepatitis Safety Studies in Humans with This Product	Viral Safety Studies in Humans with Another Product but Similar Method	FDA Approved for von Willebrand Disease
Alphanate	Alpha	Affinity chromatography / Solvent/detergent (TNBP and polysorbate 80) / Dry heat (80°C, 72 hr)	8-30	No	Yes	No
Humate-P	Aventis Behring GmbH (Marberg, Germany)	Pasteurization (60°C, 10 hr)	1-2	Yes	No	Yes
Koate-DVI	Bayer	Solvent/detergent (TNBP and polysorbate 80) / Dry heat (80°C, 72 hr)	9-22	No	Yes	No

Factor IX Products Licensed in the United States
Recombinant Factor IX Products

Product Name	Manufacturer	Method of Viral Depletion or Inactivation	Stabilizer	Human or Animal Protein Used in Culture Medium	Specific Activity (IU Factor IX/mg Total Protein)	Hepatitis Safety Studies in Humans with This Product
Benefix	Wyeth	Affinity chromatography / Ultrafiltration	Sucrose	None	≥200	Yes

Coagulation Factor IX Products Derived from Human Plasma

Product Name	Manufacturer	Method of Viral Depletion or Inactivation	Specific Activity of Final Product (IU Factor IX/mg Total Protein)	Viral Safety Studies in Humans with This Product	Viral Safety Studies in Humans with Another Product but Similar Inactivation Method
Alpha-Nine SD	Alpha	Dual affinity chromatography / Solvent/detergent (TNBP and polysorbate 80) / Nanofiltration (viral filter)	229 ± 23	Yes	Yes
Mononine	Aventis Behring	Immunoaffinity chromatography / Sodium thiocyanate / Ultrafiltration	>160	Yes	No

Prothrombin Complex Concentrates Derived from Human Plasma that Contains Factors II, VII, IX, X (for Use in Individuals with Deficiencies of Factors II, VII, IX, X; Content Varies by Lot and Product)

Product Name	Manufacturer	Method of Viral Inactivation	Specific Activity of Final Product (IU Factor IX/mg Total Protein)	Viral Safety Studies in Humans with This Product	Viral Safety Studies in Humans with Another Product but Similar Viral Inactivation Method
Bebulin VH	Baxter (Vienna)	Vapor heat (10 hr 60°C, 1190 mbar pressure plus 1 hr, 80°C, 1375 mbar)	2	Yes	No
Profilnine SD	Alpha	Solvent/detergent (TNBP and polysorbate 80)	4.5	No	Yes
Proplex T	Baxter	Dry heat (60°C, 144 hr)	3.9	No	No

Anti-inhibitor Coagulation Complex (Activated Prothrombin Complex Concentrates) Derived from Human Plasma (for Use in Individuals with Inhibitors to Factor VIII or IX)

Product Name	Manufacturer	Method of Viral Depletion or Inactivation	Specific Activity of Final Product (IU Factor/mg Total Protein)	Viral Safety Studies in Humans with This Product	Viral Safety Studies in Humans with Another Product but Similar Viral Inactivation Method
FEIBA VH	Baxter (Vienna)	Vapor heat (10 hr, 60°C, 1190 mbar plus 1 hr, 80°C, 1375 mbar)	0.8	Yes	Yes

Factor VII Products Licensed in the United States Recombinant Factor VIIa

Product Name	Manufacturer	Method of Viral Depletion or Inactivation	Stabilizer	Viral or Animal Protein Used in Culture Medium	Viral Safety Studies in Humans with This Product
NovoSeven	Novo Nordisk (Bagsvaerd, Denmark)	Affinity chromatography	Mannitol	Bovine calf serum	Yes

Desmopressin Formulations Useful in Disorders of Hemostasis

Product Name	Manufacturer	U.S. Distributor	Formulation	Recommended Dosage and Administration
DDAVP injection	Ferring AB (Malmo, Sweden)	Aventis Pharma	For parenteral use 4 mcg/mL in a 10- or 1-mL vial	0.3 mcg/kg, mixed in 30 mL normal saline solution, infused slowly over 30 min IV 0.4 mcg/kg subcutaneously; maximum dose 24 mcg once every 24 hr; may repeat after 24 hr
Stimate nasal spray for bleeding	Ferring AB	Aventis Behring (Malmo, Sweden)	Nasal spray, 1.5 mg/mL; metered dose pump delivers 0.1 mL (150 mcg) per actuation; bottle contains 2.5 mL with spray pump capable of delivering 25 150-mcg doses or 12 300-mcg doses	In individuals weighing <50 kg, one spray in one nostril delivers 150 mcg; >50 kg, give one spray in each nostril (total dose 300 mcg); may repeat after 24 hr

Fresh Frozen Plasma Products

Product Name	Manufacturer	Distributor	Method of Viral Depletion or Inactivation	Pool Size, Number of Donor Units
Donor retested fresh frozen plasma	Some community blood centers	Some community blood centers	Donors must test negative on second donation for first donation to be released	1

repeated more often than every 24 hours. The intravenous infusion dosage is 0.3 mg/kg diluted in 30 to 50 mL of normal saline and infused over 30 minutes (Franchini, 2007).

The effectiveness of this medication for various bleeding episodes depends on the rise in coagulation protein activity. Peak response is generally obtained 30 minutes after IV infusion is complete. Individuals should have a test dose of this product to determine response before using it therapeutically. The response varies among individuals, and it should be determined if an individual is a candidate for this therapy before it is used for a bleeding episode or before an invasive procedure. Individuals tend to show consistency in the degree of response over time. Desmopressin has also been given subcutaneously at a slightly higher dose with good results in some children (Franchini, 2007).

A concentrated intranasal form of desmopressin, Stimate Nasal Spray (1.5 mg/mL) provides its peak effect 1 to 2 hours after administration. Some studies have shown similar clinical response with this intranasal form in children with mild hemophilia A and VWD who responded well to the intravenous (IV) form (Mannucci, 2008). If a child has had prior desmopressin testing with the IV form, repeat laboratory testing with the intranasal form may still be indicated before clinical use, because for some individuals results may not be consistent for the two forms of administration (Franchini, 2007). The less-concentrated DDAVP Nasal Spray (0.1 mg/mL) is ineffective in treating children with bleeding disorders (Castaman, 2008). Desmopressin has an antidiuretic effect, so children and parents must be cautioned to limit fluid intake for the remainder of the day that the drug is administered (Federici, 2008; Franchini, 2007; Lozier & Kessler, 2005). For those individuals with VWD in whom desmopressin is either ineffective or contraindicated, or in instances where it is anticipated that the risk of major bleeding is high, von Willebrand factor and factor VIII levels can be restored by the infusion of plasma-derived concentrates of these proteins. These products have been shown to be free of transfusion-transmitted infectious agents (Kessler, 2007).

Hormonal Therapy

In young women with a history of heavy menstrual bleeding, the use of oral contraceptives is useful in reducing the severity of menorrhagia. Exogenous estrogens can increase the factor VIII and ristocetin cofactor activity levels in females with low factor VIII levels (hemophilia A carriers) and females with von Willibrand disease.

Oral Antifibrinolytic Agents

Children with hemophilia and VWD often have oral bleeding that requires additional medication to keep the clot stable once it has formed. Because of digestive enzymes in the saliva that lyse fibrin clots, an antifibrinolytic agent should be given orally for 7 to 10 days or until the site of oral bleeding has completely healed (Montgomery et al., 2008). The only such agent currently licensed is epsilon-aminocaproic acid (Amicar).

Topical Hemostatic Agents

Collagen hemostat (Avitene) fibers can be applied to nasal packing or salt pork pledgets to control epistaxis or at the site of frenulum tears or tooth extraction. When nasal packing is used, it is generally left in place for 24 to 36 hours to promote stable clot formation. Nosebleeds can often be prevented or diminished by using petroleum jelly or antibiotic ointment in the nares, as well as

humidification of room air. Fibrin glue has been used to promote local hemostasis in some circumcisions; cryoprecipitate is the source of fibrinogen in this treatment (Lozier & Kessler, 2005).

Pain Management

Uncontrolled bleeding into a joint or muscle can produce significant pain. Prompt replacement of the deficient coagulation protein to stop the bleeding is the most effective way to prevent severe pain. Mild pain may be treated with acetaminophen (*not* aspirin), ice, and elevation of the affected extremity. If pain is moderate or severe, acetaminophen with codeine every 4 to 6 hours is recommended. Pain medication is generally not necessary after the first day of factor replacement. Continued pain may suggest ineffective control of bleeding because of inadequate dosing of the factor concentrate, development of an inhibitor, or a more severe bleeding episode than previously thought. Swelling caused by irritation of the synovial lining may be more effectively treated with a nonsteroidal antiinflammatory agent. These agents should be used with caution, however, because they can cause GI bleeding secondary to interference with platelet aggregation (Lozier & Kessler, 2005).

Physical Therapy

Splinting and immobilization for 1 to 2 days after acute bleeding often aid in resolution of the episode. A resting splint that places the extremity in a comfortable position is recommended for night use for several days following a significant hemarthrosis to prevent further bleeding secondary to twisting during sleep and to immobilize the joint. Following severe bleeding or prolonged immobilization, a physical therapy program should be prescribed to enable children to achieve their baseline range of motion and regain muscle mass. Factor replacement is often needed with vigorous physical therapy (Beeton & Tuffley, 2005; Heijnen & Buzzard, 2005; Raffini & Manno, 2007).

Surgical Intervention

Destruction of joint cartilage secondary to repeated bleeding episodes can result in significant pain, decreased strength and range of motion, and an impaired ability to use the affected extremity. Individuals who continue to bleed despite prophylaxis and those for whom prophylaxis is not available or feasible may benefit from surgical intervention. Several orthopedic procedures have been successful in individuals with hemophilia and can provide them with significantly reduced joint pain, decrease in number of bleeding episodes, and greater range of motion and endurance. Open synovectomy is successful in reducing pain and bleeding episodes, but mobility is often lost and progression of the arthropathy continues. Arthroscopic synovectomy reduces the pain and frequency of bleeding episodes without loss of mobility. Injection of a radioactive isotope into the affected joint to eradicate overgrown and inflamed synovium, which is a less invasive procedure, has been successful in improving range of motion and decreasing bleeding episodes in individuals who are not surgical candidates (Lozier & Kessler, 2005; Raffini & Manno, 2007).

Complementary and Alternative Therapies

A review of the literature did not identify any complementary or alternative therapies for the treatment of VWD or hemophilia. Although not evidenced based, some methods to prevent epistaxis include using a cool mist humidifier while sleeping, using a nasal saline spray four times a day, and keeping the nasal openings moist with topical gels such as petroleum jelly or a triple antibiotic ointment. Some hemophilia centers recommend using knee and elbow pads to prevent hemarthrosis (again, not scientifically based).

Anticipated Advances in Diagnosis and Management

Hemophilia care is the best that it has ever been (O'Shaughnessy, Makris, & Lillicrap, 2005). Clotting factor concentrates have never been safer. In the aftermath of the human immunodeficiency and hepatitis C epidemics, the National Hemophilia Foundation has adopted a zero tolerance policy when faced with the potential of pathogen transmission. This strategy is intended to ensure that persons with hemophilia do not become infected with a recognized or an emerging pathogen as a result of treatment with a factor concentrate (Matthew, Manno, & Aledort, 2005). Although manufacturers of plasma-derived factor replacement products strive to improve the donor screening and plasma testing and to develop techniques for pathogen inactivation, the consensus in the United States is that recombinant products are preferred in the management of infants and children with hemophilia (MASAC, 2006b; Matthew et al., 2005).

Hemophilia has a number of characteristics that make it attractive as a model for gene transfer approaches. Several trials of gene therapy for hemophilia were carried out in the last decade, but none resulted in long-term expression of the missing clotting factor at therapeutic levels. Ongoing trials of gene transfer for hemophilia continue in hopes of a successful outcome within the next decade (High, 2007).

Associated Problems of Condition and Treatment

Inhibitors

The development of inhibitory antibodies is a serious complication that occurs in 20% to 33% of all persons with hemophilia A and approximately 1% to 6% of persons with hemophilia B (DiMichele, 2005). In a person with hemophilia A or B, inhibitors are directed against the child's missing clotting factor. They are created by the body following treatment with factor replacement therapy. The antibody attaches to the factor VIII or IX protein and neutralizes (inhibits) its ability to stop bleeding. The treatment of a child with antibodies can be challenging. New therapies to prevent or treat bleeding episodes have been developed to meet the challenge. These products contain other activated clotting factors that can stimulate

the formation of a clot and stop bleeding, thus bypassing the specific requirement for factor VIII or factor IX (Astermark, 2006; DiMichele, 2005). However, eradication of the antibodies is the best option. This is accomplished through "immune tolerance," in which regular infusions of factor VIII or IX are administered, usually on a daily or every-other-day basis, for a period of weeks to years; the goal is to train the immune system to better accept treatment with the missing clotting factor (Astermark, 2006; DiMichele, 2005).

Anemia

Anemia can occur as a result of slow, persistent oozing from the mouth or nose or bleeding or pooling of blood in muscle hemorrhages. In persons with VWD, excessive or prolonged menstrual bleeding or persistent or recurrent epistaxis can result in anemia.

Neurologic Problems

Intracranial hemorrhage is the most frequent cause of death in children with hemophilia. Intracranial hemorrhage also can result in spastic quadriplegia and developmental delay. In some cases of intracranial bleeding, no known prior injury is identified. Therefore any cranial injury or neurologically related symptom should be treated aggressively. There may be significant intracranial bleeding without the presence of a "goose egg" because the most significant bleeding occurs from internal shearing of the brain and cranium. The presence of a hematoma, however, indicates that the cranium may have met with significant force. Because of the high risk of rebleeding after intracranial hemorrhage, prophylactic factor treatment is continued for an extended period. Individuals with VWD also are at increased risk for this type of bleeding. Bleeding within or around the spinal column can also produce enough pressure to cause neurologic damage. Compartment syndrome resulting from nerve compression may occur after untreated bleeding into the forearm or calf (Anderson & Forsyth, 2005; Lozier & Kessler, 2005).

Airway Obstruction as a Result of Bleeding

Posterior pharyngeal bleeding increases the potential for asphyxia. This can result from a traumatic throat culture, bronchoscopy, dental extractions, or deep injection of anesthetic without pretreatment with factor concentrates or desmopressin. Intubation should only be attempted after pretreatment with factor concentrate.

Hepatitis

In the past, exposure to blood and plasma-derived products has resulted in a high incidence of infection with hepatitis B and C in the population with hemophilia. Approximately 75% of those with hemophilia have been exposed to hepatitis B; the majority have developed immunity, but a small percentage are chronic carriers. With the use of the hepatitis B vaccine series, the incidence of hepatitis B has been greatly reduced. Previous studies have identified the number of individuals with hemophilia exposed to hepatitis C to be approximately 80% to 90% (Goedert, Chen, Preiss, et al., 2007; Rustgi, 2007). Today, most clinicians consider the risk of transmission of infection through today's factor concentrates to be minimal. The viral inactivation of factor concentrates, introduced in 1985, has been highly effective in the reduction and eventual elimination of transmission of HIV and hepatitis A, B, and C (Goedert et al., 2007; Lozier & Kessler, 2005; O'Shaughnessy et al., 2005; Smith & Smith, 2006).

Associated Problems of Bleeding Disorders and Treatment

- Inhibitors
- Anemia
- Neurologic problems (intracranial hemorrhage, bleeding around spinal column, compartment syndrome compression of nerves)
- Airway obstruction as a result of bleeding
- Hepatitis
- Gastrointestinal bleeding
- Musculoskeletal problems
- Genitourinary bleeding

Gastrointestinal Bleeding

Bleeding into the GI tract may occur in children with VWD and in those with hemophilia. The fragile mucous membrane–lined digestive system is prone to bleeding that can result from ulcers, gastritis, hemorrhoids, rectal fissures, and endoscopic procedures. This type of bleeding should be considered when there is an unexplained drop in hemoglobin levels or abdominal pain.

Musculoskeletal Problems

The normally smooth synovial lining of a joint produces synovial fluid that, along with the cartilage, serves as a shock absorber for the joint (Figure 14-4). The synovium is also supplied with many blood vessels. When bleeding into a joint ceases with the administration of the deficient coagulation protein, enzymes clear away the blood from the synovial fluid; the more blood that accumulates in the joint capsule, the more enzymes that are released. These enzymes, however, do not seem to focus their destruction solely on the unwanted blood cells; they begin to eat away at the smooth synovial lining, producing breaks in the surface that can make it easier for bleeding to recur in that joint. Eventually they may destroy the cartilaginous surface of the bones. The nonintact synovial lining can cause the synovium to produce abnormal amounts of fluid in an inflammatory response known as synovitis. Even when actual bleeding into the joint does not occur, the joint may become swollen and stiff. Synovitis is differentiated from a hemarthrosis by its gradual onset, mild or absent pain, and fuller range of motion. This destructive process can ultimately lead to severe osteoarthritic-like conditions and joint contractures. A single hip hemarthrosis can produce aseptic necrosis of the femoral head if bleeding is not fully resolved. When bleeding recurs in a specific joint, it may be referred to as a "target joint." Thus a strong case is made for early detection and treatment of bleeding episodes and ultimately for the use of prophylactic treatment for children with severe hemophilia (Raffini & Manno, 2007).

Genitourinary Bleeding

Hematuria occurs most commonly in adolescents with hemophilia, is usually of short duration, is not a result of trauma, and often stops spontaneously. Determination of an actual bleeding site is often difficult. Clots can sometimes cause renal or ureteral obstruction with temporary renal colic and, at times, hydronephrosis. Treatment with epsilon-aminocaproic acid (Amicar) should be avoided during periods of hematuria because of the risk of developing clots in the genitourinary system (Montgomery et al., 2008).

Prognosis

The treatment of children with severe hemophilia has been dramatically improved by the availability of adequate quantities of viral-safe, recombinant factor VIII and IX; advances in techniques to perform venipuncture safely and effectively on a routine basis in the home; and development and wide application of protocols to prevent bleeding and the inflammatory sequelae of bleeding episodes into joints. The musculoskeletal complications that follow repeated joint bleeding can be effectively prevented with the early initiation of prophylaxis (the routine scheduled replacement of factor) (Manco-Johnson et al., 2007; Pipe & Valentino, 2007). The HIV and hepatitis C virus tragedies raised awareness in individuals with hemophilia, as well as health care providers, of the vulnerability of blood products to viral contamination and spurred progress in science leading to viral inactivation of purified proteins.

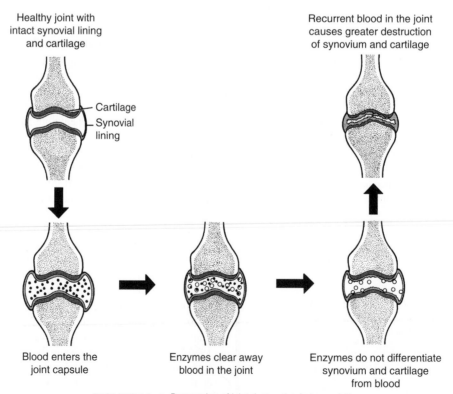

FIGURE 14-4 Progression of joint destruction in hemophilia.

Children with hemophilia can now look forward to a normal life expectancy and excellent health-related quality of life. The future of hemophilia promises a cure with gene therapy (Manco-Johnson, 2005).

PRIMARY CARE MANAGEMENT

Health Care Maintenance

Growth and Development

Monitoring the weight and height of a child with hemophilia is especially important because obesity places added stress on joints and muscles and limb length may be increased by bony overgrowth of the epiphysis on one side from chronic arthropathy. Repeated bleeding into a joint may result in a permanent contracture of that joint, with leg length discrepancy. Gait disturbances caused by scoliosis may predispose individuals with hemophilia to joint or muscle bleeding.

A thorough baseline and ongoing assessment of developmental parameters and neurologic status are useful in follow-up for head trauma and screening of potentially undiagnosed or unreported intracranial bleeding. Normal development is anticipated unless there is a history of intracranial bleeding.

Diet

It is especially important for children with bleeding disorders to meet the recommended requirements for protein and calcium intake because of their role in bone and muscle formation. A nonconstipating diet may prevent the rectal bleeding that can occur when hard stools are passed. When a child has mouth bleeding, a soft diet and avoidance of foods that are hot or have sharp edges (e.g., chips) and straws (because the sucking action can disturb the clot) are recommended. As mentioned previously, weight management to prevent obesity is important to decrease stress on weight-bearing joints.

Safety

Protection against head injury is of primary importance. Some hemophilia providers believe that a protective helmet for children with hemophilia who are learning to walk may reduce the risk of head injury. Other providers believe that it may make the child more unbalanced and lead to an increased incidence of falls. Knee pads may be used for toddlers prone to knee hematomas. From the time they start to walk, children at risk for hemarthroses should wear high-top leather sneakers and shoes; this provides physical protection against direct injury from knocks and blows, as well as reducing the tendency to indirect injury from twisting (Buzzard & Briggs, 2003). Walkers are never recommended for young children but may be particularly hazardous for children with bleeding disorders. Care must also be taken that the child is safely strapped in when using portable swings and high chairs.

Contact sports (e.g., football, soccer, hockey, wrestling, boxing, competitive basketball) are strongly discouraged because of the increased chance of head trauma and other injuries to the joints (Rice, 2008). Appropriate physical activity is encouraged, however, to maintain strong muscles that promote joint stability and normal social adjustment. Swimming is an ideal aerobic activity. Although recommended for all children, helmets are particularly important for those with bleeding disorders when riding bikes or scooters or using roller skates or in-line skates. Knee and elbow pads are also recommended for roller-skating or in-line skating and skateboarding. Activities that increase the chances for testicular trauma (dirt-bike riding, horseback riding, gymnastics) should be discouraged in boys with moderate to severe hemophilia.

Use of a medical identification emblem that includes diagnosis and treatment recommendations is required for safety. Infants can have the emblem pinned to their car seats or jackets when traveling. A wallet identification card may be used if a child or an adolescent refuses to wear the emblem. Medical information should be checked yearly and updated as necessary.

Families participating in a home infusion program should follow accepted guidelines for infection control, including the use of gloves to mix and administer factor concentrates and the disposal of infectious wastes in approved containers that are disposed of appropriately.

Arterial blood samples should only be drawn after pretreatment with factor concentrate.

Immunizations

Routine immunizations are recommended, except injectable vaccines should be given subcutaneously when possible because intramuscular injections may cause muscle bleeding (CDC, 2008). When any injectable vaccine is given, the following interventions can help prevent hematoma development: using a 25-gauge needle, applying firm pressure to the site for 5 minutes after injection, and using a factor concentrate before intramuscular injection.

Screening

Vision. Routine screening is recommended. Following an eye injury, referral to an ophthalmologist is recommended, with follow-up until resolution is obtained.

Hearing. Routine screening is recommended. Attempts at removing earwax with a curette may result in bleeing. Flushing the ear with warm water to remove cerumen is safer.

Dental. Invasive dental procedures can often be prevented through careful oral hygiene, fluoride treatments, and regular dental evaluations. An initial dental evaluation is recommended at 2 to 3 years of age, in part to help the child establish a positive relationship with the dentist, as well as to impress on parents the importance of preventive care. Hygiene should include flossing under parental supervision. Pediatric dentists with expertise in the management of persons with bleeding disorders are often associated with the local HTC. If necessary, local dentists can manage most procedures with consultation from the HTC. The HTC should be consulted about whether or not prophylactic treatment with factor concentrate or desmopressin is necessary for routine dental cleaning or anesthetic infiltrates close to the gum line for a particular child. For dental extractions, desmopressin or factor concentrate plus an antifibrinolytic agent is recommended (Brewer & Correa, 2006). If a child has an implantable port, external venous catheter, or joint replacement, some treatment centers advocate the use of subacute bacterial endocarditis (SBE) antibiotic prophylaxis (See Chapter 21).

Blood Pressure. Routine screening is recommended.

Hematocrit. Annual screening for anemia is recommended. Nosebleeds that are short in duration but occur frequently may not be regularly reported by families and may lead to significant anemia. If venipuncture is required, a 23-gauge butterfly needle should be used and firm pressure applied to the site for at least 5 minutes afterward to prevent hematoma formation. Trauma may be reduced if a skilled pediatric phlebotomist performs venipuncture. Females with VWD and females who are carriers of hemophilia and have low factor levels may have menorrhagia. This may result in a lower than normal hematocrit. Menorrhagia may be controlled by the use of birth control pills or other estrogen-containing medications or the high concentration intranasal DDAVP product, Stimate.

Urinalysis. An annual urinalysis is recommended to screen for microscopic hematuria. Hematuria may occur without a history of trauma. If this occurs the HTC should be notified, although hematuria often spontaneously resolves (see Common Illness Management).

Tuberculosis. Routine screening is recommended. No factor pretreatment is needed for purified protein derivative (PPD) skin testing.

Condition-Specific Screening

Children who have received any blood bank products (excluding factor concentrates) in the past year should have liver function studies performed. A factor VIII or IX inhibitor screen should also be performed for those with hemophilia and is usually performed during comprehensive evaluations at the HTC. HIV antibody testing with pretest and posttest counseling is recommended for individuals exposed to blood products before 1986 who have not previously been tested.

Common Illness Management
Differential Diagnosis

Headaches and Head Injury. Intracranial bleeding must be ruled out whenever there is a history of injury within the past several days, focal headaches, or vomiting without GI distress. A computed tomography (CT) scan is often helpful in ruling out intracranial bleeding. If either significant history or physical symptoms are present, however, providers often treat a child with factor concentrate prophylactically to achieve a 100% factor VIII or IX level. This conservative approach is often adopted because of the serious implications of a delay in diagnosis and treatment. Therapy may cease after the resolution of symptoms if scans remain normal. If bleeding is documented, the child would need hospitalization and factor replacement regularly for several weeks or longer.

Visual Disturbance. In the presence of acute changes in visual acuity, it is necessary to rule out intraocular bleeding by performing a thorough funduscopic examination. Documented bleeding,

---

Differential Diagnosis
- Headaches and head injury
- Visual disturbance
- Fever
- Sore throat
- Mouth bleeding
- Abdominal pain
- Gait disturbance
- Dysuria and hematuria
- Heavy menstrual bleeding
- Numbness, tingling, and pain

---

ocular injury, or persistent visual changes warrant referral to an ophthalmologist.

Fever. When children with IVADs develop a fever, blood cultures should be drawn and IV antibiotics started until the cultures are shown to be negative. These indwelling devices present a significant risk for infection even in children whose immune systems are normal.

If pretreated with factor concentrates or desmopressin, children with hemophilia may safely have lumbar punctures if required for a septic workup.

Sore Throat. If a throat culture is indicated, extreme caution must be exercised because of the potential for posterior pharyngeal bleeding. A throat culture should not be attempted in an uncooperative child. If streptococcal pharyngitis is suspected, a course of antibiotics should be initiated based on history, physical findings, and community resistance patterns.

Mouth Bleeding. Although oral bleeding may not appear to be profuse in children with hemophilia, persistent slow oozing can cause a significant drop in hemoglobin levels. Topical measures and antifibrinolytics alone are often not sufficient to control bleeding. In most cases, factor replacement or the use of desmopressin is also required. Rebleeding can be prevented with a soft diet and avoidance of placing straws, hot foods, chips, and toys in the mouth.

Abdominal Pain. Primary care practitioners should have a high suspicion of GI bleeding with acute abdominal pain or a significant drop in hemoglobin levels in the absence of other bleeding in children with hemophilia or VWD. Testing stool or emesis for blood can easily be done in the office as a screening tool. In hemophilia, iliopsoas bleeding (i.e., a combination of the iliacus muscle [origin, iliac fossa; insertion, greater trochanter] and psoas muscle [origin, thoracic and lumbar vertebrae; insertion, lesser trochanter]) can cause pain in the abdomen or in the inguinal area. Children with iliopsoas bleeding are unable to straighten their leg at the knee joint and hold their hip in a flexed position. Psoas bleeding can result in a large amount of blood loss, nerve damage, and joint destruction that may necessitates hip joint replacement later in life. Hospital admission for strict bed rest and aggressive treatment with factor concentrate is generally required for iliopsoas and GI bleeding.

Gait Disturbance. Gait disturbance may be the result of bleeding in or around the ankle, knee, hip, or iliopsoas muscle. Inability to fully extend the hip and, later, leg paresthesias are characteristics of iliopsoas bleeding. Ultrasonography is useful for confirmation. Bleeding into the hip socket, which is rare in children, is characterized by limitation of hip abduction and adduction.

Dysuria and Hematuria. Pressure within the urinary tract can cause dysuria. Testicular bleeding, however, must be ruled out. Bleeding into the testicular area is often quite pronounced with obvious bruising and swelling. Hospitalization may be required for aggressive therapy and bed rest. Hematuria may be spontaneous and directly related to the bleeding disorder. Whenever bleeding occurs, however, its origin within the urinary tract and any potential infection should be considered. Increased fluid intake, bed rest, and avoidance of antifibrinolytic agents, which may cause obstructive clots, are routinely recommended as part of a treatment plan. The benefits of treatment with factor concentrate or corticosteroids, however, are debated among clinicians.

Heavy Menstrual Bleeding. Females who are carriers of hemophilia or have VWD may have heavy menstrual flow, resulting in anemia. Once other causes have been ruled out, these individuals may benefit from treatment with estrogen therapy in the form of oral contraceptives or the high-dose form of intranasal DDAVP, Stimate.

Numbness, Tingling, and Pain. Compression of nerves caused by deep or superficial hematomas should be suspected in individuals with changes in sensation or focal pain. Bleeding in or near the calf, spine, buttock, iliopsoas muscle, and volar surface of the forearm can lead to neurologic changes.

Drug Interactions

All products that contain aspirin are contraindicated. Caution should also be exercised with prolonged use of other medications that can affect platelet aggregation (e.g., nonsteroidal antiinflammatory agents). It is important to educate parents on how to read medication labels (e.g., choosing those with acetaminophen over those with acetylsalicylic acid) and to enlist the help of the pharmacist when they are in doubt about the use of a particular product.

Developmental Issues

Sleep Patterns

Standard developmental counseling is advised. Parents are often advised to pad their child's crib rails to prevent bruising. Crib side rails should be lowered and pillows placed on the floor below as soon as the child begins to crawl out of his or her crib.

Toileting

Standard developmental counseling is advised.

Discipline

Some families tend to overprotect children with a bleeding disorder and may be more strict with unaffected siblings. Positive disciplinary techniques that are age appropriate, are developmentally appropriate, and do not include physical punishment should be recommended for all children. Pulling a child with a bleeding disorder by the arm is a specific action that may result in serious shoulder bleeding and radial head subluxation. Primary care providers should evaluate the disciplinary style of the parents and offer counseling on alternative discipline measures if potentially injurious methods are used. Families should be counseled about the use of noncontact limit-setting measures (e.g., time-outs, distraction, activity limitations).

Child Care

Contact with the proposed source of child care can help allay fears and clarify the caretaker's responsibilities with regard to the prevention and management of bleeding episodes. HTC personnel or the primary care provider may provide this service. It is helpful to emphasize that early recognition of bleeding (e.g., mild swelling or slight change in range of motion) and rapid access to medical evaluation and treatment are of primary importance for children with hemophilia. Spontaneous bleeding may occur, however, despite diligent safety efforts. Child-care providers should be discouraged from trying to make treatment decisions without the input of the parents, which is especially important when seemingly mild head "bumps" occur. To find the safest environment possible, parents may be encouraged to seek out sources of child care that have smaller numbers of children per provider, protective ground cover under outside activity spaces, and a staff willing to learn about the special needs and activity requirements of a child with a bleeding disorder. Some facilities may be fearful of admitting children with bleeding disorders because of their fear of liability. Health care providers can provide education and help allay concerns.

Schooling

Teachers, school nurses, and athletic coaches should be informed of a child's bleeding disorder. Families and children may be reticent to disclose the diagnosis to others for fear of discrimination because of the past connection between hemophilia and HIV. School personnel are more often concerned with prevention of bleeding (which may not be possible) and emergency management. Many HTCs offer school visits by the program's nurse coordinator and social worker. These educational visits are most helpful on entrance to a new school and should be done with the permission and—ideally—participation of the child and parents. It is not uncommon for children and adolescents with hemophilia to encounter peer disbelief that the disability and the need for crutches or a sling created by an acute bleeding episode can resolve in 1 to 2 days.

Alterations in body image and self-esteem may be precipitated by chronic joint arthropathy or limitations on physical activity caused by the bleeding disorder. From the time of diagnosis, parents may be assisted in guiding their child toward skills, careers, and sports that place less stress on joints and are not associated with high rates of injury. It is critical that children have activities and skills at which they can excel. The advent of prophylaxis has enabled more "normal" active play without the fear of increased injury and bleeding.

Participation in sports should be encouraged. Advances in prophylaxis have made it easier and safer for people with bleeding disorders to take part in a variety of activities; however, bleeding caused by injury is still a possibility. Anecdotal reports have demonstrated that fewer bleeding episodes are reported among children who are regularly active than among sedentary children. However, different activities carry different risks. Whenever a child is interested in participating in a sport, it should be discussed with the HTC. It is generally recommended that competitive contact sports are considered dangerous and should be avoided (Anderson & Forsyth, 2005; Rice, 2008).

Children who have learning problems resulting from intracranial bleeding must be fully evaluated and provided with appropriate support.

Sexuality

Safe-sex counseling (e.g., including decision-making skills; values clarification; and instruction in the use of condoms to prevent transmission of HIV, hepatitis B and C, and other sexually transmitted diseases) should be offered to all adolescents.

The genetic counselor at the HTC may first interact with children concerning basic education on the inheritance of the bleeding disorder and eventually include a discussion of reproductive options.

Transition to Adulthood

Arranging efficient transfer for adolescents from pediatric to adult care can be one of the greatest challenges. The transition from adolescence to adulthood can be particularly stressful for some individuals with bleeding disorders. When they approach adulthood, such individuals have their comprehensive HTC medical care transferred from the pediatric hematology service to the adult hematology service. There is also the question of whether prophylactic therapy should be discontinued as adolescents enter adulthood.

This is usually the time when the responsibility for medical care is transferred from the parents to the young adult (see Chapter 4). It is helpful if this expected transition is discussed with the child and family when the child is still young. Open and ongoing discussion about this expected transition of care may help allay some of the stress, sadness, and anger the child and family feel when they must transfer care to new providers.

Choice of college may also be influenced by the availability of specialized medical care in the area, and the individual's choice of career may be influenced by physical limitations. As adolescents make the transition to adulthood, they may no longer be eligible for medical coverage under their parents' policy and may have difficulty finding coverage that will accommodate their condition. In many states, there are special programs that cover individuals with hemophilia, or individuals may be eligible for a federal government program (e.g., Medicare, Medicaid, Supplemental Security Income [SSI]) as a result of disability (Bolton-Maggs, 2007; Valentino, Santagostino, Blanchette, et al., 2006).

Family Concerns

If a child with a bleeding disorder has excessive bruising before and after diagnosis, parents often encounter questions about suspected child abuse from health care providers or stares from friends, relatives, teachers, and strangers. Compounding the parents' distress may be guilt regarding the inheritance of the bleeding disorder.

It is difficult for parents to cope with their inability to prevent bleeding episodes despite diligent efforts to prevent injury. Fear of injury to the infant may even interfere with parent-infant bonding. When a child requires an infusion of blood products to stop bleeding, parents often continue to question the viral safety of the product despite current data on product safety.

Reimbursement for high-priced factor replacement has become an area of real concern as families reach the maximum lifetime amount of insurance reimbursement. Families who may face this problem need early intervention and counseling about insurance options. This is generally provided by the social worker at the HTC.

Different racial and ethnic groups may have varying feelings about and experiences of disability and chronic conditions. As a result, individuals with hemophilia may receive little understanding from their own ethnic community and may even encounter racial bias in the delayed diagnosis of a hemarthrosis (e.g., a black man with a swollen joint may be assumed to be having a sickle cell episode instead of being treated with a prompt infusion of factor concentrate). In many Asian cultures, it is a sign of weakness to tell others about an illness or disease. Many Hispanics are hesitant to join organized support networks for their disorder because they fear stigmatization. Women are another medically underserved group in whom the effect of bleeding disorders or carrier status has been overlooked.

Resources

The National Hemophilia Foundation (116 West 32nd St., 11th floor, New York, NY 10001; [212] 328-3700 and [800] 424-2634; www.hemophilia.org) and its local chapters disseminate information on recent advances in therapy not only for hemophilia and VWD but also for HIV and hepatitis C infection. Active members of the foundation include consumers, families, and health care providers at HTCs. The local chapters provide educational programs and support services to meet the members' needs.

Hemophilia treatment centers also provide educational programs and support groups for individuals with bleeding disorders and their families. A list of HTCs is available from the National Hemophilia Foundation in New York or from local National Hemophilia Foundation chapters.

Summary of Primary Care Needs for the Child with Bleeding Disorders: Hemophilia and von Willebrand Disease

HEALTH CARE MAINTENANCE

Growth and Development

- Monitoring and preventing obesity is important because of added stress on joints.
- Leg length discrepancy may occur due to chronic arthropathy.
- Developmental screening should be done as a follow-up for head trauma or screening for undiagnosed or unreported intracranial bleeding.

Diet

- Adequate protein and calcium intake is of particular importance because of the role of both in bone and muscle formation.
- Nonconstipating diet will help prevent rectal bleeding.
- A soft diet and avoiding foods with sharp edges is necessary when a child has mouth bleeding.
- Obesity should be avoided because it places extra stress on joints.

Safety

- A protective helmet may be recommended for children who are learning to walk to reduce the risk of head injury. Use of a helmet is controversial because it restricts peripheral vision. Some providers feel that the use of a helmet causes perceptual difficulties in children.
- Knee pads in the pants of toddlers may decrease knee hematomas.
- High-top leather sneakers and shoes are recommended for children at risk for hemarthroses from the time they start to walk.
- It is generally recommended that competitive contact sports are considered dangerous and should be avoided.
- The child should wear a medical identification emblem that includes information regarding diagnosis, treatment product, and blood type. The information should be updated annually.
- Activities that increase the chance of testicular bleeding in boys should be discouraged.

Summary of Primary Care Needs for the Child with Bleeding Disorders: Hemophilia and von Willebrand Disease—cont'd

- Families participating in a home infusion program should follow accepted guidelines for universal precautions and disposal of infectious wastes.
- Arterial blood samples should only be drawn after treatment with factor concentrate.

Immunizations

- Routine immunizations are recommended.
- Parenteral immunizations are often given subcutaneously.
- Some children may require factor replacements before immunization injections if given intramuscularly.
- Injectable vaccines should be given with a 25-gauge needle.
- Firm pressure should be applied over the immunization site for 5 minutes. Ice may be applied after pressure.

Screening

- *Vision.* Examination for eye injury should be done by an ophthalmologist. Routine screening is recommended.
- *Hearing.* Routine screening is recommended. Do not aggressively curette wax.
- *Dental.* Daily dental hygiene with supervised flossing is important. A dentist should initially be seen at 2 to 3 years of age, followed by regular routine examinations. Consult the HTC for recommendations for more extensive dental work or the need for endocarditis prophylaxis because of IVAD.
- *Blood pressure.* Routine screening is recommended.
- *Hematocrit.* Annual screening is recommended.
  - Use a 23-gauge butterfly needle for venipuncture in persons of any age.
- *Urinalysis.* Annual screening for microscopic hematuria is recommended. Hematuria should be reported to the HTC but may spontaneously resolve.
- *Tuberculosis.* Routine screening is recommended.

Condition-Specific Screening

- If blood product has been received in the past year, a factor VIII or IX inhibitor screen (i.e., specifically for persons with hemophilia) and liver function studies are indicated.

COMMON ILLNESS MANAGEMENT

Differential Diagnosis

- *Headaches and head injury.* Rule out intracranial bleeding, especially with concurrent vomiting and absence of GI symptoms.
- *Visual disturbance.* Rule out intraocular bleeding or retinal hemorrhage.
- *Fever.* If indwelling venous access device is present, blood cultures must be drawn and IV antibiotics started.
- *Sore throat.* Throat cultures present a risk for posterior pharyngeal bleeding. Cultures should not be taken from an uncooperative child.
- *Mouth bleeding.* Mouth bleeding often requires factor replacement in addition to topical measures and antifibrinolytic agents.
- *Abdominal pain.* Rule out GI bleeding. Rule out iliopsoas muscle bleeding with groin pain and decreased hip extension.
- *Gait disturbance.* Rule out bleeding in and around the ankle, knee, hip, and iliopsoas muscle. Rule out scoliosis.

- *Dysuria and hematuria.* Rule out testicular bleeding, renal or ureteral bleeding, and infection.
- *Heavy menstrual bleeding.* May occur in hemophilia carriers or women with von Willebrand disease. DDAVP or estrogen therapy may be helpful.
- *Numbness, tingling, and pain.* Rule out nerve compression caused by bleeding.
- *Drug interactions.* Products that contain aspirin are contraindicated.
  - Prolonged use of other substances that can affect platelet aggregation (e.g., nonsteroidal antiinflammatory agents) should be avoided.

DEVELOPMENTAL ISSUES

Sleep Patterns

- Standard developmental counseling is advised. Safety of sleeping environment must be assessed. Crib railings should be padded and crib lowered to floor level when infant starts to climb.

Toileting

- Counseling on prevention and management of constipation is advised to prevent possible rectal bleeding caused by straining.

Discipline

- Recognize the potential for overprotection of the affected child and the use of deferential disciplinary methods when compared with unaffected siblings.
- Pulling a child by the arm may result in shoulder or elbow joint bleeding or soft tissue bleeding.
- Physical punishment may result in internal bleeding.
- Parents should be counseled about use of time-outs, distractions, and other nonphysical methods of limit-setting.

Child Care

- Contact with the child-care provider by the primary health care provider or hemophilia treatment center staff to discuss prevention and management of bleeding episodes and trauma is advised.
- The importance of early recognition and treatment of bleeding should be stressed.
- Child-care centers with smaller numbers of children, protective ground cover, and low child-to-provider ratio are suggested.
- Recognize that the child-care provider may have fears regarding liability for injuries.

Schooling

- School visits are most helpful on enrollment in a new school and ideally include the child and parent or parents.
- Because of the difficulty in understanding acute onset and resolution of bleeding episodes, peer acceptance may initially be poor.
- Acknowledge potential fear of HIV infection among school personnel, and educate regarding transmission and current safety of treatment.
- Recognize potential alterations in body image and self-esteem because of chronic joint arthropathy or limitations on physical activity.
- Intracranial bleeding may result in learning problems.
- It is generally recommended that competitive contact sports are considered dangerous and should be avoided.

Continued

Summary of Primary Care Needs for the Child with Bleeding Disorders: Hemophilia and von Willebrand Disease—cont'd

Sexuality

- Delay circumcision until the child with a positive family history is screened for a bleeding disorder.
- Safe-sex counseling is recommended to prevent sexually transmitted diseases.
- Genetic counseling is recommended to discuss reproductive issues.

Transition to Adulthood

- The transfer of medical care from a pediatric center to an adult hemophilia center may be difficult.
- Educational and career opportunities may be restricted because of physical limitations and the need to be near a treatment center.
- Obtaining health care coverage for a bleeding disorder may be difficult and may limit employment opportunities. Individuals may be eligible for SSI if disabilities are significant.

FAMILY CONCERNS

- Child abuse may be suspected.
- Parents may experience guilt regarding the hereditary nature of a bleeding disorder.
- The fear of injury to an infant may decrease parent-infant bonding.
- Parents may fear the inability to prevent bleeding episodes despite attempts to prevent injury.
- The potential for undiscovered infectious diseases may be a concern.
- The family may experience uncertainty regarding the viral safety of blood products.
- Insurance problems may occur as children and adults reach lifetime maximum amounts of reimbursement.

REFERENCES

Anderson, A., & Forsyth, A. (2005). *Playing It Safe: Bleeding Disorders, Sports and Exercise*. New York: National Hemophilia Foundation.

Astermark, J. (2006). Basic aspects of inhibitors to factors VIII and IX and the influence of non-genetic risk factors. *Hemophilia* (Suppl 6), 8-13.

Baur, K. (2008). Rare hereditary coagulation factor abnormalities. In D.G. Nathan, S.H. Orkin, D. Ginsburg, ed al. (Eds.), *Hematology of Infancy and Childhood* (7th ed.). Philadelphia: Saunders.

Beeton, K., & Tuffley, J. (2005). Physiotherapy in the management of hemophilia. In C. Lee, D, Berntorp, & W. Hoots, (Eds.), *Textbook of Hemophilia*, Malden, MA: Blackwell.

Bolton-Maggs, P.H. (2007). Transition of care from paediatric to adult services in haematology. *Arch Dis Child, 92*, 797-801.

Brewer, A., & Correa, M.E. (2006). Guidelines for dental treatment of patients with inherited bleeding disorders. *Treatment of Hemophilia*. May 2006, no. 40.

Buzzard, B., & Briggs, P.J. (2003). Rehabilitation following ankle surgery in haemophilia. In E.C. Rodriguez-Merchan (Ed.), *The Haemophilic Joints: New Perspectives*, Malden, MA: Blackwell.

Castaman, G. (2008). Desmopressin for the treatment of haemophilia. *Haemophilia, 14*(Suppl 1), 15-20.

Centers for Disease Control and Prevention (2008). Recommended immunization schedules for persons aged 0-18 years—United States. *MMWR Morb Mortal Wkly Rep, 56*(1), Q1-Q4.

Chi, C., Lee, C.A., Shiltagh, N., et al. (2007). Pregnancy in carriers of haemophilia. *Haemophilia, 14*, 56-64.

Christie, B.A. (2002). *Nurses' Guide to Bleeding Disorders*. New York: National Hemophilia Foundation.

DiMichele, D. (2005). Inhibitors to factor VIII—epidemiology and treatment. In C. Lee, Berntorp, & W. Hoots (Eds.), *Textbook of Hemophilia*, Malden, MA: Blackwell.

Dunn, A.L., & Abshire, T.C. (2004). Recent advances in the management of the child who has hemophilia. *Hematol Oncol Clin North Am, 18*, 1249-1276.

Federici, A.B. (2008). The use of desmopressin in von Willebrand disease: The experience of the first 30 years (1977-2007). *Haemophilia, 14*(Suppl 1), 5-14.

Franchini, M. (2007). The use of desmopressin as a hemostatic agent: A concise review. *Am J Hematol, 82*, 731-735.

Goedert, J.J., Chen, B., Preiss, L., et al. (2007). Reconstruction of the hepatitis C virus epidemic in the US hemophilia population, 1940-1990. *Am J Epidemiol, 165*(12), 1443-1453.

Heijnen, L., & Buzzard, B. (2005). The role of physical therapy and rehabilitation in the management of hemophilia in developing countries. *Semin Thromb Hemost, 31*, 513-517.

Hemophilia of Georgia (2007). *The Hemophilia of Georgia Handbook*. (4th ed.). Atlanta: Author.

High, K.A. (2007). Update on progress and hurdles in novel genetic therapies for hemophilia. *Hematology Am Soc Hematol Educ Program 2007*, 466-472.

Hoots, W.K. (2003). Comprehensive care for hemophilia and related inherited bleeding disorders: Why it matters. *Curr Hematol Rep, 2*(5), 395-401.

James, P., & Lillicrap, D. (2006). Genetic testing for von Willebrand disease: The Canadian experience. *Semin Thromb Hemost, 32*, 546-552.

Jones, P. (2002). *Living with Haemophilia*. (5th ed.). Oxford: Oxford University Press.

Kadir, R.A., & Aledort, L.M. (2000). Obstetrical and gynaecological bleeding: A common presenting symptom. *Clin Lab Haematol, 22*(Suppl 1), 12-16.

Kessler, C.M. (2007). Diagnosis and treatment of von Willebrand disease: New perspectives and nuances. *Haemophilia, 13*(Suppl 5), 3-14.

Kucik, C., & Clenney, T. (2005). Management of epistaxis. *Am Fam Physician, 7*(2), 305-311.

Kulkarni, R., & Lusher, J.M. (2001). Review: Perinatal management of newborns with haemophilia. *Br J Haematol, 112*, 264-274.

Kulkarni, R., Ponder, K.P., James, A.H., et al. (2006). Unresolved issues in diagnosis and management of inherited bleeding disorders in the perinatal period: A white paper of the Perinatal Task Force of the Medical and Scientific Advisory Council of the National Hemophilia Foundation, USA. *Hemophilia, 12*, 205-211.

Lee, C.A., Chi, C., Pavord, S.R., et al. (2006). The obstetric and gynaecological management of women with inherited bleeding disorders—review with guidelines produced by a taskforce for UK Haemophilia Centre Doctors' Organization. *Haemophilia, 12*, 301-336.

Lillicrap, D. (2004). *The Basic Science, Diagnosis and Clinical Management of von Willebrand Disease*. Unpublished manuscript. Quebec: World Federation of Hemophilia.

Lillicrap, D. (2007). Von Willebrand disease—phenotype versus genotype: Deficiency versus disease. *Thromb Res, 120*(Suppl 1), S11-S16.

Lozier, J.N., & Kessler, C.M. (2005). Clinical aspects of therapy in hemophilia. In R. Hoffman, E.J. Benz, S. Shattil, et al. (Eds.), *Hematology: Basic Principles and Practice*, (4th ed.). Philadelphia: Elsevier.

Maclean, P.E., Fijnvandraat, K., Beijlevelt, M., et al. (2004). The impact of unaware carriership on the clinical presentation of haemophilia. *Haemophilia, 10*, 560-564.

Manco-Johnson, M. (2005). Hemophilia management: Optimizing treatment based on patient needs. *Curr Opin Pediatr, 17*, 3-5.

Manco-Johnson, M., Abshire, T.C., Shapiro, A.D., et al. (2007). Prophylaxis versus episodic treatment to prevent joint disease in boys with severe hemophilia. *N Engl J Med, 357*(6), 535-544.

Mannucci, P.M. (2008). Desmopressin (DDAVP): The first thirty years. *Haemophilia*, *14*(Suppl 1), 1-47.

Matthew, P., Manno, C.S., & Aledort, L.M. (2005). Therapeutic choices in the current millennium: Hemophilia workshop highlights. *Pediatr Blood Cancer*, *14*, 611-615.

Medical and Scientific Advisory Council. (2006a). *Medical and Scientific Advisory Council (MASAC) Recommendations Concerning the Treatment of Hemophilia and Other Bleeding Disorders.* New York: National Hemophilia Foundation.

Medical and Scientific Advisory Council. (2006b). *Medical and Scientific Advisory Council (MASAC) Recommendations Regarding the Treatment of von Willebrand Disease.* New York: National Hemophilia Foundation.

Montgomery, R.R., Cox-Gill, J., & DiPaola, J. (2008). Hemophilia and von Willebrand disease. In D.G. Nathan, S.H. Orkin, D. Ginsburg, et al. (Eds.). *Hematology of Infancy and Childhood* (7th ed.). Philadelphia: Elsevier.

O'Shaughnessy, D.O., Makris, M., & Lillicrap, D. (2005). *Practical Hemostasis and Thrombosis.* Malden, MA: Blackwell.

Peyvandi, F. (2005). Carrier detection and prenatal diagnosis of hemophilia in developing countries. *Semin Thromb Hemost*, *33*(5), 544-554.

Peyvandi, F., Jayandharan, G., Chandy, M., et al. (2006). Genetic diagnosis of haemophilia and other inherited bleeding disorders. *Haemophilia*, *12*(Suppl 3), 82-89.

Pipe, S.W., & Valentino, L.A. (2007). Optimizing outcomes for patients with severe haemophilia A. *Haemophilia*, *13*(Suppl 4), 1-16.

Raffini, L., & Manno, C.S. (2007). Modern management of haemophilic arthropathy. *Br J Haematol*, *136*(6), 777-787.

Rice, S. (2008). Medical conditions affecting sports participation. *Pediatrics*, *121*, 841-848.

Riddel, J.J.P., Aouizerat, B.E., Miaskowski, C., et al. (2007). Theories of blood coagulation. *J Pediatr Oncol Nurs*, *24*(3), 123-131.

Rodriguez, N.I., & Hoots, W.K. (2008). Advances in hemophilia: Experimental aspects and therapy. *Pediatr Clin North Am*, *55*, 357-376.

Rustgi, V. (2007). The epidemiology of hepatitis C infection in the United States. *J Gastroenterol*, *42*, 513-521.

Sharathkumar, A., & Pipe, S.W. (2008). Bleeding disorders. *Pediatr Rev*, *29*(4), 121–130.

Smith, A.R., Leonard, N., & Kurth, M. (2008). Intracranial hemorrhage in newborns with hemophilia: The role of screening radiologic studies in the first 7 days of life. *J Pediatr Hematol Oncol*, *30*(1), 81-84.

Smith, J., & Smith, O.P. (2006). Hemophilia A and B. In R. Arceci, I. Hann, O.P. Smith (Eds.), *Pediatric Hematology*. Malden, MA: Blackwell.

Soucie, M.J., Nuss, R., Evatt, B., et al. (2000). Mortality among males with hemophilia: Relations with source of medical care. *Blood*, *96*(2), 437-442.

Street, A.M., Ljung, R., & Lavery, S.A. (2008). Management of carriers and babies with haemophilia. *Haemophilia*, *14*(Suppl 3), 181-187.

Valentino, L., & Kapoor, M. (2005). Central venous access devices in patients with hemophilia. *Expert Rev Med Devices*, *2*(6), 699-711.

Valentino, L., Santagostino, E., Blanchette, V., et al. (2006). Managing the pediatric patient and the adolescent/adult transition. *Semin Thromb Hemost*, *32*(2), 28-31.

Warrier, I. (2005). Inhibitors in hemophilia B. In C. Lee, D. Berntorp, & W.K. Hoots (Eds.), *Textbook of Hemophilia*, Malden, MA: Blackwell.

15 Bone Marrow Transplantation

Karen Marie Kristovich and Elizabeth Callard

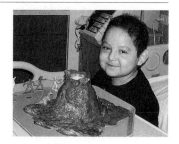

Etiology

Bone marrow transplantation, or hematopoietic stem cell transplantation (HSCT), as it is more recently referred to, is an evolving treatment option for a variety of acquired and congenital disorders that either significantly decrease life expectancy and quality of life or are potentially fatal. Initially, HSCT was developed as a potential curative therapy to replace damaged or nonfunctioning bone marrow in individuals with severe immune deficiencies or aplastic anemia. Once determined to be a viable treatment option for these disorders, other disciplines sought to incorporate the theory behind HSCT to treat additional conditions that could benefit from replacing the hematopoietic system. In particular, the field of oncology, in an effort to treat malignant conditions, was the next to benefit from this form of organ transplantation. The dose-limiting factor of excessive myelosuppressive chemotherapy was overcome by anticipating bone marrow failure and, subsequently, including HSCT as part of the treatment plan. The hematopoietic stem cells (HSCs) that were intravenously infused, rescuing the individual from lethal hematopoietic toxicity, were acquired from either donors or from the individual before myeloablative therapy. An unexpected immunotherapeutic response was observed in some people: in the graft-versus-leukemia (GVL), or graft-versus-tumor (GVT), effect, grafted donor lymphocytes were found to react against the host's malignant cells, improving the chance of cure (Gassas, Sung, Saunders, et al., 2007; Riddell, 2008).

Today, HSCT is employed to treat high-risk leukemias and other malignancies, as well as an increasing variety of disorders (including metabolic, hematologic, and immunologic disorders). Significant advances in science and medicine during the past two decades have led to improved outcomes for those undergoing HSCT. These advances can be found in the areas of supportive care, management and prevention of infectious disease, and sources of HSCs, as well as an increased understanding of human leukocyte antigens (HLAs) resulting in improved accuracy of typing for potential HSC donors.

There are two basic types of HSCT, *autologous* and *allogeneic,* and they differ with respect to the origin of the stem cells infused into children during HSCT. Autologous HSCT involves the use of the child's own stem cells, collected and stored before cytotoxic chemotherapy and then infused following the myeloablative therapy. Although there is a very low mortality rate related to this therapy and a donor search is not necessary, an autologous HSCT is not indicated for all conditions. This type of transplant is primarily used in the treatment of high-risk or recurrent solid tumors, most commonly children with high-risk neuroblastoma, recurrent Wilms' tumor, recurrent lymphomas, and some brain tumors and sarcomas. The preferred source of stem cells is from peripheral blood rather than bone marrow because of the relative ease of collection, faster engraftment time, and therefore shorter period of neutropenia. Although autologous transplants are associated with a lower transplant-related mortality (TRM) rate, they are also, unfortunately, associated with a higher incidence of recurrent disease (Levine, Harris, Loberiza, et al., 2003; Weisdorf, Bishop, Dharan, et al., 2002).

Allogeneic HSCT requires the collection of stem cells from an HLA-matched donor and is primarily used in situations where the child's own hematopoietic system is diseased or dysfunctional. HLA-identical family members, most often siblings, are the preferred source of allogeneic stem cells, because they pose the lowest risk of graft-versus-host disease (GVHD) and TRM.

There are two main classes of HLAs: class I antigens (HLA-A, HLA-B, and HLA-C) and class II antigens (HLA-DR, HLA-DQ, and HLA-DP), both of which are key in determining histocompatibility in transplantation. There are many different specific HLA proteins within each class of antigens. The genes that encode these antigens are on the short arm of chromosome 6. These genes are closely linked and inherited within families as clustered groups, or *haplotypes*. Each person has two haplotypes, one set being inherited from each parent. The best donor for an allogeneic HSCT is an HLA-identical sibling, that is, an individual who shares two sets of identical haplotypes with the recipient. Family HLA typing is obtained for children requiring an allogeneic transplant. Children receiving the same HLA haplotype from each parent would be HLA identical and express the same HLAs on the surface of their cells. There is a 25% chance that a child's sibling will be an identical HLA match. Parents should also be HLA typed because if the parents have one or more alleles in common with one another, a phenomenon known as a recombination of alleles occurs, resulting in a sharing of haplotypes, and the chance of identifying an HLA-identical family donor increases by an additional 5%. Since only 25% of individuals will have an HLA-matched sibling, the majority of allogeneic candidates require an alternate donor source. Alternate HSC sources include partially matched family members, well-matched volunteer unrelated donors, and banked umbilical cord blood (UCB). Unfortunately, an appropriate donor is not always found.

Hematopoietic conditions, both malignant and nonmalignant, as well as genetic disorders, are usually treated with allogeneic transplantation. The TRM rate is higher with this form of transplantation due, in part, to immune differences between the donor and recipient and to the immunosuppression required to achieve donor engraftment and prevent GVHD (Levine et al., 2003; Weisdorf et al., 2002). Allogeneic transplants owe their antitumor effect not only to their powerful cytotoxic therapies, but also to the potential immune effect mediated by donor lymphocytes as seen in the GVT and GVL effect (Jernberg, Remberger, Ringden, et al., 2003). Although the overall incidence of disease relapse is lower in children undergoing allogeneic transplants, there is a higher post-transplant morbidity and mortality rate among these same children. These risks are even greater when an unrelated donor or a mismatched family member is used (Jacobsohn, 2007).

Before all HSC transplants, whether autologous or allogeneic, children receive chemotherapy with or without irradiation to (1) destroy malignant cells or defective bone marrow, (2) make space in the bone marrow for the transplanted HSCs to grow, and (3) suppress the recipients' immune responses. Ultimately, the type of transplant and source of stem cells used in transplantation are primarily determined by the diagnosis, the clinical condition of the child, and the type of donor.

Although HSCT is a type of organ transplant, there are important fundamental differences between allogeneic HSCT and solid organ transplantation (see Chapter 37). In solid organ transplantation, there are a limited number of donor cells with immunologic activity transferred into the host with the transplanted organ. Without adequate immune suppression, the immune system of the recipient will recognize the organ as foreign. The primary concern after solid organ transplant is the prevention of rejection of the organ by the recipient's immune system. This usually requires lifelong administration of immunosuppressive medications. In HSCT, however, the preparative regimen that the recipient receives before transplantation, typically high-dose chemotherapy with or without total body irradiation, eliminates most elements of the host's immune system. The transplant of donor stem cells contains all of the necessary cellular elements for complete reconstitution of the hematopoietic and immunologic systems in the recipient. Thus the immune system following transplantation comes from the donor, is generated by the graft, and eventually replaces the HSCT recipient's own immune system (Martin, 2004).

After HSCT, there are four primary concerns: (1) preventing graft rejection mediated by recipient T lymphocytes that survived the preparative regimen; (2) preventing donor cells from activating an immunologic response against the recipient, thereby causing tissue injury and GVHD; (3) preventing and treating opportunistic infections and viral reactivation during the months that follow HSCT when the child is at greatest risk for life-threatening infection; and (4) allowing for immunologic reconstitution so that the donor-derived cells recognize and control pathogens in the host body. Immunosuppressive medications are used to prevent and treat GVHD. Immune tolerance between the donor and recipient can usually be achieved within 6 to 12 months, thus allowing for a taper and eventually the discontinuation of immunosuppressive medications following allogeneic HSCT in the majority of children (Hansen, Petersdorf, Lin, et al., 2007).

Incidence and Prevalence

The Center for International Blood and Marrow Transplant reports data from more than 500 centers in 54 countries and estimates that 50,000 to 60,000 HSCTs are performed annually worldwide (Pasquini, Wang, & Schneider, 2007). During the period from 2002 to 2006, bone marrow remained the primary graft source in pediatric HSCT, though use of peripheral blood and umbilical cord blood grafts is increasing. Peripheral blood grafts accounted for 27% and cord blood accounted for 19% of all allotransplants during this period. Fifty percent of allogeneic transplants in children are from unrelated donors. There has been a shift in graft source for unrelated donors toward the use of peripheral blood and cord blood rather than marrow. Among children receiving unrelated donor transplants, marrow was used for 42% of unrelated donor transplants in 2003–2006 compared to 59% in 1999–2002.

Diagnostic Criteria

Criteria for Transplant Eligibility

Referral and Consultation. Children being considered for transplantation are referred to an HSCT team by their pediatric hematologist/oncologist, immunologist, or geneticist. It is essential for potential HSC transplant recipients to be seen promptly and, in the case of metabolic disorders, during the earliest possible stage of their condition, to assess whether they are suitable candidates for HSCT. Children and their families require comprehensive evaluations and counseling by an experienced multidisciplinary team. The timing and type of transplant depend on the child's diagnosis, stage of disease, and availability of a donor. Excellent communication among the transplant team, referring physician, and primary care practitioner is essential.

Pretransplant Workup. A thorough clinical assessment of the child and donor (if applicable) takes place within 4 weeks of the proposed admission. Special attention is given to the evaluation of organ function in the child receiving the HSC transplant in an effort to determine if he or she can withstand high-dose cytotoxic therapy. The majority of the testing takes place at the referring or transplant centers, although some tests may be obtained locally. This is usually a time of anxiety and uncertainty for the child and family; these feelings are further intensified by any delays in the transplant or by unexpected problems, such as a hospital admission for infection or, possibly, even relapse of the disease.

HLA Typing. Tissue typing, or HLA typing, is used to identify genetically compatible hematopoietic stem cell donors and recipients. *Human leukocyte antigens* (HLAs) are proteins found on the surface of almost all nucleated cells in the body. These antigens regulate the immune response in specific ways and are responsible for the body's ability to recognize "self" from "nonself" on a cellular level. In addition to providing an immune response to disease, HLAs also play a role in reproduction, cancer, and autoimmunity.

If an allogeneic transplant is required and an appropriate sibling or family donor is not identified or available, an unrelated donor search is initiated. National and international donor registries are accessed by the search coordinator at the transplanting institution. The National Marrow Donor Program is the largest volunteer donor registry and has developed a network with cord blood banks as well. There are more than 7 million adult volunteer donors registered with the National Marrow Donor Program and close to 70,000 cord blood units banked with various organizations (National Marrow Donor Program, 2008).

Other factors, in addition to identifying the best HLA match, are considered when choosing a related or unrelated donor for a person needing HSCT. Age, gender, number of pregnancies or parity, and viral status, particularly cytomegalovirus (CMV) status, are other considerations during the donor search process, because all may affect the incidence of GVHD (Jernberg, Remberger, Ringden, et al.,

2004), and thereby increase the overall morbidity of the individual undergoing HSCT.

The majority of HSC transplants occur in children with malignant conditions (see Chapter 16). HSCT is also a potentially curative treatment option for some children with genetic disorders involving deficiencies or abnormalities in hematopoietically derived cells. Inherited hemoglobinopathies, such as severe beta-thalassemia and sickle cell disease (SCD) (see Chapter 40), are both associated with considerable morbidity and early death. Children with these disorders may be transplant candidates because the abnormal hemoglobin production can be corrected with donor-derived bone marrow from an allogeneic HSCT. Affected children who could benefit from HSCT are those who are transfusion dependent, as well as those with SCD and a history of acute chest syndrome or stroke. Challenges specific to these candidates include increased risk of treatment-related morbidity and death caused by organ damage from pretransplant iron overload secondary to multiple blood transfusions and the lack of suitable donors (Bhatia & Walters, 2007).

Congenital immune deficiencies, in which the defect has been traced to the stem cells, can also be corrected with allogeneic HSCT. These disorders include Wiskott-Aldrich syndrome, severe combined immune deficiency (SCID), and hemophagocytic syndromes. HSCT should be considered as soon as possible after diagnosis because these disorders often run an unpredictable course and may be rapidly fatal (Dvorak & Cowan, 2008). This is in contrast to a few inherited aplastic anemias and bone marrow failure syndromes in which supportive care therapies are used as initial treatment, reserving HSCT if the condition worsens. These disorders include Fanconi anemia, Diamond-Blackfan anemia, dyskeratosis congenita, and Kostman syndrome.

HSCT is a promising treatment option for some metabolic disorders, such as mucopolysaccharidoses (MPS). MPS disorders are caused by a deficiency in specific liposomal enzymes resulting in an inability to metabolize complex carbohydrates (mucopolysaccharidoses) into simpler molecules that the body can use. These mucopolysaccharidoses build up in all tissues, leading to progressive damage in various parts of the body including the heart valves, bones, joints, lungs, and brain with progressive deterioration and eventual death (Orchard, Blazar, Wagner, et al., 2007).

Possibly the most promising results have been observed in Hurler syndrome (MPS I) in which the missing enzyme, alpha-L-iduronidase, is needed to degrade glycosaminoglycans (GAGS). There have been encouraging preliminary results from human alpha-L-iduronidase enzyme replacement in those with the moderate phenotype; however, enzyme replacement cannot be applied in severe forms because the substitute enzyme cannot cross the blood-brain barrier (Miebach, 2005). HSCT therefore is currently the only effective intervention in severe Hurler syndrome providing donor hematopoietic stem cells to provide a source of macrophages and other marrow-derived cells that produce the deficient enzymes. Correction of the underlying enzyme deficiency prevents future deposition of abnormal storage products that are the cause of organ dysfunction in most metabolic conditions. Because of the inability of some of the transplanted hematopoietic cells to migrate into all tissue and thereby correct all of the preexisting organ-related complications, some malformations or organ dysfunction existing before transplant may not be reversible (Orchard et al., 2007). This limitation of hematopoietic cells may

help explain why HSCT does not appear to be a curative option for some metabolic disorders, including Sanfilippo syndrome (MPS III), gangliosidoses, and Niemann-Pick disease (Orchard et al., 2007). One of the greatest challenges in transplantation for genetic conditions remains the high frequency of primary and secondary graft rejection and incomplete donor chimerism.

Clinical Manifestations at Time of Diagnosis

HSCT is a treatment option for a wide variety of conditions (Box 15-1), and clinical manifestations will vary accordingly. Children with malignant conditions are often in remission or have minimal residual disease when they are referred for HSCT and therefore exhibit no clinical manifestations of their underlying condition. They may, however, exhibit treatment-related side effects, such as alopecia, anorexia, weight loss, or organ dysfunction (see Chapter 16). Children with hemoglobinopathies such as SCD (see Chapter 41) may exhibit symptoms of anemia. Children with severe aplastic anemia will be pancytopenic and may have

---

BOX 15-1

Conditions Commonly Treated with Hematopoietic Stem Cell Transplants

AUTOLOGOUS TRANSPLANTATION
Cancers
- Non-Hodgkin's lymphoma
- Hodgkin's disease
- Neuroblastoma
- Acute myeloid leukemia
- Multiple myeloma
- Ovarian cancer
- Germ cell tumors
- Other pediatric solid tumors

Other disorders
- Autoimmune disorders
- Amyloidosis

ALLOGENEIC TRANSPLANTATION
Cancers
- Acute myeloid leukemia
- Acute lymphoblastic leukemia
- Chronic myeloid leukemia
- Myelodysplastic syndromes
- Myeloproliferative disorders
- Non-Hodgkin's lymphoma
- Hodgkin's disease
- Chronic lymphocytic leukemia
- Multiple myeloma
- Juvenile chronic myeloid leukemia
- Therapy-related myelodysplastic syndrome/leukemia

Other disorders
- Aplastic anemia
- Paroxysmal nocturnal hemoglobinuria
- Fanconi anemia
- Diamond-Blackfan syndrome
- Thalassemia major
- Sickle cell anemia
- Severe combined immunodeficiency
- Wiskott-Aldrich syndrome
- Inborn errors of metabolism

From Copelan, E.A. (2006). Hematopoietic stem-cell transplantation. *N Engl J Med 354*, 1813-1826.

petechiae and bruising from thrombocytopenia. MPS and related disorders may not be apparent at birth; signs and symptoms develop within the first year, as more cells become damaged by the accumulation of cellular substrates. Clinical manifestations include coarse facies with frontal bossing, flat nasal bridge, contractures, kyphoscoliosis, short stature, and organomegaly.

Treatment

Peripheral Blood Stem Cell Collection

Children who will receive an autologous HSC transplant require peripheral blood stem cell (PBSC) collection. This process, called *apheresis,* involves the use of a commercially available automated blood cell separator, with the collection occurring weeks or months before the planned transplant. Hematopoietic stem cells normally reside in the bone marrow and are rarely detected in peripheral blood. Mobilization of the stem cells into the peripheral blood can be accomplished during the recovery phase of myelosuppressive chemotherapy and is enhanced by the administration of recombinant hematopoietic growth factors (Moog, 2006). Granulocyte colony-stimulating factor (G-CSF, also called filgrastim) is the most commonly used recombinant human growth factor and is administered daily by subcutaneous injection until collection is complete. Side effects of G-CSF include bone pain, headache, myalgia, and fatigue (American Society of Health-System Pharmacists [ASHSP], 2008b). A small percentage of children will experience poor mobilization of their HSCs, resulting in an inadequate collection for transplant. This most frequently occurs in children who have been heavily pretreated with chemotherapy or radiation. In this circumstance, the child may have to undergo a bone marrow harvest in an attempt to reach a more desirable stem cell dose in preparation for HSCT.

Treatment
- Peripheral blood stem cell (PBSC) collection
- Stem cell manipulation
  Peritransplant Phase
  - Preparative regimens
  - Chemotherapy
  - Total body irradiation
  - Total lymphoid irradiation
  - Transplant day
  Posttransplant Phase
  - Immunosuppressive management
  - Specific T lymphocyte immunosuppressive drugs
  - Nonspecific immunosuppressive drugs
  - Antibodies
  - Infection prevention
  - Tolerance and chimerism
  - Consolidative radiation therapy and chemotherapy
  - Donor lymphocyte infusion
  - Tandem transplants

Stem Cell Manipulation

Stem cells for autologous and allogeneic transplantation may be manipulated before infusion in an effort to reduce the risk of complications or disease recurrence. A blood cell separator is generally used for this purpose. For example, bone marrow products from related or unrelated donors are red blood cell depleted if the donor and recipient are ABO incompatible. In autologous PBSC collection, particular stem cells may be selected for inclusion in the infusion, allowing the remainder of the pheresis product to be discarded and thereby facilitating the removal of potential tumor cell contamination. Likewise, a technique used at some transplant centers for allogeneic transplants involves the removal of T lymphocytes from unrelated donor bone marrow to decrease the risk of GVHD. Although T lymphocyte depletion of donor marrow is an effective method of GVHD prevention, children who receive T cell–depleted grafts have been found to be at an increased risk for graft rejection, disease recurrence, and delayed immunologic recovery after HSCT (Seidel, Fritsch, Matthes-Martin, et al., 2005).

Peritransplant Phase

A child begins the conditioning or preparative regimen 5 to 10 days before his or her stem cell infusion date. Admission to the transplant unit occurs when the preparative regimen begins or on the day of transplantation, depending on the institution. Preparative regimens consist of high-dose chemotherapy with or without total body irradiation (TBI). The most common regimens use high-dose cyclophosphamide (CY) given in combination with busulfan (BU) or TBI. Other chemotherapeutic agents used in various combinations include high-dose etoposide (VP-16), carmustine (BCNU), carboplatin, melphalan, and thiotepa. Additionally, total lymphoid irradiation (TLI) may be used as an alternate form of radiation therapy (XRT).

Regimen selection is determined by the underlying condition, the HLA match and donor, and the source of stem cells and serves multiple functions: (1) tumor cytoreduction and ideally disease eradication in the case of malignancy; (2) marrow ablation to create space in the bone marrow for new stem cells while removing any remaining dysfunctional stem cells; and (3) sufficient immunosuppression to overcome host-mediated rejection of the donor cells.

On transplant day, or day 0, the stem cells are infused into the recipient, a process that is similar to a blood product transfusion. If the stem cells are from the marrow of a related donor, the bone marrow harvest takes place the same day as the HSCT. In an autologous transplant, the cryopreserved stem cell product is thawed and immediately infused into the child. When an unrelated donor is used, the freshly harvested marrow or stem cell product is escorted from the donor center, usually requiring air transportation, to the transplant center. Once the cells are infused intravenously, they migrate to the bone marrow, and within 10 to 21 days, production of bone marrow–derived cells usually begins. This is called hematopoietic *engraftment*. Children undergoing HSCT are usually confined to the transplant unit or their specific transplant rooms until they achieve an absolute neutrophil count greater than 500 to 1000 for 2 consecutive days. The relaxation of isolation guidelines may differ among transplanting centers; in fact, some institutions perform outpatient, autologous HSC transplants and may only require hospital admission if the child becomes febrile or has other more serious complications.

Posttransplant Phase

Immunosuppressive Management. Immunosuppressive regimens may vary according to the child's underlying diagnosis, stem cell source, preparative regimen, and institutional protocol. Almost all allogeneic transplant recipients receive immunosuppressive medications to prevent GVHD. Exceptions to this include syngeneic transplants, when the recipient's identical twin is the donor, and transplants for those with severe combined immune deficiency (SCID), in which little to no immunosuppression is required. Cyclosporine A (CSA, Neoral) has been the core of prophylactic therapy since the 1980s and is typically combined with a short course of posttransplant methotrexate (MTX) (Jacobsohn, 2007). Tacrolimus (FK-506, Prograf) has recently replaced CSA as the prophylactic immunosuppressive drug of choice for unrelated donor transplants at many centers after showing a lower incidence of moderate to severe GVHD (Yanada, Emi, Naoe, et al., 2004). Other common immunosuppressive agents include antithymocyte globulin (ATG), alemtuzumab (Campath), and mycophenolate mofetil (MMF, CellCept). Table 15-1 outlines toxicities of these agents.

Specific T lymphocyte immunosuppressive drugs. Cyclosporine A (CSA) interferes with the activation of T lymphocytes or T cells, the cells responsible for stimulating GVHD, by inhibiting interleukin-2 production required for T cell responses (ASHSP, 2008c; Laffan & Biedrzycki, 2006). Only steady-state trough levels are useful in determining if a therapeutic level has been achieved. Values of CSA levels drawn at other times are usually uninterpretable for drug dosing management. Although structurally different, tacrolimus (Prograf, FK-506) has the same cellular function as CSA, as it too interrupts T cell activation and function by inhibiting interleukin-2 production (ASHSP, 2008d; Laffan & Biedrzycki, 2006). Similar to CSA, it is first administered intravenously and later given orally. A third T lymphocyte immunosuppressive drug is mycophenolate mofetil (MMF), which interferes with lymphocyte proliferation while also causing less mucositis and fewer transplant-related toxicities when compared with immunosuppressive doses of methotrexate; in addition to being immunosuppressive, MMF also has antibacterial, antifungal, and antiviral properties.

Nonspecific immunosuppressive drugs. Corticosteroids can be used alone or in combination with other agents for the prevention of GVHD or treatment of acute or chronic GVHD. The mechanism of action of corticosteroids is not fully understood, but they negatively affect immune reconstitution by suppressing cellular immunity and may suppress proinflammatory cytokines (Franchimont, 2004; Iwasaki, 2004). Most often used in combination with CSA or tacrolimus, methotrexate (MTX) is a highly efficient and toxic antimetabolite. Like MMF, MTX is thought to inhibit the proliferation of lymphocytes, thereby preventing GVHD. It has been shown to induce tolerance when administered before stem cell engraftment as well. Three to four doses of MTX are usually administered within the first 2 weeks after transplant.

Antibodies. Antithymocyte globulin (ATG) is a product of serum immunoglobulins produced by injecting horses or rabbits with human thymocytes. The horse or rabbit antibodies subsequently produced are capable of reacting with and eliminating human T lymphocytes. Regimens that include ATG usually utilize these infusions both before the donor cell infusion, to decrease the incidence of graft rejection, and after the transplant, to prevent GVHD. Serum sickness, potentially involving fever, rigors, rashes, and urticaria, can occur, because ATG is a foreign xenogeneic protein; therefore premedication, and possibly treatment, with acetaminophen, corticosteroids, and H_1 and H_2 blockers may be required before and after the antibody infusions. Alemtuzumab (Campath) is a monoclonal antibody that targets CD52, a protein present on the surface of many white blood cells and mature lymphocytes but not found on stem cells. Like ATG, Campath is also infused before and after the stem cell infusion and is as effective as T cell depletion in preventing GVHD. Because some studies have shown an increase in viral reactivations and impaired immune reconstitution after transplant among HSCT recipients who received Campath as part of their conditioning therapy, research surrounding the role of Campath in HSCT continues (Avivi, Chakrabarti, Milligan, et al., 2004; Chakrabarti, Hale, & Waldmann, 2004).

Infection Prevention. Special precautions are taken to reduce the risk of infections in children who have undergone HSCT. Transplanting institutions use either high-efficiency particulate air (HEPA) filter systems or laminar airflow rooms to decrease potential environmental pathogens during the acute phase of transplantation. With no functioning immune system and alterations in mucosal integrity from treatment-related mucositis, these children are particularly at risk for bacterial, fungal, and viral infections. Several prophylactic antiinfective agents are prescribed during the acute transplant period for the prevention of *Pneumocystis jiroveci* (formerly *carinii*) pneumonia (PCP), fungal disease, and viral reactivations, including herpes simplex virus (HSV) and cytomegalovirus (CMV). Additionally, most allogeneic and some autologous HSCT recipients receive passive antibody prophylaxis with intravenous immunoglobulin (IVIG).

In an effort to further reduce the risk of infection among children undergoing HSCT, extensive counseling is provided for these children and their families regarding the prevention of infections through effective hand washing, appropriate food choices and preparation, and strict adherence to protective isolation guidelines, the details of which may vary among institutions. These guidelines

---

TABLE 15-1

Toxicities of Immunosuppressive Agents

Cyclosporine	Tacrolimus	Methotrexate	Corticosteroids	ATG	Mycophenolate Mofetil
Nephrotoxicity	Nephrotoxicity	Mucositis	Hyperglycemia	Infection risk	Leukopenia
Hypertension	Hypertension	Delayed engraftment	Muscle wasting	Fever, chills	Anemia
Decreased magnesium	Decreased magnesium	Hepatotoxicity	Infection risk	Skin reactions	Thrombocytopenia
Tremors (hand)	Tremor		GI hemorrhage	Hypersensitivity	GI effects
Neurotoxicity	Neurotoxicity		Hypertension	Serum sickness	Headaches
Hyperkalemia	Hyperkalemia				
Hirsutism	HUS				
HUS					

From Gonzales-Ryan, L., et al. (2002). Hematopoietic stem cell transplantation. In C.R. Baggot, K.P. Kelly, D. Foctman, et al. (Eds.), *Nursing Care of Children and Adolescents with Cancer* (3rd ed.). Philadelphia: Saunders, pp. 212-255. Reprinted with permission.
Key: *ATG*, antithymocyte globulin; *GI*, gastrointestinal; *HUS*, hemolytic-uremic syndrome.

typically include the use of a respirator or filter mask by the child when in the medical center or associated buildings, as well as the need to avoid crowds, public buildings, and ill contacts. Children are not allowed to return to school and therefore must use hospital-based schools or home tutors for the duration of their isolation, commonly lasting from 6 to 12 months after transplant.

Tolerance and Chimerism. Tolerance of the donor cells to the host is primarily achieved by thymic education of the donor precursor T lymphocytes that derive from donor stem cells in the marrow. Donor-derived, precursor T lymphocytes migrate to the host's thymus, where they are programmed to distinguish "self" from "nonself"; thus these new donor-derived T lymphocytes are educated to recognize the host as "self." The T lymphocytes primarily involved in activating GVHD are the mature lymphocytes infused during transplantation that were previously coded in the donor's thymus and subsequently recognize the new recipient as "nonself," thereby initiating the GVHD process.

Routine surveillance of donor- and recipient-derived hematopoiesis, using a variety of molecular methods to distinguish and quantify the percentage of donor-derived versus residual recipient-derived bone marrow, is obtained in children after allogeneic transplantation. Serial testing allows the transplant team to assess for graft rejection and relapse. Molecular techniques, using marrow and/or peripheral blood samples at specific time periods after HSCT, are applied at most transplantation centers. The institutional policy, treatment protocol, and clinical course of each transplanted child determine the frequency and timing of these studies.

Consolidative Radiation Therapy and Chemotherapy. Some children require further antineoplastic treatment after HSCT. For example, in children with high-risk neuroblastoma, improvements in remission rates after HSCT were noted with the addition of consolidative radiation therapy (XRT) to the primary tumor bed region (Fish & Grupp, 2008). Following XRT, these children also receive a 6-month treatment course of 13-*cis*-retinoic acid (isotretinoin, cisRA, Accutane), an oral retinoid that is a differentiating agent for neuroblastoma and is thought to help control minimal residual disease (Reynolds, 2004). Several pediatric oncology centers within the United States also offer posttransplant immunotherapy protocols in addition to retinoic acid for this high-risk population. Children with Hodgkin disease also usually receive post-HSCT XRT to the areas of previous disease after sufficient hematopoietic recovery. All children receiving consolidative XRT are monitored closely by the transplant team for treatment-related side effects and symptom management (see Chapter 16).

Donor Lymphocyte Infusion

For several years, donor lymphocyte infusions (DLIs) have been used with some success in treating both recurrent disease after HSCT and significant viral infections after HSCT (Comoli, Basso, Labirio, et al., 2008; Loren & Porter, 2008). DLIs are most commonly used following nonmyeloablative regimens to increase host suppression in order to engineer full donor chimerism in the recipient (Satwani, Cooper, Rao, et al., 2008).

Tandem Transplants

Dose intensification and the sequential use of chemotherapeutic agents to overcome drug resistance may benefit some children with aggressive or resistant tumors. This treatment approach attempts to reduce residual disease by repeated, closely timed courses of high-dose chemotherapy, each followed by an HSC rescue to reduce the risks associated with prolonged pancytopenia. Interest has been growing in this concept, and recent studies in children with high-risk neuroblastoma and other solid tumors show promise (George, Li, Medeiros-Nancarrow, et al., 2006; Marcus, Shamberger, Litman, et al., 2003). In the case of high-risk neuroblastoma, myeloablative therapy followed by an autologous stem cell rescue was found to be more effective than chemotherapy alone. A logical, yet still to be determined, supposition is that if one round of ablative chemotherapy followed by stem cell rescue is effective, two or three such courses may be even more effective in eradicating this tumor known for its poor prognosis (George et al., 2006).

Complementary and Alternative Treatments

Children may use a variety of complementary and alternative treatments during the conditioning phase and while recovering from HSCT to control or alleviate symptoms of their condition or treatment (i.e., pain, nausea, fatigue, depression, anxiety). Acupuncture, acupressure, imagery/relaxation, therapeutic touch, massage, and aroma therapies are the most common of these complementary therapies. These measures are employed as adjuncts to conventional medical therapy, as opposed to those that replace standard care, and are often recommended by the HSCT or oncology team managing the medical interventions.

In contrast, biologically based, natural therapies that are ingested or injected are contraindicated in children who have received HSC transplants because of multiple concerns: (1) products made from plant matter can be contaminated with fungal spores; (2) many natural products have definite biologic activity that can cause harmful side effects or interactions with other medications; and (3) the lack of product standardization and formal oversight of the herbal and dietary supplement industry fails to ensure product consistency and purity (Barnes, 2003). Families or children undergoing HSCT are encouraged to openly discuss their feelings toward and options regarding complementary and alternative medicines (CAM) in an effort to prevent any unnecessary cultural misunderstandings and unwarranted adverse effects.

Anticipated Advances in Diagnosis and Management

Research and clinical advances continue to improve the survival of children receiving HSCT; improvements in supportive care have further enhanced these children's chances of survival. Improved characterization of HLAs to identify optimal donors and novel stem cell selection technologies are examples of ongoing scientific investigations that continue to move the HSCT field forward. Additionally, treatment approaches that improve tumor kill and manipulate the immune system to decrease the risk of relapse show consistent promise (Cooper, 2008).

Peripheral Blood Stem Cells

Use of peripheral blood stem cells (PBSCs) is the preferred source of hematopoietic stem cells in autologous transplantation for both adults and children. The successful use of these faster-engrafting cells in autologous transplantation led to the investigation of this stem cell source for allogeneic transplants, in both related and unrelated donors. Healthy allogeneic donors require G-CSF to mobilize stem cells into the peripheral blood where they can be harvested by apheresis. Besides the multiple injections of G-CSF, temporary placement of a pheresis catheter may be required in young donors with small veins or in donors with insufficient vascular access for apheresis via peripheral intravenous catheters.

During the last few years, PBSCs have been used more frequently in adult allogeneic HSCT. Initial studies from adult transplantation appeared promising; however, recently published reports show an increased frequency of chronic GVHD (Urbano-Ispizua, 2007). This finding has also been documented in small pediatric studies (Nagatoshi, Kawano, Watanabe, et al., 2002; Remberger & Ringden, 2007). Further study is needed to evaluate the risk of chronic GVHD and procedure-related complications to the healthy donor, as well as the significance of the stem cell source on the graft-versus-tumor effect.

Single/Double Cord Blood Transplants

Although first attempted almost 40 years ago, umbilical cord blood transplantation (UCBT) has only become a more accepted means of HSCT since the mid-1990s. As with stem cells procured from bone marrow and peripheral blood, those found in umbilical cord blood offer yet another alternative source of potentially lifesaving HSCs for those individuals who are found to have neither an appropriate related nor unrelated HLA-matched donor. Like all sources of HSCs, using those found in umbilical cord blood has both advantages and disadvantages. UCB is relatively easily harvested without any additional risk to either the mother or newborn. In addition, there appears to be a decreased incidence of GVHD in recipients of cord blood stem cells, often despite a greater HLA mismatch between donor and recipient (Jacobsohn, 2007). Another advantage of UCBT is the decreased risk of transmitting infections and, in particular, viral infections such as CMV (Chao, Emerson, & Weinberg, 2004; Jaing, Yang, Hung, et al., 2007).

Disadvantages of UCBT include a slower rate of engraftment and therefore greater risk of morbidity and mortality associated with serious infections. Umbilical cord blood also provides a limited number of stem cells as well as the inability to procure more stem cells in the event of graft rejection or a future need for donor lymphocyte infusions or stem cell boost (Jaing et al., 2007). Another concern regarding the use of stem cells from UCB involves the lack of oversight around the harvesting and storage of the stem cells. Although the National Marrow Donor Program is involved in the banking of some UCB, there is no one agency responsible for the donation, processing, and storage of all umbilical cord blood stem cells. There has been some concern regarding these various UCB banks and the possibility of differing outcomes related to uncertain processing and storage methodologies (Moise, 2005). Because UCB donation and storage is a profitable business, there is no current movement to unite cord blood banks under one governing body.

Because of the limited stem cell dose in each cord blood unit, UCBT has, until recently, only been used in transplants involving infants and children. Studies in adult individuals have shown that 2 UCB units that are partially matched with each other and the recipient can lead to successful engraftment and should be considered as a possible stem source in those individuals without family or volunteer donor matches (Majhail, Brunstein, & Wagner, et al., 2006). Ultimately, only one of the two transplanted units engrafts and is detectable using DNA analysis. Studies in children and adolescents have now been undertaken and show promise in preventing graft rejection in those who have been heavily transfused before transplantation (Jaing et al., 2007). Further research will be needed to verify the efficacy of double UCBT in the treatment of individuals who may not have any other source of appropriate HSCs.

Reduced Intensity/Nonmyeloablative Transplants

Originally designed as a treatment option for adults not qualifying for standard ablative HSCT, reduced intensity transplants, or minitransplants, are showing promise as a therapeutic option for children. Reduced intensity transplants are being studied in the pediatric setting for both nonmalignant and malignant disorders (Kletzel, Jacobsohn, Tse, et al., 2005; Satwani et al., 2008). Unlike traditional myeloablative regimens, children receive preparative regimens that are primarily immunosuppressive. The intent is to create a partial but stable graft. In the case of malignant disorders, immune-mediated, graft-versus-tumor effect eradicates the malignancy (Chao et al., 2004). In children with sickle cell anemia or thalassemia, only a small portion of hematopoietic stem cells is needed to correct the underlying genetic defect. In children with malignancies, however, and especially those with leukemia, the goal of this approach is to achieve full donor chimerism with a nontoxic conditioning regimen. Sufficient immunosuppression is used to achieve engraftment, thereby allowing the graft-versus-leukemia/graft-versus-tumor (GVL/GVT) effect to reduce minimal residual disease and prevent relapse. The use of nonmyeloablative transplant for hematologic malignancies is currently used primarily for older adults and some children who do not qualify for standard ablative conditioning regimens because of preexisting organ toxicities (Djulbegovic, Seidenfeld, Bonnell, et al., 2003; Georges & Storb, 2003).

Natural Killer Alloreactivity

Researchers are looking for ways to select donors that are more likely to create a beneficial GVL effect in children with malignant conditions. Recent findings have shown distinct properties of natural killer (NK) cell alloreactivity in engraftment and GVL (Hsu, Keever-Taylor, Wilton, et al., 2005). Killer cell immunoglobulin-like receptors (KIRs) found on NK cells are evaluated in both the recipient and potential donor to determine if alloreactivity is likely, which could aid in donor selection.

In Utero Transplantation

Although first attempted in a human fetus more than 40 years ago, in utero transplantation (IUT) has, until recently, primarily been studied using animal models. The rationale for IUT involves several theories: (1) the fetal environment is particularly conducive to stem cell migration and proliferation; (2) by transplanting during fetal development, condition-related, irreversible organ dysfunction can be avoided; and (3) IUT would prevent the need for treatment-associated toxicities (Westgren, 2006). Although several successful in utero transplants for SCID have been documented, adequate donor chimerism has not been achieved in similar efforts using IUT for other targeted conditions. Further research is needed to identify the reason behind these failures and whether the lack of stem cell engraftment relates to HLA matching, fetal immune response, stem cell dose, or a lack of space for HSC development (Westgren, 2006).

Gene Therapy

Inherited and acquired conditions of the hematopoietic system can be cured by allogeneic HSCT, but only a small percentage of affected children will have a sibling donor. Gene-modified, autologous bone marrow transplantation represents an attractive alternative. Gene therapy is a form of investigational molecular medicine that holds promise for potentially correcting diseases caused by a single gene defect. In most gene therapy studies, a "normal" gene is inserted into the genome to replace an "abnormal," condition-causing gene. Hematopoietic stem cells appear to be ideal vehicles for gene therapy, because they can be harvested, modified ex vivo, and then infused into the individual requiring the gene therapy (Kohn, 2007). This strategy may provide new treatments for a large number of inherited conditions in the near future. Investigators have had multiple setbacks, however, including viral-vector problems, autoimmune reaction, and oncogenesis (Human Genome Project, 2007).

Associated Problems of Bone Marrow Transplantation and Treatment

Anemia and Thrombocytopenia

All children experience prolonged marrow aplasia following their pretransplant myeloablative conditioning regimen. Supportive platelet and red blood cell (RBC) transfusions are required until adequate hematopoietic function is restored by the donor's engrafting megakaryocytes and RBC precursors. The bone marrow's recovery time is affected by the child's prior therapy, source of stem cells (marrow, umbilical cord blood, peripheral blood), manipulation of the stem cells (T cell depletion, purging), infections, and GVHD. Delayed platelet engraftment is not uncommon in recipients of autologous transplants because their stem cells may lack full hematopoietic potential after extensive exposure to chemotherapy before their transplants. Packed RBC (PRBC) support is usually required for at least 2 to 4 months after transplantation. From 10% to 20% of children receiving transplants from ABO-incompatible donors may require PRBC transfusions for a longer period of time (Helbig, Stella-Holowiecka, Wojnar, et al., 2007). The ABO and HLA genes are not inherited together; therefore a child may be HLA-A, HLA-B, HLA-DR identical to the donor but have a minor or major incompatibility to the donor's RBCs. Depending on whether the conditioning regimen was nonmyeloablative or ablative, the recipient's isohemagglutinins may be present for several weeks after HSCT and thus may react against donor RBCs.

Blood products must always be irradiated to prevent transfusion-associated GVHD in immunocompromised children. Blood products may contain a small number of T lymphocytes, which, if viable, could cause a life-threatening reaction in the transfused child. Irradiation prevents these T lymphocytes from replicating and attacking host cells without altering the normal function of the transfused RBCs or platelets. CMV-negative or filtered (leuko-reduced) blood products should be used for transfusions when available, particularly in CMV-negative recipients with CMV-negative donors.

Graft-versus-Host Disease

GVHD is the major cause of morbidity and mortality in children who have received allogeneic HSC transplants and affects 11% to 28% of matching sibling donor transplant recipients and 19% to 85% of unrelated donor recipients (Jacobsohn, 2007). GVHD can be mild, with no lasting effects, or severe, with debilitating or fatal consequences. Historically, GVHD has been divided into two phases: acute and chronic.

Acute GVHD. GVHD is an immune-mediated response in which donor T lymphocytes react against host tissues after becoming sensitized to the host's antigens. The activated T lymphocytes differentiate into effector cells that then produce cytokines and mediate cytotoxic activity targeted at specific tissues, most commonly the skin, gastrointestinal tract, and liver (Jacobsohn, 2007). Typically, acute GVHD occurs within the first 100 days following transplantation and may involve one, two, or all three organs. Involvement of target organs in GVHD often follows a characteristic clinical pattern and is ultimately defined pathologically (Box 15-2). Biopsy is the definitive method of diagnosis for acute GVHD involving the skin, gastrointestinal tract, or liver. Since these children are at significant risk for bleeding with any

---

Associated Problems of Bone Marrow Transplantation and Treatment

- Anemia and thrombocytopenia
- Graft-vs.-host disease
  - Acute GVHD (<100 days after transplant)
  - Target organs: skin, gastrointestinal, liver
  - Chronic GVHD (>100 days after transplant; see Table 15-4)
- Autoimmune reactions
- Severe immunodeficiency
- Graft failure or rejection
  - Primary
  - Late or secondary
- Infection
  - Preengraftment phase
  - Postengraftment phase
  - Late phase
- Viral infections
  - Cytomegalovirus (CMV)
  - Herpes simplex virus (HSV)
  - Varicella zoster virus (VZV)
  - Fungus
  - Late effects

BOX 15-2

Acute Graft-vs.-Host Target Organs

- *Skin:* Skin is the most common organ affected by acute GVHD, with symptoms varying in intensity from mild erythematous maculopapular rash that can be pruritic to generalized erythroderma with bullous lesions and epidermal necrolysis.
- *Gastrointestinal:* Gastrointestinal symptoms are characterized by diarrhea and abdominal cramping and may include intestinal bleeding. This can be the most difficult to treat in children. Staging of gastrointestinal GVHD is usually made by quantifying daily diarrhea output, which can be quite voluminous. Providing adequate fluid and electrolyte balance can be challenging in these children. Infection must also be considered as a cause of diarrhea, and stool cultures are sent for analysis. *Rotavirus* and *Clostridium difficile* are common in children undergoing HSCT.
- *Liver:* Although a common site for acute GVHD, the liver is rarely the site of single-organ involvement. The earliest and most common sign of liver involvement is a rise in the conjugated bilirubin and alkaline phosphatase; however, there are many other causes of liver abnormalities in these children, including venoocclusive disease (VOD), hepatic infections, and drug toxicity.

invasive procedure after transplant, they often do not undergo liver biopsies, which pose the greatest risk for bleeding.

Staging and overall grading of GVHD among HSC transplant recipients are based on the extent of involvement of each organ (Jacobsohn, 2007) (Table 15-2). Grade I acute GVHD is considered mild, and grade II is moderate; both are associated with favorable outcomes. Grades III and IV are severe and have significantly higher mortality rates (Mehta, 2004a).

Chronic GVHD. Chronic GVHD (cGVHD) occurs after the first 100 days following allogeneic HSCT, usually occurring between 3 and 18 months after transplantation. Risk factors for the development of cGVHD include a history of acute GVHD, older age of donor and recipient, a female donor of a male recipient, and particular sources of stem cells (Higman & Vogelsang, 2004; Zecca, Prete, Rondelli, et al., 2002). Chronic GVHD involves target tissues that may differ from those sites affected by acute GVHD and is clinically more consistent with an autoimmune phenomenon, demonstrating features resembling lupus erythematosus, scleroderma, and rheumatoid arthritis (Ferrara & Antin, 2004) (Table 15-3). Chronic GVHD may occur as a progression of acute GVHD, often after a period of quiescence of the acute GVHD, or as "de novo" disease. Although cGVHD appears to decrease the risk of relapse-associated death after transplant (Cutler & Antin, 2006; Jernberg et al., 2004), it remains the single most significant factor determining the quality of life and extent of morbidity following allogeneic HSC transplants.

Another serious consequence of cGVHD is severe immunodeficiency. Not only is immunosuppression itself worsened by cGVHD,

it is further compounded by GVHD treatment, which invariably involves the administration of immunosuppressive agents. Treatment of both acute and chronic GVHD includes the use of steroids, CSA, tacrolimus, and other immunosuppressive agents. Prompt and aggressive treatment of moderate to severe GVHD is necessary to bring the immune response under control. Newer treatments, including extracorporeal photochemotherapy (Foss, DiVenuti, Chin, et al., 2005; Scarisbrick, Taylor, Holtick, et al., 2008) and anti-interleukin-2-receptor monoclonal antibody (Perales, Ishill, Lomazow, et al., 2007; Teachey, Bickert, & Bunin, 2005) for steroid-resistant GVHD show some promise in the ongoing effort to control both acute and chronic GVHD.

Graft Failure or Rejection

Failure or rejection of the graft is, fortunately, an infrequent complication in children following HSCT. There are generally two forms of graft failure: *primary failure*, when there are no signs of hematopoietic recovery in the weeks immediately following transplantation, and *late* or *secondary failure*, when persistent pancytopenia is seen weeks or months following initial engraftment. In a child who receives an autologous HSC transplant, graft failure can be caused by the poor function of his or her stem cells, likely caused by heavy pretreatment with chemotherapy before stem cell collection. Some drugs or infections can also damage the newly infused stem cells, thereby resulting in graft failure. The possible causes for graft failure in a child receiving an allogeneic HSC transplant include a low stem cell dose, a T cell–depleted graft, ineffective pretransplant immunosuppression of the recipient, significant HLA disparity between the donor and recipient, and damage to the marrow's microenvironment secondary to an infection or the conditioning treatment. Graft rejection is seen only in allogeneic HSCT recipients and is an immune-mediated process leading to graft failure. It is often fatal unless a second marrow infusion can be procured and engraftment achieved.

Infection

Bacterial, viral, and fungal infections are significant obstacles to both the immediate and long-term survival of children after HSCT. Although improvements in prophylaxis and treatment strategies have been numerous over the years, infections still significantly contribute to the morbidity and mortality of these children. The risk of infection even exists before transplant because many of the children are already immunocompromised secondary to previous therapy or their preexisting conditions. Their immunosuppressed state is heightened further by the cytotoxic conditioning regimen used in preparation for their stem cell infusions. High-dose chemotherapy destroys the production of white blood cells while also damaging mucosal cells, causing a temporary loss of integrity of the mucosal barrier, particularly along the gastrointestinal tract. In addition, many conditioning regimens cause vascular injury that leads to fluid retention and a decreased ability to repair tissue. All children who undergo HSCT develop cellular and humoral immunodeficiencies for at least several months after transplantation, a condition that can last even longer if they subsequently develop cGVHD, requiring additional immunosuppressive agents.

In general, phagocytic function recovers first. Lymphocytic function typically takes much longer to recover and function adequately, partially because of the need for anti-GVHD medications. Children are at risk for certain types of infections at

---

TABLE 15-2

Graft-vs.-Host Disease Staging and Grading Systems

Staging of Individual Organ System(s)		
Organ	**Stage**	**Description**
Skin	+1	Maculopapular (MP) eruption over <25% of body area
	+2	MP eruption over 25%-50% of body area
	+3	Generalized erythroderma
	+4	Generalized erythroderma with bullous formation and often with desquamation
Gut	+1	Diarrhea >30 mL/kg or >500 mL/day
	+2	Diarrhea >60 mL/kg or >1000 mL/day
	+3	Diarrhea >90 mL/kg or >1500 mL/day
	+4	Diarrhea >90 mL/kg or >2000 mL/day; or severe abdominal pain and bleeding with or without ileus
Liver	+1	Bilirubin 2.0-3.0 mg/dL; SGOT 150-750 IU
	+2	Bilirubin 3.1-6.0 mg/dL
	+3	Bilirubin 6.1-15.0 mg/dL
	+4	Bilirubin >15.0 mg/dL

Overall Grading of Acute GVHD			
Grade	**Skin Staging**	**Liver Staging**	**Gastrointestinal Staging**
I	+1 to +2	0	0
II	+1 to +3	+1 and/or	+1
III	+2 to +3	+2 to +4 and/or	+2 to +3
IV	+3 to +4	+2 to +4 and/or	+2 to +4

From Chao, N.J. (1999). *Graft-versus-Host Disease* (2nd ed.). Austin, TX: R.G. Landes, pp. 63-122. Modified with permission.
Key: *GVHD*, graft-vs.-host disease; *SGOT*, serum glutamic oxaloacetic transaminase.

TABLE 15-3

Types of Late Complications: Tissues Affected, Risk Factors, Prevention, and Treatment

Tissue/Organs	Late Complications	Risk Factors	Preventive Measures	Treatment Options
Immunity	Infections	GVHD T cell depletion Herpesvirus infection Donor source Histocompatibility of donor and recipient	Antibiotic prophylaxis Immunizations Optimization of matching PCP prophylaxis	Targeted antimicrobials for specific infectious pathogens
	Autoimmune syndromes	GVHD	Optimization of matching	IVIG for autoimmune thrombocytopenia Steroids for various autoimmune phenomena
Endocrine glands	Hypothyroidism	Radiotherapy to head, neck, and mantle TBI	Fractionation of TBI Annual thyroid screening	Thyroid replacement
	Hypoadrenalism	Prolonged corticosteroid use	Replacement steroids for surgical procedures or acute medical conditions	
	Gonadal failure	TBI, intensive chemotherapy	Sperm banking	Hormone replacement
Skeletal	Osteopenia	Prolonged corticosteroid usage, TBI, inactivity, ovarian hormonal failure	Screening densitometry, exercise, bisphosphonates, ovarian hormonal replacement	Bisphosphonates
	Avascular necrosis	Corticosteroid usage, male gender, age > 16 yr	Minimization of steroids	Joint replacement of affected weight-bearing joints
Liver	GVHD Hepatitis B or C Iron overload		Hepatitis A and B vaccines	Lamivudine or foscarnet for hepatitis B; interferon plus ribavirin for hepatitis C
Ophthalmologic	Cataracts	TBI, busulfan, corticosteroids		Extraction and lens implantation
	Keratoconjunctivitis	GVHD		Artificial tear solution and ointment
Musculature	Myopathy	Corticosteroid therapy	Minimization of corticosteroids	
	Myositis	Chronic GVHD	Exercise	
Nervous system	Leukoencephalopathy	Cranial radiotherapy Intrathecal chemotherapy Fludarabine		
	Peripheral neuropathy	GVHD		Corticosteroid therapy
Respiratory tract	Interstitial fibrosis	Intensive conditioning regimen GVHD		
	Bronchiolitis obliterans	GVHD		Immunosuppressive therapy
Growth	Short stature	CNS irradiation TBI (single dose rather than fractionated) Hypothyroidism Corticosteroid therapy Gonadal insufficiency	Periodic assessment of endocrine status	Hormone replacement
Dentition	Cavities	Chronic GVHD	Dental hygiene	
	Sicca syndrome			Artificial saliva
Bladder	Scarring after hemorrhagic cystitis	Cyclophosphamide, BK virus, adenovirus, CMV	Hyperhydration or mensa Cyclophosphamide administration	Antispasmodic for symptomatic relief
Kidneys	Neuropathy	TBI, prior platinum compounds	Angiotensin-converting enzyme inhibitors	Control of hypertension

Key: *CMV*, cytomegalovirus; *CNS*, central nervous system; *GVHD*, Graft-vs.-host disease; *IVIG*, intravenous immunoglobulin; *PCP*, *Pneumocystis jiroveci* pneumonia; *TBI*, total body irradiation.

predictable periods of time after HSCT, reflecting the predominant host-defense defect. The time line for the risk of opportunistic infections in these children is outlined in Figure 15-1.

Preengraftment Phase. For a child in the preengraftment phase, prolonged neutropenia, as well as breaks in the mucosal and cutaneous barriers, create increased risks of infection. Because of the body's inability to fight infectious organisms and balance its natural florae, bacteria and fungi normally present in the gastrointestinal tract may become potential pathogens. During this time, the risk of infection is the same for children receiving autologous and allogeneic transplantations. Translocated oral and bowel

florae, along with indwelling central venous catheters (CVCs), are the primary source of gram-positive and enteric, gram-negative bacterial infections in children undergoing HSCT. Standard practice may include the prophylactic or empiric use of antibiotics when bacteremia is suspected. The emergence of drug-resistant bacteria, such as vancomycin-resistant *Enterococcus*, however, has forced many transplant centers to rethink their practice of routine prophylaxis against bacterial infections (Sepkowitz, 2002). Superinfection with fungal organisms continues to be a serious cause of morbidity and mortality in the transplant field. *Candida* and *Aspergillus* species are the most common causes of fungal

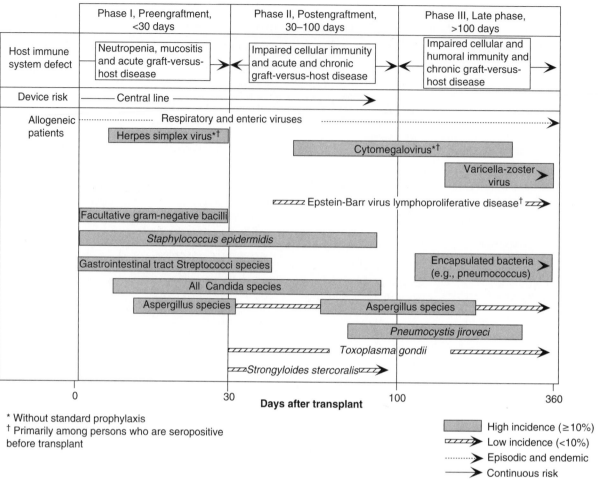

FIGURE 15-1 Phases of opportunistic infections among allogeneic HSCT recipients. From American Society of Blood and Marrow Transplantation. (2000). Guidelines for preventing opportunistic infections among hematopoietic stem cell transplant recipients. *Biol Blood Marrow Transplant, 6*(6a), 662.

infections, the latter more often resulting in serious and sometimes fatal infections.

Postengraftment Phase. During the initial period of engraftment (the first 100 days after HSCT), recipients of both autologous and allogeneic grafts have impaired cell-mediated immunity. GVHD and immunosuppressive therapy increase the risk of infection for children who have received an allogeneic transplant. Because these children lack intact T lymphocyte function, they are at particular risk for viral infections. The most common viral infections in the early posttransplant phase are herpes simplex virus (HSV), cytomegalovirus (CMV), and varicella zoster virus (VZV). Viral infections can result from a primary infection or a reactivation of a latent virus. These viruses are responsible for significant morbidity and mortality rates in children undergoing transplantation. Until recently, there were limited medicinal therapies for prophylaxis against and treatment for these infections; fortunately, new antiviral medications, including foscarnet and cidofovir, have emerged to provide clinicians with additional antiviral therapies (ASHSP, 2008a).

Pneumocystis jiroveci (formerly *carinii*) pneumonia (PCP) is a potential pulmonary pathogen that can also occur during this time. Although it was historically a frequent cause of serious infection in the immunocompromised child, it is now prevented in almost all cases by the prophylactic administration of trimethoprim-sulfamethoxazole (TMP-SMX, Septra, Bactrim).

Late Phase. During the late recovery phase (more then 100 days after transplantation), autologous recipients are at lower risk of opportunistic infections because of recovery of their immune function and the lack of need for post-HSCT immunosuppressive therapy. Children who undergo allogeneic transplantation, however, are at continued risk for viral and fungal infections until adequate immune function is restored. Although bacterial infections do not play a large role during this phase, serious bacterial infections can still occur in children, particularly those who have a CVC or cGVHD. Administration of prophylactic penicillin is highly recommended in children with cGVHD to reduce the risk of infection by encapsulated organisms (e.g., *Haemophilus influenzae, Streptococcus pneumoniae, Neisseria meningitides*). Such prophylaxis should continue as long as clinically active cGVHD is present and immunosuppressive therapy is administered.

Viral Infections

Cytomegalovirus. CMV, a common virus from the herpesvirus family, is the most frequent cause of viral-associated morbidity and mortality in children treated with HSCT. Although significant improvements in virus detection and treatment have recently been made, CMV infections remain a major infectious complication in children who receive HSC transplants (Boeckh, Fries, & Nichols, 2004). CMV, similar to other herpesviruses, can establish lifelong, latent infections after primary exposure. In children with competent immune systems, these latent infections are asymptomatic. The reactivation of latent CMV infections in children undergoing HSCT may cause severe and sometimes fatal consequences. CMV infections most commonly occur between 45 and 60 days after transplantation and can cause multiorgan disease, including pneumonia, gastroenteritis, retinitis, hepatitis, and encephalitis.

Because the outcome of therapy for disseminated CMV infection in this population is poor, prevention remains the best treatment. Primary CMV infection may be transmitted by close personal contacts, in utero from mother to child, by blood product transfusion, or by infused stem cells. Steps to prevent primary infection include using CMV-negative or leukocyte-depleted blood products, as well as by choosing a CMV-negative stem cell donor whenever possible. Ganciclovir, an antiviral medication, is used in both prophylaxis and preemptive therapy (Boeckh et al., 2004; Wingard & Anaissie, 2004). Prophylaxis with acyclovir during the first 30 days of HSCT may help decrease the risk of CMV reactivation and is incorporated into supportive care guidelines at some centers for CMV-seropositive recipients of unrelated donor HSCT.

Herpes simplex virus. In the early post-HSCT phase, HSV is the most common viral infection seen in children. Reactivation of HSV occurs in 80% of immunocompromised, seropositive children. The most common form of infection is gingivostomatitis, but dissemination can occur in the gastrointestinal tract, lungs, and liver. Prophylaxis with acyclovir is administered to children who are seropositive before transplant and is highly effective when continued for at least the first month after HSC transplants.

Varicella zoster virus. VZV can be a serious infectious risk to children undergoing HSCT. Both reactivation of the latent virus, herpes zoster, and primary VZV infections can cause severe complications from dissemination, including pneumonia, encephalitis, and hepatitis. Prompt initiation of antiviral treatment is necessary to prevent dissemination. The majority of children who are seropositive will develop herpes zoster within the first year after HSCT.

Fungus. Invasive fungal infections (IFIs) caused by opportunistic molds are a significant cause of morbidity and mortality in children undergoing HSCT. The incidence of invasive *Candida* infections has been significantly decreased by antifungal prophylaxis with triazole antimicrobials such as fluconazole and voriconazole (Wingard, 2005). The major pathogen associated with IFI is now *Aspergillosis*, although the incidence of unusual molds is increasing (Malani & Kauffman, 2007; Varkey & Perfect, 2008). Whereas *Candida* infections usually arise from gut contamination via damaged mucosa, *Aspergillus* is exogenous, airborne, and found primarily in soil. Newer triazoles (voriconazole and posaconazole) and echinocandins (caspofungin and micafungin) show promise in treating IFIs, including unusual molds (Kauffman & Carver, 2008; Strasfeld & Weinstock, 2006; Zonios & Bennett, 2008).

Late Effects

Improvements in the science of transplantation have allowed more children the opportunity for potentially curative therapy. This very aggressive form of treatment, however, has resulted in late effects for the increasing number of children who survive transplant, resulting in the need for long-term follow-up and care. The delayed or late sequelae that may develop can result from a combination of the following factors: (1) side effects of the condition for which transplantation was performed; (2) effects of previous treatment for the underlying disorder; (3) toxicities associated with the cytotoxic preparative regimen (usually high-dose chemotherapy with or without TBI); (4) toxic effects from treatment of posttransplant acute complications, especially from the prophylaxis and treatment of GVHD with immunosuppressive medications; and (5) physical effects of chronic GVHD. Most late effects of HSCT are a combination of these factors. A review of treatment-related toxicities from childhood cancer can be found in Chapter 16, as well as in "Long-Term Follow-Up Guidelines for Survivors of Childhood, Adolescent, and Young Adult Cancers" (available at www.survivorshipguidelines.org). Table 15-3 (Wingard, Vogelsang, & Deeg, 2002) outlines the types of late complications, tissues affected, risk factors, preventive measures, and treatments. Table 15-4 reviews organ involvement, clinical manifestations, evaluation, and interventions associated with cGVHD. Close attention must be paid to all previous therapies that a child has received and that can adversely affect the physical and cognitive development of that child (Dahllof, Hingorani, & Sanders, 2008; Oeffinger, Nathan, & Kremer, 2008).

The most common late effects found in children who have undergone HSCT involve the endocrine system, which is particularly vulnerable to damage caused by radiation and some chemotherapeutic drugs; as a result, children may experience impaired growth and pubertal development, as well as infertility (Ranke, Schwarze, Dopfer, et al., 2005; Sanders, 2008). Similarly, thyroid function can be affected if the child received XRT before transplantation or during the preparative regimen, resulting in overt or compensated hypothyroidism (Sanders, 2008). Bone-related late effects can be the result of both endocrine and nonendocrine issues. Osteochondromas are common after HSCT, occurring in approximately 20% of children, and are known to be associated with radiation (Bordigoni, Turello, Clement, et al., 2002; Leiper, 2002b). Avascular necrosis, most commonly in the hip joints, affects fewer than 10% of this population and should be considered in children with persistent pain and a history of corticosteroid therapy following HSCT (Leiper, 2002b). Osteoporosis and reduced bone mineral density can be a result of growth hormone deficiency, radiation, and corticosteroid use and increases the risk of osteoporotic fractures in children (Carpenter & Sanders, 2004). There are other non–endocrine-related sequelae that may not become evident for months to years after transplantation (Lieper, 2002a, 2002b). Treatment-related malignancies or second malignancies are a growing concern for the increasing number of long-term survivors of HSCT. Children are at higher risk of developing posttransplant lymphoproliferative disease, solid tumors, leukemias, or myelodysplastic syndrome (MDS) because of their long life expectancy and likely increased sensitivity of proliferating tissue to carcinogens (Lowe, Bhatia, & Somlo, 2007).

Yearly evaluation in a specialized long-term follow-up clinic at their transplanting institution is highly recommended. Multidisciplinary evaluations are necessary to fully assess sequelae related to HSCT. The schedule for follow-up and surveillance testing is often coordinated by the transplanting and referring institutions and should include the evaluation and recognition of late effects, treatment options for late organ dysfunction, and evaluation for the detection of early relapse. To ensure optimum health care for general and specialty issues, good communication is critical among the

TABLE 15-4

Clinical Manifestations of Chronic Graft-vs.-Host Disease

Organ	Clinical Manifestation	Evaluation	Intervention
Skin	Erythematous papular rash (lichenoid) or thickened, tight, fragile skin (sclerodermatous)	Clinical and biopsy to confirm the diagnosis of GVHD	Moisturize (petroleum jelly), treat local infections, protect from further trauma; topical steroid ointment may be used if it gives symptomatic relief to localized areas
Nails	Vertical ridging, fragile	Clinical	Nail polish may help decrease further damage
Sweat glands	Destruction leading to risk of hyperthermia		Avoid excessive heat
Hair	Scalp and body hair thin and fragile, can be partially or completely lost	Clinical	
Eyes	Dryness, photophobia, and burning. Progression to corneal abrasion	Regular ophthalmologic evaluation including Schirmer's test	Preservative-free tears during the day and preservative-free ointment at night
Mouth	Dry; sensitivity to mint, spicy food, tomato; whitish lacelike plaques in the cheeks and tongue identical to lichen planus; erythema and painful ulcerations, mucosal scleroderma with decreased sensitivity to temperature possible	Regular dental evaluation (with appropriate endocarditis prophylaxis; viral and fungal cultures at diagnosis and at any worsening	Avoid foods that are not tolerated; regular dental care preceded by appropriate endocarditis prophylaxis; topical steroid rinses followed by an antifungal agent for symptomatic relief
Respiratory tract	Bronchiolitis obliterans can manifest as dyspnea, wheezing, cough with normal CT scan and marked obstruction at pulmonary function tests; chronic sinopulmonary symptoms and/or infections also common; with abnormal chest CT, must rule out infections; lung biopsy if clinically indicated	Pulmonary function tests including FEV_1, FVC, DLCO, helium lung volumes; CT scan in symptomatic patients	Investigational therapy
Gastrointestinal	Abnormal motility and strictures; weight loss	Swallowing studies, endoscopy if clinically indicated; nutritional evaluation	Systemic treatment of GVHD; endoscopic/surgical treatment of strictures; nutritional intervention
Liver	Cholestasis (increased bilirubin, alkaline phosphatase); isolated liver involvement needs histologic confirmation	Liver function tests; liver biopsy if clinically indicated	No specific therapy is proven superior; FK-506 may concentrate in liver
Musculoskeletal	Fasciitis; myositis is rare; osteoporosis possible secondary to hormonal deficits, use of steroids, decreased activity	Periodical physical therapy evaluation to range of motion; bone density evaluation especially in patients using steroids	Aggressive physical therapy program
Immune system	Profound immunodeficiency; functional asplenia; high risk of pneumococcal sepsis, PCP, and invasive fungal infections; variable IgG levels	Assume all patients are severely immunocompromised and asplenic to 6 mo after GVHD has resolved	PCP prophylaxis (until 6 mo after no GVHD) and pneumococcal prophylaxis (lifetime); delay vaccinations
Hematopoietic system	Cytopenias; occasional eosinophilia	Counts; bone marrow aspirate and biopsy, antineutrophil and antiplatelet antibodies when indicated	Systemic treatment of GVHD
Others	Virtually all autoimmune disease have been described in association with chronic GVHD	As clinically indicated	

Key: *CT,* computed tomography; *DLCO,* diffusion capacity of lungs for carbon monoxide; *FEV*$_1$, forced expiratory volume in 1 sec; *FVC,* forced vital capacity; *PCP, Pneumocystis jiroveci* (formerly *carinii*) pneumonia;*IgG,* immunoglobulin G.

various subspecialties and the primary care practitioner involved in caring for the child. The goal of treatment for every child who undergoes HSCT is not only to cure the underlying disorder but also to minimize both the acute and long-term complications from the therapy.

Prognosis

In children who have received either autologous or allogeneic HSC transplants, relapse of their primary disorder is the most frequent cause of treatment failure. In malignant disorders, the vast majority of relapses occur within the first 2 years after HSCT. Since transplantation is usually the child's best option for cure, additional treatment holds only a small likelihood of restoring the child to disease-free health; however, in recent years, some success has been achieved by immunotherapy, which uses the immune system to assist with disease eradication. Most commonly, this is attempted by the discontinuation of immunosuppressive medications, if the child is still taking them, to create a GVL/GVT effect. Donor lymphocyte infusions (DLIs) may also be given, if the stem cell donor is available for the pheresis of leukocytes, in an effort to achieve a remission via immunologic mechanisms. Unfortunately, this modality has shown limited utility for the most common hematologic malignancies of childhood (Loren & Porter, 2008). If the child is more than 1 year after HSCT when relapse occurs, a second transplant may be another option for cure if a hematologic remission can be achieved, although the toxicities to the child are often significant (Shah, Kapoor, Weinberg, et al., 2002). If a child is a candidate for neither DLI nor a second HSC transplant, he or she will usually return to the care of the referring center for palliative therapy or end-of-life care.

Success of HSCT ranges from 10% to 90% and depends greatly on the child's original diagnosis and response to therapy, the status of organ function before transplant, and the type of transplant and stem cell source. From 10% to 15% of children who undergo HSCT will die within the first 1 to 2 months from transplant-related complications that may include organ toxicity, venoocclusive disease of the liver, infection, and interstitial pneumonitis. The leading cause of death, however, remains recurrent disease resulting from failure of the transplant to eradicate the underlying condition. Infection is the second leading cause of death. Both of these causes of death can occur months to years after transplant.

PRIMARY CARE MANAGEMENT

The primary care provider plays a key role in the child's and the family's return home and their adjustment toward normalcy following the intensive treatment of HSCT. Most families require some encouragement to reenter the primary health care arena following several months, and possibly years, of close management by a subspecialty and multidisciplinary team, often located hundreds of miles away from their home. Good communication between the transplant team and the primary care provider can foster an easier transition to home while decreasing the overall anxiety of the family.

Health Care Maintenance

Growth and Development

The endocrine system can be affected by chemotherapy and radiation therapy, leading to problems with growth and development. Several factors may impair growth in children after HSCT, including hypothyroidism and growth hormone deficiency. The type of HSCT preparative regimen the child receives is the most significant risk factor affecting growth (Sanders, 2008). Children receiving chemotherapy alone have little to no growth disturbance, whereas children receiving a radiation-based regimen are at the greatest risk for growth impairment. This is particularly relevant for children who receive cranial XRT before receiving TBI. Growth hormone therapy can be effective in children found to be hormonally deficient.

The majority of children who receive transplants before the onset of puberty will experience some delay in onset and progression through puberty, and many will require exogenous hormone replacement to proceed through puberty and achieve maximum growth potential. Production of sex hormones is linked to linear growth; therefore accurate documentation of sexual maturity or Tanner staging is helpful in identifying those children failing to develop secondary sexual characteristics in an age-appropriate fashion. Referral to a pediatric endocrinologist, if not already coordinated by the transplant team or referring subspecialist, is critical for the management of hormone replacement in survivors of HSCT.

Careful monitoring of growth by plotting height and weight on standardized growth charts, as well as of gonadal function by plotting Tanner stage progression, after HSCT is warranted to detect disturbances early and ensure normal pubertal development. In addition, significant or continued weight loss may be a sign of other medical conditions, including chronic GVHD, recurrent disease, secondary malignancy, or thyroid dysfunction.

Relative to other chronic conditions in childhood, survivors of HSCT are few in number. There are few published studies addressing the cognitive and behavioral impact of treatment on children after HSCT. Most information in the literature looks at childhood cancer survivors and infers similar cognitive and psychosocial effects about children having received HSCTs, since the majority of those who received transplants had an underlying malignant condition. These studies, as discussed in Chapter 16, show that children who received cranial irradiation and intrathecal chemotherapy exhibit the most frequent and severe cognitive effects and that age at treatment and dose of radiation are significant predictors of outcome. Although current published literature is lacking in children who have received HSCT, several transplant centers have neurocognitive studies underway to better understand cognitive and psychosocial sequelae in children surviving this aggressive treatment. However, one problematic factor in studying this select population that will not change is the heterogeneity of this group of children, their underlying diagnoses, conditioning therapies, and their post-transplant courses.

Assessment of both academic performance and behavior should be obtained yearly. Cognitive deficits can be subtle; questioning the parents and child specifically about school performance may provide early clues, thereby enabling prompt and appropriate intervention.

Diet

Nutrition plays a key role during and after HSCT. Optimal nutrition is required for healing and to maximize long-term growth and development potential. Children usually receive total parenteral nutrition (TPN) for a few weeks during the early transplant phase because of severe mucositis, nausea, and vomiting. Once the conditioning-related toxicities have resolved, children are usually maintained on a modified diet to reduce exposure to environmental food contaminants. These precautions may be institutional-specific and often remain in effect until adequate immune reconstitution is documented. A post-HSCT diet is instituted to reduce the child's risk of infection by avoiding unpasteurized products, aged or veined cheeses, undercooked meats or seafood, and other potential sources of infection in food products. Table 15-5 outlines foods that should be avoided while the child is immunocompromised (Lipken, Lenssen, & Dickson, 2005). Multidisciplinary transplant teams commonly include nutritionists who educate parents and children on nutrition and food safety. Parents may be required to keep daily food/fluids records until the child has attained adequate oral nutrition after HSCT. Children receiving steroids for treatment of GVHD often require a low-sodium diet to minimize hypertension and at times may require insulin because of steroid-induced hyperglycemia. Calcium supplements may also be recommended in this population to offset the risk for osteopenia. Changes in taste brought about by chemotherapy and XRT may initially be a problem for some children, although this usually normalizes within 2 to 4 months after HSCT.

Safety

Child safety should be reviewed with parents at primary care visits. First-time parents whose children become ill during infancy and who are now adjusting to the liberation of protective isolation often need additional anticipatory guidance. Infant and toddler issues that would normally have been reviewed are often ignored during the acute and often life-threatening treatment that these children require.

Children returning home after transplantation require multiple oral medications, equipment for the care of their CVC, and possibly

TABLE 15-5

Foods that Pose a High Risk for Hematopoietic Stem Cell Transplantation (HSCT) Recipients and Safer Substitutions

Foods that Pose a High Risk	Safer Substitutions
Raw and undercooked eggs and foods containing them (e.g., French toast, omelettes, salad dressings, eggnog, puddings)	Pasteurized or hard-boiled eggs
Unpasteurized dairy products (e.g., milk, cheese, cream, butter, yogurt)	Pasteurized dairy products
Fresh-squeezed, unpasteurized fruit and vegetable juices	Pasteurized juices
Unpasteurized cheeses or cheeses containing molds	Pasteurized cheeses
Undercooked or raw poultry, meats, fish, and seafood	Cooked poultry, well-done meats, cooked fish and seafood
Vegetable sprouts (e.g., alfalfa, bean, other seed sprouts)	Should be avoided
Raw fruits with a rough texture (e.g., raspberries)	Should be avoided
Smooth raw fruits	Should be washed under running water, peeled, or cooked
Unwashed raw vegetables	Should be washed under running water, peeled, or cooked
Undercooked or raw tofu	Cooked tofu (i.e., cut into 1-inch or smaller cubes and boiled for 5 min or longer in water or broth before eating or using in recipes)
Raw or unpasteurized honey	Should be avoided
Deli meats, hotdogs, and processed meats	Should be avoided unless further cooked
Raw, uncooked grain products	Cooked grain products including bread, cooked and ready-to-eat cold cereal, pretzels, popcorn, potato chips, corn chips, tortilla chips, cooked pasta, and rice
Maté tea	Should be avoided
All moldy and outdated food products	Should be avoided
Unpasteurized beer (e.g., home brewed and certain bottled or canned, or draft beer that has been pasteurized after fermentation)	Pasteurized beer (i.e., retail microbrewery beer)
Raw, uncooked brewer's yeast	Should be avoided; HSCT recipients should avoid any contact with raw yeast (i.e., they should not make bread products themselves)
Unroasted raw nuts	Cooked nuts
Roasted nuts in the shell	Canned or bottled roasted nuts or nuts in baked products

Data from Centers for Disease Control and Prevention. (1996). Outbreaks of *Salmonella* serotype enteritidis infection associated with consumption of raw shell eggs—United States, 1994-1995. *MMWR, Morb Mortal Wkly Rep, 45*(34), 737-742; Taormino, P.J., Beuchat, L.R., & Slutsker, L. (1999). Infections associated with eating seed sprouts: An international concern. *Emerg Infect Dis,* 5(5), 626-634; Herwaldt, B.L., & Ackers, M.L. (1997). Outbreak in 1996 of cyclosporiasis associated with imported raspberries. *N Engl J Med,* 336(22), 1548-1556; Centers for Disease Control and Prevention. (1998). Foodborne outbreak of cryptosporidiosis—Spokane, Washington, 1997. *MMWR, Morb Mortal Wkly Rep, 47*(27), 565-567; Centers for Disease Control and Prevention. (1999). Update: Multistate outbreak of listeriosis—United States, 1998-1999. *MMWR, Morb Mortal Wkly Rep, 47*(51), 1117-1118; Kusminksy, G., Dictar, M., Arduino, S., et al. (1996). Do not drink maté: An additional source of infection in South American neutropenic patients. *Bone Marrow Transplant,* 17(1), 127.

IV medications. All medications should be stored away from children. A sharps container should be in the home to properly dispose of any needles and syringes related to the care of the CVC or IV medications. Decreasing the risk of infection at home is important. Hand washing is the single most effective act in preventing the spread of infection. Parents should supervise the hand washing of small children. No ill contacts should be allowed in the home. Eating utensils, cups, and glasses should not be shared with the immunocompromised child; all glasses, dishes, and utensils should be washed in hot soapy water or the hot cycle of a dishwasher. The child's home should be cleaned frequently and be free of mold. Any construction on the house or surrounding property should be delayed until immune reconstitution is documented. No new pets should be brought into the household for at least 6 to 12 months following transplant. Immunocompromised children should have minimal direct contact with their household pets, wash their hands after handling them, avoid contact with animal feces, and avoid contact with reptiles (e.g., snakes, lizards, turtles, iguanas) to reduce the risk of acquiring salmonellosis.

Children are encouraged to resume normal activities that fall within the protective isolation guidelines of the transplanting center. Physical activities, however, may be restricted because of thrombocytopenia. Children with a platelet count below 100,000 are restricted from climbing, contact sports, bike riding, or other physical activities in which the risk of trauma is high. Loss of muscle mass and endurance is common after lengthy hospitalizations, and physical and occupational therapy are often necessary in the post-HSCT care of the child. Travel to developing countries is not advised until the child has demonstrated adequate immune reconstitution because of the risk of contracting opportunistic or unusual infections. The families should consult their transplant centers before planning any travel out of state or internationally for the first 1 to 2 years after transplant.

Immunizations

Most children have partial or complete loss of their immunity to vaccine-preventable diseases following HSCT. Children who are immunosuppressed may not be able to initiate an immune response to immunizations. Reimmunization is necessary, but the timing of recovery of immune function is variable. Sparse research exists in this heterogeneous population. The *Red Book* (American Academy of Pediatrics Committee on Infectious Diseases, 2006) notes the two common reimmunization strategies. Many transplant centers recommend a trial of assessing antibody response to individual toxoids to determine if (1) immunizations are required and (2) the child's immune system is capable of mounting a response. Other transplant centers have adopted the generalized immunization schedule developed by the Centers for Disease Control and Prevention (CDC), Infectious Disease Society of America, and American Society of Blood and Marrow Transplantation and published

TABLE 15-6

Recommended Vaccinations for Recipients of HSCT

Vaccine	Patient Age	Timing of Administration	Comments
Diphtheria, tetanus, pertussis (DTP)	<7 yr	12, 14, and 24 mo after transplantation	No data regarding safety and immunogenicity of pertussis vaccine in this setting. Patients with a contraindication to pertussis should receive the DT vaccine.
Diphtheria toxoid–tetanus toxoid (DT)	<7 yr	12, 14, and 24 mo after transplantation	Patients with a contraindication to pertussis should receive the DT vaccine.
Tetanus-diphtheria toxoid (Td)	≥7yr	12, 14, and 24 mo after transplantation	Patients should be reimmunized every 10 yr.
Haemophilus influenzae type B conjugate	All patients	12, 14, and 24 mo after transplantation	
Hepatitis B vaccination	Age < 18 yr: susceptible patients Adults: patients with risk factors for infection	12, 14, and 24 mo after transplantation	High-dose vaccine recommended for immunocompromised adults; no data regarding response to high-dose vaccine in children. Response to be assessed 1-2 mo following completion of series of three vaccinations. Those without response may undergo a second cycle of three vaccinations.
23-valent pneumococcal polysaccharide vaccine	≥2 yr	12 and 24 mo after transplantation	Vaccine demonstrates limited efficacy in posttransplantation setting with higher response rates later after transplantation.
7-valent pneumococcal conjugative	All patients	Use age-dependent guidelines*	Antibiotic prophylaxis encouraged in patients with chronic graft-vs.-host disease.
Influenza (inactivated)	All patients		Lifelong seasonal administration beginning before transplantation and resuming at 6 mo after transplantation. Children <9 yr old should receive 2 doses for first vaccination. Children ≤12 yr should receive split vaccine. Patients >12 yr may receive transplantation split or whole vaccine.
Inactivated poliovirus (IPV)	All patients	12, 14, and 24 mo after transplantation	IPV vaccine is immunogenic after transplantation although efficacy data are not available.
Measles, mumps, rubella (live vaccine)	All patients	≥24 mo after transplantation	Vaccination reserved for patients with recovered immunity (not for patients receiving immunosuppressive therapy).
Varicella vaccine	Contraindicated	Contraindicated	Contraindicated

*MMWR. (October 6, 2000). No. RR-9, (49)21-27.
Modified from Centers for Disease Control and Prevention, Infectious Disease Society of America, and American Society of Blood and Marrow Transplantation (2000). Guidelines for preventing opportunistic infections among hematopoietic stem cell transplant recipients. *MMWR Recomm Rep 2000, 49* (RR-10), 1-25, CE 1-7.

in 2000 (Table 15-6) (Centers for Disease Control and Prevention, 2000). It is generally recommended that HSCT recipients initiate reimmunization 1 year following HSCT if there is no evidence of cGVHD and the child is not receiving corticosteroids. Live-virus immunizations such as MMR and Varivax pose the greatest risk of infection in immunocompromised children; it is therefore recommended that these vaccines be held until 2 years after HSCT. Annual inactivated influenza vaccine should be administered to all household contacts of children undergoing transplantation, as well as for children at least 6 months after transplant. Siblings, family contacts, and health professionals should all be fully immunized to decrease the potential exposure of children undergoing or recovering from HSCT.

Screening

Vision. Both routine vision screening and annual ophthalmologic examinations are advised. Corticosteroid use and radiation can cause posterior subcapsular cataract formation that usually develops within the first 2 years after HSCT (Holmstrom, Borgstrom, & Calissendorff, 2002). Small cataracts may not initially interfere with vision but should be routinely monitored by an ophthalmologist. Similarly, chronic GVHD can result in keratoconjunctivitis. Ophthalmologic evaluation should include a Schirmer's test to assess for adequate tear production. CMV retinitis is another potential complication for children. Optimally, an ophthalmologist who is familiar with sequelae from high-dose chemotherapy and radiation therapy should be closely involved in the care of any child who has had HSCT.

Hearing. Routine screening is advised. Hearing loss, usually involving high frequency, may occur in children who receive ototoxic treatments, such as platinum-based chemotherapy, aminoglycoside antibiotics, loop diuretics, or XRT (Gurney, Ness, Rosenthal, et al., 2006; Punnett, Bliss, Dupuis, et al., 2004). It should be anticipated that many children whose pre-HSCT treatment included multiple ototoxic drugs, such as children with neuroblastoma, will require hearing aids after HSCT (Gurney et al., 2006). In addition, special educational needs associated with such hearing loss will need to be addressed with the affected children and their families.

Dental. A pretransplant dental evaluation is required to identify existing dental caries needing to be repaired and other risk factors for potential infection during HSCT. Routine dental examinations are very important and should resume once the child has adequate immune reconstitution. Chemotherapy and XRT, especially TBI, are known to cause dental and skeletal abnormalities in young children, including delay in tooth development, altered root development, enamel hypoplasia, and craniofacial abnormalities (Duggal, 2003). Children who are treated before the development of secondary dentition are at greatest risk for these complications. In addition, children who develop cGVHD involving the mouth will have oral mucosal changes that may increase their risk of oral infections (Schubert & Correa, 2008).

Blood Pressure. Children are often placed on medication for hypertension after HSCT. Hypertension is most commonly secondary to either renal insufficiency caused by nephrotoxic drugs or immunosuppressive medications, such as CSA. Parents are instructed on blood pressure monitoring and the administration of antihypertensive medication. Management of hypertension is usually coordinated by the transplant team, because the tapering of immunosuppressive medications and the discontinuation of some antiinfective agents may reduce the need for antihypertensive agents. Blood pressure monitoring and documentation by the primary care provider are important even after the child has stopped all nephrotoxic medications because a small percentage of children will develop chronic renal insufficiency after transplant, requiring long-term antihypertensive management (Leung, Ahn, Rose, et al., 2007).

Hematocrit. During the first year after HSCT, routine hematocrit by the primary care provider is not required because of the multiple CBCs and close hematologic assessment by the transplanting center. Routine screening may resume once the child is off all immunosuppressive medications.

Urinalysis. Routine urinalysis is recommended. Abnormalities should be communicated to the referring subspecialist or transplant team. Hematuria may be seen in children with cystitis or opportunistic urinary viral infections. Children without a competent immune system are at increased risk for urinary tract infections.

Tuberculosis. Routine screening for tuberculosis is advised usually after the first year post-HSCT or once the child has demonstrated immunocompetence.

Condition-Specific Screening

Physical examinations and laboratory studies are usually obtained at the transplant center or medical center of the referring subspecialist during the first year after HSCT. After the first year, annual evaluations for complications and late effects are generally requested by the transplant team and include subspecialty evaluations by the transplant team, endocrinologist, and ophthalmologist, as well as periodic echocardiograms and pulmonary function tests.

Screening for Late Complications. The primary care provider plays a key role in screening for possible complications and late effects of treatment. Once the child returns to the community, it is the primary care practitioner's familiarity with the late complications of HSCT (see Table 15-3) and clinical manifestations of cGVHD (see Table 15-4) that can aid in early recognition of potential problems and result in prompt consultation with the transplant team or referring subspecialist.

Common Illness Management

Differential Diagnosis

Infections. Immunocompromised children may not be able to mount a typical response to infection (e.g., fever, erythema, edema) and therefore may not manifest signs and symptoms despite true infection. A child who is still immunocompromised following HSCT is susceptible to complications from common community-acquired respiratory viruses, such as respiratory syncytial virus (RSV), adenovirus, influenza, parainfluenza, and even rhinovirus, all of which can result in severe and life-threatening pneumonitis. It is important to limit potential exposures to ill persons by limiting contact with large groups of people; this often involves being restricted from school, church, theaters, airplane travel, or even waiting rooms of medical offices. No rectal temperatures or medications should be given because these also increase the risk of bacteremia from local trauma.

Differential Diagnosis

- Infections
  - Asymptomatic infections
  - Fever management
  - Bacteremia
  - Central venous catheter infections
  - Viral infections
- Gastrointestinal symptoms
- Headache
- Pain
  - Infections
  - Myalgias
  - Neuropathy

Guidelines for fever management may differ according to the policy of the transplanting institution. Infection and recurrent malignancy are the key differential diagnoses. Any child who is either within the first year after HSCT or is still taking immunosuppressive medication and develops a fever requires consultation with the transplant team for management guidelines. Administration of antipyretics should be delayed until after the child is examined. Ibuprofen is contraindicated if thrombocytopenia or platelet function abnormality is suspected. For children still receiving immunosuppressive therapy and for those who have a CVC, any fever requires immediate evaluation; infection is the most likely cause and must be ruled out. Any child who has chills or rigors following flushing or administration of IV fluids or medications through his or her central catheter should be evaluated immediately for possible bacteremia. After a thorough physical examination is performed, laboratory analysis usually includes aerobic and anaerobic blood cultures peripherally and from each lumen of the CVC, urinalysis, and urine culture, as well as a chest radiograph, and a throat culture and nasal swab for rapid testing of viral pathogens if upper respiratory symptoms are present.

The primary care provider may be asked to provide the initial evaluation if the child lives more then 1 hour from the transplanting institution or subspecialty clinic setting. Admission to a hospital or transfer to the transplanting institution is usually required. Broad-spectrum IV antibiotics are initiated for a minimum of 48 hours, and if bacteremia is present, the antibiotic regimen can be modified based on positive cultures and antimicrobial sensitivities.

Viral infections are also common in children after HSCT. The herpesviruses HSV, CMV, and VZV are the most common. If the child is within the first year after HSCT or still under the direct care of the transplanting institution, the transplant team should be contacted immediately if infection with one of these viruses is suspected. Uncomplicated HSV infection is usually treated with intravenous acyclovir (250 mg/m^2/8 hr); VZV, whether primary (chickenpox) or secondary (zoster), is treated with acyclovir (500 mg/m^2/8 hr) intravenously. Administration of IV acyclovir commonly requires IV fluids in addition to oral intake because of the nephrotoxic effects of this antiviral medication. Treatment for CMV infection includes the use of ganciclovir and IVIG per transplant institutional policy.

Children who are more than 1 year after HSCT, who have demonstrated adequate immune recovery, who no longer have central line access, who are on no immunosuppressive medication, and who have no evidence of cGVHD may have less stringent fever management guidelines as directed by the child's referring subspecialist.

Gastrointestinal Symptoms. In the immunocompromised child, vomiting or diarrhea could be a sign of either opportunistic infection or GVHD, and therefore the transplant team should be involved in the child's subsequent care. For a child with diarrhea, stool cultures for rotavirus, adenovirus, *Clostridium difficile*, *Campylobacter*, *Salmonella*, and *Shigella* should be obtained. It is also helpful to ascertain the volume of diarrhea within a 24-hour period, as well as the frequency, consistency, and appearance of the stool. If the child is not able to keep down daily oral medications, and in particular, immunosuppressive therapy, because of vomiting, the transplant team should be contacted to discuss alternative forms of medication administration. Blood cultures, as described previously, should be obtained because vomiting and diarrhea may be the initial signs of bacteremia. IV hydration should be administered for children with large fluid losses, symptoms of dehydration, or inability to tolerate oral fluids.

Headaches. Headaches, although a common symptom in childhood and adolescence, can indicate a serious complication in the immunocompromised child following HSCT. The list of differential diagnoses is lengthy and includes infection, hypertension, dehydration, spinal fluid leak caused by recent lumbar puncture, strain from impaired visual acuity, and medication-induced toxicities. A thorough and recent medical history to obtain information regarding medication changes, as well as a detailed description of the headaches, is essential.

Pain. A thorough history of the location, onset, precipitating factors, and qualities of the pain will usually identify the cause of pain in most children after HSCT. Because of the immunocompromised status of these children the differential diagnosis primarily focuses on an infectious etiology. Assessments should involve examining both the skin and oral pharynx for lesions. Herpes zoster can cause neuropathy and pain in a dermatomal distribution before visible vesicle formation and should be considered in children who describe recurring pain under the skin. It is not uncommon for children to have mild myalgias after HSCT as their energy level improves and they increase their physical activity. Parents are usually instructed not to administer acetaminophen and nonsteroidal antiinflamatories for discomfort until the child has been assessed by the medical provider and the medication approved. Other pain may also be related to specific post-HSCT complications and should be discussed with the transplant team. Similarly, some children experience neuropathies secondary to previous chemotherapy treatment. This neuropathic pain often slowly resolves with time and may require pharmacotherapy.

Drug Interactions

Children are administered multiple medications following HSCT. The addition of any medication, prescriptive or over the counter, increases the risk for drug interactions. Children who have received an allogeneic transplantation are at greatest risk for drug interactions because they are usually receiving CSA or tacrolimus for immunosuppression. The addition or discontinuation of other medications can greatly affect absorption or clearance of these immunosuppressive medications, causing a change in serum drug levels that can lead to organ toxicity or GVHD. Primary care providers should consult the transplant team before prescribing or advising additional medications for these children. Likewise,

families must be open with their medical providers regarding the use of any herbal complementary therapies, because these also pose a risk to children after HSCT.

These children should not receive nonsteroidal antiinflammatory drugs (e.g., ibuprofen) because they can interfere with platelet function and increase the risk of bleeding.

Developmental Issues

Sleep Patterns

It is not uncommon for children recovering from HSCT to have disturbances in their sleep pattern, particularly if they are receiving moderate to high doses of corticosteroids. As their steroids are weaned, these sleep disturbances should also dissipate. Most children receive TPN during the first month after HSCT, and many children require nighttime supplemental IV fluids for 2 to 3 additional months. Pump malfunctions and alarms may also disturb their sleep in addition to IV hydration prompting multiple trips to the bathroom at night. Children having difficulty sleeping should avoid caffeine and other stimulants that may contribute to insomnia. Keeping a predictable bedtime routine and planning quiet activities in the evening, as well as avoiding overstimulating video games and movies, may also be helpful.

Toileting

Diarrhea can be a consequence of either GVHD or infection and may affect normal toileting habits. Regression in toileting practices may be seen in very young children during and after long hospitalizations. In general, as the child's health improves, so do his or her toileting skills.

Discipline

HSCT is often the last form of treatment children receive. Families may have been dealing with the child's condition and prognosis for months or years before transplantation. Patterns of behavior and discipline, or lack thereof, are often well established before the child is hospitalized to undergo HSCT.

During the first 6 to 12 months following the transplant, parents often continue to be very protective of their child, often indulgent, and are rarely as strict with the child as with their other children. Disciplining a child who has received an HSCT can also be challenging because normal developmental "acting out" may be difficult to distinguish from medication-induced behavioral changes (e.g., behavioral changes associated with corticosteroids). In general, children recovering from HSCT are eager to be active and interact with their family, especially their siblings, following the acute phase of transplant when they are hospitalized and feeling sick. The primary care provider can be instrumental in helping to facilitate normalcy within family by reviewing with the parents age-appropriate behavior, development, limit setting, and discipline. Parents should strive to achieve consistency in limit setting and discipline equally for all the children in the household.

Child Care

Children who have received an HSCT and are immunocompromised must avoid child-care settings because of the risk of developing common community-acquired respiratory viruses. If child care is required, in-home care is strongly recommended.

Schooling

School plays a very important role in the development of a child. The transplant team, referring center, and parents should work together to ensure alternative forms of education during the child's hospitalization, as well as the period of protective isolation after transplant. This period may last between 6 and 12 months and may be longer for children with significant post-HSCT complications. Arrangements should be made for home study or hospital-based schooling until adequate immune function has been achieved. This extended period of absence from school may result in school reentry difficulties. Maintaining contact with peers in school through a webcam, teleconference, or contact with selected friends may help with reentry. Once the child is no longer in protective isolation and can resume education with his or her peers, an annual Individualized Educational Program (IEP) including cognitive and behavioral evaluations should be obtained through the school (see Chapter 3). Members of the transplant team can provide education about the child's health at a school reentry visit. There are generally no limitations placed on children returning to school unless noted by their transplant team. They are encouraged to fully participate in all activities and classes, including physical education, to the best of their ability. A small percentage of children will be fatigued from a full day of school at reentry and a partial or half day may be more appropriate at the beginning.

Sexuality

Many physical changes occur in children and young adults during and after transplantation secondary to surgery, medication side effects, transplant-related complications, and late effects. These changes can have negative effects on self-image. Fortunately, many of these changes are temporary, lasting only months, but others may be permanent. Physical changes may include alopecia, cushingoid features, scarring, striae, significant weight gain or loss, skin dyspigmentation, short stature, and hirsutism. The physical signs and symptoms of cGVHD, however, may take years to improve or may never completely resolve (see Table 15-4).

Children who receive TBI during their preparative regimen are likely to be infertile because of the damaging effects of radiation on follicular development in ovaries and germinal epithelium in the testes. Small testicular volume and low to normal testosterone levels are seen in boys after TBI, and some boys will require testosterone therapy for pubertal progression and to maintain normal sexual function as young adults.

Delayed pubertal development may also affect self-esteem and peer acceptance. Adolescents who have received HSCT should have access to counseling. Sexually active young adults should be counseled on methods to reduce the risk of sexually transmitted infections and encouraged to practice cleanliness and safe sex with their partner. Barrier methods, particularly the use of condoms, should be encouraged. Intimate oral contact should be avoided until the mouth is completely healed.

Endocrine and fertility specialists play an important role both before and after therapy for these children and young adults, who have a high rate of treatment-related infertility. Many children are often rendered infertile before referral for transplantation because of previous chemotherapy and irradiation. At present, the success rate is low for cryopreservation of unfertilized oocytes, ovarian tissue, and testicular tissue by reproductive specialists hoping to preserve fertility (Oktay, 2006; Revel & Revel-Vilk, 2008). Genetic counseling should be offered to those young adults who underwent HSCT for hereditary conditions. Although the overwhelming majority of children and young adults are infertile after HSCT, successful pregnancies have occurred and the likelihood of infertility should not be considered adequate birth control. Appropriate birth control measures should be taken by sexually active young adults.

Transition to Adulthood

The struggle for independence for the adolescent is in sharp contrast to both the protective isolation before adequate immune recovery and the parents' need for close observation of their medically fragile adolescent. Normal adolescent issues still occur in young adults who have received HSCT. Practitioners caring for long-term survivors of HSCT should emphasize the importance of the routine use of sunscreen and abstinence from tobacco because of increased vulnerability to ultraviolet rays and carcinogens. Body piercing is not advised while the risk for developing GVHD still exists or the immune system is still incompetent. Education focusing on a healthy lifestyle is important for these young adults. Maintaining a healthy weight, staying active with routine exercise, eating a varied diet, and limiting alcohol consumption may reduce the risk of further disease and complications as they age.

There are few data regarding the ability of survivors of HSCT to obtain medical and life insurance, to achieve gainful employment, or to successfully form intimate relationships and live independently. There is information, however, on survivors of childhood cancer (a much larger population), which can be found in Chapter 16 and is largely applicable to HSCT survivors. Chapters 3 and 4 also outline the Americans with Disabilities Act of 1990, which protects any person who has had the diagnosis of cancer from discrimination in employment or housing and is applicable to the vast majority of survivors of HSCT.

Family Concerns

Owing to the rapid improvements surrounding HSCT and the relatively small number of affected individuals, particularly in comparison with other chronic conditions of childhood, there is a substantial gap in our understanding of the psychological sequelae associated with this procedure. HSCT is a very intense, complicated form of treatment. Parents and children are often balancing the choice of potential long-term survival with the up-front risk of significant morbidity and mortality. The child and family face a series of intense stressors. These stressors include the decision to accept the treatment; the search for a donor; the workup to determine the child's eligibility for transplant; enduring the cytotoxic preparative regimen followed by the anticlimactic infusion of the stem cells; the wait for blood count recovery; the potential for death from therapy-related complications; and, finally, discharge from the hospital and the eventual return home. Although the actual transplant hospitalization is very stressful, parents often experience even more anxiety after discharge. Whereas nurses and doctors have been available to assess and treat their children, they now become responsible for administering daily medications and deciding what problems necessitate calling the transplant team. When children finally are allowed to return home, they may be at a significant distance from the security of the transplant team and medical center, and although they are home their physical and social isolation has not ended. Additionally, parents must now juggle their child's complex care while also managing a household and meeting the needs of the other children and family members. Last, the threat of relapse or severe complications is ever present and looming.

More information is needed on this growing population to better understand the physical and psychosocial sequelae of HSCT. Research is ongoing to make transplant a safer, more successful treatment option to provide more children with a second chance at long-term survival. Since the number of children successfully treated with HSCT is increasing, we can expect, in the near future, more studies assessing the psychosocial issues and concerns facing these children and young adult survivors.

Resources

Organizations

American Cancer Society
(800) ACS-2345
Website: www.cancer.org
Candlelighters Childhood Cancer Foundation
(800) 366-2223
Website: www.candlelighters.org

Caring Bridge web sites
Website: www.caringbridge.org
Federation for Children with Special Needs
(617) 236-7210
Website: www.fcsn.org
Lance Armstrong Foundation
(866) 235-7205
Website: www.livestrong.org
National Cancer Institute (NCI) Childhood Cancers
Website: www.cancer.gov/cancerinfo/types/childhoodcancers
National Center for Learning Disabilities
(888) 575-7373
Website: www.ncld.org
National Childhood Cancer Foundation
(800) 458-6223
Website: www.curesearch.org
National Marrow Donor Program
Website: www.marrow.org

Summary of Primary Care Needs for the Child with Bone Marrow Transplant

HEALTH CARE MAINTENANCE

Growth and Development

- Height and weight should be measured at each visit and plotted on standard growth curve forms. Hypothyroidism and hormone deficiencies are common side effects of chemotherapy and radiation therapy.
- Children who receive transplants before puberty will often experience delay in onset and progression of puberty. Tanner staging should be done at each visit. Hormone replacement therapy may be needed for both males and females.
- Cognitive development has had limited study in children with bone marrow transplants. Risks of cognitive impairment are similar to those of children with cancer receiving similar chemotherapy and radiation, especially cranial radiation and intrathecal chemotherapy.

Diet

- Optimal nutrition is required for healing and to maximize growth.
- A post-HSCT diet is instituted to reduce the risk of infection by avoiding foods with potential vectors for infection, such as unpasteurized products and undercooked meats.
- Nutritional support via total parenteral nutrition (TPN) is often needed for a few weeks after discharge.
- Children receiving steroids may be placed on a low-sodium diet to reduce hypertension and calcium supplements to reduce the risk of osteopenia.

Safety

- Anticipatory guidance is important, especially for parents who have only parented when their child was sick and now must care for a child who is more active and mobile.
- Hand washing to prevent the spread of infections is critical. Eating utensils, cups, and glasses should not be shared.
- Avoid ill contacts and large groups of people while the child's immune system is suppressed.

- All medicines should be stored safely away from children and needles and syringes deposited in a sharps container.
- The child should have minimal direct contact with animals.
- Physical activity may be restricted in children with thrombocytopenia.
- Travel to developing countries is not advised. Travel away from the transplant center should be arranged with the knowledge of the transplant team.

Immunizations

- Most children lose their immunity to previously administered vaccines following HSCT. Reimmunization should begin 1 year after transplant if there is no evidence of graft-vs.-host disease (GVHD) and the child is not receiving steroids.
- Live-virus vaccines pose the risk of active disease.
- Influenza vaccine should be given annually to the child, all household or close contacts, and clinic and hospital personnel.

Screening

- *Vision.* An ophthalmologist familiar with sequelae of high-dose chemotherapy and radiation should be involved in care.
- Corticosteroid use can cause cataracts, cGVHD can result in keratoconjunctivitis, and cytomegalovirus (CMV) can cause retinitis.
- Vision should be screened at each primary care visit and referral made for visual changes or abnormalities.
- *Hearing.* Routine screening is advised. Hearing loss may occur as a result of ototoxic drug therapy.
- *Dental.* Dental screening and restorative care should be done before transplant to reduce potential sources of infection. Routine dental care should be resumed once the child's immune system is restored.
- *Blood pressure.* Blood pressure should be taken and recorded at each visit. Children are commonly placed on medication for hypertension after HSCT because of nephrotoxic medications. Parents may be instructed to record blood pressure at home.

Continued

Summary of Primary Care Needs for the Child with Bone Marrow Transplant—cont'd

- *Hematocrit.* Routine screening is resumed after the child is off all immunosuppressive therapy. Before this the child has frequent complete blood counts (CBCs) done by the transplant center so additional hematocrit testing is not necessary.
- *Urinalysis.* Routine screening is recommended. Abnormalities should be reported to the transplant team.
- *Tuberculosis.* Routine screening is recommended. Controls may need to be in place to determine immunocompetency.

Condition-Specific Screening

- Physical and laboratory analysis during the first year after HSCT is usually obtained by the transplant team.
- Screening for late complications needs to be done by the primary care provider (see Table 15-3).

COMMON ILLNESS MANAGEMENT

Differential Diagnosis

- *Infections.* When a child is immunocompromised, community-acquired respiratory infections can result in serious pneumonia.
- Children with central venous catheters (CVCs) or still taking immunosuppressants must have fever immediately evaluated for possible bacteremia. Initial evaluation of fever may be done by the primary care provider in conjunction with the transplant center if the child lives more than 1 hour from the transplant center.
- Rectal temperatures are not recommended.
- *Viral infections.* Herpes simplex virus (HSV), CMV, and varicella zoster virus (VZV) are common in children after HSCT.
- *Gastrointestinal symptoms.* Gastrointestinal symptoms may be caused by opportunistic infections or GVHD.
- *Headaches.* Headaches may be a symptom of serious complications in the immunocompromised child.
- *Pain.* Pain may be the result of prolonged bed rest and treatment side effects but also must be evaluated as a symptom associated with infection. Herpes zoster can cause neuropathy.

Drug Interactions

- Children are taking multiple drugs after HSCT, and additions of other medications have the potential to alter absorption or clearance of these medications, leading to possible organ toxicity or GVHD. New pharmacotherapy must be evaluated by the transplant team.
- Nonsteroidal antiinflammatory drugs (NSAIDs) are not recommended because they may interfere with platelet function.

DEVELOPMENTAL ISSUES

Sleep Patterns

- Disturbance in sleep patterns is associated with high doses of corticosteroids.
- TPN and supplemental intravenous fluids at night may interfere with sleep and increase nighttime voiding.

- Caffeine and other stimulants, including television and videos, should be avoided in the evening.
- Bedtime routines are encouraged.

Toileting

- Diarrhea can be a symptom of GVHD and affect normal toileting habits.
- Regression is common after a stressful hospitalization.

Discipline

- Family patterns of behavior and discipline are often well established before the child receives HSCT. Children have often had chronic life-threatening conditions for a long time before transplant intervention.
- Parents are encouraged to establish common discipline patterns for all children in the family.

Child Care

- In-home child care is recommended because of the risk of infection in other child-care settings.

Schooling

- In-hospital or in-home schooling is required after HSCT for 6 to 12 months until immune function has been obtained because of concern regarding infection exposure.
- An Individualized Educational Program (IEP) should be done yearly to identify learning problems. Fatigue may be an issue.
- There are no general limitations, and children are encouraged to participate fully in school activities.

Sexuality

- Many physical changes occur with treatment that may interfere with body image.
- Sex education is important, especially for infection control.
- The overwhelming majority of children are infertile after transplant, but birth control is advised.
- Oral sexual contact is discouraged until mucositis is completely healed.

Transition to Adulthood

- The development of independence is often difficult after prolonged illness and a life-threatening condition.
- Healthy life behaviors (e.g., good nutrition, regular exercise, no smoking) are important.

FAMILY CONCERNS

- There is very little information on long-term quality of life after HSCT, employment, relationships, and insurability.
- Individuals are protected under the Americans with Disabilities Act.

REFERENCES

American Academy of Pediatrics Committee on Infectious Diseases (2006). Immunocompromised children. In L.K. Pickering (Ed.), *Red Book:2006 Report of the Committee on Infectious Diseases.* Elk Grove Village, IL: American Academy of Pediatrics.

American Society of Health-System Pharmacists. (2008a). Anti-infective agents—antivirals. In *AHFS Drug Information* 2008 (pp. 803-844). Bethesda, MD: Author.

American Society of Health-System Pharmacists. (2008b). Hematopoietic agents—filgrastim. In *AHFS Drug Information 2008* (p. 1573). Bethesda, MD: Author.

American Society of Health-System Pharmacists. (2008c). Immunosuppressive agents—cyclosporine. In *AHFS Drug Information 2008* (p. 3762). Bethesda, MD: Author.

American Society of Health-System Pharmacists. (2008d). Immunosuppressive agents—tacrolimus. In *AHFS Drug Information 2008* (p. 3786). Bethesda, MD: Author.

Avivi, I., Chakrabarti, S., Milligan, D.W., et al. (2004). Incidence and outcome of adenovirus disease in transplant recipients after reduced-intensity conditioning with alemtuzumab. *Biol Blood Marrow Transplant, 10*(3), 186-194.

Barnes, J. (2003). Meeting the impact of the traditional herbal medicinal products directive: Conference organized by the British Institute of Regulatory Affairs, London, UK, January 2003. *Complementary Therapies in Medicine, 11*(2), 129-131.

Bhatia, M., & Walters, M.C. (2007). Hematopoietic cell transplantation for thalassemia and sickle cell disease: Past, present and future. *Bone Marrow Transplant, 41*(2), 109-117.

Boeckh, M., Fries, B., & Nichols, W.G. (2004). Recent advances in the prevention of CMV infection and disease after hematopoietic stem cell transplantation. *Pediatr Transplant, 8,* 19-27.

Bordigoni, P., Turello, R., Clement, L., et al. (2002). Osteochondroma after pediatric hematopoietic stem cell transplantation: Report of eight cases. *Bone Marrow Transplant, 29*(7), 611-614.

Carpenter, P.A., & Sanders, J.E. (2004). Late effects after hematopoietic cell transplantation. In P. Mehta (Ed.), *Pediatric stem cell transplantation,* Sudbury, MA: Jones & Bartlett.

Centers for Disease Control and Prevention, Infectious Disease Society of America, and the American Society of Blood and Marrow Transplantation (2000). Guidelines for preventing opportunistic infections among hematopoietic stem cell transplant recipients; recommendations of CDC. *Biol Blood Marrow Transplant, 6*(6a), 659-727.

Chakrabarti, S., Hale, G., & Waldmann, H. (2004). Alemtuzumab (Campath-1H) in allogeneic stem cell transplantation: Where do we go from here? *Transplant Proc, 36*(5), 1225-1227.

Chao, N.J., Emerson, S.G., & Weinberg, K.I. (2004). Stem cell transplantation (cord blood transplants). *Hematology, 2004,* 354-371.

Comoli, P., Basso, S., Labirio, M., et al. (2008). T cell therapy of Epstein-Barr virus and adenovirus infections after hemopoietic stem cell transplant. *Blood Cells, Molecules, and Diseases, 40*(1), 68-70.

Cooper, L.J. (2008). Adoptive cellular immunotherapy for childhood malignancies. *Bone Marrow Transplant, 41*(2), 183-192.

Cutler, C., & Antin, J.H. (2006). Chronic graft-versus-host disease. *Curr Opin Oncol, 18*(2), 126-131.

Dahllof, G., Hingorani, S.R.M., & Sanders, J.E. (2008). Late effects following hematopoietic cell transplantation for children. *Biol Blood Marrow Transplant, 14*(Suppl 1), 88-93.

Djulbegovic, B., Seidenfeld, J., Bonnell, C., et al. (2003). Nonmyeloablative allogeneic stem-cell transplantation for hematologic malignancies: A systematic review. *Cancer Control, 10*(1), 17-41.

Duggal, M.S. (2003). Root surface areas in long-term survivors of childhood cancer. *Oral Oncol, 39*(2), 178-183.

Dvorak, C.C., & Cowan, M.J. (2008). Hematopoietic stem cell transplantation for primary immunodeficiency disease. *Bone Marrow Transplant, 41*(2), 119-126.

Ferrara, J.L., & Antin, J. (2004). The pathophysiology of graft-vs.-host disease. In K.G. Blume, S.J. Forman, & F.R. Appelbaum (Eds.), *Thomas' hematopoietic cell transplantation,* Malden, MA: Blackwell.

Fish, J.D., & Grupp, S.A. (2008). Stem cell transplantation for neuroblastoma. *Bone Marrow Transplant, 41*(2), 159-165.

Foss, F.M., DiVenuti, G.M., Chin, K., et al. (2005). Prospective study of extracorporeal photopheresis in steroid-refractory or steroid-resistant extensive chronic graft-versus-host disease: Analysis of response and survival incorporating prognostic factors. *Bone Marrow Transplant, 35*(12), 1187-1193.

Franchimont, D. (2004). Overview of the actions of glucocorticoids on the immune response: A good model to characterize new pathways of immunosuppression for new treatment strategies. *Ann NY Acad Sci, 1024*(1), 124-137.

Gassas, A., Sung, L., Saunders, E.F., et al. (2007). Graft-versus-leukemia effect in hematopoietic stem cell transplantation for pediatric acute lymphoblastic leukemia: Significantly lower relapse rate in unrelated transplantations. *Bone Marrow Transplant, 40*(10), 951-955.

George, R.E., Li, S., Medeiros-Nancarrow, C., et al. (2006). High-risk neuroblastoma treated with tandem autologous peripheral-blood stem cell-supported transplantation: Long-term survival update. *J Clin Oncol, 24*(18), 2891-2896.

Georges, G.E., & Storb, R. (2003). Review of "minitransplantation": Nonmyeloablative allogeneic hematopoietic stem cell transplantation. *Int J Hematol, 77*(1), 3-14.

Gurney, J.G., Ness, K.K., Rosenthal, J., et al. (2006). Visual, auditory, sensory, and motor impairments in long-term survivors of hematopoietic stem cell transplantation performed in childhood. *Cancer, 106*(6), 1402-1408.

Hansen, J.A., Petersdorf, E.W., Lin, M.T., et al. (2007). Genetics of allogeneic hematopoietic cell transplantation. Role of HLA matching, functional variation in immune response genes. *Immunol Res,.* November 8, 2007 : (electronic publication).

Helbig, G., Stella-Holowiecka, B., Wojnar, J., et al. (2007). Pure red-cell aplasia following major and bi-directional ABO-incompatible allogeneic stem-cell transplantation: Recovery of donor-derived erythropoiesis after long-term treatment using different therapeutic strategies. *Ann Hematol, 86*(9), 677-683.

Higman, M.A., & Vogelsang, G.B. (2004). Chronic graft versus host disease. *Br J Haematol, 125*(4), 435-454.

Holmstrom, G., Borgstrom, B., & Calissendorff, B. (2002). Cataract in children after bone marrow transplantation: Relation to conditioning regimen. *Acta Ophthalmol Scand, 80*(2), 211-215.

Hsu, K.C., Keever-Taylor, C.A., Wilton, A., et al. (2005). Improved outcome in HLA-identical sibling hematopoietic stem-cell transplantation for acute myelogenous leukemia predicted by KIR and HLA genotypes. *Blood, 105*(12), 4878-4884.

Human Genome Project. (2007). Gene therapy. Available at: www.ornl.gov/hgmis. Retrieved January 5, 2008.

Iwasaki, T. (2004). Recent advances in the treatment of graft-versus-host disease. *Clin Med Res, 2*(4), 243-252.

Jacobsohn, D.A. (2007). Acute graft-versus-host disease in children. *Bone Marrow Transplant, 41*(2), 215-221.

Jaing, T.H., Yang, C.P., Hung, I.J., et al. (2007). Transplantation of unrelated donor umbilical cord blood utilizing double-unit grafts for five teenagers with transfusion-dependent thalassemia. *Bone Marrow Transplant, 40*(4), 307-311.

Jernberg, A.G., Remberger, M., Ringden, O., et al. (2003). Graft-versus-leukaemia effect in children: Chronic GVHD has a significant impact on relapse and survival. *Bone Marrow Transplant, 31*(3), 175-181.

Jernberg, A.G., Remberger, M., Ringden, O., et al. (2004). Risk factors in pediatric stem cell transplantation for leukemia. *Pediatr Transplant, 8*(5), 464-474.

Kauffman, C.A., & Carver, P.L. (2008). Update on echinocandin antifungals. *Semin Respir Crit Care Med, 2,* 211-219.

Kletzel, M., Jacobsohn, D., Tse, W., et al. (2005). Reduced intensity transplants (RIT) in pediatrics: A review. *Pediatr Transplant, 9,* 63-70.

Kohn, D.B. (2007). Gene therapy for childhood immunological diseases. *Bone Marrow Transplant, 41*(2), 199-205.

Laffan, A., & Biedrzycki, B. (2006). Immune reconstitution: The foundation for safe living after an allogeneic hematopoietic stem cell transplantation. *Clin J Oncol Nurs, 10*(6), 787-794.

Leiper, A.D. (2002a). Non-endocrine late complications of bone marrow transplantation in childhood: Part I. *Br J Haematol, 118*(1), 3-22.

Leiper, A.D. (2002b). Non-endocrine late complications of bone marrow transplantation in childhood: Part II. *Br J Haematol, 118*(1), 23-43.

Leung, W., Ahn, H., Rose, S.R., et al. (2007). A prospective cohort study of late sequelae of pediatric allogeneic hematopoietic stem cell transplantation. *Medicine, 86*(4), 215-224.

Levine, J.E., Harris, R.E., Loberiza, F.R. Jr., et al. (2003). A comparison of allogeneic and autologous bone marrow transplantation for lymphoblastic lymphoma. *Blood, 101*(7), 2476-2482.

Lipkin, A.C., Lenssen, P., & Dickson, B.J. (2005). Nutrition issues in hematopoietic stem cell transplantation: State of the art. *Nutr Clin Pract, 20*(4), 423-439.

Loren, A.W., & Porter, D.L. (2008). Donor leukocyte infusions for the treatment of relapsed acute leukemia after allogeneic stem cell transplantation. *Bone Marrow Transplant, 41*(5), 483-493.

Lowe, T., Bhatia, S., & Somlo, G. (2007). Second malignancies after allogeneic hematopoietic cell transplantation. *Biol Blood Marrow Transplant, 3*(10), 1121-1134.

Majhail, N.S., Brunstein, C.G., & Wagner, J.E. (2006). Double umbilical cord blood transplantation. *Curr Opin Immunol, 18*(5), 571-575.

Malani, A.N., & Kauffman, C.A. (2007). Changing epidemiology of rare mould infections: Implications for therapy. *Drugs, 67*(13), 1803-1812.

Marcus, K.J., Shamberger, R., Litman, H., et al. (2003). Primary tumor control in patients with stage 3/4 unfavorable neuroblastoma treated with tandem double autologous stem cell transplants. *J Pediatr Hematol Oncol, 25*(12), 934-940.

Martin, P. (2004). Overview of hematopoietic transplantation immunology. In K.G. Blume, S.J. Forman, & F.R. Appelbaum, (Eds.), *Thomas' Hematopoietic Cell Transplantation,* Malden, MA: Blackwell.

Mehta, P. (2004a). Graft-versus-host disease after stem cell transplantation in children. In P. Mehta (Ed.), *Pediatric Stem Cell Transplantation.* Sudbury, MA: Jones & Bartlett.

Miebach, E. (2005). Enzyme replacement therapy in mucopolysaccharidosis type I. *Acta Paediatr, 94*(Suppl 447), 58-60.

Moise, K.J. Jr. (2005). Umbilical cord stem cells. *Obstet Gynecol, 106*(6), 1393-1407.

Moog, R. (2006). Mobilization and harvesting of peripheral blood stem cells. *Curr Stem Cell Res Ther, 1*(2), 189-201.

Nagatoshi, Y., Kawano, Y., Watanabe, T., et al. (2002). Hematopoietic and immune recovery after allogeneic peripheral blood stem cell transplantation and bone marrow transplantation in a pediatric population. *Pediatr Transplant, 6*(4), 319-326.

National Marrow Donor Program. (2008). Outcomes and trends from the NMDP January 2008. Available at: www.marrow.org/PHYSICIAN/Outcomes_Data/index.html. Retrieved January 5, 2008.

Oeffinger, K.C., Nathan, P.C., & Kremer, L.C.M. (2008). Challenges after curative treatment for childhood cancer and long-term follow up of survivors. *Pediatr Clin North Am, 55*(1), 251-273.

Oktay, K. (2006). Spontaneous conceptions and live birth after heterotopic ovarian transplantation: Is there a germline stem cell connection?. *Hum Reprod, 21*(6), 1345-1348.

Orchard, P.J., Blazar, B.R., Wagner, J., et al. (2007). Hematopoietic cell therapy for metabolic disease. *J Pediatr, 151*(4), 340-346.

Pasquini, M., Wang, Z., & Schneider, L. (2007). Current use and outcome of hematopoietic stem cell transplantation: Part I—CIBMTR summary slides, 2007. *CIBMTR Newsletter, 13*(2), 5-9.

Perales, M.A., Ishill, N., & Lomazow, W.A., et al. (2007). Long-term follow-up of patients treated with daclizumab for steroid-refractory acute graft-vs-host disease. *Bone Marrow Transplant, 40*(5), 481-486.

Punnett, A., Bliss, B.B., Dupuis, L.L., et al. (2004). Ototoxicity following pediatric hematopoietic stem cell transplantation: A prospective cohort study. *Pediatr Blood Cancer, 42*(7), 598-603.

Ranke, M.B., Schwarze, C.P., Dopfer, R., et al. (2005). Late effects after stem cell transplantation (SCT) in children—growth and hormones. *Bone Marrow Transplant, 35*(Suppl 1), S77-S81.

Remberger, M., & Ringden, O. (2007). Similar outcome after unrelated allogeneic peripheral blood stem cell transplantation compared with bone marrow in children and adolescents. *Transplantation, 84*(4), 551-554.

Revel, A., & Revel-Vilk, S. (2008). Pediatric fertility preservation: Is it time to offer testicular tissue cryopreservation? *Mol Cell Endocrinol, 282*(1-2), 143-149.

Reynolds, C.P. (2004). Detection and treatment of minimal residual disease in high-risk neuroblastoma. *Pediatr Transplant, 8*, 56-66.

Riddell, S.R. (2008). The graft-versus-leukemia effect—breaking the black box open. *Biol Blood Marrow Transplant, 14*(Suppl 1), 2-3.

Sanders, J.E. (2008). Growth and development after hematopoietic cell transplant in children. *Bone Marrow Transplant, 41*(2), 223-227.

Satwani, P., Cooper, N., Rao, K., et al. (2008). Reduced intensity conditioning and allogeneic stem cell transplantation in childhood malignant and nonmalignant diseases. *Bone Marrow Transplant, 41*(2), 173-182.

Scarisbrick, J.J., Taylor, P., Holtick, U., et al. (2008). U.K. consensus statement on the use of extracorporeal photopheresis for treatment of cutaneous T-cell lymphoma and chronic graft-versus-host disease. *Br J Dermatol, 158*(4), 659-678.

Schubert, M.M., & Correa, M.E.P. (2008). Oral graft-versus-host disease. *Dent Clin North Am, 52*(1), 79-109.

Seidel, M.G., Fritsch, G., Matthes-Martin, S., et al. (2005). In vitro and in vivo T-cell depletion with myeloablative or reduced-intensity conditioning in pediatric hematopoietic stem cell transplantation. *Haematologica, 90*(10), 1405-1414.

Sepkowitz, K.A. (2002). Antibiotic prophylaxis in patients receiving hematopoietic stem cell transplant. *Bone Marrow Transplant, 29*(5), 367.

Shah, A.J., Kapoor, N., Weinberg, K.I., et al. (2002). Second hematopoietic stem cell transplantation in pediatric patients: Overall survival and long-term follow-up. *Biol Blood Marrow Transplant, 8*(4), 221-228.

Strasfeld, L., & Weinstock, D.M. (2006). Antifungal prophylaxis among allogeneic hematopoietic stem cell transplant recipients: Current issues and new agents. *Expert Review of Anti-infective Therapy, 4*(3), 457-468.

Teachey, D.T., Bickert, B., & Bunin, N. (2005). Daclizumab for children with corticosteroid refractory graft-versus-host disease. *Bone Marrow Transplant, 37*(1), 95-99.

Urbano-Ispizua, A. (2007). Risk assessment in haematopoietic stem cell transplantation: Stem cell source. *Best Practice Res Clin Haematol, 20*(2), 265-280.

Varkey, J.B., & Perfect, J.R. (2008). Rare and emerging fungal pulmonary infections. *Semin Respir Crit Care Med, 29*(2), 121-131.

Weisdorf, D., Bishop, M., Dharan, B., et al. (2002). Autologous versus allogeneic unrelated donor transplantation for acute lymphoblastic leukemia: Comparative toxicity and outcomes. *Biol Blood Marrow Transplant, 8*(4), 213-220.

Westgren, M. (2006). In utero stem cell transplantation. *Semin Reprod Med, 24*, 348-357.

Wingard, J.R. (2005). The changing face of invasive fungal infections in hematopoietic cell transplant recipients. *Curr Opin Oncol, 17*, 89-92.

Wingard, J.R., & Anaissie, E. (2004). Infectious complications after hematopoietic cell transplantation. In P. Mehta (Ed.), *Pediatric stem cell transplantation,* Sudbury, MA: Jones & Bartlett.

Wingard, J.R., Vogelsang, G.B., & Deeg, H.J. (2002). Stem cell transplantation: Supportive care and long-term complications. *Hematology, 2002*(1), 422-444.

Yanada, M., Emi, N., & Naoe, T., et al. (2004). Tacrolimus instead of cyclosporine used for prophylaxis against graft-versus-host disease improves outcome after hematopoietic stem cell transplantation from unrelated donors, but not from HLA-identical sibling donors: A nationwide survey conducted in Japan. *Bone Marrow Transplant, 34*(4), 331-337.

Zecca, M., Prete, A., & Rondelli, R., et al. (2002). Chronic graft-versus-host disease in children: Incidence, risk factors, and impact on outcome. *Blood, 100*(4), 1192-1200.

Zonios, D.I., & Bennett, J.E. (2008). Update on azole antifungals. *Semin Respir Crit Care Med, 29*(2), 198-210.

16 Cancer

Christina Baggott

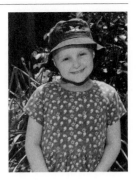

Etiology

An estimated 10,400 children and adolescents under age 14 years are diagnosed with cancer annually in the United States (American Cancer Society, 2007). Cancer results when the body fails to regulate cell production. A proliferation and spread of abnormal cells then occur, which—if left unchecked—may lead to death of the host. Common sites of malignancy in children include the blood and bone marrow, bone, lymph nodes, brain and central nervous system (CNS), kidneys, and soft tissues (Table 16-1).

Although particular genetic factors or environmental exposures are known to place children at risk of developing cancer (as outlined in Table 16-1), the specific etiology of childhood cancer is yet to be identified. The genes associated with many pediatric tumors have been discovered, and scientists are making progress in applying this knowledge to successful therapies (Kim & Hahn, 2007). Researchers are studying the deoxyribonucleic acid (DNA) point mutations, carcinogen-metabolizing enzymes, DNA repair enzymes, signal transduction, viral insertions and gene amplifications, deletions, or gene rearrangements to gain an understanding of the process of malignant transformation (Anderson, 2006; Corey, 2005; Kim & Hahn, 2007; Knudson, 2002; Mullighan, Goorha, Radtke, et al., 2007).

Incidence and Prevalence

The overall incidence of malignancy in children under 20 years of age is approximately 16.7:100,000 per year (Ries, Melbert, Krapcho, et al., 2008). Leukemia and CNS tumors account for the majority of pediatric malignancies. A comparison of the incidence of the various childhood malignancies in the United States (see Table 16-1) illustrates a wide variation depending on site. Childhood cancer incidence also varies by race. White children have the highest rates of childhood cancer, followed by Hispanic children, Asian/Pacific Islander children, and black children. American Indians have the lowest rate of childhood cancer (Ries et al., 2008).

Diagnostic Criteria

Prompt referral to a pediatric cancer treatment center ensures that specimens for staging are properly obtained and the child is enrolled in multiinstitutional treatment studies (Corrigan & Feig, 2004). The initial workup is crucial to the accurate and timely establishment of a diagnosis and treatment. A review of the studies of diagnosis delays in pediatric oncology found that age, parental level of education, type of cancer, and first medical specialty consulted were among the factors affecting the time between a child's presentation of symptoms and the diagnosis of cancer. Older children and those with bone tumors and brain tumors had much longer lag times than young children and those with other tumors (Dang-Tan & Franco, 2007). After a thorough history and physical examination and laboratory tests, the workup may include nuclear-radiologic examinations, ultrasound, bone marrow aspirate, bone marrow biopsy, or lumbar puncture, depending on the type of tumor suspected and the most frequent sites of metastases.

Whenever a biopsy is being considered, the primary care provider should consult an oncology treatment center before proceeding. Accurate staging increasingly depends on molecular genetics and the immunocytochemistry of initial diagnostic materials processed in specialty laboratories.

Clinical Manifestations at Time of Diagnosis

The signs and symptoms of a malignant disease depend on the interval between time of origin and diagnosis, as well as the type and location of the tumor. In general, cancer may manifest in one of the following three ways: (1) as a mass lesion, (2) with symptoms directly related to the tumor, or (3) with nonspecific symptoms. The presence of a mass lesion should alert the primary care provider to the possibility of a malignancy after benign conditions (e.g., constipation, a distended bladder) have been ruled out (Malogolowkin, Quinn, Steuber, et al., 2006). A biopsy of other lesions should be taken in a timely manner to rule out malignancy. Symptoms related directly to the tumor may include bone pain, limping, unexplained

> ### Clinical Manifestations at Time of Diagnosis
>
> - Mass lesion, particularly in abdomen
> - Lymph node enlargement that is unresponsive to antibiotic therapy or accompanied by nonspecific symptoms
> - Unexplained bruising, bleeding, or petechiae
> - Pallor and fatigue
> - Unexplained or persistent fevers
> - Recurrent infection
> - Bone pain or limping
> - Morning headache with vomiting
> - Swelling in the face or neck
> - White spot in pupil (leukokoria)
> - Hematuria
> - Airway or urinary tract obstruction
> - Nonspecific symptoms: weight loss, diarrhea, failure to thrive, malaise, low-grade fevers

TABLE 16-1

Common Pediatric Cancers

Type	Site	Incidence (Ages 0-14 yr)	Etiology	Signs/Symptoms	Treatment
LEUKEMIA	Bone marrow	4.1 per 100,000 children per year	*For ALL and AML:* Genetic factors Chromosomal abnormalities (trisomy 21, Bloom syndrome, Fanconi anemia, AT) Familial predisposition (ALL: infant identical twins)	*For ALL and AML:* Pallor Fatigue, headache Fever, infection Purpura, bruising Organomegaly Bone pain	Combination chemotherapy CNS prophylaxis Radiation therapy (for high-risk cases)
Acute lymphoblastic leukemia (ALL)			Environmental factors Ionizing radiation Chronic chemical exposure Use of alkylating agents for treatment of malignant disease (AML)		Intrathecal chemotherapy Combination chemotherapy CNS prophylaxis
Acute myelogenous leukemia (AML)			Possible viral infection		Single-agent intrathecal chemotherapy HSCT in first remission
CENTRAL NERVOUS SYSTEM		2.9 per 100,000 children per year	*For all CNS cancers:* Genetic factors Heritable disease (NF, VHL, LFS) Familial	*Early:* Decreased academic performance Fatigue Personality changes Intermittent headache	Anticonvulsants, if symptoms present Treatment of hydrocephalus Corticosteroids
Infratentorial Medulloblastoma	Cerebellum/brainstem Midline cerebellar		Environmental factors Chronic chemical exposure Ionizing radiation	*Late:* Morning headache Vomiting	Shunting Surgical resection (if operable) Radiation therapy
Ependymoma	Ependymal lining of ventricular system or central canal of spinal cord		Other primary malignancies Exogenous immunosuppression	Diplopia/visual changes Brainstem/cerebellar Deficits of balance/positioning	Chemotherapy for some tumors HSCT in rare cases
Brainstem glioma	Brainstem				
Supratentorial Astrocytomas	Ventricles, midline diencephalus, cerebrum			*Supratentorial:* Nonspecific headache Seizures Hemiparesis	
Craniopharyngioma	Sella turcica				
Gliomas	Visual pathway				
Pineoblastoma or germ cell tumors	Pineal region				

Type	Primary site	Incidence	Etiology/Risk factors	Clinical manifestations	Treatment
NON-HODGKIN LYMPHOMA					
Lymphoblastic lymphoma	Usually generalized Anterior mediastinum Lymph nodes Bone marrow	1.1 per 100,000 children per year	*For all non-Hodgkin lymphomas:* Immunodeficiency (HIV) Exogenous immunosuppression Viral: associated with Epstein-Barr virus	Generally rapid progression Dysphagia, dyspnea Swelling of neck, face, upper extremities Supradiaphragmatic lymphadenopathy Respiratory distress	Treatment of emergent symptoms Multiagent chemotherapy CNS prophylaxis
Small noncleaved lymphoma, Burkitt lymphoma, non-Burkitt lymphoma	Abdomen Bone marrow Lymph nodes			Abdominal pain or swelling Change in bowel habits Nausea/vomiting GI bleeding Intestinal perforation (rarely) Inguinal/iliac adenopathy Intussusception	Treatment of emergent symptoms and tumor lysis syndrome Multiagent chemotherapy CNS prophylaxis Multiagent chemotherapy
Large cell lymphoma	Lymph nodes Cutaneous lesions Mediastinum Abdomen Head, neck			As cited earlier, depending on site	
HODGKIN LYMPHOMA	Single lymph nodes or lymphatic chains Mediastinal mass Spleen	1.2 per 100,000 children per year	Genetic factors Familial predisposition Environmental influence Iatrogenic or acquired immunodeficiency (HIV, AT) Infectious etiology (Epstein-Barr virus)	Lymphadenopathy Organomegaly Fatigue Anorexia/weight loss/fever	Splenectomy, if surgical staging Multiagent chemotherapy Radiation therapy
NEUROBLASTOMA	Anywhere along the sympathetic nervous system chain Most commonly Abdomen Adrenal gland Paraspinal ganglion Thorax Neck	0.8 per 100,000 children per year	Genetic factors Autosomal dominant inherited predisposition in some children Familial predisposition Associated with fetal alcohol syndrome and fetal hydantoin syndrome	Dependent on primary site, site of metastases Metastases present in 70% of cases at diagnosis (especially in bone marrow) Presence of a mass (abdomen, thoracic, cervical, pelvic, liver) Symptoms from compression of mass (Horner syndrome, edema of upper and lower extremities secondary to vascular compression, hypertension caused by compression of renal vasculature, cord compression symptoms [paresis, paralysis, bowel/bladder dysfunction]) Diarrhea from vasoactive intestinal peptides produced by tumor cells Skin or subcutaneous nodules (infants only) Nonspecific symptoms (fever, weight loss, failure to thrive, generalized pain) Rarely syndrome of opsoclonus-myoclonus	Treatment of emergent symptoms Surgery (staging excision of tumor, evaluation of treatment) Radiation therapy Combination chemotherapy HSCT in some cases

Continued

Key: *AT,* ataxia telangiectasia; *CNS,* central nervous system; *GI,* gastrointestinal; *HIV,* human immunodeficiency virus; *HSCT,* hematopoietic stem cell transplantation; *LFS,* Li-Fraumeni syndrome; *NF,* neurofibromatosis; *VHL,* von Hippel-Lindau syndrome.

TABLE 16-1

Common Pediatric Cancers—cont'd

Type	Site	Incidence (Ages 0-14 yr)	Etiology	Signs/Symptoms	Treatment
SOFT TISSUE SARCOMAS					*For both sarcomas:*
Rhabdomyosarcoma	Head and neck (most common)	1.2 per 100,000 children per year	Genetic factors	*For both sarcomas:* Dependent on location and size of tumor	Surgical removal (if feasible)
Undifferentiated sarcoma	Abdomen		Associated with NF, LFS, Beckwith-Wiedemann syndrome		Radiation therapy for residual tumor
	Anywhere in body		Environmental factors		Multiagent systemic chemotherapy
			Parental use of recreational drugs		
			Possible viral etiology		
KIDNEY					
Wilms' tumor (nephroblastoma, renal embryoma)	Unilateral, bilateral	0.7 per 100,000 children per year	Genetic factors	Asymptomatic mass	Complete surgical excision (if bilateral, nephrectomy of more involved site, excisional biopsy/partial nephrectomy of smaller lesion in remaining kidney)
			Associated with aniridia, NF, Beckwith-Wiedemann syndrome, hemihypertrophy, Denys-Drash syndrome	Malaise, pain	Multiagent chemotherapy
			Familial predisposition	Microscopic or gross hematuria	Radiation therapy for high-risk tumors
			Environmental factors	Hypertension	
			Long-term chemical exposure (hydrocarbons/lead)		
BONE TUMORS					
Osteosarcoma	Long bones of extremities	0.8 per 100,000 children per year	Genetic factors	Pain over involved area with or without swelling (often 3-5 mo or longer)	Multiagent chemotherapy
			Familial predisposition (hereditary retinoblastoma)		Surgical excision of tumor with limb salvage or amputation if extent of disease or location does not allow complete excision
			Environmental factors		
			Ionizing radiation		
			Use of alkylating agents		
Ewing sarcoma	Bones of the extremities and central axis		Possible genetic factors	In presence of metastatic disease nonspecific symptoms (fatigue, anorexia, weight loss, intermittent fever, malaise)	Localized radiation therapy or surgical excision
			No strong or consistent association with constitution of chromosomal abnormalities or congenital diseases		Multiagent chemotherapy
RETINOBLASTOMA					
	Eye	0.3 per 100,000 per year	Genetic factors	Leukokoria (cat's eye reflex)	Surgery (resection, enucleation with extensive disease; salvage of one eye attempted in bilateral disease)
			Gene mutation (nonhereditary)	Squint	Radiation therapy
			Autosomal dominant (all bilateral retinoblastomas and 15% of unilateral)	Strabismus	Chemotherapy (usually palliative)
				Orbital inflammation	Cryotherapy
					Laser photocoagulation

Data from Ries, L.A., et al. (Eds.). (2007). *Incidence data from SEER cancer statistics review, 1975-2004.* Bethesda, MD: National Cancer Institute. Available at: http://seer.cancer.gov/csr/1975_2004/. Additional resources: Bernstein, M., Kovar, H., Paulussen, M., et al. (2006). Ewing sarcoma family of tumors: Ewing sarcoma of bone and soft tissue and the peripheral primitive neuroectodermal tumors. In P.A. Pizzo & D.G. Poplack (Eds.), *Principles and practice of pediatric oncology* (5th ed.). Philadelphia: Lippincott Williams & Wilkins. Blaney, S.M., Kun, L.E., Hunter, J., et al. (2006). Tumors of the central nervous system. In P.A. Pizzo & D.G. Poplack (Eds.), *Principles and practice of pediatric oncology* (5th ed.). Philadelphia: Lippincott Williams & Wilkins. Brodeur, G.M. & Maris, J.M. (2006). Neuroblastoma. In P.A. Pizzo & D.G. Poplack (Eds.), *Principles and practice of pediatric oncology* (5th ed.). Philadelphia: Lippincott Williams & Wilkins. Dome, J.S., Perlman, E.J., Ritchey, M.L., et al. (2006). Renal tumors. In P.A. Pizzo & D.G. Poplack (Eds.), *Principles and practice of pediatric oncology* (5th ed.). Philadelphia: Lippincott Williams & Wilkins. Golub, T.R., & Arceci, R.J. (2006). Acute myelogenous leukemia. In P.A. Pizzo & D.G. Poplack (Eds.), *Principles and practice of pediatric oncology* (5th ed.). Philadelphia: Lippincott Williams & Wilkins. Hudson, M.M., Onciu, M., & Donaldson, S.S. (2006). Hodgkin lymphoma. In P.A. Pizzo & D.G. Poplack (Eds.), *Principles and practice of pediatric oncology* (5th ed.). Philadelphia: Lippincott Williams & Wilkins. Hurwitz, R.L., Shields, C.L., Shields, J.A., et al. (2006). Retinoblastoma. In P.A. Pizzo & D.G. Poplack (Eds.), *Principles and practice of pediatric oncology* (5th ed.). Philadelphia: Lippincott Williams & Wilkins. Link, M.P., Gebhardt, M.C., & Meyers, P.A. (2006). Osteosarcoma. In P.A. Pizzo & D.G. Poplack (Eds.), *Principles and practice of pediatric oncology* (5th ed.). Philadelphia: Lippincott Williams & Wilkins. Link, M.P., & Weinstein, H.J. (2006). Malignant non-Hodgkin lymphomas in children. In P.A. Pizzo & D.G. Poplack (Eds.), *Principles and practice of pediatric oncology* (5th ed.). Philadelphia: Lippincott Williams & Wilkins. Margolin, J.F., Steuber, C.P., & Poplack, D.G. (2006). Acute lymphoblastic leukemia. In P.A. Pizzo & D.G. Poplack (Eds.), *Principles and practice of pediatric oncology* (5th ed.). Philadelphia: Lippincott Williams & Wilkins. Wexler, L.H., Meyer, W.H., & Helman, L.J. (2006). Rhabdomyosarcoma and the undifferentiated sarcomas. In P.A. Pizzo & D.G. Poplack (Eds.), *Principles and practice of pediatric oncology* (5th ed.). Philadelphia: Lippincott Williams & Wilkins.

bleeding, bruising or petechiae, morning headache and vomiting, hematuria, pallor, swelling of the face or neck, a white spot in a pupil (leukokoria), airway or urinary tract obstruction, or endocrinologic symptoms from hormone production by the tumor. Nonspecific symptoms include weight loss, diarrhea, low-grade fevers, malaise, or failure to thrive.

Treatment

Cancer treatment involves the concurrent or sequential use of surgery, chemotherapy, radiation therapy, hematopoietic stem cell transplantation, and immunotherapy. State-of-the-art treatment is provided by multiinstitutional cooperative study groups and some specialty cancer treatment centers. These centers generally employ a multidisciplinary approach combining the expertise of nurses, physicians, advanced practice nurses, nutritionists, social workers, art and child life therapists, and other specialists. More than 90% of children younger than 15 years with cancer in the United States are treated at institutions participating in National Cancer Institute (NCI)–sponsored clinical trials (Bleyer, 2002). In 2000, the Children's Oncology Group (COG) was formed from a merger of four pediatric clinical trial cooperative groups (the Children's Cancer Group, the Pediatric Oncology Group, the National Wilms Tumor Study Group, and the Intergroup Rhabdomyosarcoma Study Group). Children under 15 years of age were equally represented in these groups regardless of race (Liu, Krailo, Reaman, et al., 2003). Nurses have actively contributed to advancements in pediatric oncology through these cooperative groups (Ruccione, Hinds, Wallace, et al., 2005).

> *Treatment*
> - National Cancer Institute clinical trials
> - Surgery
>   - Biopsy
>   - Resection
>   - Palliation
> - Chemotherapy
> - Radiation therapy
> - Immunotherapy
> - Hematopoietic stem cell transplantation

Only 20% of adolescents ages 15 to 19 years, however, are treated at institutions offering clinical trials sponsored by the NCI, and only 10% are registered in clinical trials (Bleyer, 2002). Adolescents' lack of equal access to national clinical trials requires further analysis of the effect on survival and quality of life. Although at times adolescents with cancer may be referred to adult oncologists, adolescents treated in pediatric clinical trials showed improved survival over those treated with adult treatment regimens (Boissel, Auclerc, Lheritier, et al., 2003; de Bont, Holt, Dekker, et al., 2004; Ramanujachar, Richards, Hann, et al., 2006).

A child's treatment protocol, determined by the type of cancer and the extent of disease, consists of a schedule and combination of therapies shown to be effective in treating the condition. A particular disease protocol may have several treatment regimens ("arms"), which are based on an accepted standard treatment with slight variations. Because no protocol regimen is known to be more effective than another, ongoing research investigates various therapies that

maximize treatment efficacy while minimizing toxicity. Before a child is assigned to a particular protocol, informed consent is obtained from the parents and, if appropriate, the child. If a child is treated on a research protocol, the family may elect to withdraw the child from the study at any time and have the child treated according to standard therapy.

Surgery

Surgical intervention is used to (1) obtain a biopsy specimen; (2) determine the extent of disease; (3) remove primary or metastatic lesions; (4) evaluate previously unresectable tumors; (5) provide a "second look" to evaluate the effects of chemotherapy and radiation on partially or nonresected tumors; and (6) relieve symptoms. Surgical procedures are also used to place indwelling venous access devices and to displace organs outside the radiation field (e.g., ovaries during pelvic irradiation).

Chemotherapy

The goal of chemotherapy is to interrupt the cell cycle of proliferating malignant cells while minimizing the damage to normal cells. In combination chemotherapy, different drugs are used to disrupt the cell cycle at different phases, increasing the exposure of the malignant cells to cytotoxic agents. The route of chemotherapy administration includes oral, intramuscular, intravenous, intrathecal, and intraventricular routes. Although most intravenous infusions have traditionally been administered in the hospital setting, certain agents lend themselves to safe administration in the home (Frierdich, Goes, & Dadd, 2003; Lashlee & O'Hanlon Curry, 2007; Stevens, McKeever, Law, et al., 2006). Eligibility for home infusion often depends on stable utilities in the home, parental reliability, and few side effects during an in-hospital trial of the agent.

Chemotherapeutic agents may be either cycle phase specific or nonspecific. Cell cycle–specific drugs kill cells only in a certain stage of the cell's development and are most effective on rapidly growing cells. Along with malignant cells, the cells of the bone marrow, hair follicles, and intestinal epithelium are susceptible to damage from these drugs. Cell cycle–nonspecific drugs kill cells regardless of their stage of development. They act on both dormant and dividing cells. Chemotherapeutic agents are further classified by their mechanism of action. The major classifications include alkylating agents, antimetabolites, vinca alkaloids, antibiotics, and corticosteroids. Side effects and toxicities vary depending on the specific agent (Table 16-2).

Radiation Therapy

Radiation therapy is often used in conjunction with surgery and chemotherapy. Radiation causes breakage of DNA strands, thus inhibiting cell division. The goal of radiation therapy is to destroy the cancer cells while minimizing complications and long-term sequelae. External beam radiotherapy is the most common delivery method for radiation treatments. Radiation therapy may also be given by brachytherapy (radiation implants placed near the tumor). Generally the surgery is used to place the implants, but they may also be placed in body cavities, such as the vagina. The role of radiation therapy may be definitive, adjunctive, or palliative. Definitive treatment is given with curative intent to a tumor on which a biopsy has been performed or that has been partially resected. In adjunctive radiotherapy, a primary tumor—although totally resected—is at risk for a local recurrence. This area is then treated

Text continued on p. 294

TABLE 16-2

Summary of Chemotherapeutic Agents Used in the Treatment of Childhood Cancers*

Agent/Administration	Side Effects and Toxicity	Comments and Specific Nursing Considerations
ALKYLATING AGENTS	All alkylating agents: Azoospermia, ovarian failure Secondary malignancy (AML)	Sperm banking, egg donation, if feasible
Mechlorethamine (nitrogen mustard, Mustargen) IV	N/V Myelosuppression Alopecia Local phlebitis Mucositis	Vesicant†
Cyclophosphamide (Cytoxan, CTX) PO, IV	N/V Myelosuppression Alopecia Hemorrhagic cystitis Stomatitis (rare) Cardiac toxicity (high dose) Pulmonary fibrosis (high dose) Syndrome of inappropriate secretion of antidiuretic hormone (SIADH)	Give dose early in day to allow adequate fluids afterward Force fluids before administering drug and for 2 days after to prevent chemical cystitis; encourage frequent voiding even during night Warn parents to report signs of burning on urination or hematuria Mesna given with high doses to protect bladder Mesna causes false ketonuria
Ifosfamide (IFEX) IV	N/V Myelosuppression Alopecia Renal tubular damage (Fanconi-like syndrome) Hemorrhagic cystitis Peripheral neuropathy Encephalopathy	See Cyclophosphamide above Mesna given with all doses to protect the bladder
Busulfan (Myleran) PO	N/V Myelosuppression Excessive dryness of skin and mucous membranes Gynecomastia (rare) Pulmonary fibrosis (long-term therapy) Seizures at high doses	Pulmonary function tests
Melphalan (Alkeran, L-PAM) PO, IV	Myelosuppression N/V Mucositis Diarrhea Alopecia Hypersensitivity reaction Pulmonary fibrosis	Take PO on empty stomach Hydrate well for 24 hr after dose
Procarbazine (Matulane) PO	N/V Myelosuppression Lethargy Dermatitis Myalgia Arthralgia Stomatitis Neuropathy Alopecia Diarrhea Amenorrhea	CNS depressants (phenothiazines, barbiturates) enhance CNS symptoms Monoamine oxidase (MAO) inhibition sometimes occurs; therefore all other drugs are avoided unless medically approved; red wine, fava beans, broad bean pods, tea, coffee, cola, cheese, bananas are to be avoided Give medication in evening to reduce nausea
Dacarbazine (DTIC) IV	N/V Myelosuppression Alopecia Flulike syndrome Burning sensation in vein during infusion (not extravasation)	Vesicant (less sclerosive) Must be given cautiously in individuals with renal dysfunction Decrease IV rate or use cold pack on IV site to decrease burning

Data from Ettinger, A., Bond, A., & Sievers, T.D. (2002). Chemotherapy. In C.R. Baggott, K.P. Kelly, & D. Fochtman (Eds.), *Nursing Care of Children and Adolescents with Cancer* (3rd ed.). Philadelphia: Saunders, pp. 133-176; Adamson, P.C., Balis, F.M., Berg, S., et al. (2006). General principles of chemotherapy. In P.A. Pizzo & D.G. Poplack (Eds.), *Principles and Practice of Pediatric Oncology* (5th ed.). Philadelphia: Lippincott Williams & Wilkins, pp. 290-365.

Key: *AML,* acute myelogenous leukemia; *BUN,* blood urea nitrogen; *CNS,* central nervous system; *ECG,* electrocardiogram; *IM,* intramuscularly; *IT,* intrathecally; *IV,* intravenously; *N/V,* nausea and vomiting; *PO,* orally; *PT,* prothrombin time; *PTT,* partial thromboplastin time; *PVC,* polyvinylchloride; *SQ,* subcutaneously.

*Table includes principal drugs used in the treatment of childhood cancers. Other chemotherapeutic agents may be employed in treatment regimens.

†Vesicants (sclerosing agents) can cause severe cellular damage if even minute amounts of the drug infiltrate surrounding tissue. These drugs must be given through a free-flowing IV line. The infusion is stopped *immediately* if any sign of infiltration (pain, stinging, swelling, or redness at needle site) occurs. Additional interventions for extravasation vary.

TABLE 16-2

Summary of Chemotherapeutic Agents Used in the Treatment of Childhood Cancers—cont'd

Agent/Administration	Side Effects and Toxicity	Comments and Specific Nursing Considerations
ALKYLATING AGENTS—cont'd		
Carmustine (BCNU) IV	N/V Myelosuppression Burning pain along IV infusion (usually from alcohol diluent) Flushing and facial burning on pulmonary infiltration or fibrosis	Prevent extravasation; contact with skin causes brown spots Reduce IV burning by diluting drug and infusing slowly via IV drip Crosses blood-brain barrier Check pulmonary function tests
Lomustine (CCNU) PO	N/V Myelosuppression Pulmonary infiltrates or fibrosis (but more common with carmustine)	Oral form: Give on empty stomach Crosses blood-brain barrier Check pulmonary function tests
ANTIMETABOLITES		
Cytarabine (Ara-C, Cytosar, cytosine arabinoside) IV, IM, SQ, IT	N/V Myelosuppression Mucosal ulceration Hepatitis (usually subclinical) Conjunctivitis (high dose) Ara-C syndrome: fever, myalgia, malaise, rash 6-12 hr after administration Neurotoxicity with high doses	Crosses blood-brain barrier Use with caution in individuals with hepatic dysfunction Corticosteroid ophthalmic drops to prevent conjunctivitis
Mercaptopurine (6-MP, Purinethol) PO, IV	N/V Stomatitis Myelosuppression Dermatitis Elevated liver enzymes	6-MP is an analog of xanthine; therefore allopurinol (Zyloprim) delays its metabolism and increases its potency, necessitating a lower dose (1/3 to 1/4) of 6-MP
Methotrexate (MTX, amethopterin) PO, IV, IM, SC IT; may be given in conventional doses (mg/m^2) or high doses (g/m^2)	N/V Diarrhea Mucosal ulceration (2-5 days later) Myelosuppression Dermatitis Photosensitivity Alopecia Hepatitis (fibrosis) Elevated liver enzymes Nephropathy Pneumonitis (fibrosis) Neurologic toxicity with high doses and IT use— arachnoiditis, leukoencephalopathy, seizures	Side effects and toxicity are dose related Potency and toxicity increased by reduced renal function, salicylates, sulfonamides; avoid use of aspirin and ibuprofen High-dose therapy Citrovorum factor (folinic acid or leucovorin) decreases cytotoxic action of MTX; used as an antidote for overdose and to enhance normal cell recovery following high-dose therapy; avoid use of vitamins containing folic acid during MTX therapy unless prescribed by physician IT therapy Drug *must* be mixed with preservative-free diluent Report signs of neurotoxicity immediately
Thioguanine (6-TG) PO	N/V Myelosuppression Stomatitis Dermatitis Liver dysfunction	Side effects unusual
5-Fluorouracil (5-FU, fluorouracil) IV	N/V Myelosuppression Dermatitis Stomatitis	Take at least 2 hr before or after food
PLANT ALKALOIDS		
Vincristine (Oncovin, VCR) IV	Neurotoxicity—paresthesia (numbness) ataxia, weakness, footdrop, hyporeflexia, constipation (adynamic ileus), hoarseness (vocal cord paralysis); abdominal, chest, and jaw pain Fever Myelosuppression Alopecia SIADH	Vesicant Report signs of neurotoxicity because this may necessitate cessation of drug Individuals with underlying neurologic problems may be more prone to neurotoxicity Monitor stool patterns closely; administer stool softener Excreted primarily by liver into biliary system; check bilirubin before administration

Continued

TABLE 16-2

Summary of Chemotherapeutic Agents Used in the Treatment of Childhood Cancers—cont'd

Agent/Administration	Side Effects and Toxicity	Comments and Specific Nursing Considerations
PLANT ALKALOIDS—cont'd		
Irinotecan IV	Diarrhea Myelosuppression Diaphoresis Abdominal cramping N/V Alopecia Malaise Electrolyte abnormalities	Atropine or loperamide for treatment of diarrhea
Vinblastine (Velban) IV	Neurotoxicity (same as for vincristine but less severe) N/V (rare) Myelosuppression Alopecia	Same as for vincristine
Etoposide, (VP-16, Ve-Pesid) PO, IV	N/V Myelosuppression Alopecia Hypotension with rapid infusion Diarrhea May reactivate erythema of irradiated skin (rare) Allergic reaction with anaphylaxis possible Secondary malignancy (AML)	Give slowly via IV drip over at least 1 hr with child recumbent Have emergency drugs available at bedside‡ Vital signs with blood pressure every 15 min during infusion
Teniposide (VM-26) IV	Myelosuppression Alopecia N/V Hypotension with rapid infusion Mild neurotoxicity Hypersensitivity reaction with anaphylaxis possible	Irritant Have emergency drugs available at bedside
Paclitaxel (Taxol) IV	Myelosuppression N/V during infusion "Stocking-glove" peripheral neuropathy Mucositis Bradycardia Alopecia	Monitor frequently Premedicate with corticosteroids and antihistamines Avoid PVC bags and tubing
ANTIBIOTICS		
Dactinomycin (actinomycin D, Cosmegen, ACT-D) IV	N/V Myelosuppression Mucosal ulceration Diarrhea Anorexia (may last few weeks) Alopecia Erythema or hyperpigmentation of previously irradiated skin Fever Malaise Hepatic (venooclusive disease)	Vesicant Enhances cytotoxic effects of radiation therapy but increases toxic effects May cause serious desquamation of irradiated tissue
Doxorubicin (Adriamycin, ADR), IV	N/V Stomatitis Myelosuppression Local phlebitis Alopecia Cumulative-dose toxicity includes the following: 　Cardiac abnormalities 　ECG changes 　Heart failure 　Secondary malignancy (AML) when used in high doses with cyclophosphamide	Vesicant (extravasation may *not* cause pain) Use only sterile distilled water as diluent Observe for any changes in heart rate or rhythm and signs of failure; follow echocardiogram or multiple gated acquisition (MUGA) scan Recommended cumulative lifetime dose: 450 mg/m² Warn parents that drug causes urine to turn red (for up to 12 days after administration); this is normal, not hematuria
Daunomycin (Cerubidine, daunorubicin) IV	Similar to doxorubicin	Similar to doxorubicin May tolerate slightly higher cumulative lifetime dose

‡Emergency drugs include oxygen and parenteral preparations of epinephrine 1:1000, diphenhydramine or similar antihistamine, aminophylline, corticosteroids, and vasopressors.

TABLE 16-2

Summary of Chemotherapeutic Agents Used in the Treatment of Childhood Cancers—cont'd

Agent/Administration	Side Effects and Toxicity	Comments and Specific Nursing Considerations
ANTIBIOTICS—cont'd		

Bleomycin (Blenoxane) IV, IM, SQ	Allergic reaction—fever, chills, hypotension, anaphylaxis
	Fever (nonallergic)
	N/V
	Stomatitis
	Cumulative dose effects include the following:
	    Skin—rash, hyperpigmentation, thickening, ulceration, peeling, nail changes, alopecia
	    Lungs—pneumonitis with infiltrate that can progress to fatal fibrosis
	    Raynaud syndrome
		Have emergency drugs at bedside
		Should give test dose (IM) before therapeutic dose administered
		Hypersensitivity occurs with first one to two doses
		May give acetaminophen before drug to reduce likelihood of fever
		Concentration of drug in skin and lungs accounts for toxic effects
		Cumulative lifetime dose no more than 400 units
		Pulmonary function test as baseline and in follow-up

Idarubicin (Ida) IV	Similar to doxorubicin	Similar to doxorubicin
HORMONES		
Corticosteroids (prednisone, prednisolone, dexamethasone) Prednisone—PO Prednisolone—PO, IV Dexamethasone—PO, IV, IM	Moon face, mood changes, increased appetite, insomnia Immunosuppression Aseptic necrosis Pancreatitis Psychiatric disorders Amenorrhea Trunk obesity Muscle wasting and weakness Osteoporosis Poor wound healing Gastric bleeding Hypertension Diabetes mellitus Growth failure Acne	Explain expected effects, especially in terms of body image, increased appetite, and personality changes Monitor weight gain Recommend moderate salt restriction May need to disguise bitter taste (crush tablet and mix with syrup, jam, ice cream, or other high-flavored substance; use ice to numb tongue before administration; place tablet in gelatin capsule if child can swallow it) Observe for potential infection sites; usual inflammatory response and fever are absent Test stools for occult blood Monitor blood pressure Test blood for sugar and urine for acetone Observe for signs of abrupt steroid withdrawal: flulike symptoms, hypotension, hypoglycemia, shock
ENZYMES		
Asparaginase (L-ASP, Elspar) IM, IV	Allergic reactions (including anaphylactic shock) N/V Anorexia Weight loss Low fibrinogen levels Liver dysfunction Hyperglycemia (transient) Renal failure Pancreatitis Somnolence, lethargy	Have emergency drugs at bedside Record signs of allergic reaction (urticaria, facial edema, hypotension, abdominal cramps) Normally, BUN and ammonia levels rise as a result of drug—not evidence of liver damage Check urine for sugar and ketones; treat with insulin as needed Check PT, PTT, fibrinogen—may need fresh frozen plasma Check amylase levels
Pegasparaginase (Oncaspar) IM	See Asparaginase	See Asparaginase Lower incidence of hypersensitivity reaction than use of native asparaginase
OTHER AGENTS		
Cisplatin (Platinol) IV	Renal toxicity (severe) N/V Myelosuppression Ototoxicity Neurotoxicity (similar to that for vincristine) Nephrotoxicity-induced electrolyte disturbances, especially hypomagnesemia Anaphylactic reactions may occur	Renal function (creatinine clearance) must be assessed before giving drug Must maintain hydration before and during therapy (specific gravity of urine is used to assess hydration) Mannitol may be given IV to promote osmotic diuresis and drug clearance Monitor intake and output Monitor for signs of ototoxicity (e.g., ringing in ears) and neurotoxicity; report signs immediately; ensure that routine audiogram is done before treatment for baseline and routinely during treatment Do not use aluminum needle; reaction with aluminum decreases potency of drug Monitor for signs of electrolyte loss (i.e., hypomagnesemia—tremors, spasm, muscle weakness, lower extremity cramps, irregular heartbeat, convulsions, delirium) Have emergency drugs at bedside
Carboplatin (Paraplatin) IV	N/V	As for cisplatin Myelosuppression, ototoxicity (rare), neurotoxicity, renal toxicity, anaphylaxis

with a lower dose of radiation than what would be given to control the tumor without surgery. Palliative radiotherapy is used to relieve symptoms of incurable disease after more conservative methods have proved ineffective.

Some children have been treated with hyperfractionated radiation delivery. This method uses smaller individual doses of radiation two or more times daily instead of the usual daily dose to affect more of the rapidly dividing tumor cells. The total overall dosage of radiation used is higher. However, this method has failed to provide a treatment advantage compared with daily radiotherapy treatments (Donaldson, Meza, Breneman, et al., 2001; La, Meyers, Wexler, et al., 2006; Waber, Silverman, Catania, et al., 2004).

The tumor's response to radiation depends on the type of tumor, the type and dose of radiation delivered, and the size of the area irradiated. These factors also influence the type and severity of side effects and long-term sequelae. Many side effects are similar to those of chemotherapy, but, rather than a systemic response, the side effects are generally related to the irradiated area. They include nausea and vomiting, diarrhea, mucositis, cataracts, skin changes, neurocognitive deficits, and growth and endocrine abnormalities. Fatigue can also occur during radiation therapy regardless of the site being treated (Tarbell, Yock, & Kooy, 2006).

Immunotherapy

Researchers have studied the connection between the immune system and cancer for many years in hopes of discovering effective therapies. Immunotherapy encompasses both cytokines (interleukins, interferons, tumor necrosis factor) and monoclonal antibodies. Although there is evidence that a person's immune system can recognize cancer cells and mount a cellular immune response to malignant cells, the direct use of cytokines to fight cancer have not shown benefit in the pediatric population. However, scientists are now exploring the ex vivo use of cytokines in designing cancer treatments (Foster, Forrester, Li, et al., 2004; Gottschalk, Rooney, & Brenner, 2006). The use of some monoclonal antibodies has become front-line therapy, as in the use of rituximab for some types of non-Hodgkin lymphoma (Link & Weinstein, 2006).

Hematopoietic Stem Cell Transplantation

Hematopoietic stem cell transplantation is used in treating some cases of relapsed acute lymphocytic leukemia (ALL), acute myelogenous leukemia (AML), neuroblastoma, and lymphoma and is being investigated for use in recurrent Ewing sarcoma and brain tumors (see Chapter 15). Hematopoietic stem cells for transplantation come from bone marrow, peripheral blood, or umbilical cord blood. Donors of bone marrow or blood stem cells come from three sources: the affected person (autologous), an identical twin (syngeneic), or another histocompatible or incompatible donor (allogeneic) (Radeva, VanScoyoc, Smith, et al., 2005). In some institutions, transplantation is the initial therapy of choice for children with high-risk (having clinical and laboratory features at diagnosis that are known to have a poor prognosis) ALL and AML. This procedure allows for potentially lethal doses of chemotherapy and radiation to be given to rid the body of all malignant cells. The donor's marrow or blood stem cells replace the child's destroyed marrow and after engraftment should produce the donor's nonmalignant functioning cells.

An autologous transplantation may be used when there is no available histocompatible donor, the tumor is not in the marrow, or the marrow can be purged of all tumor cells. However, allogeneic transplantation offers the benefit of graft-versus-leukemia (GVL) effect, in which the immune cells of the donor attack any remaining leukemia cells (Mackall & Sondel, 2006). In allogeneic transplantation, the donor is preferably a tissue-identical relative of the child, most often a sibling.

Hematopoietic cell transplantation is a promising treatment modality for certain malignancies in children. It must be realistically viewed, however, in terms of the potentially fatal toxicities, developmental sequelae, and psychosocial and financial effects on the child and family.

Complementary and Alternative Therapies

The category of complementary therapies encompasses a variety of interventions ranging from the use of herbs and dietary supplements in hopes to fight cancer to the use of relaxation techniques, guided imagery, hypnosis, art therapy, and play therapy in the control of symptoms such as pain and nausea (Hawks, 2006; Kelly, 2007, 2008; Post-White, 2006; Post-White, Hawks, O'Mara, et al., 2006).

Parents will often inquire about the use of herbs, special diets, or other dietary interventions to speed the recovery of the blood cell counts or combat the tumor. These therapies are widely used (Fletcher & Clarke, 2004; Martel, Bussieres, Theoret, et al., 2005; Weyl Ben Arush, Geva, Ofir, et al., 2006). Any supplement or major dietary change should be viewed in terms of its potential to interact with chemotherapeutic agents. Recently, a commonly used herbal preparation, St. John's wort, was found to interfere with the metabolism of the chemotherapeutic agent irinotecan (Mathijssen, Verweij, de Bruijn, et al., 2002). Other drug interactions most likely exist, and further research on herbal preparations is needed (Kelly, 2004). The primary care provider can acknowledge and support the parents' desire to help their child while providing access to information that puts the cost and potential benefits or hazards of such treatments in perspective.

Anticipated Advances in Diagnosis and Management

Oncology is a constantly evolving field. Breakthroughs in all types of therapy occur on a daily basis. Although many new therapies are developed, only a small fraction of these treatments become front-line therapy.

Immunotherapy

Immunotherapy continues to show promise in the treatment of childhood cancer. Types of immunotherapy include monoclonal antibodies (MoAbs), cancer vaccines, and cytokines (Smith, 2006). MoAbs are hybrid cells made from the fusion of B cells from mice to cancer cells. These MoAbs are most effective in children with minimal residual disease after initial surgery, chemotherapy, or radiation therapy. MoAbs are used alone ("naked antibodies") or as conjugates with toxins (immunotoxins), or they may be radiolabeled (often with radioactive iodine as the isotope) (Smith, 2006). Examples of MoAbs include anti-GD$_2$* in the treatment of neuroblastoma and rituximab in the treatment of lymphoma. Immunotherapy has recently become front-line therapy for a limited group

---

*GD$_2$ is the disialoganglioside expressed in virtually all cases of neuroblastoma.

of pediatric malignancies (Corey, 2005; Smith, 2006). MoAb therapy can be enhanced with cytokines (e.g., the combination of the anti-GD$_2$ antibody with interleukin-2 in the treatment of neuroblastoma) or with chemotherapeutic agents, radionucleotides, toxins, or long-acting liposomal compounds (Neal, Yang, Rakhmilevich, et al., 2004; Smith, 2006).

Chemotherapy

Most new chemotherapeutic drugs currently arise from the study of molecular biology, often referred to as "targeted therapy." Scientists are examining the molecular defects in cancer cells and how cancer cells differ from normal cells in order to design treatment aimed at these defects (Stephenson, 2002). The agents used as targeted therapy can be classified as monoclonal antibodies, agents targeted toward nucleic acids (antisense agents), or small molecule agents (Smith, 2006). The small molecule agents have a variety of mechanisms, including but not limited to promoting apoptosis (programmed cell death), inhibiting angiogenesis (blood vessel formation), and inhibiting extracellular survival signaling pathways. The most extensively studied signaling pathway is the pathway initiated by the receptor tyrosine kinase family (Smith, 2006). Up to six biologic processes must occur for a cancer cell to survive (cell cycle progression, failure to undergo cell cycle arrest, escape from apoptosis, lack of senescence, cytoskeletal rearrangement to promote invasiveness, and angiogenesis) (Corey, 2005). During cancer development the genes that encode for proteins that regulate these six processes are altered or mutated. In general these mutated genes are classified as either tumor promoting (oncogenes) or tumor suppressing. Research into methods to block oncogenes or to restore the function of tumor suppressor genes now lead to effective cancer therapies (Corey, 2005; Smith, 2006).

Targeted therapies exhibit fewer systemic toxicities than traditional chemotherapy. However, the toxicities that are observed with these agents are attributed to their effects on normal cells that express their target antigens. An antibody toward GD$_2$ ganglioside can be administered to children with neuroblastoma. This antigen is expressed on nerve cells and the agent typically induces significant pain. Antibodies that target immune cells often cause allergic-type reactions. Antibodies targeting leukemia cells often induce profound immunosuppression (Smith, 2006).

Agents that inhibit angiogenesis (e.g., bevacizumab) are of interest to many researchers. However, careful study is needed when using these agents in growing children because of concern about reducing the blood supply to normal tissues, the potential for bleeding or embolism, and the agents' potential effects on growth and ovarian function. Adults who have received antiangiogenic agents have experienced these types of toxicities (Saif & Mehra, 2006). Too few children have received these agents to draw conclusions about the rates of adverse events in children (Bender, Adamson, Reid, et al., 2008).

Overexpression of human epidermal growth factor receptor 2 (HER2) is associated with a poor prognosis for individuals with osteosarcoma. Trastuzumab (Herceptin) is an antibody against the HER2 receptor and is being studied in children with osteosarcoma who have tumors that overexpress HER2 (Scotlandi, Manara, Hattinger, et al., 2005).

The targeted therapy imatinib mesylate has drastically changed the treatment and outlook for children and adults with Philadelphia chromosome–positive leukemia (Champagne, Capdeville, Krailo, et al., 2004; Millot, Guilhot, Nelken, et al., 2006). Before treatment with this therapy, children with this type of leukemia had little chance for survival. However, the ideal length of therapy with imatinib has yet to be defined, and these children may require lifelong treatment with this agent.

Many cancer therapies fail because of the development of drug resistance in the cancer cells. The initial agents used to prevent the development of drug resistance, such as verapamil and cyclosporine, have been generally ineffective. However, the study of other methods to block drug resistance is underway (Fischer, Einolf, & Cohen, 2005).

A few drugs are being revisited for cancer therapy. Thalidomide has been shown to modulate cytokines, particularly tumor necrosis factor, and to inhibit angiogenesis (Matthews & McCoy, 2003). Many other antiangiogenic drugs are in development. Arsenic, a well-known poison that was historically used to treat syphilis, is now being used to treat acute promyelocytic leukemia and is used as single-agent therapy to replace chemotherapy for some individuals (Mathews, George, Lakshmi, et al., 2006). Valproic acid is being used as cancer therapy because of its ability to inhibit histone deacetylase (Furchert, Lanvers-Kaminsky, Juurgens, et al., 2007).

Radiation Therapy

The development of fast and powerful computers along with accurate imaging software supports the delivery of radiotherapy to precise fields. Stereotactic radiosurgery (using a single, highly focused dose of radiation) is an option for some children, particularly to treat a small residual tumor or as treatment for recurrent disease in a person previously irradiated. Treatment with a new stereotactic radiation machine, the CyberKnife, is under investigation (Chang, Main, Martin, et al., 2003; Hara, Soltys, & Gibbs, 2007). Intensity-modulated radiation therapy is a new technique using many fields of radiation treatment, each with varying degrees of intensity. This therapy contrasts with conventional radiation therapy that uses only a few fields each with a fixed intensity (Tarbell et al., 2006).

Hematopoietic Stem Cell Transplantation

Advances in hematopoietic stem cell transplantation include the type of conditioning regimen and sources for stem cells. Nonmyeloablative transplants are being performed in select situations in which the recipient's immune system and marrow cells are only partially destroyed. In another type of transplant, haploidentical marrow or peripheral stem cell donors are used (three out of six antigens match). The most common donor in this situation is the child's parent (Satwani, Morris, Bradley, et al., 2008).

Surgery

Robotics is an emerging field in surgery. In oncology, robotic techniques can provide greater precision than standard surgical procedures and have been used to obtain biopsy specimens of areas difficult to access in the brain (Mendez, Hill, Clarke, et al., 2005). With Internet access, the surgeon can be located many miles away. This treatment may allow children in remote areas, who may be critically ill, to have surgery performed by experts in the field, without the burden of travel.

Supportive Care

Advances are also being made in supportive care. Chemoprotective agents are used to mitigate the toxic effects of chemotherapy. These drugs include dexrazoxane, to minimize the cardiotoxic effects of anthracyclines, and amifostine, to minimize the myelotoxicity, nephrotoxicity, and mucositis associated with chemotherapy and radiotherapy (Schuchter, Hensley, Meropol, et al., 2002). A new formulation of granulocyte colony-stimulating factor (G-CSF) is now approved for use in children who weigh more than 40 kg. This agent, peg-filgrastim, promotes an increase in the white blood cells following chemotherapy, as does standard G-CSF. However, peg-filgrastim is given as one injection following treatment as opposed to daily injections with standard G-CSF. Additional studies are needed to determine the safety and efficacy of the drug in young children (Andre, Kababri, Bertrand, et al., 2007). A new class of antiemetics, neurokinin-1 (NK1) receptor antagonists, has been developed. One such agent is now widely used with the highly emetic chemotherapy agent cisplatin. However, this agent is only approved for use in individuals who weigh greater than 40 kg and has many potential drug interactions with other chemotherapy agents (Smith, Repka, & Weigel, 2005).

Knowledge of Genetic Etiology or Treatment

Scientists are studying specific mutations that correspond to enhanced sensitivities to drug therapies or that can be used as prognostic markers to predict patient response to therapy (Kim & Hahn, 2007). The study of protein expression, or proteomics, is a guiding force in the search for new targeted therapies. Researchers steadily make progress toward the goal of developing truly personalized target therapy aimed at an individual's specific tumor characteristics (Kim & Hahn, 2007).

Associated Problems of Cancer and Treatment

Vascular Access

Children receiving prolonged, intensive treatment are required to endure frequent venipunctures for laboratory tests and the administration of chemotherapy, blood products, antibiotic therapy, and nutritional support. These children are often aided by the placement of a long-term indwelling central venous access device (VAD) that helps minimize the trauma of frequent needle sticks and vein irritation from the chemotherapy. Access devices include tunneled catheters, peripherally inserted central catheters, and subcutaneous implanted ports. Many factors must be considered in the choice of a VAD. Such factors include the child's frequency, duration, and type of therapy; the presence of a weakened immune system or other potential contraindications for surgery; the child's age; and the child's home environment (Matsuzaki, Suminoe, Koga, et al., 2006; Schultz, Durning, Niewinski, et al., 2006).

Tunneled catheters are single-, double-, or triple-lumen silicone catheters with a Dacron felt cuff that anchors the catheter under the skin and provides a barrier to infection. Tunneled catheters have an internal and external portion, whereas subcutaneous ports are totally implanted below the skin with the catheter tip at the junction of the superior vena cava and the right atrium. Venous access is achieved by puncturing the skin above the reservoir and passing a specially designed needle through the silicone membrane into the port receptacle. Topical anesthetics may be applied to port sites before accessing to reduce discomfort and fear.

The patency of all long-term VADs is maintained through periodic flushing with heparinized saline. Care of these lines is taught to the child (when appropriate) and parents. Complications of indwelling VADs include infection, occlusion of the catheter from

---

> ### *Associated Problems* of Cancer and Treatment
>
> *Vascular access:* Most children require the use of indwelling central VADs
> - All lumens must be cultured if any fever
> - SBE prophylaxis for dental procedures
>
> Therapy-related complications
> - *Nausea and vomiting:* Use antiemetics before and after chemotherapeutic administration, NOT on an "as needed" (i.e., prn) basis
> - *Anorexia and weight loss:* Monitor weight regularly, early intervention
> - *Bone marrow suppression:*
>   - Hemoglobin <7 to 8 g/dL, consider transfusion
>   - Platelets <10,000 to 20,000/mm3, consider transfusion
>   - ANC <500, high risk for infection; possible use of erythropoietins for treatment of anemia and G-CSF or GM-CSF for neutropenia
> - *Infection:* Blood cultures for all fevers
>   - IV antibiotics for fever and neutropenia or for any child with an implanted central venous access device
> - *Alopecia*
> - *Fatigue*
>
> *Late effects:* See Table 16-3
> *Relapse*
> *Death*

Key: *ANC,* absolute neutrophil count; *G-CSF,* granulocyte colony-stimulating factor; *GM-CSF,* granulocyte-macrophage colony-stimulating factor; *SBE,* subacute bacterial endocarditis; *VAD,* venous access device.

thrombus and fibrin formation, damage to the external portion of the catheter, dislodgement, and, rarely, cardiac tamponade (Barrett, Imeson, Leese, et al., 2004; Forauer, 2007).

Because a child with cancer is at risk for profound neutropenia as a result of therapy, prompt and aggressive treatment of infection at the catheter site is necessary. Most exit site infections can be cleared with oral and topical antibiotics in children without neutropenia, but tunnel infections, septicemia, or any catheter-related infection in the child with neutropenia requires intravenous antibiotics and possible catheter removal (Simon, Bode, & Beutel, 2006).

Therapy-Related Complications

Nausea and Vomiting. Nausea and vomiting are common side effects of chemotherapy and radiation. Nausea and vomiting can have profound physiologic and psychological effects on the child receiving therapy (Holdsworth, Raisch, & Frost, 2006; Robinson & Carr, 2007). Problems, including dehydration, chemical and electrolyte imbalances, and decreased nutritional intake, can lead to decreased compliance with or termination of treatment.

The mechanisms involved in nausea and vomiting are complex, and no single drug will consistently control these side effects. The situation is further complicated by the wide variation in response of the individual child to both the chemotherapeutic agent and the antiemetic. The antiemetic should be given before nausea and vomiting occur and should be continued until the symptoms have resolved. Nausea and vomiting related to the chemotherapy generally will not last longer than 48 hours after chemotherapy administration. However, some children do experience delayed nausea and vomiting, particularly if cisplatin is used in the chemotherapeutic regimen. Radiation-induced nausea is generally limited to the first few hours following treatments directed toward the head or abdomen.

Serotonin antagonists have a significant role in the management of nausea and vomiting in children. Ondansetron (Zofran) and

BOX 16-1
Calculation of Absolute Neutrophil Count (ANC)

- *White blood cell* (WBC) *count* = 7400 (also expressed as 7.4 K/mcL; $7.4 \times 10^3/mm^3$)
- *Neutrophils* (poly, segs) = 40%
- *Nonsegmented neutrophils* (bands) = 12%
  Step 1: Determine total percent neutrophils (segs + bands)
  40% + 12% = 52% (0.52)
  Step 2: Multiply WBC by percent neutrophils
  ANC = 7400 × 0.52
  ANC = 3848 (normal)
- *WBC* = 900 (0.9K/mcL; $0.9 \times 10^3/mm^3$)
- *Neutrophils* (poly. segs) = 7%
- *Nonsegmented neutrophils* (bands) = 7%
  Step 1: 7% + 7% = 14% (0.14)
  Step 2: ANC = 900 × 0.14
  ANC = $126/mm^3$ (severely neutropenic)

granisetron (Kytril) inhibit the binding of serotonin to receptors in both the CNS and the gastrointestinal system. These medications do not cause drowsiness and rarely cause extrapyramidal side effects (Olver, 2005). Adjunctive methods such as progressive relaxation and guided imagery have had some positive effects when combined with antiemetic medications (Miller & Kearney, 2004).

Anorexia and Weight Loss. During therapy, anorexia and weight loss are common and can be attributed to both the disease and its treatment. The psychological impact of cancer and the tumor's metabolic influence can contribute to weight loss. Treatment-induced nausea and vomiting, as well as changes in taste acuity, may lead to food aversion (Skolin, Wahlin, Broman, et al., 2006). Therefore the child's weight must be closely monitored throughout treatment. Oral supplements and, in some cases, nasogastric or gastrostomy feedings or hyperalimentation may be necessary (Rogers, Melnick, Ladas, et al., 2008).

Bone Marrow Suppression. Bone marrow suppression is another side effect of chemotherapy and radiation. Leukopenia, thrombocytopenia, and anemia usually begin within 7 to 10 days after drug administration, with the nadir (i.e., the point at which the blood cell counts are the lowest) occurring at approximately 14 days. The marrow then recovers by 21 to 28 days. The exact time of the nadir varies depending on the specific chemotherapeutic agent. Close monitoring is necessary to determine the extent of marrow suppression.

Leukopenia refers to the presence of a low number of all white blood cells (WBCs), whereas neutropenia refers specifically to a low neutrophil cell count. Neutrophils are the body's main defense against bacterial infection. It is necessary to determine the absolute neutrophil count (ANC) (Box 16-1) because the incidence and severity of infection are inversely related to the child's ANC. Infections are a major life-threatening complication of cancer and its treatment (Crawford, Dale, & Lyman, 2004).

Several precautions can be taken to reduce the risk of infection. Good hand-washing techniques by the child, the parents, all family members, and the caregivers are paramount to reducing the spread of pathogens. Good personal hygiene by the child, including thorough dental care, is also important. A child with neutropenia should avoid individuals who are ill, crowded situations, and anyone with a communicable disease, especially chickenpox. Rectal temperatures and suppositories should also be avoided because abrading

the rectal mucosa increases the risk of introducing bacteria into the bloodstream.

Guidelines for transfusion are based on laboratory parameters and clinical symptoms. The child who is thrombocytopenic may require transfusions of platelets because of the risk of serious hemorrhage. Transfusion is recommended if the platelet count is less than 10,000 to $20,000/mm^3$ and/or in the presence of bleeding. In a child whose hemoglobin level is less than 7 to 8 g/dL and/or who is symptomatic (e.g., shortness of breath, headache, dizziness), a transfusion is usually indicated. However, many variations in transfusion practice guidelines exist concerning transfusion thresholds, methods of minimizing exposure to cytomegalovirus (CMV), dose, prevention of RhD alloimmunization, and the use of irradiated blood products (Nathan & Selwood, 2006; Wong, Perez-Albuerne, Moscow, et al., 2005). G-CSFs and granulocyte-macrophage colony-stimulating factors (GM-CSFs) may be used in high-risk children to reduce the severity and duration of neutropenia. These agents may decrease the rates of infection among children receiving chemotherapy but have no effect on overall mortality rates (Sung, Nathan, Alibhai, et al., 2007).

Alopecia. A distinguishing therapy-related complication is alopecia. It is generally a temporary condition that results from damage to the hair follicles by chemotherapy and radiation. Although the hair usually regrows after therapy, the texture and color may be slightly different. Cutting the child's hair into a shorter style may help to reduce some distress when the hair begins to fall out. Younger children and some adolescents prefer to cover their heads with colorful hats, baseball caps, and scarves. Adolescent girls are more likely to consider the use of wigs.

Fatigue. Fatigue is now recognized as a frequent and distressing consequence of childhood cancer and its therapy. Mechanisms of fatigue and interventions to minimize the symptom are being explored (Hinds, Hockenberry, Rai, et al., 2007; Hockenberry & Hooke, 2007; Sanford, Okuma, Pan, et al., 2008).

Late Effects

As survival rates continually improve, the long-term effects of therapy are becoming evident. The goal of therapy is not merely improving survival but also reducing physiologic and developmental morbidity. A growing body of knowledge indicates that both chemotherapy and radiation have adverse effects on normal tissues that may not be manifested for months or years after therapy. The development of second malignancies, impaired growth, diminished cognitive functioning, and organ damage are the areas of greatest concern. Factors that appear to influence the development of late effects include the child's age and stage of development at the time of diagnosis, the primary tumor, socioeconomic factors, and the therapy used (Dickerman, 2007; Hudson, Mertens, Yasui, et al., 2003). Although the majority of survivors of childhood cancer in three large studies did not demonstrate symptoms of depression or somatic distress, the survivors were more likely than their healthy siblings to demonstrate such symptoms (Zebrack, Gurney, Oeffinger, et al., 2004; Zebrack, Zeltzer, Whitton, et al., 2002; Zebrack, Zevon, Turk, et al., 2007).

Secondary malignant neoplasms (SMNs) are found with greater frequency in children with a genetic predisposition based on the primary tumor or as a result of chemotherapy and radiation therapy. The highest rate of SMNs occurs in children with hereditary retinoblastoma (Kleinerman, Tucker, Abramson, et al., 2007).

Text continued on p. 302

TABLE 16-3

Late Effects of Antineoplastic Therapy on Body Systems

Adverse Effects	Causative Agent	Time Interval	Signs and Symptoms	Predisposing Factors	Preventive/Diagnostic Measures
CARDIOVASCULAR SYSTEM					
Cardiomyopathy	Anthracycline chemotherapy	Weeks to years after therapy	Abrupt onset of congestive heart failure; tachycardia; tachypnea; edema; hepatomegaly; cardiomegaly; gallop rhythms; pleural effusions; dyspnea	Increased risk with age <15 yr and females	Careful monitoring with chest radiograph, ECG, echocardiogram, MUGA scan
	Cyclophosphamide (high dose)			Anthracycline therapy; especially if lifetime cumulative dose of ≥550 mg/m²	Observation for shortness of breath, exercise intolerance, weight gain, edema
	Irradiation of mediastinum			Stresses such as growth hormone use; cocaine or excessive alcohol use; pregnancy, labor and delivery; anesthesia; isometric exercising such as heavy weight lifting	Partial shielding of mediastinum; Close monitoring of pregnant females, particularly immediately postpartum; Use of cardioprotectant drug, ICRF-187 (dexrazoxane) with anthracyclines under investigation; Referral to cardiologist
Chronic constrictive pericarditis	Mediastinal irradiation	Few months to years	Chest pain; dyspnea; fever; paradoxic pulse; venous distention; friction rub; Kussmaul sign	Most common with doses of 40-60 Gy	Partial shielding of mediastinum; Referral to cardiologist
Premature coronary artery disease	Mediastinal or spinal irradiation	Years after therapy	Chest pain with exertion; exercise intolerance; chest pressure; arm pain; heartburn, nausea, or fatigue	Sedentary lifestyle; high-fat diet	Promote healthy lifestyle with moderate aerobic exercise and diet low in fat and salt; Close monitoring with ECG, lipid panel
PULMONARY SYSTEM					
Pneumonitis followed by pulmonary fibrosis	Pulmonary irradiation	Months to years after treatment	Dyspnea; decreased exercise tolerance; pulmonary insufficiency	Increased risk with the following: Large lung volume in radiation field; Therapy during periods of pulmonary infection; Use of radiation sensitizing chemotherapy; Doses >40 Gy	Careful monitoring of status with physical examination; chest radiograph; pulmonary function tests
	Bleomycin, carmustine, high-dose cyclophosphamide, busulfan			Subsequent delivery of high levels of oxygen (as with anesthesia) may exacerbate lung injury	Yearly influenza vaccine; Pneumothorax; Avoid smoking; Encourage frequent rest periods; High-dose steroids for severe cases; Careful use of oxygen therapy after busulfan and bleomycin therapy
HEMATOPOIETIC SYSTEM					
Long-term suppression of marrow function	Extensive irradiation of marrow-containing bones; Chemotherapy	Months to years following therapy	Fall in WBC and platelet counts; hypoplastic/aplastic bone marrow aspirates; diminished uptake of radioisotopes	Radiation doses; 30-50 Gy in older individuals; Concomitant use of chemotherapy	Limitation of areas of marrow irradiated; Monitoring of child's status with periodic bone marrow aspirates and peripheral blood cell counts
Alterations in immune system	Nodal irradiation affects cellular immunity; Splenectomy or splenic irradiation affects humoral immunity	Weeks to years following therapy	Predisposition to infection	Adolescents more at risk than younger children	Pneumococcal vaccine and penicillin if splenectomy done; Monitoring of child's status with periodic blood counts and tests of immune response

GASTROINTESTINAL SYSTEM

Effect	Causative treatment	Time of occurrence	Signs and symptoms	Risk factors	Management
Hepatic fibrosis-cirrhosis	Chemotherapy	Months to years following therapy	Persistent elevation of liver function tests after cessation of therapy; hepatomegaly; cirrhosis; jaundice; spider nevi	Daily low doses of methotrexate by mouth for long periods; Long-term use of mercaptopurine	Monitor child's status with liver function tests; Perform liver biopsy if liver function test results remain persistently abnormal
Chronic enteritis	Radiation therapy	Months to years following therapy	Pain; recurrent vomiting; diarrhea; malabsorption syndrome, weight loss	Radiation doses >50 Gy; Children with previous abdominal surgery; Chemotherapy as radiation sensitizers (actinomycin, doxorubicin)	Avoid concomitant use of radiation sensitizers; Careful monitoring of height and weight; Supportive therapy when symptoms develop, including low-residue, low-fat, gluten- and milk-free diet
Hepatitis C infection	Blood transfusion before 1993	Months to years	Most patients asymptomatic	Other risk factors: IV drug use, sexual promiscuity, tattooing	Screen all recipients of transfusion before 1993 with AST/ALT and hepatitis C antibody; if positive (or negative with elevated ALT) monitor PCR-based RNA screen for hepatitis C and refer to gastroenterologist

KIDNEY AND URINARY TRACT

Effect	Causative treatment	Time of occurrence	Signs and symptoms	Risk factors	Management
Nephritis-glomerular and/or tubular dysfunction	Radiation to renal structures (20-30 Gy)—may be enhanced by chemotherapy; Cisplatin, ifosfamide, lomustine, carmustine, methotrexate (high doses)	Weeks to years after therapy	Decrease in renal function with elevated BUN and creatinine; proteinuria; anemia; hypertension; may have urinary wasting of magnesium, potassium, and calcium with cisplatin	Other nephrotoxic drugs (aminoglycosides, vancomycin, amphotericin, cyclosporine); Inadequate alkalinization of urine before methotrexate; Urinary tract infections	Periodically monitor renal status during and after therapy with blood pressure readings, urinalysis, CBC, BUN, and creatinine; Once progressive renal failure develops, treatment is supportive; Electrolyte supplementation as needed; Child should avoid rough contact sports after nephrectomy to protect remaining kidney
Renal Fanconi syndrome	Ifosfamide	Weeks to years after therapy	Urinary wasting of phosphorus, glucose, proteins and inability to acidify urine; can lead to renal rickets with inhibition of growth and bone deformity	Age <3 yr at time of treatment, prior renal dysfunction, nephrectomy	Periodically monitor renal status during and after therapy with urinalysis and electrolytes and phosphorus; Electrolyte supplementation as needed
Chronic hemorrhagic cystitis	Cyclophosphamide, ifosfamide; Radiation therapy	Months to years after treatment	Sterile, painful hematuria; urinary frequency	Inadequate hydration during cyclophosphamide or ifosfamide therapy	Techniques to reduce bladder exposure during radiation therapy; Frequent emptying of bladder during and 24 hr after therapy; Adequate hydration before, during, and after therapy; Concomitant use of mesna with chemotherapy; Treatment of bladder hemorrhage with formalin instillation or cauterization of bleeding sites

Data from Bhatia, S., Blatt, J., & Meadows, A.T. (2006). Late effects of childhood cancer and its treatment. In P.A. Pizzo & D.G. Poplack (Eds.). *Principles and Practice of Pediatric Oncology* (5th ed.). Philadelphia: Lippincott Williams & Wilkins, pp. 1490-1514; Hobbie, W. et al. (2002). Care of survivors. In C.R. Baggott, K.P. Kelly, & D. Fochtman (Eds.), *Nursing Care of Children and Adolescents with Cancer* (3rd ed.). Philadelphia: Saunders, pp. 426-464.
Key: *ALT*, alanine transaminase; *AML*, acute myelocytic leukemia; *AST*, aspartate transaminase; *BUN*, blood urea nitrogen; *CBC*, complete blood count; *CT*, computed tomography; *DEXA*, dual energy x-ray absorptiometry; *ECG*, electrocardiogram; *FSH*, follicle-stimulating hormone; *IT*, intrathecal; *IV*, intravenous; *LH*, luteinizing hormone; *MRI*, magnetic resonance imaging; *MUGA*, multiple gated acquisition; *PCR*, polymerase chain reaction; *RNA*, ribonucle ic acid; T_3, triiodothyronine; T_4, thyroxine; *TSH*, thyroid-stimulating hormone; *WBC*, white blood cell.

Continued

TABLE 16-3

Late Effects of Antineoplastic Therapy on Body Systems—cont'd

Adverse Effects	Causative Agent	Time Interval	Signs and Symptoms	Predisposing Factors	Preventive/Diagnostic Measures
MUSCULOSKELETAL SYSTEM					
Impaired skeletal growth	Irradiation of skeletal structures and abdomen	Months to years following treatment	Growth retardation, reduction in sitting height, scoliosis, altered growth of facial skeleton	Effect of spinal irradiation to vertebral bodies in doses 10-20 Gy dependent on age of child; known damage >20 Gy. Unilateral radiation results in asymmetric deformities. Symmetric growth delay during periods of chemotherapy	Careful monitoring of child's status with growth charts, radiographic studies, sitting and standing height. Dose radiation reduction during periods of rapid growth
Delayed or arrested tooth development	Irradiation of maxilla or mandible. Chemotherapy	Months to years	Teeth are small with pale enamel; malocclusion	Radiation during period of dental growth and development	Dental examinations every 6 mo. Good oral hygiene including flossing. Fluoride prophylaxis
Avascular necrosis (AVN) and osteoporosis	Radiation. Steroids (particularly dexamethasone). Methotrexate (usually resolves at end of therapy)	Months to years	AVN—joint pain often accompanied by slipped capital epiphysis of femoral head. Osteoporosis—bone fractures	Poor calcium intake. Increased body weight	Encourage calcium intake and low-impact exercise as preventive measures. DEXA scan for osteoporosis. Referral to orthopedics
ENDOCRINE SYSTEM					
Thyroid gland dysfunction	Irradiation of thyroid gland, brain, and total body irradiation	Months to years	Hypothyroidism; may be asymptomatic and have abnormal thyroid function; nodular abnormalities	Reported with varying radiation doses: 25-70 Gy	Monitor thyroid function with T_3, free T_4, and TSH. Hormonal replacement therapy for all children with abnormal thyroid tests since elevated TSH is associated with thyroid cancer
Injuries to gonads	Irradiation of gonads. Chemotherapy (alkylating agents)	Months to years	Infertility, sterility, hormonal dysfunction, azoospermia, teratogenic during first trimester of pregnancy	Testicular radiation; ovarian radiation. Chemotherapy damage dependent on drug used, dose, duration of therapy, child's gender and age	Tanner staging yearly. Protection of testes/ovaries from radiation field. Gonadal dysfunction from chemotherapy may be reversible. *Males (14 yr old):* check LH, FSH, testosterone levels. *Females (12 yr old):* check LH, FSH, estradiol levels
Decreased growth rate	Irradiation of cranium and/or spine. Total body irradiation. Chemotherapy	Months to years	Reduction in height percentile or growth rate	Radiation therapy at younger age and dose of ≥30 Gy to brain. Spinal irradiation at >35 Gy. Total body irradiation at >10 Gy	After completion of therapy, check standing and sitting heights 1-2 times each year. Thyroid function tests, bone age, and growth hormone testing to be considered if rate declines
NERVOUS SYSTEM					
Peripheral sensory or motor neuropathies	Irradiation of peripheral nerves; chemotherapy (vincristine, etoposide, cisplatin)	Months to years	Deficit in function. Pain. Decreased tendon reflexes	Radiation doses: 55-120 Gy. Chemotherapy with vinca alkaloids	Careful monitoring of child's status during and after therapy. Vinca alkaloid damage may be diminished or reversed by reducing or withholding therapy

Effect	Cause	Onset	Clinical Manifestations	Risk Factors	Management
Central neuroendocrine dysfunction of hypothalamic pituitary axis	Cranial irradiation; chemotherapy	Months to years	Growth hormone deficiency; Panhypopituitarism with short stature; hypothyroidism; Addison disease	Dependent on dose of radiation, age of child, and concomitant use of chemotherapy; Younger children who receive >25 Gy at greatest risk	Careful monitoring of child's status with growth charts, Tanner staging, bone age at 9 yr then yearly to puberty; Thyroid, hormone, insulin, and cortisol measurement may be necessary; Treatment with replacement of deficient hormones
Encephalopathy	Cranial irradiation; chemotherapy, particularly IV methotrexate (high dose) and IT methotrexate	Months to years	May be asymptomatic but demonstrate abnormalities on head CT scans; May have overt symptoms ranging from lethargy to somnolence, dementia, seizures, paralysis, and coma	Cranial radiation alone or with concomitant chemotherapy; Frequency increased with chemotherapy; Less damage with cranial radiation <18 Gy; Younger children more vulnerable	Monitor child's status with careful physical examination, head MRI/CT scans, psychometric testing; Reduce chemotherapy dose when preclinical radiographic findings appear
Intelligence deficits and/or neuropsychological dysfunctions	Radiation therapy, chemotherapy	Months to years	Abnormal psychological tests with deficits in perceptual behavior, language development, and learning abilities; Personality changes	More common in younger children, those who received cranial irradiation >18 Gy and concomitant chemotherapy; Damage may occur in all individuals who received prophylactic or therapeutic cranial radiation and/or chemotherapy	Careful monitoring with periodic neurocognitive/psychological evaluations; Early intervention with multidisciplinary approach and specialized education programs
SECONDARY (MALIGNANCY MULTIPLE SYMPTOMS)					
Leukemia, especially AML	Alkylating agents; Doxorubicin; Etoposide	Years	Leukopenia; Anemia; Thrombocytopenia; Fever; Bone pain	Hodgkin disease as primary malignancy	Monitor CBC
Thyroid cancer	Irradiation of mediastinum, spine, head, or neck		Palpable mass/nodule; Anterior cervical adenopathy	Younger age at time of radiation therapy	If thyroid nodule present obtain thyroid scintiscan, tests of thyroid function; Biopsy or bone needle aspiration of nodule or node
Breast cancer	Irradiation of mediastinum, spine, or chest wall		Palpable mass	More common with >20 Gy mantle area; Genetic form of Wilms' tumor or Hodgkin disease as primary malignancy	Teach adolescents to do breast self-examination; Consider baseline mammogram in early twenties; May consider chemoprevention for Hodgkin survivors in the future
Bone and soft tissue tumors	Irradiation of bone or soft tissue		Mass; Pain	Retinoblastoma as primary malignancy especially if treated with radiation or bilateral	

TABLE 16-4

Relative 5-Year Survival Rates (%) of Children (Ages 0-14 Years) with Malignant Disease

Site	Year of Diagnosis							
	1975-1977	1978-1980	1981-1983	1984-1986	1987-1989	1990-1992	1993-1995	1996-2004
All sites	58.1	62.6	66.9	68.2	71.4	75.7	77.3	80.0*
Bone and joint	50.6†	48.7†	56.8†	57.9†	66.8†	66.8	74.1	70.6*
Brain and central nervous system (CNS)	56.9	57.5	56.2	61.7	63.9	64.3	70.3	73.7*
Hodgkin disease	80.5	87.7	88.0	90.9	87.1	96.8	94.6	95.9*
Acute lymphocytic leukemia	57.6	66.1	71.4	72.5	77.8	83.0	83.8	88.1*
Acute myelocytic leukemia	18.8	25.8†	26.7†	30.5†	37.1†	41.0	41.7†	55.2*
Neuroblastoma	52.4	56.9	54.6	52.3	62.0	76.3	67.3	69.7*
Non-Hodgkin lymphoma	43.1	52.7	66.9	70.3	70.7	76.1	80.6	86.1*
Soft tissue	61.0	74.9	69.2	73.0	65.4	79.7	76.5	74.4*
Wilms' tumor	73.1	79.0	86.6	90.7	92.1	91.9	91.6	92.2*

From Ries L.A. et al. (Eds.). (2008). SEER *cancer statistics review, 1975-2005*. Bethesda, MD: National Cancer Institute. Available at http://seer.cancer.gov/csr/1975_2005.
Rates are from the SEER 9 areas. They are based on data from population-based registries in Connecticut, New Mexico, Utah, Iowa, Hawaii, Atlanta, Detroit, Seattle-Puget Sound, and San Francisco. Rates are based on follow-up of patients into 2005.
*The difference in rates between 1975-1977 and 1996-2005 is statistically significant ($p < .05$).
†The standard error of the survival rate is between 5 and 10 percentage points.

There may also be an increased risk of SMN in persons with the genetic forms of Wilms' tumor (bilateral), neuroblastoma, and other embryonal tumors. In children with Hodgkin disease treated with radiation and chemotherapy, there is an increased incidence of SMN—especially breast cancer and AML and solid tumors (Neglia, Friedman, Yasui, et al., 2001). Treatment with alkylating agents and etoposide increases the risk of AML. Concurrent use of dose-intensive anthracyclines with cyclophosphamide has been associated with an increased risk of SMN (Neglia et al., 2001).

Children receiving treatment directly to the CNS are at risk for negative neurologic and intellectual sequelae. Neurotoxicity is related to the number and sequence of treatment modalities used. The impact of late effects on the various organ systems is described in Table 16-3.

Relapse

Despite the advances in treatment of childhood cancer, some children will experience a relapse of their disease. Relapse, like diagnosis, is a crisis period for the family. It poses a challenge for the oncology team because the best methods of treatment were used at diagnosis. Relapse often requires more experimental modes of treatment. The primary care provider in cooperation with the oncology team can support the family—and especially the child—through this difficult time.

Death

There may come a time when all possible viable treatment options have been exhausted. The care of the child moves from focusing on a cure to providing comfort and as much quality time as possible. The collaboration between the primary care provider and the oncology team can be invaluable during this time. Families often seek guidance and support in making decisions that they can live with long after the child's death. Knowledge of the community- and hospital-based hospice programs in their area can be beneficial in meeting many of the home care and support needs of families. All families need reassurance that they will not be abandoned at this time and that multidisciplinary resources will be made available to them as required.

Prognosis

The prognosis of a malignancy depends on the age of the child, primary site, extent of the disease, and cell type. Before the 1970s the overall cure rate for pediatric malignancies was less than 50% (American Cancer Society, 2007). Over the past 20 years dramatic advances have been made in the treatment and potential cure of children with cancer (Table 16-4). The current figures estimate an overall 5-year disease-free survival rate of 80.0% for pediatric cancers in general (Ries et al., 2008).

PRIMARY CARE MANAGEMENT

Health Care Maintenance

Growth and Development

Although growth retardation secondary to chemotherapy often resolves when therapy is complete, it may persist for some children (Bhatia, Blatt, & Meadows, 2006). The effect of radiation, however, can be permanent. Radiation affects growth by damaging the epiphyseal plates of the long bones and the glands that are responsible for growth-related hormone production. A child's growth should be observed on a standardized growth curve, with growth patterns examined over time rather than as isolated measurements. Preferably both sitting and standing heights should be obtained. Growth rates should be checked every 1 to 3 months during therapy and for the first year after therapy; then measurements should be taken every 6 months until linear growth is completed. Because of the risk of significant weight loss, weight should also be monitored at each visit.

Primary care providers can play an invaluable role in providing anticipatory guidance for parents about the developmental changes children with cancer will experience. Children with cancer are often limited in their opportunities to develop independence and autonomy. The limitations come from restrictions placed by treatment regimens, therapy-related complications, and protective parents.

Ongoing developmental assessment should be performed during and after therapy. Early identification and intervention are important in assisting the child in maintaining age-appropriate development. Neuropsychological testing is recommended within the first 2 years after completion of therapy for children receiving cranial radiation. Age-standardized tests should be used to measure intellectual ability, visual perception, visual-motor and motor skills, language, memory and learning, academic achievement, and behavior and social functioning (see Chapters 2 and 3). Neuropsychological testing may need to be repeated to diagnose long-term effects.

Diet

Maintaining adequate nutrition while a child is receiving treatment is challenging because of the child's anorexia. Well-balanced, nutritious meals should be offered. Small, frequent meals may often be more appealing than the standard three meals each day. High-calorie, high-protein snacks may also be helpful.

Children receiving corticosteroids often experience an increased appetite and weight gain, but because corticosteroids usually are administered for limited periods of time, such symptoms generally are of short duration. Nutritious foods low in sodium should be encouraged.

Constipation and diarrhea are frequent side effects of chemotherapy. A stool softener or laxative may be necessary, especially with vincristine therapy. Enemas and suppositories should be avoided, especially if the child is neutropenic. Diarrhea should be monitored closely and the child evaluated for signs and symptoms of dehydration and electrolyte imbalances.

Safety

Safety issues for a child with a malignant disease involve balancing normal participation in daily activities with taking appropriate precautions imposed by the treatment of a malignant disease. For the safety of all children, chemotherapeutic agents must be stored securely out of reach. Thorough hand washing should follow the handling of any chemotherapeutic agent. Pregnant women should avoid contact with the chemotherapeutic agents and the urine of children receiving chemotherapy. If circumstances make this impossible, gloves should be worn to avoid direct contact with the medication. Unused portions of chemotherapeutic drugs should be returned to the dispensing pharmacy for disposal with other potent chemicals.

External tunneled VADs must have a clean dressing applied to the exit site and the line secured to the chest to minimize any excessive tension on the catheter. Needles, syringes, and other supplies used to maintain the line should be stored properly out of reach of children. Needles should be disposed of carefully, without recapping, in an approved container.

Children with external tunneled VADs should avoid lake or ocean swimming and hot tubs to reduce the risk of infection. They should also have an extra padded clamp available in case of damage to the catheter lumen.

Exposures to ill contacts should be minimized for all immunosuppressed children. Frequent hand washing is another important intervention to prevent infections.

If the child should have a significant fall or head injury, blood cell counts should be checked to determine the platelet count and the possible need for transfusion. Contact sports may be discouraged if the platelet count is less than 100,000/mm³.

Many chemotherapeutic agents will alter the skin's tolerance for sun exposure. It is important that children receiving chemotherapy take extra caution in using a para-aminobenzoic acid (PABA)–free sun block whenever sun exposure is anticipated. It is best to avoid sun exposure during midday. If the child has alopecia, a hat and sun block should be worn to protect the scalp.

The primary care provider can play a key role in helping the child and family set realistic expectations and limitations on activities. Limitations are influenced by immunosuppression, hematologic compromise, or extremity dysfunction because of peripheral neuropathy induced by chemotherapy or as a result of amputation or limb salvage procedures.

Immunizations

Live-virus vaccines (e.g., those preventing measles, mumps, and rubella; rotavirus, varicella, smallpox, and yellow fever; the oral polio vaccine; and live-attenuated influenza vaccine) and live-bacteria vaccines (e.g., those preventing bacille Calmette-Guérin [BCG] and Ty21a *Salmonella typhi*) are contraindicated for severely immunocompromised children because of safety reasons (American Academy of Pediatrics [AAP] Committee on Infectious Diseases, 2006). The smallpox or oral polio vaccines must also be avoided in the household contacts of any immunosuppressed individual. Household contacts may receive the vaccine for measles, mumps, and rubella (MMR) and the varicella vaccine. Although the AAP recommends administering inactivated vaccines (e.g., the diphtheria-pertussis-tetanus, hepatitis B, *Haemophilus influenzae* type B, pneumococcal, and inactivated polio vaccines) it also recognizes that children are unlikely to develop an immune response if the immunizations are delivered within 2 weeks of immunosuppressive therapy (AAP Committee on Infectious Diseases, 2006). Children typically receive courses of chemotherapy every 3 weeks and thus would not have an opportunity to receive vaccines 2 weeks or more from the time of cancer treatment. Many oncology practitioners hold all routine vaccines during immunosuppressive therapy and for the first 3 to 12 months after cancer treatment (Allen, 2007). Some clinicians use in vitro testing of children's immune function after chemotherapy is completed to determine the optimal timing of immunizations in individual patients (AAP Committee on Infectious Diseases, 2006). However, the use of the inactivated influenza vaccine is recommended for children receiving therapy and any household contacts during therapy and for up to 1 year after therapy (AAP Committee on Infectious Diseases, 2006). Persons at risk for pulmonary fibrosis may also benefit from using the vaccine throughout their lives. Normal immunologic response usually returns between 3 and 12 months after discontinuing immunosuppressive therapy (AAP Committee on Infectious Diseases, 2006). However, in one study 40% of children with leukemia who had completed chemotherapy lacked immunity to measles and 28% lacked immunity to rubella; these children had all received the MMR vaccine before starting cancer treatment (Nilsson, De Milito, Engstrom, et al., 2002). Because there is some variation in immunization recommendations among cancer treatment centers, it is best to consult the child's oncology team for specific guidance. See Chapter 15 for recommendations after bone marrow transplantation.

Varicella Exposure Prophylaxis and Vaccination. If a child who is seronegative for antibody to the varicella virus or who has not been vaccinated has a direct exposure to a person with active chickenpox or to a person who develops lesions within 48 hours of the contact, the child must receive varicella-zoster immune globulin (VZIG) if available, or intravenous immune globulin (IVIG), within 48 to 96 hours of exposure. The dose of VZIG is 125 U/10 kg, with a maximum dosage of 625 U. Once a child is exposed to chickenpox, the child must be isolated from other children who are immunocompromised from day 10 to day 28 following the exposure (Allen, 2007).

The live-attenuated varicella vaccine is not currently licensed for children with malignancies. The vaccine is available through a research protocol, however, for children with ALL who have been in remission for at least 1 year and who have an absolute lymphocyte count over 700/mm^3 (AAP Committee on Infectious Diseases, 2006). Transmission of vaccine-induced varicella from healthy children to their immunocompromised siblings is rare, and the risks of natural varicella outweigh the potential for mild vaccine-related illness (AAP Committee on Infectious Diseases, 2006).

Other Immunizations. Children with Hodgkin disease should receive the pneumococcal and meningococcal vaccines before splenectomy or splenic irradiation. In addition, these children should be given daily antimicrobial therapy to prevent pneumococcal infection (AAP Committee on Infectious Diseases, 2006).

Screening

Vision. Routine vision screening is advised. A recurring brain tumor may manifest as impaired visual acuity caused by ocular nerve compression or increased intracranial pressure or as blurred vision caused by papilledema. There may be ptosis, visual disturbances, and sixth cranial nerve dysfunction with recurrent orbital rhabdomyosarcoma. Two classic signs of recurrent retinoblastoma are the white eye reflex in place of the normal red reflex and strabismus. Cataracts are also a late effect of radiation therapy. In addition, vincristine and vinblastine may cause ptosis that can interfere with vision.

Hearing. Routine screenings of hearing are advised. Unilateral hearing loss may indicate the presence of a mass. Children receiving radiation or cisplatin or both are at increased risk for hearing loss (Coradini, Cigana, Selistre, et al., 2007; Skinner, 2004); evaluation by an audiologist every 6 to 12 months is recommended.

Dental. Routine dental care is advised during treatment and after therapy. Both radiation therapy and chemotherapy place a child at risk for stomatitis, dental caries, and periodontal disease. Ideally, dental work requiring manipulation of the oral tissues should be performed only if the ANC is greater than 1000/mm^3 and the platelet count is greater than 50,000/mm^3 (Haytac, Dogan, & Antmen, 2004). The American Heart Association recently revised the guidelines for administering prophylactic antibiotics before dental work to prevent subacute bacterial endocarditis (SBE). According to these guidelines, children with central VADs having dental manipulation do not require antibiotic prophylaxis (Wilson, Taubert, Gewitz, et al., 2007) (see Chapter 21 for SBE guidelines). Daily brushing with a soft-bristled brush and flossing are recommended. Daily fluoride rinses may be indicated in children with a high potential for caries. The promotion of good oral hygiene by an interdisciplinary team is important in preventing stomatitis and infection. Despite widespread research on numerous agents, no medication clearly shows efficacy in the prophylaxis or treatment of stomatitis (Keefe, Schubert, Elting, et al., 2007).

Blood Pressure. Blood pressure should be measured at every visit because of possible hypertension from corticosteroids, potential renal toxicity of many chemotherapeutic agents, and cardiac toxicities from anthracyclines.

Hematocrit. Because of frequent hematologic analyses, routine hematocrit screening is not necessary while a child is receiving therapy. After therapy, routine screening is recommended.

Urine. Routine urinalysis is advised because it may reveal red blood cells in children with bladder or kidney tumors. Late effects of radiation therapy may include proteinuria. Children receiving cyclophosphamide may experience hemorrhagic cystitis, although symptoms may occur months to years after the drug has been discontinued. Particular care is required to screen for and treat urinary tract infections in children who have undergone a nephrectomy.

Tuberculosis. Routine screening for tuberculosis of children off therapy is advised. Children receiving therapy may be anergic to skin testing. The placement of controls (e.g., *Candida* and diphtheria-tetanus [dT]) will help assess the individual's responsiveness. A chest radiograph may be necessary if skin testing is unsuccessful.

Children receiving immunosuppressive therapy are at risk for tuberculosis. Optimal therapy for tuberculosis in children with immunosuppression has not been established (AAP Committee on Infectious Diseases, 2006).

Condition-Specific Screening

The primary care provider must keep in mind the possibility of abnormalities because of disease recurrence or the long-term effects of treatment (see Table 16-3). Screening for these complications should be done in consultation with either the pediatric oncology team or other subspecialty team.

Common Illness Management
Differential Diagnosis

Fever. The presence of fever (i.e., 101°F [38.3°C]) adds a critical dimension to diagnosis and treatment in the face of neutropenia. If adequate therapy is not initiated promptly, the result could be life threatening. The first step in evaluating a fever is obtaining a complete blood count (CBC) with differential to determine if the child is neutropenic, blood cultures from all central VAD lumens, and cultures from other potential sites of infection as indicated by the history and physical examination. Obtaining a chest radiograph is not indicated in the absence of respiratory symptoms (McCullers & Shenep, 2001). The physical examination should focus on the skin, lungs, nose, sinuses, oral cavity, pharynx, catheter site, abdomen, joints, and perineal and perirectal areas. Expected signs of infection such as erythema and edema may be absent or diminished. A history of chills or rigors occurring within 2 hours of flushing a central VAD may indicate the presence of bacteremia (Ammann, Aebi, Hirt, et al., 2004).

The febrile child with a central VAD should have aerobic and anaerobic blood cultures obtained peripherally and from each lumen of the catheter or port. Parenteral broad-spectrum antibiotics are initiated and later modified based on culture and sensitivity results.

If, after 48 to 72 hours, the ANC is over 500/mm³, the cultures are negative, and the child is afebrile, antibiotics may be stopped. If the cultures are positive, a full 10- to 14-day course of antibiotics should be administered (Ammann et al., 2004; Sung, Feldman, Schwamborn, et al., 2004).

Admission to the hospital for treatment is generally required for the child who is febrile and neutropenic (i.e., ANC less than 500/mm³). In selected cases of moderate neutropenia (i.e., ANC 200 to 500/mm³), the child may be treated as an outpatient with daily examination by the oncologist (Orudjev & Lange, 2002). However, many factors (e.g., children's comorbidities and social factors) prevent the widespread practice of complete outpatient therapy for children with febrile neutropenia (Quezada, Sunderland, Chan, et al., 2007). After cultures are obtained, parenteral broad-spectrum antibiotics should be started immediately under the direction of the oncologic team. Antibiotic choice is based on suspected organism and institutional-regional patterns of antibiotic resistance.

Differential Diagnosis

Fever
- Bacterial, viral, fungal, or protozoal infection
- Site: Blood, VAD, nasopharynx, skin, joints, perineal, perirectal areas

Gastrointestinal Symptoms
- Diarrhea: Infectious causes or chemotherapy induced
- Constipation: Vinca alkaloids (paralytic ileus)
- Vomiting: Chemotherapy induced, anticipatory

Headaches
- Increased intracranial pressure caused by a mass lesion or shunt malfunction
- CSF leak with recent history of lumbar puncture

Pain
- Tumor related: Caused by compression of nerves or invasion of bone
- Treatment related: Mucositis, dermatitis, neurotoxicity, phantom limb pain, infection
- Procedure related: Bone marrow, lumbar puncture, venipuncture

Key: *CSF*, cerebrospinal fluid; *VAD*, venous access device.

Viral infections. The human viruses most frequently affecting children with malignant diseases are herpes simplex virus (HSV), varicella-zoster virus (VZV), and cytomegalovirus (CMV). Treatment of HSV infections in children with cancer depends on the site and severity of the infection but is most often with acyclovir (250 mg/m² every 8 hours).

In the event that the child contracts a primary (chickenpox) or secondary (shingles) VZV infection, acyclovir (500 mg/m² every 8 hours) should be administered intravenously immediately and continued for at least 7 days or until all lesions have crusted. Vigorous hydration and monitoring of blood urea nitrogen (BUN) and creatinine during acyclovir treatment are needed to prevent renal toxicity of the drug.

An acute CMV infection may cause fever, hepatosplenomegaly, retinitis, pneumonia, colitis, CNS manifestations, and a rash. Antiviral therapy for CMV includes the use of gancyclovir and immune globulin intravenously.

Other infections. Candidiasis and aspergillosis are the two most common fungal infections in children with malignant diseases. Candidiasis is more common and can involve the oral mucosa, gastrointestinal tract, urinary tract, bone, lungs, and, less frequently, the blood. Meticulous oral care and prompt identification of lesions help reduce morbidity from oral candidiasis. Once an oral infection is documented, systemic oral antifungal agents may be used. Aspergillosis is seen most frequently in the respiratory tract, gastrointestinal tract, and brain. Although amphotericin B is the standard treatment for systemic fungal infections in pediatric oncology patients, newer agents such as liposomal formulations of amphotericin, antifungal triazoles, and echinocandins may be used as safe alternatives with similar efficacy (Walsh, Roilides, Groll, et al., 2006).

The child who is immunocompromised and at risk for *Pneumocystis jiroveci* (formerly *carinii*) may take trimethoprim/sulfamethoxazole (Septra, Bactrim) prophylactically. The usual dose is 150 mg/m²/day divided and given twice daily for 3 days each week. The prophylaxis is continued for approximately 6 months after the completion of therapy. In children who cannot tolerate Septra or Bactrim, daily oral dapsone or monthly aerosolized or intravenous pentamidine may be used (Walsh et al., 2006). Pneumonitis is the most common clinical manifestation of *Pneumocystis jiroveci*. Symptoms include a dry cough, fever, tachypnea, cyanosis, and respiratory distress. Onset may be acute (a few days) or insidious (months). All significant infections in children who are immunocompromised should be managed by the oncology team.

Gastrointestinal Symptoms. Nausea, vomiting, and diarrhea, which are common side effects of cancer treatment, may be difficult to distinguish from infections caused by bacteria, protozoa, viruses, or *Clostridium difficile* toxin. The primary care provider must establish the relationship of the symptoms to the administration of chemotherapy or radiation. During these symptoms, it is important to monitor fluid intake and avoid dehydration, especially in children who are currently receiving chemotherapy. In some cases intravenous fluid replacement and antiemetics may be necessary. Stool cultures will help identify an infectious source of diarrhea. Blood chemistry values, especially BUN, creatinine, aspartate transaminase (AST), and alanine transaminase (ALT), must be monitored closely to avoid damaging vital organs from concentrated levels of the chemotherapeutics and from delayed excretion as a result of dehydration. Many families are taught how to administer antiemetics and intravenous hydration at home.

Vinca alkaloids predispose children to the development of constipation. If dietary intervention is not successful, supplementation with a stool softener or laxative will be needed to prevent paralytic ileus. This is most often needed when frequent repeated doses of vincristine are used. Suppositories and enemas should not be used without consultation with the oncology team because of the potential risk of infection related to reduced WBC counts.

Headaches. Headache pain, which is usually benign late in childhood and adolescence, is indicative of serious underlying difficulties in young children. Morning headaches associated with vomiting and minimal nausea should always arouse suspicion of increased intracranial pressure caused by a mass lesion or shunt malfunction in a child with a brain tumor. Headaches following a lumbar puncture that resolve with lying down may be caused by a slow cerebrospinal fluid leak. This type of headache is best treated by bed rest and adequate hydration. While taking a thorough history, the primary care provider should note onset, any precipitating factors or symptoms, location, severity, and what, if any, medication gives relief. A thorough neurologic examination is imperative. Many headaches may be treated at home with acetaminophen and rest; however, if the headache symptoms are unrelieved by medication or there is any change in vision or neurologic function, immediate evaluation is necessary.

Pain. Pain in children is often difficult to assess and requires understanding of normal child development and age-appropriate verbal and behavioral cues. Most important, keep in mind that children rarely fabricate the presence of pain. The child with cancer poses additional challenges because of the multiple etiologies of pain, which may result from the malignancy, treatments, or procedures (e.g., bone marrow and spinal tap).

Tumor-related pain occurs with direct tumor invasion of the bone, impingement of the tumor on nervous tissue, or metastatic lesions. Compression of the spinal cord by a tumor may result in back pain and is accentuated by maneuvers such as coughing, sneezing, and flexion of the spine. Immediate evaluation is imperative because an untreated cord compression can rapidly progress to irreversible neurologic damage (Walker, Yaszemski, Kim, et al., 2003). Treatment-related pain can occur from mucositis, infection, radiation-induced dermatitis, neurotoxicity from chemotherapy (vincristine), abdominal pain, or phantom limb pain following the amputation of a limb (Monteiro Caran, Dias, Seber, et al., 2005). Management of disease-related pain relies on pharmacologic and behavioral approaches. Systematic assessment of the child's pain is needed to design an optimal plan.

Pain resulting from procedures is greatly reduced with the use of conscious sedation (e.g., using a combination of a sedative [midazolam, diazepam] and an opioid [fentanyl, morphine]). Some children who experience great psychological or physical pain during procedures may benefit from the use of short-acting general anesthetics (Iannalfi, Bernini, Caprilli, et al., 2005).

Topical anesthetics are used in combination with sedation to reduce procedural pain. There are three primary methods of achieving topical anesthesia: subcutaneous infiltration with lidocaine, topical lidocaine creams, and use of electric current with anesthetic. Creams are most commonly used. The onset, duration, and depth of analgesia depend on the brand of cream used and the duration of application. Numby Stuff (Iomed) delivers lidocaine into the skin using a low-level electric current from a battery-powered dose control unit. Topical anesthesia for procedures is achieved in 7 to 15 minutes.

Nonpharmacologic therapies to reduce pain and distress include distraction, guided imagery, and hypnosis. Art and play therapy can also assist children and adolescents in coping with the loss of control and pain associated with invasive procedures (Rheingans, 2007).

Drug Interactions

Children receiving therapy need to avoid aspirin-containing products because they impair platelet function. Acetaminophen is generally recommended; however, its use during periods of neutropenia is discouraged because it may mask a fever. Multivitamins high in folic acid should be avoided because of the interference of folate with methotrexate. Vitamins low in folic acid are acceptable. Because of the number of drugs a child may be taking for therapy and the possibility of interaction, it is advisable that the

primary care provider contact the pediatric oncology team before prescribing additional medications.

Developmental Issues
Sleep Patterns

Disturbances in sleep patterns are common. The extent to which the child is affected will depend on the age at diagnosis, medication schedules, the frequency of hospitalizations, and the general coping patterns of the child. Maintaining a consistent bedtime ritual whenever possible provides security during a time when many routines are disrupted. Parents should also be encouraged to bring transitional objects (e.g., a teddy bear, favorite blanket) to the hospital because these may help the child with sleep during periods of hospitalization.

Toileting

Diarrhea and constipation may occur with certain chemotherapy agents. Toilet training may be delayed or regression may occur if treatment occurs during the toddler or preschool period.

Discipline

Discipline for the child with cancer should be the same as for all children. A consistent approach in establishing expectations and setting limits is important to the child's sense of security. The parents should be supported in maintaining normal patterns of discipline, although they may initially be ambivalent about disciplining their child who is ill. Cancer treatment imposes considerable role strain on parents. Those who maintain normal patterns of discipline may be judged for treating their children harshly whereas parents who are more lenient may be seen as spoiling their children (Young, Dixon-Woods, Findlay, et al., 2002). Consistency in discipline among siblings is also important.

Child Care

The intensity of certain phases of therapy may make regular daycare both impractical and potentially harmful to the child with cancer because of the increased risk of acquiring some infectious diseases in these settings. When a child has begun less intensive therapy, a home or small group situation is recommended because it minimizes exposure to the various common pediatric illnesses. The caretaker must be educated about (1) the child's disease and notifying the family immediately of any fever, signs and symptoms of infection, or increased bruising or bleeding; (2) reporting any communicable illness—especially chickenpox—in the other children; and (3) any medication or oral chemotherapeutic agent that must be administered during child-care hours. In addition, the importance of good hand washing should be emphasized, especially before and after toileting, food preparation, and meals.

Schooling

With advances in the treatment of children with cancer, more children are surviving into adulthood. The child who is too ill to participate in the regular classroom should be enrolled in a home study program. The role of health care providers, parents, and educators is to work as a team to assist the child in returning to school as soon after diagnosis as is medically possible. The return to school provides a sense of normalcy and contributes to the child's sense of hopefulness (see Chapter 3).

The child's school reentry must be carefully planned. To enhance the child's participation in school activities, anticipatory guidance should include attention to the special precautions that need to be taken for the child's safety and learning needs. Research results support a three-pronged method of school reentry: direct communication with school personnel, education of the child's classmates, and determination of the child's attitude toward school (Walker et al, 2003). This can be achieved by mutual respect between parents and school personnel, a willingness to provide needed resources such as homebound education, and advocacy on the part of parents and the oncology team to educate school personnel to the special needs created by hospitalizations, chemotherapy-induced side effects, and long-term sequelae of surgery, radiation, and chemotherapy on learning abilities.

Establishing an Individualized Educational Program (IEP) can help define and anticipate the special needs of the child. The teachers, school nurse, and school staff must be informed of the child's illness and implications that will influence attendance, social interaction, educational capacity, and the restrictions or special needs dictated by medical care. Early recognition of learning disabilities enhances prompt assessment and intervention.

With the family's and child's permission, the child's classmates are taught about the child's illness at an appropriate developmental level. The child also needs to be prepared to answer classmates' questions. The primary care provider can provide the family with support and resources to help ease the transition into school (see Chapter 3).

Sexuality

The child with cancer often struggles with an alteration in body image because of hair loss, weight loss or gain, or disfiguring surgery. A major task of these children is learning to deal with this change, be it temporary or permanent. This is especially true in adolescents, who, in addition to treatment, may be experiencing the normal pubertal changes. Ongoing monitoring of the child's development through the use of Tanner staging is important. Failure to progress through the stages warrants referral to a pediatric endocrinologist.

A young woman receiving chemotherapy may experience delayed development of secondary sexual characteristics and amenorrhea. However, she should be counseled to use appropriate methods of birth control because the effects of chemotherapy and radiation on fertility vary. Prevention of sexually transmitted infections (STIs) is critical, particularly in the immunocompromised adolescent. After the cessation of therapy, development often occurs and generally the menses will begin. Fertility status of children surviving childhood malignancies varies depending on the type and extent of treatment. Transposition of ovaries from the radiation field has been shown to help preserve ovarian function (Bhatia et al., 2006). It appears that treatment with chemotherapy does not increase the risk of congenital anomalies in the offspring of childhood cancer survivors (Meistrich & Byrne, 2002). Ongoing long-term follow-up is required.

Sperm banking should be offered to pubescent males, if feasible, before therapy because sterility and mutagenicity can occur from cancer treatment. Ongoing assessment of appropriate sexual development and functioning (e.g., libido, impotence) is important. Hormone replacement may be necessary if there is a deficiency.

Peer support groups are often useful in helping adolescents to deal with issues of sexuality and body image.

Transition to Adulthood

Because most children diagnosed with cancer are surviving into adulthood, pediatric cancer centers are attempting to create follow-up or "late effects" clinics that meet the needs of young adults or are referring them to adult oncologists who have remained current on issues specific to childhood cancer survivors. Follow-up including the same multidisciplinary approach used during treatment would benefit the young adult (Oeffinger & McCabe, 2006).

The protections provided by the Americans with Disabilities Act of 1990 apply to persons with cancer—whether it is cured, controlled, or in remission. The Department of Defense generally does not allow cancer survivors to enlist but has provided waivers on a case-by-case basis when the individual has been off therapy with no recurrence for 5 years. To avoid job discrimination, it is advisable for young adults to apply for jobs for which they are clearly qualified, be honest with employers' questions but not volunteer a prior cancer history, and supply a letter from their primary care provider about prognosis and life expectancy if a question arises (Wiener, Hersh, & Kazak, 2006). Health insurance through large employers is much less likely to create a barrier to coverage than individual or small business policies.

Family Concerns

Advances in medicine that have led to improved survival rates of children with cancer have also brought problems of chronic uncertainty. The uncertainty faced by families centers around the basic issue of the child's survival. Family concerns often reflect the phase of treatment they are experiencing. In the beginning, uncertainty is focused on whether or not remission will be obtained. If remission is achieved, will it be long term or will relapse occur? If relapse occurs, will the child enter remission again or die? At the end of treatment, families struggle with ambivalent feelings; they are grateful for the end of therapy yet fearful of the loss of their "safety net" of frequent contact with providers and the end of drugs that have maintained remission (Chanock, Kundra, Johnson, et al., 2006).

In addition to providing illness-related information, the health care team must help families cope with this uncertainty (Santacroce, 2002). Learning to cope with uncertainty is important to the health and well-being of all family members. Support for the child and family must be ongoing, not only at diagnosis but also long after completion of therapy or death of the child (see Chapter 6).

At diagnosis, parents often feel extreme guilt for not having brought the child to medical care sooner or for not being a more vocal advocate if providers did not realize the significance of the symptoms. The pediatric oncology team tries to support families through this difficult time by allowing opportunities for individual and family counseling. Siblings of the child with cancer benefit from an understanding of what happens during clinic and hospital visits and from interventions directly addressing their need for communication and support (Chanock et al., 2006; Nolbris, Enskar, & Hellstrom, 2007; Wiener et al., 2006).

Adherence becomes an issue when the child's or adolescent's chemotherapy consists primarily of oral medications taken at home. Several factors, including confusion about parental versus adolescent responsibilities, denial of the illness, and a loss of control, may affect adolescent noncompliance (Malbasa, Kodish, & Santacroce, 2007; Spinetta, Masera, Eden, et al., 2002). Adherence in younger children may encompass a parental inability to get them to take the medication because of its taste or form or because of the timing of doses (Sawyer & Aroni, 2003). There are many innovative methods that can be shared with parents if they express these difficulties in administering the chemotherapy.

Cultural issues related to how individuals regard and prepare for death are of particular interest in the care of children with cancer. In Korea, for example, dying outside the home is considered very undesirable, which has implications for the importance of home care for these children who are terminally ill. With regard to the caretaking of children who are ill, mothers most commonly take on this responsibility in Korea, Japan, and many Hispanic families, whereas in China, fathers often assume this role when the child is ill (Martinson, Kim, Yang, et al., 1995). At an appropriate time, assessing such issues as the family's feelings about disclosure of information to the child, caretaking responsibilities, death rituals, and comfort with asking questions and voicing concerns and disagreement with health care providers is important. Significant differences exist in the disclosure of a cancer diagnosis to children by physicians in the United States and those in Japan (Parsons, Saiki-Craighill, Mayer, et al., 2007).

The financial burden of a catastrophic illness is of monumental concern to the family. It not only affects the current financial status of the family but also has far-reaching implications for the child's future insurability. Insurance companies and health maintenance organizations (HMOs) vary in their reimbursement of medications and procedures they deem to be experimental. All of these factors place a tremendous amount of stress on an already taxed family unit.

Numerous local, regional, and national organizations provide information and educational resources about childhood malignant diseases. Local hospitals and cancer centers often provide support groups for family members. Informal parent-to-parent interactions based on the sense of having a common understanding of parenting a child with cancer can be a powerful source of support. Identifying local resources will provide a much-welcomed service to these families.

Resources

American Cancer Society
250 Williams St. NW
Atlanta, GA 30303
(800) ACS-2345; (404) 320-3333
Website: www.cancer.org

A volunteer organization offering educational programs, family services, rehabilitation support, and referral to local and regional resources.

Association of Pediatric Hematology/Oncology Nurses
4700 W. Lake Ave.
Glenview, IL 60025-1485
(847) 375-4724
Website: www.aphon.org

A professional organization for pediatric hematology/oncology nurses and other pediatric hematology/oncology health care professionals.

Cancer Information Service, National Cancer Institute
Blair Building, Room 414
9000 Rockville Pike
Bethesda, MD 20892
(800) 4CANCER
Website: www.cancernet.nci.nih.gov

A network of regional information centers that provide personalized answers to cancer-related questions from individuals, families, the general public, and health care professionals; also provides referral to local and regional resources.

Candlelighters Childhood Cancer Foundation, Inc.
7910 Woodmont Ave., Suite 460
Bethesda, MD 20814
(800) 366-2223; (301) 657-8401
Website: www.candlelighters.org

An international organization of parents whose children have had cancer; provides guidance and emotional support through local chapters, information, and referral to local and regional resources.

CureSearch
National Childhood Cancer Foundation
4600 East West Hiwy., Suite 600
Bethesda, MD 20814-3457
(800) 458-6223
Website: www.curesearch.org

An organization that raises funds for childhood cancer research and provides family educational materials in conjunction with the Children's Oncology Group research trials.

Leukemia and Lymphoma Society
1311 Mamaroneck Ave.
White Plains, NY 10605
(800) 955-4572; (914) 949-5213
Website: www.leukemia.org

A volunteer organization offering educational programs, information, financial assistance, and referral to local and regional resources.

Summary of Primary Care Needs for the Child with Cancer

HEALTH CARE MAINTENANCE
Growth and Development

- Growth slows because of chemotherapy and radiation.
- Closely monitor weight; child is at risk for significant weight loss because of disease and treatment and is also at risk for weight gain because of steroids.
- Periodic developmental screening is done to assess for age-appropriate behaviors.
- Neuropsychological testing is done for children who received cranial radiation.

Diet

- Maintain an adequate diet. Offer small, frequent meals if the child is experiencing anorexia. Low-sodium foods should be given to children receiving corticosteroid therapy. Increase fluid intake and high-fiber foods for constipation. Monitor diarrhea closely.

Safety

- Ensure proper handling of chemotherapeutic agents at home and proper maintenance and protection of indwelling venous access devices.
- Check platelet count after significant fall or head injury. The child may need platelet transfusion.
- Minimize roughhousing and discourage contact sports if the platelet count is less than 100,000. Because of photosensitivity, protect the child from sun. Use PABA-free sunblock.

Immunizations

- No live-virus vaccines are given while the child is receiving therapy or for the first year off therapy.
- Some centers recommend administering killed vaccines if the child is scheduled to receive them; booster doses, however, may be needed after therapy is complete. Other centers do not give killed vaccines until child has been off treatment for 6 months.
- Siblings and household contacts should not receive live polio vaccine because of transmissibility to child who is immunocompromised. Siblings and household contacts may receive measles, mumps, rubella (MMR) vaccine.
- The varicella vaccine, although not routinely recommended for children with malignancies, is available for use in some children with acute lymphocytic leukemia (ALL) who have been in remission for at least 1 year.
- Children recovering from hematopoietic stem cell transplantation require special consideration in determining immunization schedule and protocol (see Chapter 15).
- Children with Hodgkin disease should be vaccinated with the pneumococcal and *Haemophilus influenzae* type B conjugate vaccines before splenectomy or splenic irradiation.

Screening

- *Vision.* Routine screening is recommended. Thorough assessment is warranted if visual abnormalities are detected. Visual changes may occur secondary to tumor growth, radiation, or chemotherapy.
- *Hearing.* Routine screening is recommended. Children receiving ototoxic drugs should have regular evaluations by an audiologist.
- *Dental.* Routine screening is recommended. A complete blood count (CBC) should be done before an appointment to verify adequate absolute neutrophil count (ANC), platelet count. Meticulous oral hygiene is necessary to prevent infections.
- *Blood pressure.* Blood pressures should be taken at each visit to evaluate for hypertension as a result of drug toxicity.
- *Hematocrit.* Routine hematocrit testing should be performed when the child is off therapy. It is done as needed while the child is receiving therapy. Critical levels are ANC less than 500, platelets less than 20,000, and hemoglobin less than 7 to 8 g/dL.
- *Urinalysis.* Urinalysis is routine. Protein may be observed after radiation therapy, or hematuria may be seen after cyclophosphamide/ifosfamide therapy. Special UTI caution should be taken when only one kidney is present.
- *Tuberculosis.* Tuberculosis screening is routine and is done off therapy. Possible anergic status requires use of a control if child is tested on therapy. Chest x-ray may be necessary for screening.

Condition-Specific Screening

- Close assessment is required for signs and symptoms of late effects of therapy or recurrence of malignancy (see Table 16-3).

COMMON ILLNESS MANAGEMENT
Differential Diagnosis

- *Fever.* Rule out neutropenia and infection. Do septic workup as warranted. Prompt intervention is required with neutropenia or the presence of central VAD.
- *Viral and other infections.* Varicella-zoster immune globulin (VZIG) is required within 96 hours of exposure if the child does not have antibodies to varicella or has not been immunized. Acyclovir is given intravenously for chickenpox in the immunosuppressed individual. CMV and candidiasis are other common infections. Rule out dissemination of disease.
  - Give *Pneumocystis jiroveci* prophylaxis.
- *Gastrointestinal symptoms.* For chemotherapy-induced constipation, ensure adequate hydration and begin stool softeners or laxatives as needed. Avoid suppositories and enemas.
  - For nausea and vomiting, determine the relationship to chemotherapy and radiation; rule out viral and bacterial infection. Give hydration fluid and antiemetics as needed.
- *Headaches.* Perform a thorough neurologic examination. Consider possibility of a brain tumor, central nervous system (CNS) involvement, and lumbar puncture cerebrospinal fluid leak.
- *Pain.* Determine the source of pain; rule out tumor growth or cord compression. Do not treat with aspirin. Premedicate for procedures.

Drug Interactions

- No aspirin-containing products should be given. Acetaminophen is recommended except in times of neutropenia to avoid masking a fever.
- Low folic acid multivitamins may be taken. Consult with the oncology team before prescribing additional medication because of the risk of drug interaction.

Continued

Summary of Primary Care Needs for the Child with Cancer—cont'd

DEVELOPMENTAL ISSUES

Sleep Patterns

- Disturbances are common. Maintain consistent bedtime schedule and routine whenever possible. A transitional object may increase security during hospitalization.

Toileting

- Standard developmental counseling is advised. Regression may occur.
- Constipation may occur with some therapies.

Discipline

- Use normal patterns of discipline; it is important to maintain consistency for all siblings.

Child Care

- Generally a small group setting or home care is better than a large group to minimize exposure to infections. The caretaker should know the signs and symptoms that pose a concern.
- Communicable diseases must be reported.
- Frequent hand washing as infection control is recommended.

Schooling

- The child should return to school as soon as possible.
- Ongoing communication between primary care providers and teachers is necessary. Education of school staff and classmates is crucial.
- Assist the family in developing an individualized educational program (IEP). Periodically assess for school problems and learning disabilities.

- If the child is unable to participate in a regular school program, arrange for home tutoring.

Sexuality

- Give support for altered body image.
- Assess for appropriate Tanner staging. Any significant delay should be evaluated.
- Provide information about fertility preservation as appropriate. Sperm banking may be an option before an adolescent male begins chemotherapy or radiation.
- Provide contraception if appropriate and counsel regarding sexually transmitted infection (STI) prevention.

Transition to Adulthood

- It is necessary to transition care from the pediatric oncology center to an adult oncology center knowledgeable on long-term survival of children with cancer.
- Primary care providers may be of assistance in employment situations, if requested by individual, by providing factual information concerning prognosis.

FAMILY CONCERNS

- The family must deal with chronic uncertainty.
- Insurance and catastrophic financial effects are also concerns.
- Address needs of siblings.

REFERENCES

Allen, U.D. (2007). Immunizations for children with cancer. *Pediatr Blood Cancer, 49,* 1102-1108.

American Academy of Pediatrics Committee on Infectious Diseases. (2006). In L.K. Pickering (Ed.), *Red Book: 2006 Report of the Committee on Infectious Diseases* (27th ed.). Elk Grove Village, IL: American Academy of Pediatrics.

American Cancer Society. (2007). *Cancer facts and figures 2007.* Available at www.cancer.org/downloads/STT/CAFF2007PWSecured.pdf. Retrieved November 30, 2008.

Ammann, R.A., Aebi, C., Hirt, A., et al. (2004). Fever in neutropenia in children and adolescents: Evolution over time of main characteristics in a single center, 1993-2001. *Supportive Care in Cancer, 12,* 826-832.

Anderson, L.M. (2006). Environmental genotoxicants/carcinogens and childhood cancer: bridgeable gaps in scientific knowledge. *Mutat Res, 608,* 136-156.

Andre, N., Kababri, M.E., Bertrand, P., et al. (2007). Safety and efficacy of pegfilgrastim in children with cancer receiving myelosuppressive chemotherapy. *Anti-Cancer Drugs, 18,* 277-281.

Barrett, A.M., Imeson, J., Leese, D., et al. (2004). Factors influencing early failure of central venous catheters in children with cancer. *J Pediatr Surg, 39,* 1520-1523.

Bender, J.L., Adamson, P.C., Reid, J.M., et al. (2008). Phase I trial and pharmacokinetic study of bevacizumab in pediatric patients with refractory solid tumors: A Children's Oncology Group Study. *J Clin Oncol, 26,* 399-405.

Bhatia, S., Blatt, J., & Meadows, A.T. (2006). Late effects of childhood cancer and its treatment. In P.A Pizzo & D.G., Poplack (Eds.), *Principles and Practice of Pediatric Oncology* (5th ed.). Philadelphia: Lippincott Williams & Wilkins.

Bleyer, W.A. (2002). Cancer in older adolescents and young adults: Epidemiology, diagnosis, treatment, survival, and importance of clinical trials. *Med Pediatr Oncol, 38,* 1-10.

Boissel, N., Auclerc, M.F., Lheritier, V., et al. (2003). Should adolescents with acute lymphoblastic leukemia be treated as old children or young adults? Comparison of the French FRALLE-93 and LALA-94 trials. *J Clin Oncol, 21,* 774-780.

Champagne, M.A., Capdeville, R., Krailo, M., et al. (2004). Imatinib mesylate (STI571) for treatment of children with Philadelphia chromosome-positive leukemia: Results from a Children's Oncology Group Phase 1 Study. *Blood, 104,* 2655-2660.

Chang, S.D., Main, W., Martin, D.P., et al. (2003). An analysis of the accuracy of the CyberKnife: A robotic frameless stereotactic radiosurgical system. *Neurosurgery, 52,* 140-146. discussion 146-147.

Chanock, S.J., Kundra, V., Johnson, F.L., et al. (2006). The other side of the bed: What caregivers can learn from listening to patients and their families. In P.A. Pizzo & D.G. Poplack (Eds.), *Principles and Practice of Pediatric Oncology* (5th ed.). Philadelphia: Lippincott Williams & Wilkins.

Coradini, P.P., Cigana, L., Selistre, S.G., et al. (2007). Ototoxicity from cisplatin therapy in childhood cancer. *J Pediatr Hematol Oncol, 29,* 355-360.

Corey, S.J. (2005). Targeted therapy: For kids, too. *Pediatr Blood Cancer, 45,* 623-634.

Corrigan, J.J., & Feig, S.A. (2004). Guidelines for pediatric cancer centers. *Pediatrics, 113,* 1833-1835.

Crawford, J., Dale, D.C., & Lyman, G.H. (2004). Chemotherapy-induced neutropenia: Risks, consequences, and new directions for its management. *Cancer, 100,* 228-237.

Dang-Tan, T., & Franco, E.L. (2007). Diagnosis delays in childhood cancer: A review. *Cancer, 110,* 703-713.

de Bont, J.M., Holt, B., Dekker, A.W., et al. (2004). Significant difference in outcome for adolescents with acute lymphoblastic leukemia treated on pediatric vs adult protocols in the Netherlands. *Leukemia, 18,* 2032-2035.

Dickerman, J.D. (2007). The late effects of childhood cancer therapy. *Pediatrics, 119,* 554-568.

Donaldson, S.S., Meza, J., Breneman, J.C., et al. (2001). Results from the IRS-IV randomized trial of hyperfractionated radiotherapy in children with rhabdomyosarcoma—a report from the IRSG. *Int J Radiat Oncol Biol Phys, 51,* 718-728.

Fischer, V., Einolf, H.J., & Cohen, D. (2005). Efflux transporters and their clinical relevance. *Mini Rev Med Chem, 5,* 183-195.

Fletcher, P.C., & Clarke, J. (2004). The use of complementary and alternative medicine among pediatric patients. *Cancer Nurs, 27,* 93-99.

Forauer, A.R. (2007). Pericardial tamponade in patients with central venous catheters. *J Infus Nurs, 30,* 161-167.

Foster, A.E., Forrester, K., Li, Y.C., et al. (2004). Ex-vivo uses and applications of cytokines for adoptive immunotherapy in cancer. *Curr Pharm Design, 10,* 1207-1220.

Frierdich, S., Goes, C., & Dadd, G. (2003). Community and home care services provided to children with cancer: A report from the Children's Cancer Group Nursing Committee—Clinical Practice Group. *J Pediatr Oncol Nurs, 20,* 252-259.

Furchert, S.E., Lanvers-Kaminsky, C., Juurgens, H., et al. (2007). Inhibitors of histone deacetylases as potential therapeutic tools for high-risk embryonal tumors of the nervous system of childhood. *Int J Cancer, 120,* 1787-1794.

Gottschalk, S., Rooney, C.M., & Brenner, M.K. (2006). Cell and gene therapies. In P.A Pizzo & D.G. Poplack (Eds.), *Principles and Practice of Pediatric Oncology* (5th ed.). Philadelphia: Lippincott Williams & Wilkins.

Hara, W., Soltys, S.G., & Gibbs, I.C. (2007). CyberKnife robotic radiosurgery system for tumor treatment. *Expert Rev Anticancer Ther, 7,* 1507-1515.

Hawks, R. (2006). Complementary and alternative medicine research initiatives in the Children's Oncology Group and the role of the pediatric oncology nurse. *J Pediatr Oncol Nurs, 23,* 261-264.

Haytac, M.C., Dogan, M.C., & Antmen, B. (2004). The results of a preventive dental program for pediatric patients with hematologic malignancies. *Oral Health Prev Dent, 2,* 59-65.

Hinds, P.S., Hockenberry, M., Rai, S.N., et al. (2007). Nocturnal awakenings, sleep environment interruptions, and fatigue in hospitalized children with cancer. *Oncol Nurs Forum, 34,* 393-402.

Hockenberry, M., & Hooke, M.C. (2007). Symptom clusters in children with cancer. *Semin Oncol Nurs, 23,* 152-157.

Holdsworth, M.T., Raisch, D.W., & Frost, J. (2006). Acute and delayed nausea and emesis control in pediatric oncology patients. *Cancer, 106,* 931-940.

Hudson, M.M., Mertens, A.C., Yasui, Y., et al. (2003). Health status of adult long-term survivors of childhood cancer: A report from the Childhood Cancer Survivor Study. *J Am Med Assoc, 290,* 1583-1592.

Iannalfi, A., Bernini, G., Caprilli, S., et al. (2005). Painful procedures in children with cancer: Comparison of moderate sedation and general anesthesia for lumbar puncture and bone marrow aspiration. *Pediatr Blood Cancer, 45,* 933-938.

Keefe, D.M., Schubert, M.M., Elting, L.S., et al. (2007). Updated clinical practice guidelines for the prevention and treatment of mucositis. *Cancer, 109,* 820-831.

Kelly, K.M. (2004). Complementary and alternative medical therapies for children with cancer. *Eur J Cancer, 40,* 2041-2046.

Kelly, K.M. (2007). Complementary and alternative medicines for use in supportive care in pediatric cancer. *Supportive Care in Cancer, 15,* 457-460.

Kelly, K.M. (2008). Bringing evidence to complementary and alternative medicine in children with cancer: Focus on nutrition-related therapies. *Pediatr Blood Cancer, 50,* 490-493; discussion 498.

Kim, S.Y., & Hahn, W.C. (2007). Cancer genomics: Integrating form and function. *Carcinogenesis, 28,* 1387-1392.

Kleinerman, R.A., Tucker, M.A., Abramson, D.H., et al. (2007). Risk of soft tissue sarcomas by individual subtype in survivors of hereditary retinoblastoma. *J Natl Cancer Inst, 99,* 24-31.

Knudson, A.G. (2002). Cancer genetics. *Am J Med Genet, 111,* 96-102.

La, T.H., Meyers, P.A., Wexler, L.H., et al. (2006). Radiation therapy for Ewing's sarcoma: Results from Memorial Sloan-Kettering in the modern era. *Int J Radiat Oncol Biol Phys, 64,* 544-550.

Lashlee, M., & O'Hanlon Curry, J. (2007). Pediatric home chemotherapy: Infusing "quality of life." *J Pediatr Oncol Nurs, 24,* 294-298.

Link, M.P., & Weinstein, H.J. (2006). Malignant non-Hodgkin lymphomas in children. In P.A. Pizzo & D.G. Poplack (Eds.), *Principles and Practice of Pediatric Oncology* (5th ed.). Philadelphia: Lippincott Williams & Wilkins.

Liu, L., Krailo, M., & Reaman, G.H., et al. (2003). Childhood cancer patients' access to cooperative group cancer programs: A population-based study. *Cancer, 97,* 1339-1345.

Mackall, C., & Sondel, P.M. (2006). Tumor immunology and pediatric cancer. In P.A. Pizzo & D.G. Poplack (Eds.), *Principles and Practice of Pediatric Oncology* (5th ed.). Philadelphia: Lippincott Williams & Wilkins.

Malbasa, T., Kodish, E., & Santacroce, S.J. (2007). Adolescent adherence to oral therapy for leukemia: A focus group study. *J Pediatr Oncol Nurs, 24,* 139-151.

Malogolowkin, M.H., Quinn, J.J., Steuber, C.P., et al. (2006). Clinical assessment and differential diagnosis of the child with suspected cancer. In P.A. Pizzo & D.G. Poplack (Eds.), *Principles and Practice of Pediatric Oncology* (5th ed.), Philadelphia: Lippincott Williams & Wilkins.

Martel, D., Bussieres, J.F., Theoret, Y., et al. (2005). Use of alternative and complementary therapies in children with cancer. *Pediatr Blood Cancer, 44,* 660-668.

Martinson, I.M., Kim, S., Yang, S.O., et al. (1995). Impact of childhood cancer on Korean families. *J Pediatr Oncol Nurs, 12,* 11-17.

Mathews, V., George, B., Lakshmi, K.M., et al. (2006). Single-agent arsenic trioxide in the treatment of newly diagnosed acute promyelocytic leukemia: Durable remissions with minimal toxicity. *Blood, 107,* 2627-2632.

Mathijssen, R.H., Verweij, J., de Bruijn, P., et al. (2002). Effects of St. John's wort on irinotecan metabolism. *J Natl Cancer Inst, 94,* 1247-1249.

Matsuzaki, A., Suminoe, A., Koga, Y., et al. (2006). Long-term use of peripherally inserted central venous catheters for cancer chemotherapy in children. *Supportive Care in Cancer, 14,* 153-160.

Matthews, S.J., & McCoy, C. (2003). Thalidomide: A review of approved and investigational uses. *Clin Ther, 25,* 342-395.

McCullers, J.A., & Shenep, J.L. (2001). Assessment and management of suspected infection in neutropenic patients. In C.C. Patrick, (Ed.), *Clinical Management of Infections in Immunocompromised Infants and Children.* Philadelphia: Lippincott Williams & Wilkins.

Meistrich, M.L., & Byrne, J. (2002). Genetic disease in offspring of long-term survivors of childhood and adolescent cancer treated with potentially mutagenic therapies. *Am J Hum Genet, 70,* 1069-1071.

Mendez, I., Hill, R., Clarke, D., et al. (2005). Robotic long-distance telementoring in neurosurgery. *Neurosurgery, 56,* 434-440; discussion 434-440.

Miller, M., & Kearney, N. (2004). Chemotherapy-related nausea and vomiting—past reflections, present and future management. *European Journal of Cancer Care (English Language Edition), 13,* 71-81.

Millot, F., Guilhot, J., Nelken, B., et al. (2006). Imatinib mesylate is effective in children with chronic myelogenous leukemia in late chronic and advanced phase and in relapse after stem cell transplantation. *Leukemia, 20,* 187-192.

Monteiro Caran, E.M., Dias, C.G., Seber, A., et al. (2005). Clinical aspects and treatment of pain in children and adolescents with cancer. *Pediatr Blood Cancer, 45,* 925-932.

Mullighan, C.G., Goorha, S., Radtke, I., et al. (2007). Genome-wide analysis of genetic alterations in acute lymphoblastic leukaemia. *Nature, 446,* 758-764.

Nathan, M., & Selwood, K. (2006). The use of blood products in paediatric oncology units in the UK. *Paediatr Nurs, 18,* 14-17.

Neal, Z.C., Yang, J.C., Rakhmilevich, A.L., et al. (2004). Enhanced activity of hu14.18-IL2 immunocytokine against murine NXS2 neuroblastoma when combined with interleukin 2 therapy. *Clin Cancer Res, 10,* 4839-4847.

Neglia, J.P., Friedman, D.L., Yasui, Y., et al. (2001). Second malignant neoplasms in five-year survivors of childhood cancer: Childhood Cancer Survivor Study. *J Natl Cancer Inst, 93,* 618-629.

Nilsson, A., De Milito, A., Engstrom, P., et al. (2002). Current chemotherapy protocols for childhood acute lymphoblastic leukemia induce loss of humoral immunity to viral vaccination antigens. *Pediatrics, 109,* e91.

Nolbris, M., Enskar, K., & Hellstrom, A.L. (2007). Experience of siblings of children treated for cancer. *Eur J Oncol Nurs, 11,* 106-112; discussion 113-116.

Oeffinger, K.C., & McCabe, M.S. (2006). Models for delivering survivorship care. *J Clin Oncol, 24,* 5117-5124.

Olver, I.N. (2005). Update on anti-emetics for chemotherapy-induced emesis. *Intern Med J, 35,* 478-481.

Orudjev, E., & Lange, B.J. (2002). Evolving concepts of management of febrile neutropenia in children with cancer. *Med Pediatr Oncol, 39,* 77-85.

Parsons, S.K., Saiki-Craighill, S., Mayer, D.K., et al. (2007). Telling children and adolescents about their cancer diagnosis: Cross-cultural comparisons between pediatric oncologists in the US and Japan. *Psycho-Oncology, 16,* 60-68.

Post-White, J. (2006). Complementary and alternative medicine in pediatric oncology. *J Pediatr Oncol Nurs, 23,* 244-253.

Post-White, J., Hawks, R., O'Mara, A., et al. (2006). Future directions of CAM research in pediatric oncology. *J Pediatr Oncol Nurs, 23*, 265-268.

Quezada, G., Sunderland, T., Chan, K.W., et al. (2007). Medical and non-medical barriers to outpatient treatment of fever and neutropenia in children with cancer. *Pediatr Blood Cancer, 48*, 273-277.

Radeva, J.I., VanScoyoc, E., Smith, F.O., et al. (2005). National estimates of the use of hematopoietic stem-cell transplantation in children with cancer in the United States. *Bone Marrow Transplant, 36*, 397-404.

Ramanujachar, R., Richards, S., Hann, I., et al. (2006). Adolescents with acute lymphoblastic leukaemia: Emerging from the shadow of paediatric and adult treatment protocols. *Pediatr Blood Cancer, 47*, 748-756.

Rheingans, J.I. (2007). A systematic review of nonpharmacologic adjunctive therapies for symptom management in children with cancer. *J Pediatr Oncol Nurs, 24*, 81-94.

Ries, L.A.G., Melbert, D., Krapcho, M., et al. (2008). *SEER cancer statistics review, 1975-2005.* Available at http://seer.cancer.gov/csr/1975_2005/. Retrieved May 3, 2008.

Robinson, D.L., & Carr, B.A. (2007). Delayed vomiting in children with cancer after receiving moderately high or highly emetogenic chemotherapy. *J Pediatr Oncol Nurs, 24*, 70-80.

Rogers, P.C., Melnick, S.J., Ladas, E.J., et al. (2008). Children's Oncology Group (COG) nutrition committee. *Pediatr Blood Cancer, 50*, 447-450; discussion 451.

Ruccione, K.S., Hinds, P.S., Wallace, J.D., et al. (2005). Creating a novel structure for nursing research in a cooperative clinical trials group: The Children's Oncology Group experience. *Semin Oncol Nurs, 21*, 79-88.

Saif, M.W., & Mehra, R. (2006). Incidence and management of bevacizumab-related toxicities in colorectal cancer. *Expert Opin Drug Saf, 5*, 553-566.

Sanford, S.D., Okuma, J.O., Pan, J., et al. (2008). Gender differences in sleep, fatigue, and daytime activity in a pediatric oncology sample receiving dexamethasone. *J Pediatr Psychol, 33*(3), 298-306.

Santacroce, S. (2002). Uncertainty, anxiety, and symptoms of posttraumatic stress in parents of children recently diagnosed with cancer. *J Pediatr Oncol Nurs, 19*, 104-111.

Satwani, P., Morris, E., Bradley, M.B., et al. (2008). Reduced intensity and non-myeloablative allogeneic stem cell transplantation in children and adolescents with malignant and non-malignant diseases. *Pediatr Blood Cancer, 50*, 1-8.

Sawyer, S.M., & Aroni, R.A. (2003). Sticky issue of adherence. *J Paediatr Child Health, 39*, 2-5.

Schuchter, L.M., Hensley, M.L., Meropol, N.J., et al. (2002). 2002 update of recommendations for the use of chemotherapy and radiotherapy protectants: Clinical practice guidelines of the American Society of Clinical Oncology. *J Clin Oncol, 20*, 2895-2903.

Schultz, T.R., Durning, S., Niewinski, M., et al. (2006). A multidisciplinary approach to vascular access in children. *J Spec Pediatr Nurs, 11*, 254-256.

Scotlandi, K., Manara, M.C., Hattinger, C.M., et al. (2005). Prognostic and therapeutic relevance of HER2 expression in osteosarcoma and Ewing's sarcoma. *Eur J Cancer, 41*, 1349-1361.

Simon, A., Bode, U., & Beutel, K. (2006). Diagnosis and treatment of catheter-related infections in paediatric oncology: An update. *Clin Microbiol Infect, 12*, 606-620.

Skinner, R. (2004). Best practice in assessing ototoxicity in children with cancer. *Eur J Cancer, 40*, 2352-2354.

Skolin, I., Wahlin, Y.B., Broman, D.A., et al. (2006). Altered food intake and taste perception in children with cancer after start of chemotherapy: Perspectives of children, parents and nurses. *Supportive Care in Cancer, 14*, 369-378.

Smith, A.R., Repka, T.L., & Weigel, B.J. (2005). Aprepitant for the control of chemotherapy induced nausea and vomiting in adolescents. *Pediatr Blood Cancer, 45*, 857-860.

Smith, M.A. (2006). Evolving molecularly targeted therapies and biotherapeutics. In P.A. Pizzo & D.G. Poplack (Eds.), *Principles and Practice of Pediatric Oncology* (5th ed.), Philadelphia: Lippincott Williams & Wilkins.

Spinetta, J.J., Masera, G., Eden, T., et al. (2002). Refusal, non-compliance, and abandonment of treatment in children and adolescents with cancer: A report of the SIOP Working Committee on Psychosocial Issues in Pediatric Oncology. *Med Pediatr Oncol, 38*, 114-117.

Stephenson, J. (2002). Cancer studies explore targeted therapy, researchers seek new prevention strategies. *J Am Med Assoc, 287*, 3063-3067.

Stevens, B., McKeever, P., Law, M.P., et al. (2006). Children receiving chemotherapy at home: Perceptions of children and parents. *J Pediatr Oncol Nurs, 23*, 276-285.

Sung, L., Feldman, B.M., Schwamborn, G., et al. (2004). Inpatient versus outpatient management of low-risk pediatric febrile neutropenia: Measuring parents' and healthcare professionals' preferences. *J Clin Oncol, 22*, 3922-3929.

Sung, L., Nathan, P.C., Alibhai, S.M., et al. (2007). Meta-analysis: Effect of prophylactic hematopoietic colony-stimulating factors on mortality and outcomes of infection. *Ann Intern Med, 147*, 400-411.

Tarbell, N.J., Yock, T., & Kooy, H. (2006). Principles of radiation oncology. In P.A. Pizzo & D.G. Poplack (eds.), *Principles and Practice of Pediatric Oncology* (5th ed.). Philadelphia: Lippincott Williams & Wilkins.

Waber, D.P., Silverman, L.B., Catania, L., et al. (2004). Outcomes of a randomized trial of hyperfractionated cranial radiation therapy for treatment of high-risk acute lymphoblastic leukemia: Therapeutic efficacy and neurotoxicity. *J Clin Oncol, 22*, 2701-2707.

Walker, M.P., Yaszemski, M.J., Kim, C.W., et al. (2003). Metastatic disease of the spine: Evaluation and treatment. *Clin Orthop Relat Res, Oct*(415 Suppl), S165-S175.

Walsh, T.J., Roilides, E., Groll, A.H., et al. (2006). Infectious complications in pediatric cancer patients. In P.A. Pizzo & D.G. Poplack (Eds.), *Principles and Practice of Pediatric Oncology* (5th ed.), Philadelphia: Lippincott Williams & Wilkins.

Weyl Ben Arush, M., Geva, H., Ofir, R., et al. (2006). Prevalence and characteristics of complementary medicine used by pediatric cancer patients in a mixed Western and Middle-Eastern population. *J Pediatr Hematol Oncol, 28*, 141-146.

Wiener, L.S., Hersh, S.P., & Kazak, A.E. (2006). Psychiatric and psychosocial support for the child and family. In P.A. Pizzo & D.G. Poplack (Eds.), *Principles and Practice of Pediatric Oncology* (5th ed.), Philadelphia: Lippincott Williams & Wilkins.

Wilson, W., Taubert, K.A., Gewitz, M., et al. (2007). Prevention of infective endocarditis: Guidelines from the American Heart Association: A guideline from the American Heart Association Rheumatic Fever, Endocarditis, and Kawasaki Disease Committee, Council on Cardiovascular Disease in the Young, and the Council on Clinical Cardiology, Council on Cardiovascular Surgery and Anesthesia, and the Quality of Care and Outcomes Research Interdisciplinary Working Group. *Circulation, 116*, 1736-1754.

Wong, E.C., Perez-Albuerne, E., Moscow, J.A., et al. (2005). Transfusion management strategies: A survey of practicing pediatric hematology/oncology specialists. *Pediatr Blood Cancer, 44*, 119-127.

Young, B., Dixon-Woods, M., Findlay, M., et al. (2002). Parenting in a crisis: Conceptualising mothers of children with cancer. *Soc Sci Med, 55*, 1835-1847.

Zebrack, B.J., Gurney, J.G., Oeffinger, K., et al. (2004). Psychological outcomes in long-term survivors of childhood brain cancer: A report from the Childhood Cancer Survivor Study. *J Clin Oncol, 22*, 999-1006.

Zebrack, B.J., Zeltzer, L.K., Whitton, J., et al. (2002). Psychological outcomes in long-term survivors of childhood leukemia, Hodgkin's disease, and non-Hodgkin's lymphoma: A report from the Childhood Cancer Survivor Study. *Pediatrics, 110*, 42-52.

Zebrack, B.J., Zevon, M.A., Turk, N., et al. (2007). Psychological distress in long-term survivors of solid tumors diagnosed in childhood: A report from the Childhood Cancer Survivor Study. *Pediatr Blood Cancer, 49*, 47-51.

17 Celiac Disease

Kari Runge and Kaylie K. Nguyen

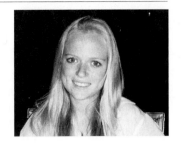

Etiology

Historically, celiac disease, or gluten-sensitive enteropathy, was called celiac sprue to describe its similarity to tropical sprue. It is classically defined as an autoimmune-mediated enteropathy occurring in genetically predisposed individuals triggered by the ingestion of gluten. "Gluten" is a broad term used to describe the proteins in grass-related grains, mainly wheat, barley, and rye. Aretaeus of Cappadocia, who lived during the second century in Greece, is credited with writing the first description of a malabsorptive syndrome characterized by chronic diarrhea. The term "celiac" is derived from the Greek word κοιλκιακος (koiliakos), meaning *abdominal*. Celiac disease was first reported in modern times as a disease entity by a British pediatrician, Samuel Gee. In 1888, he published a paper that described his clinical experience with a malabsorption syndrome in children. Gee noted that the cure to this affliction was likely related to diet. A substantial breakthrough in celiac disease research came from Dr. Willem Karel Dicke (Netherlands) in 1950 with his discovery of the harmful link between wheat and celiac disease. Later, with the advent of improved intestinal biopsy techniques, gluten was found to cause small intestinal villous atrophy and crypt hyperplasia. The finding of the association of human leukocyte antigen (HLA) with the disease has helped to expand knowledge of its genetic relevance. The discovery of gluten-dependent antibodies, in particular tissue transglutaminase, was instrumental in improving screening techniques (Maki & Lohi, 2004). These advances in screening, genetics, and diagnostics have raised celiac disease to national attention.

The pathogenesis of celiac disease is multifactorial and includes environmental triggers, immune processes, and genetic susceptibility. The exact mechanism of pathogenesis is unknown, but many hypotheses have been described. These include the missing enzyme theory, immunologic hypothesis, membrane glycoprotein defect, and mucosal permeability defect (Maki & Lohi, 2004). The environmental trigger is the ingestion of gluten-containing products. These toxic proteins trigger a complex inflammatory cascade of T cell–mediated immune events and include the proliferative production of inflammatory cytokines. Mucosal damage caused by chronic inflammation is cumulative and, in conjunction with increased intestinal permeability, distorts the absorptive capability of the small intestine.

A genetic predisposition is seen in celiac disease, with an increased prevalence among first-degree relatives (5%) (Fasano, Berti, Gerarduzzi, et al., 2003) and a concordance rate of approximately 70% in monozygotic twins (Greco, Romino, Coto, et al., 2002). One of the major advances in the understanding of the genetic aspect of celiac disease was the discovery of its association with HLA-DQ genes, for which testing is now commercially available. The HLA complex is the major human histocompatibility complex. This group of genes is located on chromosome 6 and encodes cell surface antigen–presenting proteins on white blood cells and tissue cells. These genes have an essential function in the immune process. They are also used as genetic markers to match donated organs with transplant recipients (Guyton & Hall, 2001). The *HLA-DQ2* allele combination is found in 90% to 95% of celiac disease patients and *HLA-DQ8* is present in the remaining 5% to 10%. However, 20% to 30% of people without celiac disease also have the *HLA-DQ2* gene (Hill, Bhatnagar, Cameron, et al., 2005). Thus carrying either *DQ2* or *DQ8* is necessary for the disease expression but not sufficient. In fact, in those of Western European ancestry, 30% to 40% carry *DQ2* or *DQ8* but fewer than 3% are thought to eventually develop celiac disease (Green & Jabri, 2006).

Incidence and Prevalence

Celiac disease was previously thought to be a rare disorder. However, a large landmark epidemiologic study found the prevalence of celiac disease to be surprisingly high, occurring in approximately 1% of the general population (Fasano et al., 2003). In a large longitudinal study of *HLA-DQ2* and *HLA-DQ8* characterized normal newborns from Denver, Colorado, 1 in 100 children had evidence of celiac disease by 5 years of age (Hoffenberg, MacKenzie, Barriga, et al., 2003). The incidence of celiac disease has been found to be 0.81 per 1000 live births in a study of newly diagnosed children with celiac disease in the Netherlands, with a linear increase from 1993 to 2000 (Steens, Csizmadia, George, et al., 2005). Similarly, the incidence of celiac disease among Finnish school children is at least 1 in 99 (Maki, Mustalahti, Kokkonen, et al., 2003). Celiac disease is believed to be more common in individuals of European descent and less common in black Africans, Chinese, and Japanese groups (Hill, 2002). The question remains whether the incidence and prevalence of celiac disease are really increasing or whether it is being diagnosed more frequently with the improvement in screening and endoscopic tools. There may be three to seven undiagnosed cases for each diagnosed case of celiac disease (Rewers, 2005), pointing out that only a small percentage of cases are actually recognized. The term "celiac iceberg" has been used to describe the idea that we are only diagnosing the very tip of the population (Catassi, Ratsch, Fabiani, et al., 1994). Screening strategies to identify silent and latent forms of celiac disease will help uncover the actual incidence of the disease.

Diagnostic Criteria

Despite the high prevalence of celiac disease in the United States, a survey of 132 primary care physicians in a southern California county who had been in practice for an average of 20 years revealed that only 35% had ever diagnosed a patient with celiac disease (Zipser, Farid, Baisch, et al., 2005). This finding highlights the need for education in identifying and screening potential cases of celiac disease.

The diagnostic criteria for celiac disease include positive serologic markers, characteristic intestinal biopsies, and response to a gluten-free diet (GFD). Serologic tests aid in identifying patients for whom intestinal biopsy is indicated to confirm the diagnosis of celiac disease. The currently available tests include antigliadin immunoglobulin A (IgA) and immunoglobulin G (IgG), antireticulin IgA, antiendomysial (EMA) IgA, and antitissue transglutaminase (TTG) IgA and IgG antibodies. The North American Society of Pediatric Gastroenterology, Hepatology, and Nutrition (NASPGHAN) recommends the measurement of TTG IgA in the initial screening for celiac disease (Hill et al., 2005). TTG is a normal gut enzyme released during cell injury. In those with celiac disease, it modifies gliadin peptides (toxic protein factor of gluten) in the intestinal mucosa leading to an inflammatory cascade. The sensitivity of TTG ranges from 0.92 to 1.00 and specificity from 0.91 to 1.00. EMA IgA is as accurate as TTG (sensitivity 0.88 to 1.00 and specificity 0.91 to 1.00) but is not recommended for initial screening because it is more expensive, time consuming, and prone to operator error in interpretation (Hill et al., 2005). Current recommendations suggest checking quantitative serum IgA to screen for IgA deficiency, which is more common in individuals with celiac disease (Hill et al., 2005). Thus initial screening should include TTG IgA along with total serum IgA. If a child is IgA deficient, TTG IgG should be performed (Hill et al., 2005). Antigliadin IgG and IgA and antireticulin IgA are no longer recommended because of their variability and inferior specificity and sensitivity. Nevertheless, these serologic markers continue to be drawn as part of a panel and often are found to be elevated. Elevation of antigliadin IgA or IgG antibodies in the absence of TTG or EMA antibody positivity is considered a negative celiac screen.

In addition to antibody markers, genetic typing can also aid diagnosis in that the absence of *HLA-DQ8* and *HLA-DQ2* essentially rules out celiac disease. However, HLA typing is not recommended as part of routine screening and many insurance companies may not cover its high cost. Further supportive evidence of diagnosis is the reduction or resolution of antibodies after a period on a GFD (Hill et al., 2005).

All children with positive serologic markers should be referred to a gastroenterologist for esophagogastroduodenoscopy (EGD) to obtain confirmatory biopsies. This remains the gold standard for diagnosis of celiac disease (Hill et al., 2005). There are no set guidelines for biopsy retrieval, but common practice is to obtain four to six biopsies in the duodenum, given the patchy distribution of the disease. The characteristic histologic features include mucosal inflammation, villous atrophy, crypt hyperplasia, and lymphocyte infiltration of the epithelium (Figure 17-1). Villous atrophy of the duodenum is characteristic but not specific to celiac disease. Other causes include giardiasis, collagenous sprue, common variable immunodeficiency, autoimmune enteropathy, radiation enteritis, Whipple's disease, tuberculosis, tropical sprue, eosinophilic gastroenteritis, human immunodeficiency virus (HIV) enteropathy, intestinal lymphoma, Zollinger-Ellison syndrome, Crohn's disease, and food allergies or intolerances other than to gluten (Green & Cellier, 2007). Thus the diagnosis of celiac disease should be based not only on intestinal biopsy but also on serologic testing and clinical response to a GFD. A skilled endoscopist and pathologist familiar with celiac disease morphology are essential in confirming the diagnosis (Figure 17-2).

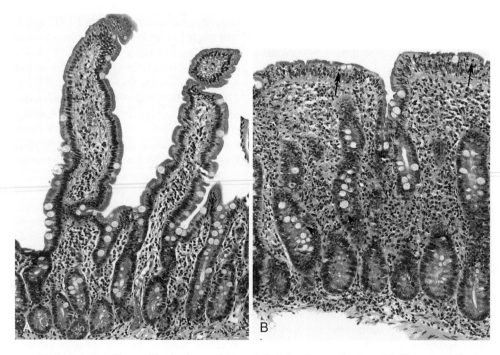

FIGURE 17-1 Biopsy of the duodenum. **A,** Normal. **B,** Celiac disease. Courtesy of Teri Longacre, MD.

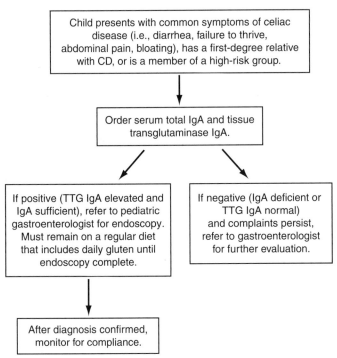

FIGURE 17-2 Diagnostic algorithm for celiac disease.

Clinical Manifestations at Time of Diagnosis

Celiac disease is thought to be one of the most common genetic disorders in the world and a frequent cause of malabsorption in children. It is important that primary care providers be aware of both the gastrointestinal and nongastrointestinal symptoms that may be an indication of celiac disease, because they vary widely among affected individuals.

Clinical Manifestations at Time of Diagnosis

- Failure to thrive
- Diarrhea
- Abdominal distention/bloating
- Nausea/vomiting
- Constipation
- Dermatitis herpetiformis
- Dental enamel defects
- Short stature
- Delayed puberty
- Osteoporosis
- Iron deficiency anemia

Data from Fasano, A (2005). Clinical presentation of celiac disease in the pediatric population. *Gastroenterology, 128,* 68-73.

Typically, infants and young children who have not yet been diagnosed with celiac disease have impaired growth, chronic diarrhea, abdominal distention, muscle wasting, poor appetite, and irritability. These signs and symptoms generally manifest between 6 and 24 months of age, depending on when adequate amounts of gluten are introduced into the diet. The longer the diagnosis is delayed, the more malnourished a child may be. However, some children, such as those who belong to high-risk groups, may have positive markers on screening but be clinically asymptomatic. Older children may present to their health care provider with gastrointestinal complaints such as recurrent abdominal pain, nausea, vomiting, bloating, and constipation. Extraintestinal manifestations of celiac disease include short stature, pubertal delay, dental enamel defects, osteopenia, osteoporosis, and anemia secondary to iron, folate, or vitamin B_{12} deficiency (D'Amico, Holmes, Stavropoulos, et al., 2005; Fasano, 2005). There also exists a cutaneous manifestation of gluten enteropathy called dermatitis herpetiformis. This is a severe erythematous pruritic skin rash that is rare in children, though cases have been reported in infants as young as 8 months (Templet, Welsh, & Cusack, 2007).

Other, less common, manifestations may include neurologic and psychiatric syndromes such as peripheral neuropathy, cerebellar ataxia, migraines, and epilepsy (Bushara, 2005). However, further studies are needed to establish possible causal relationships between these disorders and gluten sensitivity. In adults, it has been found that elevations in liver transaminases and liver biopsies revealing nonspecific reactive hepatitis improve on a GFD (Hill et al., 2005). Long-standing data demonstrate increased risk of infertility, miscarriage, delayed menarche, and amenorrhea in females with delayed diagnosis or untreated celiac disease (Hill et al., 2005).

Although providers should be aware of the classic symptoms of celiac disease—diarrhea, abdominal distention, and failure to thrive (Fasano, 2005)—as well as the atypical symptoms mentioned previously, it should be emphasized that "silent" forms of celiac disease are becoming increasingly prevalent. A retrospective medical record review of pediatric patients with the diagnosis of celiac disease by intestinal biopsy between 1986 and 2003 by Telega, Rivera Bennet, and Werlin (2008) revealed that 59.6% of the patients diagnosed with celiac disease had no gastrointestinal symptoms, but instead had associated conditions such as type 1 diabetes, thyroiditis, Down syndrome, family history of celiac disease, short stature, and iron deficiency. They also found that gastrointestinal symptoms are becoming less prevalent as presenting symptoms of celiac disease, especially in children older than 3 years. The study concluded that 11.2% of the patients diagnosed were overweight with body mass index greater than 90% at time of diagnosis. Additionally, a New Zealand study by Westerbeek, Mouat, Wesley, and colleagues (2005) found that a large number of patients (19%) in the high-risk group who were diagnosed with celiac disease were asymptomatic. This chart review found that children less than 5 years of age at time of diagnosis more often had failure to thrive and those older than 5 years more frequently had abdominal pain. Garampazzi, Rapa, Mura, and colleagues (2007) also came to similar conclusions in their chart review of Italian children diagnosed with celiac disease from 1987 to 2006: the age of diagnosis and asymptomatic forms of celiac disease have increased significantly from 2001 to 2006. These studies illustrate the importance of considering routine screening for celiac disease in children in high-risk groups (Box 17-1) who are often asymptomatic.

Last, primary care providers should also be cognizant of the rare phenomenon of celiac crisis, which can easily be mistaken for viral gastroenteritis. Signs and symptoms of celiac crisis include severe acute diarrhea, marked abdominal distention, edema, dehydration, and electrolyte imbalances (Fasano, 2005; Mones,

BOX 17-1

High-Risk Groups

- Autoimmune thyroiditis
- Down syndrome
- First-degree relatives of celiac patients
- Selective immunoglobulin A (IgA) deficiency
- Turner syndrome
- Type I diabetes
- Williams syndrome

From Hill, I., Bhatnagar, S., Cameron, D., et al. (2005). Guideline for the diagnosis and treatment of celiac disease in children: Recommendations of the North American Society for Pediatric Gastroenterology, Hepatology, and Nutrition. *J Pediatr Gastroenterol Nutr, 40,* 1-19.

Atienza, Youssef, et al., 2007). These children should be hospitalized to rule out infection and allergy, resuscitated with fluids and electrolytes, and screened for celiac disease.

Treatment

The only known treatment for celiac disease at this time is lifelong adherence to a GFD. Gluten is a combination of the proteins gliadin and glutenin, which exist along with starch in grass-related grains, mainly wheat. Gliadin is the alcohol-soluble portion of gluten that is toxic in persons with celiac disease (Green & Jabri, 2006). Rye and barley contain proteins very similar to gliadin: hordeins and secalins. Therefore a GFD excludes mainly wheat, rye, and barley. Malt, including malt syrups, extracts, and flavorings, should also be avoided, because it is a partial hydrolysate of barley proteins. Triticale (combination of wheat and rye), kamut, spelt (faro), semolina (durum wheat), farina, einkorn, bulgar, and couscous are other grains that contain gluten and should also be excluded (Hill et al., 2005).

Oats were thought to cause mucosal damage in individuals with celiac disease in the past, but recent studies have demonstrated no such effects with consumption of pure, uncontaminated oat products. The average amounts of oats consumed daily in these studies ranged from 15 to 50 grams per day (Hogberg, Laurin, Falth-Magnusson, et al., 2004; Holm, Maki, Vuolteenaho, et al., 2006, Janatuinen, Kemppainen, Julkunen, et al., 2002). A GFD with inclusion of oats was not found to prevent mucosal healing or normalization of serologic markers (Hogberg et al., 2004). The concern over oat's safety is its contamination with gluten in the harvesting, milling, and transport process. It is therefore very important that individuals confirm the product's purity before including it in their GFD.

The definition of "gluten free" is constantly undergoing revision because the exact amount of gluten that induces harm is unknown and techniques for detecting gluten can be imprecise (Akobeng & Thomas, 2008). The Codex Alimentarius Commission is a joint effort by the Food and Agriculture Organization of the United Nations (FAOUN) and the World Health Organization (WHO) charged with setting the standard amount of gluten allowed in a food product for it to be considered a "gluten-free" food for international trade. They revised the Standard for Foods for Special Dietary Uses for Persons Intolerant to Gluten in July, 2008. It dictates that gluten-free foods, either natural or specially processed to remove gluten, should not contain more than 20 mg/kg or 20 parts per million (ppm) gluten (Codex Alimentarius Commission, 2007). The U.S. Food and Drug Administration (FDA) is adopting this standard in its working proposal for voluntary

Treatment

Gluten-Free Grains and Flours and Foods Derived from Grains

Allowed on GFD

- Amaranth
- Arrowroot
- Beans
- Buckwheat
- Corn (maize)
- Distilled alcoholic beverages (e.g., wines, hard liquor)
- Distilled vinegars
- Flax
- Garfava
- Millet
- Montina
- Nut flours
- Oats (see discussion in chapter)
- Potatoes
- Quinoa
- Rice
- Sorghum
- Soy
- Tapioca
- Teff

NOT Allowed on GFD

- Barley
- Beers, ales, lagers
- Malt, malt flavoring, malt vinegar
- Nondistilled alcoholic beverages
- Rye
- Triticale
- Wheat (durham, einkorn, faro, graham, kamut, semolina, and spelt)

From www.celiac.org.
Key: *GFD,* gluten-free diet.

gluten-free food labeling. There are currently no official federal regulations to define the term "gluten-free" food (U.S. FDA Center for Food Safety and Applied Nutrition, n.d.).

Clinical improvement on a GFD can usually be noticed within several days to several weeks, but it is unclear precisely how long it takes for the intestinal mucosa to recover completely. For now, the only known treatment is a GFD for life, though a small number of patients do not show clinical or histologic improvement with a GFD. In these cases, the child needs to be followed closely by a gastroenterologist for further evaluation, including checking for compliance with the GFD, consideration of other diagnoses (eg: lactose intolerance, small bowel bacterial overgrowth, food allergies), and to screen for complications of celiac disease such as intestinal carcinoma, enteropathy-associated T cell lymphoma, or refractory sprue (Green & Cellier, 2007).

The most common pitfall to a GFD are foods with hidden gluten. Because beer is made from fermented grains, it should be avoided on a GFD. Gluten-free beers are available at specialty stores. Distilled forms of alcohol are safe to drink if they are without gluten-containing additives. Closely examine liquors and premixed drinks for unsafe ingredients. Assume all processed products contain gluten unless otherwise labeled or confirmed by the manufacturer. For example, it is possible that products such as cosmetics and toothpaste contain gluten (Box 17-2).

Potential Gluten Pitfalls*

- Breading and coating mixes
- Brown rice syrup
- Communion wafers
- Croutons
- Drugs and over-the-counter medications
- Energy bars
- Flour or cereal products
- Herbal supplements
- Imitation bacon
- Imitation seafood
- Marinades
- Nutritional supplements
- Panko (Japanese breadcrumbs)
- Pastas
- Play-Doh (This is a potential problem if hands are put on or in the mouth while playing with Play-Doh. Hands should be washed immediately after use.)
- Processed luncheon meats
- Sauces, gravies
- Self-basting poultry
- Soup bases
- Soy sauce or soy sauce solids
- Stuffings, dressing
- Thickeners (roux)
- Vitamins and mineral supplements

From www.celiac.org.
*Not a comprehensive list.

Complementary and Alternative Therapies

The only known treatment for celiac disease at this point is a life-long adherence to a GFD.

Anticipated Advances in Diagnosis and Management

Research is underway for more sensitive and specific screening techniques that may eliminate the need for intestinal biopsy (Hill et al., 2005). However, there are no published studies to prompt a change in the current recommendations for diagnosis. Capsule endoscopy is currently being explored as a way to monitor adherence and mucosal healing. Presently, the only treatment for celiac disease is the GFD. Many ideas for nondietary treatments have been proposed, including techniques to genetically detoxify grains and modify gluten during the manufacturing process. Other proposals include immunomodulators to inhibit the inflammatory response, vaccinations to induce gluten tolerance, inhibition of intestinal permeability, and oral peptidase supplementation or other recombinant enzymes that digest gliadin in the gastrointestinal tract, all of which require extensive research before their application in clinical practice (Hill, 2002; Kwon & Farrell, 2006).

Associated Problems of Celiac Disease and Treatment

The conditions most strongly associated with celiac disease in children are first-degree relatives of individuals with proven celiac disease (5% prevalence), autoimmune thyroiditis (3%), type 1 diabetes mellitus (3% to 8%), Down syndrome (5% to 12%), Turner syndrome (5%), Williams syndrome (3%), selective IgA deficiency (2%), and other autoimmune disorders, including dermatitis herpetiformis, systemic lupus erythematosus, liver disease, collagen vascular disease, rheumatoid arthritis, and Sjögren syndrome (Hill et al., 2005; National Institute of Health Consensus Development Conference on Celiac Disease, 2005). Current guidelines recommend routine periodic screening of asymptomatic children belonging to these groups beginning at age 3, after at least 1 year of adequate ingestion of gluten (Hill et al., 2005). Current literature estimates the prevalence of mucosal changes consistent with celiac disease in approximately 8% of those with type 1 diabetes, but determination of exact numbers is a challenge because seroconversion can occur over time, leaving those who initially screened negative without confirmatory biopsies (Goh & Banerjee, 2007). Similarly, in those with Down syndrome, it is estimated that between 5% and 12% have celiac disease. Adult cohorts with Down syndrome have higher prevalence rates than cohorts of children, again suggesting seroconversion over time (Hill et al., 2005). In a study of Italian children with Down syndrome, Bonamico, Mariani, Danesi, and colleagues (2001) found that one third of those with celiac disease did not have any gastrointestinal symptoms. These examples demonstrate that routine, periodic screening for celiac disease in all children at high risk for developing the condition is an important consideration in clinical practice.

The clinical manifestations of celiac disease vary widely and thus so do the differential diagnoses. Depending on the symptoms, providers should consider inflammatory bowel disease, especially Crohn's disease; small bowel bacterial overgrowth; giardiasis and other parasitic, bacterial, or viral gastroenteritis; food allergies; eosinophilic enteropathy; malabsorptive syndromes; hypothyroidism; IgA deficiency; and protein-losing enteropathy. These may exist concurrently with celiac disease. Because of the autoimmune nature of these conditions, there is a high crossover of celiac disease with inflammatory bowel disease. According to Yang, Chen, Scherl, and colleagues (2005), the prevalence ratio for Crohn's disease was 8.4 and for ulcerative colitis 3.56 in a cohort of 455 individuals with celiac disease, which is higher than that of the general population. Thus the possibility of dual diagnosis should be considered, especially if the child continues to be symptomatic on a GFD.

Prognosis

The prognosis of children diagnosed and treated in a timely manner is excellent. Clinical improvement is usually apparent within the first few weeks on a GFD, but complete restoration of intestinal mucosa may take up to 2 years (Al-toma, Verbeek, & Mulder, 2007). Complications of untreated celiac disease include short stature, dermatitis herpetiformis, dental enamel hypoplasia, recurrent stomatitis, fertility problems, osteoporosis, gluten ataxia and other neurologic disturbances, hyposplenism, refractory celiac disease, and intestinal lymphoma. The risk of reduced bone mineral density in children with untreated celiac disease is well documented, but a strict GFD improves bone mineralization in as quickly as 1 year (Kavak, Yuce, Kocak, et al., 2003). Hyposplenism is a known complication in adults with untreated celiac disease but is less commonly found in children. Individuals with untreated celiac disease have an overall risk of intestinal cancer (adenocarcinoma and enteropathy-associated T cell lymphoma) that is almost twice that of the general population (Green & Cellier, 2007). In adult studies, enteropathy-associated T cell lymphoma generally has a very poor prognosis; less than 20% of patients survive for 30 months (Green & Cellier, 2007). On a brighter note, new research shows that individuals whose celiac disease is diagnosed in childhood or adolescence have no increased lifetime cancer risk (Hill et al., 2005). Other less quantifiable symptoms for untreated or refractory celiac disease have been described, such as fatigue, generalized discomfort, lack of concentration, and personality and behavior changes, all of which can lead to a poor quality of life.

A minority of children (5%) (Green & Cellier, 2007) have refractory celiac disease, defined as "persistent or recurring villous atrophy with crypt hyperplasia and increased intraepithelial lymphocytes in spite of a strict gluten free diet for more than twelve months or when severe persisting symptoms necessitate intervention independent of the duration of dietary therapy" (Al-toma et al., 2007, p. 230). There are two categories of refractory celiac disease: type I and type II. Type I is characterized by the absence of aberrant T cells and type II by their presence. Al-toma and colleagues (2007) suggest that in these cases the diagnosis of celiac disease should first be reexamined, along with assessing dietary compliance and excluding other causes of diarrhea, villous atrophy, and malignant complications of celiac disease. Immunosuppression beginning with corticosteroid induction is the treatment for type I refractory disease. Case reports have described maintenance therapy with azathioprine, budesonide, cyclosporine, infliximab, and tacrolimus, but there is no current consensus on the best therapy (Al-toma et al., 2007). Type II refractory celiac disease is nonresponsive to medical treatment and has a poor prognosis, with a dismal 5-year survival rate of less than 50%. The most frequent cause of death in this group is the occurrence of T cell lymphoma and recurrent infection (Al-toma et al., 2007). A potential promising therapy is autologous stem cell transplantation.

PRIMARY CARE MANAGEMENT

Health Care Maintenance

The National Institute of Health Consensus Development Conference on Celiac Disease (2005) describes six key elements in the management of individuals affected by celiac disease: consultation with a skilled dietitian, education about the disease, lifelong adherence to a gluten-free diet, identification and treatment of nutritional deficiencies, access to an advocacy group, and continuous long-term follow-up by a multidisciplinary team (i.e., primary care providers, gastroenterologists, nurses, dietitians, social workers) (Box 17-3).

Growth and Development

After the diagnosis of celiac disease has been established and the GFD initiated, children should have routine visits with either the primary care provider or gastroenterologist to assess symptoms, monitor growth and development, and check nutritional status such as fat-soluble vitamin, folic acid, vitamin B_{12}, zinc and calcium levels, hematocrit, as well as celiac serology as a marker of dietary compliance. Reinforcement of the GFD is of utmost importance. A thorough physical examination should be performed

---

> **BOX 17-3**
>
> ## CELIAC: Six Key Elements in Management of Children with Celiac Disease
>
> Consultation with a skilled dietitian
> Education about the disease
> Lifelong adherence to a gluten-free diet
> Identification and treatment of nutritional deficiencies
> Access to an advocacy group
> Continuous long-term follow-up by a multidiscplinary team

From National Institute of Health Consensus Development Conference Statement on Celiac Disease, June 28-30, 2004 (2005). *Gastroenterology, 128,* S1-S9.

---

at every visit. Signs and symptoms of rickets, bone pain, tetany, acrodermatitis, coagulopathy, night blindness, dental enamel defects, muscle wasting, scant adipose tissue, protuberant abdomen, skin rash, nail abnormalities, or poor hair growth should alert the clinician to nutritional deficiencies that could represent refractory celiac disease or dietary noncompliance (Hill et al., 2005). Routine DEXA scans do not need to be routinely performed as most children achieve fully restored bone mass after one 1 year on a GFD (American Gastroenterological Association [AGA], 2006). Developmental screening and anthropometric data (length, height, body mass index) should be performed as part of routine screening at all well-child care visits and plotted to evaluate trends. Children with neurologic manifestation of celiac disease may be at hypothetical risk of developmental delay, although there are few data to support this association (Hill et al., 2005). Visits may be necessary weekly or monthly after initial diagnosis until clinical and biologic signs and symptoms improve and stabilize. Thereafter, the frequency of follow-up and serologic evaluation depends on the clinical progress of the child and is at the discretion of the health care provider in collaboration with the family. At a minimum these children should be seen on a yearly basis to monitor dietary compliance and symptoms and so that families can be provided with the most up to date information on management of celiac disease.

Diet

Treatment with a GFD is recommended for all symptomatic children with histologic changes on intestinal biopsy to reverse growth failure, diarrhea, and other gastrointestinal symptoms, normalize anemia, bone demineralization, and other nutritional deficiencies and to prevent complications (i.e., lymphoma). However, complete adherence to the GFD can be challenging, especially for children who are surrounded by gluten-containing foods in their day-to-day life. Studies from Europe indicate variable compliance rates with gluten restriction, ranging between 45% and 81% (Fabiani, Catassi, Villari, et al., 1996; Hopman, le Cessei, von Bloomberg, et al., 2006; Mariani, Viti, Montuori, et al., 1998). These self-reports may be overestimates, because some who reported full compliance had abnormal histology on small intestinal biopsy (Hill et al., 2005). A study in the Netherlands found that although dietary compliance was high (75%) among a group ages 12 to 25 years, intake of nutrients such as iron and fiber were deficient and consumption of saturated fat was much higher than in the general Dutch population (Hopman et al., 2006). Additionally, a study by Hallert, Grant, Grehn, and colleagues (2002) found evidence of folate and vitamin B_{12} deficiencies in adults who had biopsy-proven remission after 8 to 12 years on a GFD. This may be due to the fact that substitute grains are not fortified with B vitamins the way most wheat products are.

In children with chronic diarrhea and lactose intolerance, a lactose-free diet is also recommended by some clinicians as part of initial treatment to reduce gastrointestinal symptoms. Chronic inflammation of the small bowel can lead to alterations in the jejunal brush border with a reduction in the activity of the lactase enzyme, which can result in secondary lactose intolerance in some children with celiac disease. This is generally transient and resolves on a GFD unless the child has underlying primary lactose intolerance (inherited lactase deficiency). Ojetti, Gabrielli, Migneco, and colleagues (2008) observed normalization of the lactose breath test in 1 out of 15 patients (6.7%) after 6 months and in 9 of the remaining 14 (64.2%) after 12 months on a GFD. The study did not mention if the actual clinical symptoms of lactose intolerance (diarrhea, bloating, and abdominal discomfort) gradually improved before the lactose breath test becoming negative. There is no evidence that a lactose-free diet can hasten the recovery of intestinal villi or conversely that lactose ingestion prolongs recovery.

If thorough dietary analysis identifies nutritional deficiencies, vitamin or mineral supplementation should be recommended. Up to two thirds of those on a GFD have suboptimal calcium intake (Children's Digestive Health and Nutrition Foundation [CDHNF], 2005). Children with low calcium intake, including those on a lactose-free diet, should take a calcium supplement daily. Some celiac disease experts suggest supplementation with folic acid (1 mg daily) because folic acid is known to lower the risk of gastrointestinal malignancy and empirically treat the folic acid deficiency common in these individuals (CDHNF, 2005).

There is controversy about the need to delay the introduction of solid foods in infants in high-risk groups for celiac disease. According to the AGA, "early introduction of cereals into the infant diet before three months may be associated with an increased risk of developing childhood celiac disease, but there is no evidence that delaying the introduction of gluten into the diet of children at high risk for celiac disease beyond the three to six month period is beneficial" (2006, p. 1977). Additionally, various European studies have concluded breastfeeding to be protective against the development of celiac disease in at-risk children. A retrospective study of Swedish children (Ivarsson, Hernell, Stenlund, et al., 2002) found that the risk of developing celiac disease was lower in children less than 2 years of age if gluten was introduced into the diet while they were still breastfed, and reduced further if they continued to breastfeed beyond the time when gluten was first introduced. Furthermore, Norris, Barriga, Hoffenberg, and colleagues (2005) concluded, in their prospective observational study of children with increased risk of celiac disease or type 1 diabetes, that the introduction of gluten within the first 3 months of life increased the risk of celiac disease autoimmunity by five-fold as compared with children who were introduced to gluten between 4 and 6 months of age. The risk was only minimally increased if exposure to gluten was delayed until 7 months or later. This suggests that the timing of gluten introduction in susceptible children can lead to increased risk of celiac disease autoimmunity.

The reality for individuals with celiac disease on a GFD is that cross-contamination of supposedly gluten-free products is common, leading to tiny amounts of gluten ingestion on a daily basis. The exact safety threshold for prolonged exposure to trace amounts of gluten is currently unknown, but a recent double-blind, placebo-controlled study by Catassi, Fabiani, Iacono, and colleagues (2007) concluded that the ingestion of contaminating gluten should be kept lower than 50 mg per day in the treatment of celiac disease to prevent damage to intestinal villi. To put this in perspective, consider that an average 30-gram slice of wheat bread contains about 4.8 grams of gluten. Fifty milligrams of gluten is thus equivalent to about 1/96th of an average piece of wheat bread.

Safety

Children with celiac disease have no special restrictions related to physical activity. The main safety risk for children with celiac disease is the ingestion of gluten. Reactions to gluten vary considerably among individuals; some may not have any immediate or discernible reactions whereas others may have anaphylactic-type reactions with consumption of only minute amounts of gluten contaminant. Thus children and their caretakers, including parents, teachers, daycare providers, coaches, babysitters, and the like, should continually be updated on safe, gluten-free foods. Families should be especially careful when eating out at restaurants, where gluten contamination in the cooking process can easily occur. Common household items such as lipstick, toothpaste, and play dough may contain gluten. As individuals with celiac disease approach adolescence they are faced with temptations that involve risks such as alcohol consumption. Grain alcohols contain high amounts of gluten and should be avoided on the GFD. Adolescents should be counseled about this risk factor.

Immunizations

There are no contraindications to the current Centers for Disease Control and Prevention (CDC) childhood immunization schedule for children with celiac disease. However, a recent article by Nemes, Lefler, Szegedi, and colleagues (2008) concluded that nonresponse to recombinant hepatitis B vaccines may be a sign of undiagnosed, and thus untreated, celiac disease. They found adequate vaccine response in children with celiac disease treated with a GFD and recommend revaccination during a period of good compliance on a GFD. Similarly, a prospective study by Park, Markowitz, Pettel, and colleagues (2007) concluded that more than 50% of children with celiac disease do not show a response to standard vaccination regimens for hepatitis B virus. They hypothesize that ongoing exposure to gluten, nutritional deficiencies, or age may have contributed to the failure to develop immunity. Further research needs to be done before recommendations can be made for repeat hepatitis B immunization or antibody measurements to confirm immunity. Fortunately, the researchers found that the study population's response to rubella, tetanus, and *Haemophilus influenzae* type b (Hib) vaccines was not impaired (Park et al., 2007). Additionally, McKinley, Leibowitz, Bronzo, and colleagues (1995) demonstrated that even persons with hyposplenism as a complication of celiac disease were able to mount appropriate antibody response to the pneumococcal vaccine and should receive the vaccine, given the increased association of pneumococcal sepsis in persons with celiac disease. This implies that children with hyposplenism as a complication of celiac disease should receive the conjugate pneumococcal vaccine recommended for all infants and toddlers and should receive in addition the polysaccharide pneumococcal vaccine after 2 years of age (Centers for Disease Control and prevention, 2008).

Screening

No expert collaborative guidelines exist on screening individuals for coexisting conditions or complications of celiac disease. The following discussion is based on the findings of associations in the current literature.

Vision. Routine vision screening at regular well-child visits should be provided to children with celiac disease. Except for those with severe nutritional deficiencies, they have not been found to be at risk for vision impairments or ocular disease.

Hearing. Children with celiac disease should have regular hearing examinations. They are not at risk for hearing deficits greater than the general population.

Dental. Children with dental enamel defects should be screened for celiac disease because this can be the only presenting sign of celiac disease. Daily dental hygiene and regular dental cleanings and examinations should be encouraged, as with all other children.

Blood Pressure. The blood pressure of children with celiac disease should be routinely measured. They are not at risk for hypertension, although it would be interesting to document changes in pre- and post-GFD blood pressures. A large study in adults found that individuals with celiac disease have a lower prevalence of hypertension and hypercholesterolemia than the general population, probably dietary related (West, Logan, Card, et al., 2004). Other researchers have described a correlation of cardiomyopathy, heart arrhythmias, and heart failure with celiac disease that significantly improves after treatment with a GFD. A large Swedish study (Elfstrom, Hamsten, Montgomery, et al., 2007) found that celiac disease in childhood was not associated with later myocarditis, cardiomyopathy, or pericarditis greater than their general population cohort. Further research is needed in regard to cardiovascular risk factors, especially in children, to determine the need for more frequent screening. Currently there are neither formal recommendations nor routine practice for further blood pressure screening beyond routine vital signs at well-child care visits.

Hematocrit. Anemia is the most common abnormal laboratory manifestation of celiac disease. The etiology of anemia in this population may be multifactorial and include iron, folate, and vitamin B_{12} malabsorption. People with celiac disease who are vegetarians are at even greater risk for anemia because of dietary restrictions. Screening should not only include hemoglobin and hematocrit, but also mean corpuscular volume (MCV) to check for macrocytic anemia related to vitamin B_{12} or folate deficiencies. There are no set guidelines on the frequency of screening; it is at the discretion of the health care provider and depends on the clinical status of the child and the degree of anemia.

Urinalysis. Routine urinalysis should be performed. Data limited to adult populations have shown that individuals with celiac disease may face an increased risk of developing chronic renal disease and higher risk of glomerulonephritis (Ludvigsson, Montgomery, Olen, et al., 2006). The commonality of high antigliadin and antiendomysial antibodies in both celiac disease and IgA nephropathy suggests a common pathogenesis of disease

(Pierucci, Fofi, Bartoli, et al., 2002). However, no clear guidelines exist for more than the routine urinalysis.

Tuberculosis. Children with celiac disease are at a higher risk of developing active tuberculosis (TB) for unknown reasons. A recent Swedish study concluded that people diagnosed with celiac disease in adulthood had nearly four times the risk of active TB infection, and those diagnosed as children had triple the risk. The study also found that a prior diagnosis of TB nearly doubled the risk of celiac disease (Ludvigsson, 2007). The author hypothesized that the association between gluten intolerance and TB may be due to poor intake of vitamin D and calcium caused by intestinal malabsorption and the nutritional deficiencies of a GFD. These findings suggest that children with celiac disease may benefit from more frequent TB screening.

Condition-Specific Screening

The NASPGHAN Celiac Disease Guideline Committee (Hill et al., 2005) recommends rechecking TTG IgA after 6 months on the GFD. A decrease in antibody titer from initial presentation is an indirect measure of dietary compliance. Thereafter, measurement of TTG levels on a yearly basis may be helpful in monitoring long-term compliance. The committee also recommends repeating TTG levels in children with persistent symptoms despite the GFD. Levels that remain elevated may indicate contamination of gluten in the diet or nonadherence. The primary care provider can order and interpret these tests as part of well-child care visits or defer care to a gastroenterologist if one is available or if abnormalities or complications arise. Current practice guidelines do not recommend repeating an intestinal biopsy after treatment with a GFD, nor do they recommend gluten rechallenge to confirm diagnosis in straightforward cases (Hill et al., 2005; National Institute of Health Consensus Development Conference Statement on Celiac Disease, 2005). Some providers choose to screen for nutritional deficiencies after diagnosis of celiac disease is established with bone density studies and blood work, including parathyroid hormone, complete blood count, iron studies, folate, vitamins A, E, and D, electrolytes, albumin, total protein, liver enzymes, prothrombin time and vitamin K. One could also consider screening first- and second-degree relatives for celiac disease (Pietzak, 2005). This will depend on the individual family circumstances and the clinical progress of the child.

Common Illness Management

Differential Diagnosis

The classic symptoms of untreated celiac disease, including diarrhea, abdominal distention, and failure to thrive, can often be difficult to differentiate from common childhood conditions such as gastroenteritis, acquired lactose intolerance, food allergies, and various viral illnesses. The important point, however, is that the presentation of celiac disease varies widely, from asymptomatic disease to severe growth failure (Fasano, 2005; Telega et al., 2008; Westerbeek et al., 2005). Fortunately, children who are compliant with the GFD are able to remain in general good health, and exacerbations are more often related to ingestion of gluten. However, all complaints should be thoroughly evaluated to include the same differentials that might be applied to children without celiac disease.

Diarrhea. Chronic diarrhea is a common complaint in children with celiac disease, but chronicity is not always the rule. In children with undiagnosed celiac disease, parents may not perceive diarrhea to be a chronic problem if it occurred only intermittently, for example, when the child unknowingly consumed large amounts of gluten. The history, therefore, may not reveal a chronic problem. In those children previously diagnosed with celiac disease and on a GFD, acute diarrhea could indicate dietary noncompliance, intercurrent gastroenteritis, food intolerance or allergy, side effect of antibiotics, or concurrent diagnosis of inflammatory bowel disease. The practitioner should consider celiac disease if the course of diarrhea extends beyond a normal period of time or if laboratory data reveal anemia. Severe, acute diarrhea accompanied by electrolyte imbalances should prompt consideration of celiac crisis and hospitalization. Persons with celiac disease generally do not experience bloody diarrhea, so inflammatory bowel disease or infectious colitis should be considered if a child has bloody stools. Persistent diarrhea despite a GFD again should prompt further evaluation for accuracy of the diagnosis, as well as concurrent conditions such as lactose intolerance, small bowel bacterial overgrowth, underlying inflammatory bowel disease, and food allergy. Tursi, Brandimarte, and Giorgetti (2003) found that 10 out of 15 patients who had persistent gastrointestinal symptoms after 6 to 8 months on a GFD had small bowel bacterial overgrowth based on positive lactulose hydrogen breath test. Ojetti, Nucera, Migneco, and colleagues (2005) found that lactose intolerance can be the only clinical sign of an otherwise asymptomatic individual with celiac disease. The study observed a much higher prevalence of celiac disease (24%, 13 of 54) in those subjects with hydrogen breath test–proven lactose intolerance compared with the control group (2%, 1 of 50). These findings suggest that children with bloating and diarrhea related to lactose intolerance should be screened for celiac disease as well.

Failure to Thrive. Failure to thrive is a very broad diagnosis, but for the purpose of this discussion, it will comprise the following: poor weight gain, growth retardation (short stature), and decreased weight for height. The physiologic basis of failure to thrive is inadequate nutrition, the cause of which is often multifactorial and includes both organic and nonorganic reasons. It is well accepted that children with delayed diagnosis of celiac disease suffer growth retardation caused by malabsorption, but proper adherence to a GFD will usually result in catch-up and eventual normalization of growth. Damen, Boersma, Wit, and colleagues (1994) found that weight for height in children diagnosed with celiac disease before 9 years of age progressively decreased in the 12 to 18 months before diagnosis, but catch-up gain was rapid during the first 6 to12 months on a GFD, reaching normal for age after 15 months of treatment. Luciano, Bolognani, Di Falco, and colleagues (2002) evaluated 35 children diagnosed at early age (mean 1.17 years) and found most to have achieved target final height except for the child diagnosed late at 13 years of age. However, a prospective study by Patwari, Kapur, Satyanarayana, and colleagues (2005) found incomplete catch-up growth in children diagnosed with celiac disease anytime between 2 and 10 years of age. Primary care providers should be aware of the potential for short stature in children with celiac disease, especially if they had growth failure at time of diagnosis (Salardi, Cacciari, Volta, et al., 2005). The aforementioned studies found weight and weight for height to normalize on a GFD even if the child failed to catch up in height. If catch-up weight gain does not occur after initiation of treatment, a careful diet history should be performed to make sure that all foods are completely gluten free and that the child is consuming enough calories for growth. If weight gain is not achieved despite adequate caloric intake and proper adherence to gluten-free foods, other causes of malabsorption such as pancreatic insufficiency, inflammatory bowel disease, chronic parasitic infections, or food allergies should be considered. Last, the association of growth hormone deficiency with celiac disease has been documented in several studies (Bozzola, Giovenale, Bozzola, et al., 2005; Giovenale, Meazza, Cardinale, et al., 2006; Salardi et al., 2005). Thus children with celiac disease who achieve no vertical catch-up gain after a reasonable period of time on a GFD should be referred to an endocrinologist for evaluation of growth hormone deficiency. Supplementation with growth hormone in addition to a GFD has been found to improve final height (Salardi et al., 2005).

Abdominal Pain. Children with celiac disease who have abdominal pain should elicit the same broad-based evaluation as all other children because this is a common complaint that could be related to anything from stress to constipation to more serious conditions such as inflammatory bowel disease. Constipation can be a chronic and perplexing symptom, both in children with undiagnosed celiac disease and in children after diagnosis who adhere to a GFD. Telega and colleagues (2008) reported 5% of the 143 children in the study to have had constipation prior to diagnosis. Dietary nonadherence as a cause of pain is another consideration and should prompt a thorough dietary review. Recurrent abdominal pain (RAP) in children with celiac disease who are adhering to a strict GFD should again prompt reconsideration of the diagnosis in addition to evaluation of RAP separate from celiac disease. Small bowel bacterial overgrowth should also be considered, because this condition was found to be highly prevalent in adults with celiac disease with persistent abdominal pain and diarrhea despite gluten withdrawal (Tursi et al., 2003). Various studies have indicated an increased risk of celiac disease in cohorts of patients with irritable bowel syndrome (IBS) as well (Leeds & Sanders, 2007; Sanders, Carter, Hurlstone, et al., 2001). Because of the overlapping symptoms of abdominal pain, diarrhea, bloating, and constipation in both conditions, screening for celiac disease in children with IBS may be necessary as part of the evaluation. Last, dual diagnosis of inflammatory bowel disease should be considered given the high crossover rate of the two conditions (Yang et al., 2005).

Developmental Issues

Sleep Patterns

Chronic fatigue may be a symptom of untreated celiac disease. Nighttime bowel movements may also hinder the ability to get an adequate night's sleep. After diagnosis and treatment with a GFD, sleep patterns of children with celiac disease should be normal unless a coexisting condition exists.

Toileting

The chronic diarrhea, increased flatulence, and abdominal distention that may accompany undiagnosed celiac disease may increase the difficulty of toilet training. It would be preferable to delay rigorous toilet training until symptom resolution is achieved on a GFD. Poor adherence to a GFD may induce a spectrum of symptoms including abdominal pain, bloating, and diarrhea that may affect the toileting regimen or evoke embarrassment in older children. Conversely, a minority of children with celiac disease may have intractable constipation of unclear etiology.

Discipline

Behavioral expectations for children with celiac disease should be the same as their peers. As children get older they have more responsibility and power over their dietary choices and strict adherence to a GFD may be difficult, especially when they are feeling well or have no immediate symptoms. Compliance numbers may be underestimates because children may be reluctant to admit they are not following medical advice. Knowledge of reported barriers to compliance may be useful in promoting adherence. These include ability to manage emotions (depression and anxiety), ability to resist temptation and exercise restraint, feelings of deprivation, fear generated by inaccurate information, time pressures (planning and preparation of meals may take longer), competing priorities (work, job, school), assessing gluten-free content in foods (label reading), eating out (avoidance, fear, difficulty ensuring food safety), social events (not wanting to look or be different), and support of family and friends. One strategy to help with compliance may be a gluten-free household, where the entire family is gluten free for ease in grocery shopping and cooking. Children should be encouraged by positive reinforcement for healthy food choices.

Child Care

Educating child-care providers on a GFD is essential in providing a gluten-free environment for children with celiac disease.

Schooling

Children with celiac disease should be held to the same academic expectations as their peers. Special gluten-free school lunches that are nutritionally balanced should be provided for these children. The burden of chronic disease has been shown to affect school performance in studies of those with celiac disease and other chronic diseases (Calsbeek, Rijken, Bekkers, et al., 2006). There should not be significant differences in the school performance of children with well-controlled disease. These children may also face social stigma because of food choices that set them apart from their peers.

Sexuality

Delayed menarche is more prevalent in adolescent females with untreated celiac disease. Issues surrounding poor self-esteem and body image may also affect the development of sexuality. At some point in adolescence those with celiac disease should be counseled on the complications of miscarriage and infertility in poorly treated celiac. There are no contraindications to contraceptive alternatives.

Transition to Adulthood

The number of children with celiac disease is growing, increasing the need for strategies to make the transition from pediatric to adult care smooth. A small study by O'Leary, Wiencke, Healy, and colleagues (2004) of 50 individuals diagnosed with celiac disease in childhood found that most receive no medical or dietary supervision after transition to adult care. The data also showed that 32% were not compliant with a GFD, mostly due to avoidance of symptoms versus fear of complications. The bone mineral density was abnormal in 32%, pointing out the failure in avoiding preventable complications. Primary care providers can help with the transition to adult care by reinforcing adherence, educating about complications, identifying resources, and compiling a referral base of adult providers knowledgeable about celiac disease.

Family Concerns

Families with members who have celiac disease are challenged not only to keep their children safe with gluten-free foods, but also to provide the nonaffected members opportunities to enjoy their favorite foods. Offering a consultation with a dietitian who is knowledgeable about the GFD at the time of diagnosis is very important. Seeing the dietitian after several weeks or months on the GFD for follow-up might also prove useful, because families often have additional questions after initiating the GFD. Other considerations include the higher cost of gluten-free products, which might present a financial burden for some families. These families may need additional assistance with creating affordable but well-balanced meals and snacks. They should be encouraged to experiment with cuisines from other regions of the world. For example, Southeast Asian cuisine incorporates many rice-based ingredients that are often gluten free. National supermarkets such as Whole Foods and Trader Joe's are well stocked with gluten-free products, as are local health food and specialty stores. However, rural markets may not carry many gluten-free options and the availability of gluten-free foods may be a barrier for some families.

The decision as to whether or not to impose the GFD on non-affected family members is a very individual one and should be based on the common good (How many family members have celiac disease?), the family's lifestyle (Does everyone eat dinner together? Does the family eat out often?), and the personal preferences of the main food preparer and the individuals in question, as well as the ability to afford gluten-free foods in bulk.

It is imperative that the primary care provider reinforce to the entire family the importance of lifelong compliance on the GFD after the diagnosis is made, specifically for those children with positive serologic markers and biopsy-proven celiac disease who may be clinically asymptomatic. It may be especially difficult for these children and their families to find the motivation to follow through with the GFD when there are no observable improvements to track.

Resources

Many websites offer information on celiac disease and the GFD. Health care providers should be aware of reputable sites. Many of these websites offer online or local support groups to provide families with additional information and practical advice, as well as a source of emotional and psychological support.

Celiac Disease Foundation
13251 Ventura Blvd. #1
Studio City, CA 91604
(818) 990-2354; Fax: (818) 990-2379
Website: www.celiac.org

Children's Digestive Health and Nutrition Foundation
P.O. Box 6
Flourtown, PA 19031
(215) 233-0808; Fax: (215) 233-3918
Website: http://celiachealth.org

Celiac Sprue Association/USA
P.O. Box 31700
Omaha, NE 68131-0700
Toll-free number: (877) CSA-4CSA; Fax: (402) 558-1347
Website: www.csaceliacs.org

Canadian Celiac Association
5170 Dixie Rd., Suite 204
Mississauga, ON L4W 1E3
Canada
Toll-free number: (800) 363-7296
Website: www.celiac.ca

Gluten Intolerance Group of North America
31214 124th Ave. SE
Auburn, WA 98092-3667
(253) 833-6655; Fax: (253) 833-6675
Website: www.gluten.net

Summary of Primary Care Needs for the Child with Celiac Disease

HEALTH CARE MAINTENANCE

Growth and Development

- Physical growth can be impaired as a result of malnutrition if diagnosis and treatment are not prompt.
- Routine visits to health care provider to monitor growth, monitor nutritional deficiencies, and to review GFD.
- No deficits in cognition and development are specifically associated with celiac disease.

Diet

- Lifelong adherence to a GFD is the only known treatment.
- Increased risk of calcium, vitamin B_{12}, and folate deficiency caused by limitations in diet.
- No clear guidelines exist on whether or not the delayed introduction of gluten to at-risk infants will alter the risk of developing celiac disease.
- Recommend American Pediatric Association (APA) guidelines on food introduction.

Safety

- All caretakers should be educated about gluten-free foods.
- Reactions to gluten vary widely among individuals, from none to anaphylactic-type reaction; care must be taken to avoid consumption of hidden gluten in foods.
- No special restrictions related to physical activity.

Immunizations

- Routine vaccines are recommended per CDC guidelines.

Screening

- *Vision.* Routine screening at regular well-child visits.
- *Hearing.* Routine screening at well-child visits.
- *Dental.* Increased risk of dental enamel defects in untreated celiac disease. Routine screening recommended for those on GFD.
- *Blood pressure.* Routine screening at well-child visits.
- *Hematocrit.* Anemia is a common symptom in untreated celiac disease; it generally resolves on proper GFD. Currently, no set guidelines on frequency of screening exist; depends on clinical presentation and increased risk related to dietary restrictions (e.g., vegetarian GFD).
- Recommend full complete blood count (CBC) to screen for macrocytic anemia and iron deficiency.
- *Urinalysis.* Routine screening is recommended.
- *Tuberculosis.* Risk of tuberculosis is higher in persons with celiac disease for unknown reasons. No guidelines exist for more frequent screening, thus routine screening is recommended at minimum.

Condition-Specific Screening

- Recheck TTG IgA after 6 months on GFD to indirectly measure dietary compliance, then once yearly or as needed to monitor long-term compliance.
- No clear guidelines exist on nutritional screening. If diet record is suspicious for noncompliance or deficiencies, screen CBC, folate, vitamin B_{12}, albumin, and zinc.
- No surveillance endoscopies are recommended after initial diagnosis.
- No consensus exist on whether or not to routinely screen asymptomatic family members, though some clinicians advise this given increased risk.

COMMON ILLNESS MANAGEMENT

Differential Diagnosis

- *Diarrhea and abdominal pain.* Rule out gluten ingestion (noncompliance versus accidental). Reeducate on GFD if necessary. If symptoms persist on GFD, consider lactose intolerance, small bowel bacterial overgrowth (SBBO), inflammatory bowel disease (IBD), concurrent infection, food allergy, etc.
- *Failure to thrive.* Malabsorption can lead to growth retardation. Generally normalizes on GFD, but potential for short stature persists, especially with late diagnosis. If no catch-up gain on GFD, consider dietary noncompliance or other causes of malabsorption such as pancreatic insufficiency, IBS, chronic parasitic infection, or food allergies.

Continued

Summary of Primary Care Needs for the Child with Celiac Disease—cont'd

DEVELOPMENTAL ISSUES

Sleep Patterns

- Normal unless there is a coexisting condition. Chronic fatigue is possible in untreated celiac disease.

Toileting

- No special needs if well on GFD. Symptoms of diarrhea, increased flatulence, bloating, and abdominal pain can make toilet training difficult in untreated celiac disease. Delay toilet training until symptoms resolve.

Discipline

- Same as peers. May be difficult to adhere to GFD, especially in teen years when able to make own food purchases and choices. Offer positive reinforcement for making healthy food choices.

Child Care

- Essential to educate all care providers and school about celiac disease and GFD.

Schooling

- Same academic standards as peers. Food choices that set children on GFD apart from peers may lead to social stigma.

Sexuality

- No contraindications to contraceptive measures. Delayed menarche and sexual development in untreated celiac disease can alter body image.

Transition to Adulthood

- Adolescent females should be counseled on higher risk of infertility and miscarriages in untreated celiac disease.
- Lifelong dietary adherence should be emphasized, because most adults with celiac disease do not receive routine dietary screening after transfer to adult care.

FAMILY CONCERNS

A strict GFD is a lifelong commitment. The decision about whether or not to impose this diet on members without celiac disease should be considered based on family circumstances. Higher cost of gluten-free foods may be a burden on family resources. Reputable websites (see Resources) offer food ideas and support groups either locally or online. No clear guidelines exist on whether or not to routinely screen asymptomatic family members; therefore a discussion about the risks and benefits of screening may help families make informed decisions.

REFERENCES

Akobeng, A., & Thomas, A. (2008). Systematic review: Tolerable amount of gluten for people with coeliac disease. *Aliment Pharmacol Ther, 27,* 1044-1052.

Al-toma, A., Verbeek, W., & Mulder, C. (2007). Update on the management of refractory celiac disease. *J Gastrointest Liver Dis, 16,* 57-63.

American Gastroenterological Association (2006). AGA Institute medical position statement on diagnosis and management of celiac disease. *Gastroenterology, 131,* 1977-1980.

Bonamico, M., Mariani, P., Danesi, H., et al. (2001). Prevalence and clinical picture of celiac disease in Italian Down's syndrome patients: A multicenter study. *J Pediatr Gastroenterol Nutr, 33,* 139-143.

Bozzola, M., Giovenale, D., Bozzola, E., et al. (2005). Growth hormone deficiency and coeliac disease: an unusual association? *Clin Endocrinol, 62,* 372-375.

Bushara, K. (2005). Neurologic presentation of celiac disease. *Gastroenterology, 128,* S92-S97.

Calsbeek, H., Rijken, M., Bekkers, M.J., et al. (2006). School and leisure activities in adolescents and young adults with chronic digestive disorders: Impact of burden of disease. *Int J Behav Med, 13,* 121-130.

Catassi, C., Fabiani, E., Iacono, G., et al. (2007). A prospective, double-blind, placebo-controlled trial to establish a safe gluten threshold for patients with celiac disease. *Am J Clin Nutr, 85,* 160-166.

Catassi, C., Ratsch, I., Fabiani, E., et al. (1994). Coeliac disease in the year 2000: Exploring the iceberg. *Lancet, 343,* 200-203.

Centers for Disease Control and Prevention (2008). *Epidemiology and Prevention of Vaccine-Preventable Diseases* (10th ed.). Washington, DC: Public Health Foundation.

Children's Digestive Health and Nutrition Foundation. (2005). *Celiac disease evaluation and management slide set.* Available at http://celiachealth.org/pdf/Celiac_full_set_2005.pdf. Retrieved January 1, 2008.

Codex Alimentarius Commission, Joint FAO/WHO Foods Standards Programme. (2007). *Draft revised Codex standard for foods for special dietary use for persons intolerant to gluten.* Alinorm 08/31/26, Appendix III, 50-51. Available at www.codexalimentarius.net/download/report/687/nf29_01e.pdf. Retrieved February 28, 2008.

D'Amico, M.A., Holmes, J., Stavropoulos, S.N., et al. (2005). Presentation of pediatric celiac disease in the United States: Prominent effect of breastfeeding. *Clin Pediatr, 44,* 249-258.

Damen, G.M., Boersma, B., Wit, J.M., et al. (1994). Catch-up growth in 60 children with celiac disease. *J Pediatr Gastroenterol Nutr, 19,* 394-400.

Dicke, W.K. (1950). *Coeliac disease.* Investigation of the harmful effects of certain types of cereal on patients with celiac disease (thesis). University of Utrecht, the Netherlands.

Elftstrom, P., Hamsten, A., Montgomery, S., et al. (2007). Cardiomyopathy, pericarditis, and myocarditis in a population based cohort of inpatients with celiac disease. *J Intern Med, 262,* 545-554.

Fabiani, E., Catassi, C., Villari, A., et al. (1996). Dietary compliance in screening-detected celiac disease adolescents. *Acta Paediatr, 412,* 65-67.

Fasano, A. (2005). Clinical presentation of celiac disease in the pediatric population. *Gastroenterology, 128,* 68-73.

Fasano, A., Berti, I., Gerarduzzi, T., et al. (2003). Prevalence of celiac disease in at-risk and not-at-risk groups in the United States. A large multicenter study. *Arch Intern Med, 163,* 286-292.

Garampazzi, A., Rapa, A., Mura, S., et al. (2007). Clinical pattern of celiac disease is still changing. *J Pediatr Gastroenterol Nutr, 45,* 611-614.

Gee, S. (1888). On the celiac affection. *St. Bartholomew's Hospital Reports, 24,* 17-20.

Giovenale, D., Meazza, C., Cardinale, G.M., et al. (2006). The prevalence of growth hormone deficiency and celiac disease in short children. *Clin Med Res, 4,* 180-183.

Goh, C., & Banerjee, K. (2007). Prevalence of celiac disease in children and adolescents with type 1 diabetes mellitus in a clinic-based population. *Postgrad Med J, 83,* 132-136.

Greco, L., Romino, R., Coto, I., et al. (2002). The first large population based twin study of celiac disease. *Gut, 50,* 624-626.

Green, P., & Cellier, C. (2007). Celiac disease. *N Engl J Med, 357,* 1731-1743.

Green, P., & Jabri, B. (2006). Celiac disease. *Ann Rev Med, 57,* 207-221.

Guyton, A.C., & Hall, J.E. (2001). *Textbook of Medical Physiology.* Philadelphia: Saunders.

Hallert, C., Grant, C., Grehn, S., et al. (2002). Evidence of poor vitamin status in coeliac patients on a gluten-free diet for 10 years. *Aliment Pharmacol Ther, 16,* 1333-1339.

Hill, I. (2002). Celiac DiseaseWorking Group report of the First World Congress of Pediatric Gastroenterology, Hepatology and Nutrition. *J Pediatr Gastroenterol Nutr, 35,* S78-S88.

Hill, I., Bhatnagar, S., Cameron, D., et al. (2005). Guideline for the diagnosis and treatment of celiac disease in children: Recommendations of the North American Society for Pediatric Gastroenterology, Hepatology, and Nutrition. *J Pediatr Gastroenterol Nutr, 40,* 1-19.

Hoffenberg, E.J., MacKenzie, T., Barriga, K.J., et al. (2003). A prospective study of the incidence of celiac disease. *J Pediatr, 143,* 308-314.

Hogberg, L., Laurin, P., Falth-Magnusson, K., et al. (2004). Oats to children with newly diagnosed celiac disease: A randomized double blind study. *Gut, 53,* 649-654.

Holm, K., Maki, M., Vuolteenaho, N., et al. (2006). Oats in the treatment of childhood celiac disease: A 2-year controlled trial and long-term clinical follow-up study. *Aliment Pharmacol Ther, 23,* 1463-1472.

Hopman, E., le Cessie, S., von Blomberg, B.M., et al. (2006). Nutritional management of the gluten-free diet in young people with celiac disease in the Netherlands. *J Pediatr Gastroenterol Nutr, 43,* 102-108.

Ivarsson, A., Hernell, O., Stenlund, H., et al. (2002). Breastfeeding protects against celiac disease. *Am J Clin Nutr, 75,* 914-921.

Janatuinen, E.K., Kemppainen, T.A., Julkunen, R.J.K., et al. (2002). No harm from five year ingestion of oats in celiac disease. *Gut, 50,* 332-335.

Kavak, U., Yuce, A., Kocak, N., et al. (2003). Bone mineral density in children with untreated and treated celiac disease. *J Pediatr Gastroenterol Nutr, 37,* 409-411.

Kwon, J., & Farrell, R. (2006). Recent advances in the understanding of celiac disease: Therapeutic implications for the management of pediatric patients. *Pediatr Drugs, 8,* 375-388.

Leeds, J., & Sanders, D. (2007). Is there an association between celiac disease and irritable bowel syndrome? *Gut, 56,* 1326-1327.

Luciano, A., Bolognani, M., Di Falco, A., et al. (2002). Catch-up growth and final height in celiac disease. *Pediatr Med Chir, 24,* 9-12.

Ludvigsson, J.F. (2007). Celiac disease and the risk of tuberculosis: A population based cohort study. *Thorax, 62,* 23-28.

Ludvigsson, J.F., Montgomery, S.M., Olen, O., et al. (2006). Coeliac disease and risk of renal disease–a general population cohort study. *Nephrol Dial Transplant, 21,* 1809-1815.

Maki, M., & Lohi, O. (2004). Celiac disease. In W.A. Walker, R.E. Kleinman, P.M. Sherman (Eds.), *Pediatric Gastroenterology,* Ontario, CA: B.C. Decker.

Maki, M., Mustalahti, K., Kokkonen, J., et al. (2003). Prevalence of celiac disease among children in Finland. *N Engl J Med, 348,* 2517-2524.

Mariani, P., Viti, M.G., Montuori, M., et al. (1998). The gluten-free diet: A nutritional risk for adolescents with celiac disease. *J Pediatr Gastroenterol Nutr, 27,* 519-523.

McKinley, M., Leibowitz, S., Bronzo, R., et al. (1995). Appropriate response to pneumococcal vaccine in celiac sprue. *J Clin Gastroenterol, 20,* 113-116.

Mones, R.L., Atienza, K.V., Youssef, N.N., et al. (2007). Case report: Celiac crisis in the modern era. *J Pediatr Gastroenterol Nutr, 45,* 480-483.

National Institute of Health Consensus Development Conference on Celiac Disease, June 28-30, 2004. (2005). *Gastroenterology, 128,* S1–S9.

Nemes, E., Lefler, E., Szegedi, L., et al. (2008). Gluten intake interferes with the humoral immune response to recombinant hepatitis B vaccine in patients with celiac disease. *Pediatrics, 121,* e1570-e1576.

Norris, J., Barriga, K., Hoffenberg, E., et al. (2005). Risk of celiac disease autoimmunity and timing of gluten introduction in the diet of infants at increased risk of disease. *J Am Med Assoc, 293,* 2343-2351.

Ojetti, V., Gabrielli, M., Migneco, A., et al. (2008). Regression of lactose malabsorption in coeliac patients after receiving a gluten-free diet. *Scand J Gastroenterol, 43,* 174-177.

Ojetti, V., Nucera, G., Migneco, A., et al. (2005). High prevalence of celiac disease in patients with lactose intolerance. *Digestion, 71,* 106-110.

O'Leary, C., Wiencke, P., Healy, M., et al. (2004). Celiac disease and the transition from childhood to adulthood: A 28 year follow-up. *Am J Gastroenterol, 99,* 2437-2441.

Park, S.D., Markowitz, J., Pettel, M., et al. (2007). Failure to respond to hepatitis B vaccine in children with celiac disease. *J Pediatr Gastroenterol Nutr, 44,* 431-435.

Patwari, A.K., Kapur, G., Satyanarayana, L., et al. (2005). Catch-up growth in children with late-diagnosed coeliac disease. *Br J Nutr, 94,* 437-442.

Pierucci, A., Fofi, C., Bartoli, B., et al. (2002). Antiendomysial antibodies in Berger's disease. *Am J Kidney Dis, 39,* 1176-1182.

Pietzak, M.M. (2005). Follow-up of patients with celiac disease: Achieving compliance with treatment. *Gastroenterology, 128,* S135-S141.

Rewers, M. (2005). Epidemiology of celiac disease: What are the prevalence, incidence, and progression of celiac disease?. *Gastroenterology, 128,* 47-51.

Salardi, S., Cacciari, E., Volta, U., et al. (2005). Growth and adult height in atypical coeliac patients, with or without growth hormone deficiency. *J Pediatr Endocrinol Metabol, 18,* 769-775.

Sanders, D., Carter, M., Hurlstone, D., et al. (2001). Association of adult coeliac disease with irritable bowel syndrome: A case-control study in patients fulfilling ROME II criteria referred to secondary care. *Lancet, 358,* 1504-1508.

Steens, R.F., Csizmadia, C.G., George, E.K., et al. (2005). A national prospective study on childhood celiac disease in the Netherlands 1993-2000: An increasing recognition and a changing clinical picture. *J Pediatr, 147,* 239-245.

Telega, G., Rivera Bennet, T., & Werlin, S. (2008). Emerging new clinical patterns in the presentation of celiac disease. *Arch Pediatr Adolesc Med, 162,* 164-168.

Templet, J., Welsh, J., & Cusack, C. (2007). Childhood dermatitis herpetiformis: A case report and review of the literature. *Cutis, 80,* 473-476.

Tursi, A., Brandimarte, G., & Giorgetti, G. (2003). High prevalence of small intestinal bacterial overgrowth in celiac patients with persistence of gastrointestinal symptoms after gluten withdrawal. *Am J Gastroenterol, 98,* 839-843.

U.S. Food and Drug Administration Center for Food Safety and Applied Nutrition. (n.d.). Available at www.cfsan.fda.gov/~dms/glutqa.html. Retrieved February 24, 2008.

West, J., Logan, R.F., Card, T.R., et al. (2004). Risk of vascular disease in adults with diagnosed celiac disease: A population-based study. *Aliment Pharmacol Ther, 20,* 73-79.

Westerbeek, E., Mouat, S., Wesley, A., et al. (2005). Coeliac disease diagnosed at Starship Children's Hospital: 1999-2002. *N Z Med J, 118,* 1-9.

Yang, A., Chen, Y., Scherl, E., et al. (2005). Inflammatory bowel disease and patients with celiac disease. *Inflammatory Bowel Disease, 11,* 538-532.

Zipser, R.D., Farid, M., Baisch, D., et al. (2005). Physician awareness of celiac disease. A need for further education. *J Gen Intern Med, 20,* 644-646.

18 Cerebral Palsy

Wendy M. Nehring

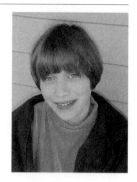

Etiology

Cerebral palsy, a condition first described by Dr. George Little in 1861, was redefined in 2005 as a group of disorders of the development of movement and posture, causing activity limitation, that are attributed to nonprogressive disturbances that occurred in the developing fetal or infant brain. The motor disorders of cerebral palsy are often accompanied by disturbances of sensation, cognition, communication, perception, or behavior, and may be accompanied by a seizure disorder (Rosenbaum, Dan, Leviton, et al., 2005, p. 572).

This revised definition was necessary because of increased knowledge of developmental neurobiology, the array of conditions that result in motor impairments that affect activities of daily living, and the antecedents and consequences of cerebral palsy in particular. In addition, advances in neuroimaging technology and the management of care for motor impairments have resulted in the need to reexamine the definition of cerebral palsy. This condition should be described by the dominant movement or tone abnormality, brain morphology, and neurologic findings. Etiologically, it is not a diagnosis but rather a clinical description of a set of multidimensional disorders that are diverse in clinical presentation (Bax, Goldstein, Rosenbaum, et al., 2005; Krageloh-Mann, 2005).

A proposed revision of the classification system also was presented in 2005 (Box 18-1) to recognize the importance of an accurate description of the child's current clinical problems and their severity, an evaluation of the child's physical and quality-of-life status across time, and a listing of short- and long-term support needs. The four types of movement disorders seen in children with cerebral palsy are spasticity, dystonia, athetosis, and ataxia. The "mixed" category should only be used when there is a clear description of each of the motor disorders present. Each primary category carries a different set of characteristics and prognoses, and any additional findings should be identified as secondary categories. It is recommended that the terms "diplegia" and "quadriplegia" not be used (although these words will appear in this chapter where they were used in the literature cited). Instead, all body regions, including the oropharynx, should be described for any tonal or postural abnormalities or impairments. The presence or absence of epilepsy and visual, hearing, or cognitive impairments should be noted (Paneth, Damiano, Rosenbaum, et al., 2005).

Spasticity

Spasticity describes the presence of increased muscle tone, which is noted through the passive range of motion of a joint. Characteristics of spastic cerebral palsy include persistent primitive reflexes,

exaggerated stretch reflexes, positive Babinski reflex, ankle clonus, and later development of contractures. This form of cerebral palsy is most distinctly divided by the extremities involved and affects the majority of people with cerebral palsy. Damage has occurred in the motor cortex and pyramidal tracts in the brain (Colver & Sethumadhavan, 2003; Odding, Roebroeck, & Stam, 2006; Pellegrino, 2007).

Dystonia

Dystonic cerebral palsy is characterized by slow and twisting abnormal movements of the trunk or extremities that may involve abnormal posturing. In other words, with a voluntary change in position, the moved extremity shifts into an abnormal position and stays in that position (Pellegrino, 2007).

Athetosis

Athetosis is a result of damage to the basal ganglia and is characterized by slow, writhing movements. Choreoathetoisis palsy is a form of athetosis and is additionally characterized by chorea (i.e., jerky, rapid, random movements). Children with this form of cerebral palsy often display rigid muscle tone when awake and normal or decreased muscle tone when asleep. This aberrant positioning is a result of the inadequate regulation of muscle tone coordination by the central nervous system, which results from insult to the basal ganglia or extrapyramidal tracts (Pellegrino, 2007).

Ataxia

The fourth motor dysfunction group of cerebral palsy is ataxia. Neurologic damage is present in the cerebellum. Ataxia includes a range of conditions marked by the degree of muscle tone and coordination of movements and balance. These conditions can range from ataxic to hypotonic to atonic. Children with ataxia walk with an unstable, wide-based gait and have some difficulty trying to move a hand or arm voluntarily or timing such movement. Increased or decreased muscle tone may be present (Pellegrino, 2007).

Mixed

This motor dysfunction group of cerebral palsy is characterized by more than one type of motor pattern, which is found as a result of many defects to various areas of the brain. The term "mixed" is also used when no one motor pattern is dominant. Spasticity and dyskinesia can exist either alone or together and each should be described in detail (Pellegrino, 2007).

Classification System for Cerebral Palsy

1. MOTOR ABNORMALITIES
A. Nature and typology of the motor disorder: the observed tonal abnormalities assessed on examination (e.g., hypertonia or hypotonia), as well as the diagnosed movement disorders present, such as spasticity, ataxia, dystonia, or athetosis.

B. Functional motor abilities: the extent to which the individual is limited in his or her motor function in all body areas, including oromotor and speech function.

2. ASSOCIATED IMPAIRMENTS
The presence or absence of associated nonmotor neurodevelopmental or sensory problems, such as seizures, hearing or vision impairments, or attentional, behavioral, communicative, and/or cognitive deficits, and the extent to which impairments interact in individuals with cerebral palsy.

3. ANATOMIC AND RADIOLOGIC FINDINGS
A. Anatomic distribution: the parts of the body (e.g., limbs, trunk, or bulbar region) affected by motor impairments or limitations.

B. Radiological findings: the neuroanatomic findings on computed tomography or magnetic resonance imaging, such as ventricular enlargement, white matter loss, or brain anomaly.

4. CAUSATION AND TIMING
Whether there is a clearly identified cause, as is usually the case with postnatal cerebral palsy (e.g., meningitis or head injury) or when brain malformations are present, and the presumed time frame during which the injury occurred, if known.

From Paneth, N., Damiano, D., Rosenbaum, P., et al. (2005). The classification of cerebral palsy. Proposed definition and classification of cerebral palsy, April 2005. *Dev Med Child Neurol, 47,* 571-576.

The etiology of cerebral palsy may be due to a number of risk factors. Sometimes a cause for the diagnosis of cerebral palsy is never clearly identified. The possible causes are delineated by the period of time when the insult to the child's brain may have occurred. Most incidences of congenital cerebral palsy are unknown (Krigger, 2006). Table 18-1 lists the risk factors for cerebral palsy according to the following time periods: prenatal, labor and delivery, perinatal, childhood (postnatal), and unknown. During the prenatal period, both maternal and gestational risk factors are given. The United Cerebral Palsy Research and Educational Foundation (2002) reported that 70% of cases of cerebral palsy occur during the prenatal period, especially in the second and third trimesters, as a result of damage during the developmental growth of the brain; 20% of cases occur during the perinatal or birthing period; and the remaining 10% occur postnatally during the first 2 years of life. This percentage varies by study (Serdaroglu, Cansu, Ozkan, et al., 2006), and future research based on large databases will yield ongoing current percentages.

Advances in neuroimaging technologies, such as magnetic resonance imaging (MRI), allow more definitive diagnoses and identification and timing of causation (Ashwal, Russman, Blasco, et al., 2004; Krageloh-Mann, 2004). Krageloh-Mann and Horber (2007), in a systematic review of the literature, found that periventricular white matter lesions were the most common finding (56% of cases) and that it was more common in preterm infants with

Risk Factors of Cerebral Palsy

Time Period	Risk Factors
Prenatal	**Maternal factors** Diabetes or hyperthyroidism Exposure to radiation or toxins Malnutrition Seizure disorder or mental retardation Infections Incompetent cervix Bleeding Polyhydramnios Genetic abnormalities Previous child with developmental disabilities Previous premature birth Previous fetal loss Medication use (e.g., thyroid, estrogen, progesterone) Inflammatory response Severe proteinuria **Gestational insults** Chromosomal abnormalities Genetic syndromes Teratogens Rh incompatibility infections Congenital malformations Fetal development abnormalities Problems in placental functioning Inflammatory response
Labor and delivery	**Labor and delivery complications** Premature delivery Prolonged rupture of membranes Fetal heart rate depression Abnormal presentations Long labor Preeclampsia Asphyxia
Perinatal	**Prematurity and associated problems** Sepsis and/or central nervous system (CNS) infection Seizures Intraventricular hemorrhage (IVH) Periventricular encephalomalacia (PVL) Meconium aspiration Days on mechanical ventilation Persistent pulmonary hypertension in newborn Intrauterine growth retardation Low birth weight
Childhood/postnatal	**Brain injury** Meningitis/encephalitis Toxins Traumatic brain injury Infections Stroke
Unknown	

Data from National Institute of Neurological Disorders and Stroke (NINDS). (2008). Cerebral palsy: Hope through research. Available at: www.ninds.nih.gov/disorders/cerebral_palsy/detail_cerebral_palsy.htm; Wood, E. (2006). The child with cerebral palsy: Diagnosis and beyond. *Semin Pediatr Neurol, 13,* 286-296; Pellegrino, L. (2007). Cerebral palsy. In M.L. Batshaw, L. Pellegrino, & N.J. Roizen (Eds.), *Children with disabilities* (6th ed., pp. 387-408). Baltimore: Brookes Publishing; Johnson, M.W., Hoon, A.H., Jr., & Kaufmann, W.E. (2008). Neurobiology, diagnosis, and management of cerebral palsy. In P.J. Accardo (Ed.), *Capute and Accardo's neurodevelopmental disabilities in infancy and childhood (Vol. II: The spectrum of neurodevelopmental disabilities)* (3rd ed., pp. 61-81). Baltimore: Brookes Publishing.

cerebral palsy. They indicated that the specific brain lesion could be identified by MRI in 75% of preterm infants. Bax, Tydeman, and Flodmark (2006) also found white matter lesions, in particular, periventricular leukomalacia, to be the most common finding from MRI findings in their study of 351 infants from Europe.

The occurrence of cerebral palsy as a result of maternal and infant infection has received increased research attention. In a study of 688 children between 1987 and 1999, the infant's risk for cerebral palsy was increased when the mother experienced any type of infection during her hospitalization for delivery, whether the infant was born prematurely or at term (Neufeld, Frigon, Graham, et al. 2005). The risk of cerebral palsy as a result of a maternal infection at any point during pregnancy is also confirmed in studies from Europe (Bax et al., 2006; Greenwood, Yudkin, Sellers, et al. 2007). Stoll, Hansen, Adams-Chapman and colleagues (2004) found an increased risk of cerebral palsy in preterm newborns as a result of acquired infections.

Two hundred twenty-five children with cerebral palsy from England were studied to identify risk factors. Term infants experienced higher risks for cerebral palsy as a result of preeclampsia, small for gestational age, placental abruption, sepsis, and intrapartum pyrexia. Preterm infants had increased risks for cerebral palsy as a result of placental abruption, premature rupture of membranes, sepsis, and chorioamnionitis. Children with cerebral palsy as a result of postnatal causes were not studied (Greenwood et al., 2007). Similar results were found in a Greek study of 78 children with cerebral palsy. Predictors of cerebral palsy in term infants were sepsis/meningitis, small for gestational age, and neonatal transfer; in preterm infants, the predictors were patent ductus arteriosus, premature rupture of membranes, and periventricular leukomalacia (Drougia, Giapros, Krallis, et al., 2006). Placental defects and inflammation were also causative or predictive in other studies (Kaukola, Herva, Perhomaa, et al., 2005; Lee, Croen, Backstrand, et al., 2005). Wu, Day, Strauss, and colleagues (2004) found birth asphyxia to be a predictor of cerebral palsy in term infants, although the rate is declining. Other researchers found that about half of the children with cerebral palsy in their studies had cerebellar as well as cerebral injury (Bodensteiner & Johnson, 2004; Johnson, Bodensteiner, & Lotze, 2005). Cerebral palsy also occurs if the infant experiences a stroke before age 3 years (Lee et al., 2005; United Cerebral Palsy Research and Educational Foundation, 2008).

Most of the time, cerebral palsy does not result from a genetic cause. In a recent Swedish study, Costeff (2004) estimated that 40% of all incidences of cerebral palsy between 1959 and 1970 had a genetic cause. More than half of the cases of term hemiplegia and ataxia were found to be genetic in origin. A number of biochemical disorders and cerebral malformations may result in motor abnormalities and may be misdiagnosed as cerebral palsy, such as hypotonia, Duchenne muscular dystrophy, arginase deficiency, metachromatic leukodystrophy, adrenoleukodystrophy, hereditary progressive spastic paraplegia, dopa-responsive dystonia, Lesch-Nyhan disease, Rett syndrome, ataxia telangiectasia, Niemann-Pick disease type C, and mitochondrial cytopathies (Gupta & Appleton, 2001; Krigger, 2006).

The apolipoprotein E genotype has received attention since its discovery for its role in identifying neurologic conditions. The presence of the apolipoprotein E e4 allele in an infant carries a 3.4-fold risk for cerebral palsy affecting multiple limbs. Children with cerebral palsy with the e4 allele have greater severity and microcephaly. The risk for cerebral palsy is further increased with the presence of the apolipoprotein E e2 allele (Kuroda, Weck, Sarwark, et al., 2007).

Incidence and Prevalence

The specific prevalence of cerebral palsy was 2.4 per 1000 live births based on a literature review of prevalence studies between 1990 and 2005 (Hirtz, Thurman, Gwinn-Hardy, et al., 2007). Another review of the prevalence literature between 1965 and 2004 found similar findings (Odding et al., 2006). Prevalence rates vary slightly across countries: (1) Sweden, 1995 to 1998, 0.69 per 1000 live births (Himmelmann, Beckung, Hagberg, et al., 2007); (2) Northern Ireland, 1981 to 1997, 2.2 per 1000 live births (Dolk, Parkes, & Hill, 2006); (3) Turkey, 1980 to 1994, 4.4 per 1000 live births (Serdaroglu et al., 2006); (4) three areas in the United States, 2002, 3.6 per 1000 live births (Yeargin-Allsopp, Van Naarden Braun, Doernberg, et al., 2008); and (5) Northern Alberta, Canada, 2001 to 2003, 22 per 1000 live births (Robertson, Watt, & Yasui, 2007). The United Cerebral Palsy Research and Educational Foundation (2008) indicates that the number of infants born each year with cerebral palsy is increasing worldwide. The statistics reported in this paragraph are increased from those found in the last edition of this text. Recurrence risks are rare.

In addition, the prevalence of cerebral palsy is higher in twins (Bonellie, Currie, & Chalmers, 2005) and in males, and approximately half of the infants born with cerebral palsy are born prematurely (Johnston & Hagberg, 2007; United Cerebral Palsy Research and Educational Foundation, 2008). In recent years, researchers have found greater prevalence of cerebral palsy in infants born to families with low socioeconomic status (Sundrum, Logan, Wallace, et al., 2005) and in black children (Bhasin, Brocksen, Avchen, et al., 2006; Yeargin-Allsopp et al., 2008). Further research on larger samples is needed to substantiate these findings.

Diagnostic Criteria

The two major elements leading to a diagnosis of cerebral palsy are nonprogressive damage to the brain and subsequent motor impairment of varying severity and type. Physical and functional disabilities are usually present. Diagnosis of cerebral palsy is based on an assessment of the child's developmental, functional, and physical abilities. The detailed health history should include the family's medical history, the mother's and fetus' health during pregnancy, the infant's health at birth and up to the present time, and the infant's development since birth. Additional testing, such as parental and infant genetic screening and testing, prenatal ultrasound or amniocentesis, cranial sonography or MRI, and other designated developmental testing and evaluations of specific impairments should further be included as warranted. When parents have related concerns, it is important for primary care providers to rule out other neurologic problems in conjunction with specialty consultations. The diagnosis of cerebral palsy is not given until after the child is 18 to 24 months of age because early muscle and motor tone abnormalities may signify another neurodevelopmental problem. Moreover, some children who initially present with symptoms of cerebral palsy no longer have

BOX 18-2
Assessment of Tone in Infants

NORMAL TONE
- Infant moves well against gravity and lacks high- or low-tone characteristics.

LOW TONE
- Infant lacks tone to move against gravity and resistance to passive movement; has low-tone postures (e.g., supine lying with arm abducted and/or legs abducted in a frog-legged position) or decreased movement.

HIGH TONE
- Infant becomes stiff when moving against gravity; the neck or extremities resist passive movement; infant has hypertonic head reactions (e.g., hyperextension of the neck when rolling over and/or head pushing when supine or when pulled to sitting position); infant has high-tone posturing (e.g., increased extension of the head when supine lying, retracted shoulder girdle, lordosis of the back of extended lower extremities).

them after 24 months of age. This change is especially true in cases of prematurity, although other communication and learning problems may persist (United Cerebral Palsy Research and Educational Foundation, 2003).

Parents are often the first to discover a child's delayed or failed attainment of motor milestones at the appropriate time, or they may complain of difficulty in diapering their child. Other specific signs that may be noted by the parents or the clinician include poor head control and clenched hands after 3 months of age, no side protective reflexes after 5 months of age, extended Moro and atonic neck reflexes past 6 months of age, no parachute reflex after 10 months of age, crossing of the midline to reach objects before 12 months of age, hand preference before 18 months of age—sometimes as early as 6 months, and leg scissoring in late infancy or the early toddler period. These signs can appear in one or both sides (Krigger, 2006; Pellegrino, 2007). An assessment of normal and abnormal muscle tone is outlined in Box 18-2.

Clinical Manifestations at Time of Diagnosis

Clinical manifestations of cerebral palsy center on abnormal motor development and behaviors and are often associated with other disabilities (Gupta & Appleton, 2001; Krigger, 2006). Behavioral manifestations during infancy that may indicate cerebral palsy include irritability, a weak cry, poor sucking ability with tongue thrust, excessive sleep patterns, and little interest in surroundings. Infants may also sleep in a rag doll or floppy position or in an arched and extended position (i.e., opisthotonos). Later signs of abnormal mobility include "bunny hopping" (i.e., when crawling, the legs are brought forward together after the hands and arms are advanced) and "W sitting" (Krigger, 2006). Children may also show signs of toe walking, crouched gait, foot deformity, flat foot, unequal leg length, or walking on the outer aspects of the feet.

Treatment

The goals of treatment of children with cerebral palsy are designed to maintain mobility and maximize joint range of motion, as well as to optimize muscle control and balance, communication, and

---

Clinical Manifestations at Time of Diagnosis

DELAYED GROSS MOTOR DEVELOPMENT
- A universal manifestation
- Delay in all motor accomplishments
- Increases as growth advances
- Delays more obvious as growth advances

ABNORMAL MOTOR PERFORMANCE
- Very early preferential unilateral hand use
- Abnormal and asymmetric crawl
- Standing or walking on toes
- Uncoordinated or involuntary movements
- Poor sucking
- Feeding difficulties
- Persistent tongue thrust

ALTERATIONS OF MUSCLE TONE
- Increased or decreased resistance to passive movements
- Opisthotonic postures (exaggerated arching of back)
- Feels stiff on handling or dressing
- Difficulty in diapering
- Rigid and unbending at the hip and knee joints when pulled to sitting position (an early sign)

ABNORMAL POSTURES
- Maintains hips higher than trunk in prone position with legs and arms flexed or drawn under the body
- Scissoring and extension of legs, with the feet plantar flexed in supine position
- Persistent infantile resting and sleeping posture
- Arms abducted at shoulders
- Elbows flexed
- Hands fisted

REFLEX ABNORMALITIES
- Persistence of primitive infantile reflexes
  - Obligatory tonic neck reflex at any age
  - Nonpersistence beyond 6 months of age
- Persistence or hyperactivity of the Moro, plantar, and palmar grasp reflexes
- Hyperreflexia, ankle clonus, and stretch reflexes elicited in many muscle groups on fast, passive movements

ASSOCIATED DISABILITIES*
- Altered learning and reasoning
- Seizures
- Impaired behavioral and interpersonal relationships
- Sensory impairment (vision, hearing)

Adapted from Jones, M.W., Morgan, E., & Shelton, J.E. (2007). Primary care of the child with cerebral palsy: A review of systems (part II). *J Pediatr Health Care, 21*, 226-237.
*May or may not be present.

---

performance of activities of daily living following the International Classification of Functioning, Disability, and Health (World Health Organization, 2001). Treatment plans should be determined by the child's present and future health, developmental, and functional needs and goals and the parent's wishes if the child is too young to speak for himself or herself (Pellegrino, 2007). A continuum of comprehensive, interdisciplinary care should prevail across the life span (Bax et al., 2005). Box 18-3 lists the different evaluations that health care professionals can use for management decisions. A developmental timeline for occupational, physical, and speech therapy, as well as orthotics, is included in Table 18-2 (Helsel, McGee, & Graveline, 2001).

Treatment

Therapies
- Physical therapy
  - Gait analysis
  - Neuromuscular electrical stimulation
- Occupational therapy
- Speech therapy
- Behavioral therapy

Orthotic Devices
- Braces
- Casting
- Splints
- Molded ankle-foot orthosis (MAFO)
- Adaptive equipment
  - Boards
  - Computers
  - For functional use (e.g., eating utensils)
  - Scooters and tricycles
  - Switches
  - Wheelchairs and standing devices

Pharmacologic Therapy
- Botulinum toxin A
- Intrathecal baclofen
- Medications for:
  - Pain
  - Constipation
  - Urinary tract infections
  - Upper respiratory tract infections
  - Decubitus ulcers
  - Other secondary complications and conditions

Surgery
- Orthopedic-corrective (e.g., tendon transfers, muscle lengthening)
- Neurologic (e.g., neurectomies)
  - Selective dorsal rhizotomy
- Feeding (e.g., gastrostomy)
- Dental

BOX 18-3

Evaluations/Instruments Used for Management Decisions

- 3-D gait analysis
- 9-hole Peg Test
- Activities Scale for Kids
- Assisting Hand Assessment
- Barry-Albright Dystonia Scale
- Bimanual Fine Motor Function (BFMF)
- Canadian Occupational Performance Measure (COPM)
- Edinburgh Visual Gait Analysis Interval Testing Scale
- Energy expenditure measures
- Gillette Functional Assessment Questionnaire
- Goal Attainment Scale (GAS)
- Gross Motor Function Measure (GMFM)
- Lifestyle Assessment Questionnaire for Cerebral Palsy (LAQ-CP)
- Manual Ability Classification System (MACS)
- Melbourne Assessment of Upper Limb Function
- Modified Ashworth Scale
- Pediatric Evaluation of Disability Inventory (PEDI)
- Pediatric Quality of Life Inventory (PedsQL)
- Physician Rating Scale, Observational Gait Scale
- Pediatric Outcomes Data Collection Instrument (PODCI)
- Range of Motion
- Quality of Upper Extremity Skills Test (QUEST)
- Spinal Alignment and Range of Motion Measure
- Tardieu Scale
- Video documentation
- WeeFIM (Functional Independence Measure)
- Wong-Baker FACES Pain Rating Scale

Adapted from Heinen, F., Molenaers, G., Fairhurst, C., et al. (2006). European consensus table 2006 on botulinum toxin for children with cerebral palsy. *Eur J Paediatr Neuroly, 10,* 215-225; Chaleat-Valayer, E., Bernard, J.-C., Morel, E., et al. (2006). Use of videographic examination for analysis of efficacy of botulinum toxin in the lower limbs in children with cerebral palsy. *J Pediatr Orthop B, 15,* 339-347; Krigger, K.W. (2006). Cerebral palsy: An overview. *Am Fam Physician, 73,* 91-100.

Physical and Occupational Therapy

During infancy and toddlerhood, when most presumptive diagnoses take place, the first line of treatment involves physical and occupational therapy. The aim of these therapies is to enhance motor development, minimize the development of contractures, and prevent deterioration or weakening of the muscles (Wood, 2006). Physical therapists have used neuromuscular electrical stimulation in tandem with standard active and passive therapies to improve joint mobility, control muscle movement and strength, and reduce spasticity. Neuromuscular electrical stimulation has been found to be useful when combined with dynamic bracing and with repeated applications of this procedure (Ozer, Chesher, & Scheker, 2006). Overall, although some positive results have been achieved with the use of neuromuscular electrical stimulation, such as stimulating impulses for ambulation (Ho, Holt, Saltzman, et al., 2006), the benefits remain inconclusive and require further research (Darrah, Walkins, Chen, et al., 2004; Ho et al., 2006). Gait analysis is also used, along with other types of evaluation, to determine treatment plans (Chang, Seidl, Muthusamy, et al., 2006; Lofterod, Terjesen, Skaaret, et al., 2007; Narayanan, 2007). Additional research is recommended to determine efficacy and standards for its use for optimal outcomes (Narayanan, 2007). Dobson, Morris, Baker, and colleagues (2007) suggested that a classification system of gait abnormalities needs to be designed and tested.

From the preschool years through adolescence, the aim of a physical or occupational treatment program is to help a child with cerebral palsy function optimally in the home and school. Gross motor skills, muscle control, balance, and coordination are needed for sitting and moving. Fine motor skills, muscle control, and coordination are needed for writing and holding materials. Motor, cognitive, and language skills also are needed for self-care activities. Bowel and bladder control and prevention of pressure ulcers are important to learn at this time. Independent ambulation may be decreased in adolescents using orthotic devices because of contractures, a lack of motivation, or weight gain, and they may choose to use a wheelchair to maximize their energy (National Institute of Neurological Disorders and Stroke, 2008). Postural management, which involves a comprehensive, multi-multimethod, individualized plan for the optimal development of function and posture across the pediatric years, is presented by Gericke (2006).

Other Therapies

Speech therapy should be recommended if an oromotor deficit exists. Augmentative communication devices may be warranted (Jones, Morgan, & Shelton, 2007; Krigger, 2006).

TABLE 18-2

Developmental Timeline for Specific Therapies and Orthotics

Age	OT	PT	Speech	Orthotics
0-3 mo Infant Hemiparetic, diparetic, or tetraparetic not usually diagnosed	Yes—developmental screening and follow-up treatment as needed Feeding addressed	Maybe—most likely involved if child has orthopedic issues	Probably not—only if severe oral motor deficit that may affect speech production	Probably not—may be involved if child has orthopedic issues
3-12 mo Infant	Yes—usually if hemiparetic or tetraparetic Fine motor development, feeding, ADL, cognitive and sensory issues	Yes—hemiparetic, diparetic, or tetraparetic Gross motor development, range of motion, etc.	Probably not—see above	Probably not—see above
1-3 yr Toddler	Yes—usually if hemiparetic or tetraparetic Usually outpatient Diparetics at times for visual motor or oral motor issues	Yes—hemiparetic, diparetic, or tetraparetic Usually outpatient	Yes—if tetraparetic Hemiparetic or diparetic if diaphragm involved or significant oral motor involvement Usually outpatient	Yes—may be for hemiparetic, diparetic, or tetraparetic as needed
3-6 yr Preschool	Yes—may also see diparetics from this age on for ADL Outpatient and/or school	Yes—outpatient and/or school	Yes—outpatient and/or school	Yes—as needed
6-12 yr School years	Yes—usually school, but may also have outpatient postsurgical treatment for "tune-ups" and skills not related to school performance	Yes—see OT description for this age-group	Yes—usually school based May require additional therapy if augmentative communication system introduced	Yes—to update orthotics as needed for growth and development
12 yr–adult Adolescent to adulthood	Yes—may continue at school and/or outpatient for specific "tune-up" or functional independence issues, adaptive equipment, or postoperatively	Yes—may continue at school and/or outpatient for specific "tune-up" or functional independence issues, adaptive equipment, or postoperatively	Possibly—at school or to introduce and train with new augmentative communication device	Yes—generally to replace worn-out equipment or postoperatively

From Helsel, P., McGee, J., & Graveline, C. (2001). Physical management of spasticity. *J Child Neurol, 16,* 25.
Key: *ADL,* activities of daily living; *OT,* occupational therapy; *PT,* physical therapy.

Living with cerebral palsy may be frustrating and difficult for many children. Behavioral therapy or counseling may be needed at any point in a child's life (Krigger, 2006).

Orthotic Devices

Orthotic devices, which include braces and splints, usually accompany therapy when it alone no longer helps the child. Orthotic devices are used to provide stability to the joints, maintain the optimal range of motion of the joints, prevent the occurrence or progression of contractures, and control involuntary movements. The most common types of orthoses are the short arm or leg cast or splint, the hand splint, and the molded ankle-foot orthosis (MAFO), which is worn inside the shoe. Other types of adaptive equipment include devices for functional use (e.g., eating utensils), switches, computers, boards for positioning a child (e.g., on his or her side or in the prone or supine positions), scooters, tricycles, and wheelchairs. In severe cases, wheelchairs and standing devices are constructed and molded for an individual child (Figure 18-1) (Pellegrino, 2007). In each case, the orthosis is designed for a child and altered as the child grows or the condition changes. Although the use of orthotic devices is largely practiced, a recent review of the research literature on the use of limb casting and orthoses found inconclusive evidence (Autti-Ramo, Suoranta, Anttila, et al., 2006). Further research involving randomized clinical trials is warranted.

Pharmacologic Therapy

Decision making in pharmacologic treatment approaches includes age, adherence, degree of spasticity, dosage, comorbidity, costs, known adverse effects, and prior health and medication history. The most commonly researched medications for the treatment of spasticity in cerebral palsy include botulinum toxin A and intrathecal baclofen. Analyses of the research completed on botulinum toxin A indicate that there is insufficient evidence to affirm or refute the effectiveness of this medication on upper limb spasticity (Park & Rha, 2006; Reeuwijk, van Schie, Becher, et al., 2006; Speth, Leffers, Janssen-Potten, et al., 2005), spasticity in general (Lannin, Scheinberg, & Clark, 2006; Weigl, Arbel, Katz, et al., 2007), and in regard to long-term effects (Gough, Fairhurst, & Shortland, 2005; Linder-Lucht, Kirschner, Herrmann, et al., 2006). Methodologic weaknesses have influenced the efficacy of current pediatric research concerning these medications (Koman, Smith, & Shilt, 2004; Park & Albright, 2006; Reeuwijk et al., 2006; Schroeder, Berweck, Lee, et al., 2006). Intrathecal baclofen has been found to improve dystonia in one third of those treated and have long-term effects (Albright & Ferson, 2006), but additional study is warranted. Withdrawal from this medication can be fatal, and steps must be taken to prevent untoward effects of withdrawal (Albright & Ferson, 2006; Zuckerbraun, Ferson, Albright, et al., 2004). Muscle relaxants are also used alone or in combination to reduce dystonia

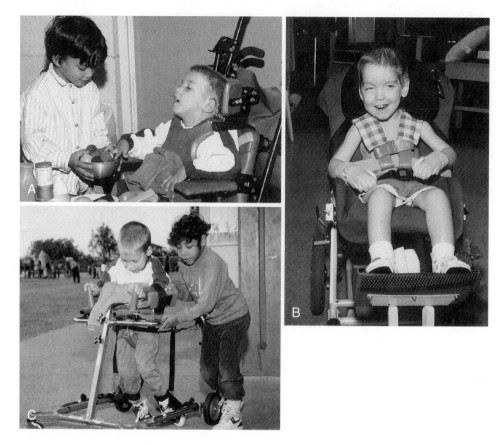

FIGURE 18-1 **A** and **B,** Individualized wheelchair. **C,** Standing device. From author's personal collection. Taken at Matheny Medical and Educational Center, Peapack, NJ.

(Koman et al., 2004; Mathew, Mathew, Thomas, et al., 2005). Bjornson, Hays, Graubert, and colleagues (2007) stressed the importance of discussing pharmacologic treatment decisions with parents specifically addressing the possible outcomes so that the child and the parents have realistic expectations of the effect of the medication(s).

Pain management in cerebral palsy is discussed less frequently, although pain is common, especially in spastic cerebral palsy. Pain is experienced most frequently in the joints of the lower extremities (National Institute of Neurological Disorders and Stroke, 2008). Heinen, Molenaers, Fairhurst, and colleagues (2006) discussed the importance of providing analgesia and sedation before the injection of botulinum toxin, due to this painful procedure. Additional research is needed to assess the pain experience in children with cerebral palsy.

Medications are also prescribed for secondary conditions as they occur. These include treatment for constipation, urinary tract infections, upper respiratory infections, decubitus ulcers, and other secondary complications and conditions.

Surgery

Surgery for cerebral palsy is not an early choice of intervention. Orthopedic and neurologic forms of surgery are the most common, but surgeries to enhance feeding, such as gastrostomy, gastroscopy, esophagoscopy, and correction of gastroesophageal reflux, as well as dental surgeries, are frequently done (Aker & Anderson, 2007). Orthopedic surgery is not usually performed until after a child is 6 years old. A child attains independent ambulation by this age if

independence is at all possible. Orthopedic surgery is performed to achieve greater leg movement and gait control, as well as to correct any extremity deformities. Orthopedic surgery is done to correct hip subluxation or dislocation and spinal deformities (e.g., scoliosis), to promote muscle balance and joint stabilization, to prevent contractures, and to reduce spasticity through muscle lengthening and tendon transfers (Murphy, Hoff, Jorgensen, et al., 2006; Steinbok, 2006). The child's degree of spasticity, the child's size, and the effect of the spasticity on the child's life should be considered when determining surgical alternatives (O'Brien & Park, 2006; Steinbok, 2006).

Selective dorsal rhizotomy is performed on many children with cerebral palsy. The outcomes of this surgery, especially decreasing the need for further orthopedic procedures, is dependent on type of cerebral palsy with those less affected having the most positive long-term effects (Kim, Steinbok, & Wickenheiser, 2006; O'Brien & Park, 2006; Park & Johnston, 2006). Spinal deformities as a result of this surgery are a common adverse effect, with 54.8% of 105 subjects in one study experiencing scoliosis with worsening of the condition in 25% of those affected at follow-up (Steinbok, Hicdonmez, Sawatzky, et al., 2005). The primary care provider, surgeon, parents, and child should carefully discuss the risks and benefits.

Potential anesthesia complications can occur in children with cerebral palsy as a result of the physiologic and motor impairments. When the child is hypotonic, preoperative sedation is contraindicated because of the risk of aspiration and potential for a decrease in airway tone. Succinylcholine should be used with caution. Narcotics can be used, but the child's airway should be closely monitored after extubation (Theroux & Akins, 2005). General and epidural anesthesia can be used safely, but careful assessment for hypothermia, seizures, spasms and contractures, and gastroesophageal reflux should be done during surgery (Aker & Anderson, 2007).

Complementary and Alternative Therapies

Complementary and alternative therapies are used most often by children with cerebral palsy who are more severely affected. Additional reasons for its use include parental use, children of younger ages, and the inability to walk alone (Hurvitz, Leonard, Ayyangar, et al., 2003; Samdup, Smith, & Song, 2006).

Recent research evidence has found insufficient or no significant gains from the use of conductive education (Darrah et al., 2004), the Feldenkrais Method (Liptak, 2005), constraint-induced movement therapy (Hoare, Imms, Carey, et al., 2007), growth hormone therapy (Ali, Shim, Fowler, et al., 2007), or the Adeli suit (Bar-Haim, Harries, Belokopytov, et al., 2006; Turner, 2006). Hyperbaric oxygenation continues to be used in children with cerebral palsy. Results, to date, do not support a benefit, and a procedure for its use has not been standardized. Common side effects are middle ear barotraumas and ear pain (Essex, 2003; McDonagh, Carson, Ash, et al., 2003; Muller-Bolla, Collet, Ducruet, et al. 2006). Therefore it is not recommended.

There are preliminary results that the use of Chinese herbs and acupuncture, alone (Sun, Ko, Wong, et al., 2004) and in combination with therapies and other alternative and complementary treatments (Zhou & Zheng, 2005), improved motor function. Additional research is warranted. In addition, aquatic exercise (Kelly & Darrah, 2005) and equine-assisted therapy (Cherng, Liao, Leung, et al., 2004) have been found to be beneficial, but appropriate research studies have not been conducted on their efficacy.

Anticipated Advances in Diagnosis and Management

MRI and ultrasonography can be used to identify pathogenesis and to facilitate early diagnosis of cerebral palsy in low birth weight and premature infants. Therefore it is a recommendation of the revised classification system to obtain neuroimaging on any child with cerebral palsy (Paneth et al., 2005) and supported by other professional neurology associations (Ashwal et al., 2004).

Documentation of the effects of medications and other specific interventions will further the continued efforts to improve the quality of life in children with cerebral palsy. For example, the use of electrophysiologic techniques, such as electromyography, and ultrasound may help to identify the optimal muscles and location for botulinum toxin treatment (Schroeder et al., 2006). Robotics and regenerative techniques offer future possibilities for optimal quality of life (United Cerebral Palsy Research and Educational Foundation, 2008).

Associated Problems of Cerebral Palsy and Treatment

Secondary conditions may be acute, chronic, or transitory and usually coexist with cerebral palsy. These secondary conditions are listed in the accompanying box (Jones et al., 2007; Krigger, 2006;

Associated Problems of Cerebral Palsy and Treatment

Cognitive Impairments
- Learning disabilities
- Intellectual and developmental disabilities
- Perceptual and attention problems

Seizure Disorders

Speech Impairments
- Vocal strength and quality
- Articulation

Sensory Deficits
- Vision
  - Refractive errors
  - Strabismus
  - Amblyopia
  - Cataracts
  - Retinopathy of prematurity
  - Cortical blindness
  - Homonymous hemianopsia (hemiplegia)
- Hearing
  - Sensorineural
  - Conductive
- Other Sensory Deficits
  - Tactile hypersensitivity or hyposensitivity
  - Dyspraxia
  - Balance and movement problems
  - Proprioception difficulties
  - Stereognosis

Motor Impairments
- Prolonged primitive reflexes
- Absence of protective reflexes
- Delayed motor milestones

- Hip subluxation and dislocation
- Scoliosis
- Contractures
- Fractures

Feeding and Eating Problems
- Chewing, sucking, and swallowing deficits
- Aspiration
- Drooling
- Gastroesophageal reflux

Bowel Problems
- Constipation
- Encopresis

Urinary Problems
- Bladder control
- Urinary retention
- Urinary tract infections

Dental Problems
- Malocclusions
- Enamel defects and caries
- Gum hyperplasia (with phenytoin)
- Reduced saliva (with sedatives and barbiturates for spasticity)

Pulmonary Effects
- Respiratory infections
- Pneumonia

Skin Problems
- Decubitus ulcers

Latex Allergy

Behavioral and Emotional Problems
- Behavioral disorders
- Attention-deficit/hyperactivity disorder, all forms

Pellegrino, 2007). Plans for treatment, education, and habilitation must consider a child's individual symptoms and complaints.

Cognitive Impairments

Learning or intellectual disabilities often occur in children with cerebral palsy. The United Cerebral Palsy Research and Educational Foundation (2008) estimate that 6 in 10 individuals with cerebral palsy have normal intelligence and 3 in 10 children experience severe learning disabilities. In addition, 1 in 9 individuals with cerebral palsy has autistic tendencies. Intellectual disabilities/mental retardation is more prevalent when epilepsy is also present (Odding et al., 2006). Intellectual and developmental disabilities are usually most profound in children with abnormal motor behavior in all extremities, wherein more than 60% of the children have a normal intelligence quotient (IQ). Even if a child's IQ is normal, perceptual impairments and learning disabilities often exist. Any associated speech articulation problems, however, should not be misconstrued as an intellectual disability (National Institute of Neurological Disorders and Stroke, 2008). Children with hemiplegia also have perceptual and attentional problems, with children with left hemiplegia experiencing more perceptual problems and inattention than children with right hemiplegia (Katz, Cermak, & Shamir, 1998). As a result of the incidence of cognitive impairments with cerebral palsy, screening for cognitive impairments should take place on a regular basis and immediate intervention should begin if identified (Ashwal et al., 2004; Cooley, 2004). The revised classification system calls for indication of the presence or absence of cognitive impairments with any assessment (Paneth et al., 2005).

Seizure Disorders

Approximately 20% to 40% of children with cerebral palsy will experience seizures (Odding et al., 2006; Pellegrino, 2007; United Cerebral Palsy Research and Educational Foundation, 2008). Seizures are most commonly seen in children with spastic quadriplegia and hemiplegia and are less common in children with dyskinesias and ataxia. Generalized tonic-clonic and minor motor types of seizures are the most common. A genetic predisposition may also be present when seizures and cerebral palsy are present in a child (Pellegrino, 2007). The revised classification system calls for indication of the presence or absence of seizures or the diagnosis of epilepsy with any assessment (Paneth et al., 2005). (See Chapter 26 for a further discussion of seizure disorders.)

Speech Impairments

The incidence of speech impairments in cerebral palsy is as high as 80% (Odding et al., 2006).The same muscle tone problems that make it difficult for children with cerebral palsy to move also create oromotor problems. Limitations in trunk movements and positioning may limit lung capacity, which is needed for strength in speaking both clearly and loudly. Problems in articulation, called dysarthrias, are caused by muscle tone deficiencies (National Institute of Neurological Disorders and Stroke, 2008). Computers and adaptive equipment (e.g., switches) have allowed individuals with speech problems to dramatically improve their communication (Figure 18-2).

Sensory Deficits

Vision. Children with cerebral palsy may develop a number of visual problems, including refractive error, strabismus, amblyopia, cataracts, retinopathy of prematurity, and cortical blindness. The

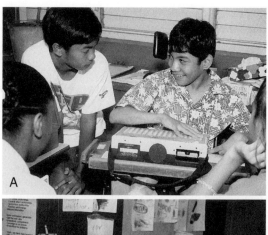
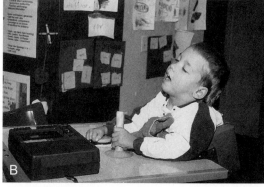

FIGURE 18-2 Child using an augmentative communication device and wheelchair switch. From author's personal collection. Taken at Matheny Medical and Educational Center, Peapack, NJ.

majority of all children with cerebral palsy develop strabismus (National Institute of Neurological Disorders and Stroke, 2008); about 75% develop some form of refractive errors (i.e., most often farsightedness) resulting in low visual acuity; and approximately 25% with hemiplegia develop homonymous hemianopsia (the inability to see toward the affected side) (Odding et al., 2006; Pellegrino, 2007). Nine percent of children with cerebral palsy are legally blind (United Cerebral Palsy Research and Educational Foundation, 2008).

Hearing. Children with cerebral palsy experience hearing impairments at a greater frequency than in the general population. The hearing loss is either sensorineural (i.e., damage to the auditory nerve or the inner ear) or, more commonly, conductive (i.e., as a result of anatomic abnormalities or frequent otitis media). Hearing impairments further add to speech and communication delays (Jones et al., 2007; Krigger, 2006). Two percent of children with cerebral palsy are deaf (United Cerebral Palsy Research and Educational Foundation, 2008).

Other Sensory Deficits. As a result of damage to the parietal lobe of the brain, children with cerebral palsy have deficits in other sensory functions. These deficits may include tactile hypersensitivity or hyposensitivity; dyspraxia (i.e., difficulty in using one's senses to plan movements); balance difficulties; and problems with proprioception, stereognosis, and movement (Krigger, 2006; Odding et al., 2006). The development of a scale to assess laryngeal and speech impairments is greatly needed. The revised classification system calls for indication of the presence or absence of speech impairments with any assessment (Paneth et al., 2005; Reddihough, 2006).

Motor Impairments

Successful attainment of motor milestones is always delayed in children with cerebral palsy. Some children's primitive reflexes persist and protective reflexes never develop, thus permanently blocking their ability to ambulate. Poor muscle tone and control often lead to secondary physical problems (e.g., hip dislocation, scoliosis, contractures, fractures), which create further motor impairment and other medical problems related to basic physiologic functioning. In the worst-case scenario, these impairments are life threatening.

Subluxation and dislocation of the hip are common in children with cerebral palsy, especially in spastic cerebral palsy and, in particular, immobile children with spastic quadriplegia. Complications can include further motor impairment, positioning difficulties, pain, chronic arthritis, scoliosis, and hygienic concerns (Jones et al., 2007; Morton, Scott, McClelland, et al., 2006).

Scoliosis can result from unequal muscle tension resulting from the cerebral palsy or from poor posture or positioning in seating and recumbent positions. The degree of scoliosis directly coincides with the amount of spasticity and neurologic damage present (Jones et al., 2007).

Shortening and misalignment of the muscles can be created by a constant pull of tight muscles or spasticity or by diminished muscle use, which may lead to contractures. Contractures in the lower extremities are most often seen in children with spastic quadriplegia and diplegia. Contractures in the upper extremities are most commonly found in children with spastic hemiplegia (Krigger, 2006).

The prevalence of fractures ranges from 4% to 50%. Fractures were found most often in children with cerebral palsy with spasticity in all limbs, who were nonambulatory, took anticonvulsants, had osteopenia, had higher body fat, had a gastrostomy, and/or experienced previous fractures (Leet, Mesfin, Pichard, et al., 2006; Presedo, Dabney, & Miller, 2007; Stevenson, Conaway, Barrington, et al., 2006). Fractures occurred most often in the lower limbs (82%), followed by the femur (48%) (Presedo et al., 2007). Additional research is needed to understand fracture risk and how best to prevent and treat the occurrence of fractures (Leet et al., 2006; Stevenson, et al., 2006).

Feeding and Eating Problems

Feeding and eating difficulties are common in children with cerebral palsy, primarily as a result of orofacial muscle impairments. Compromised cardiopulmonary functioning, as well as poor muscle tone (i.e., either hypertonic or hypotonic) in the neck, shoulders, and trunk, can impede the process of eating. Specifically, muscle tone and function deficits create problems with sucking, chewing, swallowing, and aspiration. Increased drooling and gastroesophageal reflux may also occur. Feeding and eating disabilities are most often seen in children with the athetoid type of cerebral palsy. Early and severe feeding problems are a predictor for later growth, nutritional, and developmental outcomes.

Bowel Problems

Constipation is a common and often chronic condition in children with cerebral palsy. Low muscle tone or spastic abdominal muscles can prevent contractility and pressure to adequately advance and empty the bowel contents. Further reasons for constipation include lack of exercise; inability to sense the signals of a bowel movement; painful defecations; inadequate fluid intake; a diet lacking in fruits, vegetables, and fiber; medications; a fear of toileting; poor positioning on the toilet; and behavior problems (Jones et al., 2007; Ozturk, Oktem, Kisioglu, et al., 2006). Bowel incontinence, or encopresis, can also occur in cerebral palsy. Good dietary and bowel management is imperative.

Urinary Problems

Problems with bladder control and urinary retention that occur in cerebral palsy are often the result of neurologic insults (Karaman, Kaya, Caskurlu, et al., 2005; Ozturk et al., 2006). Intellectual and developmental disabilities may reduce a child's ability to sense bladder fullness and signals to urinate. A combination of incomplete bladder emptying, infrequent voiding, severe fluid restriction, and urinary reflux increases the likelihood of frequent urinary tract infections, as do chronic constipation, improper perineal hygiene, and motor impairments (Jones et al., 2007; Krigger, 2006). Prompt treatment of urinary tract infections is imperative.

Dental Problems

Malocclusions commonly occur in children with cerebral palsy as a result of orofacial muscle tone deficiencies. An overbite or underbite can affect chewing and speech. Tooth enamel defects also occur frequently and if untreated may lead to dental caries. Children who have seizures and take phenytoin (Dilantin) often experience hyperplasia (i.e., excessive growth of the gums). Problems with gum disease and oral hygiene can occur. Other medications taken for spasticity (e.g., sedatives, barbiturates) can reduce the amount of saliva, increasing the propensity for dental caries (Keinan, Smith, & Zilberman, 2006; National Institute of Dental and Craniofacial Research, 2007).

Pulmonary Effects

Alterations in positioning caused by abnormal muscle tone and spasticity, immobility, scoliosis, and contractures can affect pulmonary function and place children with cerebral palsy at a higher risk for respiratory infections (e.g., pneumonia). When respiratory infections occur, they often linger beyond the usual period because many children have difficulty coughing and blowing their nose. Aspiration and gastroesophageal reflux can also cause pneumonia. Knowing the warning signs of respiratory infection and pneumonia is important for health professionals and families because pneumonia is a leading cause of death in children with cerebral palsy (Hemming, Hutton, & Pharoah, 2006). Children with severe dysphagia who show abnormal respiratory rates and fatigue during feeding are likely hypoxemic.

Skin Problems

Skin breakdown leading to raw and excoriated skin and decubitus ulcers is a common problem in children and adolescents with cerebral palsy—especially when mobility is compromised. Thorough skin assessment and protection of bony prominences while a child is seated or recumbent are necessary. Prompt and aggressive treatment of any evidence of skin breakdown is necessary. During infancy, when the child is in diapers, and later, in adolescence, when the girl is menstruating, are times when vigilance is needed.

Latex Allergy

An association exists between cerebral palsy and latex allergy. Primary care providers should be mindful of the risk for anaphylaxis if a child has had repeated surgeries and ventriculoperitoneal shunts (Grzybowski, Ownby, Rivers, et al., 2003).

Behavioral and Emotional Problems

As a result of exaggerated and prolonged existence of primitive reflexes, especially the startle reflex, infants and children with cerebral palsy overreact to the mildest amounts of stimulation. These children easily become tired and frustrated, and they may become demanding and uncooperative (Green, 2003). Children with cerebral palsy may also develop attention-deficit/hyperactivity disorder (Shapiro, 2004) (see Chapter 12).

Prognosis

Prognosis, similar to treatment, depends on the type and severity of the cerebral palsy. In general, the more extremities involved, the more severe the involvement, and the greater the feeding difficulties, presence of seizures, and developmental disability, the worse the prognosis (Katz, 2003). On the other hand, increased quality of life, functional status, and formal and informal social supports enhance prognosis (Strauss, Shavelle, Reynolds, et al., 2007).

Prognosis may be specifically discussed in terms of independent ambulation. If primitive reflexes are generally still present at 12 months of age and the protective reflexes are not yet present or the child has not walked by 6 to 7 years of age, the child will not ambulate independently. Prognosis for ambulation is predicted by type of cerebral palsy, motor milestones at age 2 years, and the presence of blindness (Beckung, Hagverg, Uldall, et al., 2008; Wu et al., 2004). Wu and colleagues (2004) developed probability charts for ambulation based on motor milestones at age 2 years. Day, Wu, Strauss, and colleagues (2007) found that those adolescents who were independent ambulators were most likely able to maintain their ambulatory ability over the next 15 years, but those with limited mobility usually lost function across time. The United Cerebral Palsy Research and Educational Foundation (2008) reported that one third of children with cerebral palsy are nonambulatory.

Few studies have been completed on survival statistics for persons with cerebral palsy. In infants with cerebral palsy studied in Japan from 1995 to 2002, mortality rate was affected by length of gestation and presence of infection (Sameshima & Ikenoue, 2006). In a study of adults with cerebral palsy in England, death was more frequently caused by respiratory diseases in those in their twenties and thirties, and diseases of the circulatory, digestive, and nervous systems and neoplasms in those in their forties and fifties (Hemming et al., 2006). The presence of comorbidities further affects mortality risk.

PRIMARY CARE MANAGEMENT

Health Care Maintenance

Growth and Development

Growth retardation does not occur in all cases of cerebral palsy. Children who are nonambulatory, affected in all extremities, or experience seizures are shorter in height than peers of the same age (Day, Strauss, Vachon, et al., 2007; Stevenson & Conaway, 2007; Stevenson et al., 2006). Odding and colleagues (2006) estimate that stunted growth occurs in 25% of children with cerebral palsy.

Obtaining accurate measurements for height and weight can be challenging if a child experiences motor difficulty and has contractures. When height cannot be measured in either a standing or recumbent position, the upper arm length (UAL) and lower leg length (LLL) measurements are adequate. Accurate measuring also monitors changes in spasticity, tone, contracture, and scoliosis. Triceps and subscapular skinfold thicknesses should also be obtained. The North American Growth in Cerebral Palsy Project's website (www.healthsystem.virginia.edu/internet/NAGCePP) lists full explanations for measuring using each form of anthropometric technique. Weight charts for boys and girls with cerebral palsy from ages 2 to 20 years are found in Stevenson, Conaway, Chumlea, et al., 2006. Weight may be recorded from a standing position on a standardized scale or while the child is sitting or supine on a chair or hammock scale (e.g., Hosey). Primary care providers may most easily obtain an accurate weight by having a parent hold the child and step on the scale and then subtracting the parent's weight.

An interdisciplinary team is needed to longitudinally observe the development of a child with cerebral palsy. Periodic assessments of the child's mental, motor, language, self-care, and emotional development are warranted (Cooley, 2004). Many general and specific screening instruments can be used by primary care providers and should be an important part of a child's care (see Box 18-3 and Chapter 2).

Assessment of a child's cognitive status is important because of the presence of intellectual disabilities in many children with cerebral palsy, as well as physical limitations and speech and language problems that may make determining a child's true cognitive abilities difficult. Standardized intelligence tests for infants and children are appropriate, but someone experienced in examining children with motor and language delays should conduct this assessment.

Motor assessment is most often completed by the physical or occupational therapist. Videotaping a child's movements, in combination with computer gait analysis, has greatly enhanced the abilities of the physical therapist and physiatrist to plan and treat motor deficits and complications.

Speech and language problems can be screened by using, for example, the Preschool Language Scale or the Denver Articulation Screening Examination. There are also specific screening tools that assess a child's receptive and expressive language ability (see Chapter 2). Primary care providers must accurately assess parental reports of language skills, however, because parents often overestimate the number of spoken words by counting grunts and partial words. A speech therapist is the best person to assess language skills. Because of the many feeding and eating problems in infancy, a language assessment should be done in conjunction with a nutritional assessment when solid foods are introduced at about 6 months of age.

Self-care skills should be assessed throughout childhood and adolescence during history taking at each primary health care visit. This assessment can be done through an interview, a questionnaire, or a standardized test (e.g., Functional Independence Measure for Children [WeeFIM] or the Pediatric Evaluation of Disability Inventory). The United Cerebral Palsy Research and Educational Foundation (2008) reported that 25% of children with cerebral palsy cannot dress or feed themselves.

Emotional development is another important area for periodic assessment. Although there are a number of available instruments that measure self-concept and self-esteem, a good discussion with a trusted health professional is usually adequate for obtaining an understanding of how a child is coping at home, at school, and in other environments. Pain and fatigue have been associated with decreased school functioning (Berrin, Malcame, Varni, et al., 2007) and health-related quality of life (Arnaud, White-Koning, Michelsen, et al., 2008; Dickinson, Parkinson, Ravens-Sieberer, et al., 2007). The presence of intellectual disabilities or epilepsy (Voorman, Dallmeijer, Schuengel, et al., 2006) and limited motor abilities (Morris, Kurinczuk, Fitzpatrick, et al., 2006) and type of cerebral palsy (Varni, Burwinkle, Sherman, et al., 2005; Varni, Limbers, & Burwinkle, 2007) have affected social participation and health-related quality of life.

Diet

Undernutrition is most often seen during infancy in children with cerebral palsy. After any medical reasons for such difficulty are determined, further problems must be assessed. Exercises to improve facial muscle tone can be initiated. If a child has trouble controlling the jaw or keeping the mouth closed, external assistance or supports can be applied. Children may also have oral tactile defensiveness and require a program of desensitization to different textures and a food plan developed around the foods that they will eat. Other children do not feel the food or drink in their mouths, so most of the food or liquid falls out of the mouth, creating skin problems. These children may also drool excessively. These children are also at risk for aspiration.

Nutritional status often improves over time as a result of improved oromotor, gross motor, and fine motor skills; general improvement in health status; and better nutritional intake. Decreased independent mobility in late childhood and adolescence can even lead to a child being overweight (Odding et al., 2006). This needs to be guarded against because becoming overweight can significantly affect motor performance and peer acceptance.

As a result of hypersensitivity, parents may need to try different nipples until one is found that the infant prefers. The size of the nipple hole may also need to be increased if thickened formula is prescribed. Motor problems may inhibit a child from being an independent feeder. Adaptive equipment can be designed for a growing child at each developmental stage. Most important, bottle feeding or baby foods should not be forced on an infant because there is a high risk for aspiration—a risk that is lifelong for children with severe cerebral palsy (Jones et al., 2007). A nutritionist and an occupational therapist can suggest ways to help a child with oromotor difficulties and supplement the diet to ensure that a child receives adequate calories. See Jones and colleagues (2007) for a list of suggestions that can be used by primary care providers to add calories and protein to the diet of a child with cerebral palsy.

Some children with severe cerebral palsy may eventually need a feeding tube surgically inserted in the stomach. When needed, the placement of a gastrostomy tube has resulted in improved health, a reduction in time spent in feeding, and decreased chest infections from aspiration (Craig, Carr, Cass, et al., 2006; Samson-Fang, Butler, & O'Donnell, 2003; Sullivan, Juszczak, Bachlet, et al., 2005). A temporary nasogastric tube can be prescribed during an acute illness. Whether temporary or permanent, an interdisciplinary assessment is warranted with appropriate teaching of its use (Peterson, Kedia, Davis, et al., 2006; Van der Burg, Jongerius, Van Hulst, et al., 2006). Complications include blockage, leakage, skin irritation, infection, gastrointestinal bleeding, bowel obstruction,

and ulceration (Samson-Fang et al., 2003). Careful lifelong monitoring of a child's feeding abilities and nutritional status is critically important in cerebral palsy.

Safety

Children with motor impairments and seizure disorders are at increased risk for injury. Special concern should be taken when physical activities, car seats, and environmental surroundings are chosen for children with cerebral palsy. Children with cerebral palsy may not be restricted in the type of physical activity (e.g., canoeing), but adult supervision is needed. Seizure precautions and helmets may be necessary for children with seizure disorders. Car seats should be appropriately padded and positioned to protect a child's head—especially if head control is an issue. These precautions apply to any seating arrangement. A child's environment should be free of sharp edges in case of unexpected falls and roomy enough for the child to maneuver. If the child is in a wheelchair, the home environment should be wheelchair accessible. Some engineers are specially trained to suggest adaptations to homes, daycare settings, or schools to make them more wheelchair accessible. Home emergency plans should account for a child in a wheelchair, and local police and fire departments should be alerted.

Immunizations

Pertussis. Children with seizure disorders are at increased risk of seizure after receiving the pertussis vaccine. The risks and benefits of administering the pertussis vaccine when a child is at risk for seizures should be explained to the family, and the acellular form of the vaccine should be given in conjunction with tetanus and diphtheria (Broder, Cortese, Iskander, et al., 2006). Children with cerebral palsy who do not have seizures should also receive the acellular form recommended for all children (Committee on Infectious Diseases, American Academy of Pediatrics [AAP], 2008).

Measles. Children with a seizure disorder are at risk for a seizure after receiving the measles vaccine in the form of the measles-mumps-rubella (MMR) vaccine. Because of the complications of measles, the high probability of contracting measles, and the unlikelihood of having a seizure after the immunization is administered, however, the standard schedule for measles vaccination should be followed (Committee on Infectious Diseases, AAP, 2008).

Chickenpox (Varicella). Children with cerebral palsy should be immunized against varicella. For children with severe cerebral palsy in whom complications of the disease could be life threatening, prophylactic treatment of varicella exposure in unimmunized children with varicella-zoster immunoglobulin (VariZIG) should be recommended over the vaccine (Marin, Guris, Chaves, et al., 2007).

Haemophilus influenzae Type B. The recommended immunization schedule for *Haemophilus influenzae* type B (HiB) should be followed for children and adolescents with cerebral palsy (Committee on Infectious Diseases, AAP, 2008; Kroger, Atkinson, Marcuse, et al., 2006).

Influenza Vaccine. Children with cerebral palsy are at risk for complications of influenza and should follow the recommended schedule (Committee on Infectious Diseases, AAP, 2008).

Other Immunizations. Children with cerebral palsy should receive immunizations for mumps, rubella, diphtheria, tetanus, pneumococcal infections, meningococcal infections, rotavirus, human papillomavirus, hepatitis B, and polio as recommended (Committee on Infectious Diseases, AAP, 2008). Hepatitis A vaccine should be given only if the child's place of residence is in a location of high incidence and community prophylaxis is being done (Fiore, Wasley, & Bell, 2006).

Screening

Vision. A pediatric ophthalmologist should annually assess the eyes of children with cerebral palsy because of the many types of visual impairments that may occur (Jones et al., 2007). Vision can also be screened each time the child comes for a primary care visit and a referral made to an ophthalmologist by the preschool years. When performing a visual acuity test, children with motor problems may have difficulty showing which way an E points, and those with speech problems may have difficulty naming the letters.

Glasses often are prescribed for refractive errors. Contact lenses are contraindicated in children with cerebral palsy because their motor impairments inhibit placement and removal of the lenses. Glasses should be placed correctly on a child's face, and adaptive equipment (e.g., Velcro straps) may be recommended for comfortable and correct placement. Patching and surgery may be recommended for other vision complications associated with cerebral palsy (e.g., strabismus, amblyopia).

Hearing. A pediatric audiologist should regularly check the hearing of a child with cerebral palsy. For specific diagnostic information, an audiologist will use a tympanometer and evoked response audiometry. The primary care provider should check the tympanic membranes at each visit (Jones et al., 2007).

Children with sensorineural hearing loss may be fitted with a hearing aid. A speech therapist may join the assessment team when the hearing aid is placed to facilitate language development through words or signs (National Institute of Neurological Disorders and Stroke, 2008). Proper maintenance and use of hearing aids by children and families will help a child to interact optimally with the environment.

Dental. Children with cerebral palsy need a dentist who has experience with children with movement and motor disorders. The environment of the dentist's office must be accessible, with a chair that allows for easy transfer from a wheelchair if the child uses one. The chair must also protect fragile skin and support spastic extremities. Children with cerebral palsy should visit the dentist at least every 6 months and more often if recommended (National Institute of Dental and Cranofacial Research, 2007). Sedation may be necessary for children with severe spasticity.

Malocclusions can be prevented through oromotor exercises to improve muscle tone around the oral cavity. An interdisciplinary team consisting of the nutritionist, occupational therapist, and speech-language pathologist can plan exercises to reduce the oral reflexes that can lead to development of overbites or underbites. This team can also address drooling problems and help a child to swallow saliva and keep the tongue in the mouth. If drooling persists, surgery may be warranted. Adaptive equipment (e.g., an altered toothbrush or a washcloth for washing the teeth) may be appropriate (National Institute of Dental and Craniofacial Research, 2007).

Blood Pressure. Routine screening is recommended.

Hematocrit. Routine screening is recommended.

Urinalysis. Routine screening is recommended. A referral to a pediatric urologist may be needed if the child has chronic urinary tract infections.

Tuberculosis. Routine screening is recommended.

Condition-Specific Screening

Motor and Movement Problems. A motor assessment should be done at each primary care visit. Body alignment and positioning; passive and active range of motion; and signs of hip dislocation, spinal deformities, contractures, and movement patterns (e.g., gait disturbances) should be assessed and measured when appropriate (Paneth et al., 2005). Goniometric measurements of the joint mobility and motion of the knee and ankle can assist in screening for abnormalities in tone. Radiography and electromyography (EMG) may be needed for further diagnosis (Leet & Blasco, 2008). Palisano, Rosenbaum, Bartlett, and colleagues (2007) expanded and revised their five-level classification system for gross motor function in children with cerebral palsy. This classification system can be found at www.canchild.ca/Default.aspx?tabid=195. Correct management and follow-through by the child and family are necessary to prevent the development of further complications and can be useful in planning and evaluating interventions (Cooley, 2004).

Exercise should also be encouraged. Elements of flexibility, strength, endurance, and balance can be incorporated in an individualized physical fitness program (Pellegrino, 2007).

Common Illness Management
Differential Diagnosis

Fever. Children experience many febrile episodes in their lives as a result of the many viruses and bacteria that are present in their environment. Children with cerebral palsy are prone to respiratory and urinary tract infections and may also get gastrointestinal infections. In each of these infections, fever is usually an accompanying symptom. Children with cerebral palsy must be seen by a primary care provider if they are under 6 months of age, have had a fever over 38.6°C for 3 or more days without symptoms, appear acutely ill with undefined symptoms, or have had a seizure with a fever. A physical assessment and laboratory work need to be done by the primary care provider at this time for an accurate diagnosis and treatment.

Respiratory Tract Infections. Children with cerebral palsy are susceptible to upper and lower respiratory tract infections, namely, otitis media, sore throats, rhinorrhea, sinusitis, and influenza. Asthma is more prevalent in premature infants with cerebral palsy. Routine management of these problems is warranted with careful monitoring of the resolution of the infection. Sometimes these infections are not resolved with one round of antibiotics, and complications can occur (e.g., additional hearing loss from a case of otitis media). Referral to a specialist may be recommended.

Pain with an infection is difficult to assess in children with severe cerebral palsy. For example, the typical sign of pulling on the ear for an ear infection may not be present. Parents are often able to discern subtle signs in their child (e.g., increased irritability, decreased energy, fewer vocalizations, increased drooling) or to think that the child is just not acting like himself or herself. Children can also be asked yes-or-no questions to identify the source of pain. If a child uses a communication system, signs or symbols can be used to describe pain. Children's pain scales (e.g., the Wong FACES Scale) can be used by primary care providers to further assess a child's pain.

It is important to stress the high probability of pneumonia occurring after an initial upper respiratory infection or bout of influenza in children with severe cerebral palsy. Pneumonia can also be caused by aspiration and gastroesophageal reflux. Careful monitoring must be done to prevent a life-threatening situation. Children with cerebral palsy are unable to expectorate well and handle increased secretions. Dehydration can easily occur. Hospitalization may be suggested as a preventive measure to ensure close observation of any changes in a child's health status. If a child is being cared for at home, parents must understand the importance of the treatment plan and contact their clinician if the condition worsens.

Dermatology Issues. Skin problems arise from positioning in chairs and beds when bony prominences rub against hard surfaces. Decubitus ulcers can occur quickly, and vigilant skin management is warranted, especially in nonmobile children. Protection of the bony prominences with soft protective coverings is usually enough, but medical attention should be obtained for persistent areas of redness. Assess for latex allergy.

Urinary Tract Problems. Common problems are incontinence, urgency, frequency, and retention. Urinary tract infections also occur more frequently in children with cerebral palsy. The age of the child and any communication problems may impede obtaining detailed information on pain or other symptoms experienced by the child. A urinalysis and urine cultures must be ordered if there is any suspicion of a urinary tract infection or the cause of the fever or other symptoms cannot be identified. After one or two urinary tract infections have been diagnosed and treated in a child with cerebral palsy, the parents and primary care provider may be better able to identify the signs and symptoms associated with this condition in the child. This information is especially important in a child who is nonverbal and should be recorded in the child's chart for further reference.

Antibiotic therapy and additional comfort measures (e.g., increased fluid intake, perineal hygiene after voiding, increased rest, taking acetaminophen based on body weight) are recommended for urinary tract infections. Follow-up is imperative after a urinary tract infection and should include a urine culture 2 to 3 days after initiation and at the conclusion of antibiotic therapy to assess its effect. If recurrent urinary tract infections occur, referral to a pediatric urologist is recommended.

Gastrointestinal Problems. Parents may note that a child has abdominal pain, straining with hard stools, rectal bleeding, soiled underwear, and a distended, hard abdomen when constipated. Documenting the signs and symptoms of this problem in infants or nonverbal children is especially important. Increased fluids, exercise, and a healthy diet with additional fiber are recommended. A bowel management program designed by an interdisciplinary team may be needed if constipation is an ongoing problem. A program of stool softeners, laxatives, suppositories, and enemas can be prescribed, as well as suggestions for proper positioning and seating on the toilet. The effectiveness of the program should be closely monitored and recorded.

A pattern for bowel elimination should be initiated and maintained. Urinary tract infections and impactions are complications of chronic constipation. Constipation is a very difficult long-term problem to deal with when a child is immobile and has a poor appetite. Bowel management programs must be individualized and evaluated periodically.

Drug Interactions

Medications may be prescribed to reduce spasticity. These medications should be used with caution if the adolescent with cerebral palsy is pregnant. Diazepam (Valium) and baclofen should be monitored closely if used in a child with a seizure disorder because seizure control could be altered. Dantrolene (Dantrium) and baclofen are also affected by the concurrent use of alcohol, so drinking should be strongly discouraged in the adolescent. Dantrolene should also be discouraged if a degree of spasticity is needed for daily functioning. Adverse respiratory symptoms and bowel function should also be monitored when using dantrolene (Karch, 2007). No other specific drug interactions have been noted with medications used to treat spasticity. A discussion of the drug interactions for seizure medications is included in Chapter 26. The occurrence of constipation must be examined for its cause—whether because of diet or as a side effect of medications such as anticonvulsants or iron. Overall, drug interactions need to be assessed when a child with cerebral palsy is receiving multiple medications.

Developmental Issues

Sleep Patterns

A clinical manifestation of cerebral palsy in infancy is prolonged sleeping patterns interfering with nutritional intake and developmental stimulation. A variety of other sleeping problems may also exist with cerebral palsy, such as severe hypoxemia during sleep, which may require a sleep apnea monitor, difficulty in falling asleep and staying asleep, and difficulties during the sleep-to-wake transition (Newman, O'Regan, & Hensey, 2006). A neutral body position (i.e., with the neck and head slightly flexed) is encouraged during sleep. Bolsters or wedges can be used to facilitate appropriate positions, but in one study were not found to affect sleep quality (Newman et al., 2006). A side-lying position should be used for children who drool so that excessive fluid can drain out of the mouth instead of down the throat, which may cause choking. A referral to an otolaryngologist may be needed (Jones et al., 2007).

Toileting

If children with cerebral palsy are able to be toilet trained, then—like any other children—they will give their parents clues of their physical and neurologic readiness. The potty chair or toilet must adequately support the child's body and minimize the risk of skin breakdown from extended sitting. The child's feet must be able to touch the floor to assist the abdominal muscles in pushing. Special potty chairs can be made, or current chairs can be adapted with input from a physical or occupational therapist.

Discipline

Parents often discipline children who have special health and developmental needs differently from their siblings. As a result of their special needs and possible past health care emergencies, parents are often reluctant to discipline a child with cerebral palsy. Parents must be consistent when disciplining all their children; both parents should agree with the type of discipline; and the discipline should be developmentally appropriate for a child's mental age.

Child Care

Many child care programs today include children both with and without chronic conditions. Depending on the child's degree of functional and cognitive severity, parents may choose an early intervention or an inclusive child care program. Children enrolled in an early intervention program will have an individualized family service plan (IFSP) developed for the child's development and family support. In an inclusive child care program, the providers will need instruction by the parents or a member of the child's interdisciplinary health care team on the best approaches for care and development. Parents of a child with cerebral palsy must be aware that the risk for infection is greater in settings where children are together (e.g., in daycare) (Kroger et al., 2006) and that issues of safety and accessibility are also important to consider.

Schooling

Children with cerebral palsy may need to use different augmentative communication systems (e.g., communication boards, computers, keyboard voice synthesizers; see Figure 18-2). Adaptive equipment for communicating, seating, writing, and reading may be needed and should be obtained. Occupational, physical, and speech therapy, as well as adaptive physical education, is often needed and individually planned for either group or individual sessions. An aide may be required to help a child with cerebral palsy with personal needs. A diagnosis of homonymous hemianopsia, in which the child can see straight ahead but not to the affected side, is important for a seating assignment in the front of the classroom (Pellegrino, 2007). Transportation to and from school, transfer needs between classrooms, and emergency health and safety plans must also be arranged with school personnel.

Along with an interdisciplinary health plan, which is mandatory for children with cerebral palsy, an accommodation plan or individualized educational plan (IEP) is also necessary, which may include physical, occupational, speech, and behavioral therapy and other formal and informal support services (Jones et al., 2007; Krigger, 2006; Pellegrino, 2007). (See Chapter 3 for more information on daycare and school issues and needs.) Today most children with cerebral palsy participate in inclusive education. Special attention must be paid to a child's cognitive ability and social integration into the regular classroom by assisting the child with peer relationships and self-esteem. Primary care providers can assess the school situation, including safety, performance, ambulation, and fatigue issues, during well-child visits.

During the middle and high school years, children with cerebral palsy can be enrolled in vocational or college preparation programs, depending on career interests and the presence and degree of mental retardation. Adolescents with cerebral palsy may also experience renewed social problems during these years as they cope with adolescent self-esteem issues and contemplate life after school. Work and social opportunities are not as prevalent in the adult years as they are during childhood for individuals with special health and developmental needs. Adolescents often experience depression when faced with the stigma of their condition and rejection in social situations. School performance also may decrease. Parents and professionals should look for signs that might alert them to these psychosocial issues during adolescence and offer support and professional counseling where needed.

Sexuality

Social isolation, long-term low self-esteem, and a poor body image can affect the development of intimate relationships. Sexuality education can help the adolescent develop a positive self-esteem and body image. Role modeling and exposure to social situations can be planned and executed. During their adolescent years, children do not often discuss sexuality and their feelings with parents. Therefore peers, other adults, and support groups should be available to help adolescents with cerebral palsy with these issues. In some cases, referral to a sexuality counselor may be needed.

Female adolescents should begin to receive gynecologic care if they are sexually active. Because of spasticity, contractures, or poor muscle control, a woman's position for such an examination should be adapted; the Sims position is often better than the lithotomy position. The woman may also require assistance in positioning menstrual pads or tampons. Pregnancy is possible for women with cerebral palsy.

Transition to Adulthood

The transition to adulthood in children with cerebral palsy must address medical care, equipment needs, communication, activities of daily life, mobility, nutrition, vocational decisions, transportation, housing, and social needs. Comorbidities reported in adulthood include pain, scoliosis, fractures, aspiration, vomiting, constipation, bladder dysfunction, osteopenia, dental problems (Zaffuto-Sforza, 2005), and fatigue (Jahnsen, Villien, Stanghelle, et al. 2003). Throughout life, optimal independence should be encouraged and learned helplessness avoided. Independence and self-advocacy should be stressed during the transitional period between adolescence and adulthood. Adolescents with cerebral palsy need to take an active role in choosing a primary care provider and health care interdisciplinary team. Their participation in decision making about dietary choices, medications, surgical interventions if needed, and adaptive equipment is important. Hospital admission rates and health care visits are higher in adolescents and adults with cerebral palsy in comparison to peers of the same ages (Young, McCormick, Mills, et al., 2006).

Vocational decisions should be discussed, and plans for successful employment should be determined. When deciding on a site for college or work, the physical layout, wheelchair accessibility, availability of personal aides, housing, and repair shop for wheelchairs and any other adaptive equipment must be considered and resources identified. Independence in the use of public transportation should be planned. Individuals with mild cerebral palsy may be able to drive. Independent living or assisted living arrangements must be discussed, and individuals should be placed on waiting lists early if living outside the home is desired because these lists are often years long. Social needs, including activities consistent with an individual's abilities, planned social programs, and opportunities to develop successful relationships, should be met. In a review of the literature, Wiegerink, Roebroeck, Donkervoort, and colleagues (2006) found that parental influence, transportation concerns, and physical impairments impeded development of friendships and sexual relationships. Most important, adolescents making the transition to adulthood must participate to the greatest possible extent in decisions about their lives.

Family Concerns

In incidences of mild cerebral palsy, the effects on the family may be minimal or nonexistent (see Chapter 5). Parents who were stressed reported lower health-related quality of life for their children (Arnaud et al., 2008). Also, parents were most unhappy when they received the child's diagnosis close to the child's first birthday, when the child's prognosis for physical and mental development was poorer, and when the child was born with low birth weight or prematurely (33 weeks of gestation and less). A greater degree of unhappiness or dissatisfaction was related to maternal depression (Baird, McConachie, & Scrutton, 2000). Respite care is highly recommended to give families time away from the constant responsibilities of caring for a child with cerebral palsy. Social support, identification of and intervention with stressors, presence of parenting skills for caring for a child with special needs, and the use of early intervention programs are all very important for family well-being (Pellegrino, 2007). The Centers for Disease Control and Prevention (n.d.) estimates that the lifetime costs for a person with cerebral palsy in 2003 dollars is $921,000.

There are no specific cross-cultural or religious concerns for children with cerebral palsy, although a stigma based on the diagnosis is attached to all families. The visibility of this condition may create more of a stigma in some cultures than in others, and in some cultures the child may be hidden from the outside world.

Resources

A variety of local, state, and regional services for children with cerebral palsy exist. Appropriate resources and organizations are usually listed in the local yellow pages of the telephone directory under "Social Services and Organizations." Several books and organizations can also offer assistance to families and professionals.

Books

Campbell, S.K., vander Linden, D.W., & Palisano, R.J. (Eds.). (2006). *Physical Therapy for Children* (2nd ed.). Philadelphia: Saunders. (Available from Elsevier, Inc., 1600 John F. Kennedy Blvd, Suite 1800, Philadelphia, PA 19103.)

Kennedy, M.A. (2001). *My Perfect Son has Cerebral Palsy: A Mother's Guide of Helpful Hints.* Bloomington, IN: 1stBooks Library. (Available from 1stBooks Library, 2595 Vernal Pike, Bloomington, IN 47404.)

Martin, S. (2006). *Teaching Motor Skills to Children with Cerebral Palsy and Similar Movement Disorders: A Guide to Parents and Professionals.* Bethesda, MD: Woodbine House. (Available from Woodbine House, 6510 Bells Mill Rd., Bethesda, MD 20817).

Miller, F., & Bachrach, S.J. (2006). *Cerebral Palsy: A Complete Guide for Caregiving* (2nd ed.). Baltimore: Johns Hopkins University Press. (Available from Johns Hopkins University Press, PO Box 19966, Baltimore, MD 21211.)

Parker, J.N., & Parker, P.M. (2002). *The Official Parent's Sourcebook on Cerebral Palsy: A Revised and Updated Directory for the Internet Age.* San Diego: ICON Health Publishers. (Available from ICON Group International, Inc., 7404 Trade St., San Diego, CA 92121).

Organizations

American Academy for Cerebral Palsy and Developmental Medicine
6300 North River Rd., Suite 727
Rosemont, IL 60018-4226
(847) 698-1635; Fax: (847) 823-0536
Email: woppenhe@ucla.edu
Website: www.aacpdm.org

DisABILITY Information and Resources
Provides information on products, services, computer accessibility, home automation and environmental control, governmental and legislative disability information, legal advice and advocacy, sports, travel, recreation, and assistive technology.
Website: www.makoa.org

National Disability Sports Alliance (NDSA)
25 Independence Way
Kingston, RI 02881
(401) 792-7130, (401) 792-7132 (fax)
Email: info@ndsaonline.org
Website: www.ndsaonline.org

North American Growth in Cerebral Palsy Project
UVA Children's Hospital
Kluge Children's Rehabilitation Center
2270 Ivy Rd.
Charlottesville, VA 22903
(888) 4CP-GROW (427-4769)
Email: 4CP-GROW@virginia.edu
Website: www.healthsystem.virginia.edu/internet/NAGCePP

UCP National
1660 L Street NW, Suite 700
Washington, DC 20036
(800) 872-5827 (national office), (202) 973-7197 (voice/TTY), Fax: (202) 776-0414
Email: ucpnatl@ucp.org
Website: www.ucpa.org

Summary of Primary Care Needs for the Child with Cerebral Palsy

HEALTH CARE MAINTENANCE

Growth and Development

- Different techniques should be used to obtain height, arm and leg lengths, and skinfold measurements.
- Weights may be attained via standing or sitting scales or recumbent lifts.
- Delayed development in motor and communication skills is common.
- Development strengths and weaknesses must be assessed and recorded.
- Intellectual and developmental disabilities and seizure disorders inhibit intellectual development.
- An exercise program may be individually developed.

Diet

- Undernutrition in infancy often leads to growth retardation.
- Different nipples may be tried if hypersensitivity is an issue.
- Infants can have difficulty with sucking, swallowing, and chewing.
- Overweight conditions may occur in adolescence if mobility decreases.
- Drooling and aspiration can also be problems.
- Assessment should be done early and repeatedly; referral to a nutritionist is commonly needed.
- Adaptive equipment is useful.
- Nutritional concerns may be lifelong, and placement of a gastrostomy tube may be warranted in severe cases.

Safety

- Children are at risk for injury as a result of spasticity, muscle control problems, delayed protective reflexes, and potential seizures.
- Positioning, modified car seats, and other adaptive equipment are often required.

Immunizations

- If the etiology for seizure activity is unknown, the pertussis vaccine may be deferred or an acellular vaccine used when age appropriate.
- The measles and varicella vaccines should be given as scheduled.
- Children with cerebral palsy are at risk for complications of varicella and should be immunized.
- *Haemophilus influenzae* type B (Hib) vaccine and other immunizations should be given as scheduled.
- Children with cerebral palsy are at risk for complications of influenza and should be immunized.
- Pneumococcal, meningococcal, rotavirus, hepatitis B, human papillomavirus vaccines should be given as recommended.
- Fever management is necessary to decrease the possibility of febrile seizures.

Screening

- *Vision.* A pediatric ophthalmologist should be seen during infancy because of the likelihood of vision problems.
  - Vision should be checked for acuity, refractive errors, strabismus, retinopathy of prematurity, and cataracts.
- *Hearing.* Referral to a pediatric audiologist may be necessary during infancy to check for hearing problems and loss.

- Both sensorineural and conductive hearing loss is possible.
- Routine screening for conductive hearing problems and loss should be done.
- *Dental.* Children should be evaluated by a dentist experienced with children with motor problems every 6 months.
  - Proper dental hygiene is needed.
  - Administration of phenytoin may cause hyperplasia of the gums; proper preventive care and early treatment of this condition are important.
  - Malocclusions can be prevented through oromotor exercises.
- *Blood pressure.* Routine screening is recommended.
- *Hematocrit.* Routine screening is recommended.
- *Urinalysis.* Routine screening is recommended.
  - A referral to a pediatric urologist may be needed if the child has chronic urinary tract infections.
- *Tuberculosis.* Routine screening is recommended.

Condition-Specific Screening

- A motor assessment, including assessment for scoliosis, hip dislocation, and contractures, should be done at every well-child visit.

COMMON ILLNESS MANAGEMENT

Differential Diagnosis

- *Fever.* Management of fever is routine except when the child is less than 6 months of age, has had a fever over 38.6°C for 3 or more days without symptoms, appears acutely ill with undefined symptoms, or has had a seizure with a fever, in which case the child needs to see his or her primary care provider for an accurate diagnosis and treatment.
- *Respiratory tract infections.* Respiratory infections should be promptly treated. Pneumonia may be life threatening to children with severe cerebral palsy. Follow-up is important.
- *Dermatology issues.* Vigilant skin management is warranted because of high risk for decubiti, especially those children using wheelchairs. Assess for latex allergies.
- *Urinary tract problems.* Treatment for urinary tract infections should be prompt, and follow-up is essential. Urinary tract abnormalities may also be present.
- *Gastrointestinal problems.* Constipation is a long-term problem for many children. A bowel management program may be needed.

Drug Interactions

- Diazepam (Valium) and baclofen may alter seizure control.
- Dantrolene (Dantrium) and baclofen are affected by the concurrent use of alcohol, so drinking should be strongly discouraged in the adolescent.
- Adverse respiratory symptoms and bowel function should also be monitored when using dantrolene.

DEVELOPMENTAL ISSUES

Sleep Patterns

- Correct positioning is needed during sleep because sleep apnea can occur.

Toileting

- Adaptive equipment is often needed for correct positioning on the toilet. Bladder and bowel training may be delayed.

Summary of Primary Care Needs for the Child with Cerebral Palsy—cont'd

Discipline

- It is important that consistent and age-appropriate discipline measures be taken.

Child Care

- Careful planning must be undertaken in choosing the best child care arrangements, especially regarding issues of safety, accessibility, health care needs, and increased rates of infection.

Schooling

- Use Individualized Educational Plans (IEPs) and inclusive classrooms. Specialized services and therapies for each child must be procured. Adaptive equipment and computers enhance a child's ability to learn. Behavioral and school problems can occur in adolescence as a result of poor self-esteem and body image.

Sexuality

- Opportunities for social activities should be arranged. Transportation needs are important to consider. Opportunities for same-sex and opposite-sex relationships are needed. Classes in social interaction and sexuality may be needed. Gynecologic examinations should begin for women with adaptations to the normal positioning. Reproductive issues should be discussed.

Transition to Adulthood

- A child's independence and self-advocacy should be promoted. Future residential and vocational plans need to be addressed.

FAMILY CONCERNS

- Respite care meets a family's needs.
- Effects on individual family members must be assessed and addressed. Special support groups are available for fathers and siblings.
- Family stigmas may be perceived.

REFERENCES

Aker, J., & Anderson, D.J. (2007). Perioperative care of patients with cerebral palsy. *AANA J, 75,* 65-73.

Albright, A.L., & Ferson, S.S. (2006). Intrathecal baclofen therapy in children. *Neurosurg Focus, 21,* E3.

Ali, O., Shim, M., Fowler, E., et al. (2007). Growth hormone therapy improves bone mineral density in children with cerebral palsy: A preliminary pilot study. *J Clin Endocrinol Metabol, 92,* 932-937.

Arnaud, C., White-Koning, M., Michelsen, S.I., et al. (2008). Parent-reported quality of life of children with cerebral palsy in Europe. *Pediatrics, 121,* 54-64.

Ashwal, S., Russman, B.S., Blasco, P.A., et al. (2004). Practice parameter: Diagnostic assessment of the child with cerebral palsy: Report of the Quality Standards Subcommittee of the American Academy of Neurology and the Practice Committee of the Child Neurology Society. *Neurology, 62,* 851-863.

Autti-Ramo, I., Suoranta, J., Anttila, H., et al. (2006). Effectiveness of upper and lower limb casting and orthoses in children with cerebral palsy. *Am J Phys Med Rehabil, 85,* 89-103.

Baird, G., McConachie, H., & Scrutton, D. (2000). A multivariate model of determinants of motor change for children with cerebral palsy. *Arch Dis Child, 83,* 475-480.

Bar-Haim, S., Harries, N., Belokopytov, M., et al. (2006). Comparison of efficacy of Adeli suit and neurodevelopmental treatments in children with cerebral palsy. *Dev Med Child Neurol, 48,* 325-330.

Bax, M., Goldstein, M., Rosenbaum, P., et al. (2005). Introduction. Proposed definition and classification of cerebral palsy, April 2005. *Dev Med Child Neurol, 47,* 571-576.

Bax, M., Tydeman, C., & Flodmark, O. (2006). Clinical and MRI correlates of cerebral palsy: The European Cerebral Palsy Study. *J Am Med Assoc, 296,* 1602-1608.

Beckung, E., Hagverg, G., Uldall, P., et al,. for Surveillance of Cerebral Palsy in Europe. (2008). Probability of walking in children with cerebral palsy in Europe. *Pediatrics, 121,* e187-e192.

Berrin, S.J., Malcame, V.L., Varni, J.W., et al. (2007). Pain, fatigue, and school functioning in children with cerebral palsy: A path-analytic model. *J Pediatr Psychol, 32,* 330-337.

Bhasin, T.K., Brocksen, S., Avchen, R.N., et al. (2006). Prevalence of four developmental disabilities among children aged 8 years—Metropolitan Atlanta Developmental Disabilities Surveillance Program, 1996 and 2000. *MMWR Morb Mortal Wkly Rep, 55,* 1-9.

Bjornson, K., Hays, R., Graubert, C., et al. (2007). Botulinum toxin for spasticity in children with cerebral palsy: A comprehensive evaluation. *Pediatrics, 120,* 49-58.

Bodensteiner, J.B.,& Johnson, S.D. (2004). Cerebellar injury in the extremely premature infant: Newly recognized by relatively common outcome. *J Child Neurol, 19,* 139-142.

Bonellie, S.R., Currie, D., & Chalmers, J. (2005). Comparison of risk factors for cerebral palsy in twins and singletons. *Dev Med Child Neurol, 47,* 587-591.

Broder, K.R., Cortese, M.M., Iskander, J., et al. (2006). Preventing tetanus, diphtheria, and pertussis among adolescents: Use of tetanus toxoid, reduced diphtheria toxoid and acellular pertussis vaccines. Recommendations of the Advisory Committee on Immunization Practices (ACIP). *MMWR Morb Mortal Wkly Rep, 55*(RR-3), 1-44.

Centers for Disease Control and Prevention (n.d.). *Cerebral palsy among children* Available at www.cdc.gov/cerebralpalsy. Retrieved February 16, 2008.

Chaleat-Valayer, E., Bernard, J.-C., Morel, E., et al. (2006). Use of videographic examination for analysis of efficacy of botulinum toxin in the lower limbs in children with cerebral palsy. *J Pediatr Orthop B, 15,* 339-347.

Chang, F.M., Seidl, A.J., Muthusamy, K., et al. (2006). Effectiveness of instrumented gait analysis in children with cerebral palsy—comparison of outcomes. *J Pediatr Orthop, 26,* 612-616.

Cherng, R., Liao, H., Leung, H.W.C., et al. (2004). The effectiveness of therapeutic horseback riding in children with spastic CP. *Adaptive Physical Activity Quarterly, 21,* 103-121.

Colver, A.F., & Sethumadhavan, T. (2003). The term diplegia should be abandoned. *Arch Dis Child, 88,* 286-290.

Committee on Infectious Diseases, American Academy of Pediatrics (2008). Recommended immunizations schedules for children and adolescents—United States, 2008. *Pediatrics, 121,* 219-220.

Cooley, W.C. (2004). Providing a primary care medical home for children and youth with cerebral palsy. *Pediatrics, 114,* 1106-1113.

Costeff, H. (2004). Estimated frequency of genetic and nongenetic causes of congenital idiopathic cerebral palsy in west Sweden. *Ann Hum Genet, 68,* 515-520.

Craig, G.M., Carr, L.J., Cass, H., et al. (2006). Medical, surgical, and health outcomes of gastrostomy feeding. *Dev Med Child Neurol, 48,* 353-360.

Darrah, J., Walkins, B., Chen, L., et al. (2004). Conductive education intervention for children with CP: An AACPDM evidence report. *Dev Med Child Neurol, 46,* 187-203.

Day, S.M., Strauss, D.J., Vachon, P.J., et al. (2007). Growth patterns in a population of children and adolescents with cerebral palsy. *Dev Med Child Neurol, 49*, 167-171.

Day, S.M., Wu, Y.W., Strauss, D.J., et al. (2007). Change in ambulatory ability of adolescents and young adults with cerebral palsy. *Dev Med Child Neurol, 49*, 647-653.

Dickinson, H.O., Parkinson, K.N., Ravens-Sieberer, U., et al. (2007). Self-reported quality of life of 8-12 year old children with cerebral palsy: A cross-sectional European study. *Lancet, 369*, 2171-2178.

Dobson, F., Morris, M.E., Baker, R., et al. (2007). Gait classification in children with cerebral palsy: A systematic review. *Gait and Posture, 25*, 140-152.

Dolk, H., Parkes, J., & Hill, N. (2006). Trends in the prevalence of cerebral palsy in Northern Ireland, 1981-1997. *Dev Med Child Neurol, 48*, 406-412.

Drougia, A., Giapros, V., Krallis, N., et al. (2006). Incidence and risk factors for cerebral palsy in infants with perinatal problems: A 15-year review. *Early Hum Dev, 83*, 541-547.

Essex, C. (2003). Hyperbaric oxygen and cerebral palsy: No proven benefit and potentially harmful. *Dev Med Child Neurol, 45*, 213-215.

Fiore, A.E., Wasley, A., & Bell, B.P. (2006). Prevention of hepatitis A through active or passive immunization. Recommendations of the Advisory Committee on Immunization Practices (ACIP). *MMWR Morb Mortal Wkly Rep, 55*(RR-7), 1-23.

Gericke, T. (2006). Postural management for children with cerebral palsy: Consensus statement. *Dev Med Child Neurol, 48*, 244.

Gough, M., Fairhurst, C., & Shortland, A.P. (2005). Botulinum toxin and cerebral palsy: Time for reflection? *Dev Med Child Neurol, 47*, 709-712.

Green, S. (2003). "What do you mean 'what's wrong with her?'": Stigma and the lives of families of children with disabilities. *Soc Sci Med, 57*, 1361-1374.

Greenwood, C., Yudkin, P., Sellers, S., et al. (2007). Why is there a modifying effect of gestational age on risk factors for cerebral palsy? *Arch Dis Child Fetal Neonat Educ, 90*, F141-F146.

Grzybowski, M., Ownby, D.R., Rivers, E.P., et al. (2003). The prevalence of latex-specific IgE in patients presenting to an urban emergency department. *Obstet Gynecol Surv, 58*, 229-230.

Gupta, R., & Appleton, R.E. (2001). Cerebral palsy: Not always what it seems. *Arch Dis Child, 85*, 356-361.

Heinen, F., Molenaers, G., Fairhurst, C., et al. (2006). European consensus table 2006 on botulinum toxin for children with cerebral palsy. *Eur J Paediatr Neurol, 10*, 215-225.

Helsel, P., McGee, J., & Graveline, C. (2001). Physical management of spasticity. *J Child Neurol, 16*, 24-30.

Hemming, K., Hutton, J.L., & Pharoah, P.O.D. (2006). Long-term survival for a cohort of adults with cerebral palsy. *Dev Med Child Neurol, 48*, 90-95.

Himmelmann, K., Beckung, E., Hagberg, G., et al. (2007). Bilateral spastic cerebral palsy—prevalence through four decades, motor function and growth. *Eur J Paediatr Neurol, 11*, 215-222.

Hirtz, D., Thurman, D.J., Gwinn-Hardy, K., et al. (2007). How common are the "common" neurologic disorders? *Neurology, 68*, 326-337.

Ho, C.-L., Holt, K.G., Saltzman, E., et al. (2006). Functional electrical stimulation changes dynamic resources in children with spastic cerebral palsy. *Phys Ther, 86*, 987-1000.

Hoare, B., Imms, C., Carey, L., et al. (2007). Constraint-induced movement therapy in the treatment of the upper limb in children with hemiplegic cerebral palsy: A Cochrane systematic review. *Clin Rehabil, 21*, 675-685.

Hurvitz, E.A., Leonard, C., Ayyangar, R., et al. (2003). Complementary and alternative medicine use in families of children with CP. *Dev Med Child Neurol, 45*, 364-370.

Jahnsen, R., Villien, L., Stanghelle, J.K., et al. (2003). Fatigue in adults with cerebral palsy in Norway compared with the general population. *Dev Med Child Neurol, 45*, 296-303.

Johnson, M.W., Hoon, A.H. Jr., & Kaufmann, W.E. (2008). Neurobiology, diagnosis, and management of cerebral palsy. In P.J. Accardo (Ed.), *Capute and Accardo's Neurodevelopmental Disabilities in Infancy and Childhood*, Vol. II. *The Spectrum of Neurodevelopmental Disabilities* (3rd ed.). Baltimore: Brookes Publishing.

Johnson, S.D., Bodensteiner, J.B., & Lotze, T.E. (2005). Frequency and nature of cerebellar injury in the extremely premature survivor with cerebral palsy. *J Child Neurol, 20*, 60-64.

Johnston, M.V., & Hagberg, H. (2007). Sex and the pathogenesis of cerebral palsy. *Dev Med Child Neurol, 49*, 74-78.

Jones, M.W., Morgan, E., & Shelton, J.E. (2007). Primary care of the child with cerebral palsy: A review of systems (part II). *J Pediatr Health Care, 21*, 226-237.

Karaman, M.I., Kaya, C., Caskurlu, T., et al. (2005). Urodynamic findings in children with cerebral palsy. *Int J Urol, 12*, 717-720.

Karch, A.M. (2007). *2008 Lippincott's Nursing Drug Guide*. Philadelphia: Lippincott Williams & Wilkins.

Katz, N., Cermak, S., & Shamir, Y. (1998). Unilateral neglect in children with hemiplegic cerebral palsy. *Percept Mot Skills, 86*, 539-550.

Katz, R.T. (2003). Life expectancy for children with cerebral palsy and mental retardation: Implications for life care planning. *Neurorehabilitation, 18*, 261-270.

Kaukola, T., Herva, R., Perhomaa, M., et al. (2005). Chorioamnionitis and cord serum proinflammatory cytokines: Lack of association with brain damage and neurological outcome in very premature preterm infants. *Pediatr Res, 58*, 1-6.

Keinan, D., Smith, P., & Zilberman, U. (2006). Microstructure and chemical composition of primary teeth in children with Down syndrome and cerebral palsy. *Arch Oral Biol, 51*, 836-843.

Kelly, M., & Darrah, J. (2005). Aquatic exercise for children with cerebral palsy. *Dev Med Child Neurol, 47*, 838-842.

Kim, H.S., Steinbok, P., & Wickenheiser, D. (2006). Predictors of poor outcome after selective dorsal rhizotomy in treatment of spastic cerebral palsy. *Childs Nerv Syst, 22*, 60-66.

Koman, L.A., Smith, B.P., & Shilt, J.S. (2004). Cerebral palsy (review). *Lancet, 363*, 1619-1631.

Krageloh-Mann, I. (2004). Imaging of the early brain injury and cortical plasticity. *Exp Neurol, 190*(Suppl 1), S84-S90.

Krageloh-Mann, I. (2005). Cerebral palsy: Towards developmental neuroscience. *Dev Med Child Neurol, 47*, 435.

Krageloh-Mann, I., & Horber, V. (2007). The role of magnetic resonance imaging in elucidating the pathogenesis of cerebral palsy: A systematic review. *Dev Med Child Neurol, 49*, 144-151.

Krigger, K.W. (2006). Cerebral palsy: An overview. *Am Fam Physician, 73*, 91-100.

Kroger, A.T., Atkinson, W.L., Marcuse, E.K., et al. (2006). General recommendations on immunization. Recommendations of the Advisory Committee on Immunization Practices (ACIP). *MMWR Morb Mortal Wkly Rep, 55*(RR-15), 1-48.

Kuroda, M.M., Weck, M.E., Sarwark, J.F., et al. (2007). Association of apolipoprotein E genotype and cerebral palsy in children. *Pediatrics, 119*, 306-313.

Lannin, N., Scheinberg, A., & Clark, K. (2006). AACPDM systematic review of effectiveness of therapy for children with cerebral palsy after botulinum toxin A injections. *Dev Med Child Neurol, 48*, 533-539.

Lee, J., Croen, L.A., Backstrand, K.H., et al. (2005). Maternal and infant characteristics associated with perinatal arterial stroke in the infant. *J Am Med Assoc, 293*, 723-729.

Leet, A.I., & Blasco, P.A. (2008). Orthopedic interventions in cerebral palsy. In P.J. Accardo (Ed.), *Capute and Accardo's Neurodevelopmental Disabilities in Infancy and Childhood*, Vol II. *The Spectrum of Neurodevelopmental Disabilities* (3rd ed.) Baltimore: Brookes Publishing.

Leet, A.I., Mesfin, A., Pichard, C., et al. (2006). Fractures in children with cerebral palsy. *J Pediatr Orthop, 26*, 624-627.

Linder-Lucht, M., Kirschner, J., Herrmann, J., et al. (2006). Why do children with cerebral palsy discontinue therapy with botulinum toxin A? *Dev Med Child Neurol, 48*, 319-320.

Liptak, G.S. (2005). Complementary and alternative therapies for cerebral palsy. *Ment Retard Dev Disabil Res Rev, 11*, 156-163.

Lofterod, B., Terjesen, T., Skaaret, I., et al. (2007). Preoperative gait analysis has a substantial effect on orthopedic decision making in children with cerebral palsy: Comparison between clinical evaluation and gait analysis in 60 patients. *Acta Orthop, 78*, 74-80.

Marin, M., Guris, D., Chaves, S.S., et al. (2007). Prevention of varicella. Recommendations of the Advisory Committee on Immunization Practices (ACIP). *MMWR Morb Mortal Wkly Rep, 56*(RR-4), 1-40.

Mathew, A., Mathew, M.C., Thomas, M., et al. (2005). The efficacy of diazepam in enhancing motor function in children with spastic cerebral palsy. *J Trop Pediatr, 51*, 109-113.

McDonagh, M., Carson, S., Ash, J., et al. (2003). *Hyperbaric Oxygen Therapy for Brain Injury, Cerebral Palsy, and Stroke. Evidence Report/Technology Assessment No. 85*. AHRQ Publication no. 04-E003. Rockville, MD: Agency for Healthcare Research and Quality.

Morris, C., Kurinczuk, J.J., Fitzpatrick, R., et al. (2006). Do the abilities of children with cerebral palsy explain their activities and participation? *Dev Med Child Neurol, 48*, 954-961.

Morton, R.E., Scott, B., McClelland, V.M., et al. (2006). Dislocation of the hips in children with bilateral spastic cerebral palsy, 1985-2000. *Dev Med Child Neurol, 48*, 555-558.

Muller-Bolla, M., Collet, J.-P., Ducruet, T., et al. (2006). Side effects of hyperbaric oxygen therapy in children with cerebral palsy. *Undersea Hyperb Med, 33,* 237-244.

Murphy, N.A., Hoff, C., Jorgensen, T., et al. (2006). A national perspective of surgery in children with cerebral palsy. *Pediatr Rehabil, 9,* 293-300.

Narayanan, U.G. (2007). The role of gait analysis in the orthopaedic management of ambulatory cerebral palsy. *Curr Opin Pediatr, 19,* 39-43.

National Institute of Dental and Craniofacial Research. (2007). *Practical oral care for people with cerebral palsy.* Available at www.nidcr.nih.gov/Health-Information/DiseasesandConditions/DevelopmentalDisabilitiesAndOral-Health/CerebralPalsy.htm. Retrieved February 29, 2008.

National Institute of Neurological Disorders and Stroke. (2008). *Cerebral palsy: Hope through research.* Available at www.ninds.nih.gov/disorders/cerebral_palsy/detail_cerebral_palsy.htm?css=print. Retrieved February 29, 2008

Neufeld, M.D., Frigon, C., Graham, A.S., et al. (2005). Maternal infection and risk of cerebral palsy in term and preterm infants. *J Perinatol, 25,* 108-113.

Newman, C.J., O'Regan, M., & Hensey, O. (2006). Sleep disorders in children with cerebral palsy. *Dev Med Child Neurol, 48,* 564-568.

O'Brien, D.F., & Park, T.S. (2006). A review of orthopedic surgeries after selective dorsal rhizotomy. *Neurosurg Focus, 21,* e2.

Odding, E., Roebroeck, M.E., & Stam, H.J. (2006). The epidemiology of cerebral palsy: Incidence, impairments and risk factors. *Disabil Rehabil, 28,* 183-191.

Ozer, K., Chesher, S.P., & Scheker, L.R. (2006). Neuromuscular electrical stimulation and dynamic bracing for the management of upper-extremity spasticity in children with cerebral palsy. *Dev Med Child Neurol, 48,* 559-563.

Ozturk, M., Oktem, F., Kisioglu, N., et al. (2006). Bladder and bowel control in children with cerebral palsy: Case-control study. *Croatian Med J, 47,* 264-270.

Palisano, R., Rosenbaum, P., Bartlett, D., et al. (2007). *Gross motor function classification system: Expanded and revised (GMFCS-E & R).* Available at www.canchild.ca/Default.aspx?tabid=195. Retrieved April 13, 2008.

Paneth, N., Damiano, D., Rosenbaum, P., et al. (2005). The classification of cerebral palsy. Proposed definition and classification of cerebral palsy, April 2005. *Dev Med Child Neurol, 47,* 571-576.

Park, E.S., & Rha, D. (2006). Botulinum toxin type A injection for management of upper limb spasticity in children with cerebral palsy: A literature review. *Yonsei Med J, 47,* 589-603.

Park, T.S., & Albright, L. (2006). Treatment of spasticity. *Neurosurg Focus, 21.*

Park, T.S., & Johnston, J.M. (2006). Surgical techniques of selective dorsal rhizotomy for spastic cerebral palsy. *Neurosurg Focus, 21,* e7.

Pellegrino, L. (2007). Cerebral palsy. In M.L. Batshaw, L. Pellegrino, & N.J. Roizen (Eds.), *Children with Disabilities,* (6th ed.). Baltimore: Brookes Publishing.

Peterson, M.C., Kedia, S., Davis, P., et al. (2006). Eating and feeding are not the same: Caregivers' perceptions of gastrostomy feeding for children with cerebral palsy. *Dev Med Child Neurol, 48,* 713-717.

Presedo, A., Dabney, K.W., & Miller, F. (2007). Fractures in patients with cerebral palsy. *J Pediatr Orthop, 27,* 147-153.

Reddihough, D. (2006). Measurement tools: New opportunities for children with cerebral palsy. *Dev Med Child Neurol, 48,* 548.

Reeuwijk, A., van Schie, P.E.M., Becher, J.G., et al. (2006). Effects of botulinum toxin type A on upper limb function in children with cerebral palsy: A systematic review. *Clin Rehabil, 20,* 375-387.

Robertson, C.M.T., Watt, M.-J., & Yasui, Y. (2007). Changes in the prevalence of cerebral palsy for children born very prematurely within a population-based program over 30 years. *J Am Med Assoc, 297,* 2733-2740.

Rosenbaum, P., Dan, B., Leviton, A., et al. (2005). The definition of cerebral palsy. Proposed definition and classification of cerebral palsy, April 2005. *Dev Med Child Neurol, 47,* 571-576.

Samdup, D.Z., Smith, R.G., & Song, S.I. (2006). The use of complementary and alternative medicine in children with chronic medical conditions. *Am J Phys Med Rehabil, 85,* 842-846.

Sameshima, H., & Ikenoue, T. (2006). Developmental effects on neonatal mortality and subsequent cerebral palsy in infants exposed to intrauterine infection. *Early Hum Dev, 83,* 517-519.

Samson-Fang, L., Butler, C., & O'Donnell, M. (2003). Effects of gastrostomy feeding in children with cerebral palsy: An AACPDM evidence report. *Dev Med Child Neurol, 45,* 415-426.

Schroeder, A.S., Berweck, S., Lee, S.H., et al. (2006). Botulinum toxin treatment of children with cerebral palsy—a short review of different injection techniques. *Neurotoxicity Res, 9,* 189-196.

Serdaroglu, A., Cansu, A., Ozkan, S., et al. (2006). Prevalence of cerebral palsy in Turkish children between the ages of 2 and 16 years. *Dev Med Child Neurol, 48,* 413-416.

Shapiro, B.K. (2004). Cerebral palsy: A reconceptualization of the spectrum. *J Pediatr, 145*(Suppl 1), S3-S7.

Speth, L.A.W.M., Leffers, P., Janssen-Potten, Y.J.M., et al. (2005). Botulinum toxin A and upper limb functional skills in hemiparetic cerebral palsy: A randomized trial in children receiving intensive therapy. *Dev Med Child Neurol, 47,* 468-473.

Steinbok, P. (2006). Selection of treatment modalities in children with spastic cerebral palsy. *Neurosurg Focus, 21,* e4.

Steinbok, P., Hicdonmez, T., Sawatzky, B., et al. (2005). Spinal deformities after selective dorsal rhizotomy for spastic cerebral palsy. *J Neurosurg, 102,* 363-373.

Stevenson, R.D., & Conaway, M. (2007). Growth assessment of children with cerebral palsy: The clinician's conundrum. *Dev Med Child Neurol, 49,* 164.

Stevenson, R.D., Conaway, M., Barrington, J.W., et al. (2006). Fracture rate in children with cerebral palsy. *Pediatr Rehabil, 9,* 396-403.

Stevenson, R.D., Conaway, M., Chumlea, W.C., et al. (2006). Growth and health in children with moderate-to-severe cerebral palsy. *Pediatrics, 118,* 1010-1018.

Stoll, B.J., Hansen, N.I., Adams-Chapman, I., et al. (2004). Neurodevelopmental and growth impairment among extremely low-birth-weight infants with neonatal infection. *J Am Med Assoc, 292,* 2357-2401.

Strauss, D., Shavelle, R., Reynolds, R., et al. (2007). Survival in cerebral palsy in the last 20 years: Signs of improvement? *Dev Med Child Neurol, 49,* 86-92.

Sullivan, P.B., Juszczak, E., Bachlet, A.M.E., et al. (2005). Gastrostomy tube feeding in children with cerebral palsy: A prospective, longitudinal study. *Dev Med Child Neurol, 47,* 77-85.

Sun, J.G., Ko, C.H., Wong, V., et al. (2004). Randomised control trial of tongue acupuncture versus sham acupuncture in improving functional outcome in CP. *J Neurol Neurosurg Psychiatry, 75,* 1054-1057.

Sundrum, R., Logan, S., Wallace, A., et al. (2005). Cerebral palsy and socioeconomic status: A retrospective cohort study. *Arch Dis Child, 90,* 15-18.

Theroux, M.C., & Akins, R.E. (2005). Surgery and anesthesia for children who have cerebral palsy. *Anesthesiol Clin North Am, 23,* 733-743.

Turner, A.E. (2006). The efficacy of Adeli suit treatment in children with cerebral palsy. *Dev Med Child Neurol, 48,* 324.

United Cerebral Palsy Research and Educational Foundation. (2002). *The prevention of cerebral palsy.* Available at www.ucpresearch.org/cerebral-palsy-research/prevention.php. Retrieved January 2, 2008.

United Cerebral Palsy Research and Educational Foundation. (2003). *The diagnosis of cerebral palsy.* Available at www.ucpresearch.org/cerebral-palsy-research/diagnosis-of-cerebral-palsy.php. Retrieved January 2, 2008.

United Cerebral Palsy Research and Educational Foundation. (2008). *Did you know?* Available at www.ucpresearch.org. Retrieved January 2, 2008.

Van der Burg, J.J.W., Jongerius, P.H., Van Hulst, K., et al. (2006). Drooling in children with cerebral palsy: Effect of salivary flow reduction on daily life and care. *Dev Med Child Neurol, 48,* 103-107.

Varni, J.W., Burwinkle, T.M., Sherman, S.A., et al. (2005). Health-related quality of life of children and adolescents with cerebral palsy: Hearing the voices of the children. *Dev Med Child Neurol, 47,* 592-597.

Varni, J.W., Limbers, C.A., & Burwinkle, T.M. (2007). Impaired health-related quality of life in children and adolescents with chronic conditions: A comparative analysis of 10 disease clusters and 33 disease categories/severities utilizing the PedsQL 4.0 Generic Core Scales. *Health and Quality of Life Outcomes, 5,* 43-57.

Voorman, J.M., Dallmeijer, A.J., Schuengel, C., et al. (2006). Activities and participation of 9- to 13-year-old children with CP. *Clin Rehabil, 20,* 937-948.

Weigl, D.M., Arbel, N., Katz, K., et al. (2007). Botulinum toxin for the treatment of spasticity in children: Attainment of treatment goals. *J Pediatr Orthop B, 16,* 293-296.

Wiegerink, D.J.H.G., Roebroeck, M.E., Donkervoort, M., et al. (2006). Social and sexual relationships of adolescents and young adults with cerebral palsy: A review. *Clin Rehabil, 20,* 1023-1031.

Wood, E. (2006). The child with cerebral palsy: Diagnosis and beyond. *Semin Pediatr Neurol, 13,* 286-296.

World Health Organization. (2001). *International Classification of Functioning, Disability, and Health (ICFDH).* Geneva: Author.

Wu, Y.W., Day, S.M., Strauss, D.J., et al. (2004). Prognosis for ambulation in cerebral palsy: A population-based study. *Pediatrics, 114,* 1264-1271.

Yeargin-Allsopp, M., Van Naarden Braun, K., Doernberg, N.S., et al. (2008). Prevalence of cerebral palsy in 8-year-old children in three areas of the United States in 2002: A multisite collaboration. *Pediatrics,121*, 547-554.

Young, N.L., McCormick, A., Mills, W., et al. (2006). The transition study: A look at youth and adults with cerebral palsy, spina bifida and acquired brain injury. *Phys Occup Ther Pediatr, 26*, 25-45.

Zaffuto-Sforza, C.D. (2005). Aging with cerebral palsy. *Phys Med Rehabil Clin North Am, 16*, 235-249.

Zhou, X., & Zheng, K. (2005). Treatment of 140 cerebral palsied children with a combined method based on traditional Chinese medicine (TCM) and Western medicine. *Journal of Zhejiang University Science, 6B*(1), 57-60.

Zuckerbraun, N.S., Ferson, S.S., Albright, A.L., et al. (2004). Intrathecal baclofen withdrawal: Emergent recognition and management. *Pediatr Emerg Care, 20*, 759-764.

19 Cleft Lip and Palate

Ginny Curtin and Anne Boekelheide

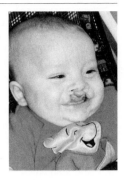

Etiology

The embryology of cleft lip with or without cleft palate is distinctly different from cleft palate alone. The cleft lip occurs when the median nasal and premaxillary prominences fail to fuse with the lateral maxillary prominences. The lip and alveolar ridge or primary palate is fully formed between 6 and 7 weeks of gestation. The presence of a cleft lip can hinder the closure of the palate. A cleft palate results from a failure of the palatine shelves to fuse between 6 and 12 weeks of gestation (Mulliken, 2004; Stanier & Moore, 2004).

Although the specific cause is usually unknown, clefts can be divided into two categories: nonsyndromic and syndromic (Box 19-1). The majority of clefts are nonsyndromic, meaning the cleft is not part of a pattern of malformation affecting other organs and systems. The term "multifactorial" (multiple genetic and environmental influences) is used to describe the etiology of nonsyndromic clefts. Examples of environmental factors that may increase the risk of a cleft occurring are maternal folic acid deficiency and teratogens such as maternal alcohol and tobacco use (Romitti, Sun, Honein, et al., 2007; Vieira, 2008). A positive family history of oral facial clefts increases the incidence of nonsyndromic clefts.

A syndrome is a collection of two or more major anomalies that occur together. There are more than 350 syndromes that include oral facial clefts. Cleft palate alone is far more often associated with a syndrome than a cleft lip or cleft lip and palate (Gorlin, Cohen, & Hennekam, 2001).

Syndromic clefts can be grouped into categories based on the underlying etiology or defect. The first category would be single-gene disorders, such as Van der Woude syndrome. This condition is recognizable by the lower lip pits and has an autosomal dominant pattern of inheritance. Another category is chromosomal syndromes, such as velocardiofacial syndrome, which is a microdeletion of chromosome 22. This syndrome with velopharyngeal insufficiency or cleft palate is associated with cardiac malformation and developmental delay. There are also teratogenic syndromes that are caused by any agent that can adversely affect embryonic development. Examples of teratogenic syndromes include fetal alcohol syndrome and fetal hydantoin syndrome.

The fourth category of syndrome is actually called a sequence, such as holoprosencephaly (underdevelopment of the premaxilla and nasal septum, brain abnormalities) and Pierre Robin (U-shaped cleft palate, micrognathia [small lower jaw], glossoptosis [posteriorly rotated tongue]). Researchers postulate that in fetal development the micrognathia is the primary problem and the cleft palate is a result of the tongue being placed superiorly, obstructing the movement of the maxillary shelves in the midline. The suboptimal mandibular growth has been thought to be caused by a variety of factors. The factors vary from positional malformation in utero, intrinsic causes from chromosomal or teratogenic influences, neurologic or neuromuscular abnormalities inhibiting the tongue from normal movement into the floor of the mouth in utero, or connective tissue disorders (St. Hilaire & Buchbinder, 2000). Both holoprosencephaly and Pierre Robin sequence can have devastating consequences in the newborn period by interfering with the airway and normal swallowing.

Known Genetic Etiology

The knowledge of genetic etiology for syndromic clefts that include single-gene mutations and chromosomal abnormalities is more advanced than the understanding of the genetic causes for nonsyndromic clefts. Genetic influences are thought to play a major role, and recently there has been considerable effort to map and identify genes that constitute risk factors for nonsyndromic clefts (Vieira, 2008). Interferon regulatory factor 6 (IRF6) has been shown to be an important contributor to cleft lip and palate, but the functional variant leading to the defect has not yet been defined. Inactivation of MSX1 and genes in the FGF family has also been shown to lead to cleft lip and palate (Vieira). As more is understood about the genetic influences on nonsyndromic clefts, the question becomes more complex.

BOX 19-1

Etiology of Cleft Lip and Palate

- Nonsyndromic—multifactorial
  - Environmental
  - Genetic
- Syndromic
  - Single-gene disorders
  - Chromosomal abnormalities
  - Teratogens
  - Sequences

Incidence and Prevalence

Cleft lip and/or palate ranks among the most commonly occurring birth defects (Centers for Disease Control and Prevention, [CDC] National Center on Birth Defects and Developmental Disabilities, n.d.). The generally accepted incidence rate of clefts worldwide is 1 in 700 births, although some ethnic differences exist (Murray, 2002). American Indians have an incidence of 3.6 in 1000 live births followed in descending order by Japanese, Chinese, whites, Hispanics, and blacks, with the lowest reported incidence of 0.3 in 1000. Incidence rates are based on varied reporting mechanisms, and problems occur with mixing together studies of live births, stillbirths, and spontaneous abortions. No registry or national database exists documenting cleft birth defects. Clefts may or may not be recorded when they are components of a known syndrome.

Cleft lip and palate makes up approximately 50% of all oral facial clefts with a unilateral cleft lip occurring more often than a bilateral cleft lip. A left-sided cleft lip occurs twice as often as a right-sided cleft lip. Cleft lip alone makes up 25% of clefts and occurs more frequently in males with or without cleft palate. Females are affected more often with cleft palate alone.

Diagnostic Criteria

Cleft lip is an obvious birth defect noted in the delivery room. It is described as unilateral or bilateral and incomplete or complete depending on whether the cleft extends into the nasal cavity (Figure 19-1). A microform cleft lip is characterized by very minor notching or the appearance of a well-healed surgical scar or "seam"; however, microform cleft lip is usually only described by a craniofacial team or plastic and reconstructive surgeon.

Cleft palate may involve the primary palate (lip and alveolus anterior to the incisive foramen) and the secondary palate (hard and soft palates) (Figure 19-2). A submucous cleft palate is characterized by a notch at the posterior spine of the hard palate, translucence at the midline, or bifid uvula. The wide spectrum of variations in the types of cleft lip and cleft palate has made standardized and inclusive classification difficult (Koul, 2007) (Figure 19-3). As a result, routinely, clinicians draw a diagram or use physical descriptors to define tissue deficiencies.

Clinical Manifestations at Time of Diagnosis

The majority of babies born with cleft lip only or with cleft lip and palate do not have associated syndromes; however, all infants with clefts need a physical examination by a dysmorphologist (Willner, 2000).

Clinical Manifestations at Time of Diagnosis

- *Cleft lip and palate:* physical findings
- *Cleft palate:* difficulty feeding because of infant's inability to create suction
- *Pierre Robin sequence:* signs and symptoms of upper airway obstruction as a result of posterior position of tongue in the airway, micrognathia
- *Submucous cleft palate:* nasal-sounding speech

Infants with cleft palate only should be examined carefully for other anomalies. Some clefts of the palate are not detected by the staff in the delivery room. Infants who are unable to successfully breastfeed, are unable to "latch on," or exhibit difficulties with bottle feedings such as prolonged (more than 30 to 45 minutes) feeding times should be reexamined carefully for the presence of a cleft. Even a small cleft of the soft palate usually produces ineffective sucking as a result of the infant's inability to create a vacuum to draw the milk out of the nipple (Curtin, 1990). The mother may initially report that the baby will nurse for 45 minutes yet does not seem satisfied. The mother's breasts may still feel engorged at the end of a feeding, and there is never a feeling that the breast is empty of milk. Frequent snacking usually results; however, urine output is inadequate and the baby continues to be fussy. After approximately 4 to 5 days of this feeding behavior, the infant becomes sleepier and lethargic and exhibits signs of dehydration, including weight loss (Livingstone, Willis, Abdel-Wareth, et al., 2000). For some bottle-fed infants, the parents report that it may take more than 1 hour for the infant to consume 1 oz of formula. It is at this time that a palatal cleft may be noted. Somnolent, dehydrated 4-day-old infants may be hard to examine because they are resistant to opening their mouth. Insertion of a water-moistened gloved finger may be useful in examining palatal integrity (American Cleft Palate–Craniofacial Association, 2004).

Pierre Robin sequence often has a rather benign presentation with the findings of cleft palate, glossoptosis, and micrognathia (Box 19-2). Airway obstruction may not become evident until the infant is 2 weeks of age or until the first upper respiratory tract infection. Therefore it is prudent to observe these infants closely during the first months of life and consider a baseline pediatric pulmonary evaluation within the first weeks of life. The infants are able to maintain adequate oxygen and carbon dioxide saturations initially after birth, but they can tire over time with increased work of breathing. As infants grow, the size of the airway cannot accommodate their body's demand for more oxygen. There is increased respiratory effort demonstrated by retractions, nasal flaring, and stridor. With increased effort the muscles of the tongue and nasopharynx or larynx collapse, especially during sleep, when the muscles of the upper airway are relaxed. The tongue is retropositioned in the mandible, and the infant has difficulty expiring carbon dioxide, which particularly occurs when the baby is placed supine, and also during sleep when the ventilatory effort is diminished (Figure 19-4). When this occurs there is complete or partial obstruction of the airway, and although it appears that the child is breathing, there are only intermittent breath sounds to auscultation. Oxygen saturation can drop and carbon dioxide levels rise, necessitating treatment (Anderson, Cole, Chuo, et al., 2007; Smith & Senders, 2006).

The presentation of a child with a submucous cleft palate is more elusive. The observation of a posterior notch in the nasal spine at the juncture of the hard and soft palates along with a translucence of the soft palate is unusual unless there are clinical symptoms to warrant closer physical examination of the soft palate. There may or may not be a bifid uvula, which can also be a normal variant, and a short soft palate with muscle separation in the midline. Submucous cleft palate is frequently undetected until the preschool years when the speech is unintelligible secondary to velopharyngeal insufficiency (Gorlin et al., 2001).

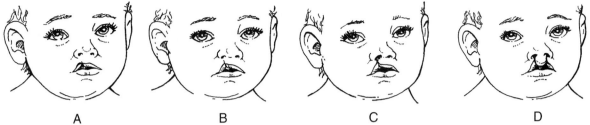

FIGURE 19-1 Varieties of lip clefts. **A, B,** and **C,** Unilateral, or one-sided, clefts in the lip and gum ridge. **D,** Bilateral, or two-sided, cleft. From Moller, K.T., Starr, C.D., & Johnson, S.A. (1990). *A Parent's Guide to Cleft Lip and Palate.* Minneapolis: University of Minnesota Press. Modified with permission.

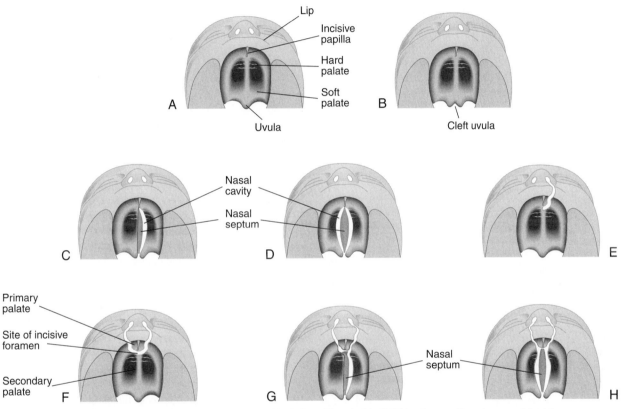

FIGURE 19-2 Various types of cleft palate with cleft lip. **A,** Normal lip and palate. **B,** Bifid uvula seen with a submucous cleft palate. **C,** Unilateral cleft of the secondary palate. **D,** Bilateral cleft of the secondary palate. **E,** Complete unilateral cleft of the lip and the primary palate. **F,** Complete bilateral cleft of the lip with bilateral cleft of the primary palate. **G,** Complete bilateral cleft of the lip with bilateral cleft of the primary palate and unilateral cleft of the secondary palate. **H,** Complete bilateral cleft of the lip, with complete bilateral cleft of the primary and secondary palates. Moore, K., & Persaud, T.V.N. (2007). *Before We Are Born,* 7e. Philadelphia: Saunders.

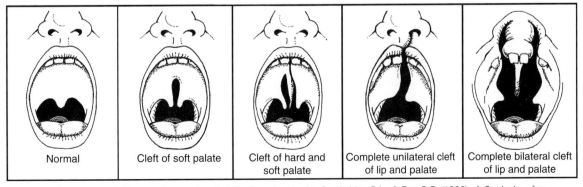

FIGURE 19-3 Types and examples of clefts. From Lynch, J.I., Brookshire, B.L., & Fox, D.R. (1993). *A Curriculum for Infants and Toddlers with Cleft Palate.* Austin, TX: Pro-Ed, Inc. Modified with permission.

BOX 19-2

Findings Apparent in Infants with Pierre Robin Sequence

- Increasing levels of carbon dioxide when measured serially as a result of carbon dioxide retention from intermittent upper airway obstruction with retropositioning of the tongue.
- Transient oxygen desaturations measured by pulse oximetry accompanied by increased work of breathing with chest wall retractions and gasping sounds as the tongue blocks the upper airway. These episodes usually self-correct within a short time as the infant repositions the tongue forward; however, the frequency may increase as the infant tires.
- Difficulty during feedings, especially when the nipple is removed from the mouth and the infant is still swallowing residual milk. The tongue becomes retropositioned easily without the stimulus of the nipple to move it forward. Gagging sounds may be heard and become worse with supine positioning.
- Deceleration on the growth curve despite adequate intake of formula or expressed breast milk. This should signal a possible worsening respiratory status.

From Monasterio, F.O., Drucker, M., Molina, F., et al. (2002). Distraction osteogenesis in Pierre Robin sequence and related respiratory problems in children. *J Craniofac Surg*, *13*, 79-83; Sidman, J.D., Sampson, D., & Templeton, B. (2001). Distraction osteogenesis of the mandible for airway obstruction in children. *Laryngoscope, 111*, 1137-1146. Reprinted with permission.

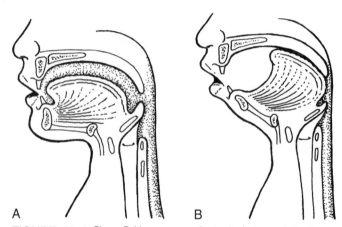

FIGURE 19-4 Pierre Robin sequence. Anatomic features of the larynx. **A,** Normal. **B,** Mandibular hypoplasia. Note that posterior placement of the tongue makes the larynx appear more anteriorly situated than normal.

Children who have nasal-sounding speech for all sounds should have a more detailed examination of their velopharyngeal mechanism. This nasal tone is often not noted until age 3 to 5 years. When the submucous cleft palate is found, a primary care provider may then retrospectively find a predictable history of nasal regurgitation of fluids, inability to breastfeed in infancy, initial feeding problems, slow weight gain, and prolonged bottle-feeding times. In addition, a child may have a history of frequent episodes of serous and acute otitis media as a result of eustachian tube dysfunction associated with the cleft palate (Aniansson, Svensson, Becker, et al., 2002). Only submucous cleft palates that are symptomatic require intervention (Ysunza, Pamplona, Mendoza, et al., 2001).

Treatment
Goals of Treatment and Team Care

Goals of treatment are (1) to achieve optimum growth and function in speech, hearing, dental, and psychosocial development and (2) to achieve optimal esthetic repair. The American Cleft Palate–Craniofacial Association believes that every individual with cleft lip or cleft palate is best served by the multidisciplinary coordinated approach offered by a cleft palate or craniofacial team (see Resources at the end of this chapter for listings). Parents may contact the team independently, or contact can be facilitated by their primary health care provider.

> *Treatment*
> - Establishment of adequate feeding
> - Airway management for infants with Pierre Robin sequence
> - Surgical reconstructive management
> - Otolaryngology treatment
> - Audiology and speech pathology management
> - Dental care and orthodontic treatment

Newborns should be referred to a team before discharge from the birthing hospital. Older children can and should be referred for team consultation because management occurs over the first 18 years of life. The team must include a qualified speech pathologist, an orthodontist, and a plastic surgeon. Other specialties on a cleft palate team often include audiology, otolaryngology, dental specialties (e.g., pediatric dentistry, prosthodontics, oral and maxillofacial surgery), genetics/dysmorphology, genetic counseling, nursing, social work, psychology, and pediatrics. Teams that care for children with more complex craniofacial deformities may also include members from anesthesia, neurosurgery, ophthalmology, radiology, and psychiatry.

Initial management of a newborn with a cleft involves diagnosis clarification (i.e., rule out associated syndromes), psychosocial support for the grieving family of the child with a congenital birth defect, feeding issues, and airway management for infants with Pierre Robin sequence.

Establishment of Adequate Feeding

The goal of feeding is to maintain optimum nutrition using a technique that is as normal as possible. Infants with an isolated cleft lip or a cleft lip and alveolus (gum) do not generally experience any feeding difficulties. Infants with cleft palate, on the other hand, require some minor adaptations to establish effective feeding. Generating intraoral negative pressure is necessary to draw milk out of a nipple, and an infant with a cleft palate is unable to accomplish this because of the air leak through the nose. There is generally no problem with the infant's ability to swallow. Despite "noisy" feeding sounds there is no increased risk of aspiration pneumonia in infants with cleft palate. Therefore the feeding technique must deliver the milk into the oral cavity so the baby can swallow it normally.

Although infants with a cleft lip or cleft lip and alveolus may be able to breastfeed with minor positioning modifications, infants with cleft palate are rarely able to breastfeed owing to the inability

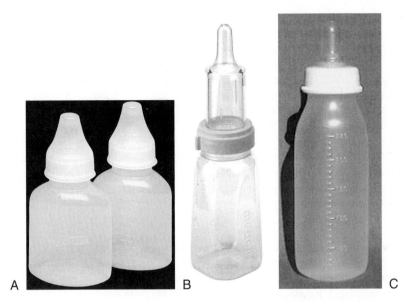

FIGURE 19-5 **A,** The Mead Johnson Cleft Palate Nurser (photo courtesy of Mead Johnson & Co.). **B,** Haberman SpecialNeeds Feeder (photo courtesy of Medela, Inc.). **C,** Pigeon nipple and bottle (photo courtesy of Children's Medical Ventures).

to create a vacuum (Reilly, Reid, Skeat, et al., 2007). The simplest adaptation is to use a large soft nipple with a fast flow of milk or open a standard nipple hole with a cross cut. This does not always deliver adequate milk in a 30-minute feeding. Therefore bottles that can be squeezed or have a one-way flow valve are used to increase the volume of milk flowing into the baby's mouth.

One of the more common feeding devices used is the Mead Johnson Cleft Lip and Palate Nurser (Figure 19-5), which has a soft plastic compressible bottle and a cross-cut nipple that is slightly longer and narrower than regular nipples. The nipple, however, is not the crucial element of this device, as evidenced by some infants' preference for an orthodontic type of nipple that is also effective. The orthodontic nipple is useful in large clefts because it can span the distance between the edges of the cleft. This large nipple can provide some tongue stabilization during the sucking process, and its single hole provides a faster flow of milk. The soft plastic bottle allows the parent to control the rate of milk delivered, with rhythmic squeezing of the bottle timed to the infant's cues of swallowing. The nipple should be aimed at the parts of the palate that are intact to take advantage of any possible nipple compression between the tongue and the palate.

Alternatives to the Mead Johnson nurser are available. The Medela Company distributes the SpecialNeeds Feeder (formerly known as a Haberman feeder), which provides milk flow when the nipple is manually compressed by the caregiver or when the infant's gums apply pressure to the silicone nipple. There are varying flow rates and also a one-way valve between the nipple and bottle to decrease the chances of air ingestion with milk.

The Pigeon nipple, with its simple one-way valve system, is less expensive than the SpecialNeeds Feeder. It is commercially available (see Resources) with instructions for use available in English and Japanese. The nipple is made of soft, easily compressible, non-latex isoprene and has a one-way valve that fits into the nipple assembly. Therefore the milk flows only into the mouth, not back into the bottle when the baby compresses the nipple.

The Ross cleft palate nipple is intended for postoperative feeding and is not appropriate for newborns because the flow rate is too fast. Likewise, the Lamb nipple is an outdated device that is bulky and causes gagging.

Whatever feeding method is chosen, there are principles or guidelines most effective in achieving appropriate weight gain. The family needs personalized teaching within the first week of life regarding assessment, feeding methodology, and evaluation of response to feeding by a practitioner experienced in management of infants with clefts (American Cleft Palate–Craniofacial Association, 2004). Ideally, this practitioner should be a member of a cleft palate or craniofacial team. Consistency with a chosen technique for a minimum of 24 hours is important to allow both parent and infant to adapt. Continuous switching of nipples is confusing. Feedings should last no longer than 30 minutes, and the frequency should not be less than every 2½ to 3 hours. These guidelines promote conservation of energy and decreased caloric expenditure during the feeding process. It is helpful for the parents to know how many ounces their child needs each day to grow normally. A quick easy guide is a minimum of 2 oz of milk per 1 lb of baby's weight every 24 hours. Therefore a 7 lb baby will need 14 oz each day.

The use of feeding appliances or presurgical orthopedic devices varies across the United States. These devices assist the infant with a cleft by creating a barrier over the palatal cleft to enable the baby to then compress a nipple against a hard surface. Some groups anecdotally report improved feeding efficiency for both bottle feeding and breastfeeding using these plates. However, Masarei, Wade, Mars, and colleagues (2007) found that the use of presurgical orthopedics does not significantly improve feeding efficiency or general body growth.

Airway Management

Infants who have Pierre Robin sequence require a careful airway assessment, and effective airway management strategies must be in place before addressing feeding issues. These strategies may include placing a temporary nasopharyngeal airway or tracheostomy for severe upper airway obstruction, lip-tongue placation, or prone positioning. A new surgical therapy involves mandibular lengthening in the neonate and is discussed under Anticipated Advances in Diagnosis and Management later in this chapter. A feeding specialist in conjunction with a craniofacial team will develop the feeding plan for oral feeding with or without a nasogastric tube or gastrostomy tube. Infants with airway distress caused by obstructive etiology are postulated to have a higher incidence of gastroesophageal reflux; however, the association between Pierre Robin sequence and gastroesophageal reflux has not been proven. If an infant does have symptoms of this condition, appropriate diagnostic studies and management are recommended.

Surgical Reconstructive Management

There is a frequent misconception that cleft lip or palate or both are merely surgical problems that are corrected in early childhood when the lip and palatal defects are closed. Parents who are very eager for the surgical repairs soon learn of the multidisciplinary rehabilitative services that must be coordinated with the surgeries. Specific timing of surgery also depends on the child's health and development.

Surgical Reconstruction of a Cleft Lip. Surgical repair of cleft lip is generally done between 3 and 5 months of age. Many surgeons use the rule of 10s—10 weeks of age, hemoglobin level of 10 g/dL, and 10 lb in body weight—in planning the repair. Occasionally, if the cleft is very wide, especially in a unilateral defect, a surgical cleft lip adhesion is done at about 1 month of age to better approximate the lip tissue in preparation for the definitive procedure at the usual age. Some centers prepare the lip before surgery by moving the premaxilla into a better position with simple taping techniques or a more precise movement with orthodontic appliances (Peterson-Falzone, Hardin-Jones, & Karnell, 2001).

Postoperative management for an infant with cleft lip has changed dramatically in recent years. Unrestricted breastfeeding or bottle feeding immediately after surgery has been shown to decrease the length of hospital stay, increase oral intake, and improve parental satisfaction without negatively affecting suture line integrity (Boekelheide, Curtin, Ursich, et al., 1992). Surgery can be performed on an outpatient basis with the infant discharged with elbow restraints. Parents are instructed to clean the suture line with normal saline followed by application of petroleum jelly or antibiotic ointment for 1 to 2 weeks. Pain management is usually adequate with oral acetaminophen.

Secondary lip revisions may be necessary before beginning school or during the school-age years. A nasal repair during the toddler years to lengthen the columella (soft tissue from nasal tip to nostril sill area) is frequently indicated for children with bilateral clefts.

Surgical Reconstruction of a Cleft Palate. Surgical repair of a cleft palate is usually done between 9 and 18 months of age. This is timed to provide the reconstructed palate needed for speech development (Figure 19-6). The repair is most commonly done at one time in one stage. The postoperative management usually dictates a 1- or 2-night hospital stay for airway monitoring and establishing adequate oral hydration. The use of elbow restraints and avoidance of straws and utensils for feeding for 2 weeks are

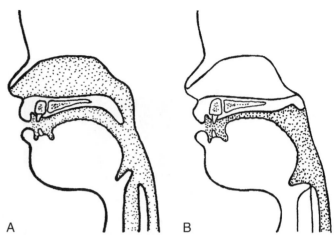

FIGURE 19-6 Anatomy of the roof of the mouth. The hard and soft palates separate the nasal cavity from the mouth. **A,** Soft palate open. Muscles relax for breathing and making certain speech sounds. **B,** Soft palate closed. Muscles in the soft palate and throat seal off the nasal cavity for swallowing foods and liquids and making certain speech sounds. From Mead Johnson & Co. (1997). *Looking Forward: A Guide for Parents of the Child with Cleft Lip and Palate.* Evansville, IN: Author. Modified with permission.

routine. The use of bottles 24 to 48 hours after palatal surgery is variable depending on the center. Cup feeding is taught for liquids and blenderized solid food. Some centers use mist tents or supplemental humidity for 1 night to liquefy dried bloody nasal and oral secretions. Good pain management usually requires a parenteral narcotic (e.g., morphine sulfate) with an enteral analgesic (acetaminophen) on the day of surgery. On the first postoperative day an enteral narcotic analgesic (e.g., acetaminophen with codeine elixir) is substituted for the parenteral narcotic. Regularly scheduled analgesia around the clock after surgery optimizes the success of oral feeding. Infants may require pain management at home with acetaminophen (with or without codeine) for up to 2 weeks after surgery.

Secondary palatal surgery may be recommended by the speech pathologist to address persistent nasal speech after a period of speech therapy. The procedures may lengthen the palate (i.e., Furlow palatoplasty), create a smaller space in all dimensions (i.e., sphincter pharyngoplasty), or create a flap of tissue in the middle (i.e., pharyngeal flap) with two side ports to produce velopharyngeal sufficiency or closure during speech. This secondary palatal surgery is done for children of preschool age to achieve clear speech before school entry (Sie, Tampakopoulou, Sorom, et al., 2001). This procedure is also used in school-age children who develop nasal speech after the adenoid pad involutes.

Repair of the bony defect along the gum or alveolar ridge appears to be optimal between maxillary growth completion and maxillary canine eruption, usually between 8 and 10 years of age (Craven, Cole, Hollier, et al., 2007). Roots of the teeth need to be anchored on bone, and generally iliac crest cancellous bone is harvested and packed into the alveolar cleft defect. Dietary restrictions and the use of blenderized food for 2 weeks by cup are indicated. Once the bone has healed it is possible to use implants to replace missing teeth in the alveolar cleft (Kramer, Baethge, Swennen, et al., 2005).

Nasal reconstructive surgery (i.e., rhinoplasty) is done when full growth has been attained (i.e., after menstruation in females and the growth spurt in males). Approximately 20% of teens with cleft lip and palate repaired in infancy also require midface oral and maxillofacial surgery (Le Fort I) to address facial imbalances that cannot be completely corrected by orthodontics (Good, Mulliken, & Padwa, 2007). Factors predisposing teenagers to the Le Fort I surgery include multiple missing teeth, secondary palate surgery for speech, and inconsistent team care (Oberoi, Chigurupati, & Vargervik, 2008).

Otolaryngology Treatment

Otolaryngology management involves monitoring persistent serous otitis media and frequently placement of ventilation tubes in the tympanic membranes (Valtonen, Dietz, & Qvarnberg, 2005). Ventilation tubes should be considered if there is fluid in the middle ear space at the time of any other surgical procedures (i.e., cleft lip or palate repair). Because of the high incidence of middle ear problems, some centers favor placement of ventilation tubes at the time of surgical palate repair for all children. Following placement of the tubes, some otolaryngologists advise the use of silicone ear plugs while bathing and swimming to prevent water from entering the middle ear; however, updated research supports use of earplugs only for diving to depths of 6 feet or greater or in the case of recurrent otorrhea (Carbonell & Ruiz-Garcia, 2002; Goldstein, Mandel, Kurs-Lasky, et al., 2005).

A small percentage of children have chronic eustachian tube dysfunction after 5 years of age and may require multiple replacements of ventilating tubes to maintain normal hearing through the school-age years. The indication for tubes may be recurrent or persistent serous otitis media or severe retraction of the tympanic membrane in which there is little air present in the middle ear space, resulting in an increased risk for cholesteatoma. The tympanic membranes may be very scarred or weak and thin, which may result in persistent perforation of the tympanic membrane after extrusion of the ventilating tube. This membrane does not need to be patched surgically on an urgent basis if the hearing is not negatively affected because the perforation is functioning like a patent ventilating tube. When the child is a teenager, it may be patched when the eustachian tube functioning improves and there are no recurrent infections (Muntz, 1993).

It is common practice to perform an adenoidectomy on the second set of middle ear ventilation tubes in the quest to avoid subsequent ear tube surgery; however, this practice is not common for children with cleft palate. The adenoidectomy is advocated for children without a cleft to prevent fluid accumulation in the middle ear and eustachian tube caused by blockage from an obstructing adenoid (Lous, Burton, Felding, et al., 2005). For children with clefts, the adenoid tissue is often a factor in establishing velopharyngeal closure during speech when the soft palate abuts the posterior pharyngeal wall at the level of the adenoid. As a result, an adenoidectomy is not usually recommended.

When children with cleft lip and palate experience obstructive sleep apnea because of tonsil and adenoid hypertrophy, a modified surgical treatment plan is advocated. A tonsillectomy and superior adenoidectomy is generally done to preserve the inferior adenoid for velopharyngeal closure. Children with cleft lip and palate are not at a risk greater than that of the population for this problem; however, the intervention is modified based on their underlying anatomic concerns for speech outcome.

Audiology and Speech Pathology Management

Diagnostic audiologic evaluation and management are an integral component of the treatment plan for infants and children with cleft palate. Speech and language development is similarly monitored and therapy provided as appropriate (see Associated Problems later in this chapter).

Dental Care and Orthodontic Treatment

Dental care should begin early (i.e., at 1 to 2 years of age) with regular dental examinations every 6 months and fluoride supplements provided in nonfluoridated areas (Cheng, Moore, & Ho, 2007) to preserve the health of the primary dentition. Children with bilateral or unilateral clefts of the alveolar ridge require considerable orthodontic management.

A child with a cleft palate alone requires regular pediatric dental care and orthodontic services. The anterior and lateral palatal growth may be restricted—especially if the cleft extends into the hard palate. Cleft palate repair results in scarring along areas that normally experience significant growth during childhood. As a result, a palatal expansion appliance may be necessary to achieve adequate dental occlusion.

Children with Pierre Robin sequence who have a significantly smaller mandible as compared with children with isolated cleft palate were studied for catch-up growth, and the results showed that the difference does not change after age 5 years (Daskalogiannakis, Ross, & Thompson, 2001). Sometimes, however, children may need orthodontic management to deal with dental crowding as a result of the small mandible.

Complementary and Alternative Therapies

Parents frequently ask the plastic surgeon if there are complementary or alternative therapies to reduce the visibility of the scar on the lip following cleft lip surgery. Some surgeons routinely cover the incision with paper tape or Steri-strips until the wound is completely healed. This stabilizes the adjoining tissue and decreases the stress on the incision with movement from crying or smiling. Another therapy that has been used is a silicone patch over the incision. There are also creams and ointments with vitamin E that do no harm as long as the wound has healed before the cream or ointment is applied; however, the effectiveness in reducing scar formation has not been substantiated. The act of massaging cream on the lip may break down some of the scar-forming fibrinogen and soften the area; however, it is difficult to get an infant to hold still for a lip massage.

Anticipated Advances in Diagnosis and Management

There has been a recent focus on fetal surgery for cleft lip and palate repair (Wagner & Harrison, 2002). Proposed advantages of such surgical intervention include decreased scar formation in fetal wound healing; decreased potential costs as a result of less need for extensive postoperative care, orthodontia, and speech therapy; and minimized psychological trauma associated with facial deformity (Lorenz & Longaker, 2003). This type of surgical repair has been done in the laboratory in fetal mice, rabbits, sheep, and monkeys. Currently, nonlethal conditions such as cleft lip and palate are not repaired in humans because of the high surgical risks. The potential risks to the mother and the early fetus are considerable and probably do not justify the intervention. Endoscopic techniques may reduce the risks of surgery in the future (Wagner & Harrison, 2002). Obvious limitations to this treatment modality include accurate prenatal diagnosis through ultrasound, which would capture some infants with cleft lip but would not include those with a cleft palate only. Nonetheless, the current research will be beneficial for an increased understanding of craniofacial development and effects of management on wound healing.

Prenatal diagnosis of a cleft lip in the second trimester with two-dimensional (2-D) and three-dimensional (3-D) ultrasonography is becoming more common as the technique and interpretation are perfected (Tonni, Centini, & Rosignoli, 2005). The 2-D ultrasound technique visualizes the baby in layers, which is beneficial for detecting anomalies of the internal organs, and 3-D ultrasound looks at the surface of the baby, which can confirm the presence of a cleft lip. It is important to define any other anomalies, such as those found with a chromosomal syndrome, which have a much different prognosis than an isolated cleft of the lip, which may or may not include a cleft of the palate as well. Families need to obtain accurate diagnostic information with follow-up genetic counseling when a prenatal diagnosis is made. Realistic and accurate preparation by the craniofacial center with emphasis on the first year of life management issues is helpful for the couple referred from the obstetric ultrasound screening process (Jones, 2002).

Potential advances in the management of children with cleft lip and palate include genetic testing to identify the genes that are transformed when an infant has a clefting disorder (Murray, 2002). Further research regarding the effects of maternal vitamin deficiencies and environmental factors on gene transformation may provide clues into preventive measures that may be used during pregnancy (Prescott, Natalie, & Malcolm, 2002).

Recently, surgical techniques that lengthen the mandible have been introduced to avoid a tracheostomy for infants with significant upper airway obstruction caused by Pierre Robin sequence. The technique is known as distraction osteogenesis and is usually undertaken only at major craniofacial centers with experienced surgeons and neonatal intensive care personnel (Monasterio, Drucker, Molina, et al., 2002; Sidman, Sampson, & Templeton, 2001; Wittenborn, Panchal, Marsh, et al., 2004). Distraction osteogenesis was pioneered by orthopedic surgeons in such procedures as long bone lengthening when a child has a leg length discrepancy. An osteotomy is created on both sides of the mandible, and hardware is attached to the bony fragments and serially expanded with an appliance at the same time as the mandible is regenerating new bony growth. Lengthening the mandible in this way draws the tongue forward and out of the airway. The enthusiasm for this new intervention must be tempered with the concerns for tooth buds that may be in the path of the distraction hardware (Zim, 2007). This procedure requires a complete otolaryngology evaluation to determine the level of obstruction (i.e., the tongue may not be the only source of the obstruction).

Associated Problems of Cleft Lip and Palate and Treatment

Audiology and Otolaryngology

Infants and children with an isolated cleft lip or cleft lip and alveolus generally do not have abnormal hearing at a rate above the general population. Infants and children with cleft palate, however, have significant hearing and middle ear problems. Audiology testing is appropriate in children with cleft palate to monitor the degree of conductive hearing loss in order to guide the clinician in providing appropriate interventions and documenting the effectiveness of management. Hearing can be tested in newborns in the nursery by a screening known as automated auditory brainstem response screening (AABR), or otoacoustic emissions (American Cleft Palate–Craniofacial Association, 2004). If an infant does not pass the hearing screen, it is appropriate to proceed with more complex testing known as auditory brainstem response (ABR) testing, which monitors the sensorineural auditory system.

Associated Problems of Cleft Lip and Palate and Treatment

- Audiology/otolaryngology
- Speech pathology
- Dental/orthodontic problems
- Psychosocial adjustment to a physical deformity

Children who are at least 6 to 9 months of age may be tested by behavioral audiologic testing. This type of testing requires some degree of cooperation and is done when an infant can sit and respond to sounds. These findings should ideally correlate with the physical examination by the otolaryngologist so that a combined approach to management can then be devised.

The dynamic functioning of the eustachian tube, which serves as the communication link between the middle ear space and the back of the throat, is controlled by the palatal musculature. The child with cleft palate has abnormal placement and underdevelopment of palatal musculature. As a result the eustachian tube functions poorly. When a child develops an upper respiratory tract infection, fluid can accumulate in the middle ear space. This fluid usually drains into the oral cavity when the infection and swelling of the eustachian tube subside (Figure 19-7). In a child with cleft palate, however, the eustachian tube may only rarely open, and as a result the fluid remains behind the tympanic membrane on a long-term basis. Infants and children with cleft palate have up to a 90% incidence of developing chronic serous otitis media associated with eustachian tube dysfunction.

Monitoring children with ear tubes in place is usually done every 6 months and more frequently as necessary for blocked, infected, or prematurely extruded tubes. It is especially important to monitor for the presence of middle ear fluid and resultant conductive hearing loss in children who are rapidly acquiring speech and language skills and are already challenged by the cleft palate, which makes this acquisition more difficult.

Many parents query the primary care provider as to why the eustachian tube dysfunction continues after the surgical repair of the cleft palate. Even though palatal tissue is restored closer to normal, the dynamic mechanisms that control the influence of the

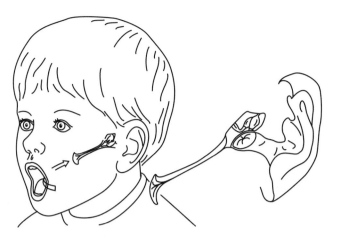

FIGURE 19-7 Ear–eustachian tube relationship and proximity to the palate. From Ross Laboratories, Columbus, OH. Reprinted with permission.

palatal musculature on eustachian tube function are not normalized (Bluestone, 2004).

Speech Pathology

Children with cleft lip only usually do not have significant speech articulation problems. These children may only require short-term therapy that focuses on bilabial sounds found in *m* and *b* and *p*, which require competent lip closure. Children with clefts of the alveolus have additional challenges with anterior sounds, as well as with managing air leakage from the front of the gums into the anterior nasal cavity before the alveolar bone graft surgery (Peterson-Falzone et al., 2001).

Children with clefts of the palate have problems with speech articulation trying to correct the nasal air escape (Henningsson, Kuehn, Sell, et al., 2008). The goal of palate surgery is to create a normally functioning palate before the emergence of compensatory mechanisms. The speech pathologist should meet the parents before surgery to explain normal speech and language development. Families must be taught the fact that babies need to receive speech input directed at them and need to reciprocate in a turn-taking fashion with the use of body language and prespeech babbling behavior. Anticipatory guidance is standard practice for such families.

Following surgical closure of the cleft palate, the speech pathologist evaluates the success of the surgery. If formal speech therapy is needed it can begin with children as young as 2 years of age. Without this intervention, these children can become frustrated in their inability to expand in expressive speech and language skills and may develop behavioral responses such as temper tantrums to communicate. In addition, the child is unable to communicate even simple desires to strangers who are unfamiliar with the child's speech repertoire.

Ongoing monitoring and parental guidance on a 6-month basis with the speech pathologist are appropriate during the toddler and preschool years. At some point during this time, the speech pathologist may determine that the child could benefit from regular speech therapy services. For children younger than 3 years of age, therapy may be provided by an infant development program that has specific speech therapy services or a speech pathologist

who is community or hospital based. After 3 years of age, the child usually receives speech therapy that is provided by the local school district. An individualized educational program (IEP) is necessary for this isolated service because it is a component of special education services (see Chapter 3). The speech pathologist at the craniofacial or cleft palate center should continue to monitor progress every 6 to 12 months and provide feedback and suggestions to the speech pathologist providing the therapy.

The desired outcome following cleft palate surgery and speech therapy is clear articulation by 4 years of age. Although many variables have been studied, including type of cleft, age of surgical repair, type of surgical technique used, initiation time, and length of speech therapy services, no one factor has been determined to provide the desired outcome (Peterson-Falzone et al., 2001). Rather, it is a combination of factors that produces the optimal outcome.

Children who do not have clear speech development by 4 years of age may require secondary surgical palatal treatment—ideally before school entry. This surgery is particularly helpful if the articulation of sounds is good but there is persistent nasal air emission as a result of a deficiency of palatal tissue or a palate that has inadequate motion. If secondary surgical or prosthetic management is done, follow-up speech therapy is usually needed to obtain maximum benefit from the intervention. It is not unusual for school-age children to receive speech therapy during school, especially because they receive active orthodontic services that may further challenge speech articulation.

Dental and Orthodontic Problems

Children with a cleft lip and/or palate generally display poorer oral hygiene and higher susceptibility to caries associated with dental anomalies and defects of the repaired lip and palate (Cheng, Moor & Ho, 2007). Care should be taken not to remove teeth in the cleft area because they maintain alveolar bone mass in a dental arch that is deficient in bone at the area of the cleft. Children often develop a crossbite from surgical closure of the palate causing collapse of the arches. The crossbite does not always need to be corrected in primary dentition, but some pediatric dentists do offer early interceptive orthodontic treatment.

At 5 to 7 years of age, it is appropriate for a child with an alveolar cleft to have an orthodontic consultation, baseline records (e.g., photographs, dental study models, radiographs, examination), and a treatment plan. Initial management focuses on expansion of the maxillary arch with a fixed active appliance in preparation for surgical grafting with iliac crest donor bone. The orthodontist usually indicates the appropriate time to perform the bone graft procedure. Following the grafting procedure, the expectation is that adjacent teeth will erupt into the arch. Dental implants combined with bone grafting can offer a reliable alternative to prosthetics for missing teeth (Kramer et al., 2005).

Orthodontic management is usually done in phases and may have periods of rest when the teeth are held in place by a passive retention type of appliance. The timing and phase of intervention depend on the maxillary and mandibular growth that occurs into the teen years. It is not uncommon for orthodontic management to span a period of 10 years. Compliance with the recommended regimen is crucial because active movement of teeth depends on keeping frequent appointments, maintaining appliances, and practicing good oral hygiene. Maintaining regular pediatric dental care services during the orthodontic treatment is also important.

Psychosocial Adjustment to a Physical Deformity

Parents of the infant with a cleft are the first clients for the long-term psychosocial management of the child. According to observations, families who positively accommodate to their child's chronic condition have children who appear to cope at a higher level than parents who exhibit negative adaptive behaviors (Klein, Pope, Getahun, et al., 2006). The degree of clefting is not predictive of the level of psychosocial functioning (Endriga & Kapp-Simon, 1999).

The first questions parents ask the primary care provider after the birth of a child with cleft lip or palate are "How did this happen?" and "Did I do something wrong?" (Bender, 2000). The parents should be reassured that clefts can occur in the healthiest of pregnancies; therefore they should not blame themselves. The birth of an infant with a facial malformation is a constant reminder of the physical condition. Bonding and attachment activities are related to the infant's face, and it takes some time to adjust and positively regard an abnormal face (Endriga & Kapp-Simon, 1999). Up to 25% of pregnant and postpartum women can experience some depressive symptoms (Bennett & Indman, 2006). With the added stress of the birth of a child with a difference, the health of the mother should be assessed by the craniofacial team social worker or psychologist or primary care provider. Most families learn over time to appreciate their infant's own personality and special way of expressing a "wide smile." Some families have a secondary grief reaction once the child's lip is repaired and express that they "miss the cleft" (Curtin, 1990). A second adjustment to the "new" face is necessary and may take 1 to 2 weeks after surgery. Parents do not regret deciding to have the lip repair done, but rather, it is a normal adjustment. Parents are reassured when the team providers give them anticipatory guidance about their feelings. The feelings of grief commonly experienced by parents at the birth of their child with a cleft can resurface at times of stress, such as hospitalization, initiation of speech, dental eruption, and school entry. It is important for parents to recognize that everyone copes with grief differently and not to expect other family members to be feeling the same emotions at the same time.

The health care provider can model acceptance of the child and encourage the parents to support the interests and talents their child exhibits in areas such as music, art, sports, or academia. One technique parents can use to communicate their acceptance of their child with a cleft is to incorporate stories about the child's adventures as a baby going to the hospital for the lip surgery with a positive outcome. That way the cleft is part of the child and the outcome is due to their innate characteristics.

Children in the preschool years gain an increased understanding of their birth defect as they develop a sense of self-awareness and experience teasing from peers. Simple explanations about the cleft can be reviewed, and strategies for deflecting the teasing can be suggested. School-age children may need support from counselors, school personnel, and their family to promote a positive self-image and to cope with teasing (Hunt, Burden, Hepper, et al., 2006). Teenagers are able to articulate their wishes and priorities in treatment planning and should participate in the decision-making process. Teenagers also have increased self-image concerns and may benefit from counseling services.

Prognosis

The long-term prognosis for children with nonsyndromic cleft lip and palate is excellent. The goals of team management are to achieve good speech articulation, functional dental occlusion, normal hearing acuity, an acceptable appearance, and a positive self-regard. In addition, children with Pierre Robin sequence have a goal of achieving adequate airway function. They are generally cared for in tertiary medical centers with cleft-craniofacial teams that work with pediatric pulmonary or pediatric otolaryngology specialists to achieve adequate airway function.

Prognosis for development can vary from normal for a child with a nonsyndromic cleft to severely delayed for a child with a chromosomal defect causing the cleft. Therefore all infants with cleft lip and palate need to be examined by a geneticist or dysmorphologist before surgery (American Cleft Palate–Craniofacial Association, 2004; Arosarena, 2007).

PRIMARY CARE MANAGEMENT

Health Care Maintenance
Growth and Development

Growth and development are not affected in children with a nonsyndromic cleft lip and palate. In the past, infant feeding devices used to provide nutrition for neonates with a cleft palate were suboptimal. With the evolution of the squeeze bottle and the proliferation of team care and trained professionals to provide teaching, this aspect of management has improved. In addition, current postoperative feeding routines are simpler and hospital stays are shorter, which all contribute to a more normalized nutritional status.

Infants with cleft lip and palate are expected to grow along the same parameters as infants without clefts. Once the feeding method has been taught by a member of the cleft-craniofacial team, the primary care provider will monitor the child's growth. All children with craniofacial abnormalities should be referred to a pediatric endocrinologist if short stature (other than constitutional) is identified. Children who have a known syndrome may have growth and developmental problems related to the syndrome.

Occasionally, infants with clefts do not grow along the expected norms. There may be extenuating psychosocial factors that challenge the parent or caretaker in feeding the infant. Initially an observation and review of the feeding method should be pursued along with a 24- to 72-hour diet record. Serial weight checks can provide both parental and health care provider reassurance. For the infant with Pierre Robin sequence, deceleration on the growth curve should prompt a careful reassessment of respiratory status and the probable finding of some degree of upper airway obstruction.

Diet

Mothers of infants with cleft palate can provide expressed breast milk for their children. Hospital-grade electric pumps work the best and can be rented from a lactation consultant who is trained to provide education and support regarding long-term pumping and storage of breast milk. Most mothers use a double pumping system attachment to decrease the amount of time spent pumping milk. Mothers with low income may be able to procure an electric pump from their local Women, Infants, and Children (WIC) agency.

Mothers who are pumping breast milk four to six times per day in addition to bottle feeding the milk six to eight times per day need support and assistance from others. It is important to balance the needs of the mother and the family with the needs of the infant with a cleft in such a way that the mother not only feels encouraged to continue but also feels support if she decides to discontinue pumping. Mothers who are able to persevere with providing their infant expressed breast milk will be encouraged by a study that linked breast milk intake to a decreased incidence of otitis media specifically in infants with clefts (Aniansson et al., 2002; Paradise, Elster, & Tan, 1994).

Upright positioning of the infant during feeding will decrease the amount of nasal regurgitation. Parents should be reassured that a small amount of nasal regurgitation is expected and should be handled by simply wiping the nose of the infant with a cloth rather than interpreted as a signal of a problem. Cleansing of the nose and mouth with water or a cotton-tipped applicator or bulb syringe is not necessary because the mouth is self-cleaning and the nasal secretions and milk will drain by gravity. The parent may need to be reassured about the anatomy of the cleft palate. The oral cavity and nasal cavity are continuous, and the parent may have an unspoken fear that the feeding will hurt the infant or that the nasal turbinates and the vomer represent brain tissue that can be injured with feeding. It is not unusual to see an ulcer on the vomer (bottom of nasal septum seen near the middle of the open cleft palate). This is caused by suckling or bottle feeding and goes away as the tissue toughens. The use of feeding plates has not been shown to improve feeding or nutritional status (Prahl, Kuijpers-Jagtman, Van't Hof, et al., 2005).

The primary care provider can offer anticipatory guidance by discouraging the use of bottles in bed, especially when filled with formula, milk, or juice. This practice causes early childhood caries. The supine position favors accumulation of the fluid into the middle ear space when the eustachian tube is open in a population that is already at risk for recurrent otitis media.

For an infant who is 4 to 6 months old, introduction of solid foods and progression to table foods is sequenced the same as for infants without clefts. There may be some nasal regurgitation as the infant learns this new skill. Varying textures can sometimes alleviate this issue. Some parents require extra encouragement to proceed with the introduction of solid foods by spoon. Delayed initiation of this normal developmental skill can create negative feeding behaviors and may interfere with the normal oral motor development that is a precursor to speech development. Using a bottle type of infant feeder or enlarging nipple holes to accommodate solid foods also delays normal development. Messy spoon feedings are expected, and nasal reflux of solids should be handled calmly. Infants and children have only minor dietary restrictions. Some tricky foods for a child with an unrepaired cleft palate include peanut butter, soft cheese, and sweets, which are all gummy in texture. Avoiding foods that are a choking risk, such as peanuts, popcorn, and pellet candy, is advised because these foods can lodge in the nasal cavity.

Safety

In addition to routine anticipatory guidance on safety issues, the child may have some restrictions during the first 2 to 4 weeks following reconstructive surgical procedures. Elbow splints are generally used for 1 to 2 weeks after reconstructive surgery in the infant and toddler. Older preschool children may need the immobilizers at nap times and bedtime as "reminders" not to put their fingers in the mouth immediately postoperatively.

Dietary restrictions that are recommended postoperatively (e.g., avoidance of utensils, straws, and textured foods) are generally only necessary for about 2 weeks after surgery to allow for nontraumatic healing of the oral tissues. Some families may need to be encouraged and reassured to advance to soft foods 2 weeks after the surgery and an unrestricted diet 1 month after the surgery.

Youngsters need to avoid contact sports for 6 weeks after alveolar bone grafting procedures, nasal reconstruction, and midface jaw procedures to prevent disruption of the surgery before bone healing.

Infants with Pierre Robin sequence who require prone positioning for adequate respiration may need a car safety bed rather than a car seat when traveling in an automobile; these beds are available commercially (see Resources at the end of this chapter).

Immunizations

Infants and children with cleft lip and palate should receive all routine immunizations at the ages recommended by the American Academy of Pediatrics (AAP) Committee on Infectious Diseases (2006). A planned surgical procedure is not a rationale for deferring routine immunizations; the child is better protected within the hospital setting when immunization status is current. Administration of immunizations within 72 hours of a planned surgical procedure is not advisable because a low-grade fever following vaccine administration may preclude surgery. Administration of the measles-mumps-rubella (MMR) or varicella vaccine within 1 week before scheduled surgery is not recommended for similar reasons. Administration of the pneumococcal vaccine is advocated for this population because of its protective effect in preventing some of the episodes of acute otitis media, although admittedly the vaccine's prime target is the more life-threatening meningitis risk (Overturf, 2000). Respiratory syncytial virus (RSV) immunoprophylaxis (Synagis) is recommended for children with conditions that compromise pulmonary function and congenital abnormalities of the airways such as Pierre Robin sequence (Committee on Infectious Diseases & Committee on Fetus and Newborn, 2003).

Screening

Vision. Routine vision screening is recommended. Children with cleft palate alone should have a pediatric ophthalmology dilated examination at approximately 1 year of age and again before school entry at age 4 or 5 years to screen for Stickler syndrome, which is associated with myopia and sometimes leads to retinal detachment (Jones, 2006).

Hearing. A high index of suspicion and prompt referral to an audiologist and otolaryngologist should be made if the child does not pass an audiologic screening in the school-age years. Detailed audiologic testing (as previously described) is done by the specialty center in the early years of life.

Dental. Routine screening is recommended for a child with an isolated cleft lip. Dental and orthodontic care is indicated for children with clefts of the alveolar ridge or the secondary palate. A pediatric dental provider is strongly advised—even if the family needs to travel some distance to obtain the service. The primary care provider should promote good oral hygiene practices, including initiation of tooth brushing or cleansing with a rough face cloth with eruption of the first tooth. Parents must be counseled on the hazards of early childhood caries (Cheng, Moor, & Ho, et al., 2007).

Dental eruption may be slightly delayed in a child with a cleft. Many families may mistakenly believe that once their child starts orthodontic care they no longer need to see the regular pediatric dentist. However, dental cleanings and topical fluoride treatment are even more important during active orthodontic management.

Blood Pressure. Routine screening is recommended.

Hematocrit. Routine screening is recommended.

Urinalysis. Routine screening is recommended.

Tuberculosis. Routine screening is recommended.

Condition-Specific Screening

Children with cleft lip and palate require particular vigilance in vision, hearing and dental screening, as previously discussed in this chapter.

Common Illness Management

Differential Diagnosis

Fever. The parents of a child with a cleft are alerted to the increased incidence of middle ear disease. The presence of a fever, increased irritability, tugging at the ears, and asking family members to repeat verbalizations all signal the need to have the ears examined for acute or serous otitis media.

Children with cleft palate are defined as an outlying population by the current AAP recommendations regarding middle ear disease, which means they favor ongoing monitoring of serous otitis media rather than aggressive surgical management (AAP, American Academy of Family Physicians [AAFP] Subcommittee on Management of Acute Otitis Media, 2004). Primary care providers are advised to refer these children to the otolaryngologist for a microscopic examination if they have persistent (i.e., 3 months or longer) middle ear fluid or recurrent (i.e., every 1 to 2 months) acute otitis media. Acute otitis media should be managed with the usual oral antibiotics. Prompt management is indicated for acute otitis media rather than the "watch and wait" approach currently in practice in the healthy child population because of the frequency of otitis media and the deleterious effects on hearing in an at-risk population. Prophylactic antibiotic use is not recommended because of development of resistant pathogens (AAP, AAFP, Subcommittee on Management of Acute Otitis Media, 2004; Gungor & Bluestone, 2001) as well as its ineffectiveness in the management of chronic serous otitis media—the main problem in children with cleft palate.

Drug Interactions

Medications are not required as part of the normal treatment regimen.

Developmental Issues

Sleep Patterns

Infants and children with a unilateral cleft lip usually have a deviated nasal septum that causes noisy breathing during upper respiratory tract infections but does not negatively affect air exchange.

Children who have secondary palatal surgery to address nasal speech have a smaller upper airway space in the nasopharynx. These children are particularly at risk for sleep state upper airway obstruction during the first 6 weeks following surgery when local edema is present. Symptoms may include chest wall retractions with or without partial ventilation, irregular snoring with pauses greater than 15 to 20 seconds, diaphoresis, nighttime waking (especially after an apnea episode), daytime somnolence, and enuresis (Muntz, Wilson, Park, et al., 2008). The child's symptoms should be reported to the specialty center physician, who may be a pediatric pulmonologist or otolaryngologist. The severity of the symptoms will be assessed, and medical management (e.g., steroid administration or inpatient observation) may be warranted. The surgical procedure rarely needs to be revised because the symptoms are usually temporary and the desired outcome is to provide a decreased nasal airflow during speech without negatively affecting the ventilatory capabilities.

An infant with Pierre Robin sequence may have a disrupted sleep experience as a result of sleep state obstructive apnea. Careful history taking, evaluation, and management by the pediatric pulmonologist or otolaryngologist are appropriate. A formal overnight pediatric polysomnogram is often ordered. Ideally, this test should be done with the infant in various sleep positions (prone position, supine position, side-lying position, and while in the intended car seat) to document tolerance to position changes.

Sleep patterns are usually disrupted following hospitalizations because of upset routines and psychological distress. Families should be told of this probable change in sleeping pattern at both the preoperative and postoperative visits.

Toileting

There is no physiologic effect on toileting. The psychological impact of stressful surgeries and hospitalization experiences can temporarily delay acquisition of toileting skills or result in regression of recently acquired skills.

Discipline

Parents of children with a congenital birth defect often feel guilty that they "caused" the problem in some way. This feeling can then translate into an altered perception of the child as being special and requiring extra attention to overcompensate for the guilt. In addition, parents are very saddened to learn of the initial surgeries that their child will require and the long-term management. Many parents report that they wish the treatment could be done on them rather than on the child. Because the initial surgeries are done in infancy, the psychological burden is thrust on the parents.

Parents must be encouraged to return to the infant's or child's normal routine following hospitalizations (Strauss, 2001). A routine is reassuring for the child and promotes normalcy and an earlier return to normal behavior. Parents who focus exclusively on the needs of the infant or child who is sick and cater to every whim soon find that this is not functional or pleasant for the child or the family. Symptoms of this phenomenon include the following: no structured feeding or meal routine; irregular nap times; nighttime waking; nighttime feedings; co-sleeping in the parental bed (only if this is not the family's usual practice); excessive fussiness, irritability, or clinginess; loss of previously achieved developmental milestones; and inability to get along with others. These are all normal reactions to a stressful experience such as a hospitalization but usually do not persist beyond 2 to 6 weeks after a 24- to 48-hour hospital stay. Parents can benefit from anticipatory guidance and encouragement to promote normalcy, which initially may appear harsh and unsympathetic. When it is presented as comforting for the child, however, most parents embrace the concept.

Issues of discipline arise again when a child with a cleft lip or palate enters school, especially if the child appears very different from peers and is teased. Overprotectiveness and lack of appropriate limits can exacerbate these problems. The child and family can often benefit from short-term counseling regarding self-image concerns and development of skills to cope with teasing from others.

Child Care

Child care in a group daycare setting can be stressful for parents of a child who is at risk for frequent ear infections. For this reason, some parents choose a setting with a more limited number of children—especially during the winter months.

Once children are old enough to attend a Head Start program or structured preschool, they should. Such programs can be helpful as an adjunct to speech therapy because a child's peers will promote expressive language development. Peers usually do not understand the elaborate gesturing system and monosyllabic vocalizations that substitute for expressive language and may encourage children to expand their repertoire by modeling.

Schooling

Children with cleft palate are eligible for special education services (i.e., speech therapy) under the Individuals with Disabilities Education Act (IDEA) of 1991, amended in 2004 (see Chapter 3). Parents should request in writing a speech evaluation focused on articulation when a child is 2 years, 9 months of age. It is helpful if the parents provide medical information and any prior speech evaluations.

Peer teasing can occur as a child progresses through school because of speech and facial appearance issues (Millard & Richman, 2001). Some parents and children use the "class presentation" approach to explain the cleft, and teachers can incorporate this into their lesson plans about differences among people. A child rarely reports teasing and ridicule so severe that school phobia and frequent absences become an issue. It is important to query parents about these issues at primary care visits and offer supportive services and coordinated efforts between the primary care providers and the school system.

Children with cleft lip and palate may have learning disabilities, particularly in the areas affected by expressive language, such as reading problems (Endriga & Kapp-Simon, 1999). Children who have an isolated cleft palate that is part of a syndrome may have a lower intellectual potential that is specifically associated with the syndrome. These children should be evaluated by special education professionals as appropriate.

Sexuality

No special sexual problems are associated with cleft lip and palate. The obvious concerns about self-image may be exaggerated during adolescence.

When discussing reproductive issues, the risks of recurrence for clefting must be addressed. The rates quoted for nonsyndromic clefts are between 2% and 7% (Gorlin et al., 2001), depending on previous family history and the severity of the cleft. A bilateral cleft lip is rare and more severe than a unilateral one and also has a slightly higher risk of recurrence. Other factors, such as gender, influence the recurrence risk as well. A complete family history and physical examination of an affected individual by a geneticist and genetic counselor are necessary to provide the most accurate information.

Women with increased risk for having a child with a cleft are eligible for a detailed ultrasound that has a better resolution of the facial features than a traditional ultrasound. Women of childbearing age are counseled to take increased folic acid and a multivitamin supplement 3 months before conception and during the first trimester in the hope of reducing the recurrence risk of a cleft condition (Prescott et al., 2002).

Transition to Adulthood

State funding for care of children with cleft lips and palates is available to financially eligible children up to age 21 years through Medicaid (see Chapter 8). Most individuals are able to complete the orthodontic and oral-maxillofacial surgical procedures by this age. Problems are encountered if there were treatment lapses or delays during crucial stages of dental development or orthodontic management that necessitated restarting the treatment. In addition, orthodontic interventions are effective during active treatment, and then the position of the teeth and the occlusion are often maintained with removable appliances (e.g., a retainer worn at night). Adolescents and their families often do not appreciate the need for these appliances, so relapse occurs. If relapse occurs before the insurance is terminated, some active management can be reinitiated. Otherwise, young adults must usually pay for these services as out-of-pocket expenses. It is difficult for young adults to gain third-party payment for follow-up lip or nasal surgery because such procedures are considered to be cosmetic by insurance carriers even though the treatment is for reconstruction of a congenital birth defect.

Family Concerns

Postpartum depression is not uncommon in the general population and is a treatable condition that may be overlooked when present in a mother who has just given birth to a child with a cleft lip and/or palate. Primary care providers should assess the mother for signs and symptoms of depression such as persistent tearfulness, isolation, and lack of social support systems (Bennett & Indman, 2006). Parents of children with a cleft lip worry about their child's physical attractiveness to others, especially strangers. Parents are sensitive to the reactions and comments of professionals and their family and look at others' facial and emotional reactions when viewing their baby with a facial deformity. Fears of feeding or hurting the face and the mouth and concern that the cleft extends into the brain are common. Demonstrating feeding techniques and promoting normal infant care routines provide opportunities for learning and allaying anxieties.

It is beneficial to recommend that parents photograph their infant with a facial cleft. The provider can discuss with parents the usefulness of retaining a photograph that will be available for the child to view when older. If the parents are resistant, stating that they prefer to forget this time of sadness and wish to defer picture taking until after cleft lip repair, it may be prudent for a professional working with the family to take a photograph to keep in the infant's chart.

Families may verbalize concerns regarding oral, auditory, and dental problems in their child. These concerns and consequent stressors recur over time with multiple hospitalizations, tooth eruption, initial speech, school entry, and adolescent self-image concerns.

Orthodontic services are a crucial component of the rehabilitation process and are covered by the local state and federal funding programs for children with birth defects if a family is financially eligible. Families who do not meet the financial eligibility often find this care very expensive. Many insurance companies do not authorize treatment by nonmedical providers who render services such as dental, orthodontic, or prosthetic care, as well as speech and psychological care.

Special cultural issues that affect families who have a child with a cleft lip and palate are mostly concerned with the etiology of the cleft condition. Superstitions about why clefts occur often originate in a family's country of origin. Hispanic and Filipino cultural folklores believe that clefting is related to the lunar cycle. A lunar eclipse or a crescent moon during a woman's pregnancy predisposes her unborn child to clefts. Some Asian cultural folklores relate construction, cutting, a fall, or moving the mother's bed during pregnancy with birth defects—especially clefting. In Chinese culture the center of a person's face is very important and integral to that person's being (i.e., instead of the heart, which is common in Western culture). This view has implications for a cleft lip and palate deformity in its central location.

Most young parents acknowledge that such beliefs are part of cultural folklores and are explanations that their parents and grandparents provided for the untoward events that happened during a pregnancy. Trying to disprove these theories is unnecessary, especially because the etiology of clefts is unknown. It is more useful to focus on the common feeling of paternal and maternal guilt associated with a birth defect and work through the grief process over time.

Some families bring with them extreme fears of surgery and hospitalization, but fear usually seems to be experience related (i.e., a relative who died after a surgical procedure) rather than related to a specific cultural framework. The concept of health care in general, especially preventive health care (e.g., the routine dental care or anticipatory guidance needed to prevent speech articulation problems), is unfamiliar to some families. The very idea of seeking nonemergent health care services is particularly unknown in families who originate from other countries outside the United States that do not have many health care resources.

Resources

Organizations

Ameriface
Provides newsletter, information, and support.
P.O. Box 751112
Las Vegas, NV 89136-1112
(888) 486-1209; Fax: (702) 341-5351
Email: info@ameriface.org
Website: www.aboutfaceusa.org

American Cleft Palate–Craniofacial Association (ACPA)
Referral to local cleft-craniofacial team; written pamphlets and fact sheets in English and Spanish; distribution of document, *Parameters for Evaluation and Treatment* (2004).
1504 East Franklin St., Suite 102
Chapel Hill, NC 27514-2820
(919) 933-9044; Cleftline: (800) 24-CLEFT
Email: info@cleftline.org

Changing Faces
Support organization and publisher of child and adult books and material on the emotional and social aspects of living with a facial difference.
Website: www.changingfaces.co.uk

Children's Medical Ventures
Specialty feeding products, cleft palate nipple (Pigeon nipple).
275 Longwater Dr.
Norwell, MA 02061
(888) 766-8443; Hospital ordering: (800) 345 6443; Fax: (724) 387 5270
Website: www.chmv.respironics.com

Cleftadvocate
Support organization for families with children born with clefts, and provides legislative advice and activity for obtaining insurance coverage for procedures.
(888) 486-1209
Website: www.cleftadvocate.org

COSCO
Dream Ride SE infant car bed/car seat is a car safety bed for infants with Pierre Robin sequence who require prone positioning.
2525 State St.
Columbus, IN 47201-7443
(800) 544-1108; (812) 372-0141
Website: www.djgusa.com

Let's Face It
Comprehensive guide to support and information on craniofacial anomalies.
University of Michigan School of Dentistry/Dentistry Library
1011 North University
Ann Arbor, MI 48109-1078
(360) 676-7325
Website: www.dent.umich.edu/faceit
Evansville, IN 47721-0001
(812) 429-5000; (800) BABY123

Mead Johnson & Co., Nutritional Division

Free booklet for cleft lip and palate nursers, *Your cleft lip and palate child: A basic guide for parents.*

Evansville, IN 47721-0001

(812) 429-5000; (800) BABY 123

Website: www.store.enfamil.com/bottles_and_nursers.html

Medela, Inc.

For breast pump rentals and SpecialNeeds Feeders (6000S).

1101 Corporate Dr.

McHenry, IL 60050-7005

(800) 435-8316

Website: www.medela.com

Wide Smiles

Online support organization for families with children born with clefts.

P.O. Box 5153

Stockton, CA 95205-0153

(209) 942-2812

Website: www.widesmiles.org

Books for Parents

Berkowitz, S. (1994). *The Cleft Palate Story.* Chicago: Quintessence Publishing.

Bristow, L., & Bristow, S. (2007). *Making Faces: Logan's Cleft Lip and Palate Story.* Oakville, Ontario: Pulsus Group Inc.

Charkins, H. (1996). *Children with Facial Difference: A Parent's Guide.* Bethesda, MD: Woodbine House.

Moller, K.T., Starr, C.D., & Johnson, S.A. (1990). *A Parent's Guide to Cleft Lip and Palate.* Minneapolis: University of Minnesota Press.

Videocassettes/Compact Discs for Parents

Feeding the Newborn with a Cleft Palate. Available from Hospital for Sick Children–Cleft Lip and Palate Program; 555 University Ave.; Toronto, Ontario M5G1X8; Canada. (416) 813-7490; fax: (416) 813-6637.

Feeding Your Baby. Available from Cleft Palate Foundation; 1504 East Franklin St., Suite 102; Chapel Hill, NC 27514. (800) 24-CLEFT.

Teasing and How to Stop It. Available from British Columbia's Children's Hospital; 4480 Oak St.; Vancouver, BC V6H 3V4; Canada. (604) 875-2345.

Understanding Cleft Lip and Palate—A Guide for New Parents. Excellent videotape for new parents in the nursery; free and in English and Spanish. Available from Foundation for Faces of Children; 258 Harvard St., #367; Brookline, MA 02446.

Summary of Primary Care Needs for the Child with Cleft Lip and Palate

HEALTH CARE MAINTENANCE

Growth and Development

- Expectations for physical growth and development are the same as those for the noncleft population.
- Syndromic clefts may be associated with poor growth and developmental delay.

Diet

- Use of squeeze bottle, cleft palate nurser, or special nipples enhances bottle feeding. Provision of expressed breast milk with use of an electric pump is desirable in infants with cleft palate.
- Introduction of solids by spoon is possible at the same time as in unaffected infants.
- Gummy or sticky foods or foods that can cause choking should be avoided.

Safety

- Elbow splints are needed following surgical procedures to prevent baby's hands from disrupting repaired lip or palate.
- Avoidance of utensils, straws, and textured foods is recommended for approximately 2 weeks after surgical procedures to allow for nontraumatic oral healing.
- Contact sports should be avoided for 6 weeks after surgeries.
- Prone positioning for infants with Pierre Robin sequence may require car safety bed vs. car seat.

Immunizations

- All routine immunizations should be given on schedule.
- May elect not to administer DTaP within 72 hours of a surgical procedure and MMR/varicella 1 week before a surgery.

- Administer pneumococcal vaccine as additional protective effect in preventing otitis media.
- RSV immunoprophylaxis for children with Pierre Robin sequence under age 2 years.

Screening

- *Vision.* Routine screening is recommended. Children with isolated cleft palate or Pierre Robin sequence need a dilated eye examination by a pediatric ophthalmologist at 1 year of age and 4 to 5 years of age to rule out myopia, which is found in Stickler syndrome.
- *Hearing.* Audiology screening for children with cleft lip and alveolus is recommended with the same guidelines as for the unaffected population. Ongoing close monitoring for conductive hearing loss in children with cleft palate is required because of eustachian tube dysfunction.
- *Dental.* Screening for early childhood caries is important to preserve dentition and prevent alveolar bone loss. Routine pediatric dental care is given for children with cleft lip. In addition, children with cleft alveolus and palate need an orthodontic evaluation by age 5 to 7 years.
- *Blood pressure.* Routine screening is recommended.
- *Hematocrit.* Routine screening is recommended.
- *Urinalysis.* Routine screening is recommended.
- *Tuberculosis.* Routine screening is recommended.

COMMON ILLNESS MANAGEMENT

Differential Diagnosis

- *Fever.* Rule out acute otitis media. Chronic serous otitis media or recurrent acute otitis media must be aggressively treated.
- *Drug interactions.* There are no drug interactions.

Continued

Summary of Primary Care Needs for the Child with Cleft Lip and Palate—cont'd

DEVELOPMENTAL ISSUES

Sleep Patterns

- Unilateral cleft lip and palate and deviated septum result in noisy breathing, especially with upper respiratory infection.
- There is an increased risk of sleep state obstructive apnea following secondary palatal surgical procedures.
- Disruption of sleep patterns may occur following surgical procedures and hospitalization.
- Signs of sleep state obstructive apnea require careful pulmonary evaluation and management in infants with Pierre Robin sequence.

Toileting

- Temporary regression may occur following surgical procedure and hospitalization.

Discipline

- Discipline expectations are normal, with allowances during hospitalizations and 1 to 2 weeks after surgery.
- Overprotectiveness or lack of limit setting may result if family pities child.

Child Care

- Child care may need to be in a smaller group setting during winter months because of increased risk of otitis media.
- Speech therapy sessions need to be coordinated with child care arrangements.

Schooling

- Speech therapy may begin at age 3 years for children with cleft palate, and they require an Individualized Educational Program (IEP). They may also require assistance with expressive language development.

- Peer teasing may negatively affect performance.
- Teasing may occur because of lip, nose, and dentition appearance or speech articulation problems.

Sexuality

- Genetic counseling is recommended to discuss recurrence risks.
- It is recommended that women of childbearing age take folic acid in an attempt to reduce recurrence risk of clefts.
- During pregnancy a detailed level 2 ultrasound is available for women affected with a cleft condition to ascertain whether the fetus has a cleft lip.

Transition to Adulthood

- Treatment plan should be completed by age 21 years.
- There is difficulty in procuring third-party payment for any orthodontic, oral-maxillofacial, or plastic surgical services in adulthood.

FAMILY CONCERNS

- There is heightened awareness of physical appearance.
- Presurgical photographs are important.
- Speech, audiology, and dental issues are challenging for families.
- Orthodontic treatment may span over 10 years.
- Cultural superstitions are common regarding the etiology of clefts.
- Multiple surgical procedures during childhood are stressful for families.

REFERENCES

American Academy of Pediatrics (AAP), American Academy of Family Physicians (AAFP), Subcommittee on Management of Acute Otitis Media. (2004). Diagnosis and management of acute otitis media. *Pediatrics, 113,* 1451-1465.

American Academy of Pediatrics (AAP) Committee on Infectious Diseases (2006). In L.K.Pickering (Ed.), *Red Book: 2006 Report of the Committee on Infectious Diseases* (27th ed). Elk Grove, IL: Author.

American Cleft Palate–Craniofacial Association. (2004). *Parameters for Evaluation and Treatment of Patients with Cleft Lip/Palate or Other Craniofacial Anomalies.* Official publication of the American Cleft Palate–Craniofacial Association (rev. ed.). Chapel Hill, NC: Author.

Anderson, K.D., Cole, A., Chuo, C.B., et al. (2007). Home management of upper airway obstruction in Pierre Robin sequence using a nasopharyngeal airway. *Cleft Palate Craniofac J, 44*(3), 269-273.

Aniansson, G., Svensson, H., Becker, M., et al. (2002). Otitis media and feeding with breast milk of children with cleft palate. *Scand J Plast Reconstr Surg Hand Surg, 36*(1), 9-15.

Arosarena, O. (2007). Cleft lip and palate. *Otolaryngol Clin North Am, 40,* 27-60.

Bender, P.L. (2000). Genetics of cleft lip and palate. *J Pediatr Nurs, 15,* 242-249.

Bennett, S., & Indman, P. (2006). *Beyond the Blues: A Guide to Understanding and Treating Prenatal and Postpartum Depression.* San Jose, CA: Moodswings Press.

Bluestone, C.D. (2004). Studies in otitis media: Children's Hospital of Pittsburgh–University of Pittsburgh progress report—2004. *Laryngoscope, 114,* 1-26.

Boekelheide, A., Curtin, G., Ursich, C., et al. (1992). *Comparison of postsurgical feeding techniques following cleft lip repair on suture line integrity, volume of oral fluid intake and length of hospital stay: A multicenter study.* Presented at the American Cleft Palate–Craniofacial Association Annual Meeting, Portland, OR.

Carbonell, R., & Ruiz-Garcia, V. (2002). Ventilation tubes after surgery for otitis media with effusion or acute otitis media and swimming. Systematic review and meta-analysis. *Int J Pediatr Otorhinolaryngol, 66*(3), 281-289.

Centers for Disease Control and Prevention, National Center on Birth Defects and Developmental Disabilities. (n.d.). *Birth defects: Frequently asked questions.* Available at www.cdc.gov/ncbddd/bd/faq1.htm. Retrieved January 15, 2009.

Charkins, H. (1996). *Children with Facial Differences: A Parent's Guide.* Bethesda, MD: Woodbine House.

Cheng, L., Moor, S., & Ho, C. (2007). Predisposing factors to dental caries in children with cleft lip and palate: A review and strategies for early prevention. *Cleft Palate Craniofac J, 44*(1), 67-72.

Committee on Infectious Diseases & Committee on Fetus and Newborn. (2003). Policy statement revised indications for the use of palivizumab and respiratory syncytial virus immune globulin intravenous for the prevention of respiratory syncytial virus infections. *Pediatrics, 112*(6), 1442-1446.

Craven, C., Cole, P., Hollier, L., et al. (2007). Ensuring success in alveolar bone grafting: A three-dimensional approach. *J Craniofac Surg, 18*(4), 855-859.

Curtin, G. (1990). The infant with cleft lip or palate: More than a surgical problem. *J Perinat Neonatal Nurs, 3,* 80-89.

Daskalogiannakis, J., Ross, R., & Tompson, B. (2001). The mandibular catch-up growth controversy in Pierre Robin sequence. *Am J Orthod Dentofacial Orthop, 120*(3), 280-285.

Endriga, M.C., & Kapp-Simon, K.A. (1999). Psychological issues in craniofacial care, state of the art. *Cleft Palate Craniofac J, 36*(1), 3-11.

Goldstein, N.A., Mandel, E.M., Kurs-Lasky, M., et al. (2005). Water precautions and tympanostomy tubes: A randomized, controlled trial. *Laryngoscope, 115*(2), 324-330.

Good, P., Mulliken, J., & Padwa, B. (2007). Frequency of Le Fort I osteotomy after repaired cleft lip and palate or cleft palate. *Cleft Palate Craniofac J, 44*(4), 396-401.

Gorlin, R.Y., Cohen, M.M., & Hennekam, R.C. (2001). Orofacial clefting syndromes: General aspects. In R.Y. Gorlin, M.M. Cohen, & R.C. Hennekam, (Eds.), *Syndromes of the Head and Neck* (4th ed.). New York: Oxford University Press.

Gungor, A., & Bluestone, C.D. (2001). Antibiotic theory in otitis media. *Curr Allergy Asthma Rep, 1*(4), 364-372.

Henningsson, G., Kuehn, D., Sell, D., et al. (2008). Universal parameters for reporting speech outcomes in individuals with cleft palate. *Cleft Palate Craniofac J, 45*(1), 1-17.

Hunt, O., Burden, D., Hepper, P., et al. (2006). Self-reports of psychosocial functioning among children and young adults with cleft lip and palate. *Cleft Palate Craniofac J, 43*(5), 598-605.

Jones, K.L. (2006). *Smith's Recognizable Patterns of Human Malformation.* (6th ed.). Philadelphia: Elsevier Saunders.

Jones, M.C. (2002). Prenatal diagnosis of cleft lip and palate: Detection rates, accuracy of ultrasonography, associated anomalies, and strategies for counseling. *Cleft Palate Craniofac J, 39*(2), 169-173.

Klein, T., Pope, A., Getahun, E., et al. (2006). Mothers' reflections on raising a child with a craniofacial anomaly. *Cleft Palate Craniofac J, 43*(5), 590-597.

Koul, R. (2007). Describing cleft lip and palate using a new expression system. *Cleft Palate Craniofac J, 44*(6), 595-597.

Kramer, F., Baethge, C., Swennen, G., et al. (2005). Dental implants in patients with orofacial clefts: A long-term follow-up study. *Int J Oral Maxillofac Surg, 34*(7), 715-721.

Livingstone, V.H., Willis, C.E., Abdel-Wareth, L.O., et al. (2000). Neonatal hypernatremic dehydration associated with breast-feeding malnutrition: A retrospective survey. *Can Med Assoc J, 162*(5), 647-652.

Lorenz, H., & Longaker, M. (2003). In utero surgery for cleft lip/palate: Minimizing the "ripple effect" of scarring. *J Craniofac Surg, 14*(4), 504-511.

Lous, J., Burton, M.J., Felding, J.U., et al. (2005). Grommets (ventilation tubes) for hearing loss associated with otitis media with effusion in children. *Cochrane Database of Systematic Reviews, Issue 1.* Art. no: CD0011801. DOI: 10.1002/14651858. CD001801.pub2.

Masarei, A., Wade, A., Mars, M., et al. (2007). A randomized control trial investigating the effect of presurgical orthopedics on feeding in infants with cleft lip and/or palate. *Cleft Palate Craniofac J, 44*(2), 182-193.

Millard, T., & Richman, L.C. (2001). Different cleft conditions, facial appearance, and speech: Relationship to psychological variables. *Cleft Palate Craniofac J, 38*(1), 68-75.

Moller, K.T., Starr, C.D., & Johnson, S.A. (1990). *A Parent's Guide to Cleft Lip and Palate.* Minneapolis: University of Minnesota Press.

Monasterio, F.O., Drucker, M., Molina, F., et al. (2002). Distraction osteogenesis in Pierre Robin sequence and related respiratory problems in children. *J Craniofac Surg, 13,* 79-83.

Mulliken, J. (2004). The changing faces of children with cleft lip and palate. *N Engl J Med, 351*(8), 745-747.

Muntz, H.R. (1993). An overview of middle ear disease in cleft palate children. *Facial Plast Surg, 9,* 177-180.

Muntz, H.R., Wilson, M., Park, A., et al. (2008). Sleep disordered breathing and obstructive sleep apnea in the cleft population. *Laryngoscope, 118,* 348-353.

Murray, J.C. (2002). Gene/environment causes of cleft lip and/or palate. *Clin Genet, 61*(4), 248-256.

Oberoi, S., Chigurupati, R., & Vargervik, K. (2008). Morphologic and management characteristics of individuals with unilateral cleft lip and palate who require maxillary advancement. *Cleft Palate Craniofac J, 45*(1), 42-49.

Overturf, G.D. (2000). American Academy of Pediatrics Committee on Infectious Diseases technical report: Prevention of pneumococcal infections, including the use of pneumococcal conjugate and polysaccharide vaccines and antibiotic prophylaxis. *Pediatrics, 106,* 367-376.

Paradise, J.L., Elster, B.A., & Tan, L. (1994). Evidence in infants with cleft palate that breast milk protects against otitis media. *Pediatrics, 94,* 853-860.

Peterson-Falzone, S., Hardin-Jones, M., & Karnell, M. (2001). *Cleft Palate Speech* (3rd ed.). St. Louis: Mosby.

Prahl, C., Kuijpers-Jagtman, A., Van't Hof, M., et al. (2005). Infant orthopedics in UCLP: Effect on feeding, weight, and length: A randomized clinical trial (Dutchcleft). *Cleft Palate Craniofac J, 42*(2), 171-177.

Prescott, N.J., Natalie, J., & Malcolm, S. (2002). Folate and the face: Evaluating the evidence for the influence of folate genes on craniofacial development. *Cleft Palate Craniofac J, 39*(3), 327-331.

Reilly, S., Reid, J., Skeat, J., & Academy of Breastfeeding Medicine Clinical Protocol Committee. (2007). ABM protocols. *Breastfeeding Med, 2*(2), 243-248.

Romitti, P., Sun, L., Honein, M., et al. & National Birth Defects Prevention Study. (2007). Maternal periconceptional alcohol consumption and risk of orofacial clefts. *Am J Epidemiol, 166*(7), 775-785.

Sidman, J.D., Sampson, D., & Templeton, B. (2001). Distraction osteogenesis of the mandible for airway obstruction in children. *Laryngoscope, 111,* 1137-1146.

Sie, K.C., Tampakopoulou, D.A., Sorom, J., et al. (2001). Results with Furlow palatoplasty in management of VPI. *Plast Reconstr Surg, 108,* 17-25.

Smith, M.C., & Senders, C.W. (2006). Prognosis of airway obstruction and feeding difficulty in the Robin sequence. *Int J Pediatr Otorhinolaryngol, 70*(2), 319-324.

Stanier, P., & Moore, G. (2004). Genetics of cleft lip and palate: Syndromic genes contribute to the incidence of non-syndromic clefts. *Hum Mol Genet, 13*(review issue 1), 73-81.

St. Hilaire, H., & Buchbinder, D. (2000). Maxillofacial pathology and management of Pierre Robin sequence. *Otolaryngol Clin North Am, 33*(6), 1241-1258.

Strauss, R.P. (2001). "Only skin deep": Health, resilience, and craniofacial care. *Cleft Palate Craniofac J, 38*(3), 226-230.

Tonni, G., Centini, G., & Rosignoli, L. (2005). Prenatal screening for fetal face and clefting in a prospective study on low risk population: Can 3- and 4-dimensional ultrasound enhance visualization and detection rate? *OOOOE, 100,* 420-426.

Valtonen, H., Dietz, A., & Qvarnberg, Y. (2005). Long-term clinical, audiologic, and radiologic outcomes in palate cleft children treated with early tympanostomy for otitis media with effusion: A controlled prospective study. *Laryngoscope, 115*(8), 1512-1516.

Vieira, A. (2008). Unraveling human cleft lip and palate research. *J Dent Res, 87*(2), 119-125.

Wagner, W., & Harrison, M.R. (2002). Fetal operations in the head and neck area: Current state. *Head Neck, 24*(5), 482-490.

Willner, J.P. (2000). Genetic evaluation and counseling in head and neck syndromes. *Otolaryngol Clin North Am, 33*(6), 1159-1169.

Wittenborn, W., Panchal, J., Marsh, J.L., et al. (2004). Neonatal distraction surgery for micrognathia reduces obstructive apnea and the need for tracheostomy. *J Craniofac Surg, 15*(4), 623-630.

Ysunza, A., Pamplona, M.C., Mendoza, M., et al. (2001). Surgical treatment of submucous cleft palate: A comparative trial of two modalities for palatal closure. *Plast Reconstr Surg, 107*(1), 9-14.

Zim, S. (2007). Treatment of upper airway obstruction in infants with micrognathia using mandibular distraction osteogenesis. *Facial Plastic Surg, 23*(2), 107-112.

20 Congenital Adrenal Hyperplasia

Angelique M. Champeau

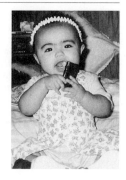

Etiology

Congenital adrenal hyperplasia (CAH) encompasses a family of autosomal recessive disorders involving impaired synthesis of cortisol from cholesterol by the adrenal cortex (New & Nimkarn, 2006; Stewart, 2003). The most common is 21-hydroxylase deficiency (21-OHD), accounting for 95% of all forms of CAH (Miller, 2002; Stewart, 2003). Other forms are rare and will not be discussed here.

The adrenal cortex synthesizes mineralocorticoids (mainly aldosterone), glucocorticoids (primarily cortisol), and androgens (male hormones) through three separate metabolic pathways (Figure 20-1). Cortisol, aldosterone, and adrenal androgens play a crucial role in maintaining homeostasis by helping to regulate the body's blood pressure; glucose, sodium, and water levels; sexual development; and other metabolic processes (New, 1995; New & Nimkarn, 2006; Speiser, 2001). Cortisol is particularly crucial in mediation of the body's response to stress.

Adrenal production of glucocorticoids is regulated by a feedback system to the hypothalamus and pituitary gland (Figure 20-2). The hypothalamus secretes corticotropin-releasing factor (CRF), which causes the pituitary gland to produce adrenocorticotropic hormone (ACTH), which in turn stimulates the adrenals to produce cortisol. Cortisol feeds back to the hypothalamus and pituitary, reducing release of CRH and ACTH and thus the level of adrenal stimulation. In CAH, the "block" at 21-hydroxylase leads to decreased cortisol production, which means less feedback and therefore ever-increasing stimulation of the adrenals by ACTH, causing hypertrophy of the gland. Since the androgen pathway is "upstream" of the block, androgens (dehydroepiandrosterone [DHEA], Δ^4-androstenedione) are overproduced.

In severe cases of CAH, where the 21-hydroxylase enzyme is completely—or nearly completely—inactive, these high levels of androgens lead to in utero virilization of females, causing them to be born with ambiguous genitalia (Figure 20-3). Males are generally normal in appearance. Without treatment in the first several weeks after birth, the lack of cortisol and aldosterone can result in salt loss, hypovolemic shock, and death—so-called adrenal crisis.

Classification

21-OHD CAH occurs in classic and nonclassic forms. In the classic form prenatal exposure to potent androgens such as testosterone and Δ^4-androstenedione at critical stages of sexual differentiation virilizes the external genitalia of genetic females, often resulting in genital ambiguity at birth. The classic form is further divided into the simple virilizing form (approximately 25%) and the

salt-wasting form, in which aldosterone production is inadequate (approximately 75%) (Stewart, 2003).

Individuals with the nonclassic form of 21-OHD CAH have only mild to moderate enzyme deficiency and postnatally have signs of hyperandrogenism; females with nonclassic form are not virilized at birth (Merke, Bornstein, Avila, et al., 2002; New & Nimkarn, 2006; Speiser, 2003; Stewart, 2003).

This classification system is somewhat arbitrary and even misleading in the sense that it suggests a qualitative difference among the groups. In reality, there is a continuum of severity, from mild to severe, based on the specific combination of 21-hydroxylase gene defects. The term "non–salt wasting" should be used with caution because it is now well appreciated that all affected children are salt wasters to some extent (Frisch, Battelino, Schober, et al., 2001). Neonatal mass screening is not sufficient for detecting nonclassic CAH, and most are found after puberty because of symptoms of androgen excess or in the course of family studies (Merke et al., 2002).

Genetic Etiology

CAH is an autosomal recessive disease—two defective genes must be inherited (one from the mother, one from the father) for the disease to become manifest. Most children with CAH are compound heterozygotes (Krone, Braun, Roscher, et al., 2000), having inherited a different mutation from each of their parents. If a "null" mutation is inherited from both parents the child will be severely affected (classic salt wasting). If two mild defects are inherited, the child will be mildly affected (nonclassic). Those that inherit a "null" mutation from one parent and a less severe mutation from the other will fall somewhere in between (Gunther & Bukowski, 1999; Miller, 1994).

The gene for adrenal 21-hydroxylase, *CYP 21A2*, and a pseudogene, *CYP 21A2p*, are located on chromosome 6p21.3 within the human leukocyte antigen (HLA) gene cluster and are about 30 kb apart (Forest, 2004; Miller, 2002; Stewart, 2003).

The major mechanism by which the active gene acquires defects is via transfer of segments from the pseudogene to the active gene. To date, approximately 100 different *CYP 21* mutations have been reported, mostly point mutations, but small deletions or insertions have also been described, as well as complete gene deletions and complex rearrangements of the gene (Forest, 2004).

No other phenotypes are known to be associated with mutations in *CYP 21A2* (Nimkarn & New, 2007).

Parents

Most parents are heterozygotes with one normal allele and one mutated allele. Heterozygotes are asymptomatic but may have slightly elevated 17-hydroxyprogesterone (17-OHP) levels when stimulated with ACTH, as compared with individuals with two

*The author gratefully ackowledges the contribution of Betty Flores and Judy Ruble, the authors of this chapter in previous editions.

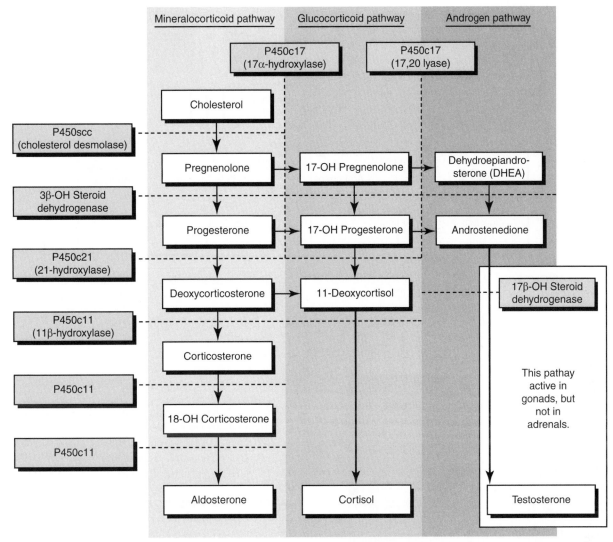

FIGURE 20-1 Adrenal steroid pathway for mineralocorticoids, glucocorticoids, and androgens. From Gunther, D.G., & Bukowski, T.P. (1999). Congenital adrenal hyperplasia: A spectrum of disorders. *Contemp Urol, 11*(1), 54. Reprinted with permission.

normal alleles. Approximately 1% of mutations occur de novo, and thus 1% of affected children have only one parent who is heterozygous (Krone et al., 2000). In some instances, a parent who was previously not known to be affected may be found to have the nonclassic form of 21-OHD CAH. It is appropriate to evaluate both parents with molecular genetic testing and hormonal profiling to determine if either has nonclassic 21-OHD CAH.

Siblings

If the parents of an affected child are both heterozygotes, each sibling has a 25% chance of inheriting both altered alleles and being affected, a 50% chance of inheriting one altered allele and being an unaffected carrier, and a 25% chance of inheriting both normal alleles and being unaffected. Once an at-risk sibling is known to be unaffected, the risk of his or her being a carrier is two thirds. If one parent is heterozygous and the other has 21-OHD CAH, each sibling has a 50% chance of inheriting both mutated alleles and being affected and a 50% chance of inheriting one mutated allele and being a carrier.

Offspring of an Affected Individual

An affected individual transmits one disease-causing allele to each child. Given the high carrier rate for 21-OHD CAH, it is appropriate to offer molecular genetic testing of the *CYP21A2* gene to the reproductive partner of an affected individual. If the reproductive partner is determined not to be a carrier, the prospective child is at significantly decreased risk of having 21-OHD.* If the reproductive partner is determined to be heterozygous for an identified mutation, the risk to each prospective child of being affected is 50%.

Carrier Detection

Carrier testing using molecular genetic testing of the *CYP21A2* gene is available to at-risk relatives when one or both disease-causing mutations have been identified in the affected individual.

---

*Since targeted mutation analysis does not detect 100% of altered alleles, there is a slight residual risk that the reproductive partner may carry a mutant allele that might be detected if the entire gene had been sequenced.

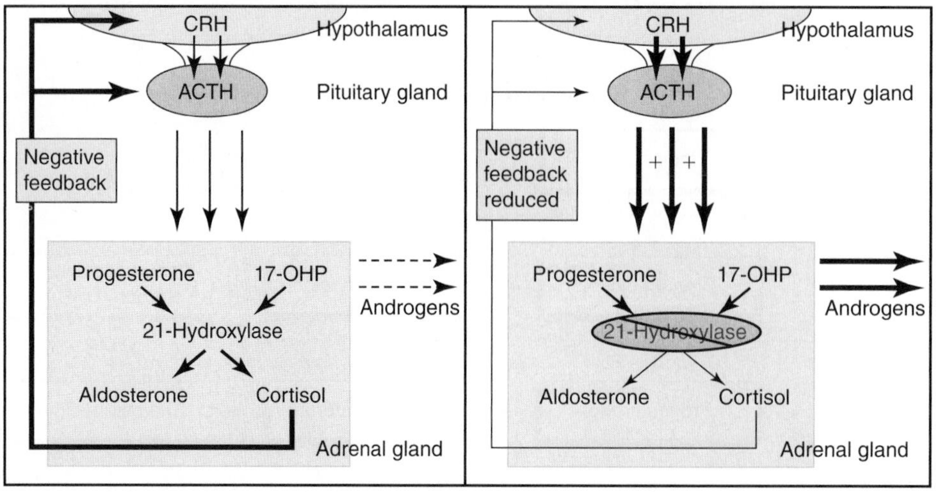

Normal Adrenal Feedback   **Disordered Feedback in CAH**

FIGURE 20-2 Hypothalamic/pituitary/adrenal feedback loop in normal subjects and in those with CAH. Note that in CAH corticotropin-releasing hormone (CRH) and adenocorticotropic hormone (ACTH) are increased because of decreased cortisol feedback. This leads to adrenal gland hypertrophy and a buildup of "upstream" steroids—progesterone and 17-hydroxyprogesterone (17-OHP), which are then shunted toward androgen production.

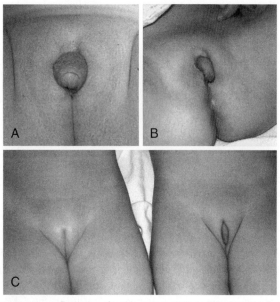

FIGURE 20-3 Examples of ambiguous genitalia in **(A)** a female infant with CAH, and **(B)** a toddler with CAH. **C,** 3-year-old fraternal twins, one with CAH and the other unaffected, highlight the difference in clitoral development.

Incidence and Prevalence

Classic 21-Hydroxylase Congenital Adrenal Hyperplasia

Analysis of data from almost 6.5 million newborns worldwide has demonstrated an overall incidence of 1:15,000 live births for the classic form of 21-OHD (Pang & Shook, 1997). This was confirmed in Texas through screening of 1.9 million newborns (Therrell, Berenbaum, Manter-Kapanke, et al., 1998), where the incidence was found to be

1:16,000. The breakdown ethnically was 1:15,600 whites, 1:14,500 Hispanics (primarily Mexican American), and 1:42,300 blacks[*] (Miller, 2002). More recently, estimates based on case surveys have varied from 1:12,099 to 1:23,044, except in Asian countries where it is 1:43,764 (Forest, 2004). Two populations, the Yupik Eskimos (Alaska) at 1:282 and the people of La Réunion (France) at 1:2141, have been reported with higher than usual frequency (Forest, 2004).

Nonclassic 21-Hydroxylase Congenital Adrenal Hyperplasia

Nonclassic 21-OHD CAH is much more common, but the data are more variable. It is estimated that nonclassic CAH is the most common autosomal recessive disease in humans (Levine, 2000). The prevalence of nonclassic 21-OHD CAH in the general heterogeneous population of New York City was estimated to be 1:100 (Miller, 2002). Furthermore, the nonclassic prevalence was broken down and found to vary depending on ethnic background: 1:27 among Ashkenazi Jews, 1:53 among Hispanics, 1:63 among Yugoslavs, 1:333 among Italians, and 1:1000 for other Caucasians (Forest, 2004). Other studies have shown carrier rates of 1.2% to 6% for white populations (Miller, 2002).

Diagnostic Criteria

A diagnosis of 21-OHD should be considered in any newborn infant who has genital ambiguity, salt wasting, or hypotension (Stewart, 2003).

A multidisciplinary team of specialists in pediatric endocrinology, pediatric urology, medical genetics, and psychology is essential for the diagnosis and management of the individual with ambiguous genitalia (Hughes, 2007).

---

[*]Because about 20% of the black (African American) gene pool is of European descent, the calculated incidence in individuals of wholly African ancestry is about 1:250,000 (Miller, 2002).

The evaluation of an infant with ambiguous genitalia includes a complete history, a physical examination, a reliable ultrasound of the internal genitalia and adrenals, and a genitogram; however, the diagnosis of 21-OHD CAH is made by biochemical findings.

17-Hydroxyprogesterone

Newborns with either form of classic CAH will have significantly elevated 17-hydroxyprogesterone (17-OHP) levels by 24 to 36 hours of age. False-positive results are possible in premature or low birth weight infants; therefore, in these infants, serial measurements of 17-OHP may be necessary (New & Nimkarn, 2006; Pang & Shook, 1997).

Plasma Renin

Plasma renin activity (PRA) is markedly elevated in individuals with salt-wasting 21-OHD and can also be elevated in some with simple virilizing 21-OHD. Direct measurement of active renin can also be used. In salt-wasting 21-OHD, the serum concentration of aldosterone is inappropriately low compared with the degree of PRA elevation.

Other Adrenal Steroids

Δ^4-Androstenedione and progesterone are increased in males and females. Serum concentrations of testosterone and adrenal androgen precursors are increased in affected females and prepubertal males.

ACTH Stimulation Test

The serum concentration of 17-OHP and Δ^4-androstenedione measured at baseline and at 60 minutes after intravenous administration of a standard bolus of synthetic ACTH are plotted on a nomogram. Although the ACTH stimulation test provides far more reliable diagnosis of 21-OHD CAH than a test of baseline values alone, the results must be confirmed with molecular genetic testing (New & Nimkarn, 2006).

Electrolytes

Children with untreated or poorly controlled salt-wasting CAH may have decreased levels of sodium, chloride, and carbon dioxide; increased potassium; and an inappropriately increased urine concentration of sodium.

Karyotype

Females have normal 46,XX and males have normal 46,XY chromosomes.

Molecular Genetic Testing

Molecular genetic analysis is not essential for the diagnosis but may be helpful to confirm the basis of the defect, carrier testing, prenatal testing, genotype/phenotype correlation for management, preimplantation genetic diagnosis, and to establish the diagnosis in uncertain cases (New & Nimkarn, 2006).

Genetic testing methods include targeted mutation analysis, deletion/duplication analysis, and sequence analysis. In targeted mutation analysis testing of the *CYP21A2* gene is done for a panel of common mutations and gene deletions. This detects 80% to 98% of disease-causing alleles in affected individuals (Koppens, Hoogenboezem, & Degenhart, 2002; Krone et al., 2000; Mao, Nelson, Kates, et al., 2002). Deletion/duplication analysis detects about 20% of mutant alleles (White & New, 1988) and uses Southern blot analysis to detect large deletions. Last, entire gene sequencing (sequence analysis) may detect rare alleles not detected by targeted mutation analysis or deletion/duplication analysis (New & Nimkarn, 2006).

Genotype-Phenotype Correlations

A strong correlation between the severity of the clinical disease and the mutation is generally observed. However, for reasons that are not understood, genotype does not always predict phenotype within mutation-identical groups or even within the same family (Forest, 2004; Miller, 2002; New & Nimkarn, 2006) (Box 20-1).

Prenatal Screening

As of December, 2008, all 50 states within the United States, as well as Washington, D.C., and Guam, are screening for CAH at birth (National Newborn Screening and Genetics Resource Center, 2008). Additionally, half of all Canadian provinces include CAH testing in their newborn screening programs.

Neonatal mass screening for 21-OHD identifies both male and female affected infants, prevents incorrect sex assignment, and decreases mortality and morbidity rates; therefore newborn screening for CAH is beneficial and is recommended (Clayton, Miller, Oberfield, et al., 2002; Speiser, 2007).

Newborn screening is sufficiently specific and sensitive to detect almost all infants with classic CAH and some infants with nonclassic CAH. Sampling of blood spots should be performed, ideally between 48 and 72 hours of age, and sent to the screening laboratory without delay. At present, direct binding assays for blood-spot 17-OHP are the only practical method for screening. The concentration of 17-OHP is measured on a filter paper blood-spot sample obtained by the heel-stick technique as used for newborn screening for other disorders (Pang & Shook, 1997; Speiser, 2007).

The cost of screening is estimated to be about $20,000 per quality-adjusted life-year per case of CAH diagnosed, which is considered reasonable (Caroll & Downs, 2006). Case studies conducted retrospectively in the United Kingdom revealed a 4:1 predominance of females to males, suggesting that males are dying

---

BOX 20-1

Evaluations at Initial Diagnosis to Establish the Extent of Disease

To assess for salt wasting:
- Plasma renin activity (PRA) or direct renin assay
- Serum electrolytes

To distinguish classic and nonclassic forms of 21-OHD CAH:
- Baseline 17-OHP, Δ^4-androstenedione, cortisol, and aldosterone
- ACTH stimulation test to compare stimulated concentration of 17-OHP to the baseline level

To assess the degree of prenatal virilization in females:
- Careful physical examination of the external genitalia and its orifices
- Genitogram* to assess the anatomy of urethra, vagina, common urogenital sinus (high vs. low confluence)

To assess the degree of postnatal virilization in both males and females:
- Bone maturation assessment by bone age
- Serum concentration of adrenal androgens (unconjugated dehydroepiandrosterone [DHEA], Δ^4-androstenedione, and testosterone)

*A genitogram is a radiologic procedure that can help identify internal genital structures, as well as define the level of the confluence (location where the urethra and vagina connect) of the common urogenital sinus in virilized females. If the confluence is closer to the bladder ("high"), the surgery to correct will be more complicated; if the confluence is closer to the perineum ("low"), the surgery will be less complicated.

in infancy when screening is not implemented (Nordenström, Ahmed, Jones, et al., 2005). The infant mortality rate for CAH is estimated at about 3% of diagnosed cases.

Only laboratories with excellent internal and external quality control, demonstrated accuracy, and a rapid turnaround time on a large number of samples should be used. The laboratory should report immediately any abnormal result to the practitioner responsible for the patient. A positive screening result needs to be confirmed.

There are potential false screening results. Samples taken in the first 24 hours of life are elevated in all infants and may give false positives (Allen, Hoffman, Fitzpatrick, et al., 1997; Therrell et al., 1998). In addition, a false positive may occur in premature or in low birth weight infants (Allen et al., 1997). Conversely, false negatives may occur in neonates receiving dexamethasone for management of unrelated problems.

Clinical Manifestations at Time of Diagnosis

The diagnosis of 21-OHD CAH is suspected in females who are virilized at birth (Figure 20-4), who become virilized postnatally, or who have precocious puberty or adrenarche. In males, CAH is suspected with virilization in childhood and in infants of either sex with a salt-wasting crisis in the first 4 weeks of life (New & Nimkarn, 2006).

Classic Simple Virilizing

Excess adrenal androgen production in utero results in genital virilization at birth in 46,XX females. In affected females the excess androgens result in varying degrees of enlargement of the clitoris, fusion of the labial scrotal folds, and formation of a common urogenital sinus (CUGS). A CUGS occurs when the vagina, because of internal fusion with the urethra, does not extend all the way to the perineum. In males, antimüllerian hormone (AMH) is secreted by the testicles, preventing the development of internal female reproductive organs. In CAH, there is no AMH secretion, and the müllerian ducts develop normally into the uterus and fallopian tubes. The examiner cannot differentiate between simple virilizing classic and salt-wasting classic CAH based on degree of virilization at birth.

After birth, both males and females with classic simple CAH who do not receive glucocorticoid replacement therapy develop signs of androgen excess such as precocious development of pubic and axillary hair, acne, rapid linear growth, and advanced bone age. Untreated males have progressive penile enlargement and small testes. Untreated females have clitoral enlargement, hirsutism, male pattern baldness, menstrual abnormalities, and reduced fertility.

Clinical Manifestations at Time of Diagnosis

CLASSIC
Virilization
- Elevated 17-OHP (hydroxyprogesterone)

Electrolyte instability
- Vomiting, dehydration
- Failure to thrive
- Metabolic alkalosis

Adrenal crisis

NONCLASSIC
Female: virilization
Male: early beard browth, enlarged hallus with small testes
Both: accelerated growth, advanced bone age, premature adrenarche

---

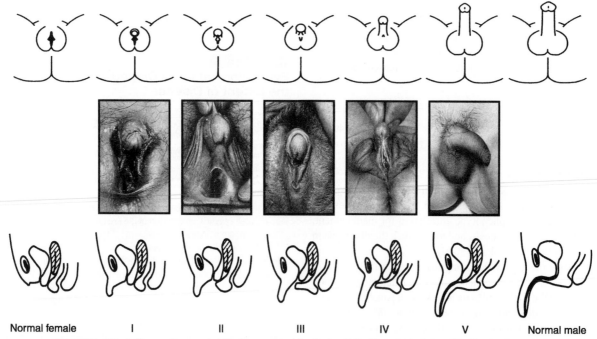

Normal female   I   II   III   IV   V   Normal male

FIGURE 20-4 The continuum of virilization proposed by Prader. Virilization ranges from mild clitoral enlargement (Prader I) to male-appearing phallus with penile urethra (Prader V). From Gunther, D., & Bukowski, T.P. (1999). Congenital adrenal hyperplasia: A spectrum of disorders. *Contemp Urol, 11*(1), 63. Reprinted with permission.

Classic Salt-Wasting Congenital Adrenal Hyperplasia

Infants with renal salt wasting have poor feeding, weight loss, failure to thrive, vomiting, dehydration, hypotension, and hyponatremic-hyperkalemic metabolic acidosis progressing to adrenal crisis (azotemia vascular collapse, shock, and death). Adrenal crisis can occur as early as age 1 to 4 weeks.

Affected males who are not detected in the newborn screening program are at high risk for a salt-wasting adrenal crisis because their normal genitalia do not alert medical professionals to their condition; they are often discharged from the hospital after birth without diagnosis and experience a salt-wasting crisis at home. Conversely, the ambiguous genitalia of females with salt-wasting form usually prompts diagnosis and treatment.

Nonclassic Congenital Adrenal Hyperplasia

Nonclassic 21-OHD CAH may manifest anytime postnatally with symptoms of androgen excess, including acne, premature pubic hair, accelerated growth, and advanced bone age. These children may have reduced adult stature as a result of premature epiphyseal fusion.

Females with nonclassic CAH are born with normal genitalia; postnatal symptoms may include hirsutism, temporal baldness, delayed menarche, menstrual irregularities, and infertility. Among adult females with nonclassic CAH, about 60% have hirsutism only, about 10% have hirsutism and menstrual disorder, and 10% have menstrual disorder only. The fertility rate among untreated females is reported to be 50% (Pang, 1997). Many females with nonclassic forms develop polycystic ovaries.

Males with nonclassic CAH have early beard growth and enlarged phallus with relatively small testes.

Mildly reduced synthesis of cortisol is not clinically significant in nonclassic forms (Table 20-1).

Growth

The initial growth in a child with CAH is rapid; however, potential height is reduced from premature epiphyseal fusion. Even if cortical replacement therapy is started at an early age and secretion of excess androgens is controlled, individuals do not usually achieve expected adult height. Actual bone age remains advanced compared with chronologic bone age.

Pubertal Development

In males and females with proper therapy, onset of puberty usually occurs at appropriate chronologic age. However, even when well controlled there are exceptions. In some previously untreated children, the start of glucocorticoid replacement therapy triggers true precocious puberty. This central precocious puberty may occur when glucocorticoid treatment releases the hypothalamic pituitary axis from inhibition by estrogens derived from excess adrenal androgen secretion.

Fertility

Females may have issues with fertility because of elevated androgens leading to ovarian dysfunction.

In males the main cause of subfertility is presence of testicular adrenal rest tumors, which are thought to originate from aberrant adrenal tissue and to respond to treatment with glucocorticoids. Further, gonadotropic hypogonadism may result from suppression of luteinizing hormone (LH) secretion by the pituitary by excessive adrenal androgens and their aromatization product (Ogilvie, Crouch, Rumsby et al., 2006).

Classic deficiency of cortisol also affects the development and function of adrenal medulla resulting in lower epinephrine and metanephrine concentrations than those in unaffected individuals (Merke, Keil, Jones, et al., 2000).

Treatment
Classic Congenital Adrenal Hyperplasia

The goal of treatment of classic 21-OHD CAH is to replace deficient steroids while minimizing adrenal sex hormone and glucocorticoid excess, preventing virilization, optimizing growth, and

> **Treatment**
>
> *Classic*
> - Glucocorticoid replacement
> - Mineralocorticoids and sodium chloride replacement
> - Stress treatment
> - Genital surgery
> - Psychological assessment and support
>
> *Nonclassic*
> - Female: pregnancy

TABLE 20-1

Evaluation at Initial Diagnosis to Establish Extent of Condition

Age at Diagnosis	Newborn to 6 mo	Newborn to 2 yr (Female) 2-4 yr (Male)	Child to Adult
Genitalia	Males normal Females ambiguous	Males normal Females ambiguous	Males normal Females virilized
Incidence	1:20,000	1:60,000	1:1000
Hormones			
Aldosterone	Reduced	Normal	Normal
Renin	Increased	Normal or increased	Normal
Cortisol	Reduced	Reduced	Normal
17-OHP	>5000 nmol/L	2500-5000 nmol/L	500-2500 nmol/L (ACTH stimulation)
Growth	−2 to −3 SD	−1 to −2 SD	Probably normal
21-Hydroxylase Activity	0%	1%	20%-50%

protecting potential fertility (Clayton et al., 2002; Stewart, 2003). Treatment does not always mimic physiologic secretion and outcome is not always ideal.

Glucocorticoid Replacement. Treatment for CAH principally involves glucocorticoid replacement therapy, usually in the form of hydrocortisone. Glucocorticoid therapy for children involves balancing suppression of adrenal androgen secretion against iatrogenic Cushing syndrome to maintain a normal linear growth rate and normal bone maturation. During infancy, initial reduction of markedly elevated adrenal sex hormones may require higher dosing.

Excessive doses, especially during infancy, may cause persistent growth suppression, obesity, and other cushingoid features (Grumbach, Hughes, & Conte, 2003). Therefore complete adrenal suppression should be avoided. Insufficient data exist to recommend higher morning or evening dosages. Overtreatment resulting in cushingoid features often occurs when serum concentration of 17-OHP is reduced to the physiologic range for age. An acceptable range for serum concentration of 17-OHP in the treated individual is higher (100 to 1000 ng/dL) than normal, providing androgens are maintained in an appropriate range for gender and pubertal status.

Undertreatment will cause signs of adrenal insufficiency, impair the individual's response to stress, and lead to overproduction of adrenal androgens, which will hasten epiphyseal maturation and closure, thus compromising ultimate adult height (Grumbach et al., 2003).

During periods of stress (e.g., surgery, febrile illness, shock), all individuals with classic 21-OHD CAH require increased amounts of glucocorticoid. Typically, two to three times the normal dose is administered orally or by intramuscular (IM) injection when oral intake is not tolerated.

Affected individuals should carry medical information regarding emergency steroid dosing.

Individuals with classic 21-OHD CAH require lifelong administration of glucocorticoid. After linear growth is complete, a more potent glucocorticoid can be used (such as prednisone and dexamethasone). These should not be used in childhood because they tend to suppress growth. Prednisone and prednisolone need to be given twice daily. Prednisolone may be preferable, because this is the active drug. Monitoring of these more potent glucocorticoids should include blood pressure, in addition to weight, and other clinical and laboratory variables. These steroids have minimal mineralocorticoid effect, compared with hydrocortisone. In children with advanced bone age, such as in boys with non–salt-losing CAH, initiation of therapy may precipitate central precocious puberty, requiring treatment with a gonadotropin-releasing hormone (GnRH) agonist.

Mineralocorticoids and Sodium Chloride Replacement. Replacement therapy with mineralocorticoids is indicated for children with salt-losing CAH (Grumbach et al., 2003). All children with classic CAH should be treated with fludrocortisones at diagnosis in the newborn period. Dosage requirements in early infancy may be higher than typical maintenance doses. The dose depends on the sodium intake. Such therapy will reduce vasopressin and ACTH levels and lower the dosage of glucocorticoid required. The need for continuing mineralocorticoid should be assessed based on PRA and blood pressure. Sodium chloride supplements are often needed in infancy distributed in several feedings. Sodium chloride supplementation may not be necessary after infancy, and the amount of mineralocorticoid required daily may likewise decrease with age.

Monitoring Treatment for Classic Congenital Adrenal Hyperplasia. Monitoring may be accomplished based on physical and hormonal findings suggestive of excessive or inadequate steroid therapy. Laboratory measurements may include serum/plasma electrolytes, serum 17-OHP, androstenedione and/or testosterone, and PRA or direct renin, every 3 months during infancy and every 4 to 12 months thereafter. The time from the last glucocorticoid dose should be noted. The diurnal rhythm of the adrenal axis should be taken into account.

Children receiving adequate replacement therapy may have hormone levels above the normal range. Alternative measurements include urinary metabolites (pregnanetriol) or filter paper blood and salivary hormones. Ideally, laboratory data will indicate a need for dosage adjustments before physical changes, growth, and skeletal maturation indicate inadequate or excessive dosing.

Bone age to assess osseous maturation should be done at 6- to 12-month intervals.

Stress Treatment. Children with CAH should carry medical identification and information concerning therapy for stress. Caregivers should have an emergency supply of intramuscular hydrocortisone or glucocorticoid suppositories. Because circulating levels of cortisol normally increase during stress, children should be given increased doses of glucocorticoids during febrile illness (greater than 38.5°C [101°F]), when vomiting or when unable to take oral feedings, after trauma, and before surgery. Participation in endurance sports may also require extra steroid dosing. Evidence has not shown that individuals need increased dosing for mental and emotional stress, such as school examinations. Stress dosing should be two to three times the maintenance glucocorticoid dose for children able to take oral medications. Glucose concentrations should be monitored, and intravenous (IV) sodium and glucose replacement may be required.

Genital Surgery. Deciding when, what type, and even if genital surgery should be performed in infants with genital ambiguity is the subject of continuing debate. Some adults with disorders of sexual development (not specific to 21-OHD CAH) who are unhappy with their gender assignment, as well as some medical professionals, advocate postponing genital surgery until the affected individual is able to provide informed consent. Others advocate that all children should have genital surgery early in life in order to match their gender of rearing and obviate any gender dysphoria (Meyer-Bahlburg, Migeon, Berkovitz, et al., 2004; White & Speiser, 2000; Wilson & Reiner, 1998). With better surgical techniques (Pippi Salle, Braga, Macedo, et al., 2007; Poppas, Hochsztein, Baergen, et al., 2007; Rink, Metcalfe, Cain, et al., 2006), better knowledge of the neuroanatomy of the genitalia (Baskin, 2004), and further knowledge with regard to sexual function, the answer may lie somewhere in between these two views.

Unfortunately, current adult outcomes data are not particularly useful because the surgical techniques have changed.

It is important to remember that genital surgery is irreversible. Although concerns about undergoing irreversible genital surgery at a young age are valid, also valid are concerns regarding how families would accept raising a child with ambiguous genitalia and whether children reared in a gender not congruent with their external genitalia would be able to develop a clear gender identity.

Furthermore, each specific disorder of sexual differentiation has different levels of clarity with regard to future gender identity. Clinicians must be careful not to lump disorders of sexual development into one category when making decisions regarding genital surgery. For the purposes of this chapter we will only be discussing 21-OHD CAH, which is, as previously mentioned, not only the most common form of CAH, but is also the most common cause of ambiguous genitalia. Because males born with this condition have normal anatomy, we will only discuss virilized females with 21-OHD with regard to genital surgery.

In general, 46,XX females with 21-OHD CAH born with ambiguous genitalia grow up with a fairly consistent female gender identity. In these cases, current opinion would recommend genital surgery to repair the common urogenital sinus, and at the same time consider minor cosmetic surgery to "hide" an enlarged clitoris, preserving the erectile tissue and nerves of the clitoris. At a later date, adulthood or adolescence, individuals who find the enlarged clitoris to be functionally problematic or are not happy with its appearance can choose to have the clitoris reduced. At the same time, in adolescence or adulthood, the individual can choose to have vaginoplasty, if desired. In 2005, 50 different medical experts met to review the state of the science and to establish recommendations based on what little is known about children born with disorders of sexual differentiation (Lee, Houk, Ahmed, et al., 2006). Table 20-2 outlines these recommendations and others and includes only information specific to congenital adrenal hyperplasia.

The most difficult decision making lies with the 46,XX 21-OHD CAH females who are completely virilized (appear phenotypically male with bilateral undescended testicles). Though rare, these children have a much less clear course and outcome for two reasons: (1) despite prenatal screening, some infants/children may present at a later age, having been reared male since birth; and

---

TABLE 20-2

Evidence and Recommendations Regarding Genital Surgery for 46, XX 21-OHD CAH

Evidence	Recommendations
CLITORAL SURGERY AND REPAIR OF THE CUGS	
• Clitoral surgery affects orgasmic function and erectile sensation. • Outcomes from clitoroplasty identify problems related to decreased sexual sensitivity, loss of clitoral tissue, sexual function, and cosmetic issues (Creighton, 2004; Crouch et al., 2008; Minto et al., 2003; Warne, Grover, Hutson, et al., 2005; Yang, Felsen, & Poppas, 2007). • Parents now are less inclined to choose surgery for less severe clitoromegaly (Lee & Witchel, 2002). • Newer techniques preserve clitoral structures (Pippi Salle et al., 2007; Poppas et al., 2007; Rink et al., 2006). *These have not been tested.* • Anatomic studies describe the innervation of the clitoris (Baskin, 2004; Baskin, Erol, Li, et al., 1999; Yucel, De Souza, & Baskin, 2004).	• Emphasis should be on functional outcome rather than a strictly cosmetic appearance. • Surgery should only be considered in cases of severe virilization (Prader III-V) and be performed in conjunction with repair of the common urogenital sinus. • Genital surgery should be anatomically based to preserve erectile function and the innervation of the clitoris (Baskin, 2004). • Only surgeons with expertise in the care of children and specialty training in genital surgery should perform these procedures.
TIMING OF GENITAL SURGERY	
• According to the American Academy of Pediatrics, elective genital surgery should be performed in infancy. • Surgery between age 12 months and adolescence is not recommended in the absence of complications causing medical problems. *The basis for this statement is not clear.* • There are beneficial effects of estrogen on tissue in early infancy. • The recommended time for surgery is 2-6 months (Clayton et al., 2002). • Early surgery may avoid complications from connection between the urinary tract and the vagina, fallopian tubes. • Surgery in infancy is technically easier than at later stages. • There is inadequate evidence to stop the current practice of early separation of the vagina and urethra. • There is no evidence to support the common belief that surgery that is performed for cosmetic reasons in the first year of life relieves parental distress and improves attachment between the child and the parents.	• Early reconstruction of common urogenital sinus (CUGS) in infancy.
VAGINOPLASTY	
• Surgical reconstruction in infancy will need to be refined at the time of puberty. *This may change with newer surgical techniques.* • An absent or inadequate vagina (with rare exceptions) requires vaginoplasty. • No one vaginoplasty technique has been universally successful; self-dilation, skin substitution, and bowel vaginoplasty each have specific advantages and disadvantages. • There are no controlled clinical trials that show the efficacy of early (<12 months of age) versus late (in adolescence and adulthood) surgery. • Techniques for vaginoplasty carry the potential for scarring at the introitus, necessitating repeated modification before sexual function can be reliable. • Surgery to construct a neovagina may carry a risk of neoplasia (Steiner & Woernie, 2002).	• Vaginoplasty should be performed in adolescence when the patient is psychologically motivated and a full partner in the procedure. • Other than separation of the CUGS, further vaginoplasty should be postponed until adolescence or older. • Vaginal dilation should not be undertaken before puberty.

Data from Lee, P.A., Houk, G.P., Ahmed, S.F., et al. (2006). International Consensus Conference on Intersex. Consensus statement on management of intersex disorders. *Pediatrics, 118*(2), 488-499 or as noted.

(2) these individuals may have more gender identity issues than less virilized individuals (Woelfle, Hoepffner, Sippell, et al., 2002). These infants need to be assessed and addressed on a case-by-case basis with an experienced team of experts. Currently, there is insufficient evidence to support rearing Prader 5 (see Figure 20-4) as male. Consideration for sex reassignment must be undertaken only after performing a thorough psychological evaluation of patient and family, and any surgery should be undertaken after a period of endocrine treatment (Clayton et al., 2002).

Psychological Assessment and Support. Females with CAH show behavioral masculinization, most pronounced in gender role behavior, less so in sexual orientation, and rarely in gender identity. Even in females with psychosexual problems, general psychological adjustment seems to be similar to that of females without CAH. Although studies of women whose surgery was performed 20 to 30 years ago indicate a range of psychosexual difficulties (Crouch et al., 2008; Hagenfeldt, Janson, Holmdahl, et al., 2008; Minto et al., 2003), there is reason for optimism that outcomes will be better with current surgical and medical treatment.

Psychological assessment and support of the patient and his or her family should be a routine component of the comprehensive care and management of these patients. Parents and patients should be offered the option of age- and sex-appropriate psychological counseling at the time of the initial diagnosis. Counseling regarding sexual function, future surgeries, gender role, and issues related to living with a chronic disorder should be addressed.

Gender Role Assignments

Prenatal exposure to androgens correlates with a decrease in self-reported femininity by adult females, but not an increase in self-reported masculinity by adult females (Long, Wisniewski, & Migeon, 2004).

Changes in childhood play behavior correlate with reduced female gender satisfaction and reduced heterosexual interest in adulthood. In contrast, males with 21-OHD do not show an alteration in childhood play behavior or sexual orientation (Hines, Brook, & Conway, 2004).

Nonclassic Congenital Adrenal Hyperplasia

Individuals with nonclassic 21-OHD CAH do not always require treatment. Many are asymptomatic throughout their lives, or symptoms may develop during puberty, after puberty, or postpartum. Treatment is only recommended for symptomatic patients: those with an advanced bone age coupled with a poor height prediction (compared with the family target height), hirsutism, severe acne, menstrual irregularities, testicular masses, and (in the young adult) infertility (Degitz, Placzek, Arnold, et al., 2003).

Management of Women with Congenital Adrenal Hyperplasia in Pregnancy

Pregnant women with CAH should be monitored and delivered in a tertiary center equipped and experienced to handle such pregnancies. Glucocorticoids that do not cross the placenta, such as hydrocortisone and prednisolone, should be used. Dexamethasone should be avoided (except when used in prenatal therapy). Glucocorticoid doses should be adjusted to maintain maternal serum testosterone concentrations near the upper range of normal for pregnancy. When reconstructive surgery has been performed, elective cesarean section should be considered if there is risk to the genital tract.

When cesarean section is performed, dosage of hydrocortisone has to be increased before and tapered after delivery. A pediatrician should be present during delivery to take care of the newborn and to initiate diagnostic procedures when an affected child is expected according to the results of prenatal testing.

Complementary and Alternative Therapies

There are currently no known complementary or alternative therapies for the treatment of CAH.

Anticipated Advances in Diagnosis and Management

Prenatal Treatment

Prenatal treatment has been advocated for fetuses at risk for classic 21-OHD CAH. However, the appropriateness, ethics, and outcomes of the prenatal treatment of CAH remain controversial.

Based on more than 200 fetuses treated to term and more than 1000 partially treated fetuses, it is clear that early prenatal administration of dexamethasone decreases the genital ambiguity in all affected females and eliminates it in more than 85% (New, 2001; New, Carlson, Obeid, et al., 2003). No consistent untoward effects on the infants have been reported. The maternal complications of prenatal management are variable and include striae, weight gain, and edema (New & Nimkarn, 2006).

The controversy primarily lies with the fact that adrenal hormone secretion and genital differentiation begin at 7 to 8 weeks, before our current abilities to obtain diagnostic samples (about 10 to 12 weeks for chorionic villus sampling). Thus treatment must be started before the diagnosis has been made. As a consequence, seven out of eight pregnancies will be treated unnecessarily to prevent one case of virilized genitalia in an affected female. Furthermore, few treated fetuses have reached adulthood and long-term prospective studies have not been done. In addition, although glucocorticoids have not been shown to cause any congenital malformations in humans, animal studies have shown some adverse outcomes (Clayton et al., 2002; Hughes, 2006; Seckl & Miller, 1997; Speiser, 2007; Stewart, 2003).

Most researchers agree that the results to date are very good, but long-term safety has not yet been proven in patients treated to term or in the seven of eight fetuses in whom treatment is stopped because they are male or unaffected (Clayton et al., 2002; Speiser, 2007).

Prenatal treatment, at this time, is a research endeavor and should be undertaken by designated teams consisting of a pediatric endocrinologist, an expert in high-risk obstetrics, a genetic counselor, and a reliable molecular genetics laboratory following institutional review board (IRB)–approved protocols. Treatment is continued to term in the affected female fetus and discontinued in all other fetuses.

The treatment of seven out of eight fetuses who cannot be helped by prenatal treatment creates an ethical dilemma for which there is no clear answer, and parents should be aware of this.

Most important, prenatal therapy does not "cure" the disease; it merely allows for decreased virilization, obviating the need for surgery. Extensive review of the risks and benefits must be done with the family and informed consent must be obtained. As part of the consent process, families should be obligated to continue long-term follow-up whether they have CAH or not (New & Nimkarn, 2006).

Adrenalectomy in Congenital Adrenal Hyperplasia

Bilateral adrenalectomy by laparoscopy is effective in decreasing adrenal androgens and the likelihood of iatrogenic hypercortisolism (Clayton et al., 2002; Gmyrek, New, Sosa, et al., 2002; Van Wyk & Gunther, 1996; White & Speiser, 2000). Proponents believe it should be considered in severe cases where conventional therapy is failing, whereas others believe it is too radical a step.

Although some patients have been managed with adrenalectomy, further data are needed before deciding whether it is a viable therapeutic alternative. The procedure should only be carried out where long-term follow-up is secured, and in the form of ethically approved clinical studies. It should only be considered in severe cases that are refractory to standard treatment. Vigilance in maintaining regular substitution of hydrocortisone and fludrocortisone is mandatory, with prompt institution of stress dosages at the onset of illness. The patient must be monitored, throughout life, for activation of ectopic adrenal rest tissue (Clayton et al., 2002; New & Nimkarn, 2006; White & Speiser, 2000).

Corticotropin-Releasing Hormone Antagonists for Adrenal Suppression

Rat studies have shown that antalarmin effectively decreases ACTH and cortisol secretion without causing adrenal insufficiency. Adrenal size is reduced with chronic treatment, and it is well tolerated (Merke et al., 2002). The use of corticotropin-releasing hormone (CRH) antagonists in CAH is promising on theoretical grounds but awaits future investigation before CRH antagonists are applied to patient treatment. Further development of drugs with improved pharmacologic properties is needed (Clayton et al., 2002).

Aromatase Inhibitors and Antiandrogens

It was hypothesized that the deleterious effects of elevated androgens on adult height could be prevented by using an antiandrogen to block androgen action or an aromatase inhibitor to block conversion of androgen to estrogen. Aromatase inhibitors (medications that inhibit the conversion of androgens to estrogens) and antiandrogens (medications that block androgen receptors) used with lower-than-usual dosing of hydrocortisone and fludrocortisone have shown some benefit in short-term studies. Children receiving new treatment regimens had normalization of growth rate, normalization and slowing of bone maturation, and less weight gain at reduced glucocorticoid dosage. After 2 years there was further improvement in biochemistry studies.

However, no long-term safety data are available and reproductive effects are not known. Liver function must be monitored carefully (Clayton et al., 2002; Forest, 2004; Merke et al., 2000; Merke et al., 2002; White & Speiser, 2000). Considerations include the high cost and the difficulty for an average family to cope with administration of a complicated regimen.

Gene Therapy

Gene therapy is currently not possible in humans with this disorder. Gene therapy represents a potential cure for CAH, but achieving safe and effective methods has proven to be challenging. There is much deliberation about the ethical and moral issues involved with this research because current medical therapy, though imperfect, is effective and relatively inexpensive (Clayton et al., 2002).

Preimplantation genetic diagnosis for CAH is possible, but further research is required to determine its utility.

DHEA Replacement

CAH patients on glucocorticoid treatment have low DHEA levels. Studies in adult patients with Addison's disease have shown beneficial effects of DHEA replacement, but the relevance in CAH is unknown at this time (Clayton et al., 2002).

11 Beta-Hydroxysteroid Dehydrogenase Inhibitors

The 11 beta-hydroxysteroid dehydrogenase (11β-HSD) inhibitors may have potential to decrease the dose of glucocorticoids (i.e., hydrocortisone) needed for treatment of 21-OHD CAH. At present, its use is not recommended outside research, due to limited availability/knowledge of 11β-HSD inhibitors and significant adverse side effects (Clayton et al., 2002; Walker & Stewart, 2000; White & Speiser, 2000).

Growth Hormone Treatment

An acceptable height is achieved by many patients with CAH, and the mean adult height deficit is substantially less than previously thought (Eugster, Dimeglio, Wright, et al., 2001). Regardless, some CAH patients fail to reach normal adult height. A small group of short CAH patients were treated with growth hormone (GH) for 2 years, either alone or in combination with a GnRH agonist, and there was significantly improved growth rate and predicted final height (Quintos, Vogiatzi, Harbison, et al., 2001). Adult height data are not yet available. Further investigation is needed.

Adrenomedullary Dysfunction/Epinephrine Deficiency

Patients with CAH suffer from varying degrees of dysfunction of the adrenal medulla primarily expressed by epinephrine deficiency (Merke et al., 2000). This may play a role in response to stress (Clayton et al., 2002). More studies are needed on the risk of low blood glucose in CAH, as well as the function of the adrenal medulla in patients with nonclassic CAH (Clayton et al., 2002; Merke et al., 2000).

Congenital Adrenal Hyperplasia and the Brain

An MRI study found that the structure and function of the amygdala (the part of the brain that regulates emotion and fear) is affected in patients with CAH (Merke, Fields, Keil, et al., 2003). The implications need to be further studied.

DNA Banking

Deoxyribonucleic acid (DNA) banking is the storage of DNA for possible future use. Understanding of the genetics of 21-OHD CAH will certainly improve in the future. Some consideration should be given to banking DNA of affected individuals.

Associated Problems of Congenital Adrenal Hyperplasia and Treatment

The problems associated with CAH are limited in children receiving appropriate therapy. However, primary care providers must be aware of the potential for acute adrenal insufficiency, growth disorders, virilization, and problems surrounding issues of sexuality.

Precocious Puberty

The true precocious puberty that may occur in 21-OHD CAH can be treated with analogs of luteinizing hormone–releasing hormone (LHRH) (Dacou-Voutetakis & Karidis, 1993).

Fertility

For females treated, menses are normal and pregnancy is possible (Lo, Schwitzgebel, Tyrrell, et al., 1999). Overall fertility rates are low, though (Hagenfeldt et al., 2008). Reported reasons include inadequate introitus, elevated androgens leading to ovarian dysfunction, and psychosexual behaviors around gender identity and selection of sexual partners (Gastaud, Bouvattier, Duranteau, et al., 2007; Hagenfeldt et al., 2008; Jäskeläinen, Hippeläinen, Kiekara, et al., 2000; Meyer-Bahlburg, 1999; Otten, Stikkelbroeck, Claahsen-van der Grinten, et al., 2005).

Male subfertility arises from suppression of gonadotropins by adrenal testosterone and adrenal "rests" stimulated by adrenocorticotrophic hormone, both the result of poor compliance with glucocorticoid treatment (Conway, 2007). Further, gonadotropic hypogonadism may result from suppression of luteinizing hormone (LH) secretion by the pituitary by excessive adrenal androgens and their aromatization product (Miller, 2002). Serum LH is probably the single most important endocrine parameter to monitor in men. Some centers have raised the possibility of storing sperm in the event a patient is lost to follow-up or a low sperm count is slow to respond to better management.

In a Swedish study by Hagenfeldt and colleagues in 2008, 62 women with CAH were compared with 62 age-matched controls. Pregnancy and delivery rates were significantly lower in women with CAH than controls, and the severity of the 21-hydroxylase mutation correlated with the reduced number of children born. More women with salt-wasting CAH were single and had not attempted pregnancy. Pregnancies were normal except for a significantly increased incidence of gestational diabetes in CAH patients. The children had normal birth weight and normal formations were observed. Later follow-up of children showed normal intellectual and social development. The sex ratio of the offspring differed significantly, with 25% boys in the CAH group and 56% among controls. Women with CAH had more gynecologic problems during menopause.

Congenital Anomalies

The incidence of congenital anomalies associated with CAH is not thought to be significantly increased over that of the general population. Although there have been reports of an increased incidence of upper urinary tract abnormalities associated with CAH, these have not been clearly established (Bacon, Spencer, Hopwood, et al., 1990; Nabhan & Eugster, 2006).

Prognosis

The major risk for children with CAH is death from an unrecognized salt-losing crisis early in infancy or from inadequately treated acute adrenal insufficiency during stress. Screenings of individuals with a family history of CAH for the carrier state, prenatal screenings, and routine neonatal screenings have the potential to greatly reduce the number of children who die of CAH (Therrell, 2001).

Nearly all female infants with classic CAH have morbidity associated with prenatal virilization and the surgical procedures necessary to correct it.

PRIMARY CARE MANAGEMENT

Health Care Maintenance

Growth

Because abnormal linear growth is an indication of inappropriate treatment or poor compliance, careful monitoring of growth is essential. Linear growth should be measured every 1 to 4 months for infants and every 3 to 6 months for children older than 2 years of age. These measurements should be done carefully, using an infantometer for lengths and a stadiometer for heights. The standard scale-mounted measuring device is not accurate enough to detect slight variations in growth. Measurements should be plotted on a standardized growth chart and assessed for changes in growth rate.

Poor Linear Growth. Linear growth is acutely sensitive to excessive levels of hydrocortisone; therefore any decrease in height percentile on the growth chart should prompt a reassessment of the hydrocortisone dosage. A child's hydrocortisone therapy will occasionally be increased based on a high laboratory 17-OHP result when the result was high because of acute illness, stress from an unusually traumatic venipuncture, or frequently missed hydrocortisone doses before sampling. To avoid unnecessary and possibly harmful increases in hydrocortisone doses, clinicians must rule out these other causes of high 17-OHP values before increasing medication doses. Clinicians can do this by taking a careful history and comparing the prescribed dose of hydrocortisone with the established dose ranges. The primary care provider may be in a position to identify the problem and should contact the endocrinologist with this information.

Another cause of poor linear growth in children with CAH is chronically inadequate mineralocorticoid levels (Migeon & Wisniewski, 2001). A plasma renin activity level that is abnormally high indicates that a child needs additional mineralocorticoid or dietary sodium. A careful history and comparison with established dose ranges will determine if this problem is one of compliance or inadequately prescribed doses.

A child with poorly controlled CAH, or one who was not diagnosed until preschool or school age, may have early cessation of growth because of premature closure of the epiphyses. If such premature closure is suspected, radiographic studies of bone age should be done to assess skeletal maturity.

Excessive Growth. Inadequate hydrocortisone replacement will cause excessive androgen synthesis by the adrenals, resulting in accelerated linear growth. An elevated serum 17-OHP level or clinical findings of increased virilization (e.g., pubic and axillary hair, oily skin, acne, enlargement of the phallus) confirm the cause of excessive growth. Clinicians must be careful to assess whether the inadequate hydrocortisone replacement is secondary to an inappropriately prescribed dose or to poor adherence.

Excessive Weight Gain. Glucocorticoid replacement therapy—even at doses within the accepted therapeutic range—has been associated with obesity (Cornean, Hindmarsh, & Brook, 1998). Clinicians must closely monitor weight gain, avoid overtreatment with glucocorticoids, and encourage good dietary and activity habits to reduce any tendency toward obesity.

Development. Children with CAH who are diagnosed in infancy or very early in childhood and receive consistently adequate treatment should develop normally (Lim, Batch, & Warne, 1995). However, if the diagnosis of CAH is not made until late childhood, the child will be much taller and more mature looking than their peers. When these children stop growing early because of premature epiphyseal closure, they will go from being the tallest to the shortest children in their peer group. Short stature has an effect on behavior and social relationships and probably has an even greater effect on someone who spent early childhood as the tallest person in any group of peers (Holmes, Karlsson, & Thompson, 1986; Young-Hyman, 1986).

Parents, school personnel, child-care workers, and others who regularly interact with these children should be given clear, frequently reinforced guidelines on age-appropriate expectations to avoid demanding too much of tall but immature children or too little of short adolescents.

Diet

The main modification to a normal diet is an allowance for adequate sodium intake. Although an appropriate dose of mineralocorticoid prevents significant sodium depletion in children with salt-losing CAH, these children should be offered salty foods and allowed to salt their food to taste. This recommendation also applies to children with non–salt-losing CAH because they may have a mild salt deficit when compared with unaffected children. As mentioned previously, good dietary habits are essential to reduce the tendency to gain excessive weight (Cornean et al., 1998). The advice of a dietitian can be helpful in identifying nutritionally dense foods that meet a child's dietary needs without excessive calories.

Safety

Children with CAH are not physically impaired or at increased risk for any of the usual physical hazards of childhood, but they are at risk for having their special needs neglected when away from home. Injuries such as a broken bone may not be recognized as potentially life-threatening events. Teachers, child-care personnel, coaches, and others in regular contact with the child should have written information describing the condition and the need for prompt treatment in an emergency. The child should wear a Medic-Alert bracelet with this information on it.

The decision of whether to keep injectable hydrocortisone at school or daycare depends on the situation and must be made on a case-by-case basis. Factors to consider are as follows: (1) Can the primary care provider or emergency department be reached in 5 to 10 minutes? (2) Is a parent always available at short notice? (3) Are there trained personnel at the site who are willing to give an IM injection? (4) Does the child engage in activities with a high risk of serious injury?

Participation in sports is a normal part of childhood and should be encouraged. If possible, some believe, children with CAH should be directed toward activities with a low risk of serious injury (e.g., swimming, track, tennis); however, this needs to be considered on a case-by-case basis, and ultimately the decision lies with the parents after risks and benefits have been explored. Minor injuries (e.g., bruises, mild or moderate sprains, abrasions) are not cause for special concern. If these children are involved in high-risk sports (e.g., football), parents should meet with the coach to explain their child's special needs in an emergency, as well as to provide appropriate written materials, instructions, and authorization for treatment. A parent or team clinician should ideally be present and have hydrocortisone for IM injection on hand during competition. Their presence should be mandatory if the activity takes place more than 15 minutes away from a source of emergency care.

Immunizations

Children with CAH are not immunosuppressed and should receive all standard immunizations at the usual ages (American Academy of Pediatrics Committee on Infectious Diseases, 2006). There is currently no recommendation for or against giving additional immunizations, but the benefits of immunity to these diseases must be weighed against the possibility of adverse reactions to the vaccine. In weighing these factors, many clinicians believe that giving additional immunizations is worthwhile to reduce the risk of acute adrenal insufficiency triggered by illness.

It is not necessary to increase the basal dose of hydrocortisone before immunizations are given unless there is a history of adverse reactions to previous immunizations with that vaccine. A common but discretionary recommendation is to give a child acetaminophen a few hours before giving an immunization that is likely to produce a rapid-onset febrile reaction and continue it for 24 to 48 hours afterward.

For new vaccines or new combinations of vaccines, the package insert should be referred to for information on the type and timing of possible reactions and families should be counseled to observe their child closely on the days when reactions are likely to occur (e.g., 5 to 12 days after measles vaccination).

Stress doses of hydrocortisone should be given when a child develops a temperature of more than 38.4°C (101.1°F) or is fussy or lethargic after an immunization. Any immunization reaction should be documented so that stress doses of hydrocortisone can be given before subsequent immunizations with the same vaccine.

Screening

Vision. Routine screening is recommended.

Hearing. Routine screening is recommended.

Dental. Routine screening is recommended.

Blood Pressure. Blood pressure should be checked at each primary care visit. Every effort should be made to relax and quiet children so that readings are accurate.

Elevated blood pressure in a quiet child may indicate excessive mineralocorticoid or hydrocortisone dosage, whereas low blood pressure may indicate an inadequate mineralocorticoid or hydrocortisone dosage. Either situation should prompt an evaluation of the replacement therapy regimen and compliance.

Hematocrit. Routine screening is recommended.

Urinalysis. Routine screening is recommended.

Tuberculosis. Routine screening is recommended.

Condition-Specific Screening

Serum 17-OHP. Primary care providers may want to order additional screening tests to more closely monitor the adequacy of replacement therapy in children who have difficulty with adherence. The serum 17-OHP level is widely accepted as a measure of hydrocortisone therapy, even though it has the disadvantage of being influenced by temporary stress (e.g., traumatic venipuncture), the length of time since the last hydrocortisone dose, and diurnal fluctuations. To help evaluate the significance of 17-OHP results, clinicians should note on the specimen the time of day (i.e., preferably morning) and the time of the last dose of hydrocortisone.

Androstenedione and testosterone levels can be evaluated along with 17-OHP to monitor adequacy of hydrocortisone therapy. Some clinicians rely on 24-hour urinary 17-ketosteroid and pregnanetriol levels to monitor hydrocortisone therapy because of the lack of short-term fluctuations, despite the difficulty in collecting a 24-hour specimen. Serum 17-OHP levels should be no more than three times above normal (i.e., preferably less than 200 ng/dL). Urinary 17-ketosteroid and pregnanetriol levels should also be in the normal to near-normal range for age, as should plasma renin activity. Specimens ordered by the primary care provider should be coordinated with the endocrinologist and sent to the same laboratory to ensure consistency.

Plasma Renin Activity. Mineralocorticoid therapy is monitored by measuring plasma renin activity level. The primary care provider who is monitoring 17-OHP levels should include a plasma renin activity assay for individuals with salt-losing CAH.

Bone Age. The frequency of radiographic studies of bone age depends on the clinical course. Bone-age evaluations are not helpful in newborns. Initial bone age should be determined early in childhood (i.e., at 2 to 3 years of age or at the time of diagnosis if the diagnosis is delayed) and can be used as a baseline for future studies. If a child is growing normally and has consistently acceptable 17-OHP and plasma renin activity levels, routine screening should not be necessary more than every few years.

If a child has growth acceleration, physical findings of increased virilization, or consistently high 17-OHP laboratory results, bone age should be determined to further assess the effects of androgen excess. If bone age is accelerated, this finding can be used to help impress on the family the serious and permanent consequences of poor adherence. All bone-age studies should ideally be read by the same person to avoid inconsistencies in interpretation.

Monitoring for Testicular Abnormalities in Males. Periodic imaging of the testes either by ultrasonography or magnetic resonance imaging (MRI) should begin after puberty.

Common Illness Management

Children with CAH are not immunosuppressed and their susceptibility to common childhood illnesses is no different from that of their peers; it is their ability to withstand the stress of illness that is impaired. During periods of illness, these children must be observed closely; consultation with an endocrinologist is necessary if a child shows any signs or symptoms of acute adrenal insufficiency (Box 20-2).

The primary care provider caring for a child with CAH should keep injectable hydrocortisone in the office for emergencies. In addition to a Medic-Alert bracelet or necklace, the child and family should carry written materials (e.g., a wallet card) with the diagnosis, a stress dose of hydrocortisone, indications for administering the stress dose, and the name and telephone number of the endocrinologist. This emergency information should be updated regularly.

Upper Respiratory Infections and Allergies

If the symptoms are mild and the child does not have fever or marked malaise, no specific treatment or increase in basal dose of hydrocortisone is necessary for upper respiratory infections or allergies. Parents should watch for worsening of symptoms, fever, or unusual lethargy, and school-age children should know to report these symptoms to their teacher and contact their parents. If symptoms worsen or complications develop, children should be promptly treated with a stress dose of hydrocortisone and seen by the primary care provider for assessment and specific therapy for the illness.

Acute Illnesses

Any known or suspected bacterial illness (e.g., acute otitis media, urinary tract infection, streptococcal pharyngitis, cellulitis) should be treated aggressively with the appropriate antibiotic and stress doses of hydrocortisone during the acute phase of the illness if fever, pain, and malaise are present. When the diagnosis is uncertain or there is a significant risk for secondary infections or complications (e.g., a suspicious but not clearly inflamed tympanic membrane, viral pneumonia, prolonged or marked nasal congestion in a child with a history of frequent acute otitis media or sinusitis), it is wise to treat the child with antibiotics rather than wait for the situation to worsen. The child must be observed closely, with an initial office visit for diagnosis and assessment of the child's overall condition and daily telephone progress reports until the acute phase of the illness has passed. Follow-up office visits should be scheduled as for any other child.

BOX 20-2

Signs and Symptoms of Acute Adrenal Insufficiency

- Nausea or vomiting
- Pallor
- Cold, moist skin
- Weakness
- Dizziness or confusion
- Rapid heart rate
- Rapid breathing
- Abdominal, back, or leg pain
- Dehydration
- Hypotension

Fever

Although fever is a physiologic response to illness, it is also a stress. Therefore fever in a child with CAH should be treated with acetaminophen in the recommended dose for age. Stress doses of hydrocortisone should be given. It is important to advise families that reducing the fever does not cure the illness and that other treatments (e.g., antibiotics, stress doses of hydrocortisone) should continue to be given as directed. The child must be observed closely (i.e., as described for bacterial and viral illnesses) until the illness has resolved.

Vomiting

If a child with CAH vomits once but otherwise appears well, three times the usual oral dose of hydrocortisone should be given about 20 minutes later, and the child should be closely observed. If a child appears weak or lethargic after vomiting once or vomits more than once, the family should give injectable hydrocortisone IM and contact the endocrinologist immediately. If family members are not able to give injectable hydrocortisone, they must immediately take the child to the nearest emergency department to receive parenteral hydrocortisone and appropriate fluid and electrolyte therapy because this can be a life-threatening situation. The emergency department staff should contact the endocrinologist but should not delay hydrocortisone therapy while awaiting consultation. A wallet card or other written information on the child's diagnosis, emergency treatment, and endocrinologist can facilitate prompt and appropriate care.

Injury

A child with a significant injury (e.g., fracture, concussion, injury from an automobile accident) should immediately be given hydrocortisone IM and evaluated further for acute adrenal insufficiency at an emergency department. Emergency department personnel should contact the endocrinologist but not delay hydrocortisone therapy while awaiting consultation.

Differential Diagnosis: Acute Adrenal Insufficiency

Acute adrenal insufficiency is a life-threatening situation. Symptoms of acute adrenal insufficiency include weakness, nausea, abdominal discomfort, vomiting, dehydration, and hypotension. Any of these signs or symptoms in a child with CAH should be presumed to indicate acute adrenal insufficiency and be treated with hydrocortisone IV or IM at three to five times the basal dose. This administration should be done at home—or in the primary care setting if the child is there—instead of delaying initial treatment until the child arrives at an emergency department. Further work up can be done after the initial hydrocortisone treatment.

The diagnosis of acute adrenal insufficiency can be confirmed by laboratory values showing hyponatremia and hyperkalemia. Although consultation with an endocrinologist should be sought, treatment should not be delayed.

An IM injection of hydrocortisone or IV therapy in an emergency department is a frightening experience that no one wants to go through unnecessarily. In this type of situation, however, it is always best to err on the side of aggressive treatment.

Drug Interactions

Medications for CAH replace hormones normally present in the body; therefore concern about using other medications is limited to their effect on the absorption or rate of metabolism (Box 20-3).

BOX 20-3
Drug Interactions

- Barbiturates
- Phenytoin
- Rifampin

Barbiturates (e.g., phenobarbital [Donnatal], phenytoin [Dilantin], and rifampin [Rifadin, Rifamate, Rimactane]) increase the rate of metabolism of glucocorticoids. Therefore children with CAH who are taking any of these medications for more than a few weeks may require a higher than usual dose of hydrocortisone for adequate cortisol replacement (Bello & Garrett, 1999). A serum 17-OHP level done approximately 2 weeks after the start of any of the medications listed here will show if an adjustment in the hydrocortisone dose is necessary. Short-term use of barbiturates perioperatively or prophylactic use of rifampin for *Haemophilus influenzae* meningitis should not require a change in hydrocortisone dose.

Antibiotics, decongestants, antihistamines, cough preparations, analgesics, antipyretics, and topical preparations have no unusual adverse effects.

Varicella-Zoster Virus (Chickenpox)

Affected children who come down with varicella-zoster virus should still be given stress doses despite concerns with regard to steroid use in the presence of the virus. Complications of acute adrenal insufficiency outweigh concerns with steroid use in varicella-zoster virus infections. Prevention with immunization is the best defense.

Developmental Issues
Sleep Patterns

Children with CAH do not differ from their peers in their sleep patterns or needs. Unusual fatigue may indicate an illness or inadequate cortisol replacement and should be evaluated.

Toileting

Children who have obvious virilization of their external genitalia should be given privacy when using the toilet to avoid teasing. The initial corrective surgery for girls who experience virilization is usually done at an early age to avoid problems related to looking different. However, some parents will postpone surgery until the children are older and can give informed consent. In these cases, notes should be written for physical education classes allowing changing clothes privately, in addition to a private restroom. Although boys who experience excessive virilization may have some regression in pubic hair and penile size once they establish consistently adequate treatment, they will be noticeably different from their peers until adolescence.

Girls with a CUGS will be prone to vaginal voiding and vaginitis caused by vaginal voiding. Vaginal voiding is when, during urination, urine refluxes into the vagina because of the close proximity of the vagina and urethra. The symptoms are urinary "leaking" after voiding and mildly wet underwear and "smelly" urine. Vaginal voiding can easily be treated with leg abduction with voiding (sitting backward on the toilet for younger girls) and sitting on the toilet a few seconds after urination has stopped. The associated vaginitis can be treated with sitz baths and prevented with leg abduction with voiding.

These children are otherwise no different in toileting readiness or skills than their peers and are not unusually prone to constipation, other types of incontinence, enuresis, polyuria, or other disorders related to toileting.

Discipline

Children with CAH should be expected to behave appropriately for their age. The only special consideration has to do with children who appear older than their actual age. Parents, teachers, and others must be given clear guidelines on appropriate expectations for a child's developmental stage if it is different from his or her appearance.

Another area that raises disciplinary issues is adherence with taking medication, especially during toddlerhood and adolescence when children struggle with issues of dependency and autonomy. Parents should be advised from the beginning to use a matter-of-fact approach and avoid negotiating something that is nonnegotiable. During infancy and early school years, parents have full responsibility for giving medications. As children mature and are able to assume more responsibility, parents should encourage their child's active participation (e.g., by remembering when it is "pill time," marking off the calendar for each dose, or filling a pillbox). Adolescents should have the primary responsibility for taking the medication with the parents offering support. Using a watch with a beeper is helpful for adolescents, as is a pillbox, which also provides an unobtrusive way for a parent to see if the medication disappears on schedule.

Clinicians can help make older children and adolescents aware of the consequences of poor adherence by pointing out signs of virilization to girls and slowed growth to both genders and emphasizing that it is within their power to "get back to normal." The risks of acute adrenal insufficiency and impaired fertility associated with poor adherence should also be discussed with adolescents, again with emphasis that such things are avoidable.

An adolescent will occasionally choose to make adherence to medications the focus of serious rebellion. Every effort should be made to explain the purpose and necessity of medication, and counseling should promptly be sought if the problem is severe or chronic.

Child Care

Parents should meet with child-care personnel before enrollment to explain their child's special needs. Child-care personnel do not require detailed knowledge of CAH but should be given a clear explanation that a child has a metabolic disorder that requires simple but important treatment.

Written information for the child-care center should include written authorization to give hydrocortisone orally with instructions on the dose, time, and purpose; instructions on when to call parents, the telephone numbers where they can be reached, and what symptoms or events require emergency care; where to take the child for care; authorization for treatment; and the name and telephone number of the primary care provider and endocrinologist. It is neither necessary nor desirable to have special rules or restrictions on activities at school or child care for children with CAH. The usual policies on safety and appropriate play are sufficient to avoid serious injury.

Because hydrocortisone is usually given every 8 hours, many children will need at least one dose while at daycare. Mineralocorticoid is given once daily to children with salt-losing CAH and can be administered at home. Although most child-care providers are conscientious, they may occasionally miss or delay doses of hydrocortisone if they do not understand its importance or are distracted by other demands on their attention. A routine that ties medication time to a regular activity (e.g., rest period or story time) can be established, or the child can wear a watch programmed to beep at the desired time. A letter from the primary care provider or the endocrinologist is helpful in making this invisible condition real to the people caring for these children.

Schooling

Children with CAH may have more absences than usual because of their need for close observation at home during acute illnesses. Concerns about excessive absences should be brought to the attention of the primary care provider, who can assess their appropriateness. Legitimate absences include any illness that would keep other children at home. In addition, symptoms such as a scratchy throat and malaise that might be ignored in other children should be initially observed at home.

Studies of cognitive abilities and school function in children with CAH have shown inconsistent results. Although earlier studies found normal or above-normal cognitive function in individuals with CAH (Ehrhardt & Baker, 1977; Galatzer & Laron, 1989; Nass & Baker, 1991), later studies found an increased prevalence of cognitive impairment or learning disabilities (Helleday, Bartfai, Ritzen, et al., 1994; Plante, Boliek, Binkiewicz, et al., 1996). More current research does not support either the concept of an overall intellectual advantage or an increased risk of learning disabilities in children with CAH, when compared with unaffected relatives. Females with CAH do seem to have enhanced spatial abilities as a result of exposure to androgens in early development (Berenbaum, 2001).

Although it is not possible to identify what influence CAH itself has on cognitive and educational function with the information currently available, it is clear that acute CAH crises have a deleterious effect. Not surprisingly, children who had episodes of acute adrenal insufficiency with hypoglycemia or convulsions have a significantly higher prevalence of learning difficulties than children—with or without CAH—who did not experience such events (Donaldson, Thomas, Love, et al., 1994). Because hypoglycemia and convulsions are associated with learning difficulties, these findings may represent a complication of poor management rather than the biochemical abnormality inherent in CAH. A child with CAH who has had severe hypoglycemia and convulsions should be assessed for learning difficulties and referred for special education intervention if indicated.

Sexuality

Because of the considerable attention paid to the genital examination during clinic visits, girls with CAH may get the message that there is something "wrong" with them and that it has to do with their genitalia. It is important to reassure these girls that they have all the normal female organs, hormones, and chromosomes, and that any surgeries are simply to correct a cosmetic mistake that happened before they were born. Frequent genital examinations in females, unless there is concern about poor control or to assess pubertal progression, should be limited and genital photography should be done only with informed consent from the parents (Clayton et al., 2002; Lee et al., 2006).

Children with CAH should be regularly evaluated for premature sexual development to determine the adequacy of therapy. Clinicians should include appropriate counseling regarding sexual development to the child and family.

Menstrual irregularities caused by androgen excess are common in adolescent girls with CAH. Androgen excess can also cause hirsutism and acne in children and adolescents of either gender and may contribute to impaired fertility (Lo & Grumbach, 2001; Speiser, 2001).

Although many observers have noted "tomboyish" behavior (e.g., rough-and-tumble play) or increased activity levels in girls with CAH, most early studies are difficult to interpret because of small sample size, lack of data on adequacy of treatment, and lack of control groups (Ehrhardt & Baker, 1977; Galatzer & Laron, 1989; Hines & Kaufman, 1994; Hochberg, Gardos, & Benderly, 1987; Money, Schwartz, & Lewis, 1984). Stereotyping behavior as "masculine" or "feminine" also remains controversial. Some recent studies using better methodology have shown significant differences between the gender-stereotypic activities and sexual behaviors of girls and women with CAH and those of their unaffected sisters. Investigators attribute these differences to prenatal exposure to high levels of adrenal androgens (Berenbaum, 1999; Berenbaum, Duck, & Bryk, 2000; Dittmann, Kappes, & Kappes, 1992; Dittmann, Kappes, Kappes, et al., 1990; Zucker, Bradley, Oliver, et al., 1996). The data suggest that, compared with their unaffected sisters, more women with CAH delay or fail to establish intimate heterosexual relationships (Dittmann et al., 1992; Kuhnle, Bullinger, & Schwartz, 1995). However, the data are conflicting on whether there is an increased prevalence of homosexual orientation among women with CAH (Dittmann et al., 1992; Kuhnle et al., 1995). Prenatal androgen exposure is considered to be a predisposing—rather than a causative—factor in gender behavior, and all aspects of psychosocial development must be considered in the care of girls with CAH (Dittmann et al., 1992). Primary care providers must use caution when interpreting these data and base discussions of sexuality on an individualized assessment of each child and family.

Women with CAH—particularly those with the salt-losing form—may not have an adequate introitus for vaginal penetration, in spite of surgical intervention (Lo & Grumbach, 2001). In addition, women who become pregnant may require cesarean delivery because of a small birth canal (Lo & Grumbach, 2001). One study evaluated fertility in eight heterosexual women with CAH who were diagnosed early, were generally compliant with treatment, had an introitus that was adequate for intercourse, and were sexually active (Premawadhara, Hughes, Read, et al., 1997). Five of the eight women conceived (i.e., three of this five had salt-wasting CAH and two had non–salt-wasting CAH), for an overall fertility rate of slightly greater than 60%. It is important to note that a significant number of women had successful pregnancies in spite of late diagnosis and treatment of CAH, inadequate reconstruction of the introitus, and poor compliance with replacement therapy (Lo & Grumbach, 2001). Other studies have shown that genital sensitivity is impaired in areas where surgery has been performed and, in addition, impairment of sensitivity is linearly related to difficulties in sexual function (Crouch et al., 2008; Minto et al., 2003).

For treated females, menses are normal and pregnancy is possible (Lo et al., 1999), but overall fertility rates are low (Hagenfeldt et al., 2008). Reported reasons include inadequate introitus, elevated androgens leading to ovarian dysfunction, and psychosexual behaviors around gender identity and selection of sexual partners (Hagenfeldt et al., 2008; Jäskeläinen et al., 2000; Meyer-Bahlburg, 1999; Otten et al., 2005).

There are no published studies on sexual function of women with classic CAH who did not have surgery. In addition, the surgery that was performed on women with CAH who are currently adults is very different from the surgical techniques performed on infants today, so the relevance of adult outcomes studies to children with CAH is questionable. There is some optimism that the outcomes will be improved for today's infants when they reach adulthood; however, we will not know for another 20 or more years. (See Table 20-2 on genital surgery.) Males with CAH generally do not have problems with erectile function or fertility. In males, the main cause of subfertility is the presence of testicular adrenal rest tumors, which are thought to originate from aberrant adrenal tissue and respond to treatment with glucocorticoids (Otten et al, 2005)

Transition to Adulthood

Improved care for individuals with 21-OHD CAH has resulted in good prognosis and normal life expectancy (New & Nimkarn, 2006). During the transition from adolescence into adulthood, youths with CAH assume the primary responsibility for managing the condition and the medical issues change from a focus on growth and development to long-term health preservation (Conway, 2007). Sexuality and fertility issues become a focus. Educating the adolescent (not just the parent) on the principles of adrenal suppression and the diurnal rhythm of the adrenal glands requires time and encouragement (Conway, 2007). Consideration should be given to leaving parents in the waiting room for part or all of visits. Transition affords the young adult the opportunity for an educational review of CAH. Although the primary management will be with the endocrinologist, increasingly it should involve a multidisciplinary team including gynecology, urology, fertility specialists, dietitians, sex therapists, biochemists, geneticists, clinical psychologists, and nursing Ogilvie et al., 2006).

Changes in Requirements for the Adolescent. At present, evidence-based treatment protocols for adults are lacking (Kruse, Riepe, Krone, et al., 2004).

Glucocorticoids. Glucocorticoid treatment in adolescence has to be adjusted according to individual goals because there is no "perfect regimen." In contrast to the pediatric agenda of optimizing final height, the adult concerns relate to long-term consequences of glucocorticoid use. A common strategy is to find the minimal effective dose of a glucocorticoid for an adult maintenance based on a combination of clinical and biochemical markers. The goal is to achieve a glucocorticoid regimen that fails to fully suppress 17-OHP but maintains androgens in the midnormal range (Conway, 2007).

Mineralocorticoids. Mineralocorticoids require precise monitoring in adulthood. The sensitivity to salt loss noted in childhood diminishes throughout the teen years, and in adults salt wasting is a far less precarious situation (Conway, 2007). In addition, the tendency to develop hypertension with age means that many adults are better off on progressively lower doses of fludrocortisone. To avoid hypertension one must use renin as a guide to fludrocortisone dosing adjustments.

Males are often lost to follow-up during transition (Conway, 2007), and permanent infertility may result from neglected care. As children with CAH approach adulthood, the primary care provider needs to help their families identify an internist or family practice provider to assume primary care responsibilities. If a child has had specialty care through a pediatric endocrinologist, the transition must also be made to adult endocrine care; the pediatric endocrinologist usually has a list of names available. Counseling for early prenatal care (i.e., prenatal screening, diagnosis, and potential treatment) should be provided as well.

Unfortunately, insurance may become a problem when children reach an age when they are no longer covered by government-sponsored insurance for children with disabilities or their parents' insurance. Medicaid—for those who meet the criteria—and group insurance through employment—for those with medical benefits—will cover care for CAH. Information about other programs and resources can be sought from county social services agencies, health departments, and state insurance commissions.

Family Concerns

The parents of an infant girl with CAH must cope with the effect of ambiguous genitalia and of possibly a delayed or even incorrect gender assignment. The initial explanations and reassurances that health care personnel give to the family must be both sensitive and accurate to prevent serious misperceptions of the child's condition and prognosis. Discussions with parents should focus on listening to the parents' concerns and reinforcing the normality of their daughter's internal female organs and chromosomes and explaining that the appearance of the external genitalia is correctable and the underlying condition treatable.

People tend to blame the occurrence of an abnormality in a baby on something the mother or father did. It is important to discuss this issue with the parents and the extended family and to repeatedly reinforce the lack of fault. Even after the best of explanations and reassurances, these families continue to have much anxiety and guilt about their child's condition, so constant reinforcement and support are necessary.

Families must be taught to be assertive in communicating the urgency of their child's need for hydrocortisone to health care personnel who are not familiar with the child or CAH. Unfortunately, treatment is commonly delayed because of a lack of understanding of the implications of acute illness in children with CAH. Primary care providers can help avoid delays in treatment by alerting other health care personnel (e.g., call group, emergency department staff) to a child's special needs. The endocrinologist should be consulted for any questions about treatment. In addition, the child should wear a Medic-Alert bracelet or necklace, and the family should carry written information on the child's condition (e.g., wallet card) to facilitate prompt treatment.

Parents have initial difficulty believing the seriousness of CAH unless the diagnosis was made during an episode of acute adrenal insufficiency. Once parents experience the rapidity with which their child can change from being robustly healthy to being deathly ill, they may be fearful of future episodes. It is difficult for these parents to find a balance between protecting their child from serious harm and allowing the child to have an active, normal life. This balance must be assessed at each primary care visit by asking about the child's social and academic progress, outside interests and activities, and special concerns. Any problem areas should then be discussed.

Children with CAH may experience emotional disturbances related to multiple factors involved in having this chronic condition. Such factors include being concerned about sexuality and fertility; being perceived and treated as different by others, including their parents; receiving mixed or confusing messages from health care personnel; being overprotected by their parents; and dealing with their own fears related to life-threatening crises they may have experienced. Psychotherapy is indicated for significant emotional disturbance and behavioral problems. Newborn siblings should be screened for CAH, and if the screening results are positive, confirming tests should be done. Because nonclassic CAH can cause virilization or accelerated growth, all older siblings with these findings should be screened.

Although prenatal diagnosis and treatment are still being refined, they should be discussed in detail with parents. Testing for the carrier state is also available and should be explained to unaffected siblings and other first-degree relatives.

The effect of CAH on a family varies with their cultural beliefs about the cause of congenital disorders and their attitudes toward sexuality. Primary care providers must determine what these beliefs are in order to provide sensitive and successful care to the child and family. Families will usually tell providers their beliefs if asked.

Individuals from cultures in which sexual topics are not openly discussed can be expected to have difficulty asking questions about CAH. Primary care providers and endocrinologists are faced with the challenge of presenting information on a sensitive subject without offending a family's values. In some cultures it may be helpful to have a male health care provider speak to the men in the family and a female provider speak separately to the women in the family.

Families are often afraid of giving their child steroids because of negative publicity in the popular press. It is important to stress to families that the hydrocortisone and fludrocortisone medications their child takes for CAH are replacing substances normally produced in the body and that the recommended doses are calculated to match normal blood levels as closely as possible. This is very different from taking high doses of glucocorticoids to treat inflammatory diseases. Families may have read stories of athletes having severe side effects from using steroids to increase muscle mass, so they should be told that anabolic steroids are completely different from hydrocortisone in actions and side effects. Replacement therapy for CAH is also an entirely different situation from taking a foreign substance such as an antibiotic.

Resources

Informational Pamphlets for Patients and Families

Congenital Adrenal Hyperplasia Due to 21 Hydroxylase Deficiency: A Guide for Patients and Their Families. Recommended by the Lawson Wilkins Pediatric Endocrine Society and the European Society for Paediatric Endocrinology. Downloadable version available from the Division of Pediatric Endocrinology at Johns

Hopkins Children's Center. Website: www.hopkinsmedicine. org/pediatricendocrinology/cah.

Connaughty, S. (1996). *Congenital Adrenal Hyperplasia.* Available from Patient/Parent Education Department of British Columbia's Children's Hospital; 4480 Oak St.; Vancouver, British Columbia, V6H 3V4, Canada.

Pang, S. *Congenital Adrenal Hyperplasia.* Available from The Magic Foundation; 1327 N. Harlem Ave.; Oak Park, IL 60302. (708) 383-0808; (708) 383-0899 (fax); (800) 3MAGIC 3 (parent help line). Website: www.magicfoundation.org.

Hormones and Me: Congenital Adrenal Hyperplasia (CAH). A 29-page booklet for families of children with CAH. Available from Serono Symposia Australia: Unit 3-4; 25 Frenchs Forest Rd. East; Frenchs Forest NSW 2086; Australia.

Your Child with Congenital Adrenal Hyperplasia. Recommended by the Lawson Wilkins Pediatric Endocrine Society and the European Society for Paediatric Endocrinology. Downloadable version available from the Royal Children's Hospital, Melbourne, Australia. Website: www.rch.unimelb.edu.au/cah_book.

Pamphlets with Medication Information

Congenital Adrenal Hyperplasia. Explains CAH and its management. Available from University of Wisconsin Hospital; Department of Education; 600 Highland Ave.; Madison, WI 53792.

Guidelines for the Child Who Is Cortisol Dependent. Provides parents with information on cortisone replacement and illness management. Available from University of Wisconsin Hospital; Department of Education; 600 Highland Ave.; Madison, WI 53792.

How to Mix and Inject Injectable Hydrocortisone. Gives parents a clear description of this procedure. Available from University of Wisconsin Hospital; Department of Education; 600 Highland Ave.; Madison, WI 53792.

The Hydrocortisone/Florinef Handout. A concise 2-page handout for parents that includes information on illness management. Available from Pediatric Endocrinology; CB 7220, Burnett-Womack; University of North Carolina at Chapel Hill; Chapel Hill, NC 27599.

Medication Instructions for Patients with Congenital Adrenal Hyperplasia: Instructions for Families. Available from Pediatric Endocrinology Nursing Society; PO Box 2933; Gaithersburg, MD 20886-2933. Website: www.pens.org also describes dosages.

Organizations

CARES (Congenital Adrenal Hyperplasia Research, Education, and Support) Foundation Inc.

Nonprofit organization formed in 2001 to educate the public, physicians, and legislators about CAH and to provide support to families of children with CAH. Provides useful information about CAH and links to other related sites.

Website: www.caresfoundation.org

National Adrenal Diseases Foundation (NADF)

Nonprofit organization dedicated to providing support, information, and education to individuals having Addison disease, as well as other diseases of the adrenal glands.

Erin A. Foley, MPH, President/Director
National Adrenal Diseases Foundation
505 Northern Blvd.
Great Neck, NY 11021
(516) 487-4992
Website: www.medhelp.org/nadf

Pediatric Endocrinology Nursing Society (PENS)

Organization with professional members in many regions who are willing to speak to parent, school, professional, or other groups.

P.O. Box 2933
Gaithersburg, MD 20886-2933
Website: www.pens.org

Products

Medic-Alert bracelets and necklaces (recommended for all children with CAH)

Available from Medic-Alert Foundation; PO Box 1009; Turlock, CA 95381-1009.

Website: www.medicalert.org (in the United States) or www.medicalert.ca (in Canada).

Summary of Primary Care Needs for the Child with Congenital Adrenal Hyperplasia

HEALTH CARE MAINTENANCE

- A temperature greater than 101.1°F (38.4°C), significant malaise, pain, lethargy, or persistent vomiting (regardless of cause) should be covered by stress doses of hydrocortisone in addition to appropriate specific therapy.
- If the child has hypertension, excessive dietary sodium intake and overtreatment with mineralocorticoids or glucocorticoids should be ruled out.
- If the child has hypotension, inadequate mineralocorticoid and glucocorticoid dosage should be ruled out.
- If the child has nausea or vomiting; pallor; cold, moist skin; weakness; dizziness or confusion; rapid heart rate; rapid breathing; abdominal, back, or leg pain; dehydration; or hypotension, acute adrenal insufficiency should be ruled out.

Growth and Development

- If CAH is diagnosed in infancy and adequately and consistently treated, growth and development are normal.
- Accelerated linear growth occurs if CAH is inadequately treated.
- Accelerated bone age advancement and early closure of epiphyses with reduced final adult height will occur if CAH is inadequately treated.
- Stunted linear growth will occur if CAH is overtreated with hydrocortisone.
- Precocious puberty may occur with improved treatment.

Diet

- Children should be allowed to salt food to taste and eat salty foods.
- Good dietary and activity habits are necessary to counteract the tendency for hydrocortisone therapy to promote excessive weight gain.

Continued

Summary of Primary Care Needs for the Child with Congenital Adrenal Hyperplasia—cont'd

Safety

- These children have no increased susceptibility to injury.
- There is a risk of acute adrenal insufficiency with a serious injury (e.g., fracture, concussion).
- A Medic-Alert bracelet or necklace should be worn and written information should be carried stating the diagnosis, stress dosage of hydrocortisone, and the name and telephone number of the endocrinologist.

Immunizations

- Routine immunizations are recommended.
- Increased stress doses of hydrocortisone are not prophylactically necessary unless the child has a history of previous adverse reaction to the vaccine.
- Give increased stress dose of hydrocortisone for immunization reactions involving fever, unusual malaise, and lethargy.
- Giving acetaminophen before immunization with likelihood of febrile reaction is discretionary.

Screening

- *Vision.* Routine screening is recommended.
- *Hearing.* Routine screening is recommended.
- *Dental.* Routine screening is recommended.
- *Blood pressure.* Blood pressure should be checked at each visit (including infants). Children with abnormal findings should be referred to an endocrinologist.
- *Hematocrit.* Routine screening is recommended.
- *Urinalysis.* Routine screening is recommended.
- *Tuberculosis.* Routine screenings is recommended.

Condition-Specific Screening

- Screening serum 17-OHP levels or 24-hour urine pregnanetriol values may be indicated and should be coordinated with the endocrinologist.
- Checking plasma renin activity levels may be indicated and should be coordinated with the endocrinologist.
- Bone age should be checked every 2 to 3 years or more often if there are indications of androgen excess.
- Imaging of tests by ultrasound or MRI after puberty.

COMMON ILLNESS MANAGEMENT

- If the child has nausea or vomiting; pallor; cold, moist skin; weakness; dizziness or confusion; rapid heart rate; rapid breathing; abdominal, back, or leg pain; dehydration; or hypotension, acute adrenal insufficiency should be ruled out.
- A temperature greater than 101.1°F (38.4°C), significant malaise, pain, lethargy, or persistent vomiting (regardless of cause) should be covered by stress doses of hydrocortisone in addition to appropriate specific therapy.
- If the child has hypertension, excessive dietary sodium intake and/or overtreatment with mineralocorticoids or glucocorticoids should be ruled out.
- If the child has hypotension, inadequate mineralocorticoid and glucocorticoid dosage should be ruled out.

Drug Interactions

- Long-term use of barbiturates, phenytoin, or rifampin increases the rate of metabolism of glucocorticoids. Adjustments in dosage may be required.

DEVELOPMENTAL ISSUES

Sleep Patterns

- Unusual fatigue or lethargy may indicate the need for increased doses of hydrocortisone.

Toileting

- Increased vaginal voiding symptoms (e.g., urinary "leaking" after voiding and vaginitis) are easily treated with leg abduction with voiding and sitz baths. There is no impairment in readiness or functioning. Children with obvious virilization should be allowed privacy.

Discipline

- Expectations are normal based on age and developmental level.
- Physical appearance may differ from age and developmental level, leading to inappropriate expectations.

Child Care

- Child-care providers must be aware of special needs with illness and injury and the importance of routine and stress medication.

Schooling

- Children with CAH who have a history of acute adrenal insufficiency or hypoglycemic seizures should be assessed for learning difficulties.
- School personnel should be aware of special needs of the child's illness and injury.

Sexuality

- Virilization of infant girls requires surgical correction.
- Inadequate treatment results in continued virilization, acne, hirsutism, menstrual irregularities, infertility in girls, and—eventually—impairment of fertility in boys.
- Most children will be fertile.

Transition to Adulthood

- Transition to providers of adult primary care and endocrine care should be accomplished.
- Source of medical insurance must be identified.

FAMILY CONCERNS

- Rapid onset of acute adrenal insufficiency is possible.
- Appropriate emergency treatment may be delayed because of health care providers' lack of awareness or knowledge of CAH.
- The normality of girls should be stressed.
- Others in the family may be affected (e.g., siblings, children of affected child). Genetic counseling, prenatal screening, diagnosis, and treatment are available.
- Family members may have difficulty speaking openly about sexuality and genitalia.

REFERENCES

Allen, D., Hoffman, G., Fitzpatrick, P., et al. (1997). Improved precision of newborn screening for congenital adrenal hyperplasia using weight-adjusted criteria for 17-hydroxyprogesterone levels. *J Pediatr, 130*(1), 128-133.

American Academy of Pediatrics Committee on Infectious Diseases (2006). *Red Book: 2006 Report of the Committee on Infectious Diseases.* (27th ed.). Elk Grove Village, IL: American Academy of Pediatrics.

Bacon, G.E., Spencer, M.L., Hopwood, N.J., et al. (1990). *A Practical Approach to Pediatric Endocrinology.* (3rd ed.). Chicago: Year Book Medical Publishers.

Baskin, L.S. (2004). Anatomical studies of the female genitalia: Surgical reproductive implications. *J Pediatr Endocrinol Metab, 17*(4), 581-587.

Baskin, L.S., Erol, A., Li, Y.W., et al. (1999). Anatomical studies of the human clitoris. *J Urol, 162*, 1015.

Bello, C., & Garrett, S. (1999). Therapeutic issues in oral glucocorticoid use. *Lippincott's Primary Care Practice, 3*(3), 333-344.

Berenbaum, S. (1999). Effects of early androgens on sex-typed activities and interests in adolescents with congenital adrenal hyperplasia. *Horm Behav, 35*, 102-110.

Berenbaum, S. (2001). Cognitive function in congenital adrenal hyperplasia. *Endocrinol Metab Clin North Am, 30*(1), 173-192.

Berenbaum, S., Duck, S., & Bryk, K. (2000). Behavioral effects of prenatal versus postnatal androgen excess in children with 21-hydroxylase-deficient congenital adrenal hyperplasia. *J Clin Endocrinol Metab, 85*, 727-733.

Caroll, A.E., & Downs, S.M. (2006). Comprehensive cost-utility analysis of newborn screening strategies. *Pediatrics, 117*(5 pt 2), 287-295.

Clayton, P.E., Miller, W.L., Oberfield, S.E., et al. (2002). Consensus statement on 21-hydroxylase deficiency from the European Society for Paediatric Endocrinology and the Lawson Wilkins Pediatric Endocrine Society. *Horm Res, 58*(4), 188-195.

Conway, G.S. (2007). Congenital adrenal hyperplasia: Adolescents and transition. *Horm Res, 68*(Suppl), 90-92.

Cornean, R., Hindmarsh, P., & Brook, C. (1998). Obesity in 21-hydroxylase deficient patients. *Arch Dis Child, 78*, 261-263.

Creighton, S.M. (2004). Long-term outcome of feminization surgery: The London experience. *BJU Int, 93*(Suppl 3), 44-46.

Crouch, N.S., Liao, L.M., Woodhouse, C.R., et al. (2008). Sexual function and genital sensitivity following feminizing genitoplasty for congenital adrenal hyperplasia. *J Urol, 179*(2), 634-638.

Dacou-Voutetakis, C., & Karidis, N. (1993). Congenital adrenal hyperplasia complicated by central precocious puberty: Treatment with LHRH-agonist analog. *Ann N Y Acad Sci, 687*, 250-254.

Degitz, K., Placzek, M., Arnold, B., et al. (2003). Congenital adrenal hyperplasia and acne in male patients. *Br J Dermatol, 148*(6), 1263-1266.

Dittmann, R., Kappes, M., Kappes, M., et al. (1990). Congenital adrenal hyperplasia I: Gender-related behavior and attitudes in female patients and sisters. *Psychoneuroendocrinology, 15*, 401-420.

Dittmann, R., Kappes, M., & Kappes, M. (1992). Sexual behavior in adolescent and adult females with congenital adrenal hyperplasia. *Psychoneuroendocrinology, 17*, 153-170.

Donaldson, M.D., Thomas, P.H., Love, J.G., et al. (1994). Presentation, acute illness, and learning difficulties in salt wasting 21-hydroxylase deficiency. *Arch Dis Child, 70*, 214-218.

Ehrhardt, A., & Baker, S. (1977). Males and females with congenital adrenal hyperplasia: A family study of intelligence and gender-related behavior. In P. Lee, L. Plotnick, & A. Kowarski (Eds.), *Congenital Adrenal Hyperplasia.* Baltimore: University Park Press.

Eugster, E.A., Dimeglio, L.A., Wright, J.C., et al. (2001). Height outcome in congenital adrenal hyperplasia caused by 21-hydroxylase deficiency: A meta-analysis. *J Pediatr, 138*(1), 26-32.

Forest, M.G. (2004). Recent advances in the diagnosis and management of congenital adrenal hyperplasia due to 21-hydroxylase deficiency. *Hum Reprod Update, 10*, 469-485.

Frisch, H., Battelino, T., Schober, E., et al. (2001). Salt wasting in simple virilizing congenital adrenal hyperplasia. *J Pediatr Endocrinol Metab, 14*(9), 1649-1655.

Galatzer, A., & Laron, Z. (1989). The effects of prenatal androgens on behavior and cognitive functions. In M. Forest (Ed.). *Androgens in Childhood.* Basel Switzerland: Karger AG.

Gastaud, F., Bouvattier, C., Duranteau, L., et al. (2007). Impaired sexual and reproductive outcomes in women with classic forms of congenital adrenal hyperplasia. *J Endocrinol Metabol, 92*, 1391-1396.

Gmyrek, G.A., New, M.I., Sosa, R.E., et al. (2002). Bilateral laparoscopic adrenalectomy as a treatment for classical congenital adrenal hyperplasia attributable to 21-hydroxylase deficiency. *Pediatrics, 109*(2), E28.

Grumbach, M.M., Hughes, I.A., & Conte, F.A. (2003). Disorders of sex differentiation. In P.R. Larson, H.M. Kronenberg, S. Melmed, et al. (Eds.), *Williams Textbook of Endocrinology* (10th ed.). Heidelberg, Germany: Saunders.

Gunther, D., & Bukowski, T. (1999). Congenital adrenal hyperplasia: A spectrum of disorders. *Contemp Urol, 11*(1), 52-69.

Hagenfeldt, K., Janson, P.O., Holmdahl, G., et al. (2008). Fertility and pregnancy outcome in women with congenital adrenal hyperplasia due to 21-hydroxylase deficiency. *Hum Reprod Adv Access*, 1-7.

Helleday, J., Bartfai, A., Ritzen, E.M., et al. (1994). General intelligence and cognitive profile in women with congenital adrenal hyperplasia (CAH). *Psychoneuroendocrinology, 19*(4), 343-356.

Hines, M., Brook, C., & Conway, G.S. (2004). Androgen and psychosexual development: Core gender identity, sexual orientation and recalled childhood gender role behavior in women and men with congenital adrenal hyperplasia (CAH). *J Sexual Res, 41*(1), 75-81.

Hines, M., & Kaufman, F. (1994). Androgen and the development of human sex-typical behavior: Rough-and-tumble play and sex of preferred playmates in children with congenital adrenal hyperplasia (CAH). *Child Dev, 65*, 1042-1053.

Hochberg, Z., Gardos, M., & Benderly, A. (1987). Psychosexual outcome of assigned females and males with 46XX virilizing congenital adrenal hyperplasia. *Eur J Pediatr, 146*, 497-499.

Holmes, C., Karlsson, J., & Thompson, R. (1986). Longitudinal evaluation of behavior patterns in children with short stature. In B. Stabler & L. Underwood (Eds.), *Slow Grows the Child.* Hillsdale, NJ: Lawrence Erlbaum Associates.

Hughes, I. (2006). Prenatal treatment of congenital adrenal hyperplasia: Do we have enough evidence?. *Treatments in Endocrinology, 5*(1), 1-6.

Hughes, I. (2007). Congenital adrenal hyperplasia: A lifelong disorder. *Horm Res, 68*(Suppl 5), 84-89.

Jäskeläinen, J., Hippeläinen, M., Kiekara, O., et al. (2000). Child rate, pregnancy outcome and ovarian function in females with classical 21-hydroxylase deficiency. *Acta Obstet Gynecol Scand, 79*(8), 687-692.

Koppens, P.F., Hoogenboezem, T., & Degenhart, H.J. (2002). Duplication of the CYP21A2 gene complicates mutation analysis of steroid 21-hydroxylase deficiency: Characteristics of three unusual haplotypes. *Hum Genet, 111*(4-5), 405-410.

Krone, N., Braun, A., Roscher, A.A., et al. (2000). Predicting phenotype in steroid 21-hydroxylase deficiency? Comprehensive genotyping in 155 unrelated, well defined patients from southern Germany. *J Clin Endocrinol Metab, 85*(3), 1059-1065.

Kruse, B., Riepe, F.G., Krone, N., et al. (2004). Congenital adrenal hyperplasia—how to improve the transition from adolescence to adult life. *Exp Clin Endocrinol Diabetes, 112*(7), 343-355.

Kuhnle, U., Bullinger, M., & Schwartz, H. (1995). The quality of life in adult female patients with congenital adrenal hyperplasia: A comprehensive study of the impact of genital malformations and chronic disease on female patients' life. *Eur J Pediatr, 154*, 708-716.

Lee, P.A., Houk, G.P., Ahmed, S.F., et al. (2006). International Consensus Conference on Intersex. Consensus statement on management of intersex disorders. *Pediatrics, 118*(2), 488-499.

Lee, P.A., & Witchel, S.F. (2002). Genital surgery among females with congenital adrenal hyperplasia: Changes over the past 5 decades. *J Pediatr Endocrinol Metab, 15*, 1473-1477.

Levine, L.S. (2000). Congenital adrenal hyperplasia. *Pediatr Rev, 21*(5), 159-170.

Lim, Y., Batch, J., & Warne, G. (1995). Adrenal 21-hydroxylase deficiency in childhood: 25 years' experience. *J Paediatr Child Health, 31*(3), 222-227.

Lo, J., Schwitzgebel, V.M., Tyrrell, J.B., et al. (1999). Normal female infants born of mothers with classic congenital adrenal hyperplasia due to 21-hydroxylase deficiency. *J Clin Endocrinol Metab, 84*(3), 930-936.

Lo, J., & Grumbach, M. (2001). Pregnancy outcomes in women with congenital virilizing adrenal hyperplasia. *Endocrinol Metab Clin North Am, 30*(1), 207-229.

Long, D.N., Wisniewski, A.B., & Migeon, C.J. (2004). Gender role across development in adult women with congenital adrenal hyperplasia due to 21-hydroxylase deficiency. *J Pediatr Endocrinol Metab, 17*(10), 1367-1373.

Mao, R., Nelson, L., Kates, R., et al. (2002). Prenatal diagnosis of 21-hydroxylase deficiency caused by gene conversion and rearrangements: Pitfalls and molecular diagnostic solutions. *Prenat Diagn, 22*(13), 1171-1176.

Merke, D., Bornstein, S., Avila, N., et al. (2002). Future directions in the study and management of congenital adrenal hyperplasia due to 21-hydroxylase deficiency. *Ann Intern Med, 136*(4), 320-334.

Merke, D., Fields, J., Keil, M.F., et al. (2003). Children with classic congenital adrenal hyperplasia have decreased amygdale volume: Potential prenatal and postnatal hormone effects. *J Clin Endocrinol Metab, 88*(4), 1760-1765.

Merke, D., Keil, M.F., Jones, J.V., et al. (2000). Flutamide, testolactone, and reduced hydrocortisone dose maintain normal growth velocity and bone maturation despite elevated androgen levels in children with congenital adrenal hyperplasia. *J Clin Endocrinol Metab, 85*(3), 1114-1120.

Meyer-Bahlburg, H.F. (1999). What causes low rates of child-bearing in congenital adrenal hyperplasia?. *J Clin Endocrinol Metab, 84*(6), 1844-1847.

Meyer-Bahlburg, H.F., Migeon, C.J., Berkovitz, G.D., et al. (2004). Attitudes of adult 46, XY intersex persons to clinical management policies. *J Urol, 171*, 1615-1619.

Migeon, C.J., & Wisniewski, A.B. (2001). Congenital adrenal hyperplasia owing to 21-hydroxylase deficiency: Growth, development, and therapeutic considerations. *Endocrinol Metab Clin North Am, 30*(1), 193-206.

Miller, W.L. (1994). Genetics, diagnosis, and management of 21-hydroxylase deficiency. *J Clin Endocrinol Metab, 78*, 241-246.

Miller, W.L. (2002). The adrenal cortex. In Sperling M.A. (Ed.), *Pediatric Endocrinology* (2nd ed.). Philadelphia: Saunders.

Minto, C.L., Liao, L., Woodhouse, R.J., et al. (2003). The effect of clitoral surgery on sexual outcome in individuals who have intersex conditions with ambiguous genitalia cross-sectional study. *Lancet, 361*, 1252-1257.

Money, J., Schwartz, M., & Lewis, V. (1984). Adult herotosexual status and fetal hormonal masculinization and demasculinization: 46XX congenital virilizing adrenal hyperplasia and 46XY androgen-insensitivity syndrome compared. *Psychoneuroendocrinology, 9*, 405-414.

Nabhan, Z.M., & Eugster, E.A. (2006). Upper-tract genitourinary malformations in girls with congenital adrenal hyperplasia. *Pediatrics, 120*, 304-307.

Nass, R., & Baker, S. (1991). Learning disabilities in children with congenital adrenal hyperplasia. *J Child Neurol, 6*, 306-312.

National Newborn Screening and Genetics Resource Center (2008). National newborn screening status report. Available at http://genes-r-us.uthscsa.edu/nbdisorders.pdf. Retrieved January 7, 2009.

New, M.I. (1995). Congenital adrenal hyperplasia. In L. DeGroot, M. Besser, H.G. Burger, et al. (Eds.), *Endocrinology* (3rd ed.). Philadelphia: Saunders.

New, M.I. (2001). Prenatal treatment of congenital adrenal hyperplasia. *Endocrinol Metab Clin North Am, 30*(1), 1-13.

New, M.I., Carlson, A., Obeid, J., et al. (2003). Update: Prenatal diagnosis for congenital adrenal hyperplasia in 595 pregnancies. *Endocrinologist, 3*, 233-239.

New, M.I., & Nimkarn, S. (2006). 21-Hydroxylase-deficient congenital adrenal hyperplasia. *Gene Reviews, 3*, 1-38.

Nimkarn, S., & New, M.I. (2007). Prenatal diagnosis and treatment of congenital adrenal hyperplasia. *Horm Res, 67*(2), 53-60.

Nordenström, A., Ahmed, S., Jones, J., et al. (2005). Female preponderance in congenital adrenal hyperplasia due to CYP21 deficiency in England: Implications for neonatal screening. *Horm Res, 63*(1), 22-28.

Ogilvie, C.M., Crouch, N.S., Rumsby, G., et al. (2006). Congenital adrenal hyperplasia in adults: A review of medical, surgical and psychological issues. *Clin Endocrinol, 64*(1), 2-11.

Otten, B.J., Stikkelbroeck, M.M., Claahsen-van der Grinten, H.L., et al. (2005). Puberty and fertility in congenital adrenal hyperplasia. *Endocrine Development, 8*, 54-66.

Pang, S. (1997). Congenital adrenal hyperplasia. *Endocrinol Metab Clin North Am, 26*(4), 853-891.

Pang, S., & Shook, M. (1997). Current status of neonatal screening for congenital adrenal hyperplasia. *Curr Opin Pediatr, 9*(4), 419-423.

Pippi Salle, J.L., Braga, L.P., Macedo, N., et al. (2007). Corporeal sparing dismembered clitoralplasty: An alternative technique for feminizing genitoplasty. *J Urol, 178*, 1796-1801.

Plante, E., Boliek, C., Binkiewicz, A., et al. (1996). Elevated androgen, brain development and language/learning disabilities in children with congenital adrenal hyperplasia. *Dev Med Child Neurol, 38*, 423-437.

Poppas, D.P., Hochsztein, A.A., Baergen, R.N., et al. (2007). Nerve sparing ventral clitoralplasty preserves dorsal nerves in congenital adrenal hyperplasia. *J Urol, 178*, 1802-1806.

Premawadhara, L.D., Hughes, I.A., Read, G.F., et al. (1997). Longer term outcome in females with congenital adrenal hyperplasia (CAH): The Cardiff experience. *Clin Endocrinol, 46*, 327-332.

Quintos, J.B., Vogiatzi, M.G., Harbison, M.D., et al. (2001). Growth hormone therapy alone or in combination with gonadotropin-releasing hormone analog therapy to improve the height deficit in children with congenital adrenal hyperplasia. *J Clin Endocrinol Metab, 86*(4), 1511-1517.

Rink, R.C., Metcalfe, P.D., Cain, M.P., et al. (2006). Use of the mobilized sinus with total urogenital mobilization. *J Urol, 176*(5), 2205-2211.

Seckl, J.R., & Miller, W.L. (1997). How safe is long-term prenatal glucocorticoid treatment?. *J Am Med Assoc, 277*(13), 1077-1079.

Speiser, P.W. (2001). Congenital adrenal hyperplasia owing to 21-hydroxylase deficiency. *Endocrinol Metab Clin North Am, 30*(1), 31-59.

Speiser, P.W. (2007). Prenatal and neonatal diagnosis and treatment of congenital adrenal hyperplasia. *Horm Res, 68*(Suppl), 90-92.

Steiner, E., & Woernie, F. (2002). Carcinoma of the neovagina: Case report and review of the literature. *Gynecol Oncol, 84*, 171-175.

Stewart, P.M. (2003). The adrenal cortex. In P.R. Larson, H.M. Kronenberg, S. Melmed, et al. (Eds.), *Williams Textbook of Endocrinology* (10th ed.). Philadelphia: Saunders.

Therrell, B. (2001). Newborn screening for congenital adrenal hyperplasia. *Endocrinol Metab Clin North Am, 30*(1), 15-30.

Therrell, B.L. Jr., Berenbaum, S.A., Manter-Kapanke, V., et al. (1998). Results of screening 1.9 million Texas newborns for 21-hydroxylase-deficient congenital adrenal hyperplasia. *Pediatrics, 101*(4 pt 1), 583-590.

Van Wyk, J., & Gunther, D. (1996). The use of adrenalectomy as a treatment for congenital adrenal hyperplasia. *J Clin Endocrinol Metab, 81*(9), 3180-3182.

Walker, B.R., & Stewart, P.M. (2000). Carbenoxolone effects in congenital adrenal hyperplasia. *Clin Endocrinol, 52*(2), 246-248.

Warne, G., Grover, S., & Hutson, J., et al. (2005). A long-term outcome study of intersex conditions. *J Pediatr Endocrinol Metab, 18*, 555-567.

White, P.C., & New, M.I. (1988). Molecular genetics of congenital adrenal hyperplasia. *Baillière's Clin Endocrinol Metab, 2*(4), 941-965.

White, P.C., & Speiser, P.W. (2000). Congenital adrenal hyperplasia due to 21-hydroxylase deficiency. *Endocr Rev, 21*(3), 245-291.

Wilson, B.E., & Reiner, W.G. (1998). Management of intersex: A shifting paradigm. *J Clin Ethics, 9*(4), 360-368.

Woelfle, J., Hoepffner, W., Sippell, W.G., et al. (2002). Complete virilization in congenital adrenal hyperplasia: Clinical course, medical management and disease-related complications. *Clin Endocrinol, 56*, 231-238.

Yang, J., Felsen, D., & Poppas, D.P. (2007). Nerve sparing ventral clitoroplasty: Analysis of clitoral sensitivity and viability. *J Urol, 178*, 1598-1601.

Young-Hyman, D. (1986). Effects of short stature on social competence. In B. Stabler and L. Underwood (Eds.). (1986). *Slow Grows the Child*. Hillsdale, NJ: Lawrence Erlbaum Associates.

Yucel, S., De Souza, A. Jr., & Baskin, L.S. (2004). Neuroanatomy of the human female lower urogenital tract. *J Urol, 172*(1), 191-195.

Zucker, K.J., Bradley, S.J., Oliver, G., et al. (1996). Psychosexual development of women with congenital adrenal hyperplasia. *Horm Behav, 30*, 300-318.

21 Congenital Heart Disease

Elizabeth H. Cook and Sarah S. Higgins

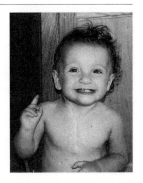

Etiology

Congenital heart disease (CHD) results from the abnormal development of the heart or related vascular structures during embryologic development. CHD is one of the most common forms of birth defects, and is the leading cause of death from congenital malformations. The causes of CHD are still poorly understood. The majority of congenital heart defects have a multifactorial cause, in which there is interplay of a genetic predisposition for abnormal cardiac development with an environmental trigger (e.g., an infection, a maternal condition, or ingestion of substances) at the vulnerable time of cardiac development.

Some form of chromosomal abnormality or syndrome accounts for approximately 20% of CHD (Bentham & Bhattacharya, 2008). Also, a growing number of cardiac conditions have been found to be associated with mutations in single or multiple genes. Many defects are associated with a syndrome in which other systems also are affected. One of the most common genetic associations with CHD is Down syndrome; over 40% of these children have some form of cardiac malformation (see Chapter 24). Approximately 90% of children with DiGeorge, or velocardiofacial, syndrome have microdeletion of 22q11 chromosome (Jenkins, Correa, Feinstein, et al., 2007). Other syndromes that do not have an identified chromosomal defect (e.g., asplenia syndrome and VACTERL syndrome, which is a constellation of anatomic defects involving *v*ertebral, *a*nal, *c*ardiac, *t*racheal, *e*sophageal, *r*enal, and *l*imb systems) often have CHD as one of many anomalies.

Though purely environmental causes of CHD are less understood than genetic factors, there is a developing body of knowledge regarding the cardiac teratogenicity of certain substances. Cardiac development occurs between the eighteenth and forty-fifth days of gestation, and the fetus is vulnerable to cardiac defects from teratogens from 2 to 10 weeks of gestation. This exposure may be from a maternal infection, a health condition, or maternal ingestion of drugs (Jenkins et al., 2007). There is also emerging evidence that possibly a woman's intake of multivitamins containing folic acid periconceptually may reduce the risk of offspring with congenital heart defects. As more information about genetic and environmental effects on the developing heart is discovered, more specific identification of cause is being determined. Table 21-1 lists these factors frequently associated with cardiac malformations.

Incidence and Prevalence

CHD generally occurs in approximately 0.8% to 1% of live births (Hoffman & Kaplan, 2002), making it one of the most common birth defects. The incidence of specific heart defects is shown in Table 21-2. Gender distribution is equal for CHD as a whole, but boys tend to have a higher incidence of some severe defects (such as transposition of the great arteries and left-sided heart defects).

The risk of CHD recurring in the same family depends on several factors. The risk of recurrence is greatest if the mother or full sibling—instead of the father or half-sibling—has the heart defect. If the defect is part of a syndrome or chromosomal abnormality, the recurrence risk of the heart lesion is related to the recurrence risk of the syndrome. With left-sided defects (such as hypoplastic left heart syndrome and aortic valve abnormalities), the rate of another defect of the same spectrum recurring may be as high as 22% (Hinton, Martin, Tabangin, et al., 2007; Loffredo, Chokkalingam, Sill, et al., 2004).

Though there are many ways of categorizing congenital cardiac malformations, one broad method separates the defects into acyanotic or cyanotic, depending on the hemodynamic changes that occur as a result of the specific heart anomaly. In acyanotic heart disease, the systemic circulation is not exposed to unoxygenated blood; in cyanotic heart disease, unoxygenated blood mixes in the systemic circulation (Figure 21-1). A brief description of the intracardiac pressure-flow relationship may clarify this classification of CHD.

Depleted of oxygen, blood returns to the heart from the venous system and enters the right atrium. From the right atrium, blood flows through the tricuspid valve into the right ventricle, where it is pumped through the pulmonary arteries into the lungs to pick up oxygen. Therefore the oxygen saturation in the right side of the heart is low (SaO_2 of 70% to 75%). The pressure in the right-sided circulation is also relatively low (i.e., approximately 25/2 mm Hg in the right ventricle and 25/10 mm Hg in the pulmonary arteries).

The blood that enters the left atrium from the lungs is rich in oxygen, with the oxygen saturation reaching 95% to 100%. The blood flows through the mitral valve into the left ventricle, where it is pumped into the systemic circulation via the aorta. Blood in the left ventricle is under high pressure (approximately 100/5 mm Hg), as is that in the aorta (i.e., approximately 100/60 mm Hg).

Because the pressure in the left side of the heart is greater than that in the right side, blood flows from the left to the right side of the heart if there is an abnormal connection between the two sides. This flow is called left-to-right shunting. Because the oxygen saturations are significantly higher in the left side of the heart than the right side of the heart, defects that cause left-to-right shunting are acyanotic. Left-to-right shunts commonly cause overcirculation of

TABLE 21-1

Factors Commonly Associated with Cardiac Malformations

Condition	Associated Defect
INFANT SYNDROME	
Genetic Disorders	
Trisomy 13	ASD, VSD, TOF
Trisomy 18	VSD, PDA, PS, TGA
Trisomy 21	AVSD, VSD, ASD
Turner's syndrome (XO)	COTA, ASD, AS, bicuspid aortic valve
DiGeorge/velocardiofacial syndrome (deletion 22q11)	Interrupted aortic arch, TOF, truncus arteriosus, VSD
Marfan syndrome (autosomal dominant)	Great artery aneurysms, aortic insufficiency, mitral regurgitation
Noonan syndrome (multiple gene mutation)	PS, ASD, hypertrophic cardiomyopathy
Williams syndrome (deletion 7q11.23)	Supravalvular subaortic stenosis, branch pulmonary artery stenosis
Ellis–van Crieveld syndrome (EVC and EVC2 gene mutations)	ASD, single atrium
Holt-Oram syndrome (TBX5 mutation)	ASD, VSD, single atrium
Alagille syndrome (deletion 22p12)	PPH, TOF, PS
Cri du chat syndrome (deletion 5p)	VSD, PDA, ASD
Genetic Disorder Not Identified	
Osteogenesis imperfecta	Aortic valve disease
Treacher Collins syndrome	VSD, PDA, ASD
Asplenia syndrome	VSD, single ventricle, common AV valve, TGA
VACTERL syndrome	TOF, VSD
MATERNAL CONDITION	
Rubella	PDA, ASD, VSD, peripheral pulmonary stenosis
Diabetes	TGA, VSD, AVSD, COTA, ASD, HLHS, cardiomyopathy
Lupus erythematosus	Heart block
Phenylketonuria	TOF, VSD, COTA, HLHS
Febrile illness	R or L obstructive defects, TA, COTA, VSD
Influenza	TGA, VSD, TA, COTA, R or L obstructive defects
MATERNAL INGESTION	
Alcohol	VSD, PDA, ASD, pulmonary atresia, DORV. TOF
Amphetamines	VSD, PDA, ASD, TGA
Cocaine	VSD, ASD, congenital complete heart block
Marijuana	VSD, Ebstein's anomaly
Smoking	Septal and right-sided obstructive defects
Organic solvents	HLHS, COTA, TGA, PS, TOF, TAPVR, AVSD
Hydantoin	PS, AS, COTA, PDA, VSD, ASD
Ibuprofen	TGA, VSD
Lithium	Ebstein's anomaly
Retinoic acid	VSD, varied CHD
Sex hormones	VSD, TGA, TOF
Thalidomide	TOF, truncus arteriosus, VSD, ASD
Trimethadione	ASD, PDA, VSD
Valproic acid	TOF, VSD, AS, PDA
Vitamin A	Outflow tract defects, PS
Warfarin	TOF, VSD

Data from Jenkins, K., Correa, A., Feinstein, J., et al. (2007). Noninherited risk factors and congenital cardiovascular defects: Current knowledge: A scientific statement from the American Heart Association Council on Cardiovascular Disease in young. *Circulation, 115,* 2995-3014; Pierpoint, M., Basson, C., Benson, W., et al. (2007). Genetic basis for congenital heart defects: Current knowledge: A scientific statement from the American Heart Association Council on Cardiovascular Disease in the Young. *Circulation, 115,* 3015-3038.
Key: *AS,* aortic stenosis; *ASD,* atrial septal defect; *AVSD,* atrioventricular septal defect; *COTA,* coarctation of the aorta; *HLHS,* hypoplastic left heart syndrome; *L,* left; *PDA,* patent ductus arteriosus; *PPH,* peripheral pulmonary hypoplasia; *PS,* pulmonary stenosis; *R,* right; *TA,* tricuspid atresia; *TGA,* transposition of the great arteries; *TOF,* tetralogy of Fallot; *VSD,* ventricular septal defect.

the lungs and strain on the right side of the heart, which often result in congestive heart failure (CHF).

Cyanosis usually results from one or both of the following physiologic problems: (1) right-to-left shunting, which results from obstruction of blood flow to the lungs plus an intracardiac communication; or (2) intracardiac mixing of oxygenated and deoxygenated blood. Figure 21-2 summarizes and illustrates the most common defects.

Diagnostic Criteria

Approximately 40% of the infants born with CHD will become symptomatic within the first year of life (Pierpont, Basson, Benson, et al., 2007). Methods of diagnosing include a thorough history and physical examination (with particular attention paid to signs and symptoms referable to the cardiovascular system), as well as multiple diagnostic procedures. Echocardiography is the most common tool used for diagnosing cardiac malformations. Cardiac catheterization may be used to help identify specific anatomy and physiology. Cardiac magnetic resonance imaging (MRI) plays an important role in identifying certain cardiac malformations, particularly aortic arch anomalies (Cantinotti, Hegde, Bell, et al., 2008). Cardiac disease can also be diagnosed in utero through fetal echocardiogram. This is an important method of diagnosis, because the early identification of fetuses with CHD may improve their outcomes (Hameed & Sklansky, 2007).

Clinical Manifestations at Time of Diagnosis

The clinical presentation of a child with CHD varies depending on the specific defect. Symptoms usually relate to the degree of CHF or cyanosis.

Congestive Heart Failure

CHD is the most common cause of CHF in children. CHF occurs when there is a strain on the myocardium from pressure or volume overload severe enough to reduce cardiac output to a level insufficient to meet the body's metabolic demands. Symptoms of CHF

TABLE 21-2		
Incidence of Specific Heart Defects		
Defect	**CHD (%)**	**Prevalence (per 10,000 Live Births)**
Ventricular septal defect (VSD)	15 to 25	15.57
Tetralogy of Fallot (TOF)	10	2.6
Pulmonary stenosis (PS)	8 to 12	3.78
Coarctation of the aorta (COTA)	8 to 10	1.39
Patent ductus arteriosus (PDA)	5 to 10 (excluding premature)	0.88
Atrial septal defect (ASD)	5 to 10	2.35
Transposition of the great arteries (TGA)	5	2.64
Aortic stenosis (AS)	3 to 6	0.81
Atrioventricular septal defect (AVSD)	2	3.27
Tricuspid atresia (TA)	1 to 3	3.6
Pulmonary atresia (PA)	1 to 2	5.8
Hypoplastic left heart syndrome (HLHS)	1 to 2	1.78
Total anomalous pulmonary venous return (TAPVR)	1	0.66
Ebstein's anomaly	<1	0.52
Truncus arteriosus	<1	0.69

Data from Park, M.K. (2008). *Pediatric Cardiology for Practitioners* (5th ed.). St Louis: Mosby; Clark, E.B. (2001). Etiology of congenital cardiovascular malformations: Epidemiology and genetics. In H.D. Allen, H.P. Gutgesell, E.B. Clark, et al. (Eds.), *Moss and Adams' Heart Disease in Infants, Children, and Adolescents Including the Fetus and Young Adult* (6th ed.). Philadelphia: Lippincott Williams & Wilkins.

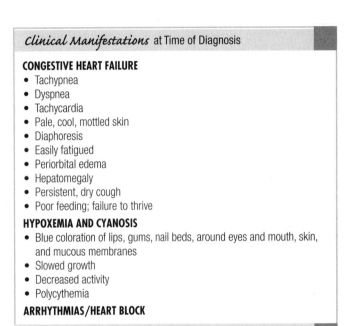

Clinical Manifestations at Time of Diagnosis

CONGESTIVE HEART FAILURE
- Tachypnea
- Dyspnea
- Tachycardia
- Pale, cool, mottled skin
- Diaphoresis
- Easily fatigued
- Periorbital edema
- Hepatomegaly
- Persistent, dry cough
- Poor feeding; failure to thrive

HYPOXEMIA AND CYANOSIS
- Blue coloration of lips, gums, nail beds, around eyes and mouth, skin, and mucous membranes
- Slowed growth
- Decreased activity
- Polycythemia

ARRHYTHMIAS/HEART BLOCK

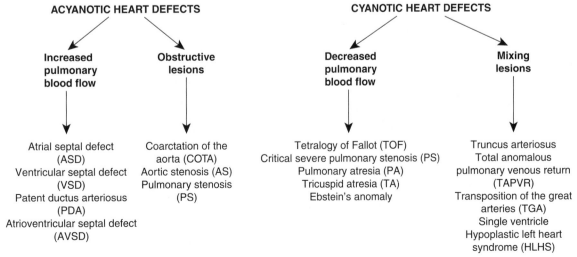

FIGURE 21-1 Classification of congenital heart defects.

result from the decreased cardiac output and the body's compensatory mechanisms, which include cardiac hypertrophy, cardiac dilation, and stimulation of the sympathetic nervous system. Initially, the compensatory mechanisms serve to improve cardiac performance. Over time, however, these compensatory mechanisms may actually exacerbate the decreased cardiac output. Infants with CHF are tachypneic, dyspneic, tachycardic, pale, cool, mottled, diaphoretic, and easily fatigued. Additional symptoms include periorbital edema, hepatomegaly, and a persistent cough. A history of difficult feeding and decreased food intake is a classic sign of CHF. Therefore growth failure is a common consequence of CHF in infancy and childhood (Da Silva, de Oliveira Lopes, & de Araujo, 2007). Clinical manifestations of CHF depend on the severity of the defect and pulmonary vascular resistance. CHF is manifested in neonates with a severe cardiac defect (e.g., transposition of the great arteries, hypoplastic left heart syndrome, critical aortic stenosis, or total anomalous pulmonary venous return, especially with pulmonary venous obstruction) or large left-to-right shunts in a premature infant (e.g., patent ductus arteriosus [PDA], ventricular septal defect [VSD], atrioventricular septal defect [AVSD]). Premature infants with a left-to-right shunt may develop symptoms of CHF earlier than term infants because their pulmonary vascular resistance drops faster than that of term infants. Infants with defects causing moderate left-to-right shunts (e.g., moderate VSD) do not usually develop symptoms until 4 to 8 weeks of age, when the high pulmonary vascular resistance of the fetal period drops low enough to cause increased pulmonary blood flow. The onset of symptoms is usually gradual; tachypnea, changes in feeding patterns, and poor weight gain are often early clues for parents. Children with small VSDs, small PDAs, or atrial septal defects (ASDs) generally are asymptomatic.

Hypoxemia and Cyanosis

Hypoxemia is the presence of an arterial oxygen saturation that is below normal. Cyanosis is the blue coloration of the skin and mucous membranes caused by deoxygenated hemoglobin. This coloration is usually seen in the lips, gums, and nail beds and around the eyes and mouth. Cyanosis is best perceived in children of all ethnicities by observing mucous membranes and nail beds in natural light. Children with cyanosis often have slowed growth, although they are not usually poor feeders. Polycythemia occurs in children who are chronically hypoxemic, because the body attempts to increase its oxygen-carrying capacity. Toddlers who are cyanotic (most commonly seen in children requiring staged repair of a complex lesion) usually limit their activity but still become easily fatigued and breathless if running, climbing stairs, or playing for long periods of time. Increasing cyanosis may be subtle and difficult to discern; monitoring increasing hemoglobin may facilitate the determination of progressive hypoxemia.

Arrhythmias/Heart Block

In infants and children who have not had cardiac surgery, there is an increased incidence of supraventricular tachycardia with Ebstein's anomaly, tricuspid atresia, hypertrophic cardiomyopathy, and double-outlet right ventricle. Anatomically corrected transposition of the great arteries (L-TGA) is a rare congenital heart defect that may also lead to supraventricular tachycardia (SVT) or varying degrees of heart block (Park, 2008).

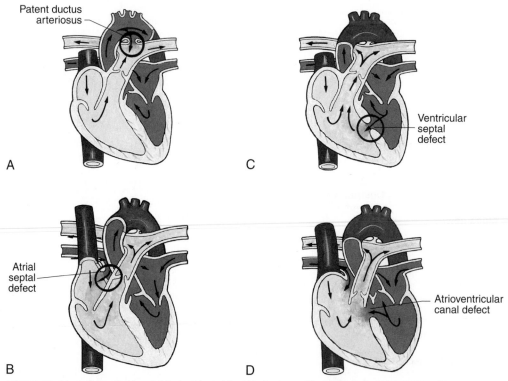

FIGURE 21-2 Congenital heart defects. Adapted from Hockenberry, M., & Wilson, D. (Eds.). (2006). *Wong's Nursing Care of Infants and Children* [8th ed.]. St. Louis: Mosby.

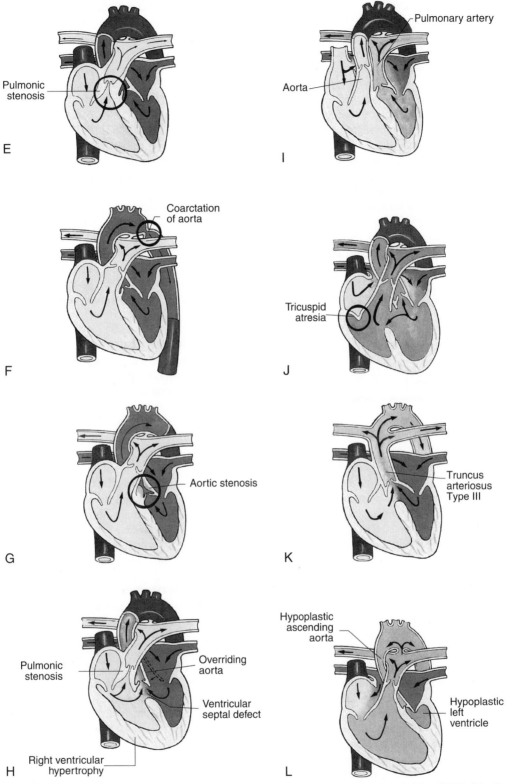

FIGURE 21-2, cont'd Congenital heart defects. Adapted from Hockenberry, M., & Wilson, D. (Eds.). (2006). *Wong's Nursing Care of Infants and Children* [8th ed.]. St. Louis: Mosby.

Treatment

Corrective Surgery

The natural history of some congenital heart defects (e.g., small VSD, ASD) is such that spontaneous closure of the defect may occur, avoiding intervention. These children have few if any symptoms. Most lesions, however, require surgery. For most defects, echocardiogram provides all of the information needed to perform surgery (Kimball & Meyer, 2001). For some cardiac defects, however, cardiac catheterization, perfusion scan, or MRI may also be performed before surgery to determine the precise anatomy and physiology of a child's heart. As techniques in surgical intervention, cardiopulmonary bypass, cardiac preservation, and postoperative care are refined, the trend in treating children with CHD is toward definitive repair at a very young age (frequently early infancy). Early corrective surgery decreases the negative consequences of longstanding hypoxemia, myocardial strain, and pulmonary overcirculation.

Treatment
- Corrective surgery
- Staged surgery
- Interventional cardiac catheterization
- Control of congestive heart failure
- Prevention of pulmonary hypertension

Staged Surgery

There is a population of children with complex CHD (e.g., children with single ventricle physiology) where staged repair is the treatment of choice. The child may undergo one or multiple palliative procedures as a neonate or infant followed by definitive repair after infancy. Interventional cardiac catheterization is frequently indicated to close collateral pulmonary circulation or anomalous vessels as the child is prepared for definitive repair. In children requiring a staged repair, symptoms of cyanosis and CHF may exist until the definitive repair is performed, sometimes into toddlerhood.

Interventional Cardiac Catheterization

For an increasing number of defects, interventional cardiac catheterization has replaced surgery as the treatment of choice. Some forms of aortic and pulmonary valvular or vascular stenosis can be repaired through balloon valvuloplasty and angioplasty. Vascular stents can be placed within the vessel to maintain the patency of stenosed vessels in conjunction with balloon angioplasty. Closure of PDAs, septal defects, and unnecessary collateral blood vessels is being performed via placement of various occlusive devices within the defect (Holzer & Hijazi, 2004; Patel & Hijazi, 2005). Clinical results of PDA closure with transcatheter coils are comparable to surgical closure, with no significant long-term complications and a significant decrease in cost.

Electrophysiologic studies are used in conjunction with cardiac catheterization to identify cardiac arrhythmias, evaluate the effectiveness of certain drugs under controlled circumstances, and abolish or ablate the accessory pathway causing the arrhythmia (Hanisch, 2001). Catheter therapy has now been applied to cure or modify most pediatric arrhythmias, including atrioventricular (AV) node reentry tachycardia, ectopic atrial tachycardia, and some forms of ventricular tachycardia (Berul & Dubin, 2006; Samii & Cohen, 2004). Implantable pacemaker/cardioverter-defibrillators (ICDs) may be indicated for children with long QT syndrome, cardiomyopathy, ventricular tachycardia, and other lethal arrhythmias (Hanisch, 2001). The broad field of therapeutic cardiac catheterization has become a valuable tool in managing many children with CHD.

Control of Congestive Heart Failure

Control of CHF is usually achieved with the use of diuretics and inotropes and afterload reducers. Since failure to thrive is a common complication of CHF (alone or in combination with cyanosis), feeding support is also a priority in management. Support may include methods of decreasing fatigue during feeding, increasing the caloric concentration of formula, or providing gavage feeding.

Infants who are cyanotic additionally require monitoring for progressive cyanosis, anemia, and dehydration. Parents of children who are cyanotic must learn to identify increasing blueness and cyanotic spells. Infants awaiting surgery are closely followed by a cardiologist to manage CHF or cyanosis and to time surgery.

Prevention of Pulmonary Hypertension

Crucial factors in determining the timing of surgery include preventing irreversible pulmonary hypertension and the development of aortopulmonary collateral vessels, as well as maintaining adequate ventricular function. Large left-to-right shunts rarely cause irreversible changes in the pulmonary vasculature before 12 months of age. Once these irreversible changes occur, however, surgery is contraindicated and the child becomes progressively cyanotic.

To aid the cardiologist in following the progress of the child's disease, communication between the cardiologist and the primary care provider is important. Signs or symptoms of increasing tachycardia, tachypnea, decreasing feeding, slowed weight gain, edema, hepatomegaly, worsening perfusion, or increased cyanosis should be reported to the cardiologist.

Complementary and Alternative Therapies

There is no alternative to surgical correction of congenital heart disease, and most surgeries are done while the child is very young. Parents need to be cautioned about complementary therapies because some may interfere with medications used to manage heart conditions. Products containing ginkgo interact with warfarin (Coumadin). Herbal and dietary supplements have not undergone the rigorous review of the U.S. Food and Drug Administration. Because there is no standardization related to dosage, side effects, and drug interactions with herbal products, their use is not recommended.

Anticipated Advances in Diagnosis and Management

Many aspects of pediatric cardiology continue to benefit from advances in technology, genetics, and research. Imaging techniques, fetal cardiology, interventional cardiology, arrhythmia management, and surgical techniques have shown significant developments (Duran, Brotons, Aeguelles, et al., 2008). The ability to diagnose CHD by echocardiogram has expanded beyond major centers through tele-echocardiography. Advances in devices and techniques associated with interventional cardiac catheterization continue to expand treatment options for children with CHD (Majunke & Sievert, 2007). Fetal surgery and interventional cardiac catheterization both show promise in preventing minor defects in utero from developing into critical ones once the heart is fully formed and the child is born.

For infants and children with the most complex defects (primarily single ventricle physiology), recent advances in diagnosis, surgical technique, and postoperative management have continued to improve outcomes. In an attempt to further reduce the mortality and morbidity risks associated with complex cardiac surgery, a recent approach to the first stage of repair for neonates with high-risk hypoplastic left heart syndrome incorporate interventional cardiac catheterization with palliative surgery (the Hybrid procedure) (Pigula, Vida, Del Nido, et al., 2007). Tissue engineering of prosthetic valves and conduits has great potential to create devices with the ability to grow with the child (Leyh, Wilhelmi, Rebe, et al., 2006). This technique would be a major breakthrough for pediatric cardiac surgery, in which a significant proportion of surgeries are performed to replace devices children have "outgrown."

Clinical electrophysiology (i.e., including pacemaker therapy) is another growing field. Various types of transcatheter ablations are playing an important role for managing children with supraventricular tachycardias (De Santis, Fazio, Silvetti, et al., 2008). Rhythm control—whether accomplished via advanced antiarrhythmic drugs, ablative therapy, or implantable devices—continues to evolve as more clinical experience is gained, new technologies are refined, and adult treatments are adapted for use in children.

Associated Problems of Congenital Heart Disease and Treatment

Hematologic Problems

Children with cyanotic heart disease develop polycythemia to increase the oxygen-carrying capacity of the blood. If the hematocrit reaches 65% or higher, there is a marked increase in the viscosity of the blood, resulting in an increased tendency for thrombus formation (Park, 2008). Bleeding disorders are also seen in children with polycythemia, most commonly thrombocytopenia and defective platelet aggregation, but also prolonged prothrombin time and partial thromboplastin time and lower levels of factors V and VIII. These children may bruise easily or develop petechiae, gingival bleeding, or epistaxis.

Anemia can be a special problem in children with CHD. In children with existing CHF, decreased hemoglobin may exacerbate myocardial strain. Therefore children with an acyanotic heart defect should have a hemoglobin level within the normal range for their age. Supplemental iron may be prescribed if their hemoglobin falls below normal levels or after surgery if their hemoglobin falls as a result of blood loss. In cyanotic infants, iron deficiency anemia has been associated with cerebral venous thrombosis (Park, 2008). Children who are cyanotic with a low hematocrit may exhibit hypoxic spells more readily than if the oxygen-carrying capacity of the blood were normal. Cyanosis will not be as obvious in children with anemia as in children with normal or elevated hemoglobin.

It is important for children with cyanosis who have a low hematocrit to receive iron therapy. It is equally important to monitor their response to the therapy to prevent the hematocrit from rising

to undesirably high levels, thus increasing blood viscosity. Adequate hydration must be maintained in children with cyanotic heart disease to avoid increased hemoconcentration. Problems associated with fever and exposure to hot weather, as well as vomiting and diarrhea, can cause dehydration. The problem of dehydration can be exacerbated if any of these conditions causing excessive volume loss occur in an infant or child who is on diuretic therapy.

Associated Problems of Congenital Heart Disease

- Hematologic problems
- Polycythemia
- Bleeding disorders
- Anemia
- Infectious processes
- Respiratory tract infections
- Bacteremia
- Infective endocarditis
- CNS complications
- Brain abscess
- CVA
- Arrhythmias/heart block
- Failure to thrive
- Obesity
- Slowed development
- Vulnerable child syndrome

Key: *CNS*, central nervous system; *CVA*, cerebrovascular accident.

Infectious Processes

Children with significant heart defects are at high risk for developing a variety of infections. Recurrent respiratory tract infections are especially common in children with lesions causing increased pulmonary blood flow. Infections can significantly affect a child's health in the following ways: (1) severe respiratory tract infections can exacerbate hypoxemia in cyanotic children; (2) fever can increase metabolic rate and oxygen demands, thus precipitating myocardial decompensation; (3) dehydration in a child with polycythemia can lead to thrombus formation; and (4) electrolyte imbalances from vomiting, diarrhea, or fever can impair cardiac performance or lead to digoxin toxicity in the child receiving digoxin.

Children with asplenia syndrome (i.e., a condition that includes absence of the spleen and complex cardiac defects) are extremely susceptible to bacteremia with an associated high mortality rate. *Streptococcus pneumoniae* and *Haemophilus influenzae* type B are the most common pathogens. Routine immunizations are recommended (see Immunizations, later in this chapter). Daily antimicrobial prophylaxis against pneumococcal infections is recommended for children less than 5 years of age with asplenia syndrome. Some experts continue prophylaxis throughout childhood and into adulthood in particularly high-risk individuals with asplenia. Recommended treatment for prophylaxis is oral penicillin V 125 mg twice a day for children under 5 years, and 250 mg twice a day for children 5 years and older (Committee on Infectious Diseases, 2006). Recently, the percentage of pneumococcal organisms that show some degree of resistance to penicillin has increased. Administration of conjugate pneumococcal vaccine reduces the penicillin-nonsusceptible vaccine strains of pneumococcus (Committee on Infectious Diseases, 2006). Because of the risk of infection, close observation and prompt intervention for symptoms of infection is critical.

Infective Endocarditis

Infective endocarditis (IE) may occur because of blood-borne bacteria that lodge on damaged, synthetic, or abnormal heart valves, prosthetic material, or the endocardium near congenital anatomic defects. Over the long term, individuals with the following conditions are at the greatest risk of developing IE: (1) prosthetic cardiac valve or prosthetic material used for cardiac valve repair; (2) previous infectious endocarditis; (3) unrepaired cyanotic heart defects; (4) surgically constructed shunts and conduits; (5) completely repaired defects with prosthetic material or device (surgical or interventional cardiac catheterization) within the first 6 months after the procedure; and (6) repaired CHD with residual defect (Wilson, Taubert, Gewitz, et al., 2007). Most cases of IE are not caused by an invasive procedure, but rather from random bacteremias from normal daily activities. The most common organisms responsible

for IE are *Streptococcus viridans, Staphylococcus aureus,* and enterococcus. However, there has been an increase in the incidence of endocarditis caused by such organisms as fungi, *Haemophilus,* and *Actinobacillus* (Park, 2008).

Recommendations for IE prophylaxis were revised in 2007 by the American Heart Association to include prophylaxis only for those individuals at highest risk (Box 21-1). For these children, dental procedures that manipulate the gingival tissue, respiratory tract procedures, and procedures on infected skin, skin structures, or musculoskeletal tissues must be preceded by antibiotic prophylaxis. Genitourinary (GU) and gastrointestinal (GI) procedures no longer require antibiotic prophylaxis. Maintaining good oral hygiene is a critical component of IE prevention. The current recommendation for prophylaxis for dental, oral, or respiratory tract procedures is amoxicillin (50 mg/kg for children; 2.0 g for adults) given orally 1 hour before the procedure (Box 21-2).

Central Nervous System Complications

In children with cyanosis caused by right-to-left intracardiac shunting, the normally effective phagocytic filtering action of the pulmonary capillary bed is bypassed. As a result, these children are at increased risk for brain abscess, most commonly after 2 years of age. Infants who are cyanotic with iron deficiency anemia are prone to develop cerebrovascular accidents (CVAs). A possible explanation for this finding is that relative anemia secondary to cyanosis leads to increased blood viscosity and increased coagulability and thus venous thrombosis (Park, 2008). Additionally, intracardiac thrombus from cardiac catheterization or surgery may embolize, leading to a CVA.

Arrhythmias/Heart Block

Rhythm disturbances can occur in children with CHD as a direct result of the cardiac defect, electrolyte imbalances, medications, or the surgical repair. Atrial arrhythmias are more common than

---

BOX 21-1

Infective Endocarditis Prophylaxis*

Endocarditis prophylaxis is recommended only for the following conditions:
- Prosthetic cardiac valve or prosthetic material used for cardiac valve repair
- Previous history of infective endocarditis
- CHD
  - Unrepaired cyanotic CHD, including palliative shunts and conduits
  - Completely repaired CHD with prosthetic material or device, whether placed surgically or by interventional cardiac catheterization, for the first 6 months after the procedure
  - Repaired CHD with residual defects at the site or near the site of a prosthetic patch or prosthetic device
  - Patients who receive a cardiac transplant who develop cardiac valvulopathy

Procedures for which endocarditis prophylaxis is recommended:
- Dental procedures that involve manipulation of the gingival tissue or the periapical region of the teeth or perforation of the oral mucosa
- Tonsillectomy and/or adenoidectomy
- Surgical procedures that involve intestinal or respiratory mucosa
- Bronchoscopy involving incision of the respiratory tract mucosa

Procedures for which endocarditis prophylaxis is not recommended:
- Dental procedures not likely to cause gingival bleeding (e.g., simple adjustment of orthodontic appliances or fillings above the gum line, restorative dentistry)
- Any GU or GI tract procedures
- Shedding of deciduous teeth
- Insertion of tympanostomy tubes
- Bronchoscopy without biopsy
- Endotracheal intubation
- Transesophageal echocardiography
- Cardiac catheterization
- Implanted cardiac pacemakers or defibrillators
- Endoscopy
- Cesarean section
- Uncomplicated vaginal delivery
- Vaginal hysterectomy

Adapted from Wilson, W., Taubert, K., Gewirtz, M., et al. (2007). Prevention of infective endocarditis: Guidelines from the American Heart Association. *Circulation, 116,* 1736-1754.
*This box lists common pediatric conditions and procedures but is not meant to be all-inclusive.
Key: *CHD,* congenital heart disease; *GI,* gastrointestinal; *GU,* genitourinary.

BOX 21-2

Endocarditis Prophylaxis Recommendations

FOR DENTAL, ORAL, AND RESPIRATORY TRACT PROCEDURES
1. For most patients: amoxicillin 50 mg/kg (maximum 2.0 g) orally 30 to 60 minutes before procedure
2. For patients unable to take oral medications: ampicillin 50 mg/kg (maximum 2.0 g) IM or IV 30 to 60 minutes before procedure
3. For patients allergic to amoxicillin, ampicillin, and/or penicillin: clindamycin 20 mg/kg (maximum 600 mg) orally 30 to 60 minutes before procedure
   or
   cephalexin or cefadroxil 50 mg/kg (maximum 2.0 g) orally 30 to 60 minutes before procedure
   or
   azithromycin or clarithromycin 15 mg/kg (maximum 500 mg) orally 30 to 60 minutes before procedure
4. For individuals allergic to amoxicillin, ampicillin, and/or penicillin who are unable to take oral medications: clindamycin 20 mg/kg (maximum 600 mg) IV 30 to 60 minutes before the procedure
   or
   cefazolin 25 mg/kg (maximum 1.0 g) IM or IV 30 to 60 minutes before the procedure

Adapted from Wilson, W., Taubert, K., Gewirtz, M., et al. (2007). Prevention of infective endocarditis: Guidelines from the American Heart Association. *Circulation, 116,* 1736-1754.

ventricular rhythm disturbances in children. Postoperatively, disturbances in atrial rhythms may be seen in children after surgical manipulation of the atrium (e.g., the Fontan procedure, repair of total anomalous pulmonary venous return [TAPVR], ASD repair). Intraarterial baffling procedures (e.g., the Mustard procedure) for transposition of the great arteries have been replaced by arterial switch procedure, in part, because of the incidence of arrhythmias in over 50% of children and adolescents. However, practitioners may still be seeing adolescents or young adults who have had the Mustard or Senning procedure in the past. Both atrial and ventricular arrhythmias are a growing problem in adolescents and young adults with CHD with associated increasing morbidity and mortality rates (Warnes, Liberthson, Danielson et al., 2001). Postoperative second- or third-degree heart block may occur in surgeries involving the ventricular septum (e.g., repair of VSD, AVSD, and tetralogy of Fallot), or with subaortic resection and aortic valve replacement. In addition, children who have had a complete repair of tetralogy of Fallot can develop ventricular ectopy, which can infrequently lead to sudden death (Hanisch, 2001).

Digoxin toxicity generally manifests as atrioventricular block, but it can also produce a wide variety of arrhythmias (Artman, 2001). A low serum potassium concentration potentiates the effects of digoxin. A child receiving a non–potassium-sparing diuretic (e.g., furosemide [Lasix]) without potassium replacement may be at particular risk of hypokalemia or digoxin toxicity. A therapeutic digoxin level is generally 1.0 to 2.0 ng/mL, although toxicity has been seen at lower levels and may not be seen at higher levels in some infants. A sound rule is to assume that an arrhythmia noted in a child on digoxin therapy is caused by digoxin until proved otherwise. If extra beats or an abnormal rhythm—including bradycardia and tachycardia—is identified by the primary care provider, an electrocardiogram should be obtained and the child should be referred to the cardiologist for further evaluation as soon as possible.

Failure to Thrive

Growth failure has frequently been observed in children with CHD. The decreased growth is usually more pronounced in weight than in height. CHF is one of the most potent factors in the development of failure to thrive because of inadequate caloric intake, malabsorption, increased resting energy expenditure, and pulmonary hypertension (Da Silva et al., 2007; Nydegger, Walsh, Penny, et al., 2007). Growth failure is especially problematic in children with single ventricle physiology, particularly those with hypoplastic left heart syndrome after their first palliative surgery (Davis, Davis, Cotman, et al., 2008; Kelleher, Laussen, Teixeira-Pinto, et al., 2006).

A new onset of slowed growth is particularly important to recognize because it may suggest significant hemodynamic compromise, necessitating an alteration in the drug regimen or surgery. Corrective surgery—particularly in infancy—generally restores a normal growth pattern. Weight usually improves more quickly than height. Palliative surgery generally improves growth, although not to the same degree as corrective surgery. As the age of corrective surgery decreases, the recovery of height, weight, and head circumference improves.

Obesity

In addition to the problems of failure to thrive, obesity has also become a significant problem among children with CHD (Pinto, Marino, Wernovsky, et al., 2007). This may develop from sedentary lifestyle resulting from appropriate or inappropriate activity restrictions or poor feeding habits as a result of failure to thrive during infancy. Children with coronary artery abnormalities (transposition of the great arteries [TGA]) or obstructive lesions of the aorta or left ventricle (coarctation of the aorta [COTA] or aortic stenosis) have a higher than normal risk of developing atherosclerotic cardiovascular disease (Kavey, Allada, Daniels, et al., 2006).

Slowed Development

The majority of children with CHD show cognitive performance within the range of normal. However, as a group they tend to have more neurodevelopmental problems. Those at highest risk are children with complex cardiac anatomy necessitating deep hypothermic circulatory arrest as a neonate in surgery and children with single ventricle physiology, particularly hypoplastic left heart syndrome (Hövels-Gürich, Konrad, Skorenski, et al., 2006; Mahle, 2001; Tabbutt, Nord, Jarvik, et al., 2008; Wernovsky, Shillingford, & Gaynor, 2005). Structural brain abnormalities, abnormal cerebral blood flow, chromosomal abnormalities, and cerebral ischemic and embolic lesions contribute to a decrease in neurodevelopmental functioning (Holm, Fredriksen, Fosdahl, et al., 2007; Mahle, Tavani, Zimmerman, et al., 2002; McQuillen, Barkovich, Hamrick, et al., 2007; Shillingford, Glanzman, Ittenbach, et al., 2008). Clinically, decreases in cognitive functioning, motor skills, language, attention, and memory are more common in children with complex congenital heart disease than healthy children. Learning disabilities are common (Bellinger, Wypij, Kuban et al., 2000; Shillingford et al., 2008). Other factors, such as a decrease in the child's ability to physically interact with his or her environment, parental overprotection, and prolonged hospitalization and illness, may contribute to neurodevelopmental delay (McCusker, Doherty, Molloy, et al., 2007).

CHF and cyanosis may significantly affect gross motor development. Children with CHD may sit, crawl, and walk much later than their peers (Mahle, 2001; Smith, 2001).

Vulnerable Child Syndrome

Children with a heart defect are at high risk for overprotection and altered parent-infant attachment. Parental anxiety and psychosocial stress can occur as a result of the disturbing array of clinical symptoms and feeding problems of a child with CHD, the fear of a sudden catastrophic event, and the paradox of becoming attached while dealing with fears about a child's vulnerability and potential death (Carey, Nicholson, & Fox, 2002). The mere presence of the defect unrelated to the severity of the heart disease, however, can produce severe anxiety leading to overprotection and placement of inappropriate limits on a child (Morelius, Lundh, Nelson et al., 2002; Uzark & Jones, 2003). Additionally, children with CHD, regardless of the severity of defect, report a decreased psychosocial quality of life (Uzark, Jones, Slusher, et al., 2008). Social adjustment and the development of independence is a challenge for children from school age to adolescents, and may be related to parental overprotection (Brosig, Mussatto, Kuhn, et al., 2007). Because overprotection may delay development in children with existing physical impediments to development, primary care providers should be aware of feelings of vulnerability in parents and children and reinforce the importance of treating these children normally. Practitioners should also routinely ask parents about parental stress, family functioning, and behavioral expectations for the child (Brosig et al., 2007).

Prognosis

The prognosis for children with CHD is good for the majority of lesions. Only the most complex defects require multiple surgeries. Most children have had definitive repair by their first year. Improved preoperative diagnosis, medical management, and surgical techniques have contributed to the significant decrease in surgical mortality rate of almost all congenital cardiac defects to approximately 5% to 6% (Chang, Rodriguez, Lee, et al., 2006). Low birth weight and female gender are associated with an increased mortality rate (Dimmick, Walker, Badawi, et al., 2007; Klitzner, Lee, Rodriguez, et al., 2006). The notable exception is hypoplastic left heart syndrome (HLHS), which has historically had a mortality rate significantly higher than other cardiac defects. In the past decade, changes in surgical approach and refinement of preoperative and postoperative management have improved the survival of infants with HLHS to as high as 93% for stage one and approximately 85% for the first two stages of repair (Tabbutt, Dominguez, Ravishankar, et al., 2005). The majority of children after cardiac surgery require long-term follow-up for potential problems related to myocardial changes, ventricular failure, deteriorating or outgrown prosthetic materials, arrhythmias, and infective endocarditis.

PRIMARY CARE MANAGEMENT

Health Care Maintenance
Growth and Development

Significant delays in both height and weight are seen in children with symptomatic CHD (Da Silva et al., 2007; Nydegger et al., 2007). Infants with single ventricle defects are at particular risk of growth failure (Davis et al., 2008; Kelleher et al., 2006). Height is generally not affected as much as weight, and head circumference should not be affected. If growth is slowed to a point where a child's growth curve flattens, the child should be referred to the cardiologist for an evaluation of worsening CHF. Because growth of a child with well-controlled CHF may still be slow, it is important to look at trends of weight gain, as well as make comparisons with the norms. There are also some syndromes associated with CHD (e.g., Turner syndrome, Down syndrome) that display slowed growth independent of a heart defect.

In assessing the developmental and emotional status of children with CHD, primary care providers must take into account factors such as preexisting neurologic abnormalities, hypoxemia, CHF, extended hospitalization, parental overprotection, and physical incapacity. Preoperatively, infants with CHF are often too exhausted to pass all of the developmental tasks in screening tests. If a child is developing at a slower but progressive rate, referral for additional developmental testing is not immediately warranted. If there appear to be significant alterations in the level of alertness or if there is no progress in mastering developmental tasks, further assessment is advised. If CHD is part of a syndrome that involves developmental delay, early referral and enrollment in an infant-stimulation program is important.

Infants and children who have been hospitalized may display developmental regression as an adaptation to the stress of hospitalization. Parents may notice that after surgery there are disturbances in their child's patterns of sleep, feeding, behavior, toilet training, and speech. Though this regression can be very concerning for

parents, it is a common response to the stress of hospitalization. It usually resolves within a few weeks and does not warrant further developmental follow-up. If there are other neurologic symptoms, such as change in level of consciousness, seizures, or weakness, the child should be examined and referred as needed.

When discussing developmental concerns with parents, the practitioner should help the parents normalize their responses to their child with a chronic condition. Primary care providers can guide parents in treating their child normally by reinforcing that children who are symptomatic will limit themselves naturally.

Diet

Feeding is often a major problem for children with CHD, particularly if they have a complex defect or are experiencing CHF. During feeding, symptomatic infants often have difficulty coordinating sucking, swallowing, and breathing. The distribution of calories in these infants is similar to the recommended dietary allowances, but the caloric needs of symptomatic infants with failure to thrive are about 150 kcal/kg/day (Abad-Sinden & Sutphen, 2001; Leitch, 2000). If infants are not adequately gaining weight, their caloric intake may need to be increased by concentrating breast milk or formula. Concentrating the breast milk or formula to 24 to 30 calories per ounce will elevate the total calories without increasing the total volume. If breast milk or formula is concentrated by adding powder formula to breast milk or decreasing the amount of water added to powder or concentrate, the increased renal solute load the infant receives must be considered. An alternative is to add low-osmolarity glucose polymers or oils to standard formulas to increase the caloric density. A diet providing increased carbohydrates and fats may lead to increased retention of nitrogen for growth. Consulting a nutritionist and the cardiologist is advised if nutritional manipulations are used.

Breastfeeding children with even a hemodynamically significant heart defect is not contraindicated if growth is adequate. Breast milk is the best source of nutrition for infants with a chronic condition, such as CHD (Kleinman, 2004). The physiologic stress of breastfeeding is less than the stress related to bottle feeding (Barbas & Kelleher, 2004; Marino, O'Brien, & LoRe, 1995). Methods to decrease the work of feeding during breastfeeding or bottle feeding include holding infants at a 45-degree angle to minimize tachypnea; feeding them for no longer than 40 minutes at a time to minimize fatigue; allowing them to develop their own rhythm of feeding and resting; and following their cues for hunger, satiety, and tiring.

A child with complex disease or CHF may not gain weight despite aggressive feeding and breast milk or formula concentration. Such children may need gavage feedings to minimize the calories used with feeding. Using a pacifier during gavage feeding helps an infant develop a strong suck, facilitates the transition to oral feeding after surgery, and promotes future language development.

Some children require manipulation of feeding regimens as a result of operative complications. Children who develop chylous pleural effusions because of damage to the thoracic duct are often discharged home on a low-fat formula or diet, which may need to be followed for several weeks (Chan, Russell, Williams, et al., 2005).

Parents often need a tremendous amount of support for feeding a child with CHD. Children with symptomatic CHD and tachypnea have difficulty consuming enough calories to satisfy hunger and may be irritable. Both infants and mothers may contribute to a less than optimal feeding situation. Infants with CHD give fewer feeding cues and respond less to caregivers, and mothers of infants with CHD may exhibit less fostering behavior (e.g., eye contact, smiling, and cuddling) during feeding. Parents may also feel the pressure of getting a child to gain weight for surgery. In addition, a parent's self-esteem may be tied to the feeding and growth of the child. Primary care providers should stress to parents that feeding can be a positive time for bonding and nurturing. Ongoing support includes teaching the parents to be sensitive to the infant's cues for hunger, satiety, and distress; pointing out the positive aspects of the child; and reinforcing feeding skills. Through feeding, the parent and child are developing their relationship. A primary care provider who understands the potential problems of feeding can be instrumental in fostering a positive feeding relationship by providing support and counseling.

Safety

In addition to standard safety precautions, children with CHD have unique safety needs. For example, digoxin elixir has a pleasant taste and attractive color, which increases the potential for accidental ingestion by the child or siblings. Therefore safe storage and administration of medications is essential. Marking a syringe at the correct dose, giving written and pictorial instructions on medication administration and allowing parents to practice drawing the medication will help ensure the safe use of all medications.

Electrical safety is critical for children with permanent pacemakers. An electric shock may irreparably damage the pacemaker, requiring immediate surgical replacement. There is no risk of electromagnetic interference between a permanent pacemaker and common household items such as electrical appliances, radios, cellular phones, or electronic equipment. Both microwave ovens and pacemakers have filtering systems that prevent interference with the pacemaker's function. Large magnets placed directly over the pacemaker will temporarily change its function; therefore MRI is contraindicated for children with a permanent pacemaker. Metal detectors should also be avoided because they have an electromagnetic field that may temporarily alter a pacemaker's function, as well as set off the alarm as a result of the metal in the pacemaker. Small magnet toys, however, will not alter a pacemaker's function. A pacemaker identification card or letter from the primary care provider should be sufficient to allow a child to avoid metal detectors or airport security.

Activity recommendations for children with CHD are published by the American Heart Association for competitive and recreational sports activities (Maron, Chaitman, Ackerman, et al., 2004; Maron, Thompson, Ackerman, et al, 2007). Children with permanent pacemakers, with cardioverters/defibrillators, or on anticoagulants for prosthetic valves can maintain most normal activities. They should discuss with their cardiologist recommendations for contact sports because bodily trauma may disrupt the lead system or cause excessive bleeding. Older children with pacemakers and children on anticoagulants should wear Medic-Alert bracelets for emergencies. Some conditions such as hypertrophic cardiomyopathy, Marfan syndrome, and prolonged QT syndrome have been associated with sudden death during exercise among adolescents and young adults. The decision of what sport is acceptable for these people should be discussed at length with their cardiologist (Maron et al., 2004).

Air travel may need to be altered for children with CHD. Altitudes of 5000 feet or higher are not recommended for children with moderate to severe pulmonary hypertension, severe CHF, or significant hypoxemia (i.e., PO_2 of 50 mm Hg). These children may require precautions to fly on an airplane because cabin pressure is usually equivalent to an altitude of 5000 to 7500 feet. The child's cardiologist can determine if supplemental oxygen will be needed during a flight. Families should check with individual airlines about their policy regarding availability of in-flight oxygen.

Training parents of children with CHD in cardiopulmonary resuscitation (CPR) may be effective and particularly warranted for certain problems. Suggesting CPR training to parents as a skill that is worthwhile for any parent to know can allay potential concerns about the importance of learning CPR. The American Red Cross or the American Heart Association may offer CPR training to families.

Immunizations

The standard immunization protocol (including the pneumococcal, meningococcal, and yearly influenza vaccines) is recommended for children with CHD (Committee on Infectious Diseases, 2006). A significant percentage of children with CHD, however, are behind in their immunization schedule. Some cardiologists are hesitant to give the full complement of vaccines to infants with single ventricle physiology because of the potential for cardiovascular compromise due to fever, irritability, or dehydration. However, research has not identified an association between routine immunizations and adverse events in these infants (McAlvin, Clabby, Kirshbom, et al., 2007). For children with CHD who are either unrepaired or palliated up to 2 years of life, immunization against respiratory syncytial virus (Synagis) is recommended. Monthly intramuscular injections usually begin in fall and continue until spring.

The timing of immunizations in children having heart surgery requires several considerations. Immunizations should not be given soon before cardiac catheterization or surgery because a fever would delay the procedure. Measles vaccine has been shown to cause a significant increase in the rate of thrombocytopenia, which could exacerbate the decreased platelet count and function seen after cardiopulmonary bypass. In addition, blood transfusion may affect immune response to vaccines for several weeks. After surgery, immunizations should be delayed approximately 6 weeks so that a fever from an immunization is not confused with a postoperative infection.

For children with asplenia or hemodynamically significant CHD who have received the full complement of the pneumococcal vaccine, an additional dose is recommended at 24 months of age and an additional dose is recommended to be given 3 to 5 years after the first dose (Committee on Infectious Diseases, 2006).

Screening

Vision. Routine screening is recommended.

Hearing. Routine screening is recommended.

Dental. Dental care should be meticulously followed to prevent caries and gum disease, which may predispose a child to bacteremia if left untreated. Children with high-risk cardiac defects need endocarditis prophylaxis before all dental procedures except simple adjustment of braces and shedding of deciduous teeth (see Infective Endocarditis, earlier in this chapter, and Boxes 21-1 and 21-2)

(Wilson et al., 2007). Because oral procedures (e.g., dental cleaning, drilling at the gum level, or pulling a permanent tooth) produce a higher inoculum of bacteria over a longer period of time than the shedding of deciduous teeth, antibiotic coverage is recommended for these procedures. The specific antibiotic depends on the child's sensitivity to penicillin. The child's cardiologist should communicate this information to the dentist and primary care provider. Wallet-size cards that outline specific prophylactic regimens are available from the American Heart Association.

Blood Pressure. Blood pressure should be obtained in the upper and lower extremities for children with preoperative or postoperative repair of the aorta to identify discrepancies in pressure readings that may indicate progression of the heart defect. A child who has had a Blalock-Taussig shunt procedure to increase blood flow to the lungs or a subclavian flap repair of coarctation of the aorta will have a diminished or absent pulse in the upper extremity on the side of the surgical scar.

Hematocrit. A rise in hemoglobin and hematocrit may indicate progressive hypoxemia in the child with a cyanotic heart defect. Furthermore, because of the problems associated with anemia in the child with cyanosis or CHF, hemoglobin and hematocrit levels should be checked regularly. Iron supplementation should be prescribed if the hemoglobin level is low for a child's specific condition. Because the child's cardiologist will be checking these values periodically, communication with the cardiologist may save a child the pain and expense of repeated laboratory tests.

Urinalysis. Routine screening is recommended.

Tuberculosis. Routine screening is recommended.

Condition-Specific Screening. Drugs and electrolytes: Infants and children on digoxin or warfarin (Coumadin) may need to have serum blood levels measured periodically. If the child is on diuretics, electrolytes may be routinely monitored by the cardiologist and may need to be checked if the child develops gastroenteritis.

Common Illness Management
Differential Diagnosis

Children with CHD may be susceptible to common pediatric problems that can be more severe than in children with structurally normal hearts. Therefore it is important for primary care providers to know the common problems that can lead to serious complications. It is equally important, however, that they treat these children normally and look for common, uncomplicated problems. Families need reinforcement that these children are normal but have special medical needs. Children who have had heart surgery are often scared or hesitant of examinations, particularly of their chest. If the child's trust is gained before the examination, visits will be less stressful for the child and more productive for the primary care provider.

Fever. Although febrile illnesses can have serious consequences in children with CHD, an acute fever may also be caused by a common, uncomplicated childhood illness. Primary care providers should investigate and treat fever the same way they would for any child the same age, while being mindful of the more serious possibilities. The chronic use of antibiotics without a diagnosis just because the child has CHD is not warranted and will put the child at risk of developing infections from resistant organisms.

Differential Diagnosis

Fever
- *Focus found:* common intercurrent illness unrelated to CHD postoperatively versus:
  - *Wound infection:* wound erythema, drainage
  - *Postpericardiotomy syndrome:* pericardial friction rub, malaise, chest pain

Infective Endocarditis
- Malaise, anorexia, night sweats, new murmur

Respiratory Compromise
- *URI or LRI:* fever, productive cough, infiltrates on chest radiograph versus:
  - *CHF:* poor feeding, sweating, dry cough, cardiomegaly

Gastrointestinal Symptoms
- Acute gastroenteritis versus:
  - Digoxin toxicity
  - Worsening CHF

Neurologic Symptoms
- Brain abscess
- CVA

Chest Pain
- Musculoskeletal problems, pulmonary conditions versus:
  - Cardiac etiology

Syncope
- Autonomic nervous system, seizures, hyperventilation versus:
  - Cardiac abnormalities

Key: *CHD*, congenital heart disease; *CHF*, congestive heart failure; *CVA*, cerebrovascular accident; *LRI*, lower respiratory infection; *URI*, upper respiratory infection.

A fever within a few weeks after heart surgery may be a sign of an operative infection or postpericardiotomy syndrome (i.e., an inflammatory reaction of the pericardial sac after heart surgery). A careful and complete examination is necessary to identify a source of infection. If no focus of infection (e.g., otitis media or pharyngitis) is found, the primary care provider should obtain a complete blood count (CBC) with differential and a blood culture and should refer the child to the cardiologist or surgeon. In addition, if there are any signs of a superficial surgical wound infection, the child should be referred to the cardiologist or surgeon. Postpericardiotomy syndrome should be suspected by the presence of a fever between 7 and 10 days after surgery, with a pericardial friction rub, chest pain, malaise, irritability, or enlargement of the cardiac silhouette on a chest radiograph. It is seen fairly frequently after surgery in which the pericardium has been opened, but is rarely seen in children less than 2 years of age (Rheuban, 2001; Wernovsky et al., 2005). The condition is usually self-limited, and treatment consists of antiinflammatory agents (aspirin, nonsteroidal antiinflammatory agents, or occasionally steroids) and rest.

A fever will increase the metabolic demands and thus the work of the heart. It is therefore important to evaluate a febrile child with symptomatic CHD for the development or worsening of CHF. Children with asplenia must be seen by the primary care provider immediately on developing a fever for a complete workup to identify the cause and initiate antibiotic therapy.

Infective Endocarditis. Primary care providers should be alert to signs of endocarditis in children with CHD who have a sustained, unexplained fever because symptomatology may be nonspecific and insidious. Fever may be associated with decreased activity, anorexia, malaise, night sweats, petechiae, splenomegaly, or a new murmur. Children with an unexplained fever and any of these symptoms should be referred to their cardiologist for evaluation, including an echocardiogram, to look for vegetations within the heart. Blood cultures should be drawn before initiating antibiotics. Children who have prosthetic cardiac valve or prosthetic material used for cardiac valve repair, previous infectious endocarditis, unrepaired cyanotic heart defects, surgically constructed shunts and conduits, completely repaired defects with prosthetic material or device (surgical or interventional cardiac catheterization) within the first 6 months after the procedure, and repaired CHD with residual defect may develop endocarditis (Wilson et al., 2007). Parental knowledge of measures to prevent endocarditis is limited. Therefore primary care providers must reinforce instructions on endocarditis prophylaxis at each visit.

Respiratory Compromise. Children with CHD—particularly those with a defect causing left-to-right shunting—may have frequent or significant upper and lower respiratory infections. It is important to evaluate the degree of respiratory compromise compared with the child's baseline respiratory status. If there is an increase in respiratory effort or the presence of adventitious breath sounds, a chest radiograph should be obtained to rule out pneumonia or worsening CHF. Infiltrates evident by radiograph, fever, and productive cough could indicate a lower respiratory infection. Cardiomegaly, poor feeding, sweating, and a dry cough would indicate CHF and require referral to the cardiologist. The primary care provider should have follow-up contact with a family 24 hours after initial contact to evaluate the child's progress.

Respiratory syncytial virus (RSV) can have especially serious effects in a child with symptomatic CHD. In addition, performing cardiac surgery in a child still recuperating from RSV can increase the risk of postoperative complications, particularly pulmonary hypertension.

Gastrointestinal Symptoms. Gastrointestinal symptoms may also occur. Vomiting or anorexia may occur secondary to gastroenteritis, worsening CHF, or digoxin toxicity. If the history and physical findings are not compatible with more common causes of GI symptoms, the child must be evaluated for other symptoms of CHF and a serum digoxin level obtained.

Excessive fluid losses from vomiting, diarrhea, or anorexia can lead to dehydration and thrombus formation in children who are cyanotic and polycythemic. Replacement fluids or consultation with the cardiologist to hold diuretic therapy may be necessary until the GI disturbance is resolved.

Neurologic Symptoms. A child with unexplained fever, headache, focal neurologic signs, or seizures must be immediately referred to a medical center because of the risk of a brain abscess (most common in children younger than 2 years of age) or CVA (most common in children older than 2 years of age).

Chest Pain. Only a very small percentage of children complaining of chest pain have symptoms caused by significant cardiovascular abnormality (Driscoll, 2001). The most common cause of chest pain is conditions involving the musculoskeletal structures of the chest wall (e.g., costochondritis, idiopathic chest wall pain, trauma, muscle strain, or sickle cell–related chest-wall bone pain). Less common causes include asthma, pneumonia, and gastroesophageal reflux. Cardiac etiologies of chest pain include pericarditis, aortic stenosis, obstructive hypertrophic cardiomyopathy, coronary artery ischemia, or arrhythmias (i.e., particularly in toddlers unable to differentiate pain from unusual sensations of arrhythmias). The mean age of all children complaining of chest pain is 12 to 14 years.

Critical components in a child's history that may clarify the cause can be determined with the following questions: (1) Is the chest pain related to exercise, eating, or breathing? (2) Is there related light-headedness or syncope? (3) Are there any other serious medical problems? (4) Is there unusual stress at home or school? (5) Is there a family history of sudden death or heart disease? and (6) Did the child experience recent physical trauma or new physical activity? The practitioner should be concerned if the chest pain is associated with symptoms such as syncope, light-headedness, or dyspnea. A careful history and physical examination can usually differentiate benign conditions from dangerous ones. An electrocardiogram and referral to a cardiologist should occur if the primary care provider identifies chest pain in conjunction with syncope, dizziness, easy fatigue, palpitations, exertion, drug use, fever, or associated medical problems (e.g., lupus erythematosus, diabetes, Marfan syndrome, or Kawasaki disease).

Syncope. Syncope is the transient loss of consciousness, usually from decreased cerebral blood flow. The most common causes of syncope in pediatrics involve the autonomic nervous system. These conditions may be caused by emotional stress, breath holding, hypovolemia, or anemia. Other causes include arrhythmias, seizures, pulmonary hypertension, hypercyanotic spells, or psychogenic reaction (often with hyperventilation). As with chest pain, a thorough history and physical examination are critical. Particular attention should be paid to the activity and position of the child before the event, as well as associated symptoms. Practitioners should pay special attention to syncope during or following activity because it may be a marker for sudden death (Scott, 2001). Family history of syncope, seizures, deafness, sudden death, or long QT syndrome should be noted. Physical examination should concentrate particularly on neurologic and cardiovascular systems. Diagnostic workup may include an electrocardiogram, and referral to a cardiologist may be recommended for further evaluation (i.e., including an exercise test and tilt-table test).

Drug Interactions

Children with CHF or arrhythmias often receive combinations of digoxin, diuretics, and other medications. The addition of any drug to a child's regimen when he or she is receiving cardiac medications should receive close attention and consultation with a pharmacist or cardiologist if there are questions about interaction. Coadministration of digoxin and quinidine (Cin-Quin), verapamil (Calan, Isoptin), or amiodarone (Cordarone) may elevate digoxin plasma concentrations (Trujillo & Nolan, 2000). Aminoglycosides can affect renal function and alter excretion of digoxin. Children with severe CHF may require medications (e.g., captopril [Capoten] or enalapril [Vasotec]) to decrease resistance to left ventricular ejection (i.e., afterload), thus decreasing the workload on the heart. These drugs may increase serum potassium. Therefore a potassium-sparing diuretic (e.g., spironolactone [Aldactone]) should be used with caution if a child is on captopril, and serum potassium should be followed closely. The combination of adenosine (Adenocard) and carbamazine (Tegretol) may act synergistically and cause heart block. Concurrent use of clonidine (Catapres) and verapamil (Calan, Isoptin) may lead to severe hypotension AV block. There are many well-documented interactions between cardiac and psychotropic drugs; consultation with the cardiologist is vital before beginning these drugs.

Warfarin (Coumadin) may be used in children with a propensity for clotting (i.e., those with prosthetic valves, pulmonary hypertension, or after the Fontan procedure). When children are on warfarin, their bleeding status is followed by periodic measurements of the International Normalized Ratio (INR). This value can be altered with concomitant use of warfarin and many medications (e.g., erythromycin). Any time a child on warfarin requires antibiotics or other medications, the primary care provider should consult with the cardiologist before administering them to prevent possibly altering the INR. There is no interaction with warfarin and immunizations.

When advising parents on the use of over-the-counter (OTC) medications for their child, the practitioner should stress the importance of using the simplest preparation of medication and to avoid multiple-ingredient products if possible. Decongestants, sympathomimetics, and drugs containing caffeine should be avoided in a child with a rapid heart rhythm (e.g., supraventricular tachycardia or atrial fibrillation) or hypertension because they may exacerbate tachyarrhythmias or increase blood pressure. Aspirin may be used in children requiring mild anticoagulation (i.e., after the Fontan procedure or aortopulmonary shunts). It should be avoided for 1 week before surgery because of its anticoagulant properties, and it should be avoided altogether in children receiving warfarin (Coumadin). It is important for the primary care provider to counsel parents to read labels of OTC medications because they may contain aspirin. Nonsteroidal antiinflammatory drugs (NSAIDs) can decrease the effectiveness of beta-blockers and angiotensin-converting enzyme (ACE) inhibitors (Smith, 2001). The primary care provider may be monitoring certain drug levels (digoxin, antiarrhythmics) or response to drugs (INR in the child taking anticoagulants) in close association with the cardiologist.

Developmental Issues

Sleep Patterns

Infants with CHF who are tachypneic may be unable to satisfy their hunger and thus have a difficult time sleeping through the night. Referral to the cardiologist is advised if a child's respiratory status is deteriorating to the point of interfering with feeding and sleeping. When discussing sleep with parents, primary care providers should ask them where the child sleeps. Parents may be keeping the child in their bed because of fears of their child's stability. Primary care providers should reinforce the stability of a child to help parents deal with their anxiety. The transition to the child's bed should not occur when the child's routine or security has been disrupted (e.g., around the time of hospitalization or surgery).

Toileting

Children on diuretic therapy may have difficulty with toilet training. If a child is receiving diuretics for a short period of time, parents may want to delay toilet training until the medication has been discontinued. If a child is on chronic diuretic therapy, the timing of the diuretic may need to be adjusted to facilitate toilet training. Toilet training, as with other developmental milestones, may be affected by the regression frequently seen after a child has been hospitalized.

Discipline

Behavioral expectations of children with CHD should be similar to those for children without a heart defect. It is not uncommon for parents to overprotect and pamper children with CHD. The diagnosis of CHD may cause changes in a family's approach and attitudes toward discipline, not only to the child with the disease but also to the normal siblings. Primary care providers can play a key role in reinforcing the importance of setting limits and disciplining children as if there were no heart disease, as well as helping to normalize family dynamics in light of the risk of overprotection.

On the other hand, infants with CHF who are irritable, hard to console, and difficult to feed may present a very stressful situation for parents. Primary care providers must be aware of family stressors and infant characteristics that may lead to abuse of a child with a chronic condition.

Child Care

Some parents choose to stop working when they have a child with a cardiac condition, but many do not. Child care is necessary for most families. Several factors that must be balanced when parents are deciding to return to work include the following: (1) the financial and emotional need to return to work; (2) parental anxiety about leaving the child; (3) the increased incidence of infection for children in child care and the effect of infection on a child's cardiovascular status; and (4) parental confidence in a child-care provider's ability to recognize symptoms, give medications properly, and respond to emergencies appropriately.

Before surgery or cardiac catheterization, parents may be counseled to take their child out of child care to avoid exposure to infections that would cancel the procedure. Children with asplenia or DiGeorge syndrome are at the highest risk of infection. For these children who are prone to infection, home or small group daycare is advised. For 6 weeks after surgery, parents should limit activities that stress the child's sternum (e.g., climbing, pulling, heavy lifting, rough playing, or lifting the child under the arms). Parents must communicate these restrictions to the child-care provider to see if it is realistic or safe for the child to return to daycare before normal activity is allowed. Primary care providers can play a key role in educating child-care providers about a child's condition, as well as in reinforcing activity limits—and lack of limits.

Schooling

Most school-age children with CHD can attend school with their peers, although children with complex heart disease are at risk for having learning disabilities, including attention disorders, hyperactivity, and language, motor, and intelligence quotient (IQ)/performance discrepancies (Miatton, de Wolf, Francois, et al., 2007; Shillingford et al., 2008). Since learning problems may be more subtle than a significant decrease in IQ, the practitioner should be particularly alert to signs of learning disabilities. Special education is often warranted for children with CHD. Missed school is often related to hospitalization, recuperation from surgery, and visits to the cardiologist. Primary care providers can play an important role in assessing the need for home or in-hospital schooling for prolonged absences and facilitating services. Absenteeism may also be associated with parental perception of a child's vulnerability and their lack of control over improving their child's health status.

As children enter junior high and high school, they may have body image concerns related to their scar, small stature, or ability to keep up with peers. Parents often underestimate their child's activity tolerance, and adolescents with heart disease may have a distorted conception of their disease and their abilities and limitations related to physical activity (Canobbio, 2001). The American Heart Association (Kavey et al., 2006) recommends a combination of moderate and vigorous physical activity for adults and children to decrease the long-term risks of developing stroke, coronary artery disease, hypertension, and obesity. Specific to CHD, detailed recommendations have been established for determining the level of activity related to each congenital cardiac lesion, arrhythmia, or acquired heart disease. The issue in prescribing specific activities to children with congenital heart disease is that it is difficult to quantify the degree of myocardial demand for specific activities related to the hemodynamic consequences of specific defects and each repair (Canobbio, 2001). Because of this potential problem, children should generally be encouraged to participate in physical activity to their tolerance based on an individualized plan formulated from discussions with the child, primary care provider, cardiologist, parents, and school professionals.

A standard letter of recommendations for activity (Figure 21-3) will clarify expectations and limits so that children can participate in physical activities to their highest potential. The cardiologist may perform stress testing to develop an individualized activity plan. This information should be relayed to the primary care provider. An ongoing discussion with parents and children will reinforce the realistic goals for activity and help prevent overprotection and resulting cardiac deconditioning.

Sexuality

Technologic and surgical advances have enabled the majority of young women with CHD to reach childbearing age. Many can successfully carry a pregnancy through delivery. A woman with complex congenital heart defects, however, warrants a careful evaluation of maternal and fetal risk. The increased risk of CHD in the offspring of individuals with CHD should be discussed with a cardiologist or a genetic counselor before conception if possible.

The issues of contraception and safety of pregnancy must be discussed with parents before their daughter becomes an adolescent, as well as when she is in early adolescence. Communication with the cardiologist will give the primary care provider critical information about a young woman's risk factors for contraception and pregnancy given her particular physical status.

RECOMMENDATIONS FOR PHYSICAL ACTIVITY IN SCHOOL FOR CHILDREN WITH HEART DISEASE

DATE_____

To Whom it May Concern:

_____ is a patient of mine for a congenital heart condition. The following recommendations are guidelines for physical activity in school. The child's cardiac diagnosis is
_____
_____.

____(1) May participate in the entire physical education program, including varsity competitive sports without any restriction.

____(2) May participate in the entire physical education program EXCEPT for varsity competitive sports where there is strenuous training and prolonged physical exertion, such as football, hockey, wrestling, soccer, basketball, etc. Less strenuous sports such as baseball and golf are acceptable at varsity level. All activities during the regular physical education program are acceptable.

____(3) May participate in the physical education program EXCEPT for restrictions from all varsity sports and from excessively stressful activities such as rope climbing, weight lifting, sustained running (i.e., laps) and fitness testing. MUST be allowed to stop and rest when tired.

____(4) May participate only in mild physical activities such as walking, golf, and circle games.

____(5) Restricted from the entire physical education program.

____(6) Additional remarks: (see other side)

____(7) Duration of recommendations: _____

If there are any additional questions about these recommendations, please contact me.

Sincerely,

_____ (Cardiologist's signature)

FIGURE 21-3 Sample letter or recommendation for activity.

Because of the problem with estrogen-containing oral contraceptives and thromboembolism, they are not recommended for women who are cyanotic and those with right-to-left shunts, pulmonary vascular disease, or prosthetic valves or conduits (Canobbio, Perloff, & Rapkin, 2005). Injectable (medroxyprogesterone acetate [Depo-Provera]) or oral contraceptives that contain only progestin are suitable for these women. Because of the potential for cervicitis and subsequent bacteremia, intrauterine devices (IUDs) are contraindicated in women at risk for developing infective endocarditis (Canobbio et al., 2005). Barrier methods (e.g., condoms and diaphragms with spermicidal cream) are safe methods of birth control from a cardiac standpoint but are not as effective in preventing pregnancy. For women at very high risk for cardiac compromise with pregnancy, surgical sterilization should be discussed. The social, emotional, and ethical considerations regarding sterilization make it a very controversial topic that should be discussed at length with the young woman and possibly her family. Tubal ligation in women with longstanding pulmonary hypertension leading to Eisenmenger syndrome carries with it a high surgical risk and should not be performed unless absolutely necessary. If tubal ligation is recommended, it is best to wait, if possible, until young adulthood when a woman has gained maturity and can participate in the decision.

Experts often look at an individual's cardiovascular status based on the New York Heart Association (NYHA) functional classification to determine the relative risk of pregnancy. Adolescents with mild heart disease that has not been operated on or those with well-repaired cardiac defects (NYHA class I or II) are generally at no higher risk from pregnancy than the general population (Canobbio, 2001). Adolescents in class III or above with CHF need special attention during pregnancy. Pregnancy in adolescents with pulmonary vascular disease carries a high risk for morbidity and mortality and may need to be terminated for the safety of the mother (Canobbio, 2001). It is important for primary care providers to discuss the risks of pregnancy with the cardiologist so that the recommendation can be reinforced to the adolescent. A multidisciplinary approach involving the cardiologist, the high-risk obstetrician, and the primary care provider should be used for adolescents with CHD who are pregnant.

Transition to Adulthood

There are approximately 800,000 adults with CHD in the United States (Betz, 2004). Current recommendations are that about half of adults with CHD should be followed by a cardiologist with CHD expertise at adult centers every 1 to 2 years. These individuals are at risk for serious sequelae related to arrhythmias, need for reoperation, and premature death (Reid, Irvine, McCrindle, et al., 2004). Key problems associated with the care of the adult with CHD have been identified by Dearani, Connolly, Martinez and colleagues (2007) as poor follow-up and weak infrastructure of care. These problems are primarily related to lack of transitional programs from pediatric to adult cardiology care, inadequate education of the individual and family with respect to future medical and surgical needs, and practitioners who have not received specialized training in the complexity of CHD. Bjornsen (2004) further identifies the following barriers for successful transition of the adolescent with CHD to adult centers: (1) pediatricians can be unwilling to transfer or lack confidence in transferring patients; (2) individuals and their families may be resistant to moving to an adult setting; and (3) lack of adequate preparation of the adolescent for the transfer of care.

Specific issues for adolescents with CHD as they transition into adult health care include the following: (1) lack of confidence in the care given to them from unknown providers; (2) fear of future invasive procedures; (3) insecurity about their ability to advocate for themselves; and (4) inadequate education about their condition and the specific details of immediate and long-term care needs (Higgins & Tong, 2003).

Recommendations for transitioning the care of the adolescent with CHD into adulthood as outlined in the 32nd Bethesda Conference convened by the American College of Cardiology include the following: (1) organizing the care for adults with CHD; (2) improving access to care; and (3) addressing the special needs of adults with congenital heart problems (Webb & Williams, 2001). A recommendation for the delivery of care to adolescents and adults with CHD was to establish adult congenital heart disease regional centers. These centers include a multidisciplinary team of pediatric and adult cardiologists, congenital heart surgeons, and advanced practice nurses who would coordinate care (Landzburg, Murphy, Davidson et al., 2001).

Recommendations were further made to develop a structured plan for the adolescent transitioning from a pediatric cardiology setting into an adult cardiology practice. This plan includes a "health care passport" designed to accompany the adolescent into the new cardiology setting. The specific "passport" information includes the adolescent's diagnosis, surgical procedures, medications with side effects, endocarditis prophylaxis, exercise prescription, contraception, frequency of medical follow-up, and insurance coverage (Foster, Connelly, Martinez et al., 2001).

Children with CHD should be oriented to the transition process to adult care during the preteen years. Staged discussions that are developmentally appropriate should be done with and without parents to potentially help the adolescent with a more effective transfer from the pediatric setting (Reid et al., 2004).

Facilitating the effective coordination of care from pediatrics to adult health care is central to maximizing the lifelong function and potential of an increasing number of children surviving CHD (Bjornsen, 2004). Management of these individuals by a core interdisciplinary team with expertise in congenital heart conditions, as well as the social and psychological impact of growing up with CHD, is paramount throughout their adulthood (Higgins & Tong, 2003).

Family Concerns

The family of a child with CHD may have ongoing concerns about symptoms, feeding problems, sudden death, finances, and the long-term physical and emotional effects of multiple surgeries. When parents are counseled about symptoms, it is important that primary care providers convey that the parents will be watching for trends over time rather than minute-by-minute. Reinforcing the fact that parents become the experts in observing their child for changes decreases their feelings that only health care providers can adequately monitor their child.

Some parents of children with CHD believe that their primary care provider is unable to meet many of their child's illness needs, whereas other parents of adolescents with mild heart disease would prefer to see their primary care provider for all routine health care needs and many cardiovascular health needs (Miller, Forrest, & Kan, 2000). Parental information needs related to caring for their infant after cardiac surgery are significant, and the parent's level of understanding may be limited. A review of postoperative instructions by the primary care provider and ongoing, careful evaluation of the child will help solidify the parent's knowledge base and reinforce the health provider's position as a valuable asset to the child's care.

The insurability of a child with heart disease depends on the particular defect and repair. As children become older, they often lose their parents' coverage and have difficulty obtaining insurance as adults (Foster et al., 2001). Parents must investigate the options for extended coverage of the child on their health insurance plan well before the policy's coverage expires for the child. Depending on their parents' income and the level of disability, children with CHD may qualify for Supplemental Security Income (see Chapter 8).

Parents may also be concerned about the occurrence of CHD in subsequent children. The cardiologist or genetic counselor should advise a family about specific risks to future children, and the primary care provider should reinforce this information and support the family in their decision making. Early prenatal diagnosis of CHD is possible through ultrasound of the fetal heart (i.e., fetal echocardiogram).

Resources

Parent support groups are valuable resources and provide an important network for families who are coping with anxieties related to caring for a child with CHD. Newsletters and special interest groups often develop from parent networking. The primary care provider should contact the local American Heart Association (AHA) or the pediatric cardiology department to see if such groups exist. Written information on many aspects of CHD is also available through the AHA. Public health or home health nursing may be an additional source of support, especially for families learning to identify symptoms, give multiple medications, provide adequate nutrition to a newly diagnosed infant with CHD, or care for a child with complex home care needs. Summer camps for children with CHD are available in several locations across the country.

The Internet has a wealth of information about heart defects, surgical procedures, and support for families of children with heart defects. Parents should be advised to use websites from the AHA and medical centers with pediatric cardiology subspecialty departments for medical information regarding their child's disease. Other websites may be valuable for support and information sharing to help families cope with the stressors of having a child with CHD.

Informational Materials

The following resource booklets and pamphlets are available for families through the local or national chapter of the AHA (this is not a complete listing of resources):

- *If Your Child Has a Heart Defect—A Guide for Parents*
- *Feeding Infants with Heart Disease—A Guide for Parents*
- *Dental Care for Children with Heart Disease*
- *Abnormalities of Heart Rhythm—A Guide for Parents*
- *Caring for a Child with a Heart Condition—A Guide for Parents* (San Francisco chapter)
- *Marfan Syndrome*
- *Kawasaki's Disease*
- *Coumadin*
- *AHA Scientific Statement: Guidelines for Parent Support Groups*

Organizations

The following list is a small sampling of the support/information networks available to families online. It is by no means complete but will provide information, as well as links to other resources. There are many online and in-person parent support groups and child/family resources across the nation.

American Heart Association
Website: www.americanheart.org
Congenital Heart Information Network
Websites: www.tchin.org; www.pediheart.org
Medlineplus: congenital heart disease
Website: www.nlm.nih.gov/medlineplus/congenitalheartdisease. html

---

Summary of Primary Care Needs for the Child with Congenital Heart Disease

HEALTH CARE MAINTENANCE

Growth and Development

- Significant delays in weight and height are common in children with symptomatic CHD preoperatively; corrective surgery improves growth.
- Intellectual development is not significantly impaired by CHD; cyanosis, parental overprotection, and CHF may contribute to delayed development.
- Behavioral regression during or after hospitalization is common.

Diet

- Feeding is a major problem for children with CHD—especially for a child in CHF; required daily allowances are normal, but caloric needs may be higher.
- Breastfeeding is encouraged if growth is adequate.

- May need to concentrate formula or breast milk if growth is inadequate. Gavage feeding may be necessary to conserve energy.
- Parents should be taught methods to decrease work of feeding.
- Feeding is a major source of stress for parents, who will need much support.

Safety

- Safe storage of medications is critical.
- For the child with a pacemaker, electrical safety is critical. There is no risk of damage with usual household appliances, including microwaves. Children with pacemakers should not have MRIs and should avoid metal detectors and wear a Medic-Alert bracelet.
- Children on anticoagulants or with permanent pacemakers should avoid contact sports.

Continued

Summary of Primary Care Needs for the Child with Congenital Heart Disease—cont'd

- Air travel and altitude may need to be limited depending on the defect.
- Cardiopulmonary resuscitation training for parents is warranted for certain defects.

Immunizations

- Standard immunization protocol including meningococcal, pneumococcal, and influenza vaccines is recommended; delay should occur only around cardiac catheterization or surgery.
- With asplenia syndrome or hemodynamically significant CHD, after receiving the full complement of the pneumococcal vaccine, additional doses are recommended at 24 months of age and an additional dose is recommended to be given 3 to 5 years after the first dose.

Screening

- *Vision.* Routine screening is recommended.
- *Hearing.* Routine screening is recommended.
- *Dental.* Dental care is important to prevent caries, which predispose a child to bacteremia and endocarditis. Endocarditis prophylaxis is recommended for all dental procedures except routine adjustment of braces and shedding of deciduous teeth (see Boxes 21-1 and 21-2).
- *Blood pressure.* Check blood pressure in all four extremities for children with aortic abnormalities preoperatively and postoperatively. Children with a Blalock-Taussig shunt or subclavian flap repair of coarctation of the aorta will have low or absent blood pressure values in the arm on the side of surgery.
- *Hematocrit.* A rise in hematocrit may indicate worsening cyanosis. Anemia is problematic in children with CHF or cyanosis. Monitor hemoglobin levels closely in coordination with the cardiologist.
- *Urinalysis.* Routine screening is recommended.
- *Tuberculosis.* Routine screening is recommended.

Condition-Specific Screening

- Serum levels of digoxin, warfarin, and diuretics may need to be monitored.
- Complete blood counts and electrolytes are also monitored frequently before surgery.

COMMON ILLNESS MANAGEMENT

Differential Diagnosis

- *Fever.* Postoperatively rule out (1) wound infection and (2) postpericardiotomy syndrome. If no focus is found, obtain a CBC and blood culture, and consult with the cardiologist. The child with asplenia with fever must be seen immediately. Fever may worsen CHF.
- *Infective endocarditis.* Symptoms are often vague; a high level of suspicion is needed for diagnosis. It is rarely seen in children less than 2 years of age. The child should be referred to the cardiologist for evaluation.
  - Refer to the cardiologist if fever, malaise, anorexia, splenomegaly, or night sweats are present.
- *Respiratory infection.* Frequent or significant upper and lower respiratory infections may occur; rule out CHF or pneumonia. RSV can cause significant morbidity.

- *Gastrointestinal symptoms.* Rule out digoxin toxicity and CHF; excessive fluid losses are dangerous in children who are cyanotic or taking diuretics and digoxin.
- *Neurologic symptoms.* Cyanotic children are at increased risk for brain abscess (if >2 years) or CVA (if <2 years); unexplained fever, headaches, seizures, or focal neurologic signs require immediate referral to a medical center.
  - Children with CHD are at increased risk of neurologic abnormalities (e.g., seizures, muscle tone abnormalities, and motor asymmetry).
- *Chest pain.* Most chest pain is caused by noncardiac problems. Careful history and physical examination usually differentiate benign from dangerous conditions.
- *Syncope.* There are many cardiac and noncardiac causes.
  - Close attention should be paid to head, eyes, ears, nose, and throat to rule out vestibular disease.
  - An electrocardiogram may be useful to rule out cardiac causes.

Drug Interactions

- The addition of any drug to a child's regimen should be preceded by consultation with a pharmacist or cardiologist.
- Accurate administration of digoxin is critical. Many medications can alter plasma levels of digoxin.
- Potassium levels need to be monitored in children on diuretics and digoxin.
- Aminoglycosides may decrease renal function and increase the digoxin level.
- Digoxin or anticoagulant dosages may need to be monitored.
- Children on warfarin (Coumadin) may have prothrombin time (PT) and INR altered when placed on antibiotics.
- Interactions between antiarrhythmia drugs and psychotropic drugs may occur.
- Decongestants are not recommended for children with rapid heart arrhythmias or hypertension.

DEVELOPMENTAL ISSUES

- *Sleep patterns.* Children may have difficulty sleeping through the night if they are tachypneic and unable to satisfy their hunger.
- *Toileting.* Toilet training children receiving diuretics may be difficult.
- *Discipline.* Normal behavior should be expected from children regardless of CHD. Parents often overprotect and pamper children with CHD.
  - Infants with CHF may be irritable and hard to console. The stress and coping of caregivers must be assessed.
- *Child care.* The child-care provider must understand medications, be able to recognize symptoms, and know emergency procedures.
  - Infants with DiGeorge syndrome or asplenia syndrome are prone to infection, so home daycare or small-group daycare is recommended.
  - Vigorous activity should be limited for 6 weeks after surgery.
- *Schooling.* Learning disabilities are common in children with CHD. Children may need home tutoring around hospitalization and surgery time.
  - Children may develop self-image concerns about their scar, ability to keep up with peers, and small stature.

Summary of Primary Care Needs for the Child with Congenital Heart Disease—cont'd

- The AHA publishes guidelines for activity limits based on each defect. Generally, children limit themselves. Children who have a pacemaker or are taking anticoagulants should avoid rough contact sports.
- Parents frequently underestimate their child's activity tolerance.
- *Sexuality.* Estrogen-containing oral contraceptives are not recommended for individuals with pulmonary hypertension, cyanotic CHD, or prosthetic valves.
  - An intrauterine device is not recommended for individuals at risk for developing endocarditis.
- An individual's heart defect and functional ability (i.e., as assessed by the cardiologist) determine risks associated with pregnancy; teens need early and thorough counseling.

Transition to Adulthood

- The transition process should begin during the preteen years.
- Adolescents and adults with CHD should be followed every 1 to 2 years by a cardiologist with CHD experience.

FAMILY CONCERNS

- Families have ongoing concerns about symptoms, multiple surgeries, and sudden death.
- Children and adults with CHD have difficulty finding insurance coverage.
- Parents may be concerned that CHD will occur in subsequent children and may want genetic counseling; prenatal diagnosis of CHD is possible through fetal echocardiography.

REFERENCES

Abad-Sinden, A., & Sutphen, J.L. (2001). Growth and nutrition. In H.D. Allen, H.P. Gutgesell, E.B. Clark, (Eds.) (2001). *Moss and Adams' Heart Disease in Infants, Children, and Adolescents Including the Fetus and Young Adult,* 6th ed. Philadelphia: Lippincott Williams & Wilkins.

Artman, M. (2001). Pharmacologic therapy. H.D. Allen, H.P. Gutgesell, E.B. Clark, (Eds.) (2001). *Moss and Adams' Heart Disease in Infants, Children, and Adolescents Including the Fetus and Young Adult,* 6th ed. Philadelphia: Lippincott Williams & Wilkins.

Barbas, K.H., & Kelleher, D.K. (2004). Breastfeeding success among infants with congenital heart disease. *Pediatr Nurs, 30*(4), 285-289.

Bellinger, D.C., Wypij, D., Kuban, K.C.K. et al. (2000). Eight-year neurodevelopmental status: The Boston circulatory arrest study (abstract). *Circulation, 102*(Suppl 2), II-497.

Bentham, J., & Bhattacharya, S. (2008). Genetic mechanisms controlling cardiovascular development. *Ann N Y Acad Sci, 1123,* 10-19.

Berul, C., & Dubin, A. (2006). Rhythm management in pediatric heart failure. *Congenital Heart Disease, 1*(4), 140-147.

Betz, C.L. (2004). Adolescents in transition of adult care: Why the concern?. *Nurs Clin North Am, 39*(4), 681-713.

Bjornsen, K.D. (2004). Health care transition in congenital heart disease: The providers' view point. *Nurs Clin North Am, 39*(4), 715-726.

Brosig, C., Mussatto, K., Kuhn, E., et al. (2007). Psychosocial outcomes for preschool families after surgery for complex congenital heart disease. *Pediatr Cardiol, 28*(4), 255-262.

Canobbio, M. (2001). Health care issues facing adolescents with congenital heart disease. *J Pediatr Nurs, 16,* 363-370.

Canobbio, M., Perloff, J., & Rapkin, A. (2005). Gynecological health of females with congenital heart disease. *Int J Cardiol, 98,* 379-387.

Cantinotti, M., Hegde, S., Bell, A., et al. (2008). Diagnostic role of magnetic resonance imaging in identifying aortic arch anomalies. *Congenital Heart Disease, 3,* 117-123.

Carey, L., Nicholson, B., & Fox, R. (2002). Maternal factors related to parenting young children with congenital heart disease. *J Pediatr Nurs, 17*(3), 174-183.

Chan, E., Russell, J., Williams, W., et al. (2005). Postoperative chylothorax after cardiothoracic surgery in children. *Ann Thorac Surg, 80,* 1864-1870.

Chang, R., Rodriguez, S., Lee, M., et al. (2006). Risk factors for deaths occurring within 30 days and 1 year after hospital discharge for cardiac surgery among pediatric patients. *Am Heart J, 152,* 386-393.

Committee on Infectious Diseases. (2006). *Report of the Committee on Infectious Diseases.* (27th ed). Elk Grove Village, IL: American Academy of Pediatrics.

Da Silva, V., de Oliveira Lopes, M., & de Araujo, T. (2007). Growth and nutritional status of children with congenital heart disease. *J Cardiovasc Nurs, 22*(5), 390-396.

Davis, D., Davis, S., Cotman, K., et al. (2008). Feeding difficulties and growth delay in children with hypoplastic left heart syndrome versus d-transposition of the great arteries. *Pediatr Cardiol, 29*(2), 328-333.

Dearani, J.A., Connolly, H.M., Martinez, R., et al. (2007). Caring for adults with congenital cardiac disease: Successes and challenges for 2007 and beyond. *Cardiology in the Young, 17*(2), 87-96.

De Santis, A., Fazio, G., Silvetti, M.S., et al. (2008). Transcatheter ablation of supraventricular tachycardias in pediatric patients. *Current Pharmaceutical Design, 14,* 788-793.

Dimmick, S., Walker, K., Badawi, N., et al. (2007). Outcomes following surgery for congenital heart disease in low-birth weight infants. *J Pediatr Child Health, 43,* 370-375.

Driscoll, D.J. (2001). Chest pain in children and adolescents. In H.D. Allen, H.P. Gutgesell, E.B. Clark, (Eds.) (2001). *Moss and Adams' Heart Disease in Infants, Children, and Adolescents Including the Fetus and Young Adult,* 6th ed. Philadelphia: Lippincott Williams & Wilkins.

Duran, R.M., Brotons, D.A., Aeguelles, I.Z., et al. (2008). Advances in pediatric cardiology and congenital heart diseases. *Rev Esp Cardiol, 61*(Suppl 1), 15-26.

Foster, E., Connelly, H.M., Martinez, R. et al. (2001). Task force 2: Special health care needs of adults with congenital heart disease. *J Am Coll Cardiol, 37,* 1176-1183.

Hameed, A.B., & Sklansky, M.S. (2007). Pregnancy: Maternal and fetal heart disease. *Curr Probl Cardiol, 32,* 419-494.

Hanisch, D. (2001). Pediatric arrhythmias. *J Pediatr Nurs, 16,* 351-362.

Higgins, S.S., & Tong, E. (2003). Transitioning adolescents into adult health care. *Prog Cardiovas Nurs, 18*(2), 93-98.

Hinton, R., Martin, L., Tabangin, M., et al. (2007). Hypoplastic left heart syndrome is heritable. *J Am Coll Cardiol, 16,* 1590-1595.

Hoffman, J., & Kaplan, S. (2002). The incidence of congenital heart disease. *J Am Coll Cardiol, 39,* 1890-1900.

Holm, I., Fredriksen, P., Fosdahl, M., et al. (2007). Impaired motor competence in school-age children with complex congenital heart disease. *Arch Pediatr Adolesc Med, 161,* 945-950.

Holzer, R., & Hijazi, Z. (2004). Interventional approach to congenital heart disease. *Curr Opin Cardiol, 19*(2), 84-90.

Hövels-Gürich, H., Konrad, K., Skorenski, D., et al. (2006). Long-term neurodevelopmental outcome and exercise capacity after corrective surgery for tetralogy of Fallot or ventricular septal defect in infancy. *Ann Thorac Surg, 81,* 958-967.

Jenkins, K., Correa, A., Feinstein, J., et al. (2007). Noninherited risk factors and congenital cardiovascular defects: Current knowledge. *Circulation, 115,* 3015-3038.

Kavey, R., Allada, V., Daniels, S., et al. (2006). Cardiovascular risk reduction in high risk pediatric patients: A scientific statement from the American Heart Association. *Circulation, 114,* 2710-2738.

Kelleher, D., Laussen, P., Teixeira-Pinto, A., et al. (2006). Growth and correlates of nutritional status among infants with hypoplastic left heart syndrome after stage 1 Norwood procedure. *Nutrition, 22*, 237-244.

Kimball, T.R., & Meyer, R.A. (2001). Echocardiography. In H.D., Allen, Gutgesell, H.P., Clark, E.B.(eds.) (2001). *Moss and Adams' Heart Disease in Infants, Children, and Adolescents Including the Fetus and Young Adult*, 6th ed. Philadelphia: Lippincott Williams & Wilkins.

Kleinman, R. (2004). *Pediatric Nutrition Handbook*. (2nd ed.) Elk Grove Village, IL: American Academy of Pediatrics.

Klitzner, T., Lee, M., Rodriguez, S., et al. (2006). Sex-related disparity in surgical mortality among pediatric patients. *Congenital Heart Disease, 1*(3), 77-88.

Landzburg, M.J., Murphy, D.J., Davidson, W.R. et al. (2001). Task Force 4: Organization of delivery systems for adults with congenital heart disease. *J Am Coll Cardiol, 37*, 1187-1193.

Leitch, C.A. (2000). Growth, nutrition and energy expenditure in pediatric heart failure. *Prog Pediatr Cardiol, 11*(3), 195-202.

Leyh, R.G., Wilhelmi, M., Rebe, P., et al. (2006). Tissue engineering of viable pulmonary arteries for surgical correction of congenital heart defects. *Ann Thorac Surg, 81*, 1466-1470.

Loffredo, C.A., Chokkalingam, A., Sill, A.M., et al. (2004). Prevalence of congenital cardiovascular malformations among relatives of infants with hypoplastic left heart, coarctation of the aorta, and d-transposition of the great arteries. *Am J Med Genet Assoc, 124*, 225-230.

Mahle, W.T. (2001). Neurologic and cognitive outcomes in children with congenital heart disease. *Curr Opin Pediatr, 13*, 482-486.

Mahle, W.T., Tavani, F., Zimmerman, R., et al. (2002). An MRI study of neurologic injury before and after congenital heart surgery. *Circulation, 106*(Suppl), I109-I114.

Majunke, N., & Sievert, H. (2007). ASD/PFO devices: What is in the pipeline? *J Interventional Cardiol, 20*, 517-523.

Marino, B.L., O'Brien, P., & LoRe, H. (1995). Oxygen saturations during breast and bottle feedings in infants with CHD. *J Pediatr Nurs, 10*, 360-364.

Maron, B., Chaitman, B., Ackerman, M., et al. (2004). Recommendations for physical activity and recreational sports participation for young patients with genetic cardiovascular diseases. *Circulation, 109*, 2807-2816.

Maron, B., Thompson, P.D., Ackerman, M., et al. (2007). Recommendations and considerations related to participation screening for cardiovascular abnormalities in competitive athletes: 2007 update: A scientific statement from the American Heart Association Council on Nutrition, Physical Activity, and Metabolism: Endorsed by the American College of Cardiology Foundation. *Circulation, 115*, 1643-1655.

McAlvin, B., Clabby, M., Kirshbom, P., et al. (2007). Routine immunizations and adverse events in infants with single ventricle physiology. *Ann Thorac Surg, 84*, 1316-1319.

McCusker, C., Doherty, N., Molloy, B., et al. (2007). Determinants of neuropsychological and behavioural outcomes in early childhood survivors of congenital heart disease. *Arch Dis Child, 92*(2), 137-141.

McQuillen, P., Barkovich, A., Hamrick, S., et al. (2007). Temporal and anatomic risk profile of brain injury with neonatal repair of congenital heart defects. *Stroke, 38*(2 Suppl), 736-741.

Miatton, M., de Wolf, D., Francois, K., et al. (2007). Neuropsychological performance in school-age children with surgically corrected congenital heart disease. *J Pediatr, 151*, 73-78.

Miller, M.R., Forrest, C.B., & Kan, J.S. (2000). Parental preferences for primary and specialty care collaboration in the management of teenagers with congenital heart disease. *Pediatrics, 106*(2), 264-269.

Morelius, E., Lundh, U., Nelson, E.F., et al. (2002). Parental stress in relation to the severity of congenital heart disease in the offspring. *Pediatr Nurs, 28*(1), 28-34.

Nydegger, A., Walsh, A., Penny, D., et al. (2007, November 14). Changes in resting energy expenditure in children with congenital heart disease. *Eur J Clin Nutr (epub ahead of print.).*

Park, M.K. (2008). *Pediatric Cardiology for Practitioners.* (5th ed.). St. Louis: Mosby.

Patel, H., & Hijazi, Z. (2005). Pediatric catheter interventions: A year in review 2004-2005. *Curr Opin Cardiol, 17*, 568-573.

Pierpont, M., Basson, C., Benson, W., et al. (2007). Genetic basis for congenital heart defects: Current knowledge: A scientific statement from the American Heart Association Congenital Cardiac Defects Committee, Council on Cardiovascular Disease in the Young. *Circulation, 115*, 3015-3038.

Pigula, F., Vida, V., Del Nido, P., et al. (2007). Contemporary results and current strategies in the management of hypoplastic left heart syndrome. *Semin Thorac Cardiovasc Surg, 19*(3), 238-244.

Pinto, N., Marino, B., Wernovsky, G., et al. (2007). Obesity is a common comorbidity in children with congenital and acquired heart disease. *Pediatrics, 120*, 1157-1164.

Reid, G.J., Irvine, M.J., McCrindle, B.W., et al. (2004). Prevalence and correlates of successful transfer from pediatric to adult health care among a cohort of young adults with complex congenital heart defects. *Pediatrics, 113*(3), 197-205.

Rheuban, K.S. (2001). Pericardial disease. In H.D. Allen, H.P. Gutgesell, E.B. Clark, (eds.) (2001). *Moss and Adams' Heart Disease in Infants, Children, and Adolescents Including the Fetus and Young Adult*, 6th ed. Philadelphia: Lippincott Williams & Wilkins.

Samii, S., & Cohen, M. (2004). Ablation of tachyarrhythmias in pediatric patients. *Curr Opin Cardiol, 19*, 64-67.

Scott, W.A. (2001). Syncope and the assessment of the autonomic nervous system. In H.D. Allen, H.P. Gutgesell, E.B. Clark, (eds.) (2001). *Moss and Adams' Heart Disease in Infants, Children, and Adolescents Including the Fetus and Young Adult*, 6th ed. Philadelphia: Lippincott Williams & Wilkins.

Shillingford, A., Glanzman, M., Ittenbach, R., et al. (2008). Inattention, hyperactivity, and school performance in a population of school-age children with complex congenital heart disease. *Pediatrics, 121*, 759-767.

Smith, P. (2001). Primary care in children with congenital heart disease. *J Pediatr Nurs, 16*, 308-319.

Tabbutt, S., Dominguez, T., Ravishankar, C., et al. (2005). Outcomes after stage I reconstruction comparing the right ventricular to pulmonary artery conduit with the modified Blalock Taussig shunt. *Ann Thorac Surg, 80*, 1582-1591.

Tabbutt, S., Nord, A., Jarvik, G., et al. (2008). Neurodevelopmental outcomes after staged palliation for hypoplastic left heart syndrome. *Pediatrics, 121*, 476-483.

Trujillo, T.C., & Nolan, P.E. (2000). Antiarrhythmic agents: Drug interactions of clinical significance. *Drug Saf, 26*, 509-532.

Uzark, K., & Jones, K. (2003). Parenting stress and children with heart disease. *J Pediatr Health Care, 17*(4), 163-168.

Uzark, K., Jones, K., Slusher, J., et al. (2008). Quality of life in children with heart diseases as perceived by children and parents. *Pediatrics, 121*, 1060-1067.

Veldtman, G.R., Matley, S.L., Kendall, L., et al. (2001). Illness understanding in children and adolescents with heart disease. *West J Med, 174*, 171-175.

Warnes, C.A., Liberthson, R., Danielson, G.K., et al. (2001). Task force 1: The changing profile of congenital heart disease in adult life. *J Am Coll Cardiol, 37*, 1170-1175.

Webb, G.D., & Williams, R.G. (2001). Care of the adult with congenital heart disease. *J Am Coll Cardiol, 37*, 1166.

Wernovsky, G., Shillingford, A., & Gaynor, W. (2005). Central nervous system outcomes in children with complex congenital heart disease. *Curr Opin Cardiol, 20*, 94-99.

Wilson, W., Taubert, K., Gewitz, M., et al. (2007). Prevention of infective endocarditis: Guidelines form the American Heart Association. *Circulation, 116*, 1736-1754.

22 Cystic Fibrosis

Leslie A. Hazle

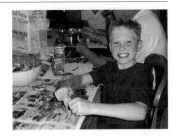

Etiology

Cystic fibrosis (CF), a condition characterized by complex multisystem involvement, is the most common life-shortening genetic illness among white children, adolescents, and young adults. Significant advances in genetic and biomedical research have been made over the past 20 years that have influenced health professionals' understanding of the condition, its cause, its clinical management, and approaches to diagnosis. Although still without a cure, CF is no longer considered a terminal childhood disease but a chronic condition with a median life expectancy of more than 37 years of age (Cystic Fibrosis Foundation, 2008b). Experts expect that further advances in CF will extend the median life expectancy and the quality of life of affected individuals in the future.

After a succession of scientific breakthroughs in genetics, in 1989 the CF gene was isolated on the long arm of chromosome 7, which encodes a protein product (i.e., cystic fibrosis transmembrane conductance regulator [CFTR]) (Davis, 2006). More than 1500 unique mutations in the CFTR gene have been reported, the most common of which is the delta F508 mutation, which accounts for approximately 70% of CF alleles (Cystic Fibrosis Foundation, 2008b). CF genetic mutations have been divided into five classes based on their influence on CFTR manufacture and function at the cellular level. These defects include lack of CFTR production, trafficking, conductance and regulation problems, and reduction in synthesis of the protein (Davis, 2006; Gibson, Burns, & Ramsey, 2003; Langfelder-Schwind, Kloza, Sugarman, et al., 2005). The specific class of defect, in part, may explain the phenotypic expression of the disease. However, the variability in disease severity is influenced by the presence of environmental, therapeutic, and other gene modifiers (Davis, 2006). Significant scientific inquiry is underway to further understand the CFTR defect and to develop therapeutic pharmacologic approaches to change its function at the cellular level.

Although identifying the relationship between specific mutations and defects in CFTR function is important, so also is an understanding of how abnormal CFTR function produces the clinical picture of pancreatic dysfunction, persistent respiratory infection, and inflammation. At this time, this relationship and the host responses to infection and inflammation are not fully understood. For example, why is the CF airway such an inviting environment for bacterial colonization, and what factors contribute to the damage and deterioration of lung parenchyma from host response to the bacteria? What is the CFTR dysfunction that causes CF liver disease? Current research is targeting ways to restore chloride or sodium ion transport, to promote the repair and function of the CFTR protein, to determine the reason for the hyperinflammatory response and ways to control it, and to understand and change the airway environment that fosters colonization and infection (Cystic Fibrosis Foundation, 2008a).

At least one function of CFTR appears to be as a chloride ion channel regulated by cyclic adenosine monophosphate (cAMP) (Davis, 2006). An impermeability to chloride ions, as well as increased sodium reabsorption, leads to decreased water movement across cell membranes. This defect causes secretions to become viscous and less well hydrated and lumens of airways and ducts to be obstructed (Davis 2006; Gibson et al., 2003). The pathogenesis of an ion-transport defect leads to pathologic sequelae of mucus-obstructing ducts in various body organs. Progressive pathologic changes are produced in nearly every organ of the body. The most consistent changes occur in the exocrine glands (e.g., pancreatic acini, bile ducts and gallbladder, prostatic glands, salivary and lacrimal glands, mucous glands of the tracheobronchial tree, upper respiratory tract, and intestinal wall, and the sweat glands) (Rosenstein, 2006). Table 22-1 is an overview of CF that delineates organ system pathogenesis, clinical manifestations, complications, and management.

Incidence and Prevalence

The transmission of CF follows an autosomal recessive mode with an incidence in whites of approximately 1 in 3500 (Farrell, Rosenstein, White, et al., 2008). The incidence in other races is usually lower: in blacks, it is about 1 in 17,000; in Asians, it is about 1 in 32,000. Native Americans have a higher incidence than any other group; Sontag, Hammond, Zielenski, and colleagues (2005) reported an incidence of 1 in 2717 in Colorado. Occurrence is possible in any race, however. The Hispanic ethnic group is the fastest growing and has an incidence of about 1 in 8000. In addition, CF is found in the Ashkenazi Jews and Amish groups. With a gene frequency in whites of approximately 1 in 25, it is estimated that for 1 in 400 to 500 couples, both partners are carriers of this recessive trait, with a subsequent 1 in 4 risk of bearing an affected child with each pregnancy (Langfelder-Schwind et al., 2005). The 2007 Cystic Fibrosis Foundation's Patient Registry reported about 24,500 individuals living with CF in the United States with approximately 700 new diagnoses during that year (Cystic Fibrosis Foundation, 2008b).

Diagnostic Criteria

Diagnosis of CF requires a positive sweat test in the presence of either (1) clinical symptoms consistent with CF, (2) a family history of CF, or (3) a positive neonatal screening test or for the individual to have two CF-causing mutations (Farrell et al., 2008). Sweat testing is done by pilocarpine iontophoresis with quantitative analysis of sweat chloride. Box 22-1 provides indications for sweat testing,

TABLE 22-1

Overview of Cystic Fibrosis

System	Pathogenesis	Clinical Manifestations	Complications	Management
Sweat glands	Abnormal electrolytes	High rate of salt loss; salt depletion	Heat prostration	Dietary salt replacement, sweat test
Lungs	Thick, tenacious mucus	Cough; decreased exercise tolerance	Infection, inflammation	Airway clearance techniques, antibiotics
	Mucous plugging	Air trapping: increased anteroposterior chest diameter	Fibrosis, bronchiectasis	
	Obstruction	Hyperresonance	Atelectasis	Bronchodilators
	Decreased mucociliary clearance	Wheezing, fine and coarse crackles, clubbing	Hypoxia, respiratory failure	Dornase alfa
			Pneumothorax	Hypertonic saline
			Hemoptysis	Antiinflammatories
			Cor pulmonale	Ibuprofen
			Allergic bronchopulmonary aspergillosis	Steroids: oral, inhaled
			Failure to thrive (increased energy expenditure	High-calorie diet
Upper airway	Viscous mucus	Chronic sinusitis	Obstruction, mouth breathing	Decongestants (intermittent use)
		Nasal polyposis		Nasal cromolyn sodium or corticosteroids
				Antibiotics
				Surgery
Gastrointestinal (GI) tract	Inspissated tenacious meconium	No passage of meconium	Obstruction: meconium ileus	Enema, surgery
	Maldigested food and viscous mucus in gut	Abdominal distention	Distal ileal obstruction syndrome (DIOS)	Pancreatic enzymes
		Cramping abdominal pain	Fecal mass in colon	Dietary changes to avoid complications
			Volvulus, intussusceptions	Laxatives
				Gastrografin with Tween 80 enema or GoLYTELY; Miralax
Pancreas	Viscous secretions, obstructions, fibrosis	Maldigestion; bulky, foul-smelling stools	Pancreatitis	Enzyme replacement
			Fibrosis	Antacids
				H$_2$ antagonists, Proton pump inhibitor
	Abnormal electrolytes	Fat malabsorption (including fat-soluble vitamins)	Failure to thrive	High-energy diets
	Suboptimal enzyme function		Delayed maturation	Normal fat intake
			Rectal prolapse	Concentrated dietary supplements
			Vitamin deficiency	Aggressive nutrition supplementation
				Vitamin and mineral supplement
			Glucose intolerance	Insulin preferred
Biliary tract	Obstruction	Subclinical cirrhosis	Cirrhosis	Ursodiol (Actigall)
	Fibrosis		Portal hypertension	Cholecystectomy
			Cholelithiasis	
Salivary glands	Abnormal electrolyte concentrations	Probably not clinically significant		
Reproductive tract	Abnormal viscous secretions	Male: absence of vas deferens, infertility		Genetic and reproductive counseling
		Female: thick vaginal and decreased cervical secretions		

which is the gold standard test for diagnosing CF. Sweat should only be collected and assayed through a qualified laboratory (LeGrys, Yankaskas, Quittell, et al., 2007). All of the 115 regional Cystic Fibrosis Foundation–accredited care centers have clinical chemistry laboratories that meet CF-specific standards for the accuracy and reliability of sweat tests. Sweat chloride concentrations at or above 60 mmol/L collected on two separate occasions are consistent with a diagnosis of CF. A value of 30 to 59 mmol/L is considered borderline and should be repeated, or a basic CFTR gene mutation panel looking for two CF-causing mutations should be done (Farrell et al.,

2008; LeGrys et al., 2007). Adequate quantities of sweat may be difficult to obtain from infants under 2 weeks of age, so CF centers may do CF mutation panels to help with early diagnosis in these infants when sweat collections yield an inadequate quantity (Parad, Comeau, Dorkin, et al., 2005). Once the diagnosis has been established in a child, all siblings should be sweat tested. In a small number of individuals with clinical symptoms suggestive of CF, the sweat test may be borderline or even high normal. In these situations, the primary care provider should consult with CF specialty providers who can use expanded laboratory criteria and methods (e.g., identifying

BOX 22-1

Indications for Sweat Testing

Positive newborn screen
Respiratory
- Chronic cough
- Recurrent or chronic pneumonia, especially with *Pseudomonas*
- Wheezing, hyperinflation, tachypnea, retractions—if persistent
- Atelectasis focused in the right upper lobe
- Bronchiectasis
- Hemoptysis
- Nasal polyps
- Pansinusitis
- Digital clubbing
Gastrointestinal
- Meconium ileus
- Meconium plug syndrome
- Prolonged neonatal jaundice
- Steatorrhea
- Rectal prolapse
- Mucoid-impacted appendix
- Late intestinal obstruction
- Intussusceptions at an uncommon age
- Cirrhosis and portal hypertension
- Recurrent pancreatitis
Metabolic and miscellaneous
- Family history of CF, including first cousins
- Failure to thrive
- Salt crystals or salt taste on the skin
- Hyponatremia
- Metabolic alkalosis
- Vitamin K, A, or E deficiency
- Absence of the vas deferens
- Hypoproteinemia and edema

Adapted from Rosenstein, B. (2006). Cystic fibrosis. In J. McMillian (Ed.), *Oski's Pediatrics* (4th ed.). Philadelphia: Lippincott Williams & Wilkins.

Clinical Manifestations at Time of Diagnosis (If Not by Newborn Screening)

- Meconium ileus in the neonate
- Malabsorption with failure to thrive
- Chronic or recurrent upper and/or lower respiratory infections

---

CF mutations by deoxyribonucleic acid [DNA] analysis and abnormal bioelectric properties of nasal epithelium) to diagnose CF (Davis, 2006; Farrell et al., 2008; Gibson et al., 2003).

In 2004, the Cystic Fibrosis Foundation and the Centers for Disease Control and Prevention (CDC) convened a working group and determined that the benefit from early diagnosis and treatment of CF would support a recommendation for states to add CF to their newborn screening panels (Comeau, Accurso, White, et al., 2007). Screening is done using immunoreactive trypsinogen (IRT) as the first tier. Levels of IRT, a pancreatic protein, are typically elevated in infants with CF; however, this is not sufficient for diagnosis, and a second tier of screening by a second IRT or DNA is required. If the second IRT is elevated or a CFTR mutation is found, the child should be referred to a CF care center for diagnostic sweat chloride or full mutation testing (Comeau et al., 2007).

Clinical Manifestations

The pathophysiologic hallmarks of CF are as follows: (1) pancreatic enzyme deficiency from duct blockage by viscous mucus; (2) progressive chronic obstructive lung disease associated with viscous infected mucus and subsequent interstitial destruction; and (3) sweat gland dysfunction, resulting in abnormally high sodium and chloride concentrations in the sweat (Davis, 2006; Gibson et al., 2003).

There are three common clinical presentations. The first is meconium ileus or intestinal obstruction in neonates, which occurred in 14% of newly diagnosed infants in 2007 (Cystic Fibrosis Foundation, 2008b). The occurrence of meconium ileus should be presumed to be CF until testing confirms or rules out the diagnosis. Meconium plug syndrome—although less frequently associated with the diagnosis of CF—should also raise the primary care provider's suspicion.

The second common clinical presentation is failure to thrive with malabsorption as a result of lost or diminished exocrine pancreatic function, which occurs in 80% to 90% of children with CF. These children exhibit varying degrees of weight loss or poor growth patterns, usually in the presence of a normal to voracious appetite; frequent foul-smelling, greasy, bulky stools; rectal prolapse (in about 3% of children); and a protuberant belly with decreased subcutaneous tissue in the extremities. In 2007, failure to thrive with malnutrition was the clinical presentation in 18.1% of individuals diagnosed with CF (Cystic Fibrosis Foundation, 2008b).

The third common clinical presentation is the occurrence of chronic or recurrent upper and lower respiratory infections. This occurred in approximately 31% of newly diagnosed individuals in 2007 (Cystic Fibrosis Foundation, 2008b). Manifestations include the following: nasal polyps, chronic sinusitis, recurrent pneumonia and bronchitis, bronchiectasis, and atelectasis. Children with these manifestations have a chronic cough that persists after a respiratory infection and may become paroxysmal and productive, provoking choking and vomiting. Auscultatory findings may include fine crackles and expiratory wheezes—particularly in the upper lobes and right middle lobe. Some children, however, have no findings on auscultation. Infants may have recurrent episodes of wheezing and tachypnea. *Staphylococcus aureus,* which is often seen initially, and subsequently *Pseudomonas aeruginosa* and *Haemophilus influenzae* are frequent isolates in a respiratory tract culture. Fungi—including *Candida albicans* and *Aspergillus fumigatus*—are also often cultured from the respiratory tract (Gibson et al., 2003; Saiman, Siegel, & Cystic Fibrosis Foundation Consensus Conference on Infection Control Participants., 2003; Stevens, Moss, Kurup, et al., 2003). Box 22-2 lists pathogens found in CF respiratory sputum. Chest radiographic changes include air trapping and peribronchial thickening, followed by atelectasis, infiltrates, and hilar adenopathy (Rosenstein, 2006). Without treatment, these early signs and symptoms progress and complications occur (Davis, 2006; Gibson et al., 2003). Additionally, the institution of newborn screening for CF should help identify children with CF early and allow for early intervention before obvious symptoms occur. Box 22-3 and Figure 22-1 summarize the clinical progression of changes in CF lung disease.

Although these presentations are most common, CF's multisystem involvement (see Table 22-1) may lead to the presentation of variable and subtle symptoms, possibly leading to diagnostic delays and creating an anxious and difficult period for the family and the

---

BOX 22-2

Cystic Fibrosis Sputum Pathogens

- *Staphylococcus aureus*
- *Haemophilus influenzae*
- *Pseudomonas aeruginosa*
- Methicillin-resistant *Staphylococcus aureus* (MRSA)
- *Burkholderia cepacia* complex
- *Stenotrophomonas maltophilia*
- *Achromobacter (Alcaligenes) xylosoxidans*
- *Aspergillus* spp.
- *Candida albicans*
- Nontuberculous *Mycobacterium*

BOX 22-3

Progressive Changes in the Clinical Picture of Cystic Fibrosis

1. Early
   a. Voracious appetite
   b. Dry, hacking, nonproductive cough
   c. Increased respiratory rate
   d. Decreased activity
2. Moderate
   a. Increased cough, increased sputum production
   b. Rales, musical rhonchi, scattered or localized wheezes
   c. Repeated episodes of respiratory tract infection
   d. Signs of obstructive lung disease
       (i) Increased anteroposterior diameter
       (ii) Depressed diaphragm
       (ii) Palpable liver border
   e. Decreased appetite
   f. Failure to gain weight or grow or weight loss
   g. Decreased exercise tolerance
3. Advanced
   a. Chronic paroxysmal, productive cough
   b. Increased respiratory rate, shortness of breath on exertion, orthopnea, dyspnea
   c. Diffuse and localized fine and coarse crackles
   d. Signs of severe obstructive lung disease
       (i) Marked increase in anteroposterior (barrel chest, pigeon breast)
       (ii) Limited respiratory excursion of thoracic cage
       (iii) Depressed diaphragm
       (iv) Hyperresonance over entire chest
       (v) Decreased ventilation, persistent hypoxemia
   e. Noisy respirations
   f. Marked decrease in appetite
   g. Muscular weakness
   h. Cyanosis
   i. Digital clubbing
   j. Rounded shoulders
   k. Fever, tachycardia
   l. Hemoptysis
   m. Pneumothorax
   n. Lung abscess
   o. Signs of cardiac failure (cor pulmonale, edema, enlarged tender liver)
   p. Bone pain and osteoarthropathy

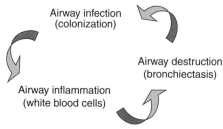

FIGURE 22-1 Cystic fibrosis: cycle of infection/inflammation/ destruction.

associated with CF. However, the primary care provider must keep CF in mind with the differential diagnosis, because some children may not be diagnosed through newborn screening.

CF newborn screening (NBS) by immunoreactive trypsinogen (IRT) is now recommended by both the CDC and the Cystic Fibrosis Foundation. IRT-positive screens are followed by either a second IRT or DNA analysis before the newborn is referred to an accredited CF care center for testing for CF. The CF diagnosis consensus conference (Farrell et al., 2008) states that sweat testing remains the gold standard for the diagnosis. Statewide screening programs in Colorado and Wisconsin have been in place for over 15 years. As of the end of 2008, all but one state have either mandated CF NBS or it was being voluntarily done statewide by health organizations (Cystic Fibrosis Foundation, Newborn Screening for Cystic Fibrosis, 2008). There is clear evidence that early diagnosis of CF is beneficial in the area of improved growth and nutrition. If a child with CF can grow and develop at the national average for healthy children, the child's lungs are larger, thus opening the possibility of a longer and healthier life with CF (Peterson, Jacobs, & Milla, 2003). As more targeted therapies are developed, early diagnosis may become even more beneficial to a child. Both carrier detection and CF newborn screening are advances in genetics. However, they can provide further confusion for primary care providers and parents. Because there are more than 1500 known CF mutations, a person may receive a negative carrier test but have a newborn with a positive IRT, requiring further testing for CF. It is important for primary care providers to clearly explain to families that carrier testing for a CF mutation is not a guarantee that their newborn will have a negative CF screen at birth. It is important that individuals clearly understand what carrier testing and what a newborn screen for CF mean in relation to life choices for themselves and for their children.

Treatment

Nutritional Management

Closely monitored nutritional management for children with CF allows them to grow and develop at the normal rates. Current recommendations from the Cystic Fibrosis Foundation Clinical Practice Guidelines Subcommittee on Growth and Nutrition (Stallings, Stark, Robinson, et al., 2008) state that children with CF, ages 2 to 20 years, should have the goal of a body mass index (BMI) of the 50th percentile or greater. Experts in CF nutrition note that "there are three specific times when special attention should be focused on growth and nutritional status within the scope of usual clinical care. These are: (1) the first 12 months after diagnosis of CF; (2) birth to 12 months of age for infants diagnosed prenatally or at birth, until a normal pattern of growth (head circumference, weight and

primary care provider. Manifestations may be minimal or absent during childhood. In 2007, 10% of new diagnoses were made in individuals over 10 years of age (Cystic Fibrosis Foundation, 2008b). Diagnostic delays may be decreased if primary care providers maintain a high level of suspicion of the various symptoms length) is clearly established; and (3) the peripubertal growth period (girls about 9 to 16, and boys about 12 to 18 years of age)" (Borowitz, Baker, & Stallings, 2002). The goal of focused interventions during these periods is to establish and support normal growth and development during periods of physiologic stress from growth and the disease process. Successful nutritional management of CF can be achieved with the use of pancreatic enzyme replacements, high-calorie diets, and supplementation of fat-soluble vitamins.

Treatment

Nutritional management
- Pancreatic enzyme replacement
- High-calorie diet
- Vitamin, mineral, and sodium supplementation

Respiratory management
- Antimicrobials: oral, inhaled, IV
- Airway clearance
- Exercise
- Antiinflammatory therapy
- Mucolytics/other pulmonary therapies
- Bilateral lung transplantation

Pancreatic Enzyme Replacement. The principal treatment for the resulting malabsorption in CF is oral pancreatic enzyme replacement. Enteric coating of enzyme preparations decreases the likelihood of inactivation by gastric acid, and doses may be adjusted to achieve weight gain and one to two formed stools per day. Concerns have been raised, however, by reports of colonic strictures in children with CF. These strictures have occurred in children under 12 years of age receiving enzyme doses of more than 6000 lipase units/kg/meal. Current recommendations are that pancreatic enzyme doses should be reduced to the lowest effective dose that allows for continued normal growth without altering a child's diet. Dosing guidelines of 500 to 2500 lipase units/kg/meal are now used by most CF centers as a safe range. The safety of doses between 2500 and 6000 lipase units/kg/meal is not known, and such doses should be used with caution (Stallings et al., 2008).

Children often experience continued problems with malabsorption despite reasonable coverage with enzymes. Table 22-2 lists factors that contribute to a poor response to pancreatic enzyme therapy. Initial assessment and intervention should address adherence, enzyme storage, and a child's eating habits (e.g., small frequent snacks without taking enzymes). Neutralizing gastric acid with antacids or inhibiting its production with histamine-receptor antagonists can improve the efficacy of the enzyme preparation. If the problem persists, consultation with the CF center and specifically the CF dietitian may be helpful.

High-Calorie Diet. Caloric and protein requirements are increased in children with CF because of malabsorption related to pancreatic insufficiency, inadequate enzyme replacement, and progressive pulmonary disease. For children with CF 2 years of age and older, the recommended energy intake is 110% to 200% greater than the usual recommended daily allowance (Stallings et al., 2008).

With progression of pulmonary disease, children usually have chronic weight and nutrition problems as a result of their increased pulmonary energy requirements and decreased appetites. Calories are encouraged in both complex carbohydrates and fats. Dietary fat is the highest-density source of calories and also improves the palatability of foods and maintains normal essential fatty acid status. Energy-boosting tips are found in Box 22-4. When an individual

---

TABLE 22-2

Factors Contributing to a Poor Response to Pancreatic Enzyme Therapy

Enzyme factors	Generic pancreatic enzymes used
	Expired medications
	Enzymes not stored in cool place
Dietary factors	Excessive juice intake
	Parental perception that enzymes are not needed with milk or snacks
	"Grazing" eating behavior
	High-fat fast foods
Poor adherence to prescribed enzyme regimen	Toddler's willful refusal
	Chaotic household, multiple meal givers
	Anger or desire to be "normal"
	Teenage girls' desire to be slim
Acid intestinal environmental	Poor dissolution of enteric coating
	Microcapsule contents released all at once
Concurrent gastrointestinal disorder	Biliary disease, cholestasis
	Crohn disease

Adapted from Borowitz, D., Grand, R.J., & Durie, P.R. (1995). Use of pancreatic enzyme supplements for patients with cystic fibrosis in the context of fibrosing colonopathy. *J Pediatr, 127*, 681-684.

BOX 22-4

Maximizing Calories for the Healthy Individual with Cystic Fibrosis

ADDING CALORIES TO FOODS
- Add fats such as butter, gravy, cheese, or dressings to starches, fruits, and vegetables.
- Use whipped cream on fruits and desserts
- Make "super" milk: ½ cup whole milk + ½ cup half and half
- Flavor milk with syrups or powders (chocolate, strawberry, etc.) or add whole-milk yogurt to milk
- Add eggs to hamburger meat or casseroles (never serve raw eggs)
- Use extra salad dressing; avoid low-calorie or reduced-calorie dressings
- Serve gravies and cheese sauces

HIGH-CALORIE FOODS AND SNACKS*
- Full-fat ice cream, puddings
- Cookies and milk
- Cheese or peanut butter crackers
- Muffins or bagels with cream cheese or butter
- Cheese breadsticks
- Chips and dip
- French fries
- Whole-milk yogurt
- Egg salad, tuna salad, cheese or avocado slices with crackers
- Trail mixes, nuts, and granola (after age 2 years)
- Cold cuts, pizza
- Fresh vegetables with salad dressing or dip

*Assess age appropriateness, especially with respect to choking risk in young children, before recommending.

has difficulty with certain high-fat foods, these may be limited. However, children with CF should generally be encouraged to cover high fat intake with additional enzymes. As the CF population ages, questions have been raised related to the impact on the gastrointestinal and cardiovascular systems of a diet high in fats and the type of fats eaten. This is an issue without answers; however, a discussion about dietary fats provides an opportunity for the practitioner to discuss the importance of healthy diets for siblings of the child with CF.

Aggressive nutritional supplementation (i.e., oral, enteral, and parenteral) is routinely used for children with weight loss or growth delays despite a reasonable intake. The Cystic Fibrosis Foundation's Patient Registry (2008b) shows a strong correlation between growth at or above the 50th percentile BMI and improved pulmonary function as measured by forced expiratory volume in 1 second (FEV_1) percent predicted. However, long-term studies using appropriate control group methodology have not been done. Nutritional status and pulmonary function, as well as quality of life, adverse effects, cost, and adherence, would be important outcomes for evaluation (Conway, Morton, & Wolfe, 2002).

Vitamin, Mineral, and Sodium Supplementation. Optimal dietary intake also includes attention to fat-soluble vitamins, essential fatty acids, calcium, iron, zinc, and sodium. Because fat malabsorption is particularly problematic in CF and deficiencies in fat-soluble vitamins are not unusual, CF centers recommend a standard age-appropriate dose of non–fat-soluble multivitamins plus supplementation of vitamins A, D, E, and K at an age-appropriate dose. Consultation with the CF center dietitian can be helpful in establishing the appropriate doses of vitamins. Water-miscible preparations combining the fat-soluble vitamins A, D, E, and K are available, providing the convenience of supplementation with a single vitamin preparation for most children (Borowitz et al., 2002).

There is a high prevalence of osteopenia and osteoporosis in children and adults with CF. Aris, Merkel, Bachrach, and colleagues (2005) recommend that dietary intake of calcium and vitamin D, as well as encouraging regular weight-bearing exercise for the general population, be emphasized in people with CF, and their vitamin D levels should be assessed annually. Table 22-3 outlines the recommended calcium intake per day for people with CF. The use of bisphosphonates in adults with CF has been shown to be effective in increasing bone density in small studies, but larger clinical trials are needed. There is limited information about their use in children (Aris et al., 2005).

Children with CF lose more salt in their sweat than other children because of the basic CF defect of chloride ion transport. It is recommended that people with CF have a higher level of salt intake to maintain electrolyte balances. This is especially important in hot weather and when participating in sports or other activities that increase sweat.

Respiratory Management

Interventions are designed to interrupt or slow the cascade of pathophysiologic phenomena by either preventing the development of abnormal airway secretions and lung infections or treating the existing infection and inflammation (Figure 22-2). Progressive lung disease is the major cause of morbidity and mortality in CF. The pathophysiologic basis of CF lung disease is impaired

TABLE 22-3

Dietary Reference Intakes for Calcium*

Age	Calcium (mg/day)
Infants	
0-6 mo	210
7-12 mo	270
Children	
1-3 yr	500
4-8 yr	800
9-18 yr	1300
Adults	1300-1500

From Cystic Fibrosis Foundation. (2002). Bone health and disease in cystic fibrosis consensus conference report. *CF Foundation Consensus Conferences, X*(4), 32.
*Values given represent Adequate Intakes (AI).

mucociliary clearance of dehydrated mucus followed by endobronchial infection. Children with CF become chronically colonized with gram-negative organisms that may be quantitatively decreased with antimicrobial therapy but cannot be eradicated. The respiratory tract environment in CF that promotes bacterial growth is not fully understood, and there is widespread controversy over the optimal approach to the long-term treatment of sequelae to this bacterial growth. General agreement exists, however, that bacterial infection—especially from *Pseudomonas aeruginosa* and other gram-negative bacilli with their virulence factors—and the intense host inflammatory response to infection (i.e., antibody response and neutrophil influx) lead to chronic bronchiectasis (see Figure 22-2). CF centers recognize that antimicrobial therapy is of primary importance in decreasing the rate of this deterioration. Additionally, therapies to help clear the airways, thin mucus, and diminish the intense inflammatory response all play a role in the increased survival of individuals with CF (Accurso, 2007; Weiner, 2002). Table 22-4 lists the recommend chronic pulmonary therapies for people with CF.

Antibiotic/Antimicrobial Therapy. Pulmonary exacerbations often follow mild viral illnesses, particularly upper respiratory tract infections. It has been hypothesized that viruses may suppress host defenses, although this mechanism has not been clearly proven (Davis, 2006). It can be argued that an early course of oral antibiotic therapy should be used with viral illness symptoms to prevent exacerbation of the bacterial pulmonary infection during the viral illness. Continuous oral antibiotic coverage to reduce the frequency of exacerbations in young children is questioned. In a multicenter trial of continuous *Staphylococcus* prophylaxis with cephalexin versus a placebo over a 5- to 7-year period, there were no differences in the pulmonary and nutritional outcomes of each group; however, the group treated with antibiotics had a higher rate of *Pseudomonas aeruginosa* colonization (Gibson et al., 2003).

Traditional concerns about the development of resistant organisms with overuse of antibiotics must be balanced against the concern for progressive bronchiectasis and parenchymal damage. The initial choice of antibiotic and dosage should provide broad-spectrum coverage, specifically for *Staphylococcus aureus, Streptococcus pneumoniae,* and *Haemophilus* species. Accurate identification of pathogens with appropriate antibiotic sensitivity testing is important to successful treatment of infections (Weiner, 2002). Further considerations in children whose pulmonary infections do not respond to initial therapy include antibiotic resistance, lack of

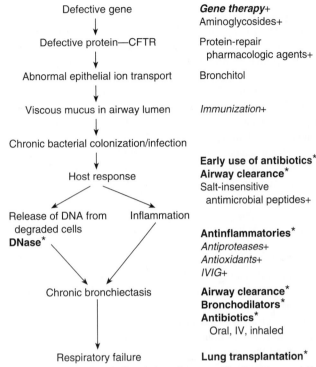

Use of **Standard*** and *Experimental+* therapy
to alter the pathologic sequence of CF lung disease

FIGURE 22-2 Pathologic sequence of cystic fibrosis lung disease and the therapies used. Use of standard (*) and experimental (+) therapy to alter the pathologic sequence of CF lung disease.

TABLE 22-4

Recommended Chronic Pulmonary Therapies for People with Cystic Fibrosis

Strong Recommendation for	Recommendation for
Inhaled tobramycin: for people with moderate to severe disease	Inhaled tobramycin: for people with asymptomatic to mild disease
Dornase alfa: for people with moderate to severe disease	Dornase alfa: for people with asymptomatic to mild disease
	Hypertonic saline
	Ibuprofen
	Macrolides
	Inhaled beta-agonists

Adapted from Flume, P.A., O'Sullivan, B.P., Robinson, K.A., et al. (2007). Cystic fibrosis pulmonary guidelines: Chronic medications for maintenance of lung health. *Am J Respir Crit Care Med, 176,* 957-969. First published online August 29, 2007, as doi:10.1164/rccm.200705-6640C.

adherence to pharmacologic therapy, or abnormal pharmacokinetics (Gibson et al., 2003).

Aerosolization delivers high concentrations of antibiotics to the site of infection while decreasing the risk of systemic absorption and toxicity. This approach has been used most effectively as suppressive therapy in individuals chronically colonized with *Pseudomonas aeruginosa.* Aminoglycosides and colistin (Coly-Mycin M Parenteral) have been the most consistent choices. High-dose tobramycin for inhalation has been the most extensively studied antibiotic for nebulization and approved by the Food and Drug Administration (FDA). High-dose tobramycin used as suppressive therapy twice a day every other month has been associated with slowed decline of pulmonary function, improved quality of life, and improved weight gain (Quittner & Buu, 2002).

Because of the potential for developing resistant strains of *Pseudomonas* species, the clinical expertise of the CF team is recommended in selecting appropriate individuals for therapy and in monitoring their therapy (Flume, O'Sullivan, Robinson, et al., 2007).

When oral and aerosolized antibiotics do not control pulmonary exacerbations, intravenous antibiotics may be necessary. A pulmonary and nutritional "tune-up" or "clean-out" may be initiated in the hospital or home. These 2-week—or longer—courses of therapy allow the CF center team to employ more aggressive strategies to contain infection and maintain or supplement nutrition. Such strategies include using intravenous antibiotics (i.e., often an aminoglycoside with either a semisynthetic penicillin or third-generation cephalosporin), as well as increased pulmonary toilet, physical therapy, exercise, and nutritional support measures. Intravenous antibiotics are chosen for their effectiveness in treating *Pseudomonas aeruginosa,* which is less responsive to oral therapy. Quinolone antibiotics are currently the only available oral preparations that effectively treat *Pseudomonas* species; of these, ciprofloxacin (Cipro) has been the most extensively studied in CF. In clinical trials of Cipro in children with CF, the antibiotic was well tolerated and without reports of side effects, although federal approvals are not yet in place. Many CF centers use it judiciously in children. Clinicians should be aware that *Pseudomonas aeruginosa* rapidly develops resistance to oral quinolones; frequent use and use in more severely affected individuals is often associated with a suboptimal response (Flume et al., 2007).

Airway Clearance. Other pulmonary therapeutic interventions are aimed at relief of bronchial obstruction through clearance of pulmonary secretions. Chest physical therapy (e.g., postural drainage and cupping and/or clapping and/or vibration two to four times a day) has been effective and has been standard therapy for years. Other techniques of airway clearance have been developed for school-age children and adolescents; such techniques include active cycle of breathing technique (ACBT) and forced expiration technique (FET), autogenic drainage (AD), positive expiratory pressure (PEP), airway oscillating devices (AODs, e.g., Flutter, Acapella), and high-frequency chest wall oscillation (e.g., vest) (Lannefors, Button, & McIlwaine, 2004). The common advantage of these techniques is that they allow the child and teen independence in clearing the airway of mucus. Cumulative data of short-term trials indicate that airway clearance, whatever the specific technique, when compared with no airway clearance is associated with improved outcomes. In 2007, the Cystic Fibrosis Foundation's Pulmonary Guidelines committee reviewed the medical literature and found no advantage for any airway clearance technique over another. It is recommended that airway clearance techniques are individualized based on age, quality of life, severity of pulmonary disease, and individual preference. There may be benefit for definitive long-term studies that compare the effectiveness of specific techniques in people with CF (Flume, Robinson, O'Sullivan, et al., 2008; van der Schans, Prasad, & Main, 2002).

Routine airway clearance is recommended for all children with pulmonary involvement; the specific regimen recommended for an individual with CF should be made by the CF center's physician and respiratory or physical therapist. Because more newborns are diagnosed as a result of newborn screening when symptomatic pulmonary disease is not evident, there is discussion as to when airway clearance should be started, with the first pulmonary symptom or at diagnosis. Some consider that, although there may not be clinical evidence of pulmonary involvement, there is pulmonary disease and thick CF mucus in the lungs. The debate will continue as to when to begin airway clearance techniques, but it is agreed that the method to clear the mucus from the lungs is a key therapy for everyone with CF.

Exercise. Exercise (i.e., particularly an aerobic conditioning program) is recommended for people with cystic fibrosis and because it positively influences general health, cardiopulmonary and musculoskeletal function, and airway clearance (Cystic Fibrosis Foundation, 2007a). Schneiderman-Walker, Pollock, Corey, and colleagues (2000) demonstrated a slowing of decline in forced vital capacity (FVC) and FEV_1 percent predicted, as well as an improved sense of well-being in the group that exercised regularly versus the control group. Clinicians should be aware that reactive airways disease (RAD) in CF may result from chronic inflammation and infection.

Bronchodilators often are used if a clinical response can be observed or if a beneficial response of a more than 10% increase in FEV_1 after bronchodilator use is shown by pulmonary function testing (Flume et al., 2007; Gibson et al., 2003). Many children with CF use an aerosolized bronchodilator before airway clearance as a part of their chronic pulmonary therapies.

Antiinflammatory Therapy. The immune systems of children with CF mount an intense inflammatory response to chronic bronchial infection, which contributes to parenchymal destruction and disease progression. Adolescents and adults with mild CF lung disease who appear clinically healthy are often found to have evidence of bacterial infection and significant local inflammatory response on bronchoalveolar lavage. Infants have early markers for pulmonary inflammation (Flume, 2008). Studies have been done to address the effectiveness of ibuprofen therapy in CF. These studies show that children and adolescents treated with high-dose ibuprofen had a slower rate of FEV_1 decline than children not on this therapy. Ibuprofen use requires serum drug levels to be monitored so that the therapeutic dosage can be established and maintained. Additionally, it is suggested that subtherapeutic levels may result in an increase in the inflammatory response (Konstan, Schluchter, Xue, et al. 2007). Individuals most likely to benefit from this therapy should be selected and their ibuprofen regimen monitored by the CF center team.

Clinicians have long recognized the clinical efficacy of antiinflammatory therapy and have used short courses of oral and inhaled corticosteroids, as well as cromolyn sodium, to treat reactive airway disease associated with CF. The chronic use of systemic corticosteroids in people with CF improves lung function but is associated with significant side effects, including cataracts, growth retardation, and glucose abnormalities. Inhaled corticosteroid use has shown no benefit for people with CF. The Cystic Fibrosis Foundation's 2007 guidelines for chronic pulmonary therapies recommend against using either oral steroids in children with CF or inhaled corticosteroids in anyone with CF (Flume et al., 2007).

Mucolytics and Other Pulmonary Therapies. Pharmacotherapies that clear airways of thick, tenacious secretions may indirectly improve inflammation. Dornase alfa cleaves extracellular DNA, which is present in high concentrations in purulent CF airway mucus, and reduces its viscosity to a more liquid form. It is efficacious in improving pulmonary function, as well as decreasing the frequency of hospitalizations, school or work absenteeism, and CF-related symptoms in individuals with mild to moderate pulmonary disease (i.e., FVC greater than 40% predicted). Side effects were limited to upper airway irritation (i.e., resulting in hoarseness, rash, chest pain, and conjunctivitis) and were usually mild and transient (Flume et al., 2007). Serial pulmonary function testing and clinical markers of morbidity should be used to monitor children started on dornase alfa. Quan, Tiddens, Sy, and colleagues (2001) reported that young children with mild disease on dornase alfa had better pulmonary outcomes and fewer pulmonary exacerbations over the 96-week study period than did those on placebo. The long-term effectiveness of dornase alfa in CF may be preventing early disease progression.

Nebulized hypertonic saline has also been shown to improve mucociliary clearance. In a clinical trial of 164 people with CF, inhalation of 7% hypertonic saline preceded by a bronchodilator improved pulmonary function and lessened exacerbation (Elkins, Robinson, Rose, et al., 2006). It works by increasing the airway surface liquid. Routine use is now recommended for individuals with CF ages 6 years and older.

Individuals with CF ages 6 years and older who received chronic macrolide therapy showed improved FEV_1 and weight and decreased pulmonary exacerbations and hospitalization as compared with the control group (Saiman, Marshall, Mayer-Hamblett, et al., 2003). Three times a week dosing of 250 mg or 500 mg of azithromycin showed benefit. It is hypothesized that it works not as an antibiotic but as an antiinflammatory. However, individuals who have nontuberculosis mycobacterium or *Burkholderia cepacia* complex should not be on this therapy. Further studies are needed to determine the benefit, if any, in young children, the impact on antibiotic resistance, and if it would be a viable therapy for individuals with *Burkholderia cepacia* complex.

Bilateral Lung Transplantation. Bilateral lung transplantation has emerged as a viable therapeutic option for individuals with end-stage CF lung disease. As of 2008, estimates of overall 5-year survival rate after transplantation are approximately 60%. Improved surgical techniques and antirejection drugs have had—and will continue to have—a marked impact on survival statistics. The biggest impediment to more widespread use of this intervention is the critical shortage of suitable organ donors (Yankaskas, Marshall, Sufian, et al., 2004). Although this procedure offers hope to individuals with end-stage disease and their families, it also presents them with significant psychosocial and financial challenges. In 2005, the United Network for Organ Sharing (UNOS) put into place a new lung allocation system to lessen wait times for people with more severe pulmonary disease. This appears to have lessened the waiting time for people with CF. Because such complex decisions are involved, consideration of transplantation, individual and family counseling, and referral for evaluation should be coordinated through the CF center.

Anticipated Advances in Diagnosis and Management

The effect of genetic discoveries on understanding etiology and pathophysiology is only beginning to unfold while approaches to detection are changing and reflect new technologic advances. Carrier screening is available and reliable for siblings and family members of a child with CF whose mutations have been identified. Appropriate studies of DNA deletion and linkage analysis are highly complex, and any family member contemplating such a screening should be referred to a regional CF center with a genetics center for counseling.

Prenatal diagnosis is available to parents of a child affected with CF and other at-risk couples. As a result, increasing numbers of at-risk families are using these diagnostic resources and confronting the ethical dilemma of having a therapeutic abortion versus continuing the pregnancy. Such decision making occurs while the science of treatment is advancing and clinicians observe the variability of the phenotypic expression of CF in individual children. Chorionic villus sampling (CVS) performed at 8 to 10 weeks of gestation or amniocentesis done at 12 to 16 weeks of gestation may provide information on CF mutations in the fetus. Prenatal diagnosis services, along with related counseling, are an area of specialization and should be coordinated by the regional CF center (Langfelder-Schwind et al., 2005).

Heterozygote (carrier) detection of the general population is technically possible and being implemented. Specialized genetic laboratories now offer screening for up to 97 of the most common CF mutations, which account for about 85% to 90% of mutant CF genes in North America. The American College of Medical Genetics and the American College of Obstetricians and Gynecologists have adopted standards and guidelines for implementation of CF genetic screening for any couple planning a pregnancy or seeking prenatal care. Zoler (2003) estimated that by early 2003 about 500,000 women were being screened yearly. As population-based carrier screening programs are being developed, many issues have not been completely addressed, including the burden of widespread screening on existing genetic counseling resources, the limited options available to at-risk couples who undergo testing during pregnancy, the large number of mutations, and numerous other issues (Grody, Cutting, Klinger, et al., 2001).

New breakthroughs in pharmacologic interventions that focus on the treatment of CF lung disease, which is the major determinant of morbidity and mortality in CF, are currently being tested (Cystic Fibrosis Foundation, 2008a; Zeitlin, 2007). Some of the more promising areas of research are as follows:

1. Novel therapeutic approaches directed at the common defects of CFTR (e.g., protein-repair therapy). For all of these therapies, clinical studies of safety, efficacy, and methodology are in progress in research centers across the United States. Individuals with CF, their families, and their health care providers ultimately hope that these therapies will eventually be collectively realized in a cure for CF.
   a. These approaches include PTC-124 that promotes readthrough of nonsense mutations in messenger ribonucleic acid (mRNA) and correctors and potentiators. Correctors will transport the CFTR protein to the epithelium where a potentiator will assist with the opening of the chloride channel. Both of these compounds are in varying stages of clinical trials (Zeitlin, 2007).
   b. Gene therapy has received the most attention by the lay CF community. The first human trial of gene therapy for CF was initiated at the National Institutes of Health (NIH) in April 1993. The goal of this therapy is to insert coding for normal CFTR protein in airway epithelial cells.
2. *Restore ion transportation:* Clinical trials are currently underway to discover alternative chloride channels that can be activated and inhibition of sodium absorption in the airway epithelium of children with CF, thus bypassing the CFTR protein chloride channel. This will lead to more hydrated airways and allow mucociliary clearance to be more effective.
3. *Antiinflammatories:* Interruption of the neutrophil-mediated inflammatory cascade with agents. Studies are in progress to determine if oral n-acetylcysteine, docosahexaenoic acid (DHA), methotrexate, or simvastatin can quiet the inflammatory response in CF.
4. *Antimicrobials:* Currently, a multicenter trial is underway looking at the time to acquisition of *Pseudomonas aeruginosa,* the impact of eradication, and the continuous use of antibiotics on the health of children with CF. Clinical trials testing aerosolized antibiotics in people with CF continue to find medications to effectively control CF pathogens.

5. A number of therapies being used in clinical care have shown promise. For example, early evidence of improved growth and clinical status with the use of growth hormone and megestrol acetate in CF in small samples has been reported (Hardin, Ellis, Dyson, et al., 2001). These therapies are experimental and should only be considered in consultation with the CF team and subspecialists in endocrinology.

Associated Problems of Cystic Fibrosis and Treatment

Salt Depletion: Hyponatremia and Dehydration

Children with CF have abnormal sodium and chloride loss in their sweat and are therefore at risk for dehydration secondary to electrolyte imbalance. Risk factors include hot weather, febrile illnesses with or without vomiting and diarrhea, and strenuous physical activity. Excessive salt loss may lead to listlessness, vomiting, heat prostration, and dehydration. Infants are at particular risk because of the low salt content of breast milk, commercial infant formulas, and infant foods. Prevention includes supplementing salt in infant formulas of at least 4 mEq/kg/day of sodium and adding salt to an older child's diet (Borowitz et al., 2002).

Associated Problems of Cystic Fibrosis and Treatment

- Salt depletion: hyponatremia and dehydration
- Rectal prolapse
- Nasal polyps and parasinusitis
- Distal ileal obstruction syndrome (DIOS)/constipation
- Hemoptysis
- Gastroesophageal reflux disease
- Cystic fibrosis–related diabetes mellitus (CFRD)
- Other serious complications

Rectal Prolapse

Rectal prolapse may be the initial symptom and may occur only once or be a recurrent problem. Initiation of appropriate enzyme replacement or adjustment of enzyme dosage often prevents its reoccurrence. Persistent or recurrent prolapse may rarely require surgical intervention. The first episode of rectal prolapse is frightening for both parents and child, and its reduction usually requires both immediate guidance (i.e., via phone) and assistance in the primary care provider's office or emergency department.

If a child experiences recurrent episodes of rectal prolapse, parents may learn to manually reduce a prolapse. With the child lying on his or her side, a parent (i.e., using a glove and lubricant jelly) is usually able to gently invert the mucosa through the rectal opening.

Nasal Polyps and Pansinusitis

Nasal polyps occur in 10% of children with CF and, if found on physical examination of any child, should raise the suspicion of CF. The upper respiratory tract (i.e., including sinuses) is lined with respiratory epithelial cells similar to the lining in the lungs and is therefore also affected by CF pathology. Sinuses are often chronically infected, producing symptoms such as frontal headaches, tenderness on palpation, purulent nasal discharge, and postnasal discharge that further contributes to the chronic cough. Treatment includes extended use of antibiotics and nasal cromolyn sodium or steroids, as well as intermittent use of nasal decongestants. Children may also find warm mist and saline nasal rinses to be comfort measures; some CF clinicians and otolaryngologists recommend sinus irrigations with saline. Surgical interventions for polyposis and sinusitis are sometimes necessary and are usually followed by stringent postsurgical nasal and/or sinus hygiene regimens.

Distal Ileal Obstruction Syndrome and/or Constipation

Although the prevalence of distal ileal obstruction syndrome (DIOS) is higher in adolescents and young adults, young children with CF are also at risk for developing total or partial intestinal obstruction. Constipation is often the result of a combination of malabsorption (i.e., from inadequate pancreatic enzyme doses or failure to take enzymes), decreased intestinal motility, and abnormally viscous intestinal secretions. DIOS is seen when intestinal contents accumulate at the ileocecum. Abdominal cramping with either diarrhea or the absence of stool and anorexia occurs. A stool mass may be palpable in the right lower quadrant. If the obstruction becomes complete, vomiting and increased pain and distention occur. Appendicitis, intussusception, and volvulus occur more frequently in children with CF and must be considered. A plain abdominal film may help confirm the diagnosis of DIOS. Contrast enemas (e.g., gastrografin with Tween 80) may be both diagnostic and therapeutic and are the treatment of choice for children with complete obstruction. Children with partial obstruction may be treated with polyethylene-glycol solutions (GoLYTELY, Colyte) or gastrografin given orally or by nasogastric tube. Miralax, a polyethylene glycol product, has proven useful in early intervention of a partial obstruction and long-term therapy to prevent reoccurrence. Follow-up should include long-term use of some combination of stool softener, mild stimulant, and bulk laxative, as well as the addition of bulk to the diet, consistent enzyme use, and exercise.

Hemoptysis

It is not uncommon in CF for blood-streaked sputum and small quantities of bright red blood to be expectorated from the lungs. Although initially alarming to the child and family, this bleeding is usually self-limited. Bleeding reflects increased bronchial infection, inflammation, and irritation, which require treatment that is more aggressive. Initiation or change of antibiotic therapy should be considered in addition to increasing routine pulmonary toilet. Massive hemoptysis (i.e., usually 240 mL/24 hr), however, requires immediate referral to the CF center team for management.

Gastroesophageal Reflux Disease

Heartburn and regurgitation is reported by more than 19% of individuals with CF (Cystic Fibrosis Foundation, 2008b), although the frequency with which reflux exacerbates pulmonary disease is unknown. Reflux is probably related to chest hyperinflation and increased abdominal pressure from coughing. Infants with failure to thrive and regurgitation and older children with dysphagia and epigastric pain should be evaluated for reflux and treated appropriately. In addition to pharmacologic management with a histamine-receptor antagonist and motility agent, dietary measures and an upright position after feedings and/or meals should be instituted. Postural drainage should always be done before feedings and/or meals and no longer include the head-down position (Lannefors et al., 2004).

Cystic Fibrosis–Related Diabetes Mellitus

The prevalence of CF-related diabetes (CFRD) is increasing as individuals with CF live longer. It is the leading comorbidity in cases reported in the 2007 Cystic Fibrosis Foundation's Patient Registry (2008b). CFRD results from both insulin deficiency and resistance and its management is complicated by the high caloric requirements of CF. CF centers routinely screen for CFRD and have well-developed guidelines for treatment, including nutritional management. The primary care provider should maintain a high suspicion for glucose intolerance, particularly in the adolescent and in children with more severe disease; when CFRD is suspected, consultations with the CF center and an endocrinologist familiar with CFRD are strongly recommended.

Other Serious Complications

Cystic fibrosis is a multisystem condition with an increased rate of complications and morbidity with age and disease progression. The complications listed in Box 22-5 are more serious and usually require the expertise of the CF center team. Primary care providers must recognize the early signs and symptoms of these complications so that timely referral for evaluation and treatment is possible.

BOX 22-5

Serious Complications of Cystic Fibrosis

- Colonization with highly resistant bacteria and other organisms
- Cor pulmonale
- Massive hemoptysis
- Pneumothorax
- Allergic bronchopulmonary aspergillosis (ABPA)
- Pancreatitis
- Hypertrophic pulmonary osteoarthropathy
- Liver disease including portal hypertension
- Gallbladder disease

Colonization with *Burkholderia cepacia* complex has emerged as a perplexing problem in CF. This organism is highly resistant to antibiotic therapy and has been implicated in the rapid progression of lung disease resulting in death. Other resistant organisms, particularly methicillin-resistant *Staphylococcus aureus* (MRSA) and *Stenotrophomonas maltophilia*, are also becoming more prevalent in the CF population. Following an extensive review of the evidence, a multidisciplinary team of experts in CF microbiology and clinical care has made evidence-based recommendations for prevention of cross-infection among individuals with CF (Saiman et al., 2003). These guidelines, which recommend minimizing close contact between individuals with CF, are rapidly becoming the standard of care in CF centers throughout North America.

Prognosis

Despite over 50 years of remarkable progress and a recent surge of new approaches to treatment, CF remains a progressive disease without cure. The median survival age is rapidly approaching 40 (Figures 22-3), and survival has markedly increased over the past 20 years. This change is likely a result not only of an improved understanding of pathophysiology and treatment but also of an appreciation and detection of the milder phenotypic expressions of the disease. With continued improvement in survival, CF is becoming a chronic condition of children, adolescents, and a growing population of adults (Yankaskas et al., 2004) (Figure 22-4).

PRIMARY CARE MANAGEMENT

Health Care Maintenance
Growth and Development

The achievement of adequate nutrition and normal growth in children with CF is the goal and a continual challenge for health care providers and families. Malnutrition and growth retardation are common complications of CF and may be the initial clinical

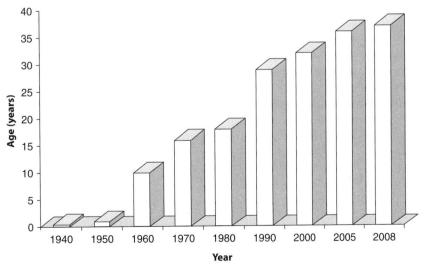

FIGURE 22-3 Median survival age of people with CF.

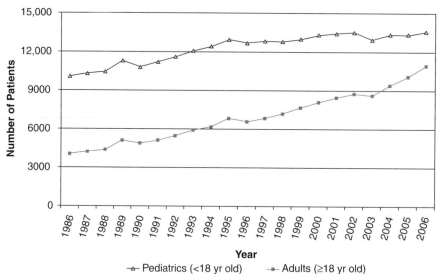

FIGURE 22-4 Number of adults compared with children with CF (1986-2006).

signs both in infancy and early adolescence; however, catch-up growth is often observed after diagnosis and initiation of pulmonary and nutritional therapy (Farrell, Kosorok, Rock, et al., 2001). Nutritional growth retardation is a significant independent prognostic indicator of survival as highlighted in the longitudinal data from the Cystic Fibrosis Foundation's Patient Registry (Cystic Fibrosis Foundation, 2008b). Other organic causes of malnutrition can be present and contribute to the need for increased caloric needs such as CFRD, reflux, and hepatobiliary disease (Rosenstein, 2006).

It is important to detect suboptimal growth of children with CF early so appropriate intervention strategies can be taken. First, adequate surveillance of growth by appropriate measurement and plotting of head circumference, weight, length or height, and BMI percentile at routine visits is essential (Borowitz et al., 2002; Stallings et al., 2008). Head circumference should be measured with a nonstretchable tape with the infant lying down. Weight should be measured on an electronic digital scale with infants unclothed and minimal clothing without any shoes for older children. For length, the infant should be measured on a length board until 24 months of age and then on a stadiometer after 2 years of age for the most accurate height. It is important to plot the measurements using the CDC growth charts for appropriate age and sex. The CF center will do specific growth measurements such as anthropometrics (triceps skin fold thickness, midarm circumference) and laboratory assessment annually (Borowitz et al., 2002).

Pubertal development is often delayed in adolescents with CF. This delay is usually related to poor nutritional status and pulmonary infections (Orenstein, 2004). Primary care providers may be able to help adolescents understand that this delay is not unusual or unexpected and that sexual development—though delayed—will occur. Pubertal development of individuals with CF can be assessed by a standardized method of self-assessment or physical examination using Tanner stages starting at age 9 for girls and 12 for boys (Borowitz et al., 2002).

Studies demonstrate that this period of pubertal growth is critical to achieving peak bone mass and adult bone health (Aris et al., 2005). Bone health can be evaluated by history, physical examination, and laboratory and radiologic assessment and is important for those individuals with CF who have specific risk factors such as chronic use of corticosteroids, poor nutrition, and delayed pubertal development. Primary care providers should communicate these concerns to the CF care team so the appropriate evaluation can be done (Aris et al., 2005; Borowitz et al., 2002).

Diet

The goal of nutritional therapy in children with CF is to promote normal growth. Their diet is usually a well-balanced, high-protein diet with unrestricted fat that provides 110% to 200% of standard energy need for the healthy general population (Stallings et al., 2008). Each individual with CF has a unique set of nutritional problems depending on his or her age and disease progression. It is important to remember that the nutritional intervention must be individualized and take into account the child's age, severity of lung disease, degree of maldigestion and malabsorption, dietary preferences, and financial resources (Borowitz et al., 2002).

In infancy, breastfeeding should be continued whenever possible for the immunologic, nutritional, and emotional advantages it offers. Conventional formulas can also meet the nutritional needs of infants, but often a caloric density greater than the standard 20 kcal/oz may be needed. This can be achieved by concentrating the formula, fortifying the breast milk, or adding fat and/or carbohydrates. Either breast milk or formula should be given until 12 months of age, at which time an infant with CF who has maintained normal growth can switch to whole milk. The primary care provider can also provide guidance on the introduction of solid foods at 4 to 6 months according to the recommendations of the American Academy of Pediatrics (AAP) for children with uncomplicated CF (Borowitz et al., 2002).

As toddlers and preschoolers experience developmentally appropriate changes in eating patterns, parents are often anxious about providing adequate food intake to maintain the child's well-being and growth. Maintaining growth at this developmental stage can be achieved by routinely adding calories to table foods with fats such as butter, sour cream, cheese, peanut butter, and whole milk. In toddlers, self-feeding skills begin to develop as do eating problems. Primary care providers can help parents understand how to provide appropriate nutritious foods, set limits for mealtimes, and encourage child feeding autonomy. Parents should avoid mealtime battles, force feeding, and grazing behavior (Powers, Jones, Ferguson, et al., 2005). In a study of families of toddlers with CF, Powers, Patton, Byars, and associates (2002) found that toddlers with CF and healthy peers did not differ on the rate of mealtime behaviors (i.e., amount of talking or reinforcements given). However, parents of toddlers with CF differed on the types of strategies used to manage meals. They also found that toddlers with CF were not getting the necessary calories for normal growth and that parents may need additional support in learning how to manage their child's mealtime behavior.

School-age children with CF need to have a basic understanding about their disease, including the importance of good nutrition and enzyme therapy. This age-group presents additional nutritional challenges that include "taste-fatigue" with oral nutritional supplements, resistance to taking enzymes in the presence of peers, and decreased time to complete treatments (Borowitz et al., 2002).

Adolescence is a time of increased energy requirements resulting from puberty, changes in lifestyle, and increased physical activity along with the potential progression in lung disease. All of these factors increase the need for calories at a time when there can be denial about one's disease, poor adherence to treatments, rebellion, and altered body perceptions, especially in females. During this developmental stage, it is vital that dietary intake, growth velocity, and nutritional status are monitored every 3 months by either the CF care center or the primary care provider (or both) (Borowitz et al., 2002) To be most effective, nutritional interventions to increase caloric needs should be planned with the teenagers themselves. Adolescents are most receptive to the idea that the nutritional interventions will promote pubertal development, muscular strength, and energy rather than improving their CF and weight gain. Primary care providers should monitor adolescents with CF for signs of eating disturbances. Shearer and Bryon (2004) state that CF may be a risk factor for eating disorders or disturbances because adolescents with CF experience many of the same risk factors. They concluded that eating disorders were not prevalent in the study group, but eating disturbances were present in 24% of the study with no difference in occurrence between males and females.

Parents often have questions about pancreatic enzyme doses. Enzymes are given with each meal and most snacks except those that have very little or no fat. Enzymes are also necessary with breast milk and any of the predigested formulas. Doses are adjusted by the CF care team according to the growth curve, stool pattern, and signs of malabsorption (i.e., abdominal cramping, flatulence). The enzyme beads should not be chewed or crushed; destroying the enteric coating inactivates the enzymes and may excoriate the oral mucosa (Borowitz et al., 2002). For infants and younger children who cannot swallow the enzyme capsule, it can be opened and the beads mixed with applesauce or other nonalkaline food that can be consumed immediately. Finally, generic enzymes are not bioequivalent to proprietary enzymes, and this should be investigated whenever one is demonstrating signs of malabsorption and/or growth failure; the 2008 recommendations for the nutritional management of CF state that only proprietary preparations of pancreatic enzymes should be used (Stallings et al., 2008).

Supplementation of fat-soluble vitamins, essential fatty acids, calcium, iron, zinc, and sodium, should be strongly considered for any child with CF. Consultation with the CF care center dietitian can be helpful in establishing the appropriate doses of vitamins. There are recommended dosages of non–fat-soluble multivitamins plus supplementation of vitamins A, D, E, and K at age-appropriate levels. These are based on the "Consensus Report on Nutrition for Pediatric Patients with Cystic Fibrosis" (Borowitz et al., 2002).

Primary care providers should remember that nutritional issues in children and adolescents with CF are unique and may not respond to the traditional interventions. Whenever difficult nutritional problems arise, the multidisciplinary team at the CF center should be consulted.

Safety

In addition to age-appropriate anticipatory guidance about safety issues, primary care providers should emphasize safe storage and handling of the large quantities of medications often used by children with CF and how to avoid germs to lessen the risk of infections. Medications are to be kept out of reach and have safety caps on all medication containers. The issue of accidental ingestion of pancreatic enzymes by another child may arise because ample supplies of these enzymes are often available at mealtimes in the home and carried by the child for use. Enzymes are not likely to be harmful if small quantities are ingested; they are activated in the small intestine and excreted in stool.

Many of the antibiotics that individuals with CF take for an exacerbation or on a chronic basis will alter the skin's tolerance for sun exposure. It is important for all children to use sunscreen, but for those who are on antibiotics such as ciprofloxacin, avoidance of the sun and artificial ultraviolet light is recommended.

Hand hygiene is the single most important practice to prevent transmission of infectious agents. Hand hygiene includes cleaning one's hands with soap and water or waterless antiseptic hand rubs. For individuals with CF, hand hygiene should be done after toileting, coughing, sneezing, and nose blowing; before medications; and after inhaled therapies and airway clearance. The Cystic Fibrosis Foundation's infection control recommendations (Saiman et al., 2003) stress the importance of good hand hygiene and minimizing the exposure to others with CF to prevent the spread of CF-specific pathogens such as *Burkholderia cepacia* complex. Additionally, coughing into a tissue and then disposing of it in a covered trash receptacle and keeping a minimum distance of 3 feet between others with CF and/or a respiratory infection are recommended.

Immunizations

Infants and children with CF should receive all routine immunizations at the ages recommended by the CDC (AAP, 2008; CDC, 2008a). In a few instances, the CF team may recommend a brief delay to stabilize an acute pulmonary or nutritional problem, but there is no evidence to support delay of routine immunizations (Orenstein, Winnie, & Altman, 2002).

Immunization with an annual influenza vaccine is also recommended, following CDC guidelines for the type and dose of vaccine for all children with CF who are 6 months and older. It should be administered during the autumn of each year before the start of the influenza season. For those children with CF who are on high doses of corticosteroids for a prolonged period, influenza administration should be deferred temporarily (AAP, 2008). Inter-nasal influenza vaccine is not recommended for individuals with chronic lung disease, including CF. It is also important for the primary care provider to encourage all household contacts to also be immunized against influenza to help reduce the individual's risk of exposure (Rosenstein, 2006).

Because respiratory syncytial virus (RSV) can be a risk to one with CF, RSV immunization is an appealing notion, but the safety and efficacy of palivizumab injections remains debated among CF health care providers. A 2007 Cystic Fibrosis Foundation infant care workshop states that in infants with CF with additional risk factors for acquiring RSV or for severe RSV disease, palivizumab should be considered during the first winter of life. These risk factors include previous lower respiratory tract illness, older siblings, daycare, smoke exposure, and/or malnutrition, among others (Cystic Fibrosis Foundation, 2007b). This is an area where further research is needed.

Screening

Vision. Routine screening is recommended. A pediatric ophthalmologist should monitor steroid-dependent children annually for early detection of cataracts or glaucoma. For individuals with CFRD, retinal screening should be done annually.

Hearing. Routine screening is recommended. Children should be monitored by an audiologist for occurrence of high-frequency hearing loss after every 2 to 4 courses of intravenous aminoglycosides or 180 accumulated days of aerosolized aminoglycoside.

Dental. Routine screening is recommended. Precautions for the use of tetracycline before permanent tooth formation are advised. Orthodontia work can cause some difficulty in eating, and nutritional supplements may need to be added if there is growth failure.

Blood Pressure. Blood pressure should be measured at every visit for those on corticosteroids because of possible hypertension side effects.

Hematocrit. Routine screening is recommended. Anemia may result from other organic causes such as protein deficiencies or chronic infection, and further studies may be warranted to differentiate between iron deficiency and anemia of chronic illness.

Urinalysis. Routine screening is recommended.

Tuberculosis. Routine screening is no longer recommended for all children with CF, only those who are at increased risk of acquiring tuberculosis infection and disease. Active disease caused by *Mycobacterium tuberculosis* is probably no more prevalent in individuals with CF than in the general population. Olivier, Weber, Wallace, and associates (2003) reported a prevalence of nontuberculous mycobacteria of 13% in people with CF.

Condition-Specific Screening

Primary care providers and the CF care team should communicate their findings of each visit, including the physical examination and any laboratory and radiologic assessment, to all health care providers. This will not only provide continuity of care but also eliminate the repetition of screening evaluations and laboratory work because many of the routine screening tests recommended by the AAP may also be part of the annual screening that is done by the CF care centers (i.e., urinalysis, hematocrit, etc.).

Pulmonary function testing (PFT) is used to measure lung function and is routinely performed in children over 5 years of age at every CF center visit and hospitalization. PFT and chest roentgenography monitor the progression of pulmonary disease and identify acute problems.

Other screenings routinely performed at CF center visits include sputum cultures with antibiotic sensitivities; blood and urine assays of liver and renal function; complete blood counts; serum measures of nutritional status; and screening for CFRD. People with CF are known to have reduced bone mass and an increasing number of people with CF have osteoporosis or osteopenia. Because of this, it is recommended that a dual x-ray absorptiometry (DXA) scan be done at age 18 years and repeated every 2 to 5 years depending on bone density and health (Aris et al., 2005). Depending on the individual's age, medications, and disease progression, more intensive laboratory monitoring maybe indicated.

Common Illness Management
Differential Diagnosis

Symptoms associated with common pediatric illnesses also may be symptoms specific to CF, and questions about their cause and management often arise. Parents often need to hear that their child will develop common, minor childhood illnesses and will usually respond to routine management. Parents should be reassured that the CF center team is available to the primary care provider whenever questions about the cause and treatment of an acute illness arise. Thorough history taking and examination are not only necessary for primary care providers to make a differential diagnosis but are also reassuring to parents and the child.

Differential Diagnosis

- *Gastrointestinal symptoms:* Common vs. distal ileal obstruction syndrome (DIOS), rule out appendicitis, volvulus, intussusceptions, gallstones, pancreatitis, fibrosing colonopathy
- *Fever:* Viral illness with exacerbation of chronic infection
- *Chest pain:* Pneumothorax vs. muscle pull vs. gastroesophageal reflux (GER)
- *Cough:* Sinusitis vs. lower respiratory tract exacerbation
- *Wheezing:* Heightened bronchial reactivity caused by chronic infection and inflammation

---

Gastrointestinal Symptoms. Abdominal pain is a relatively common complaint in individuals with CF and can be caused by a variety of conditions, not all which are CF related. Diarrhea, constipation, and abdominal cramping may be the initial complaints of a partial or complete intestinal obstruction. A history of intermittent cramping pain and changes in stool pattern in the absence of other acute gastrointestinal and systemic symptoms is suggestive of DIOS. Abdominal pain may also be suggestive of gallstones or pancreatitis, and a careful pain history is essential. Appendicitis, intussusception, peptic ulcer disease, fibrosing colonopathy, necrotizing enterocolitis (for those on antibiotics), and volvulus should always be in the differential diagnosis (Orenstein et al., 2002). Children who have gastrointestinal symptoms that coincide with those of others with whom they have had close contact and suggest infectious causes not related to CF should be treated appropriately. Finally, children with CF have a high prevalence of gastroesophageal reflux disease (GERD), which is associated with regurgitation, failure to thrive, dysphagia, epigastric pain, esophageal ulcerations, blood loss in older individuals, chronic respiratory symptoms, and feeding problems (Boesch & Acton, 2007; Rosenstein, 2006). In treating GERD in infants, conservative measures should be tried first, including the use of the prone, upright position postfeeding, and thickening formula feeds. Head-down positioning for chest physical therapy is not recommended for individuals with CF because of GERD (Cystic Fibrosis Foundation, 2007b). The administration of prokinetic agents to increase lower esophageal sphincter tone and promote gastric emptying may be indicated in those who do not respond to conservative measures (Orenstein et al., 2002). Boesch and Acton (2007) looked at the outcomes of fundoplication in children with CF and found that symptoms of GERD recurred in about 48% of children and there was little apparent nutritional or pulmonary benefit.

Fever. Fever associated with a CF pulmonary exacerbation is a relatively uncommon presentation, and evaluation of fever in children with CF should elicit the same broad-based approach used with other children. An initial brief febrile period with a viral illness can be anticipated in children with CF and symptomatically treated per usual practice protocols. When a viral illness exacerbates lower respiratory tract symptoms—as often occurs with upper respiratory tract infections—an increase in frequency of airway clearance and a 2- to 4-week course of oral or aerosolized antibiotics, or both, are usually recommended (Rosenstein, 2006). Prevention of hyponatremia and dehydration during febrile illness includes adding salt and increasing fluids to a child's intake and reviewing warning signs of dehydration with parents. When a rehydration solution is indicated, electrolyte-balanced clear liquids (e.g., Pedialyte [Ross Laboratories]) may be used. One must also evaluate the fever that could be symptomatic of influenza. In younger children and infants, the manifestations are similar to common respiratory viral illnesses whereas with older children they may have additional complaints of headache, chills, myalgia, and malaise. Approved treatment of influenza includes one of the recommended antiviral drugs such as amantadine or rimantadine, which should be initiated within 48 hours of onset of illness (AAP, 2008).

Chest Pain. Children with lung disease occasionally complain of chest pain. These complaints should always be evaluated because of the potential occurrence of pneumothorax. Complaints associated with pneumothorax are typically an abrupt onset of sharp pain unilaterally followed by dull aching and accompanied by profound shortness of breath and activity intolerance. This complication, confirmed by physical examination and chest roentgenogram, is best managed at the regional CF center following local emergency stabilization as indicated.

Other causes of chest pain include musculoskeletal strains, especially from prolonged paroxysmal coughing episodes. These chest pains are usually bilateral, not associated with dyspnea, and reproduced by palpitation. This pain usually responds to rest and antiinflammatory agents. Chest pain, especially during pulmonary exacerbations, can be pleural inflammation. This type of chest pain increases with deep breaths and is not reproducible on palpitation. Since this chest pain is usually secondary to underlying infection, treatment should include an increase in airway clearance, antibiotics, and nonnarcotic analgesics (Flume, 2008). People with CF experience midline chest and epigastric burning related to

GERD and esophagitis. If antacids are not effective, the CF center team should be consulted regarding the use of histamine-receptor antagonists and proton pump inhibitors (Tipnis & Rudolph, 2007).

Cough. The respiratory tract is usually involved in CF, even in those children whose initial presentation is not pulmonary related. The most prominent feature of pulmonary involvement is a chronic cough. Initially, the cough can be dry, but as the disease progresses or in an acute exacerbation, it becomes paroxysmal and productive. An increase in cough is always of significance and requires intervention even if the chest is clear to auscultation (Orenstein et al., 2002). Nighttime coughing and/or wheezing may develop and can be associated with reactive airway disease, increased pulmonary infection and inflammation, or postnasal discharge from sinusitis or rhinitis (Rosenstein, 2006). Delineating a clear cause of the cough can be challenging. Both antibiotic therapy and initiation of or increase in the use of aerosolized bronchodilators and antiinflammatory agents may be helpful. Cough suppressants are generally contraindicated and should only be used after consultation with the CF center team. A trial of decongestants may be useful. Antihistamines may be used when allergy plays a role in symptomatology, but primary care providers should be aware that antihistamines might increase the viscosity of mucus, inhibiting its mobilization.

Wheezing. Wheezing is a common manifestation of CF—particularly in infancy—that is most often attributed to heightened bronchial reactivity from chronic infection and inflammation. This often makes it difficult to distinguish airway symptoms caused by infection from those caused by asthma. One who has recurrent wheezing (not just a cough), a family history of asthma, a personal history of atopy, or responses to antiasthma medications is most likely to have asthma (Balfour-Lynn, 2003). The 2007 Cystic Fibrosis Foundation's Patient Registry (2008b) reports that 17% of children less than 18 years of age have asthma. Bronchodilators have been used in individuals with CF for many years and can increase airflow significantly in those who also have asthma, although responses typically vary over time and with degree of illness (Rosenstein, 2006). In children with CF where clinical data support the diagnosis of asthma, inhaled corticosteroids should be the first-line prophylaxis, but doses should not escalate (Balfour-Lynn, 2003). It is imperative that antibiotics also be used during acute asthma exacerbations if there is underlying respiratory infection. Finally, there are other underlying causes of wheezing that should be included in the differential diagnosis, including foreign body aspiration (especially in toddlers), allergic bronchopulmonary aspergillus, other medications that could induce bronchospasm (e.g., aerosolized antibiotics), GERD, and RSV infection.

Drug Interactions

Although very few drug interactions have been studied specifically in individuals with CF, primary care providers should be cognizant that certain drugs commonly used to manage CF lung disease may interact with other medications. With the use of corticosteroids, there is an increase risk for gastrointestinal ulceration if the child with CF is also on high-dose nonsteroidal antiinflammatory drugs (NSAIDs) such as ibuprofen. Itraconazole and ketoconazole can decrease the clearance of corticosteroids; decrease the absorption of antacids, cimetidine, ranitidine, and famotidine; and interact with phenytoin (MedlinePlus.gov, 2007). Children using ciprofloxacin, an antibiotic that is used frequently in CF, should be advised not to take antacids, zinc, or calcium supplements concurrently. For those individuals who have had a lung transplant, antirejection medications, such as cyclosporin, have multiple drug interactions, and the primary care provider should consult the transplant center before prescribing any new medications. The use of herbal supplements has been increasing in the general population, as well as in individuals with CF. A detailed medication history including oral or inhaled nutritional supplements and over-the-counter vitamins and medications can help alleviate potential drug interactions. Health care providers should provide education about the medications that are prescribed.

Primary care providers routinely include anticipatory guidance about substance abuse to children, adolescents, and parents. The harmful effects of tobacco smoke, both active and passive, have been well documented in reports such as the 2004 Surgeon General's report *The Health Consequences of Smoking* (www.cdc.gov). Smoking is closely tied with heart disease, lung cancer, cataracts, and dental disease. Children who have a chronic respiratory disease such as CF are most vulnerable to passive smoking or secondhand smoke. Collaco, Vanscoy, Bremer, and associates (2008) determined that any exposure to secondhand smoke negatively affected lung function in people with CF.

Tyc and Throckmorton-Belzer (2006) reported that 21.1% of adolescents with CF said they had ever smoked, and almost 3% reported smoking more than 2 days within the previous 30 days. This corresponds to Verma, Clough, McKenna, and associates (2001), who reviewed the literature and determined that 20% of youths with CF had tried other substances, including marijuana. For those persons with CF who actively smoked, there was a dose-dependent relationship between the number of cigarettes smoked and the severity of the disease (Verma et al., 2001). It is important for the primary care provider to discuss the health risks of smoke and secondhand smoke exposure with children and adolescents with CF. Education about the harmful effects of smoking, with referral to smoking cessation programs, should be provided and reinforced by primary care providers.

Alcohol can have detrimental effects on anyone who abuses it, but it can be worse for someone with CF. Malnutrition is a common complication of CF and alcohol in excess can worsen one's nutritional status. It can also increase the risk for liver damage to those with CF who already have the potential for hepatobiliary disease. Alcohol use in individuals on NSAIDs or corticosteroids can greatly increase the risk for gastrointestinal ulceration and bleeding.

Developmental Issues

Sleep Patterns

Sleep patterns may be altered by either an acute exacerbation or a gradual progression of disease that increase cough and/or decrease oxyhemoglobin saturation. Nighttime coughing can interfere with the child's sleep, as well as that of family members. Children with CF also have a busy morning routine, which requires early rising for school-age children and adolescents to get in their multiple medications, treatments, and nutrition. They are often more vulnerable to fatigue because of their increased basal metabolic rate. Difficulty falling asleep and remaining asleep are associated somatic symptoms of depression. Although sleep requirements are not necessarily greater in these children, sleep should not be reduced. All health care providers should include a detailed sleep history as part of the individual's evaluation. It is also important to help families maintain a consistent bedtime ritual that is appropriate for their child's developmental level. When a child with CF is hospitalized, the child should be encouraged to bring transitional objects (e.g., blankets, stuffed animals, music) from home to help the child sleep.

Toileting

As in other children, toilet training should proceed when cues of developmental readiness are noted in a child. Many children with CF, however, continue to have stools more than once a day and may have some abdominal cramping before stooling, even with adequate enzyme therapy. These problems may impede the child's interest in toileting, and parents should allow for this delay.

Even though enzymes improve digestion of nutrients, some maldigested food passes through the intestine. As a result, stools may be excessive, urgent, malodorous, and an embarrassment for children and adolescents. Parents, teachers, and friends' parents should be aware of the need for privacy during toileting.

Stress urinary incontinence occurs in individuals with CF. Moraes, Carpenter, and Taylor (2002) surveyed 6- to 17-year-olds and found that stress urinary incontinence was reported by 14% of the children and that it was more common in females. Females with CF have a prevalence of stress incontinence of 33%, compared to healthy females with a rate of 7% (Prasad, Balfour-Lynn, Carr, et al., 2006). Urinary leakage was usually associated with coughing, sneezing, laughing, pulmonary exacerbations, daily airway clearance and exercise, and more severe lung disease. Primary care providers should be assessing degree of urinary incontinence for all people with CF because it is a problem that can cause anxiety and psychosocial issues. Pelvic floor muscle exercises, such as Kegel exercises, reduce incontinence and improve muscle strength compared with other interventions (Dodd & Langman, 2005).

Discipline

From the time of diagnosis, parents of children with CF not only grieve the loss of a healthy child but also feel guilty about their genetic contribution. Parents struggle to redefine a future for their child and family. The primary care provider can provide ongoing support and counseling during this difficult adjustment period especially since they often already have an established relationship with the parents and/or child.

Improved medical treatments have increased life expectancy for those with CF, but also increased the time and complexity of the daily home regimen. This time commitment of daily therapy may not only create conflicts between parents and children but also be viewed by siblings as an inequity in parental attention. There have been reports of enuresis, headaches, depression, abdominal pain, and poor school performances in siblings of children with chronic conditions (Bluebond-Langner, 2001). Conscious efforts by parents to give individual attention to each child may prevent feelings of jealousy and guilt. Effective parental coping strategies—including assigning meaning to the illness, sharing the burden, and incorporating therapy into a schedule—help parents to set limits and encourage similar responsibilities for the child with CF and siblings, making it easier to maintain a consistent family life.

Parents of adolescents with CF are often frustrated and anxious about disease progression, particularly when they have difficulty maintaining their child's adherence to the treatment plan on one hand and seek to promote independence on the other. Factors influencing adherence with CF regimens include inadequate knowledge and psychosocial difficulties (Angst, 2001). Normal adolescent behavior (i.e., testing limits, perceiving themselves as invincible, and taking risks) is complicated by the chronicity and morbidity of CF. Therapies that are burdensome and do not result in any clear-cut short-term benefit, such as airway clearance, are more likely to be missed than treatments that have a more immediate effect (e.g., aerosols, enzymes). Parents who begin to transfer responsibility for management of CF to their child beginning in the early school years often report fewer problems in adolescence. Adolescents with CF may also be more adherent if allowed to control parts of their treatment regimen, such as which type of airway clearance or at what time to do it. Encouraging school-age children and adolescents to actively participate in clinic visits by specifically asking them questions and asking for their answer in addition to the parental response can provide the opportunity for the child to learn and be involved in his or her health care. Answering the questions and involving them in decision making is essential to their development of accountability, independence, and learning how to partner with the health care provider to manage CF for their lifetime. Behavioral contracts may be useful tools for families and health care providers who are experiencing problems with an adolescent (D'Angelo & Lask, 2001).

Part of every visit should be dedicated to psychosocial issues such as discipline and coping of the child with CF and the rest of the family. Referral for individual and family counseling may be necessary to assist with the particular challenges that arise.

Child Care

Parents of children with CF often struggle with child-care issues, especially at the time of diagnosis. Certain factors should be remembered when health care providers assist parents in making the appropriate choice for child care. First, the financial needs of the family are critical to determine what type of child care they can afford. Second, one must examine what is available to the family in their area (e.g., private home or a licensed child-care center). Ideally, the best child-care setting would be in the child's own home, or in another home setting with few children, because this decreases their exposure to illnesses. Whatever setting is selected, it is important to address any guilt feelings parents have about placing their child with CF in child care. When a child-care program has been selected, child-care providers should be specifically educated on issues such as the following: (1) the child's individual nutritional and pulmonary treatment plan; (2) the child's chronic cough and lack of contagion; and (3) methods to prevent the spread of illness in the setting. (See the educational materials at the end of this chapter.)

Schooling

School officials, including principals, teachers, coaches, and the school nurse, should be educated about several issues with the child with CF in the school setting. (See educational resources at the end of the chapter.) First, the child will need to take medications during school, including enzymes with lunch and snacks and, at times, inhalers, aerosols, or antibiotics. It is helpful if the school can allow the older child to carry his or her medications with him or her instead of going to the office. This allows the child to not

miss out on activities and to educate his or her peers about the treatments for CF.

A student with CF may be fatigued because of malnutrition, early morning treatments, and, as the disease progresses, interruption of sleep from coughing. Education of the school personnel and parents about options such as altering the school-day schedule or establishing an individualized educational program (IEP) to fit the individual needs of the student can help keep a child in school. Home instruction may be necessary for the child who is too ill, but these children will still need the social interaction that friends can provide.

Coughing is another school issue that is often misunderstood by the school personnel and classmates. Children with CF are encouraged to cough, because it is the body's way of clearing secretions. It is important for these students to be given the privacy, if needed, to cough and not suppress it. Classmates and their families should understand that their cough is not contagious.

The most sensitive school issue for children with CF is related to their bowel movements. These can be foul smelling, excessive, and urgent. The student with CF will need extra restroom privileges and preferably the use of a private restroom (i.e., teacher's lounge or nurse's office).

Full participation in school activities, including physical education and athletic activities, is desirable for children with CF. How much the student can participate in physical education will depend on the severity of CF and how the child is feeling that day. It is important to remind both the student and the teacher that children with CF lose an abnormally high amount of salt through their sweat and this can cause an increased risk of dehydration, electrolyte imbalance, and even heat prostration. Thus the student should be encouraged to carry water or sports drinks and eat salty snacks when he or she exercises, especially during hot weather (Fulton, Casey, Luder, et al., 2006).

Children with CF do not show any evidence of impairment in their intellectual/academic performance when compared with their peers. Problems in school performance are more likely related to absenteeism as a result of physical illness, fatigue, and/or psychological reactions to the disease, such as lowered self-esteem or depression (Morris, Ryan, Williams, et al., 2002). Further evaluation may be necessary to determine the cause of poor school performance so that the appropriate interventions can be prescribed.

Sexuality

The majority of male adults with CF (98%) have obstruction or absence of the vas deferens resulting in azoospermia and infertility. A sperm count should be offered routinely for purposes of counseling (Rosenstein, 2006). Male adolescents and young adults need reassurance that this condition does not indicate impotence and will not diminish their ability to have normal sexual relations (Sawyer, Farrant, Cerritelli, et al., 2005). Recent advances in fertility medicine have given males with CF the opportunity to biologically father children. Health care providers do need to educate teens about the use of condoms to decrease the risk of sexually transmitted diseases despite the fact that they are most likely infertile.

Although fertility in females with CF is decreased due to thickened cervical mucus, many women are still able to have children (Rosenstein, 2006). In contemplating pregnancy, women with CF need to be counseled as to the potential risk to their health, the genetic risk and health of their offspring, and the challenges of child-care responsibilities in light of deteriorating health and shortened life expectancy. Contraception alternatives for adolescent and young adult women with CF can be a sensitive issue to discuss for both the health care provider and the individual, but it needs to be assessed at regular visits. A variety of contraceptive methods have been used in females with CF, and the results are similar to those of the general population. Oral contraceptives have been reported to have side effects of headaches, heartburn, and breakthrough bleeding, and their effectiveness may be decreased when certain antibiotics are taken at the same time. Because of the comparative risk of pregnancy, many CF center providers recommend oral contraceptives or another form of birth control after fully discussing these issues with a young woman. Reproductive issues in CF should be managed in consultation with the CF center team and a high-risk obstetrician/gynecologist familiar with the disease.

Frequent antibiotics can cause fungal vaginitis in women with CF. This causes vaginal itching, irritation, discomfort, and pain with urination and intercourse. Conventional treatment with antifungal cream or suppositories can be used, but many women need oral antifungal agents (Sawyer, 2001).

The primary health care provider should make sure that any adolescent or young adult with CF who is considering having biologic children should consider genetic risks, as well as the physical and financial challenges that both CF and parenthood entail.

With the advances in the field of fertility, many couples known to carry two CF mutations are opting to use in vitro fertilization to eliminate the possibility of having a child with CF. Additionally, over 45% of people with CF in the United States are age 18 years and older (Cystic Fibrosis Foundation, 2008b). The aging of the CF population has increased the number of adults with CF consulting fertility clinics to biologically conceive children without CF, although a CF carrier.

Transition to Adulthood

Advances in CF treatment have led to improved outcomes and greater life expectancy. In 2007 more than 45% of people with CF in the United States were age 18 years or older (Cystic Fibrosis Foundation, 2008b). Transition programs to move adolescents from the pediatric setting to the care of adult providers have been developed in many CF centers. These programs include a committed team of adult providers who have developed expertise in CF care. Many transitions include a visit by the CF adult health care team in the pediatric clinic. This can begin at any time during adolescence. The timing of the completed transition to the adult program has usually been between 18 and 21 years of age, although some individuals may be ready earlier than 18. Additionally, others who are in the terminal phase of their disease may never be transitioned to maintain care consistency. Preparation of adolescents for transition to adult care begins by increasing their independence early in adolescence. This begins by maximizing opportunities for independence, including time during a clinic visit without a parent present, prompting responsibility for their own daily medical regimen, and educating them on how to communicate with their health care team (e.g., calling for prescription refills, discussing their concerns). Some adolescents and their families may find this transition difficult because of the long-established relationship they have had with the pediatric CF center and their primary care providers. For others, it is seen as a significant "rite of passage" into adulthood (Yankaskas et al., 2004).

Family Concerns

Families who deal with CF have a multitude of special concerns, including the stress of its prognosis, added financial burden of chronic medical care, and maintenance of family life despite the uncertainty of exacerbations, hospitalizations, and disease progression. There have been a myriad of studies in the past that examine how families, including mothers, fathers, and well siblings, cope with CF in their family member. Families who are dealing with CF, like any chronic condition, need and appreciate the consistency and open communication that they develop with health care professionals. The health care team should be sensitive to the individual needs of each family member and the coping mechanisms they embrace. From the time of diagnosis, through the first exacerbation, hospitalization, and disease progression, questions should be answered honestly and directly but within a framework of cautious optimism (Rosenstein, 2006). CF is a complex disease and needs the support of the multidisciplinary team including not only those health care providers at the CF center but the home care team, community support groups, and primary care provider.

Care for children with CF is a significant burden on families, especially with the advent of additional treatment options and improved life expectancy. This coincides with increasing medical costs and shrinking insurance benefits. Families often need assistance with unraveling prescription coverage, medical bills, government benefits, appeals, and referrals. The social worker at the CF center is often the best person to assist the families in the jargon used in insurance matters such as co-payment, deductible, authorization, PPO, HMO, and POS (see Chapter 8). It is also the CF center staff who can guide the families to additional resources such as the state-funded program for the medically handicapped that is offered in many states for children with chronic diseases such as CF. All health care providers can be strong advocates in helping children with CF and their families with financial planning issues.

Despite all recent advances (the median predicted age of survival is over 37; Cystic Fibrosis Foundation, 2008b), many children with CF still face end-of-life issues. Most will die from respiratory failure. Mechanical ventilation for respiratory failure in individuals with CF has generally been ineffective and is usually not recommended unless there is clearly a reversible component. More recently, noninvasive positive pressure ventilation has been used in end-stage CF primarily in those individuals awaiting lung transplantation. Care provided at the end of life is often a mix of preventive, therapeutic, and palliative treatments depending on values and preferences of both the individual with CF and the family (Yankaskas et al., 2004). Together, primary care providers and the CF care team can help prepare individuals with CF and their families for the types of decisions they will face at the end of life.

Resources

The Cystic Fibrosis Foundation is a national organization that was formed in 1955 by a committed group of parents whose children had CF. It now operates as a nonprofit, voluntary health organization that raises money to assure the development of the means to cure and control CF and improve the quality of life for those with the disease. This is done by funding CF research, supporting drug discovery and development and CF care centers, training medical professionals, and educating the public about CF. A network of local chapters in the United States raises money to support CF programs and research through a variety of fundraising events. Involvement in the local fundraising events is one way to help families participate in the fight to find a cure for this dreadful disease.

There are approximately 115 Cystic Fibrosis Foundation–accredited care centers in the United States that offer a multidisciplinary health care team approach in the care and management of CF. The Cystic Fibrosis Foundation's Therapeutic Development Program is an innovative resource for drug discovery and development that involves many of the CF care centers throughout the United States. The Cystic Fibrosis Foundation has also supported the development of CF clinical practice guidelines and their subsequent implementation, as well as education for health care professionals, individuals with CF, and their families. These are written care guidelines based on a review of the published medical literature and the best available scientific information, and are supplemented by clinical experience and expert consensus. These clinical practice guidelines are the foundation for care centers, using quality improvement (QI) tools, to improve quality of care and thus the clinical outcomes for people with CF (Britton, Thrasher, & Gutierrez, 2008). Parents of children with CF should be encouraged to establish an ongoing relationship with a Cystic Fibrosis Foundation–accredited care center.

Years ago, the primary care provider might not have been involved in the care of the child with CF. Today, with the increasing number of newly diagnosed individuals with CF, both by newborn screening and later in life, and the ongoing education of medical professionals, primary care providers are an integral part of the health care team. Together, each health care provider brings a unique emphasis and expertise to a complex disease.

Educational Materials

People with CF, families, and health care professionals can access vast arrays of educational materials available on websites, Web casts, videos, pamphlets, books, and interactive CD-ROMs.

In 2001, the Cystic Fibrosis Foundation formed an education committee whose mission is to improve the understanding and knowledge for patients and families about CF and to standardize the educational materials available for people with CF. Educational materials that have been reviewed and approved by the Cystic Fibrosis Education Committee display its logo.

The Cystic Fibrosis Foundation has available on its website (www.cff.org), as well as on request, information related to nutrition, respiratory, insurance, and other issues, including the following:

- *An Introduction to Cystic Fibrosis for Patients and Families* (5th ed.)
- Nutrition series
  - *Nutrition and Cystic Fibrosis: Changes Through Life*
  - *Nutrition: How to Encourage Healthy Eating*
  - *Nutrition: Pancreatic Enzyme Replacement in People with Cystic Fibrosis*
  - *Nutrition for Your Infant (Birth to One) with Cystic Fibrosis*
  - *Nutrition for Your Toddler (One to Three) with Cystic Fibrosis*
  - *Nutrition for Your Child (Four to Seven) with Cystic Fibrosis*
  - *Nutrition: School, Enzymes, and Sports for the Child with Cystic Fibrosis*
  - *Nutrition for Teens with Cystic Fibrosis*

- Respiratory
  - *Stopping the Spread of Germs*
  - *What You Should Know about Germs*
  - *Which Nebulizer for Which Drug?*
- Day-to-day
  - A *Teacher's Guide to CF*
  - *School and CF*
  - *Know Your Health Insurance Coverage*
- *Advocacy Manual: A Clinician's Guide to the Legal Rights of People with Cystic Fibrosis.* A manual with information about health insurance, education, employment, and government benefit programs for people with CF.

These monographs, a large resource guide, and more are available from the Cystic Fibrosis Foundation.

The Cystic Fibrosis Foundation
6931 Arlington Road, Suite 200
Bethesda, MD 20814
(800) FIGHT CF; fax: (301) 951-6378
E-mail: info@cff.org
Website: www.cff.org

Many other educational materials are published by pharmaceutical companies, hospitals, universities, and individuals. The following are a few:

- *An Introduction to CF and Your Healthcare Team.* A video showing the different members of the CF health care team interacting with parents of a newly diagnosed infant with CF. Available from Digestive Care; 1120 Win Drive; Bethlehem, PA 18017-7059. (610) 882-5950. Website: www.digestivecare.com.
- Bluebond-Langner, M., Lask, B., & Angst, D. (Eds.). (2001). *Psychosocial Aspects of Cystic Fibrosis.* New York: Oxford University Press. A detailed book for health care professionals on a myriad of psychosocial issues of people with CF and their families.
- *Can We Talk? My Sibling Has CF.* Pamphlet about CF for well siblings. Available from Solvay Pharmaceuticals; 901 Sawyer Road; Marietta, GA 30062.
- *Fitting Cystic Fibrosis into Life Every Day.* An interactive Web or CD-ROM video for 10- to 15-year-olds about CF, including information on IV lines and radiology. Available from Starlight Starbright Children's Foundation; 5757 Wilshire Blvd., Suite M100; Los Angeles, CA 90036. (310) 479-1212; fax: (310) 479-1235. Email: info@starlight.org.
- *Jeremy Bishop Explains CF: Children's Guide for Learning about CF.* Pamphlet and video that are appropriate for school-age children with CF. Available from Axcan Scandipharm Inc.; 22 Inverness Center Parkway; Birmingham, AL 35242. (800) 615-4393.
- *Mallory's 65 Roses.* Delightful book for children with CF ages 3 to 6 years old. Available from Axcan Scandipharm Inc.; 22 Inverness Center Parkway; Birmingham, AL 35242. (800) 615-4393.
- Orenstein, D. (2003). *Cystic Fibrosis: A Guide for Patient and Family* (3rd ed.). New York: Lippincott-Raven. Comprehensive book for patients and families.

Summary of Primary Care Needs for the Child with Cystic Fibrosis

HEALTH CARE MAINTENANCE

Growth and Development

- Malnutrition and growth retardation are common complications, but catch-up growth can be achieved with proper nutritional therapy and treatment for pulmonary complications.
  - Careful surveillance of growth is essential.
- Pubertal development often is delayed; mean age of menarche for females is 14.5 years and a 2- to 4-year lag for males.
- Assessment of bone health is essential, especially for those with specific risk factors.

Diet

- Goal is to promote normal growth.
- Breastfeeding is encouraged.
- Diet is a well-balanced, high-protein, high-calorie diet with unrestricted fat that promotes 110% to 200% of recommended dietary allowances (RDAs).
- Nutritional issues correlate with age of the child and severity of the child's disease.
- Pancreatic enzyme replacement and vitamin supplementation are necessary in most children with CF.

Safety

- Emphasize safe storage of multiple medications.
- Use sunscreen or avoid sun when on antibiotics.
- Perform hand hygiene at routine times, such as before and after coughing, as well as with therapies that expose others with CF.

Immunizations

- All routine immunizations should generally be given on schedule.
- Influenza vaccine should be given annually per CDC guidelines, internasal vaccine is not recommended.
- RSV immunizations for those with additional risk factors should be used in CF.
- Pneumococcal vaccine should be administered to all children with CF, 2 years and older.

Screening

- *Vision.* Routine screening is recommended. Annual retinal screening should be done for children with CFRD.
- *Hearing.* Routine screening is recommended. An auditory screen for high-frequency hearing loss should be done with aminoglycoside therapy.
- *Dental.* Routine care. Cautious use of tetracycline before permanent teeth are formed.
- *Hematocrit.* Routine screening is recommended with full review of iron status as indicated.
- *Blood pressure.* Measure at every visit for those on corticosteroids.
- *Tuberculosis.* Screen only those who are at increased risk of acquiring TB.
- *Condition-specific screening.* PFT, chest roentgenography, sputum culture with antibiotic sensitivities, blood and urine assays of liver and renal function, DXA bone scan, oral glucose tolerance test (OGTT), complete blood counts, and serum and anthropometric measures of nutritional status are monitored at routine CF center visits.

COMMON ILLNESS MANAGEMENT

Differential Diagnosis

- *Constipation or diarrhea.* Rule out DIOS.
- *Abdominal pain.* Rule out DIOS, gallstones, pancreatitis, appendicitis, intussusception, fibrosing colonopathy, volvulus.
- *Fever.* Prevention of hyponatremia and dehydration. Influenza treatment if indicated.
- *Chest pain.* Rule out pneumothorax, musculoskeletal strain, pleural inflammation, GERD.
- *Cough/wheezing.* Differentiation between asthma, exacerbation of CF, rhinitis, and/or sinusitis will help select treatment.

Drug Interactions/Substance Abuse

- *Corticosteroids.* Increased risk for GI ulceration with high-dose nonsteroidal antiinflammatory drugs, such as ibuprofen. Itraconazole, and ketoconazole, can decrease clearance of steroids.
- *Ciprofloxacin.* Avoid antacids, zinc, or calcium supplements concurrently. Avoidance of UV exposure.
- *Herbal supplements.* Many can have potential side effects or interactions.
- *Tobacco smoke.* Those with chronic respiratory disease are most vulnerable to passive smoke.
- *Alcohol.* Detrimental effects if abused, especially since people with CF have increased liver disease and malnutrition.

DEVELOPMENTAL ISSUES

Sleep Patterns

- Sleep patterns may be altered with acute exacerbation or progression of disease because of increased cough and decreased oxyhemoglobin saturation.
- Early morning routines may require adjustment of bedtime.
- Difficulty falling asleep may be a sign of depression.
- Snoring may be related to obstructive sleep apnea.

Toileting

- Delayed bowel training may occur, secondary to increased frequency of stools and associated abdominal cramping.
- Provide privacy for toileting.
- Stress urinary incontinence is common in CF.

Discipline

- Expectation should be normal with allowances during periods of acute illnesses.
- Encourage independence in CF management with child/adolescent having some control over treatment choices.
- Individual and family counseling, as indicated.

Child Care

- Assist parents in making appropriate child-care choices and educational providers.
- In-home or small group childcare preferred to reduce exposure to infectious diseases.

Summary of Primary Care Needs for the Child with Cystic Fibrosis—cont'd

Schooling

- Education of school officials is imperative. Development of an IEP yearly is beneficial.
- Allow child to carry his or her own enzymes, if possible.
- School schedule may need to be altered as the disease progresses.
- Provide privacy for coughing episodes and toileting.
- Avoid dehydration with physical activities and sports.
- School performance may be affected by fatigue and coughing related to impending pulmonary exacerbation.
- CF does not affect one's intellectual/academic performance.

Sexuality

- The majority of males are infertile; sperm count recommended for males.
- Provide education about sexually transmitted diseases (STDs) and prevention.
- Genetic counseling for anyone with CF considering having a biologic child.
- Females contemplating pregnancy need counseling regarding their and their child's risks.
- Frequent use of antibiotics can cause fungal vaginitis.

Transition to Adulthood

- Prepare for transition by increasing independence and self-management in pre- and adolescence.
- Transition to adult primary care provider and CF care center.

FAMILY CONCERNS

- Despite a multitude of special concerns, including the stress of its prognosis, financial burden, and uncertainty of illness, most families adjust well.
- Provide open and honest communication.
- Provide multidisciplinary team support.
- End-of-life care often is a mix of preventive, therapeutic, and palliative treatments.

RESOURCES

- CF specific care for children with CF should be provided by a Cystic Fibrosis Foundation–accredited CF center.
- Primary care providers provide a wealth of expertise and anticipatory guidance to the care of children and families dealing with CF.

REFERENCES

Accurso, F.J. (2007). Update in cystic fibrosis 2006. *Am J Respir Crit Care Med, 175,* 754-757.

Akanli, L., & Wheeler-Dobrota, N. (2002). Cystic fibrosis and sleep related problems. *Pediatr Pulmonol, 34*(Suppl 24), 305.

American Academy of Pediatrics (2008). Committee on Infectious Diseases, recommended immunization schedules for children and adolescents United States. *Pediatrics, 121,* 219-220.

Angst, D. (2001). Working with families to enhance adherence. *Pediatr Pulmonol, 32*(Suppl 22), 143-144.

Aris, R.M., Merkel, P.A., Bachrach, L.K., et al. (2005). Guide to bone health and disease in cystic fibrosis. *J Clin Endocrinol Metab, 90*(3), 1888-1896. Epub 2004 Dec 21.

Balfour-Lynn, I. (2003). Asthma in cystic fibrosis. *J R Soc Med, 96*(Suppl 43), 30-34.

Bluebond-Langner, M. (2001). The well siblings of children with cystic fibrosis. In M. Bluebond-Langner, B. Lask, & D. Angst (Eds.), *Psychosocial Aspects of Cystic Fibrosis*. London: Arnold Press & New York: Oxford University Press.

Boesch, R.P., & Acton, J.D. (2007). Outcomes of fundoplication in children with cystic fibrosis. *J Pediatr Surg, 42*(8), 1341-1344.

Borowitz, D., Baker, R.D., & Stallings, V. (2002). Consensus report on nutrition for pediatric patients with cystic fibrosis. *J Pediatr Gastroenterol Nutr, 35*(3), 246-259.

Borowitz, D., Grand, R.J., & Durie, P.R. (1995). Use of pancreatic enzyme supplements for patients with cystic fibrosis in the context of fibrosing colonopathy. *J Pediatr, 127,* 681-684.

Britton, L.J., Thrasher, S., & Gutierrez, H. (2008). Creating a culture of improvement experience of a pediatric cystic fibrosis center. *J Nurs Care Qual, 23*(2), 115-120.

Centers for Disease Control and Prevention. (2008a). *Vaccines and immunizations: For specific groups of people.* Available at www.cdc.gov/vaccines/spec-grps/default.htm. Retrieved December 22, 2008.

Centers for Disease Control and Prevention. (2008b). *Smoking and tobacco use: 2004 Surgeon General's report*—The health consequences of smoking. Available at www.cdc.gov/tobacco/data_statistics/sgr/sgr_2004/index.htm. Retrieved June 12, 2008.

Collaco, J.M., Vanscoy, L., Bremer, L., et al. (2008). Interactions between secondhand smoke and genes that affect cystic fibrosis lung disease. *J Am Med Assoc, 299*(4), 417-424.

Comeau, A.M., Accurso, F.J., White, T.B., et al. (2007). Guidelines for implementation of cystic fibrosis newborn screening programs: Cystic Fibrosis Foundation workshop report. *Pediatrics, 119*(2), e495-e518.

Conway, S.P., Morton, A., & Wolfe, S. (2002). Enteral tube feeding for cystic fibrosis. *Cochrane Database of Systematic Reviews,* CF001198.

Cystic Fibrosis Foundation (2002). Bone health and disease in cystic fibrosis consensus conference report. *CF Foundation Consensus Conferences, X*(4), 1-35.

Cystic Fibrosis Foundation (2007a). *Management of Infants Diagnosed with Cystic Fibrosis Through Newborn Screening. Cystic Fibrosis Foundation Workshop Report.* Bethesda MD: Author.

Cystic Fibrosis Foundation (2007b). *Patient Registry 2006 Annual Data Report to the Center Directors.* Bethesda, MD: Author.

Cystic Fibrosis Foundation. (2008a). *CFFT drug development pipeline.* Available at www.cff.org/research/DrugDevelopmentPipeline. Retrieved December 22, 2008.

Cystic Fibrosis Foundation (2008b). *Patient Registry 2007 Annual Data Report to the Center Directors.* Bethesda, MD: Author.

Cystic Fibrosis Foundation (2008c). *Personal communication.*

Cystic Fibrosis Foundation. (2008d). *Newborn screening for cystic fibrosis.* Available at www.cff.org/GetInvolved/Advocate/WhyAdvocate/NewbornScreening. Retrieved December 21, 2008.

D'Angelo, S., & Lask, B. (2001). Approaches to problems of adherence. In M. Bluebond-Langner, B. Lask, & D. Angst (Eds.), *Psychosocial aspects of cystic fibrosis.* London: Arnold Press & New York: Oxford University Press.

Davis, P.B. (2006). Cystic fibrosis since 1938. *Am J Respir Crit Care Med, 173,* 475-482.

Dodd, M.E., & Langman, H. (2005). Urinary incontinence in cystic fibrosis. *J R Soc Med, 98*(Suppl 45), 28-36.

Elkins, M.R., Robinson, M., Rose, B.R., et al. (2006). A controlled trial of long-term inhaled hypertonic saline in patients with cystic fibrosis. *N Engl J Med, 354,* 3.

Farrell, P., Kosorok, M.R., Rock, M.J., et al. (2001). Early diagnosis of cystic fibrosis through neonatal screening prevents severe malnutrition and improves long-term growth. *Pediatrics, 107,* 1-13.

Farrell, P., Rosenstein, B., White, T.B., et al. (2008). Guidelines for diagnosis of cystic fibrosis in newborns through older adults: Cystic Fibrosis Foundation Consensus Report. *J Pediatr 153*(2), S4-S14.

Flume, P. (2008). Personal communication.

Flume, P., O'Sullivan, B.P., Robinson, K.A., et al. (2007). Cystic fibrosis pulmonary guidelines: Chronic medications for maintenance of lung health. *Am J Respir Crit Care Med, 176*, 957-969.

Flume, P., Robinson, K.A., O'Sullivan, B.P., et al. (2008). Cystic fibrosis pulmonary guidelines: Airway clearance therapies. Cystic Fibrosis Foundation, Bethesda MD accepted for publication for 2009 in *Respiratory Care*.

Fulton, J., Casey, S., Luder, E., et al. (2006). *Nutrition: School, Enzymes and Sports for the Child with Cystic Fibrosis*. Bethesda, MD: Authors.

Gibson, R.L., Burns, J.L., & Ramsey, B.W. (2003). Pathophysiology and management of pulmonary infections in cystic fibrosis. *Am J Respir Crit Care Med, 168*, 918-951.

Grody, W.W., Cutting, G.R., Klinger, K.W., et al. (2001). Laboratory standards and guidelines for population-based cystic fibrosis carrier screening. *Genet Med, 3*(2), 149-154.

Hardin, D.S., Ellis, K.J., Dyson, M., et al. (2001). Growth hormone decreases protein catabolism in children with cystic fibrosis. *J Clin Endocrinol Metab, 86*, 4424-4428.

Konstan, M.W., Schluchter, M.D., Xue, W., et al. (2007). Clinical use of ibuprofen is associated with slower FEV_1 decline in children with cystic fibrosis. *Am J Respir Crit Care Med, 176*(11), 1084-1089.

Langfelder-Schwind, E., Kloza, E., Sugarman, E., et al., & NSGC Subcommittee on Cystic Fibrosis Carrier Testing. (2005). Cystic fibrosis prenatal screening in genetic counseling practice: Recommendations of the National Society of Genetic Counselors. *J Genet Counseling, 14*(1), 1-15.

Lannefors, L., Button, B.M., & McIlwaine, M. (2004). Physiotherapy in infants and young children with cystic fibrosis: Current practice and future developments. *J R Soc Med, 97*(Suppl 44), 8-25.

LeGrys, V.A., Yankaskas, J.R., Quittell, L.M., et al. (2007). Diagnostic sweat testing: The Cystic Fibrosis Foundation guidelines. *J Pediatr, 151*, 85-89.

MedlinePlus.gov. (2007). Drugs, supplements and herbal information. Available at www.nlm.nih.gov/medlineplus/druginfo/medmaster/a692049.html. Retrieved June 12, 2008.

Moraes, T., Carpenter, S., & Taylor, L. (2002). Cystic fibrosis and incontinence in children. *Pediatr Pulmonol, 34*(Suppl 24), 315.

Morris, K., Ryan, C., Williams, T., et al. (2002). Neuropsychological correlates of CF in adolescence. *Pediatr Pulmonol, 34*(Suppl 24), 349.

Naqvi, S., Sawnani, H., Vlasic, V., et al. (2002). Sleep complaints and sleep quality in patients with cystic fibrosis. *Pediatr Pulmonol, 34*(Suppl 24), 305.

Olivier, K.N., Weber, D.J., Wallace, R.J. Jr., et al. (2003). Nontuberculous mycobacteria. I: Multicenter prevalence study in cystic fibrosis. *Am J Respir Crit Care Med, 167*(6), 828-834.

Orenstein, D. (2004). *Cystic Fibrosis: A Guide for Patient and Family* (3rd ed.). Philadelphia: Lippincott Williams & Wilkins.

Orenstein, D., Winnie, G., & Altman, H. (2002). Cystic fibrosis: A 2002 update. *J Pediatr, 140*, 156-164.

Parad, R.B., Comeau, A.M., Dorkin, H.L., et al. (2005). Sweat testing infants detected by cystic fibrosis newborn screening. *J Pediatr, 147*(3 Suppl), S69-S72.

Peterson, M.L., Jacobs, D.R., & Milla, C.E. (2003). Longitudinal changes in growth parameters are correlated with changes in pulmonary function in children with cystic fibrosis. *Pediatrics, 112*(3), 588-592.

Powers, S., Jones, J.S., Ferguson, K.S., et al. (2005). Randomized clinical trial of behavioral and nutrition treatment to improve energy intake and growth in toddlers and preschoolers with cystic fibrosis. *Pediatrics, 116*(6), 1442-1450.

Powers, S., Patton, S., Byars, K., et al. (2002). Parent and child mealtime behaviors in families of toddlers with cystic fibrosis. *Pediatr Pulmonol, 34*(Suppl 24), 346.

Prasad, S.A., Balfour-Lynn, I.M., Carr, S.B., et al. (2006). A comparison of the prevalence of urinary incontinence in girls with cystic fibrosis, asthma, and healthy controls. *Pediatr Pulmonol, 41*(11), 1065-1068.

Quan, J.M., Tiddens, H., Sy, J., et al. (2001). A two-year randomized, placebo-controlled trial of dornase alfa in young patients with cystic fibrosis with mild lung function abnormalities. *J Pediatr, 139*, 813-820.

Quittner, A.L., & Buu, A. (2002). Effects of tobramycin solution for inhalation on global ratings of quality of life in patients with cystic fibrosis and *Pseudomonas aeruginosa* infection. *Pediatr Pulmonol, 33*, 269-276.

Rosenstein, B. (2006). Cystic fibrosis. In J. McMillian, (Ed.), *Oski's Pediatrics* (4th ed.). Philadelphia: Lippincott Williams & Wilkins.

Saiman, L., Marshall, B.C., Mayer-Hamblett, N., et al. (2003). Azithromycin in patients with cystic fibrosis chronically infected with *Pseudomonas aeruginosa*. *J Am Med Assoc, 290*(13), 1749-1756.

Saiman, L., Siegel, J., and the Cystic Fibrosis Foundation Consensus Conference on Infection Control Participants. (2003). Infection control recommendations for patients with cystic fibrosis: Microbiology, important pathogens and infection control practices to prevent patient-to-patient transmission. *Infect Control Hosp Epidemiol, 24*(5 Suppl), S2-S53.

Sawyer, S. (2001). Sexual and reproductive health in CF: Don't ask, won't tell. *Pediatr Pulmonol, 22*, 113-114.

Sawyer, S., Farrant, B., Cerritelli, B., et al. (2005). A survey of sexual and reproductive health in men with cystic fibrosis: New challenges for adolescent and adult services. *Thorax, 60*(4), 326-330.

Schneiderman-Walker, J., Pollock, S., Corey, M., et al. (2000). A randomized controlled trial of a 3-year home exercise program in cystic fibrosis. *J Pediatr, 136*(3), 304-310.

Shearer, J.E., & Bryon, M. (2004). The nature and prevalence of eating disorders and eating disturbance in adolescents with cystic fibrosis. *J R Soc Med, 97*(Suppl 44), 36-42.

Sontag, M.K., Hammond, K.B., Zielenski, J., et al. (2005). Two-tiered immunoreactive trypsinogen-based newborn screening for cystic fibrosis in Colorado: Screening efficacy and diagnostic outcomes. *J Pediatr, 147*(3 Suppl), S83-S88.

Stallings, V.A., Stark, L.J., Robinson, K.A., et al., & Clinical Practice Guidelines on Growth and Nutrition Subcommittee and Ad Hoc Working Group. (2008). Evidence-based practice recommendations for nutrition-related management of children and adults with cystic fibrosis and pancreatic insufficiency: Results of a systematic review. *J Am Diet Assoc, 108*(5), 832-839.

Stevens, D.A., Moss, R.B., Kurup, V.P., et al. (2003). Allergic bronchopulmonary aspergillosis in cystic fibrosis—state of the art: Cystic Fibrosis Foundation consensus conference. *Clin Infect Dis, 37*(Suppl 3), S225-S264.

Tipnis, N.A., & Rudolph, C.D. (2007). Treatment options in pediatric GERD. *Curr Treat Opt Gastroenterol, 10*, 391-400.

Tyc, V.L., & Throckmorton-Belzer, L. (2006). Smoking rates and the state of smoking interventions for children and adolescents with chronic illness. *Pediatrics, 118*(2), e471-e487.

van der Schans, C., Prasad, A., & Main E. (2002). Chest physiotherapy compared to no chest physiotherapy for cystic fibrosis. *The Cochrane Library*, issue 3, Oxford.

Verma, A., Clough, D., McKenna, D., et al. (2001). Smoking and cystic fibrosis. *J R Soc Med, 94*(Suppl 40), 29-34.

Weiner, D.J. (2002). Respiratory tract infections in cystic fibrosis. *Pediatr Ann, 31*(2), 116-123.

Yankaskas, J.R., Marshall, B.C., Sufian, B., et al. (2004). Cystic fibrosis adult care: Consensus conference report. *Chest, 125*(1 Suppl), 1S-39S.

Zeitlin, P.L. (2007). Emerging drug treatments for cystic fibrosis. *Exp Opin Emerg Drugs, 12*(2), 329-336.

Zoler, M.L. (2003). Still below target levels, cystic fibrosis screening soars. *OB/GYN News, 38*(6), 1.

23 Diabetes Mellitus (Types 1 and 2)

Elizabeth A. Doyle and Margaret Grey

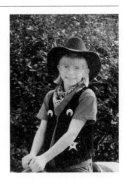

Etiology

Diabetes mellitus was first described in the Egyptian Ebers Papyrus in 1500 BC. Type 1 diabetes mellitus, or insulin-dependent diabetes mellitus, most commonly occurs in young people and is characterized by beta cell failure. In type 2 diabetes mellitus, or non–insulin-dependent diabetes mellitus, individuals are often overweight and usually more than 30 years of age, overproduce insulin, and have a receptor-site defect. In recent years, however, type 2 diabetes has become increasingly common in children and youth, with up to 43% of new cases of diabetes under age 20 being type 2 (American Diabetes Association [ADA], 2000; Shaw, 2007). Individuals with type 2 diabetes can often be treated with oral hypoglycemic agents, but those with type 1 diabetes must be treated with insulin.

The cause of type 1 diabetes is unknown, but many factors have been hypothesized to contribute to the cause of the disease. Type 1 diabetes is an autoimmune disease. In autoimmunity, "self" antigens are no longer recognized as such, so a self-destructive process occurs. Islet cell antibodies can be detected in a majority of individuals newly diagnosed with type 1 diabetes, and evidence of an autoimmune response may be present up to 9 years before the onset of clinical symptoms (Bingley, Bonfacio, & Gale, 1993). Genetic susceptibility is a necessary precursor to the development of type 1 diabetes. Certain human leukocyte antigen (HLA) genes are thought to play a role in the genetic inheritance of the tendency to develop type 1 diabetes. Individuals with type 1 diabetes have an increased frequency of HLA genes *B8, B15, DR3,* and *DR4.* The *HLA-DR* genes are known to be associated with autoimmunity. Evidence of autoimmunity is necessary but not sufficient for the development of type 1 diabetes. It is hypothesized that without genetic susceptibility, other factors will not initiate the autoimmune process. Other factors (e.g., host and environment factors) may influence the development of the condition because the concordance rate is only 50% in identical twins. Such factors include stress and infectious agents (Leslie & Elliot, 1994).

The genetic and pathologic processes leading to the development of type 2 diabetes are multiple and not yet well defined. There is an interplay of genetic and environmental factors, with a significant hereditary component that appears to be polygenic. A total of 83% of children with type 2 diabetes in the SEARCH for Diabetes in Youth study had a positive family history (Gilliam, Liese, Block, et al., 2007). It is not clear, however, how genetic factors work in type 2 diabetes. Other factors are also associated with higher risk: obesity (especially central obesity), sedentary lifestyle, diet high in fat and low in fiber, minority group, family history of type 2 diabetes, use of psychotropic drugs, insulin resistance,

puberty, and female gender (Pihoker, Scott, Lensing, et al., 1998). Those most likely to be affected include Native American, black, and Hispanic children (Fagot-Campagna, Pettitt, Engelgau, et al., 2000). Peripheral insulin resistance is the primary metabolic defect associated with type 2 diabetes, and it is associated with hyperinsulinemia, glucose intolerance, nonalcoholic fatty liver, and dyslipidemia. Insulin resistance is also associated with acanthosis nigricans, a thickening and darkening of skin usually seen on the neck and axilla. Insulin resistance is considered an independent risk factor for the development of type 2 diabetes, hypertension, and atherosclerosis. The combination of obesity, insulin resistance, hypertension, dyslipidemia, and atherosclerosis is known as the metabolic syndrome (Pinhas-Hamiel & Zeitler, 2007). In addition, insulin resistance is associated with polycystic ovary syndrome and is thereby associated with infertility.

The problem of insulin resistance and its relationship to obesity and other comorbid conditions has been well established in adults, but it is only relatively recently that it has been described in substantial numbers of youths. A study of obese minority youths ages 5 to 10 years demonstrated a significant relationship between obesity and the presence of the metabolic syndrome, particularly in African American girls (Young-Hyman, Schlundt, Herman, et al., 2001). A comparison of type 1 and type 2 diabetes is shown in Table 23-1.

Incidence and Prevalence

Type 1 diabetes mellitus is the most common metabolic disorder of childhood, affecting 0.22% of individuals younger than 20 years of age, or about 176,500 children in the United States. About 1 in every 400 to 600 children and adolescents has type 1 diabetes (ADA, 2008b). The true incidence and prevalence of type 2 diabetes in children is unknown. Until completion of the SEARCH trial (SEARCH Study Group, 2004), the true rate of type 2 diabetes in the population will remain unknown. Among youths ages 10 to 19 years in the SEARCH study, prevalence ranged from 1.74 per 1000 in American Indian youths, to 1.05 per 1000 in African American youths, to 0.19 per 1000 in non-Hispanic white youths. Nonetheless, it is known that the incidence is on the rise, and because the condition is often silent, as many as twice the number of children diagnosed with type 2 may have the condition. Recent data suggest that the incidence is low in the 0- to 9-year-old age-group, rising to 8.1 per 100,000 in the 10- to 14-year-old age-group and 11.8 per 100,000 in the 15- to 19-year-old age-group (Shaw, 2007). In a report from a single site, Sinha, Fisch, Teague, and colleagues (2002) demonstrated that in a multiethnic cohort of obese children and adolescents who underwent oral glucose tolerance tests, 25% of

TABLE 23-1

Comparison of Type 1 and Type 2 Diabetes in Youths

	Type 1 Diabetes	Type 2 Diabetes
Age	Throughout childhood	Puberty
Onset	Acute, severe	Mild to severe, often insidious
Insulin secretion	Very low	Variable
Insulin dependence	Permanent	Variable
Genetics	Polygenic	Polygenic
Race/ethnic distribution	All (low frequency in Asians)	African American, Hispanic, Asian, Native American
Frequency (of all diabetes in children and youths)	60%-70%	30%-40%
ASSOCIATION		
Obesity	No	Strong
Acanthosis nigricans	No	Yes
Autoimmunity	Yes	Unclear

the obese children and 21% of the obese adolescents had impaired glucose tolerance, and 4% had silent type 2 diabetes. The average age of onset of type 2 diabetes in youths is 12 to 14 years, but cases have been reported in children as young as 5 years of age (Glaser, 1997).

Diagnostic Criteria

The diagnosis of diabetes is easily established. Any children with the classic symptoms should have their levels of blood and urinary glucose and urine ketone levels determined. If the blood glucose level is more than 200 mg/dL (11.1 mmol/L) and symptoms of diabetes are present, the diagnosis of type 1 diabetes is established. Alternatively, if fasting blood glucose (i.e., no calories in 8 hours before the test) is greater than or equal to 126 mg/dL (7 mmol/L) or the 2-hour plasma glucose level is greater than or equal to 200 mg/dL on a glucose tolerance test, the diagnosis is established (ADA, 2008a). Hyperglycemia that is not sufficient to meet diagnostic criteria for diabetes is categorized as either impaired fasting glucose (IFG), when the glucose level is greater than or equal to 100 to 125 mg/dL (5.6 to 6.9 mmol/L), or impaired glucose tolerance (IGT), when the 2-hour plasma glucose level is 140 to 199 mg/dL (7.8 to 11 mmol/L) (ADA, 2008a).

Type 2 diabetes can usually be differentiated from type 1 at diagnosis by the presence of obesity. In addition, insulin and C-peptide levels are elevated. The presence of antibodies to the pancreatic islet cell (antiinsulin, antityrosine phosphatases ICA-2 and IAA-2) (Borg, Gottsater, Landin-Olsson, et al., 2001) and anti–glutamic acid decarboxylase (GAD) antibodies may indicate type 1 diabetes in an overweight child, but may be present also in a relatively small percentage of youths with type 2 diabetes (Pinhas-Hamiel & Zeitler, 2007). Further, separation of acute-onset diabetes with ketosis or frank ketoacidosis from insidious-onset diabetes and cases of nonketotic severe hyperglycemia can be helpful. The child with newonset diabetes whose glucose is greater than 750 to 1000 mg/dL in the absence of significant ketosis or ketoacidosis is unlikely to have type 1 diabetes.

Clinical Manifestations at Time of Diagnosis

Despite the fact that the autoimmune process may be longstanding before the diagnosis of type 1 diabetes is made, the signs and symptoms of type 1 diabetes are usually present for a short period of time. Once the autoimmune process has destroyed enough of the pancreatic beta, or islet, cells to produce clinical evidence of diabetes, the classic symptoms (i.e., polydipsia, polyuria, polyphagia) of diabetes occur. As can be seen in Figure 23-1, the lack of insulin production leads to disturbances in metabolism of carbohydrate, protein, and fat.

Clinical Manifestations at Time of Diagnosis

Type 1 diabetes
- Polydipsia
- Polyuria
- Polyphagia

Type 2 diabetes
- Obesity
- Acanthosis nigricans
- Polydipsia
- Polyuria
- Polyphagia

The hormone insulin, produced by the pancreatic beta cells (i.e., islets of Langerhans), is responsible for the use of glucose in the cell. In the absence of insulin, there are three general alterations: (1) reduced entry of glucose into the cell; (2) unavailability of carbohydrate as a substrate for energy needs; and (3) the cell's use of alternate substrates (i.e., fatty acids derived from adipose stores and amino acids from body protein). Thus when there is lack of insulin, glucose cannot be used in the cell for energy, and hyperglycemia results. The extraordinary concentration of glucose in the blood promotes an osmotic diuresis, so that large amounts of urine are produced. This osmotic diuresis is responsible for the symptom of polyuria, and as the body struggles to maintain homeostasis, polydipsia ensues.

If glucose is not available as a source of energy, alternative sources must be used. The body relies on lipolysis, as well as proteolysis. When this occurs, polyphagia becomes prominent as the body tries to avoid starvation. If these symptoms go uncorrected, the hyperglycemia and ketonemia secondary to increased lipolysis will progress to severe levels, and diabetic ketoacidosis (DKA) will occur.

The primary defect in type 2 diabetes is peripheral insulin resistance, with obesity and sedentary lifestyle contributing to its development. Weiss (2007) has demonstrated that severe obesity contributes to insulin resistance, partially because of abnormalities in lipid partitioning, with greater fat deposition in intramyocellular and intraabdominal compartments. Once there is insulin resistance, there is initially a compensatory increase in insulin secretion. There is also a decrease in the first-phase insulin response, and a state of chronic hyperglycemia ensues. There is also inappropriate hepatic gluconeogenesis, causing fasting hyperglycemia. This further worsens peripheral insulin resistance and beta cell dysfunction. Most affected individuals have marked peripheral insulin resistance with high serum insulin levels, but insufficient to maintain

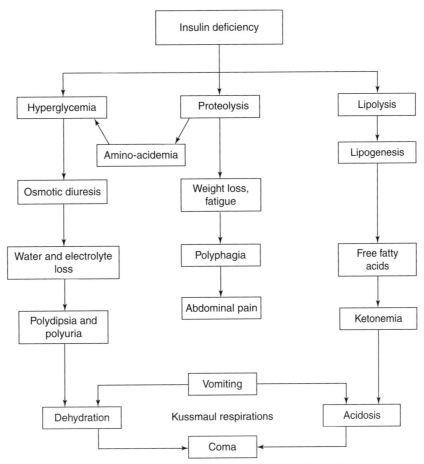

FIGURE 23-1 Signs and symptoms of type 1 diabetes mellitus.

normoglycemia (Callahan & Mansfield, 2000). Pancreatic beta cell function eventually declines and insulin secretion decreases. Because the onset of type 2 diabetes is gradual and insidious compared with type 1 diabetes, the condition may go undetected for months or years. Clinical manifestations that suggest type 2 diabetes include obesity and acanthosis nigricans, in addition to polydipsia and polyuria. High-risk youths (those who are obese and have additional risk factors for type 2 diabetes, including a family history of type 2 diabetes) should be screened every 2 years beginning at age 10 years or at the onset of puberty if it occurs before age 10 years. Screening should be with a fasting plasma glucose or an oral glucose tolerance test. The criteria for diagnosis of diabetes are described previously and shown in Box 23-1. If a child meets the criteria for impaired glucose tolerance (or prediabetes), she or he should be referred for intensive lifestyle management to prevent type 2 diabetes from developing. If symptoms of diabetes occur, they will be similar to those of type 1, including polyphagia, polydipsia, and polyuria.

Treatment

Type 1 Diabetes

Diabetes Control and Complications Trial. The Diabetes Control and Complications Trial (DCCT) was a multicenter, randomized clinical trial of 1441 people with type 1 diabetes designed to compare intensive diabetes therapy with conventional therapy to

---

BOX 23-1

Diagnostic Criteria for Diabetes Mellitus

- Classic symptoms of diabetes, including polydipsia, polyuria, polyphagia, and weight loss with random plasma glucose >200 mg/dL
  OR
- Fasting plasma glucose level >126 mg/dL
  OR
- One oral glucose tolerance test (OGTT) with the 2-hour plasma glucose >200 mg/dL, using 1.75 g/kg to maximum of 75 g glucose load

Data from American Diabetes Association. (2008). Clinical practice recommendations 2008. *Diabetes Care, 31*(Suppl 1), entire issue.

determine its effects on the development and progression of early microvascular and neurologic complications of type 1 diabetes (DCCT Research Group, 1993b). The goals of intensive therapy were to reduce glucose to the normal range and keep glycosylated hemoglobin in the normal range. Intensive therapy consisted of insulin pump therapy (otherwise known as continuous subcutaneous insulin infusion [CSII]) or three or more injections per day of insulin with frequent blood glucose monitoring; conventional therapy consisted of one or two insulin injections per day. Study results showed that in the group without retinopathy, the risk for developing it decreased 76% with intensive therapy, and in the secondary prevention group, the progression of retinopathy was slowed by

54%. Further, microalbuminuria was reduced by 39%, albuminuria by 54%, and clinical neuropathy by 60%. Intensive therapy, however, was associated with a two- to three-fold increase in severe hypoglycemia and clinically significant weight gain. Based on these findings, the researchers and the ADA recommended that for individuals with type 1 diabetes, "a primary treatment goal should be blood glucose control at least equal to that achieved in the intensively treated cohort" (ADA, 1993).

Treatment

Type 1 diabetes
- Insulin to achieve near-normal blood glucose
- Diet and activity for glucose control and growth
- Monitoring of blood glucose at least four times daily
- Continuous glucose monitoring
- Monitoring by diabetic treatment team with use of glycosylated hemoglobin (HbA$_{1c}$)

Type 2 diabetes
- Initial treatment to correct diabetic ketoacidosis
- Life style intervention
  - Diet lower in fats and calories
  - Decreased sedentary activity
- Pharmacologic treatment
  - Insulin
  - Metformin

There were 195 adolescents (i.e., 13 to 17 years of age at entry) in the DCCT, 125 with no retinopathy and 70 with mild retinopathy. Similar positive results of intensive treatment were also found in this group: the risk of retinopathy, retinopathy progression, microalbuminuria, and clinical neuropathy decreased by 53% to 70%. Thus the DCCT Research Group (1994) recommended that most teens with diabetes be treated with intensive therapy because the potential for reduction of long-term complications was substantial. Based on these results, many diabetes providers recommend intensive therapy regimens (now called flexible regimens) to achieve the goals of treatment (i.e., to return the blood glucose levels to near normal and to prevent complications for most young people with diabetes) (ADA, 1999). The ADA (2008a) guidelines recommend that the blood glucose level be normalized using intensive treatment regimens as the goal of treatment for children and adolescents. Insulin doses are often adjusted according to frequent blood glucose monitoring (i.e., at least four times per day), monitored dietary intake, and anticipated exercise. Treatment goals may be slightly more relaxed in children under 7 years of age because of the risk of severe hypoglycemia. The concern with severe hypoglycemia in young children is the potential effect of lowered blood sugar on brain development and functioning. These regimens require frequent and careful monitoring by the diabetes team (i.e., physician, nurse, dietitian, behaviorist) and are difficult to accomplish in a primary care setting.

Insulin Therapy. There are multiple approaches to providing insulin to children and adolescents with type 1 diabetes. The appropriate regimen should be determined with the child and the family. The available types of insulin shown in Table 23-2 can be combined to create a regimen that fits the child's lifestyle and the provider's and family's goals. Most children use genetically engineered human insulin preparations.

TABLE 23-2

Types and Actions of Insulin Preparations

Class/Name	Approximate Action Curves		
	Onset	Peak	Duration
Quick acting			
Insulin lispro	0.25 hr	1 hr	2-4 hr
Insulin aspart	10-20 min	1-3 hr	3-5 hr
Rapid acting			
Regular	0.5-1 hr	2-4 hr	4-6 hr
Intermediate acting			
NPH	1.5-2 hr	6-12 hr	18-24 hr
Long acting			
Glargine	1-2 hr	None	24 hr
Detemir	~1-2 hr	None	~14-16 hr

Insulin replacement results in a dramatic reversal of diabetes symptoms. At diagnosis, most children are hospitalized for correction of the metabolic derangement. Although a recent study (Rewers, Klingensmith, Davis, et al., 2008) has shown that only one in four children actually have DKA at diagnosis, another important purpose of this hospitalization is for education in the management of the condition, and therefore children even not in DKA are often hospitalized. Some centers have been able to provide this education successfully in an ambulatory setting, if the child is not severely ill (i.e., in DKA) (Siminerio, Charron-Prochownik, Banion, et al., 1999). Once any acidosis is corrected, subcutaneous treatment with insulin is the mainstay of therapy. Diabetes in most children is adequately controlled on an initial regimen of two injections of insulin per day: one before breakfast and one before the evening meal. These injections usually consist of rapid-acting and intermediate-acting insulin. Based on the blood glucose response, the dose is titrated to achieve blood glucose levels as close to normal as possible.

Shortly after the diagnosis is made, many children experience a significant reduction in the insulin requirement. Commonly, the doses of rapid insulin are sharply reduced or discontinued during this time. Many children are managed well with two injections of intermediate-acting insulin, and some may not require an evening injection. The insulin requirement eventually returns, and children should be cautioned that this "honeymoon period" (the duration of which is highly variable) does not indicate that the diabetes has gone away. Once destruction of the beta cells is complete—usually within 2 years of diagnosis—most children will require insulin replacement of approximately 1 U/kg of body weight per day, although 2 U/kg of body weight or more may be necessary, particularly in adolescents.

Once the honeymoon phase is over, it is difficult to achieve optimal metabolic control without using flexible insulin regimens. These regimens consist of three or more daily injections or the use of an insulin pump. Multiple daily injection (MDI) regimens usually consist of rapid or quick-acting insulin (regular, aspart, or lispro) before meals with intermediate insulin (NPH) twice per day, or a long-acting insulin once or twice a day. Two long-acting insulins have recently been developed. Glargine is a nearly peakless, clear insulin that lasts for 22 to 24 hours, and is usually taken once a day.

It has been approved for children ages 6 years and older. Insulin detemir is another peakless, clear, long-acting insulin, with a 12- to 16-hour insulin duration, that has been shown to have less variability than the intermediate-acting insulin, NPH (Danne, Lange, & Kordonouri, 2007). Insulin detemir is taken once or twice a day. Both of these insulins cannot be mixed with other insulins and therefore must be taken as separate injections. When these peakless, long-acting insulins are used, quick-acting insulin is taken before each meal and large snack, based on the carbohydrate amount in the meal. Such regimens more closely mimic the body's normal response to a carbohydrate meal. These regimens are referred to as basal bolus therapies.

Insulin pump therapy, or CSII, is the other option for flexible therapy (Figure 23-2). The pumps are battery powered and are about the size of a pager. A reservoir containing quick-acting insulin is inserted into the pump, and connects to fine tubing, connected to an infusion set, that is inserted into the hip or the abdomen area every other day. Multiple different infusion sets are available for use. Many of the sets are inserted at a 90-degree angle, and others can be inserted at a 30- to 45-degree angle, which seems to work better for very young children and those with very little subcutaneous fat. These infusion sets are inserted with a spring-loaded device, making insertion easy for the parent or older child. They also have "quick-release" or disconnect mechanisms allowing the pump to be easily removed for bathing, sports, and so on, while leaving the catheter in place under the skin. There are now shorter cannula infusion sets making these more attractive for younger children. Additionally, there are other sets that use a very small (6 mm) needle that is inserted at 90 degrees and left in place. These have worked very well for toddlers and young children who experience problems with even the smaller cannulas "crimping" because of little subcutaneous fat. Some may prefer them to the sets inserted at a 30- to 45-degree angle because of their ease of use.

The pump delivers small amounts of quick-acting insulin at a basal rate, which can be varied throughout the 24-hour day based on personal needs, and larger bolus doses are programmed in by the child or family to cover all meals and snacks. Bolus doses are varied based on the amount of carbohydrate in the planned meal or snack, current blood glucose level, and any anticipated exercise.

Over the past few years there have been many improvements in insulin pumps. They are smaller, the programming is simpler, they have more alarms, and some pumps have a "child lock" feature that can be set by parents to prevent younger children from inadvertently giving themselves an insulin dose. The child (or parent) enters the amount of carbohydrate he or she plans on eating along with his or her current blood sugar level, and the pump calculates the appropriate dose based on a preprogrammed insulin to carbohydrate ratio and a blood glucose correction factor.

Recently, a different insulin pump system called the Omnipod (Insulet, Bedford, MA) was released. This system does not have any tubing. The Omnipod system consists of a lightweight, self-enclosed, watertight "pod" that is filled with rapid-acting insulin. It is disposable and has a spring-loaded automated cannula insertion. The pod delivers insulin according to preprogrammed instructions that are wirelessly transmitted from a handheld device. The device calculates meal and correction doses in a similar manner as the other pumps and communicates this information to the pod for insulin delivery. Zisser and Jovanovic (2006) compared use of this system with a more conventional insulin pump in 20 adults, who were established pump wearers. Over a 30-day trial period, they found the system to be well received with 90% of subjects preferring the Omnipod system to their conventional insulin pump. Studies are still needed in pediatrics to determine if younger children and adolescents would have similar satisfaction with this system.

Although less frequently used by children in the past, many more pediatric providers are recommending CSII therapy for children and adolescents. National and international pediatric endocrine societies recently released a consensus statement on the use of insulin pumps in children and concluded that although there are very few published long-term studies on pump use in children, CSII therapy may be appropriate for children of all ages, provided that there is adequate support personnel available (Philip, Baltelino, Rodriguez, et al., 2007). One earlier report in adolescents (Boland, Grey, Oesterle, et al., 1999) showed that adolescents who used insulin pumps were able to achieve better metabolic control than those on MDI regimens (hemoglobin A_{1c} [HbA_{1c}] levels 7.5% vs. 8.3%). Most impressive, the rate of severe hypoglycemia was 50% lower with CSII compared with MDI regimens. A later report by Ahern, Boland, Doane, and colleagues (2002) demonstrated that pump treatment can be both safe and successful in the treatment of children of all ages with diabetes. These authors described the clinical outcomes of 161 children (26 preschoolers, 76 school-age children, and 59 adolescents) who had used CSII for at least 12 months. There was a significant and consistent reduction in mean HbA_{1c} (by 0.6% to 0.7%) and a 32% decrease in severe hypoglycemic events. Continued follow-up of the infants and toddlers in this group has revealed that the benefits of CSII have been sustained for more than 4 years (Weinzimer, Ahern, Doyle, et al., 2004). Other studies in very young children have found that the use of CSII can greatly reduce the incidence of severe hypoglycemia (Tubiana-Rufi, deLonlay, Bloch, et al., 1996) and can also result in improved metabolic control and greater parent satisfaction (Buckingham, Paguntalan, Fassl, et al., 2001) in this challenging age-group, whereas others have shown no difference in HbA_{1c} levels

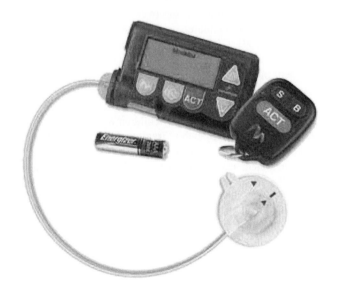

FIGURE 23-2 Example of an insulin pump used for continuous subcutaneous insulin infusion, with the real-time glucose sensor. Courtesy Medtronic MiniMed, Northridge, CA.

between CSII and MDI in this age-group (Fox, Buckloh, Smith, et al., 2005; Wilson, Buckingham, Kunsekman, et al., 2005).

Diet and Activity. Because replacement of insulin does not mimic the minute-to-minute response to blood glucose, attention to both diet and activity help minimize variation in blood glucose levels. Routine activity should be encouraged for all children, including those with type 1 diabetes. However, insulin doses often have to be adjusted or an extra snack may be necessary to help prevent hypoglycemia, which can occur with prolonged activity.

Children with type 1 diabetes—unlike individuals with type 2 diabetes—are often slender. Therefore the goal of dietary therapy is to provide sufficient calories for normal growth and development. Initially, a meal plan based on an individual's usual intake pattern is used to integrate insulin therapy into typical eating and exercise patterns. Such a meal plan helps avoid hyperglycemia, prevent hypoglycemia, and maintain metabolic balance. Consistent with the current recommendations of the American Academy of Pediatrics, American and Canadian Diabetes Associations, and the American Dietetic Association, a meal plan should comprise 55% to 60% carbohydrate, 10% to 20% protein, and 10% to 20% fat, with less than 10% saturated fat (ADA, 2008a). As discussed in the later section on diet, carbohydrate counting is an approach that allows for more flexibility in dietary management.

Daily caloric requirements can be estimated to be 1000 calories for the first year of life with approximately 100 calories added each year until age 10 to 12 years. Thereafter, unless they are exceptionally active on a regular basis, females may need their total calories reduced to the common adult level of 1400 to 1600 calories daily. Males, however, will continue to need approximately 2000 calories daily. Shortly after diagnosis, children may need an additional 200 to 700 kcal per day to make up the negative energy balance at diagnosis.

Glucose Monitoring. Maintenance of near-normal or normal blood glucose levels requires constant self-monitoring. Self-monitored blood glucose (SMBG) levels allow people with diabetes to have more precision in monitoring than with urine testing. Glucose is not found in the urine until the blood glucose level rises above the renal threshold (i.e., usually about 180 mg/dL). The goal of therapy is to maintain blood glucose levels from 70 to 130 mg/dL before meals (ADA, 2008a). Most pediatric providers aim for bedtime glucose levels to be between 100 and 140 mg/dL because of concerns of nocturnal hypoglycemia. Therefore self-monitoring of blood glucose levels lets children know exactly what the blood glucose level is at any moment and adjust the dose of insulin in response to their actual blood glucose level.

Most children are advised to test their blood at least four times daily, at various times throughout the day, and when symptoms are present. The results of SMBG testing are used to identify asymptomatic hypoglycemia, determine patterns in insulin action, and appropriately alter the insulin dose. For example, if a child consistently has high blood glucose levels before lunch, the morning intermediate-acting insulin (i.e., NPH) is increased to prevent this effect. If the child is using a basal bolus therapy regimen, the morning rapid-acting insulin may need to be increased to normalize the lunch values.

Continuous Glucose Monitoring. Real-time continuous glucose sensors hold great promise for improving diabetes care in individuals of all ages, particularly children. They measure interstitial glucose levels and are inserted just under the skin with a spring-loaded device and changed periodically (every 3 to 7 days, dependent on the sensor used). The sensor is plugged into a small transmitter that is taped to the skin that communicates glucose data wirelessly to a receiver. With the Medtronic (Northbridge, CA) system, if the youth uses a Medtronic pump, the receiver software is incorporated into the pump, so that glucose data are displayed on the pump screen when selected (see Figure 23-2). If the youth does not wear a Medtronic pump, the Guardian unit is the receiver and is worn on the belt or in a pocket much like a pump. Similarly, both the Free-Style Navigator and the DexCom 7 system consist of a subcutaneous sensor that attaches to a transmitter that is taped to the skin. Glucose data are communicated wirelessly to a receiver, which is the size of a small pager.

The receiver of the continuous glucose sensors is calibrated with a few finger-stick glucose measurements done every 24 hours. The receiver emits alarms when the glucose levels go above or below targets set by the user to alert the user to hypoglycemia and hyperglycemia.

Although the first-generation systems lacked the accuracy and precision of commonly used glucose meters (DirecNet Study Group, 2003a, 2003b), newer sensors (e.g., modified Medtronic CGMS sensor) have been shown to be more accurate (DirecNet Study Group, 2005). Additionally, the accuracy of another continuous real-time sensor, the FreeStyle Navigator (which recently gained Food and Drug Administration [FDA] approval for adults) was studied, and though it was not as accurate as the current home glucose meters, the authors concluded that its accuracy was sufficient to believe that this device could potentially be an important adjunct in the treatment of children with diabetes (DirecNet Study Group, 2007b).

Several studies both in children (DirecNet Study Group, 2007a; Halvorson, Carpenter, Kaiserman, et al., 2007) and adults (Bailey, Zisser, & Garg, 2007; Garg, Zisser, Schwartz, et al., 2006) have shown that use of real-time continuous glucose sensors is associated with improved metabolic control and significantly improved glucose excursions in adults (Garg et al., 2006) and children (Halvorson et al., 2007). Earlier generations of the Medtronic device have been shown to help clinicians discover undetected hypoglycemia and hyperglycemia in children and adolescents (Boland, Monsod, Delucia, et al., 2001; Gandrud, Xing, Kollman, et al., 2007). Larger, randomized trials in children are underway to further demonstrate their benefit in children and adolescents. Although the use of real-time continuous glucose sensors outside of a research setting is gradually increasing, their use is still limited. This technology may be a great asset in the care of many children with diabetes.

Monitoring by the Diabetes Treatment Team. Children and adolescents with diabetes are evaluated every 3 months by the diabetes treatment team. Quarterly visits correspond to the rate at which the glycosylated hemoglobin levels can be expected to change. Glycosylated hemoglobin, or HbA_{1c} (often referred to as A_{1c}), is a measure of the attachment of glucose to the circulating hemoglobin molecule. In individuals without diabetes, HbA_{1c} makes up 3% to 6% of the total hemoglobin; those with diabetes, however, have levels in excess of 6% that vary in proportion to the blood glucose levels. The HbA_{1c} level reflects the average blood glucose level over the most recent 3 months because the life span of the hemoglobin molecule is approximately 90 to 120 days. This level is not affected by short-term fluctuations and is considered to be an objective and accurate measure of long-term diabetes control (ADA, 2008a; Goldstein, Little, Lorenz, et al., 1995). A home HbA$_{1c}$ test is available for purchase, although a recent study found it relatively inaccurate in children when compared with a laboratory value, and therefore the authors did not recommend its use (DirecNet Study Group, 2003, 2005, 2007).

Type 2 Diabetes

Initial Treatment. At diagnosis, youths with type 2 diabetes may have DKA, but much less commonly. They may need insulin initially to correct the metabolic derangement at diagnosis. Treatment with insulin, as with type 1, rapidly improves the symptoms of diabetes.

Lifestyle Intervention. Because the underlying pathology is insulin resistance, the initial approach to treatment focuses on improving insulin sensitivity. The cornerstone of treatment for type 2 diabetes in youths is intensive lifestyle intervention that focuses on decreasing adiposity, increasing activity, and behavior change approaches to improve these lifestyle behaviors. Demonstrable improvement in insulin sensitivity occurs with moderate, gradual weight loss (Ludwig & Ebbeling, 2001; Pinhas-Hamiel & Zeitler, 2007). It is believed that modest weight loss or weight maintenance as a child grows, with improvement in physical fitness, can delay or prevent the need for pharmacologic treatment (Upchurch, Anding, & Brown, 1999). Unfortunately, there have been few large-scale studies of this approach in children and adolescents, but one is currently underway (Treatment Options for Diabetes Type 2 in Adolescents and Youth—The TOD^{2}AY Study Group, 2007). Trials on the reduction of obesity in children and youths suggest that interventions that incorporate nutritional counseling with a focus on decreasing fat and caloric density (Epstein, Wing, Penner, et al., 1985; Stolley & Fitzgibbon, 1997), physical activity to increase lean muscle mass and decrease adiposity (Epstein et al., 1985; McMurray, Bauman, Harrell, et al., 2000), and behavior modification with goal setting and problem solving (Grey, Berry, Davidson, et al., 2004) are more likely to succeed than other approaches. Physical activity that decreases sedentary behavior and encourages aerobic activity is favored, especially activity that can be sustained over the long term. Long-term behavior change of diet and physical activity is difficult, and pharmacologic intervention may be necessary.

Pharmacologic Treatment. If lifestyle intervention fails, pharmacologic treatment is necessary. Once, insulin was the only choice, but treatment with insulin was often counterproductive, because insulin promotes fat deposition and children often gained more weight. Metformin has been evaluated for safety and efficacy in children (Jones, Arslanian, Peterokova, et al., 2002) and has been approved for use in children ages 10 and older (Jones, 2002). Metformin improves metabolic control by reducing hepatic glucose production, increasing insulin sensitivity, and reducing intestinal glucose absorption, without increasing insulin secretion. Metformin has been found to significantly improve metabolic control compared with placebo and does not have a negative effect on body weight or lipid profiles. Further, the rates of adverse events in children (mostly gastrointestinal symptoms, especially diarrhea) were consistent with adverse event rates reported with adults and tend to decrease over the first few weeks of treatment (Jones et al., 2002).

Other oral medications, such as insulin sensitizers, are frequently used in adults in combination with metformin with good results.

Unfortunately, there have been only small studies in children, and these drugs are not approved for use with children. Insulin secretagogues, such as the sulfonylureas, are also not approved for use with children (Pinhas-Hamiel & Zeitler, 2007).

Once there is beta cell failure in type 2 diabetes, metformin will no longer be effective, and insulin becomes the only effective treatment. As with type 1 diabetes, all treatments must be monitored with blood glucose monitoring and quarterly glycosylated hemoglobin and weight measurements.

Complementary and Alternative Therapies

Type 1 Diabetes. Although insulin is necessary for the treatment of type 1 diabetes, there is some suggestion that additional behavioral, biofeedback-assisted relaxation may help improve glucose control (McGrady, Bailey, & Good, 1991). The rationale behind this is that stress in itself can raise glucose levels, and therefore therapies aimed at decreasing stress may help overall glucose control.

Type 2 Diabetes. Although complementary therapies such as hypnosis are commonly used by adults with diabetes to achieve weight loss, there is little in the literature about their use in children and adolescents. The mineral chromium has been studied in adults for weight loss and control of type 2 diabetes with mixed results (Althius, Jordon, Ludington, et al., 2002), but there have not been studies in children. Families also may resort to "fad diets" in an attempt to help youths with type 2 diabetes lose weight.

Recent and Anticipated Advances in Diagnosis and Management

Researchers are developing artificial insulin delivery systems and transplantation of beta cells as new methods of treatment. The artificial insulin delivery systems will improve on the CSII by incorporating a feedback loop that will alter the insulin delivered according to the glucose level, based on data from a subcutaneous continuous glucose sensor. This is referred to as a "closed loop system." Steil, Rebrin, Darwin, and colleagues (2006) have reported success with a 30-hour session of closed loop insulin delivery in adults. Weinzimer, Steil, Swan, and colleagues (2008) recently used a closed loop system in 17 adolescents and were able to achieve near-normal glucose concentrations during the overnight period. Furthermore, they used a "hybrid closed loop" in nine of these youths, where a small manual priming bolus dose was given before the meal. The adolescents who received the hybrid treatment were able to achieve better postprandial glucose levels than those with the complete closed loop. Although these studies are preliminary, and adolescents need to be admitted to a clinical research unit for the closed loop insulin delivery for monitoring, the success of these studies is extremely exciting as we look toward a true "artificial pancreas" as a treatment option for type 1 diabetes in the future.

Transplantation of beta cells or the whole pancreas results in a reduction of insulin requirements for people with diabetes who are already on immunosuppression therapy for previous organ transplants (Sutherland & Gruessner, 1997). The remaining challenge is to prevent autoimmune destruction of these cells in individuals who are not immunosuppressed. More recently, there has been successful experience with islet cell transplantation for people with labile diabetes (Edmonton protocol). These people received immunosuppressive therapy as well, and insulin independence was obtained for 11 of 12 adults studied (Sutherland & Gruessner, 1997). This protocol has since been repeated in nine different centers internationally, and 36 adults with labile diabetes received islet cell transplants with immunosuppression. After 1 year, 16 (44%) remained completely insulin independent, and 5 of these 16 remained insulin independent after 2 years. The authors concluded that for individuals seeking complete insulin independence, whole pancreas transplantation may be a more robust option at this time (Shapiro, Ricordi, Hering, et al., 2006). Further research to determine effective, safe immunosuppressive therapies, as well as other potential sources for insulin-producing cells, is needed so that islet cell transplantation may result in an eventual cure for type 1 diabetes.

New insulin delivery systems are also being tested. A study of 226 adults demonstrated that use of inhaled insulin (Exubera) with meals and intermediate or long-acting insulin for basal needs was as effective as a more conventional injection regimen with quick- or rapid-acting insulin (Thompson, Coovert, Richards, et al., 1995). Although one formulation of inhaled insulin (Exubera) has been approved by the FDA, its manufacturer announced in December 2007 that it will no longer be making this product (because too few individuals were using it), and it is no longer available. Implantable insulin pumps that deliver insulin intraperitoneally have also been used in adults, but not routinely in children (Dunn, Nathan, Scavini, et al., 1997).

New pharmacologic treatments for type 2 diabetes are currently being evaluated in children. The TOD^{2}AY trial is assessing the relative efficacy of metformin with an insulin sensitizer or an intensive lifestyle management program. Other treatments, such as meglitinide analogs and glucosidase inhibitors, require further testing in children and adolescents. In addition, advances in the pharmacologic and surgical treatment of obesity will likely affect treatment for type 2 diabetes in children and adolescents as well (see Chapter 36).

Recently, bariatric surgery has been advocated as an approach to the management of severe obesity and type 2 diabetes in adults (Meneghini, 2007). Although such surgery is occasionally performed in children, current research reveals no controlled studies on bariatric surgery in youths with type 2 diabetes. Of concern is that although gastric bypass surgery results in significant and sustained weight loss, it is also associated with greater morbidity and nutritional/metabolic issues than that seen with lifestyle intervention and metformin.

Associated Problems of Diabetes Mellitus and Treatment

Diabetic Ketoacidosis and Hypoglycemia

Figure 23-1 shows the physiologic process that results in diabetic ketoacidosis (DKA) when there is a lack of insulin. Any potential stressor (e.g., illness, fever, injury, and psychosocial stress) can increase the risk of metabolic derangement caused by disturbances in counterregulatory hormones and lead to DKA. Thus any stressor in a child with diabetes must be managed with care.

It should be noted that children with type 2 diabetes can have DKA, but once they are stabilized after diagnosis, DKA becomes rare in these children. What can occur is nonketotic severe hyperglycemia (nonketotic hyperosmolar coma), which is usually associated with significant dehydration and is characterized by

Associated Problems of Diabetes Mellitus and Treatment		
	Type 1	**Type 2**
Diabetic ketoacidosis or nonketotic severe hyperglycemia	Yes	Yes
Hypoglycemia	Common	Rare
Monilial vaginitis	Yes	Yes
Cardiovascular complications		
Hyperlipidemia	Yes	Common
Hypertension	Yes	Common
Nonalcoholic fatty liver disease	No	Yes
Polycystic ovary syndrome	No	Yes
Long-term complications		
Renal failure	Yes	Yes
Retinopathy	Yes	Yes
Neuropathie	Yes	Yes
Vascular insufficiency	Yes	Yes
Depression/psychosocial problems	Yes	Unknown

BOX 23-2

Comparison of Hyperglycemia and Hypoglycemia

Diabetic ketoacidosis (hyperglycemia)
- Slow onset
- Increased thirst and urination
- High blood and urine glucose levels
- Urinary ketones
- Weakness and abdominal pain
- Heavy, labored breathing
- Anorexia
- Nausea and vomiting
- Monilial vaginitis

Hypoglycemia
- Rapid onset
- Excessive sweating
- Fainting
- Headache
- Trembling and shaking
- Hunger
- Unable to wake
- Irritability
- Personality change

---

very high plasma glucose levels (greater than 750 mg/dL) without ketosis or ketoacidosis. Treatment with intravenous hydration and insulin is required.

Children with well-controlled diabetes will occasionally experience episodes of hypoglycemia, especially when treated with insulin. Because the symptoms of hyperglycemia and hypoglycemia can sometimes be confused, they are compared in Box 23-2. Hypoglycemia may be caused by too much insulin, too little food, too much activity, or a combination of these. Although hypoglycemia is easily treated, prevention is the best approach. Again, self-monitored blood glucose (SMBG) determination is helpful. With SMBG testing, children can identify patterns of lower blood glucose levels that may indicate periods of increased risk. During these periods, the insulin dose can be altered to prevent the hypoglycemia. If a child anticipates unusual physical activity, both insulin and diet can be adjusted to prevent low glucose levels. Hypoglycemia can occur with the sulfonylureas, an older treatment for type 2 diabetes. Changing to metformin is associated with lower incidence of hypoglycemia in people with type 2 diabetes.

Hypoglycemia

Hypoglycemia presents particular problems at different ages. Infants and toddlers are unable to express the feelings associated with hypoglycemia, so they must be observed for listlessness, sleepiness, or irritability. Parents should be instructed that unusual behavior at any time is an indication for blood glucose levels to be measured. If the result is less than 70 mg/dL, a conscious infant should be given 2 to 4 oz of sweet liquids or a small amount of cake frosting (gel) and an unconscious or convulsing infant should be given 0.25 to 0.5 mL of glucagon by injection. Older children can be taught the symptoms of hypoglycemia and how to prevent its occurrence. They should also be instructed to carry high-sugar foods with them at all times. All children with diabetes should wear medical identification so that they can be diagnosed and treated appropriately if they lose consciousness while away from home. In the DCCT, intensive regimens were associated with a three-fold increase in the incidence of severe hypoglycemia (DCCT Research Group, 1995), so extra care must be taken by children on intensive regimens.

Some substances can increase the likelihood of hypoglycemia. Adolescents need to know that alcohol augments the glucose-lowering effects of insulin and that the symptoms of alcohol intoxication and hypoglycemia are similar. Low blood glucose levels can increase the body's sensitivity to alcohol, and many experimenting teenagers have found themselves in the emergency department with profound hypoglycemia. Stimulants such as amphetamines and cocaine may increase metabolism and decrease appetite, so hypoglycemia may occur.

Monilial Vaginitis

Once healthy girls are toilet trained, monilial infections of the perineum are rare until adolescence, when the estrogenation of the vagina provides a potential environment for growth of candida. Hyperglycemia also leads to increased glucose levels in vaginal secretions, providing an ideal medium for candida. Thus girls with poorly controlled diabetes (either type 1 or type 2) are at increased risk for monilial vaginitis; any complaint of vaginal discharge and itching should be investigated with a potassium hydroxide preparation and treated appropriately.

Cardiovascular Complications

Hyperlipidemia and hypertension are common in youths with type 2 diabetes. Blood lipids (total cholesterol, low-density lipids [LDLs], high-density lipids [HDLs], and triglycerides) should be measured yearly in all youths with type 2 diabetes. Although there have been few studies of children with type 2 diabetes and hyperlipidemia, aggressive treatment is recommended. Blood pressure should be obtained at every quarterly visit and recorded as hypertension is common, especially in youth with type 2 diabetes.

Nonalcoholic Fatty Liver Disease

Nonalcoholic fatty liver disease (NAFLD) is a long-term complication of obesity, hyperlipidemia, and diabetes. Elevations in liver enzymes, especially alanine aminotransferase (ALT), may be an indication of NAFLD. Children and youth with NAFLD are usually asymptomatic. Weight loss, diet, exercise and lipid control with cholesterol-lowering medication in older children is often recommended.

Polycystic Ovary Syndrome

Insulin resistance and type 2 diabetes are also associated with polycystic ovary syndrome (POS) in girls. This disorder is associated with increased ovarian or adrenal androgen production. Symptoms include menstrual irregularities and evidence of hyperandrogenism, especially hirsutism. Girls with POS should be referred to a reproductive endocrinologist for care. Treatment with low-dose birth control pills along with insulin sensitizers may be necessary. Metformin may also be used to control hyperglycemia.

Long-Term Complications

Long-term complications of type 1 diabetes (renal failure, eye degeneration, neuropathies, vascular insufficiency) are well known. Little has been known until recently about the long-term complications of type 2 diabetes in youths. Unfortunately, recent data suggest that complications follow a more rapid trajectory than in adults. This risk is present because those with type 2 diabetes also have hyperinsulinemia and obesity, both risk factors for cardiovascular disease. Dean and Sellers (2007) have reported that in a population of Native American young people who developed type 2 diabetes in youth, complications such as renal disease, microvascular and macrovascular disease, and retinopathy were already present when the youths were in their early twenties. Thus the recommendations of the United Kingdom Prospective Diabetes Study (UKPDS) (Clarke, Gray, Adler, et al., 2001) to aggressively treat both glucose control and blood pressure control are accepted as the current standards for management of type 2 diabetes in youths.

Depression and Other Psychosocial Complications

It is generally accepted that type 1 diabetes is a risk factor for adolescent psychiatric disorders (Kovacs, Goldston, Obrosky, et al., 1997). Approximately three times more adolescents with diabetes have psychiatric disorders than their age-mates, with rates as high as 33% (Blanz, Rensech-Riemann, Fritz-Sigmund, et al., 1993). This increased morbidity is primarily associated with the incidence of major depression (approximately 27.5%) and generalized anxiety disorder (18.4%), rather than psychiatric behavioral disorders (Kovacs et al., 1997). A substantial number of adolescents with diabetes consider suicide after the onset of the condition (Goldston, Kelley, Reboussin, et al., 1997). The rate of suicidal ideation has been found to be higher than would be expected (26.4%), but in contrast, the number of suicide attempts was only 4.4%, which is a rate comparable with the general population of adolescents (Goldston et al., 1997). In addition, adolescents who have recurrent DKA may be more likely to have psychiatric disorders, especially anxiety and depression, than those without recurrent hospitalization (Liss, Waller, Kennard, et al., 1998). Although it is unclear whether diabetes causes depression or vice versa, the ADA has recently recommended that children ages 8 years and older with type 1 diabetes be screened for depression yearly (Silverstein, Klingensmith, Copeland, et al., 2005).

Although a smaller percentage of adolescents with diabetes manifest significant psychiatric problems, many have difficulty in psychosocial adjustment. The presence of diabetes in adolescence may hinder normal adolescent development by limiting the development of independence. One study examined the personal meaning and perceived impact of diabetes on 54 adolescents and found that youths felt that diabetes controlled or limited their freedom and independence

(Kyngas & Barlow, 1995). Girls have been found to report more symptoms of anxiety and depression related to these restrictions and to be in worse metabolic control than boys (Glasgow, Fisher, Anderson, et al., 1999). Interventions such as coping skills training (Grey, Boland, Davidson, et al., 2000) and parent-child conflict prevention (Anderson, Brackett, Ho, et al., 1999) may be helpful in reducing these problems. Appropriate referral to behavioral treatment should not be delayed if problems in adjustment are suspected.

Obesity in youths is associated with body dissatisfaction and lower self-esteem (Caldwell, Brownell, & Wilfley, 1997; Strauss, 2000), altered body image (Kolody & Sallis, 1995; Thompson et al., 1995), decreasing preference for physical activity (Kolody & Sallis, 1995), self-efficacy for activity (Kolody & Sallis, 1995), and depression (Falkner, Neumark-Sztainer, Story, et al., 2001). Although studies of the psychosocial consequences of type 2 diabetes in youths are just beginning, there is every reason to believe that the psychosocial consequences of type 2 will be similar to those found in type 1 and in obesity (see Chapter 36).

Prognosis

Diabetes is the sixth leading cause of death in the United States. For the most part, this high mortality rate is a result of the long-term complications of the condition. The risk of death among people with diabetes is about two times that of their same-age peers without diabetes (ADA, 2008b). Because diabetes treatment and technology is continuing to improve, however, and because individuals with diabetes are managed more aggressively since the DCCT was completed, there is hope that children diagnosed post-DCCT will have lower rates of long-term complications, and therefore may have a better prognosis.

Complications can range from asymptomatic mild proteinuria to blindness, renal failure, painful neuropathies, cardiovascular disease, and death. Hyperglycemia is a necessary—but not sufficient—factor for the development of complications. In addition to hyperglycemia, genetic factors seem to influence the development of complications. In the United States, diabetic retinopathy causes 12,000 to 24,000 cases of blindness each year, and diabetes is also the leading cause of kidney failure, accounting for 44% of new cases in 2002 (ADA, 2008b). Although the DCCT showed that improvement in metabolic control to near-normal levels delays the onset or progression of complications, complications were not eliminated. It is clear, however, that the better the metabolic control, the better the chance of avoiding complications. As noted earlier, complications appear to occur earlier in the course of type 2 diabetes in youths, but no long-term follow-up studies are yet available. Nonetheless, aggressive blood glucose control, blood pressure control, and lifestyle change are essential in youths with type 2 diabetes.

PRIMARY CARE MANAGEMENT

Health Care Maintenance
Growth and Development
Because type 1 diabetes is a metabolic disorder affecting metabolism, growth and sexual development may be slowed. Children and adolescents whose diabetes is less well controlled may fail to grow

normally. Therefore accurate measurements of height and weight and comparison with growth norms are imperative.

Even when children have normal linear growth, there may be delays in the onset and progression of puberty if glycemic control is inadequate. At each visit, Tanner stages should be assessed and recorded. Any deviation from the normal pattern should be investigated. In girls, menarche may be delayed. Loss of regular menses once cycling has been established may indicate a further degeneration in metabolic control and should be investigated.

Obesity can occur in children and adolescents with type 1 diabetes, especially in those on flexible regimens. In the DCCT, intensive therapy was associated with a 73% higher risk of becoming overweight (DCCT Research Group, 1995). Management of this obesity should be done carefully, with attention to the need to maintain self-monitoring, because glucose levels may change dramatically when a weight loss program is followed.

Adolescents who manipulate weight by overeating or reducing or omitting insulin are another concern. Some adolescent girls with type 1 diabetes engage in insulin withholding to maintain body shape or lose weight (Pollock, Kovacs, & Charron-Prochownik, 1995). Researchers have studied the incidence of eating disorders in adolescents with type 1 diabetes with conflicting results. Some found that adolescents with diabetes are at higher risk for eating disorders than those without diabetes (Polonsky, Anderson, Lohrer, et al., 1994), but others have not found differences between the two groups of adolescents (Striegel-Moore, Nicholson, & Tamborlane, 1992). Nevertheless, alterations in insulin dosage may affect an adolescent's ability to grow and develop normally and should be considered in evaluation of children with growth difficulties.

In type 2 diabetes, obesity is often associated with early puberty, as well as accelerated linear growth. Height and weight should be measured at each visit and body mass index (BMI) calculated. BMI should be plotted and followed as an indicator of the effectiveness of treatment. Tanner staging should be completed at each visit, and unusually rapid progression noted and referred. Calculation of BMI z-score, which shows how far above or below normal the BMI is, at every primary care visit can be used to help prevent obesity and the development of type 2 diabetes.

Diet
Although insulin therapy is the cornerstone of treatment for type 1 diabetes, a dietary plan is important in maintaining near-normoglycemia without wide swings in blood glucose levels. Long-term adherence to the dietary plan is probably the most difficult aspect of management for families.

All dietary management plans for type 1 diabetes have the goal of providing adequate calories and nutrients for normal growth and maintaining blood glucose as normal as possible. The consistency of daily intake with regular meals and snacks is important. Families, in consultation with the diabetes team, should select the appropriate meal plan because they are in the best position to judge the approach that will work. Imposing a rigid approach on an unwilling family only leads them not to adhere to the diet. In addition, most children will not adhere without question to a diet perceived as different from that of peers. Thus primary care providers must be understanding in their approach and work with families to ensure as much dietary consistency as possible.

Most diabetes clinicians advocate carbohydrate counting for the dietary management. The family is taught which foods have carbohydrates (often based on the principles of the exchange system [Table 23-3]) and how to read nutrition labels to determine the carbohydrate count for different foods. If the child is using an injection regimen other than a basal bolus therapy, the dietitian and family will determine specific amounts of carbohydrates the child should consume at meals and snacks. The youth can vary what kinds of carbohydrates he or she may have at a particular meal, as long as the total remains constant.

A more flexible carbohydrate counting approach is used most frequently by those on flexible insulin regimens (DCCT Research Group, 1993a). This method provides more flexibility in the diet by providing for varying amounts of carbohydrates at meals and snacks with appropriate coverage with rapid-acting insulin. Protein and fat intake are not controlled, but efforts to stay within low-fat guidelines are encouraged. For example, adolescents who choose to eat a second sandwich at lunch (i.e., 30 g of extra carbohydrate in the bread) may need to take 5 to 10 units of rapid-acting insulin before the meal, depending on their regimen.

The wide availability of artificially sweetened foods and drinks has eased some of the difficulties children with diabetes faced in following the meal plan. Parents sometimes express concern, however, that extensive use of artificial sweeteners will be problematic for their children. There are four nonnutritive sweeteners approved for use by the FDA in the United States: saccharine, aspartame, sucralose, and acesulfame K. For these and all other additives, the FDA determines an acceptable daily intake (ADI) (i.e., the amount that can be safely consumed on a daily basis over a person's lifetime without any adverse effects), which includes a 100-fold safety factor. Average intake is actually much less than the acceptable daily intake. For example, the average aspartame consumption in the general population (i.e., including children) is 2 to 3 mg/kg/day or approximately 4% of the U.S. ADI of 50 mg/kg.

As noted previously, dietary management is the cornerstone of treatment for type 2 diabetes. A multidisciplinary approach involving dietary modification, increased physical activity, decreased sedentary time, and behavior modification offers the best hope for a successful outcome. Traditionally, dietary approaches have emphasized individualization and reduction in dietary fat intake. Often, reducing calories from sodas and fruit drinks can result in

substantial improvement. Often the dietary approach is based on the same exchange system (see Table 23-3) with reductions of 200 to 500 calories per day to achieve weight loss. The exchange system allows for variety in the meal plan from day to day. Carbohydrate counting can help youths prevent hyperglycemia after meals as well.

Physical activity is to be encouraged for all children. Regular exercise and active participation in organized sports have positive effects on both the psychosocial and physical well-being of children with type 1 diabetes. Parents and their children should be advised that different types of exercise may have different effects on blood glucose levels. For example, sports that involve short bursts of activity may increase glucose levels, whereas a more prolonged activity is more likely to decrease blood glucose levels. Parents and their children also need to be warned that a prolonged session of physical activity during the day may lead to hypoglycemia while the child is sleeping during the night, and therefore an extra bedtime snack or a change in the evening insulin may be necessary. Additionally, if the blood glucose level before exercise is greater than 240 mg/dL, urinary ketones should be checked; if they are present, the child should not exercise, because the presence of ketones means the child has considerably insufficient insulin levels.

For children with type 2 diabetes, physical activity is strongly encouraged to enhance weight management. Activities that decrease sedentary behavior and increase aerobic capacity (McMurray et al., 2000) have been demonstrated to lower insulin and glucose levels. Physical activity should be aimed at establishing lifelong habits, rather than youth sports alone. Encouraging families to participate in activities together may help establish an exercise habit.

Safety

The safety issues faced by families with a child or adolescent with diabetes are two-fold. As discussed earlier, hypoglycemia is a significant risk for all affected children on insulin, so families and others in a child's social sphere should be prepared to respond appropriately. Children should wear medical identification so proper treatment can be instituted quickly. Older children need to know how to prevent severe hypoglycemia, especially when exercising. Children should be taught to eat a snack of complex carbohydrate and protein (e.g., peanut butter and crackers) before exercise, not to inject insulin into an exercising muscle, and to carry glucose with them at all times. Furthermore, the use of uncooked corn starch in convenient snack bars (e.g., Extend Bar) has been advocated for a preexercise snack or a bedtime snack by some diabetes clinicians. Uncooked corn starch is a complex carbohydrate that is slowly hydrolyzed by the enzyme amylase and is slowly absorbed by the gastrointestinal tract. When traveling or on school day trips, children or their parents should carry the supplies with them—not in checked baggage—and always have food available in case a meal is delayed. Airlines require insulin and syringes to be carried in the box with the pharmacy label to bring them on board an airplane.

Parents or caretakers of children with type 1 diabetes must learn to treat episodes of severe hypoglycemia with glucagon. Glucagon is the antagonist hormone to insulin and releases glycogen from the liver. When a child or adolescent cannot take sugar by mouth, glucagon is administered by intramuscular injection to rapidly raise the blood glucose. The dose for infants or toddlers is 0.5 mg (0.5 mL), and the dose for older children is 1 mg (1.0 mL).

TABLE 23-3
Dietary Exchange System

Food Exchange	Calories	Approximate Content g/Serving		
		Carbohydrate	Protein	Fat
Fruit	60	12	0	0
Vegetable	25	5	2	0
Starch	68	15	2	0
Milk				
Whole	170	12	8	10
Skim	90	12	8	Trace
Meat				
Lean	55	0	7	3
Medium fat	75	0	7	5
High fat	95	0	7	8
Fat	45	0	0	5
Free*	0	Negligible	0	0

*Foods with less than 5 g CHO, which would have little or no impact on glucose levels.

Another important safety issue is the proper disposal of syringes. Children and parents must be taught the importance of proper disposal of syringes to reduce the risk of injury to themselves and others.

For youths with type 2 diabetes on oral medications, care should be taken to ensure that medications are taken as prescribed. As with all medications, safety containers should be used so that young children do not accidentally ingest them. Should an accidental ingestion occur, children should be watched for hypoglycemia and a poison control center contacted.

Immunizations

Routine immunizations are recommended. Children with diabetes are potentially at an increased risk for developing complicated influenza illness; therefore they should receive a yearly influenza vaccination after age 6 months (ADA, 2008b). Some providers also recommend that youths with diabetes receive the 23 Valent pneumococcal vaccine (PPV 23), but with improved metabolic control, there is less risk for overwhelming infection.

Screening

Vision. Vision screening is particularly important in children with diabetes because visual problems are common. A small number of children develop cataracts early in the course of the condition; therefore observing the normalcy of the red reflex during the ophthalmic examination is very important. Fluctuations in blood glucose levels can also affect visual acuity. Children experiencing hypoglycemia may complain of visual disturbances, and those with hyperglycemia may also complain of blurred vision. Thus it is important to relate the results of routine visual screening to the level of metabolic control, because improvement in metabolic control may improve the results of the visual testing.

Parents and children are often most concerned about the risk of diabetic retinopathy. Retinopathy of diabetes is the leading cause of blindness. The ADA (2008b) recommends that funduscopic examination be performed in individuals with diabetes at each primary care visit. Furthermore, an annual examination with dilation by a pediatric ophthalmologist is recommended for children over 10 years of age within 3 to 5 years after the onset of diabetes, and then repeated annually. Less frequent (every 2 to 3 years) examinations may be considered following one or more normal examinations (ADA, 2008a). Because type 2 diabetes may have been present for some time before it is diagnosed, dilated retinal examination should be done at the time of diagnosis and then yearly.

Hearing. Routine screening is recommended.

Dental. Routine screening is recommended. If metabolic control is poor, children may experience increased dental caries and gingivitis caused by increased glucose in saliva. Thus those with poorer control should have frequent dental screening and appropriate treatment.

Blood Pressure. Screening should be performed at each visit. Hypertension has been reported in up to 45% of all individuals with diabetes. Thus the ADA (1993) recommends that orthostatic measurements be performed and recorded routinely. Aggressive blood pressure control may significantly improve the long-term outcome for youths with both type 1 and type 2 diabetes. Current treatment guidelines suggest that the use of angiotensin-converting enzyme (ACE) inhibitors to achieve and maintain normotension

may also improve the risk for microvascular kidney complications (Clarke et al., 2001).

Hematocrit. Routine screening is recommended.

Urinalysis. Screening is performed yearly, with examination for levels of ketones, glucose, and protein. After 5 years of type 1 diabetes, and once the child is 10 years old, total urinary protein excretion should be measured yearly by the microalbuminuria method to screen for renal complications. The albumin-to-creatinine ratio in a random spot collection is the preferred method (ADA, 2008b). If proteinuria is detected, serum creatinine clearance or blood urea nitrogen concentration should be measured and glomerular filtration assessed. In youths with type 2 diabetes, screening should be done at diagnosis and yearly thereafter.

Tuberculosis. Routine screening is recommended.

Condition-Specific Screening

Lipids. Individuals with type 1 or type 2 diabetes are at risk for disorders of lipid metabolism, and these disorders may increase the risk of macrovascular complications. Children with type 1 diabetes should be screened with blood lipid profiles yearly after puberty (10 years of age). If a child has other risk factors, including a family history, or has type 2 diabetes, lipid screening should begin earlier, with the first fasting lipid profile being done soon after diagnosis (after glucose control is established) in children older than 2 years of age (ADA, 2008b).

Thyroid. Because type 1 diabetes is an autoimmune disease, it is associated with other autoimmune diseases—especially Hashimoto's thyroiditis. Youths should be screened for thyroid peroxidase and thyroglobulin antibodies at diagnosis. Thyroid-stimulating hormone (TSH) should be measured after glucose control has been established, and if normal, they should be rechecked every 1 to 2 years (ADA, 2008b). Children and adolescents who show any change in growth pattern or develop signs and symptoms of hypothyroidism (e.g., fatigue, dry skin, constipation) or hyperthyroidism (e.g., heat intolerance, tremor, diarrhea) should be tested with thyroid function studies.

Celiac. Celiac disease is another immune-mediated condition (see Chapter 17) that is seen in increased frequency with type 1 diabetes. Symptoms include diarrhea, weight loss, poor weight gain, abdominal pain, fatigue, malnutrition, and unexplained hypoglycemia or erratic blood glucose control. Children with type 1 diabetes who exhibit any symptoms of celiac disease should be tested by measuring tissue transglutaminase or antiendomysial antibodies (with documentation of normal serum immunoglobulin A [IgA] levels). If the test is positive, the child should be referred to a gastroenterologist for evaluation. Once the diagnosis is confirmed, the child should be placed on a gluten-free diet, and the family should be referred to a nutritionist for guidance (ADA, 2008b).

Nonalcoholic Fatty Liver Disease. Many obese adolescents with type 2 diabetes have elevations in alanine aminotransferase (ALT), suggestive of nonalcoholic fatty liver disease (NAFLD). Obese youths with type 2 diabetes should be screened yearly. It is not yet clear whether weight loss will reverse NAFLD, but small studies in adults suggest that it is possible.

Depression. Due to the increased incidence of depression or anxiety in children and adolescents with diabetes they should be screened on a regular basis for mental health concerns or symptoms (see Chapter 33).

Common Illness Management

Differential Diagnosis

Management of Vomiting and Diarrhea and Prevention of Diabetic Ketoacidosis. Provided that their diabetes is under reasonable metabolic control, children and adolescents with diabetes are not at higher risk than their peers for most common infectious diseases of childhood. Because any stressor may lead to DKA in a child with type 1 diabetes, infections and other stressors must be managed with care.

Regardless of the stress, there are several important principles for management; the need to continue to take insulin even when unable to eat a normal diet is of utmost importance because the excess of counterregulatory hormones released in response to the stressor will more than offset the decreased oral intake. Thus, even though dietary intake may be decreased, the insulin requirement may be increased.

Differential Diagnosis

- Stressors, including illness, can lead to DKA
- "Sick day" management needed for common illnesses and stress
- Important to maintain hydration during illness
- Vaginal discharge may be monilial infection
- Skin manifestations may require referral
- Weight loss may indicate poor metabolic control
- Gastroparesis may be the cause of prolonged vomiting

The principles of management include monitoring glucose and ketone levels, maintaining hydration, preventing hypoglycemia, and preventing DKA and non-ketotic hyperosmolar coma. For these principles to work effectively, it is imperative that the child and family know that any illness or insult involving fever, gastrointestinal symptoms, congestion in the head or chest, or urinary symptoms should be managed as a "sick day." Once a day is identified as a "sick day," the usual rules for self-monitoring are altered to reflect the need for closer monitoring. Blood glucose levels should be tested every 1 to 4 hours, and individuals with blood glucose levels greater than 200 mg/dL should test their urine for ketones. Blood glucose levels of more than 400 mg/dL on two or more determinations and moderate or high ketone levels in the urine that do not decrease with additional insulin, along with any persistent vomiting, regardless of the blood glucose level, should be viewed as an indication that the child should be seen and evaluated by either the primary care provider or the specialist.

Maintaining hydration is important to help clear extra glucose and ketones, and hydration must be carefully monitored if vomiting or diarrhea is present. If children cannot eat their usual diet, a large fluid intake should be maintained. In adolescents, this amount should be more than 8 oz of fluid hourly. Such fluids should contain adequate amounts of carbohydrate (i.e., 50 to 75 g in 6 to 8 hours) to maintain the usual caloric intake. Children often drink regular (i.e., not diet) sodas, drink flavored gelatin water, or suck on ice pops when ill. If a child is vomiting or has diarrhea, broth or electrolyte solutions help replace sodium losses.

A child with type 1 diabetes may need additional insulin to prevent DKA, and a child with type 2 may need insulin to treat DKA or to prevent non-ketotic hyperosmolar coma. If the blood glucose

---

BOX 23-3

Indications for Evaluation by a Health Care Provider

- Vomiting for more than 6 hours or more than five diarrheal stools in 1 day
- Any change in mental status
- Syncope
- Temperature greater than 102.2°F (38.9°C) for 12 hours
- Blood glucose levels more than 400 mg/dL twice
- Moderate or high ketone levels that do not decrease with extra insulin intake
- Dysuria or other symptoms of urinary tract infection
- Decreased urinary output

---

level is greater than 300 mg/dL, the family should generally administer the usual dose of insulin and add up to 20% of the total daily dose as rapid-acting insulin every 4 hours. Such management should be undertaken in careful consultation with the child's diabetes team. Studies have shown that treatment with the quick-acting insulin lispro during ketosis and hyperglycemia may result in more rapid correction than with conventional rapid-acting insulin (Attia, Jones, Holcombe, et al., 1998).

Box 23-3 lists the indications for which children or adolescents should be seen and evaluated. Most important is the need for children with any alteration in mental status to be evaluated. Primary care providers should never assume that sleepiness in children with diabetes is merely the result of the fatigue associated with an illness.

Other Conditions

Vaginal Discharge. Young women with diabetes are prone to monilial infections when glucose control is inadequate. Treatment with an antifungal agent is warranted in young girls if vaginal discharge with itching exists without evidence of sexual activity. If there has been sexual contact of any kind, the vagina should be examined, and testing for other infections (e.g., *Chlamydia*) should be performed.

Other Skin Manifestations. Children and adolescents with diabetes may develop skin lesions associated with diabetes (e.g., necrobiosis diabeticorum). If scaly lesions develop—usually on extensor surfaces—treatment by a dermatologist is warranted. Children with thyroid disease may have alopecia.

Acanthosis nigricans is a marker for insulin resistance. If acanthosis is present, the child should be referred for oral glucose tolerance testing and appropriate treatment. Girls with POS often have hirsutism. Referral to a reproductive endocrinologist and treatment with low-dose estrogen birth control pills will often correct the hirsutism.

Weight Loss. The most common cause of weight loss in youths with type 1 diabetes is worsening metabolic control. Therefore evaluation of weight loss should include assessment of overall glucose control. If control is inadequate and attempts to improve control are not successful, deliberate withholding of insulin for weight control should be investigated. Weight loss could also be related to the development of celiac disease, so this should be considered as well. Individuals with diabetes may also develop bulimic characteristics as a method of weight control, but vomiting and abdominal distress in youths with longstanding diabetes may also be a symptom of diabetic gastroparesis. Evaluation for gastroparesis includes radiographic gastric emptying studies that should be done under the direction of a specialist.

Drug Interactions

Many over-the-counter medications and antibiotics contain glucose, and some contain alcohol or traces of gluconeogenic substances, such as sorbitol or glycerine (Kumar, Weatherly, & Beaman, 1991). In the amounts usually ingested, these compounds may raise blood glucose levels slightly but should not markedly impair metabolic control.

Developmental Issues

Sleep Patterns

Children with diabetes whose metabolic control is good should have no problems sleeping. Those who are hyperglycemic overnight, however, will have difficulty sleeping because of the recurrent need to urinate. This problem can be managed by improving metabolic control.

Nighttime hypoglycemia is a concern of parents of children on insulin. A child may not wake with the usual early signs and symptoms, and the first sign may be a severe event with nightmares or seizures. Therefore it is important to prevent nighttime hypoglycemia by appropriately adjusting the evening insulin dose and offering a bedtime snack with carbohydrate and protein or fat. Parents should also be instructed in the use of the counterregulatory hormone glucagon in case the child is not able to be aroused.

Nightmares are common in young children and may be caused by hypoglycemia. Parents should determine the blood glucose level before assuming the cause of a nightmare. If the cause is hypoglycemia, treatment includes administration of glucose. If the nightmares are not related to hypoglycemia, appropriate comfort measures should be instituted. Prevention is the key, however, and significant nighttime hypoglycemia is to be avoided as much as possible by careful adjustment of diet and insulin.

Toileting

Several issues related to toileting are important in the management of diabetes in children. Many children have secondary enuresis at the time of diagnosis. It is important to tell children who were previously dry that diabetes is the cause of their enuresis and that the enuresis should remit when the diabetes is adequately controlled. Enuresis can occur, however, with well-controlled diabetes. Other methods of diagnostic confirmation and treatment should be explored with these families.

Although testing urine for glucose is not as critical to management as it was before SMBG testing was available, urinary ketone levels are important indicators of status when a child with diabetes is ill. Parents should know how to obtain such samples from infants and toddlers. Cotton balls tucked into a diaper can provide an adequate sample for use on a dipstick to determine ketone levels in children who are not yet toilet-trained. Urine is readily obtainable when a child uses a potty chair during toilet training. When children begin to use the bathroom commode, parents need to teach them to urinate into a paper cup so that the urine can be tested. If taught when a child is feeling well, this task can be made into a game so that, when necessary, the behavior has been learned.

Discipline

Although the issues related to discipline of a child with diabetes are not different from those of all children with a chronic condition, parents of children with diabetes report that their second most common concern in raising the child is discipline (Hodges & Parker, 1987). Parents most often worry that a hypoglycemic episode will be missed by attributing the unruly behavior to lack of discipline. It is appropriate for parents to test the blood glucose level at any time hypoglycemia is suspected; if the result is within the normal range, the child can be appropriately disciplined. Blood testing should be performed matter-of-factly, so that children do not misinterpret the test as a punishment. Some parents also worry that the stress of imposed discipline will raise the blood glucose level because of the presence of counterregulatory hormones. Although severe stressors may increase blood glucose levels, no evidence suggests that usual disciplinary measures increase blood glucose levels or worsen metabolic control. Indeed, some authors (Grey & Tamborlane, 2003) have suggested that parents who set reasonable limits for their children are more likely to have children in good metabolic control.

Child Care

Toddlers and preschoolers with diabetes benefit from the socialization of preschool programs, as do all children, and they do not need specialized medical daycare. Preschool teachers should be informed of parental expectations, such as blood glucose testing and insulin administration. Snack and lunch intake are very important, so preschool teachers must be aware of the child's need to eat and what should be served at each mealtime. They should be aware of appropriate food substitutions when food is refused. All caregivers should be told how to manage symptoms of hypoglycemia. Emergency telephone numbers should always be available and should include telephone numbers of the parents, another emergency contact, the primary care provider, and the diabetes specialists. The ADA has specific guidelines for diabetes care in the school and daycare setting in its standards of care document, which is updated annually (ADA, 2008b). This can be an excellent resource for parents and school personnel.

Parents of children with diabetes often express concerns about the abilities of baby-sitters or daycare workers to manage a young child's type 1 diabetes. Parents of young children can begin by leaving the child for only short periods of time, thus reassuring themselves that the sitter can successfully care for the child. Clear instructions on the child's meal plan and management of hypoglycemia should be provided in writing. Parents should be encouraged to train sitters in blood glucose monitoring and recognition of hypoglycemic symptoms.

Schooling

Children whose diabetes is adequately controlled should attend school regularly and participate in any activities for which they are otherwise suited. Parents should be encouraged to inform the school nurse and the child's teachers when the diabetes is diagnosed. It is important that school personnel are knowledgeable about the child's care so that hypoglycemia or illness can be appropriately managed. The need for other involvement (e.g., SMBG testing or injections) depends on the child's usual regimen. For youths with type 2 diabetes, the school can be invaluable in providing support and follow-up in a weight loss program.

With older children, providers need to work with the child, family, and school personnel to arrange a school schedule that fits the child's diabetes regimen. For example, a child who has had regular and NPH insulin at 7:00 AM should probably have a snack before a gym class that precedes a late lunch period. Arrangements must be made so that the child can always have access to glucose-containing foods or tablets in case of a hypoglycemic episode. The child should always have food available on field trips. A sack lunch with all food groups serves nicely as a substitute if a meal is unexpectedly delayed.

Sports are also encouraged. For youths with type 1 diabetes, coaches should be aware of the diabetes and keep foods containing glucose on hand. Depending on the degree of exercise on extra-activity days, the insulin dose may be lowered or the diet increased, or both, in an attempt to prevent hypoglycemia. Hypoglycemia following exercise may occur up to 12 hours after the event, so children should be carefully monitored when any new activity is undertaken. Children should be advised that insulin is absorbed more rapidly from exercising muscle; therefore if a muscle is to be exercised, insulin should be injected in another site. For example, if a child will run track, the insulin could be administered in the arm or the abdomen instead of the leg. For youths with type 2 diabetes, physical activity is crucial to improving outcomes. These youths should be encouraged to participate fully in physical activities in the school and at home.

Children with type 1 or type 2 diabetes whose diabetes is in poor control may experience difficulties in school performance. Because hypoglycemia can cause a child to lose the ability to concentrate when the blood glucose level is low, learning can be a problem. When the blood glucose level is consistently too high, many children experience difficulties in concentration and grades may suffer. Any child with diabetes whose school performance changes should be carefully assessed for alterations in metabolic control. Unless there are other problems, children with diabetes should not require special education or an individual learning plan. Indeed, several class action suits have been brought against school districts that required otherwise well children with diabetes to attend special education classes.

Because children and adolescents with diabetes are encouraged to participate fully in sports and other activities, they may be encouraged to go to camp as well. There are specialized camps for children with diabetes, which may help young people to learn about their diabetes and meet peers who also have diabetes. Children and adolescents with diabetes may also safely attend regular camps. Whether the camp is a diabetes-specific camp or not, care should be taken to adjust the insulin dose and food intake to account for the markedly increased physical activity at camp. Extra blood glucose monitoring may be necessary.

As with all children with chronic conditions, emphasis should be on the normality of the child—not on the diabetes. Such an approach helps minimize the sense of being different that is experienced by all affected children.

Sexuality

Achievement of normal growth and development is a goal of therapy for type 1 diabetes. If the diabetes is adequately controlled, sexual development should be normal. If sexual development is delayed, however, normal concerns about self-adequacy and physical adequacy may be amplified. Primary care providers need to monitor secondary sexual development carefully in children with diabetes, and any deviation from normal should be investigated. Tightening the metabolic control often improves growth. If not, the cause should be investigated.

All sexually active teenagers need information about birth control. Such information is especially important for those with type 1 and type 2 diabetes because the risks for complications of pregnancy are at least five times greater than the already high risk for adolescents. Because of the risk for acquired immunodeficiency syndrome (AIDS), many providers encourage condoms over all other birth control methods. Unfortunately, as with all teenagers, proper and consistent use of condoms is variable. Other barrier methods (e.g., diaphragms, foams, and creams) may also be used by those with diabetes but share the same disadvantages as condoms and do not prevent sexually transmitted diseases.

Teenagers who are willing to use contraceptives often find using the birth control pill acceptable. Earlier versions of the combination pill (i.e., containing both estrogen and progesterone) carried risks for cerebral ischemia, myocardial infarction, and rapid progression of retinopathy and were not recommended for adolescents with diabetes. Newer low-dose estrogen combination pills, however, seem to be reasonably well tolerated and are the oral contraceptive of choice. These medications are also used to threat amenorrhea associated with POS in youths with type 2 diabetes.

Although avoidance of adolescent pregnancy is clearly preferred for youths with type 1 or type 2 diabetes, some teenagers express the desire to become pregnant. It has been clearly demonstrated, however, that pregnancy outcomes can be dramatically improved if euglycemia is maintained both in the months preceding conception and throughout the pregnancy. Therefore female adolescents at risk for pregnancy or contemplating pregnancy should receive preconception counseling.

Male adolescents often express concern about the well-known complication of impotence in adult men. Impotence is thought to be a result of both vascular and neurologic compromise in those with longstanding diabetes. Fortunately, impotence caused by diabetes is very rare in adolescence, so most of these individuals can be reassured.

Transition to Adulthood

The challenges of making the transition to adulthood may be more complex for adolescents with type 1 diabetes because of the extraordinary demands of diabetes self-management on the adolescent and the family. Wysocki, Hough, Ward, and associates (1992) found that older adolescents had worse adjustment to diabetes and metabolic control than younger children. In addition, difficulties in adjustment in early adolescence tended to persist into young adulthood. Additional studies have suggested that young adults with type 1 diabetes have more difficulty with vocational adjustment and marital relationships (Bryden, Peveler, Stein, et al., 2001) than other young adults. Insabella, Grey, Knafl, and associates (2007) have recently shown that youths managed with flexible regimens following the DCCT findings have better outcomes in young adulthood compared with other youths. The care provided during this crucial time may be important for long-term quality of life.

Care provided in early adolescence with attention to improving psychosocial adjustment is just as important as providing quality transitional care. Little empirical work on the provision of care in the transition from adolescence to adulthood has been accomplished, but Court (1993) surveyed adolescents on their views about the transfer process from pediatric to adult care. Court found that adolescents value continuity of care by a provider they trust, as well as expect confidentiality and privacy, informality, and waiting rooms tailored to their needs. In addition, young adults and late adolescents may be less capable of insulin self-regulation than providers assume. Therefore transition to adult care must be designed to respect the wishes of these young adults and to support their assumption of self-care and development in their vocational and social roles.

Another concern of young adults is the increasing risk of complications. Dunning (1995) found that concerns about complications were common among young adults with diabetes and included concerns about eye disease, pregnancy and childbirth, hypoglycemia, and loss of independence. It is clear that these young adults need help implementing intensive regimens and self-care management styles that will help delay complications.

Studies of youths with type 2 diabetes transitioning to young adulthood are just beginning. Little is known about their care requirements or the process of transition.

Family Concerns

Families of children with type 1 diabetes worry about the appropriate assumption of self-care because of its importance in preventing long-term complications. Recommendations for understanding the developmental levels at which children should assume various self-care activities are available. There is, however, broad disagreement among professionals as to the appropriate age for management of skills (Wysocki, Meinhold, Cox, et al., 1990), and too-early assumption of self-management is associated with poorer psychological and metabolic outcomes. Therefore decisions about the assumption of self-care activities should be made with the family, child, and providers working together. Until more data on the effect of assuming self-care at different ages are available, providers' strict regulation of such activities may be unwarranted.

In studies of parental concerns in type 1 diabetes (Hauenstein, Marvin, Snyder, et al., 1989; Hodges & Parker, 1987), several issues are prominent: first is the adherence to the diabetes regimen—especially diet and the assumption of self-care; second is the question of genetics and inheritance. Parents frequently also express concerns about long-term complications and the risk of hypoglycemia. As noted earlier, the risk of severe hypoglycemia is three to four times greater in children on intensive treatment regimens. Parents may be more concerned about their child participating in sports, going on field trips, or spending the night at a friend's house if he or she is on an intensive treatment regimen.

Parents of very young children describe the care of these children as requiring "constant vigilance" to prevent the swings of blood glucose from high to low (Sullivan-Bolyai, Deatrick, Gruppuso, et al., 2003). These parents often feel isolated and overwhelmed initially, but eventually learn to manage the condition.

Guilt is often of concern to parents of children with type 1 diabetes, particularly because the condition may be inherited. Families must be provided with appropriate genetic counseling so that they are aware of the risks to other family members and to offspring of the individual with diabetes. Such information often helps to assuage the guilt present at diagnosis because the risk for first-degree relatives is low. The sibling of a child with type 1 diabetes has about a 5% to 10% risk, and an offspring of one parent with diabetes has about a 1% to 2% risk, as compared with a 0.05% risk for the general population. In the Diabetes Prevention Trial for type 1 diabetes, parents of at-risk youth were likely to engage in lifestyle management behaviors to prevent the development of diabetes

(Johnson, Baughcum, Hood, et al., 2007). The risk for type 2 diabetes is higher in families, with the risk as high as 50%.

Considerable attention has been paid to family problems and their effect on metabolic control in children with diabetes. Studies of the influence of family life on diabetes control have been inconclusive. Some families, however, exhibit psychosomatic characteristics that clearly have an adverse effect on the child with diabetes. Poorly functioning families have been shown to be associated with poorer metabolic control (Kovacs, Kass, Schnell, et al., 1989). Such families should be referred for family therapy.

Social issues (e.g., cultural differences) may also influence adaptation to diabetes in youths, but little work on these questions has been done with adolescents with type 1 diabetes. Delamater, Shaw, Appelgate, and associates (1999) found that minority children and adolescents had worse metabolic control than white children. Differences in metabolic control between these families may be because of cultural dietary factors (e.g., eating more foods that affect blood glucose swings or participating in less exercise). Because eating behaviors and participation in sports may be influenced by cultural values, families should be assessed for their beliefs and values about food and exercise.

Although some of these family issues may also be true for youths with type 2 diabetes, there has been limited research on these families. There are, however, studies that deal with the profound influence of the family on dietary and activity levels. Based on a comprehensive review of the literature on family determinants of health behavior, Sallis and Nadler (1988) concluded that physiologic and behavioral risk factors for chronic conditions such as obesity and hypertension, as well as behavioral patterns related to dietary intake and physical activity, are aggregated within families. Several studies have shown that having more than one overweight parent is closely tied to youthful obesity (Fisher & Birch, 1995; Klesges, Klesges, Eck, et al., 1995; Whitaker, Wright, Pepe, et al., 1997). Moreover, parents exert a powerful influence on their children's health behaviors, including those behaviors that put youths at risk for type 2 diabetes. Youths' dietary and activity patterns have been linked to the family environment (Dowda, Ainsworth, Addy, et al., 2001; Dunning, 1995; Fisher & Birch, 1995). In particular, parental control of the youth's diet and the parents' own eating behaviors have been associated with excess body fat in youth.

Resources

Two national organizations provide help for families coping with diabetes in a child: the American Diabetes Association (ADA) and the Juvenile Diabetes Research Foundation International (JDRFI) (see the list of organizations that follows). The ADA is the largest such organization, composed of both lay individuals and professionals. The ADA supports research, education, fundraising, and camps, and it provides lobbying efforts related to diabetes. It publishes several pamphlets and books for families to use in understanding diabetes. At the local level, many affiliates provide support and educational programs for families and children. The ADA deals with all types of diabetes, not only type 1 diabetes.

Research toward a cure for type 1 diabetes is the primary focus of the JDRFI. The organization does provide some support for families, but its major effort is devoted to fundraising for research to find a cure for type 1 diabetes. Some families find that working toward the cure helps them deal with the condition in their family.

Organizations

American Diabetes Association
1660 Duke St.
Alexandria, VA 22314
(800) ADA-DISC
Website: www.diabetes.org

Juvenile Diabetes Research Foundation International
120 Wall St.
New York, NY 10005-4001
(800) 533-CURE
Website: www.jdfcure.org

Relevant Websites

CDC Diabetes home page: www.cdc.gov/Diabetes
National Institute of Diabetes and Digestive and Kidney Disease (NIDDK): www.nih/niddk.gov

Children with Diabetes: www.childrenwithdiabetes.com
Diabetes Book Store: www.members.aol.com/ healthbook/diabetes
Diabetes Monitor: www.mdcc.com
KidsRPumping: www.members.aol.com/CamelsRFun/index.html
Insulin pumpers: www.insulin-pumpers.org/index.html/
Health; Diseases and Conditions; Diabetes: www.yahoo.com/Health/Diseases_and_Conditions/Diabetes

News and Chat Groups

misc.health.diabetes: This is the place to find people to talk with about diabetes.
alt.support.diabetes.kids: A support group for parents with children with diabetes.

Summary of Primary Care Needs for the Child with Diabetes Mellitus (Types 1 and 2)

HEALTH CARE MAINTENANCE

Growth and Development

- Height and weight are normal in type 1 unless diabetes control is less than adequate.
- Secondary sexual development may be delayed.
- Rapid weight gain may require intervention.
- Weight loss usually indicates poor control or insulin omission.
- Weight and body mass index (BMI) are elevated in type 2.
- Secondary sexual development may be accelerated in type 2 diabetes with hirsutism if polycystic ovaries are present.

Diet

- Maintenance of normoglycemia is critical.
- Stress the importance of regular distribution of meals and snacks.
- In type 1, sufficient calories for growth is paramount.
- In type 2, reduction in calories and fat is a cornerstone of treatment to reduce obesity.
- Physical activity is encouraged in type 1 with modification of insulin as needed.
- Increasing aerobic capacity while decreasing sedentary behaviors is the focus in children with type 2 diabetes.
- Celiac disease is more common in children with type 1 disbetes.

Safety

- Prevent hypoglycemia with careful monitoring; be sure a glucose source is always available.
- Dispose of syringes properly.
- Use glucagon for severe hypoglycemic episodes.
- Ensure safe storage of oral medications.
- A medical identification bracelet should be worn to ensure appropriate prompt treatment.

Immunizations

- Routine immunizations are recommended.
- Yearly influenza vaccine is recommended.

Screening

- *Vision.* Check red reflex and perform funduscopic examination at each visit.
- A thorough pediatric ophthalmologic examination yearly for 3-5 years or longer in children with diabetes ages 10 and older. In type 2 diabetes, examination should occur at diagnosis and yearly.
- Cataracts are possible at diagnosis.
- *Hearing.* Routine screening is recommended.
- *Dental.* Routine screening is recommended. Poor metabolic control can lead to increased cavities and gingivitis.
- *Blood pressure.* Blood pressure and orthostatic variation should be checked at each visit. Hypertension should be aggressively managed.
- *Hematocrit.* Routine screening is recommended.
- *Urinalysis.* Perform urinalysis yearly for ketones, glucose, and protein determinations; after 5 years screen for microalbuminuria yearly. Youths with type 2 diabetes should be screened at diagnosis and yearly.
- *Tuberculosis.* Routine screening is recommended.

Condition-Specific Screening

- Lipid screening should be done yearly after 10 years of age or earlier if other risk factors are present.
- Hemoglobin A_{1c} levels should be checked every 3 months by the diabetes treatment team.
- Perform thyroid function studies at diagnosis, yearly, and if a change in growth patterns occurs or symptoms of hypothyroidism develop.
- Screen for celiac disease if symptoms are present.
- Screen youths with type 2 diabetes for nonalcoholic fatty liver disease.
- Screening for depression has been recommended for children and adolescents 8 years or older.
- Perform other studies as indicated.

Continued

Summary of Primary Care Needs for the Child with Diabetes Mellitus (Types 1 and 2)—cont'd

COMMON ILLNESS MANAGEMENT

Differential Diagnosis

- Common illnesses and stress requires "sick day" management.
- It is important to maintain hydration during illness.
- It is most important to evaluate for hypoglycemia with changes in mental status.
- Monilial vaginal infections are more common in adolescent females.
- Skin lesions must be evaluated.
- Weight loss in type 1 diabetes and weight gain in type 2 diabetes may indicate poor metabolic control.
- Diabetic gastroparesis may cause vomiting or abdominal pain.

Drug Interactions

- Beware that many over-the-counter (OTC) medications and antibiotics contain glucogenic substances or alcohol.

DEVELOPMENTAL ISSUES

Sleep Patterns

- Prevention of nighttime hypoglycemia is important.
- Nightmares may be the result of hypoglycemia.

Toileting

- Enuresis may be present when control is poor.
- Measurement of urinary ketones is important when blood glucose levels are high or when the child is ill.

Discipline

- Unruly behavior may be caused by hypoglycemia.
- The potential for conflict over diet, blood testing, and insulin administration should be recognized.
- Stress associated with discipline should not elevate blood glucose.

Child Care

- Teachers and babysitters need training in management of dietary needs and hypoglycemia.

Schooling

- Full attendance and participation are expected.
- School personnel must be aware of the child's special needs.
- If metabolic control is poor, performance may be affected.

Sexuality

- If diabetes is adequately controlled, sexual development should be normal.
- Pregnancy prevention is very important because of combined risks of diabetes and adolescent pregnancy.
- Low-dose estrogen combination oral contraceptives are recommended because of the risk for complications with birth control pills (BCPs) or oral contraceptives containing estrogen.
- Pregnancy outcomes are dramatically improved if euglycemia is maintained preceding and during pregnancy.
- Impotency caused by long-term vascular and neurologic compromise is a rare problem during adolescence.
- Type 2 diabetes is associated with polycystic ovary syndrome.
- Depression and psychosocial adjustment problems may be present.

Transition to Adulthood

- Challenges in the transition to adulthood may be more complex for adolescents with type 1 diabetes because of the extraordinary demands of the disease self-management.

FAMILY CONCERNS

- Assumption of self-care activities and adherence to the regimen are prime concerns.
- Parents often experience guilt about the inheritance of type 1 diabetes.
- Minority children and children from single-parent homes are at highest risk for poor metabolic control.
- Minority children and adolescents tend to have worse metabolic control than white children and adolescents. Differences in metabolic control may be from cultural dietary factors or participation in less exercise, both of which may be influenced by cultural values.
- Food preferences and adiposity are associated with family eating and activity patterns. Families should be encouraged to adopt healthy eating and activity behaviors.
- Depression, anxiety, and psychosocial difficulties are not uncommon in children and adolescents with diabetes.

REFERENCES

Ahern, J.H., Boland, E.A., Doane, R., et al. (2002). Insulin pump therapy in pediatrics: A therapeutic alternative to safely lower HbA$_{1c}$ levels across all age groups. *Pediatr Diabetes, 3,* 10-15.

Althius, M.D., Jordon, N.E., Ludington, E.A., et al. (2002). Glucose and insulin responses to dietary chromium supplements: A meta-analysis. *Am J Clin Nutr, 72,* 148-155.

American Diabetes Association (1993). Position statement: Implications of the Diabetes Control and Complications Trial. *Diabetes, 42,* 1555-1558.

American Diabetes Association (1999). Clinical practice recommendations 1999. *Diabetes Care, 22*(Suppl 1), S1-S114.

American Diabetes Association (2000). Type 2 diabetes in children and adolescents. *Diabetes Care, 23,* 381-389.

American Diabetes Association. (2008a). Clinical practice recommendations. *Diabetes Care, 25*(Suppl 1), entire issue.

American Diabetes Association. (2008b). *Diabetes facts.* Available at www.diabetes.org Retrieved February 23, 2008.

Anderson, B.J., Brackett, G., Ho, J., et al. (1999). An office-based intervention to maintain parent-adolescent teamwork in diabetes management. *Diabetes Care, 22,* 713-721.

Attia, N., Jones, T.W., Holcombe, J., et al. (1998). Comparison of human regular and lispro insulins after interruption of continuous subcutaneous insulin infusion and the treatment of acutely decompensated IDDM. *Diabetes Care, 21,* 817-821.

Bailey, T.S., Zisser, H.C., & Garg, S.K. (2007). Reduction in hemoglobin A$_{1c}$ with real-time continuous glucose monitoring: Results from a 12-week observational study. *Diabetes Technol Ther, 9,* 203-210.

Bingley, P.J., Bonfacio, E., & Gale, E.A.M. (1993). Can we really predict IDDM?. *Diabetes, 42*, 213-220.

Blanz, B.J., Rensech-Riemann, B.S., Fritz-Sigmund, D.I., et al. (1993). IDDM is a risk factor for adolescent psychiatric disorders. *Diabetes Care, 16*, 1579-1587.

Boland, E.A., Grey, M., Oesterle, A., et al. (1999). Continuous subcutaneous insulin infusion: A new way to achieve strict metabolic control and lower the risk of severe hypoglycemia in adolescents. *Diabetes Care, 22*(11), 1779-1784.

Boland, E.A., Monsod, T., Delucia, M., et al. (2001). Limitations of conventional methods of self-monitoring of blood glucose: Lessons learned from three days of continuous glucose sensing in pediatric patients with type 1 diabetes. *Diabetes Care, 24*, 1858-1862.

Borg, H., Gottsater, A., Landin-Olsson, M., et al. (2001). High levels of antigen-specific islet antibodies predict future beta-cell failure in patients with onset of diabetes in adult age. *J Clin Endocrinol Metab, 86*, 3032-3038.

Bryden, K.S., Peveler, R.C., Stein, A., et al. (2001). Clinical and psychological course of diabetes from adolescence to young adulthood: A longitudinal cohort study. *Diabetes Care, 24*, 1536-1540.

Buckingham, B.A., Paguntalan, H., Fassl, B., et al. (2001). Continuous subcutaneous insulin infusion (CSII) in children under five years of age. *Diabetes, 50*(Suppl 2), A107.

Caldwell, M.B., Brownell, K.D., & Wilfley, D.E. (1997). Relationship of weight, body dissatisfaction, and self-esteem in African American and white female dieters. *Int J Eat Disord, 22*, 127-130.

Callahan, S.T., & Mansfield, M.J. (2000). Type 2 diabetes in adolescents. *Curr Opin Pediatr, 12*, 310-315.

Clarke, P., Gray, A., Adler, A., et al. (2001). United Kingdom Prospective Diabetes Study. Cost-effectiveness analysis of intensive blood-glucose control with metformin in overweight patients with type II diabetes. *Diabetologia, 44*, 298-304.

Court, J.M. (1993). Issues of transition to adult care. *J Pediatr Child Health, 29*(Suppl 1), S53-S55.

Danne, T., Lange, K., & Kordonouri, O. (2007). New developments in the treatment of type 1 diabetes in children. *Arch Dis Child, 92*, 1015-1019.

Dean, H.J., & Sellers, E.A.C. (2007). Comorbidities and microvascular complications of type 2 diabetes in children and adolescents. *Pediatr Diabetes, 8*(Suppl 9), 35-41.

Delamater, A.M., Shaw, K.H., Appelgate, E.B., et al. (1999). Risk for metabolic control problems in minority youth with diabetes. *Diabetes Care, 22*, 700-705.

Diabetes Control and Complications Trial Research Group. (1993a). Expanded role of the dietitian in the DCCT: Implications for clinical practice. *J Am Diet Assoc, 93*, 758-767.

Diabetes Control and Complications Trial Research Group. (1993b). The effect of intensive treatment of diabetes on the development and progression of long-term complications in insulin-dependent diabetes mellitus. *N Engl J Med, 329*, 435-459.

Diabetes Control and Complications Trial Research Group (1994). Effect of intensive diabetes treatment on the development and progression of long-term complications in adolescents with insulin-dependent diabetes mellitus: DCCT. *J Pediatr, 125*, 177-188.

Diabetes Control and Complications Trial Research Group (1995). Adverse events and their association with treatment regimens in the Diabetes Control and Complications Trial. *Diabetes Care, 18*, 1415-1427.

DirecNet Study Group. (2003a). The accuracy of the CGMS in children with type 1 diabetes: Results of the diabetes research in children network (DirecNet) accuracy study. *Diabetes Technol Ther, 5*, 781-789.

DirecNet Study Group. (2003b). The accuracy of the Glucowatch G biographer in children with type 1 diabetes: Results of the diabetes research in children network (DirecNet) accuracy study. *Diabetes Technol Ther, 5*, 791-800.

DirecNet Study Group. (2005). Accuracy of the modified Continuous Glucose Monitoring System (CGMS) sensor in an outpatient setting: Results from the diabetes research in children network (DirecNet) study. *Diabetes Technol Thera, 7*, 109-114.

DirecNet Study Group. (2007a). Continuous glucose monitoring in children with type 1 diabetes. *J Pediatr, 151*, 388-393.

DirecNet Study Group. (2007b). The accuracy of the Freestyle Navigator continuous glucose monitoring system in children with type 1 diabetes. *Diabetes Care, 30*, 59-64.

Dowda, M., Ainsworth, B.E., Addy, C.L., et al. (2001). Environmental influences, physical activity, and weight status in 8- to 16-year-olds. *Arch Pediatr Adolesc Med, 155*, 711-717.

Dunn, F.L., Nathan, D.M., Scavini, M., et al. (1997). The implantable insulin pump trial study group. *Diabetes Care, 20*, 59-63. 1997.

Dunning, P.L. (1995). Young-adult perspectives of insulin-dependent diabetes. *Diabetes Educ, 21*, 58-65.

Epstein, L.H., Wing, R.R., Penner, B.C., et al. (1985). A comparison of lifestyle exercise, aerobic exercise, and calisthenics on weight loss in obese children. *Behav Ther, 16*, 345-356.

Fagot-Campagna, A., Pettitt, O.J., Engelgau, M.M., et al. (2000). Type 2 diabetes among North American children and adolescents: An epidemiologic review and a public health perspective. *J Pediatr, 136*, 664-672.

Falkner, N.H., Neumark-Sztainer, D., Story, M., et al. (2001). Social, educational, and psychological correlates of weight status in adolescents. *Obesity Res, 9*, 32-42.

Fisher, J., & Birch, L. (1995). Fat preferences and fat consumption of 3- to 5-year-old children are related to parental adiposity. *J Am Diet Assoc, 95*, 759-764.

Fox, L., Buckloh, L.M., Smith, S.D., et al. (2005). A randomized controlled trial of insulin pump therapy in young children with type 1 diabetes. *Diabetes Care, 28*, 1277-1281.

Fox, L., Dontchev, M., Ruedy, K. , et al., for the DirecNet Study Group (2007). Relative inaccuracy of the A1cNow in children with diabetes. *Diabetes Care, 30*(1), 135-137.

Gandrud, L.M., Xing, D., Kollman, C., et al. (2007). The Medtronic MiniMed Gold continuous glucose monitoring system: An effective means to discover hypo- and hyperglycemia in children under 7 years of age. *Diabetes Technol Ther, 9*, 307-316.

Garg, S., Zisser, H., Schwartz, S., et al. (2006). Improvement in glycemic excursions with a transcutaneous, real-time continuous glucose sensor: A randomized controlled trial. *Diabetes Care, 29*, 44-50.

Gilliam, L.K., Liese, A.D., Block, C.A. et al., the SEARCH for Diabetes in Youth Study Group (2007). Family history of diabetes, autoimmunity, and risk factors of cardiovascular disease among children with diabetes in the SEARCH for Diabetes in Youth Study. *Pediatr Diabetes, 8*, 354-361.

Glaser, N.S. (1997). Non-insulin-dependent diabetes mellitus in childhood and adolescence. *Pediatr Clin North Am, 44*, 307-333.

Glasgow, R.E., Fisher, E.B., Anderson, B.J., et al. (1999). Behavioral science in diabetes. Contributions and opportunities. *Diabetes Care, 22*(5), 832-843.

Goldstein, D.E., Little, R.R., Lorenz, R.A., et al. (1995). Tests of glycemia in diabetes (technical review). *Diabetes Care, 18*, 896-909.

Goldston, D.B., Kelley, A.E., Reboussin, D.M., et al. (1997). Suicidal ideation and behavior and noncompliance with the medical regimen among diabetic adolescents. *J Am Acad Child Adolesc Psychiatry, 36*, 1528-1536.

Goldston, D.B., Kovacs, M., Ho, V.Y., et al. (1994). Suicidal ideation and suicide attempts among youth with insulin-dependent diabetes mellitus. *J Am Acad Child Adolesc Psychiatry, 33*, 240-246.

Grey, M., Berry, D., Davidson, M., et al. (2004). Preliminary testing of a program to prevent type 2 diabetes in high-risk youth. *J School Health, 74*, 10-15.

Grey, M., Boland, E.A., Davidson, M., et al. (2000). Coping skills training has long-lasting effects on metabolic control and quality of life in adolescents on intensive therapy. *J Pediatr, 137*, 107-113.

Grey, M., & Tamborlane, W.V. (2003). Behavioral and family aspects of treatment of children and adolescents with type 1 diabetes. D. porte, R.S.Sherwin, & A.Baron (Eds.), *Ellenberg and Rifkins Diabetes Mellitus.*, New York: McGraw-Hill.

Halvorson, M., Carpenter, S., Kaiserman, K., et al. (2007). A pilot trial in pediatrics with the sensor-augmented pump: Combining real-time continuous glucose monitoring with the insulin pump. *J Pediatr, 150*, 103-105.

Hauenstein, E.J., Marvin, R.S., Snyder, A.L., et al. (1989). Stress in parents of children with diabetes mellitus. *Diabetes Care, 12*, 18-23.

Hodges, L.C., & Parker, J. (1987). Concerns of parents with diabetic children. *Pediatr Nurs, 13*, 22-24.

Insabella, G., Grey, M., Knafl, G., et al. (2007). The transition to young adulthood in youth with type 1 diabetes on intensive treatment. *Pediatr Diabetes, 8*, 228-234.

Johnson, S.B., Baughcum, A.E., Hood, K., et al., & DPT-1 Study Group (2007). Participant and parent experiences in the parenteral insulin arm of the diabetes prevention trial for type 1 diabetes. *Diabetes Care, 30*, 2193-2198.

Jones, K.L. (2002). Treatment of type 2 diabetes mellitus in children. *J Am Med Assoc, 287*, 716.

Jones, K.L., Arslanian, S., Peterokova, V.A., et al. (2002). Effect of metformin in pediatric patients with type 2 diabetes: A randomized controlled trial. *Diabetes Care, 25*, 89-94.

Klesges, R.C., Klesges, L.M., Eck, L.H., et al. (1995). A longitudinal analysis of accelerated weight gain in preschool children. *Pediatrics, 95*, 126-130.

Kolody, B., & Sallis, J.F. (1995). A prospective study of ponderosity, body image, self-concept, and psychological variables in children. *J Dev Behav Pediatr, 16*, 1-5.

Kovacs, M., Goldston, D., Obrosky, D.S., et al. (1997). Psychiatric disorders in youth with IDDM: Rates and risk factors. *Diabetes Care, 20*, 36-44.

Kovacs, M., Kass, R.E., Schnell, T.M., et al. (1989). Family functioning and metabolic control of school-aged children with type 1 diabetes. *Diabetes Care, 12*, 409-414.

Kumar, A., Weatherly, M., & Beaman, D.C. (1991). Sweeteners, flavorings, and dyes in antibiotic preparations. *Pediatrics, 87*, 352-360.

Kyngas, H., & Barlow, J. (1995). Diabetes: An adolescent's perspective. *J Adv Nurs, 22*, 941-947.

Leslie, D.G., & Elliot, R.G. (1994). Early environmental events as a cause of IDDM: Evidence and implications. *Diabetes, 43*, 843-850.

Liss, D.S., Waller, D.A., Kennard, B.D., et al. (1998). Psychiatric illness and family support in children and adolescents with diabetic ketoacidosis: A controlled study. *J Am Assoc Child Adolesc Psychiatry, 37*, 536-544.

Ludwig, D.S., & Ebbeling, C.B. (2001). Type 2 diabetes mellitus in children: Primary care and public health considerations. *J Am Med Assoc, 286*, 1427-1430.

McGrady, A., Bailey, B.K., & Good, M.P. (1991). Controlled study of biofeedback-assisted relaxation in type 1 diabetes. *Diabetes Care, 14*, 360-365.

McMurray, R.G., Bauman, M.J., Harrell, J.S., et al. (2000). Effects of improvement in aerobic power on resting insulin and glucose concentrations in children. *Eur J Appl Physiol, 81*, 132-139.

Meneghini, L.F. (2007). Impact of bariatric surgery on type 2 diabetes. *Cell Biochemistry and Biophysics, 48*, 97-102.

Philip, M., Baltelino, T., Rodriguez, H., et al. (2007). Use of insulin pump therapy in the pediatric age group: Consensus statement from the European Society for Pediatric Endocrinology, the Lawson Wilkins Pediatric Endocrine Society, and the International Society for Pediatric and Adolescent Diabetes, endorsed by the American Diabetes Association and the European Association for the Study of Diabetes. *Diabetes Care, 30*, 1653-1662.

Pihoker, C., Scott, C.R., Lensing, S.Y., et al. (1998). Non-insulin dependent diabetes mellitus in African-American youth of Arkansas. *Clin Pediatr, 37*, 97-102.

Pinhas-Hamiel, O., & Zeitler, P. (2007). Clinical presentation and treatment of type 2 diabetes in children. *Pediatr Diabetes, 8*(Suppl 9), 16-27.

Pollock, M., Kovacs, M., & Charron-Prochownik, D. (1995). Eating disorders and maladaptive dietary/insulin management among youths with childhood-onset insulin dependent diabetes mellitus. *Am Acad Child Adolesc Psychiatry, 34*, 291-296.

Polonsky, W.H., Anderson, B.J., Lohrer, P.A., et al. (1994). Insulin omission in women with IDDM. *Diabetes Care, 17*, 1178-1185.

Rewers, A., Klingensmith, G., Davis, C., et al. (2008). Presence of diabetic ketoacidosis at diagnosis of diabetes mellitus in youth: The search for diabetes in youth study. *Pediatrics, 121*, e1258-e1266.

Sallis, J., & Nader, P. (1988). Family determinants of health behavior. In D. Gochman (Ed.), *Health Behavior: Emerging Research Perspectives.* New York: Plenum.

SEARCH Study Group. (2004). SEARCH for diabetes in youth: A multicenter study of the prevalence, incidence, and classification of diabetes in youth. *Clin Trials, 25*, 458-471.

Shapiro, A.M., Ricordi, C., Hering, B.J., et al. (2006). International trial of the Edmonton protocol for islet transplantation. *N Engl J Med, 355*(13), 1318-1330.

Shaw, J. (2007). Epidemiology of childhood type 2 diabetes and obesity. *Pediatr Diabetes, 8*(Suppl 9), 7-15.

Silverstein, J., Klingensmith, G., Copeland, K., et al., & American Diabetes Association, (2005). Care of children and adolescents with type 1 diabetes: A statement of the American Diabetes Association. *Diabetes Care, 28*(1), 186-212.

Siminerio, L.M., Charron-Prochownik, D., Banion, C., et al. (1999). Comparing outpatient and inpatient diabetes education for newly diagnosed pediatric patients. *Diabetes Educ, 25*(6), 895-906.

Sinha, R., Fisch, G., Teague, B., et al. (2002). Prevalence of impaired glucose tolerance among children and adolescents with marked obesity. *N Engl J Med, 346*, 802-810.

Steil, G.M., Rebrin, K., Darwin, C., et al. (2006). Feasibility of automating insulin delivery for the treatment of type 1 diabetes. *Diabetes, 55*, 3344-3350.

Stolley, M.R., & Fitzgibbon, M.L. (1997). Effects of an obesity prevention program on the eating behavior of African American mothers and daughters. *Health Educ Behav, 24*, 152-164.

Strauss, R.S. (2000). Childhood obesity and self-esteem. *Pediatrics, 105*, E15-E25.

Striegel-Moore, R.H., Nicholson, T.J., & Tamborlane, W.V. (1992). Prevalence of eating disorder symptoms in preadolescent and adolescent girls with type 1 diabetes. *Diabetes Care, 15*, 1361-1368.

Sullivan-Bolyai, S., Deatrick, J., Gruppuso, P., et al. (2003). Constant vigilance: Mothers' work parenting young children with type 1 diabetes. *J Pediatr Nurs, 18*(1), 21-29.

Sutherland, D.E.R., & Gruessner, R.W.G. (1997). Current status of pancreas transplantation for the treatment of type 1 diabetes mellitus. *Clin Diabetes, 15*, 152-156.

Thompson, J.K., Coovert, M.D., Richards, K.J., et al. (1995). Development of body image, eating disturbance, and general psychological functioning in female adolescents: Covariance structure modeling and longitudinal investigations. *Int J Eat Disord, 18*, 221-236.

The TOD[2]AY Study Group, Zeitler, P., Epstein, L. et al. (2007). Treatment options for type 2 diabetes in adolescents and youth: A study of the comparative efficacy of metformin alone or in combination with rosiglitazone or lifestyle intervention in adolescents with type 2 diabetes. *Pediatr Diabetes, 8*(2), 74-87.

Tubiana-Rufi, N., de Lonlay, P., Bloch, J., et al. (1996). Remission of severe hypoglycemia incidents in young diabetic children treated with subcutaneous infusion. *Arch Pediatr, 3*, 969-976.

Upchurch, S.L., Anding, R., & Brown, S.A. (1999). Promoting weight loss in persons with type 2 diabetes: What do we know about the most effective dietary approaches? *Practical Diabetology, 18*(9), 22-28.

Weinzimer, S.A., Ahern, J.H., Doyle, E.A., et al. (2004). Persistence of benefits of continuous subcutaneous insulin infusion in very young children with type 1 diabetes: A follow-up report. *Pediatrics, 114*, 1601-1605.

Weinzimer, S.A., Steil, G.M., Swan, K.L., et al. (2008). Fully automated closed-loop insulin delivery vs. semi-automated hybrid control in pediatric patients with type 1 diabetes using an artificial pancreas. *Diabetes Care, 31*, 934-939.

Weiss, R. (2007). Impaired glucose tolerance and risk factors for progression to type 2 diabetes in youth. *Pediatr Diabetes, 8*(Suppl 9), 70-75.

Whitaker, R.C., Wright, J.A., Pepe, M.S., et al. (1997). Predicting obesity in young adulthood from childhood and parental obesity. *N Engl J Med, 337*, 869-873.

Wilson, D.M., Buckingham, B.A., Kunsekman, E.L., et al. (2005). A two-center randomized controlled feasibility trial of insulin pump therapy in young children with diabetes. *Diabetes Care, 28*, 15-19.

Wysocki, T., Hough, B.S., Ward, K.M., et al. (1992). Diabetes mellitus in the transition to adulthood: Adjustment, self-care, and health status. *Dev Behav Pediatr, 13*, 194-201.

Wysocki, T., Meinhold, P., Cox, D.J., et al. (1990). Survey of diabetes professionals regarding developmental changes in diabetes self-care. *Diabetes Care, 13*, 65-68.

Young-Hyman, D., Schlundt, D.G., Herman, L., et al. (2001). Evaluation of insulin resistance syndrome in 5- to 10-year-old overweight/obese African American children. *Diabetes Care, 24*, 1359-1364.

Zisser, H., & Jovanovic, L. (2006). Omnipod Insulin Management System: Patient perceptions, preference, and glycemic control. *Diabetes Care, 29*, 2175.

24 Down Syndrome

Wendy M. Nehring

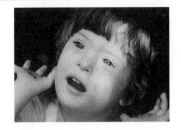

Etiology

Down syndrome, which was first described by Jean Etienne Esquirol in 1838 and promulgated by John Langdon Down in 1866, is a condition that is associated with a recognizable phenotype and limited intellectual endowment because of extra chromosome 21 material. It is the most frequent autosomal chromosomal anomaly and the primary chromosomal cause of intellectual and developmental disabilities. Chromosome 21 was the initial chromosome to be completely mapped with the deoxyribonucleic acid (DNA) sequence fully determined (Hattori, Fujiyama, Taylor, et al., 2000). The long arm of chromosome 21 contains over 400 genes, but it is a subset of these genes that have been implicated in Down syndrome. It has been designated the "Down syndrome critical region" located at 21q22 to qter. However, even though this critical region has been identified, until the functions of each of the genes and proteins are understood, the pathology of Down syndrome remains unknown.

Nondisjunction

Nondisjunction of chromosome 21 is responsible for the majority of cases (approximately 95%) of trisomic Down syndrome, with approximately 90% of maternal meiotic origin; this form is not inherited (Roizen, 2007). Nondisjunction (i.e., the uneven division of chromosomes) can occur during anaphase 1 or 2 in meiosis (i.e., reduction and division of germ cells) or in anaphase of mitosis (i.e., somatic cell division). In nondisjunction, the pair of chromosomes fails to separate and migrate properly during cell division. When this occurs in meiosis, the haploid number for the respective daughter cells is unequal. If the cell receiving 24 rather than 23 chromosomes is fertilized, a trisomic zygote results (Figure 24-1). Mosaicism, though associated with fewer phenotypic features and defined by the presence of a percentage of cell lines with trisomy 21, is also most often caused by maternal mitotic nondisjunction (see Figure 24-1) (Lashley, 2005; Roizen, 2007).

The recurrence risk for nondisjunction Down syndrome is approximately 1%. For older mothers, the risk is 1% plus the percentage of risk for chronologic age (Tolmie, 2002).

Translocation

In Down syndrome caused by translocation (approximately 4% to 5% of cases), there are also three copies of chromosome 21. The third copy does not occur independently, however, but is attached to another chromosome—usually to one of the D or G group. Robertsonian translocations, where the long arms of chromosome 21 attach to the long arms of chromosome 14, 21, or 22, are the most common translocations, although other forms can occur (Lashley, 2005; Roizen, 2007).

The total chromosome count in Down syndrome is 46, even though material for 47 chromosomes is present. Although the phenotype for Down syndrome caused by translocation is the same as that for nondisjunction, the inheritance pattern is quite different. With translocation, the disorder may recur in future pregnancies. If one parent has 45 chromosomes—including a translocation of chromosome 21—the gametes produced could result in a trisomic zygote. Although six combinations are theoretically possible, three are nonviable. Of the three that are viable, one is normal (i.e., $N = 46$), one results in a balanced translocation (i.e., $N = 45$), and one is an unbalanced translocation resulting in Down syndrome (i.e., $N = 46$) (Figure 24-2). The recurrence risk for a second child with translocation Down syndrome (usually 14;21) is approximately 10% at the lowest probable maternal age and very low for the mother older than 35 years. If the translocation carrier is the father, the risk is approximately 5% (Aitken, Crossley, & Spencer, 2002; Tolmie, 2002). If the translocation involves both copies of chromosome 21 (21;21), the recurrence risk is 100% (Aitken et al., 2002).

A variety of hypotheses as to the cause of Down syndrome have been offered over the years, including the following: (1) a genetic predisposition to nondisjunction; (2) autoimmunity; (3) hormonal alterations in aging women; (4) advanced age of the maternal grandmother; (5) environmental and chemical factors such as irradiation before conception, smoking, and drug exposure; (6) chromosomal damage; (7) gestational diabetes; and (8) frequency of coitus (Coppede, Colognato, Bonelli, et al., 2007; Malini & Ramachandra, 2006). No one factor has been confirmed, although new genetic findings suggest that the cause is probably multifactorial.

Incidence and Prevalence

The prevalence rate for Down syndrome is 1.3 per 1000 live births (Centers for Disease Control and Prevention, 2006), with the incidence rate at around 4000 children born each year with Down syndrome in the United States (National Dissemination Center for Children with Disabilities, 2004). Prenatal diagnosis of women of advanced maternal age explains this difference over time. Prevalence rates vary by inheritance pattern. Nondisjunction is found in the majority of Down syndrome conceptions. Approximately 90% of these cases are of maternal meiotic causation, with 75% of this number occurring at maternal meiosis I. Only about 8% of total cases of nondisjunction are of paternal origin. Translocation occurs in about 4% to 5% of cases, and mosaicism occurs in approximately 2% of cases (Roizen, 2007).

Down syndrome caused by translocation is independent of parental age. The incidence is also stable across age cohorts, although one third of the cases of translocation Down syndrome are inherited from parents (Tolmie, 2002).

For women in their early twenties, the incidence of having a child with Down syndrome is approximately 1 in every 1667

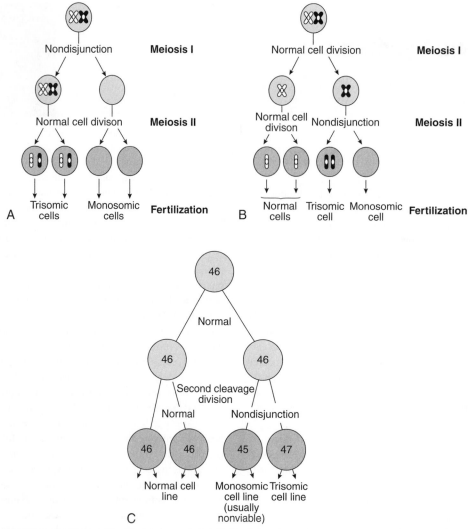

FIGURE 24-1 A, Nondisjunction during meiosis I. **B,** Nondisjunction during meiosis II. **C,** Nondisjunction following fertilization, during mitosis, resulting in mosaicism. From Hockenberry, M.J. (2002). *Wong's Nursing Care of Infants and Children* (7th ed.). St. Louis: Mosby.

births. The incidence rises gradually until maternal age surpasses 35 years and then climbs to approximately 1 in every 30 live births for 45-year-old women (Hecht & Hook, 1996). Advanced paternal age (i.e., age 55 years and older) has also been shown to affect the incidence of nondisjunction Down syndrome (Lashley, 2005). Although the extra chromosome is paternal in origin, nondisjunction still occurs after fertilization. Because an overwhelming percentage of cases of Down syndrome are caused by nondisjunction, parental age directly affects the overall incidence (Figure 24-3).

Down syndrome is found in all races and ethnic groups. Although the incidence rates of Down syndrome vary little among whites, blacks, and Hispanic infants born to mothers under 35 years of age, rates are significantly higher in Hispanic infants and moderately higher in black infants born to mothers over 35 years of age. Differences in these rates may reflect differences in early prenatal care, prenatal diagnosis, and views on abortion (Khoshnood, Pryde, & Wall, 2000).

Diagnostic Criteria

Down syndrome is most often diagnosed through karyotyping of fetal cells after chorionic villus sampling or amniocentesis after positive screening results (Palomaki, Bradley, McDowell, et al., 2005). Karyotyping can also be done postnatally if either the prenatal screening produced a false-negative result or no prenatal screening or testing was done. In such cases with infants of color or those born very prematurely, diagnosis may be delayed because the clinical features may not be as clearly recognized. Although more than 50 physical characteristics can be identified at birth, no one feature is considered diagnostic. Features vary in their expression and are not always present. Some of the most commonly associated features, however, include generalized hypotonia, brachycephaly, epicanthal folds, palpebral fissures, single transverse palmar creases, incurved fifth finger, neck skinfold, and widely spaced first and second toes.

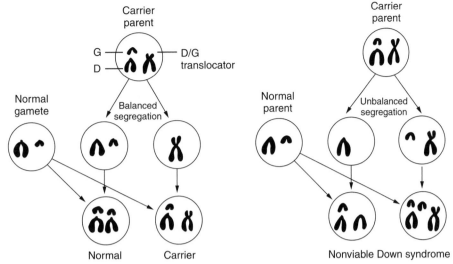

FIGURE 24-2 Possible zygotes from the union of a somatically normal carrier of D/G translocation and a genetically and somatically normal individual. From Wong, D.L., et al. (1999). *Whaley and Wong's Nursing Care of Infants and Children* (6th ed.). St. Louis: Mosby. Reprinted with permission.

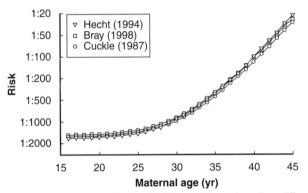

FIGURE 24-3 Age-specific risks for Down syndrome from three different studies. From Aitken, D.A., et al. (2002). Prenatal screening for neural tube defects and aneuploidy. In D.L. Rimoin et al. (Eds.), *Emory and Rimoin's Principles and Practices of Medical Genetics* (4th ed.). New York: Churchill Livingstone, pp. 763-801. Reprinted with permission.

Clinical Manifestations at Time of Diagnosis

A variety of congenital anomalies are commonly associated with Down syndrome. Congenital cardiac disease is seen in approximately 44% of children with Down syndrome, with endocardial cushion defects accounting for about 20% and septal defects making up another 19% of cardiac malformations (American Academy of Pediatrics [AAP], Committee on Genetics, 2001; Cohen, 1999). Gastrointestinal (GI) malformations are seen in 5% of children with Down syndrome; among the most common problems are duodenal or esophageal atresia, congenital megacolon (Hirschsprung disease), imperforate anus, tracheoesophageal fistula, and pyloric stenosis (Roizen & Patterson, 2003). Anomalies can usually be surgically corrected in the neonatal period. Although many children experience total correction of the anomaly, others will experience untoward sequelae throughout their lives.

Treatment

No treatment can eliminate the chromosomal defect that causes Down syndrome. Extensive interdisciplinary services and research over the last 45 years have, however, transformed society's view of children with Down syndrome and accepted treatment protocols. Accepted approaches include genetic counseling, prompt referral for surgical correction of congenital anomalies, prevention of secondary conditions, enrollment in an early intervention program, and inclusion from preschool through high school (ages 3 to 21 years).

Genetic Counseling

Pregnant women are given the option of prenatal screening. Current practice for the prenatal screening for Down syndrome consists of an ultrasound to measure nuchal translucency and maternal blood work for free beta human chorionic gonadotropin (β-hCG) and pregnancy-associated plasma protein (PAPP-A) at 11 to 13 weeks of gestation (American College of Obstetricians and Gynecologists, 2004; Lashley, 2007). Further blood work can be done during the second trimester, or diagnostic testing can be done. Cuckle, Malone, Wright, and colleagues (2008) suggest that first trimester positive results be diagnostically tested and those women with borderline results undergo further blood work for alpha-fetoprotein, hCG, inhibin, and unconjugated estriol (uE_3) at 15 to 18 weeks of gestation. Although this validation will not affect a child's treatment or prognosis, it has significant implications for the genetic counseling of family members. Because translocation is the cause of about 5% of cases, parents and siblings must be tested to determine their carrier status, as well as have the risk of recurrence in future pregnancies carefully explained to them. Researchers have recently explored the impact of ethnic differences (Fransen, Essink-Bot, Oenema, et al., 2007) and ethical beliefs (Garcia, Timmermans, & van Leeuwen, 2007) on prenatal screening decisions and provide suggestions for tailoring information given on prenatal screening.

Clinical Manifestations at Time of Diagnosis

SKULL
- False fontanel
- Flat occipital area
- Brachycephaly
- Separated sagittal suture
- Hypoplasia of midfacial bones
- Reduced interorbital distance
- Underdeveloped maxilla
- Obtuse mandibular angle

Eyes
- Oblique narrow palpebral fissures
- Epicanthal folds
- Brushfield spots
- Strabismus
- Nystagmus
- Myopia
- Hypoplasia of the iris

Ears
- Small, shortened ears
- Low and oblique implantation
- Overlapping helices
- Prominent antihelix
- Absent or attached earlobes
- Narrow ear canals
- External auditory meatus
- Structural aberrations of the ossicles
- Stenotic external auditory meatus

Nose
- Hypoplastic
- Flat nasal bridge
- Anteverted, narrow nares
- Deviated nasal septum

Mouth
- Prominent, thickened, and fissured lips
- Corners of the mouth turned downward
- High-arched, narrow palate
- Shortened palatal length
- Protruding, enlarged tongue
- Papillary hypertrophy (early preschool)
- Fissured tongue (later school years)
- Periodontal disease
- Partial anodontia
- Microdontia
- Abnormally aligned teeth
- Anterior open bite
- Mouth held open

NECK
- Short, broad neck
- Loose skin at nape

CHEST
- Shortened rib cage
- Twelfth rib anomalies
- Pectus excavatum or carinatum
- Congenital heart disease

ABDOMEN
- Distended and enlarged abdomen
- Diastasis recti
- Umbilical hernia
- Muscle tone and musculature
  - Hyperflexibility
  - Muscular hypotonia
  - Generalized weakness
- Integument
  - Skin appears large for the skeleton
  - Dry and rough
  - Fine, poorly pigmented hair

EXTREMITIES
- Short extremities
- Partial or complete syndactyly
- Clinodactyly
- Brachyclinodactyly

Upper Extremities
- Short, broad hands
- Brachyclinodactyly
- Single palmar transverse crease
- Incurved, short fifth finger
- Abnormal dermatoglyphics

Lower Extremities
- Short and stubby feet
- Gap between first and second toes
- Plantar crease between first and second toes
- Second and third toes grouped in a forklike position
- Radial deviation of the third to fifth toes

PHYSICAL GROWTH AND DEVELOPMENT
- Short stature
- Increased weight in later life

OTHER FINDINGS SEEN IN NEWBORNS
- Enlarged anterior fontanel
- Delayed closing of sutures and fontanels
- Open sagittal suture
- Nasal bone not ossified, underdeveloped
- Reduced birth weight

Treatment
- Genetic counseling
- Surgical correction of abnormalities
- Prevention or treatment of secondary conditions
- Early intervention programs
- Choosing appropriate educational settings (e.g., inclusion)

Surgery

Surgical corrections of most major cardiac, GI, and genitourinary anomalies are now performed routinely, although not without risk. The risk for upper airway compromise during and after surgery is increased in Down syndrome because of clinical features such as subglottic stenosis, smaller middle and lower face skeleton, adenoid and tonsil volume, tracheal stenosis, hypotonia, and a narrow nasopharyngeal inlet. Atlantoaxial instability also poses a surgical risk, and it is recommended that the necks of all children with Down syndrome, with or without normal cervical spine radiographs, should be treated carefully when undergoing surgical procedures. An endotracheal tube two sizes smaller than normal for the child's age should be used for children with Down syndrome (Cohen, 2006; Shott, 2006). Further, bradycardia, airway obstruction, and postextubation stridor (Borland, Colligan, & Brandom, 2004) are common, and a longer hospital stay is recommended for children with Down syndrome.

In addition to lifesaving surgeries, some children with Down syndrome also undergo plastic surgery to alter their phenotypic appearance. As these children continue to become more integrated into society, they may be stigmatized because of their physiognomy. Some parents, concerned about their child's social acceptance, seek plastic surgery for the child (e.g., partial glossectomies, neck resections, Silastic implants for the chin and nose, and reconstruction of dysplastic helices). Better articulation of speech, less mouth breathing, fewer and less severe upper respiratory tract infections, and improved mastication and swallowing may be realized, especially if a pathologic condition exists that warrants corrective surgery. The degree of success, however, may be small or nonexistent. There are surgical risks, surgery is expensive, and it is most often not covered by insurance. Any parents or children with Down syndrome wanting to undergo plastic surgery should talk at length with their primary care provider and surgeon before the procedure so that they understand the risks.

Prevention and Treatment of Secondary Conditions

Children with Down syndrome are susceptible to a number of secondary conditions, including but not limited to feeding problems, vision and hearing abnormalities, constipation, upper respiratory infections, thyroid disorders, and skin problems. Regular visits to the primary health care provider and a Down syndrome clinic, if available, and comprehensive anticipatory guidance can help prevent these problems. If they do occur, intervention and treatment can begin early. Referring the family to a support group composed of other families with a child with Down syndrome can also provide a means for information and support to prevent such conditions.

Early Intervention

Infant stimulation programs and continued early childhood education are designed to optimize a child's rate of development and minimize the amount of developmental lag that will occur between children with Down syndrome and their developmentally normal peers. Specific therapeutic exercises are devised to stimulate an infant's cognitive, social, motor, and language domains. These exercises are incorporated in the individualized family service plan (IFSP) that is mandated by the Individuals with Disabilities Education Improvement Act (IDEA) of 2004 (Public Law 108-446). Researchers have found motor and cognitive improvement in infants after their participation in an early intervention program (Crocker, 2006; Van Cleve & Cohen, 2006). Parents are usually taught these skills by special education teachers, physical therapists, occupational therapists, and speech pathologists so that therapy can be conducted at home. Timing seems to be a critical factor, however, with earlier interventions correlated with greater developmental gains. These children will later be referred to a specialized program designed to continue these intervention strategies and then integrated into generic child care or school (see Chapter 3).

Inclusion

With inclusion, children ages 3 to 21 years are included in the regular classroom, including preschool programs, under IDEA of 2004 (see Chapter 3). The individualized education program (IEP), developed by the child (if age appropriate), his or her parents, and an interdisciplinary team at the school, gives direction to the child's preferences, interests, and academic and developmental needs (Betz & Nehring, 2007). The primary health provider should be a part of this process.

Complementary and Alternative Therapies

Such therapies that have been reported to be used by children with Down syndrome are nutritional supplements, herbal therapies, massage therapy, and diet modifications (Prussing, Sobo, Walker, et al., 2005). Prussing and colleagues (2005) found that parents used such therapies to counteract illness and prevent secondary conditions. They also chose to use these therapies to enhance their child's well-being and development. Parents felt that by using these therapies, they were doing everything possible to assist their child. In another study (Prussing, Sobo, Walker, et al., 2004), parents indicated that they often did not inform their pediatricians about the use of complementary and alternative therapies with their children with Down syndrome.

Numerous other approaches (e.g., patterning, cell therapy, growth hormone, megavitamin therapy, combinations of enzymes, minerals, and vitamins, such as Haps Caps and NuTriVene-D) designed to improve the developmental outcomes of children with Down syndrome have been tried. Unfortunately, the results of these interventions have been disappointing. The drug piracetam, which some consider to be a cognitive enhancer, has received the most attention, but has never shown statistically significant positive findings (Roizen, 2005).

Anticipated Advances in Diagnosis and Management

Advances in Knowledge of Genetic Etiology or Treatment

Pregnant women must be aware of the screening options available to them (e.g. biochemical screening, ultrasound, chorionic villi sampling, amniocentesis). A variety of serum markers have been studied for their use in detecting Down syndrome. ADAM12s (a disintegrin and metalloprotease) is currently being explored as an early first trimester (before 10 weeks of gestation) marker for Down syndrome (Spencer, Cowans, Uldbjerg, et al., 2008; Spencer, Vereecken, & Cowans, 2008). Additional research is warranted with larger samples before recommendations can be made for general practice.

Associated Problems of Down Syndrome and Treatment

Intellectual and Developmental Disabilities

The intellectual capabilities of children with Down syndrome vary dramatically. Most of these children have moderate intellectual limitations (i.e., intelligence quotient [IQ] of 40 to 55, standard deviation [SD] of 15), but a small percentage are either mildly affected (i.e., IQ of 56 to 69, SD of 15) or severely impaired (i.e., IQ of 39, SD of 15). For a few children, their IQs are not consistent with a diagnosis of an intellectual and developmental disability. Known correlates to the intelligence and adaptive behavior skills of children are their physical condition, home environment, and individualized early intervention. Unfortunately, cognitive function often deteriorates with age, and significant

---

Associated Problems of Down Syndrome and Treatment

- Intellectual and developmental disabilities
- Cardiac defects
- Gastrointestinal tract anomalies
- Musculoskeletal and motor abilities
- Immune system deficiency
- Sensory deficits
- Vision problems
- Hearing loss
- Growth retardation
- Altered respiratory function
- Thyroid dysfunction
- Malignancies
  - Leukemia
  - Tumors
- Celiac disease
- Sleep-disordered breathing
- Skin conditions
- Dental changes
- Seizure disorders

---

losses in intelligence, memory, and social skills are seen earlier (i.e., often by age 40 years) than in persons without Down syndrome (Roizen, 2007).

Behavior disorders may also be present, such as social withdrawal, noncompliance, aggression, inattention, hyperactivity, or a thought disorder. It has been estimated that the prevalence of behavioral problems is 18% to 40% (Capone, Goyal, Ares, et al., 2006; Capone, Grados, Kaufmann, et al., 2005; Nicham, Weitzdorfer, Hauser, et al., 2003; Visootsak & Sherman, 2007). Depression, autistic-like behavior, and psychotic episodes have been reported. Neurologic deterioration, disturbed family life, and stress associated with inclusion may affect the mental health of children with Down syndrome.

Cardiac Defects

Approximately 44% of children with Down syndrome have congenital heart defects. In order of decreasing frequency, the most common heart anomalies include atrioventricular septal defect (i.e., endocardial cushion defect and atrioventricular canal defect), ventricular septal defect, patent ductus arteriosus, and atrial septal defect (see Chapter 21). Other heart or cardiac-associated conditions that may occur in Down syndrome include tetralogy of Fallot, polycythemia, and pulmonary artery hypertension (AAP, Committee on Genetics, 2001; Cohen, 1999). Folic acid taken by mothers during pregnancy was not found to protect against the incidence of cardiac anomalies in infants with Down syndrome (Meijer, Werler, Louik, et al., 2006). Vida and Castaneda (2006) speculate that geographic and ethnic factors may influence the incidence of cardiac defects in children with Down syndrome and call for further research to test this possibility.

Children with Down syndrome and cardiac defects requiring surgery also are at risk for developing subacute bacterial endocarditis (Van Cleve & Cohen, 2006). In addition, children with Down syndrome who do not have congenital heart disease are at risk for developing mitral valve prolapse with age; by the end of adolescence, mitral valve prolapse has been detected in more than 50% of the individuals tested (National Institute of Dental and Craniofacial

Research, 2007). The use of echocardiography and a cardiac evaluation during the newborn period has greatly enhanced detection rates, early management, and survival rates (Roizen, 2007).

Gastrointestinal Tract Anomalies

Common congenital GI tract anomalies include tracheoesophageal fistula, Hirschsprung disease, pyloric stenosis, duodenal atresia, annular pancreas, aganglionic megacolon, and imperforate anus, with duodenal atresia and imperforate anus occurring most commonly (Roizen & Patterson, 2003). Most of these anomalies require immediate surgical correction and careful follow-up throughout life.

Musculoskeletal and Motor Abilities

Orthopedic problems are second only to cardiac defects as a cause of morbidity in Down syndrome. Flaccid muscle tone and ligamentous laxity occur to some extent in all children with Down syndrome, possibly because of an intrinsic defect in their connective tissue (Concolino, Pasquzzi, Capalbo, et al., 2006). Among these conditions are pes planus, patellar subluxation, scoliosis, dislocated hips, atlantoaxial subluxation, joint and muscle pain, and rapid muscle fatigue. These problems may occur throughout a child's life, and the primary care provider should carefully screen for them at each visit.

Another significant disorder associated with Down syndrome is atlantoaxial instability. Atlantoaxial instability results from a "loose joint" between C1 and C2 and increased space between the atlas and odontoid process and affects approximately 15% of children with Down syndrome (Cohen, 2006; Nader-Sepahi, Casey, Hayward, et al., 2005). At least 98% to 99% of affected children are asymptomatic. Subluxation or dislocation may result, and early manifestations may include neck pain, torticollis, deteriorating gait, or changes in bowel or bladder function. If left untreated, symptoms may progress to frank neurologic findings associated with spinal cord compression, which occurs in about 2% of children and can be a life-threatening condition.

Immune System Deficiency

Children with Down syndrome have altered immune function. Immune system deficits directly contribute to the increased incidence and severity of numerous other conditions, including—but not limited to—periodontal disease, respiratory problems, thyroid disorders, lymphocytic thyroiditis, leukemia, diabetes mellitus, alopecia areata, adrenal dysfunction, vitiligo, and joint problems (Cohen, 2006; Roizen, 2007). Children with Down syndrome who also have type 1 diabetes have been found to have increased human leukocyte antigen (HLA) class II genotypes, which are indicative of islet autoimmunity. Further genetic studies are needed to explore the link between type 1 diabetes and chromosome 21 anomalies (Gillespie, Dix, Williams, et al., 2006).

Sensory Deficits

Vision Problems. An increased prevalence of numerous ocular deviations is associated with Down syndrome and occurs in approximately 60% of these children, with most experiencing more than one ocular problem. The most commonly occurring abnormalities are, in order of decreasing frequency, slanted palpebral fissures, spotted irises, refractive errors, strabismus, nystagmus, cataracts, blepharitis, pseudopapilledema, and keratoconus (Haargaard & Fledelius,

2006; Stephen, Dickson, Kindley, et al., 2007; Stewart, Woodhouse, Cregg, et al., 2007; Van Cleve & Cohen, 2006). A significant loss in visual acuity will result if many of these conditions are not diagnosed and treated in early childhood. Moreover, visual problems—especially refractive errors—increase with age (Stephen et al., 2007) and may interfere with cognitive development. Bianca and Bianca (2004) found an association between atrial septal defects and congenital cataract and nystagmus, as well as between severe congenital heart defects and myopia. Additional research is needed to verify these findings.

Hearing Loss. The incidence of hearing loss in children with Down syndrome is approximately 40% to 75%. Structural deviations of the skull, foreface, external auditory canal, middle and inner ears, and throat accompanied by eustachian tube dysfunction are associated with congenital and acquired hearing loss that can be sensorineural or conductive or both and occur unilaterally or bilaterally (Shott, 2006). Hearing loss may greatly affect speech and cognitive development if not treated promptly and correctly.

Growth Retardation

At birth, infants with Down syndrome weigh less, are typically shorter, and have smaller occipital-frontal circumferences than unaffected children. The velocity of linear growth is also reduced, with the most marked reductions between 6 and 24 months of age. This reduction in velocity recurs during adolescence, when the growth spurt—which is less vigorous than would normally be expected—occurs earlier in adolescents with Down syndrome (Roizen, 2007). Other causes for the reduction in linear growth may be congenital heart disease, hypothalamic dysfunctions, thyroid disorders, and nutrition problems, and each should be evaluated if suspected (Cohen, 1999).

Children with Down syndrome tend to be overweight. Beginning around 2 years of age, these children often have untoward weight gain that persists throughout their lives. For virtually every age, more than 30% of children with Down syndrome are above the 85th percentile for weight/height ratios, but some researchers have found this percentage to be as high as 50%. Children of school age show the greatest propensity for weight/height percentile gain (Cohen, 1999). In a study to develop growth charts for children with Down syndrome in Europe, it was found that European boys with Down syndrome are taller than their American counterparts, and European girls with Down syndrome are thinner than their American counterparts, but the girls are roughly the same weight (Myrelid, Gustafsson, Ollars, et al., 2002). Geographic and ethnic differences should continue to be studied.

Altered Respiratory Function

Combined with a compromised immune system, pulmonary hypertension and hyperplasia, fewer alveoli, a decreased alveolar blood capillary surface area, and associated upper airway obstruction (e.g., lymphatic hypertrophy in the Waldeyer ring) predispose children with Down syndrome to respiratory tract infections, as well as high-altitude pulmonary edema (Durmowicz, 2001). If recurrent severe respiratory tract infections occur, they will have a significant effect on a child's development. Bloemers, van Furth, Weijerman, and colleagues (2007) identified the presence of Down syndrome as a risk for respiratory syncytial virus (RSV) bronchiolitis and found that if children with this condition needed to be hospitalized, their conditions were much worse than other children. Prophylaxis for this condition should be considered for children with Down syndrome.

Thyroid Dysfunction

Thyroid dysfunction in Down syndrome is commonly associated with autoimmune dysfunction (Cohen, 2006) and occurs more often than in the general population. Cohen (2006) states that a screening algorithm is needed for appropriate treatment of thyroid disorders and ethnic differences must be considered. Thiel and Fowkes (2007) advocate for nutritional thyroid support over medications as a first step in treatment for children with Down syndrome who have identified thyroid dysfunction.

Malignancies

Leukemia. Children with Down syndrome are approximately 150-fold more likely to acquire acute myeloid leukemia (AML) and approximately 500-fold more likely to acquire acute megakaryoblastic leukemia (AMKL) than children without Down syndrome (Vyas & Roberts, 2006), and this is probably due to having trisomy 21, a mutation of *GATA1*, and another genetic alteration as of yet unidentified (Cushing, Clericuzio, Wilson, et al., 2006; Vyas & Crispino, 2007; Vyas & Roberts, 2006). The focus of current research continues to be on the epidemiology and pathogenesis of leukemia in Down syndrome (Ravindranath, 2005).

Children with Down syndrome with AML appear to have a better clinical outcome than children without Down syndrome with AML. Researchers hypothesize that this difference is due to a higher sensitivity to the chemotherapy drugs, and it is suggested that children with Down syndrome less than 2 years of age should receive less intensive chemotherapy regimens in both dose and duration. It is further thought that children with Down syndrome who are 2 years of age or older when diagnosis occurs show a disease picture that is more similar to those children without Down syndrome who acquire the disease (Gamis, 2005; Tomizawa, Tabuchi, Kinoshita, et al., 2007).

Although the incidence of AMKL in children with Down syndrome is greater than in children without Down syndrome, children with Down syndrome who acquire AMKL have a better prognosis and respond to treatment better than other children. AMKL primarily occurs in children with Down syndrome before age 4 years (Vyas & Roberts, 2006).

Acute lymphatic leukemia (ALL) also occurs at a higher rate (i.e., 10- to 20-fold increase than in the general population) in children with Down syndrome. ALL does not occur in children with Down syndrome before age 1 year (Rajantie & Siimes, 2003). Today, children with Down syndrome with ALL survive at similar rates as children without Down syndrome with this condition; this was not always the case. This is largely due to improvements in treatment and making changes based on biologic differences. Children with Down syndrome with ALL, similar to children with Down syndrome with AML, experience greater sensitivity to methotrexate and also are at higher risk for infections while taking the chemotherapy (Whitlock, 2006; Whitlock, Sather, Gaynon, et al., 2005). Alderton, Spector, Blair, and colleagues (2006) found a link between ALL in children with Down syndrome and maternal exposure to chemicals, pesticides, and professional pest exterminations. Further research is needed to confirm this relationship.

A final form of leukemia, transient leukemia (TL), occurs most often in infants with Down syndrome (approximately 10%). This form of leukemia occurs during the newborn period and disappears within the first 3 months. In approximately 20% of these cases, the child develops AMKL before age 4 years (Massey, Zipursky, Chang, et al., 2006; Vyas & Roberts, 2006) (see Chapter 16).

Tumors. Individuals with Down syndrome appear to be at lower risk of developing solid tumors (Dixon, Kishnani, & Zimmerman, 2006; Sullivan, Hussain, Glasson, et al., 2007), although the incidence of testicular germ cell tumors may be increased in males with Down syndrome. Because they can occur at an early age, ongoing assessment of the gonads is warranted (Dixon et al., 2006) (see Chapter 16).

Celiac Disease

The frequency of celiac disease in children with Down syndrome is 1% to 7%; in the general population, celiac disease generally occurs in 3 to 13 per 1000 live births. Since Down syndrome is an at-risk condition for celiac disease, it is recommended that children with Down syndrome be tested after age 3 years, when they would have had a gluten diet for at least 1 year, with the immunoglobulin A (IgA) class tissue transglutaminase (tTG) (Hill, Dirks, Liptak, et al., 2005). Researchers have called for randomized controlled trials to ascertain an appropriate protocol for screening of children with Down syndrome for this condition (Cohen, 2006; Kaatu & LeLeiko, 2008; Swigonski, Kuhlenschmidt, Bull, et al., 2008) (see Chapter 17).

Sleep-Disordered Breathing

Anatomic and physiologic differences (e.g., midfacial hypoplasia, glossoptosis) predispose children with Down syndrome to obstructive sleep apnea and other sleep-disordered breathing problems. This may occur in all children with Down syndrome (Shott, 2006). Age, obesity, and cardiac disease do not affect the incidence of these problems (Fitzgerald, Paul, & Richmond, 2007).

Skin Conditions

Several skin conditions—most of an immune origin—are common in individuals with Down syndrome. These conditions include atopic dermatitis, fissured tongue, premature graying, chelitis, seborrheic dermatitis, xerosis, ichthyosis, and vitiligo (Daneshpazhooh, Nazemi, Bigdeloo, et al., 2007).

Dental Changes

Children with Down syndrome seem to develop caries less often than unaffected children. Numerous other dental problems (e.g., bruxism, malocclusion, defective dentition, microdontia, periodontal disease), however, are more prevalent in these children because of anatomic anomalies of the oral cavity and immunologic dysfunction. Primary teeth can stay in place until the child reaches age 14 or 15 years (Lee, Kwon, Song, et al., 2004; National Institute of Dental and Craniofacial Research, 2007). Lee and colleagues (2004) found that children with Down syndrome have higher concentrations of the salivary *Streptococcus mutans*–specific IgA than children without Down syndrome, and this may be the reason why these children have fewer caries. Keinan, Smith, and Zilberman, (2006) found less enamel in the primary teeth of children with Down syndrome. Mouth breathing and consumption of a diet high in soft foods—two common occurrences in children with Down syndrome—also contribute to their dental problems.

Seizure Disorders

Children with Down syndrome have an increased frequency of seizure disorders, with approximately 6% of these children being diagnosed with epilepsy (AAP, Committee on Genetics, 2001; Cohen, 1999) (see Chapter 26). Structural differences and biochemical changes associated with Down syndrome have been implicated but have not been confirmed. The distribution of the onset of seizures is bimodal, occurring before age 3 years and after 13 years. Of the affected children, 40% begin to have seizures (i.e., generally infantile spasms and generalized tonic-clonic seizures) before 1 year of age. The prognosis of infantile spasms in children with Down syndrome is better than in the general population (Roizen, 2007). The onset of seizures again peaks in adults in their thirties, with tonic-clonic seizures and partial simple and partial complex seizures being the most common. Seizures in adulthood can be indicative of Alzheimer's disease (Tolmie, 2002).

Prognosis

Because Down syndrome is associated with numerous anatomic and physiologic aberrations, life expectancy is reduced, with approximately a 7% mortality rate in the first year of life that rises to 11% by 10 years of age (Rasmussen, Wong, Correa, et al., 2006). The number and severity of congenital anomalies significantly decrease life expectancy for some of these children. Premature aging and a high incidence of Alzheimer's disease may reduce life expectancy for adults. With correct medical, educational, and social interventions, most individuals live well into adulthood and have satisfying, productive lives. Today, the median age for death in a review of death certificates in the United States for whites with Down syndrome from 1983 to 1997 was 49 years. The median age was less for persons with Down syndrome of other races. Primary causes of death were congenital heart disease, dementia, hypothyroidism, and leukemia (Yang, Rasmussen, & Friedman, 2002). In a review of causes of death in persons with Down syndrome in California from 1988 to 1999, Day, Strauss, Shavelle, and colleagues (2005) found that blacks had the shortest life expectancy, fewer children died from congenital heart defects than they had in earlier periods, and the most frequent causes of death included circulatory diseases, congenital anomalies, leukemia, and respiratory illnesses. In an Australian study from 1953 to 2000, leading causes of death in childhood and adulthood were congenital heart defects. In old age, the leading causes of death were coronary heart disease and cardiac, respiratory, and renal failure (Bittles, Bower, Hussain, et al., 2007). Additional factors that need to be examined in relationship to mortality risk in persons with Down syndrome are ethnicity, socioeconomic status, type of residence, health status, and access to appropriate health care (Rasmussen et al., 2006). Successful outcomes heavily depend on the early interventions children and their families receive. If children with Down syndrome are to reach their full potential, aggressive, interdisciplinary management is paramount.

PRIMARY CARE MANAGEMENT

Health Care Maintenance

Primary care providers are encouraged to consult the *Health Care Guidelines for Individuals with Down Syndrome: 1999 Revision* (Cohen, 1999; currently under revision by the AAP, Committee on Genetics) (Figures 24-4 and 24-5), the *Health Supervision Guidelines for Children with Down Syndrome* (AAP, Committee on Genetics, 2001), and clinical practice guidelines for children with Down syndrome ages birth to 12 years (Van Cleve & Cohen, 2006) and ages 12 to 21 years (Van Cleve, Cannon, & Cohen, 2006).

Name:_____   Birthdate:_____

Medical issues	At birth or at diagnosis	6 mo	1	1½	2	2½	3	4	5	6	7	8	9	10	11	12
Karyotype and genetic counseling	___															
Usual preventative care	___	___	___	___	___	___	___	___	___	___	___	___	___	___	___	___
Cardiology	Echo															
Audiologic evaluation	ABR or OAE	___	___	___	___	___	___	___	___	___	___	___	___	___	___	___
Ophthalmologic evaluation	Red reflex	___	___		___		___	___	___	___	___	___	___	___	___	___
Thyroid (TSH and T4)	State screening	___	___		___		___	___	___	___	___	___	___	___	___	___
Nutrition	___	___	___	___	___	___	___	___	___	___	___	___	___	___	___	___
Dental examination[1]					___	___	___	___	___	___	___	___	___	___	___	___
Celiac screening[2]					___											
Parent support	___	___	___	___	___	___	___	___	___	___	___	___	___	___	___	___
Developmental and educational services	Early Intervention	___	___	___	___	___	___	___	___	___	___	___	___	___	___	___
Neck x-rays and neurologic examination[3]							X-ray	___	___	___	___	___	___	___	___	___
Pneumococcal conjugate vaccine series		___	___													

Instructions: Perform indicated examination/screening and record date in blank spaces. The grey or shaded boxes mean no action is to be taken for those ages.

[1]Begin dental examinations at 2 years of age, and continue every 6 months thereafter.
[2]IgA antiendomysium antibodies and total IgA.
[3]Cervical spine x-rays: flexion, neutral, and extension, between 3-5 years of age. Repeat as needed for Special Olympics participation. Neurologic examination at each visit.

FIGURE 24-4 Down Syndrome Health Care Guidelines (1999 revision). Record Sheet #1: Birth to Age 12 Years. From *Down Syndrome Quarterly, 4,* no. 3 (1999, September). Reprinted with permission.

Growth and Development

Evaluating the growth of children with Down syndrome is a detailed process. When linear growth is assessed, primary care providers must take into account the variations in velocity. Whereas growth adequacy is often determined by maintaining a particular percentile rank, variations in growth velocity affect the growth curves of these children during early childhood. Growth velocities for children with and without Down syndrome are similar during the school-age period, however, and stability is then seen in percentile curves.

Measurements should be plotted on both the National Center for Health Statistics (NCHS) growth charts and growth charts with specific norms for children with Down syndrome (Figures 24-6 to 24-11). The NCHS growth charts allow children with Down syndrome to be compared with their chronologic-age peers and also provide a frame of reference for parents. The weight/height percentiles on the NCHS growth charts are independent of a child's age and are also useful in determining appropriate weight in children before adolescence. The specialty charts, in which all percentiles for stature are less than their analogous percentiles on the NCHS charts, provide an excellent reference point for comparing growth among children with Down syndrome and determining those at risk for failure to thrive or obesity. The methodology used in obtaining the growth charts for children with Down syndrome has been questioned, but it is recommended that these charts be consulted until future charts are available (Cohen & Patterson, 1998).

Because inappropriate growth and excessive weight gain have ramifications for motor performance and social acceptance for children with Down syndrome, yearly assessments are required.

Name:____________________ **Birthdate:**____________________

	Age (yr)							
Medical issues	13	14	15	16	17	18	19	20-29
Usual preventative care	___	___	___	___	___	___	___	___
Audiologic evaluation	___	___	___	___	___	___	___	___
Ophthalmologic evaluation	___	___	___	___	___	___	___	___
Thyroid (TSH and T4)	___	___	___	___	___	___	___	___
Nutrition	___	___	___	___	___	___	___	___
Dental examination[1]	___	___	___	___	___	___	___	___
Parent support	___	___	___	___	___	___	___	___
Developmental and educational services	___	___	___	___	___	___	___	___
Neck x-rays and neurologic examination[2]	___	___	___	___	___	___	___	___
Pelvic examination[3]				___	___	___	___	___
Assess contraceptive need[3]				___	___	___	___	___

Instructions: Perform indicated examination/screening and record date in blank spaces. The grey or shaded boxes mean no action is to be taken for those ages.

[1]Begin dental examinations at 2 years of age and continue every 6 months thereafter.
[2]Cervical spine x-rays: flexion, neutral, and extension, between 3-5 years of age. Repeat as needed for Special Olympics participation. Neurological examination at each visit.
[3]If sexually active.

FIGURE 24-5 Down Syndrome Health Care Guidelines (1999 revision). Record Sheet #2: 13 Years to Adulthood. From *Down Syndrome Quarterly, 4,* no. 3 (1999, September). Reprinted with permission.

Interventions for weight management may be introduced as necessary. Caloric reduction and increased exercise incorporated into a behavior management program are likely to be the most effective approach to decrease cardiovascular risk factors of obesity, hypertension, and other issues associated with a sedentary lifestyle (Van Cleve & Cohen, 2006).

Virtually all children will have an intellectual and developmental disability.; the most difficulty is with language development, especially with expressive language. Males appear to have more difficulties (Barnes, Roberts, Mirrett, et al., 2006; Roberts, Long, Malkin, et al., 2005). The transition from one- to two-word sentences has been found to be delayed in children with Down syndrome (Iverson, Longobardi, & Caseli, 2003). The presence of hearing impairments also affects speech and language development in children with Down syndrome (Miolo, Chapman, & Sindberg, 2005). Paul (2007) found that adolescents with Down syndrome had difficulty asking for clarification in a conversation. In an interesting study by Bird, Cleave, Trudeau, and colleagues (2005), children with Down syndrome who were bilingual were compared to children with Down syndrome who were monolingual, children without Down syndrome who were monolingual, and children without Down syndrome who were bilingual. They found that language development was not harmed by being exposed to two languages if exposure was ongoing, although not all children with Down syndrome were successful in speaking two languages. Therefore children with Down syndrome should have their language skills frequently assessed across all domains (Roberts, Price, & Malkin, 2007). Success has been found with responsivity education/prelinguistic milieu teaching (RE/PMT) in which the child with Down syndrome is taught to interact with gestures, eye contact, and vocalizations and parents are instructed on how to respond to their child's words, sounds, and communicative gestures (Fey, Warren, Brady, et al., 2006). Further research is needed to identify the oral motor patterns and examine the progression of gestures and vocalizations to speech and language in children with Down syndrome (Roberts et al., 2007).

Children with Down syndrome will pass through the normal developmental milestones but at a much slower rate than expected. The primary care provider can assist in a child's development by referring the family to an early intervention program as soon as possible after the child's birth. As the child grows older, a variety of activities that are known to assist in development (e.g., Special

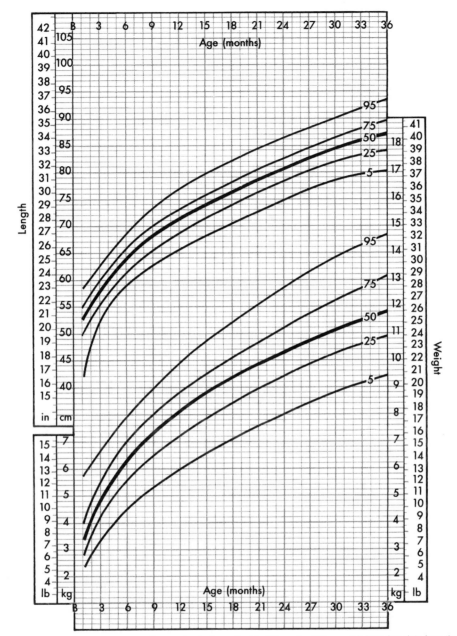

FIGURE 24-6 Boys with Down syndrome: physical growth: 1 to 36 months. This graph is based on data from the Developmental Evaluation Clinic of the Children's Hospital, Boston; the Child Development Center of Rhode Island Hospital; and the Clinical Genetics Service of the Children's Hospital of Philadelphia (supported by March of Dimes grant 6-449).

Olympics, summer camp) can be encouraged. If a child has significant congenital anomalies, program personnel will need guidance as to the intensity of activity the child is allowed. A child's progress should be carefully documented on standardized developmental schedules at each primary care visit. Since Down syndrome is associated with global developmental delay, most children with Down syndrome will have IQs below the second standard deviation on standardized tests, such as the Wechsler Intelligence Scale for Children–Revised or the Bayley Scales of Infant Development.

Normal childhood and adolescent stressors are also of concern. For example, adolescents with Down syndrome often desire to date other adolescents of normal intelligence. When they are rejected, along with their inability to drive to social events, adolescents with Down syndrome can become depressed. Therefore social and behavioral concerns should be assessed and addressed at each health care visit.

Diet

Among the most significant concerns are feeding difficulties in young children and obesity in older children. Feeding problems may be encountered because of the disproportionately large tongue, muscle flaccidity, poor coordination, significantly delayed social maturation, thyroid or pituitary disorders, and congenital heart disease.

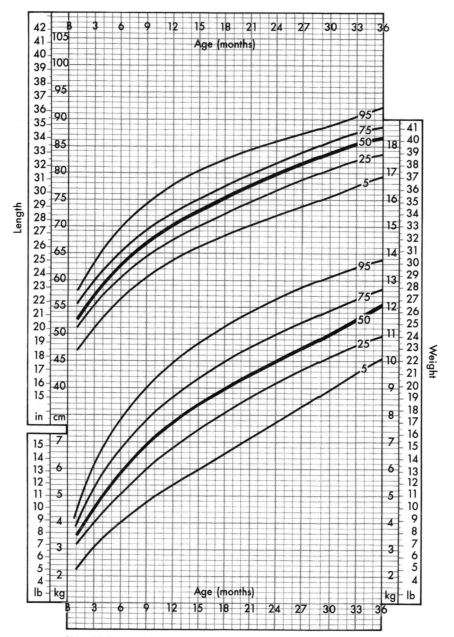

FIGURE 24-7 Girls with Down syndrome: physical growth: 1 to 36 months. This graph is based on data from the Developmental Evaluation Clinic of the Children's Hospital, Boston; the Child Development Center of Rhode Island Hospital; and the Clinical Genetics Service of the Children's Hospital of Philadelphia (supported by March of Dimes grant 6-449).

For infants, breastfeeding should be encouraged. The immunogenic qualities of breast milk offer additional protection against upper respiratory tract infections and other illnesses. The extra effort required of infants who are breastfeeding also helps them to develop orofacial muscles and tongue control and promotes greater jaw stability. Breastfeeding may take longer at first, and mothers will need to be encouraged in their efforts. The LaLeche League of America has material on breastfeeding infants with Down syndrome.

Blended and chopped foods and shallow-bowl, latex-covered spoons may help children who are learning to eat solids. If significant problems (e.g., aspiration) occur, an occupational therapist or other developmental therapist should be consulted in designing an individualized feeding program (Van Cleve & Cohen, 2006).

There are no routine dietary restrictions for older children. Care should be taken to avoid excessive caloric intake if inappropriate weight gain is a problem. A balanced diet, a program of physical exercise, and vitamin and mineral supplementation are recommended as necessary (Van Cleve et al., 2006).

The only dietary restriction for children with Down syndrome is for those diagnosed with celiac disease. These children must be on a gluten-free diet to relieve symptoms and protect against future malignancy (Cohen, 2006).

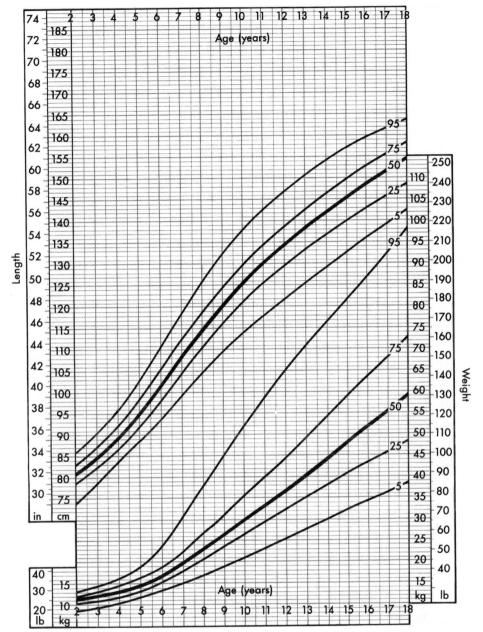

FIGURE 24-8 Boys with Down syndrome: physical growth: 2 to 18 years. This graph is based on data from the Developmental Evaluation Clinic of the Children's Hospital, Boston; the Child Development Center of Rhode Island Hospital; and the Clinical Genetics Service of the Children's Hospital of Philadelphia (supported by March of Dimes grant 6-449).

Safety

Safety issues for children with Down syndrome are the same as for their developmental, not chronologic, peers. Primary care providers must adjust their normal schedule for providing anticipatory guidance to the development of children with Down syndrome. If information is given too far in advance of a child's developmental progression, parents may forget or find the information to be a painful reminder that their child is progressing more slowly than unaffected children.

Children with Down syndrome are more likely to sustain joint injuries as a result of their musculoskeletal problems. For children with atlantoaxial instability or those who have not yet been adequately evaluated, contact sports, somersaults, or other activities that may result in cervical injury should be restricted. Documentation that the child is not in danger of subluxation may be required for children participating in the Special Olympics.

Immunizations

There are no contraindications for immunizations for children with Down syndrome. If they have a cell-mediated disorder, live-viral vaccines are contraindicated. In most cases, the national immunization schedule should be followed (AAP, Committee on Infectious Diseases, 2008; Kroger, Atkinson, Marcuse, et al., 2006; Marin, Guris, Chaves, et al., 2007).

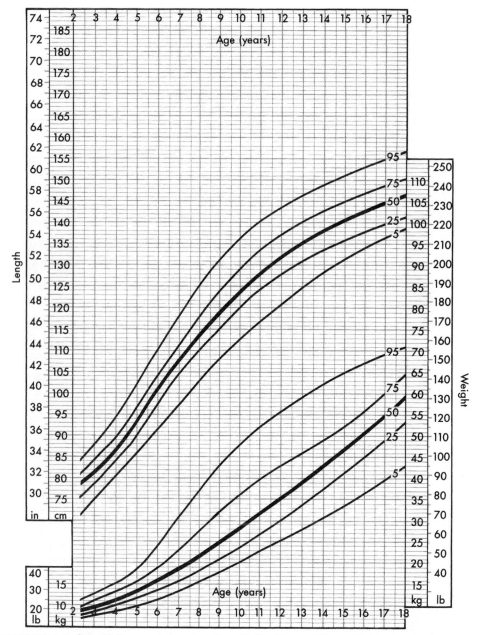

FIGURE 24-9 Girls with Down syndrome: physical growth: 2 to 18 years. This graph is based on data from the Developmental Evaluation Clinic of the Children's Hospital, Boston; the Child Development Center of Rhode Island Hospital; and the Clinical Genetics Service of the Children's Hospital of Philadelphia (supported by March of Dimes grant 6-449).

It is recommended that children with Down syndrome should receive palivizumab (Synagis) injections monthly during RSV season in the first 2 years (Van Cleve & Cohen, 2006).

Hepatitis A vaccination should not be given to children with Down syndrome unless warranted because their place of residence has a high incidence rate and community prophylaxis is being done (Fiore, Wasley, & Bell, 2006).

Screening

Vision. Because of the large number of ocular defects associated with Down syndrome, all children should be evaluated by an ophthalmologist by 6 months of age and every 2 years to assess

for strabismus and cataracts. Early referral is critical considering the synergistic effects that diminished vision and hearing have on development. Significant visual impairment is usually preventable because the conditions common in Down syndrome (e.g., strabismus, myopia) are treatable (Roizen, 2007). Future screening recommendations should be determined in conjunction with the ophthalmologist according to the status of the child's eyes. At minimum, the primary care provider should screen for visual problems at each well-child visit. Such screening should include testing acuity, examining the red reflex and optic fundi, and checking alignment and oculomotor functions. Because children with Down syndrome may have difficulty using a Snellen or lazy E

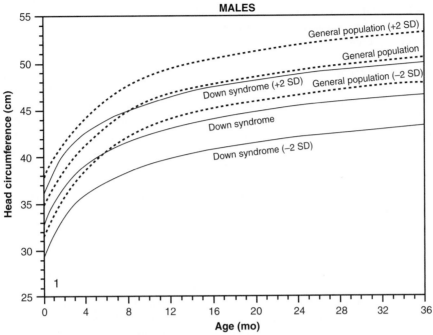

FIGURE 24-10 Head circumference growth curves for males with Down syndrome (solid line) compared with those for males in the general population (dotted line). From Palmer, C.G., et al. (1992). Head circumference of children with Down syndrome 0 to 36 months. *Am J Med Genet, 42,* 61-67. Reprinted with permission.

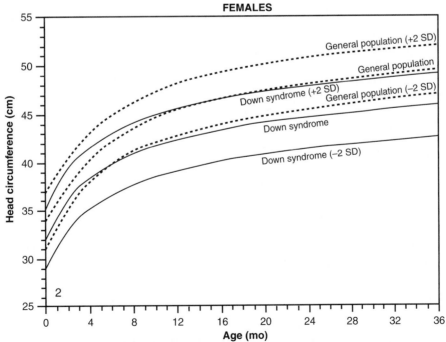

FIGURE 24-11 Head circumference growth curves for females with Down syndrome (solid line) compared with those for females in the general population (dotted line). From Palmer, C.G., et al. (1992). Head circumference of children with Down syndrome 0 to 36 months. *Am J Med Genet, 42,* 61-67. Reprinted with permission.

chart, acuity screening performed with the Titmus picture test or Teller acuity cards will yield more valid results.

Many children with Down syndrome have difficulty keeping their glasses in place, so parents should be counseled that purchasing glasses with lightweight plastic lenses and using an elastic strap around the child's occiput to secure them will help correct this problem. Contact lenses are not routinely recommended but may be appropriate for children with keratoconus.

Hearing. Because good hearing is a requisite for cognitive, social, and language development and because these children are at high risk for conductive hearing loss, careful assessment is necessary. The health care provider should use the smallest size speculum (2 mm) for the examination because of typically tiny ear openings. It is recommended that all infants be evaluated for auditory brainstem responses (ABRs) or otoacoustic emission (OAE) during the first 3 months of life (Shott, 2006). Behavioral audiograms should take place every 6 months until the child is 3 years of age and yearly thereafter (Shott, 2006; Van Cleve & Cohen, 2006). If the external ear orifice is stenotic or there are other difficulties that preclude adequate pneumo-otoscopic examination, alternative methods of evaluation must be used. Tympanometry provides one useful adjunct to assessment but is not reliable in children under 1 year of age. Because of the importance of early intervention, infants between 9 and 12 months of age should be referred for micro-otoscopy if examination is difficult. The accumulation of cerumen leading to impacted canals is common; removal of cerumen every 6 months is recommended for children with this problem. When middle ear disease occurs, it deserves aggressive intervention and close follow-up if further developmental insult is to be prevented. Therefore a hearing evaluation by an otolaryngologist should take place every 6 months until the child is 3 years old and then on an annual basis (Shott, 2006; Van Cleve & Cohen, 2006).

If hearing aids are required, those that fasten onto the earpiece of eyeglasses may be better than ear molds. Hearing aids dependent on ear molds are hard to fit for children who are just beginning to wear them. These children often do not like the increased sound. Parents may need help finding methods (e.g., behavior management) to help improve their child's compliance for leaving the hearing aid in place. Parents must also be cautioned to devise mnemonic cues for remembering to change the batteries routinely because it is unlikely that their child will be able to realize that the hearing aid is malfunctioning.

Dental. Because of the extremely high prevalence of dental problems in young children, aggressive dental care is necessary. Primary care providers must document and carefully observe the dental problems of these children. All children with Down syndrome should be evaluated before age 18 months by a dentist or pedodontist skilled in caring for children with developmental disabilities. Locating such dentists is often difficult for parents, and specific referrals to professionals may be warranted.

Good dental hygiene—including twice-daily brushing and flossing—is indicated to reduce the amount of periodontal disease. If good dental hygiene is difficult to achieve, using a Water Pik or an electric toothbrush should be considered. Effective tooth-brushing techniques may be difficult to achieve because of the child's limited manual dexterity, enlarged tongue, and small mouth. Close supervision is required, and independent tooth brushing and mouth care may not be feasible until the child is at least of preschool age.

Weaning children from a bottle by 18 months and diets that contain low-sugar, crunchy foods (e.g., fresh vegetables) also help deter dental deterioration and should be encouraged. In areas where the water supply is nonfluoridated, fluoride supplementation should be initiated. If periodontal disease is severe, chemical plaque control may be necessary. For children with congenital heart disease, prophylactic antibiotics may be warranted for dental interventions (National Institute for Dental and Craniofacial Research, 2007; Van Cleve & Cohen, 2006) (see Chapter 21).

Blood Pressure. Routine screening is recommended. If there is a history of cardiac disease or a positive family history of cardiac disease or hypertension, more careful assessment is required. A cardiac evaluation, including an echocardiogram, however, is warranted during infancy to rule out congenital heart disease or cardiac defects (Van Cleve et al., 2006; Van Cleve & Cohen, 2006).

Hematocrit. Routine screening is recommended. Consider obtaining a complete blood count (CBC) on all neonates with Down syndrome because neutrophilia was found in 80% of 158 newborns with Down syndrome in a recent study (Henry, Walker, Wiedmeier, et al., 2007). It has also been recommended to check for polycythemia and thrombocytopenia (Van Cleve & Cohen, 2006).

Urinalysis. Routine screening is recommended.

Tuberculosis. Routine screening is recommended. No special precautions must be taken unless the child is or has been institutionalized.

Condition-Specific Screening

Thyroid Dysfunction. Because the abnormalities seen in Down syndrome are similar to some seen in thyroid dysfunction, it is difficult to diagnose thyroid problems by clinical examination. Thyroid-stimulating hormone levels (TSH, T4) should be assessed at 6 and 12 months of age and annually thereafter (Van Cleve & Cohen, 2006). If there are any signs or symptoms suggestive of thyroid dysfunction, a complete thyroid panel should be drawn.

Atlantoaxial Instability. Primary care providers must appraise the risk of atlantoaxial subluxation for all children with Down syndrome who are planning to engage in physically active exercise or the Special Olympics or who are to undergo surgical or rehabilitative procedures (Cohen, 2006). Currently, the need for cervical spine radiographic studies in children with Down syndrome is controversial (Tolmie, 2002).

Hip Dislocation. Assessing hip stability through age 10 years is indicated because early detection (i.e., before the dislocation is fixed and acetabular dysplasia occurs) allows for optimal surgical correction. Early signs of habitual dislocation are an increasing limp, decreasing activity, and an audible click. Pain does not usually occur unless the dislocation is acute. In older children, radiographic studies may be necessary for assessment.

Mitral Valve Prolapse. Screening should begin in adolescence. Echocardiographic evaluations are recommended before surgical or dental procedures (Cohen, 1999).

Celiac Disease. Although screening is not mandatory for individuals with Down syndrome, increased attention has been brought to the incidence of celiac disease in persons with Down syndrome. IgA-antiendomysium antibodies (AEAs) and IgA tTG have been found to be good immunologic markers in screening for this disease (Cohen, 2006).

Common Illness Management

Differential Diagnosis

Immune Dysfunction. The significant changes in the immune systems of children with Down syndrome have significant implications for primary care providers. Specifically, all infections must be treated aggressively because negative sequelae are more likely to develop. The incidence of many autoimmune diseases (including insulin-dependent diabetes mellitus and chronic arthritis) is also much greater in this population. If a child exhibits signs and symptoms compatible with a diagnosis of any of these diseases, a thorough evaluation is indicated. Parents must be educated about the signs and symptoms of conditions and the need to seek medical advice promptly (see Chapters 23 and 31).

Differential Diagnosis

- Infectious diseases require aggressive treatment due to underlying immune dysfunction.
- Upper respiratory tract infections and sequelae are common.
- Behavioral changes may have physical cause.
- Gastrointestinal symptoms in infants may be due to congenital anomalies.
- Leukemia is 18 to 20 times more likely to be acquired than in the general population.

Upper Respiratory Tract Infections. Children with Down syndrome are prone to upper respiratory tract infections. These infections should be managed aggressively because untoward sequelae—including otitis media and pneumonia—are apt to develop. Children with congenital heart disease should be examined at the first signs of illness because these children are more likely to develop secondary problems and parents may confuse an upper respiratory tract infection with early congestive heart failure. These children may also need to be given subacute bacterial endocarditis prophylaxis (see Chapter 21).

Behavioral Changes. Behavioral changes may be caused by a variety of physiologic and psychological problems, including the following: (1) thyroid dysfunction, (2) obstructive sleep apnea, (3) neurodegeneration (primarily in older individuals), (4) declining physical competence (e.g., congestive heart failure), (5) disturbed home environment, and (6) overstimulation. Interventions must be cause specific. Trials with stimulants, antidepressants, or antipsychotic drugs may be indicated in some cases after a thorough evaluation, although diagnosis of mental illness should not be given based solely on the fact that the child has Down syndrome.

Gastrointestinal Symptoms. Because pyloric stenosis and Hirschsprung disease are more common in children with Down syndrome, primary care providers should carefully pursue reports of persistent vomiting, constipation, or chronic diarrhea in infants.

Leukemia. Children with Down syndrome acquire leukemia 18 to 20 times as often as other children. Easy bruising, unusual pallor, or listlessness must be fully evaluated. Parents must be alerted to immediately seek health care for their child if any of these signs or symptoms develops.

Drug Interactions

Because children with Down syndrome are at risk for health problems affecting any organ or system of their body, they may often be taking medications. It is important that family members understand how to administer the medications, what the side effects are, and to report any allergic reactions to the primary care provider. Over-the-counter medications are often ineffective (e.g., with skin problems), and prescription medications may be needed.

Developmental Issues

Sleep Patterns

Sleep disorders are uncommon in children with Down syndrome, with the exception of obstructive sleep apnea and related conditions. Anatomic and immunologic differences predispose school-age children in particular to this condition. The primary care provider should have a high index of suspicion if the child has a history of snoring, restless sleep, abnormal sleep positions, being awake for hours during the night, night terrors, or daytime somnolence, as well as if failure to thrive, pulmonary hypertension, or behavioral problems are present. As a result, a thorough history and physical examination is warranted, especially an examination of the oral and nasal passages. Referral to a sleep laboratory for periodic overnight polysomnography evaluation may be warranted. Options for treatment may include saline spray, oxygen at night, or continuous positive airway pressure (CPAP) also delivered at night. Surgical treatment can range from tonsillectomy and adenoidectomy to a combination of skeletal and soft tissue alterations to eliminate the specific cause of obstruction. It is recommended that a sleep study be conducted after recovery from surgery to verify that the cause of obstruction was eliminated (Shott, 2006).

Toileting

The median age for toilet training children with Down syndrome is approximately 36 months. Parents must be advised of this to reduce frustrations associated with unrealistic expectations. Routine toilet training techniques are effective. It takes longer, however, to train a child with Down syndrome, and additional positive reinforcement is necessary.

Constipation, a common problem, may also be related to inadequate peristalsis, poor diet, lack of exercise, or thyroid dysfunction. The cause of constipation must clearly be assessed so that the correct interventions are initiated. It is important for the child to maintain a healthy diet with fruits and vegetables, to exercise regularly, and use an osmotic agent such as polyethylene glycol if needed (Van Cleve & Cohen, 2006).

Discipline

Children with Down syndrome are usually not more difficult to discipline than other children. Parents must be encouraged to remember that discipline needs to be appropriate for the child's developmental, not chronologic, age. Children with Down syndrome should not receive special compensation just because they have Down syndrome. Parental expectations should be consistent, and limits should be set for all children in the family. Behavior management programs can be developed for specific discipline problems when a child has not been responsive to the parents' usual methods.

Child Care

Daycare should provide appropriate social, cognitive, and physical stimulation for a child with Down syndrome. When selecting the type of daycare setting, parents should be encouraged to consider the child's personality and medical needs, as well as their own philosophy about inclusion. Many generic daycare centers include children with Down syndrome into their programs and are sufficiently staffed to provide an excellent experience for these children. If a child has significant medical problems, specialized daycare, which is often available through the school system, may be a better option. If a child is highly susceptible to infections, a home care setting (i.e., with fewer than six children) is recommended. Primary care providers should be aware of resources in their community to assist parents with daycare placement. Local parent groups for children with Down syndrome, as well as the local affiliates of the Arc of the United States (see Resources) and other specialty agencies, may also help with placement.

Schooling

A variety of options—from total inclusion to residential placement—for academic placement exist. If circumstances permit, children with Down syndrome do best in an environment fully integrated with nondisabled peers. Children with Down syndrome, however, need support from their families while they deal with being exceptional and with social pressures from peers. Parents and teachers working together to create a supportive environment can ensure that a child has some social and academic successes. Otherwise, the child may become frustrated and demoralized, which can lead to disruptive behavior and poor self-esteem.

Families may need assistance in choosing the school setting they deem most appropriate for their child. Primary care providers can be instrumental in helping families locate appropriate community services to assist in educational placement. All children with Down syndrome are eligible for educational provisions under Public Law 108-446 (IDEA) (see Chapter 3). Parents should be encouraged to contact their social worker or local office of mental retardation shortly after the child's birth so that they can receive the educational, vocational, and supportive services for which the child is eligible.

Sexuality

Pubertal changes in adolescents with Down syndrome occur at approximately the same time as in their unaffected peers. Accompanying these physical changes, adolescents will have social interests and biologic drives similar to those of their chronologic-age peers and must be given the opportunity to participate in social activities with their peers. For parents who are highly protective, the social education and sexual education that must accompany their child's increasing independence are often difficult and sensitive issues (Roizen, 2007; Van Cleve et al., 2006). Primary care providers need to help parents recognize their responsibility in ensuring that children can handle themselves in a socially and sexually appropriate manner.

Individualized instruction about self-care skills, biologic changes, social implications, and contraception is paramount to minimizing both the appearance of sexual impropriety and the risk of being sexually exploited. Routine pelvic examination is not recommended for females who are not sexually active, and the young woman, her parents, and the primary care provider should discuss the frequency of this examination (Van Cleve et al., 2006). Genetic counseling for both the parents and the child is necessary. Although men are virtually always sterile, women are capable of reproducing. Planned Parenthood, the Arc of the United States, and parent support groups offer printed and audiovisual materials specifically designed for use with these families.

The age at onset of menses for females is similar to that of their mothers. Handling pubertal changes is difficult for some female adolescents. Family members must be helped to recognize the behavior changes that may be related to normal hormonal cycles. For those women who are menstruating and are unable to manage their own hygienic care, parents and other caregivers must follow Universal Precautions.

Some parents may request that their daughter with Down syndrome be sterilized. The right to procreative choice is protected by law, and statutes regarding sterilization vary greatly from state to state. Primary care providers are strongly suggested to consult their state office of mental retardation for current guidelines because sterilization is illegal in some jurisdictions. If sterilization is to be pursued, the adolescent must participate in the decision to the extent possible (Committee on Bioethics, 1999).

Transition to Adulthood

The life expectancy for individuals with Down syndrome has increased dramatically with most living well into middle age, creating the need to address independent living, sexuality, vocational choices, and health maintenance in adulthood and older adulthood.

Individuals with Down syndrome vary in their abilities to live independently; some require ongoing, consistent supervision, and others merely need minimal guidance with complex tasks. Most individuals remain at home until a crisis forces different arrangements. Because individuals with Down syndrome often have aged parents, families can help plan for a smooth transition to a different living situation within the context of normal development. For example, some parents may help their son or daughter move to a group home at about the same age as their other children left for college. Recreational activities, such as bowling, swimming, and dancing, are encouraged because they promote social relationships and physical fitness. Registering to vote is also an important function of adulthood.

Vocational choices are directed by an individual's cognitive abilities, social skills, and adaptive abilities. Many persons with Down syndrome can seek competitive employment in custodial work, offices, housekeeping, restaurants, landscaping, or other occupations where the required skills are not too difficult and are fairly repetitive, and there is ongoing supervision. The skills necessary to survive in the workforce (e.g., basic money management, telling time, using public transportation) must be mastered before such positions are sought. For others, working in sheltered workshops is a better option because this type of job requires fewer adaptive abilities.

Generally, the overall health of most individuals with Down syndrome is good. Premature aging may occur as early as the twenties with dental changes often seen first. Dermatologic, thyroid, cardiac, and sensory problems are the most troublesome and worsen with age. Changes in mental health may also be a concern after children complete formal schooling at 21 years of age. Depression and obsessive-compulsive behaviors continue to be seen in adulthood (Ailey, 2005). Of concern is Alzheimer's disease, which occurs in a sizable proportion of adults (approximately 40%) with Down syndrome over 40 years of age (Crocker, 2006). The actual percentage differs among studies, but the minimum percentage is generally considered to be 25%. The incidence rises as the person ages. IQ levels and adaptive functioning also decline over time. Further longitudinal study of adults with Down syndrome—especially documentation of health status changes—is warranted.

Family Concerns

Parents of children with Down syndrome will experience joy and pride in their child, although they will be faced with many challenges throughout their child's life. Most parents meet these challenges with resilience and adaptive functioning (Van Riper, 2007). For some parents, however, raising these children can become overwhelming. Locating and coordinating acceptable medical, educational, and ancillary personnel may produce stress. Primary care providers may be of tremendous assistance to the families in identifying appropriate resources (e.g., respite care) and helping parents become their child's best lifelong advocate. Mothers in particular may find it difficult to balance their time and responsibilities among their children and spouse. Siklos and Kerns (2006) found that the greatest unmet parental needs were information about special services and programs, friends for their child with Down syndrome, and getting a break from responsibilities.

Down syndrome parent support groups have also been invaluable to families, especially in the first year after a child with Down syndrome is born. Support groups for families of Hispanic and other ethnicities are becoming increasingly common throughout the country (Martorell & Martorell, 2006).

Many families are interested in adopting infants and children with Down syndrome, and the demand continues to be greater than the available children. A recent survey found the average time to adopt a child with Down syndrome was 1 to 2 years (Lindh, Steele, Page-Steiner, et al., 2007).

Siblings are also important members of any family, and their adjustment to a child with Down syndrome has been researched over the past several years. Currently, researchers have found their adjustment to be primarily positive and their own development has not been negatively influenced by having a brother or sister with Down syndrome (Cuskelly & Gunn, 2006; Skotko & Levine, 2006). Skotko and Levine (2006) recommend that parents maintain honestly and openness about the child with Down syndrome and explain the condition to their other children as soon as possible, encourage expression of feelings, recognize that all interactions will not be positive (as with any siblings), reduce the amount of time that the brother or sister has to care for the sibling with Down syndrome, recognize each child's uniqueness, and offer informal or formal support when needed for the sibling(s) without Down syndrome.

Although many concerns are similar for all families who have a child with special needs, one notable issue for families of children with Down syndrome is the need for long-range planning. Most individuals with Down syndrome never become totally self-sufficient, and families must plan for a child's lifetime through, for example, estate planning and custody arrangements. They must also enroll an adult child to receive Supplemental Security Income (SSI) (see Chapter 8). Other individuals with Down syndrome, however, may marry and live semi-independent lives. The degree of the child's limitations, the internal strengths of the family, and the support from extended family and community networks all affect a family's adjustment.

Resources

Caring for a child with Down syndrome is a complex task because of the physical, cognitive, and social concerns that must be addressed. Additional resources for professionals and parents of children with Down syndrome are given here.

Informational Materials

Bruni, M. (2006). *Fine Motor Skills in Children with Down Syndrome: A Guide for Parents and Professionals* (2nd ed.). Bethesda, MD: Woodbine House.

Couwenhoven, T. (2007). *Teaching Children with Down Syndrome About Their Bodies, Boundaries, and Sexuality: A Guide for Parents and Professionals.* Bethesda, MD: Woodbine House.

Kumin, L. (2003). *Early Communication Skills for Children with Down Syndrome: A Guide for Parents and Professionals.* Bethesda, MD: Woodbine House.

McGuire, D., & Chicoine, B. (2006). *Mental Wellness in Adults with Down Syndrome: A Guide to Emotional and Behavioral Strengths and Challenges.* Bethesda, MD: Woodbine House.

Pueschel, S.M. (2006). *Adults with Down Syndrome.* Bethesda, MD: Woodbine House.

Schermerhorn, W. (2004). *Down Syndrome: The first 18 months* (DVD). Bethesda, MD: Woodbine House. Available from Woodbine House; 6510 Bells Mill Rd., Bethesda, MD 20817. Website: www.woodbinehouse.com.

Cohen, W.I., Nadel, L., & Madnick, M.E. (Eds.). (2002). *Down Syndrome: Visions for the 21st Century.* New York: Wiley. Available from Wiley;111 River St.; Hoboken, NJ 07030. Website: www.wiley.com.

Pueschel, S.M. (Ed.). (2000). *A Parents Guide to Down syndrome: Toward a Brighter Future* (rev. ed.). Baltimore: Brookes Publishing Co. Available from Brookes Publishing Co.; PO Box 10624; Baltimore, MD 21285-0624. Website: www.brookespublishing.com.

Organizations

The Arc of the United States
1010 Wayne Ave., Suite 650
Silver Spring, MD 20910
(301) 565-3842; Fax: (301) 565-3843
Website: info@thearc.org; www.thearc.org

Canadian Down Syndrome Society
811-14 St. NW
Calgary, Alberta, Canada T2N 2A4
(403) 270-8500; Fax: (403) 270-8291
Email: dsingo@cdss.ca
Website: www.cdss.ca

Commission on Mental and Physical Disability Law
American Bar Association
740 15th St., NW
Washington, DC 20005
(202) 662-1570; Fax: (202) 662-1032
Email: cmpdl@abanet.org
Website: www.abanet.org/disability

National Down Syndrome Congress
1370 Center Drive, Suite 102
Atlanta, GA 30338
(800) 232-6372 (NDSC); Fax: (770) 604-9500
Email: info@ndsccenter.org
Website: www.ndsccenter.org

National Down Syndrome Society
666 Broadway, 8th Floor
New York, NY 10012-2317
(800) 221-4602; Fax: (212) 979-2873
Email: Info@ndss.org
Website: www.ndss.org/

Summary of Primary Care Needs for the Child with Down Syndrome

HEALTH CARE MAINTENANCE

Growth and Development

- Children usually have a shorter stature and increased weight (after infancy).
- Children should have height and weight measured at each visit and plotted on NCHS growth charts and growth charts for children with Down syndrome.
- Caloric reduction and increased exercise are recommended with untoward weight gain.
- Virtually all children will have an intellectual and developmental disability.
- Expressive language problems are common.
- Normal progression of developmental milestones occurs, but at a slower rate.
- Early intervention programs are recommended.
- *Diet.* Feeding support is needed in infancy to ensure adequate weight gain.
  - Breastfeeding is encouraged in infancy.
  - Adaptive equipment and occupational therapy may be needed when teaching feeding skills.
  - Diets may need to be tailored to help correct constipation or obesity in childhood and adulthood.
  - Vitamin and mineral supplementation is often recommended.
  - Children with celiac disease require a gluten-free diet.
- *Safety.* Anticipatory guidance needs to be based on a child's developmental—not chronologic—age.
  - There is increased incidence of musculoskeletal or joint injuries from laxity.
  - Atlantoaxial instability is a hazard and must be ruled out before active sports programs.
- *Immunizations.* Routine immunizations are recommended.
  - Live-viral vaccines may be contraindicated in children with cell-mediated disorders.
  - RSV immunoprophylaxis should be considered in the first 2 years.

Screening

- *Vision.* The incidence of ocular defects is high. All infants should be evaluated by an ophthalmologist by 6 months of age and at 2 years.
  - Acuity and alignment testing and examination of the red reflex and optic fundi should be done at each visit.
- *Hearing.* Anatomic abnormalities of the ears are common.
  - Auditory brainstem response or otoacoustic emission testing is recommended by 3 months of age.
  - Behavioral audiograms are recommended every 6 months until age 3 years and then annually.
  - Tympanometry is often a useful adjunct over 1 year of age.

- Evaluation by a specialist is recommended every 6 months until age 3 years and then annually.
- Cerumen impaction and otitis media are common.
- A majority of children have hearing loss. Many will require hearing aids.
- *Dental.* Dental screening should be done a minimum of every 6 months from age 18 months because of the high incidence of periodontal disease.
  - Good dental hygiene is important. If not in water, fluoride is recommended.
  - Children should be weaned from the bottle by 18 months to prevent dental deterioration.
  - Children with congenital heart disease (CHD) may require antibiotic prophylaxis to prevent endocarditis.
- *Blood pressure.* Routine screening is recommended.
  - A full cardiac evaluation with echocardiogram should be done in infancy.
- *Hematocrit.* Routine screening is recommended. Consideration should be given to obtaining a CBC in the first week of life to assess for neutrophilia, polycythemia, and thrombocytopenia.
- *Urinalysis.* Routine screening is recommended.
- *Tuberculosis.* Routine screening is recommended.

Condition-Specific Screening

- Obtain karyotype in neonatal period if prenatal diagnostic tests for Down syndrome are not done.
- Thyroid-stimulating hormone levels should be checked at 6 and 12 months of age and yearly thereafter.
- Atlantoaxial instability risk should be assessed before surgery or athletic involvement.
- Screening for hip dislocation is necessary through age 10 years or whenever a gait abnormality occurs.
- Screening for mitral valve prolapse should start in adolescence.
- Screening for celiac disease should be done with IgA AEA and IgA tTG.

COMMON ILLNESS MANAGEMENT

Differential Diagnosis

- *Immune dysfunction.* Children with Down syndrome are more susceptible to infections and autoimmune disorders.
- *Upper respiratory tract infections.* Upper respiratory tract infections are often associated with otitis media and pneumonia and should be managed aggressively, especially when a child has CHD.
- *Behavioral changes.* Thyroid dysfunction, obstructive sleep apnea, neurodegeneration, declining physical functioning, disturbed home environment, and overstimulation should be ruled out as a cause for behavioral changes.

Summary of Primary Care Needs for the Child with Down Syndrome—cont'd

- *Gastrointestinal symptoms.* Pyloric stenosis and Hirschsprung disease should be ruled out.
  - Constipation is a common problem and may be due to decreased peristalsis, poor diet, lack of exercise, or thyroid dysfunction.
- *Leukemia.* Unusual pallor, easy bruising, and listlessness should be fully evaluated.

Drug Interactions

- Children may be taking different medications for different conditions, so primary care providers should be aware of drug interactions and side effects and inform family members who are administering the medications.

DEVELOPMENTAL ISSUES

Sleep Patterns

- Obstructive sleep apnea may occur; it is a problem primarily of school-age children. Surgical intervention may be necessary. Refer for periodic overnight polysomnography if history warrants further assessment.

Toileting

- Delayed bowel and bladder training may occur as a result of developmental lag; constipation is common because of low activity level, decreased peristalsis, and poor diet.

Discipline

- Discipline must be developmentally appropriate; behavior management programs are often successful.

Child Care

- Small-group daycare lessens the risk of repeated infections.
- Children may be eligible for specialized daycare programs; infants up to 3 years of age may be eligible for early intervention programs.

Schooling

- Children and youths are eligible for special education services through Public Law 108-446 (IDEA).

Sexuality

- Sex education must be taught so that children with Down syndrome are not abused and do not display inappropriate sexual behaviors.
- Girls may need assistance with menstrual hygiene.
- Boys are usually infertile, but girls may be fertile.

Transition to Adulthood

- Emphasis should be on independent living, vocational skills, and health maintenance.
- Premature aging is present and signs appear in the twenties with dental changes.
- Mental health problems (e.g., depression, obsessive-compulsive disorder [OCD], Alzheimer's disease) may be problematic.

FAMILY CONCERNS

- Special family concerns may include long-term care and prolonged adaptation to the diagnosis.

REFERENCES

Ailey, S. (2005). Behavior management and mental health. In W.M. Nehring (Ed.), *Core Curriculum for Specializing in Intellectual and Developmental Disability: A Resource for Nurses and Other Health Care Professionals.* Boston: Jones & Bartlett.

Aitken, D.A., Crossley, J.A., & Spencer, K. (2002). Prenatal screening in neural tube defects and aneuploidy. In D.L. Rimoin, J.M. Connor, R.E. Pyeritz, (Eds.) *Emery and Rimoin's Principles and Practices of Medical Genetics* (4th ed.). New York: Churchill Livingstone.

Alderton, L.E., Spector, L.G., Blair, C.K., et al. (2006). Child and maternal household chemical exposure and the risk of acute leukemia in children with Down's syndrome: A report from the Children's Oncology Group. *Am J Epidemiol, 164,* 212-221.

American Academy of Pediatrics, Committee on Genetics. (2001). Health supervision guidelines for children with Down syndrome. *Pediatrics, 107,* 442-448.

American Academy of Pediatrics, Committee on Infectious Diseases. (2008). Recommended immunization schedules for children and adolescents–United States, 2008. *Pediatrics, 121,* 219-220.

American College of Obstetricians and Gynecologists (2004). First-trimester screening for fetal aneuploidy. ACOG opinion no. 297. *Obstetr Gynecol, 104,* 423-424.

Barnes, E.F., Roberts, J.E., Mirrett, P., et al. (2006). A comparison of oral motor structure and function in young males with fragile X syndrome and Down syndrome. *J Speech Lang Hear Res, 49,* 903-917.

Betz, C.L., & Nehring, W.M. (2007). Integrating health-related needs into individualized education programs and 504 plans. In C.L. Betz & W.M. Nehring, (Eds.) *Promoting Health Care Transitions for Adolescents with Special Health Care Needs and Disabilities,* Baltimore: Paul H. Brookes.

Bianca, S., & Bianca, M. (2004). Heart and ocular anomalies in children with Down's syndrome. *J Intellect Disabil Res, 48*(pt 3), 281-282.

Bird, E.K., Cleave, P., Trudeau, N., et al. (2005). The language abilities of bilingual children with Down syndrome. *Am J Speech-Lang Pathol, 14,* 187-199.

Bittles, A.H., Bower, C., Hussain, R., et al. (2007). The four ages of Down syndrome. *Eur J PublicHealth, 17,* 121-225.

Bloemers, B.L.P., van Furth, A.M., Weijerman, M.E., et al. (2007). Down syndrome: A novel risk factor for respiratory syncytial virus bronchiolitis—a prospective birth-cohort study. *Pediatrics, 120,* e1076-e1081.

Borland, L.M., Colligan, J., & Brandom, B.W. (2004). Frequency of anesthesia-related complications in children with Down syndrome under general anesthesia for noncardiac procedures. *Pediatr Anesth, 14,* 733-738.

Capone, G., Goyal, P., Ares, W., et al. (2006). Neurobehavioral disorders in children, adolescents, and young adults with Down syndrome. *Am J Med Genet C (Semin Med Genet), 142,* 158-172.

Capone, G., Grados, M.A., Kaufmann, W.E., et al. (2005). Down syndrome and comorbid autism-spectrum disorder: Characterization using the Aberrant Behavior Checklist. *Am J Med Genet A, 134,* 373-380.

Centers for Disease Control and Prevention (2006). Improved national prevalence estimates for 18 selected major birth defects—United States, 1999-2001. *MMWR Morb Mortal Wkly Rep, 54,* 1301-1305.

Cohen, W.I. (2006). Current dilemmas in Down syndrome clinical care: Celiac disease, thyroid disorders, and atlanto-axial instability. *Am J Med Genet C (Semin Med Genet), 142C,* 141-148.

Cohen, W.I.(Ed.). (1999). Health care guidelines for individuals with Down syndrome: 1999 revision. *Down Syndr Q, 4,* 1-16.

Cohen, W.I., & Patterson, B. (1998). News from the Down syndrome medical interest group. *Down Syndr Q, 3*(3), 15.

Committee on Bioethics (1999). Sterilization of minors with developmental disabilities. *Pediatrics, 104,* 337-347.

Concolino, D., Pasquzzi, A., Capalbo, G., et al. (2006). Early detection of podiatric anomalies in children with Down syndrome. *Acta Paediatr, 95,* 17-20.

Coppede, F., Colognato, R., Bonelli, A., et al. (2007). Polymorphisms in folate and homocysteine metabolizing genes and chromosome damage in mothers of Down syndrome children. *Am J Med Genet A, 143A*, 2006-2015.

Crocker, A.C. (2006). Down syndrome. In I.L. Rubin, & A.C. Crocker, (Eds.) *Medical Care for Children and Adults with Developmental Disabilities.* Baltimore: Paul H. Brookes.

Cuckle, H.S., Malone, F.D., Wright, D., et al. (2008). Contingent screening for Down syndrome—results from the FaSTER trial. *Prenat Diagn, 28*, 89-94.

Cushing, T., Clericuzio, C.L., Wilson, C.S., et al. (2006). Risk for leukemia in infants without Down syndrome who have transient myeloproliferative disorder. *J Pediatr, 148*, 687-689.

Cuskelly, M., & Gunn, P. (2006). Adjustment of children who have a sibling with Down syndrome: Perspectives of mothers, fathers, and children. *J Intellect Disabil Res, 50*, 917-925.

Daneshpazhooh, M., Nazemi, T.M., Bigdeloo, L., et al. (2007). Mucocutaneous findings in 100 children with Down syndrome. *Pediatr Dermatol, 24*, 317-320.

Day, S.M., Strauss, D.J., Shavelle, R.M., et al. (2005). Mortality and causes of death in persons with Down syndrome in California. *Dev Med Child Neurol, 47*, 171-176.

Dixon, N., Kishnani, P.S., & Zimmerman, S. (2006). Clinical manifestations of hematologic and oncologic disorders in patients with Down syndrome. *Am J Med Genet C (Semin Med Genet), 142C*, 149-157.

Durmowicz, A.G. (2001). Pulmonary edema in 6 children with Down syndrome during travel to moderate altitudes. *Pediatrics, 108*, 443-447.

Fey, M.E., Warren, S.F., Brady, N., et al. (2006). Early effects of responsivity education/prelinguistic milieu teaching for children with developmental delays and their parents. *J Speech Lang Hear Res, 49*, 526-547.

Fiore, A.E., Wasley, A., & Bell, B.P. (2006). Prevention of hepatitis A through active or passive immunization. Recommendations of the Advisory Committee on Immunization Practices (ACIP). *MMWR Morb Mortal Wkly Rep, 55*(RR-7), 1-23.

Fitzgerald, D.A., Paul, A., & Richmond, C. (2007). Severity of obstructive apnoea in children with Down syndrome who snore. *Arch Dis Child, 92*, 423-425.

Fransen, M.P., Essink-Bot, M.-L., Oenema, A., et al. (2007). Ethnic differences in determinants of participation and non-participation in prenatal screening for Down syndrome: A theoretical framework. *Prenat Diagn, 27*, 938-950.

Gamis, A.S. (2005). Acute myeloid leukemia and Down syndrome evolution of modern therapy—state of the art review. *Pediatr Blood Cancer, 44*, 13-20.

Garcia, E., Timmermans, D.R.M., & van Leeuwen, E. (2007). The impact of ethical beliefs on decisions about prenatal screening tests: Searching for justification. *Soc Sci Med, 66*, 753-764.

Gillespie, K.M., Dix, R.J., Williams, A.J.K., et al. (2006). Islet autoimmunity in children with Down's syndrome. *Diabetes, 55*, 3185-3188.

Haargaard, B., & Fledelius, H.C. (2006). Down's syndrome and early cataract. *Br J Ophthalmol, 90*, 1024-1027.

Hattori, M., Fujiyama, A., Taylor, T.D., et al. (2000). The DNA sequence of human chromosome 21: The chromosome 21 mapping and sequencing consortium. *Nature, 405*, 311-319.

Hecht, C.A., & Hook, E.B. (1996). Rates of Down syndrome at live birth at one-year maternal age intervals in studies with apparent close to complete ascertainment in populations of European origin: A proposed revised rate schedule for use in genetic and prenatal screening. *Am J Med Genet, 62*, 376-385.

Henry, E., Walker, D., Wiedmeier, S.E., et al. (2007). Hematological abnormalities during the first week of life among neonates with Down syndrome: Data from a multihospital healthcare system. *Am J Med Genet A, 143A*, 42-50.

Hill, I.D., Dirks, M.H., Liptak, G.S., et al. (2005). Guidelines for the diagnosis and treatment of celiac disease in children: Recommendations of the North American Society for Pediatric Gastroenterology, Hepatology, and Nutrition. *J Pediatr Gastroenterol Nutr, 40*, 1-19.

Iverson, J., Longobardi, E., & Caseli, M.C. (2003). Relationship between gestures and words in children with Down's syndrome and typically developing children in the early stages of communicative development. *Int J Lang Communication Disord, 38*, 179-197.

Kaatu, D., & LeLeiko, N.S. (2008). Screening for celiac disease in asymptomatic children with Down syndrome: Cost-effectiveness of preventing lymphoma. *Pediatrics, 118*, 816-817.

Keinan, D., Smith, P., & Zilberman, U. (2006). Microstructure and chemical composition of primary teeth in children with Down syndrome and cerebral palsy. *Arch Oral Biol, 51*, 836-843.

Khoshnood, B., Pryde, P., & Wall, S. (2000). Ethnic differences in the impact of advanced maternal age on birth prevalence of Down syndrome. *Am J Public Health, 90*, 1778-1781.

Kroger, A.T., Atkinson, W.L., Marcuse, E.K., et al. (2006). General recommendations on immunization: Recommendations of the Advisory Committee on Immunization Practices (ACIP). *MMWR Morb Mortal Wkly Rep, 55*(RR-15), 1-48.

Lashley, F.R. (2005). *Clinical Genetics in Nursing Practice.* (3rd ed.). New York: Springer.

Lashley, F.R. (2007). *Essentials of Clinical Genetics in Nursing Practice.* New York: Springer.

Lee, S.R., Kwon, H.K., Song, K.B., et al. (2004). Dental caries and salivary immunoglobulin A in Down syndrome children. *J Paediatr Child Health, 40*, 530-533.

Lindh, H.L., Steele, R., Page-Steiner, J., et al. (2007). Characteristics and perspectives of families waiting to adopt a child with Down syndrome. *Genet Med, 9*, 235-240.

Malini, S.S., & Ramachandra, N.B. (2006). Influence of advanced age of maternal grandmothers on Down syndrome. *BMC Med Genet, 7*, 4.

Marin, M., Guris, D., Chaves, S.S., et al. (2007). Prevention of varicella. Recommendations of the Advisory Committee on Immunization Practices (ACIP). *MMWR Morb Mortal Wkly Rep, 56*(RR-4), 1-40.

Martorell, S.J., & Martorell, G.A. (2006). Bridging uncharted waters in Georgia: Down Syndrome Association of Atlanta outreach to Latino/a families. *Am J Community Psychol, 37*, 219-225.

Massey, G.V., Zipursky, A., Chang, M.N., et al. (2006). A prospective study of the natural history of transient leukemia (TL) in neonates with Down syndrome (DS): Children's Oncology Group (COG) study POG-9481. *Blood, 107*, 4606-4613.

Meijer, W.M., Werler, M.M., Louik, C., et al. (2006). Can folic acid protect congenital heart defects in Down syndrome?. *Birth Defects Res (Part A), 76*, 714-717.

Miolo, G., Chapman, R.S., & Sindberg, H.A. (2005). Sentence comprehension in adolescents with Down syndrome and typically developing children: Role of sentence voice, visual context, and auditory-verbal short-term memory. *J Speech Lang Hear Res, 48*, 172-188.

Myrelid, A., Gustafsson, J., Ollars, B., et al. (2002). Growth charts for Down's syndrome from birth to 18 years of age. *Arch Dis Child, 87*, 97-103.

Nader-Sepahi, A., Casey, A.T.H., Hayward, R., et al. (2005). Symptomatic atlantoaxial instability in Down syndrome. *J Neurosurg (Pediatr 3), 103*, 231-237.

National Dissemination Center for Children with Disabilities (2004). *Disability Fact Sheet, No. 4, Down Syndrome.* Washington, DC: Author.

National Institute of Dental and Craniofacial Research. (2007). *Practical oral care for people with Down syndrome.* Available at www.nidcr.nih.gov/HealthInformation/DiseasesAndConditions/DevelopmentalDisabilitiesAndOral Health/DownSyndrome.htm. Retrieved August 18, 2008.

Nicham, R., Weitzdorfer, R., Hauser, E., et al. (2003). Spectrum of cognitive, behavioral and emotional problems in children and young adults with Down syndrome. *J Neural Transm, 67* (Suppl), 173-191.

Palmer, C.G., Cronk, C., Pueschel, S.M., et al. (1992). Head circumference of children with Down syndrome 0 to 36 months. *Am J Med Genet, 42*, 61-67.

Palomaki, G.E., Bradley, L.A., McDowell, G.A., Down Syndrome Working Group, & ACMG Laboratory Quality Assurance Committee. (2005). Technical standards and guidelines: Prenatal screening for Down syndrome. *Genet Med, 7*, 344-354.

Paul, R. (2007). *Language Disorders from Infancy Through Adolescence: Assessment and Intervention* (3rd ed.). Philadelphia: Elsevier.

Prussing, E., Sobo, E.J., Walker, E., et al. (2004). Communicating with pediatricians about complementary/alternative medicine: Perspectives from parents of children with Down syndrome. *Ambulatory Pediatr, 4*, 488-494.

Prussing, E., Sobo, E.J., Walker, E., et al. (2005). Between "desperation" and disability rights: A narrative analysis of complementary/alternative medicine use by parents for children with Down syndrome. *Soc Sci Med, 60*, 587-598.

Rajantie, J., & Siimes, M.A. (2003). Long-term prognosis of children with Down's syndrome and leukaemia: A 34-year nation-wide experience. *J Intellect Disabil Res, 47*, 617-621.

Rasmussen, S.A., Wong, L.-Y, Correa, A., et al. (2006). Survival in infants with Down syndrome, metropolitan Atlanta, 1979-1998. *J Pediatr, 148*, 806-812.

Ravindranath, Y. (2005). Down syndrome and leukemia: New insights into the epidemiology, pathogenesis, and treatment. *Pediatr Blood Cancer, 44*, 1-7.

Roberts, J.E., Long, S.H., Malkin, C., et al. (2005). A comparison of phonological skills of boys with fragile X syndrome and Down syndrome. *J Speech Lang Hear Res, 48*, 980-995.

Roberts, J.E., Price, J., & Malkin, C. (2007). Language and communication development in Down syndrome. *Ment Retard Dev Disabil Res Rev, 13*, 26-35.

Roizen, N.J. (2005). Complementary and alternative therapies for Down syndrome. *Ment Retard Dev Disabil Res Rev, 11*, 149-155.

Roizen, N.J. (2007). Down syndrome. In M.L. Batshaw, L. Pellegrino, & N.J. Roizen, (Eds.). *Children with Disabilities* (6th ed.)., Baltimore: Paul H. Brookes.

Roizen, N.J., & Patterson, D. (2003). Down's syndrome. *Lancet, 361*, 1281-1289.

Shott, S.R. (2006). Down syndrome: Common otolaryngologic manifestations. *Am J Med Genet C (Semin Med Genet), 142C*, 131-140.

Siklos, S., & Kerns, K.A. (2006). Assessing need for social support in parents of children with autism and Down syndrome. *J Autism Dev Disord, 36*, 921-933.

Skotko, B.G., & Levine, S.P. (2006). What the other children are thinking: Brothers and sisters of persons with Down syndrome. *Am J Med Genet C (Semin Med Genet), 142C*, 180-186.

Spencer, K., Cowans, N.J., Uldbjerg, N., et al. (2008). First-trimester ADAM12s as early markers of trisomy 21: A promise still unfulfilled? *Prenat Diagn, 28*, 338-342.

Spencer, K., Vereecken, A., & Cowans, N.J. (2008). Maternal serum ADAM12s as a potential marker of trisomy 21 to 10 weeks of gestation. *Prenat Diagn, 28*, 209-211.

Stephen, E., Dickson, J., Kindley, A.D., et al. (2007). Surveillance of vision and ocular disorders in children with Down syndrome. *Dev Med Child Neurol, 49*, 513-515.

Stewart, R.E., Woodhouse, J.M., Cregg, M., et al. (2007). Association between accommodative accuracy, hypermetropia, and strabismus in children with Down's syndrome. *Optom Vis Sci, 84*, 149-155.

Sullivan, S.G., Hussain R., Glasson, E.J., et al. (2007). The profile and incidence of cancer in Down syndrome. *J Intellect Disabil Res, 51*, 228-231.

Swigonski, N.L., Kuhlenschmidt, H.L., Bull, M.J., et al. (2008). Screening for celiac disease in asymptomatic children with Down syndrome: Cost-effectiveness of preventing lymphoma. *Pediatrics, 118*, 594-602.

Thiel, R., & Fowkes, S.W. (2007). Down syndrome and thyroid dysfunction: Should nutritional support be the first-line treatment? *Med Hypotheses, 69*, 809-815.

Tolmie, J.L. (2002). Down syndrome and other autosomal trisomies. In D.L. Rimoin, J.M. Connor, R.E. Pyeritz, et al. (Eds.) *Emery and Rimoin's Principles and Practices of Medical Genetics (4th ed.).* New York: Churchill Livingstone.

Tomizawa, D., Tabuchi, K., Kinoshita, A., et al. (2007). Repetitive cycles of high-dose cytarabine are effective for childhood acute myeloid leukemia: Long-term outcome of the children with AML treated on two consecutive trials of Tokyo Children's Cancer Study Group. *Pediatr Blood Cancer, 49*, 127-132.

Van Cleve, S.N., Cannon, S., & Cohen, W.I. (2006). Part II: Clinical practice guidelines for adolescents and young adults with Down syndrome: 12 to 21 years. *J Pediatr Health Care, 20*, 198-205.

Van Cleve, S.N., & Cohen, W.I. (2006). Part 1: Clinical practice guidelines for children with Down syndrome from birth to 12 years. *J Pediatr Health Care, 20*, 47-54.

Van Riper, M. (2007). Families of children with Down syndrome: Responding to "a change in plans" with resilience. *J Pediatr Nurs, 22*, 116-128.

Vida, V.L., & Castaneda, A.R. (2006). Types of cardiac defects in children with Down's syndrome. *Cardiology of the Young, 16*, 197.

Visootsak, J., & Sherman, S. (2007). Neuropsychiatric and behavioral aspects of trisomy 21. *Curr Psychiatr Rep, 9*, 135-140.

Vyas, P., & Crispino, J.D. (2007). Molecular insights into Down syndrome-associated leukemia. *Curr Opin Pediatr, 19*, 9-14.

Vyas, P., & Roberts, I. (2006). Down myeloid disorders: A paradigm for childhood preleukaemia and leukaemia and insights into normal megakaryopoiesis. *Early Hum Dev, 82*, 767-773.

Whitlock, J.A. (2006). Down syndrome and acute lymphoblastic leukaemia. *Br J Haematol, 135*, 595-602.

Whitlock, J.A., Sather, H.N., Gaynon, P., et al. (2005). Clinical characteristics and outcome of children with Down syndrome and acute lymphoblastic leukemia: A Children's Cancer Group study. *Blood, 106*, 4043-4049.

Yang, Q., Rasmussen, S.A., & Friedman, J.M. (2002). Mortality associated with Down's syndrome in the USA from 1983 to 1997: A population-based study. *Lancet, 359*, 1019-1025.

25 Eating Disorders

Barbara E. Wolfe, Adrian T. Smith, and Donna L. Cullinan

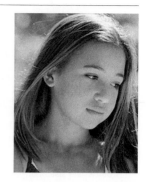

ALTERED eating patterns during childhood and adolescence can include a variety of behaviors ranging from the finicky 5-year-old who will only eat peanut butter and jelly sandwiches, to the 11-year-old who refuses to eat broccoli, to the teenager who tries to adopt a vegan diet. Such behaviors are not uncommon, nor are they pathologic. Eating disorders, however, are specific conditions that involve disturbed eating patterns associated with significant distress and impairment. These disorders are coupled with deleterious psychosocial and medical consequences. In addition, eating disorders are often chronic psychiatric conditions with symptoms that typically develop during childhood or adolescent years.

The *Diagnostic and Statistical Manual of Mental Disorders* (*DSM-IV-TR*; American Psychiatric Association [APA], 2000) classifies eating disorders into three distinct categories: anorexia nervosa (AN), bulimia nervosa (BN), and eating disorder not otherwise specified (EDNOS). AN is characterized by the cardinal feature of a low weight for age and height, often a result of significant weight loss brought on by severe dietary restriction or compensatory behaviors directed at weight control (e.g., self-induced vomiting, laxative or diuretic abuse, excessive exercising). In contrast to AN, BN occurs in individuals who are at or above a normal weight for age and height who experience the hallmark feature of recurring binge eating episodes followed by compensatory behaviors to control body weight. EDNOS is a diagnostic category used to classify individuals with sub-threshold AN or BN or those who exhibit other disordered eating that causes distress or impairment. An example of the latter category includes binge eating disorder (BED), a diagnostic category currently deemed provisional and in need of further research (APA, 2000). Characteristics of BED include regular binge eating with no compensatory behaviors to prevent weight gain.

Children and adolescents with an eating disorder are challenged by the psychological distress of the condition, as well as the toll of the negative physical health effects, particularly during a time of developmental growth (Kreipe & Birndorf, 2000). These youth may be at a dangerously low weight and/or a state of severe malnutrition. They may have serious electrolyte imbalances, delayed onset of menstruation, and/or engage in the use of risky compensatory behaviors. Medical and psychological sequelae put youth at risk during this vulnerable period of growth and development (Watkins & Lask, 2002). For these reasons, both primary and specialty (e.g., mental health) health care are important for the child or adolescent struggling with an eating disorder.

Primary care providers (PCPs) often are the first clinicians to assess and detect the presence of an eating disorder. Similarly, the PCP may be the initial health care professional to whom the individual discloses disordered eating. Thus, PCP awareness and cognizance of the signs and symptoms of eating disorders, the need for referral to mental health services, and the ongoing need for primary health care monitoring are crucial to the care of the child.

Etiology

Over the years, several theories have emerged pertaining to the cause of eating disorders. Many of these theories reflect the state of science at the time of their inception, and many continue to have limited empirical support. A single cause of an eating disorder is unlikely; rather, the cause is anticipated to be multifaceted. The following section reviews some of the major theories on the development of an eating disorder. However, it is important to remember that most empirical studies of these theories have been conducted in adults. Thus, caution for generalization of these findings to children and adolescents is warranted.

Psychological Theories

One of the earlier theories of the development of an eating disorder, particularly that of AN, was that individuals starve themselves as a defense mechanism in response to sexual fantasies of oral impregnation (Waller, Kaufman, & Deutsch, 1940). Early theories of BN suggested that binge eating episodes reflect a fantasy of incestuous impregnation (Schwartz, 1988). Although these explanations have surfaced episodically over the years, there has been little actual research testing them.

Additional psychological theories have focused on other underlying psychological conflicts. Bruch (1982) theorized that early life experiences, including the mother-child interaction, provided a foundation for later behaviors leading to the development of an eating disorder. She noted that AN typically occurs during a time of developmental crisis, although faulty experiences occurred long before the actual onset of illness. Bruch suggested that inconsistent and repeated maternal failures to attend to a child's needs lead to the child's self-imposed starvation as a means of controlling her or his immediate environment. Thus, children with eating disorders are characteristically overachieving, obedient, and overly compliant in an effort to meet the mother's needs rather than their own. This jeopardizes the child's ability to successfully experience autonomy and self-identity. Thus, according to Bruch, the symptoms of the disorder reflect an expression of a deficit in self-concept.

Other theories have focused on the potential role of child abuse, particularly sexual abuse, in the development of an eating disorder. This theory has been an area of debate in the literature with regard to the specificity of a cause-and-effect relationship. As reviewed by Brewerton (2007), research suggests that childhood sexual abuse is a "nonspecific" risk factor for the development of an eating disorder. Thus, it is also a risk factor for other psychiatric disorders, hence the "nonspecific" designation. These findings have been extended to suggest an association with a wider range of childhood traumatic events, including childhood neglect and bullying (Brewerton). Trauma histories are reportedly more frequent in persons with bulimic symptoms (e.g., binge-purge behavior) compared with persons with the restricting subtype of AN (Brewerton).

Family Theories

Earlier family theories focused on the role of family dynamics in the development and maintenance of a child's eating disorder. In the classic work by Minuchin and colleagues (1975), the child's symptoms were viewed as psychosomatic, playing a homeostatic role in a system of family conflict. Families of a child with AN have been characterized as enmeshed (e.g., overly involved, intrusive, or lacking boundaries), overprotective (e.g., both parents are protective of the child, and the child is protective of the family), rigidity (e.g., avoidance of change), and limited in conflict resolution (e.g., conflict avoidance) (Minuchin et al.). The child's disorder enables family members in avoiding the real underlying family issues. Researchers have tried to discern the extent to which these types of interactions are unique to families of a person with AN or reflect families of a person with a psychiatric illness in general.

More contemporary studies have focused on understanding familial risk factors in persons with AN, persons with a non-eating psychiatric disorder, and persons without a psychiatric disorder (Pike, Hilbert, Wilfley, et al., 2008). Individuals with AN demonstrated increased rates and greater severity of family discord and parental demands than the other two groups. Recent efforts have been extended to include an understanding of the influence of parent-child relationships on sibling adaptation to a sister with AN (Honey & Halse, 2006).

For individuals with BN, low family closeness/cohesion, low familial independence, and high family achievement orientation are associated with eating disorder symptoms (Ackard & Neumark-Sztainer, 2001). Negative family communication, external control of food intake, and rules related to family mealtimes also have been observed to be predictive of the severity of BN symptoms (Crowther, Kichler, Sherwood, et al., 2002).

Although the literature often has focused on the role of the mother in the cause of an eating disorder, Agras, Bryson, Hammer, and colleagues (2007) more recently have examined the influence of fathers in children's preoccupation with body weight and desire to be thin. These researchers found that girls with higher rates of "thin body preoccupation and social pressure to be thin" were more likely to have fathers who were dissatisfied with their own body weight or had a high drive for thinness.

Sociocultural Theories

The focus on thinness as an ideal body shape in Western cultures has been theorized as a possible contributor to the development of an eating disorder. Western countries have greater prevalence rates of eating disorders than non-Western countries, although rates in non-Western countries are on the rise (Makino, Tsuboi, & Dennerstein, 2004). The reason for such increase may be related to growing exposure to Western ideals. This rationale is best illustrated by studies showing an increase of eating disorders following globalization of Western media exposure. For example, Becker and colleagues (2002) found a 58% increase in disordered eating after 3 years of television exposure in Fijian schoolgirls. Others have found a positive relationship between exposure to Western culture (e.g., media or travel) and eating disorder symptoms among East African women (Eddy, Hennessey, & Thompson-Brenner, 2007). Additional theories suggest that differences in eating disorders and culture need to be examined within the context of cultural change. DiNicola (1990) proposed that AN is a "cultural-change syndrome," emerging in environments undergoing rapid economic and sociocultural change.

Although cultural differences exist in the prevalence of eating disorders, other important factors may play a contributory role. Lee and Lock (2007) observed that Asian-American adolescents with AN are from families with higher income and orientation toward achievement than their non-Asian peers. In addition, the Asian adolescents scored significantly lower on measures of restrained eating and weight concerns compared with the non-Asian cohort, suggesting that they may underreport symptoms. Cultural differences in family orientation toward achievement may inhibit the reporting of symptoms and hence contribute to lower prevalence rates observed in some of the non-Western cultures.

The role of sociocultural ideals beyond those of a geographical culture also may be important. For instance, subcultures that idealize thinness exist among ballet dancers, fashion models, jockeys, and wrestlers. These groups also exhibit a higher risk for disordered eating (Dale & Landers, 1999; Ringham, Klump, Kaye, et al., 2006; Santonastaso, Mondini, & Favaro, 2002). The "female athlete triad," a term characterizing the clustered relationship among reduced energy availability, amenorrhea, and osteoporosis, highlights another group of individuals that may have increased risk for eating disorders and possibly contribute to gender differences seen in the occurrence of these disorders (Nattiv, Loucks, Manore, et al., 2007). Sexual orientation is yet another factor that may be associated with greater risk for an eating disorder, particularly for males. Feldman & Meyer (2007) found that gay and bisexual men had higher prevalence estimates of eating disorders compared with heterosexual men, whereas no such differences were observed among lesbian and bisexual women compared with heterosexual women.

Biologic Theories

The role of neurobiology in the onset, maintenance, and recovery of an eating disorder has been an area of intense investigation. Studies have focused on the role of neurotransmitters, particularly serotonin, because of its involvement in appetite regulation. Investigation of the serotonin metabolite, 5-hydroxyindole acetic acid, and neuroendocrine responsivity suggests that persons with AN and BN have dysregulated serotonergic functioning in the central nervous system (CNS) (Jimerson & Wolfe, 2006). It is still unclear whether the dysregulation is a contributing factor or a consequence of the illness. In addition to neurotransmitter systems, other biologic substrates involved in the regulation of feeding behavior have been implicated. These include the neuropeptides cholecystokinin, corticotropin-releasing hormone, ghrelin, leptin, and neuropeptide Y. For example, decreased plasma levels of leptin, a hormone thought to play a role in the regulation of food intake and energy expenditure, have been found in women with

BN (Jimerson, Mantzoros, Wolfe, et al., 2000) and in those with AN (Mantzoros, Flier, Lesem, et al., 1997). Interestingly, plasma leptin levels appear to return to normal in persons with AN during weight recovery with treatment even though normal body weight has not yet been achieved (Mantzoros et al.). The authors note that normalization of leptin levels before weight restoration may play a role in resistance to weight gain during this critical recovery period.

Related to serotonin function is the role of dietary intake (or lack there of) on neurotransmitter functioning. Dieting in healthy women has been shown to decrease the availability of the essential amino acid tryptophan (Wolfe, Metzger, & Stollar, 1997). Plasma tryptophan competes with other large neutral amino acids for transport into the CNS, where it then is converted into the neurotransmitter serotonin. Thus, severe dietary restriction in persons with eating disorders may influence CNS serotonin and subsequent regulation of appetite.

Familial aggregation studies also suggest a biologic heritability of eating-related psychopathology. Family members of people with the diagnosis of AN or BN are 7 to 12 times more likely to have a diagnosis of EDNOS, compared with families in which no family member has an eating disorder (Lilenfeld, Kaye, Greeno, et al., 1998). Although family studies indicate a biologic heritability of eating disorders, they do not rule out the possibility of environmental influences. Twin studies, which provide an opportunity to examine both genetic and environmental effects, suggest a heritability of approximately 33% to 84% for AN (Wade, Bulik, Neale, et al., 2000) and 28% to 83% for BN (Bulik, Sullivan, Wade, et al., 2000). Interestingly, Klump, Burt, McGue, and colleagues (2007) observed a significant change in genetic and environmental influences on disordered eating during early to mid adolescence, with genetic influences having an increased effect between the ages of 14 and 18 years and environmental influences having a decreased effect during this period.

Neuroanatomic studies have been yet another source of investigation into the cause of eating disorders. Earlier studies of AN using computed tomography and subsequent studies using magnetic resonance imaging show cerebral ventricular enlargement with return to normal after weight restoration (Jimerson, Wolfe, & Naab, 2006). Findings during active illness may be related to a host of factors, including hydration and body mass index (BMI), which render it difficult to determine whether they are antecedents or consequences of the disorder. Several functional imaging studies in patients with AN and BN have implicated several possible brain regions; however, findings have been inconsistent and the clinical significance remains unclear.

Incidence and Prevalence

The lifetime prevalence of eating disorders, although obtained from adults and not necessarily indicative of childhood prevalence rates, provides a crude index of the lifetime occurrence of the disorder. The lifetime prevalence for AN is estimated to be 0.9% in women and 0.3% in men; the prevalence of BN is approximately 1.5% in women and 0.5% in men; and the prevalence of BED is 3.5% in women and 2% in men (Hudson, Hiripi, Pope, et al., 2007). The average age of onset is typically late adolescence to young adulthood—age 18.9 years for AN, 19.7 for BN, and 25.4 for BED (Hudson et al.). However, the disorders and prodromal symptoms can occur much earlier.

Studies are beginning to parse out the prevalence of eating disorders in children and adolescents from that in their adult counterparts. In an investigation of the prevalence of AN, BN, and EDNOS among youths 12 to 21 years of age in Spain, 3.4% of the sample met criteria for an eating disorder (5.3% of females and 0.6% of males) (Fernandez, Labrador, & Raich, 2007). For both females and males who met diagnostic criteria for an eating disorder, EDNOS was the most common category, followed by BN, and then AN. When looking at lifetime prevalence of eating disorders in a group of Norwegian adolescents 14 to 15 years of age, 17.9% of the girls reported a history of an eating disorder (Kjelsas, Bjørnstrøm, & Götestam, 2004). For the girls in this sample, EDNOS (excluding BED) was the most common category (14.6%), followed by BED (1.5%), BN (1.2%), and then AN (0.7%). The adolescent boys reported a 6.5% lifetime prevalence of an eating disorder, with EDNOS (5%) the most common, followed by BED (0.9%), BN (0.4%), and then AN (0.2%). No reports have focused specifically on the prevalence of eating disorders in young children; however, the disorders are considered rare in prepubertal youth (Watkins & Lask, 2002) but are slowly growing more prevalent (Peebles, Wilson, & Lock, 2006). Although it may be premature to generalize these findings, they do point to the occurrence of eating disorders during childhood and adolescence and the related struggles that these youth endure. Additionally, it is possible that the overall understanding of prevalence is further limited by the denial and minimization of symptoms that may contribute to underreporting of the disorders (Couturier & Lock, 2006).

Recent attention has focused on the possibility that children and adolescents with certain types of chronic medical conditions may be at increased risk for eating disorders. A significantly higher incidence of binge eating and compensatory behaviors has been observed in adolescents with insulin-dependent diabetes mellitus (Smith, Latchford, Hall, et al., 2008). Yet others have found that youths with type 1 diabetes do not appear to be at increased risk for eating disorders and, relative to their healthy adolescent counterparts, are less likely to engage in unhealthy weight control practices and more likely to be satisfied with their body weight (Ackard, Vik, Neumark-Sztainer, et al., 2008).

Diagnostic Criteria
Anorexia Nervosa

The cardinal feature of AN is a body weight significantly lower than one would expect. Such low weight can involve a severe or dangerous weight loss or the refusal to maintain a healthy weight. The low weight state is defined as weight approximately at or below 85% of the expected body weight for age and height (APA, 2000; see Box 25-1 for diagnostic criteria). For adults, this is a BMI less than 18.5 kg/m^2 (APA, 2006). In children who are still developing, this criterion is adjusted and defined as refusal to meet expected or average weight gain over a period of time (APA, 2000). For children and adolescents, an age-adjusted BMI is calculated. Tables for age-adjusted BMI values can be found at www.cdc.gov/nchs/about/major/nhanes/growthcharts/clinical_charts.htm. Children with weights below the BMI 5th percentile are considered underweight (APA, 2006).

Amenorrhea is a cardinal feature for the diagnosis of AN in postmenarcheal females, although evidence to support its use as

DSM-IV-TR Criteria for Anorexia Nervosa

A. Refusal to maintain body weight at or above a minimally normal weight for age and height (e.g., weight loss leading to maintenance of body weight less than 85% of that expected; or failure to make expected weight gain during period of growth leading to body weight less than 85% of that expected).
B. Intense fear of gaining weight or becoming fat, even though underweight.
C. Disturbance in the way in which one's body weight or shape is experienced, undue influence of body weight or shape on self-evaluation, or denial of the seriousness of the current low body weight.
D. In postmenarcheal females, amenorrhea, i.e., the absence of at least three consecutive menstrual cycles. (A woman is considered to have amenorrhea if her periods occur only following hormones, e.g., estrogen, administration.)

SPECIFY TYPE

Restricting Type: During the current episode of Anorexia Nervosa, the person has not regularly engaged in binge-eating or purging behavior (i.e., self-induced vomiting or the misuse of laxatives, diuretics, or enemas).
Binge-Eating/Purging Type: During the current episode of Anorexia Nervosa, the person has regularly engaged in binge-eating or purging behavior (i.e., self-induced vomiting or the misuse of laxatives, diuretics, or enemas).

Reprinted with permission from the America Psychiatric Association. (2000). *Diagnostic and Statistical Manual of Mental Disorders* (4th ed., Text Revision). Washington DC, The Association.

DSM-IV-TR Criteria for Bulimia Nervosa

A. Recurrent episodes of binge eating. An episode of binge eating is characterized by both of the following:
(1) Eating, in a discrete period of time (e.g., within any 2-hour period), an amount of food that is definitely larger than most people would eat during a similar period of time and under similar circumstances.
(2) A sense of lack of control over eating during the episode (e.g., a feeling that one cannot stop eating or control what or how much one is eating).
B. Recurrent inappropriate compensatory behavior in order to prevent weight gain, such as self-induced vomiting; misuse of laxatives, diuretics, enemas, or other medications; fasting; or excessive exercise.
C. The binge eating and inappropriate compensatory behaviors both occur, on average, at least twice a week for 3 months.
D. Self-evaluation is unduly influenced by body shape and weight.
E. The disturbance does not occur exclusively during episodes of Anorexia Nervosa.

SPECIFY TYPE

Purging Type: During the current episode of Bulimia Nervosa, the person has regularly engaged in self-induced vomiting or the misuse of laxatives, diuretics, or enemas.
Nonpurging Type: During the current episode of Bulimia Nervosa, the person has used other inappropriate compensatory behaviors, such as fasting or excessive exercise, but has not regularly engaged in self-induced vomiting or the misuse of laxatives, diuretics, or enemas.

Reprinted with permission from the America Psychiatric Association. (2000). *Diagnostic and Statistical Manual of Mental Disorders* (4th ed., Text revision). Washington DC, The Association.

a diagnostic criterion is limited because of the questionable specificity to active AN (Smith & Wolfe, 2008). For example, amenorrhea can occur with dieting, before low weight is achieved, after weight restoration, and during BN. *Amenorrhea* is defined as the absence of three successive menstrual cycles (termed *secondary amenorrhea*). For pubescent female adolescents, the delay of onset of menstruation is termed *primary amenorrhea*. This criterion can be particularly difficult to assess in girls who are just starting to menstruate because of its irregular course in early puberty for most girls, regardless of eating pathology (Kotler & Walsh, 2000). It is important to note that adolescent girls at low weight and receiving hormonal therapy or oral contraceptives to induce menstruation, with fear of fat and body image distortion, are exempt from this criterion.

AN Subtypes. Individuals at low weight who struggle with AN are typically classified into one of two subtypes: restricting and binge eating/purging. Those in the restricting type engage in severe dieting, fasting, and excessive exercise. Those in the binge eating/purging type regularly engage in binge eating and/or self-induced vomiting, abuse of laxatives and diuretics, and/or use of enemas (APA, 2000).

Bulimia Nervosa

BN is particularly difficult to detect because affected children and adolescents are typically normal weight for their age and height, with some individuals above a normal weight range (Kreipe & Birndorf, 2000). Thus, obtaining a thorough history from the child and family is particularly important. The core feature of BN is the cycle of recurring binge eating episodes followed by compensatory behaviors to prevent weight gain (see Box 25-2 for BN diagnostic criteria). Similar to persons with AN, these individuals experience a preoccupation with body dissatisfaction and place a great deal of importance on their body weight and shape. BN does not occur during an episode of AN.

Binge eating episodes occur over a discrete period during which an individual eats an excessively large amount of food. The amount of food is "objectively" large, meaning that it exceeds what someone else would eat in a similar situation (APA, 2000). This amount can be somewhat complicated to quantify, particularly when energy intake needs vary across the developmental span of childhood and adolescents. Binge foods are typically high in calories and easily ingested. Anecdotally, binges tend to occur separately from regular meals, although meals can evolve into binge episodes.

Currently, binge eating episodes and compensatory actions must occur at least twice a week for three months or longer to meet the diagnostic criteria for BN (APA, 2000). However, empirical validation of this frequency is needed (Wilfley, Bishop, Wilson, et al., 2007).

BN Subtypes. Children and adolescents with BN are subtyped based on their compensatory behaviors, which include either "purging" type or "nonpurging" type. The purging type relies on methods to eliminate or rid the body of excess food and calories. The most common method of purging is self-induced vomiting, which often relieves physical pain and facilitates further binge eating. Fingers or other devices (e.g., spoon or toothbrush) are used to stimulate the uvula to trigger a gag reflex and induce vomiting. Some individuals can elicit a vomiting reflex at will, without stimulation of the uvula—this is usually quieter, can be less painful, and may therefore be harder to detect. Purging comes in other forms (or combinations of use), such as laxative abuse, diuretic abuse, syrup of ipecac use, and enema use, although these methods are less common in children and adolescents than adults with BN (Fisher, Schneider, Burns, et al., 2001).

Nonpurging type BN involves the use of compensatory mechanisms to "even out" or "make up for" the calories consumed during the binge episode. These include fasting, excessive exercise, and strict dieting. In addition to duration of time considerations, exercise is usually defined as excessive if it interferes or takes precedence over important activities, is excessively ritualistic, or both (APA, 2000). Because exercise is often less secretive than other compensatory behaviors, this behavior can serve as an important flag to clinicians, and it may be a source of conflict when youths are ill or injured and refuse to stop exercising. Additionally, the extent of excessive exercising can be difficult to assess when youths are involved in rigorous athletic activities.

Eating Disorder Not Otherwise Specified

The EDNOS designation is used to classify abnormal eating patterns and/or body perceptions in association with significant distress and impairment that do not meet the criteria for AN or BN. Currently, more children than adults fall into the EDNOS category, because the AN and BN criteria are not as applicable to the developmental manifestations of an eating disorder in children (Fisher et al., 2001; Chamay-Weber, Narring, & Michaud, 2005). Examples include the adolescent who binge eats and purges but not at a minimum frequency of twice a week for three months (e.g., sub-threshold BN), a postmenarcheal adolescent obsessed with her food intake who has recent severe weight loss (e.g., <85% of average body weight) but still menstruates (e.g., sub-threshold AN), the young normal-weight child who purges after meals and reports subjective binge eating episodes, or the adolescent who regularly chews her food for taste but routinely spits it out before ingestion (APA, 2000).

Food avoidance emotional disorder and functional dysphagia are additional EDNOS conditions described in the literature that are specific to children. Food avoidance emotional disorder is characterized by anxiousness, phobias, or depressed mood elicited by food (Watkins & Lask, 2002). The avoidance of food is severe, not purposeful, obsessive, and can be a product of preoccupation with weight and shape. Functional dysphagia describes a condition in which an intense fear of swallowing, choking, or vomiting prevents a child from eating (Watkins & Lask).

Binge Eating Disorder. One specific example of EDNOS that has gained significant attention in the past decade is BED. It is a provisional diagnosis in *DSM-IV-TR* (APA, 2000) and is recognized as occurring in children and adults (Shapiro, Woolson, Hamer, et al., 2007). BED is defined by distressing and frequent episodes of binge eating that are not routinely followed by compensatory behaviors (APA, 2000). Because the binge episodes, in the absence of regular compensatory behaviors, lead to excessive calorie consumption, individuals with BED are often above average weight, overweight, or obese (although this is not a diagnostic criterion for the disorder) (Box 25-3).

Binge eating episodes are similarly defined as those characteristic of BN and must also be associated with significant psychological or physical distress (APA, 2000). This distress is manifested in unpleasant feelings during and after the binge episode and concern about the long-term physical effects of frequent binge eating. The binge episodes are associated with a lack of control and occur for at least 6 months to be considered diagnostic (APA, 2000).

BOX 25-3

DSM-IV-TR Research Criteria for Binge Eating Disorder

A. Recurrent episodes of binge-eating. An episode of binge eating is characterized by both of the following:
   (1) Eating, in a discrete period of time (e.g., within any 2-hour period), an amount of food that is definitely larger than most people would eat in a similar period of time under similar circumstances
   (2) A sense of lack of control over eating during the episode (e.g., a feeling that one cannot stop eating or control what or how much one is eating)
B. The binge-eating episodes are associated with three (or more) of the following:
   (1) Eating much more rapidly than normal
   (2) Eating until feeling uncomfortably full
   (3) Eating large amounts of food when not feeling physically hungry
   (4) Eating alone because of being embarrassed by how much one is eating
   (5) Feeling disgusted with oneself, depressed, or very guilty after overeating
C. Marked distress regarding binge eating is present.
D. The binge eating, on average, at least 2 days a week for 6 months. NOTE: The method of determining frequency differs from the used for Bulimia Nervosa; future research should address whether the preferred method of setting a frequency threshold is counting the number of days on which binges occur or counting the number of episodes of binge eating.
E. The binge eating is not associated with the regular use of inappropriate compensatory behaviors (e.g., purging, fasting, excessive excursive) and does not occur exclusively during the course of Anorexia Nervosa or Bulimia Nervosa.

Reprinted with permission from the America Psychiatric Association. (2000). *Diagnostic and Statistical Manual of Mental Disorders* (4th ed., Text revision). Washington DC, The Association.

Clinical Manifestations at Time of Diagnosis

Although early detection of eating disorders is associated with a better long-term prognosis or prevention of full disorder development (Le Grange & Loeb, 2007), it is important to realize that the detection of these disorders can be particularly difficult. PCPs often overlook the potential diagnosis of an eating disorder in pediatric settings (Le Grange & Loeb). Patients struggling with an eating disorder are often high functioning, high achieving, and may be essentially normal-looking children or adolescents (i.e., with the exception of low weight in AN). Furthermore, patients with an eating disorder often rationalize and try to normalize their eating behaviors, weight, and other destructive habits. This deception may be purposeful denial, genuine disconnection, or a function of embarrassment. Nonetheless, the denial prevents this group of children and youth from seeking help or recognition of their problem (Viglione, Muratori, Maestro, et al., 2006). These youth are therefore particularly resistant to the idea of seeing specialists (e.g., nutritionists and psychiatric mental health practitioners) who are perceived as manipulative or threatening to their "way of being." Thus the PCP may be the only health care provider who sees a child or adolescent struggling with an eating disorder, and it is particularly important that PCPs remain vigilant of signs and symptoms, as well as the diagnostic criteria, for these disorders. Additionally, it is essential to plan for referrals for psychiatric care with a mental health specialist and ongoing care with the PCP for their physical health monitoring needs.

Clinical Manifestations at Time of Diagnosis

ANOREXIA NERVOSA
- Refusal to maintain normal weight
- Dietary: Constant calorie counting, episodic or persistent fasting, ritualistic eating patterns
- Avoidance of new foods, refusal to eat between meals
- Acting out, stress, anxiety or tantrums at meal time
- Distorted body image
- Excessive checking of appearance and weight throughout the day

BULIMIA NERVOSA
- Binge episodes typically secret, planned, involve similar foods
- Binge episodes may be triggered by stress, dysphoria, dieting

PHYSICAL HEALTH ASSESSMENT
- Weight concealed by wearing many layers of clothing
- Body mass index (BMI) low (AN) to normal (AN, BN) or high (BN)
- Bradycardia or tachycardia from dehydration, arrhythmias
- Orthostatic hypotension
- Skeletal frame with rib cage and iliac crests visible
- Pale skin color or yellow skin (carotenemia)
- Dry, rough skin, poor skin turgor, brittle nails, dull or thinning hair
- Lanugo
- Russell's sign: Skin abrasions or callus areas on knuckles (BN)
- Parotid gland enlargement
- Discoloration of teeth, enamel erosion
- Normal or delayed sexual development

Anorexia Nervosa

Weight loss or refusal to maintain a normal weight is driven and maintained by the diagnostic criterion of an "intense fear of fat or weight gain" (APA, 2000). These fears motivate the child or adolescent to severely restrict his or her dietary intake. Dietary restriction typically involves the avoidance of "high fat" or "unhealthy" foods until a severely limited diet remains. Dietary restriction is evident in constant calorie counting, episodic or persistent fasting, and ritualistic menus and/or eating patterns. The fear can also be seen in the youth's rigid adherence to these rituals and eating habits, including the absolute refusal to break any of these rules, avoidance of eating new and different foods, and/or inability to eat between regular mealtimes. In children and adolescents, expressing and understanding a cognitive "fear" can be difficult, and therefore this is manifested in acting-out behavior, tantrums, or stress and anxiety around eating and mealtime (Workgroup for Classification of Eating Disorders in Children and Adolescents [WCEDCA], 2007).

Importantly, weight loss and even emaciation do not quell these fears or stop the severe dieting behavior, but may, in fact, augment them. One reason is that children and adolescents struggling with AN also have distorted body image (APA, 2000). This symptom is seen when the child or adolescent excessively complains of being "too chubby" or becomes preoccupied with disliked areas of his or her body (e.g., stomach, thighs, "double chin"), even when body weight is extremely low. These youths also may obsessively check their appearance in the mirror and weigh themselves often (e.g., several times a day) because their self-esteem and identity may depend greatly on their ability to achieve or maintain a low body weight. Often when one weight goal is met, a new lower goal is immediately put in place. This obsession makes it difficult for the youth to understand the medical severity of their condition. However, in children, it is important to note that an understanding of medical severity and risk may not be present based on developmental stage or educational background (Watkins & Lask, 2002).

Bulimia Nervosa

Binge eating is often premeditated, yet described as out of control. Individuals often plan what they will eat and typically select the same types of foods. Similarly, they typically plan where the episode will occur, usually in secret. The actual binge is characterized by eating fast with an inability to slow down or stop the episode. During the episode, some individuals describe feeling numb and oblivious to events occurring in the surrounding environment. Because of the loss of control, children and adolescents may eat until they are painfully full.

In addition to stress, binge eating episodes in BN are often triggered by dysphoria, starvation, and dieting (Kjelsas, Børsting, & Gudde, 2004). Individuals more commonly stop eating because of stomach pain, dysphoria, vomiting, and by being interrupted by others (Kjelsas, et al.). After the eating episode, feelings of guilt, shame, and self-disgust usually occur, leading to compensatory behaviors to keep the weight off.

Physical Health Assessment

A physical examination can provide key information on the diagnosis and assessment of clinical manifestations of eating disorders. Physical appearance can range from normal to severely emaciated in the case of AN. The adolescent with AN may attempt to camouflage the severity of weight loss by wearing layers of clothing (which also may be worn because of endocrine changes that lead to persistence of feeling cold). Height and weight should be obtained and BMI calculated. Vital signs should be monitored, including orthostatic pulse and blood pressure (BP). Heart rate is often slowed and bradycardia is common. Tachycardia can occur with dehydration or cardiomyopathy arrhythmias associated with ingestion of syrup of ipecac (historically used to induce vomiting). Hypotension is frequently observed and orthostasis suggests dehydration. For children and adolescents, a resting heart rate of about 40 beats per minute (bpm), BP < 80/50 mm Hg, and orthostatic BP change (>10 mm Hg drop or >20 bpm increase in heart rate) are signs of medical instability and hospitalization should be considered (APA, 2006).

Visual inspection and palpation of the individual reveals dry rough skin, brittle nails, dull or thinning hair, and poor skin turgor in the presence of severe dehydration and malnutrition. Individuals with AN may have lanugo—a fine, downy hair covering the face and neck, trunk, and limbs—caused by endocrine changes. For those with severe weight loss, the skeletal frame becomes more apparent with the rib cage and iliac crests visible. Inspection of the hands can reveal Russell's sign—skin abrasions or callus areas on the knuckles—that occur as a result of scraping the fingers against the teeth during digit-induced vomiting. Skin color is often pale but may have a yellow overtone in the presence of hypercarotenemia. Parotid gland enlargement may be visible and is associated with binge/self-induced vomiting behavior. Discoloration of the teeth occurs with enamel erosion, a result of the effects of hydrochloric acid during self-induced vomiting. Depending on age, normal expected sexual development may be delayed (e.g., breast development, appearance of pubic hair, onset of menarche).

Treatment

Several levels of psychiatric care are available for children and adolescents with an eating disorder, including outpatient psychotherapy, intensive outpatient day or partial hospitalization programs, residential programs, and hospitalization (APA, 2006). The level of care needed is largely determined by the child's medical stability, risk for suicide, percent of ideal body weight, coexisting conditions, and motivation for recovery (APA, 2006). Hospitalization should be considered for children and adolescents who are not medically stable, as well as for those who are suicidal, severely depressed, at a low body weight, and in need of nutritional stabilization or a highly structured environment to contain the level of symptomatology (APA, 2006). Specialized inpatient units are preferred if they are geographically available. Outpatient therapy typically involves individual, group, and/or family psychotherapy with a mental health care specialist. Both inpatient and outpatient treatment can involve adjunct therapies, including nutritional counseling, medications, and supportive therapies. In addition, primary health care monitoring is often a key component during outpatient treatment, particularly for individuals susceptible to weight loss and medical instability. The least restrictive environment is the preferred level of care for children and adolescents, provided that it can optimally meet their medical, psychological, and overall safety needs.

Treatment

Levels of Care
- Outpatient psychotherapy
- Day treatment
- Medical and/or psychiatric hospitalization
- Vigilant monitoring in primary care

Types of Therapy
- Individual, group, family
  - Cognitive behavioral therapy
  - Interpersonal therapy
  - Dialectical behavioral therapy
- Medication
  - SSRIs (BN) (limited evidence in BED)

Psychotherapy

Anorexia Nervosa. Treatment of children and adolescents with AN can be particularly challenging as these individuals characteristically do not think that they have a problem. Although there is general consensus that psychotherapy is valuable for the person with AN, some forms of psychotherapy may be more promising at different stages of illness. For example, traditional insight-oriented, cognitive-behavioral, or interpersonal talk therapies may be less effective during the acute stage of illness when the child is likely to have greater cognitive impairment.

Although a wide range of therapies exist, family therapy is the most effective form of psychotherapy for children and adolescents (Eisler, Dare, Hodes, et al., 2000). Family therapy has been shown to be helpful when conducted with the patient and the family together, or the patient and family seen separately by the same therapist (Eisler, Simic, Russell, et al., 2007).

Short-term family therapy (i.e., 10 sessions over 6 months) is as beneficial as long-term family therapy (i.e., 20 sessions over 1 year) (Lock, Couturier, & Agras, 2006), although chronic and more complicated cases may require longer individual and family therapy. As weight restoration progresses, the child may be more cognitively present and the parents may be more receptive to listening, as they no longer see their child on the brink of disaster or death.

Bulimia Nervosa. Children and adolescents with BN are typically more receptive to treatment from the time of initial recognition of the disorder than those with AN. In studies of adults with BN, cognitive behavioral therapy (CBT) has been shown to effectively reduce both binge eating and purging behavior (APA, 2006). The goal of CBT is to restructure the illogical thought patterns (cognitions) that lead to maladaptive behaviors. It is thought to be effective in adolescents with BN when adapted to fit their developmental needs, age, and specific triggers (e.g., peer interaction and influence), and when paired with parental monitoring of behaviors in the early stages (Schapman-Williams, Lock, & Couturier, 2006). Self-guided CBT, often used as a first-line strategy with adults struggling with BN, has also been shown to be helpful with adolescents (Schmidt, Lee, Beecham, et al., 2007). When CBT does not appear beneficial, switching to interpersonal therapy (IPT) may be useful. IPT focuses on assisting the person to understand the sources and reason for poor coping skills. It is not uncommon for mental health clinicians to use aspects of both IPT and CBT in the treatment of BN (APA, 2006). As with AN, family therapy is useful for the treatment of children and adolescents with BN.

Psychotherapy for EDNOS and BED. Treatment of patients with EDNOS is enhanced by recognizing which eating disorder their behavior most closely mirrors, and following the treatment recommendations for this condition (APA, 2006). With the addition of BED as a provisional diagnosis in the *DSM-IV-TR,* research is beginning to shed light on possible treatment strategies for this subcategory of EDNOS. Moreover, little is known on the best approach for the treatment of BED in adolescents and children; however, CBT and dialectical behavioral therapy (DBT) are modalities used with the adult population (APA, 2006). DBT is based on many of the same principles as CBT but emphasizes the concept of mindfulness. These findings are promising and can guide treatment for younger patients with BED, although further studies on adapting these therapies to children and adolescents are needed (Bulik, Brownley, & Shapiro, 2007). As with other child and adolescent eating disorders, family involvement and group therapies are likely to be beneficial.

Psychopharmacologic Interventions

Most studies on psychopharmacologic interventions have been conducted with adults, and there is a dearth of knowledge on prescribing for eating disorders in children and adolescents. Therefore prescribing is most often "off-label," which can be risky, particularly with young children. It is very important to be cognizant of the fragile and unstable state of both AN and BN, and to be aware of potential adverse effects of different drugs in persons with these disorders.

Anorexia Nervosa. Medications may be useful as an adjunct intervention in the treatment of AN (APA, 2006). Sometimes, for example, drugs may be helpful for treating co-occurring disorders, although concurrent depressive symptoms tend to remit with weight restoration. When medications are used in AN, they are often prescribed in lower doses (APA, 2006). Given that affected individuals have low body weight and malnutrition, they are at greater risk for side effects, as well as possibly a lowered seizure threshold (APA, 2006). Selective serotonin reuptake inhibitors (SSRIs) have little effect on the core psychopathology during low weight AN in adolescents (Holtkamp, Konrad, Kaiser, et al., 2005), as also observed in adults (Attia, Haiman, Walsh, et al., 1998). Preliminarily, medications do appear to have a possible beneficial effect in relapse prevention after weight gain (Kaye, Nagata, Weltzin, et al., 2001). Tricyclic agents do not appear particularly helpful and are avoided in low-weight children and adolescents because of the significant side effects in this population (Couturier & Lock, 2007). Other less frequently prescribed drugs, such as second-generation antipsychotic agents (e.g., olanzapine), have been thought to be mildly helpful with AN symptoms, although further research is needed (Reinblatt, Redgrave, & Guarda, 2008; Spettigue, Buchholz, Henderson, et al., 2008). Antipsychotic agents are sometimes used for their ability to induce weight gain in adults with AN, but they have other significant side effects that merit serious consideration before use in a vulnerable population such as children and adolescents (Powers & Santana, 2002; Couturier & Lock, 2007). These effects include extrapyramidal symptoms, prolonged QTc interval, and hyperlipidemia. Other medications include the use of anxiolytic drugs such as benzodiazepines immediately before meals, as they may help to prevent excessive anxiety triggered by eating (Kotler & Walsh, 2000). Additionally, care is essential in treating individuals who may have coexisting attention-deficit/hyperactivity disorder with medications, because stimulant abuse may occur as a result of desired drug-induced weight loss.

Bulimia Nervosa. Unlike AN, there is more empirical support for the use of pharmacologic interventions in adults with BN, but there are few studies of children and adolescents. In BN, various antidepressants have been shown to reduce the frequency of binge eating and purging, as well as to help alleviate comorbid depressive symptoms. Only the SSRI fluoxetine, however, is approved by the Food and Drug Administration (FDA) for the treatment of BN in adults and it is prescribed in higher doses than those typical for the treatment of depression (APA, 2006). It is preferred over other antidepressant agents because of its more favorable side effect profile, and is FDA-approved for the treatment of depression in children and adolescents. However, antidepressants are accompanied by an FDA "black box" warning regarding an increased risk for suicidal thoughts and behavior in children and adolescents (see Chapter 33). Tricyclic drugs and monoamine oxidase inhibitors (MAOIs), at doses similar to those used for depression, have been shown to decrease BN symptoms in adults, but they are rarely used because of their side effect profiles. MAOIs are risky because following the specific dietary restrictions required on this drug regimen (e.g., low-tyramine diet) can be particularly difficult for the patient with BN. Mood stabilizers and anticonvulsants are not first-line agents because of side effects (APA, 2006). Lithium, in particular, is not recommended because of its ineffectiveness (APA, 2006).

EDNOS and BED. Children and adolescents with EDNOS should be treated based on the extent to which their symptomatology reflects the features of AN or BN. Treatment for BED, much like that for BN, has not been specifically tested in adolescents and children. However, in adults, SSRIs have been shown to reduce the frequency of binge eating and symptoms of depression, although they have not been observed to result in any significant weight loss (APA, 2006). Studies of sibutramine, topiramate, and zonisamide suggest that they can reduce frequency of binge eating and also positively effect weight loss in adults (APA, 2006); however this has not been studied in children and adolescents. Thus, inference to children and adolescents with eating disorders is premature. To date, there are few data to inform medication strategies for relapse preventions in BED.

Complementary and Alternative Therapies

Other modalities of psychotherapy may be beneficial, although they have received relatively little study in the child and adolescent population. Nonverbal communication psychotherapies provide a possible alternative or complementary modality for young children and adolescents. Examples include movement therapy, yoga, art therapy, psychodrama, and/or occupational therapy (APA, 2006; Diamond-Raab & Orrell-Valente, 2002).

Anticipated Advances in Diagnosis and Management

The *DSM-IV-TR* (APA, 2000) is created to guide diagnoses for the purpose of moving toward evidence-based treatment for optimally informed practice. It is a fluid document—changes are made with each version to reflect the latest advances in diagnoses and treatment of psychiatric disorders. The lack of research pertaining to eating disorders in children and adolescents leaves room for many advances in the diagnoses and management of these disorders. One area in need of further examination is the diagnostic category of EDNOS and the extent to which it is clinically informative. ED-NOS accounts for 40% to 60% of child cases of eating disorders (WCEDCA, 2007). This means that 40% to 60% of children with an eating disorder are diagnosed with a condition for which efficacious treatments are moderately ambiguous. At present, it is unclear that EDNOS has enough specificity to inform treatment strategies in the clinical arena and is therefore in great need of further investigation.

Another diagnostic area in question by the WCEDCA (2007) includes the extent to which eating disorder diagnostic criteria are age sensitive. For example, it is unclear how a child expresses the "fear of fat" or defines "distorted body image" when developmentally the child may not yet fully understand the experiences and the labels attributed to them. Similarly, it is unclear whether parental observations might be accepted for endorsing a child's preoccupation with weight and shape rather than assuming that the child will be able to verbalize his or her "self-evaluation" to others (WCEDCA, 2007). Also in question is whether the intent of engaging in binge-purge behaviors might be indicative of eating pathology in younger children rather than the actual frequency, given the lack of independence afforded to children. In addition, cross-cultural variation needs further examination, as it may have implications for diagnoses, understanding of risk factors, manifestations of illness, management strategies and responsivity, as well as relapse prevention (Becker, 2007). For example, "fear of becoming fat" is a criterion not commonly experienced among a group of Asian females who seem to meet all of the other diagnostic criteria for AN (Lee, Ho, & Hsu, 1993).

Associated Problems of Eating Disorders and Treatment

Eating disorders are associated with a number of coexisting conditions that occur with increased frequency in this population. They are often accompanied by a sense of low self-esteem. Some evidence suggests that self-esteem is higher in those who recover from the disorder, although it is unclear if this means that it improved with recovery or if individuals with a higher level of self-esteem are those most likely to recover (Daley, Jimerson, Heatherton, et al., 2008). Low self-esteem, as well as effects from malnutrition, can contribute to clinical depression in this population. More than half of all individuals being treated for an eating disorder have concurrent depressive symptoms (O'Brien & Vincent, 2003). The low self-esteem and increased risk for depression make the need for assessment of suicidal ideation critically important.

Associated Problems of Eating Disorders and Treatment

- Depression
- Anxiety
- Obsessive-compulsive disorder
- Substance abuse disorders
- Suicidal ideation and attempts
- Refeeding syndrome (AN)
  - Electrolyte shifts
  - Severe hypophosphatemia
  - Fluid overload

In children and adolescents with AN, anxiety and obsessive-compulsive behaviors tend to co-aggregate. These individuals are often high achievers striving for an endless perfection, not only in relation to their body image but also in other facets of their life. They characteristically have an image of being "the good" child or the "obedient" and "compliant" one. On the other hand, individuals with BN are more typically described as impulsive. Both patients with AN and those with BN have increased risks for co-occurrence of substance abuse problems. For the group with AN, stimulants may be abused to enhance weight loss. For those with BN, alcohol can be a problem, with as many as 26% meeting criteria for alcohol dependence and 25% meeting criteria for alcohol abuse (Bulik, Klump, Thornton, et al., 2004).

The treatment of co-existing conditions typically occurs concurrently with the treatment of the eating disorder. The exception is if the individual's safety is compromised (e.g., suicidal ideation) or if the severity of symptoms requires immediate intense treatment (e.g., detoxification from substance dependence). Some coexisting psychiatric symptoms in children and adolescents with AN tend to improve with weight recovery (e.g., depression).

During hospitalization for the severely malnourished child or adolescent with AN, significant dangers can occur with refeeding (Gowers, 2008). Specifically, "refeeding syndrome" is a condition associated with electrolyte shifts that can result in severe hypophosphatemia. This syndrome typically occurs during the first few days on reinitiation of feeding. There is a risk for excess fluid volume. Thus, careful monitoring of the patient's vital signs, presence or absence of edema, fluid intake and output, urine specific gravity, and serum electrolytes is essential.

Prognosis

Overcoming an eating disorder is a difficult and sometimes life-long battle. In fact, eating disorders are considered one of the most deadly psychiatric disorders (Harris & Barraclough, 1998). AN has a profoundly high mortality risk for suicide—32 times that expected (Harris & Barraclough). A review of the literature found that among adults *and* adolescents with an eating disorder, 50% generally recover over time, 30% do reasonably well but continue to have eating disorder symptoms, and 20% remain diagnosable or significantly impaired (Fisher, 2003). Additionally, it is not uncommon for individuals with eating disorders to switch between AN and BN. Individuals recovering from AN often report experiencing BN-like symptoms on the way to weight recovery while they are learning to readapt to normal amounts of food intake and hunger and satiety cues. In one study of a 7-year follow-up of adolescents who were hospitalized for AN, 3% continued to have AN, 12% had switched to a diagnosis of BN, and the remaining percentage had a diagnosis of EDNOS (Herpertz-Dahlmann, Wewetzer, Schulz, et al., 1996).

Factors associated with prognosis have not always led to consistent findings. Studies suggest that younger age of onset and shorter duration of illness are associated with a better prognosis (Fisher, 2003). Coexisting psychiatric conditions and poor psychosocial adaptation have also been associated with less favorable outcomes (Herpertz-Dahlmann, Müller, Herpetz, et al., 2001).

Adolescents with a diagnosed eating disorder generally have a better long-term prognosis than their adult counterparts (Fisher, 2003). Early detection and intervention for an eating disorder that begins in childhood or adolescence is associated with better prognosis for an otherwise potentially chronic condition (Kotler, Cohen, Davies, et al., 2001).

PRIMARY CARE MANAGEMENT

Eating disorders are a significant adolescent health problem that also may occur in young children. They have the potential for severe or life-threatening physical manifestations. Therefore screening and early identification of those with the disorder or those at risk is critical. An eating disorder should be considered whenever a child or adolescent fails to attain age-appropriate weight, height, body composition, or stages of sexual development. Routine and urgent care office visits provide an opportunity for ongoing assessment of growth and development, as well as signs and symptoms of an eating disorder, again emphasizing the importance of early identification for early intervention and better long-term outcomes. Information should be obtained from the child *and* the parent or care provider. Discussions with the latter assist in engaging the family in the child's treatment, as well as obtaining corroborating and supplementary information.

Establishing a therapeutic alliance is essential. This is often the case for primary care clinicians who have a long-term established relationship in place with the patient. However, during active illness, establishing and maintaining the therapeutic alliance can be challenging because of the defensive, sometimes manipulative, suspicious, and controlling nature associated with the eating disorder. It is therefore important to proceed in a nonjudgmental manner, engaging the child or adolescent in a way that allows him or her to feel a sense of some control over the interaction.

It is particularly important that the clinician ask about, and listen for, physical complaints; these can be important clues that an individual is in the midst of denial and is, in fact, actively struggling with an eating disorder. For example, unconcerned reporting of vomiting blood may suggest denial of the severity of self-induced vomiting. Fatigue and easy bruising may be indicative of dietary malnutrition. If the child is identified as being at risk or having an eating disorder, the focus of the assessment should be on health and the exploration of underlying factors (Kreipe & Birndorf, 2000). Denial of symptoms is common, particularly if the child or adolescent is confronted directly with the issue. However, this denial can be diffused with a focus on the assessment of health behaviors such as asking them about their nutritional habits and physical symptoms.

For the child or adolescent with suspected AN, the initial focus should be to determine whether weight loss is intentional or desired, as opposed to having a medical cause. Although many patients present with symptoms that mirror those of an eating disorder, differential diagnoses (see below) must be considered and ruled out to ensure the absence of a medical cause.

Health Care Maintenance

Growth and Development

Growth and development can be severely compromised in children or adolescents with an eating disorder. It is important to obtain an accurate measurement of height and weight. This should be done with the patient in a gown after voiding to ensure that no layers of clothes or other concealed items add weight. Weighing the individual after voiding prevents an erroneous higher weight measurement that results from purposeful consumption of excessive water before data collection. The BMI can be calculated by dividing the weight (in kilograms) by the youth's height (in meters squared) (BMI = kg/m^2). This figure then can be age-adjusted (www.cdc.gov/nchs/about/major/nhanes/growthcharts/clinical_charts.htm) for children and youth ages 2 to 20 years (APA, 2006). For children, a BMI less than the 5th percentile is considered significantly underweight (APA, 2006).

Some individuals will want to know their weight and others prefer to not be told. To date, no studies have empirically examined whether—and under what conditions and situations—it is best to disclose (or not disclose) patients weight measurements to them. Thus, unfortunately there are relatively few data to inform the clinician of which option is best. For some patients, withholding their body weight can be stressful and induce further anxiety. For others, however, knowledge of their weight has the potential of inducing further preoccupation. Optimally, with consideration given to development and severity of symptoms, letting the patient know his or her weight encourages engagement in the treatment goals and recovery process. However, anxiety is a common fear expressed by individuals with AN during the weight-recovery phase.

A body weight history should be obtained. The history includes assessment of previous high and low weights and duration at the respective weights, extent of weight fluctuations, weight loss patterns, and methods for achieving weight loss goals (e.g., compensatory behaviors). The type, amount, duration, frequency, and intensity (as in exercise) of compensatory methods should be queried.

Assessment of social and developmental milestones is important. Challenging developmental tasks include progression to independence and establishing and maintaining appropriate boundaries. These normal developmental tasks may be influenced by a number of factors including family dynamics. Developmental milestones can be delayed in the presence of severe symptoms or prolonged hospitalization. For adolescents, preoccupation with body image and weight, low self-esteem, and co-occurring depressive symptoms may influence peer relations and lead to increased isolation. For others who are obese or overweight, social functioning may be hampered by stigma or a history of ongoing peer teasing.

Diet

Nutritional patterns and dietary intake are key areas of assessment. Food intake should be explored, including frequency of meals, where they occur (e.g., at family meals), types of food consumed (e.g., macronutrient content), and any associated patterns such as eating when stressed or lonely. See Box 25-4 for types of questions to ask when assessing eating and weight patterns.

It is beneficial to start by asking patients to recall what they ate in the past 24 hours. The daily caloric intake (including both foods and fluids) should be estimated and interpreted according to their developmental growth needs for their age and height. Additionally, patients should be queried about episodes of subjective and objective binge eating, fasting, and dieting behavior. Daily fluid intake should be assessed for volume, frequency, type, and associated intake patterns should be explored. Many individuals with eating disorders are dehydrated, resulting from dietary restriction or through fluid loss associated with compensatory behaviors (e.g., self-induced vomiting, diarrhea associated with laxative abuse).

BOX 25-4

Questions to Assist in Assessment of Eating and Weight Patterns

EATING PATTERNS
- Over the past week, how many days have you eaten breakfast (lunch, dinner)?
- How many snacks do you eat a day?
- What time of day do you eat breakfast (lunch, dinner, snacks)?
- Where do you eat breakfast (lunch, dinner, snacks)?
- What did you eat yesterday? (e.g., note type and amount of food)
- Do you count calories? If so, how many calories do you consume a day?
- Do you follow any special diets?
- How many times have you been on a diet in the past year?
- Have you ever had a binge episode?
- Is there anything that triggers eating for you?
- Ever feel like your eating has been out of control?

WEIGHT PATTERNS
- What is your current weight?
- What is the most you have weighed in the past month? in past 3 months? 6 months)?
- What is the least you have weighed in the past month? in past 3 months? 6 months)?
- What weight would you like to be at? (e.g., ideal weight)
- Are you currently trying to lose weight? If so, how much and how?
- Do you do anything specific to maintain your weight or lose weight? (e.g., self-induced vomiting, laxative use, diuretic use, enema use, excessive exercising, fasting, strict dieting)

A 1-week food diary is often a useful tool to obtain a comprehensive picture of food intake. It is important to keep in mind, however, that persons with AN may overestimate their food intake, whereas persons with BN may fail to report their actual intake because of embarrassment over the amount of food consumed during a binge episode. Food models are helpful in teaching serving sizes and helping recalibrate food intake estimates.

Safety

Medical instability is a primary safety concern for persons with an eating disorder. Risk for electrolyte imbalances, cardiac arrhythmias and arrest, other emergency medical complications (e.g., esophageal tear associated with binge/purge episodes), and effects of severe dietary restriction and starvation require ongoing monitoring (see "Screening" below). For low-weight patients, hospitalization may be necessary, especially if the body weight is <75% of ideal body weight (Gonzalez, Kohn, & Clarke, 2007). Ideally, hospitalization should occur before medical instability ensues, although in the present health care climate, this decision may be influenced by insurance coverage. Over the long term, patients with AN are at increased risk for stress fractures, which can pose a safety risk, particularly when malnutrition and amenorrhea are prolonged.

Risk for suicide is another area of safety that should be taken seriously. Clinicians may feel awkward asking about suicidal ideation, particularly if the patient appears stable outwardly, and the clinician may feel that asking may jeopardize the therapeutic relationship. However, such individuals are not likely to provide this information unsolicited. Individuals should be assessed for current or past history of suicidal thoughts, plan, and/or attempt. Obtaining details about the thoughts, plan, and/or attempts provides clues about the level of intent and access to potentially harmful devices. For children and adolescents with current suicidal ideation, a referral to a psychiatric clinician or emergency department is warranted for further evaluation.

Immunizations

Routine immunizations are recommended. Immunization schedules are available at www.cdc.gov/vaccines/recs/schedules/child-schedule.htm (Centers for Disease Control & Prevention, 2007).

Screening

Routine child and adolescent health screening for vision, hearing, and tuberculosis is recommended.

Vision. Routine screening is recommended.

Hearing. Routine screening is recommended.

Dental. The provider should check for discoloration and sensitivity at each visits that could be signs of enamel erosion related to self-induced vomiting.

Blood Pressure. Orthostatic blood pressures and pulses should be checked at each visit. Adolescents may exercise just before the visit in hopes of bringing low pulses and blood pressures up to normal, and provider should ensure adequate rest before beginning vital signs. Unstable blood pressures or resting heart rate below 50 during the day can be criteria for hospitalization.

Hematocrit. Numerous hematologic abnormalities can occur with eating disorders. See Condition-specific screening.

Urinalysis. Check at each visit. Some centers check urine ketones as a measure of adequate dietary intake. Specific gravity can be a sign that the child or adolescent is water loading in order to falsely increase weight at the visit.

Tuberculosis. Routine screening is recommended.

Condition-Specific Screening

A comprehensive medical history and physical examination should be conducted. Other condition-specific screening is detailed in the following text.

Focused Review of Systems. Symptoms commonly reported by patients include fatigue and general weakness secondary to malnutrition or, in some cases, excessive exercising. Hematemesis is sometimes reported with self-induced vomiting. Abdominal pain, bloating, and gastric distention may be related to binge eating or constipation. Syncope can occur with dehydration. Another neurologic symptom is poor concentration. Individuals who have been at a low weight are particularly vulnerable to osteoporosis and therefore skeletal stress fractures. For postmenarcheal adolescents, irregular menstrual cycles are common in BN; amenorrhea is diagnostically characteristic of AN.

Laboratory Tests: Chemistries. Laboratory findings provide an additional assessment of physical health. Electrolyte abnormalities include low sodium, potassium, magnesium, and phosphorus. Hypokalemia, hypophosphatemia, and increased sodium bicarbonate (i.e., alkalosis) are associated with frequent self-induced vomiting, whereas low sodium bicarbonate (i.e., acidosis) is associated with laxative abuse. Serum glucose is low following fasting or strict dieting. Blood urea nitrogen is elevated with dehydration.

Laboratory Tests: Hematology. Hematologic findings include low serum hematocrit and albumin, which are observed with poor dietary intake. Leukopenia, thrombocytopenia, and low eosinophilia sedentary rate can also occur.

Laboratory Tests: Endocrine. Other laboratory findings may include endocrine changes resulting from severe weight loss. This includes decreased serum estrogen, follicle-stimulating hormone (FSH), luteinizing hormone (LH), and testosterone. Serum thyroids are low in individuals with AN but return to normal with weight restoration.

Adolescents who are amenorrheic should have a urine or serum human chorionic gonadotropin (HCG) test to exclude pregnancy, as well as thyroid stimulating hormone (TSH) and prolactin levels, to exclude thyroid abnormalities or a prolactinoma as potential causes.

Electrocardiogram (ECG). An ECG should be done on patients who are bradycardic. Findings can include a variety of abnormalities including prolonged QTc intervals, non-specific S-T wave changes, and cardiomyopathy associated with syrup of ipecac emetine toxicity.

Bone Density (DXA). As previously mentioned, prolonged amenorrhea increases vulnerability to decreased bone density. While there are age-matched norms for dual energy X-ray absorptiometry (DXA) scans, the benefits in actual patient management are unclear.

Common Illness Management
Differential Diagnosis

Several symptoms that might initially appear to be related to an eating disorder may in fact reflect other medical or psychiatric conditions. Weight loss is a common symptom observed in autoimmune deficiency disorders, cancer, peptic ulcer disease, hyperthyroidism, and adrenocortical insufficiency (Wolfe & Gimby, 2003). It is also a feature often seen in depression and substance use disorders. Excessive or uncontrolled eating is characteristic of Kleine-Levin syndrome (Arnulf, Lin, Gadoth, et al., 2008), Prader-Willi syndrome (Benarroch, Hirsch, Genstil, et al., 2007), and some brain tumors. Preoccupations limited to a single body part and not directly related to weight or shape may be more reflective of body dysmorphic disorder rather than an eating disorder. For preoccupations that are not focused on body shape and weight, obsessive-compulsive disorder should be explored.

Differential Diagnosis

Weight loss
- Autoimmune deficiency disorders
- Cancer
- Peptic ulcer disease
- Hyperthyroidism
- Adrenocortical insufficiency
- Depression
- Substance use disorders

Excessive or uncontrolled eating
- Kleine-Levin syndrome
- Prader-Willi syndrome
- Brain tumor

Preoccupations
- Body dysmorphic disorder
- Obsessive-compulsive disorder

Arnulf, I., Lin, L., Gadoth, N., et al. (2008). Kleine-Levin syndrome: A systematic study of 108 patients. *Ann Neurol, 63,* 482-493; Benarroch, F., Hirsch, H.J., Genstil, L., et al. (2007). Prader-Willi syndrome: Medical prevention and behavioral challenges. *Child Adolesc. Psychiatr Clin North Am, 16*(3), 695-708; Wolfe, B.E., & Gimby, L.B. (2003). Caring for hospitalized patient with an eating disorder. *Nurs Clin North Am, 38,* 75-99.

Developmental Issues

Sleeping Patterns

Altered sleep patterns are not typically attributable to the presence of an eating disorder. Rather, sleeping too much or too little can occur because of co-occurring depression. Fatigue is often present because of malnutrition.

Toileting

Eating disorders are not associated with issues of toileting. Individuals who routinely engage in self-induced vomiting may exhibit regular use of the bathroom immediately after consumption of meals or binge foods.

Discipline

Because of the characteristic nature of both AN and BN, these disorders are more closely associated with compliant and obedient behavior in childhood. Disciplinary problems, if they occur, are likely to be related to co-occurring issues (e.g., substance abuse, manipulative behavior). For individuals with AN, struggles may ensue during meal times with regard to food intake.

Child Care

Eating disorders are not associated with any particular child-care issues. However, it may be advisable to educate child-care providers about the disorder to prevent struggles with the child or adolescent around meals, diet, or other related routines.

Schooling

Although they are often overachievers, children and adolescents with an eating disorder can experience difficult times with peers during school years. Such difficulties may include teasing about weight (i.e., underweight and overweight states), issues pertaining to body image, and embarrassment related to binge eating or purging behaviors if these become disclosed.

Sexuality

For individuals with AN, sexual development can be delayed because of the physical halt in maturation that occurs with significant weight loss and malnutrition. Additionally, negative body image can influence sense of self-worth and affect intimacy. Of particular note relative to sexuality is that the occurrence of amenorrhea observed in AN and that occurs episodically in BN may give the sexually active adolescent a false sense of protection from pregnancy; thus, education on adequate contraception is needed in this cohort.

Transition to Adulthood

Much of the psychodynamic formulation of both AN and BN revolves around issues of separation, individuation, autonomy, and control. These conditions may partially reflect the struggles encountered with these issues that are central to independent adult functioning. Thus, periods of transition may be anticipated as a time of increased stress, exacerbation of symptoms, or increased risk for relapse.

Puberty presents major physical and emotional changes, with body weight and shape self-cognitions predicting adolescent girls' emotional health (Stein & Hedger, 1997). Although the transition to college may contribute to exacerbation of symptoms because of increased stress, evidence indicates that disordered eating and related attitudes are already rooted before college (Vohs, Heatherton, & Herrin, 2001). For individuals who move away from their families that may be characteristically described as enmeshed, going to college may be difficult in that it involves a significant loss of the role of the patient's illness for both the family and affected person. Alternatively, such separation provides new opportunities for growth and development, for both adolescent and family, which would not easily occur otherwise (e.g., geographically diffusing enmeshed families). A child making the transition to young adulthood prompts the need for consideration of a referral from a child mental health specialist to an adult eating disorder specialist (Arcelus, Bouman, & Morgan, 2008).

Family Concerns

Eating disorders can be very trying on families and are particularly daunting for family members who constantly face evidence of the problem. Some individuals are often literally watching their child or sibling waste away in front of them. Others are constantly confronted with seeing their loved one head for the bathroom to purge after dinner. This constant stress of dealing with the disorder can leave family members feeling angry, guilty, shameful, or even in denial. Additionally, families may feel on the brink of disintegration, unable to cope, and socially isolated (Hillege, Beale, & McMaster, 2006). This is particularly difficult because family involvement is critically important in the treatment of children and adolescents with eating disorders (APA, 2006).

During active illness, individuals with an eating disorder can be manipulative, competitive, needy, and hostile, particularly with family members who are aware of their shame-inducing behaviors or who are attempting to assist them in getting help. This scenario can be especially hard for siblings to handle. Furthermore, siblings can often feel inadvertently ignored or forgotten because of the commanding presence an eating disorder takes in a household.

It is often difficult for family members or friends to understand the condition or the associated behaviors. Thus, families often feel uneducated and without the necessary skills to support and help a family member living with an eating disorder (Treasure, Supulveda, MacDonald, et al. 2008). This disempowerment augments the family's fear and frustration surrounding these stubborn, seemingly irrational, and persistent disorders. This fear and frustration feeds a cycle that may perpetuate the eating disorder and causes further stress on the family (Treasure et al.).

Other family concerns include financial worries (Hillege et al., 2006), as insurance coverage for eating disorders (an often chronic condition) is often limited (Kalisvaart & Hergenroeder, 2007). Furthermore, eating disorders are particularly expensive to treat because of the psychological and medical interface. As with all mental illness, the stigma associated with eating disorders can be a burden for the patient and the family (Whitney, Haigh, Weinman, et al., 2007). It is important to encourage and support families to seek help and resources as they cope with these difficulties.

Resources

Several resources are available for families and friends of children and adolescents with an eating disorder. Box 25-5 highlights Internet and organizational resources that focus on helping, educating, and advocating for children, adolescents, and their families.

Adolescents with an eating disorder often avoid effective treatment because of shame and embarrassment concerning the symptoms (e.g., BN), refusal to gain weight (e.g., AN), denial of symptoms, or stigmatization associated with mental disorders. With access and ease of Internet use, adolescents have the ability to frequent websites that glorify eating disorders. Such sites are known as "pro-anorexia" or "pro-ana" sites and give individuals "tips and tricks" for example, on how to pretend to be compliant and/or hide the extent of weight loss (Norris, Boydell, Pinhas, et al., 2006). Additionally, these websites promote "control," "success," and "perfection" through motivational materials directed at encouraging weight loss by including photo galleries, endorsing

lifestyle descriptions, and providing other words of encouragement (Norris et al., 2006). Not surprisingly, initial data suggest that individuals who view pro-ana websites have greater disturbance in self-esteem–related cognitions and negative affect (Bardone-Cone & Cass, 2007), as well as body image and eating disturbances (Harper, Sperry, & Thompson, 2008). Additionally, "silent browsers" who frequent such sites to sustain the disorder are particularly vulnerable to the harmful effects (Csipke & Horne, 2007).

Internet Resources
Anorexia Nervosa and Related Eating Disorders (ANRED)
Website: www.ANRED.com
Mirror-Mirror Eating Disorder Information
Website: www.mirror-mirror.org/eatdis.htm
Something Fishy: Website on Eating Disorders
(866) 690-7239
Website: www.something-fishy.org

Organizations
Academy for Eating Disorders (AED)
111 Deer Lake Rd.
Suite 100
Deerfield, IL 60015
(847) 498-4274
Website: www.aedweb.org
Alliance for Eating Disorders Awareness
P.O. Box 13155
North Palm Beach, FL 33408-3155
(561) 841-0900
Website: www.eatingdisorderinfo.org
Eating Disorders Anonymous (EDA)
P.O. Box 55876
Phoenix, AZ 85078-5876
Website: www.eatingdisordersanonymous.org
Multi-service Eating Disorder Association (MEDA)
92 Pearl St.
Newton, MA 02458
Business office: (866) 343-MEDA
Website: www.medainc.org
National Eating Disorders Association (NEDA)
603 Stewart St., Suite 803
Seattle, WA 98101
Business office: (206) 382-3587
Toll-free information and referral helpline: (800) 931-2237
Website: www.myneda.org

Summary of Primary Care Needs for the Child or Adolescent with an Eating Disorder

HEALTH CARE MAINTENANCE

Growth and Development

- Growth and development can be severely compromised for the child or adolescent with an eating disorder.
- Accurate height and weight measurements should be obtained. A body weight history should be obtained, including assessment of previous high and low weights, duration at the respective weights,

and extent of weight fluctuations, weight loss patterns, and methods for attempting weight loss.

- The BMI can be calculated by dividing the weight (in kilograms) by the youth's height (in meters squared) (BMI = kg/m^2). This then can be age-adjusted (www.cdc.gov/nchs/about/major/nhanes/growth-charts/clinical_charts.htm)

Summary of Primary Care Needs for the Child or Adolescent with an Eating Disorder—cont'd

Diet

- Nutritional patterns and dietary intake are key areas of assessment.
- The daily caloric intake (including foods and fluids) should be estimated and interpreted according to the person's developmental growth needs for their age and height.
- Persons with AN may overestimate their food intake, whereas those with BN may fail to report their actual intake because embarrassment over the amount of food consumed during a binge episode.
- Food models are helpful in teaching serving sizes and recalibrating food intake estimates.

Safety

- Medical instability is a primary safety concern for persons with an eating disorder.
- Individuals are at risk for electrolyte imbalances, cardiac arrhythmias and arrest, other emergency medical complications, and effects of severe dietary restriction and starvation.
- Individuals require ongoing physical health monitoring.
- Hospitalization should occur before medical instability ensues.
- Risk for suicide should be routinely assessed.

Immunizations

- Routine immunizations are recommended.

Screening

- *Vision.* Routine screening is recommended.
- *Hearing.* Routine screening is recommended.
- *Dental.* Check at each visit for signs and symptoms of enamel erosion.
- *Blood pressure.* Orthostatic blood pressure (and pulse) should be checked at each visit, with adequate rest before beginning screen.
- *Hematocrit.* See condition-specific screening below.
- *Urinalysis.* Check specific gravity for water loading.
- *Tuberculosis.* Routine screening is recommended.

CONDITION SPECIFIC SCREENING

- *Serum and hematologic.* Check for abnormalities of chemistries (sodium, potassium, magnesium, phosphorus, bicarbonate, glucose, blood urea nitrogen, albumin). Check for low hematocrit, leucopenia, thrombocytopenia, eosinophils.
- *Endocrine.* Low estrogen, FSH, LH, abnormal thyroid function. For amenorrhea, check urine or serum HCG, thyroid, prolactin levels
- *ECG.* If bradycardic, check for prolonged QTc intervals, S-T wave changes.

COMMON ILLNESS MANAGEMENT

Differential Diagnosis

- Weight loss is a common symptom observed in autoimmune deficiency disorders, cancer, peptic ulcer disease, hyperthyroidism, adrenocortical insufficiency, depression, and substance use disorders.
- Excessive or uncontrolled eating is characteristic of Kleine-Levin syndrome, Prader-Willi syndrome, and some brain tumors.

- Preoccupations that are limited to a single body part may be more reflective of body dysmorphic disorder.
- Preoccupations not focused on body shape and weight may be more related to obsessive-compulsive disorder.

DEVELOPMENTAL ISSUES

Sleeping Patterns

- Sleeping too much or too little can occur because of co-occurring depression.

Toileting

- Eating disorders are not associated with issues of toileting. Individuals who routinely engage in self-induced vomiting may exhibit regular use of the bathroom immediately after consumption of meals or binge foods.

Discipline

- Because of the characteristic nature of both AN and BN, these conditions are more closely associated with compliant and obedient behavior in childhood. Disciplinary problems, if they occur, are likely to be related to co-occurring issues (e.g., substance abuse, manipulative behavior). For individuals with AN, struggles may ensue during mealtimes with regard to food intake.

Child Care

- It may be advisable to educate child-care providers about the condition to prevent struggles with the child or adolescent about meals, diet, or other related routines.

Schooling

- Although they often are overachievers, children and adolescents with an eating disorder can experience difficult times with peers during school years by being teased about weight.

Sexuality

- For patients with AN, sexuality can be delayed because of the physical halt in maturation that occurs with significant weight loss and malnutrition.
- The occurrence of amenorrhea observed in AN and episodically in BN may give the sexually active adolescent a false sense of protection from pregnancy; thus, education on adequate contraception is needed.

Transition to Adulthood

- Promoting self-esteem and positive body weight and shape self-cognitions enhance young girls' emotional health.
- Referral to an adult eating disorder specialist is indicated during transition to early adulthood.
- Referral should be made to university health center for medical and mental health follow-up with transition to college.
- The need for continuous care after transitions and periods of increased stress should be reinforced.
- Transitions may be anticipated as a time of increased stress, exacerbation of symptoms, or increased risk for relapse.

Continued

Summary of Primary Care Needs for the Child or Adolescent with an Eating Disorder—cont'd

FAMILY CONCERNS

- Eating disorders can be daunting for family members.
- The constant stress of dealing with the disorder can leave family members feeling angry, guilty, shameful, or even in denial.
- Siblings can often feel inadvertently ignored or forgotten because of the commanding presence an eating disorder takes in a household.
- Families often feel undereducated and without the necessary skills to support and help a member living with an eating disorder.

- Other family concerns include financial worries and the stigma associated with psychiatric illnesses.

RESOURCES

- Several resources are available for families and friends of children and adolescents with an eating disorder (see Box 25-5).

REFERENCES

Ackard, D.M., Neumark-Sztainer, D. (2001). Family mealtime while growing up: Associations with symptoms of bulimia nervosa. *Eat Disord, 9,* 239-249.

Ackard, D.M., Vik, N., Neumark-Sztainer, D., et al. (2008). Disordered eating and body dissatisfaction in adolescents with type 1 diabetes and a population-based comparison sample: comparative prevalence and clinical implications. *Pediatr Diabetes, 9*(4 Pt 1), 312-319.

Agras, W.S., Bryson, S., & Hammer, L.D., et al. (2007). Childhood risk factors for thin body preoccupation and social pressure to be thin. *J Am Acad Child Adolesc Psychiatry, 46,* 171-178.

American Psychiatric Association (2000). Eating disorders. In *Diagnostic and Statistical Manual of Mental Disorders* (4th ed., revised). Washington, DC: American Psychiatric Association.

American Psychiatric Association Workgroup on Eating Disorders (2006). *Practice Guideline for the Treatment of Patients with Eating Disorders* (3rd ed.). Washington, DC: Author, 2006.

Arcelus, J., Bouman, W.P., & Morgan, J.F. (2008). Treating young people with eating disorders: transition from child mental health to specialist adult eating disorder services. *Eur Eat Disord Rev, 16,* 30-36.

Arnulf, I., Lin, L., & Gadoth, N., et al. (2008). Kleine-Levin syndrome: A systematic study of 108 patients. *Ann Neurol, 63,* 482-493.

Attia, E., Haiman, C., & Walsh, T., et al. (1998). Does fluoxetine augment the inpatient treatment of anorexia nervosa? *Am J Psychiatry, 155,* 548-551.

Bardone-Cone, A.M., & Cass, K.M. (2007). What does viewing a pro-anorexia website do? An experimental examination of website exposure and moderating effects. *Int J Eat Disord, 40,* 537-548.

Becker, A.E. (2007). Culture and eating disorders classification. *Int J Eat Disord, 40,* S111-S116.

Becker, A.E., Burwell, R.A., Gilman, S.E., et al. (2002). Eating behaviors and attitudes following prolonged exposure to television among ethnic Fijian adolescent girls. *Br J Psychiatry, 180,* 509-514.

Benarroch, F., Hirsch, H.J., Genstil, L., et al. (2007). Prader-Willi syndrome: Medical prevention and behavioral challenges. *Child Adolesc Psychiatr Clin North Am, 16*(3), 695-708.

Brewerton, T.D. (2007). Eating disorders, trauma, and comorbidity: Focus on PTSD. *Eat Disord, 15,* 285-304.

Bruch, H. (1982). Anorexia nervosa: Therapy and theory. *Am J Psychiatry, 139,* 1531-1538.

Bulik, C.M., Brownley, K.A., & Shapiro, J.R. (2007). Diagnosis and management of binge eating disorder. *World Psychiatry, 6,* 142-148.

Bulik, C.M., Klump, K.L., Thornton, L., et al. (2004). Alcohol use disorder comorbidity in eating disorders: multicenter study. *J Clin Psychiatry, 65,* 1000-1006.

Bulik, C.M., Sullivan, P.F., Wade, T.D., et al. (2000). Twin studies of eating disorders: A review. *Int J Eat Disord, 27,* 1-20.

Centers for Disease Control and Prevention. Atkinson, W., Hamborsky, J., McIntyre, L., et al., (Eds.). (2007). *Epidemiology and Prevention of Vaccine-Preventable Diseases* (10th ed.). Washington, DC: Public Health Foundation. Available at www.cdc.gov/vaccines/recs/schedules/child-schedule. htm. Retrieved January 22, 2009.

Chamay-Weber, C., Narring, F., & Michaud, P.-A. (2005). Partial eating disorders among adolescents: A review. *J Adolesc Health, 37,* 417-427.

Couturier, J.L., & Lock, J. (2006). Denial and minimization in adolescents with anorexia nervosa. *Int J Eat Disord, 39,* 212-216.

Couturier, J., & Lock, J. (2007). A review of medication use for children and adolescents with eating disorders. *J Can Acad Child Adolesc Psychiatry, 16,* 173-176.

Crowther, J.H., Kichler, J.C., Sherwood, N.E., et al. (2002). The role of familial factors in bulimia nervosa. *Eat Disord, 10,* 141-151.

Csipke, E., & Horne, O. (2007). Pro-eating disorder websites: users' opinions. *Eur. Eat Disord Rev, 15,* 196-206.

Dale, K.S., & Landers, D.M. (1999). Weight control in wrestling: eating disorders or disordered eating?. *Med Sci Sports Exerc, 31,* 1382-1389.

Daley, K.A., Jimerson, D.C., Heatherton, T.F., et al. (2008). State self-esteem ratings in women with bulimia nervosa in remission. *Int. J Eat Disord, 41,* 159-163.

Diamond-Raab, L., & Orrell-Valente, J.K. (2002). Art therapy, psychodrama, and verbal therapy. An integrative model of group therapy in the treatment of adolescents with anorexia nervosa and bulimia nervosa. *Child Adolesc Psychiatr Clin North Am, 11,* 343-364.

DiNicola, V.F. (1990). Anorexia multiforme: Self-starvation in historical and cultural context. *Transcult Psychiatr Res Rev, 27,* 245-286.

Eddy, K.T., Hennessey, M., & Thompson-Brenner, H. (2007). Eating pathology in East African women. The role of media exposure and globalization. *J Nerv Ment Dis, 195,* 196-202.

Eisler, I., Dare, C., Hodes, M., et al. (2000). Family therapy for adolescent anorexia nervosa: The results of a controlled comparison of two family interventions. *J Child Psychol Psychiatry, 41,* 727-736.

Eisler, I., Simic, M., Russell, G.F.M., et al. (2007). A randomized controlled treatment trial of two forms of family therapy in adolescent anorexia nervosa: a five-year follow-up. *J Child Psychol Psychiatry, 48,* 552-560.

Feldman, M.B., & Meyer, I.H. (2007). Eating disorders in diverse lesbian, gay, and bisexual populations. *Int J Eat Disord, 40,* 218-226.

Fernandez, M.A.P., Labrador, F.J., & Raich, R.M. (2007). Prevalence of eating disorders among adolescent and young adult scholastic population in the region of Madrid (Spain). *J Psychosom Res, 62,* 681-690.

Fisher, M. (2003). The course and outcome of eating disorders in adults and in adolescents: a review. *Adolesc Med, 14,* 149-158.

Fisher, M., Schneider, M., Burns, J., et al. (2001). Differences between adolescents and young adults at presentation to an eating disorders program. *J Adolesc Health, 28,* 222-227.

Gonzalez, A., Kohn, M.R., & Clarke, S.D. (2007). Eating disorders in adolescents. *Aust Fam Physician, 36,* 614-619.

Gowers, S.G. (2008). Management of eating disorders in children and adolescents. *Arch Dis Child, 93,* 331-334.

Harper, K., Sperry, S., & Thompson, J.K. (2008). Viewership of pro-eating disorder websites: association with body image and eating disturbances. *Int J Eat Disord, 41,* 92-95.

Harris, E.C., & Barraclough, B. (1998). Excess mortality of mental disorders. *Br J Psychiatry, 173,* 11-53.

Herpertz-Dahlmann, B.M., Müller, B., Herpertz, S., et al. (2001). Prospective 10-year follow-up in adolescent anorexia nervosa—course, outcome, psychiatric comorbidity, and psychosocial adaptation. *J Child Psychol Psychiatry, 42,* 603-612.

Herpertz-Dahlmann, B.M., Wewetzer, C., Schulz, E., et al. (1996). Course and outcome in adolescent anorexia nervosa. *Int J Eat Disord, 19,* 335-345.

Hillege, S., Beale, B., & McMaster, R. (2006). Impact of eating disorders on family life: individual parents' stories. *J Clin Nurs, 15,* 1016-1022.

Holtkamp, K., Konrad, K., Kaiser, N., et al. (2005). A retrospective study of SSRI treatment in adolescent anorexia nervosa: Insufficient evidence for efficacy. *J Psychiatr Res, 39,* 303-310.

Honey, A., & Halse, C. (2006). Looking after well siblings of adolescent girls with anorexia: an important parental role. *Child Care Health Dev, 33,* 52-58.

Hudson, J.I., Hiripi, E., Pope, H.G., et al. (2007). The prevalence and correlates of eating disorders in the national comorbidity survey replication. *Biol Psychiatry, 61,* 348-358.

Jimerson, D.C., Mantzoros, C., Wolfe, B.E., et al. (2000). Decreased serum leptin in bulimia nervosa. *J Clin Endocrinol Metabol, 85,* 4511-4514.

Jimerson, D.C., & Wolfe, B.E. (2006). Psychobiology of eating disorders. In S.Wonderlich, J.Mitchell, M. de Zwaan, et al, (Eds.), *Eating Disorders Review: Part II,* Oxford, UK: Radcliffe Publishing.

Jimerson, D.C., Wolfe, B.E., & Naab, S. (2006). Eating disorders. Coffey, C., Brumback, R.A., Rosenberg, D.R.(eds.) (2006). *Pediatric Neuropsychiatry,* Philadelphia, PA: Lippincott Williams & Wilkins.

Kalisvaart, J.L., & Hergenroeder, A.C. (2007). Hospitalization of patients with eating disorders on adolescent medical units is threatened by current reimbursement systems. *Int J Adolesc Med Health, 19,* 155-165.

Kaye, W.H., Nagata, T., Weltzin, T.E., et al. (2001). Double-blind placebo-controlled administration of fluoxetine in restricting- and restricting-purging-type anorexia nervosa. *Biol Psychiatry, 49,* 644-652.

Kjelsas, E., Bjørnstrøm, C., Gotestam, G. (2004). Prevalence of eating disorders in female and male adolescents (14-15 years). *Eat Behav, 5,* 13-25.

Kjelsas, E., Børsting, I., & Gudde, C. (2004). Antecedents and consequences of binge eating episodes in women with an eating disorder. *Eat Weight Disord, 9,* 7-15.

Klump, K.L., Burt, S.A., McGue, M., et al. (2007). Changes in genetic and environmental influences on disordered eating across adolescence: a longitudinal twin study. *Arch Gen Psychiatry, 64,* 1409-1415.

Kotler, L.A., Cohen, P., Davies, M., et al. (2001). *J Am Acad Child Adolesc Psychiatry, 40,* 1434-1440.

Kotler, L.A., Walsh, B.T. (2000). Eating disorders in children and adolescents: pharmacological therapies. *Eur Child Adolesc Psychiatry, 9*(Suppl 1), 108-116.

Kreipe, R.E., & Birndorf, S.A. (2000). Eating disorders in adolescents and young adults. *Med Clin North Am, 84,* 1027-1049.

Le Grange, D., & Loeb, K.L. (2007). Early identification and treatment of eating disorders: prodrome to syndrome. *Early Interv Psychiatry, 1,* 27-39.

Lee, H.-Y., & Lock, J. (2007). Anorexia nervosa in Asian-American adolescents: Do they differ from their non-Asian peers? *Int J Eat Disord, 40,* 227-231.

Lee, S., Ho, T.P., & Hsu, L.K. (1993). Fat phobic and non-fat phobic anorexia nervosa: a comparative study of 70 Chinese patients in Hong Kong. *Psychol Med, 23,* 999-1017.

Lilenfeld, L.R., Kaye, W.H., Greeno, C.G., et al. (1998). A controlled family study of anorexia nervosa and bulimia nervosa. Psychiatric disorders in first-degree relatives and effects of proband comorbidity. *Arch Gen Psychiatry, 55,* 603-610.

Lock, J., Couturier, J., & Agras, W.S. (2006). Comparison of long-term outcomes in adolescents with anorexia nervosa treated with family therapy. *J Am Acad Child Adolesc Psychiatry, 45,* 666-672.

Makino, M., Tsuboi, K., & Dennerstein, L. (2004). Prevalence of eating disorders: A comparison of western and non-western countries. *Med Gen Med, 6*(3), 49.

Mantzoros, C., Flier, J.S., Lesem, M.D., et al. (1997). Cerebrospinal fluid leptin in anorexia nervosa: Correlation with nutritional status and potential role in resistance to weight gain. *J Clin Endocrinol Metab, 82,* 1845-1851.

Minuchin, S., Baker, L., Rosman, B.L., et al. (1975). A conceptual model of psychosomatic illness in children. Family organization and family therapy. *Arch Gen Psychiatry, 32,* 1031-1038.

Nattiv, A., Loucks, A.B., Manore, M.M., et al. (2007). American College of Sports Medicine position stand. The female athlete triad. *Med Sci Sports Exerc, 39,* 1867-1882.

Norris, M.L., Boydell, K.M., Pinhas, L., et al. (2006). Ana and the Internet: a review of pro-anorexia websites. *Int J Eat Disord, 39,* 443-447.

O'Brien, K.M., & Vincent, N.K. (2003). Psychiatric comorbidity in anorexia and bulimia nervosa: Nature, prevalence, and causal relationships. *Clin Psychol Rev, 23,* 57-74.

Peebles, R., Wilson, J.L., & Lock, J.D. (2006). How do children with eating disorders differ from adolescents with eating disorders at initial evaluation?. *J Adolesc Health, 39,* 800-805.

Pike, K.M., Hilbert, A., Wilfley, D.E., et al. (2008). Toward an understanding of risk factors for anorexia nervosa: A case control study. *Psychol Med, 10,* 1443-1453.

Powers, P.S., & Santana, C.A. (2002). Childhood and adolescent anorexia nervosa. *Child Adolesc Psychiatr Clin North Am, 11,* 219-235.

Reinblatt, S.P., Redgrave, G.W., & Guarda, A.S. (2008). Medication management of pediatric eating disorders. *Int Rev Psychiatry, 20,* 183-188.

Ringham, R., Klump, K., Kaye, W., et al. (2006). Eating disorder symptomatology among ballet dancers. *Int J Eat Disord, 39,* 503-508.

Santonastaso, P., Mondini, S., & Favaro, A. (2002). Are fashion models a group at risk for eating disorders and substance abuse?. *Psychother and Psychosom, 71,* 168-172.

Schapman-Williams, A.M., Lock, J., & Couturier, J. (2006). Cognitive-behavioral therapy for adolescents with binge eating syndromes: A case series. *Int J Eat Disord, 39,* 252-255.

Schmidt, U., Lee, S., Beecham, J., et al. (2007). A randomized controlled trial of family therapy and cognitive behavior therapy guided self-care for adolescents with bulimia nervosa and related disorders. *Am J Psychiatry, 164,* 591-598.

Schwartz, H.J.(Ed.) (1988). *Bulimia: Psychoanalytic Treatment and Theory,* Madison, CT: International University Press.

Shapiro, J.R., Woolson, S.L., Hamer, R.M., et al. (2007). Evaluating binge eating disorder in children: Development of the Children's Binge Eating Disorder Scale (C-BEDS). *Int J Eat Disord, 40,* 82-89.

Smith, A.T., & Wolfe, B.E. (2008). Amenorrhea as a diagnostic criterion for anorexia nervosa: A review of the evidence and implications for practice. *J Am Psychiatr Nurses Assoc, 14,* 209-215.

Smith, F.M., Latchford, G.J., Hall, R.M., et al. (2008). Do chronic medical conditions increase the risk of eating disorder? A cross-sectional investigation of eating pathology in adolescent females with scoliosis and diabetes. *J Adolesc Health, 42,* 58-63.

Spettigue, W., Buchholz, A., Henderson, K., et al. (2008). Evaluation of the efficacy and safety of olanzapine as an adjunctive treatment for anorexia nervosa in adolescent females: A randomized, double-blind, placebo-controlled trial. *BMC Pediatr, 8.* [Open Access].

Stein, K.F., & Hedger, K.M. (1997). Body weight and shape self-cognitions, emotional distress, and disordered eating in middle adolescent girls. *Arch Psychiatr Nurs, 11,* 264-275.

Treasure, J., Sepulveda, A.R., MacDonald, P., et al. (2008). The assessment of the family of people with eating disorders. *Eur Eat Disord Rev, 16*(4), 247-255.

Viglione, V., Muratori, F., Maestro, S., et al. (2006). Denial of symptoms and psychopathology in adolescent anorexia nervosa. *Psychopathology, 39,* 255-260.

Vohs, K.D., Heatherton, T.F., & Herrin, M. (2001). Disordered eating and the transition to college: a prospective study. *Int J Eat Disord, 29,* 280-288.

Wade, T.D., Bulik, C.M., Neale, M., et al. (2000). Anorexia nervosa and major depression: Shared genetic and environmental risk factors. *Am J Psychiatry, 157,* 469-471.

Waller, J.V., Kaufman, M.R., & Deutsch, F. (1940). Anorexia nervosa: A psychosomatic entity. *Psychosom Med, 11,* 3-16.

Watkins, B., & Lask, B. (2002). Eating disorders in school-aged children. *Child Adolesc Psychiatr Clin North Am, 11,* 185-199.

Whitney, J., Haigh, R., Weinman, J., et al. (2007). Caring for people with eating disorders: Factors associated with psychological distress and negative caregiving appraisals in carers of people with eating disorders. *Br J Clin Psychology, 46*(Pt 4), 413-428.

Wilfley, D.E., Bishop, M.E., Wilson, G.T., et al. (2007). Classification of eating disorders; Toward DSM-V. *Int J Eat Disord, 40,* S123-S129.

Wolfe, B.E., & Gimby, L.B. (2003). Caring for hospitalized patient with an eating disorder. *Nurs Clin North Am, 38,* 75-99.

Wolfe, B.E., Metzger, E.D., & Stollar, C. (1997). The effect of dieting on plasma tryptophan concentration and food intake in healthy women. *Physiol Behav, 61,* 537-541.

Workgroup for Classification of Eating Disorders in Children and Adolescents [WCEDCA] (2007). Classification of child and adolescent eating disturbances. *Int J Eat Disord, 40,* S117-S122.

26 Epilepsy and Seizure Disorders

Joan L. Blair

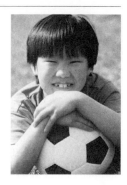

Etiology

Epilepsy and seizures are the most common serious neurologic disorders in the world and affect both children and adults (Brodie, Schachter, & Kwan, 2005; Leppik, 2006). *Epilepsy* is a brain disorder characterized by recurrent and unpredictable interruptions of normal brain function that result in a predisposition to recurrent seizures. A history of at least one seizure must be present to diagnose epilepsy. In addition, neurobiologic, cognitive, psychological, and social disturbances/consequences accompany the disorder. A *seizure* is a sudden, time-limited event with clinical manifestations with a distinct start and finish (Fisher, van Emde Boas, Eger, et al., 2005). A seizure is stereotypical and repetitive and causes an alteration in at least one of the following: autonomic, sensory or motor function; consciousness; emotional state; memory; cognition; or behavior. A seizure is the result of abnormal and excessive synchronized discharges of a group of cortical neurons in the brain (Brodie et al., 2005). Seizures are caused by multiple factors, including (but not limited to) the location of the onset of abnormal discharges in the brain, patterns of reproduction, brain maturity, additional disease processes, sleep-wake cycles, and medications (Fisher et al., 2005). Seizures are further characterized as epileptic and nonepileptic. *Epileptic seizures* are associated with abnormal electrical activity in the brain. They can arise either from a general dysfunction of the biochemical mechanisms of the brain (generalized seizures) or from distinct areas of the brain (localization-related seizures) (Leppik, 2006). *Nonepileptic seizures,* conversely, are clinical events that can mimic epileptic seizures. They can be a response to a physiologic event, such as fever, toxins, or hypoxia, or a reaction to some type of psychic stressor *(psychogenic seizures)* (Brodie et al., 2005; Leppik, 2006).

The International League Against Epilepsy (ILAE) developed a classification of epileptic seizures in 1969, revised it in 1981, and updated the classification in 1989 to add epileptic syndromes (Engel, 2001). This classification is still used today. The ILAE grouped the underlying causes of epilepsy into three classifications. *Symptomatic epilepsies* reveal no immediate cause for the seizure, however, a prior central nervous system (CNS) or systemic insult to the brain has occurred (i.e., asphyxia, severe electrolyte disturbance, stroke, meningitis, trauma, vascular lesion, CNS degenerative conditions) or a static form of encephalopathy is present (i.e., cerebral palsy, intellectual disability) (Foldvary-Schaefer, 2006; Hauser & Banerjee, 2008; Prasad & Prasad, 2008). *Idiopathic epilepsies* represent a mostly benign course of epilepsy with a presumed inherited origin (Foldvary-Schaefer, 2006), such as in benign rolandic epilepsy and childhood absence epilepsy. In *cryptogenic epilepsies,* no cause is identified but an underlying pathologic cause that may

be subsequently discovered is presumed (Jain & Morton, 2008). Cryptogenic epilepsies occur with or without accompanying neurologic abnormalities (Foldvary-Schaefer, 2006).

Because of the many advances in epilepsy since these classifications were first accepted, the ILAE agreed to review and revise the current system. To better address clinical and research needs, a new diagnostic scheme to describe affected individuals that includes five levels or axes, was proposed in 2001. The axes include a description of the ictal semiology, seizure type(s), syndrome identification, etiology, and degree of impairment. Axis 1, *ictal semiology,* uses standardized descriptive terminology to describe the ictal event. Axis 2, *seizure type or types,* is derived from a list of accepted seizure types representing diagnostic entities with etiologic, therapeutic, and/or prognostic implications. Axis 3, *syndrome identification,* is derived from a list of accepted syndromes. It is widely accepted that a diagnosis of a syndrome for epilepsy is not always possible. Axis 4, *etiology,* is specified when it is known. Axis 5, *impairment,* is an optional designation (Engel, 2001; ILAE, 2008). Although the five axes seems to improve the classification of seizures and seizure syndromes, this diagnostic scheme has not yet been fully adopted by the neuroscience community and still requires further development.

Understanding the molecular pathogenesis of human epilepsy has been studied for the past two decades. Epilepsy can result from genetic and genomic influences. Some epilepsy syndromes are monogenic, resulting from changes in known ion channel genes. Others include numerous autosomal or X-linked genetic disorders in which epilepsy is predominantly phenotypic. Clear links between altered gene sequence and seizures are frequently reported, yet the molecular mechanisms that underlie epilepsy remain a challenge (Crino, 2007).

It is known that mutations in single genes can lead to distinct epilepsy syndromes, such as generalized epilepsy with febrile seizures plus (GEFS+), in which a mutation occurs in a sodium channel gene. GEFS+ is associated with febrile seizures that may or may not cease with age (Avanzini, Franceschetti, & Mantegazza, 2007). The syndrome later progresses to afebrile generalized seizures that are sometimes associated with absence, myoclonic, and focal seizures. It has been suggested that in some families, the model of inheritance of GEFS+ may actually involve two or more genes, as opposed to a single-gene defect (Bonanni, Malcarne, Moro, et al., 2004). Mutations of the *SCN1A* gene have been found in severe myoclonic epilepsy of infancy (SMEI), otherwise known as Dravet syndrome, even in the absence of a family history of the disorder. SMEI is characterized by prolonged tonic, clonic, and tonic-clonic seizures, with or without fever, followed later in life by absence, tonic-clonic, simple partial seizures, and complex partial seizures (Avanzini et al., 2007). Other known epilepsy syndromes associated with single-gene channelopathies include (but are not limited to) benign familial neonatal-infantile convulsions (BFNIC), some simple febrile seizures, and familial absence seizures (Avanzini et al., 2007; Brodie et al., 2005).

However, idiopathic epilepsies are rarely inherited as single-gene disorders. Instead, they are more often complex genetic diseases with simultaneous involvement of multiple genes (Kaneko, Okada, Iwasa, et al., 2002b). Abnormalities in different genes and different mutations (genetic heterogeneity) may cause the same epilepsy phenotype (Berkovic & Ottman, 2000; Kaneko, Iwasa, Okada, 2002a). This characteristic is seen in benign familial neonatal convulsions (BFNCs), in which a mutation in two potassium channel genes *(KCNQ2* and *KCNQ3)* is responsible for the majority of individuals with the disorder (Avanzini et al., 2007; Brodie et al., 2005). Autosomal dominant nocturnal frontal lobe epilepsy (ADNFLE), in which mutations in the neuronal nicotinic acetylcholine receptors alpha$_4$- and beta$_2$-subunit genes have been identified as a cause for the syndrome (Avanzini et al., 2007), is another example of mutations of ion channels that cause idiopathic epilepsies. In most cases, however, how these channelopathies lead to recurrent seizures is still unclear (Brodie et al., 2005).

Evidence suggests that altered gene expression is associated with recurrent seizures. Studies of gene expression analysis are performed to identify either a single gene or a panel of genes associated with epileptogenesis. *Genomics* refers to gene sequence alterations that may predict clinical outcomes or phenotype. These influences may explain the types of epilepsy that occur in individuals with no obvious structural abnormality or an inherited cause of their seizures (Crino, 2007).

Abnormal cortical development is a major cause of epilepsy. Severe malformations in cortical development can result in profound developmental delays and epilepsy. In some of these malformations, a clear pattern of inheritance is evident, whereas in others a sporadic pattern exists. Some cortical malformations with an explained or suspected genetic basis include some of the malformation syndromes of lissencephaly (smooth brain), schizencephaly (cleft brain), and polymicrogyria (excessive small, prominent convolutions spaced by shallow, enlarged sulci) (Guerrini & Carrozzo, 2001).

Incidence and Prevalence

Active prevalence is often used to measure the affected population with epilepsy. It is a measurement of individuals who are currently being treated or have had a seizure within a specified period (Berg, 2006).

Epilepsy develops in approximately one third of individuals who have a seizure (Leppik, 2006). Approximately 50 million people in the world have epilepsy (Epilepsy Foundation of America [EFA], 2008). The prevalence is about 1% of the population in both developing and developed countries (Brodie et al., 2005). Approximately 10% of the population will experience one or more seizures at some time in their life (Schneker & Fountain, 2003). Approximately 5% of children and adolescents will have a seizure by 20 years of age (Hauser & Banerjee, 2008). The risk of recurrence after a first unprovoked seizure in untreated individuals is about 40% to 50% within the first 2 years. Treatment may reduce the risk by half (Berg, 2008). Many researchers also believe that after two seizures, the risk of a third seizure is about 80% (Camfield & Camfield, 2005). Those with abnormal electroencephalograms (EEGs) or

an identifiable neurologic condition (or symptoms consistent with one) are at greatest risk (Berg, 2008).

The incidence of epilepsy varies with age; rates are higher in early childhood. The incidence is highest in the first year of life: approximately 100 per 100,000 children (Hauser & Banerjee, 2008). The rates then decrease into adult life, with a second peak in adults older than 65 years (Brodie et al., 2005). The incidence is also slightly higher in males. When etiology of epilepsy is reported in incidence studies, the cause is unknown in 60% to 80% of cases. With regard to seizure type, generalized seizures seem highest in the first year of life (Hauser & Banerjee, 2008). In the United States, epilepsy affects more than 326,000 children younger than 15 years of age, and more than 90,000 have intractable seizures (EFA, 2008). Later in life, partial seizures are more common (Hauser & Banerjee, 2008). The majority of adults with active epilepsy had a childhood onset (Shinnar & Pellock, 2002).

Most epilepsies in childhood are benign; however, most catastrophic secondarily generalized epilepsies begin in infancy (Camfield & Camfield, 2002). Certain events, such as brain tumors, brain traumas, CNS infections, and cerebrovascular disease, greatly increase the risk of epilepsy. In addition, neurologic events from birth, such as cerebral palsy (CP) and intellectual disability (ID), are associated with a high incidence of epilepsy. About 15% to 30% of new cases of epilepsy in children are associated with neurologic problems from birth, CP, ID, or a combination of these (Hauser & Banerjee, 2008; Shinnar & Pellock, 2002).

Diagnostic Criteria

The diagnosis of epilepsy relies on the correct classification of seizures and epilepsy syndromes. The diagnosis is based on obtaining an accurate history of the event, a complete medical and social history, a physical and neurologic examination, and ancillary tests and consultations as necessary. The most important information is obtained through a thorough and accurate history obtained from the individual and/or family. Information should include details of the events before, during, and after the episode. In addition, information should include factors that may lower the seizure threshold (Brodie et al., 2005; Schneker & Fountain, 2003). Box 26-1 lists the key elements in obtaining a history of a suspected seizure. It is important to determine when the event occurred, if there was a warning, what signs and symptoms occurred during the event, and specifically what part or parts of the body were involved and how. Whether the episode was stereotypical is also important in determining the diagnosis of epilepsy. In addition, the duration of the event, whether consciousness was intact, the frequency of the episodes, and the presence of a postictal phenomenon are important (Arzimanoglou, 2002; Schneker & Fountain, 2003). Precipitating factors should be evaluated (Box 26-2). The history should also include questions about febrile seizures, birth complications, development, serious infections, head trauma, drug or alcohol abuse, and family history of epilepsy (Browne, 2000). A complete physical and neurologic examination should be performed to determine any abnormalities.

An EEG is performed during the diagnostic workup for epilepsy. Only about 40% of individuals have an epileptiform EEG on the initial test. Sleep deprivation before the test to capture sleep on the EEG, activation procedures (e.g., photic stimulation, hyperventilation), and prolonging the length of the study may increase the yield on the EEG (Prego-Lopez & Devinsky, 2002). Ambulatory

Pertinent History of a Suspected Seizure

PRECEDING OR PRECIPITATING THE EVENT

- Fatigue
- Sleep deprivation
- Hyperventilation
- Recent illness (fever, vomiting, diarrhea)
- Dehydration
- Electrolyte imbalance
- Unusual stress/emotional trauma
- Unusual stimuli (e.g., flickering lights, visual stimuli, thinking, reading, eating, hot water, startle)
- Somatosensory stimuli
- Proprioceptive stimuli
- Use of medications
- Excessive stimulant use
- Use of alcohol
- Withdrawal from sedative drugs or alcohol
- Use of recreational drugs
- Toxin or heavy metal exposure
- Activity immediately before event (e.g., change in posture, exercise)

THE EVENT ITSELF

- Symptoms at onset (e.g., aura)
- Motor symptoms
- Sensory symptoms
- Mode of onset: gradual versus sudden

- Duration: brief (ictal phase <5 minutes) versus prolonged (ictal phase >5 minutes)
- Stereotypy: duration and features of episodes nearly identical versus frequently changing
- Irregular respirations or pauses in respirations
- Presence of cyanosis
- Single event versus clusters
- Time of day: related to sleep or occurring on awakening
- Level of awareness/responsiveness
- Ability to talk and respond appropriately
- Ability to comprehend
- Ability to recall events during the seizure
- Abnormal movements of the eyes, mouth, face, head, arms, and legs
- Gaze deviation
- Bowel or bladder incontinence
- Forced eye closure (suggests nonepileptic event)
- Forced clenching of mouth (suggests pseudoseizure)
- Random thrashing (suggests pseudoseizure)

AFTER THE EVENT

- Confusion
- Lethargy
- Abnormal speech
- Focal weakness or sensory loss (i.e., Todd's paralysis)
- Headache, muscle soreness, or physical injury
- Duration of postseizure symptoms

Adapted from Brodie, M.J., Schachter, S.C., & Kwan, P. (2005). *Fast Facts: Epilepsy* (3rd ed.). Oxford: Health Press; Jain, S.J., & Morton, L.D. (2008). Evaluating the child with seizure. In J. Pellock, B. Bourgeois, & W. Dodson (Eds.), *Pediatric Epilepsy: Diagnosis and Therapy* (3rd ed.). New York: Demos; Leppik, I. (2006). *Contemporary Diagnosis and Management of the Patient with Epilepsy* (6th ed.). Newtown, PA: Handbooks in Health Care.; Prego-Lopez, M., & Devinsky, O. (2002). Evaluation of a first seizure: Is it epilepsy? *Postgrad Med, 111*(1), 34-48.

Precipitating Factors for Seizures

- Sleep deprivation
- Antiepileptic drug noncompliance
- Epileptogenic drugs
- Excessive stimulant use
- Alcohol or sedative drug withdrawal
- Barbiturate or benzodiazepine withdrawal
- Recreational drugs/substance abuse
- Menstrual cycle
- Dehydration
- Hyperventilation
- High fever
- Hypoglycemia
- Electrolyte imbalance
- Hypoxia
- Flickering/flashing lights
- Specific "reflex" triggers
  - Eating
  - Hot water
  - Music
  - Praxis
  - Reading
  - Startle
  - Thinking
- Intense exercise
- Emotional stress
- Diet and missed meals

Data from Brodie, M.J., Schachter, S.C., & Kwan, P. (2005). *Fast Facts: Epilepsy* (3rd ed.). Oxford: Health Press; Jain, S.J., & Morton, L.D. (2008). Evaluating the child with seizure. In J. Pellock, B. Bourgeois, & W. Dodson (Eds.), *Pediatric Epilepsy: Diagnosis and Therapy* (3rd ed.). New York: Demos; Leppik, I. (2006). *Contemporary Diagnosis and Management of the Patient with Epilepsy* (6th ed.). Newtown, PA: Handbooks in Health Care.

EEGs and inpatient video EEGs are performed at the discretion of the treating physician.

Medical imaging studies also may be performed during the diagnostic workup. Computed tomography (CT) scans can detect gross structural abnormalities or bleeding. Magnetic resonance imaging (MRI) is more sensitive and specific for evaluating brain parenchyma and structural abnormalities (Prego-Lopez & Devinsky, 2002). These and other studies (e.g., single photon emission computed tomography [SPECT] scans) are performed at the discretion of the treating physician.

See Table 26-1 for the full range of diagnostic procedures. Box 26-3 provides specific guidance for neonatal seizures.

Clinical Manifestations at Time of Diagnosis

Classification of Seizures

The first and most important step in the treatment of epilepsy is the correct diagnosis, thereby correctly classifying the seizure or the epilepsy syndrome (Brodie et al., 2005). The classification of epileptic seizures and epileptic syndromes that is widely used today is that developed by the ILAE. This classification system groups seizures with similar clinical presentations.

Partial Seizures. *Partial* (focal or localization-related) *seizures* are characterized by seizure activity that begins in specific loci in the cortex of the brain in one hemisphere (Nordli, 2008; Foldvary-Schaefer, 2006). Partial seizures are the most common seizure type in people with epilepsy (EFA, 2008). Partial seizures are then divided into simple partial seizures, complex partial seizures, and partial seizures with secondary generalization (Kellinghaus, Luders, & Wyllie, 2006).

Basis for Laboratory Studies

History and Physical Examination	Seizure Types	Type of Evaluation
Normal	Generalized	Routine EEG; serum glucose, calcium, magnesium
Normal	Partial (focal)	Routine or sleep-deprived EEG; brain scan (CT or MRI); serum glucose, calcium, magnesium
Suggests a chronic neurologic insult not previously evaluated with focal physical findings	Generalized or partial	Routine or sleep-deprived EEG; brain scan (CT or MRI); serum glucose, calcium, magnesium
Presence of mental retardation or slow development without focal signs	Generalized or partial	Routine EEG; serum glucose; calcium; serum and urine amino acids; chromosome studies, if otherwise indicated; TORCH titers, if <age 12 mo; if seizure is partial, brain imaging is indicated
Normal other than for presence of fever ± vomiting or diarrhea	—	—
Acute symptoms	Generalized or partial	LP; serum glucose, calcium, electrolytes, BUN; EEG
Child seen some days later when recovered	Generalized	Fasting glucose, calcium; EEG
Normal other than for a clouded sensorium	Generalized or partial	Brain imaging (CT or MRI); if scan normal, an LP, glucose, calcium, electrolytes; if these are normal, liver chemistries, including a serum ammonia, urine ketones, drug screen; EEG; AIDS testing
Presence of increased ICP ± focal signs	Generalized or partial	Brain imaging with contrast enhancement (CT or MRI); calcium, electrolytes, urinalysis; LP if scan is normal; EEG; if no cause is found, an MRI may be indicated at a later date
Presence of focal signs of recent onset	Generalized or partial	Contrasted brain scan (CT or MRI); LP if scan is normal; EEG; glucose, calcium, electrolytes; if CT scan is normal, cardiac evaluation; screen for hemoglobinopathies and coagulation defects, sedimentation rate, antinuclear antibodies, serum cholesterol, triglycerides; anticardiolipin antibodies if an infarct is seen on imaging

From Prensky, A. (2001). An approach to the child with paroxysmal phenomenon with emphasis on nonepileptic disorders. In J. Pellock, W. Dodson, & B. Bourgeois (Eds.), *Pediatric Epilepsy: Diagnosis and Therapy* (2nd ed.). New York: Demos. Reprinted with permission.
Key: *AIDS,* acquired immunodeficiency syndrome; *BUN,* blood urea nitrogen; *CT,* computed tomography; *EEG,* electroencephalogram; *ICP,* intracranial pressure; *LP,* lumbar puncture; *MRI,* magnetic resonance imaging; *TORCH,* toxoplasmosis, other agents, rubella, cytomegalovirus, herpes simplex virus.

Evaluation of a Neonatal Seizure

With a history that suggests a probable cause (intrauterine insult, hypoxia, etc.):
- Serum chemistries: Glucose, calcium, magnesium, electrolytes, blood urea nitrogen, or creatinine
- Serum pH, Po_2 (arterial or capillary)
- Urine screen for toxic substances
- Lumbar puncture: CSF protein, glucose, cells, smear, and culture
- Cranial ultrasound or noncontrast CT scan of the brain
- EEG

Without a probable cause also include:
- TORCH titers
- Quantitative urine and amino acids
- Serum and urine organic acids
- AIDS testing
- Drug screen

From Prensky, A. (2001). An approach to the child with paroxysmal phenomenon with emphasis on nonepileptic disorders. In J. Pellock, W. Dodson, & B. Bourgeois (Eds.), *Pediatric Epilepsy: Diagnosis and Therapy* (2nd ed.). New York: Demos. Reprinted with permission. Key: *AIDS,* acquired immunodeficiency virus; *CSF,* cerebrospinal fluid; *CT,* computed tomography; *EEG,* electroencephalogram; *TORCH,* toxoplasmosis, other (congenital syphilis and viruses), rubella, cytomegalovirus, and herpes simplex virus.

cause motor symptoms (jerking, twitching, shaking) that are usually unilateral, somatosensory symptoms (change in vision, sound, smell, or taste), autonomic symptoms (dilated pupils, altered heart or breathing rate, flushing), or psychic symptoms (fear, anger, hallucinations, déjà vu) (American Epilepsy Society [AES], 2000; Kellinghaus et al., 2006).

Clinical Manifestations at Time of Diagnosis

Manifestations vary by seizure type but may contain the following:
- Impaired consciousness
- Aura
- Automatisms
- Motor symptoms
  - Clonic—rhythmic, repetitive muscle contractions
  - Tonic—stiffening, rigidity
  - Flexor or extensor spasms
  - Loss of muscle tone
- Autonomic symptoms (e.g., flushing, pallor, pupil dilation, hypersalivation, incontinence, altered cardiac or respiratory rates)
- Psychic symptoms (e.g., fear, anger, visual and auditory hallucinations, déjà vu)

Simple partial seizures arise from the isocortex (Nordli, 2008). A simple partial seizure refers to seizure activity in which consciousness has been preserved and the individual recalls the event (for those who are able to verbalize) (Pellock & Duchowny, 2005). During a simple partial seizure, the individual remains alert, can understand what is happening in the environment, and can respond appropriately to questions or direction. Simple partial seizures can

It is believed that *complex partial seizures* involve the limbic system of the brain and therefore can lead to early bilateral dysfunction, affecting the frontal or temporal lobes of the brain (AES, 2000; Nordli, 2008). However, complex partial seizures can also occur in other lobes of the brain (Pellock & Duchowny, 2005). The clinical manifestations are determined by the location of the focus. A *complex partial seizure* refers to seizure activity in which consciousness has been impaired. A complex partial seizure can follow a simple partial seizure, or it can begin as a complex partial seizure with altered consciousness at the onset (AES, 2000; Nordli, 2008). During a complex partial seizure, the individual's ability to pay attention or respond to questions or direction is impaired or lost. Complex partial seizures can have all the same symptoms of a simple partial seizure, but in addition, the individual is confused, disoriented, or unresponsive. Automatisms (automatic movements) can occur, including mouth movements (lip smacking, chewing), upper extremity movements (picking at things), vocalization (grunting, repeating), or complex motor acts (AES, 2000). Automatisms are a more reliable manifestation of a complex partial seizure in childhood and older individuals. In infancy, oroalimentary movements such as sucking and simple repetitive gestures may be observed (Pellock & Duchowny, 2005). The individual may be aware of the seizure or have no recollection of the event (AES, 2000).

Some individuals experience an aura (or warning) before a complex partial or generalized seizure. The aura (sensory, autonomic, or psychic disturbance) is actually a simple partial seizure (So, 2006). *Todd's paralysis* can occur after a complex partial or secondarily generalized seizure. Weakness (associated with the affected region of the brain) of a part or whole side of the body can last from minutes to hours after a seizure (AES, 2000).

Partial seizures can begin as a simple partial seizure or a complex partial seizure and then progress to a generalized seizure. Secondarily, generalized seizures are more common in younger children with complex partial seizures, especially in infants. In these individuals, motor spread may be so rapid that the onset is undetected or localization is difficult to determine. Children with brain injuries can experience secondary generalized seizures well into their adult years (Pellock & Duchowny, 2005).

Generalized Seizures. *Generalized seizures* are characterized from the onset by abnormal activity that involves large parts of the brain, usually both cerebral hemispheres simultaneously or almost simultaneously. They can be convulsive (violent shaking of the entire body) or nonconvulsive (brief staring). The initial manifestations are bilateral with loss of consciousness. The individual has no memory of the seizure. Various types of generalized seizures exist, including absence, tonic, tonic-clonic, myoclonic, akinetic, atonic, and infantile spasms (Nordli, 2008; Pellock & Duchowny, 2005).

Absence seizures are described as typical and atypical. The *typical absence seizures* are characterized by a brief (up to 20 seconds) stare that begins and ends suddenly, with a total impairment of consciousness. A blank facial expression occurs (Pearl & Holmes, 2008). These expressions are often so brief that they go undetected (EFA, 2008). Associated features include clonic movements (eye blinking, mild jerking of extremities), change in tone (increased or decreased), subtle automatisms (oral, vocal, gestural), and autonomic signs or symptoms (change in skin color, urinary incontinence, pupillary dilation) that accompany the seizure. There is no warning, and the individual is totally attentive when the seizure ends. The child has no memory of the event. Hyperventilation or flashing lights can provoke absence seizures. The EEG shows a characteristic 3-Hz spike and wave pattern (AES, 2000; Hadjiloizou & Bourgeois, 2005; Pearl & Holmes, 2008).

Atypical absence seizures vary slightly in that they can begin and end gradually, they are generally not provoked by hyperventilation, and they can last slightly longer (up to 30 seconds).

Automatisms are less likely to occur in an atypical absence seizure, which has a longer recovery period. Atypical absence seizures are usually associated with diffuse or multifocal structural abnormalities of the brain. These seizures are less responsive to antiepileptic drug (AED) therapy (AES, 2000; Hadjiloizou & Bourgeois, 2005; Pearl & Holmes, 2008).

Tonic seizures are characterized by body stiffening and rigidity. Slight tremors or fine shaking may occur. Tonic seizures are usually brief, lasting from 1 to 20 seconds (AES, 2000; Hadjiloizou & Bourgeois, 2005). They usually involve the extensor muscles and have an abrupt onset with rapid return to baseline (Hadjiloizou & Bourgeois, 2005).

Clonic seizures are characterized by rhythmic, repetitive muscle contractions. They may involve any muscle groups but are most common in the arms, neck, and face. Generalized clonic seizures are accompanied by total impairment of consciousness. The duration of clonic seizures is variable. Postictal confusion does not occur after the seizure (Hadjiloizou & Bourgeois, 2005).

Tonic-clonic seizures usually begin abruptly with no warning. However, some individuals have described premonitory symptoms, such as headache, insomnia, and irritability, for hours or days before the seizure. This prodrome stage is not an aura; auras are associated with partial seizures (Hadjiloizou & Bourgeois, 2005). In a tonic-clonic seizure, the body stiffens initially (the tonic phase). Often a short cry occurs as the air is forced through contracted vocal cords. The tonic stage averages about 10 to 30 seconds. This stage often is accompanied by apnea, cyanosis, hypersalivation, bowel or bladder incontinence, and upper eye deviation. The body then jerks in a rhythmic pattern (the clonic phase), which lasts an average of 30 to 60 seconds. As the seizure continues, the clonic phase progressively slows until the individual becomes completely limp after the last clonic jerk. During the postictal period the individual is flaccid and unarousable. A period of confusion or agitation may follow the seizure (AES, 2000; Hadjiloizou & Bourgeois, 2005).

Myoclonic seizures are very brief (<1 second), very quick, shock-like, muscle jerks that are uncontrollable. They often involve the arms or face, but they may also involve the entire body. These seizures resemble a quick startle but are not precipitated by an event, such as a loud noise, light, or movement. Myoclonic seizures can occur as isolated events or in succession (clusters) (AES, 2000; Hadjiloizou & Bourgeois, 2005).

Akinetic seizures are also known as drop attacks. The individual suddenly and forcefully drops to the ground but immediately recovers (AES, 2000; Hadjiloizou & Bourgeois, 2005). Some researchers believe that the majority of akinetic seizures are brief tonic seizures (Hadjiloizou & Bourgeois, 2005). *Atonic seizures*, on the other hand, consist of a sudden loss of muscle tone. The individual suddenly drops (or melts) to the ground and is limp for some time (AES, 2000; Hadjiloizou & Bourgeois, 2005; Morita & Glauser, 2008). Some professionals use the terms *akinetic* and *atonic seizures* interchangeably, but they are actually two different seizure types.

Infantile spasms are very quick seizures that usually occur in clusters. There are three varieties of infantile spasms: flexor, extensor, and mixed. *Flexor spasms,* often called jackknife or salaam seizures, are characterized by abrupt flexing (bending) spasms of the neck, trunk, arms, and legs. *Extensor spasms,* often called cheerleading spasms, are the least common. They are characterized by extensor (straightening) spasms involving abrupt movements of the neck, trunk, and legs. *Mixed infantile spasms* are the most common type and are characterized by flexion of the neck, trunk, and arms and extension of the legs (Curatolo, 2005; Wong & Trevathan, 2001). Infantile spasms are not easily recognized or reported by parents, so diagnosis is often delayed. In addition, the primary care physician may misdiagnose the spasms as colic, a startle response, or normal infant behavior. Any repetitive, stereotypic movement in infancy should arouse suspicion of infantile spasms. The EEG shows a characteristic pattern called hypsarrhythmia, but a modified version of this reading (modified hypsarrhythmia) can also be seen (Curatolo, 2005).

Classification of Epileptic Syndromes

Epilepsy syndromes are classified into the following categories: localization-related, generalized, undetermined, and special syndromes (Leppik, 2006). The syndromes are defined by clinical features related to age of onset, family history of epilepsy, seizure type(s), and associated neurologic signs and symptoms (Brodie et al., 2005). Epilepsy syndromes are either benign or catastrophic disorders. Benign epilepsy disorders involve mild, infrequent seizures; the disorder resolves fairly quickly and is not associated with psychological or cognitive delays that affect long-term development (Camfield & Camfield, 2002; Shields, 2002). The catastrophic disorders consist of disorders with very frequent, intractable (difficult to control) seizures that are treatment resistant and associated with significant cognitive and psychosocial issues that affect long-term development. If catastrophic epilepsies begin in a young child during the developmental stages, the long-term effects are permanent (Camfield & Camfield, 2002). The primary goal is to obtain the best seizure control possible in catastrophic epilepsies so there is a positive effect on the child's development. The more common epilepsy syndromes are discussed in the following text.

Localization-Related Idiopathic Epilepsies and Syndromes. *Benign childhood epilepsy with centrotemporal spikes* (BECTS), also known as benign rolandic epilepsy, is one of the most common epilepsy syndromes in childhood, representing approximately 15% of childhood epilepsies. The age of onset of seizures typically occurs between 3 and 13 years of age, with a peak of 5 to 9 years of age. The seizures usually occur within hours of the child falling asleep and begin with simple partial seizures characterized by hemifacial motor seizures (twitching of the face and tongue). BECTS and the simple partial seizures are frequently associated with somatosensory symptoms. The seizures progress to the limbs and can then secondarily generalize, but this is uncommon. The EEG is consistent with bilateral centrotemporal spikes. The etiology is an autosomal dominant genetic disorder. The prognosis is good—BECTS usually resolves during adolescence. Treatment is optional since the seizures usually occur at night (Camfield & Camfield, 2002; Leppik, 2006; Pellock & Duchowny, 2005). Nearly all affected children enter remission by 16 years of age (Pellock & Duchowny, 2005).

Benign childhood epilepsy with occipital spikes (Panayiotopoulos syndrome) is less common than BECTS and typically presents in the later part of the first decade of life. Children with this type of epilepsy have normal cognition. About two thirds of such seizures occur in sleep or during daytime naps and are usually prolonged (30 minutes or longer). The seizures usually begin with nausea, retching, or vomiting. If a seizure occurs during wakefulness, it can be accompanied by behavioral changes (i.e., restlessness, agitation, and/or terror). Other autonomic features can occur (i.e., pallor,

cyanosis, flushing, papillary abnormalities [mydriasis or miosis], urinary or fecal incontinence, elevated temperature as an ictal phenomenon, headache, hypersalivation, and coughing). If the seizure begins when the child is awake, it starts as a simple partial seizure and then progresses to impairment of consciousness. Seizure frequency is low, and remission is usually obtained in these children (Ferrie, Nordli, & Panayiotopoulos, 2008).

Benign occipital epilepsy usually consists of visual hallucinations of small, multicolored circular patterns, or less commonly, formed shapes and faces, or visual illusions. The child then experiences ictal blindness, which may be bilateral, unilateral, or part of a hemifield. The child describes the vision as everything going black or white. Other symptoms can include eye pain, a feeling of the eye being tugged, forced eye closure, and eye blinking. The child may experience a headache during or after the seizure, which is migrainous in character. Consciousness is usually preserved during the seizure (Ferrie et al., 2008). There is no clear etiology. The prognosis for most individuals is favorable, with remission occurring by the end of the second decade of life (Pellock & Duchowny, 2005).

Localization-Related Symptomatic Epilepsies and Syndromes. These epilepsy syndromes are less common in children compared with adults, and they have a variety of specific, identifiable causes (Box 26-4). The seizures are usually partial and can secondarily

---

BOX 26-4

Some Causes of Symptomatic Localization-Related Epilepsies

VASCULAR
- Stroke
- Infantile hemiplegia
- Arteriovenous malformations
- Sturge-Weber syndrome
- Aneurysms (subarachnoid hemorrhage)
- Venous thrombosis
- Cerebral embolisms
- Hypertensive encephalopathy
- Blood dyscrasias (sickle cell anemia)

INFECTIOUS
- Abscess
- Meningitis and encephalitis
- Toxoplasmosis
- Cytomegalovirus
- Syphilis
- Parasitic
- Rubella
- Rasmussen syndrome (presumed viral)
- Central nervous system

TUMORS
- Meningiomas
- Gliomas

- Hamartomas
- Metastatic tumors

DEGENERATIVE
- Multiple sclerosis

TRAUMATIC
- Prenatal injuries
- Perinatal injuries
- Head injuries
- Birth trauma
- Anoxia

BRAIN MALFORMATIONS
- Cysts
- Calcifications
- Cortical dysplasias
- Hippocampal malformations
- Lissencephaly
- Schizencephaly
- Tuberous sclerosis
- Neurofibromatosis
- Mesial temporal sclerosis

CRYPTOGENIC
- No cause identified

Data from Foldvary-Schaefer, N. (2006). Symptomatic focal epilepsies. In E. Wyllie (Ed.), *The Treatment of Epilepsy: Principles and Practice* (4th ed.). Philadelphia: Lippincott Williams & Wilkins; Kotagal, P. (2008). Localization-related epilepsies: Simple partial seizures, partial seizures, complex partial seizures, and Rasmussen syndrome. In J. Pellock, B. Bourgeois, & W. Dodson (Eds.), *Pediatric Epilepsy: Diagnosis and Therapy* (3rd ed.). New York: Demos; Leppik, I. (2006). *Contemporary Diagnosis and Management of the Patient with Epilepsy* (6th ed.). Newtown, PA: Handbooks in Health Care.

generalize if untreated (Leppik, 2006). An example of a syndrome in this category is *epilepsia partialis continua* (EPC). The seizures are characterized by muscular twitches that affect a particular part of the body, usually the distal limb and face, but they can also involve the trunk, diaphragm, neck, and throat muscles. The seizure lasts for a minimum of 1 hour and does not stop spontaneously. The duration, rhythm, amplitude, and the limb involved, as well as the extent of involvement, can change throughout the episode (Deray, Resnick, & Alvarez, 2001). This syndrome usually indicates an underlying cerebral disorder; therefore the prognosis depends on the etiology of EPC (Fenichel, 2005).

Generalized Idiopathic Epilepsies and Syndromes with Age-Related Onset. *Benign neonatal familial convulsions* is a disorder characterized by generalized seizures that usually occur on the third day of life, but seizures can begin at 24 hours to 1 month after delivery. The seizures begin as tonic posturing of trunk and limbs, a shrill cry, abnormal ocular movements, and cyanosis as a result of apnea. Clonic movements, whether they affect one part of the body or are generalized, often occur after the initial symptoms. Remission usually occurs within the first week of life in 70% of affected infants. The disorder is autosomal dominant with incomplete penetrance with two known foci: one on chromosome 20q13.3 and one on chromosome 8q. A clear family history is usually present. Epilepsy develops later in life in about 14% of these infants (Abdel-Hamid, Alvin, & Painter, 2005; Mizrahi, 2008).

Benign neonatal convulsions are also known as *benign idiopathic neonatal convulsions* because of the lack of an identifiable etiology, and *fifth-day fits,* because they usually occur on the fifth day of life. The seizures are characterized by partial clonic or apneic seizures that are usually brief (lasting 1 to 3 minutes). The self-limiting seizures can recur during a 24- to 48-hour period. Etiology is unknown. Affected infants have a normal neurologic examination, normal laboratory findings, and no family history of seizures. Prognosis is good with no recurrence of seizures and no developmental problems (Abdel-Hamid et al., 2005; Mizrahi, 2008).

Childhood absence epilepsy (CAE) is also known as pyknolepsy (referring to crowding) because the seizures can occur many times in an hour and usually occur daily (Leppik, 2006). Age of onset is 5 to 10 years of age; CAE occurs more frequently in girls. Generalized tonic-clonic seizures also develop in approximately 30% of affected individuals. Both seizures and the EEG reading are consistent for typical absence seizures and can be activated by hyperventilation in approximately 80% of cases. Children with CAE are neurologically normal, and a family history of idiopathic generalized epilepsy may exist. These seizures are usually fairly easy to control and remit in approximately 80% of individuals. Remission rates are lower in those individuals in whom generalized tonic-clonic seizures develop (Hadjiloizou & Bourgeois, 2005; Pearl & Holmes, 2008).

Juvenile absence epilepsy (JAE) is similar to CAE; however, age of onset is during puberty and both genders are affected equally. Typical seizures that occur in JAE happen sporadically and occur less frequently than in CAE. Generalized tonic-clonic seizures are common and usually occur on awakening; they occur in up to 80% of youths affected. Often the tonic-clonic seizures are recognized before the absences. Myoclonic seizures can also be seen. Individuals usually respond well to treatment. JAE can persist into adulthood, and the rate of remission is not as good as in CAE (Behrouz & Benbadis, 2008; Hadjiloizou & Bourgeois, 2005).

Juvenile myoclonic epilepsy (JME) is one of the most common forms of idiopathic generalized epilepsies. Age of onset is in adolescence. Initial seizures are single or repetitive myoclonic jerks that involve primarily the shoulders and arms. Seizures usually occur on awakening, often as a result of sleep deprivation, stress, fatigue, or alcohol use. The seizure can be intense and cause the individual to drop objects. If the myoclonic jerks occur in the legs, the individual can suddenly fall. Consciousness does not change noticeably during the seizures (Behrouz & Benbadis, 2008; Hadjiloizou & Bourgeois, 2005). The individual often complains of being clumsy or jittery (Leppik, 2006). Generalized tonic-clonic seizures associated with JME often occur later in the disease course in a large majority of untreated individuals, which is usually the motivating factor to obtain the initial medical evaluation. The tonic-clonic seizures usually occur in the morning and are often preceded by myoclonic jerks. Absence seizures are seen in approximately one fifth to one third of individuals with JME. Both myoclonic and tonic-clonic seizures are precipitated by sleep deprivation, alcohol consumption, and stress (Behrouz & Benbadis, 2008; Hadjiloizou & Bourgeois, 2005). Individuals can have photosensitive seizures (Behrouz & Benbadis, 2008), which can diagnosed using strobe lights during an EEG.

Generalized Cryptogenic or Symptomatic Epilepsies and Syndromes. *West syndrome* is the most common catastrophic epilepsy in children (Shields, 2000). West syndrome consists of infantile spasms (occurring up to hundreds of times per day), hypsarrhythmia on the EEG, and psychomotor retardation, although this may be absent (Curatolo, 2005; Hadjiloizou & Bourgeois, 2005). West syndrome occurs in the first year of life, with a peak between 4 and 7 months of age (Curatolo, 2005). Infant development is usually normal up to this point (Leppik, 2006). The etiology of West syndrome includes structural abnormalities (i.e., tuberous sclerosis), metabolic diseases (i.e., phenylketonuria, hypoxia), perinatal causes (i.e., hypoxic-ischemic encephalopathy, porencephaly), or cryptogenic etiologies (Curatolo, 2005; Shields, 2002; Wong & Trevathan, 2001). Prognosis depends on the underlying brain disorder and response to treatment. Intellectual disability is seen in approximately 75% to 93% of cases. Approximately 50% of children with West syndrome have epilepsy in later years, and Lennox-Gastaut syndrome (LGS) develops in about half of this group (Leppik, 2006).

Lennox-Gastaut syndrome is also a catastrophic epilepsy; approximately 1% to 4% of all childhood epilepsies are attributable to this syndrome. LGS consists of intractable mixed seizures, cognitive impairment that deteriorates over time, and a slow spike-and-wave pattern on the EEG (Hadjiloizou & Bourgeois, 2005; Morita & Glauser, 2008). Onset is usually between 1 and 8 years of age, but it primarily begins in the preschool-age child. Boys are affected more often than girls (Hadjiloizou & Bourgeois, 2005; Nordli, 2008). Typically, LGS consists of tonic, atonic, myoclonic, atypical absence, tonic-clonic, and focal seizures (Golumbek, 2004; Nordli, 2008). Most children with this syndrome are intellectually disabled; however, a few (<10%) remain intellectually normal (Camfield & Camfield, 2002). The etiology of LGS varies. Infantile spasms have previously occurred in 9% to 30% of individuals with LGS. Most etiologies (30% to 75%) are symptomatic, and about 33% of the cases are cryptogenic (Crumrine, 2002). Seizures are very difficult to control and the prognosis for these children is poor; 90% or more have persistent seizures and/or intellectual delay (Hadjiloizou & Bourgeois, 2005).

Undetermined Epilepsies and Syndromes. *Landau Kleffner syndrome* (LKS) is a rare syndrome also known as *acquired epileptic aphasia* (Brodie et al., 2005; RamachandranNair & Snead, 2008). Onset is usually between 2 and 11 years of age, with 75% of the cases occurring between 3 and 10 years (Fenichel, 2005). Typically children with LKS previously have normal cognition with normal speech development (Camfield & Camfield, 2002). Then language regression develops with verbal auditory agnosia (the inability to know the meaning of words) and rapid reduction of spontaneous oral expression (Camfield & Camfield, 2002; Nordli, 2008). Speech often stops altogether, and behavioral and psychomotor problems often develop. Approximately 50% of individuals with LKS have a severe language delay or mental handicap that continues throughout life. About 40% to 50% can lead a normal social and professional life if speech returns before adulthood (Camfield & Camfield, 2002). Epileptic seizures, either complex partial or generalized tonic-clonic, occur in approximately two thirds of individuals with LKS; and the seizures usually remit by 15 years of age (Nordli, 2008). Etiology is unknown but reflects an underlying cerebral disorder. AEDs improve some individuals' seizures but do not improve speech. The EEG may become normalized if corticosteroids are used early in the course of treatment. Corticosteroids can also provide long-lasting seizure and aphasia remission. However, despite corticosteroid treatment, 50% to 80% of children have long-term language dysfunction. Most individuals often require intensive language therapy for speech (Fenichel, 2005; Riviello & Hadjiloizou, 2008).

Special Syndromes: Situation-Related Seizures. *Febrile seizures* occur in approximately 2% to 5% of children in the United States; this type of seizure is the most common seizure disorder in childhood. Approximately 9% to 10% of Japanese children experience at least one febrile seizure, indicating a possible genetic predisposition in this population (Wolf & Shinnar, 2005).

Onset of febrile seizures is usually between 3 months and 5 years of age and is associated with an acute febrile illness (Brodie et al., 2005). The onset of febrile seizures usually peaks between 18 and 22 months of age. Febrile seizures rarely develop after 5 years of age; however, they can occur up to 10 years of age (Wolf & Shinnar, 2005). Seizures are either simple febrile seizures or complex febrile seizures. *Simple febrile seizures* are generalized and brief, lasting less than 15 minutes. They do not recur during the same illness. *Complex febrile seizures* have at least one of the following features: duration longer than 15 minutes, focal onset, and possible recurrence during the same febrile illness (Shinnar & Glauser, 2002; Wolf & Shinnar, 2005). Children can experience a seizure before or within an hour of the recognized fever. However, most children experience the seizure 1 to 24 hours after the fever. Some children experience the seizure more than 24 hours after the onset of the fever (Wolf & Shinnar, 2005).

The overall risk of recurrence of febrile seizures is approximately 34%; about one third of children have at least one recurrence (Leppik, 2006; Wolf & Shinnar, 2005). In children who have their first febrile seizure before 12 months of age, the recurrence is higher, approximately 50% (Leppik, 2006). In children older than 12 months of age, the recurrence for a second

seizure is lower, approximately 30%. In addition, of those 30% who experience a second febrile seizure, 50% have the possibility of having another (Steering Committee on Quality Improvement and Management, Subcommittee on Febrile Seizures [Steering Committee], 2008). The risk factors for recurrent febrile seizures include a family history of febrile seizures, first febrile seizure before 18 months of age, a lower temperature, and an interval less than 1 hour between the onset of the fever and the seizure. Fifty percent of all recurrences occur within the first 6 months, and 90% of recurrences occur within 2 years (Wolf & Shinnar, 2005). Febrile seizures are relatively benign and are not associated with any long-term consequences, such as intellectual disability or serious neurologic impairment (Leppik, 2006; Steering Committee, 2008).

Epilepsy occurs in approximately 2% to 10% of children with febrile seizures. The risk factors for the development of epilepsy after febrile seizures include multiple simple febrile seizures, complex febrile seizures, an interval less than 1 hour between the onset of the fever and the seizure, preexisting neurologic abnormality, and a family history of epilepsy (Steering Committee, 2008; Wolf & Shinnar, 2005). Children with simple febrile seizures have about the same risk as the general population for developing epilepsy (Steering Committee, 2008).

Treatment of febrile seizures is a controversial issue with two approaches to treatment. The first approach is that these seizures are harmful and may lead to the individual developing epilepsy. Those who believe in this approach use either intermittent or chronic treatment with medications aimed at seizure prevention. The second approach follows the premise that febrile seizures are benign, and treatment is directed only at very prolonged febrile seizures. Those who believe in this approach will treat to abort febrile seizures when they occur to prevent status epilepticus (Wolf & Shinnar, 2005).

The American Academy of Pediatrics (AAP) and its Provisional Committee on Quality Improvement, in collaboration with neurologists, pediatricians, and research methodologists, developed a practice parameter for the *evaluation of a child with a first simple febrile seizure*. The source of the fever should be evaluated and treated, and the fever should be treated with antipyretics. A lumbar puncture (LP) should be performed based on the circumstances. If meningeal signs are present, an LP should be performed. If the child is younger than 12 months, an LP should be strongly considered, since the symptoms associated with meningitis can be minimal or absent at this age. If the child is between 12 and 18 months, an LP should be considered, because the symptoms associated with meningitis can be subtle at this age. If the child is older than 18 months, an LP is recommended if meningeal signs are present, since clinical signs of meningitis are more reliable in a child 18 months and older. An LP is recommended in the child with a first complex febrile seizure or if symptoms warrant one. If LP findings are consistent with meningitis, then the infection should be treated with the proper antibiotics. If the LP is abnormal, but not consistent with meningitis, then further evaluation of the abnormalities on the LP and possible treatment is warranted. An EEG and medical imaging studies are not recommended for a normal healthy child with a first simple febrile seizure. Laboratory studies (serum electrolytes, glucose, calcium, phosphate, magnesium, complete blood count, and serum glucose) are not routinely recommended for a first simple febrile seizure in a child older than 6 months, unless specific indications are present. In the younger child, laboratory studies may be helpful in come cases (Provisional Committee on Quality Improvement, Subcommittee on Febrile Seizures, 1996; Wolf & Shinnar, 2005). These practice parameters are still used today, however, emergency departments may develop their own guidelines based on these principles.

Status epilepticus (SE) is a common, potentially life-threatening medical emergency that must be treated immediately. Most cases occur in children. SE consists of 30 minutes or more of either continuous seizure activity or recurrent seizures without recovery of consciousness between the seizures (Riviello, Ashwal, Hirtz, et al., 2006; Wheless & Clarke, 2005). This time period is based on the fact that in animal studies after 30 minutes of seizure activity physiologic changes fail to compensate for the increase in cerebral metabolism, resulting in harmful effects on the neurons (Brodie et al., 2005; Wheless & Clarke, 2005). Generalized convulsive status epilepticus (GCSE) is the most common form, but nonconvulsive status epilepticus (NCSE) can also occur (Leppik, 2006). NCSE consists of seizures that do not have convulsive motor activity, such as absence status, simple partial status, or complex partial status (Leszczyszyn & Pellock, 2008). Of the approximately 100,000 to 150,000 cases of SE that occur each year in the United States, the highest proportion occur in children. The longer the seizures persist, the more difficult they are to treat, which leads to a higher mortality rate. Death after SE is usually due to the underlying cause of the prolonged seizure, as opposed to the seizure itself. Although children are at a higher risk of development of SE compared with adults, the morbidity and mortality rates are lower (Wheless & Clarke, 2005).

Treatment

Decision to Treat

The question continues to be whether to treat (or not treat) a child with seizures. Discussion with the child and family should include the risk and benefits of both choices. Topics should include the chance of a successful outcome with treatment and the likelihood of remission. Diagnosing the epilepsy syndrome when possible not only aids the clinician in providing the prognosis and recommending genetic counseling when appropriate, but also aids in choosing the most appropriate antiepileptic drug (AED) for the seizure type or types (Brodie et al., 2005).

Treatment

Decision to treat
Pharmacologic therapy (antiepileptic drugs [AEDs])
Nonpharmacologic interventions
• Ketogenic diet
• Vagus nerve stimulator (VNS)
Epilepsy surgery
   Resective surgery
   • Temporal lobectomy
   • Extratemporal resection
   • Hemispherectomy
   Functional surgery
   • Corpus callosotomy
   • Multiple subpial transection

Other factors to consider in making this decision include kindling, the recurrence rate, the fear of brain damage and other physical injury, and the possibility of death (Camfield & Camfield, 2002). The premise of *kindling,* documented only in animal studies, is that the abnormal activity that occurs in a particular part of the brain that causes the seizure will eventually spread to other areas, resulting in worsening seizures that are more difficult to control, if not treated. *Recurrence rate* refers to whether a seizure recurs or is a one-time event, whether it is a febrile or afebrile seizure. This will affect treatment. Recurrent seizures often require treatment, whereas one-time seizures often do not require treatment. The fear of injury with a seizure must take into account the seizure type, age of the child, and the activity in which the child is involved. Individuals at a continued risk for neurologic (brain) or other body injuries because of seizure activity need to be treated. Brain injury is usually caused by the loss of consciousness and the resulting fall (Shinnar & O'Dell, 2008); the seizure itself is usually not the actual cause of the brain damage.

Status epilepticus (SE) can sometimes cause brain damage, but it rarely causes brain damage in children (Camfield & Camfield, 2002). In rare cases, however, SE can result in death. Sudden unexplained death in epilepsy (SUDEP) is also a concern. SUDEP refers to a sudden death in an individual with confirmed epilepsy without an identifiable cause found on autopsy but who is otherwise in good health. Probable SUDEP refers to the same, without an autopsy (Nei, Ho, Abou-Khalil, et al., 2004). SUDEP is responsible for approximately 2% to 17% of deaths in individuals with epilepsy (Ficker, 2000).

Treatment Options

Once the decision to treat is made, treatment options vary. Pharmacologic treatment consists of AEDs. Nonpharmacologic treatment consists of the ketogenic diet, vagus nerve stimulation (VNS), and epilepsy surgery. Some parents have elected to treat their child's epilepsy with alternative therapies, such as herbal preparations and supplements. The decision to treat should be made after considering the risks and benefits of the option chosen.

Pharmacologic Therapy. *Pharmacologic therapy* is usually the first course of action in treating epilepsy. The discussion with the family must include common side effects, including the risk of teratogenesis in an affected female's future pregnancies. Other issues to discuss include fears and misconceptions about drug treatment and the importance of complete adherence with the medication regimen (Brodie et al., 2005). The goal of therapy is maximum seizure control with minimum or no side effects. Approximately 60% to 70% of individuals with newly diagnosed epilepsy remain seizure free while receiving monotherapy, whereas 30% or more continue to have seizures and require additional medications. The localization-related epilepsies are more difficult to control. Approximately 60% of individuals can become seizure free with the first or second AED, and the response to the first AED is a good predictor of the prognosis for seizure control. When seizure control is not possible with monotherapy, then polytherapy must be considered (Brodie & Kwan, 2002; Brodie et al., 2005).

A variety of established AEDs are used in the United States for seizures; these were marketed between 1912 and 1981. From 1993 to 2005, a second generation of AEDs was approved for the adjunctive treatment of intractable epilepsy. A list of all approved

AEDs is provided in Table 26-2. Although some AEDs have not been approved for use in children, nor have they been approved as first-line treatment of seizures, many epilepsy centers use the newer AEDs in children as first-line treatment of seizures or as adjunctive therapy for seizures. The efficacy of the established and newer AEDs on common seizure types and epilepsy syndromes is presented in Table 26-3.

The American Academy of Pediatrics (AAP) and its Steering Committee on Quality Improvement and Management, in collaboration with other experts, concluded that long-term therapy for simple febrile seizures is not warranted, despite evidence that treatment with phenobarbital, primidone, and valproic acid, as well as intermittent treatment with oral diazepam, is effective in preventing recurrence of further febrile seizures. The potential toxic effects of these drugs outweighed the minor risks associated with simple febrile seizures. For families with extreme anxiety about recurrence, oral diazepam can be used at the onset of a febrile illness to try to prevent recurrence of a febrile seizure. Antipyretics can be used to try to reduce fever and make the child more comfortable; however, no studies have demonstrated that antipyretics, without AEDs, reduce the risk of recurrent febrile seizures (Steering Committee, 2008).

Nonpharmacologic Interventions

Ketogenic diet. The ketogenic diet is another treatment for epilepsy. It is a rigid, mathematically calculated, physician-supervised diet that is high in fat and low in carbohydrate and protein. The diet usually contains three to four times as much fat as carbohydrate and protein combined (Freeman, Kossoff, Freeman, et al., 2007; Hartman & Vining, 2007). A ratio of 5:1 can be used, but the diet is so restricted with this ratio that it is not usually used for longer than 6 months. Calories and liquid intake are limited. The human body normally burns glucose and glycogen to meet its energy needs. If no new sources of glucose are provided within 24 to 36 hours, then the body burns energy that is stored as fat. However, the body cannot do this indefinitely, because once it depletes fat stores, it burns its own muscle protein. The ketogenic diet therefore simulates the metabolism of a person who is fasting and primarily burns the fat in the diet for energy. The diet allows the individual to maintain

---

TABLE 26-2

Antiepileptic Drugs

Drug	Approved Children/Adults	Dosage and Interval	Plasma Half-life	Therapeutic Plasma Level	Side Effects
Adrenocorticotropic hormone (ACTH)	Children ≥6 yr	Varied: high dose is 60 IU/day to 150 IU/m²/day			Intracranial hemorrhage Irritability Gastrointestinal disturbances/ bleeding Fluid retention Electrolyte disturbance Immune system and adrenal suppression Hypertension Cushingoid facies
Bromides (triple bromide elixir)		Children <6 yr: 300-600 mg tid Children >6 yr: 300 mg to 1 g tid	12-14 days	750-1250 mg/mL (10-15 mEq/L)	Sedation Anorexia Rash Dementia Delirium
Carbamazepine (Tegretol, Tegretol-XR, Carbatrol) (1974)	Children Adults	15-30 mg/kg/day bid or tid	12-17 hr	4-12 mg/L	Lethargy Ataxia Gastrointestinal upset Weight gain Pancreatitis Leukopenia Rash/Stevens-Johnson syndrome Arrhythmias in patients with conduction defects
Clonazepam (Klonopin) (1975)	Children Adults	0.1-0.2 mg/kg/day qd or tid	18-50 hr	20-80 mg/L	Sedation Ataxia Hyperactivity Increased salivation Rash Increased bronchial secretions

Data from Bourgeois, B.F.D. (2006). Phenobarbital and primidone. In E. Wyllie (Ed.), *The Treatment of Epilepsy: Principles and Practice* (4th ed.). Philadelphia: Lippincott Williams & Wilkins; Brodie, M.J., Schachter, S.C., & Kwan, P. (2005). *Fast Facts: Epilepsy* (3rd ed.). Oxford: Health Press; Garnett, W.R., & Cloyd, J.C. (2008). Dosage form considerations in the treatment of pediatric epilepsy. In J. Pellock, B. Bourgeois, & W. Dodson (Eds.), *Pediatric Epilepsy: Diagnosis and Therapy* (3rd ed.). New York: Demos; Holmes, G.L., & Pearl, P.L. (2008). Gabapentin and pregabalin. In J. Pellock, B. Bourgeois, & W. Dodson (Eds.), *Pediatric Epilepsy: Diagnosis and Therapy* (3rd ed.). New York: Demos; Kyllonen, K.C. (2006). Appendix: Indications for antiepileptic drugs sanctioned by the United States Food and Drug Administration. In E. Wyllie (Ed.), *The Treatment of Epilepsy: Principles and Practice* (4th ed.). Philadelphia: Lippincott Williams & Wilkins; Leppik, I. (2006). *Contemporary Diagnosis and Management of the Patient with Epilepsy* (6th ed.). Newtown, PA: Handbooks in Health Care; Nolan, M.A., & Snead, O.C. (2006). Adrenocorticotropin and steroids. In E. Wyllie (Ed.), *The Treatment of Epilepsy: Principles and Practice* (4th ed.). Philadelphia: Lippincott Williams & Wilkins; Uthman, B.M., & Beydoun, A. (2006). Less commonly used antiepileptic drugs. In E. Wyllie (Ed.), *The Treatment of Epilepsy: Principles and Practice* (4th ed.). Philadelphia: Lippincott Williams & Wilkins.

Key: *MHD,* 10-Monohydroxyl metabolite (active metabolite); Year: The year that the AED was marketed in the United States; not all AEDs are approved for use in children.

Continued

TABLE 26-2

Antiepileptic Drugs—cont'd

Drug	Approved Children/Adults	Dosage and Interval	Plasma Half-life	Therapeutic Plasma Level	Side Effects
Ethosuximide (Zarontin) (1960)	Children: ≥6 yr Adults	15-20 mg/kg/day bid or tid	30-60 hr	40-100 mg/L	Sedation Headache Nausea/vomiting Rash/erythema multiforme Stevens-Johnson syndrome
Felbamate (Felbatol) (1993)	Children: ≥2 yr with Lennox-Gastaut Adults	15-45 mg/kg/day tid or qid	15-23 hr	30-80 mg/L	Headache Drowsiness Insomnia Anorexia/weight loss Nausea/vomiting Rash/Stevens-Johnson syndrome Liver and renal failure Aplastic anemia
Fosphenytoin sodium (Cerebyx) (1996)	Children Adults	Loading dose: 15-20 mg/kg IV or IM Maintenance: 4-8 mg/kg/day IV or IM, qd or tid	12-29 hr	10-25 mg/L	Paresthesias Ataxia Nystagmus Lethargy Liver failure Hypotension Burning/itching Stevens-Johnson syndrome Toxic epidermal necrolysis
Gabapentin (Neurontin) (1993)	Children: ≥3 yr Adults	30-60 mg/kg/day tid or qid	4-6 hr	2-12 mg/L	Fatigue/somnolence Dizziness Ataxia Eye problems Weight gain Hypertension/hypotension
Lamotrigine (Lamictal) (1994)	Children: ≥2 yr Adults	With valproate: 1-5 mg/kg/day bid With monotherapy or enzyme inducer: 5-15 mg/kg/day bid	11-61 hr	4-20 mg/L	Lethargy Dizziness Nausea Pancreatitis Thrombocytopenia Rash/Stevens-Johnson syndrome/ toxic epidermal necrolysis
Oxcarbazepine (Trileptal) (2000)	Children: ≥4 yr Adults	10-60 mg/kg/day	8-10 hr	MHD 12-30 mg/L	Headache Dizziness Tiredness/somnolence Nausea/vomiting Hyponatremia
Phenobarbital (1912)	Children Adults	3-7 mg/kg/day bid Neonates: 2-5 mg/kg/day bid	24-110 hr	15-40 mg/L	Hyperactivity Drowsiness/sedation Behavioral problems Subtle cognitive changes Hepatic dysfunction Rash/Stevens-Johnson syndrome
Phenytoin (Dilantin) (1938)	Children Adults	4-8 mg/kg/day bid or tid	7-42 hr	10-20 mg/L Unbound: 0.5-3 mg/L (nonlinear kinetics)	Ataxia Nystagmus Lethargy Hirsutism Coarse facies Gingival hyperplasia Movement disorder Neuropathy Rash/Stevens-Johnson syndrome Bone marrow suppression Lupus

TABLE 26-2
Antiepileptic Drugs—cont'd

Drug	Approved Children/Adults	Dosage and Interval	Plasma Half-life	Therapeutic Plasma Level	Side Effects
Pregabalin (Lyrica) (2005)	Adults	1-2 mg/kg; increase 1-2 mg/kg/wk until seizure control or adverse events	6-8 hr	Not known	Dizziness Somnolence Asthenia Headache Ataxia Weight gain
Primidone (Mysoline) (1954)	Children: >8 yr Adults	10-25 mg/kg/day tid	8-80 hr	5-12 mg/L	Sedation Ataxia Hyperactivity Cognitive dysfunction Thrombocytopenia Rash/Stevens-Johnson syndrome
Tiagabine (Gabitril) (1997)	Adolescents: ≥12 yr Adults	20-32 mg/day bid or qid Increase every 2-4 days by 0.1-0.2 mg/kg to max 3 mg/kg/day	4-9 hr	0.1-0.3 mg/L	Dizziness Insomnia Somnolence Ataxia Nausea Increased appetite Concentration Loss Rash/Stevens-Johnson syndrome
Topiramate (Topamax) (1996)	Children: >2 yr Adults	5-15 mg/kg/day bid 24 mg/kg/day in infantile spasms	19-23 hr	4-10 mg/L	Lethargy Ataxia Psychomotor slowing Paresthesias Anorexia/weight loss Rash Renal stones Pancreatitis
Valproic acid, divalproex sodium, valproate sodium (Depakene, Depakote) (1978) (Depacon) (Depakote ER)	Children: ≥10 yr Adults	15-60 mg/kg/day bid or qid 1.5-3 mg/kg/min When converting from Depakote to Depakote ER, increase dosage by 14%-20%	9-12 hr	50-130 mg/L	Tremor Hyperactivity Sedation Gastrointestinal disturbances Pancreatitis Hepatotoxicity Thrombocytopenia Rash/Stevens-Johnson syndrome Polycystic ovary syndrome (PCOS)
Zonisamide (Zonegran) (2000)	Adults: ≥16 yr	8-12 mg/kg/day	60 hr	15-40 mg/L	Fatigue Dizziness Somnolence Ataxia Memory impairment Anorexia Rash/Stevens-Johnson syndrome Renal stones

this state over an extended period (Freeman et al., 2007). Although ketones suppress seizures and carbohydrates interfere with this suppression, the mechanism of the diet's effects on seizures is unknown (Freeman et al., 2007; Leppik, 2006).

More than 50% of children who have been tried on the ketogenic diet had improved seizure control; in some their AEDs could be reduced and some became medication free. This diet is effective in all seizure types and is particularly effective in controlling the absence, atonic, and myoclonic seizures associated with Lennox-Gastaut syndrome. It should not be tried without the supervision of a health care provider and dietitian, both of whom are knowledgeable in the diet (Freeman et al, 2007).

Vagus nerve stimulator (VNS). The VNS device uses the Neuro Cybernetic Prosthesis (NCP) system as a treatment option to reduce seizure frequency. Its use was approved in July 1997 as adjunctive treatment for refractory partial-onset seizures in children older than 12 years and adults. Many epilepsy centers also use VNS in children younger than 12 years. The mechanism of action is unknown, but it has been hypothesized that VNS inhibits seizure activity by using projections from the nucleus solitarius to the limbic structures. The nucleus solitarius is the main afferent nucleus of the vagus nerve and has projections to a number of areas in the forebrain and brainstem that are important for epileptogenesis. VNS affects the locus ceruleus (LC), a region in the

TABLE 26-3

Efficacy of AEDs against Common Seizure Types and Epilepsy Syndromes

Drug	Status Epilepticus	Partial	Secondarily Generalized	Atonic/ Tonic	Tonic-Clonic	Absence	Myoclonic	Lennox-Gastaut	Infantile Spasms
Carbamazepine		+	+	0	+	−	−	0	0
Clonazepam		+	+	?+	+	?+	+	?+	?+
Diazepam	+	?	?	?	?	?	+	?+	?
Ethosuximide		0	0	0	0	+	0	0	0
Felbamate		+	+	+	?+	?+	?+	+	?+
Gabapentin		+	+	0	?+	−	−	?	?
Lamotrigine		+	+	+	+	+	+	+	?+
Leviteracetam		+	+	?	+	?+	+	?	?
Lorazepam	+	?	?	?	?	?	+	?	?
Oxcarbazepine		+	+	0	+	−	−	0	0
Phenobarbital	+	+	+	?	+	0	+	?	?
Phenytoin	+	+	+	0	+	0	0	0	0
Pregabalin		+	+	?+	?	?	?	?	?
Primidone		+	+	?	+	0	?	0	?
Tiagabine		+	+	0	?	−	?	?	?+
Topiramate		+	+	+	+	+	+	+	?+
Valproate sodium	+	+	+	+	+	+	+	+	+
Zonisamide		+	+	?+	+	?+	+	?+	?+

Data from Bourgeois, B.F.D. (2006). Phenobarbital and primidone. In E. Wyllie (Ed.), *The Treatment of Epilepsy: Principles and Practice* (4th ed.). Philadelphia: Lippincott Williams & Wilkins; Brodie, M.J., Schachter, S.C., & Kwan, P. (2005). *Fast Facts: Epilepsy* (3rd ed.). Oxford: Health Press; Farrell, K., & Michoulas, A. (2008). Benzodiazepines. In J. Pellock, B. Bourgeois, & W. Dodson (Eds.). *Pediatric Epilepsy: Diagnosis and Therapy* (3rd ed.). New York: Demos; Faught, R.E. (2006). Felbamate. In E. Wyllie (Ed.). *The Treatment of Epilepsy: Principles and Practice.* Philadelphia: Lippincott Williams & Wilkins; Gilliam, F.G., & Gidal, B.E. (2006). Lamotrigine. In E. Wyllie (Ed.). *The Treatment of Epilepsy: Principles and Practice.* Philadelphia: Lippincott Williams & Wilkins; Morita, D.A., & Glauser, T.A. (2006). Phenytoin and fosphenytoin. In E. Wyllie (Ed.), *The Treatment of Epilepsy: Principles and Practice* (4th ed.). Philadelphia: Lippincott Williams & Wilkins; Privitera, M.D. (2006). Topiramate. In E. Wyllie (Ed.). *The Treatment of Epilepsy: Principles and Practice* (4th ed.). Philadelphia: Lippincott Williams & Wilkins.
Key: +, effective; ?+, probably effective; 0, ineffective; -, worsens control; ?, unknown; blank places indicate that the drug is not used for that seizure type.

brain associated with seizure activity. Another hypothesis is that intermittent stimulation of the vagus nerve alters the limbic activity in the brain and decreases epileptogenesis, thereby limiting seizure activity (Kennedy & Schallert, 2001).

The VNS is effective in treating all seizure types and is available to individuals for whom treatment with several AEDs has failed or those unable to tolerate AEDs and who are not candidates for epilepsy surgery. The NCP generator usually is implanted in the left side of the chest area, with the bipolar leads threaded under the skin and wrapped around the left vagus nerve. The pulse generator is then programmed through a computer to stimulate the vagus nerve. A neurology health care provider can adjust these parameters when the individual visits the office. A special, very strong magnet is provided to the family and can be swiped across the device to prevent or stop a seizure (Brodie et al., 2005; Leppik, 2006). The pulse generator can also be turned off by taping the magnet over the device. Side effects include incisional pain and possible infection at the incision site after surgery. In addition, some people experience hoarseness, coughing, gagging, or tingling in the neck when the stimulus is activated (Brodie et al., 2005; Kennedy & Schallert, 2001). The VNS is a treatment for seizures that actually gives children and families some sense of control over the seizures.

Epilepsy surgery. Children who have epilepsy of a focal origin and are refractory to other treatment methods should be evaluated for *epilepsy surgery*. Early evaluation is important to ensure that the child has the correct epilepsy diagnosis and to consider optional therapies to stop seizures. Sometimes changes in medical management of the seizures are all that is needed. In addition, not everyone is a candidate for surgery. The goal of epilepsy surgery is to stop seizures as quickly as possible with minimal or acceptable side effects and to optimize cognitive development to improve the child's quality of life. Seizure control with epilepsy surgery can range from 60% to 70%, depending on the procedure. Operative morbidity and mortality is less than 5% (Mathern & Delalande, 2008).

An evaluation is performed to determine if a definable focal site for the seizures exists and if removal of that particular area will affect function. Surgery is classified as either resective or functional surgery. Focal resection of the seizure focus is performed when the seizures originate in an exact focus in the brain. Temporal lobectomy, removal of the temporal lobe, is the most common procedure. Extratemporal resection is considered in some children with the help of advances in neuroimaging techniques. Hemispherectomy is the complete or partial removal of one hemisphere of the brain (Cross, 2002).

The goal of functional procedures is to modify brain function. Corpus callosotomy and multiple subpial transection are two procedures that may be considered. In corpus callosotomy, either a two-thirds or complete division of the corpus callosum is performed to stop the spread of the seizure from one side of the brain to the other. Multiple subpial transection is a procedure performed in children with Landau-Kleffner syndrome (LKS) who have epileptic aphasia. The transverse fibers over the leading side of the Wernicke area in the brain are transected, leaving the longitudinal fibers intact. This procedure results in improved or normal speech in some children (Cross, 2002).

When considering epilepsy surgery the risks and benefits of the procedure must be discussed. Possible risks include perioperative or postoperative mortality, postoperative neurologic deficits, and failure to gain seizure control. The benefits of epilepsy surgery include improved or complete seizure control with resultant improvement in development and dysfunctional behavior (Gupta, Wyllie, & Bingaman, 2006).

Complementary and Alternative Therapies

More families are using alternative therapies, such as *herbal preparations* and *supplements*, to treat medical conditions. Often people use multiple herbal preparations in conjunction with prescription drugs, and polypharmacy is becoming a common practice (Fugh-Berman, 2000). A number of herbs have been described as effective or possibly effective in the treatment of seizures: American hellebore, betony, blue cohosh, kava, mistletoe, mugwort, pipsissewa, and skullcap (Blumenthal, Goldberg, & Brinckmann, 2000; Fetrow & Avila, 2001; Skidmore-Roth, 2001). However, none are recommended in the pediatric age-group (Skidmore-Roth, 2001).

All ingested substances have the potential to interact or result in an adverse reaction (Fugh-Berman, 2000). As a result, the herbal preparation may have a positive effect on seizures but may adversely affect another condition. Children and families must be aware of these issues when using herbal preparations.

Anticipated Advances in Diagnosis and Management

Significant advances in the diagnosis and subsequent management of pediatric epilepsy have been made in the past 15 years. The greatest advances have been in understanding the molecular genetics of epilepsy, including the familial idiopathic epilepsies and the many inherited symptomatic epilepsies (Kaneko et al., 2002b). In addition, the pharmacogenetics of epilepsy, another area of study, is still a relatively undiscovered field. The genetic factors that influence drug response in people with epilepsy include genes that affect pharmacokinetics, genes that influence pharmacodynamics, and genetic factors relating to epilepsy itself. Hopefully the advances in this area will lead to improved, more effective, and less harmful treatment for epilepsy. In addition, the study of pharmacogenetics can lead to a faster and more efficient approval process for new AEDs. Finally, advances in this area can target the development of new AEDs for individuals with intractable epilepsy. Future studies in the genetics of epilepsy can also lead to other new and improved treatment options, such as gene therapy. Gene therapy may lead to the need for fewer treatment modalities or an eventual cure for epilepsy (Depondt & Shorvon, 2006; Kaneko et al., 2002b).

Research to develop new AEDs to treat those with intractable epilepsy continues. Some new compounds are derived from analogs of existing compounds. Others are being considered from the point of view of novel mechanisms, and for some the mechanism of action is less clear. Newer AEDs being studied include brivaracetam, seletracetam, eslicarbazepine acetate, fluorofelbamate, ganaxalone, isovaleramide, lacosamide, retigabine, rufinamide, carisbamate, stiripentol, talampanel, and valrocemide (Pollard & French, 2008). The development of these new products may help to improve the management and quality of life of those with epilepsy.

The success and safety of deep brain stimulation (DBS) for movement disorders and VNS for seizures has prompted a renewed look at DBS for the treatment of epilepsy. DBS is the direct administration of electrical impulses to nervous tissue in the brain.

The most common belief is that high-frequency electrical stimulation in deep structures of the brain has an inhibitory effect. Neurostimulation of the thalamus, hippocampus, subthalamic nucleus, cerebellum, and caudate, to name a few, has been studied. Continued research is needed in this area (Boon, Vonck, De Herdt, et al., 2007; Kim, 2004).

Associated Problems of Epilepsy and Seizure Disorders and Treatment

The etiology, age of onset, seizure type, frequency of occurrence, and success of treatment influence problems related to epilepsy.

> **Associated Problems** with Epilepsy and Treatment
> - Injuries
> - Cognitive dysfunction
> - Psychiatric complications

Injuries

Injury during a seizure is always possible. Children with epilepsy are at a higher risk for accidents than the general population (van den Broek & Beghi, 2004). The seizure type, age of the child, and the activity in which the child is involved must be considered. Seizures can lead to abrupt falls as a result of loss of consciousness during a seizure. Because the child does not use his or her protective reflexes to brace the fall, the child may sustain subsequent injury, such as a head injury, dental injury, soft tissue injury, or broken bones. If the child falls onto a hot surface, the child may sustain burns. Complex partial seizures and absence seizures result in a loss of consciousness, which prevents the individual from responding to dangerous situations (Wirrell, 2006).

An elevated risk of mortality also exists in a child with seizures. The mortality rate for individuals with epilepsy is two to three times higher than the general population (CURE, 2008). The risk may be associated with the underlying cause of the epilepsy, but it is also associated in some cases with accidents that occur during a seizure (Berg & Chadwick, 2000), such as death from drowning or as a result of a motor vehicle accident. Automobile drivers with epilepsy have a higher risk of fatal crashes compared with those with other conditions such as cardiovascular disease (Wirrell, 2006). The risk of sudden death from epilepsy is 24 times greater than in the general population (CURE, 2008). In addition, a child may aspirate during a seizure, especially if he or she is eating. Parents and teachers must be knowledgeable about the appropriate precautions (i.e., fitted helmet for a child with uncontrolled akinetic, atonic, or tonic-clonic seizures; water safety; care when using electrical devices or appliances; driving limitations) and first aid measures to minimize injury during a seizure (Box 26-5).

Cognitive Dysfunction

Most individuals with epilepsy have normal intelligence. However, children with epilepsy are at increased risk for cognitive dysfunction and learning disabilities (Beghi, Cornaggia, Frigeni, et al., 2006). Numerous factors can affect cognitive function in children with epilepsy, including etiology of seizures; cerebral lesions; seizure type and age of onset; severity, frequency, and duration of the

First Aid for Seizures

GENERALIZED SEIZURES
- Gently lower the child to the floor, if not already there.
- Position the child on his or her side to prevent aspiration.
- Support the child's head so it is in straight alignment with the body by using a small pillow, towel, jacket, or hand.
- Do not put anything into the child's mouth to prevent injury (e.g., aspiration of broken object, broken tooth, bite to the individual providing aid).
- Loosen any tight clothing around the neck, chest, or abdomen of the child.
- Do not restrain the child.
- Move furniture away from the child.
- Remain with the child.
- If the seizure is prolonged, there are respiratory difficulties, or there is any concern, contact emergency medical services (EMS).

COMPLEX PARTIAL SEIZURES
- Remain with the child.
- Do not restrain the child.
- Speak softly to the child.
- If the child is walking, gently guide the child by placing hands on the child's shoulders from behind to prevent injury.
- If the seizure progresses to a generalized seizure, follow the first aid guidelines for a generalized seizure.

ABSENCE SEIZURES
- Stay with the child.
- Do not restrain the child.
- Guide the child from behind as necessary to prevent injury.
- Reorient the child to his or her surroundings after the seizure is over.

seizures; physiologic dysfunction as seen on the EEG; structural brain damage caused by prolonged or repetitive seizures; hereditary factors (e.g., the intelligence quotient [IQ] of the parents); psychosocial issues; and the result of treatment for epilepsy, including AEDs and epilepsy surgery (Beghi et al., 2006; Meador, 2002).

Austin, Huberty, and Huster et al. (1999) found that academic achievement in children with epilepsy remained stable over time. They found that children with low-severity seizure disorders had average school performance. Children with high-severity seizure disorders did not show improvement in their academic achievement, even when seizures improved. They concluded that children with high-severity seizure disorders are at high risk for academic underachievement.

Cognitive effects can be associated with AEDs. Factors affecting cognition include polytherapy, high doses of AEDs, and higher AED blood levels (Meador, 2002). Health care providers should treat epilepsy with the lowest possible dose of an AED and as few drugs as possible to limit untoward effects.

Epilepsy surgery is not usually associated with cognitive decline because the goal of surgery is to remove dysfunctional tissue in the brain. Cognition may improve after surgery because of the reduction of seizures and the need for fewer treatment modalities. However, cognitive deficits such as memory and language deficits may occur postoperatively. The most common epilepsy surgery is temporal lobectomy, and cognitive deficits are usually related to the language-dominant hemisphere for individuals who undergo this procedure (Meador, 2002). Improved neuropsychological testing and medical imaging techniques result in better identification of the language-dominant hemisphere and consequently the predictive risk of these adverse effects.

Psychiatric Complications

Approximately 50% of individuals with epilepsy have psychiatric syndromes accompanying the different stages of brain activity associated with seizures. Determining whether the disorder is associated with the ictal, periictal, or postictal state is important in assessing for psychiatric disorders in individuals with epilepsy (Marsh & Rao, 2002).

Various affective and behavior disorders occur as a result of seizure activity (ictal phase). Anxiety is the most common. However, depressed feelings, ictal psychosis phenomena, violence (extremely rare), and aggression may also be seen during this time. Adequate seizure control with AEDs and nonpharmacologic treatments (e.g., observation, education) are the recommended therapies for these disorders (Marsh & Rao, 2002).

Periictal disturbances are either preictal (before the seizure) or postictal (after the seizure). Preictal disturbances include irritability, apprehension, mood swings, depression, psychosis, or aggression that can last from minutes to days before a seizure occurs. Postictal psychiatric disturbances include delirium, psychosis, mania, and violence. Postictal disturbances usually resolve quickly, but they can also last from several hours to weeks. Treatment includes maintaining safety, environmental support, and behavioral redirection. Sometimes medications are necessary; medications include neuroleptics (in severe cases), sedatives (for a calming effect), and diuretics (if associated with changes in gonadal hormones and fluid balance) (Marsh & Rao, 2002).

Interictal (between seizure events) psychiatric disorders are common in epilepsy, especially in those with temporal lobe epilepsy (Marsh & Rao, 2002). Mood disorders (ranging from short-lived episodes of low or elevated mood to persistent mood disturbances) and anxiety disorders (intensity and duration of anxiety are greater than expected) are the most common (Hermann, Seidenberg, & Bell, 2000; Marsh & Rao, 2002). Depression develops in more than 33% of people with epilepsy, and people with depression have a higher risk of developing epilepsy (CURE, 2008). Dysthymic and atypical depressive syndromes, adjustment disorders with depressed mood, bipolar disorder, generalized anxiety disorders (worrying about a number of minor matters, along with having impaired functioning), phobias, panic disorders, obsessive-compulsive disorder (OCD), and psychotic disorders are also seen. In addition, medication-induced psychiatric disorders can occur because of the positive or negative psychotropic effects of various AEDs (Marsh & Rao, 2002).

Jones, Austin, Caplan, and colleagues (2008) reported that in children with epilepsy the most common interictal psychiatric disorders include attention-deficit/hyperactivity disorder (ADHD), depressive disorders, and anxiety disorders (see Chapters 12 and 33). Psychosis has also been found in children with epilepsy but occurs infrequently. ADHD is the most common psychiatric comorbidity in children with epilepsy, ranging from 15% to 40%. Epileptiform activity, medication, repeated seizures, and cognitive dysfunction can influence attention problems in these children. In children with epilepsy, the inattentive type of ADHD has a higher rate of predominance; attention deficit with hyperactivity/impulsivity (combined typed) has a high rate of predominance as well. In contrast, in the general population the combined type of ADHD has the highest incidence overall. In addition, in the general population ADHD is more common in boys, whereas in the epilepsy group it is equally distributed.

The prevalence of depression in children and adolescents with epilepsy is about 10% to 30%. Depression often is unrecognized or untreated in this population. Depression is not linked to seizure syndrome, seizure type, or seizure frequency in affected children; however, it has been strongly associated with family problems and negative attitudes toward epilepsy in affected individuals. For children in whom a depressive episode develops, the average time of an episode ranges from 7 to 9 months. Within 2 years of an event, 40% experience relapse (Jones et al., 2008).

Anxiety disorders include separation anxiety, specific phobias to a situation, generalized anxiety, social phobias, panic disorder, posttraumatic stress disorder, and OCD. The rate of occurrence is about 13% to 49%. It is important to distinguish between the ictal fear that can accompany a simple partial seizure, complex partial seizure, or secondarily generalized seizure and a true anxiety disorder (Jones et al., 2008).

Interictal psychosis is rare in children with epilepsy, although it is more common than ictal and postictal psychosis. An increase in illogical thinking and hallucinations has been reported in children with chronic epilepsy and complex partial seizures. Psychotic symptoms that occur during a seizure usually are stereotyped and children are unable to recall the event, whereas a true psychotic event usually differs every time and children can describe the hallucinations. A postictal psychotic event can occur after a prolonged seizure or cluster of seizures. They last several days and resolve spontaneously. When evaluating for psychosis in children with epilepsy, it is important to note the child's antiepileptic medication. Psychotic reactions have been reported with phenytoin, ethosuximide, zonisamide, topiramate, lamotrigine, felbamate, and vigabatrin (Jones et al., 2008).

Therefore treatment of comorbid conditions in children with epilepsy consists of improved seizure control, psychiatric and psychological therapy, and psychotherapeutic management (Hermann et al., 2000; Marsh & Rao, 2002).

Prognosis

The majority of children with epilepsy become seizure free with AEDs within a few years of diagnosis (Shinnar & Pellock, 2002), achieve long-term remission, and continue in remission with the discontinuation of treatment (Sander & Pal, 2000; Shinnar & Pellock, 2002). Children with a single seizure have also done well without treatment (Shinnar & Pellock, 2002).

About 30% to 40% of individuals continue to be refractory to treatment. Factors that indicate a poor prognosis include a family history of epilepsy, generalized epileptiform activity on the EEG, symptomatic etiology for the seizures, high seizure frequency before treatment, and generalized tonic-clonic seizures (Brodie et al., 2005). After the first seizure onset, approximately 40% achieve remission within 5 years, either with or without medication. At 10 years, approximately 61% achieve remission, and at 20 years, approximately 70% achieve remission (Shinnar & Pellock, 2002). Factors that influence achievement of remission include etiology, epilepsy syndrome, childhood onset at younger than age 10 years, monotherapy, seizure frequency before and after treatment, early treatment response, seizure freedom for many years, normal

neurologic findings, and absence of structural lesions noted on brain imaging (Brodie et al., 2005; Shinnar & Pellock, 2002). Those with childhood-onset epilepsy and cryptogenic epilepsy have a better prognosis (Shinnar & Pellock, 2002).

Approximately 60% to 75% of children who have remained seizure free with medication for 2 to 4 years continue to be seizure free after discontinuation of seizure medication (Leppik, 2006). Factors that influence recurrence risk of seizures include etiology, age of onset, and EEG findings. The rate of seizure recurrence after the withdrawal of all AEDs is approximately 15% in those with no major risk factors. This group includes children with cryptogenic or idiopathic seizures, a normal EEG before discontinuation of the AEDs, and onset of seizures before 12 years of age. Children with remote symptomatic epilepsy have a worse prognosis, yet approximately 50% of such children who remained seizure free with AEDs continue to remain seizure free once medication is stopped (Shinnar & Pellock, 2002).

PRIMARY CARE MANAGEMENT

Health Care Maintenance
Growth and Development

Obtaining regular height and weight measurement for children with epilepsy is particularly important. These children are at risk for significant changes in growth (i.e., loss or gain in weight) either because of medication or associated problems (e.g., intellectual disability, cerebral palsy [see Chapter 18]). In addition, medication dosages are based on children's weight and their response to the AED dose.

Some children with epilepsy are at risk for developmental delays because of frequent seizures, epilepsy syndrome, or other associated disorders. The primary care provider must monitor development in with regard to the child's social, cognitive, and motor development (see Chapter 2). If a delay is noted, referrals should be made for appropriate screening and treatment (i.e., physical therapy, occupational therapy, speech therapy, psychoeducational testing, early intervention or infant stimulation programs, and/or learning support in the school setting).

Diet

Feeding issues in children with epilepsy are more often related to the associated problems such children may have. Monitoring the child's growth pattern using growth charts is vital. If a significant change occurs in the child's weight, it is important to determine whether the change is associated with the AED in use or other factors. Once this determination is made, then appropriate measures can be taken. If the change is due to an increase or decrease in appetite because of the AED, the primary care provider should discuss this with the child's specialist. The medication dose may need to be reduced or the medication may need to be changed altogether. If the change is due to other factors, then a nutritional evaluation with referral to a dietitian may be indicated. Dietary supplements may be needed if the issue is one of weight loss. A weight management program may be needed if the issue is excessive weight gain. In children who are compromised by other problems such as CP, a gastrostomy tube may need to be considered to ensure proper nutrition.

Weight gain is a significant issue in infants with infantile spasms who are treated with adrenocorticotropic hormones (ACTH). The child's weight must be monitored closely while this medication is taken. Children usually return to a normal weight after ACTH treatment is discontinued.

Children using the ketogenic diet do not usually have significant weight fluctuations. However, the nutritional status of these children must be carefully monitored, and a dietitian knowledgeable in the ketogenic diet must be closely involved throughout therapy. These children require vitamin and mineral supplements recommended by the dietitian while they follow the ketogenic diet.

Safety

Awareness of the many safety issues particular to infants and children with epilepsy is important. In addition, parents and families of children with epilepsy must be educated regarding first aid for seizures (see Box 26-5). Emergency medical services should be called in situations of prolonged seizure activity, respiratory compromise, or whenever there is a concern for the child's safety. Parents and child-care providers of children with life-threatening seizures should be certified to perform cardiopulmonary resuscitation in case of respiratory or cardiac arrest.

The potential for injury always exists during a seizure. Children and families should be educated about the appropriate type of seizure precautions. With regard to *water*, the child should take showers instead of baths, if old enough, ensuring the water drains well from the tub. If the child is taking a bath, watchful attendance by an adult is necessary at all times to prevent drowning if a seizure occurs while the child is in the water. The child should not lock the bathroom door or take a shower or bath when home alone. The child should never swim alone. The child should have one-to-one adult supervision while in the water so the adult can remove the child from the water immediately if a seizure occurs. If a seizure does occur in the water, the child should be evaluated for aspiration pneumonia.

Children with uncontrolled seizures should not be allowed to climb in *high places* (e.g., rope climbing, mountain climbing, rock climbing, tree climbing, parallel bars). Children should be securely strapped into amusement park rides and should not ride alone. When playing on park equipment, there should be soft ground (e.g., mulch) beneath the equipment. The child should not mountain ski or water ski if seizures are uncontrolled.

The child must take precautions around *heat* (e.g., fire, electricity, heating devices). Pot and pan handles on the stove should be turned toward the center of the stove during cooking. If the child is cooking or grilling food, an adult should always be present. The child should never use the stove when home alone but may use a microwave when alone. If the child is near a campfire or bonfire, he or she should stand or sit away from the fire to prevent the child from falling into the fire if a seizure occurs.

If seizures are uncontrolled, the child should not use *electrical/mechanical equipment* (e.g., lawn mower, power tools). An adult should supervise the child at all times during use of such equipment.

Caution must be taken with *sport activities*. A child who has seizures and sustains a head injury has the potential to develop worsening seizures that are difficult to control. The child should wear a fitted helmet at all times when bike riding, horseback riding, ice skating, roller skating, and roller blading. The child should not participate in contact sports, such as ice hockey, and boxing. Participation in other sports should be determined on an individual basis.

Children and adolescents with epilepsy cannot participate in piloting a plane, sky diving, or scuba diving. If a seizure occurs during any of these activities, the result can be fatal. Driving laws vary by state. The health care provider can contact the Department of Motor Vehicles for each state to determine the laws for that particular state in regard to driving restrictions for an individual with epilepsy. In addition, the Epilepsy Foundation of America (EFA) lists driving requirements by all states on their website. As in all cases, each person should be evaluated individually with regard to seizure precautions.

Immunizations

Infants and children with an underlying seizure disorder or a family history of seizures are at increased risk of seizures after receiving the measles vaccine (usually MMR [measles, mumps, rubella]). The risk of fever is less with the DTaP (diphtheria, tetanus toxoid, acellular pertussis) vaccine. Seizures that occur after immunization are usually brief, self-limiting, generalized, and associated with a fever (febrile seizures). No evidence suggests that such seizures cause permanent brain damage or epilepsy, worsen already present neurologic disorders, or affect the prognosis of children with underlying disorders (AAP, 2006).

Because the DTaP vaccine is given in early infancy, the side effects of the pertussis immunization may be confused with the development of a neurologic disorder associated with seizures and may cause confusion as to the etiology of the disorder. The measles vaccine, on the other hand, is given at an older age when neurologic disorders of infancy most likely have already been established (AAP, 2006). Consequently, there is less confusion when side effects are noted.

The incidence of seizures usually occurs after the third or fourth dose of the vaccine series, within 48 hours after DTaP vaccine administration, and usually is associated with fever. The recommendations of the AAP (2006) in regard to immunization with DTaP vaccine in infants and children with recent or active seizures are as follows: (1) administration of the pertussis vaccine should be deferred until a progressive neurologic disorder has been excluded; (2) administration of the pertussis vaccine should be deferred in children with a known or suspected neurologic condition that predisposes the child to seizures (i.e., tuberous sclerosis, inherited metabolic or degenerative diseases) or unstable neurologic disorders; (3) development of an encephalopathy (a severe acute CNS disorder unexplained by any other cause, which may include major alterations of consciousness and focal seizures that last for more than a few hours without recovery within 24 hours) within 7 days of a pertussis-containing immunization would be a possible contraindication to additional doses of the pertussis vaccine; those individuals should receive DT for subsequent doses; (4) if a seizure occurs, with or without fever, within 3 days of the DTaP vaccine, then the decision to administer additional doses of pertussis vaccine should be considered carefully; (5) children with well-controlled seizures or those children in whom a recurring seizure is unlikely may be immunized; (6) administration of an antipyretic at the time of the immunization and every 4 hours for 24 hours should be considered; (7) all infants and children should be evaluated on an individual basis at each immunization visit to determine whether they can be immunized; and (8) a family history of seizures is not a contraindication for the child to receive the pertussis vaccine; DTaP vaccine is recommended.

Post–measles vaccine fevers usually occur within 1 to 2 weeks after the vaccine is administered. Therefore prevention of vaccine-related febrile seizures that may occur is difficult. The recommendations of the AAP (2006) in regard to immunization with measles vaccine in infants and children with active seizures are as follows: (1) children with a history of seizures may be at a slightly increased risk of having a post-vaccine seizure, but they should be immunized with the measles vaccine because the benefits outweigh the risks; (2) children whose first-degree relatives have a history of seizures may be at a slightly increased risk of having a post-vaccine seizure, but they should be immunized with the measles vaccine because the benefits outweigh the risks; (3) a family history of seizures is not a contraindication for the child to receive the measles vaccine; and (4) all infants and children should be evaluated on an individual basis to determine whether they can be immunized.

If any question or concern exists in regard to providing immunizations to children with seizures, the health care provider should contact the child's specialist. All other immunizations should be given according to the routine schedule.

Screening

Vision. Routine screening is recommended. Glaucoma has been reported rarely in those who take topiramate (Fenichel, 2005). Therefore, a child who takes topiramate should have an evaluation by an ophthalmologist if any eye pain/visual complaints are reported. Concentric visual field defects may develop (in up to 40% of individuals) in children taking vigabatrin (not approved in the United States) (Brodie et al., 2005). Therefore, children taking vigabatrin should have formal visual-field monitoring performed regularly.

Hearing. Routine screening is recommended.

Dental. Routine dental care is recommended. Children taking phenytoin (Dilantin) should have routine dental care at least every 6 months. Gingival hyperplasia is a potential side effect of phenytoin (Leppik, 2006); therefore children taking phenytoin require more frequent brushing and flossing with particular attention to the gums. The dentist should be informed of an individual's use of phenytoin so that frequent dental cleaning can be performed.

Blood Pressure. Routine screening is recommended. Hypertension is a potential side effect of ACTH therapy (Curatolo, 2005). Infants treated with ACTH therapy require blood pressure monitoring at least twice weekly. Children receiving home ACTH therapy usually have a visiting nurse who can monitor the child's blood pressure. In addition, parents can be taught how to take and monitor the infant's blood pressure between the nurse's visits.

Hematocrit. Routine screening is recommended.

Urinalysis. Routine screening is recommended.

Tuberculosis. Routine screening is recommended.

Condition-Specific Screening

Drug Toxicity Screening. Therapies used in the treatment of epilepsy have adverse effects that may affect body systems. The PCP should consult with the specialist in determining the frequency of monitoring throughout therapy.

ACTH. Electrolytes and glucose levels should be monitored for electrolyte imbalance. Guaiac testing of all stools should be done to look for blood.

Bromides. Perform complete blood count (CBC), electrolytes, and liver function tests (LFTs).

Carbamazepine (Carbatrol, Tegretol). Perform CBC and LFTs.

Felbamate (Felbatol). Full hematologic evaluation should be done before therapy, frequently throughout therapy, and for a significant time after completion of therapy *(Epilepsy: Disease Management Guide,* 2000).

Ethosuximide (Zarontin). Perform CBC and LFTs.

Oxcarbazepine (Trileptal). Hyponatremia is a rare side effect. If seizure activity increases suddenly in a child taking this medication, consider obtaining a serum sodium level.

Prednisone. Measure electrolytes and serum glucose.

Valproic Acid, Divalproex Sodium, and Valproate Sodium (Depakene, Depakote). Perform CBC with platelets and LFTs.

AED Drug Levels. Serum drug levels are measured throughout therapy at varying intervals. For many second-generation AEDs, drug levels are not recommended. Efficacy is based on the individual's response to the drug.

Ketogenic Diet. Perform CBC; LFTs, renal, and lipid functions; electrolytes; CO_2; calcium; and urinalysis. A baseline electrocardiogram (ECG) is performed. If bruising occurs or surgery is pending, performing platelet aggregation or platelet function tests, prothrombin time (PT), and partial thromboplastin time (PTT) is recommended.

Electroencephalogram. An EEG is performed during the diagnostic workup for epilepsy. Repeat EEGs should be performed at the discretion of the treating physician and before discontinuation of therapy.

Medical Imaging Studies. Medical imaging studies are repeated throughout therapy as warranted and at the discretion of the physician.

Common Illness Management

Common Illnesses

Various precipitating events can trigger a seizure (see Box 26-2), including sleep deprivation and illness or fever. When a child is ill with a fever, the child can have an increase in seizure activity. Upper respiratory tract infections, viral illnesses, otitis media, and streptococcal infection of the throat are just a few of the common illnesses that can cause a fever in children. Aggressive fever management with antipyretics and increased fluids to keep the elevated temperature down is important, as is antibiotic management of bacterial infections. The family should be educated to treat the fever early in the course of an illness.

Vomiting and diarrhea are often seen with a viral illness. The child should continue taking the prescribed AED throughout the illness. Routine management of vomiting and diarrhea should be provided. For example, the parent or caregiver can be instructed to keep the child NPO (nothing by mouth) for 2 to 4 hours after vomiting. When starting fluids, the parent or caregiver can begin with 1 teaspoon or 1 ounce (depending on the age of the child) of clear fluids every 10 to 15 minutes for the first 1 to 2 hours and then increase the fluids every hour by 1 teaspoon or 1 ounce every 10 to 15 minutes, if tolerated. The dose of AED can be divided over 1 hour and placed in the clear fluids for the child to take. If the vomiting continues and the child cannot keep fluids or the medication down, then the parent or caregiver should be instructed to take the child to the local emergency department for intravenous (IV) administration of the AED (or substitute AED).

Children following the ketogenic diet must have their diet managed by a dietitian who is knowledgeable in the diet. These children are kept in ketosis and a partially dehydrated state at all times. If vomiting and diarrhea develop in a child following the ketogenic diet, the family must maintain close contact with the dietitian for dietary instructions. If the vomiting and diarrhea continue despite micromanagement by the dietitian, then the child needs to go to a local emergency department for IV management. No glucose can be added in the IV line because the child must continue in the state of ketosis while managing the illness.

There is no research to support that constipation causes an increase in seizure activity. However, many parents and caregivers have reported increased seizures in their child with constipation. Chronic constipation is common in children with disabilities (Elawad & Sullivan, 2001) and therefore can be seen in many children with epilepsy who have associated problems, such as cerebral palsy (Miller & Bachrach, 2006). It is important to provide adequate treatment for the child with constipation.

Head Trauma

Head trauma can permanently alter the brain and trigger mechanisms that can eventually result in the development of epilepsy. Seizures that occur with trauma are classified as immediate, early, or late types. The immediate seizures are probably due to the direct stimulation of cerebral tissue that has a low seizure threshold. Early posttraumatic seizures occur during the first week after an injury and are due to cerebral edema, intracranial hemorrhage, contusion, laceration, or necrosis. Late posttraumatic seizures occur within 2 years after a head injury. Such seizures occur as a result of cerebromeningeal scarring and the focus is localized to grossly normal brain tissue. The incidence of late posttraumatic seizures is increased by the presence of acute trauma, depressed skull fracture, or early posttraumatic seizures (Menkes & Ellenbogen, 2005).

In the child or adolescent who already has a seizure disorder, a head injury can result in worsening of the seizures. It is important for the person with epilepsy to follow the safety precautions necessary to prevent a head injury (e.g., wearing a fitted helmet when warranted). If a child has a head injury, the child should immediately be evaluated by his or her health care provider or at the closest emergency department.

Differential Diagnosis

Nonepileptic Events. Also known as *nonepileptic paroxysmal disorders,* these are common in the pediatric population (Paolicchi, 2002). These disorders can produce behaviors similar to that exhibited by an individual with epilepsy (Box 26-6). Nonepileptic paroxysmal disorders can develop in children with epilepsy, and differentiation of them from the child or adolescent's seizure disorder is important so that AED dosages are not increased or the AED changed unnecessarily. Most such disorders are benign; some require no treatment and resolve on their own, and some require medication other than AEDs (Paolicchi, 2002; Prensky, 2008). Some of the more common paroxysmal disorders are discussed below.

Nonepileptic Seizures of Psychogenic Origin. Nonepileptic seizures are a common symptom of conversion disorder or somatization disorder (AES, 2008). They are more common in the adolescent population compared with young children and are more common in females (Fenichel, 2005). When events are refractory

to medication, nonepileptic seizures should be considered (AES, 2008). Nonepileptic seizures generally have three patterns: (1) unilateral or bilateral motor activity consisting of thrashing or jerking; (2) expression of distress or discomfort followed by semi-purposeless, nonstereotypical behaviors; and (3) periods of unresponsiveness during events that can be precipitated or ended by suggestion. Individuals experiencing nonepileptic seizures of psychogenic origin do not usually harm themselves or experience incontinence. Often individuals with nonepileptic seizures also have true epileptic seizures (Fenichel, 2005). A video EEG during the event is necessary to make the proper diagnosis (Kronenberger & Dunn, 2005). True nonepileptic seizures should be treated as a serious psychiatric illness that requires intense treatment (AES, 2008).

Benign Neonatal Sleep Myoclonus. This event, the most common paroxysmal event in infancy, usually occurs during sleep and onset is usually in the first weeks to months of life (Paolicchi, 2002; Prensky, 2008). Quick, forceful jerks usually recur every 2 to 3 seconds and can last up to 30 minutes. They resolve only to recur again throughout the night (Prensky, 2008). They do not resolve when the infant is gently restrained, and they do stop on arousal. The EEG shows no abnormal activity other than movement artifact

---

BOX 26-6
Nonepileptic Events

MOVEMENTS
- Jitteriness
- Shuddering
- Benign neonatal sleep myoclonus
- Tics
- Pseudoseizures
- Masturbation
- Paroxysmal torticollis
- Hyperekplexia (excessive startle response)
- Self-stimulation
- Eye/head movements
- Dystonia
- Tremors

LOSS OF TONE OR CONSCIOUSNESS
- Syncope
- Narcolepsy
- Attention deficit
- Daydreaming
- Staring spells
- Stereotypes
- Acute hemiplegia

RESPIRATORY
- Apnea
- Breath-holding spells
- Hyperventilation

PERCEPTUAL DISTURBANCES
- Headache/pain
- Dizziness

- Vertigo
- Hallucinations

BEHAVIOR DISORDERS
- Head banging
- Rage
- Confusion
- Fear

SLEEP DISORDERS
- Sleepwalking
- Nightmares
- Pavor nocturnus (night terrors)
- Somniloquy (sleep-talking)

FEATURES OF SPECIFIC DISORDERS
- Tetralogy spells
- Cardiac arrhythmias
- Sandifer syndrome
- Migraines
- Cyclic vomiting
- Benign paroxysmal vertigo
- Recurrent abdominal pain

OTHER EVENTS
- Phobias
- Panic attacks
- Munchausen by proxy
- Drug reactions
- Transient global amnesia
- Withholding, constipation

Data from Paolicchi, J. (2002). The spectrum of nonepileptic events in children. *Epilepsia, 43*(Suppl 3), 60-64; Pellock, J.M. (2006). Other nonepileptic paroxysmal disorders. In E. Wyllie (Ed.), *The Treatment of Epilepsy: Principles and Practice* (4th ed.). Philadelphia: Lippincott Williams & Wilkins.

(Paolicchi, 2002). If the disorder develops early in infancy, it usually resolves within 3 to 4 months. However, some children continue to exhibit this disorder until the second year of life (Prensky, 2008). A small dose of clonazepam (Klonopin) before bed can reduce the events if necessary (Paolicchi, 2002).

Sandifer Syndrome. Sandifer syndrome can present as posturing in infants that can be mistaken for tonic seizures. The syndrome consists of abnormal posturing of the neck, trunk, and limbs usually because of gastroesophageal reflux (GER). The symptoms may also be the result of a hiatal hernia or esophageal dysmotility. Posturing is usually associated with feedings, occurring within about 30 minutes of a feeding. In addition, there is often a history of "spitting up" or intolerance of formula. These infants need a gastrointestinal tract evaluation (Paolicchi, 2002; Turner, 2005).

Migraines. There is a fine line between migraines and seizures. Migraines are usually characterized by headache and accompanying focal neurologic deficits. Clinical features of the aura can include visual, sensory, and motor symptoms. Features can include hemiplegia, ophthalmoplegia, confusion, loss of consciousness, and language dysfunction such as aphasia. The migraine phenomena can be confused with epileptic seizures. In addition, an EEG can be abnormal (Turner, 2005). Diagnosis is based on a thorough clinical history.

Narcolepsy. Narcolepsy is a sleep disorder that is often confused with epilepsy. Because of an abnormally short period from sleep onset to rapid eye movement (REM) sleep, the individual achieves REM sleep in less than 20 minutes instead of the usual 90 minutes. Affected individuals usually have excessive daytime sleepiness. The four components that characterize this sleep disorder include narcolepsy (short, sudden sleep attacks that occur during the day), cataplexy (sudden loss of muscle tone that can be triggered by startle, excitement, or laughter), hypnagogic hallucinations (vivid visual and auditory hallucinations that are usually frightening, and occur during the transition from sleep to wakefulness), and sleep paralysis (the inability to move as a result of hypotonia that occurs during the transition between sleep and wakefulness). Not all individuals with narcolepsy have all four components. Narcolepsy can occur anytime from early childhood to middle adulthood but is more common in teens and those in their 20s. It is rarely seen before the age of 5 years. The EEG will remain normal during a narcoleptic event (Brown, 2005). The diagnosis is made when the child's history reveals one or more of the associated symptoms and the child has a positive multiple sleep latency test (Fenichel, 2005).

Sleepwalking. Approximately 15% of all children have at least one episode of sleepwalking in their lifetime. Sleepwalking usually begins between age 5 and 10 years and can continue into the adult years. Episodes usually occur 1 to 3 hours after the child falls asleep. The child's eyes are open, and he or she walks around the house, can perform semi-purposeful behaviors, mumbles, and can walk back to bed unassisted. If restrained, these children can become agitated. The child has no memory of the event in the morning. The behaviors are often confused with complex partial seizures (Prensky, 2008).

Nightmares and Night Terrors. *Nightmares* usually occur during REM sleep. The child may be restless but does not usually scream. He or she usually remembers the dream in the morning and can develop a fear of sleeping alone (Prensky, 2008). On the other hand, *night terrors* occur from 30 minutes to several hours after onset of sleep, during stage 3 or 4 of slow-wave sleep. Night terrors are more common between 5 and 12 years of age (Pellock, 2006). The child sits up in bed, seems terrified, screams, and is inconsolable. Symptoms of increased sympathetic activity (diaphoresis, dilated pupils) occur during the event. Night terrors can last up to 15 minutes, and then the child falls back to sleep. There is no memory of the event in the morning, and the EEG during the event is generally normal (Prensky, 2008).

Staring Spells. Commonly seen in children, staring spells often reflect daydreaming or inattention. These episodes can be misdiagnosed as absence seizures or complex partial seizures. With daydreaming and inattention, the individual may not respond to verbal stimuli but usually responds immediately to noxious tactile stimulation (Fenichel, 2005). The EEG does not show epileptic activity during these events.

Tics. Tics often occur while the individual is awake but resolve during sleep (Fenichel, 2005). They can involve one muscle group or many, are stereotypic and repetitive, and appear intermittently. They can be simple or complex. *Simple tics* are stereotypic movements involving one or two muscle groups, usually of the face and neck (Filloux & McMahon, 2005). The most common simple motor tics include eye blinking, forceful eyelid closure, ocular gaze deviations, lip smacking, facial grimacing, and shoulder shrugging. The most common simple vocal tics include clearing of the throat, snorting, sniffing, and a coughlike noise (Fenichel, 2005; Filloux & McMahon, 2005). *Complex tics* involve a number of muscle groups and have more complex movements, such as squatting to the ground, kissing objects, or sniffing objects. They often have a compulsive quality to them. *Tourette syndrome* occurs when the individual has both motor and vocal tics that wax and wane for longer than 1 year (Filloux & McMahon, 2005) (see Chapter 41). The EEG is normal.

Breath-Holding Spells. Breath-holding is common in the younger child; the age of onset for breath-holding spells is typically between 6 and 24 months of age, peaking in frequency between 2 and 3 years of age. The spells usually resolve between 5 and 6 years of age (DeMyer, 2005). There are two types: cyanotic breath-holding spells and pallid breath-holding spells. *Cyanotic breath-holding spells* are usually precipitated by fear, frustration, anger, or pain (DeMyer, 2005; Fenichel, 2005). The child cries vigorously, develops apnea on expiration, turns blue, becomes limp, and loses consciousness. The spells can be accompanied by tonic posturing of the body and trembling of the hands or arms. Cyanotic spells are due to a disturbance in central autonomic regulation. *Pallid breath-holding spells* occur as a result of a minor injury or fright. Crying is usually absent. The child simply becomes white, limp, and then loses consciousness. The body then may stiffen and clonic movements of the arms may occur. The child is alert on arousal. Pallid spells are due to reflex asystole (Fenichel, 2005). If there is no clear history, a video EEG may be necessary to capture an event. The EEG will not show epileptiform activity during a breath-holding spell.

Syncope. Syncopal events are the most common events that are confused with epilepsy (Leppik, 2006). Types of syncopal events include vasovagal syncope, reflex asystolic syncope, stretch syncope, cardiac syncope, and cerebral syncope, to name a few (Stephenson, 2005). There can be stiffening and trembling of distal extremities (Fenichel, 2005). Rarely does it cause tonic-clonic activity (Leppik, 2006). Prodromal symptoms are often associated with syncope such as lightheadedness, blurred vision with blacking out, alteration in hearing (i.e., fading of sounds, tinnitus), pallor, and diaphoresis (Fenichel, 2005; Stephenson, 2005). Most syncopal events are provoked by stimuli; therefore environmental factors, such as dehydration, change in position or posture, hunger, or heat exposure, also play a role in the individual with syncope (Fenichel, 2005; Paolicchi, 2002; Stephenson, 2005). A thorough history is important in distinguishing syncope from seizures.

Drug Interactions

Most AEDs are metabolized by the liver and therefore can interact with other AEDs and other commonly used drugs. The drug interactions occur because of induction or inhibition of the hepatic enzymes. The primary enzymes involved are the CYP 450 (cytochrome P450) and the UGT (UDP-glucuronosyltransferase) enzymes. Each enzyme is then subdivided into multiple isoenzymes (Anderson, 2004).

Many newer AEDs do not induce or inhibit metabolic enzymes significantly, but they are affected by drugs that do alter this system. Phenytoin, carbamazepine, phenobarbital, and primidone are some older AEDs that are significant hepatic enzyme inducers and affect a wide range of CYP 450 isoenzymes. Lamotrigine and oxcarbazepine are two newer AEDs that induce only selected enzymes. Valproate is a significant enzyme inhibitor, inhibiting a wide range of isoenzymes. Oxcarbazepine and topiramate are two of the newer AEDs that inhibit selective enzymes. Gabapentin, levitiracetam, tiagabine, and zonisamide are several of the new AEDs with no induction or inhibition effects (Anderson, 2004).

Other medications may be affected by or affect AEDs. Enzyme-inducing AEDs increase the metabolism and clearance of *oral contraceptive hormones*, therefore making contraceptive hormones less effective. For those females taking enzyme-inducing AEDs, ethinyl estradiol should be started at 50 mcg/day. It may need to be increased to 75 to 100 mcg/day in females with breakthrough bleeding. Contraceptive efficacy cannot be guaranteed even if a higher dose of oral contraceptives is used. Depo-medroxyprogesterone acetate (Depo-Provera), an injectable synthetic progestin derived from progesterone, has no drug interactions with AEDs. However, it is recommended that females receive this injection every 10 weeks as opposed to 12 weeks when used with enzyme-inducing AEDs (Crawford, 2005).

Macrolide antibiotics, such as e*rythromycin* and *clarithromycin,* can increase the plasma concentration of carbamazepine (Anderson, 2004); therefore when these medications are used together, carbamazepine levels must be closely monitored. *Antiviral agents* (e.g., nevirapine, indinavir, ritonavir, saquinavir) used in conjunction with enzyme-inducing AEDs result in insufficient plasma concentrations of the antiviral agent. *Fluconazole* (antifungal agent), an enzyme inhibitor, when coadministered with phenytoin, can result in increased plasma concentrations of phenytoin. Concomitant use of *griseofulvin* and an enzyme-inducing AED may increase the metabolism of griseofulvin, thereby reducing the antifungal efficacy of the drug. In addition, these AEDs may decrease the gastrointestinal absorption of griseofulvin (Patsalos, Froscher, Pisani, et al., 2002).

Antacids have been shown to reduce the serum concentrations of carbamazepine, gabapentin, phenobarbital, and phenytoin. *Omeprazole* can increase the plasma concentration of phenytoin, resulting in increased phenytoin levels. When omeprazole is

discontinued, the phenytoin levels can drop if no dose adjustment is made, resulting in increased seizures. *Cimetidine* can prolong the half-lives of the AEDs metabolized by the CYP 450 system, such as phenytoin, carbamazepine, phenobarbital, and primidone. These AEDs may also be affected by cimetidine (Patsalos et al., 2002).

Enzyme-inducing AEDs can stimulate the metabolism of *tricyclic antidepressants* (TCAs), such as nortriptyline, imipramine, nomifensine, and trazodone. In addition, the TCAs inhibit the metabolism of some AEDs, resulting in a reduced plasma concentration of the TCA and an increase of the plasma concentration of the AED. *Fluoxetine* (a serotonin reuptake inhibitor) may cause an increase in the plasma concentration of carbamazepine and phenytoin. *Sertraline* (a 5-hydroxytryptamine [5-HT]-reuptake inhibitor) can cause lamotrigine toxicity. The effect of the *anxiolytic benzodiazepines* on AEDs depends on whether the isoenzyme is induced or inhibited. For example, carbamazepine and phenytoin decrease the plasma concentrations of midazolam, but sodium valproate increases the concentration of lorazepam (Patsalos et al., 2002).

Enzyme-inducing AEDs may reduce the therapeutic effect of *corticosteroids* by increasing the metabolism of the corticosteroid. When an individual is taking *cyclosporine* for immunosuppression in conjunction with an enzyme-inducing AED, the plasma concentration of the cyclosporine may re reduced. Changing to a second-generation AED that is not an enzyme inducer of the same system (e.g., tiagabine, levetiracetam, lamotrigine, gabapentin) may be beneficial if the individual must continue taking cyclosporine (Patsalos et al., 2002).

Phenobarbital and phenytoin can enhance drug clearance of *anticancer agents* up to threefold. Theoretically, drugs that do not undergo metabolism or affect the CYP 450 system should not interact with anticancer drugs (Patsalos et al., 2002).

Promethazine, an antihistamine, can lower the seizure threshold (Micromedex Healthcare Series, 2003), resulting in seizures. If use of this medication is necessary, the lowest dose needed should be prescribed and it should be given as infrequently as required.

Phenytoin used with digoxin may cause reduced plasma concentration of digoxin; therefore digoxin levels must be closely monitored. When topiramate is used in conjunction with digoxin, the plasma level of the digoxin may be reduced slightly (Patsalos et al., 2002).

The hepatic enzyme-inducing AEDs increase the metabolism of active *vitamin D* to inactive metabolites. This decreased vitamin D can lead to decreased calcium absorption in the gut. In individuals taking older AEDs, it has been found that decreased bone mineral density (BMD) occurs with normal vitamin D metabolism. This suggests that older AEDS may have a direct affect on bone cells. Decreased active vitamin D, hypocalcemia, hypophosphatemia, and increased serum alkaline phosphatase and parathyroid hormone have been seen in individuals receiving carbamazepine, phenytoin, and phenobarbital. Valproic acid has also been associated with decreased BMD. Little or no information is available on the effects of the newer AEDs on vitamin D and BMD (Anderson, 2004).

All first-generation AEDs, with the exception of valproic acid, are known to increase high-density lipoprotein (HDL) cholesterol. Valproic acid decreases total cholesterol (TC) and low-density lipoprotein (LDL) cholesterol. The first-generation AEDs have also been associated with an increase TC and LDL cholesterol. No information is available in regard to second-generation AEDs and their effect on lipid function. Taking into consideration that the second-generation AEDs have decreased enzyme-inhibiting properties, their effects on lipid levels may be substantially less (Anderson, 2004).

Developmental Issues

Sleep Patterns

Seizures that occur at night may affect a child's sleep pattern. In addition, seizures that occur during the day followed by a prolonged postictal state characterized by sleep can affect the child's sleep pattern at night. Sleep deprivation may also cause an increase in seizure activity. Instructing parents or caregivers to continue with normal bedtime routines is very important. A two-way baby monitor, intercom, or video monitor can be used in the child's room to alert parents or caregivers to nighttime seizures or sleep disturbances.

Parents or caregivers of children with seizures may be very anxious at night. They often change their previous sleeping arrangements and bring the child into their room to sleep at night. It is important to counsel the family on the pros and cons of this sleeping arrangement. Once the family begins to feel comfortable with the child's diagnosis of seizures, previous sleeping arrangements should be encouraged. This is important for both the child and the parents or caregivers.

Toileting

There are no particular concerns about toileting the child with seizures or epilepsy. Toilet training should be appropriate for the child's developmental age. Although bowel or bladder incontinence may occur with particular seizures (usually generalized tonic-clonic), these are not controllable. If incontinence does occur with a seizure, the child should be cleaned and clothes changed as soon as the child's condition is stable. The child should be assured that he or she did not have control over this occurrence.

Discipline

Parents or caregivers of a child with epilepsy often treat the child as if he or she is sick. Illnesses are transient; however, epilepsy can continue for years or a lifetime. Parents and caregivers may think that they can make the epilepsy worse. They may fear disciplining their child, believing that if the child gets upset a seizure will occur. Children learn quickly how to play on parental fears. The child learns how to manipulate a parent or caregiver and may threaten the parent or caregiver that a seizure will occur. Families should be instructed that disciplining a child will not provoke a seizure. Parents and caregivers should continue to discipline the child when warranted, in keeping with the expectations for other children.

Supervision. Parents and caregivers are often frightened by their lack of control over their child's seizures. They often compensate by trying to extend their influence and protection over various aspects of the child's life. Many parents of children with epilepsy believe that the child needs constant supervision and will try to regulate friendships, travel, activities, and play. This overprotection may affect the child's development in regard to self-esteem, self-reliance, and initiative. Often the child eventually rebels against a parent who is too restrictive. It is important to instruct the family to allow the child to live a normal life, taking into consideration the safety precautions necessary for children

with a seizure disorder. Encouragement of a child's developing independence should be an ongoing process.

Child Care

Finding appropriate daycare can present a challenge for parents, especially if the child has seizures. Primary care providers can assist the family in this endeavor by helping to identify local agencies or providers familiar with the care involved for a child with epilepsy or by providing the necessary education about epilepsy to child-care agencies or providers willing to support these children's special needs. In addition, local chapters of the EFA often have staff willing to visit child-care centers to educate the staff about epilepsy.

Child-care providers should be educated with regard to the particular seizure type the child has, appropriate seizure precautions, and first aid procedures. If medication must be administered at the child-care facility, the providers should be informed of the following: (1) rationale for use of the AED; (2) dosage and proper administration of the AED; and (3) potential side effects of the AED. All medications should be stored properly out of the reach of children to prevent accidental ingestion.

If the child is following the ketogenic diet, the child-care provider should be instructed on the administration of the diet. Often the child-care provider is invited to meet with the nutritionist when the diet is initiated to learn about the diet. For children with the VNS device, the provider should be instructed on use of the magnet to prevent or stop a seizure.

All federally funded child-care programs must accept children with disabilities such as epilepsy under the Individuals with Disabilities Education Act (IDEA) (see Chapter 3) if space is available. An Individualized Family Service Program (IFSP) should be established to identify goals and services needed by the child and family. Staff from early intervention or infant stimulation programs should be consulted if the child with a seizure disorder has an associated delay in development. Early assessment allows appropriate interventions to begin, maximizing learning potentials.

Schooling

Children with epilepsy may have social, intellectual, and cognitive difficulties. These difficulties must be assessed and identified so that interventions for a child's particular learning needs can be individualized and addressed. If needed, the IFSP can be carried into the formal educational program as a child ages. Core evaluations by individual school systems are necessary and appropriate for children at risk. The individualized education plan (IEP) should be evaluated and updated at intervals throughout the child's schooling (see Chapter 3).

Exercise may improve epilepsy. Epileptiform discharges on EEG have been noted to decrease during exercise. Two mechanisms, compensatory hyperventilation and beta-endorphins released during exercise, may be responsible for the improved EEG. Increased attention and awareness during exercise also may have a positive antiepileptic effect, reducing seizure activity. A feeling of well-being, which may be achieved through exercise, may also help to reduce the frequency of seizures (Sirven & Varrato, 1999). It is therefore important for the child to participate in physical education class in the school setting within the limitations of the safety precautions for the child's particular seizure type to prevent serious injury.

As in the child-care setting, if the child is following the keto-genic diet or has a VNS device, the school staff should be educated about these therapies. Contact people in the specialist's office should be provided to the school staff in the event of questions or concerns about these modalities.

Establishing a supportive, well-informed environment for a child is important. School staff should be informed of a child's medical diagnosis even if the child progresses well and does not require special educational classes. This information allows teachers to help in assessing behavioral side effects of AED therapy. A teacher who is informed of the potential for seizure occurrence and who has been instructed by the parents and the primary care provider on proper interventions is more apt to be calm and intervene appropriately if necessary.

The primary care provider must recognize the stress the diagnosis of epilepsy can place on a child and its effect on the child's self-esteem and relationships with peers, as well as on the educational system. The unpredictability and lack of control of seizure activity can add to this stress. Primary care providers should explore opportunities to educate the faculty and children in the school about epilepsy. As in child-care settings, local chapters of the EFA often have staff willing to visit schools and educate the staff about epilepsy. A greater understanding of epilepsy may help to erase the social stigma that can accompany epilepsy. Health care providers should facilitate communication between themselves and the nurse or teacher at the child's school.

Sexuality

Sexual dysfunction is common in men with epilepsy, with estimates of 30% to 70% of males being affected. Both seizures and epileptiform discharges can alter sex hormones in males. In addition, structural brain abnormalities may affect sexual functioning. Enzyme-inducing AEDs increase the hepatic metabolism of sex hormones, which results in a decrease of biologically active testosterone in males. These AEDs also increase the conversion of testosterone to other steroids such as estradiol (Herman, 2008).

Epilepsy in women affects sexual development, the menstrual cycle, contraception, fertility, and reproduction. The prevalence of polycystic ovarian syndrome (PCOS) in females with epilepsy is thought to be higher than in those without epilepsy (4% to 19%) or in those not taking AEDs. In women taking valproate, the incidence of PCOS is higher. Lamotrigine or levetiracetam may reverse the symptoms of PCOS caused by valproate (Crawford, 2005). In addition, females with epilepsy have a higher rate of reproductive and endocrine disorders, as well as an increased incidence of menstrual abnormalities (e.g., fertility problems, amenorrhea, oligomenorrhea, anovulation, prolonged or irregular menstrual cycles, PCOS) (Yerby, 2008).

Catamenial epilepsy refers to seizures that occur in relation to the female menstrual cycle (Crawford, 2005). Seizure exacerbation occurs either perimenstrually, at the time of ovulation, or throughout the second half of the menstrual cycle as a result of fluctuations of naturally occurring estrogen and progesterone. Estrogen promotes seizures and progesterone inhibits them (Yerby, 2008).

No interactions occur between the non–enzyme-inducing AEDs and the combined oral contraceptive pill (COCP). The enzyme-inducing AEDs cause a reduction in steroid concentrations of the COCP, which may lead to a failure in contraception. In women receiving lamotrigine, a decrease of norethisterone concentrations can occur, resulting in risk of unplanned pregnancies (Crawford, 2005).

For females taking enzyme-inducing AEDs, contraceptive efficacy cannot be guaranteed even with a higher dose of oral contraceptives. Depo-medroxyprogesterone acetate (Depo-Provera), an injectable synthetic progestin derived from progesterone, has no drug interactions with AEDs. However, it is recommended that females receive this injection every 10 weeks instead of 12 weeks when used with enzyme inducing AEDs. The progesterone-only pill is probably ineffective in women taking enzyme-inducing AEDs. In addition, a high failure rate with the levonorgestrel implant has been noted in women taking enzyme-inducing AEDs (Crawford, 2005).

Some seizures may resolve during menarche, and some may be exacerbated. During pregnancy, some females have seizures for the first time and they occur only during pregnancy. About one third of females have an increase in seizures during pregnancy. Conversely, approximately one sixth of women have a decrease in seizure frequency during pregnancy (Klein & Herzog, 2000).

Teratogenesis is a problem for many women with epilepsy. Women with epilepsy have a higher incidence of birth malformations even if they are not being treated with AEDs at the time of pregnancy. The incidence of congenital malformations is increased with polytherapy. Undesired outcomes reported in the offspring of women with epilepsy include impaired cognitive development, growth retardation, minor anomalies and dysmorphisms, and congenital malformations (Tomson & Battino, 2008). Careful consideration with the specialist is needed in regard to AED use and pregnancy. It is recommended that all females of childbearing age should take folic acid daily.

Transition to Adulthood

Adolescence is a time when young persons strive for independence on their way to adulthood. This is also a critical time in life for the development of self-esteem. Having a chronic condition such as epilepsy can make that transition more difficult. The young adult may fear peers witnessing a seizure and therefore not be willing to participate in social events. The young adult wants to "fit in" with peers, which is an important element of socialization. He or she may believe that taking medication makes him or her different, which may interfere with medication compliance. In addition, adolescents who have active social lives may forget to take their medication, which can result in uncontrolled seizures. Individuals with uncontrolled seizures are less likely to be allowed to participate in activities outside the home. The young adult with uncontrolled seizures will also not be allowed to drive, which results in dependence on family and friends and may further restrict participation in social events. These restrictions can have a devastating effect on the young adult's ability to test limits and explore the boundaries of independence, which is critical at this stage of development. This in turn affects the young adult's self-esteem (Nordli, 2001; Sheth, 2002).

As the adolescent moves toward adulthood, numerous issues should be considered. Will he or she be able to drive? Can the adolescent pursue further education? Can he or she live away from home during college? Can the adolescent live independently? Can he or she gain useful employment? Will he or she be able to enlist in the military if desired? Will the adult be able to get health insurance? For the young adult with a significant delay or other associated problems, the parent may need to find residential placement. For many young adults with epilepsy, this is also the time to transfer care to an adult specialist rather than the pediatric specialist who may have cared for the adolescent, which may provoke anxiety.

Children and adolescents with epilepsy are at risk of not being able to achieve their goals in regard to education, vocation, and socialization. The primary care provider can assist the adolescent during this time of transition. Psychological health can be improved through education, counseling, and advocacy (Nordli, 2001).

Family Concerns

Family Adjustment

The child and family members will experience many different feelings as they learn to adjust to the diagnosis of epilepsy. These feelings occur in stages that may include the following: shock and disbelief, anger, depression/fear, hope/defense-building, acceptance/understanding, and adjustment/effective coping. It is often difficult for family members to hear information during the stages of shock and disbelief, anger, and depression/fear. Health care providers must realize the need to repeat information many times to family members during these stages of adjustment. As family members experience the various stages of adjustment, they may project their feelings onto others in either positive or negative ways. The health care provider must understand that different family members progress through different stages at different times. Family members must be educated about the stages of adjustment and be informed that this may be a difficult time for all. They must be encouraged to be understanding of each other during this stressful time.

Cultural Differences

Normative cultural values, folklores, language issues, or parent/caregiver/child health beliefs that may affect care should be considered in the care of a child with epilepsy. Cultural issues may have an adverse effect on treatment if the health care provider is unaware of them. For example, a family may believe that the cause of the seizures is related to disfavor by the gods and choose increased religious activity over prescribed medication therapy. The ability to communicate with families of varying cultures, respect their cultural health beliefs, and educate them in regard to the treatment of epilepsy is very important.

Resources

Health care providers must be empathetic to the many needs of children with epilepsy and their families. Health care workers provide the physical, emotional, and social care that individuals with epilepsy may need. Nevertheless, no one understands or feels the problems these children and families face in their day-to-day lives as well as another child or family with the same disorder. For this reason, parent and peer support groups are available to provide a network of support within the community. Such resources not only are necessary but also have proven to be a major factor in coping and adaptation for families. Individuals and families can obtain further information about epilepsy from the following associations:

Epilepsy Foundation of America
8301 Professional Pl.
Landover, MD 20785
(800) 332-1000 (state and local associations); (800) 332-4050
   (library for medical referrals)
Websites: www.epilepsyfoundation.org; www.efa.org
Epilepsy Information Service (EIS)
Department of Neurology
Wake Forest University School of Medicine
Medical Center Blvd.
Winston-Salem, NC 27157
(800) 642-0500
Website: www.wfubmc.edu/neuro/epilepsy/information
The Epilepsy Therapy Project
www.epilepsy.com
CURE: Citizens United for Research in Epilepsy
730 North Franklin St.
Suite 204
Chicago, IL 60611
(312) 255-1801; (800) 765-7118
Website: www.cureepilepsy.org

Summary of Primary Care Needs for the Child with Epilepsy

HEALTH CARE MAINTENANCE

Growth and Development
- Measure height and weight at each visit. Children are at risk for significant growth changes because of medication or associated problems.
- Medications are based on the child's weight.
- Monitor the child's development with regard to social, cognitive, and motor development. Provide referrals for appropriate evaluations and treatment as necessary.

Diet
- Feeding issues are usually due to associated problems the child may have.
- Pharmacologic and nonpharmacologic interventions may cause an increase or decrease in the child's appetite and weight.
- Consider dietary supplements as necessary.
- Consider nutritional evaluation with a dietitian or referral to weight management program as necessary.

Safety
- Provide instructions for first aid/emergency interventions for seizure activity.
- Provide instructions for seizure precautions, including height, heat, water, and mechanical/electrical equipment.
- Use caution with sports activities. Limitations are based on types and frequency of seizures.
- Use protective equipment during specific activities as indicated.
- Provide instruction on state laws with regard to driving a motor vehicle.

Immunizations
- An increased risk of a seizure exists after a DTaP or measles (usually MMR) vaccination for those children with an underlying seizure disorder or family history of seizures. Fever management is suggested.
- Follow the American Academy of Pediatrics (AAP) recommendations for childhood immunizations.

Continued

Summary of Primary Care Needs for the Child with Epilepsy—cont'd

- Contact the child's specialist if there are any questions or concerns regarding immunizations.

Screening
- *Vision.* Routine screening is recommended.
- *Hearing.* Routine screening is recommended.
- *Dental.* Routine care is recommended. Phenytoin (Dilantin) may cause gingival hyperplasia. For children taking phenytoin, more frequent brushing and flossing is necessary. In addition, they need frequent teeth and gum cleaning by a dental hygienist. Routine dental care is recommended every 6 months for those taking phenytoin.
- *Blood pressure.* Routine screening is recommended. If the child is taking adrenocorticotropic hormone (ACTH), monitor blood pressure at least twice weekly.
- *Hematocrit.* Routine screening is recommended.
- *Urinalysis.* Routine screening is recommended.
- *Tuberculosis.* Routine screening is recommended.

Condition-Specific Screening
- *Drug toxicity screening.* Treatment-specific blood tests are recommended routinely for children who take particular antiepileptic drugs (AEDs) or follow the ketogenic diet.
- *AED blood levels.* Serum drug levels are performed for particular AEDs at varying intervals.
- *Electroencephalography.* EEGs are often performed during the diagnostic workup for epilepsy. EEGs are repeated at the discretion of the child's specialist.
- *Medical imaging studies.* Studies may be performed during the diagnostic workup for epilepsy and repeated throughout therapy at the discretion of the child's specialist.

COMMON ILLNESS MANAGEMENT

Common Illnesses
- *Fever* can be a precipitating factor for seizures. Treat fevers early in the course of an illness with antipyretics and increased fluids. Certain antibiotics can affect certain AEDs (e.g., the effect of macrolides on carbamazepine).
- *Vomiting and diarrhea.* The child or adolescent must continue to take prescribed AEDs during this time. If the child is vomiting, nothing should be given by mouth for 2 to 4 hours. Then small amounts of clear liquids can be given, such as 1 teaspoon (or 1 ounce, depending on the age of the child) every 10 minutes for 1 hour, and then increased by 1 teaspoon (or 1 ounce) every 1 to 2 hours. The AED can be given over 1 hour in small amounts of clear liquids. If vomiting and/or diarrhea continue, then the child or adolescent must go to the local emergency department for intravenous (IV) administration of the AED (or another AED).
- If diarrhea and vomiting develop in a child following the ketogenic diet, the family must contact the dietitian who manages the diet for further dietary instruction. If the vomiting or diarrhea continues despite management by the dietitian and specialist, then the child must go to a local emergency department for IV management. No glucose can be added to the IV line.

- *Constipation.* Parents or caregivers often report an increase in seizure activity when a child has constipation, although no evidence exists to support this. Manage constipation appropriately.
- *Head trauma* can cause a worsening of seizures in an individual who already has a seizure disorder. The individual should follow the seizure precautions necessary to prevent a head injury. If a head injury does occur, the individual should be evaluated by the health care provider immediately or go to the local emergency department for evaluation.

Drug Interactions
- Most AEDs are metabolized by the liver and can interact with other AEDs and other commonly used drugs.
- Carbamazepine, phenytoin, phenobarbital, and primidone are significant hepatic enzyme-inducers.
- Felbatol, lamotrigine, oxcarbazepine, and topiramate have some enzyme-inducing activity.
- Valproate sodium and felbatol are enzyme inhibitors.
- Enzyme-inducing AEDs can make contraceptive hormones ineffective. Increasing the estrogen in the contraceptive hormones to 50 to 100 mcg/day may prevent failure. However, contraceptive efficacy cannot be guaranteed even with higher doses.
- Depo-Provera (injectable synthetic progestin) has no drug interactions with AEDs. It is recommended that the injection be administered every 10 weeks instead of 12 weeks when the child is taking an enzyme-inducing AED.
- Macrolide antibiotics such as erythromycin and clarithromycin can increase the plasma concentration of carbamazepine.
- AEDs can decrease the plasma concentration of antiviral agents.
- Fluconazole can increase the plasma concentration of phenytoin.
- Enzyme-inducing AEDs can increase the metabolism of griseofulvin.
- Enzyme-inducing AEDs may decrease the gastrointestinal absorption of griseofulvin.
- Enzyme-inducing AEDs can stimulate the metabolism of tricyclic antidepressants (TCAs).
- TCAs inhibit the metabolism of some AEDs, causing decreased plasma concentration of the TCA and increased plasma concentration of the AED.
- Fluoxetine can increase the plasma concentration of carbamazepine and phenytoin.
- Sertraline can cause lamotrigine toxicity.
- Anxiolytic benzodiazepines: carbamazepine and phenytoin decrease the plasma concentration of midazolam; valproate sodium increases the plasma concentration of lorazepam (Ativan).
- Enzyme-inducing AEDs may increase the metabolism of corticosteroids.
- Enzyme-inducing AEDs can cause decreased plasma concentrations of cyclosporine.
- Phenobarbital and phenytoin increase the clearance of anticancer drugs.
- Promethazine can lower the seizure threshold. Use the lowest dose necessary and administer as infrequently as necessary.
- Digoxin: phenytoin decreases the plasma concentration of digoxin; topiramate may slightly decrease the plasma concentration of digoxin.
- Antacids can decrease the plasma concentration of carbamazepine, gabapentin, phenobarbital, and phenytoin.

Summary of Primary Care Needs for the Child with Epilepsy—cont'd

- Omeprazole can increase the plasma concentration of phenytoin.
- Cimetidine can prolong the half-life of AEDs metabolized by the CYP450 system (e.g., phenytoin, carbamazepine, phenobarbital, primidone).
- Enzyme-inducing AEDs can increase the metabolism of active vitamin D to inactive metabolites. These AEDs have an effect on bone mineral density.
- The older AEDs with the exception of valproic acid increase high-density lipoprotein (HDL) cholesterol. Valproic acid decreases total cholesterol and low-density lipoprotein cholesterol. No information is available regarding the effect of newer AEDs on lipid function.

DIFFERENTIAL DIAGNOSIS

- There are numerous disorders that produce behavior that are similar to that exhibited by an individual with epilepsy. Seizure activity must be distinguished from nonepileptic events such as nonepileptic seizures of psychogenic origin, benign neonatal sleep myoclonus, Sandifer syndrome, migraines, narcolepsy, sleepwalking, nightmares/night terrors, staring spells, tics, breath holding spells, and syncope.

DEVELOPMENTAL ISSUES

Sleep Patterns

- Sleep patterns may be affected if seizures occur at night or seizures occur during the day followed by a prolonged postictal state.
- Sleep deprivation can cause an increase in seizure activity.
- Increased anxiety occurs in family members after a child experiences a seizure. Counseling in support of independent sleeping is recommended.

Toileting

- Toileting is reflective of the child's developmental age. Incontinence of bowel or bladder can occur with some seizures.

Discipline

- Parents or caregivers should continue to discipline their child without the fear of provoking a seizure or making the child's seizures worse.

Supervision

- The family should be encouraged to allow the child to lead a normal life, with some safety precautions. Independence should be encouraged.

Child Care

- Children may be eligible for individualized family service programs (IFSPs) and federally funded daycare programs as per the Individuals with Disabilities Education Act (IDEA).
- Appropriate epilepsy education should be provided to the child-care staff.

Schooling

- Learning needs must be assessed and identified.
- Early intervention plans should be incorporated into the formal education program as needed.

- An individualized education plan (IEP) should be constructed to determine the need for special education or related services.
- Appropriate epilepsy education should be provided to the school staff.
- Ongoing open communication between the health care provider and the school staff should establish a supportive, well-informed environment in the school setting.
- The child should participate in physical education classes within the limitations of the seizure precautions for the child's seizure type.

Sexuality

- Sexual dysfunction is common in men with epilepsy.
- Epilepsy in females affects sexual development, the menstrual cycle, contraception, fertility, and reproduction.
- The prevalence of polycystic ovarian syndrome (PCOS) is thought to be higher in females with epilepsy.
- Catamenial seizures, caused by fluctuations of hormones during the menstrual cycle, develop in some women with epilepsy.
- There are no contraindications to use of nonhormonal contraceptives in females with epilepsy.
- Enzyme-inducing AEDs cause a reduction in steroid concentrations of the combined oral contraceptive pill, which may lead to a failure in contraception. In females taking these AEDs, a higher dose of ethinyl estradiol is necessary although contraceptive efficacy is still not guaranteed.
- Females should receive Depo-Provera every 10 weeks instead of 12 weeks when using enzyme-inducing AEDs.
- Approximately one third of females experience worsening of seizures during pregnancy; approximately one sixth of females have a decrease in seizure activity during pregnancy.
- Reproductive and endocrine problems are common in females with epilepsy.
- Some AEDs are teratogenic. It is recommended that all females of childbearing age should take folic acid daily.

Transition to Adulthood

- Restrictions can affect the young person's independence, goals for education, vocation, socialization, and self-esteem.
- Education, counseling, and advocacy should be provided for the adolescent as needed to assist with the transition to adulthood.

FAMILY CONCERNS

- Family members experience different stages of adjustment at different times and must be understanding of this in each other.
- Health care providers may need to repeat information about seizures and management several times when family members are adjusting to a diagnosis of epilepsy.
- The individual's cultural health beliefs should be respected as the child and family are educated in the treatment of epilepsy.

COMMUNITY RESOURCES

- Epilepsy Foundation of America
- Epilepsy Information Services
- The Epilepsy Therapy Project
- Citizens United for Research in Epilepsy

REFERENCES

Abdel-Hamid, H.Z., Alvin, J., & Painter, M.J. (2005). Neonatal seizures. In B.L. Maria (Ed.), *Current Management in Child Neurology* (3rd ed.). Ontario: BC Decker.

American Academy of Pediatrics Committee on Infectious Diseases (2006). Red book: 2006 *Report of the Committee on Infectious Diseases.* (27th ed.) L.K.Pickering, Ed.). Elk Grove Village, IL: American Academy of Pediatrics.

American Epilepsy Society (AES). (2000). *Medical education program—residents version*; Available at www.aesnet.org/edu_pub/med_edu_residents.cfm.

American Epilepsy Society (AES). (2008). *Professional development: Educational Opportunities: Epilepsy education program: Clinical epilepsy.* (revised 2004). Available at www.aesnet.org/go/professional-development/educational-opportunities/epilepsy-education-program/clinical-epilepsy. Retrieved December 21, 2008.

Anderson, G.D. (2004). Pharmacogenetics and enzyme induction/inhibition properties of antiepileptic drugs. *Neurology, 63*(Suppl 4), S3-S8.

Arzimanoglou, A. (2002). Treatment options in pediatric epilepsy syndromes. *Epileptic Disord, 3*, 217-225.

Austin, J., Huberty, T., Huster, G., et al. (1999). Does academic achievement in children with epilepsy change over time? *Dev Med Child Neurol, 41*, 473-479.

Avanzini, G., Franceschetti, S., & Mantegazza, M. (2007). Epileptogenic channelopathies: Experimental models of human pathogenesis. *Epilepsia, 48* (Suppl 2), 51-64.

Beghi, M., Cornaggia, C.M., Frigeni, B., et al. (2006). Learning disorders in epilepsy. *Epilepsia, 47*(Suppl 2), 14-18.

Behrouz, R., & Benbadis, S.R. (2008). Idiopathic generalized epilepsy of adolescence. In J. Pellock, B. Bourgeois, &, W. Dodson, (Eds.), *Pediatric Epilepsy: Diagnosis and Therapy*, (3rd ed.). New York: Demos.

Berg, A. (2006). Epidemiologic aspects of epilepsy. In E. Wyllie (Ed.), *The Treatment of Epilepsy: Principles and Practice* (4th ed.). Philadelphia: Lippincott Williams & Wilkins.

Berg, A. (2008). Risk of recurrence after a first unprovoked seizure. *Epilepsia, 49*(Suppl 1), 13-18.

Berg, A., & Chadwick, D. (2000). Starting antiepileptic drugs. In D. Schmidt & S.Schachter (Eds.), *Epilepsy: Problem Solving in Clinical Practice.* London: Martin Dunitz.

Berkovic, S.F., & Ottman, R. (2000). Molecular genetics of the idiopathic epilepsies: The next steps. *Epileptic Disord, 2*(4), 179-181.

Blumenthal, M., Goldberg, A., & Brinckmann, J.(Eds.). (2000). *Herbal Medicine: Expanded Commission E Monographs.* Newton, MA: Integrative Medicine Communications.

Bonanni, P., Malcarne, M., Moro, F., et al. (2004). Generalized epilepsy with febrile seizures plus (GEFS+): Clinical spectrum in seven Italian families unrelated to *SCN1A, SCN1B,* and *GABRG2* gene mutations. *Epilepsia, 45*(2), 149-158.

Boon, P., Vonck, K., De Herdt, V., et al. (2007). Deep brain stimulation in patients with refractory temporal lobe epilepsy. *Epilepsia, 48*(8), 1551-1560.

Brodie, M., Kwan, P. (2002). Staged approach to epilepsy management. *Neurology, 58*(8, Suppl 5), S2-S8.

Brodie, M., Schachter, S.C., & Kwan, P. (2005). *Fast Facts: Epilepsy* (3rd ed.). Oxford: Health Press.

Brown, L.W. (2005). Sleep disorders. In B.L. Maria (Ed.), *Current Management in Child Neurology* (3rd ed.). Ontario: BC Decker.

Browne, T. (2000). Managing epilepsy: Diagnostic and clinical strategies. In *Epilepsy: Disease Management Guide.* Montvale, N.J: Medical Economics.

Camfield, P., & Camfield, C. (2002). Epileptic syndromes in childhood: Clinical features, outcomes, and treatment. *Epilepsia, 43*(Suppl 3), 27-32.

Camfield, P., & Camfield, C. (2005). What is epilepsy? In B.L. Maria(Eds.), *Current Management in Child Neurology* (3rd ed.). Ontario: BC Decker.

Crawford, P. (2005). Best practice guidelines for the management of women with epilepsy. *Epilepsia, 46*(Suppl 9), 117-124.

Crino, P. (2007). Gene expression. Genetics, and genomics in epilepsy: Some answers, more questions. *Epilepsia, 48*(Suppl 2), 42-50.

Cross, J. (2002). Epilepsy surgery in childhood. *Epilepsia, 43*(Suppl 30), 65-70.

Crumrine, P. (2002). Lennox-Gastaut syndrome. *J Child Neurol, 17*(Suppl 1), S70-S75.

Curatolo, P. (2005). Infantile spasms (West's syndrome). In B.L. Maria (Ed.), *Current Management in Child Neurology*, (3rd ed.). Ontario: BC Decker.

CURE: Citizens United for Research in Epilepsy. (2008). *About epilepsy: Epilepsy facts.* Available at www.cureepilepsy.org. Retrieved December 21, 2008.

DeMyer, W. (2005). Breath-holding spells. In B.L. Maria (Ed.), *Current Management in Child Neurology* (3rd ed.). Ontario: BC Decker.

Depondt, C., & Shorvon, S.D. (2006). Genetic association studies in epilepsy pharmacogenomics: Lessons learnt and potential applications. *Future Medicine, 7*(5), 731-745.

Deray, M., Resnick, T., & Alvarez, L.(Eds.). (2001). *Complete Pocket Reference for the Treatment of Epilepsy*, Miami: C.P.R. Educational Services.

Elawad, M., & Sullivan, P. (2001). Management of constipation in children with disabilities. *Dev Med Child Neurol, 43*, 829-832.

Engel, J., Jr. (2001). A proposed diagnostic scheme for people with epileptic seizures and with epilepsy: Report of the ILAE task force on classification and terminology. *Epilepsia, 42*(6), 796-803.

Epilepsy: Disease Management Guide. (2000). Montvale, N.J.: Medical Economics.

Epilepsy Foundation of America (EFA). (2008). *About Epilepsy: Epilepsy Fact Sheet.* Available at www.epilepsyfoundation.org. Retrieved December 21, 2008.

Fenichel, G.M. (2005). *Clinical Pediatric Neurology: A Signs and Symptoms Approach* (5th ed.). Philadelphia: Elsevier.

Ferrie, C.D., Nordli, D.R., Jr, & Panayiotopoulos, C.P. (2008). Benign focal epilepsies of childhood. In J. Pellock, B.Bourgeois, & W. Dodson (Eds.), *Pediatric Epilepsy: Diagnosis and Therapy*, (3rd ed.). New York: Demos.

Fetrow, C., & Avila, J.(Eds.). (2001). *Professional's Handbook of Complementary and Alternative Medicines*, (2nd ed.). Springhouse, PA: Springhouse.

Ficker, D. (2000). Sudden unexplained death and injury in epilepsy. *Epilepsia, 41*(Suppl 2), S7-S12.

Filloux, F.M., & McMahon, W.M. (2005). Tic disorders. In B.L. Maria (Ed.), *Current Management in Child Neurology*, (3rd ed.). Ontario: BC Decker.

Fisher, R.S., van Emde Boas, W., Eger, C., et al. (2005). Epileptic seizures and epilepsy: Definitions proposed by the International League against Epilepsy (ILAE) and the International Bureau for Epilepsy (IBE) *Epilepsy, 46*(4), 470-472.

Foldvary-Schaefer, N. (2006). Symptomatic focal epilepsies. In E. Wyllie (Ed.), *The Treatment of Epilepsy: Principles and Practice* (4th ed.). Philadelphia: Lippincott Williams & Wilkins.

Freeman, J.M., Kossoff, E.H., Freeman, J.B., et al. (2007). *The Ketogenic Diet: A Treatment for Children and Others with Epilepsy* (4th ed.). New York: Demos.

Fugh-Berman, A. (2000). Herb-drug interactions. *Lancet, 355*(2), 134-138.

Golumbek, E.T. (2004). Immunomodulation of Epilepsy. In J.M. Rho, R. Sankar, & J.E. Cavazos (Eds.), *Epilepsy: Scientific Foundations of Clinical Practice.* New York: Marcel Dekker.

Guerrini, R., & Carrozzo, R. (2001). Epileptic brain malformations: Clinical presentation, malformative patterns, and indications for genetic testing. *Seizure, 10*, 532-547.

Gupta, A., Wyllie, E., & Bingaman, W.E. (2006). Epilepsy surgery in infants and children. In E. Wyllie (Ed.), *The Treatment of Epilepsy: Principles and Practice* (4th ed.). Philadelphia: Lippincott Williams & Wilkins.

Hadjiloizou, S.M., & Bourgeois, B.F.D. (2005). Generalized seizures. In B.L. Maria (Ed.), *Current Management in Child Neurology* (3rd ed.). Ontario: BC Decker.

Hartman, A.L., & Vining, E.P.G. (2007). Clinical aspects of the ketogenic diet. *Epilepsia, 48*(1), 31-42.

Hauser, W.A., & Banerjee, P.N. (2008). Epidemiology of epilepsy in children. In J. Pellock , B. Bourgeois, & W. Dodson (Eds.), *Pediatric Epilepsy: Diagnosis and Therapy* (3rd ed.). New York: Demos.

Herman, S. (2008). Sex hormones and epilepsy: No longer just for women. *Epilepsy Currents, 8*(1), 6-8.

Hermann, B., Seidenberg, M., & Bell, B. (2000). Psychiatric comorbidity in chronic epilepsy: Identification, consequences, and treatment of major depression. *Epilepsia, 41*(Suppl 2), S31-S41.

International League Against Epilepsy (ILAE). (2008). *Proposed Diagnostic Scheme for People with Epileptic Seizures and with Epilepsy.* Available at www.ilae-epilepsy.org/Visitors/Centre/ctf. Retrieved December 21, 2008.

Jain, S.J., & Morton, L.D. (2008). Evaluating the child with seizure. In J. Pellock, B Bourgeois, & W. Dodson (Eds.), *Pediatric Epilepsy: Diagnosis and Therapy* (3rd ed.). New York: Demos.

Jones, J.E., Austin, J.K., Caplan, R., et al. (2008). Psychiatric disorders in children and adolescents who have epilepsy. *Pediatr Rev, 29*(2), e9-e14.

Kaneko, S., Iwasa, H., & Okada, M. (2002a). Genetic identifiers of epilepsy. *Epilepsia, 43*(Suppl 9), 16-20.

Kaneko, S., Okada, M., Iwasa, H., et al. (2002b). Genetics of epilepsy: Current status and prospectives. *Neurosci Res, 44*, 11-30.

Kellinghaus, C., Luders, H.O., & Wyllie, E. (2006). Classification of seizures. In E. Wyllie (Ed.), *The Treatment of Epilepsy: Principles and Practice* (4th ed.). Philadelphia: Lippincott Williams & Wilkins.

Kennedy, P., Schallert, G. (2001). Practical issues and concepts in vagus nerve stimulation: A nursing review. *J Neurosci Nurs, 33*(2), 105-112.

Kim, R.B. (2004). Deep brain stimulation: Why should this work? In J.M. Rho, R. Sankar, & J.E. Cavazos, (Eds.), *Epilepsy: Scientific Foundations of Clinical Practice*, New York: Dekker.

Klein, P., & Herzog, A. (2000). Hormones and epilepsy. In D. Schmidt & S. Schachter (Eds.), *Epilepsy: Problem Solving in Clinical Practice.* London: Martin Dunitz.

Kronenberger, W.G., & Dunn, D.W. (2005). Conversion reaction. In B.L. Maria (Ed.), *Current Management in Child Neurology*, (3rd ed.). Ontario: BC Decker.

Leszczyszyn, D.J., & Pellock, J.M. (2008). Status epilepticus and acute seizures. In J. Pellock, B. Bourgeois, & W. Dodson (Eds.), *Pediatric Epilepsy: Diagnosis and Therapy* (3rd ed.). New York: Demos.

Leppik, I. (2006). *Contemporary Diagnosis and Management of the Patient with Epilepsy* (6th ed.). Newtown, PA: Handbooks in Health Care.

Marsh, L., & Rao, V. (2002). Psychiatric complications in patients with epilepsy: A review. *Epilepsy Res, 49*, 11-33.

Mathern, G.W., & Delalande, O. (2008). Surgical treatment of therapy-resistant epilepsy in children. In J. Pellock, B. Bourgeois, & W. Dodson (Eds.), *Pediatric Epilepsy: Diagnosis and Therapy* (3rd ed.). New York: Demos.

Meador, K. (2002). Cognitive outcomes and predictive factors in epilepsy. *Neurology, 58*(8, Suppl 5), S21-S25.

Menkes, J.H., & Ellenbogen, R.G. (2005). Traumatic brain and spinal cord injuries in children. In B.L. Maria (Ed.), *Current Management in Child Neurology*, (3rd ed.). Ontario: BC Decker.

Micromedex Healthcare Series (March, 2003). Vol. 115 *(Drug-reax interactive drug interaction)*. Available to subscribers only.

Miller, F., & Bachrach, S. (2006). *Cerebral Palsy: A Complete Guide for Caregiving.* (2nd ed.). Baltimore: Johns Hopkins University Press.

Mizrahi, E.M. (2008). Neonatal seizures. In J. Pellock, B. Bourgeois, & W. Dodson (Eds.), *Pediatric Epilepsy: Diagnosis and Therapy* (3rd ed.). New York: Demos.

Morita, D.A., & Glauser, D.T. (2008). Lennox-Gastaut syndrome. In J. Pellock, B. Bourgeois, & W. Dodson (Eds.), *Pediatric Epilepsy: Diagnosis and Therapy* (3rd ed.). New York: Demos.

Nei, M., Ho, R.T., Abou-Khalil, B.W., et al. (2004). EEG and EKG in sudden unexplained death in epilepsy. *Epilepsia, 45*(4), 338-345.

Nordli, D., Jr. (2001). Special needs of the adolescent with epilepsy. *Epilepsia, 42*(Suppl 8), 10-17.

Nordli, D., Jr. (2008). Classification of epilepsies in childhood. In J. Pellock, B. Bourgeois, W. Dodson (Eds.). *Pediatric Epilepsy: Diagnosis and Therapy* (3rd ed.). New York: Demos.

Paolicchi, J. (2002). The spectrum of nonepileptic events in children. *Epilepsia, 43*(Suppl 3), 60-64.

Patsalos, P., Froscher, W., Pisani, F., et al. (2002). The importance of drug interactions in epilepsy therapy. *Epilepsia, 43*(4), 365-385.

Pearl, P., & Holmes, G. (2008). Childhood absence epilepsies. In J. Pellock, B. Bourgeois, & W. Dodson (Eds.), *Pediatric Epilepsy: Diagnosis and Therapy* (3rd ed.). New York: Demos.

Pellock, J.M. (2006). Other nonepileptic paroxysmal disorders. In E. Wyllie (Ed.), *The Treatment of Epilepsy: Principles and Practice* (4th ed.). Philadelphia: Lippincott Williams & Wilkins.

Pellock, J.M., & Duchowny, M. (2005). Partial seizures. In B.L. Maria (Ed.), *Current Management in Child Neurology* (3rd ed) Ontario: BC Decker.

Pollard, J.R., & French, J.A. (2008). Antiepileptic drugs in development. In J. Pellock, B. Bourgeois, W. Dodson, & (Eds.), *Pediatric Epilepsy: Diagnosis and Therapy* (3rd ed.). New York: Demos.

Prasad, A.N., & Prasad, C. (2008). Genetic influences on the risk for epilepsy. In J. Pellock, B. Bourgeois, & W. Dodson (Eds.), *Pediatric Epilepsy: Diagnosis and Therapy* (3rd ed.). New York: Demos.

Prego-Lopez, M., & Devinsky, O. (2002). Evaluation of a first seizure: Is it epilepsy? *Postgrad Med, 111*(1), 34-48.

Prensky, A. (2008). An approach to the child with paroxysmal phenomena. In J. Pellock, B. Bourgeois, & W. Dodson (Eds.), *Pediatric Epilepsy: Diagnosis and Therapy* (3rd ed.). New York: Demos.

Provisional Committee on Quality Improvement, Subcommittee on Febrile Seizures. (1996). Practice parameter: The neurodiagnostic evaluation of the child with a first simple febrile seizure. *Pediatrics, 97*(5), 769-772.

RamachandranNair, R., & Snead, O.C. (2008). ACTH and steroids. In J. Pellock, B. Bourgeois, & W. Dodson (Eds.) *Pediatric Epilepsy: Diagnosis and Therapy* (3rd ed.). New York: Demos.

Riviello, J.J., Ashwal, S., Hirtz, D., et al. (2006). Practice parameter: Diagnostic assessment of the child with status epilepticus (an evidence-based review). *Neurology, 67*, 1542-1550.

Riviello, J.J. Jr., & Hadjiloizou, S. (2008). The Landau-Kleffner syndrome and epilepsy with continuous spike-waves during sleep. In J. Pellock, W. Dodson, B. Bourgeois (Eds.), *Pediatric Epilepsy: Diagnosis and Therapy* (3rd ed.). New York: Demos.

Sander, J., & Pal, D. (2000). Long-term prognosis of epilepsy. In D. Schmidt & S. Schachter (Eds.), *Epilepsy: Problem Solving in Clinical Practice.* London: Martin Dunitz.

Schneker, B.F., & Fountain, N.B. (2003). Epilepsy. *Dis Mon, 49*, 426-478.

Sheth, R. (2002). Adolescent issues in epilepsy. *J. Child Neurol, 17*(Suppl 2). 2S23-2S27.

Shields, W. (2000). Catastrophic epilepsy in childhood. *Epilepsia, 41*(Suppl 2), S2-S6.

Shields, W. (2002). West's syndrome. *J Child Neurol, 17*(Suppl 1), S76-S79.

Shinnar, S., & Glauser, T. (2002). Febrile seizures. *J Child Neurol, 17*(Suppl 1), S44-S52.

Shinnar, S., & O'Dell, C. (2008). Treatment decisions in childhood seizures. In J. Pellock, B. Bourgeois, & W. Dodson (Eds.), *Pediatric Epilepsy: Diagnosis and Therapy* (3rd ed.). New York: Demos.

Shinnar, S., & Pellock, J.M. (2002). Update of the epidemiology and prognosis of pediatric epilepsy. *J Child Neurol, 17*(Suppl 1), S4-S17.

Sirven, J., & Varrato, J. (1999). Physical activity and epilepsy: What are the rules? *Phys Sportsmed, 27*(3), 63-70.

Skidmore-Roth, L. (2001). *Mosby's Handbook of Herbs and Natural Supplements.* St. Louis: Mosby.

So, N.K. (2006). Epileptic auras. In E. Wyllie (Ed.), *The Treatment of Epilepsy: Principles and Practice* (4th ed.). Philadelphia: Lippincott Williams & Wilkins.

Steering Committee on Quality Improvement and Management, Subcommittee on Febrile Seizures. (2008). Febrile seizures: Clinical practice guideline for the long-term management of the child with simple febrile seizures. *Pediatrics, 121*(6), 1281-1286.

Stephenson, J.B.P. (2005). Fainting and syncope. In B.L. Maria (Ed.), *Current Management in Child Neurology* (3rd ed.). Ontario: BC Decker.

Tomson, T., & Battino, D. (2008). Teratogenic effects of antiepileptic medications. In J. Pellock, B. Bourgeois, & W. Dodson (Eds.), *Pediatric Epilepsy: Diagnosis and Therapy* (3rd ed.). New York: Demos.

Turner, R.T. (2005). Paroxysmal, nonepileptic disorders of childhood. In B.L. Maria (Ed.), *Current Management in Child Neurology* (3rd ed.). Ontario: BC Decker.

van den Broek, M., & Beghi, E. (2004). Accidents in patients with epilepsy: Types, circumstances, and complications: A European cohort study. *Epilepsia, 45*(6), 667-672.

Wheless, J.W., & Clarke, D.F. (2005). Status epilepticus. In B.L. Maria (Ed.), *Current Management in Child Neurology* (3rd ed.). Ontario: BC Decker.

Wirrell, E.C. (2006). Epilepsy-related injuries. *Epilepsia, 47*(Suppl 1), 79-86.

Wolf, P., & Shinnar, S. (2005). Febrile seizures. In B.L. Maria (Ed.), *Current Management in Child Neurology* (3rd ed.). Ontario: BC Decker.

Wong, M., & Trevathan, E. (2001). Infantile spasms. *Pediatr. Neurol., 24*(2), 89-98.

Yerby, M.S. (2008). The female patient and epilepsy. In J. Pellock, B. Bourgeois, W. Dodson, & (Eds.), *Pediatric Epilepsy: Diagnosis and Therapy* (3rd ed.). New York: Demos.

27 Fragile X Syndrome

Randi Hagerman

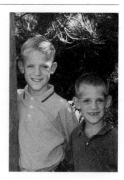

Etiology

Genetics

Fragile X syndrome is a genetic disorder that causes cognitive impairment ranging from mild learning disabilities to severe mental retardation. This condition derives its name from the presence of a fragile site or break in the X chromosome at Xq27.3 (Figure 27-1), which is identifiable by chromosome analysis. Because of the phenotypic variability among children with fragile X syndrome and because this condition was only recently discovered, most individuals with fragile X syndrome remain undiagnosed.

Fragile X syndrome is caused by a mutation in the gene called the fragile X mental retardation 1 gene *(FMR1),* which is located at Xq27.3. The *FMR1* gene was discovered and sequenced in 1991 by an international collaborative effort (Verkerk, Pieretti, Sutcliffe et al., 1991). The *FMR1* gene has a unique trinucleotide expansion located within the gene. This expansion is the source of the mutation that causes fragile X syndrome. All individuals have the *FMR1* gene, but when the trinucleotide repeat expansion (CGG)n increases in size dramatically, this expansion causes silencing of the gene, which leads to a deficiency or lack of the FMR1 protein. Normal individuals in the general population have between 6 and 44 CGG repeats within their *FMR1* gene. Individuals who are carriers for fragile X syndrome have an expansion of the CGG repetitive sequence from 55 to 200. This change in the DNA is called a *premutation* and causes an increased instability of this region and an elevation of the messenger RNA (mRNA); this sometimes can lead to clinical involvement in premutation carriers, including premature ovarian failure (POF) and the fragile X–associated tremor/ataxia syndrome (FXTAS) (Amiri, Hagerman, & Hagerman, 2008; Wittenberger et al., 2007). Further expansion can occur when this premutation is passed on to the next generation through a female carrier. Individuals who are significantly affected by fragile X syndrome have more than 200 repeats (i.e., *full mutation*). This full mutation is usually associated with methylation, which is a process of silencing the gene so that no FMR1 protein is produced from a full mutation. The absence of protein production actually causes the physical, behavioral, and cognitive problems that comprise fragile X syndrome.

Fragile X syndrome is inherited in an X-linked fashion. Males are typically affected by any deleterious gene that they carry on the X chromosome. Females, on the other hand, are usually normal because the abnormal gene on one X chromosome is compensated for by the normal gene on the other X chromosome. Heterozygous females have a 50% chance of passing the abnormal gene to their children. Males who carry the fragile X gene, however, will pass the premutation to all of their daughters but none of their sons.

Males who are carriers have the premutation, which is a CGG repeat between 55 and 200. When males pass on this premutation to all their daughters, only minimal changes occur in the CGG repeat number and it never increases to the full mutation. All sperm of affected males have only the premutation. When the premutation is passed on by a female, however, there is a high probability that the premutation will increase to a full mutation in the offspring who inherit the fragile X chromosome. The larger the size of the premutation in the carrier mother, the greater the chance that expansion will progress to a full mutation. In women with a premutation of 100 CGG repeats or larger, the expansion to the full mutation occurs 100% of the time when the fragile X chromosome is passed on to the next generation (McConkie-Rosell, Abrams, Finucane et al., 2007).

Incidence and Prevalence

Fragile X syndrome is the most common cause of inherited mental retardation known. Down syndrome, which rarely is inherited, has an incidence of approximately 1 per 1000. In comparison, fragile X syndrome causes mental retardation in approximately 1 per 3600 individuals in the general population (Crawford, Meadows, Newman et al., 2002; Turner, Webb, Wake et al., 1996). However, the frequency of the full-mutation allele in the general population is approximately 1 per 2500 because some individuals with the full mutation do not have mental retardation but instead have learning disabilities or emotional problems without significant intellectual disability (P.J. Hagerman, 2008). Studies by Dombrowski, Levesque, Morel and colleagues (2002) have shown that approximately 1 in 250 females and 1 in 800 males in the general population carry the premutation. Other studies have found a frequency of 1 in 130 females and 1 in 250 males with the premutation (P.J. Hagerman). Screenings of individuals with mental retardation in institutional and other residential settings have shown that 2% to 10% (Sherman, 2002) of this high-risk population have fragile X syndrome as the cause of their mental impairment. Screenings of individuals with autism find approximately 2% to 6% with fragile X syndrome, making fragile X the most common single-gene cause of autism (Hagerman, Rivera, & Hagerman, 2008). Testing for fragile X with *FMR1* DNA testing is recommended for all children with autism or autism spectrum disorders.

Diagnostic Criteria

When most health care providers hear the word *syndrome,* they think of someone who appears phenotypically abnormal. Similarly, most syndromes have consistent cognitive and physical features

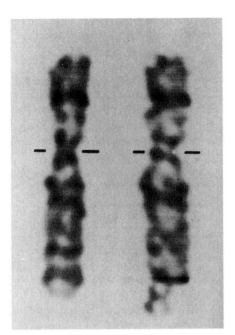

FIGURE 27-1 A normal X chromosome and a fragile X chromosome demonstrating the fragile X site at Xq27.3.

TABLE 27-1
Fragile X Checklist

Symptom	Score		
	0 (Not Present)	1 (Borderline or Present in the Past)	2 (Definitely Present)
Mental retardation			
Perseverative speech			
Hyperactivity			
Short attention span			
Tactile defensiveness			
Hand flapping			
Hand biting			
Poor eye contact			
Hyperextensible finger joints			
Large or prominent ears			
Large testicles			
Simian crease or Sydney line			
Family history of mental retardation			
TOTAL SCORE:			

From Hagerman, R.J. (1987). Fragile X syndrome. *Curr Probl Pediatr, 17,* 621-674. Reprinted with permission.

that succinctly describe the clinical manifestations (see the box in the Clinical Manifestations section). Although most individuals with fragile X syndrome share certain clinical findings, there is much variability. Health care providers should note that children with this syndrome may not be immediately recognizable by their phenotype.

To improve diagnosis in fragile X syndrome, primary care providers must be familiar with the characteristic gestalt that defines this common condition. None of the physical, behavioral, or psychological characteristics individually is diagnostic of fragile X syndrome. However, the finding of one or more of the typical features, such as prominent ears, hyperextensible finger joints, and poor eye contact, in combination with developmental delay or mental retardation of unknown cause, should alert the clinician to order a DNA study for the *FMR1* mutation.

The fragile X syndrome checklist (Table 27-1) was designed to assist primary care providers with screening children who have developmental delays or mental retardation. A child receives a score of 0 for each feature not present, 1 point for those present in the past or questionably present, and 2 points for those definitely present; thus, the higher the score, the greater the risk for fragile X syndrome (Hagerman, 2002b).

Clinical Manifestations at Time of Diagnosis

Males

Most males with fragile X syndrome have intelligence quotients (IQs) in the mild to moderate range of mental retardation. A significantly smaller percentage of affected males have severe to profound retardation. Approximately 13% of males with fragile X syndrome have an IQ above 70 and therefore are not mentally retarded (Bennetto & Pennington, 2002; Hagerman, 2002b). Most of these males have a variant pattern on DNA testing, including a lack of complete methylation of the full mutation or a

mosaic pattern, some cells with the premutation, and some cells with the full mutation. The cognitive profile of males with fragile X syndrome includes difficulty with abstract reasoning, math, and attention.

Clinical Manifestations at Time of Diagnosis

MALES
- Severe learning disabilities or mental retardation
- Delayed onset of language
- Long or narrow face
- Prominent or cupped ears
- Enlarged testicles from puberty onward
- Hyperextensible finger joints, pes planus
- Hyperactivity or attention-deficit/hyperactivity disorder
- Perseveration in speech

FEMALES
- Mild cognitive deficits to mental retardation
- Language delays
- Shyness, social anxiety
- Prominent ears
- Long, narrow face or high-arched palate
- Hyperextensible finger joints, pes planus
- Attentional problems but less prominent hyperactivity than in males

---

Delayed onset of language skills is present in approximately 85% of males with fragile X syndrome. In some children, particularly females or males with normal IQs, difficulties are only evidenced by language problems related to weaknesses in abstract reasoning. Other children as young as 18 months have delayed speech and significant deficits in receptive and expressive language (Roberts, Chapman, & Warren, 2008). Perseveration and echolalia (i.e., repetitive speech) are common speech characteristics of

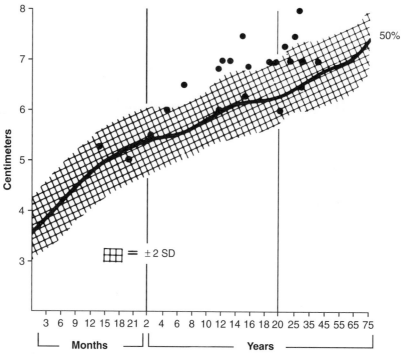

FIGURE 27-2 Mean ear length. From Hagerman, R., Smith, A.C., & Manner, R. (1983). *Clinical Features of the Fragile X Syndrome. The Fragile X Syndrome: Diagnosis, Biochemistry and Intervention.* Dillon, CO: Spectra. Reprinted with permission.

individuals with fragile X syndrome. A fast rate of speech, cluttering, mumbling, rambling, and poor topic maintenance are also frequent findings (Bennetto & Pennington, 2002; Scharfenaker, O'Connor, Stackhouse et al., 2002).

The three classic physical features associated with the fragile X syndrome phenotype are a long, narrow face; prominent or large ears; and, in males, enlarged testicles. Approximately 80% of males with fragile X syndrome exhibit one or more of these features (Hagerman, 2002b). A long, narrow face is a common feature in adults and less common in young children. Large ears (i.e., >2 SD above the norm) are seen in 50% of boys with fragile X syndrome (Figure 27-2). Prominent or cupped ears are often a more useful discriminating feature among this younger group. This finding is observed in 60% to 70% of boys and is often the only obvious physical feature associated with fragile X syndrome (Hagerman, 2002b).

Enlarged testicles are often seen in males with mental retardation; 70% to 90% of men with fragile X syndrome have a testicular volume greater than 30 mL (Hagerman, 2002b). An orchidometer (Figure 27-3) consisting of ellipsoid shapes of varying size is a useful instrument to measure testicular volume. However, most young children with fragile X syndrome do not have enlarged testicles. Macroorchidism begins to develop between 8 and 10 years of age; the largest testicle size is reached in late puberty with a mean volume of 50 mL (Lachiewicz & Dawson, 1994).

Other more subtle physical features noted in the population with fragile X syndrome include a prominent jaw, prominent forehead, and long palpebral fissures (Hagerman, 2002b). A high-arched palate, mitral valve prolapse, hypotonia, hyperextensible finger joints, and flat feet suggest the possibility of an underlying connective tissue disorder (Hagerman, 2002b).

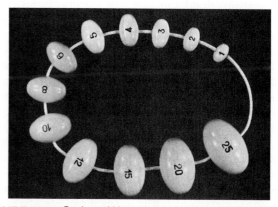

FIGURE 27-3 Prader orchidometer used to measure testicular volume.

It is important to recognize that the majority of males with fragile X syndrome—especially younger boys—appear physically normal (Figure 27-4). The behavioral characteristics are often of more concern to parents. Hyperactivity is observed in more than 70% of boys with fragile X syndrome but it frequently disappears after puberty. Poor attention span, often combined with impulsivity, is also problematic for all boys with fragile X syndrome, regardless of the level of cognitive functioning (Cornish, Turk, Wilding, et al., 2004; Sullivan, Hatton, Hammer et al., 2006). Approximately 90% have poor eye contact, and 60% to 70% display unusual hand mannerisms, including hand flapping and hand biting (Hagerman, 2002b).

Males with the premutation typically have a normal IQ, but attention problems, shyness, and social deficits are relatively

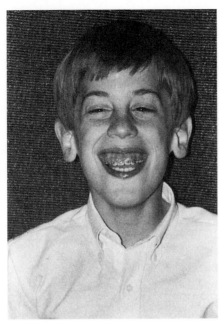

FIGURE 27-4 Prepubertal male with fragile X syndrome.

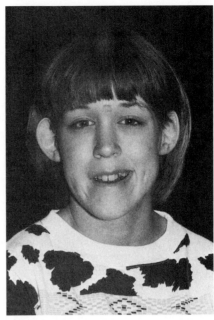

FIGURE 27-5 Young heterozygous female with fragile X who is affected physically and cognitively by fragile X.

common (Farzin, Perry, Hessl et al., 2006). Occasionally a premutation carrier has features of fragile X syndrome, including full autism and mental retardation (Hagerman, 2006). FXTAS is seen in approximately 40% of older male carriers and about 4% to 8% of older female carriers (Coffey, Cook, Tartaglia et al., 2008; Jacquemont, Hagerman, Hagerman et al., 2007). The tremor in FXTAS is typically an action tremor, and the ataxia is often characterized by frequent falling. These symptoms are usually slowly progressive and may include cognitive decline in the 60s or 70s.

Females

Overall, females affected by fragile X syndrome display milder phenotypic features than males, although some have been described with moderate and severe retardation (Figure 27-5). Females who carry the premutation are usually unaffected intellectually by fragile X syndrome. Females with the full mutation, however, are often affected to a mild or severe degree. Approximately 70% of females with the full mutation have cognitive deficits, including borderline IQ or mild to moderate mental retardation (Bennetto, Pennington, Taylor et al., 2001; de Vries, Wiegers, Smits et al., 1996). Executive function deficits—including attention and organizational difficulties—are common in most females with the full mutation but with an overall normal IQ. In addition, math difficulties, shyness, social anxiety, and poor eye contact are also common in females with the full mutation (Braden, 2002; Hagerman, 2002b).

The physical characteristics in females are less obvious than those for males with fragile X syndrome. Prominent ears; a long, narrow face; a prominent forehead and jaw; and hyperextensible finger joints have been described (Hagerman, 2002b). The degree of involvement in individuals with the full mutation correlates to the level of FMR1 protein (FMRP) (Loesch, Huggins, & Hagerman, 2004).

Treatment

Few health care professionals are knowledgeable about the diagnosis and treatment of fragile X syndrome. It is not uncommon, however, for a child with undiagnosed fragile X syndrome to be seen by the primary care provider for one of several associated medical problems, including repeated ear infections, strabismus, hyperactivity, delayed language, tantrums, violent outbursts, seizures, or hypotonia. Although much of the medical intervention is approached as it would be with any child, certain treatment options specific to the diagnosis of fragile X syndrome can significantly improve the developmental outcome for these children (Hagerman, 2006).

Treatment

- Medications for hyperactivity
  - Methylphenidate (Ritalin, Concerta, Metadate, Daytrana)
  - Dextroamphetamine (Dexedrine) or dextroamphetamine/amphetamine (Adderall, Vyvanase)
  - Clonidine (Catapres) or guanfacine (Tenex)
- Medications for aggression or severe mood lability
  - Atypical antipsychotics: aripiprazole (Abilify) and risperidone (Risperidal)
  - Anticonvulsants: carbamazepine (Tegretol), or valproic acid and derivatives (Depakote)
  - Selective serotonin reuptake inhibitors (SSRIs)
- Special education support, including speech and/or language therapy, occupational therapy, and assistive technology therapy
- Genetic counseling for all extended-family members at risk

Any signs that indicate developmental delay, sensory integration dysfunction, or language delays deserve immediate and aggressive treatment in a child with fragile X syndrome. All areas of a child's presenting signs and symptoms should be addressed, and thus a multidisciplinary approach to evaluation and therapy is essential.

Pharmacologic Therapy

Management of hyperactivity and attentional problems with medication can augment learning and behavioral management at home and in school. Central nervous system (CNS) stimulant medication has proved the most reliable, with improvements in as many as two thirds of affected children (Hagerman, 2002a). No single drug is effective for all children. Methylphenidate (Ritalin, Concerta, Metadate) is most commonly prescribed, but dextroamphetamine (Dexedrine) or dextroamphetamine/amphetamine equivalents (Adderall or Vyvanase) are also beneficial (Berry-Kravis & Potanos, 2004; Hagerman, 2002a) (see Chapter 12).

Clonidine (Catapres) has been beneficial in approximately 80% of children with fragile X syndrome who have significant hyperactivity. Clonidine is an antihypertensive medication that lowers plasma and CNS norepinephrine levels. This medication is particularly helpful for children with severe hyperactivity, overexcitability, and aggression, which are typical problems in fragile X syndrome, so clonidine is often used before stimulants. Clonidine has an overall calming effect on hyperactivity and can be used in conjunction with stimulants (Berry-Kravis & Potanos, 2004; Hagerman, 2002a).

Individuals with significant mood lability, mood instability, or aggression may benefit from the mood-stabilizing effects of aripiprazole (Abilify), an atypical antipsychotic (Hagerman, 2006) or an anticonvulsant (e.g., carbamazepine [Tegretol] or valproic acid and derivatives [Depakote]) (Hagerman, 1999, 2002a). In our clinical experience, gabapentin has not been helpful for individuals with fragile X syndrome.

Aggression in childhood or adolescence may be related to anxiety; the use of a selective serotonin reuptake inhibitor (SSRI) (e.g., fluoxetine [Prozac], sertraline [Zoloft], escitalopram [Lexapro] or citalopram [Celexa]) has been helpful in fragile X syndrome (Berry-Kravis & Potanos, 2004). SSRIs are widely known as antidepressant medications but may also be helpful in decreasing obsessive-compulsive behavior and anxiety. The side effects of fluoxetine can include gastrointestinal upset or nausea and an activation effect, which can sometimes exacerbate hyperactivity. Rarely, a child may experience an increase in obsessive-compulsive behavior, aggression, or suicidal ideation while taking an SSRI. For this reason, close follow-up (preferably weekly) is recommended in children who start taking this medication.

Educational Intervention

Whenever possible, children should be mainstreamed into a regular school classroom and receive speech and language and occupational therapy as well as special education support on an individual basis (see "Schooling" section for further details). Studies have indicated that IQ declines with age in children with fragile X syndrome (Bennetto & Pennington, 2002). However, follow-up in some males whose IQs have remained stable over time has shown that occasionally IQ may remain within the normal range. This finding has been associated with a novel pattern revealed by DNA testing: an unmethylated or partially unmethylated full mutation that is producing a significant level

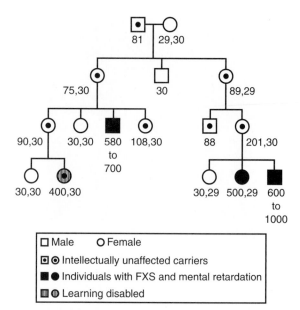

FIGURE 27-6 A family tree with individuals affected by fragile X syndrome *(FXS)*. The numbers underneath the circles and squares represent the CGG repeat number in the *FMR1* gene.

of FMRP (Loesch et al., 2004). Individuals with fragile X syndrome tend to perform better on some academic tests than their IQs would predict. Children with fragile X syndrome are typically better visual than auditory learners, which may be related to their ADHD symptoms. Significant memory abilities and well-developed skills in recognizing visual gestalts make reading, spelling, and vocabulary obvious areas of strength for many (Braden, 2002; Roberts, Price, Barnes et al., 2007; Roberts et al., 2008; Scharfenaker et al., 2002).

Because children with fragile X syndrome are easily overstimulated, occupational therapy should be geared toward helping them reorganize, interpret, and adjust to sensory stimulation. For this reason, sensory integration therapy is the method of choice for these children. When this form of treatment is used, improvements should be noticeable in motor skills, balance, coordination, movement, sequencing, and attention (Scharfenaker et al., 2002).

Genetic Counseling

Fragile X syndrome affects generation after generation, and many families have two or more children affected by this condition (Figure 27-6). Early diagnosis can provide relatives with important information about fragile X inheritance, recurrence risks, carrier testing, and family planning options (Gane & Cronister, 2002; McConkie-Rosell et al., 2007).

Because fragile X syndrome is inherited, obtaining a thorough family history or pedigree is essential. Questions about intellectual deficits, learning disabilities, emotional problems, and physical features associated with fragile X syndrome should be asked. Any relative with positive findings should be suspected as either a carrier or an affected individual. Questions regarding premutation-specific conditions including POF or FXTAS problems including tremor, ataxia, neuropathy, or cognitive decline should also be asked (McConkie-Rosell et al., 2007).

Prenatal diagnosis is available to all families with a confirmed diagnosis of fragile X syndrome or with a history of mental retardation. This testing includes amniocentesis (performed at 14 to 18 weeks' gestation), chorionic villus sampling (performed at 9½ to 12 weeks' gestation), and percutaneous umbilical blood sampling (performed at 18 to 22 weeks' gestation). Each procedure has specific benefits and drawbacks that should be carefully discussed with a genetic counselor before pregnancy or testing is pursued (Gane & Cronister, 2002; McConkie-Rosell et al., 2007). The accuracy of prenatal diagnostic testing has improved significantly (i.e., >98% accurate) with DNA-FMR1 studies. All family members who are at risk to carry either the premutation or the full mutation should have DNA testing, which is done by blood sampling. DNA testing is available throughout the United States and at large genetic centers internationally. For a list of laboratories that can perform DNA testing for fragile X syndrome, contact the National Fragile X Foundation (see Resources at the end of this chapter).

Complementary and Alternative Treatments

Folic acid therapy appears to be helpful for approximately 50% of prepubertal boys with fragile X, although the reason for this is unknown (Hagerman, 2002a). Its use is controversial, however, and several studies have shown a lack of efficacy. Other studies have shown noticeable improvements in activity level, attention span, unusual mannerisms, and coping skills. The mechanism of action of folate is unclear, but it does not appear to be specific to fragile X syndrome. Because harmful side effects are rare, many families request folic acid as a trial. A prepubescent child can use a regimen of 10 mg/day (i.e., divided twice daily) for 3 to 6 months. Regardless of the dosage, careful follow-up is warranted to monitor vitamin B_6 and zinc serum levels, which may become deficient. If improvements are not noticeable within the trial period, the clinician should consider an alternative treatment. Acetylcarnitine has been helpful for ADHD symptoms in children with fragile X syndrome according to parental reports (Torrioli, Vernacotola, Peruzzi et al., 2008).

Anticipated Advances in Diagnosis and Management

Advances in the neurobiology of fragile X syndrome have demonstrated that the metabotropic glutamate 5 system (mGluR5) is up-regulated without the FMRP that normally inhibits this system. The enhanced mGluR5 activity leads to weakened synaptic connections and therefore cognitive deficits in fragile X (Bear, Huber, & Warren, 2004). Use of an mGluR5 antagonist should be helpful in treatment for fragile X syndrome and benefits have been seen in animal models of fragile X with such intervention (Dolen, Osterweil, Rao et al., 2007). Targeted treatment trials with mGluR5 antagonists are now under way in centers of fragile X research; the results of these trials in adults will facilitate the beginning of trials in children with fragile X syndrome (Hagerman, Berry-Kravis, Kaufmann et al., 2009) Lithium can also down-regulate the mGluR5 system. An initial open trial of lithium in children and adults with fragile X syndrome demonstrated benefits in behavioral measures and on limited measures of cognition (Berry-Kravis, Sumis, Hervey et al., 2008).

Associated Problems of Fragile X Syndrome and Treatment

Speech and Language Difficulties

Speech and language difficulties are noted in both males and females with a full mutation. Although more work is needed in this area, receptive and expressive language deficits (i.e., difficulties with auditory processing, inappropriate and tangential speech, poor topic maintenance, and written language difficulties) have been reported (Bennetto & Pennington, 2002; Roberts et al., 2007; Scharfenaker et al., 2002).

Associated Problems of Fragile X Syndrome and Treatment

- Speech and language difficulties
- Otitis media
- Connective tissue problems
  - Pes planus
  - Scoliosis
  - Mitral valve prolapse
- Vision problems
  - Strabismus
  - Nystagmus
- Seizures
- Oral problems; dyspraxia
- Autistic-like features (e.g., hand flapping, hand biting)
- Psychiatric manifestations including anxiety and mood instability
- Sensory integration difficulties

Otitis Media

Recurrent otitis media has been reported in 45% to 60% of all children with fragile X syndrome. Approximately 40% of these children will require myringotomy tube insertions (Hagerman, 2002b). There has been some speculation that this may be caused by an unusual angle or collapsibility of the eustachian tube. Appropriate intervention for recurrent otitis media infections is critical to avoid conductive hearing loss, which could add to the language deficits typical of fragile X syndrome.

Connective Tissue Problems

Fifty percent of all individuals with fragile X syndrome have pes planus. In addition, joint laxity is seen in approximately 70% of children 10 years or younger (Hagerman, 2002b). Rarely, an individual with a clubfoot has been reported, which may be related to hypotonia in utero (Hagerman, 2002b). For reasons not clearly understood, hypotonia tends to disappear with age. Scoliosis may be present, and hernias appear to be more common in children with fragile X syndrome than in the general population. Gastroesophageal reflux is also common in infancy and is thought to be attributed to an underlying connective tissue disorder (Hagerman, 2002b). Routine intervention is recommended.

Cardiac problems have also been noted in individuals with fragile X syndrome and may be secondary to a connective tissue disorder. Mitral valve prolapse has been diagnosed in 22% to 55% of affected adult individuals, but it is rarely seen in children (Hagerman, 2002b). Although usually benign, mitral valve prolapse can predispose a person to arrhythmias, and prophylactic antibiotics before surgery or dental procedures may be recommended (see Chapter 21).

Mild dilation of the base of the aorta has also been observed with ultrasound studies in as many as 50% of this population, but the dilation does not appear to be progressive.

Vision Problems

Strabismus (i.e., either esotropia or exotropia) may be present in approximately 8% to 30% of those with fragile X syndrome. Other eye problems, such as myopia, nystagmus, and ptosis, have been observed with and without strabismus (Hagerman, 2002b).

Seizures

Seizures have been documented in approximately 20% of individuals with fragile X syndrome. Generalized seizures and partial complex seizures have been reported (Berry-Kravis, 2002). A careful history should be obtained and if clinical seizures are present, treatment with an anticonvulsant such as carbamazepine or valproic acid is warranted (Hagerman, 2002a) (see Chapter 26).

Oral Problems

A high-arched palate is seen with greater frequency among the fragile X population and can explain the increased incidence of dental malocclusion. Several reports of Pierre Robin syndrome (micrognathia and cleft palate) have also been noted in combination with fragile X syndrome (Hagerman, 2002b) (see Chapter 19).

Autistic-like Tendencies

An association between autism and fragile X syndrome has been mentioned frequently. Studies have estimated that approximately 30% of individuals with fragile X syndrome meet the *Diagnostic and Statistical Manual of Mental Disorders (DSM-IV-TR)* criteria for autism (Hagerman et al., 2008; Hatton, Sideris, Skinner et al., 2006; Kaufmann, Cortell, Kau et al., 2004; Loesch, Bui, Dissanayake et al., 2007). Most individuals, however, are interested in social interactions but have autistic-like features, such as poor eye contact, unusual hand mannerisms, tactile defensiveness, and obsessive interests. Those who have autism and fragile X syndrome have a lower IQ, more severe language deficits, and a history of more frequent secondary medical problems, including seizures (Garcia-Nonell, Ratera, Harris et al., 2008; Loesch et al., 2007). Anxiety can also interfere with social interactions, and social anxiety is obvious at times in most children with fragile X syndrome (Sullivan, Hooper, & Hatton, 2007). However, many children with fragile X syndrome can be quite sociable intermittently, demonstrating a spontaneous and natural sense of humor (Hagerman et al., 2008).

Psychiatric Manifestations

Researchers have only recently investigated the psychiatric manifestations of the fragile X gene in females. As with males with fragile X syndrome, social anxiety is a common complaint. Many affected girls appear shy, withdrawn, and have poor eye contact (Franke, Leboyer, Gansicke et al., 1998; Hagerman, 2002b). Women with normal cognition occasionally recall that their childhood was burdened by similar types of problems. Poor self-image, schizotypal features, and depression have also been described (Franke et al., 1998; Hagerman, 2002b). The schizotypal features appear to be related to the executive function or frontal deficits present in most females with the full mutation (Bennetto & Pennington, 2002; Bennetto et al., 2001).

Sensory Integration Difficulties

Other behavioral concerns include a child's inability to calm himself or herself when overstimulated or overwhelmed. New stimuli or novel situations can be frightening. Many parents describe their child as being hypersensitive to touch or tactilely defensive. An enhanced sympathetic response to a variety of sensory stimuli has been documented in research studies (Miller, McIntosh, McGrath et al., 1999; Roberts, Boccia, Bailey et al., 2001). Sensory integration difficulties are evidenced by an inability to screen out noises, lights, or confusion. Common responses to sensory overload can include tantrums or outburst behavior, aggressive behavior, and emotional instability (Hagerman, 2002b; Scharfenaker et al., 2002).

Prognosis

Individuals with fragile X syndrome are expected to live a normal life span regardless of their intellectual functioning. However, reports of sudden death have occurred and may be related to rare cardiac arrhythmias (Hagerman, 2002b; Sabaratnam, 2000).

PRIMARY CARE MANAGEMENT

Health Care Maintenance

Growth and Development

Growth parameters usually fall within the normal range, although head circumference greater than 75% has been reported (Hagerman, 2002b). Large heads in early childhood are more common in children who have both fragile X syndrome and autism (Chiu, Wegelin, Blank et al., 2007). Sometimes the large head circumference may lead to a misdiagnosis of Sotos syndrome.

In addition to deficits in cognitive functioning and speech, children with fragile X syndrome may be delayed in meeting other age-appropriate developmental milestones. Hypotonia is usually obvious in infancy. Developmental delay is evident with early developmental testing, such as the Bayley Scales of Infant Development (see Chapter 2). Other early warning signs are clumsiness and poor balance. Toe walking, unusual gait, lack of flow of movement, and trouble with motor planning may also occur secondary to hypotonia, joint laxity, and sensory integration difficulties (Scharfenaker et al., 2002). These children are easily overstimulated, and tantrums are common particularly during shopping or visiting a mall. Children usually like to watch their favorite videotapes over and over again.

Diet

Obsessive-compulsive behavior can be seen in children with fragile X syndrome and may involve food cravings. Obesity has been a problem for a small subgroup of children with fragile X syndrome, which may be secondary to perseverative eating or hypothalamic dysfunction. A subgroup of children with fragile X syndrome may have a Prader-Willi–like phenotype or general overgrowth (Nowicki, Tassone, Ono et al., 2007). The Prader-Willi–like phenotype of fragile X syndrome is associated with a low level of a related protein expression called CYFIP (cytoplasmic FMR1 interacting protein). Parents of obese children should be encouraged to use appropriate diets for their children coupled with intensive behavioral programs regarding food intake as has been done with Prader-Willi syndrome (Hagerman et al., 2009). Exercise programs and exercise videos may also be beneficial for older children, because they encourage children to use their visual and mimicking abilities. Failure to thrive is not uncommon in infants with fragile X syndrome but may be the result of gastroesophageal reflux, aversion to some food textures, frequent infections, or problematic mothering skills (i.e., if the mother herself is affected by the syndrome) (Hagerman, 2002b).

Safety

Families and educators should not expect every child with fragile X syndrome to be able to learn age-appropriate safety; this depends on each child's individual strengths and weaknesses. Many children can be taught to follow safety tips with strong visual and mimicking abilities and through the use of repetition.

Hyperactivity may lead to increased accidents, so affected children should be monitored closely. Home safety precautions, such as safety cabinet latches and switchplate covers, should be based on the child's developmental rather than chronologic age. Because children with fragile X syndrome can be overstimulated by their environment, the home setting—particularly the child's playroom and bedroom—should be a calm and uncluttered environment. The use of bean bag chairs, vibrating pillows, musical tapes, and appropriate environmental changes can be discussed with an occupational therapist (Miller, 2006; Scharfenaker et al., 2002). Use of tools and motorized equipment requires additional precautions. (See Chapter 12 on ADHD for further impulsive/inattention safety issues.)

Parents also may be concerned about their child's safety if self-injurious behavior is displayed. Head banging is rare but can be harmful to the child; hand biting usually causes a callus and rarely scarring. Behavior management therapies to decrease the frequency of these behaviors are often helpful (Hills-Epstein, Riley, & Sobesky, 2002; Scharfenaker et al., 2002). Safety issues are a concern when the parents are also affected. Recommendations in such situations include referral to a public health nurse and early infant stimulation programs to get professionals into the home to evaluate safety. Parents and professionals should also be advised of possible seizure activity and taught appropriate intervention (see Chapter 26).

Immunizations

The vaccination regimen is the same as for any infant or child (CDC, 2009). Prevnar (for *Pneumococcus*) can decrease otitis media by 8% to 20%, which is important in patients with fragile X syndrome because of the increased frequency of otitis. The presence of mental retardation increases risk for oral and fecal contamination, so immunization for hepatitis A and B is important. If a child has a seizure disorder, the American Academy of Pediatrics (2006) guidelines for administering pertussis and measles vaccinations to those with seizures should be followed (see Chapter 26).

Screening

Vision. An eye examination is recommended as early as possible after fragile X syndrome is diagnosed to rule out strabismus and the less-frequent findings of myopia, hyperopia, astigmatism, nystagmus, and ptosis. The evaluation should include a complete case history, visual acuity evaluation, refractive error determination, oculomotor assessment, and funduscopy. Other

---

BOX 27-1

Screening

- Vision
- Hearing
- Dental
- Cardiac examination
- Speech and/or language delays
- Connective tissue problems
- Seizures

---

testing may include an assessment of focusing function and visual developmental-perceptual skills. Yearly screening is sufficient unless visual difficulty is suspected. Early intervention is encouraged to prevent the development of blurred vision, amblyopia, or diplopia as a result of an uncorrected refractive error or strabismus. Treatment for many of the ophthalmologic problems includes corrective lenses, patching, or both (i.e., relatively inexpensive and noninvasive treatment). For some cases of strabismus, however, surgery may be the treatment of choice. Corrected vision maximizes a child's learning potential.

Hearing. Because of the increased risk of recurrent ear infections, hearing evaluations are strongly recommended in newly diagnosed children. Audiometry testing is usually sufficient to assess hearing. Any child with a history of recurrent ear infections is best referred to an ear, nose, and throat specialist (otorhinolaryngologist) to determine whether pressure-equalizing tubes are warranted.

Dental. Routine dental screening by the practitioner may reveal a high-arched palate, rare cleft palate, or dental malocclusion, all of which compound speech problems. Although it is not always possible, families should be referred to a pediatric dentist experienced in working with children who are developmentally delayed or hyperactive.

Blood Pressure. Routine screening is recommended.

Hematocrit. Routine screening is recommended.

Urinalysis. Routine screening is recommended.

Tuberculosis. Routine screening is recommended.

Condition-Specific Screening

Cardiac Examination: Mitral Valve Prolapse. Children with fragile X syndrome are at increased risk of mitral valve prolapse. Careful auscultation for a click or murmur is essential to detect this problem or any other cardiac involvement. Any child or adult with an abnormal cardiac examination should be referred to a cardiologist for formal evaluation.

Speech and Language. Some children have early speech delays that are so subtle that they go undetected by parents or teachers. An early and annual speech and language evaluation should be performed to detect any speech or language deficits that can be improved through early intervention. Because of the diversity of speech and language difficulties in children with fragile X syndrome, no single screening tool is recommended. Each child should be approached on an individual basis. Children identified with fragile X syndrome should have a formal evaluation by a licensed speech and language pathologist, preferably one who is experienced with fragile X syndrome. Speech evaluation should be included in each individualized education plan in school to determine the benefit of speech therapy.

Connective Tissue Problems. Early detection of scoliosis can often prevent further sequelae. Screening should also include a careful examination for excessive joint laxity and other complications of loose connective tissue (e.g., hernias).

Seizures. When the clinical history suggests seizures, an electroencephalogram is indicated. Unusual findings can include a slow background rhythm and spike-wave discharges, which often are similar to rolandic spikes (Berry-Kravis, 2002). Any child who appears to be having seizures should be treated with anticonvulsant medication with close follow-up by a pediatric neurologist (Hagerman, 2002a). If a child is taking medication to control seizures, anticonvulsant serum levels should be monitored.

Common Illness Management
Differential Diagnosis

Recurrent Otitis Media. Children with fragile X syndrome must be vigorously monitored and treated for recurrent otitis media to avoid sequelae that could further compromise language development and learning. Parents of young children may not recognize otitis as the cause of their child's irritability. It may be helpful to inform parents of children with fragile X that recurrent otitis media is a common problem and review signs or symptoms that indicate infection (Hagerman, 2002a).

> *Differential Diagnosis*
>
> - Attention-deficit/hyperactivity disorder (ADHD)
> - Autism
> - Pervasive developmental disorder, not otherwise specified (PDD NOS)
> - Sotos syndrome or cerebral gigantism
> - Prader-Willi syndrome
> - X-linked mental retardation
> - Fetal alcohol syndrome
> - Tourette syndrome

Families of a child with a new diagnosis of fragile X syndrome should be referred to a health care team with expertise in fragile X syndrome for a thorough evaluation and consultation. Such referral will best determine a child's individualized medical management.

Drug Interactions
Carbamazepine is a commonly prescribed anticonvulsant that is also used to control behavior problems (e.g., violent outbursts, aggression, and self-injurious behavior). Concurrent treatment with macrolide antibiotics (azithromycin [Zithromax], erythromycin), cimetidine (Tagamet), propoxyphene (Darvon), and isoniazid (INH) can interfere with the breakdown of carbamazepine, causing nausea, vomiting, and lethargy. Carbamazepine interacts with oral contraceptive pills and renders them ineffective. Folic acid therapy may worsen seizure frequency in children with epilepsy. When co-prescribed with aripiprazole (Abilify), the dosage of aripiprazole should be increased. Aripiprazole also interacts with oral antifungal medications and the SSRI fluoxetine, and doses of aripiprazole should be reduced when prescribing these medications concurrently.

Developmental Issues
Sleep Patterns
Frequent wakefulness in early childhood is a common problem in children with fragile X syndrome. Overstimulation can often interfere with sleeping, and calming techniques (e.g., music) are useful in quieting the child in preparation for bedtime. Melatonin also helps sleep disturbances in a dose of 1 to 3 mg at bedtime. Behavioral interventions can also be helpful for sleep disturbances (Weiskop, Richdale, & Matthews, 2005).

Toileting
Parents of children with fragile X syndrome often need help setting realistic expectations about toilet training. Some children achieve this milestone on time, but delayed training is more common. Parents should not be discouraged if a child takes longer to learn self-toileting. Establishing a predictable routine and consistent positive reinforcement are general principles that are helpful for children with fragile X syndrome (Crepeau-Hobson & O'Connor, 2002). As with parents of any child having toilet-training difficulties, parents are discouraged from being overly critical or reprimanding.

Discipline
Children with fragile X syndrome are especially noncompliant in response to an unexpected event or change in routine and therefore require a highly structured environment. Sending the child to school the same way each day, eating meals on a scheduled basis, and using the same nightly routines are encouraged. Behavior problems should be anticipated if a child is faced with an unexpected event. The prevention of unpredictable events in the home or at school is obviously an unrealistic expectation and should not be overemphasized. On the other hand, change and transitions should be gradually programmed into the child's learning and home environment. Setting limits, giving the child timeouts, and being consistent are appropriate responses when disciplinary action is required (Hills-Epstein et al., 2002; Reiss & Hall, 2007).

Child Care
Issues related to child care are common concerns for parents of a child with fragile X syndrome. Because of the short attention span and hyperactivity of children with fragile X syndrome, their child care providers should be knowledgeable about behavior modification techniques. The environment in which a child is placed is also important. Colors, noise level, and the amount of light can be altered to avoid overstimulation both at home and in a child-care setting. New events can be programmed slowly but gradually into a child's day. Setting a common time each week to introduce a new game, playing in a new space, or meeting a new daycare provider can help a child anticipate and deal more effectively with change. If these aspects of daycare are well managed, nothing precludes placing a child with fragile X syndrome in full-day or half-day programs. Placement with unaffected children is helpful for modeling appropriate behavior. Children also can be mainstreamed in preschool programs, but providers should be experienced in specialized education. Children with fragile X syndrome are eligible for early intervention from birth to age 3 years in addition to special education from age 3 onward, so preschool programs affiliated with a school system should be able to provide special services such as speech and language and occupational therapy.

Schooling

Most children with fragile X syndrome who have been identified are receiving special education (Roberts et al., 2008). Inclusion is a potential goal as described under the treatment section in this chapter (also see Chapter 3). Speech therapy, occupational therapy, learning assistance, and psychological counseling can all be accessed through special education. A program that provides for individualized attention and a high teacher/student ratio is best. The success of any approach depends on a number of factors specific to each child, including the child's level of cognitive functioning, distractibility, impulsivity, the structure of the class, classroom environment, and appropriate role models. All children with fragile X syndrome need a consistent routine and help with transitions in school (Braden, 2002). Sometimes their behavior problems require taking medication (e.g., stimulants or clonidine) during school hours. It is important for the school nurse to be familiar with these medications and their use in children with fragile X syndrome (Hagerman, 2002a).

Because few educators are knowledgeable about fragile X syndrome, the health care professional can play an active role in helping families educate teachers and therapists about the specialized needs of an affected child and why an integrative approach that emphasizes a child's overall strengths and remediates weaknesses is essential for effective learning. Parents should be encouraged to become actively involved in their child's program. Frequent visits to the classroom and observing therapy sessions help establish open communication among parents, teachers, and support personnel.

A child's overall intellectual abilities must be considered when developing an educational program. Inclusion is a realistic goal for some children, but others may need a more structured and specialized program. Children with fragile X syndrome will experience more significant improvement if they are shown appropriate role models. Educational intervention strategies should emphasize a child's strengths (e.g., imitating abilities, memory, computer skills, visual skills, vocabulary). The curriculum should focus on areas of a child's interest (Braden, 2002; Scharfenaker et al., 2002). Logo reading is an example of a learning tool developed to capitalize on a child's strength for incidentally acquired knowledge (Braden). This concept uses logos from popular television commercials and advertisements as the basis for a sight word vocabulary. The logos are gradually faded away so that only the word, phrase, or number remains.

Another successful learning tool is the use of computers for learning enhancement. This medium may be used to enhance language ability and academic progress in reading, spelling, and math. Computers can improve visual matching skills and help focus attention with colorful programs (Braden, 2002). Computer learning programs can enhance academic progress. Word prediction programs, such as Write:Out Loud or Co:Writer, that can enhance written language on the computer for children and adults with fragile X syndrome are just one example (Greiss-Hess, Lemons-Chitwood, Harris et al., 2009).

Speech and language and occupational therapy intervention are critical components of the education program and are recommended for all children with fragile X syndrome. Therapy is most effective when it incorporates a child's primary areas of interest. When possible, speech and language therapy sessions should include one or two other children who function at a higher level. Again, early intervention and vigorous treatment can optimize a child's speech and language abilities (Scharfenaker et al., 2002).

Sexuality

Masturbation and other forms of self-stimulatory behavior are common among individuals with mental retardation and are sometimes problematic for adolescents with fragile X syndrome. Families can be supportive by providing appropriate sex education and talking openly about sexuality issues. This need can also be met through family or individual counseling (Hills-Epstein et al., 2002). Counseling or therapy can also train new behaviors that can replace socially inappropriate behavior (e.g., masturbation in public). Most important, counseling provides adolescents a place to discuss and deal with issues of sexuality in a supportive environment. See the Adolescent and Adults Program at www.fragilex.org for guidance specific to therapists and parents for sexuality education.

Fertility is usually normal in men with fragile X syndrome, although reproduction is rare because of cognitive deficits (Hagerman, 2002b). Most males with fragile X syndrome are not sexually active but they may obsess on women they like and on rare occasions can become physically aggressive toward these women. All female children of males with fragile X syndrome will have the premutation because only the premutation—not the full mutation—is carried in the sperm. Ovarian problems and premature menopause have been reported in women with the premutation (Wittenberger, et al., 2007). Females with the full mutation are more likely to reproduce than males because they have higher cognitive abilities. However, they have an approximately 50% risk of having a child affected by fragile X syndrome or a carrier, unlike males. Sex education and genetic counseling should be available to them (McConkie-Rosell et al., 2007).

Transition to Adulthood

The transition to adulthood is usually difficult for adolescents with fragile X syndrome because living independently is a problem as a result of mental retardation. Adequate vocational training is important for adolescents. Most individuals affected by fragile X syndrome can perform jobs in the community that are consistent with their level of mental functioning. Many individuals require a job trainer who can work with them for the first several days or weeks when a new job is started. A focus on daily living skills is also critical for young adults with fragile X syndrome if they are to be successful in living independently or semi-independently. Individuals with mild or moderate mental retardation can learn to use public transportation and successfully perform activities in the home, including laundry, self-care, and cooking. Most adults affected by fragile X syndrome do well with limited supervision in an apartment setting.

Females affected by fragile X syndrome have greater difficulty trying to raise their children who are affected by fragile X syndrome. This role can be extremely stressful and may overwhelm their limited resources, particularly if the mother is mildly retarded. Additional help from family or social services agencies is usually necessary. Affected mothers should be referred to a public health nurse and parenting classes, and their children affected by fragile X should have intervention from birth onward. Adults with fragile X syndrome should also have protection under the Americans with Disabilities Act for employment and housing issues (see Chapter 4).

The connective tissue problems associated with fragile X syndrome usually improve in adulthood, and medical complications are uncommon. Hernia and mitral valve prolapse are more common in adulthood than childhood. Follow-up with a cardiologist is recommended. Most adults with fragile X syndrome and cognitive deficits can receive Supplemental Social Security income and therefore can obtain health care and counseling through Medicaid, Medicare, or both programs. Such coverage is important for ongoing care and medication.

Approximately 30% of young adults—particularly males—with fragile X syndrome may have difficulty with episodic outburst behavior. This behavior should be treated with medications (such as SSRIs with or without atypical antipsychotic agents) in addition to counseling. Remarkable benefits have been seen with the use of a new atypical drug, aripiprazole (Abilify) at low doses (i.e., 2 to 5 mg per day) (Hagerman, 2006; Hagerman et al., 2009). Counseling can help with development of calming techniques and recognition of environmental situations that can lead to outburst behavior (Hills-Epstein et al., 2002). The occupational therapist can also help with calming techniques in adults with fragile X syndrome.

Family Concerns

Perhaps the most frustrating aspect of having a child with fragile X syndrome is realizing that few professionals have a good understanding of this disorder and how it can affect a child and other family members. As a consequence, many parents become their child's primary advocate in both the educational and medical settings. Health care professionals who are unfamiliar with fragile X syndrome should make every effort to listen carefully to families. It is also the parents' responsibility to educate themselves about this unique disorder so that they too appreciate the specialized needs of these children, as well as their own needs if they require additional support because they may also be affected by the fragile X mutation.

Fragile X syndrome occurs in all ethnic and racial groups that have been studied. No evidence exists of increased prevalence in any individual group. In some cultural groups, such as certain Asian populations, genetic counseling in extended family members can be difficult because of the negative cultural implications of knowing about a genetic disorder that affects many members within the extended family. When such cultural concerns exist, permission is often denied to inform extended family members about this genetic disorder. It is helpful to write an explanatory letter about fragile X syndrome that the immediate family can distribute to other family members who may be affected or be carriers for fragile X syndrome (McConkie-Rosell et al., 2007).

The National Fragile X Foundation was established to educate parents, professionals, and the public on the diagnosis and treatment of fragile X syndrome; extensive treatment information can be found at www.fragilex.org. All parents with a child who has a diagnosis of fragile X syndrome would benefit from local contact with another family affected by fragile X syndrome. This information can be found through the foundation, which has established parent support groups throughout the United States and internationally.

Resources

Foundations

National Fragile X Foundation
P.O. Box 190488
San Francisco, CA 94119
(925) 938-9300
Website: www.fragilex.org

FRAXA Research Foundation
P.O. Box 935
West Newbury, MA 01985-0935
(978) 462-1866; Fax: (978) 463-9985
Email: info@fraxa.org
Website: www.fraxa.org

Fragile X Research Foundation of Canada
167 Queen St. West
Brampton, ON
Canada L6Y 1M5
(905) 453-9366
Email: FXRFC@ibm.net
Website: www.fragile-x.ca (e-mail)

The Fragile X Society (England)
53 Winchelsea Ln.
Hastings, East Sussex
TN35 4LG
(011) 424-813147

The International Fragile X Alliance (Australia)
263 Glen Elra Rd.
Nth Caulfield 3161
Melbourne, Australia
(03) 9528-1910; Fax: (03) 9532-9555
Email: jcohen@netspace.net.au

Fragile X Association of Australia, Inc.
15 Bowen Close
Cherrybrook
New South Wales, Australia
(019) 987012
Email: fragilex@ozemail.com.au

Newsletters

National Fragile X Foundation Newsletter—Call the National Fragile X Foundation at (800) 688-8765.

FRAXA Research Foundation Newsletter—Subscriptions through FRAXA, PO Box 935, West Newbury, MA 01985

Reading for Children

Heyman, C (2003). *My eXtra Special Brother.* Decatur, GA: Fragile X Association of GA. 404-778-8524.

O'Connor, R. (1995). *Boys with Fragile X Syndrome.* Can be obtained from the National Fragile X Foundation: (800) 688-8765

Steiger, C. (1998). *My Brother Has Fragile X Syndrome.* Chapel Hill: Avanta Publishing. (800) 434-0322.

Summary of Primary Care Needs for the Child with Fragile X Syndrome

HEALTH CARE MAINTENANCE

Growth and Development

- Physical growth is usually within normal limits, although often tall in childhood and short in adulthood.
- Some children, particularly those with autism, are reported to have large heads for body size.
- Deficits in cognitive function and speech are common.
- Developmental delays in gross motor and fine motor skills are common.

Diet

- Obsessive eating may result in obesity in older children.
- Stuffing of mouth with food is common.
- Infants may have failure to thrive related to reflux or recurrent emesis.

Safety

- Cognitive dysfunction may limit these children's awareness of safety issues.
- Hyperactivity may make these children more accident-prone.
- Self-injurious behavior may occur; parents can be taught behavior management therapies.
- If seizures are present, seizure precautions are necessary.
- Home safety may be further compromised if the parents also have fragile X syndrome.

Immunizations

- Routine immunizations are recommended.
- AAP guidelines for immunizations in children with seizures should be followed where indicated.

Screening

- *Vision.* Eye examination for strabismus, refractive errors, and visual perceptual skills is recommended at the time of diagnosis. If no problems are found, annual vision screening is recommended.
- *Hearing.* An increased risk of otitis media warrants audiometric testing. A child may need referral to an ear, nose, and throat specialist for pressure-equalizing tubes.
- *Dental.* Screening for palate and dental abnormalities is recommended. If mitral valve prolapse is present, prophylactic antibiotics will be needed for dental work or other surgery.
- *Blood pressure.* Routine screening is recommended.
- *Hematocrit.* Routine screening is recommended.
- *Urinalysis.* Routine screening is recommended.
- *Tuberculosis.* Routine screening is recommended.

Condition-Specific Screening

- *Cardiac examination: Mitral valve prolapse.* If cardiac examination is abnormal, mitral valve prolapse must be evaluated by a cardiologist.
- *Speech and language.* Speech and language evaluation should be done annually, with early intervention if a problem is detected.
- *Connective tissue problems.* Children should be screened for flat feet, scoliosis, hernias, and excessive joint laxity.
- *Seizures.* A clinical history suggestive of seizures should be evaluated by electroencephalography. If a child is taking anticonvulsants, blood levels must be monitored.

COMMON ILLNESS MANAGEMENT

Differential Diagnosis

- Recurrent otitis media is common.

Drug Interactions

- Carbamazepine is altered by macrolide antibiotics, cimetidine, propoxyphene, and isoniazid. Carbamazepine interacts with oral contraceptives and makes them ineffective.
- Aripiprazole doses should be increased if the child is taking carbamazepine and should be reduced if oral antifungal medications or fluoxetine are being used.
- See Chapter 26 for drug interactions with seizure medications.

DEVELOPMENTAL ISSUES

Sleep Patterns

- Frequent wakefulness in early childhood is not uncommon.
- Overstimulation should be avoided.

Toileting

- Delayed continence is not uncommon.

Discipline

- Children behave better in highly structured environments.
- Consistent limit setting is beneficial.
- Positive reinforcement is essential.

Child Care

- Short attention span and hyperactivity may be modified by subdued environments.
- New activities must be introduced slowly.

Schooling

- Most children receive special education services. The provider can help educate the school system personnel on condition and treatment.

Sexuality

- Self-stimulatory behaviors are common. Counseling may help decrease inappropriate behavior.
- Fertility is normal in men, but reproduction is rare because of cognitive delay.
- Carrier females may experience premature menopause.
- Sex education, birth control, and genetic counseling are necessary.

Transition to Adulthood

- Living independently is difficult; individuals will likely need support from others. Housing and employment opportunities are protected under the Americans with Disabilities Act.
- Connective tissue problems usually improve.
- Outburst behavior may be a problem and should be treated with medication and counseling.

FAMILY CONCERNS

- Families may have difficulty adjusting to the diagnosis; parents may also be affected.
- Genetic counseling is warranted.
- Because the condition is not well known, care may be nonspecific.

REFERENCES

American Academy of Pediatrics (L.K. Pickering, Ed.). (2006). *Red Book: 2006 Report of the Committee on Infectious Diseases*, (27th ed). Elk Grove Village, IL: American Academy of Pediatrics.

Amiri, K., Hagerman, R.J., & Hagerman, P.J. (2008). Fragile X-associated tremor/ataxia syndrome: an aging face of the fragile X gene. *Arch Neurol*, 65, 19-25.

Bear, M.F., Huber, K.M., & Warren, S.T. (2004). The mGluR theory of fragile X mental retardation. *Trends Neurosci*, 27, 370-377.

Bennetto, L., & Pennington, B.F. (2002). Neuropsychology. Hagerman, R.J., Hagerman, P.J. (Eds.) (2002). *Fragile X syndrome: Diagnosis, Treatment, and Research* (3rd ed). Baltimore: Johns Hopkins University Press.

Bennetto, L., Pennington, B.F., Taylor, A., et al. (2001). Profile of cognitive functioning in women with the fragile X mutation. *Neuropsychology*, 15, 290-299.

Berry-Kravis, E. (2002). Epilepsy in fragile X syndrome. *Dev Med Child Neurol*, 44, 724-728.

Berry-Kravis, E., & Potanos, K. (2004). Psychopharmacology in fragile X syndrome—present and future. *Ment Retard Dev Disabil Res Rev*, 10, 42-48.

Berry-Kravis, E., Sumis, A., Hervey, C., et al. (2008). Open-label treatment trial of lithium to target the underlying defect in fragile X syndrome. *J Dev Behav Pediatr*, 29(4), 293-302.

Braden, M. (2002). Academic interventions in fragile X. In R.J. Hagerman, & P.J. Hagerman (Eds.), *Fragile X Syndrome: Diagnosis, Treatment, and Research*, (3rd ed.). Baltimore: The Johns Hopkins University Press.

Centers for Disease Control and Prevention (CDC) (2009). Recommendations and Guidelines: 2009 child and adolescent immunization schedules for persons aged 0-6 years, 7-18 years, and "catch up" schedule. Available at www.cdc.gov/vaccines/recs/schedules/child-schedule.htm. Retrieved March 16, 2009.

Chiu, S., Wegelin, J.A., Blank, J., et al. (2007). Early acceleration of head circumference in children with fragile x syndrome and autism. *J Dev Behav Pediatr*, 28, 31-35.

Coffey, S.M., Cook, K., Tartaglia, N., et al. (2008). Expanded clinical phenotype of women with the FMR1 premutation. *Am J Med Genet A*, 146, 1009-1016.

Cornish, K.M., Turk, J., Wilding, J., et al. (2004). Annotation: Deconstructing the attention deficit in fragile X syndrome: a developmental neuropsychological approach. *J Child Psychol Psychiatry*, 45, 1042-1053.

Crawford, D.C., Meadows, K.L., Newman, J.L., et al. (2002). Prevalence of the fragile X syndrome in African-Americans. *Am J Med Genet*, 110, 226-233.

Crepeau-Hobson, F., & O'Connor, R. (2002). Appendix 4. Toilet training the child with fragile X syndrome. In R.J., Hagerman & P.J. Hagerman (Eds.), *Fragile X Syndrome: Diagnosis, Treatment, and Research* (3rd ed.). Baltimore: Johns Hopkins University Press.

de Vries, B.B., Wiegers, A.M., Smits, A.P., et al. (1996). Mental status of females with an FMR1 gene full mutation. *Am J Human Genet*, 58, 1025-1032.

Dolen, G., Osterweil, E., Rao, B.S., et al. (2007). Correction of fragile X syndrome in mice. *Neuron*, 56, 955-962.

Dombrowski, C., Levesque, M.L., Morel, M.L., et al. (2002). Premutation and intermediate-size FMR1 alleles in 10,572 males from the general population: loss of an AGG interruption is a late event in the generation of fragile X syndrome alleles. *Human Mol Genet*, 11, 371-378.

Farzin, F., Perry, H., Hessl, D., et al. (2006). Autism spectrum disorders and attention-deficit/hyperactivity disorder in boys with the fragile X premutation. *J Dev Behav Pediatr*, 27(2 Suppl), S137-S144.

Franke, P., Leboyer, M., Gansicke, M., et al. (1998). Genotype-phenotype relationship in female carriers of the premutation and full mutation of FMR-1. *Psychiatry Res*, 80, 113-127.

Gane, L., & Cronister, A. (2002). Genetic counseling. In R.J. Hagerman & P.J. Hagerman (Eds.). *The Fragile X Syndrome: Diagnosis, Treatment, and Research*, (3rd ed.). Baltimore: Johns Hopkins University Press.

Garcia-Nonell, C., Ratera, E.R., Harris, S.W., et al. (2008). Secondary medical diagnosis in fragile X syndrome with and without autism spectrum disorder. *Am J Med Genet A*, 146A(15), 1911-1916.

Greiss-Hess, L., Lemons-Chitwood, K., Harris, S.W., et al. (2009). Assistive technology use by persons with fragile X syndrome: There case reports. *Technology: Special Interest Section Quarterly*, 19(1).

Hagerman, P.J. (2008). The fragile X prevalence paradox. *J Med Genet*, 45, 498-499.

Hagerman, R.J. (1999). Psychopharmacological interventions in fragile X syndrome, fetal alcohol syndrome, Prader-Willi syndrome, Angelman syndrome, Smith-Magenis syndrome, and velocardiofacial syndrome. *Ment Retard Dev Disabil Res Rev*, 5, 305-313.

Hagerman, R.J. (2002a). Medical follow-up and pharmacotherapy. In R.J. Hagerman & P.J. Hagerman (Eds.), *Fragile X Syndrome: Diagnosis, Treatment, and Research* (3rd ed.). Baltimore: Johns Hopkins University Press.

Hagerman, R.J. (2002b). Physical and behavioral phenotype. In R.J. Hagerman & P.J. Hagerman (Eds.), *Fragile X Syndrome: Diagnosis, Treatment, and Research* (3rd ed.). Baltimore: Johns Hopkins University Press.

Hagerman, R.J. (2006). Lessons from fragile X regarding neurobiology, autism, and neurodegeneration. *J Dev Behav Pediatr*, 27, 63-74.

Hagerman, R.J., Berry-Kravis, E., Kaufmann, et al. (2009). Advances in the treatment of fragile X syndrome. *Pediatrics*, 123, 378-390.

Hagerman, R.J., Rivera, S.M., & Hagerman, P.J. (2008). The fragile X family of disorders: A model for autism and targeted treatments. *Curr Pediatr Rev*, 4, 40-52.

Hatton, D.D., Sideris, J., Skinner, M., et al. (2006). Autistic behavior in children with fragile X syndrome: Prevalence, stability, and the impact of FMRP. *Am J Med Genet A*, 140, 1804-1813.

Hills-Epstein, J., Riley, K., & Sobesky, W. (2002). The treatment of emotional and behavioral problems. In R.J.,Hagerman, P.J. Hagerman (Eds.), *Fragile X Syndrome: Diagnosis, Treatment, and Research* (3rd ed.). Baltimore: Johns Hopkins University Press.

Jacquemont, S., Hagerman, R.J., Hagerman, P.J., et al. (2007). Fragile-X syndrome and fragile X-associated tremor/ataxia syndrome: Two faces of FMR1. *Lancet Neurol*, 6, 45-55.

Kaufmann, W.E., Cortell, R., Kau, A.S., et al. (2004). Autism spectrum disorder in fragile X syndrome: communication, social interaction, and specific behaviors. *Am J Med Genet*, 129A(3), 225-234.

Lachiewicz, A.M., & Dawson, D.V. (1994). Do young boys with fragile X syndrome have macroorchidism? *Pediatrics*, 93(6 Pt 1), 992-995.

Loesch, D.Z., Bui, Q.M., Dissanayake, C., et al. (2007). Molecular and cognitive predictors of the continuum of autistic behaviours in fragile X. *Neurosci Biobehav Rev*, 31, 315-326.

Loesch, D.Z., Huggins, R.M., & Hagerman, R.J. (2004). Phenotypic variation and FMRP levels in fragile X. *Ment Retard Dev Disabil Res Rev*, 10, 31-41.

McConkie-Rosell, A., Abrams, L., Finucane, B., et al. (2007). Recommendations from multi-disciplinary focus groups on cascade testing and genetic counseling for fragile X-associated disorders. *J Genet Couns*, 16, 593-606.

Miller, L.J. (2006). *Sensational Kids: Hope and Help for Children with Sensory Processing Disorder*. London: Penguin Books.

Miller, L.J., McIntosh, D.N., McGrath, J., et al. (1999). Electrodermal responses to sensory stimuli in individuals with fragile X syndrome: A preliminary report. *Am J Med Genet*, 83, 268-279.

Nowicki, S.T., Tassone, F., Ono, M.Y., et al. (2007). The Prader-Willi phenotype of fragile X syndrome. *J Dev Behav Pediatr*, 28, 133-138.

Reiss, A.L., & Hall, S.S. (2007). Fragile X syndrome: Assessment and treatment implications. *Child Adolesc Psychiatr Clin North Am*, 16, 663-675.

Roberts, J.E., Boccia, M.L., Bailey, D.B., et al. (2001). Cardiovascular indices of physiological arousal in boys with fragile X syndrome. *Dev Psychobiol*, 39, 107-123.

Roberts, J.E., Chapman, R.S., & Warren, S.F. (2008). *Speech and Language Development and Intervention in Down Syndrome and Fragile X Syndrome*. Baltimore: Paul H. Brookes.

Roberts, J.E., Price, J., Barnes, E., et al. (2007). Receptive vocabulary, expressive vocabulary, and speech production of boys with fragile X syndrome in comparison to boys with Down syndrome. *Am J Ment Retard*, 112, 177-193.

Sabaratnam, M. (2000). Pathological and neuropathological findings in two males with fragile X syndrome. *J Intellect Disabil Res*, 44, 81-85.

Scharfenaker, S., O'Connor, R., Stackhouse, T., et al. (2002). An integrated approach to intervention. In R.J., Hagerman & P.J. Hagerman (Eds.), *Fragile X Syndrome: Diagnosis, Treatment, and Research*, (3rd ed.). Baltimore: Johns Hopkins University Press.

Sherman, S. (2002). Epidemiology. In R.J. Hagerman & P.J. Hagerman (Eds.), *. Fragile X Syndrome: Diagnosis, Treatment, and Research* (3rd ed.). Baltimore: Johns Hopkins University Press.

Sullivan, K., Hatton, D., Hammer, J., et al. (2006). ADHD symptoms in children with FXS. *Am J Med Genet A*, 140, 2275-2288.

Sullivan, K., Hooper, S., & Hatton, D. (2007). Behavioural equivalents of anxiety in children with fragile X syndrome: parent and teacher report. *J Intellect Disabil Res*, 51(Pt 1), 54-65.

Torrioli, M.G., Vernacotola, S., Peruzzi, L., et al. (2008). A double-blind, parallel, multicenter comparison of L-acetylcarnitine with placebo on the attention deficit hyperactivity disorder in fragile X syndrome boys. *Am J Med Genet A*, 146, 803-812.

Turner, G., Webb, T., Wake, S., et al. (1996). Prevalence of fragile X syndrome. *Am J Med Genet*, 64, 196-197.

Verkerk, A.J., Pieretti, M., Sutcliffe, J.S., et al. (1991). Identification of a gene (FMR-1) containing a CGG repeat coincident with a breakpoint cluster region exhibiting length variation in fragile X syndrome. *Cell*, 65, 905-914.

Weiskop, S., Richdale, A., & Matthews, J. (2005). Behavioural treatment to reduce sleep problems in children with autism or fragile X syndrome. *Dev Med Child Neurol*, 47, 94-104.

Wittenberger, M.D., Hagerman, R.J., Sherman, S.L., et al. (2007). The *FMR1* premutation and reproduction. *Fertil Steril*, 87, 456-465.

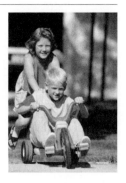

28 HIV Infection and AIDS

Rita Fahrner and Sostena Romano

Etiology

The human immunodeficiency virus (HIV) causes a continuum of infection to occur, the end stage of which is acquired immunodeficiency syndrome (AIDS). HIV type 1 (HIV-1) is a member of the *Lentivirus* genus of the Retroviridae family; its viral RNA is copied into DNA using reverse transcriptase. This virus selectively infects the T-helper (i.e., T4 or CD4) subset of T cell lymphocytes. Other cells that express CD4 (e.g., monocytes, macrophages, and glial cells) and some cells without detectable cell surface CD4 can also become infected. Through a process of replication, HIV perpetuates and integrates itself into the genetic material of the organism it infects. Full intracellular viral life cycling requires the generation of a DNA copy of the HIV-1 RNA genome; integration of this proviral DNA into the host genomic DNA permits viral persistence and impedes the eradication of virus from infected individuals (Luzuriaga & Sullivan, 1998a). The primary pathologic condition of HIV causes specific immunodeficiency that destroys the host's ability to withstand infection. In addition, the HIV directly invades other major organ systems, including the peripheral and central nervous system (CNS), lungs, heart, kidneys, and gastrointestinal (GI) tract.

Although HIV infection in children and adults share a common pathology, infants with perinatally acquired HIV infection represent a distinctive immunologic host with a developing, immature immune system (Kamani & Douglas, 1991). The fetus and neonate have a well-developed T cell, or cell-mediated, immune system, whereas their B cell, or humoral, immune system, is physiologically immature. Although the function of both B and T cells is altered in children with HIV, the consequences of B cell dysfunction, including hypergammaglobulinemia and failure to form functional antibodies, are often problematic early in the course of disease. For this reason, children with HIV are more susceptible to bacterial infections than their adult counterparts. T cell defects, allowing for opportunistic infections (OIs) such as *Pneumocystis jiroveci* (formerly *carinii*) pneumonia (PCP), are also often seen in young infants. In addition, the degree of lymphopenia, percentage of T4 (CD4) cells, absolute T4 (CD4) count, and degree of reversal of the helper-suppressor (T4/T8) ratio are more variable in infants. Depletion of T cell numbers and inversion of the helper/suppressor ratio generally occurs at a later stage of disease in children than in adults. Another major difference between adults and children with HIV is that the time from infection to development of signs and symptoms seems to be shorter in children.

HIV is transmitted to children by a variety of modes (Centers for Disease Control and Prevention ([CDC], 2006b) (Table 28-1). In the United States, perinatal transmission is the most common (92%) mode of transmission and may occur transplacentally in utero (vertically from mother to fetus), during delivery by exposure to infected maternal blood and vaginal secretions, and by postpartum ingestion of infected breast milk (CDC, 2008h). Many factors (i.e., maternal, fetal, viral, placental, obstetric, and neonatal) appear to influence mother-to-infant transmission of the virus. The success of the Pediatric AIDS Clinical Trials Group (PACTG) 076 study showed that when zidovudine (AZT) was administered during pregnancy and labor, as well as to the newborn, the risk for perinatal HIV transmission was reduced by two thirds; infection rates were 25% in the placebo group compared with 8% in the treatment group (Stiehm, Lambert, Mofenson et al., 1999) (Box 28-1). Since then, in developed countries such as the United States and Europe, early testing of pregnant women, treatment of those who are infected with triple-antiretroviral regimens during pregnancy, intravenous (IV) administration of AZT during labor, and the use of AZT orally to the infant for 6 weeks after delivery have resulted in a dramatic decline in the number of children perinatally infected with HIV. Although these advances have reduced the number of new pediatric cases in the United States, much work remains. About 100 to 200 infants in the United States are infected with HIV annually. Most infections involve women who were not tested early enough in their pregnancies or who did not receive preventive services (CDC, 2008h). In November 2008, the American Academy of Pediatrics (AAP) issued a policy statement affirming documented universal "opt-out" HIV testing of pregnant women as the key to primary prevention of mother-to-child transmission, and the use of antiretroviral prophylaxis for the mother and her infant as secondary prevention (AAP, 2008).

The achievements in reducing pediatric HIV cases in the United States are not mirrored in developing countries. The United Nations (UN)AIDS 2008 Report estimates that 370,000 children younger than 15 years of age became infected with HIV in 2007 (Figure 28-1). The number of new HIV infections among children worldwide has declined since 2002 as a result of expanded treatment to reduce mother-to-child transmission, whereas the number of children younger than age 15 living with HIV infection has increased substantially (UNAIDS, 2008). Additionally, almost half of the 500,000 new cases of HIV each year are a result of transmission through infected breast milk (Gray & Saloojee, 2008; Kumwenda, Hoover, Mofenson et al., 2008). This continuing problem in developing countries is primarily caused by lack of general resources and health care infrastructures and exceeds the scope of this chapter.

Many children were infected with HIV from contaminated blood and blood products, tissues, and factor concentrates received

TABLE 28-1

Reported AIDS Cases in Children <13 Years of Age by Transmission Category, 2006, and Cumulative United States and Dependent Areas

	2006		Cumulative	
Transmission Category	**Number**	**%**	**Number**	**%**
Perinatally acquired	74	86	8738	92
Transfusion-associated	1	1	387	4
Hemophilia	0	0	229	2
Undetermined/not reported	11	13	168	2
TOTAL	86	100	9522	100

From Centers for Disease Control and Prevention. (2006). *HIV/AIDS surveillance report, year-end 2006.* Vol 18.Atlanta: U.S. Department of Health and Human Services, CDC, 2007, 1-55.

between 1978 and 1985. The risk for infection was extremely high during these years; HIV infection was estimated to occur in up to 95% of those receiving contaminated products. Because of the safeguards instituted in blood and tissue collection and heat treatment of factor concentrates during the mid-1980s, few new cases of infection from blood and blood products, tissues, and factor concentrates have been reported.

A small number of children become infected with HIV as a result of sexual abuse. Practitioners caring for children who have experienced abuse must include HIV infection in the differential diagnosis of sexually transmitted diseases. HIV has also rarely been transmitted through blood exposure within household settings (e.g., via sharing razor blades or toothbrushes), but no cases of transmission within daycare or school settings have been reported (CDC, 2008c).

Of the HIV infection cases reported by the 35 states that tracked HIV infection in 2004, adolescents and young adults aged 13 through 24 years comprised 13% of all new HIV infections (CDC, 2005). Adolescent females accounted for 43% of the AIDS cases reported among 13- to 19-year-olds through 2005 (Henry-Reid & Martinez, 2008). The average time from HIV infection to the development of AIDS is about 11 years; thus most young adults

BOX 28-1

AZT to Reduce Vertical Transmission (from ACTG 076 Protocol)

MATERNAL
Antepartum
- Begin after 14 weeks gestation
- Zidovudine 100 mg PO five times daily

Intrapartum
- Zidovudine loading dose 2 mg/kg IV over 1 hr then 1 mg/kg/hr continuous IV infusion until delivery
- Zidovudine 1000 mg should be diluted with 250 mg D_5W to prepare a final concentration of 4 mg zidovudine per milliliter D_5W

INFANT
- Begin as soon as possible within the first 12 hours of life

For PO Infant
- Zidovudine 2 mg/kg PO q6hr for 3 to 6 weeks plus extra week's supply

For NPO Infant
- Zidovudine 1.5 mg/kg IV q6h infused over 30 to 60 minutes
- Zidovudine should be diluted with D_5W to prepare a final concentration of 0.5 mg zidovudine per milliliter D_5W

with AIDS were infected as teenagers. Teenagers are especially at risk for HIV because many of the behaviors that increase risk for HIV begin during adolescence, including unprotected sexual activity and injection substance use. In addition, as the management and therapeutic treatments for children with perinatally acquired HIV infection continue to improve, most infected children reach adolescence before a formal AIDS diagnosis is made and will need continuing care throughout these years and into adulthood.

No evidence exists of any genetic predisposition to HIV/AIDS. Because it is an infectious disease, a person must be infected with the virus for the condition to develop. Nothing specific is known about genetic susceptibility, nor do any data exist to suggest genetic defense against development of the infection. Host factors may play

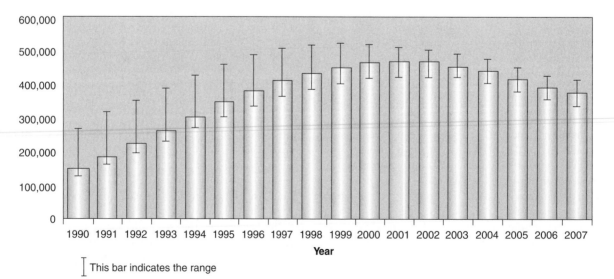

⊥ This bar indicates the range

FIGURE 28-1 New infections among children, 1990-2007. From UNAIDS 2008. *Report on the Global AIDS Epidemic Executive Summary.*

TABLE 28-2

Estimated Number of Perinatally Acquired AIDS Cases by Mother's Transmission Category and Year of Diagnosis, 1981-1996 and 1997-2006: United States and Dependent Areas

Transmission Category	1981-1996		1997-2006	
	Number	**%**	**Number**	**%**
Injection drug use	3118	41	255	19
High-risk heterosexual contact*	2,809	37	591	43
Transfusion	139	2	13	1
Mother with HIV infection (risk factor not specified)	1493	20	502	37

From Centers for Disease Control and Prevention. (2006). *HIV/AIDS surveillance report, year-end 2006.* Vol 18. Atlanta: U.S. Department of Health and Human Services, CDC, 2007, 1-55.

NOTE: Data have been adjusted for reporting delays, and cases without risk factor information were proportionally redistributed.

*Heterosexual contact with a person known to have, or to be at high risk for, HIV infection.

---

a role because cases have occurred in discordant twins in which one twin is infected and the other is not. Another theory regarding discordant twins born to mothers with HIV infection is that birth order may be relevant; the first-born twin seems more likely to be infected.

Incidence and Prevalence

Although pediatric and adolescent AIDS is a reportable condition, the actual incidence and/or prevalence is unknown because AIDS cases are underreported both in the United States and worldwide. The actual incidence and/or prevalence of HIV infection in children, however, is becoming increasingly known as national confidential HIV infection reporting continues to increase; it now occurs in 35 states as well as 4 U.S. dependencies, possessions, and associated nations. The occurrence of AIDS in children was established as early as 1982; AIDS was diagnosed in 20 children younger than 13 years of age by the end of 1981 (CDC, 1994). By the end of 2006, the cumulative estimated number of cases of AIDS in children younger than 13 years was 9144 (CDC, 2006b).

Because most children with AIDS have been perinatally infected, the demographics of this group closely parallel those of women with AIDS (Table 28-2). In this population, HIV is a condition primarily associated with poverty and drug use and continues to be clustered in inner cities and ethnic minority communities. On the other hand, parenteral cases have a broader geographic distribution and a wider ethnic apportionment.

Diagnostic Criteria

Developing a clinical definition of HIV infection and AIDS in children is a complex task (Pizzo & Wilfert, 1998). The AIDS case definition is used for purposes of surveillance and reporting. A separate pediatric classification system was developed by the CDC in 1987 to describe the spectrum of HIV disease. As more information about pediatric HIV became available, however, the 1987 classification system became inadequate. In 1994, the CDC again revised the classification system for children younger than 13 years. In the United States,

BOX 28-2

Antiretroviral Therapy to Prevent Mother-to-Child Transmission (MTCT) of HIV

MATERNAL

Antepartum
- Continue regular ARVs; include zidovudine, avoid efavirenz
- If not currently on ARVs, can defer prophylaxis to second trimester

Intrapartum
- IV zidovudine recommended during labor; continue other oral ARVs, discontinue d4T
- If no antepartal maternal ARV therapy, give IV zidovudine during labor and continue 6 weeks of infant zidovudine
- Cesarean delivery if viral load >1000 copies/mL

NEONATE
- 6-week zidovudine prophylaxis recommended for all HIV-exposed infants
  - Initiate within 6 to 12 hours of delivery
  - Adjust dosage for premature infants
  - Combination therapy efficacy not proven

From Centers for Disease Control and Prevention. (2008). Recommendations for use of antiretroviral drugs in pregnant HIV-infected women for maternal health and interventions to reduce perinatal HIV transmission in the United States. Available at www.cdc.gov/mmwr/preview/mmwrhtml/rr5118a1.htm. Retrieved January 28, 2009.

---

the HIV nucleic acid (DNA and RNA) assays are used most widely for diagnosis of HIV infection in infancy. Testing should be performed in the immediate newborn period. The presence of passively acquired maternal antibodies limits the use of HIV antibody testing in infants up to 18 months of age in whom perinatal infection is suspected. For this reason, two definitions of infection in children are necessary: one for infants up to 18 months and one for older children (CDC, 2008e; CDC, 2008i Read & The Committee on Pediatric AIDS, 2007) (Box 28-2).

Children who meet the definition of HIV exposure or infection may be further grouped into one of 12 mutually exclusive classes based on clinical signs, symptoms, and immunologic status (see Table 28-3). This classification system is helpful for health care planning and for epidemiologic purposes.

Pediatric HIV/AIDS centers can use more specific laboratory tests to determine infection in perinatally exposed infants. HIV blood culturing was considered the gold standard in virologic testing of infants. Blood culturing is very expensive and labor intensive, however, and results are not usually available for 4 to 6 weeks after specimen processing. The p24 antigen assay is another virologic test that is rather inexpensive and has been available for many years. In the presence of HIV antibodies, however, an immune complex is formed with the p24 antigen, rendering detection of the antigen itself impossible. The results of this test become more accurate in children at 6 months when maternal antibody titers in infants begin to decline. A third type of test, the HIV nucleic acid (DNA and RNA) assays, have proved superior to viral culture and p24 antigen assay. Nucleic acid detection is a method of gene amplification that directly detects proviral sequences of HIV within DNA using small amounts of blood. Nucleic acid testing is less expensive than viral culture and more sensitive than p24 antigen assays. In addition, results are usually available within 1 week of specimen processing.

TABLE 28-3

Pediatric HIV Classification*

	Clinical Categories			
Immunologic Categories	N: No S/S	A: Mild S/S	B: Moderate S/S	C: Severe S/S
1. No evidence of immune suppression	N1	A1	B1	C1
2. Evidence of moderate immune suppression	N2	A2	B2	C2
3. Severe immune suppression	N3	A3	B3	C3

From Centers for Disease Control and Prevention (1994). *MMWR Morb Mortal Wkly Rep, 43,* 2-3.
Key: *S/S,* signs/symptoms
*Children whose HIV infection status is not confirmed are classified by using the above grid with a letter E (for perinatally exposed) placed before the appropriate classification code (e.g., EN2).

Use of HIV culture, nucleic acid detection, or both methods can determine an infant's infection status with 90% to 100% certainty by 3 to 6 months of age (CDC, 2008e; Khoury & Kovacs, 2001). Although these tests are becoming more widely available, many community clinicians caring for infants with possible perinatal exposure may not have direct access to them; children should be referred to the closest pediatric HIV specialty center or clinicians should contact the National Institute of Allergy and Infectious Diseases or the Maternal-Child Health Bureau for the nearest participating research group. Many developing countries do not have access to these more advanced testing methods.

HIV is diagnosed in adolescents 13 years and older by the same testing method as adults: HIV antibody testing is the gold standard. Because enzyme-linked immunosorbent assay (ELISA) testing is highly sensitive but less highly specific, repeat ELISA testing is always warranted when the initial test result is positive. If the repeat ELISA result is positive, confirmatory testing with the Western blot technique or indirect fluorescent antibody (IFA) test is necessary for a diagnosis of HIV infection (CDC, 2008d). In this era of rapid blood and saliva testing, it is imperative that preliminary positive test results be clearly communicated to adolescents and their families as being preliminary results that require confirmation before a diagnosis is made. When the preliminary results have been confirmed as positive, the diagnosis of HIV infection should be communicated to the teen in a timely manner.

Clinical Manifestations at Time of Diagnosis

HIV infection is a multisystem condition. Infants and children with HIV present to care with a wide range of signs and symptoms. The clinical manifestations during early infection are often nonspecific and frequently are similar to those in uninfected children and children with other illnesses. Children with chronic HIV infection, however, can experience more severe signs and symptoms and often fail to respond to appropriate therapy. Some children with advanced HIV have acute OIs with the same protozoal, viral, fungal, and bacterial pathogens that are indicator diseases for adult AIDS diagnoses. Others may present with more severe symptoms, such as nephropathy, hepatitis, cardiomyopathy, and hematologic abnormalities

In most children the diagnosis of HIV infection is now made before they exhibit any signs or symptoms of illness. The general

recommendation for offering HIV testing to all pregnant women as a routine part of their prenatal care is identifying many women with HIV infection early in their pregnancies. This early identification affords the initiation of highly active antiretroviral treatment (HAART), as well as the development of plans for delivery and antiretroviral treatment of the neonate. The dramatic advances in medical management of pregnant women with HIV infection have decreased perinatal HIV transmission by more than 80% to 90% (CDC, 2008e). Furthermore, the development of HIV nucleic acid detection assay testing has allowed early diagnosis of infection in infants before symptoms develop. These advances have contributed to the dramatic reduction in pediatric HIV cases in Western and European countries and the transition of HIV from an acute illness to a chronic condition.

Clinical Manifestations at Time of Diagnosis

- Failure to thrive
- Chronic or recurrent diarrhea
- Fever of unknown origin
- Atopic dermatitis
- Persistent or recurrent fungal infections (e.g., thrush or diaper dermatitis)
- Thrombocytopenia
- Hepatosplenomegaly
- Parotitis
- Frequent infections
- Developmental delay; loss of milestones

Unlike early in the HIV epidemic when infants and children were infected through contaminated transfusions and factor concentrates, virtually no current new cases of HIV occur through this route of infection (see Chapter 14).

Treatment

With the approach of the third decade of the HIV epidemic, HIV infection has become a chronic, treatable, life-threatening condition. The most significant treatments are those aimed at interfering with the replicative process of HIV in an attempt to reduce the body's burden of HIV and thereby reduce the destruction of the individual's immune system (Palumbo, 2000). Combination antiretroviral therapy, or HAART, has become standard therapy (CDC, 2008e) and has demonstrated long-term safety and effectiveness in children (Rudin, Burri, Shen et al., 2008). Currently, highly active combination regimens including at least three drugs from two differing classes are recommended (Box 28-3). Mortality has declined 76% from 1994 to 2006 with the introduction of HAART for treatment of pediatric HIV disease (Patel, Hernan, Williams et al., 2008). The advances in combination antiretroviral therapy have provided substantial clinical benefit to children with HIV with immunologic and/or clinical symptoms of disease (Luzuriaga & Sullivan, 2002). Studies have shown definite improvements in neurodevelopment, growth, and immunologic and/or virologic status, as well as improved quality of life, with HAART (Chiriboga, Fleishman, & Chamion, 2005; CDC, 2008e).

Although the pathogenesis of HIV infection and the general virologic and immunologic principles for the use of antiretroviral

---

2008 Revised Surveillance Case Definition of HIV Infection in Children

CHILDREN AGED <18 MONTHS

A. A child <18 months of age who is known to be HIV seropositive or born to an HIV-infected mother and:
  1. Has positive results on two separate specimens (excluding cord blood) from any of the following HIV virologic tests:
    • HIV isolation (culture)
    • HIV nucleic acid (DNA or RNA) detection
    • HIV antigen (p24), including neutralization assay, in children ≥1 month
  or
  2. Meets criteria for AIDS diagnosis based on the 1987 AIDS surveillance case definition

CHILDREN AGED 18 MONTHS TO <13 YEARS

B. A child >18 months of age born to an HIV-infected mother or any child infected by blood, blood products, or other known modes of transmission (e.g., sexual contact) who:
  1. Has a positive result from a screening test for HIV antibody (e.g., reactive EIA) confirmed by a positive result from a supplemental test for HIV antibody (Western blot or immunofluorescence assay)
  or
  2. Meets any of the criteria in A

From Centers for Disease Control and Prevention. (2008). Revised surveillance case definitions for HIV infection among adults, adolescents, and children ages <18 months and for HIV infection and AIDS among children aged 18 months to <13 years—United States, 2008. *MMWR Morb Mortal Wkly Rep, 57(RR10); 1-8.*

Treatment

• Antiretroviral drugs (e.g., HAART)
• Prophylactic antibiotics, antifungals, and antivirals
• Intravenous immune globulin
• Therapies for concurrent infectious and other clinical manifestations

---

therapy are similar for all individuals with HIV, there are unique considerations for their use in infants, children, and adolescents. These considerations include the following: (1) perinatal transmission; (2) in utero, intrapartum, and/or postpartum neonatal exposure to antiretroviral drugs; (3) differences in diagnostic evaluations in perinatal infection; (4) differences in immunologic markers in young children; (5) changes in pharmacokinetics with age caused by the continuing development and maturation of organ systems involved in drug metabolism and clearance; (6) differences in the clinical and virologic manifestations of perinatal HIV infection in relation to the occurrence of primary infection in growing, immunologically immature bodies; and (7) special issues associated with treatment adherence for children and adolescents (CDC, 2008e).

Many questions regarding the use of antiretroviral drugs in children are now being answered because of the growing number of investigational treatment protocols for children that address issues such as the optimal time to start treatment, when and how to modify dosage, and how to determine disease progression. Rather than awaiting proof of their efficacy in adults before children are allowed access to them, new drugs are now simultaneously tested in adults and children. This process parallels the approval process for new chemotherapeutic agents used in cancer therapy.

Intravenous immune globulin (IVIG) continues to be used in some pediatric HIV centers in an attempt to reconstitute the immune systems of children with HIV infection. IVIG has been shown to reduce serious bacterial infections in children with HIV but has not increased survival time (Wood, 1998). The earliest studies were performed before the introduction of antiretroviral treatment. In 1994, broader studies indicated that these data did not hold true in children receiving zidovudine (AZT) in addition to trimethoprim-sulfamethoxazole (TMP-SMX) as PCP prophylaxis (Spector, Gelber, McGrath et al., 1994). Therefore the utility of IVIG in preventing bacterial infections in children with HIV who are receiving HAART and antimicrobial prophylaxis is questionable and is currently rarely used as part of treatment regimens (Darabi, Omar, & Walter, 2006).

Without a definitive cure for HIV infection, children with HIV are treated with comprehensive, multidisciplinary care, including prompt diagnosis, initiation of aggressive therapy with HAART, and treatment of concurrent infections. Recurrent and severe systemic bacterial infection, which can progress to pneumonia, meningitis, and sepsis, is one of the most frequent problems in children with HIV infection. Although bacterial infection contributes greatly to morbidity, it is potentially preventable and treatable. Treatment strategy is focused on early initiation of HAART to help preserve the child's immune system, as well as clinical and antimicrobial interventions to reduce the frequency and intensity of bacterial infections.

Most children with HIV, even those with symptomatic disease, are active, playful, functional children who consider themselves healthy and normal. They may take medications and spend time in the hospital and in outpatient clinics, but they also attend daycare, elementary, middle, and high schools, and engage in many after-school activities. It is important for primary care providers to remember that these children will develop common childhood illnesses and that all symptoms are not necessarily related to their underlying immunodeficiency. Children with HIV, however, must be quickly assessed and aggressively managed when the possibility of intercurrent illness or complications related to their antiretroviral treatments occur (CDC, 2008e; Luzuriaga & Sullivan, 1998b). A wait-and-see attitude is rarely appropriate. Children with HIV and their families must develop strong partnerships with their primary care provider and HIV specialists to ensure prompt evaluation and treatment. Infants, children, and adolescents with HIV are best treated by pediatric and adolescent HIV specialists as rapidly evolving treatment is becoming increasingly complex. Effective management requires a multidisciplinary team approach of providers, including nurses, physicians, dentists, nutritionists, psychologists, social workers, pharmacists, and community outreach workers (CDC, 2008e). Treatment centers ensure access to clinical trials and the most up-to-date information and expertise, as well as to other children and families living with this condition. Clear lines of responsibility and access to the primary care provider and the center team must be developed for each family.

Adult treatment guidelines are appropriate for postpubertal adolescents who have been infected by sexual activity or needle-sharing behaviors because their clinical course is more similar to that of adults than to that of children who were infected perinatally (CDC, 2008e). Adolescents who are long-term survivors of perinatal HIV infection or transfusion-related infection as young children, however, may have a unique clinical course. Dosages of medications for HIV infection and OI should be based on Tanner staging of puberty rather than age; adolescents in early puberty should be given dosages based on pediatric schedules, and those in late puberty should follow adult dosing schedules (CDC, 2008d).

Complementary and Alternative Therapies

Complementary and/or alternative treatments are frequently used in chronic conditions, and adults with HIV/AIDS have been at the forefront of this movement. These therapies may be used alone but are more frequently used in combination with traditional treatments. Forms of therapy include massage, acupuncture, exercise, and dietary and vitamin supplements, (MacIntyre, Holzemer, & Philippek, 1997; Standish, Greene, Bain et al., 2001). Although no studies have been completed in the pediatric populations, those that involved adolescents have shown an improved sense of well-being when alternative therapies are used in conjunction with traditional medicine (Duggan, Peterson, Schutz et al., 2001). Enhanced immune function was seen after 12 weeks in some individuals using complementary therapies (Diego & Field, 2001; Leyes, Martinez, & Forga, 2008). Another area of interest includes the use of probiotics to potentially alter the vaginal mucosa of sexually active females, thereby reducing mucosal irritation, which is associated with increased risk of HIV transmission with exposure (Bolton, Van der Straten & Cohen, 2008). No recommendations can be made, but future research may shed more light on the subject.

Anticipated Advances in Diagnosis and Management

Before the development and availability of antiretroviral drugs for children, HIV care focused on prevention and management of HIV-related complications, as well as provision of palliative care. Combination therapy has been the hallmark of HIV treatment for the past decade (McKinney, Johnson, Stanley et al. 1998). In 2007 the CDC published an update to the 1994 Public Health Service guidelines for the use of antiretroviral drugs—both for maternal health and for reducing perinatal transmission of HIV—in pregnant women with HIV (CDC, 2008h). These guidelines continue to build on the AIDS Clinical Trials Group (ACTG) 076 protocol and confirmation of the efficacy of AZT for reducing perinatal transmission. In addition to the substantial advances in the understanding of the pathogenesis of HIV infection and in the treatment and monitoring of HIV disease, standard antiretroviral therapy for adults with HIV now comprises more aggressive combination drug regimens that maximally suppress viral replication. Pregnancy is not a reason to defer standard therapy; therefore offering antiretroviral therapy to infected pregnant women—whether to primarily treat the disease, to reduce the risk of perinatal transmission, or both—is strongly recommended. Treatment discussions should include the known and unknown short- and long-term benefits and risks of such therapy for infected women and their infants (CDC, 2008h).

Advances in the early diagnosis of infants at risk for HIV infection have been dramatic. More recently, the use of repeated nucleic acid testing has made diagnosis of HIV possible as early as 1 month and in virtually all infants by 4 months of age. Additionally, the CDC will be releasing information regarding a new technology and methodology for HIV testing that will provide information as to timing of infection. The new testing technique may possibly benefit children and teens who are infected by means other than maternal exposure. The importance of this technique is related to timing of initiation of treatment to prevent damage to the immune system (Hall, Song, Rhodes et al., 2008).

HIV drug resistance assays, including genotyping and/or phenotyping of an individual's HIV strain, are useful in guiding initial antiretroviral therapy and regimen changes by identifying specific viral mutations, which may indicate HIV resistance. Expert clinical interpretation with pediatric/adolescent HIV specialists is required for appropriate evaluation of these data (CDC, 2008e).

Associated Problems of HIV/AIDS and Treatment

Although the use of HAART has significantly altered the clinical course of pediatric HIV, the need remains for understanding the signs and symptoms unique to HIV and the complications of the treatments.

Associated Problems of HIV/AIDS and Treatment

Failure to Thrive
- Chronic diarrhea
  - Infectious causes
    - Parasites
    - Protozoa
  - Noninfectious causes
    - HIV direct infiltration of GI mucosa
- *Candida* sp. esophagitis
- Malnutrition

Neurologic Manifestations
- HIV encephalopathy
  - Developmental delay
  - Deterioration of motor skills and/or cognitive functions
- CNS
  - Impaired brain growth
    - Cortical atrophy
    - Calcifications
- Gait disturbances
- Deficits in expressive language

Opportunistic Infections (OIs)
- Major cause of death
- PCP most common OI

Pulmonary Disease
- Noninfectious causes
  - PLH/LIP
  - Nonspecific pulmonary fibrosis
  - Aspiration pneumonia
  - Reactive airway disease
  - Pulmonary hypertension
- Infectious causes
  - *Pneumocystis jiroveci* (formerly *carinii*) pneumonia (PCP)
  - Cytomegalovirus (CMV)
  - Respiratory syncytial virus (RSV)
  - *Mycobacterium avium-intracellulare* infection (MAI)
  - *Mycobacterium* tuberculosis
  - Varicella

Pancytopenia
- Thrombocytopenia
- Anemias
- Leukopenia
  - Neutropenia
  - Lymphopenia

Fungal Infections
- Candidiasis
- Drug exposure
- Delayed development
- Learning/behavioral difficulties

Prenatal and Perinatal Drug Exposure

Failure to Thrive

In 1994, failure to thrive was the fourth leading cause of hospitalization among children with HIV infection; with the advent of HAART, however, the number of hospitalizations has decreased dramatically and significant improvements in nutritional status have occurred in these children (Kourtis, Bansil, Posner et al., 2007). However, nutrition continues to be a significant problem for children with HIV, particularly those with chronic diarrhea and *Candida* ssp. esophagitis. Many infants and children with symptomatic disease demonstrate poor weight gain and often fall below the fifth percentile on the National Center for Health Statistics growth curves for weight (Arpadi, 2000).

Specific causes of chronic diarrhea (e.g., *Cryptosporidium*, *Giardia*, and *Mycobacterium avium-intracellulare* [MAI] spp.) are rarely found, even after exhaustive GI and stool examinations. Some children thrive better on lactose-free diets, whereas others experience cyclical diarrhea unresponsive to dietary manipulations. The GI tract is a major target for HIV because it constitutes 60% of all the lymphocytes in the body. Therefore these problems are thought to be caused by changes in the GI tract secondary to direct invasion by HIV (Miller & Garg, 1998). HIV-associated malnutrition is no different from malnutrition of other causes. Children with chronic conditions who experience malabsorption may also have malnutrition-induced immunodeficiency, which creates an atmosphere in which enteric pathogens are likely to thrive. Therefore malabsorption, malnutrition, immunodeficiency, and enteric infections appear to be interrelated (Miller & Garg, 1998).

Additionally, many medications used in the treatment of HIV have significant associated GI side effects, including nausea, vomiting, and diarrhea (CDC, 2008e). Because the newer HAART regimens often include protease inhibitors, cardiometabolic problems have also begun to emerge in treated children; such problems include abnormal lipid profiles, insulin resistance, truncal adiposity, facial wasting, cardiovascular inflammation, and vascular stiffness (Miller, Grant, Almeida et al., 2008). Preventive care and appropriate surveillance and intervention in terms of nutrition, diet, and exercise is becoming standard care for children with HIV disease.

Neurologic Manifestations

The brain is a target site for HIV infection in infants and children, and a variety of clinical patterns of neurodevelopmental involvement emerge (Pearson, McGrath, Nozyce et al., 2000; Willen, 2006). In most children, the neurologic dysfunction appears to be a result of direct infection of the CNS by HIV. HIV encephalopathy may result in developmental delay, deterioration of motor skills and cognitive functioning, and behavioral abnormalities. This course may be static, progressive, or episodic with plateaus of relative stability that last for months alternating with intervals of marked deterioration that last for weeks. The degree of neurologic deficit is variable and related to an individual's age at first symptom, stage of disease, rate of disease progression, and current age (Smith, Malee, Leighty et al., 2006). Early HAART therapy has promoted better neurologic development. However, children infected with HIV are at increased risk for poor cognitive outcomes. Those who experience an early severe illness and advanced disease are most at risk for significant impairment.

Computed tomography (CT) scanning and magnetic resonance imaging (MRI) often show impaired brain growth with diffuse cortical atrophy and basal ganglia calcifications in severely affected children. Cerebrospinal fluid (CSF)—even if positive for HIV culture—usually shows normal glucose and protein levels and normal cell count.

Opportunistic Infections

The natural history of OIs in children is probably different than that among adults with HIV; adults generally reactivate a previously acquired OI disease, whereas children more often have a primary infection with the pathogen. Additionally, children with perinatally acquired HIV infection probably become infected with the opportunistic pathogen after HIV infection has already been established and the child is immunocompromised. This scenario can lead to manifestations of infection that are different from those in adults. Laboratory diagnosis can be more difficult in children because of a myriad of factors, including issues of maternal antibody transfer and the child's inability to describe symptoms of the infection (CDC, 2004). In the pre-HAART era, the frequency of bacterial, mycobacterial, fungal, protozoal, and viral infections varied by age and immunologic status and were the major cause of death for children with HIV infection (Dankner, Lindsey, & Levin, 2001; Hines, 2000).

Currently, the use of HAART has substantially decreased the numbers of children with OIs as a result of their improved immune status. Management and treatment of OIs continues to be critical despite the changes with HAART because an OI is frequently the presenting illness for a child who was not identified as infected at birth. The treatment and prevention of OIs is an ever-evolving science, and new agents and data analyses may improve therapeutic options and preferences. Initial and secondary prophylaxis with the use of systemic antifungal, antiviral, and/or antimicrobials is commonly indicated to prevent clinical disease in children with moderate to severe immunosuppression (CDC, 2008g).

Pulmonary Disease

Pulmonary disease and resultant respiratory failure contribute significantly to the morbidity and mortality of HIV infection in children. Despite successful trends in the treatment of HIV disease, pulmonary disease remains a common clinical manifestation of pediatric HIV disease (Perez Mato & Van Dyke, 2002). Lung disease develops in more than 80% of children with HIV during the course of their condition (Andiman & Shearer,1998). Even with HAART, with children infected with HIV-1 living longer and healthier lives, pulmonary morbidity continues to be a problem (Berman, Mafut, Djokic et al., 2007). Pulmonary complications of pediatric HIV infection may be divided into noninfectious and infectious etiologies. The lymphoid infiltrates represent a continuum from focal lymphocytic hyperplasia in lung parenchyma (PLH) to more diffuse infiltration of alveolar septa and interstitial tissue (LIP) and then to neoplastic lymphoproliferative disease (Andiman & Shearer). Symptoms may be subtle and include tachypnea, dyspnea, cough, and exercise intolerance. Treatment is generally symptomatic and supportive but also depends on antiretroviral therapy aimed at the underlying HIV infection, as well as the use of corticosteroids. PLH/LIP may be complicated by superinfection with viral, bacterial, or other pathogens.

PCP, which is a diffuse, desquamative alveolopathy that results in hypoxia, is the most frequent OI in pediatric AIDS (CDC, 2008g). The clinical manifestations of children with PCP are age and immune status dependent. Symptoms are likely to be acute with fever, dyspnea, dry cough, cyanosis, and hypoxemia. Treatment of acute infection usually begins with TMP-SMX (Bactrim, Septra) and corticosteroids. Prophylaxis, both primary and secondary, with oral TMP-SMX is extremely effective.

Other pathogens that cause pulmonary infection include cytomegalovirus (CMV); respiratory syncytial virus (RSV); *Mycobacterium tuberculosis* ssp.; MAI; rubeola; varicella; and other viral, fungal, and bacterial sources. Reactive airway disease is common and considered to be chronic airway inflammation associated with frequent and persistent infection. Bronchiectasis as a result of recurrent bacterial and viral pneumonias and reactive airway disease is also becoming more prevalent in pediatric HIV disease.

Pancytopenia

Hematologic abnormalities, occurring because of HIV infection or as an adverse effect of treatment, are common in children with HIV. Some children have thrombocytopenia, which is usually an immune response to circulating platelets, because their bone marrow produces megakaryocytes, which break down into platelets in the peripheral blood. IVIG is sometimes effective in raising the platelet count. An alternative treatment is administering pulses of high-dose corticosteroids. Platelet transfusions are rarely required. Anemias of chronic disease, drug-induced bone marrow suppression, and iron deficiency are common in this population and often require iron supplementation (Calis, Van Hensbroek, De Haan et al., 2008). Red blood cell (RBC) transfusions are sometimes indicated—especially in AZT-induced anemia. CMV-negative, washed, and irradiated RBCs and platelets are used to avoid introducing new infection and to protect against graft-versus-host (GVH) disease. Abnormalities of the white blood cell (WBC) line (i.e., neutropenia, lymphopenia, and leukopenia) are also often noted. Newer drugs that increase RBC production (erythropoietin) and WBC production are used routinely in pediatric HIV disease.

Fungal Infections

Candidiasis occurs frequently and may be manifested as either oral thrush and/or diaper dermatitis. Mucosal *Candida* sp. is the most prevalent OI in all individuals with HIV (Walsh & Butler, 1998). First-line treatments for oral thrush usually include topical nystatin (Mycostatin) and clotrimazole (Mycelex) oral troches. Clotrimazole suppositories (100 or 200 mg) used orally are often more effective because they are more potent than oral suspensions or troches. Infants can be treated either by placing the suppository into the nipple of a bottle, allowing the infant to suck formula through it, or by dissolving the suppository in warm water and swabbing the mouth. Older children can suck the suppositories. Both nystatin and clotrimazole creams are available for skin infections. Refractory cases of mucous membrane and dermatologic infections may be treated systemically with oral ketoconazole (Nizoral), fluconazole (Diflucan), or itraconazole; IV amphotericin B may be necessary for refractory cases of mucosal candidiasis.

Prenatal and Perinatal Drug Exposure

Children with HIV born to mothers with HIV who have had drug and/or alcohol exposure are often premature, small for gestational age, and have very immature immune systems. Their development is often delayed, and learning and behavioral difficulties are common (see Chapters 12, 39).

Prognosis

Studies indicate that since the introduction of HAART, death rates from AIDS have been declining, indicating that children are living longer with HIV/AIDS (CDC, 2006b); many of these children are now reaching adolescence and adulthood. When studies of the cumulative death statistics since the AIDS epidemic began, 1% of AIDS deaths are pediatric (CDC, 2006b). Although the prognosis initially was an average of 10 years from diagnosis of HIV infection to an AIDS-related death, currently long-term prognosis and length of life are unknown because of rapidly changing medical treatments and their improved effectiveness.

Pediatric HIV infection in developed countries is now a chronic manageable condition. However, in developing countries, pediatric HIV disease continues as a fast-moving epidemic. Recent estimates from UNAIDS suggest that 90% of the estimated 2.1 million children younger than age 15 who have HIV live in sub-Saharan Africa (UNAIDS, 2008). Worldwide, 14% of all new HIV infections occurred in children (UNAIDS).

Progression and prognosis for individuals infected with HIV depends on a complex variety of factors. The viral load (or amount of HIV measured as cell-free virum in blood), time to onset of symptoms, availability of treatment, medical management and adherence to medication regimens, the body's response to medical management, and the restoration of the immune system all affect progression of the infection. Children with HIV, however, should be encouraged to lead fully active, well-rounded lives and prepare for a healthy future.

PRIMARY CARE MANAGEMENT

Health Care Maintenance

All children, including children treated at HIV centers, must also have a primary care provider. The HIV specialty care providers and primary care providers must work together, collaborating with the child and family, to provide the highest level of care.

Growth and Development

The poor growth of children with symptomatic HIV disease appears to be related more to the general failure to thrive associated with the underlying HIV infection than to specific problems with caloric intake or GI losses. A health care practitioner or a skilled assistant should carefully measure height, weight, and body mass index at least monthly and plot the findings on the child's individual National Center for Health Statistics growth chart. The same scale should be used at each visit if possible. Because the status of HIV disease has changed to a chronic condition, quality of life is becoming an increasingly addressed issue.

Adequate nutrition is required for healthy development of all children. Poor nutrition further compromises the immune system of a child with HIV and can lead to increased disease progression and the development of OIs. The metabolic needs of a child's body may also be higher as a result of the physiologic stress of HIV infection. When the caloric needs of a child infected with HIV are calculated, the *ideal* weight and not the actual weight of the child should be used (Samour, Helm, & Lang, 2003). Antiretroviral therapy improves growth and survival in children with HIV infection (Kabue, Kekitiinwa, Maganda et al., 2008).

Standard developmental screening tests used by primary care providers (e.g., the Denver Developmental Screening Test II) are of little value in assessing children with HIV disease. Developmental delay is a hallmark of pediatric HIV infection, and early intervention seems to produce significant results; therefore, a skilled clinical psychologist must regularly assess children as part of the comprehensive team approach. It is important for the primary care provider and the psychologist to discuss their developmental assessments and formulate a collaborative action plan.

Intervention strategies must begin as early as possible to maximize a child's capabilities. Infant stimulation programs that focus on motor and language skills and additional specialties (e.g., physical, occupational, and speech therapy) can be provided at home, in the hospital, or in clinic or group settings. Preschool and school-aged children with the necessary physical stamina can best be mainstreamed into regular programs with special services added (Hochhauser, Gaur, Marone et al., 2008).

Diet

Children with HIV need a well-balanced diet with emphasis on adequate calories to maintain and increase their weight with growth. Nutritionists must be part of the multidisciplinary primary care team to obtain dietary histories and perform nutritional assessments to guide clinical decisions. HIV infection does not involve any special dietary recommendations or restrictions. Because failure to thrive is common in infected children, however, early nutritional intervention before wasting occurs is important (Samour et al., 2003). Dietary supplementation and special formulas are often beneficial for weight stabilization and potential gain. Enteral feedings and IV alimentation may be used acutely, intermittently, or chronically for children with severe anorexia, vomiting, diarrhea, and/or other GI problems. Families should regularly consult the primary care provider regarding the child's particular needs. Oral megestrol (Megace) has increased appetite in some children (Samour et al., 2003).

Safety

Primary care providers must teach families safety precautions for children with neutropenia and thrombocytopenia, as well as how to evaluate a child with neutropenia for signs and symptoms of infection (see Chapter 16).

Caretakers may benefit from education on infectious disease transmission and control (e.g., the need for frequent handwashing and avoiding people with known contagious infections). Children with HIV and their household contacts must learn universal/standard blood and body substance precautions; daycare and school personnel also must be knowledgeable regarding infection control issues. Because concern about casual contagion continues in the community, families must be well educated and able to withstand the apprehension of others if they choose to disclose the condition. Several prospective studies of family and school contacts have found no evidence of the spread of HIV within these settings (CDC, 1999, 2008f; Courville, Caldwell, & Brunell, 1998). Although HIV has been isolated in a variety of body fluids (including blood, CSF, pleural fluid, breast milk, semen, cervical secretions, saliva, and urine), only blood, semen, cervical secretions, and human milk have been implicated in its transmission.

It is important to counsel the child's caretakers about the safe storage of medications and equipment in the home. Families may have many potentially hazardous medications at home. Children with HIV may be developmentally delayed or exhibit neurologic regression as the infection progresses, and safety precautions must be adjusted accordingly. If an HIV-infected parent cares for the child, the parent's ability to provide safe care must be frequently assessed because of the dementia often associated with HIV infection in adults.

Immunizations

In the past, live-virus vaccines were not recommended for children with congenital or drug-induced immunodeficiencies because of the concern that live, attenuated vaccine viruses may produce infection in an immunocompromised host. Prospective studies, however, failed to reveal such problems in children with HIV (CDC, 2008a).

In addition, the dysfunction of the B cell system typical of infants with HIV disease, which includes markedly elevated immunoglobulins, reflects nonspecific stimulation that is suggestive of a poor immune response to antigens and therefore to vaccines. This immunologic dysfunction may lower immunogenicity and efficacy of vaccines in infected children. In general, children with symptomatic HIV infections have poor immunologic responses to vaccines and therefore should be considered susceptible regardless of history of vaccination. They should receive passive immunoprophylaxis if indicated when they are exposed to a vaccine-preventable disease such as measles or tetanus (CDC, 2008a). Because live-virus, attenuated immunizations may be ineffective in children who have received IVIG within the past 3 months, the general practice is to administer these vaccinations at the midpoint between monthly IVIG infusions.

The routine immunization schedule for infants and children continues to be the standard of care. Most immunizations follow the standard pediatric schedule without regard for the child's HIV status in terms of stage of infection and/or symptoms; others have specific considerations, and a few immunizations are contraindicated. Current recommendations are as follows (CDC, 2008g):

- *Hepatitis B virus (HBV):* Routine of immunization is recommended.
- *Rotavirus (Rota):* Immunization is now recommended for infants with HIV disease (CDC, 2008g).
- *DTaP, Dt, TdaP:* Routine immunization is recommended. Children with HIV should receive human tetanus immune globulin (TIG) regardless of vaccine status after an injury that places them at risk for tetanus infection (CDC, 2008a).
- *Haemophilus influenzae type B (HiB):* Routine immunization is recommended. *H. influenzae* organisms are common and serious pathogens in children with HIV, which increases the importance of immunization. Even children who have had one or more episodes of documented infection with *H. influenzae* before 2 years of age may not produce enough antibody to prevent subsequent infections, making vaccination imperative. Prophylaxis with rifampin (Rifadin) is required even after vaccination if there is a known contact with HIB (CDC, 2006a, 2008a).
- *Pneumococcal:* Routine immunization is recommended. Pneumococci are prevalent pathogens in children with HIV. The heptavalent pneumococcal conjugate vaccine (Prevnar) should be given to infants on schedule, and the 23-valent pneumococcal vaccine (PPV23) is recommended for all

children at 24 months and then repeated 3 to 5 years after the first dose (CDC, 2008a).

- *Inactivated polio (IPV):* Routine immunization is recommended.
- *Influenza:* Routine immunization is recommended. The trivalent inactivated vaccine (TIV) is recommended for children older than 6 months with HIV exposure or infection and their household contacts (CDC, 2007b, CDC, 2008a, CDC, 2008g). Caretakers and primary care providers must remember to have the child receive the annual influenza vaccine as soon as available to provide prolonged protection. In addition, all people who have contact with individuals with HIV infection should be strongly encouraged to receive annual influenza vaccination to limit the exposure of persons with compromised immune systems to influenza. Primary care providers should ensure that children with HIV and their caretakers receive the influenza vaccine as soon as it is available each year (CDC, 2008a).
- *Measles, mumps, and rubella (MMR):* Routine immunization is recommended for all asymptomatic HIV-infected children who are not severely immunosuppressed as well as some symptomatic children (CDC, 2008g). The. monovalent measles vaccine can be used for infants 6 to 11 months old, with MMR revaccination at 12 months of age or older (CDC, 2008a). Regardless of vaccination status, children with both asymptomatic and symptomatic HIV infection should receive prophylaxis with immune globulin (IG) after exposure to measles (CDC, 2006a). IG prophylaxis may help prevent or minimize measles if it is administered within 6 days of exposure and is indicated for household contacts of children with HIV disease who are measles susceptible, especially infants younger than 12 months. IG may be unnecessary if a child is receiving regular IVIG infusions and the last dose was within 3 weeks of exposure (CDC, 2006a).
- *Varicella:* Routine immunization is recommended except for children who are severely immunocompromised (CDC, 2008g). Varicella (VZV) poses significant risks for dissemination, encephalitis, and pneumonia in children who are immunosuppressed. Data on varicella vaccination in HIV-positive children have shown it to be safe and effective for asymptomatic or mildly symptomatic children with HIV with age-specific CD4+ percentages of 15% or greater (CDC, 2007a). Children with HIV who are susceptible to varicella should receive varicella-zoster immune globulin (VZIG) intramuscularly within 72 hours of exposure if they have not received IVIG within the past 3 weeks (CDC, 2007a).
- *Hepatitis A virus (HAV):* Routine immunization is recommended.
- *Meningococcal:* Routine immunization is recommended. Children with HIV may be at increased risk for meningococcal disease, although vaccine efficacy in this group of children is unknown (CDC, 2008g).
- *Human papillomavirus vaccine (HPV):* No data are available, but because it is a noninfectious vaccine, it can safely be administered to HIV-infected females (CDC, 2008g).

Screening

Vision. Because of the incidence of CMV retinitis in adults with HIV disease and therefore the theoretical risk of a similar process affecting children, primary care providers must elicit a thorough visual history and provide a careful visual and funduscopic examination. Comprehensive pediatric HIV centers may recommend that all children with HIV be referred to a knowledgeable pediatric ophthalmologist for baseline screening and annual follow-up. If the findings are normal, the primary care provider can then continue to provide regular follow-up.

Hearing. Because of frequent acute suppurative otitis media (OM) in children with HIV infection and the possibility of hearing loss, periodic audiometry and tympanometry should be performed. Children who require myringotomy tube placement must use special precautions for swimming and showers (e.g., regular use of well-fitting earplugs).

Children with severe neurologic disease, some children with chronic OM, and those receiving maintenance aminoglycoside therapy need baseline brainstem, auditory-evoked response hearing testing if routine acuity testing cannot be done or test results are abnormal.

Dental. Early screening (i.e., starting at 2 to 3 years of age) is strongly recommended because dental caries can create a focus of infection. Fluoride treatments are recommended if the community water supply does not contain adequate amounts to protect enamel. Severe dental caries and gingivitis, as well as dental abscesses, are reported in some infected children (Ramos-Gomez, 1997). Clinicians must educate families regarding appropriate oral hygiene and encourage regular dental care. Liquid medications contain sweeteners to increase drug palatability, which also increases the risk of caries.

Blood Pressure. Blood pressure measurements should be taken every 3 to 6 months unless changes warrant more frequent measurements. Increased blood pressure can indicate renal disease.

Hematocrit. Routine screening is deferred because of the need for frequent assessment of complete blood cell (CBC) counts.

Urinalysis. Children with HIV require urinalysis with microscopic examination at least every 6 months because urine abnormalities can be the first sign of illness. Findings can include hematuria and proteinuria and can result in azotemia and nephrotic syndrome. Children taking the protease inhibitor indinavir (Crixivan) need frequent (i.e., at least monthly) urinalysis with microscopic examination for blood and crystals because this drug is known to cause renal stones.

Tuberculosis. Yearly screening is strongly advised. Because tuberculosis is being diagnosed more often in adults with HIV, more children in households with infected adults are at risk for tuberculosis. Because many individuals infected with HIV demonstrate anergy to skin testing, close surveillance of families may include regular chest radiographic studies. MAI is a common bacterium of the same family as *M. tuberculosis,* which is prevalent in individuals with HIV. Unlike *M. tuberculosis,* MAI is not contagious by the respiratory route but may be transmitted through infected GI secretions. Because it can invade many organ systems, including the bone marrow and the GI system, MAI may be responsible for significant morbidity.

Condition-Specific Screening

Vital Signs. Vital signs should be assessed and documented at each visit. Children can be asymptomatic yet febrile, needing a workup. Elevations in heart and respiratory rates can indicate pulmonary or cardiac dysfunction.

Complete Blood Count. Because of bone marrow suppression caused by HIV and some OIs, as well as by many of the drugs used in treatment, children with HIV require regular CBC counts—with differential and platelet counts. Asymptomatic children should have a CBC performed every 3 to 6 months; symptomatic children usually need them at least monthly. This blood work can be performed by the primary care provider or at the pediatric HIV center.

If anemia is present, its cause should be investigated because children with iron-deficiency anemia usually benefit from oral iron supplementation. A specific cause, however, is not often discovered. Children taking antiretrovirals need frequently assessment of CBC and reticulocyte counts because anemia is a common adverse effect of HAART. CBCs are usually performed every 2 weeks for the first 2 months and then done every 3 months as long as children are stable. Some children taking antiretrovirals require RBC transfusions. Neutropenia and thrombocytopenia are also common side effects of antiretroviral treatment. Dosages of antiretrovirals may be modified based on the degree of bone marrow suppression. Bone marrow–stimulating drugs such as erythropoietin stimulators, including Epogen, Procrit, and Aranesp; and leukocyte stimulators, including filgrastim (Neupogen) and granulocyte colony–stimulating factor (G-CSF), may be used.

Immunologic Markers. Baseline T and B cell counts and percentages and quantitative immunoglobulin (QUIG) determinations are necessary to assess immunologic status. T cell subset values and T4/T8 ratios are usually checked every 3 to 6 months. T4 counts below 350/mm^3 generally indicate that antiretroviral drugs should be prescribed. Clinicians must consider age as a variable in interpreting immunologic markers for children. These markers are used in conjunction with other markers to guide antiretroviral treatment decisions and primary prophylaxis for PCP and other OIs after 1 year of age.

HIV Markers. Viral burden can be determined by using quantitative HIV RNA viral load assays of peripheral blood. During primary infection in adults and adolescents, the HIV RNA viral load rises to high peak levels and then—coinciding with the body's humoral and cell-mediated immune response—declines by 2 to 3 logs to a stable lower level some 6 to 12 months later. This leveling reflects the balance, or steady state, between ongoing viral production and immune elimination (CDC, 2008e). This pattern differs in perinatally infected infants in that high HIV RNA levels usually persist during the first year of life and then gradually decline over the next few years. This pattern may reflect an immature but developing immune system's lower efficiency in containing viral replication and more HIV-susceptible cells.

Trends in HIV RNA levels are helpful in determining initiation of antiretroviral therapy and when the agents should be changed. Because of the complexities of testing and the age-related changes in values, interpretation of HIV RNA levels for clinical decision making should be done by or in consultation with pediatric HIV experts.

Chemistry Panel. Routine serum chemistry panels (including electrolytes, blood urea nitrogen [BUN], creatinine, glucose, hepatic transaminases, calcium, and phosphorus), pancreatic enzyme evaluations, and serum lipid evaluation should be obtained every 3 to 6 months and more often for symptomatic children or those taking medications (i.e., AZT, didanosine [ddI]) that might affect liver or kidney function. Children taking ddI, d4T, and/or 3TC must also be monitored for pancreatitis by regular monitoring of amylase and lipase levels. Children taking protease inhibitors need regular lipid panels (including lipase, cholesterol, triglyceride, and glucose levels). Many children with HIV have elevated baseline liver function test results, often with both aspartate aminotransferase (AST) and alanine aminotransferase (ALT) enzyme levels two to three times normal levels.

Pulmonary Function. Children with chronic lung disease need baseline pulmonary function testing with oxygen saturation and regular serial testing based on disease severity. When available, pulse oximetry—a noninvasive technique—is used in place of arterial blood gas sampling. A baseline radiograph is useful as a comparison study for later pulmonary complaints. Children with either acute infection or chronic pneumonitis often have no adventitious sounds. Pulmonary consultation is a useful adjunct for the primary care provider in follow-up of these children.

Antiretroviral Medication Adherence Assessment. Medication adherence is fundamental to the success of HAART therapy. The degree of viral suppression achieved and restoration of the immune system is related to the degree of medication adherence (Saitoh, Hsia, & Fenton, 2002). Adherence is a complex issue that is influenced by many factors, including the regimen prescribed, patient factors (e.g., age, ability to swallow, behavioral factors), family issues (supportive or distant), and characteristics of the health care providers (supportive and engaging or distant and prescriptive). Multiple methods to assess adherence are recommended. These include self-report, verbal description of medication regimen, pill counts, checking pharmacy refills, and use of electronic monitoring devices. A nonjudgmental attitude and trusting relationship are the most valuable tools for all providers (CDC, 2008d,e).

Common Illness Management
Differential Diagnosis

Fever. Fever is often a sign in children with HIV disease and can be caused by the HIV itself or can indicate a separate infectious process. Practitioners must ensure that families have a thermometer that they can use accurately, in addition to clear guidelines about when to contact their primary care provider. Whenever a child's temperature is 101°F (38.5°C) or higher, the child needs to be examined and a treatment plan initiated based on the objective and subjective findings.

Differential Diagnosis

Fever
- HIV infection vs. other infectious processes such as bacteremia, sepsis, or opportunistic infectious agent (MAI, CMV)

Respiratory Distress
- LIP versus PCP
- Cardiomyopathy
- Reactive airway disease

Otitis Media
- Referral to ear, nose, and throat specialist for tube placement

Sinusitis
- Untreated infection can lead to meningitis

Varicella/Zoster
- Risk of dissemination high

A thorough interval history and complete physical examination are the most important part of the workup of a febrile child with

HIV. Some children will have OM, sinusitis, pneumonia, or sepsis; others will have common colds and other viral infections that can be traced to school or household contacts.

In consultation with the infectious disease specialist or the HIV center, the primary care provider can order cultures of blood and other body fluids as indicated for aerobic, anaerobic, and fungal organisms. Cultures are essential to identifying the infectious process. Cultures are often negative—even in seriously ill children, but positive cultures will determine specific antibiotic therapy. Chest radiographic studies may be an important part of the workup of a febrile child with HIV.

Respiratory Distress. A variety of respiratory conditions may occur in children with HIV. History and physical examination are paramount to the differential diagnosis. A dry, hacking cough is common in children with LIP but can also be a sign of PCP. Children with acute onset of respiratory distress require prompt evaluation because the condition can progress extremely rapidly—sometimes within hours. Pulmonary consultation is often necessary. Children with cardiac disease occasionally have respiratory symptoms and need cardiologic consultation and diagnosis.

Children with known reactive airway disease may benefit from equipment and medications for aerosol delivery at home. The primary care provider must evaluate the family's ability to provide such sophisticated assessment and treatment; if parents are capable, they can be taught the necessary skills.

Otitis Media. OM is one of the most common infectious diseases in children with HIV and is often diagnosed on routine physical examination when no pain or fever is present, even when the tympanic membrane may be ruptured with pus filling the external canal. Children with presumptive infection, rather than noninfectious effusion, should be promptly treated with antibiotics using standard treatments. Follow-up must be done after treatment is completed because the OM may not resolve and complications may occur. Children who have persistent and refractory OM should be referred to an ear, nose, and throat (ENT, otorhinolaryngologist) specialist for evaluation for placement of myringotomy tubes.

Sinusitis. Although sinusitis is uncommon in children, it is common in children with HIV disease and often occurs after a viral respiratory tract infection. Primary care providers can teach families to report changes in nasal mucus from clear or white to yellow or green, which may indicate infection; other signs and symptoms may include fever, headache and/or facial pain, and prolonged nasal discharge and congestion. If not appropriately treated, sinusitis can lead to mastoiditis and directly extend into the brain, causing meningitis.

Varicella. Because of the risk of dissemination as a result of immunocompromise, varicella is potentially life threatening in children with HIV. Because these children may not respond adequately to vaccines and the general herd immunity to varicella will not be high until the vaccine has been widely distributed for many years, herpes zoster virus (HZV) will continue to cause chickenpox as a primary manifestation and zoster as a secondary manifestation of infection in most children with HIV. If primary prevention with VZIG fails or if a child was not known to be exposed until the rash occurs, the usual practice at most centers is to quickly evaluate these children and immediately start oral treatment with acyclovir regardless of their immune status. Some children require hospitalization for treatment with IV acyclovir. With this treatment, few children progress to disseminated disease, and most go home

within 5 days of starting therapy, continuing with oral therapy to complete a 7- to 10-day course.

Drug Interactions

Antiretroviral Drugs. The antiretroviral (HAART) medications used in children with HIV are listed in Box 28-4 (CDC, 2008e). Many of these drugs have significant drug interactions. It is best to identify the specific potential interactions of every drug to be prescribed in primary care before prescribing the medication. The primary care provider can contact the HIV treatment center for consultation if questions regarding medication prescription arise.

TMP-SMX. Two major toxicities of this sulfa combination are hematologic: neutropenia and thrombocytopenia. Children receiving PCP prophylaxis or treatment regimens in whom persistent neutropenia develops secondary to TMP-SMX either alone or with AZT must often discontinue TMP-SMX treatment. Dapsone, atovaquone, and intravenous or aerosolized pentamidine can be used as alternatives in older children. Allergic reactions to sulfa are not uncommon, and primary care providers must teach families how to recognize the symptoms of skin rash and hives as part of the reaction complex. Several studies have shown successful treatment using TMP-SMX despite a history of previous adverse reactions (Simonds & Orejas, 1998).

IVIG. There are no specific drug interactions noted with IVIG. Allergic reactions have been documented but appear to be rare.

BOX 28-4

Currently Used HAART Medications

NUCLEOTIDE REVERSE TRANSCRIPTASE INHIBITORS
- Zidovudine (AZT)
- Lamivudine (Epivir)
- Emtricitabine (Emtriva)
- Tenofovir (Viread)
- Stavudine (Zerit)
- Didanosine (Videx)
- Abacavir (Ziagen)

NONNUCLEOSIDE REVERSE TRANSCRIPTASE INHIBITORS
- Nevirapine (Viramune)
- Delavirdine (Rescriptor)
- Efavirenz (Sustiva)
- Etravirine (Intelence)

PROTEASE INHIBITORS
- Atazanavir (Reyataz)
- Darunavir (Prezista)
- Ritonavir (Norvir)
- Fosamprenavir (Lexiva)
- Nelfinavir (Viracept)
- Indinavir (Crixivan)
- Amprenavir (Agenerase)
- Saquinavir (Invirase)
- Tipranavir (Aptivus)
- Lopinavir/ritonavir (Kaletra)

ENTRY AND FUSION INHIBITORS
- Maraviroc (Selzentry)
- Enfuvirtide (Fuzeon)

INTEGRASE INHIBITORS
- Raltegravir (Isentress)

Developmental Issues

Sleep Patterns

HAART generally is given during waking hours. Frequent dosing is no longer required as was necessary in the early days of HIV therapy. Other medications may require night dosing schedules that interrupt sleep; however, children whose normal sleeping hours must be interrupted for treatment may experience difficulty in returning to sleep. Therefore parents may need to try a variety of schedules to find one that works best for them and their child to minimize interruptions in their child's sleeping.

Toileting

Children with HIV who are in diapers may experience diaper dermatitis, which is often associated with candidiasis and with chronic and cyclic diarrhea. Impeccable perineal care—including frequent diaper changes, exposure of the perineum to air, and the use of topical medications—can significantly reduce morbidity. When the perineum is bloody or the child has hematuria or diarrhea, caretakers should wear gloves to protect themselves during diapering. Neurologic deterioration can lead to incontinence in children who have previously stopped using diapers.

Discipline

Discipline is often difficult for the family of a child with a chronic, life-threatening condition. Some parents are unable to set developmentally appropriate and necessary limits and need guidance and information from their primary care provider. Discipline needs and appropriate expectations will vary as the illness progresses and neurologic and motor deterioration occurs, so caretakers must be given anticipatory guidance in these areas. Other factors (e.g., homelessness, chaotic lifestyle, and parental illness) can make consistent discipline difficult. Practitioners may need to help families and caregivers understand the child's needs for safety and limits.

Child Care

Child care, respite care, and preschool placement are difficult issues for families of children with HIV. Primary care providers must advise parents that children in group settings are at increased risk for exposure to infectious diseases and common childhood illnesses compared with children who stay at home. The particular care setting must be individualized for each child based on the child and family's needs and resources. Practitioners can provide education on universal infection control and infectious disease guidelines for these agencies.

Child care and respite care are important resources for families of children with chronic conditions. Some foster families have access to respite hours through their social services division, but others do not. In some areas few, if any, child care or respite workers are willing to care for infants and children with HIV, which is an enormous problem for families who need time to care for their own HIV, as well as for their infected and uninfected children. The regular availability of respite care and other support services may allow many infected mothers to continue to care for their children. It is important to note that uninfected parents and caregivers also need respite care.

The Individuals with Disabilities Education Act (2004), Americans with Disabilities Act, and Lanterman Act may offer valuable services for children with HIV (see Chapter 3). Head Start, a federal preschool program that provides preschool for economically deprived children, is specifically mandated to enroll children with HIV.

Because daycare and preschool are not a legal requirement for children, individual daycare providers may develop their own policies in accordance with local, state, and federal regulations. Many private daycare centers and preschools do not accept children with HIV, probably because of their fears of casual contagion, litigation, and loss of enrollment if other families discover the diagnosis. Some areas of the country with a high prevalence of pediatric HIV have daycare programs developed specifically for these children. Such services are directed toward children who are too ill to attend regular daycare programs.

Daycare and preschool personnel and families should be educated before a child with HIV is enrolled. It may be useful for the primary care provider to call the preschool, stating that a family is interested in enrolling their child with HIV. The school is notified that there is no "duty to inform" and that the child will not be identified. Feelings about children with HIV infection are explored, and an offer is made to provide in-service training about pediatric HIV and control of general infection.

Some families choose to conceal the diagnosis of HIV in their family, but other families openly discuss it. As more children with HIV take HAART and other medications that must be administered frequently, it is becoming more difficult to conceal HIV infection from daycare providers. Many families schedule dosing around school hours and create unusual stories about their reasons to know immediately about chickenpox or other contagious illnesses in the classroom. Clinicians have an important role in helping families decide how, when, and to whom information about HIV disease should be disclosed. Nondisclosure may be an appropriate consideration in some cases when there is no duty to disclose.

Schooling

The major school issues faced by young children with HIV have little to do with their educational needs and much to do with concerns about confidentiality, information sharing, and infection control. These issues have created strife in many communities nationwide. As children with HIV age, however, their needs for special education programs will undoubtedly increase. Primary care providers can help families secure appropriate services (see Chapter 3).

Because AIDS is recognized as a handicap, Public Law 101-476 supports attendance of individuals with AIDS in public schools. The American Academy of Pediatrics (AAP) took the position that because of the mandated use of universal precautions, no child with HIV should be denied access to school or the ability to be involved in contact sports (AAP, 1999). Furthermore, in many states, HIV is not required to be disclosed by provider or family. In some rare cases, when a child may be banned from attending school, the school district must provide home teaching. Children benefit greatly from attending school, so this option should be strongly discouraged. When children are too ill to attend, home teaching is a viable alternative for that time only. As a child's condition progresses, particularly with neurologic deterioration, frequent meetings of school resource personnel, health care providers, and family members are needed to ensure that appropriate services are provided.

The legal duty to inform school officials about a child's HIV diagnosis varies from state to state. As more children become aware of their own HIV infection, more discussion among these children will ensue, which will increase awareness in the school and larger community that a child with HIV is in attendance. Providers should be available to the school (i.e., students, faculty, and parents) for educational discussion sessions.

Teenagers with HIV often have difficulty in school. Rumors circulating about HIV infection and students thought to be infected can cause tremendous anxiety for an infected adolescent—regardless of the route of infection (Chabon & Futterman, 1999). Primary care providers can support their teenaged clients, helping them to gain more knowledge and determine with whom they might trust this sensitive information. It may be helpful for infected teens to meet in face-to-face groups and/or in online groups to work together in developing strategies for dealing with school-based problems. Referral to the school nurse or counselor may be appropriate.

The risk of blood contamination during sports, particularly contact sports, as well as related to accidents, is an issue to consider for children and adolescents with HIV. Universal precautions should be stressed so that infected children can lead healthy, active lives both in and out of school.

Sexuality

Children and adolescents with HIV need to learn about all modes of transmission of this infection, with an emphasis on sexual, injection-drug use, and perinatal transmission. Adolescence is the time for sexual experimentation and the emergence of sexual identity; sexual activity increases steadily throughout these years, and many HIV-infected adolescents will become sexually active. Teens with HIV face much difficulty in attaining a healthy, integrated sexual identity because of the risks of oral and genital sexual transmission (Ledlie, 2002). Some teens deny the reality of their HIV, refusing to practice safe sex. Teens with cognitive delays stemming from neurologic effects of HIV may have a particularly difficult time in understanding transmission risks. Primary care providers must be comfortable discussing transmission and sexual risk–reduction strategies, as well as demonstrating the proper use of condoms and dental dams in developmentally appropriate and cognitively limited teens. Health care providers must be able to have regular discussions about sex and drugs with their teen clients.

Schools can provide an important service by providing health education to students, families, and staff. Educating students can help reduce the prevalence of sexual risk behaviors among teens, while appropriate school health policies can help protect the rights and health of students with HIV-infection and staff members and reduce the probability of HIV transmission to others (CDC, 2008c). Unfortunately, recent studies have shown that teens have not continued to reduce their risk behaviors for HIV infection during the past few years (CDC, 2008b).

Transition to Adulthood

The advent of new and more effective HIV therapies has transformed HIV infection from a terminal illness to a chronic but manageable condition. Survival times have continued to increase; there are now long-term survivors among children who were perinatally infected (CDC, 2008g). Individuals with HIV will continue to need a vast array of medical and psychosocial services throughout their childhood and transition to adulthood (Ledlie, 2002). Children born to mothers with HIV are at risk of losing their mothers, as well as other infected family members, to HIV while they are young. Adult caretakers may not be available to help assist the adolescent into adulthood.

Children and teenagers who are infected with HIV have many other concerns to face in their transition to adulthood. Some issues facing these children include the risk of sexual transmission, intimacy, and stigma. As HIV infection becomes a more chronic, life-threatening disease integrated into the mainstream of health care, these special issues may gradually decline.

Facilitating a smooth transition for adolescents with HIV to adult care facilities can be complicated. Pediatric HIV care models are family centered, with input from a multidisciplinary team of providers. The relationships of these providers with the adolescent with HIV are typically long-standing and include the adolescent and their family members. Adult HIV care facilities tend to provide more individual-centered care and can be busier and less inviting and comfortable for adolescents. General guidelines for transitional plans and the benefits of using them are available to assist primary providers (CDC, 2008e; Rosen, Blum, & Britto, 2003) (see Chapter 4).

Family Concerns

When HIV infection is diagnosed in a child, a family crisis results. Many children with HIV have infected mothers who are ill, dying, or deceased and they also may have an infected father and siblings. Most mothers who transmit HIV to their children experience tremendous guilt. The physical and emotional burden of caring for a child who requires frequent medical and supportive treatments, who have developmental delay, and who will probably die as a result of the illness is enormous for all parents and caregivers, regardless of whether the adults are infected.

The most significant psychosocial issue facing children with HIV and their families is the social stigmatization associated with the condition. Many families initially feel isolated and unable to rely on their usual support systems for fear of rejection and retaliation. Fears of transmission by casual contact continue despite scientific knowledge to the contrary, and these fears affect stigma associated with HIV. In a recent study of families with an HIV-infected parent, two-thirds of the family members expressed fears about transmission within the family (Cowgill, Bogart, Corona et al., 2008). Intervention by healthcare personnel can help to educate and allay family fears, and information about transmission prevention is a useful and important component of anticipatory guidance for adolescents.

Infected families may also lack other resources; they are primarily poor, of minority heritage, undereducated, and burdened by the social ills of inner-city life. With support, affected families may reach out to extended family, friends, and community agencies. Noninfected parents and caregivers also need support in caring for their children and in obtaining the available community support.

During the early years of the HIV epidemic, many children were not told of their diagnosis because of family concerns that the child would become depressed, angry, or might tell others and expose the family to discrimination or stigmatization. Now that infected children are surviving into adolescence and adulthood, disclosure is becoming a common clinical issue. Recommendations and guidelines for disclosure are available through the American Association of Pediatrics and national AIDS groups. Nondisclosure can result in anxiety and depression. The process of disclosure should take into account the child's age, psychological maturity, and family dynamics.

Medication adherence is an issue currently being studied by a variety of researchers (Vreeman, Wiehe, Pearce et al., 2008; Williams, Storm, Montepiedra et al., 2006). Some studies have found that medication adherence is often lower than necessary for appropriate viral suppression (Martin, Elliott-DeSorbo, Wolters et al., 2007). Family and caregivers must understand the importance of pharmacotherapy adherence, and interventions to support successful transition of medication responsibility from family and caregivers to older children and youth are imperative in improving health outcomes (Narr-King, Montepiedra, Nichols et al., 2008).

The majority of children who were perinatally infected with HIV are of African-American and Latino descent. Some children are placed in foster or adoptive care after birth if the birth mother is unable to care for them. Others later are placed with caregivers outside the home when resources cannot support their parents' ability to care for them. Foster and adoptive parents need considerable support (i.e., ongoing education, financial support, respite care, emotional support and counseling, and social and legal counseling) to provide optimal care for children with HIV. Because children in foster care are wards of the juvenile court, decisions about consent for investigational drugs and experimental protocols, as well as do-not-resuscitate orders, must be court ordered. Working relationships among the primary care provider, HIV center, and social services must be developed and maintained to ensure that children with HIV receive optimal care in the child welfare system.

Helping children and families face a chronic life-threatening illness that may ultimately lead to death is a pivotal role for primary care providers. Counseling about the physical and emotional issues of death and the dying process, options for hospital or home death, hospice services, funeral plans, and bereavement are an integral part of the clinician's role. Support groups are invaluable resources for networking, keeping current, and decreasing social isolation. Most pediatric HIV/AIDS comprehensive treatment centers offer such groups on an ongoing basis. Primary care providers should become familiar with the local, national, and international organizations (see the following list of organizations).

Resources

Camps

The National Pediatric AIDS Network has current lists of camps available at their website: www.npan.org/CampsFrame. asp?anchor=Camps.

National Organizations

CDC National AIDS Network
P.O. Box 6003
Rockville, MD 20849-6003
(800) 458-5231
Website: www.cdcnpin.org

HIV and AIDS Malignancy Branch (HAMB), National Cancer Institute
(301) 496-0328
Website: http://ccr.cancer.gov/Labs/Labs.asp?LabID=63

National AIDS Hotline
(800) CDC-INFO; (800) 232-4636; TTY: (888) 232-6348
Email: cdcinfo@cdc.gov
Website: www.ashastd.org/nah

National Center for Youth Law
114 Sansome St., Suite 900
San Francisco, CA 94104-3820
(415) 543-3307
Website: www.youthlaw.org

National Foundation for Children with AIDS
3505 South Ocean Dr.
Hollywood, FL 33019

National Pediatric and Family HIV Resource Center
15 South 9th St.
Newark, NJ 07107
(800) 362-0071
Website: www.pedhivaids.org

NIAID Intramural Trials for HIV Infection and AIDS
(866) 284-4107

The Safe Haven Project
P.O. Box 24
Vineyard Haven, MA 02568
(508) 627-1767; Cell: (508) 939-1662
Website: http://safehavenproject.org

Sunshine for HIV Kids, Inc
c/o Richard Merck
PO Box 3537
Kingston, NY 12402
Website: www.sunshine.com

The Elizabeth Glaser Pediatric AIDS Foundation
2950 31st St., #125
Santa Monica, CA 90405
(310) 314-1459; Fax: (310) 314-1469
E-mail: info@pedaids.org
Website: www.pedaids.org

Local and State Resources

County health department
State health department
AIDS task forces
AIDS hotlines

Summary of Primary Care Needs for the Child with HIV/AIDS

HEALTH CARE MAINTENANCE

Growth and Development

- Growth in both weight and height should be measured and plotted quarterly; if <5th percentile on growth curve, measure and plot monthly.
- Body composition surveillance.
- Standard developmental screening tests are not useful; if available, serial screening by a psychologist is recommended.
- Early intervention programs are recommended to maximize developmental potential.

Diet

- A balanced high-calorie diet should be emphasized.
- Nutritionist to collaborate in care.
- Nutritional supplements and medications to increase appetite are often beneficial.

Safety

- The risk of infection because of immunocompromise is increased. Frequent hand washing and avoiding people with known infections is recommended.
- The risk of bleeding because of thrombocytopenia is increased.
- Universal/Standard blood and body substance precautions should be taught to the family and caregivers.
- Safe storage of medication in the home is important.
- Developmental delay or regression may alter safety requirements.
- Parents with HIV must be evaluated for safe care practices because of symptoms of dementia.
- Uninfected parents may also benefit from home evaluation especially as medications/treatments become more complex.

Immunizations

- General poor immune response to vaccines; passive immunoprophylaxis may be indicated when exposure occurs.
- Routine vaccine schedules for:
  - HBV
  - Rotavirus is now recommended
  - DTaP, DT, TdaP
  - HiB
  - Pneumococcal; should have both Prevnar and PPV-23
  - IPV
  - Influenza, inactivated (TIV)
  - MMR
  - HAV
  - Meningococcal
  - HPV

Special Considerations

- Tetanus immunoglobulin (TIG) should be given to children at risk for infection related to injury.
- Can give monovalent measles vaccine in infants 6 to 11 months old, with MMR revaccination at 12 months or older.
- Give immune globulin within 6 days of measles exposure to prevent or modify course unless child has received IVIG within the previous 3 weeks.

- Known exposure to HiB requires prophylaxis with rifampin.
- Varicella vaccine is recommended if CD4+ T-lymphocyte percentage >15%. Varicella-zoster immune globulin (VZIG) recommended within 72 hours of varicella exposure.

Screening

- *Vision.* Consider baseline funduscopic examination by ophthalmologist with practitioner follow-up every 3 to 6 months; consider ophthalmologist follow-up every 1 to 2 years.
- *Hearing.* Periodic audiometry and tympanometry screenings are recommended. Frequent acute OM and treatment with aminoglycosides may affect hearing. A brainstem evoked-response (BSER) hearing test should be given to children with chronic OM or abnormal screening.
- *Dental.* Early screening is recommended to prevent dental infections; should be followed up at least every 6 months to prevent and/or treat dental caries.
- *Blood pressure.* Measure every 3 to 6 months. Increased BP may indicate renal disease.
- *Hematocrit.* Routine screening is deferred because of the need for frequent CBCs.
- *Urinalysis.* Urinalysis with microscopic examination should be done at least every 3 months to rule out renal disease; monthly for children taking indinavir (Crixivan).
- *Tuberculosis.* Yearly screening is recommended. Chest radiographic studies may be needed if a child is anergic. MAI infections are responsible for significant morbidity.

Condition-Specific Screening

- *Vital signs.* Temperature, heart rate, and respiratory rate should be checked at each visit.
- *Complete blood cell count.* A CBC should be assessed at baseline and then every 3 to 6 months if a child is asymptomatic; every 2 to 4 weeks when child is starting HAART or other myelosuppressive agents; those who are stable on HAART therapy may require only quarterly blood counts. Anemia, neutropenia, and thrombocytopenia are common side effects of HAART.
- *Immunologic markers.* Baseline T and B cell percentage and absolute count, QUIG values, repeat T cell subset levels, and T4/T8 ratios should be checked every 3 to 6 months.
- *HIV markers.* HIV RNA viral load assays are taken at baseline and quarterly to determine disease progression and response to HAART.
- *Chemistry panel.* Serum chemistry panels should be obtained at baseline and then every 3 to 6 months if child is asymptomatic/stable; more often if a child is symptomatic or taking liver or kidney toxic agents. Serum amylase and lipase should be obtained for children taking d4T/3TC/ddI. Lipid panel and glucose should be obtained for children taking protease inhibitors.
- *Pulmonary function.* Baseline pulmonary function testing, including pulse oximetry if available, is recommended for children with lung disease.
- *HAART adherence assessment.* Adherence, toxicity, and efficacy assessments need to be done at least quarterly, including blood counts, chemistry panels, CD4 count/percentage, and HIV viral load. Some medications require additional regular monitoring.

Summary of Primary Care Needs for the Child with HIV/AIDS—cont'd

COMMON ILLNESS MANAGEMENT
Differential Diagnosis
- *Fever.* Rule out bacterial, viral, fungal infections, and OIs.
- *Respiratory distress.* Rule out LIP, PCP, other respiratory diseases and cardiac disease.
- *Otitis media.* Rule out tympanic membrane perforation.
- *Sinusitis.* Rule out bacterial sinusitis, mastoiditis, and meningitis.
- *Varicella.* Use VZIG as primary prevention and acyclovir as secondary prevention even with history of varicella vaccine.

Drug Interactions
- *HAART medications.* Determine drug interactions and adverse reactions known with each prescribed drug.
- *TMP-SMX.* Bone marrow suppression (neutropenia, thrombocytopenia) and allergic reactions may occur.
- *IVIG.* No specific drug interactions and allergic reactions are rare.

DEVELOPMENTAL ISSUES
Sleep Patterns
- Sleep patterns may be disturbed because of medications needed around the clock.

Toileting
- Impeccable perineal care is necessary to reduce morbidity of diaper dermatitis. Caretakers should use gloves for blood or diarrhea. Neurologic deterioration can lead to incontinence.

Discipline
- Discipline is often difficult for the family; help caregivers to develop appropriate expectations of the child.
- Lifestyle issues can exacerbate problems.

Child Care
- Participation in child care and preschool increases the risk of infections. The child care program should be individualized to meet the child and family's needs.
- IDEA 2004 and the Lanterman Act cover early intervention services; all babies born to infected mothers are potentially at risk and qualify for services until the age of 3.
- Head Start is mandated to enroll children with HIV.
- Child care personnel need education on condition, infection control, and medications.

Schooling
- Public Law 101-476 aids public school attendance.
- There is no duty to inform school officials of a child's HIV status.
- The school community may benefit from education.
- Children are allowed to engage in contact sports.
- Teens may need extra support from the school nurse or counselor.

Sexuality
- Children, adolescents, and families need to understand sexual and perinatal transmission risks.
- Safer sex techniques and the use of condoms and dental dams should be demonstrated on a regular basis.

Transition to Adulthood
- With improved treatment, HIV disease has become a chronic condition.
- Parents may have died from HIV while child was very young.
- Individuals must be educated about the possible transmission of HIV to others.
- Care and attention needs to be given to preparing the adolescent for transition to adult HIV care.

FAMILY CONCERNS
- HIV infection may be present in multiple family members.
- Many families lack adequate social resources and support systems.
- HIV is an enormous physical and emotional burden.
- Stigmatization continues as a major issue.
- Many children with HIV are placed in foster or adoptive homes.
- Counseling regarding death, dying, and bereavement is helpful.
- Many children with HIV are of color; care providers must be sensitive to specific cultural issues.

REFERENCES

American Academy of Pediatrics (AAP). (1999). Issues related to human immunodeficiency virus transmission in schools, child care, medical settings, the home and community. Committee of Pediatric AIDS and Committee on Infectious Diseases. *Pediatrics, 104*(2), 318-324.

American Academy of Pediatrics (AAP). (2008). HIV testing and prophylaxis to prevent mother-to-child transmission in the United States. *Pediatrics, 122*(5), 1127-1134.

Andiman, W.A., & Shearer, W.T. (1998). Lymphoid interstitial pneumonitis. In P.A. Pizzo & C.M Wilfert (Eds.), *Pediatric AIDS: The challenge of HIV Infection in Infants, Children and Adolescents* (3rd ed.). Baltimore: Williams & Wilkins.

Arpadi, S.M. (2000). Growth failure in children with HIV infection. *J Acquir Immune Defic Syndr, 15*(Suppl 1), S37-S42.

Berman, D., Mafut, D., Djokic, B., et al. (2007). Risk factors for the development of bronchiectasis in HIV-infected children. *Pediatr Pulmonol, 42*:871-875.

Bolton, M., Van der Straten, A., & Cohen, C. (2008). Probiotics: Potential to prevent HIV and sexually transmitted infections in women. *Sex Transm Dis, 35*(3), 214-225.

Calis., J., Van Hensbroek, M., De Haan, R., et al. (2008). HIV-associated anemia in children: A systematic review from a global perspective. *AIDS, 22*(10), 1099-1112.

Centers for Disease Control and Prevention. (1994). 1994 revised classification system for human immunodeficiency virus infection in children less than 13 years of age. *MMWR Morb Mortal Wkly Rep, 43*(RR-12), 1-10.

Centers for Disease Control and Prevention. (1999). *HIV and its transmission.* Available at www.cdc.gov/hiv/resources/factsheets/PDF/transmission.pdf. Retrieved January 28, 2009.

Centers for Disease Control and Prevention. (2004). Treating opportunistic infections among HIV-exposed and infected children. *MMWR Morb Mortal Wkly Rep, 53*(RR14), 1-63.

Centers for Disease Control and Prevention. (2005). *HIV/AIDS Surveillance Report, Cases of HIV infection and AIDS in the US and dependent areas,* 2005. Vol 17, Rev. ed. Atlanta: U.S. Department of Health and Human Services, CDC, 2007, 1-54.

Centers for Disease Control and Prevention. (2006a). General recommendations on immunizations: Recommendations of the advisory committee on immunization practices (ACIP). *MMWR Morbid Mortal Wkly Rep, 55*(RR15), 1-48.

Centers for Disease Control and Prevention. (2006b). *HIV/AIDS Surveillance Report, Cases of HIV infection and AIDS in the US and dependent areas*, 2006. Vol. 18. Atlanta: U.S. Department of Health and Human Services, CDC. 2007, 1-55.

Centers for Disease Control and Prevention. (2007b). Prevention of varicella: Recommendations of the Advisory Committee on Immunization Practices (ACIP). *MMWR Morbid Mortal Wkly Rep, 56*(RR04), 1-40.

Centers for Disease Control and Prevention. (2007b). Prevention and control of influenza: Recommendations of the Advisory Committee on Immunization Practice (ACIP). *MMWR Morbid Mortal Wkly Rep, 56*(RR06), 1-54.

Centers for Disease Control and Prevention. (2007c). Recommendations from the Advisory Committee on Immunization Practices (ACIP) for use of quadrivalent meningococcal conjugate vaccine (MCV4) in children aged 2-10 years at increased risk of invasive meningococcal disease. *MMWR Morbid Mortal Wkly Rep, 56*, 1265-1266.

Centers for Disease Control and Prevention. (2008a). Recommended immunization schedule for persons aged 0-18 years—United States. *MMWR Morbid Mortal Wkly Rep, 57(01)*, Q1-Q4.

Centers for Disease Control and Prevention. (2008b). Trends in HIV- and STD-related risk behaviors among high school students—United States, 1991-2007. *MMWR Morbid Mortal Wkly Rep, 57*(30), 817-822.

Centers for Disease Control and Prevention. (2008c). HIV prevention education and HIV-related policies in secondary schools—selected sites, United States, 2006. *MMWR Morbid Mortal Wkly Rep, 57*(30), 822-825.

Centers for Disease Control and Prevention. (2008d). *Guidelines for the use of antiretroviral agents in HIV-1-infected adults and adolescents.* Available at www.aidsinfo.nih.gov/ContentFiles/AdultandAdolescentGL.pdf. Retrieved November 3, 2008.

Centers for Disease Control and Prevention. (2008e). *Guidelines for the use of antiretroviral agents in pediatric HIV infection.* Available at http://aidsinfo.nih.gov/ContentFiles/PediatricGuidelines.pdf. Retrieved July 29, 2008.

Centers for Disease Control and Prevention. (2008f). *Can I get HIV from casual contact (shaking hands, hugging, using a toilet, drinking from the same glass, or the sneezing or coughing of an infected person)?* Available at www.cdc.gov/hiv/resources/qa/qa31.htm. Retrieved August, 2008.

Centers for Disease Control and Prevention. (2008g). *Guidelines for prevention and treatment of opportunistic infections among HIV-exposed and HIV-infected children.* Available at http://AIDSinfo.nih.gov. Retrieved June 20, 2008.

Centers for Disease Control and Prevention. (2008h). *U.S. Public Health Service Task Force recommendations for use of antiretroviral drugs in pregnant HIV-1-infected women for maternal health and interventions to reduce perinatal HIV-1 transmission in the United States.* Available at www.cdc.gov/mmwr/preview/mmwrhtml/rr5118a1.htm. Retrieved January 28, 2009.

Centers for Disease Control and Prevention. (2008i). Revised surveillance case definitions for HIV infection among adults, adolescents, and children ages <18 months and for HIV infection and AIDS among children aged 18 months to <13 years—United States, 2008. *MMWR Morbid Mortal Wkly Rep, 57*(RR10), 1-8.

Chabon, B., & Futterman, D. (1999). Adolescents and HIV. *AIDS Clinical Care, 11*, 1.

Chiriboga, C., Fleishman, S., & Chamion, S. (2005). Incidence and prevalence of HIV encephalopathy in children with HIV infection receiving highly active anti-retroviral therapy (HAART). *J Pediatr, 146*(3), 402-7.

Cowgill, B.O., Bogart, L.M., Corona, R., et al. (2008). Fears about HIV transmission in families with an HIV-infected parent: a qualitative analysis. *Pediatrics, 122*(5), 950-958.

Courville, T.M., Caldwell, B., & Brunell, P.A. (1998). Lack of evidence of transmission of HIV-1 to family contacts of HIV-1 infected children. *Clin Pediatr, 37*, 175-178.

Dankner, W.M., Lindsey, J.C., & Levin, M.J. (2001). The Pediatric AIDS Clinical Trials Group Protocol Teams 051, 128, 138, 144, 152, 179, 190, 220, 240, 245, 254, 300 and 327. *Pediatr Infect Dis J, 20*(1), 40-48.

Darabi, K, Omar, A., & Walter, D. (2006). Current usage of intravenous immune globulin and the rationale behind it: The Massachusetts General Hospital data and a review of the literature. *Transfusion, 46*, 741-753.

Diego, M., & Field, T. (2001). HIV adolescents show improved immune function following massage therapy. *Int J Neurosci, 106*(1/2), 35-44.

Duggan, J., Peterson, W., Schutz, M., et al. (2001). Use of complementary and alternative therapies in HIV-infected patients. *AIDS Patient Care STDS, 15*(3), 159-167.

Gray, G.E., & Saloojee, H. (2008). Breast-feeding, antiretroviral prophylaxis, and HIV. *N Engl J Med, 359*(2), 189-191.

Hall, H., Song, R., Rhodes, P., et al. (2008). Estimation of HIV incidence in the United States. *J Am Med Assn, 300*(5), 520-529.

Henry-Reid, L.M., & Martinez, J. (2008). Care of the adolescent with HIV. *Clin Obstet Gynecol, 51*(2), 319-328.

Hines, S. (2000). Primary care for HIV-exposed and infected children: translating progress into practice. *Lippincotts Prim Care Pract, 4*(1), 43-65.

Hochhauser, C.J., Gaur, S., & Marone, R., et al. (2008). The impact of environmental risk factors on HIV-associated cognitive decline in children. *AIDS Care, 20*(6), 692-699.

Kabue, M.M., Kekitiinwa, A., & Maganda, A., et al. (2008). Growth in HIV-infected children receiving antiretroviral therapy at a pediatric infectious diseases clinic in Uganda. *AIDS Patient Care STDS, 22*(3), 245-251.

Kamani, N.R., & Douglas, S.D. (1991). Structure and development of the immune system. In D.P. Sites & A.F.Terr (Eds.), *Basic and Clinical Immunology* (7th ed.). Norfolk, CT: Appleton & Lange.

Khoury, M., & Kovacs, A. (2001). Pediatric HIV infection. *Clin Obstet Gynecol, 44*(2), 243-275.

Kourtis, A., Bansil, P., Posner, S., et al. (2007). Trends in hospitalizations of HIV-infected children and adolescents in the United States: Analysis of data from the 1994-2003 nationwide inpatient sample. *Pediatrics, 120*, e236-e243.

Kumwenda, N.I., Hoover, D.R., Mofenson, L.M., et al. (2008). Extended antiretroviral prophylaxis to reduce breast-milk HIV-1 transmission. *N Engl J Med, 359*, 119-129.

Ledlie, S. (2002). The psychological issues of children with perinatally acquired HIV disease becoming adolescents: a growing challenge for providers. *AIDS Patient Care STDS, 12*(5), 231-236.

Leyes, P., Martinez, E., & Forga, M. (2008). Use of diet, nutritional supplements and exercise in HIV-infected patients receiving combination antiretroviral therapies: a systematic review. *Antiviral Therapies, 13*(2), 149-159.

Luzuriaga, K., & Sullivan, J.L. (1998a). Viral and immunopathogenesis of vertical HIV-1 infection. In P.A. Pizzo & C.M. Wilfert (Eds.), Pediatric AIDS: The Challenge of HIV Infection in Infants, Children and Adolescents (3rd ed.). Baltimore: Williams & Wilkins.

Luzuriaga, K., & Sullivan, J.L. (1998b). Prevention and treatment of pediatric HIV infection. *J Am Med Assn, 280*, 17-18.

Luzuriaga, K., & Sullivan, J.L. (2002). Pediatric HIV-1 infection: Advances and remaining challenges. *AIDS Review, 4*(1), 21-26.

MacIntyre, R.C., Holzemer, W.L., & Philippek, M. (1997). Complementary and alternative medicine and HIV-AIDS. Part I: issues and context. *J Assoc Nurses AIDS Care, 8*, 23-31.

Martin, S., Elliott-DeSorbo, D.K., & Wolters, P.L., et al. (2007). Patient, caregiver and regimen characteristics associated with adherence to highly active antiretroviral therapy among HIV-infected children and adolescents. *Pediatr Infect Dis J, 26*(1), 61-67.

McKinney, R.E., Johnson, G.M., & Stanley, K., et al. (1998). A randomized study of combined zidovudine-lamivudine versus didanosine monotherapy in children with symptomatic therapy-naïve HIV-1 infection: The Pediatric AIDS Clinical Trials Group protocol 300 study team. *J Pediatr, 133*, 500-508.

Miller, T.L., & Garg, S. (1998). Gastrointestinal and nutritional problems in pediatric HIV disease. In P.A. Pizzo & C.M. Wilfert (Eds.), *Pediatric AIDS: The Challenge of HIV Infection in Infants, Children and Adolescents* (3rd ed.). Baltimore: Williams & Wilkins.

Miller, T.L., Grant, Y.T., & Almeida, D.N., et al. (2008). Cardiometabolic disease in human immunodeficiency virus-infected children. *J Cardiometab Syndr, 3*(2), 98-105.

Narr-King, S., Montepiedra, G., & Nichols, S., et al. (2008). Allocation of family responsibility for illness management in pediatric HIV. *J Pediatr Psychol*, June 27 (epub ahead of print).

Palumbo, P.E. (2000). Antiretroviral therapy of HIV infection in children. *Pediatr Clin North Am, 47*(1), 155-169.

Patel, K., Hernan, M., & Williams, P., et al. (2008). Long term effectiveness of the highly active antiretroviral therapy on survival of children and adolescents with HIV infection: A 10 year follow-up study. *Clin Infect Dis, 46*(4), 507-515.

Pearson, D.A., McGrath, N.M., & Nozyce, M., et al. (2000). Predicting HIV disease progression in children using measures of neuropsychological and neurological functioning. Pediatric AIDS clinical trials 152-study team. *Pediatrics, 106*(6), E76.

Perez Mato, S., & Van Dyke, R.B. (2002). Pulmonary infections in children with HIV infection. *Semin Respir Infect, 17*(1), 33-46.

Pizzo, P.A., & Wilfert, C.M.(Eds.). (1998). *Pediatric AIDS: The Challenge of HIV Infection in Infants, Children and Adolescents* (3rd ed.). Baltimore: Williams & Wilkins.

Ramos-Gomez, F.J. (1997). Oral aspects of HIV infection in children. *Oral Disease*(Suppl 1), S31-S35.

Read, J.S., The Committee on Pediatric AIDS. (2007). Diagnosis of HIV-1 Infection in children younger than 18 months in the United States. *Pediatrics, 120*(6), 1547-1561.

Rosen, D., Blum, R., & Britto, M. (2003). Society for Adolescent Medicine: Transition to adult health care for adolescents and young adults with chronic conditions: Position paper of the Society for Adolescent Medicine. *J Adolesc Health 33*(4), 309-311.

Rudin, D., Burri, M., Shen, Y., et al. (2008). Long-term safety and effectiveness of ritonavir, nelfinavir, and lopinavir/ritonavir in antiretroviral-experienced HIV-infected children. *Pediatr Infect Dis J, 27*(5), 431-437.

Saitoh, A., Hsia, K., & Fenton, T. (2002). Persistence of human immunodeficiency virus (HIV) type 1 DNA in peripheral blood despite prolonged suppression of plasma HIV-1 RNA in children. *J Infect Dis, 185*(10), 1409-16.

Samour, P., Helm, K., & Lang, C. (2003). *Handbook of Pediatric Nutrition.* Boston: Jones and Barlett.

Simonds, R.J., & Orejas, G. (1998). *Pneumocystis carinii* pneumonia and toxoplasmosis. In P.A. Pizzo & C.M. Wilfert (Eds.), *Pediatric AIDS: The Challenge of HIV Infection in Infants, Children and Adolescents* (3rd ed.). Baltimore: Williams & Wilkins.

Smith, R., Malee, K., Leighty, R., et al. (2006). Effects of perinatal HIV infection and associated risk factors on cognitive development among young children. *Pediatrics, 117*(3), 851-862.

Spector, S.A., Gelber, R.D., McGrath, N., et al. (1994). A controlled trial of intravenous immune globulin for the prevention of serious bacterial infections in children receiving zidovudine for advanced human immunodeficiency virus infection. *N Engl J Med, 331*, 1181-1187.

Standish, L.J., Greene, K.B., Bain, S., et al. (2001). Alternative medicine use in HIV-positive men and women: demographics, utilization patterns and health status. *AIDS Care, 13*(92), 197-208.

Stiehm, E.R., Lambert, J.S., Mofenson, L.M., et al. (1999). Efficacy of zidovudine and human immunodeficiency virus (HIV) hyperimmune immunoglobulin for reducing perinatal HIV transmission from HIV-infected women with advanced disease: results of pediatric AIDS clinical trials group protocol 185. *J Infect Dis, 179*(3), 567-575.

UNAIDS (2008). *2008 Report on the Global AIDS Epidemic: Executive Summary.* Available at: www.unaids.org/en/KnowledgeCentre/HIVData/ GlobalReport/2008. Retrieved July 29, 2008.

Vreeman, R.C., Wiehe, S.E., Pearce, E.C., et al. (2008). A systematic review of pediatric adherence to antiretroviral therapy in low- and middle-income countries. *Pediatr Infect Dis J, 27*(8), 686-691.

Walsh, T.J., & Butler, K.M. (1998). Fungal infections in children with HIV. In P.A. Pizzo & C.M. Wilfert (Eds.), *Pediatric AIDS: The Challenge of HIV Infection in Infants, Children and Adolescents*, (3rd ed.). Baltimore: Williams & Wilkins.

Willen, E. (2006). Neurocognitive outcomes in pediatric HIV. *Ment Retard. Dev Disabil Res Rev, 12*, 223-228.

Williams, P.L., Storm, D., and Montepiedra, G., et al. (2006). Predictors of adherence to antiretroviral medications in children and adolescents with HIV infection. *Pediatrics, 118*(6), e1745-e1757.

Wood, L.V. (1998). Immunomodulation and immune reconstitution. In P.A. Pizzo & C.M. Wilfert (Eds.), *Pediatric AIDS: The Challenge of HIV Infection in Infants, Children and Adolescents*, (3rd ed.). Baltimore: Williams & Wilkins.

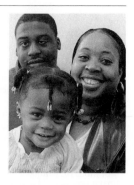

29 Hydrocephalus

Lisa V. Duffy

Etiology

Cerebrospinal fluid (CSF) is a clear fluid that circulates through the ventricles of the brain, around the spinal cord, and in the subarachnoid space. CSF functions as a shock absorber to protect the brain and spinal cord. CSF is continuously produced by the choroid plexus within the lateral, third, and fourth ventricles and as a by-product of cerebral and spinal cord metabolism. CSF forms at a rate of approximately 0.35 to 0.4 ml/min or 500 ml/day in adults and children (Johnston, 2003). The rate of CSF production is relatively constant among individuals and within the same individual over time. Premature and small infants do produce less CSF than adults, but these differences are negligible after about 1 year of age (Albright, Pollack, & Adelson, 2008). Under normal circumstances, an equal amount of CSF is absorbed from the subarachnoid space into the venous system by projections called *arachnoid villi*. To reach the subarachnoid space and villi, CSF passes through a series of channels and pathways propelled by pulsations of the choroid plexus (Figure 29-1). From the lateral ventricles, CSF flows into the third ventricle via the foramen of Monro. It then passes from the third ventricle into the fourth ventricle through the aqueduct of Sylvius and exits the fourth ventricle through either the lateral foramina of Luschka or the foramen of Magendie. CSF exits the ventricular system and travels around the brainstem and spinal cord and over the surface of the brain, where it is absorbed by the arachnoid villi. Alternate pathways for CSF absorption may come into play when ICP is increased. CSF may travel into the paranasal sinuses and lymphatics, as well as along the cranial or spinal nerves, before absorption into the systemic circulation (Rekate, 2008).

Hydrocephalus is a condition that results from an imbalance between the production and absorption of cerebrospinal fluid (CSF), leading to an increase in the volume of intracranial CSF, enlargement of the ventricular system, and possible increased intracranial pressure (ICP). Hydrocephalus is most commonly caused by an obstruction in the normal circulation and absorption of CSF.

Hydrocephalus is classified as either noncommunicating or communicating (Box 29-1). Noncommunicating hydrocephalus is characterized by failure of CSF to flow through its normal pathways from one ventricle to another or from the ventricles to the subarachnoid cisterns. CSF, therefore, does not reach the arachnoid villi where it would normally be absorbed. This results in an enlargement of the ventricles proximal to the site of the obstruction. An example of non-communicating hydrocephalus would be an obstruction of the aqueduct of Sylvius in which the lateral and third ventricles are enlarged but the fourth ventricle is normal

sized. Non-communicating hydrocephalus can be further classified as congenital or acquired. Conditions that occur congenitally include Chiari malformation, aqueductal stenosis, Dandy-Walker malformation, X-linked hydrocephalus, arachnoid cysts, tumors, and vascular malformations (Nielson, Pearce, Limbacher et al., 2007). Noncommunicating hydrocephalus can also be acquired through a head injury, tumor, cyst, or gliosis resulting from hemorrhage or infection (Nielson et al.).

Aqueductal stenosis causes obstruction of the flow of CSF through the aqueduct of Sylvius and is the most common form of non-communicating hydrocephalus. X-linked hydrocephalus occurs as a result of stenosis of the aqueduct of Sylvius (Panay, Gokhale, Mansour et al., 2005). The incidence is approximately 1 in every 30,000 live male births. Although congenital hydrocephalus is an X-linked disorder, female carriers may be mildly affected (Panay et al.). X-linked hydrocephalus with associated stenosis of the aqueduct of Sylvius is caused by mutations in the gene for neural cell adhesion molecule, *L1CAM*. The *L1CAM* gene is located at the chromosomal region Xq28 (Cinalli, Maixner, Sainte-Rose et al., 2004). Couples with one previous child with hydrocephalus have a recurrence risk of 4% for male births and 2% for female births (Cinalli et al.). Primary care practitioners should recommend genetic counseling to couples with one child with hydrocephalus before they attempt to conceive a second child. Those couples who have conceived should be offered prenatal diagnosis in the second trimester for all subsequent pregnancies.

Communicating hydrocephalus occurs when CSF flows freely through the normal pathways but cannot be absorbed through the subarachnoid spaces, the basal cisterns, or the arachnoid villi. Common causes of communicating hydrocephalus are meningitis, intrauterine infection, intraventricular hemorrhage, trauma, or congenital malformation of the subarachnoid spaces. Rarely, communicating hydrocephalus may be related to an overproduction of CSF, which occurs as a result of a choroid plexus papilloma or carcinoma (Nielson et al., 2007). Choroid plexus papillomas can produce excessive volumes of CSF (von Koch, Gupta, Sutton et al., 2003). This overproduction of CSF may result in hydrocephalus and ventricular enlargement that can be successfully treated by removing the intraventricular tumor (Cinalli et al., 2004).

Incidence and Prevalence

Hydrocephalus is the most frequent neurosurgical problem encountered in the pediatric age group. Its estimated incidence rate is 1 in 500 live births; in half of these cases a diagnosis of congenital hydrocephalus will be made (National Hydrocephalus Foundation [NHF], 2007). Hydrocephalus is often associated with neural

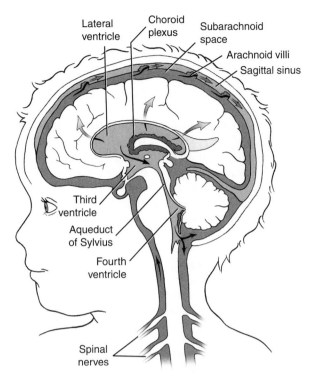

FIGURE 29-1 CSF circulatory pathway showing a view of the center of the brain. Solid arrows show the major pathway of CSF flow; broken arrows show additional pathways. (Illustration © Lynne Larson 1986-2009. Reprinted with permission.)

BOX 29-1

Classification of Hydrocephalus

NONCOMMUNICATING
Congenital
- Chiari malformation
- Aqueductal stenosis
- Dandy-Walker malformation
- X-linked hydrocephalus
- Arachnoid cysts
- Tumors
- Vascular malformations

Acquired
- Head injury
- Tumor
- Cyst
- Gliosis resulting from hemorrhage or infection

COMMUNICATING
- Meningitis
- Intrauterine infection
- Intraventricular hemorrhage
- Trauma
- Congenital malformation of the subarachnoid spaces
- Overproduction of CSF

Data from Nielson, N., Pearce, K., Limbacher, E., et al. (2007). Hydrocephalus. In C.C. Cartwright & D.C. Wallace (Eds.), *Nursing Care of the Pediatric Neurosurgery Patient.* New York: Springer.

---

tube defects, and 70% to 90% of children with a diagnosis of spina bifida will also have hydrocephalus (NHF). It is also a common complication of virtually any insult to a child's nervous system, including intraventricular hemorrhage, brain tumors, infections, and head injury (see Chapters 39 and 42). CSF shunting procedures comprise roughly half of most modern pediatric neurosurgical practices (McLone, 2001).

Accurate prevalence rates for hydrocephalus are difficult, if not impossible, to obtain because reporting is based on the *International Classification of Diseases,* 9th Revision (ICD-9) and *Current Procedural Terminology* (CPT) codes. These codes reflect an overall diagnosis that may *not* be hydrocephalus; an example is the diagnosis of a brain tumor resulting in hydrocephalus that may or may not need shunting. Although current statistics are not available to indicate the exact number of cases of hydrocephalus, shunting procedures account for approximately $100 million in health care spending each year in the United States alone (NHF, 2007). Each year in the United States, approximately 36,000 new shunts are placed and 14,000 shunt revisions are performed (Rekate, 2008).

Diagnostic Criteria

Neuroimaging of the brain is essential for the diagnosis and management of hydrocephalus. The three major imaging modalities include ultrasonography, computed tomography (CT) scanning, and magnetic resonance imaging (MRI). Ultrasonography is possible in infants only while the anterior fontanelle is open. CT scans are most commonly obtained if acute hydrocephalus or shunt malfunction is suspected. However, multiple CT scans raise concern about the amount of radiation exposure of children with hydrocephalus. Currently discussion at some pediatric institutions centers on whether MRI would be beneficial in evaluating ventricle size when shunt malfunction is suspected. MRI is also useful in determining the success of endoscopic third ventriculostomy (ETV) in restoring CSF circulation.

Clinical Manifestations at Time of Diagnosis
Clinical Manifestations in Infancy

Rapidly increasing head circumference in the premature or term infant should strongly suggest the diagnosis of hydrocephalus. Normal head circumference at birth is 33 to 38 cm. During the first few weeks of life, a newborn may have enlarged ventricles without exhibiting an increase in head size or signs and symptoms of increased ICP (Volpe, 2008). This is because the infant skull and sutures can expand to accommodate increasing ventricular size, thereby minimizing an elevation in ICP. If the accumulation of excessive CSF occurs slowly, an infant or young child may be asymptomatic until the hydrocephalus is advanced. A newborn with a head circumference greater than the 95th percentile should be evaluated promptly for hydrocephalus. In a newborn with suspected hydrocephalus, the head circumference should be measured at least daily with rapid increases evaluated by ultrasonography. Other associated findings in the infant include bulging of the anterior fontanelle and splitting of the cranial sutures. The skin over the skull can appear shiny with distention of the scalp veins. The setting-sun phenomenon (persistent downward gaze), coupled with an infant's inability to look up, is attributed to dysfunction of the tectal plate. Although rare, infants also present with papilledema, poor feeding, vomiting, drowsiness, irritability, apnea, bradycardia, and seizures (American Association of Neurological Surgeons [AANS], 2005) (see Clinical Manifestations box).

Clinical Manifestations in Children

Hydrocephalus in children beyond infancy is usually associated with a neoplasm, a mass secondary to obstruction of the flow of CSF, or history of traumatic brain injury (see Chapter 42). The ability of the brain to compensate for intracranial hypertension is limited if the sutures are closed. Macrocephaly is not necessarily a component of the presentation in older children. For this reason, the presentation of hydrocephalus in older children is typically acute. The classic history involves rapid onset of headache that is most pronounced in the morning, vomiting, and alterations of consciousness. Seizures may be a presenting symptom.

Children with acquired hydrocephalus may present with less acute symptoms of hydrocephalus, including blurred or double vision, fever, ataxia, irritability, lethargy, developmental delays, poor coordination, changes in personality, an inability to concentrate, or poor appetite (AANS, 2005).

Treatment

The ultimate goal of treatment of hydrocephalus is to prevent or reverse the neurologic damage caused by distortion of the brain from increased ICP and accumulation of CSF. Intermediate goals include allowing the actual brain tissue volume to increase and reconstitution of the mantle. Secondary goals of treatment include the prevention of complications and the avoidance of shunt dependency if possible (Albright et al., 2008).

Clinical Manifestations at Time of Diagnosis

Manifestations are determined by degree of hydrocephalus, degree of increased ICP, and etiology.

ASSOCIATED SYMPTOMS
Infants
- Macrocephaly
- Bulging fontanelle
- Split cranial sutures
- Distention of scalp veins
- Setting-sun phenomenon
- Ophthalmoplegia
- Papilledema
- Poor feeding
- Vomiting
- Drowsiness
- Irritability
- Apnea
- Bradycardia
- Seizures

Children >18 months
Acute onset
- Headache
- Vomiting
- Alteration in level of consciousness
- Seizures
Chronic onset
- Blurred or double vision
- Fever
- Ataxia
- Irritability
- Lethargy
- Developmental delays
- Poor coordination
- Changes in personality
- Inability to concentrate
- Decreased appetite

Data from American Association of Neurological Surgeons. (2005). *What is hydrocephalus?* Available at www.neurosurgerytoday.org. Retrieved December 18, 2007.

Treatment

Treatment is determined by the cause. The goal is to restore CSF flow by removing the obstruction or creating a new pathway.
- Pharmacologic treatment
  - Furosemide (Lasix)
  - Acetazolamide (Diamox)
- Surgical treatment
  - Ventriculoperitoneal
  - Ventriculoatrial
  - Ventriculopleural
  - Complications of surgical treatment
    - Shunt failure
    - Shunt infection
      - External ventricular drainage
      - Prophylactic antibiotics
- Neuroendoscopy
- Spontaneously resolving hydrocephalus

Pharmacologic Treatment

Drugs that reduce CSF formation have been used to delay or avoid shunting. Furosemide interferes with chloride transport in the apical cells of the choroid plexus and has decreased CSF production in animal models by as much as 50% to 60% (Matthews, 2008). Acetazolamide decreases the production of CSF by inhibiting carbonic anhydrase, thereby preventing sodium ions from crossing the choroids plexus (Matthews). The combination of these two drugs can decrease CSF production by as much as 75% of its original volume. These two modalities have been useful as temporizing measures but have been abandoned as treatment of chronic hydrocephalus. Randomized controlled trials have demonstrated that furosemide and acetazolamide do not decrease the need for shunt placement and are ineffective in preventing hydrocephalus in children with posthemorrhagic hydrocephalus (DelBigio, 2004; Poca & Sahuquillo, 2005).

Surgical Treatment

Surgical treatment for hydrocephalus is directed at restoring CSF flow by either removing the obstruction to CSF flow or creating a new CSF pathway. In most cases, the obstruction to CSF flow cannot be effectively or safely removed; therefore, surgical shunting is required. Shunting involves placement of a ventricular catheter or shunt to divert CSF flow to another body cavity where it can be absorbed. The peritoneal cavity is the preferred location and most commonly used. If the peritoneal cavity is not appropriate for placement of the distal tubing—either because of abdominal malformation, postsurgical adhesions, infection, or inadequate absorption—the shunt may be placed in the atrium of the heart (i.e., ventriculoatrial [VA] shunt) or the pleural space (i.e., ventriculopleural [VP] shunt). The distal portion is tunneled under the child's skin to the designated location, where a small incision is made and the shunt is inserted either through the peritoneum into the peritoneal cavity (i.e., VP shunt) or through the neck into the superior vena cava and into the right atrium (i.e., VA shunt)

(Figure 29-2). The distal end of the VP shunt is guided subcutaneously to an area just below the nipple, where an incision is made and the tube is inserted into the pleural space.

CSF shunts regulate flow by means of a one-way valve. Valves can be grouped into four general design categories: differential pressure valves, siphon-resisting valves, flow-regulating valves, and adjustable valves (Anderson, Garton, & Kestle, 2008). Differential pressure valves are considered "standard" valves that have been used for decades; these valves simply open or close depending on the pressure across them. The pressure at which they open is termed the *opening pressure;* typically designations of low, medium, and high correspond to 5, 10, and 15 cm of H_2O pressure (Anderson et al.). With siphon-resisting valves, flow of CSF through the valve is dependent on the position of the child. Flow-regulating valves have three flow stages to help regulate the flow of CSF if the ICP becomes elevated. Finally, adjustable valves are becoming more popular because the neurosurgeon is able to externally adjust the pressure of the valve according to the clinical assessment of the child (Anderson et al.) No single type of shunt is superior over another. The choice of shunt type is the preference of the neurosurgeon based on training and personal experience. No data exist to support a recommendation of one particular shunt design over another.

The reservoir and tubing for the shunt are palpable from the burr hole in the skull to the tube's insertion at either the abdomen or chest. Identification of and access to the shunt reservoir are important in evaluating shunt infection and/or malfunction. The reservoir should be easy to depress and should rebound readily when released. A small 25-gauge needle can be inserted into the reservoir

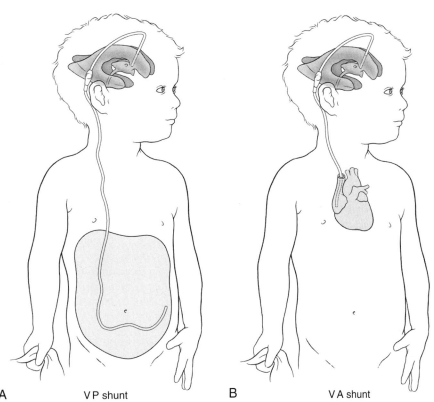

FIGURE 29-2 Pathway used for **A,** ventriculoperitoneal shunt and, **B,** ventriculoatrial shunt. (Illustration © Lynne Larson 1986-2009. Reprinted with permission.)

A   V P shunt   B   V A shunt

to collect CSF for culture, to obtain ICP readings, or to inject radio-isotopes for shunt-flow studies (Nielson et al., 2007).

Complications of Surgical Treatment

Shunt failure. Although CSF shunting has dramatically improved the prognosis for children with hydrocephalus, shunts still have inherent problems. Shunt mechanical complications may occur at any time from immediately after shunt placement to years later. Forty percent to 50% of shunts malfunction within the first 2 years after initial shunt placement (Browd, Gottfried, Ragel, et al., 2006). The incidence of mechanical shunt malfunction is approximately 30% over 1 year. Shunt occlusion is the most common shunt complication in the pediatric population; approximately 90% of these shunt occlusions occur at the site of the ventricular catheter (Grinsberg & Drake, 2004). Shunt revisions are necessary at some time in almost all children who have shunted hydrocephalus. Shunt obstruction may occur as a result of chronic or acute inflammation, overgrowth of the choroid plexus, accumulation of cellular debris or blood, or occlusion of either the distal or proximal end of the shunt as a result of the child's growth. Repeated shunt failure requiring multiple revisions is a problem for some children; it has been hypothesized that age, etiology, and interval between malfunctions may predict whether a child will require multiple shunt revisions over the course of his or her lifetime (Daszkiewicz & Barszcz, 2007). The primary pathology that resulted in hydrocephalus in these children elicits a reactive inflammatory process that is perpetuated by repeat shunt procedures.

CT and MRI studies are used to evaluate shunt failure and the need for shunt revision. These scans must be compared with prior imaging studies and reviewed in conjunction with clinical findings of probable shunt failure, as assessed by an experienced clinician. In some cases, ventricular enlargement is noted only when the latest imaging is compared with prior studies. CT imaging may not show increased ventricle size in every child with a possible shunt malfunction. Therefore, a shunt series should be obtained to identify any areas of disconnection along the shunt tract (Pitetti, 2007). A shunt series consists of a lateral radiograph of the skull, neck, chest, and abdomen to ascertain the location and continuity of the shunt apparatus. Primary care providers must remember that negative or stable CT scan findings do not rule out shunt malfunction.

Other diagnostic tools to evaluate shunt function include radionuclide CSF shunt studies, shunt tap for CSF for culture, and ICP monitoring. A measurement of ICP can be obtained either intermittently via the shunt reservoir or by placement of an ICP monitor. Keeping in mind the morbidity associated with delayed diagnosis of a shunt malfunction, primary care providers must have a low threshold for ordering a CT scan or referring a child to a neurosurgeon when symptoms of increased ICP or shunt infection are apparent.

Shunt infection. The incidence of shunt infections has decreased significantly over the past decade but continues to be a major source of shunt malfunction and potential morbidity. Most shunt infections are diagnosed within the first few months after surgery, supporting a basic premise of direct contamination at the time of surgery (Mukhida, Sharma, & Shilpakar, 2004). As a foreign body, the implanted shunt creates a medium in the host where normal phagocytosis is impaired, allowing a child to be susceptible to infection of the shunt and CSF. There seems to be consensus that very young children have a higher incidence of shunt infection than older individuals. This is important since it has been noted that

shunt infections that occur within the first year of life predispose children to cognitive problems in the future (Rekate, 2008). Risk factors for shunt infections have been identified as age of the child at shunt insertion, experience of surgeon, prematurity, or the underlying cause of hydrocephalus (Vinchon & Dhellemmes, 2006). A shunt infection is identified when a bacterial pathogen or pathogens are isolated from ventricular CSF. Although shunt infections have been as high as 40% in the past three decades, most recent studies have reported shunt infection rates at 8% (Rekate, 2008).

More than two thirds of all bacterial shunt infections are caused by staphylococcal species, with coagulase-negative *Staphylococcus* isolated in 60% of all infections and *S. aureus* the next most common organism, occurring in 18% (Campbell, 2008). Anaerobic organisms, such as *Propionibacterium acnes,* are responsible for 10% of shunt infections. Gram-negative enteric organisms, usually *Escherichia coli* and *Pseudomonas* are responsible for 6% of infections. Gram-positive organisms, like *Streptococcus,* are identified in approximately 6% of shunt infections (Campbell). Although shunt malfunction has not been associated with cognitive deficits, shunt infections—especially resulting from gram-negative organisms—can have significant detrimental effects on cognition in the host.

The treatment of shunt infections varies among neurosurgeons. The most popular treatment strategies for the management of shunt infections involve surgical removal of the infected shunt followed by a period of external drainage until CSF cultures are sterile, and finally surgical replacement of a new shunt (Simpkins, 2005; Turgut, Alabaz, Erbey, et al., 2005). Other treatment methods that involve antibiotic therapy only or the immediate removal and replacement of the shunt during the same surgery are seldom used.

Prevention of shunt infections is the key to improving outcomes in children with shunted hydrocephalus and in decreasing the cost of their care. The one approach to prevention of postoperative shunt infections that has been sufficiently studied and proven to reduce shunt infections in the adult population is the use of prophylactic intraventricular antibiotics including gentamycin and vancomycin (Ragel, Browd, & Schmidt, 2006). This practice is gaining popularity in the pediatric population as well. Many surgeons now use perioperative intraventricular vancomycin in addition to systemic antibiotics such as cefazolin (Campbell, 2008). Further research efforts in this area are needed to gain evidence to support techniques helpful in decreasing the incidence of shunt infection.

Neuroendoscopy

A significant development in pediatric neurosurgery during the past decade has been the evolution of neuroendoscopy and its application to the management of childhood hydrocephalus. Before this evolution, the standard treatment for all types of hydrocephalus was the implantation of ventriculoextracranial shunts. Although many children were spared the devastating effects of uncontrolled hydrocephalus with these shunt systems, a variety of problems emerged that prompted continued refinement of shunt systems or alternative therapies with similar if not superior results (McLone, 2001).

A decade ago few pediatric neurosurgical centers in the world offered endoscopic third ventriculostomy (ETV) as an alternative to shunting for obstructive hydrocephalus. Today, however, few major centers in the United States are without a neurosurgeon skilled in this procedure. ETV is now recommended by some centers as the preferred method of treatment for children with aqueductal stenosis (de Ribaupierre, Riliet, Vernet, et al., 2007). The procedure was first described by Dandy in 1922 but was not widely practiced because of the many complications and unacceptable failure rates (Hellwig, Grotenhuis, Tirakotai, et al., 2005). The renewed enthusiasm for this surgical procedure arises from the expectation that approximately half or more of appropriately selected individuals may remain or become shunt free. Previous studies have indicated that ETV may have lower success rates for hydrocephalus associated with myelomeningocele, infection, or hemorrhage. However, more recent studies have not replicated these findings (Kadrian, van Gelder, Florida et al., 2005). Studies have demonstrated ETV success rates between 58% and 78% at 5 years (de Ribaupierre et al., 2007; Kadrian et al., 2005). Furthermore, the safety of the procedure compared with approaches used in the past has greatly increased related to the availability of high-quality endoscopes, light sources, camera equipment, and instrumentation. The ability to visualize the oscillatory flow of CSF, as well as obstruction in the ventricular system through MRI has improved selection as well as preoperative and postoperative monitoring of children. Evidence suggests that children younger than 6 months of age may not benefit from this procedure (Kadrian et al). The arachnoid villi in these infants may not be mature enough to successfully absorb CSF, and premature closure of the ventriculostoma may occur (Wagner & Koch, 2005).

Spontaneously Resolving Hydrocephalus

Children with communicating hydrocephalus occasionally outgrow the need for a shunt. Alternative pathways for absorption are thought to be established as a result of persistent increased ICP, thereby compensating for the diminished absorption from the arachnoid villi. This compensated or resolved hydrocephalus usually occurs during the first year of life, although it may not be identified until later when lengthening of the shunt appears necessary as a result of growth. Compensated hydrocephalus is accompanied by stable ventricular size despite documented shunt obstruction. Shunt failure may be verified by the absence of flow after injection of a radioisotope into the shunt reservoir (i.e., shunt function study) or by radiologic confirmation of shunt disconnection (i.e., radiographic shunt series) or, where available, an MRI CSF flow study. When it is determined that the child is no longer shunt dependent, the shunt is left in place unless the risk of infection is high. The child is monitored by periodic CT scans and neuropsychological examinations. Annual neuropsychological testing is recommended because intellectual deterioration has been associated with arrested hydrocephalus (Iborra, Pages, Cuxart, et al., 2000).

Complementary and Alternative Treatments

No evidence is available in the current literature regarding complementary or alternative treatment of hydrocephalus.

Anticipated Advances in Diagnosis and Management

Fetal shunting was first performed in the early 1980s with the hope that early intervention would improve the outcome for children with fetal hydrocephalus. Unfortunately, knowledge about the natural history and outcome of the fetus with hydrocephalus was limited. Imaging compared with today's techniques was suboptimal and other brain anomalies were missed at the time of diagnosis and fetal shunting. Theoretically, fetal shunting would be most beneficial in cases of isolated hydrocephalus and therefore, a moratorium on fetal surgery was initiated. Because of today's improved diagnostics and surgical techniques, there may now be a place for fetal shunting. The key to positive outcomes will depend on careful selection of the appropriate fetus (Harrison, 2001).

Advances in obstetric and neonatal intensive care have decreased the incidence of hydrocephalus as a result of intraventricular hemorrhage and meningitis. In addition, nutritional guidelines recommending supplementation of folic acid in women of childbearing age have lowered the incidence of hydrocephalus by decreasing the number of children born with myelomeningocele and other neural tube defects.

Neural tube defects may be identified by fetal ultrasound and elevated levels of maternal alpha-fetoprotein (AFP). Prenatal evaluation (i.e., including high-resolution ultrasound scanning and measures of AFP) has increased the number of fetal anomalies identified. Assessment for other congenital anomalies and follow-up ultrasound scans to detect progressive ventricular enlargement are essential when counseling families. If severe brain dysfunction or other congenital anomalies are suspected, parents may decide to terminate the pregnancy; otherwise pregnancy can be continued as close to term as possible and a shunt or ventricular access device placed soon after birth.

Neuroendoscopic treatment of children with hydrocephalus is now an established surgical modality. Open MRI technology introduces new imaging features that, in combination with endoscopy, seem particularly valuable for performing these operations. "Near" real-time production of MR images in three dimensions during the procedure allows real-time neuronavigation, thus facilitating guidance of an endoscope.

The use of programmable shunts has increased over the past decade. The programmable shunt system was designed to relieve underdrainage and overdrainage problems in hydrocephalus. Slit ventricle syndrome and nonhemorrhagic postshunting subdural collections are examples of overdrainage problems for which the programmable shunt is now being used successfully (Andersson, Persson, Aring, et al., 2008). The system allows a neurosurgeon to adjust the opening pressure of the CSF by using an external device, decreasing the need for an operation to be performed to revise the shunt. The CODMAN® HAKIM® valve (Johnson & Johnson Co., Raynham, MA) is one example of a programmable valve that can be adjusted to 3 to 20 cm H_2O (Grinsberg & Drake, 2004). A newer programmable valve, the Medtronic Strata (Medtronic, Inc., Minneapolis, MN), has the added benefits of not requiring an x-ray film to confirm the pressure setting and has an antisiphon device (Ahn, Bookland, Carson et al., 2006). These programmable shunts have been useful in reducing the need for shunt revision for headache (Kay, Fisher, O'Kane, et al., 2002). Programmable shunts are sensitive to magnets; therefore the primary care practitioner must notify the child's primary neurosurgeon when ordering a diagnostic MRI study.

Associated Problems of Hydrocephalus and Treatment
Intellectual Deficits

Intellectual function is difficult to predict early after diagnosis of hydrocephalus. Some infants with severe hydrocephalus and virtually no cortical mantle visible on the initial imaging studies have experienced normal growth and development. Serial imaging studies of infants with hydrocephalus often show dramatic reconstitution of the brain over time, and the mechanism of this process remains a topic of active investigation (Harrison, Evans, Adzick et al., 2001). Although the precise nature of the neuropsychological deficits in hydrocephalus are not completely known, several factors such as etiology, raised ICP, ventricular size, and timing of diagnosis and treatment initiation have been shown to influence cognition (Futagi, Suzuki, Toribe et al., 2002). In a study by Lindquist, Carlsson, Persson and colleagues (2005), approximately 33% of the children with hydrocephalus had intelligence quotients (IQs) in the normal range (above 85); 33% had mild to moderate mental retardation (IQs 70 to 84); and 33% had severe retardation (IQs <70). An increased risk of mental retardation has been associated with gestational age at birth and the presence of hydrocephalus at birth (Lindquist et al.). The younger the individual is when hydrocephalus is diagnosed, the greater the risk for intellectual impairment. Children in whom hydrocephalus is diagnosed in utero have the poorest outcome intellectually. Children with certain comorbid conditions associated with hydrocephalus, including cerebral palsy and epilepsy, also tend to have lower intellectual function (Lindquist et al.). Children with hydrocephalus also have been found to have difficulty with reading comprehension. Specifically, these children have problems identifying irrelevant meanings in text and often cannot use an earlier sentence to help them determine the larger meaning of the passage (Barnes, Faulkner, Wilkinson, et al., 2004).

Associated Problems of Hydrocephalus and Treatment
- Intellectual deficits
- Ocular abnormalities
- Motor disabilities
- Seizures

Children and young adults with spina bifida and hydrocephalus are at greater risk for cognitive deficits than those who have hydrocephalus without spina bifida (see Chapter 35). This combination of problems causes significant dysmorphology of the cerebellum. As a result, these children and young adults have more motor and speech deficits than those individuals without spina bifida and hydrocephalus (Huber-Okrainec, Dennis, Brettschneider, et al., 2002). Children with spina bifida and shunted hydrocephalus were shown to have deficits in working memory and processed information more slowly than their healthy counterparts (Boyer, Yeates, & Enrile, 2006). Children with spina bifida and hydrocephalus who are walking tend to have higher IQs compared with those who must use a wheelchair for mobility (Rendeli, Salvaggio, Sciascia-Cannizzaro, et al., 2002). This may be due in part to the necessity of spatial organization when learning new skills (Rendeli et al.).

As with most developmental measures, social risk factors also affect cognitive outcomes. The importance of both social and biologic factors in developmental outcomes must be remembered in counseling families and planning intervention strategies. Preschool and school counseling with neuropsychological evaluations must be completed early to identify areas of learning disability and resources for intervention.

Ocular Abnormalities

Ocular abnormalities are often found at the time of diagnosis or during episodes of shunt malfunction. Increased ICP results in pressure on the optic nerve, limited upward gaze, extraocular muscle paresis, and papilledema. Without prompt treatment for acute hydrocephalus or shunt malfunction, permanent visual damage is a definite risk. Before the era of successful CSF shunting, optic atrophy secondary to hydrocephalus was the leading cause of blindness from congenital malformations. Even with a functioning shunt and controlled hydrocephalus, however, visual problems are common: Seventy percent to 80% of children with hydrocephalus have visual problems, including decreased visual acuity, visual field defects, strabismus, optic atrophy, or ocular motility abnormalities (Andersson, et al., 2006; Aring, Andersson, Hard, et al., 2007). The degree of visual impairment seems to be unrelated to the cause of the hydrocephalus, number of shunt revisions, or size of ventricular dilation (Aring et al.). However, Ricci, Luciano, Baranello and colleagues (2006) found that children with grade IV intraventricular hemorrhages and those whose hydrocephalus was associated with seizures before the age of 1 year had the worst visual impairments. These children may eventually require the use of large-print and increased-contrast work materials, as well as placement of work items within their visual field. Abnormalities in vision are associated with lower intelligence scores and may help identify children at risk for cognitive delay. Correctable visual problems should be addressed as soon as possible so that poor vision does not interfere with learning potential. Children with slit ventricle syndrome are at increased risk for significant visual loss. Therefore these children require special attention and prompt treatment when increased ICP is discovered (Nguyen, Polomeno, Farmer, et al., 2002).

Motor Disabilities

Unfortunately, as many as 60% of the children with hydrocephalus have some form of motor disability (Nielson et al., 2007). These disabilities vary from severe paraplegia to mild imbalance or weakness. Delayed walking (starting to walk at 16 to 22 months) is not unusual in children with infantile hydrocephalus (Persson, Hagberg, & Uvebrant, 2006). The severity of the motor deficit is most often related to the diagnosis; conditions such as porencephaly, Dandy-Walker malformation, and myelomeningocele portend more serious motor defects than simple congenital hydrocephalus. About half of children with myelomeningocele need wheelchair assistance by adolescence (Persson et al.). Hydrocephalus also affects fine motor control. The kinesthetic-proprioceptive abilities of the hands are often negatively affected and—coupled with the impaired bimanual manipulation and frequent visual deficits—make it difficult for children with hydrocephalus to perform well on time-limited, nonverbal intelligence tests.

Seizures

Since the introduction of shunting for individuals with hydrocephalus, controversies have arisen regarding the likelihood of the development of epileptic seizures as a result of the shunting itself and/or its complications. Hydrocephalus is not commonly recognized as a cause of seizures in general, although epilepsy is reported to be frequently associated with shunt-treated hydrocephalus, especially in children. Bourgeois, Sainte-Rose, Cinalli and colleagues (2004) found that 71% of children had seizures that began after shunt placement and were difficult to control despite treatment with antiepileptic drugs.

The insult to the brain at the time of ventricular catheter insertion, the presence of the shunt tube itself as a foreign body, the burr hole location, the number of shunt revisions after malfunction, associated infection, the cause of hydrocephalus, and associated developmental delay are thought to be related to the risk of epilepsy (see Chapter 26). Age at the time of initial shunt placement also seems to be an important factor. Early shunting is a well-known determinant of risk in shunt obstruction, and children younger than 2 years old are consequently at a higher risk of developing epilepsy than older children. It is reported that antiepileptic drug treatment is not as efficacious as might be expected. Routine electroencephalogram (EEG) recordings in children treated with antiepileptic medications may be beneficial during follow-up. Although ventriculoperitoneal shunts have been the standard treatment for hydrocephalus for decades, the long-term morbidity, including postshunt epileptic seizures, must be seriously considered. (See Chapter 26 for further discussion on seizure disorders.)

Prognosis

Hydrocephalus is the result of some event on the nervous system. A child's prognosis is ultimately determined by the underlying cause of hydrocephalus, severity of symptoms, and the time between diagnosis and the onset of treatment (AANS, 2005). The prognosis for successful management of hydrocephalus is excellent. Shunt dependency may carry with it a mortality rate as high as 1% per year, with most of the mortality related to delays in accessing a responsive system in time to prevent death. Primary care providers should remember that children with hydrocephalus are still at risk for increased morbidity and early mortality after years of excellent progress and shunt function. Early detection and treatment of shunt malfunction and complications can reduce morbidity and mortality significantly.

Research and experience show that children with hydrocephalus have excellent opportunities to attain their full potential through comprehensive integrated medical care and programs that stimulate their development (Fudge, 2000).

PRIMARY CARE MANAGEMENT

Health Care Maintenance
Growth and Development

Measurements of children seen in a primary care practice are typically done by minimally trained office or clinic personnel. If a child is suspected of having hydrocephalus or known to have hydrocephalus, the primary care provider should measure the head circumference and plot it on a head circumference chart appropriate for age. Until the cranial sutures are completely fused, which is often delayed in these children, head circumference is a major diagnostic tool in evaluating a child's condition. Normal head circumference at birth is 33 to 36 cm. During the first year, head circumference increases 2 cm/month during the first 3 months, 1.5 cm/month from 4 to 6 months, and 0.5 cm/month from 7 to 12 months (Nielson et al., 2007). A diagnosis of hydrocephalus is indicated more by increases across growth percentiles than by a normal rate of growth paralleling the 95th percentile. Increasing head circumference from hydrocephalus is usually associated with a full fontanelle, splayed sutures, and frontal bossing.

Once the diagnosis of hydrocephalus has been made and a shunt inserted, head circumference may decrease 1 to 2 cm as the pressure is relieved. The sutures may become overriding and the fontanelle sunken. After this initial decrease, the head should grow only in proportion to the child's body. Therefore, a newborn whose weight and height are in the 50th percentile for age and who has a head size of 40 cm when a shunt is placed shortly after birth may not resume head growth for 2 to 4 months. Resumption of growth before that time might indicate shunt malfunction. The significance of head size measurements in a child with a shunt cannot be overestimated, and daily measurements may be necessary during evaluation of shunt-dependent infants for possible shunt malfunction. Weight gain must be assessed carefully because the increasing weight of the head of the infant with hydrocephalus may mask failure to thrive.

Hydrocephalus may cause disorders of growth and puberty. Short stature in children with hydrocephalus is frequently due to meningomyelocele, but is rarely caused by a primary growth hormone deficiency (Cholley, Trivin, Sainte-Rose et al., 2001). Central early puberty is premature hypothalamic-pituitary-gonadal maturation and is the most frequent endocrine disorder found in children with hydrocephalus (Cholley et al.). Treatment is available and the primary care practitioner should refer the child to a pediatric endocrinologist should a question of precocious puberty arise.

The standard early infant developmental assessment tools used in primary care practice (e.g., Denver Developmental Screening Test II) are of little help in assessing infants with hydrocephalus. Tasks that require head control (e.g., elevating the head while the child is in the prone position, rolling over, pulling to a sitting position without head lag, and even sitting unassisted) will be delayed in infants with macrocrania. It is important for primary care providers to interpret developmental findings in light of other clinical observations to help parents set reasonable expectations for their infant.

Other motor delays can be expected during infancy and childhood given that approximately 60% of children with hydrocephalus have some form of motor disability. For children younger than 3 years of age, referral to an early intervention program is often appropriate to evaluate and treat motor delays. Primary care providers must carefully document motor skill acquisition, even in older school-aged children, because a loss of skill may indicate shunt malfunction or progression of the primary cause. Ataxia, slurred speech, lack of progression in school, incontinence, or other regression in developmental ability may indicate a deterioration in neurologic status and need for further evaluation.

In children surgically treated for hydrocephalus, the IQ is normal or nearly normal in approximately one third of affected individuals. As a rule, verbal IQ is higher than performance IQ, and the classic cocktail chatter of a child with hydrocephalus is common. Verbal skills are usually commensurate with intellectual abilities, and these children perform better on verbal tests than on fine motor–visual perception tests. There is some evidence to support the idea that the number of shunt revisions may have an adverse effect on IQ. Hetherington, Dennis, Barnes and colleagues (2006) found an association between multiple shunt revisions and lower cognitive ability in young adults with spina bifida and hydrocephalus. Primary care providers must assess speech carefully with each health care visit. These children often benefit from infant stimulation programs and speech therapy. Primary care providers should become familiar with the program offerings in the family's community to help them identify services that would be most beneficial for their child.

Diet

Children with hydrocephalus have no special dietary requirements. Many parents become overly concerned about the episodes of regurgitation or vomiting that are common in all infants, and clarification as to what is considered normal and what is pathologic vomiting should be made soon after the diagnosis of hydrocephalus. Parents may be hesitant to burp their infant because of poor head control or concern over dislodging the shunt. Alternate positions for burping can be demonstrated. If repeated regurgitation does occur, parents should be advised on how to use an infant seat for postfeeding positioning and introduction of solids (if age appropriate). The primary care provider can be supportive of the parents of a child with newly diagnosed hydrocephalus by reassuring them that their concerns are valid and helping to clarify symptoms common in newborns that may indicate increased ICP or some other condition such as gastroesophageal reflux. Neurosurgical practitioners reassure these same parents that it is better to notify early and too often regarding a symptom of possible shunt malfunction than to miss something and cause the child harm. Eventually, the majority of parents of children with shunted hydrocephalus become expert at recognizing shunt problems.

Safety

Primary care providers play a major role in educating parents and children about safety. Families may be so overwhelmed with the task of parenting a child with a chronic condition that routine safety measures are overlooked. Children with hydrocephalus may have trouble with head control as a result of low motor tone, which predisposes these children to head injury. In such situations use of a car seat developed for children with special needs may be appropriate. The health care provider plays a crucial role in helping families choose the best safety seat for the child. If an infant has poor head control and is unable to sit unsupported, it may be necessary to use a rear-facing convertible car seat so that the infant's head is maintained in a reclined position. The child can further be supported by placing rolled blankets or towels around the trunk, head, and under the legs so that the child maintains proper body and head alignment (American Academy of Pediatrics [AAP], 1999). Children with hydrocephalus and physical disabilities may require special devices and individualized fitting to ensure safety while being transported in a vehicle. For instance, once children outgrow the convertible infant seat, special equipment such as the E-Z-ON vest (E-Z-ON Products, Inc. of Florida; Jupiter, FL) may be necessary to provide additional trunk support (AAP, 1999). A pediatric physical therapist may help determine the appropriate equipment. The AAP lists types of car seats for children with special needs at www.aap.org/family/SpecialCarSeats Chart.pdf (AAP, 2005).

For additional assistance with car seat safety, parents may call 866-SEATCHECK to find a location where they may obtain a child safety seat inspection (AAP, 2007). Additional information may also be obtained at the National Highway Traffic Safety Administration (NHTSA) website www.nhtsa.dot.gov/people/injury/childps/contacts (NHTSA, 2008).

As the child grows, activities should be limited as little as possible to encourage normal development and peer relationships. Many parents of children with shunted hydrocephalus become overly concerned about head injuries. Parents may ask about the child wearing a helmet at all times to protect the shunt in the event of a fall or head injury. Children with shunts need only wear helmets for the same reasons all children should wear helmets while riding scooters, bicycles, skateboards, etc. unless they have difficulty with head control or seizures. It is important for the primary care provider to encourage parents not to be overly protective of their child with a shunted hydrocephalus.

A child's neurologic disabilities and visual perceptual integration may make competitive sports difficult and operation of motor vehicles hazardous. Few sports are absolutely contraindicated in children with hydrocephalus. Contact sports such as wrestling, tackle football, and hockey might increase the risk of shunt damage or head trauma, so participation in these sports may need to be restricted. Each individual's ability must be regularly assessed so that the risks and benefits of activities can be determined.

Immunizations

Routine immunizations are recommended (Centers for Disease Control and Prevention [CDC], 2009). Some precautions should be considered before administering the diphtheria and tetanus toxoids and acellular pertussis vaccine (DTaP). According to the CDC, DTaP is contraindicated only in cases of a progressive neurologic disorder or if the child experienced an episode of encephalopathy within 7 days of a previous dose (CDC, 2007). Generally infants and children with stable neurologic conditions, including well-controlled seizures and/or developmental delay, should be vaccinated. Seizures may be present in the infant with hydrocephalus, and it may be difficult to determine which of these infants has a progressive neurologic disorder. An infant's neurologic status should be evaluated at each primary care visit to determine whether the DTaP vaccine is contraindicated. Use of acellular pertussis vaccine is associated with fewer neurologic side effects and is recommended for children with hydrocephalus. Because outbreaks of pertussis still occur in the United States, deferral of the vaccine must be weighed against the potential for disease and disease-related complications. Children in daycare, attending special developmental programs, or receiving care in residential centers are exposed to other children who also may not be immunized and are therefore at increased risk for developing pertussis. In such difficult situations, consultation with the child's neurosurgeon or neurologist may help in assessing the child's seizure potential. If the primary care provider, with parental consent, decides early in infancy that the pertussis immunization will be withheld, diphtheria and tetanus vaccines should be given on schedule.

The *Haemophilus influenzae* type B (Hib) and pneumococcal conjugated vaccine (Prevnar) are particularly important for children with shunted hydrocephalus. Because of the increased risk of CNS infections in children with shunts, children with shunted hydrocephalus should be vaccinated on time for *H. influenzae* type B and pneumococcal bacteria (CDC, 2009; Pickering, 2006).

Screening

Vision. Because of the high incidence of visual defects in children with hydrocephalus, practitioners must pay particular attention to visual screening. The Hirschberg light reflex, cover test, tracking, and funduscopic examinations should be performed at each office visit and the results carefully documented in the child's record. At approximately 6 months of age, the child should be referred to a pediatric ophthalmologist for a thorough examination. Yearly examinations should be scheduled thereafter. Children with hydrocephalus often need surgery on their eye muscles to correct esotropia or exotropia. Practitioners can be instrumental in completing preoperative examinations and preparing the families for surgery. The primary care provider must remember that alterations in the funduscopic examination, eye muscle control, or visual ability may be associated with shunt malfunction and must be evaluated carefully when shunt malfunction or infection is part of the differential diagnosis. Referral to a neurologist or neurosurgeon for evaluation of an infant or young child for papilledema or evidence of increased pressure may help to differentiate benign headaches from those caused by shunt malfunction.

Hearing. In addition to routine newborn and office screening for hearing acuity, brainstem auditory evoked responses (BAERs) should be ordered if an infant has a history of CNS infection or antibiotic treatment with aminoglycosides. Subsequent shunt malfunctions or CNS infections require reassessment of hearing. Periodic evaluation by an audiologist is recommended.

Dental. Routine dental care is recommended. If a child is taking phenytoin (Dilantin) for seizure control, more frequent dental care may be needed because of hyperplasia of the gums. Poor dental hygiene and periodontal disease may produce bacteremia—even without dental procedures (Wolf, Rateitschak, Rateitschak, et al., 2004). Because intravascular foreign bodies are susceptible to bacterial colonization, any episode of transient bacteremia places a child with a VA shunt at risk for infection. However, evidence does not support the routine use of antibiotic prophylaxis for children with intraventricular shunts before dental procedures (Lockhart, Loven, Brennan, et al., 2007). The spontaneous shedding of primary teeth or simple adjustment of orthodontic appliances also does not require prophylaxis to prevent bacterial endocarditis. For further information on bacterial endocarditis and recommended antibiotic use, refer to Chapter 21.

Blood Pressure. Blood pressure readings should be recorded on each clinic or office visit. Elevations in blood pressure with a widening pulse pressure are a late sign of increased ICP. An established baseline reading can help the practitioner assess a child for possible shunt malfunctions or progression of disease process.

Hematocrit. Routine screening is recommended.

Urinalysis. Routine screening is recommended.

Tuberculosis. Routine screening is recommended.

Condition-Specific Screening

Head Circumference. Head circumference measurements should be taken at every clinic or office visit until a child's sutures are completely fused (see the discussion of growth and development earlier in this chapter).

Common Illness Management
Differential Diagnosis

Unfortunately, many symptoms of shunt malfunction or infection are the same as those commonly found with routine childhood illness (see box). It is important to remember that children with hydrocephalus experience otitis media, gastrointestinal (GI) illnesses, headaches, and viral infections with fever just like their unaffected peers. Primary care providers must approach these children as they would children without hydrocephalus. A calm manner and a thorough history and examination are reassuring to parents and productive for the primary care provider.

Differential Diagnosis

- Shunt malfunction
- Fever: concern about shunt infection
- Gastrointestinal symptoms: concern about:
  - Peritoneal shunt malfunction
  - Constipation that may result in distal peritoneal shunt malfunction
  - Abdominal pseudocyst
  - Migration of shunt tubing into inguinal or umbilical hernia
  - Brain tumors may metastasize to abdomen via shunt
- Headaches: concern about increased ICP
- Scalp infections: concern about spread of infection to shunt reservoir
- Alterations in behavior: concern about shunt malfunction

Shunt Malfunction. The most frequent symptoms of shunt malfunction include irritability, headache, nausea, vomiting, lethargy, and delays or loss of developmental milestones. Other symptoms include personality changes, diplopia, new seizures or a change in seizure pattern, worsening school performance, decreased level of consciousness, loss of upward gaze, nuchal rigidity, sixth nerve palsy, papilledema, and hemiparesis or loss of coordination and balance. With a shunt malfunction, the shunt reservoir may not pump and refill as expected, although the sensitivity and predictive value of a shunt pumping are questionable. If the shunt is infected, it may continue to work properly and therefore the child may not exhibit signs of increased ICP. Children who present with shunt infections may complain of low-grade and intermittent fevers, redness, tenderness and swelling along the shunt tract, abdominal pain, nuchal rigidity, headache, and seizures. Infections associated with VA shunts may present with glomerulonephritis (Duhaime, 2006).

Fever. There is no characteristic combination of signs and symptoms of shunt infections. Perhaps the most important clinical aspect of identifying a shunt infection is to understand that the presentation is highly variable and the diagnosis of shunt infection must be sought rather than simply found. Early in an infant's first year when shunt infections are most common, parents should be encouraged to consult the primary care provider whenever the infant has a temperature above 101.3°F (38.5°C). The practitioner, with the consulting physician, can then evaluate the child early in the course of illness and note progression of symptoms. If a focus of infection other than the shunt is identified, it should be treated appropriately. No studies indicate that frequent antibacterial therapy for illnesses of questionable origin reduces the incidence of shunt malfunction. Children being treated for bacterial infections (e.g., otitis media, pneumonia, or streptococcal sore throat) should be carefully reassessed in the office or clinic 24 to 48 hours after treatment is initiated. Continued or worsening symptoms may indicate progression of the infection into bacteremia or a CNS infection caused by the increased susceptibility resulting from the shunt; the primary care provider should obtain a complete blood cell (CBC) count, urinalysis, and blood cultures if a shunt infection is suspected and then immediately consult the child's neurosurgeon.

If a child has a mild or moderate fever of unknown origin with other symptoms compatible with a common childhood illness and no obvious signs of shunt malfunction, the primary care provider can adopt a wait-and-see attitude. Arrangements for telephone follow-up or a return appointment in 24 hours should be made. The parents must be instructed to report symptoms such as lethargy, confusion, or recurrent vomiting (more than three times within 24 hours) immediately if they occur.

In children with very high temperatures (i.e., >101.3°F [38.5°C]) and symptoms of moderate to severe illness, a shunt infection must be assumed until proven otherwise. Consultation with the neurosurgeon is advised. Blood cultures for aerobic and anaerobic organisms should be obtained, although results often are not initially positive. A CBC count is also indicated, but minimal leukocytosis does not rule out shunt infection. The neurosurgeon should obtain CSF for culture through the shunt reservoir. Although a shunt infection can be present despite normal CSF cell count, Lan, Wong, Chen and colleagues (2003) found several factors predictive of shunt infection; these include an increased C-reactive protein level, CSF leukocytosis (>100/mm^3), CSF neutrophils (>10%), decreased CSF glucose level, and an increased CSF protein level. Shunt aspiration should be done with meticulous aseptic technique so as not to contaminate a sterile shunt system or introduce a second organism into an already infected shunt. A lumbar puncture is not advised in a child with a shunt because of the possibility of downward brain herniation and death if ventriculomegaly with increased ICP is present.

A chest radiograph and urine culture are recommended to rule out pneumonia or urinary tract infection. However, if the history and physical findings strongly suggest shunt involvement, these may be omitted. The neurosurgeon may prefer that all tests be done at the hospital because hospitalization is often required to complete the evaluation and treatment process. Throughout the workup for the source of fever, the primary care practitioner should be in close communication with the primary neurosurgeon.

Gastrointestinal Symptoms. Nausea and vomiting are common clinical symptoms during childhood and often accompany such diverse conditions as influenza, otitis media, and urinary tract infections. Diarrhea and abdominal pain are also frequent complaints in childhood. Children with hydrocephalus can be expected to have these common complaints as often as other children. When a child has mild GI symptoms, the practitioner must consider the presence or absence of other symptoms and the history of exposure to GI illness. The diagnostic workup should include an evaluation for shunt infection and GI disease. The primary care provider must recognize that abdominal symptoms may be the presenting symptom of peritoneal shunt malfunction or an acute condition in the abdomen in children with shunts (Kim, Stewart, Voth, et al., 2006). Children with shunt-dependent hydrocephalus should follow a regimen to maintain normal bowel movements since chronic constipation has been shown to lead to distal shunt obstruction (Muzumdar & Ventureyra, 2007).

Children with a peritoneal shunt infection may have mild to moderate fever, abdominal pain, anorexia, nausea, vomiting, and diarrhea. They may guard their abdomen and be unwilling to ambulate. Swelling, redness, or inflammation along the catheter tract or at the incision site is highly suggestive of shunt involvement. Abdominal ultrasound and CSF cultures should help differentiate between an acute condition in the abdomen and a shunt infection. Specific signs of appendicitis can be demonstrated by a CT scan of the abdomen, but identification of an abdominal pseudocyst is more characteristic of a distal shunt infection (Browd et al., 2006). Abdominal pseudocysts may develop around the peritoneal end of the VP shunt and usually result from past or current shunt infection. A history of recent or recurrent shunt revisions also substantially

increases the risk for infection. The primary care practitioner may not be able to differentiate the symptoms of an acute condition in the abdomen from peritoneal shunt malfunction. Consultation with and referral to the attending neurosurgeon is advised.

Another abdominal concern relates to infants with inguinal or umbilical hernias and the potential for CSF or shunt tubing to migrate into the hernia. If this occurs, the hernia becomes enlarged with a collection of CSF; treatment includes repair of the hernia and possible shunt revision.

Metastasis of brain tumor cells from the ventricular cavities into the abdominal cavity is a possible side effect of ventriculoperitoneal shunts (Donovan & Prauner, 2005). This side effect must be considered when a differential diagnosis is made in children with chronic or recurring abdominal symptoms if these children also have a history of a brain tumor. Appropriate referral is required to rule out this possibility after more common reasons for the complaint have been eliminated.

Headaches. Children often report headaches, which can also occur in children with a shunt and may have the same origin as in children without hydrocephalus. If routine treatment of headaches with mild analgesics and rest does not relieve the symptom or if the headaches become frequent, affect school attendance, or are associated with lethargy or irritability, then evaluation by the neurologist and/or neurosurgeon is required. Repetitive and vigorous investigation of shunt malfunction may not be necessary in the absence of other symptoms.

Shunt malfunction can be partial or variable, depending on cerebral blood flow, CSF production, and a child's activity, and may result in periodic episodes of increased ICP. Children with shunts occasionally experience headaches and vomiting in the early morning after sleeping all night. These symptoms may be caused by temporary partial blockage of the shunt from cellular debris, inactivity, and the horizontal sleeping position, which negates the beneficial effect of gravity for ventricular drainage. These symptoms usually subside after children have been up for a few hours. If these episodes are infrequent and self-limited, they do not require treatment other than acetaminophen or ibuprofen for pain. Parents should be instructed to call the primary care provider if these symptoms continue for more than 6 hours or are associated with a decrease in the child's level of consciousness or loss of motor ability.

Scalp Infections. A thin layer of skin covers the shunt reservoir on the scalp. If the skin around the shunt reservoir becomes infected, the integrity of the skin barrier may be broken and infection of the shunt is possible. The primary care provider should manage scalp infections aggressively in collaboration with the neurosurgeon.

Alterations in Behavior. All children experience mood swings and temporary behavior changes. Parents of children with hydrocephalus may comment on them not being themselves; school performance may falter, normal interest in activities may dwindle, and lethargy or irritability may develop. If these changes persist beyond a few days, a child should be seen by the neurosurgeon for an evaluation. Subtle changes in behavior, cognition, or motor ability may be symptoms of shunt malfunction.

Drug Interactions

No routine medications are prescribed for children with hydrocephalus. (See Chapter 26 for drug interactions with anticonvulsant therapy.)

Developmental Issues

Sleep Patterns

Parents may be concerned about their infant or child sleeping in a position that might adversely affect the shunt. During the immediate period after shunt placement, these children should be positioned off the reservoir site to avoid skin breakdown. With the exception of this brief period after shunt placement or revision, parents and caretakers must be reassured that their child can sleep in any comfortable position without fear of affecting the shunt. Infants and young children should be encouraged to assume a normal sleep pattern at night. Children who seem to be sleeping or napping more than usual should be evaluated for possible increased ICP.

Toileting

Children with neurologic deficits associated with hydrocephalus may have a delayed ability to develop bowel and bladder control. Parents need to be counseled on the possibility of this difficulty, and the methods of toilet training should be reviewed. The neurologist, neurosurgeon, and physiatrist (if applicable) monitoring a child's development should be consulted about the child's neurologic capability to attain satisfactory toilet training. Chronic constipation may exert pressure on the peritoneal shunt, resulting in a malfunction. Maintenance of regular stool patterns may prevent unnecessary hospitalization and need for shunt revision. If necessary, special bowel training and clean intermittent catheterization education should be provided. These techniques can usually be obtained through referral to a pediatric urologist or physiatrist (see Chapter 35).

Discipline

Discipline for children with hydrocephalus should be managed as for other children, recognizing the limitations of cognitive and motor development of the individual child. Some parents may have difficulty understanding the discrepancy between their child's verbal and performance skills and may have expectations that are too high for the child to attain, which may lead to inappropriate discipline. On the other hand, parents may be afraid to discipline their child and must be encouraged to set appropriate limits.

Practitioners must always be concerned with the increased possibility of child abuse in children with chronic conditions. Head injuries and abdominal injuries are common in child abuse and may result in further brain injury or shunt malfunction in children with hydrocephalus.

Child Care

Most parents work outside the home. Child care and preschool placement are major issues for all working parents but are even more problematic when a child has a chronic condition. Fortunately, the current shunt systems are self-maintained and do not require special care (e.g., pumping periodically) throughout the day. Children with hydrocephalus have no special care needs unless other disabilities (e.g., cerebral palsy with spasticity or dystonia, seizures, or developmental delay) are present. If a child has significant disabilities, child care arrangements must be evaluated for their ability to meet the child's needs. Public Law 108-446 (Individuals with Disabilities Education Improvement Act, 2004), extends services to children with disabilities from birth to school entry, so federally funded programs are accessible to children with disabilities

(see Chapter 3). Parents of children with disabilities such as spina bifida and hydrocephalus may visit the website http://idea.ed.gov/ for more information about the law and current amendments.

Children with shunted hydrocephalus, however, are at greater risk for CNS infections than their peers. Parents must understand that children who attend daycare or preschool are exposed to childhood infections and have illnesses (i.e., usually respiratory tract or GI) more often than those who stay at home. Children up to 2 years of age should receive child care at home or in a small daycare program to minimize exposure to common pediatric pathogens.

Schooling

Children with hydrocephalus have a greater risk of cognitive delays including learning disabilities (Cartwright & Wallace, 2007). Primary care providers can help families plan their child's individualized educational program (IEP) to ensure appropriate interventions for the child (see Chapter 3). Although Public Law 108-446 requires the school district to assess a child's needs, the district's financial constraints may limit neuropsychological testing. Therefore results of any testing before the child attends school may be beneficial and should be forwarded to the school district. Parents may need help obtaining medical records to facilitate formulation of their child's IEP and the primary care practitioner can assist the family during this process.

Some children with hydrocephalus qualify for separate special education classes because of physical or intellectual limitations. Other children can be mainstreamed into regular classrooms and receive special services (e.g., adaptive physical education to help with motor control and balance, occupational therapy to assist with kinesthetic-proprioceptive deficits, speech therapy, or psychological counseling to address emotional issues). As these children reach junior high school and high school, some limitations may be made on competitive, high-impact sports. Tackle football, boxing, wrestling, and ice hockey have a much higher risk of head and abdominal injury than track, swimming, tennis, or golf. If a child has mild to moderate neuromotor deficits, an evaluation by a sports medicine professional may help identify sports activities that the child can successfully perform. Involvement in sports activities or formal group activities such as scouting are often beneficial to a child's self-esteem and encourages peer relationships, both of which may be problematic areas for children with hydrocephalus.

Children with less severe disabilities may experience psychosocial difficulty because they may have a difficult time fitting in with nondisabled peers but also do not fit in with more disabled children. Their disabilities may not be recognized by teachers and peers unable to understand why these individuals have difficulty in school or sports. Adolescents who are trying not to be different may not disclose their learning or motor deficit but will not be able to successfully compete with unaffected peers. The resulting incongruity between expectations and ability can lead to a sense of failure and lowered self-esteem.

Primary care providers should routinely ask parents and children about school progress. If academic difficulties develop, these children should be referred for repeat neuropsychological testing to rule out medical reasons for these problems. Shunt malfunction may result in gradual changes in cognition, fine motor abilities, or personality and must be ruled out as a contributing factor. If difficulties are assessed to be more emotional, which often happens during adolescence when children struggle with their body image and identity, children should be referred for counseling. This referral should be made to a professional experienced in working with children with disabilities.

Sexuality

As previously mentioned, delayed or precocious puberty may occur in children with hydrocephalus. Their progression through puberty must be assessed and monitored; counseling may be indicated to support them during this period. Children with precocious puberty may have lowered self-esteem, poor peer relationships, and a higher incidence of sexual abuse than normally developing children. Sexuality and reproductive issues should be managed the same as with other children. Female adolescents receiving anticonvulsant therapy should be informed of the possible teratogenic effects of the medications they are taking (see Chapter 26). It is universally recommended that all women of childbearing age should take 400 mcg (LD) of folic acid daily to help prevent serious birth defects (CDC, 2005; Lindsey, Hamner, Prue et al., 2007). Adolescents with associated motor disabilities may have additional needs (see Chapter 18).

Transition to Adulthood

Shunt dependency will always be a "preexisting condition," making it difficult for the individual with hydrocephalus to maintain health insurance coverage. A disproportionate number of these individuals, particularly young adults, are living either at or below the poverty line and are dependent on governmental programs for their health care, or they are unable to obtain any insurance until they have difficulties with their shunts, become bankrupt because of the experience, and then become indigent. Guaranteed access to a responsive system is just not a "good idea" for people with hydrocephalus; it is literally a matter of life and death because shunt malfunction can result in death if not treated early and appropriately. Health professionals must be advocates for the continued care of children as they transition into adolescent and adult care. Professionals must be involved in the creation of and constant fine-tuning of a responsive system to ensure access for all individuals with hydrocephalus (Albright et al., 2008).

Since the 1970s, improvements in shunt techniques and management of shunt complications have resulted in a dramatic increase in the survival of individuals with hydrocephalus. Unique issues have arisen as young people with hydrocephalus make their transition into adulthood. These individuals and their families now find themselves dealing with vocational training, career placement, sexuality, and family roles. Social outcomes are often highly influenced by one's associated disabilities, especially developmental delay and motor handicaps. Many adults who were shunted during childhood have achieved full-time employment and successful personal relationships because either their disabilities were minor or they were able to overcome them. Oakeshott and Hunt (2006) found that the employment rate of young adults with hydrocephalus associated with spina bifida has been less promising, with as many as 70% to 80% unable to maintain employment. Some of these individuals have been described as lacking drive or initiative, but more accurately, episodes of shunt malfunction may play a role in an individual's inability to maintain employment (Oakeshott & Hunt).

A supportive climate that encourages independence, maturity, and responsibility is essential if young adults with hydrocephalus are to complete school, maintain employment, and function as adults. Professional guidance is often necessary to create this environment. Health professionals should emphasize a positive prognosis for young adults with hydrocephalus. Parents must be prepared to face the normal problems of adolescence and let their young children develop independence. The National Dissemination Center for Children with Disabilities (NICHCY) can provide information and referrals for social skills programs that may be useful to parents, teachers, and others (see the organization's listing and website under Resources). Young adults dependent on a shunt should be cautious about living alone because they could become acutely ill, confused, or even comatose during a shunt malfunction. These individuals should form a buddy system to ensure their well-being, thereby minimizing their risk of permanent brain injury from an unrecognized shunt malfunction. At the college level, vocational training and special education resources are also available to help young adults prepare for job placement.

Hydrocephalus alone should not interfere with a woman's ability to conceive, but approximately 50% of pregnant women with shunted hydrocephalus will experience a shunt malfunction. As the pregnancy progresses, intraabdominal pressure increases, which may result in increased ICP for women with ventriculoperitoneal shunts. This risk may continue for up to 6 months after childbirth (Qaiser & Black, 2007). Prenatal counseling and assessment should include genetic counseling and a review of family history for neural tube defects. A complete assessment of shunt function should be obtained if pregnancy is being considered. In addition, maternal supplementation with folic acid significantly diminishes the number of infants born with neural tube defects (Lindsey et al., 2007); therefore women of childbearing age must be strongly encouraged to supplement their folic acid intake before conception.

Family Concerns

Parents of children with hydrocephalus constantly worry about continued shunt function. With every malfunction there is the need for surgery and the perceived threat of further brain damage. This constant worry and the daily responsibility and stress of caring for a child who may have multiple medical problems is stressful for families. The financial strain from numerous medical visits or surgical procedures may deplete a family's financial reserves. Private insurance may not be obtainable unless offered through a large group employment policy. Concern about a child's future ability to be self-supporting and independent is also an issue for parents as their child grows into adolescence and adulthood.

Parent-to-parent support groups can offer support by publishing newsletters and hosting major medical conferences for both health professionals and parents. These organizations also provide a network for children with hydrocephalus, offering them the opportunity to make new friends, develop peer support, and exchange knowledge. Support groups are now readily available on the Internet for both adolescents with hydrocephalus and their parents (see websites listed in the Resources). Primary care providers should become familiar with the organizations in the community and Web connections so that appropriate referrals can be made. It is better to make such referrals soon after a child's diagnosis than to wait to see how the parents cope; all parents need support above and beyond what is reasonable for a physician or nurse to provide.

Resources

Organizations and Websites

The Cleveland Clinic
Website: www.clevelandclinic.org

Hydrocephalus Foundation, Inc.
910 Rear Broadway, Route 1
Saugus, MA 01906
(781) 942-1161; Fax: (781) 231-5250
Website: www.hydrocephalus.org

HOPE (Hydrocephalus Opens People's Eyes)
104-47 120th St.
Richmond Hill, NY 11419

Hydrocephalus Association
870 Market St., Suite 705
San Francisco, CA 94102
(415) 732-7040 or (888) 598-3789; Fax: (415) 732-7044
Website: www.hydroassoc.org

Individuals with Disabilities Education and Improvement Act
Website: http://idea.ed.gov

National Hydrocephalus Foundation
12413 Centralia Rd.
Lakewood, CA 90715-1623
(562) 924-6666 or (888) 857-3434
Website: http://nhfonline.org

National Dissemination Center for Children with Disabilities (NICHCY)
P.O. Box 1492
Washington, DC 20013
(800) 695-0285; Fax: (202) 884-8441
Website: www.nichcy.org

National Organization for Rare Disorders (NORD)
55 Kenosia Ave.
P.O. Box 1968
Danbury, CT 06813-1968
(203) 744-0100 or (800) 999-6673 (voice mail only); Fax: (203) 798-2291
Website: www.rarediseases.org

Spina Bifida Association of America
4590 MacArthur Blvd. NW, Suite 250
Washington, DC 20007-4226
(202) 944-3285 or (800) 621-3141; Fax: (202) 944-3295
Website: www.sbaa.org; sbaa@sbaa.org

United Cerebral Palsy Association, Inc.
1660 L St., Suite 700
Washington, DC 20036
(800) 872-5827; Fax: (202) 776-1414
Website: www.ucp.org

Summary of Primary Care Needs for the Child with Hydrocephalus

HEALTH CARE MAINTENANCE

Growth and Development

- The head should be measured at each visit until the sutures are fused.
- If enlarged head size is diagnosed in infancy and a shunt is placed, head size should follow the normal growth curve.
- Carefully assess weight gain at each visit as a larger head size may mask failure to thrive.
- Evaluate for signs of central early puberty (most common endocrine disorder).
- Standard infant development tests may indicate delay because of poor head control.
- 60% of all children with hydrocephalus will have some motor disability.
- Verbal skills are usually higher than performance skills.
- Cognitive ability varies and is determined by cause and treatment of hydrocephalus.
- Early stimulation/intervention programs are recommended.

Diet

- A normal diet is indicated.
- Assessment of infant vomiting as normal or as a sign of increased ICP may be difficult.

Safety

- The risk of head injury is increased because of poor head control.
- A rear-facing car seat should be recommended until a child can sit unsupported.
- A helmet should be used for bicycle and skateboard riding.
- Neurologic deficits may make competitive sports difficult or unadvisable and operation of motor vehicles hazardous.

Immunizations

- Routine immunizations are recommended.
- Pertussis vaccine may be deferred in infants with a progressive neurologic disorder or history of encephalopathy after previous DTaP dose.
- *Haemophilus influenzae* type B conjugated vaccine and pneumococcal conjugate vaccine are strongly recommended.

Screening

- *Vision.* Hirschberg examination, cover test, ability to track, and funduscopic examination should be done at each visit. Children should be examined by an ophthalmologist at 6 months of age and then yearly thereafter.
  - Alterations in eye examination may be associated with shunt malfunction.
- *Hearing.* A routine office screening is recommended. An auditory-evoked response test should be given to children with a history of CNS infection or those who have been treated with aminoglycosides. Periodic screening by an audiologist is recommended.
- *Dental.* Routine dental care is recommended.
  - Dental hygiene is important to reduce risk of bacteremia.
  - Antibiotic prophylaxis is not recommended for dental work.
  - Children receiving phenytoin therapy require more frequent dental care.
- *Blood pressure.* Blood pressure should be recorded at each visit.
  - Blood pressure increases with increased ICP.
- *Hematocrit.* Routine screening is recommended.
- *Urinalysis.* Routine screening is recommended.
- *Tuberculosis.* Routine screening is recommended.

Continued

Summary of Primary Care Needs for the Child with Hydrocephalus—cont'd

Condition-Specific Screening

- *Head circumference.* Head circumference should be measured at each visit until the sutures are completely fused.

COMMON ILLNESS MANAGEMENT

Differential Diagnosis

- *Shunt malfunction.* Shunt malfunction needs to be ruled out acutely.
- *Fever.* Shunt or CNS infection should be ruled out.
- *Gastrointestinal symptoms.* Increased ICP with nausea and vomiting should be ruled out.
  - Peritonitis with abdominal pain or acute diarrhea should be ruled out.
  - Shunt infection caused by abdominal infection should be ruled out.
  - Constipation should be ruled out as cause of shunt malfunction.
  - Metastatic abdominal tumor should be ruled out in children with primary brain tumors and ventriculoperitoneal shunts.
- *Headaches.* Shunt malfunction should be ruled out as the cause of acute or chronic headaches.
- *Scalp infections.* Possible infection spread to shunt reservoir should be ruled out.
- *Alterations in behavior.* Alterations in behavior should be ruled out as a symptom of shunt malfunction.

Drug Interactions

- No routine medications are prescribed.

DEVELOPMENTAL ISSUES

Sleep Patterns

- Standard developmental counseling is advised.

Toileting

- Delayed bowel and bladder training may occur because of neurologic deficit.
- Constipation may cause peritoneal shunt malfunction.

Discipline

- Expectations are normal with recognition of the possible discrepancy between verbal and motor abilities. Physical punishment is a hazard because it may cause head or abdominal injury.

Child Care

- No special care needs are required except when a child has a severe motor disability or seizures.
- Home care or small daycare programs are recommended during a child's first 2 years of life to reduce exposure to infections.

Schooling

- Associated problems are often covered by Public Law 108-446 (IDEA).
- Families should be assisted in IEP hearings.
- Children may have possible adjustment problems during adolescence.
- Children may need psychometric testing for poor school performance.
- Low-impact sports should be selected to prevent head trauma and abdominal injury.
- Minor, unseen disabilities should not be overlooked.

Sexuality

- Children should be evaluated for delayed or precocious puberty.
- Standard developmental counseling is advised unless associated problems warrant additional care.

Transition to Adulthood

- Research has identified difficulty with vocational training, career, sexuality, and family roles associated with hydrocephalus and mental retardation and motor handicaps.
- Independence must be fostered from an early age to prepare young adults for independence.
- Shunt-dependent individuals should develop a buddy system to ensure that shunt malfunction leading to acute illness, confusion, or coma does not go unrecognized.
- Pregnancy may interfere with peritoneal shunt drainage. Securing independent health and life insurance may be difficult for individuals with hydrocephalus.

FAMILY CONCERNS

- Families are concerned about continued shunt function and the possibility of brain damage caused by shunt failure or infection.

REFERENCES

Ahn, E., Bookland, M., Carson, B.S., et al. (2006). The Strata programmable valve for shunt-dependent hydrocephalus: The pediatric experience at a single institution. *Child Nerv Syst, 23*(3), 297-303.

Albright, A.L., Pollack, I.F., Adelson, P.D. (2008). *Principles and Practice of Pediatric Neurosurgery.* New York: Thieme.

American Academy of Pediatrics. (1999). *Transporting Children with Special Health Care Needs.* Available at http://aappolicy.aappublications.org/cgi/reprint/pediatrics;104/4/988.pdf. Retrieved May 23, 2008.

American Academy of Pediatrics. (2005). *Special needs car safety seats/restraints product information.* Available at www.aap.org/family/SpecialCarSeatsChart.pdf. Retrieved May 10, 2008.

American Academy of Pediatrics. (2007). *Infant passenger safety: Guidance for parents.* Available at www.aap.org/family/infantpassengersafety.htm. Retrieved June 9, 2008.

American Association of Neurological Surgeons (AANS). (2005). *What is hydrocephalus?* Available at www.neurosurgerytoday.org. Retrieved December 18, 2007.

Anderson, R.C., Garton, H.J., & Kestle, J.R. (2008). Treatment of hydrocephalus with shunts. In A.L. Albright, I.F. Pollack & P.D. Adelson (Eds.), *Principles and Practice of Pediatric Neurosurgery.* New York: Thieme.

Andersson, S., Persson, E., Aring, E., et al. (2006). Vision in children with hydrocephalus. *Dev Med Child Neurol, 48,* 836-841.

Aring, E., Andersson, S., Hard, A., et al. (2007). Strabismus, binocular functions and ocular motility in children with hydrocephalus. *Strabismus, 15*(2), 79-88.

Barnes, M.A., Faulkner, H., Wilkinson, M., et al. (2004). Meaning construction and integration in children with hydrocephalus. *Brain Lang, 89,* 47-56.

Bourgeois, M., Sainte-Rose, C., Cinalli, G., et al. (2004). Epilepsy in child-hood shunted hydrocephalus. In G. Cinalli, W.J. Maixner, & C. Sainte-Rose (eds.), *Pediatric Hydrocephalus*, New York: Springer.

Boyer, K.M., Yeates, K.O., & Enrile, B.G. (2006). Working memory and information processing speed in children with myelomeningocele and shunted hydrocephalus: Analysis of the Children's Paced Auditory Social Addition test. *J Int Neuropsychol Soc, 12*, 305-313.

Browd, S.R., Gottfried, O.N., Ragel, B.T., et al. (2006). Failure of cerebrospinal fluid shunts: Part I: obstruction and mechanical failure. *Pediatr Neurol, 34*, 83-92.

Campbell, J.W. (2008). Shunt infections. In A.L. Albright, I.F.Pollack, & P.D. Adelson (Eds.), *Principles and Practice of Pediatric Neurosurgery*, New York: Thieme.

Cartwright, C.C., & Wallace, D.C.(Eds.) (2007). *Nursing Care of the Pediatric Neurosurgery Patient*, New York: Springer.

Centers for Disease Control and Prevention. (2005). *Folic acid*. Available at www.cdc.gov/ncbddd/folicacid/health_recomm.htm. Retrieved March 10, 2008.

Centers for Disease Control and Prevention. (2007). *Guide to contraindications for vaccinations*. Available at www.cdc.gov/vaccines/recs/vac-admin/contraindications.htm. Retrieved May 23, 2008.

Centers for Disease Control and Prevention. (2009). Recommended immunization schedules for persons aged 0 through 18 years—United States, 2009. MMWR, 57(51&52), 1-11.

Cholley, F., Trivin, C., Sainte-Rose, C., et al. (2001). Disorders of growth and puberty in children with non-tumoral hydrocephalus. *J Pediatr Endocrinol Metab, 14*(3), 319-327.

Cinalli, G., Maixner, W.J., & Sainte-Rose, C. (Eds.) (2004). *Pediatric Hydrocephalus*, New York: Springer.

Daszkiewicz, P., & Barszcz, S. (2007). Multiple shunt system revisions in patients with hydrocephalus—causes, effects, regularities, and prognostic factors. *Neurol Neurochir Pol, 41*(5), 404-410.

DelBigio, M. (2004). Cellular damage and prevention in childhood hydrocephalus. *Brain Pathol, 14*(3), 317-324.

de Ribaupierre, S., Riliet, B., Vernet, O., et al. (2007). Third ventriculostomy versus ventriculoperitoneal shunt in pediatric obstructive hydrocephalus: Results from a Swiss series and literature review. *Child Nerv Syst, 23*(5), 527-533.

Donovan, D.J., & Prauner, R.D. (2005). Shunt-related abdominal metastases in a child with choroid plexus carcinoma: Case report. *Neurosurgery, 56*(2), E412.

Duhaime, A. (2006). Evaluation of management of shunt infections in children with hydrocephalus. *Clin Pediatr, 45*(8), 705-713.

Fudge, R.A. (2000). *About Hydrocephalus—A Book for Parents*. San Francisco: Hydrocephalus Association.

Futagi, Y., Suzuki, Y., Toribe, Y., et al. (2002). Neurodevelopmental outcome in children with fetal hydrocephalus. *Pediatr Neurol, 27*(2), 111-116.

Grinsberg, H.J., & Drake, J.M. (2004). Shunt hardware and surgical technique. In G. Cinalli, W.J. Maixner, & C.Sainte-Rose (Eds.), *Pediatric Hydrocephalus*, New York: Springer.

Harrison, M.R., Evans, M.I., Adzick, N.S., et al. (2001). *The Unborn Patient. The Art and Science of Fetal Therapy*. (3rd ed.). Philadelphia: Saunders.

Hellwig, D., Grotenhuis, J.A., Tirakotai, W., et al. (2005). Endoscopic third ventriculostomy for obstructive hydrocephalus. *Neurosurg Rev, 28*(1), 1-34.

Hetherington, R., Dennis, M., Barnes, M., et al. (2006). Functional outcome in young adults with spina bifida and hydrocephalus. *Child Nerv Syst, 22*(2), 117-124.

Huber-Okrainec, J., Dennis, M., Brettschneider, J., et al. (2002). Neuromotor speech deficits in children and adults with spina bifida and hydrocephalus. *Brain Lang, 80*(3), 592-602.

Iborra, J., Pages, E., Cuxart, A., et al. (2000). Increased ICP in myelomeningocele (MMC) patients never shunted: Results of a prospective preliminary study. *Spinal Cord, 38*(8), 495-497.

Individuals with Disabilities Education Act. (2004). *Building the Legacy: IDEA 2004*. Available at http://idea.ed.gov. Retrieved January 9, 2009.

Johnston, M. (2003). The importance of lymphatics in cerebrospinal fluid transport. *Lymphat Res Biol, 1*(1), 41-45.

Kadrian, D., van Gelder, J., Florida, D., et al. (2005). Long-term reliability of endoscopic third ventriculostomy. *Neurosurgery, 56*(6), 1271-1278.

Kay, A.D., Fisher, A.J., O'Kane, C., et al. United Kingdom and Ireland Medos Shunt Audit Group. A clinical audit of the Hakim programmable valve in patients with complex hydrocephalus. *Br J Neurosurg, 14*(6), 535-542.

Kim, T.Y., Stewart, G., Voth, M., et al. (2006). Signs and symptoms of cerebrospinal fluid shunt malfunction in the pediatric emergency department. *Pediatr Emerg Care, 22*(1), 28-34.

Lan, C.C., Wong, T.T., Chen, S.J., et al. (2003). Early diagnosis of ventroperitoneal shunt infections and malfunctions in children with hydrocephalus. *J Microbiol Immunol Infect, 36*(1), 47-50.

Lindsey, L.L., Hamner, H.C., Prue, C.E., et al. (2007). Understanding optimal nutrition among women of childbearing age in the United States and Puerto Rico: Employing formative research to lay the foundation for national birth defects prevention campaigns. *J Health Commun, 12*(8), 733-757.

Lindquist, B., Carlsson, G., Persson, E., et al. (2005). Learning disabilities in a population-based group of children with hydrocephalus. *Acta Paediatr, 94*(7), 878-883.

Lockhart, P.B., Loven, B., Brennan, M.T., et al. (2007). The evidence base for the efficacy of antibiotic prophylaxis in dental practice. *J Am Dent Assoc, 138*(4), 458-474.

Matthews, Y.Y. (2008). Drugs used in childhood idiopathic or benign intracranial hypertension. *Arch Dis Child, 93*(1), 19-25.

McLone, D.G. (2001). *Pediatric Neurosurgery: Surgery of the Developing Nervous System*. (4th ed.). Philadelphia: Saunders.

Mukhida, K., Sharma, M.R., Shilpakar, S.K. (2004). Management of hydrocephalus with ventriculoperitoneal shunts: Review of 274 cases. *Nepal J Neurosci, 1*(2), 104-112.

Muzumdar, D., & Ventureyra, E.C. (2007). Transient ventriculoperitoneal shunt malfunction after chronic constipation: Case report and review of literature. *Child Nerv Syst, 23*, 455-458.

National Hydrocephalus Foundation. (2007). *Hydrocephalus facts*. Available at www.nhfonline.org. Retrieved May 23, 2008.

Nguyen, T.N., Polomeno, R.C., Farmer, J.P., et al. (2002). Ophthalmic complications of slit-ventricle syndrome in children. *Ophthalmology, 109*(3), 520-524.

NHTSA. (2008). *Child passenger safety*., Available at www.nhtsa.dot.gov/people/injury/childps/contacts. Retrieved January 5, 2008.

Nielson, N., Pearce, K., Limbacher, E., et al. (2007). Hydrocephalus. Cartwright, C.C., Wallace, D.C.(eds.) (2007). *Nursing Care of the Pediatric Neurosurgery Patient*, New York: Springer.

Oakeshott, P., & Hunt, G.M. (2006). Predictors of employment in people with open spina bifida at the mean age of 35 years. *Cerebralspinal Fluid Res 3*(Suppl 1), S42.

Panay, M., Gokhale, D., Mansour, S., et al. (2005). Prenatal diagnosis in a family with X-linked hydrocephalus. *Prenat Diagn, 25*(10), 930-933.

Persson, E.K., Hagberg, G., & Uvebrant, P. (2006). Disabilities in children with hydrocephalus—a population-based study of children aged between four and twelve years. *Neuropediatrics, 37*(6), 330-336.

Pickering, L.K.(Ed.). (2006). *Red Book: 2006 Report of the Committee on Infectious Diseases*. (27th ed.), New York: American Academy of Pediatrics.

Pitetti, R. (2007). Emergency department evaluation of ventricular shunt malfunction: Is the shunt series really necessary? *Pediatr Emerg Care, 23*(3), 137-141.

Poca, M.A., & Sahuquillo, J. (2005). Short-term medical management of hydrocephalus. *Expert Opin Pharmacother, 6*(9), 1525-1538.

Qaiser, R., & Black, P. (2007). Neurosurgery in pregnancy. *Semin Neurol, 27*(5), 476-482.

Ragel, B.T., Browd, S.R., & Schmidt, R.H. (2006). Surgical shunt infection: Significant reduction when using intraventricular and systemic antibiotic agents. *J Neurosurg, 105*(2), 242-247.

Rekate, H.L. (2008). Treatment of hydrocephalus. In A.L. Albright, I.F. Pollack, & P.D. Adelson, (Eds.), *Principles and Practice of Pediatric Neurosurgery*. New York: Thieme.

Rendeli, C., Salvaggio, E., Sciascia-Cannizzaro, G., et al. (2002). Does locomotion improve the cognitive profile of children with myelomeningocele?. *Child Nerv Syst, 18*, 231-234.

Ricci, D., Luciano, R., Baranello, G., et al. (2006). Visual development in infants with prenatal post-haemorrhagic ventricular dilation. *Arch Dis Child, 92*, F255-F258.

Simpkins, C.J. (2005). Ventriculoperitoneal shunt infections in patients with hydrocephalus. *Pediatr Nurs, 31*(6), 457-462.

Turgut, M., Alabaz, D., Erbey, F., et al. (2005). Cerebrospinal fluid shunt infections in children. *Pediatr Neurosurg, 41*(3), 131-136.

Vinchon, M., & Dhellemmes, P. (2006). Cerebrospinal fluid shunt infection: Risk factors and long-term follow up. *Child Nerv Syst, 22*(7), 692-697.

Volpe, J.J. (2008). *Neurology of the Newborn*. (5th ed.). Philadelphia: Saunders.

von Koch, C.S., Gupta, N., Sutton, L.N., et al. (2003). In utero surgery for hydrocephalus. *Child Nerv Syst, 19*(7-8), 574-586.

Wagner, W., & Koch, D. (2005). Mechanisms of failure after endoscopic third ventriculostomy in young infants. *J Neurosurg Pediatr, 103*, 43-49.

Wolf, H.F., Rateitschak, E.M., Rateitschak, K.H., et al. (2004). *Color Atlas of Periodontology (Color Atlas of Dental Medicine)*. (3rd ed.). New York: Thieme.

30 Inflammatory Bowel Disease

Betsy Haas-Beckert and Melvin B. Heyman

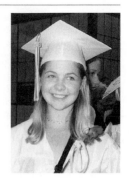

Etiology

Inflammatory bowel disease (IBD) refers to a constellation of inflammatory disorders of the gastrointestinal (GI) tract that currently are categorized into two principal diagnoses: Crohn's disease (CD) and ulcerative colitis (UC). These two forms of IBD are commonly discussed together in the literature because they share many of the same presenting symptoms and approaches to diagnosis and management, but they are two distinctly different illnesses.

CD is a chronic inflammatory disease of the bowel that may involve any portion of the GI tract—from mouth to anus. CD is characterized by inflammation that is transmural (extending through the entire wall of the intestine). It may begin as mild superficial disease and subsequently may slowly extend from the intestinal mucosal lining through the serosal layer, or it may present with severe disease in large segments of small and/or large intestine. In CD, diseased segments of the bowel may border segments of healthy tissue, giving it an uneven appearance with "skip areas." CD most commonly affects the terminal ileum in up to 70%, involves the ileum and colon in 60%, and is limited to the colon in 10% to 20% of cases (Hyams, Markowitz, & Wyllie, 2000; Nickolaus & Schreiber, 2007). Ten percent to 15% of children have diffuse small bowel disease involving the more proximal ileum or jejunum. Gastroduodenal involvement was previously thought to be less common but has recently been reported in 30% to 40% of all individuals with CD when these areas are examined for endoscopic or histologic evidence of disease (Griffiths & Hugot, 2004). Perianal disease in children with CD ranges from 25% to 30% (Griffiths & Hugot). Affected children may have skin tags, fissures, and/or fistulas.

UC is also a chronic inflammatory disease but is limited to the colonic mucosa. The inflammatory process starts in the rectum and typically extends proximally in an uninterrupted pattern to involve parts or all of the large intestine. Inflammation limited to the rectum is found in 10% of pediatric cases (termed *ulcerative proctitis*), is found in the sigmoid and descending colon, distal to the splenic flexure *(left-sided colitis)* in 30%, or may involve the entire colon from cecum to rectum *(pancolitis)* in 40% to 50% of affected individuals (Diefenbach & Breuer, 2006; Heyman, Kirschner, Gold et al., 2005; Hyams et al., 2000; Nikolaus & Schreiber, 2007). Recently, children with UC have been reported to present with rectal sparing, but these studies should be interpreted with caution as the children may have Crohn's colitis (Dubinsky, 2008).

Children with disease limited to the colon but whose condition cannot be clearly categorized as CD or UC are described as having *indeterminate colitis* (IC) and may comprise 10% to 15% of cases. Usually after 1 to 2 years, many cases (approximately 50%) can be reclassified as UC or CD (Nikolaus & Schreiber, 2007; Present, 2002). It is thought that children with IC are ultimately more likely to be diagnosed with UC than CD, although the reverse may be true for very young children (Mamula, Mascarenhas, & Baldassano, 2002).

Despite research progress over the past two decades, the etiology and pathogenesis of IBD still remain to be clearly defined. Investigators hypothesize that IBD results from an unregulated immune response to environmental and bacterial triggers, probably in a genetically susceptible host. Advances in the immunologic and genetic factors associated with CD and UC suggest that these IBDs are not simply two disorders that share similar clinical manifestations, but more likely are composed of a group of diseases triggered and sustained by a variety of interacting diverse genetic, environmental, and immunologic risk factors (Oliva-Hemker & Fiocchi, 2002). Genetics is thought to play an even greater role in disease onset and susceptibility in the pediatric age group than in adults, and efforts to identify a gene specific to the pediatric-onset disease are ongoing (Dubinsky, 2008; Nieuwehuis & Escher, 2008; Xavier & Pololsky, 2007). Investigators have found an area of apparent linkage on chromosome 16 (Ogura, Bonen, Inohara et al., 2000; Cuthbert, Fisher, Mirza, et al., 2002; Podolsky, 2002). Detailed mapping of chromosome 16 has resulted in the identification of the *NOD2* gene (also designated *CARD15* and *IBD1*) that correlates strongly with CD (Kugathasan & Amre, 2006). A second gene that has been recently identified in individuals with IBD is the interleukin-23 (IL-23) receptor gene (Bousvaros, Murray, Leichtner, 2008b). At least 30 genetic susceptibility loci have been recently reported and further advances in this area are imminent (Barrett, Hansoul, Nicolae, et al., 2008). The fundamental basis of IBD is currently hypothesized to be a genetic predisposition leading to overreactivity of the mucosal immune system to normal microflora found in the gut or to environmental triggers (Bousvaros, Morley-Fletcher, Pensabene, et al., 2008a).

Incidence and Prevalence

The incidence of IBD in children and adolescents has significantly increased over the latter half of the twentieth century (Fish & Kugathasan, 2004; Heyman, et al., 2005; Rufo & Bousvaros, 2007). Approximately 1.4 million Americans are estimated to have IBD (Bousvaros, Sylvester, Kugathasan, et al., 2006). Of all individuals with IBD, 20% to 30% have symptom onset and 10% to 20%

of them have disease diagnosed before 18 years of age (Heyman et al., 2005). The overall incidence of IBD is estimated to be 0.2 to 8.5 per 100,000 for CD disease and 0.5% to 4.3% per 100, 000 for UC (Diefenbach & Breuer, 2006). In a multicenter Pediatric IBD Consortium (six referral centers in the United States) from 2000 to 2002, data on the 1370 enrolled children showed the mean age at diagnosis among pediatric referral centers was 10.3 ± 4.4 years with 6.1% confirmed diagnosis before 3 years of age; 15.4% diagnosed before 9 years; 48% at 6 to 12 years, and 37% at 13 to 17 years (Heyman et al., 2005; Higuchi & Bousvaros, 2007) The report also provides evidence that, not uncommonly, IBD can begin very early—before 1 year of age (Heyman et al., 2005). As in previous studies, UC was more common in the younger children (3 to 5 years old), whereas the prevalence of CD in this cohort increased after 8 years of age (Heyman et al., 2005; Higuchi & Bousvaros, 2007; Rufo & Bousvaros, 2007).

The incidence and frequency of IBD vary greatly depending on geographic location and racial or ethnic background. The highest rates are found in the Northern Hemisphere and in industrialized nations: Scandinavia and Scotland, then England and North America, followed with lower rates in Central and Southern Europe, Asia, and Africa (Diefenbach & Breuer, 2006; Oliva-Hemker, & Fiocchi, 2002). The risk of having IBD is greater in urban compared with rural areas, in higher versus lower socioeconomic classes, and in developed compared with less-developed countries (Oliva-Hemker, & Fiocchi). However, probably the single greatest risk factor for developing IBD is a first-degree relative, especially among those who have siblings with IBD (Oliva-Hemker & Fiocchi; Podolsky, 2002). Children diagnosed with IBD show a 30% greater family history compared with those without IBD. The Pediatric IBD Consortium reported that 44% of children younger than 3 years with UC had a first-degree relative with IBD (Heyman et al., 2005). The family risk pattern appears to be greater for CD compared with UC. Additionally, high rates of CD have been observed in monozygotic twins compared with dizygotic twins (Podolsky, 2002). Although monozygotic twins share identical genomic material, they may be disconcordant for CD, leading investigators to hypothesize that multiple gene products contribute to a person's risk of IBD (Podolsky).

The risk for UC and CD is greater for Jewish people of Middle European origin living in the United States than for those living in Israel. African Americans are less commonly affected with CD than whites. Men and women appear to be equally affected, although recent studies have suggested a predominance of a worse course of disease among female children with CD (Gupta, Bostrom, Kirschner, et al., 2007).

Diagnostic Criteria

The diagnosis of IBD is often difficult or delayed because of the subtle manner in which it presents. Before an astute pediatric practitioner refers the child to a pediatric gastroenterologist, presenting symptoms often mimic many other disease entities that prompt referrals to different pediatric specialists: the endocrinologist for growth or pubertal delay; the rheumatologist for joint swelling or pain; the hematologist for iron deficiency anemia; and the dermatologist for skin rashes (Fish & Kugathasan, 2004).

The diagnosis of IBD should include a history and physical examination; screening laboratory tests (including both blood and stool studies), radiologic studies of the GI tract, and upper and lower endoscopy with biopsy. An in-depth history about each of these symptoms may reveal important information to not only differentiate UC from CD, but also from other diseases that resemble IBD. If the abdominal pain is also associated with other symptoms, such as growth failure, anorexia, diarrhea, or other extraintestinal manifestations of IBD (described below), then a more extensive evaluation for IBD should be performed. "Red flags" that should raise suspicion for IBD or other organic etiologies include pain distant from the umbilicus, pain that interferes with normal sleep patterns, discrete episodes of pain of acute onset, pain precipitated by eating, rectal bleeding, and dysphagia or odynophagia (Fish & Kugathasan, 2004).

Growth curves should be reviewed and growth parameters including weight and height should be plotted on growth charts. Growth failure in stature and concomitant delay in sexual maturation may precede the development of overt intestinal manifestations by years in children with CD. At the time of initial diagnosis, 85% of children with CD and 65% of children with UC have lost weight. However, over the past two decades, the body mass index (BMI) of North American children has been increasing and children with IBD may be affected by this current trend (Kugathasan, Nebel, Skelton, et al., 2007). Deceleration in linear growth may be the only presenting clinical finding in children and adolescents with CD (Fish & Kugathasan, 2004).

Increased frequency of stools, urgency and the presence of blood and painful defecation (tenesmus) are all symptoms of rectal involvement with inflammation (proctitis). Diarrhea, which is common, may not need to be present, especially if the disease is localized to the small intestine. Nonspecific symptoms may surface during the interview and careful attention should be paid to children and adolescents with fever of unknown origin; arthritis, skin lesions, and perianal symptoms (pain and/or drainage) may be isolated and early symptoms or signs that can be associated with IBD. A top-to-bottom physical examination should be performed considering symptoms and signs of extraintestinal manifestation of IBD (see Clinical Manifestations section). The abdomen should be assessed for bowel sounds, distention, bloating, masses, and tenderness. A perianal and digital examination is critical to assess for evidence of external skin tags, fissures, fistulas and/or abscesses, and internal lesions, including anal stenosis, pelvic tenderness, and the presence or absence of blood.

Common laboratory findings associated with IBD include increased erythrocyte sedimentation rate (ESR) and C-reactive protein (CRP) (both nonspecific measures of inflammation), thrombocytosis, low serum iron level, low hematocrit value, and low hemoglobin level. Hypoalbuminemia and a decreased total serum protein value may also be noted, particularly in CD that affects the small bowel and in moderate to severe UC (Mack, Langton, Markowitz, et al., 2007). Serologic markers (antibodies against the yeast *Saccharomyces cerevisiae* [ASCA] and against neutrophils/peripheral antinuclear antibodies [pANCA], anti-12, antibodies to Cbir1 flagellin [anti-Cbir1], and outer membrane C [anti-OmpC]) for IBD may occasionally be helpful to confirm diagnosis of IBD in selected individuals and to distinguish CD from UC, but these tests should be reserved for the pediatric gastroenterologist to obtain if deemed necessary (Davis, Andres, Christopher, 2007; Targan & Karp, 2007). Fecal markers (calprotectin) are also now being used to aid in the differential diagnosis in children presenting with symptoms compatible but not diagnostic of IBD (Dubinsky, 2008; Nikolaus & Schreiber, 2007).

Infectious conditions of the GI tract, such as *Salmonella, Shigella, Campylobacter, Yersinia, Aeromonas, Escherichia coli* O157/H7, and *Clostridium difficile,* and the parasite *Entamoeba histolytica,* can mimic IBD and must be ruled out. Most laboratories can perform cultures for these organisms with routine stool collections.

Radiologic contrast studies, including upper GI series with a small bowel follow-through, are still the gold standard in the diagnostic process in IBD, especially CD, as they allow for direct visualization of mucosal patterns, presence of narrowing or strictures, and obstruction and fistulization in parts of the small bowel not able to be visualized by either upper endoscopy or colonoscopy. Computed tomography (CT) scanning may be useful to delineate small intestinal wall thickening, extramural extension of inflammation by fistulization to adjacent structures, and the presence of abscesses. Magnetic resonance imaging (MRI), particularly MR enterography, can differentiate active inflammation from fibrosis and detect anorectal fistulas and abscesses. Ultrasound scanning may be used to assess for abscesses or extraintestinal manifestations (gallstones) but at this time is rarely used for primary diagnosis. Colonoscopy and upper GI endoscopy are the preferred methods to evaluate the intestinal tract. They can identify mucosal inflammation, assess the extent of the disease, and permit mucosal biopsies to obtain histologic assessment to differentiate UC from CD. Endoscopic evidence of ulcers, erythema, loss of vascular pattern, friability (spontaneous bleeding), pseudopolyps, and continuous disease from the rectum and extending more proximally, biopsies showing crypt distortion, and abscess are consistent with a diagnosis of UC. Cobblestoning (nodularity) or linear ulceration in the ileum, or in particular, skip lesions throughout the colon, can be seen in CD.

Clinical Manifestations at Time of Diagnosis

The most common presenting symptoms of UC are diarrhea, abdominal pain, and rectal bleeding with blood and mucus. Children with UC may present with one of several patterns, differing by the extent and severity of mucosal inflammation. Mild disease, characterized by insidious diarrhea progressing to hematochezia, is seen in 50% to 60% of affected children (Diefenbach & Breuer, 2006). In mild disease the inflammation is usually confined to the rectum or distal colon; children may just present with blood in their stool. Thirty percent of children, however, present with moderate disease, characterized by bloody diarrhea, cramping pain, tenesmus, urgency, and abdominal tenderness (Diefenbach & Breuer). Other systemic symptoms are observed, such as anorexia, weight loss, fever, and mild anemia. Physical examination may reveal abdominal tenderness, and stool analysis will show various amounts of blood. Severe colitis with an acute, fulminant presentation is seen in only 10% of children (Diefenbach & Breuer). These children appear moderately to severely toxic, have more than six bloody stools per day, cramping abdominal pain, fever, anemia, leukocytosis, and hypoalbuminemia. Physical examination may reveal diffuse tenderness and distention. Serious complications, such as toxic megacolon, life-threatening hemorrhage, and perforation, are rare in the pediatric population.

Clinical Manifestations at Time of Diagnosis

- Often insidious onset
- GI symptoms
  - Diarrhea
  - Abdominal pain
  - Rectal bleeding
- Weight loss
- Delayed sexual maturation
- Decreased linear growth
- Extraintestinal manifestations
  - Skin
  - Musculoskeletal
  - Hepatobiliary
  - Ophthamologic

Presenting symptoms and signs of CD are determined primarily by the location and extent of disease involvement. CD may have an insidious onset with abdominal pain and weight loss that may contribute to a delay in diagnosis. Nonspecific symptoms of abdominal pain, anorexia, weight loss, delayed sexual maturation, and decreased linear growth may or may not all be present or not immediately recognized to prompt a workup for IBD (Diefenbach & Breuer, 2006; Ponsky, Hindle, & Sandler, 2007). If chronic diarrhea or rectal bleeding is present, diagnosis may be more expeditious (Diefenbach & Breuer, 2006). Abdominal pain is the most common single symptom at presentation: It is most often periumbilical but may localize to the right lower quadrant or be diffuse in the lower abdomen. Diarrhea may not be present if the disease is confined to the small intestine. The following clinical manifestations are diagnostic of CD from the initial workup: growth failure and/or pubertal delay; perianal abscesses and fissures; upper GI series with mucosal ulceration; nodularity; ileal and cecal narrowing; enteric fistula or obstruction; and abnormalities in the oral and/or perianal area. An unusual but relevant issue to pediatric practitioners is the observation that children's presenting symptoms can sometimes be limited to abnormalities of the anogenital region. Children with CD have presented with histories of chronic constipation, even encopresis; often a thorough perianal examination provides clues to the correct diagnosis. Although physical findings consistent with sexual abuse must be appropriately investigated, organic causes of anogenital disease must also be properly evaluated. The course of the signs and symptoms of illness observed at diagnosis (e.g., the extraintestinal manifestations previously noted) may remain, disappear with treatment, reappear with exacerbations of the disease, or may never return. New symptoms (i.e., GI or extraintestinal) may also appear with exacerbations. See Table 30-1 for a comparison of presenting symptoms for CD and UC.

An exacerbation of CD or UC sometimes is preceded by an intercurrent illness or emotional stress or may occur for no apparent reason. Intercurrent GI infections may also trigger exacerbation of disease activity, with *C. difficile* and viral infections (e.g., rotavirus and adenovirus) often implicated. Exacerbations of symptoms may occur after dietary indiscretions, but such indiscretions are not considered a cause of genuine flare-ups of disease activity because they are not accompanied by changes in histologic, radiographic, or laboratory parameters. Children with IBD often become adept at anticipating which activities are likely to trigger a flare-up of their disease.

TABLE 30-1
Comparison of Crohn's Disease and Ulcerative Colitis: Presenting Symptoms

	Crohn's Disease	Ulcerative Colitis
Diarrhea	Common	Common often with urgency
Constipation	Occasional	Rare without obstruction
Blood in stool	Occult common Gross blood indication for colonic disease	Very common
Abdominal pain	Typically mid-abdomen and right lower quadrant pain	Cramping pain often with stools
Fever	Common	Rare
Weight loss/growth failure	Common May occur for many months to years before diagnosis	Rare
Perianal disease	Common for: Fistula/fissures Abscesses/skin tags Skin tags	Rare

Extraintestinal manifestations of IBD have been found in almost every organ system (Jose & Heyman, 2008) (Figure 30-1). Extraintestinal symptoms or signs of an underlying IBD may be clinically significant and prevalent in about 6% to 68% of children with IBD (Fish & Kugathasan, 2004; Jose & Heyman, 2008). The pathogenic mechanism of extraintestinal manifestations in IBD are not known, and may or may not be related to bowel disease activity (Fish & Kugathasan). Many extraintestinal manifestations are hypothesized to be due to immune reactions, intestinal bacteria, or genetic factors. The most common target organs are the skin, joints, bone, liver, and eyes. In children, extraintestinal manifestations may precede the onset of GI disease by years (Diefenbach & Breuer, 2006).

Skin manifestations of IBD are erythema nodosum (raised, red, tender nodules that appear primarily on the anterior surfaces of the leg), affecting 3% of children with CD and pyoderma gangrenosum (chronic ulcer), affecting 1% of children with UC and even fewer with CD (Jose & Heyman, 2008). Aphthous ulceration in the mouth is the most common oral manifestation in CD, occurring in 20% to 30% of children with CD and in 5% to 10% of those with UC (Jose & Heyman).

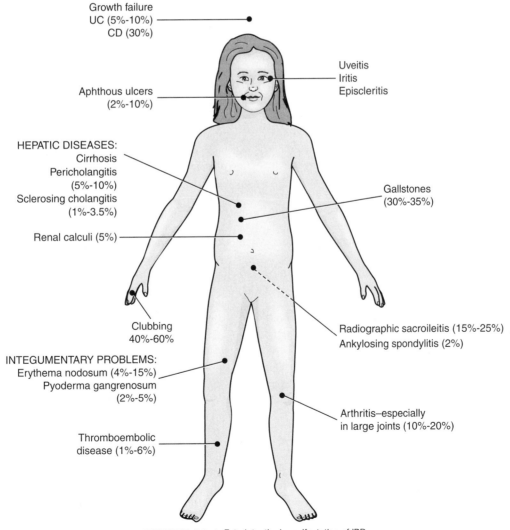

Growth failure
UC (5%-10%)
CD (30%)

Aphthous ulcers
(2%-10%)

HEPATIC DISEASES:
Cirrhosis
Pericholangitis
(5%-10%)
Sclerosing cholangitis
(1%-3.5%)

Renal calculi (5%)

Clubbing
40%-60%

INTEGUMENTARY PROBLEMS:
Erythema nodosum (4%-15%)
Pyoderma gangrenosum
(2%-5%)

Thromboembolic
disease (1%-6%)

Uveitis
Iritis
Episcleritis

Gallstones
(30%-35%)

Radiographic sacroileitis (15%-25%)
Ankylosing spondylitis (2%)

Arthritis–especially
in large joints (10%-20%)

FIGURE 30-1 Extraintestinal manifestation of IBD.

Musculoskeletal manifestations are the most common extra-intestinal manifestation in IBD. Arthritis is the most common extra-intestinal manifestation, occurring in 7% to 25% of children with IBD. Two types of arthritis are described: peripheral arthritis, sometimes referred to as *colitis arthritis;* and the axial form, *ankylosing spondylitis* or *sacroiliitis* (Jose & Heyman, 2008). Peripheral arthritis tends to track the bowel disease and can respond to medical or surgical treatment of the IBD, whereas the axial form of the disease does not seem to remit with treatment of IBD (Ephgrave, 2007). Arthritis is more commonly observed when the colon is affected for unknown reasons (Fish & Kugathasan, 2004) (see Chapter 31).

Hepatobiliary disease, both intrahepatic and extrahepatic, is relatively common and is among the more serious extraintestinal manifestations of IBD. Liver disorders may be present before or during active disease, or they may even develop after surgical resection of diseased bowel. Primary sclerosing cholangiitis (PSC) is reported in 1.6% to 7.4% of children with UC and fewer than 1% of children with CD (Jose & Heyman, 2008). Of note, up to 90% of children with PSC eventually have a diagnosis of IBD, most commonly UC.

Ophthalmologic findings for UC and CD usually appear when the condition is active. The most common ocular findings are episcleritis and anterior uveitis; glaucoma has been reported in some teenagers, independent of corticosteroid usage.

Treatment

Treatment of IBD includes pharmacologic (Table 30-2), nutritional, and surgical therapies. The goals of treatment for IBD include clinical and laboratory control of inflammation, alleviation of symptoms with the fewest, least severe possible adverse effects from medications, optimal growth and development through nutrition, avoidance of long-term disease-related complications, and facilitation of normal social development and involvement with a good/normal quality of life (QoL). The specific treatment plan depends on the location and severity of the disease, the effect of the disease on growth and development, and the degree of debilitation experienced by the child. Surgical intervention is indicated when medical therapies do not adequately control symptoms or complications (e.g., toxic megacolon, severe hemorrhage, strictures leading to obstruction, fistulas, or abscesses) or symptoms do not respond to medical management. Children with severe disease who are experiencing incapacitating symptoms accompanied by abnormal laboratory values require aggressive medical intervention, including hospitalization, restricted diets, intravenous corticosteroid therapy, or total parenteral nutrition (TPN).

Specialists now have tools to categorize disease activity and assess response to medical treatment. The Pediatric Crohn Disease Activity Index (PCDAI) and the more recent PCDAI-2 were developed to give clinicians a uniform system to stratify children and adolescents into categories of disease activity: inactive, mild, moderate, or severe activity and to assess response to treatment (Hyams, Markowitz, Otley, et al, 2005). A new noninvasive activity index of pediatric ulcerative colitis (PUCAI) also has been developed using two separate cohorts of children with UC at five pediatric IBD centers in North America and appears to accurately differentiate disease activity states without the need for colonoscopic assessment (Turner, Otley, Mack, et al., 2007).

> *Treatment*
>
> *Pharmacologic Therapy.* See Table 30-2.
> - Antiinflammatory therapy
> - Immunosuppressive therapy
> - Biologic immunotherapy
> - Novel therapies with unique modes of action
>
> *Nutritional Therapy*
> - An elemental diet is less effective in achieving remission than corticosteroids but can improve nutritional status.
> - Total parenteral nutrition is generally reserved for individuals with severe disease who cannot tolerate enteral feedings.
> - Probiotics
>
> *Surgical Intervention*
> - Surgical intervention is indicated when disease activity or complications do not respond to medical management.
> - *Ulcerative colitis:* Colectomy is the procedure of choice with the creation of an ileal pouch anal anastomosis (IPAA).
> - *Crohn's disease:* Procedures are limited resection of diseased bowel segment or colectomy with permanent ileostomy. Perianal abscesses and fistulas may need to be drained or debrided surgically.

Pharmacologic Therapy

Pharmacologic therapy is the mainstay of treatment of disease and maintenance of remission of IBD. The goals of medical therapy can be categorized as induction and remission maintenance with the fewest side effects from the medications. Because the known pathophysiology of IBD is thought to be the result of an overactive immune response at the gut level, almost all currently accepted therapies are antiinflammatory or immunosuppressive (Tamboli, 2007). The medications are often classified as antiinflammatory, immunosuppressive, and the newer biologic immunotherapeutic agents. The 5-aminosalicylic acid (5-ASA) preparations, corticosteroids, and antibiotics usually are considered antiinflammatory; whereas 6-mercaptopurine, azathioprine (AZA), methotrexate, cyclosporine A, and tacrolimus are classified as immunosuppressive therapies (see Table 30-2). The newer biologic agents are therapies that can target specific immune-related actions to block specific immune modulators or pathways. Biologic agents include antibody-based therapies, recombinant proteins, and nucleic acid–based therapies (see Table 30-2). Most clinicians currently use a step-up approach to therapy, using increasingly more potent agents to the regimen if less active drugs fail to achieve or sustain remission. This approach takes into account medication safety as the more milder/less toxic medications are used first, letting affected individuals declare treatment failures themselves before necessitating a step up to more aggressive antiinflammatory agents (Dubinsky, 2008).

Controversy exists about choosing a step-down versus a step-up approach to medical therapy in the treatment of CD (Tamboli, 2007). The step-down approach uses aggressive therapy with the newer biologic agents in hope of preventing future complications with early disease stabilization. This approach has not become standard of care in the medical community because of concern about unknown long-term toxic effects. A combination of drugs from the different categories may be necessary for treatment depending on the child or adolescent's response. Treatment regimens vary by individual clinician; each physician/

TABLE 30-2

Drugs Used for Treatment of Inflammatory Bowel Disease

Drug (Brand Name)/Dosage	Uses in IBD	Side Effects	Special Considerations
Sulfasalazine* (Azulfidine) 50-80 mg/kg/day	Treatment of UC and Crohn's colitis	*Common:* headache, malaise, GI upset, decreased sperm production *Less common:* skin eruption, hepatitis, pancreatitis, pneumonia, hemolysis, allergic reaction 5-ASA side effects (see below)	Fewer adverse reactions may be noted if the dosage is gradually increased to reach the planned therapeutic dosage. Enteric-coated tablets may alleviate GI upset. Monitor WBC count over first 3 mo of treatment. Impairs folic acid absorption; give folic acid 1 mg/day.
Olsalazine* (Dipentum) 30-50 mg/kg/day	Treatment of UC and Crohn's colitis (not used often in pediatrics because of diarrhea)	For all 5-ASAs: *Common:* GI upset, abdominal pain, dizziness, headache, diarrhea, rash, hair loss *Less common:* pancreatitis, pericarditis, aplastic anemia, allergic reaction	For all 5-ASAs: Fewer adverse reactions than sulfasalazine; useful for individuals unable to tolerate sulfasalazine Dipentum, Pentasa, and Colazal capsules may be opened and mixed in food for younger children
Balsalazide* (Colazal) 40-60 mg/kg/day	Treatment of UC and Crohn's colitis	5-ASA side effects	5-ASA special considerations
Mesalamine* (Asacol) 40-80 mg/kg/day	Treatment of UC and ileocolonic CD	5-ASA side effects	5-ASA special considerations
Mesalamine* (Pentasa) 40-80 mg/kg/day	Treatment of small intestinal and colonic CD	5-ASA side effects	5-ASA special considerations
Mesalamine* (Lialda) 40-80 mg/kg/day	Can be used to treat UC	5-ASA side effects	5-ASA special considerations
Mesalamine* (Rowasa enema) 60 mL/4 g nightly(Canasa suppository) 500mg once daily or bid	Topical therapy for proctitis and distal	5-ASA side effects *Common:* perianal irritation, pruritus, colitis *Less common:* pancreatitis, pericarditis	5-ASA special considerations Child should be instructed to try to retain the suppository or enema overnight.
Corticosteroids: prednisone, prednisolone 1-2 mg/kg/day up to 40-80 mg/day	Useful in children who do not respond adequately to 5-ASAs Useful in moderate to severe disease Also available as foam (Cortifoam) and retention enemas (Cortenema) for rectal disease	*Common:* adrenal suppression, growth retardation, cushingoid facies, weight gain, striae, mood swings, acne, impaired calcium absorption, osteoporosis, hypertension, hyperglycemia *Less common:* cataracts, aseptic necrosis of the femoral head	Alternate-day therapy at lowest possible dose is often used to minimize adverse effects once in remission. Child should be warned to not discontinue corticosteroid use suddenly; this could result in an adrenal crisis and a flare-up of symptoms. Ophthalmic examination, urine dipstick, and blood pressure monitoring should be done at each visit. Child should see an ophthalmologist once or twice a year if they are taking corticosteroids.
Budesonide* (Entocort) 9 mg/day	Mild to moderate CD	*Common (much less than corticosteroids):* headache, respiratory infection, nausea, cushingoid facies, acne, and bruising	90% of drug does not go into the bloodstream; it is a nonsystemic corticosteroid. Avoid eating grapefruit during administration. Recommended duration of therapy is 8 wk.
Metronidazole* (Flagyl) 10-15 mg/kg/day Divided into three or four doses/day	Effective adjunct treatment for CD Useful in the management of perianal disease, fistulas, abscesses	*Common:* GI upset, metallic taste in mouth, paresthesias	Assess for paresthesias at each office visit; these are usually reversible after discontinuation of the medication. Disulfiram-like effect (i.e., vomiting) occurs if taken with alcohol or products containing alcohol.
Ciprofloxacin* (Cipro) 10-20 mg/kg/day Divided into two doses/day	Effective adjunct treatment for CD	*Common:* headache; rash; GI upset; perianal disease, fistulas, and anemia Useful in the management of abscesses	Ciprofloxacin has caused damage to growing bone in some laboratory animals, but to date no such adverse reactions have been observed in children.
Rifaximin* (Xifaxin) 200-400 mg bid	May be effective adjunct treatment in CD	*Common :* GI upset	Nonsystemic

Continued

TABLE 30-2

Drugs Used for Treatment of Inflammatory Bowel Disease—cont'd

Drug (Brand Name)/Dosage	Uses in IBD	Side Effects	Special Considerations
6-Mercaptopurine* (6-MP) (Purinethol) 1.5-2.0 mg/kg/day	Used as a primary therapy in CD and UC, when 5-ASA therapy and corticosteroids have failed, or when child cannot be weaned from corticosteroids	*Common:* leukopenia, pancreatitis, hepatitis, allergic reactions, increased risk of infection	If fever develops, drug should be discontinued until illness resolves. It may take 3 to 4 mo to see response.
Azathioprine (Imuran) 2.0-2.5 mg/kg/day	Same as 6-MP	*Common:* GI upset, leukopenia, hepatitis, pancreatitis, allergy, risk of infection	CBC count, transaminases, amylase, and lipase levels should be monitored during therapy.
Methotrexate 15-25 mg/m²/wk SQ or IM	Steroid-dependent CD Refractory UC	*Common:* malaise, fatigue, headache, rash, GI upset, stomatitis, myelosuppression *Less common, serious:* toxic reactions, death, encephalopathy, cortical blindness *Less common:* tuberculosis, sepsis, malignancies, and formation of human antichimeric antibody (HACA)	Folate may decrease drug response.
Cyclosporine (Sandimmune, Neoral) 1-2 mg/kg/day IV 4-8 mg/kg/day PO	Used in steroid refractory UC, difficult to treat CD and indeterminate colitis when colectomy is suggested and family is not ready	*Common:* immunosuppression, increased risk for malignancy (lymphomas, lymphoproliferative disorder, and squamous cell tumor), nephrotoxicity, hypertension, seizure, hirsutism, acne, GI upset, gingival hyperplasia, and headache *Less common:* encephalopathy, convulsions, vision and movement disturbances, and impaired consciousness	Trough levels (before am dose) should be drawn periodically. Grapefruit juice increases absorption.
Tacrolimus (Prograf, FK506) 0.1 mg/kg/day	Same as cyclosporine Available in topical ointment	Cyclosporine side effects	Cyclosporine special considerations Many drugs can increase or decrease serum levels. Topical ointment should not be used in occlusive dressing.
Infliximab (Remicade) 5-10 mg/kg/dose at 0, 2, 6 wk, then every 8 wk IV	Used with moderate to severe active CD in children or adolescents who have inadequate response to active fistulas in CD	*Common:* headache, itching, fatigue, nausea, dizziness, fever, upper respiratory infection, autoimmune antibody formation conventional therapy	The concomitant treatment with AZA, 6-MP, methotrexate, or corticosteroid (or pretreatment) appears to reduce the frequency of formation of HACA antibodies. HACA is associated with loss of clinical response to infliximab or increased infusion reactions. Methotrexate may decrease absorption, but no adjustment to the dose is needed when methotrexate is given concomitantly.
Adalimumab* (Humira) 160 mg SQ first dose, 80 mg SQ at wk 2, then 40 mg SQ weekly	Used with moderately severe–to-conventional therapy, reaction to infliximab CD, and when inadequate response	*Common:* redness, itching, bruising, pain, or swelling at site of injection, GI upset, rash, nausea, headache, back pain, minor infections *Less common:* tuberculosis, sepsis, fungal infections, worsened nervous system symptoms, cancer, aplastic anemia	
Certolizumab* (Cimzia) 400 mg SQ at 0, 2 4 wk, then every 4 wk	Used with moderately severe–to-conventional therapy, reaction to infliximab, and when inadequate response	*Common:* redness, itching, bruising, pain, or swelling at site of injection, GI upset, rash, nausea, headache, back pain, minor infections, arthralgias *Less common:* tuberculosis, sepsis, fungal infections, worsened nervous system symptoms, cancer, aplastic anemia	No live vaccines.

*Not FDA approved for children—dosage may need to be adjusted for pediatrics.
Key: *SQ,* subcutaneously.

nurse practitioner relies on her or his experience, clinical knowledge, and the observed clinical response of the child. In addition, nutritional therapies are used as a primary therapy for CD and as adjunctive therapy for either UC or CD; these approaches are discussed below.

Antiinflammatory Therapy. The 5-ASA preparations include the oral agents: sulfasalazine (Azulfidine), olsalazine disodium (Dipentum), balsalazide (Colazal), and mesalamine (Asacol, Pentasa, Lialda, Apriso). Enema and suppository forms of mesalamine (Rowasa, Canasa) are also available as the first step in treatment of distal colonic IBD. For many years, sulfasalazine was the primary drug used to treat colonic disease. Sulfasalazine is a combination of 5-ASA and sulfapyridine. Sulfapyridine is primarily used as a delivery agent which—when bound to 5-ASA—inhibits absorption in the proximal GI tract. Unfortunately, up to 20% to 25% of individuals who take sulfasalazine experience significant allergic or other adverse side effects, which are mostly related to the sulfapyridine component (Griffiths & Buller, 2004). Although generally well tolerated, 5-ASA medications are reported to cause occasional headache, malaise, nausea, vomiting, anorexia, heartburn, and/or diarrhea. Less common but more severe reactions include skin eruptions, hepatitis, pancreatitis, pneumonia, hemolysis or bone marrow suppression, and allergic reactions (Physicians' Desk Reference [PDR], 2008). Sulfasalazine (because of the sulfapyridine) may also interfere with folate absorption, which can lead to megaloblastic anemia; this problem may be prevented by co-administering 1 mg of folic acid per day (Griffiths & Buller, 2004; PDR, 2008; Tamboli, 2007).

Sulfasalazine or one of the other 5-ASA medications may be used as primary therapy in mild to moderate UC. Sulfasalazine can be formulated into a suspension, and balsalazide and Apriso powder (from an opened capsule) can be sprinkled onto food for children who cannot take pills or capsules. When initiating therapy, a child's dose is gradually increased to the therapeutic range to alleviate or avoid the dose-dependent side effects of sulfasalazine. During initiation of therapy, leukopenia and hemolytic anemia should be monitored at least monthly by a complete blood cell count (CBC). If either of these becomes apparent, the dose should be decreased or stopped until the blood values return to normal. The dose may then be slowly returned to the therapeutic range. If this approach is unsuccessful, the drug should be discontinued and therapy with another 5-ASA preparation attempted (Griffiths & Buller, 2004). Eighty percent to 90% of people who do not tolerate or are allergic to sulfasalazine tolerate another oral 5-ASA preparation (Griffiths & Buller).

The 5-ASA drugs have the advantages of more site-specific activity and a lower incidence of side effects and are equally effective compared with sulfasalazine in prolonging remission in UC (Katz, 2002; Griffiths, & Buller, 2004; Tamboli, 2007). Adverse effects with the newer 5-ASA preparations occur less frequently than those associated with sulfasalazine but include nausea, vomiting, dizziness, headache, abdominal pain, worsening of diarrhea and rectal bleeding, rash, and hair loss. Pancreatitis, pericarditis, aplastic anemia, and hypersensitivity reactions are rare but more worrisome (Griffiths & Buller, 2004). Although pediatric doses of mesalamine have not been fully established, it has been recommended to start at 30 to 70 mg/kg/day, but doses are often increased even to 80 to 100 mg/kg/day for some children and generally tolerated (Hyams & Markowitz, 2005; Fish & Kugathasan, 2004). Recommended monitoring for toxicity includes monthly (CBC) counts, liver function tests, blood urea nitrogen (BUN) and creatinine levels, and urinalysis for 3 months, then every 3 to 6 months (Hyams & Markowitz, 2005). Asacol is available only in enteric-coated tablet form, which is difficult for children who cannot swallow pills; Dipentum, Colazal, and Pentasa capsules may be opened and mixed in food to ease administration. Colazal powder has been administered to children as young as 5 years.

Mesalamine enemas (Rowasa) and suppositories (Canasa) can be effective in treating distal colonic (left-sided disease) and rectal disease (proctitis). Rectal therapy enhances the efficacy and rapidity of oral therapy in achieving remission when given concomitantly (Katz, 2002). Enemas are typically instilled at bedtime with the goal of retaining the fluid overnight. Suppositories are inserted once or twice a day and are especially useful to treat proctitis. Treatment may be provided for a few weeks or longer. Adverse effects of these topical preparations include perianal irritation, pruritus and, rarely, pancreatitis and pericarditis (Physicians' Desk Reference, 2008). Approximately one third of individuals with IBD do not achieve remission with 5-ASA medications alone and require the addition of corticosteroids to the regimen (Ponsky et al., 2007). This may be due in large part to poor therapeutic adherence secondary to the large number of pills necessary. The newer addition of Lialda (1.2 g/cap) and Apriso (325 mg/cap), mesalamine derivatives that can be taken once a day, may help with the adherence problem.

In moderate to severe disease and during disease exacerbations, corticosteroids are often used to induce remission but must be used judiciously. No other class of medications used in the treatment of IBD works as rapidly and with such consistent results to control disease activity and improve symptoms, but unfortunately no other class of medication produces such diverse and difficult to manage side effects (Katz, 2004). Corticosteroids are of no benefit for maintenance therapy. Corticosteroid suppositories, foams, and enemas can deliver the corticosteroid directly to the rectum, sigmoid, and left colon providing relief of tenesmus and urgency associated with distal colitis but with less systemic absorption than when administered intravenously or orally (Markowitz, 2008). Pediatric IBD centers are steering away from the use of corticosteroids because of their serious, long-term side effects and the availability of new agents. Unfortunately, corticosteroid dependency is seen in 30% to 40% of children and adolescents who use them (Markowitz, 2008).

Corticosteroids are prescribed as prednisone, prednisolone, methylprednisolone, hydrocortisone, and the newest form, budesonide. The various agents differ in duration of action, strength of glucocorticoid, and relative mineralocorticoid activity. Children are started with a prednisone equivalent dosage ranging from 1 to 2 mg/kg/day, usually with a maximum dose of up to 60 to 80 mg/day. Intravenous therapy is used for severe disease and disease refractive to oral therapy. Treatment with daily prednisone at high doses should continue for 2 to 3 weeks until remission is achieved. A tapering regimen is then carefully prescribed, decreasing the dose gradually in 5- to 7-day intervals. Occasionally, if tapering is difficult, the prednisone can be tapered to an alternating-day cycle and then gradually discontinued (Griffiths & Buller, 2004). The dose is then gradually tapered while a child's symptoms and laboratory values, especially ESR, CBC count, and albumin, are monitored.

Budesonide is a synthetic steroid that has decreased adverse systemic effects compared with the other group of corticosteroids (Katz, 2002, 2004; Griffiths & Buller, 2004; Levine, Broide, Stein, et al., 2002). Budesonide exerts a strong topical antiinflammatory effect in the distal small intestine and proximal colon, but when absorbed, it is rapidly metabolized by the liver and in low dose has minimal effect on adrenal suppression (Katz, 2002, 2004; Griffiths & Buller). Because of its low bioavailability, the incidence of prednisone-like side effects is much lower (Griffiths & Buller). Some recent studies have suggested that to achieve efficacy, the higher dose needed causes systemic reactions similar to prednisone (Katz, 2004; Griffiths & Hugot, 2004).

Side effects of corticosteroids are related to the amount administered and duration of therapy or the total dose to which the child is exposed. The major side effects include acute reactions: "moon" facies, weight gain, fluid retention with hypertension, hyperglycemia, acne, striae, hirsutism, and mood swings. Long-term effects include growth retardation, calcium depletion (and osteoporosis), immunosuppression, cataract formation, glaucoma, and aseptic necrosis of the hip or knees (Fish & Kugathasan, 2004; Griffiths & Buller, 2004). Growth inhibition is a major problem in children and adolescents with daily therapy as a result of direct suppression of insulin-like growth factor-I (IGF-I) and consequent inhibition of linear growth (Fish & Kugathasan, 2004; Griffiths & Buller, 2004). Alternate-day steroid dosing allows IGF-I to normalize and preserve normal growth rates (Katz, 2004). Corticosteroid-induced bone disease results from decreased calcium absorption, increased urinary calcium excretion, increased bone reabsorption and diminished bone formation. Trials are currently under way to test the efficacy of bisphosphonates to prevent bone demineralization in children exposed to large doses of corticosteroids. Adequate calcium, vitamin D, and physical activity may reduce the rate of bone disease.

Long-term use also leads to adrenal suppression that persists for 6 to 12 months after corticosteroid therapy has been completed. Rapid cessation (often inadvertently) of prednisone during therapy or stressful incident (e.g., an accident, serious infection, or surgery) in the year following treatment with prednisone may precipitate acute adrenal insufficiency. Symptoms of acute adrenal insufficiency include fever, hypotension, dehydration, vomiting, electrolyte abnormalities, hypoglycemia, severe abdominal pain, and lethargy (see Chapter 20). Treatment consists of intravenous hydrocortisone administration until oral therapy can be resumed and if needed, fluid replacement is initiated to treat dehydration. Children should also be given stress doses of corticosteroids during episodes of significant illness or for scheduled surgical procedures.

Antibiotic therapy has been used as a primary treatment, as an adjunct to other treatments, or as specific treatment for complications of CD; antibiotics are used less frequently in individuals with UC. Although their mechanism of action is unclear, antibiotics are hypothesized to affect the enteric bacterial flora implicated in the pathophysiology of intestinal inflammation in CD. Metronidazole, ciprofloxacin, and rifaxamin are all used. Metronidazole is effective in the treatment of perianal disease, fistulas, and abscesses, and when its dose is lowered or it is discontinued, perianal disease commonly relapses (Tamboli, 2007). The effects of long-term use of metronidazole are not known, but concern has been raised that it may potentially be carcinogenic or mutagenic. However, no cases have been reported in which either cancer or chromosomal aberrations have been proven to be attributable to metronidazole use in humans (*PDR*, 2008). Side effects of metronidazole include GI upset and a metallic taste. A more worrisome side effect is peripheral neuropathy, which appears to be related to dose and duration of therapy (*PDR*). Adolescents should be warned of the disulfiram-like effect if they ingest alcohol while taking metronidazole. Ciprofloxacin is used alone or in combination with metronidazole to treat perirectal disease. The newest antibiotic currently being studied for treating IBD is rifaximin. It is an oral antibiotic that is not absorbed into the bloodstream but instead directly affects the digestive tract (Tamboli, 2007).

Immunosuppressive Therapy. Immunomodulators, 6-mercaptopurine (6-MP) and azathioprine (AZA), are now widely used to treat IBD in children. Metabolism of the two drugs is similar because AZA is converted in vivo into 6-MP (Markowitz, 2008). Initially, 6-MP was used as a steroid-sparing agent and was prescribed as a third-line therapy in children for whom more conservative medical management had failed or for those who could not be weaned from corticosteroids. Because of the increased experience using these medications, immunomodulators are prescribed much earlier in the course of treatment, even in some cases on initial presentation (because it takes several months to achieve efficacy). They improve symptom control, reduce corticosteroid requirements in 60% to 70% of children, and prevent relapses (Griffiths & Buller, 2004; Katz, 2002). They are among the most effective treatment available for the long-term maintenance of both UC and CD and they also reduce the risk of postoperative recurrence of CD after intestinal resection (Markowitz, 2008). Initiation of the drugs should be slow with close laboratory monitoring because of the risk of serious side effects, in particular leukopenia and abnormal liver function. Response to these agents is not immediate, averaging 3 to 4 months.

AZA-induced toxicity is genetically based on the availability of the enzyme thiopurine methyltransferase (TPMT), which is needed to metabolize AZA. TPMT can be detected by blood test, although the importance of screening is subject to debate. Determining an individual's enzyme activity may be useful as it allows for more rapid dosage increases to achieve medication effect within 4 to 6 weeks (rather than 3 to 4 months). Toxicities many occur regardless of TPMT activity (Nikolaus & Schreiber, 2007). Routine CBC counts and hepatic enzyme checks need to be performed as long as the child takes the drug (Tamboli, 2007).

The most commonly cited complications of 6-MP and AZA are GI irritation manifested by vomiting and abdominal pain, leukopenia, fever, hepatitis, and pancreatitis. All immunomodulators predispose individuals to an increased risk of infection because of bone marrow suppression or toxicity. Concern about the possible increased risk of lymphoma for individuals treated with these agents continues and is supported by a meta-analysis that suggests an increased risk of lymphoma in adults with CD treated with a 6-MP or AZA (Markowitz, 2008). This risk in children and adolescents has not been calculated. During the first several months of therapy a CBC count with differential (to monitor for leukopenia and lymphopenia), liver enzyme levels, and amylase and lipase levels should be checked every 2 weeks to assess for adverse reactions. These parameters should be checked monthly for several months and then every 3 months thereafter (Griffiths & Hugot, 2004). The dose is reduced or therapy discontinued if the total white blood cell count falls below 2500/mm^3 or the transaminases rise (>2 times normal). Levels of the active metabolites (6-thioguanine [6-TG]) may be useful to monitor for compliance and possibly efficacy and safety. Hepatotoxicity appears to correlate with elevated levels of another metabolite (6-methylmercaptopurine [6-MMP] levels), although the clinical relevance and usefulness of this test is controversial. Therapy may be reattempted after the liver enzyme levels return to normal. Elevation of amylase and/or lipase levels may signify pancreatitis, but this laboratory finding may also be transient, so the significance of this observation must be taken cautiously and in the context of the clinical setting (Griffiths & Buller, 2004; Markowitz, Grancher, Kohn et al., 2000, & Markowitz, 2008).

The primary care provider, family, and child must be aware that any febrile illness during therapy with 6-MP or AZA is an indication for concern and must be evaluated. Temporary discontinuation of the drug may be necessary until the illness resolves. Exposure to varicella infection in those who have not been vaccinated or had prior varicella infection and who are taking 6-MP or AZA warrants administration of varicella zoster immune globulin (VZIG) within 48 hours of exposure, and 6-MP or AZA should then be temporarily discontinued.

Methotrexate is a second-line immunosuppressant for children with IBD. Methotrexate interferes with DNA synthesis and also induces production of antiinflammatory cytokines and lymphocyte apoptosis (Kozuch & Hanauer, 2008). Methotrexate has been used in CD to treat children and adults who have been steroid-dependent and who are intolerant of or unresponsive to 6-MP (Markowitz, 2008; Podolsky, 2002). Onset of action can be shorter that that of 6-MP or AZA, so it has a place as an induction or maintenance therapy (Diefenbach & Breuer, 2006; Markowitz, 2008). Methotrexate is administered as a weekly intramuscular or subcutaneous injection (up to 25 mg per week): recently oral administration has also been used effectively. Response may take several weeks. Side effects include nausea, which can be so severe that children will refuse to continue treatment; vomiting; diarrhea; stomatitis; rash; arthralgias; leukopenia; and hepatotoxicity (Diefenbach & Breuer, 2006; Markowitz, 2008). It is also terataogenic (Markowitz, 2008).

Cyclosporine (Sandimmune) and tacrolimus (Prograf) are potent inhibitors of cell-mediated immunity and are sometimes administered to selected individuals with refractory UC (to prevent imminent colectomy) or in fistulizing CD, and are occasionally used in cases of severe indeterminate colitis (Markowitz, 2008). Response to cyclosporine therapy is inconsistent. Treated individuals have had a significant incidence of relapse while receiving therapy and recurrence when discontinuing the drug (Markowitz, 2008). Cyclosporine and tacrolimus have been used to induce remission in children and adolescents with severe UC who are hospitalized, when standard medical management has failed, and those who otherwise are in need of urgent proctocolectomy but are psychologically or emotionally unprepared to accept the surgical option (Podolosky, 2002). A recent study by Ziring, Wu, Mow and colleagues (2007) found the use of tacrolimus with steroid-resistant or steroid-dependent UC provided a rapid clinical response similar to infliximab. If remission can be achieved using either agent, other therapies such as 6-MP or AZA are used to sustain remission and cyclosporine or tacrolimus, as well as any corticosteroids, are weaned. No maintenance role for either of these two agents has been demonstrated because of their high risk of toxicity; thus they are most often used as a "bridge" therapy to ultimate maintenance with 6-MP, AZA, or methotrexate (Markowitz, 2008). Tacrolimus in steroid-resistant colitis may be capable of inducing short- to medium-term remission, but no long-term benefit has been demonstrated—all affected individuals eventually progress to colectomy (Ziring et al., 2007).

Side effects of cyclosporine and tacrolimus include hypertension, tremor, paresthesias, hirsutism, seizures, nausea and vomiting, and the potential for renal insufficiency. Careful monitoring of children and adolescents for serious infections—especially those who are taking concurrent corticosteroids and 6-MP—is essential. Prophylaxis with oral trimethoprim-sulfamethoxasole is suggested for those taking cyclosporine or tacrolimus. Frequent monitoring of vital signs, serum laboratory studies (including BUN and creatinine), and drug levels is mandatory during treatment (Jani & Regueiro, 2002). Multiple drug interactions occur with cyclosporine and tacrolimus, thus further complicating the management of children and adolescents with these medications (Irving, Shanahan, & Rampton, 2007; Markowitz, 2008). Toxicity of these agents, especially cyclosporine, limits their use, particularly in UC, which is "curable" with surgery.

Biologic Immunotherapy. Biologic agents are becoming a standard therapy in children with CD and more recently are being applied as treatment for UC (De Ridder, Benninga, Taminiau, et al., 2007; Sands, 2006). These newer therapies are directed toward specific targets of the inflammatory reaction, rather than the broad-based approach of the commonly used immunosuppressive and immunomodulatory medications.

The first genetically engineered product to be approved by the Food and Drug Administration (FDA) in 2006 for its use in pediatric CD is infliximab (Remicade), a tumor necrosis factor–alpha (TNF-α) antibody. First approved for use in CD with active fistulas, infliximab is now also being used in individuals with medically resistant, moderate to severe CD. Infliximab has been FDA approved to treat refractory adult UC and is used off-label in the treatment of children with steroid-refractory UC (Rufo & Bousvaros, 2007). Large multicenter trials are needed (and ongoing) in pediatric UC to clarify the indications for and long-term benefit of infliximab. It has shown control of many of the extraintestinal manifestations of IBD, such as pyoderma gangrenosum, arthritis, and granulomatous pneumonitis (De Ridder et al., 2007; Markowitz, 2008). Infliximab can improve growth in children with CD (De Ridder et al., 2007).

Infliximab is administered as a series of intravenous infusions at a dose of 5mg/kg/dose at baseline and at 2 and 6 weeks and then every 8 weeks thereafter. The exact duration of long-term maintenance dosing is not known and is a significant concern because of its high cost and potential side effects when altering the immune response. Studies have found that initiation of infliximab therapy early in CD may be more advantageous, as early in the disease course individuals with IBD may be more susceptible to immunomodulation (De Ridder et al., 2007). Whether this will alter the natural history of CD and prolonged duration of response remains to be determined. The side effects of infliximab therapy include infections (activation of latent tuberculosis and sepsis with opportunistic and unusual infections), acute or delayed infusion reactions, autoimmune phenomena such as positive antinuclear antibody and anti–double-stranded DNA, autoantibody formation, and malignancies (Reddy & Loftus, 2006; Sands, 2006). The preponderance of current evidence supports scheduled maintenance treatment with infliximab, primarily because of the concerns of loss of response and inferior disease outcomes with episodic therapy (Markowitz, 2008; Sands, 2006). Unfortunately, recent reports have documented the occurrence of a rare, fatal hepatosplenic T cell lymphoma in adolescents and young adults treated with a combination of infliximab and thiopurine (Markowitz, 2008). Although all cases to date have been associated with concomitant use of 6-MP or AZA (and no cases with methotrexate or infliximab alone), the role of infliximab in the development of this rare malignancy merits further investigation (Markowitz, 2008; Rufo & Bousvaros, 2007).

The recent successes with infliximab have spurred the development of other biologic agents. Adalimumab (Humira) is a fully human anti–TNF-α monoclonal IgG1 antibody, in contrast to inflix-imab, which has mouse protein fractions. It is the second TNF to be approved by the FDA for adults as induction and maintenance therapy for moderate to severe CD in those with inadequate response to conventional therapy (Tamboli, 2007). Theoretically, adalimumab should induce less antibody formation and fewer adverse reactions; long-term studies and pediatric studies of the efficacy are needed to demonstrate immunogenicity of this drug (Tamboli, 2007).

Natalizumab (Tysabri) is a humanized monoclonal antibody against alpha-4-integrins. It inhibits the recruitment of inflammatory blood cells and recall of cells to the areas of inflammation. It has been approved for use in certain forms of multiple sclerosis through a restricted distribution program secondary to the concern of progressive multifocal leukoencephalopathy. It has been investigated in the treatment of adults with CD but has not yet been approved at this time for this population.

Certolizumab pegol (Cimzia) is another humanized monoclonal antibody to TNF-α and was recently approved by the FDA in adults with CD. Certolizumab does not induce in vitro complement activation, antibody-dependent cellular cytotoxicity, or apoptosis (Sanborn, Feagan, Stoinov, et al., 2007).

Novel Therapies with Unique Modes of Action. Many novel therapies are currently being used as alternate ways of modifying the immune response in the treatment of IBD. Growth hormone (somatropin) has a host of "downstream" effects on various tissues including the gut (Sands, 2006). Its administration has not only been found beneficial in growth failure associated with IBD (Heyman, Garnett, Wojcicki et al., 2008), but in small, blinded, randomized controlled trials in combination with a high-protein diet, it also showed impressive reduction of disease activity (Sands). Granulocyte colony-stimulating factor (filgrastim) and sargramostim (Leukine) are novel therapies that boost the immune system by enhancing neutrophil function and have been used for years with individuals receiving chemotherapy. The new theory is that a person's immune system may not have been active enough to suppress the inflammatory response that often leads to the debilitating symptoms found in CD. Several studies have been conducted to determine the efficacies of subcutaneous injections of these medications. Although results have been promising, injection site reactions and bone pain have been problematic for some individuals (Sands).

Nutritional Therapy

Nutritional therapy has been used for primary management of disease activity, to induce remission, as adjunctive therapy to correct or avoid malnutrition, to facilitate growth in children and adolescents with IBD, and to replenish micronutrient deficiencies. The nutritional status of children with IBD is usually already affected by the time of diagnosis and worsens with disease progression. Nutritional deficits and malnutrition can be compounded by the child or adolescent's fear of abdominal pain and diarrhea with eating. Caloric supplementation—whether provided as nutritious meals, oral supplements, enteral nasogastric or gastrostomy feedings, or parenteral nutrition—should be incorporated into any treatment regimen. Three major classes of formulas have been used: elemental, semi-elemental, and polymeric. Elemental diets are composed of amino acids, and are hypoallergenic. However, they are not very palatable and often require the use of a nasogastric or gastrostomy tube. Semi-elemental formulas contain peptides and may be minimally allergenic, but they are more likely to be

tolerated orally. Polymeric diets are lactose free but contain intact proteins. The role of nutritional therapy as a primary method of treating IBD is controversial, but successful primary treatment with total parenteral nutrition (TPN) or enteral nutrition has been promising with CD (Borrelli, Cordischi, Cirulli et al., 2006; Karp & Koch, 2006; Markowitz, 2008). The underlying theory is to eliminate intraluminal factors that can induce or maintain intestinal inflammation. Elemental formulas were first proposed and successfully used as an acceptable and equivalent alternative to corticosteroid therapy for treating intractable small bowel CD. While aggregate studies suggest that enteral therapy with elemental formula is less effective than corticosteroids in achieving remission in active CD with distal or colonic involvement or in those who have severe anorectal involvement, small bowel disease appears to be almost equally amenable to enteral therapy as corticosteroids, thus avoiding potential adverse effects of the corticosteroid medications (Borrelli et al., 2006; Karp & Koch, 2006).

The newer oligopeptide or semi-elemental formulas are more palatable than earlier formulas, and many children are able to drink them without the need for a nasogastric tube. Many insurance carriers refuse to cover these costly formulas, and the burden of this expense must be shouldered by the families. Some studies and meta-analyses have supported the position that the composition of the formula used for nutritional replenishment may not be critical (Graham & Kandil, 2002).

Enteral nutrition offers important benefits for children experiencing growth failure—particularly when disease affects the small intestine. The "ideal" child for enteral nutrition would be an adolescent with newly diagnosed CD limited to the ileum but complicated by growth failure and delayed maturation (Ruemmele, Roy, Levy, et al., 2000). Another suitable management strategy for these children may be the combined use of steroids and nutritional therapy for faster induction. In this situation, the nutritional therapy is useful to maintain remission by permitting rapid tapering of the corticosteroids to a lower dose (Borrelli et al., 2006). Enteral nutrition also can be used in children who refuse corticosteroids or who refuse repeat courses because of their concerns about adverse effects.

TPN also can be instituted as a primary therapy and is used to provide bowel rest, theoretically reducing intestinal inflammation and thereby decreasing disease activity. TPN has been documented to diminish disease activity and reverse growth failure (Graham & Kandil, 2002; Griffiths & Buller, 2004). TPN is used to provide nutritional support in individuals with fulminant IBD who cannot tolerate enteral feedings and is necessary in individuals with short bowel syndrome as a result of multiple surgical resections. Risks of TPN include sepsis, mechanical complications of central lines (right atrial catheters), and thrombosis, particularly in children and adolescents with IBD who have an underlying risk for a hypercoagulable state. The implementation of TPN in any child must be done by considering the risks versus benefits of the therapy.

Individual nutrients have shown therapeutic promise in the adjunct treatment of IBD, but additional research is still needed to substantiate the findings (Razack & Seidner, 2007). Omega-3(ω-3) fatty acids have been investigated for their antiinflammatory effect on the GI tract and their potential ability to prevent relapse and supplementing the diet with fish oil (high in ω-3 fatty acids) has shown some therapeutic promise, but research has been inconsistent because of differences in preparation and annoying side effects (MacDonald, 2006). Short-chain fatty acids have also been investigated for their antiinflammatory response. They are derived from the fermentation of dietary fiber by the microflora of the gut and are the preferred and primary fuel for the colonic mucosa (Razack & Seidner, 2007). Enemas with short-chain fatty acids have been used in diversion colitis and have shown promise in individuals with left-sided UC (Razack & Seidner, 2007).

Probiotics

Probiotics are a useful adjunct therapy in IBD, especially in those who want to use "natural" physiologic approaches to treating IBD. Probiotics are "healthy" bacteria (*Bifidobacterium, Lactobacillus, Escherichia, Enterococcus, Bacillus,* and the yeast, *Saccharomyces boulaardi)* that when ingested in adequate amounts, alter the enteric microflora and may prevent an overgrowth of pathogenic bacteria and maintain the integrity of the mucosal barrier. The rationale for using probiotics in IBD is based on evidence that implicates intestinal bacteria in the pathogenesis of these disorders that involves genetically influenced dysregulation of the mucosal immune response to antigens present in the normal bacterial flora, thus leading to inflammation and disease (Zocco, Zileri Dal Verme, Cremonini, et al., 2006). Probiotics ostensibly fulfill this role, but evidence at this time indicates that their ability to decrease gut inflammation is limited (Boirivant & Strober, 2007; Szajewska, Setty, Mrukowicz, et al., 2006). Many individuals with UC who have ileoanal pouches after colectomy develop pouchitis and may benefit from probiotics.

Surgical Intervention

Ulcerative Colitis. Indications for surgical intervention for children with UC include intractable disease, refractory growth failure, toxic megacolon, hemorrhage, perforation, and cancer prophylaxis (Fish & Kugathasan, 2004; Griffiths & Buller, 2004) After 10 years of disease, UC carries a 10% to 20% risk of colon cancer per decade (Ponsky et al., 2007). The most commonly performed surgery is the ileal pouch anal anastomosis (IPAA). The IPAA procedure offers individuals an alternative to a permanent stoma, preserves body image, and allows somewhat normal bowel function. However, the surgery is not without its known morbidities: bleeding, infection, nerve injury, increased stool frequency, nocturnal leakage, reduced fertility in women, and pouchitis.

This curative procedure can be performed either as a primary operation or in a two-stage approach, laparoscopically or by open surgery. If surgery is urgent, an open two-stage procedure with a total colectomy, rectal mucosectomy, ileal pull-through, and creation of a diverting loop ileostomy is the procedure of choice. Creating a temporary loop ileostomy allows fecal diversion during the early weeks after surgery, which not only allows ileal pouch and ileoanal anastomotic healing, but also significantly reduces the incidence of postoperative complications, such as pelvic sepsis and anastomotic dehiscence (Stucchi, Aarons, & Becker, 2006). Many surgeons routinely perform the two-stage procedure rather than a primary operation. The one-stage surgery is commonly performed when the colectomy is elective and no temporary diverting ileostomy is performed.

Although many variations of ileal reservoirs have been tried, the most commonly performed is the J-pouch. The colon is removed and the ileum is brought down into the pelvis and sutured using an end-to-end anastomosis to the anus. A J-pouch is created by looping the ileum on itself and creating a side-to-side enterostomy in the shape of a J proximal to the ileoanal anastomosis. To preserve sphincter function and continence and reduce the potential injury to the pelvic sympathetic and parasympathetic nerves responsible for sexual functions, most surgeons remove only the rectal mucosa and leave the distal 4 to 5 cm of rectal muscle layer intact (Fish & Kugathasan, 2004).

Benefits of the pouch procedure are resumption of rectal continence and avoidance of a permanent ostomy, which makes it much easier for children and their parents to accept. Bowel movements initially occur frequently with possible fecal soiling at night, but in time frequency decreases to four to six times a day. It generally takes between 3 and 12 months to achieve this outcome (Fish & Kugathasan, 2004).

Of the long-term complications after IPAA, pouchitis, an inflammatory process in the ileal pouch, is the most common single, long-term complication; it occurs in 10% to 30% of cases and is the most problematic in children and adolescents (Griffiths & Buller, 2004). Pouchitis can present with any number of colitis-like symptoms, including increased stool frequency and/or diarrhea, tenesmus, abdominal cramping, fever, malaise, and bleeding (Stucchi et al., 2006). Episodes respond well to antibiotics (metronidazole, ciprofloxacin, and rifaximin), and maintenance may be achieved using a probiotic agent. Long-term follow-up is still needed with regular endoscopic surveillance of the pouch, especially if residual rectal mucosa is present, which can still be a risk factor for dysplastic changes (Griffiths & Buller, 2004; Shen, 2007). Increased risk of infertility is one potential complication now reported with colectomy and IPAA for young females with UC (Waljee, Waljee, Morris, et al., 2006). Although the reported estimates of both the relative risk of infertility after IPAA and the actual rate of infertility vary widely in the literature (Waljee et al., 2006). It is estimated that UC alone can cause up to a 15% increase in infertility. Currently, most practitioners advocate yearly surveillance with colonoscopy and biopsy as an effective alternative to prophylactic colectomy (Ponsky et al., 2007).

Crohn's Disease. Indications for surgery in CD include intractable disease, hemorrhage, toxic megacolon, bowel perforation, stricture with obstruction, and abscesses and fistulas unresponsive to medical management (Beattie, Croft, Fell, et al., 2006; Diefenbach & Breuer, 2006; Fish & Kugathasan, 2004). Surgery may also be indicated for prepubertal children or early adolescents who have growth failure and relatively localized disease, including stenotic segments of bowel (Diefenbach & Breuer, 2006). Surgery will not cure CD as it does UC, so the major surgical goal is to provide effective, definitive treatment while preserving as much intestinal length as possible (Fish & Kugathasan, 2004). A large pediatric IBD registry found the risk for surgery to be 17% at 5 years and 28% at 10 years from the diagnosis of CD (Gupta, Cohen, Bostrom, et al., 2006, Gupta et al., 2007). In adults with CD, approximately 58% to 92% are reported to eventually require surgery during their lifetime, depending on the location of the disease (Ponsky et al., 2007). The most common indication for surgery of the small bowel is intestinal obstruction caused by fibrosis and stricture (Ponsky et al.). Recurrence of disease is common in CD after surgery and has been reported to be 17% at 1 year, 38% at 3 years, and as high as 50% to 60% at 5 years in children after their first surgery. Prophylactic postoperative treatment with 6-MP or AZA may help to delay recurrence of disease.

Despite the risk of recurrent disease after resection, surgery is still an attractive option for children because of the potential for a significant asymptomatic interval during which normal growth and development can occur. In one pediatric study, children undergoing intestinal resection within 1 year of onset of symptoms had a delayed recurrence of active disease compared with children whose preoperative duration of symptomatic disease was greater than 1 year (Ponsky et al., 2007).

The surgical procedure required is based on the location of the disease and the complication resulting from the surgery. Surgical management should limit the resection to the grossly diseased intestinal segment with primary anastomosis involving the small intestine in most cases. An isolated, nonprogressive area of bowel may be removed, of which ileocecal resection is the most common operation performed in the pediatric population. For isolated obstruction from a stricture, strictureplasty may be performed. A greater percentage of children have surgery for intractability, fulminant disease, or anorectal disease. In cases of fulminant colitis, a total proctocolectomy with a loop ileostomy may suffice, or a permanent ileostomy may be necessary. Children with CD are not good candidates for pouch procedures because of the high rate of disease recurrence (Griffiths & Buller, 2004).

Perianal disease consisting of fistulas and abscesses is typically managed medically first because of the high rate of recurrence of fistulas and abscesses. Fistulas are initially managed medically before surgery is contemplated. Perirectal abscesses should be treated with antibiotics; if no response occurs, they require surgical drainage. Most abscesses have an associated fistula. The type of surgery depends on the depth of invasion of the fistula through the sphincter muscles. A simple fistulotomy with debridement of the tract should be performed; if more than 30% of the sphincter complex is involved, a seton should be placed (Ponsky et al., 2007). Recent studies have shown promise with infliximab combined with surgery to prevent refistulization (Ponsky et al.). Skin tags are rarely excised during surgery. Possible complications after surgery for CD include wound infection, anastomotic leak or stricture, fistula, recurrence of disease, bleeding, and small bowel obstruction.

Complementary and Alternative Therapies

Complementary alternative medicine (CAM) for IBD can incorporate chiropractic, homeopathy, naturopathy, acupuncture, aromatherapy, massage, biofeedback, probiotics, herbal medicines, and dietary supplements. In 2000, a multicenter international study was conducted in Boston, Detroit, and London to examine the use of CAM in children and young adults with IBD. The investigators found a 41% frequency of CAM use. The most common therapies were megavitamin therapy (19%), dietary supplements (17%), and herbal medicine (14%). The most common reasons cited for using CAM were side effects from prescribed medicines, lower than expected results from prescribed medicines, and wish for a cure (Heuschkel, Afzal, Wuerth, et al., 2002). A study of Scottish children with IBD found 61% reported prior use of CAM for the management of IBD and 37% were using some form of CAM on recruitment (Gerasimidis, McGrogan, Hassan, et al., 2008).

The most common therapies from this study were probiotics, dairy-free diet, omega-3/fish oils, and aloe followed by gluten-free diet, homeopathy, massage, and over-the counter multivitamins and megavitamins. Interestingly, parents reported that they received their information about CAM from personal recommendations, magazines, newspapers, and the Internet (Gerasimidis et al., 2008). The main reasons for using CAM included an attempt to

complement conventional medicine, a personal experience with CAM use, frustration with conventional medication side effects, and the belief that CAM is natural and harmless. The increased use of probiotics parallels the increase in the number of published studies suggesting a beneficial effect in IBD.

Few individuals told health care providers they were using CAM (Gerasimidis et al., 2008). This lack of disclosure may have undesirable side effects, especially when herbal therapy is being practiced. Toxicity from herbal therapies has included fatal liver and renal failure (Langmead & Rampton, 2006). Individuals with a medication history should be routinely asked if they are also using any type of CAM, including supplements. Because many CAM therapies do not simply address a problem with the body but instead focus on the entire person—body, mind and spirit—other categories may be beneficial to individuals with IBD. Stress has been identified as a factor that may contribute to the exacerbation of IBD symptoms; some children find it helpful to use acupuncture, acupressure, and massage for managing daily stressors, as well as for controlling or preventing flare-ups of their disease. Primary care providers may help families find programs that promote the development of stress management and problem-solving skills.

Anticipated Advances in Diagnosis and Management

Advances in IBD therapy now center on rapidly replacing old ideas with new knowledge in genetics, gut ecology and microflora, immune mechanisms, and newer targeted biologic therapies (Fish & Kugathasan, 2004). Many new therapies for the treatment of IBD have been developed over the past decade and are undergoing further clinical trials. Almost all data on their effectiveness are from research in adults; clinical trials are just beginning with children and many obstacles still remain. The newer therapies are aimed at either selectively blocking detrimental mucosal immune response or decreasing the levels of luminal antigens found to be partly involved in the pathogenesis of IBD (Fish & Kugathasan,).

Over the past several years, advances in immunology have led to the discovery of novel therapeutic modalities now consisting of monoclonal antibodies, small-molecule inhibitors, peptides, and vaccines (Bousvaros et al., 2008a). New humanized drugs are being designed to target and interfere at various levels within the immune complex. Many agents are under investigation or in use but have not yet been subjected to random controlled trials; these include mycophenolate mofetil, onercept, and CDP571.

The most unusual novel treatment explored in clinical trials is the therapeutic use of helminthic infestation in IBD (Sands, 2006). The reasoning for their use comes from the lack of helminthic infestation over the past century (helminths have historically modified mucosal and systemic immune response to foster a down-regulated response). Without them, the immune system may allow overly aggressive mucosal immune responses seen in IBD (Sands). Iatrogenic infestation with *Trichuris suis* (pig whipworm) was used in a few recent reports that appeared to demonstrate benefit by decreasing disease activity of CD and UC.

Despite these advances in understanding IBD and its pathophysiologic mechanisms enabling the development of powerful therapies, treatment remains difficult and only a few individuals benefit completely from the new therapies. In addition to new drugs being investigated, new imaging modalities have been developed to assist the health care professional in determining the type of disease, extent of involvement, and severity of activity. Bowel MRI, bowel ultrasound scanning, technetium-99m scanning, and video capsule endoscopy are all new imaging studies now used in children.

Associated Problems of Inflammatory Bowel Disease and Treatment

Growth Failure and Delayed Sexual Development

Growth failure and delayed sexual development associated with IBD in childhood affects children with CD more than those with UC. Deceleration in linear growth may be the only clinical presentation in children and adolescents with CD. The prevalence of growth failure is reportedly as high as 40% of children with CD but is less than 10% in those with UC (Dubinsky, 2008; Fish & Kugathasan, 2004). In a retrospective cohort study of 989 consecutive children who had CD, Gupta and colleagues (2007) found girls to be at decreased risk for growth failure compared with boys. The cumulative affect of growth failure in their cohort with CD was 9.8% at 10 years from time of diagnosis. Activity of disease was thought to be the major determinant of adequacy of growth, but reports have been contradictory (Griffiths & Buller, 2004; Gupta et al., 2007). It may be a combination of disease severity and gender.

Proposed etiologies for growth failure include inadequate nutritional intake (anorexia) and/or malabsorption, prolonged

---

Associated Problems of IBD and Treatment

- Growth failure and delayed sexual development
- Musculoskeletal problems
  - Peripheral arthritis
  - Ankylosing spondylitis
  - Bone demineralization and osteoporosis
- Dermatologic manifestations
  - Erythema nodosum
  - Pyoderma gangrenosum
- Visual changes
  - Episcleritis
  - Uveitis
  - Iritis
  - Conjunctivitis
  - Cataracts
- Hepatobiliary complications
  - Primary sclerosing cholangitis
  - Pericholangiitis
  - Gallstones
- Renal changes
  - Renal calculi
- Perianal and perirectal disease
  - Fistulas, abscesses
  - Fissures, skin tags
- Fulminant colitis or toxic megacolon
  - Intestinal malignancy
- Lactose intolerance
- Anemia
  - Vitamin B_{12} deficiency
  - Iron deficiency as a result of chronic blood loss
- Hypercoagulability
- Carcinoma
- Psychosocial issues

---

corticosteroid administration, and the growth-retarding effects of chronic inflammatory mediators (e.g., TNF-α) (Ahmed, Wong, McGrogan, et al., 2007; Fish & Kugathasan, 2004). Inadequate calorie intake resulting from disease-related symptoms and anorexia (caused by circulating pro-inflammatory cytokines such as TNF-α) or food fears related to the association of food intake with exacerbation of GI symptoms such as pain or diarrhea most likely account for the malnutrition in children with IBD (Diefenbach & Breuer, 2006; Fish & Kugathasan, 2004). Nutrient malabsorption or a protein-losing enteropathy can contribute to nutritional deficiencies.

Undernutrition delays epiphyseal fusion of long bones and progression through puberty (Diefenbach & Breuer, 2006). Ongoing inflammation with release of specific cytokines that suppress growth factors is a key determinant of growth failure. Evidence reveals that IL-6 mediates growth failure in children with CD by suppressing IGF-I production at the hepatocyte level (Dubinsky, 2008). Delay in the onset and progression through puberty may deleteriously affect not only the normal pubertal growth spurt, but also contribute to deficits in final adult heights (Fish & Kugathasan, 2004).

As in growth failure, inflammatory mediators can also have a direct adverse influence on progression of puberty. Growth hormone therapy has recently been shown to significantly increase fat-free mass, bone mineral accretion, and linear growth in individuals with CD (Hardin, Kemp, & Allen, 2007; Heyman et al., 2005). The mechanism of action is thought to derive from the enhancement of the benefit of supplemental protein on the gut by increased uptake of amino acids and electrolytes, decreased intestinal permeability, and increased protein synthesis (Newby, Sawczenko, Thomas, et al., 2005). Case reports show some efficacy of testosterone in boys and ethinyl estradiol in girls, but controlled studies in IBD have not been conducted (Fish & Kugathasan, 2004).

Musculoskeletal Problems

Musculoskeletal problems associated with IBD include peripheral arthritis, ankylosing spondylitis (see Chapter 31), and sacroiliitis. Arthritis is the most likely of the extraintestinal manifestations to precede the GI manifestations of CD (see p. 564). Symptoms include pain/discomfort, swelling, erythema and "hot" joints, especially those of the hips, knees, and ankles, and is typically asymmetric. Unlike the other musculoskeletal manifestations of IBD, the arthritic symptoms may fluctuate with the activity of the bowel disease and respond to treatment of the disease. Nonsteroidal antiinflammatory agents may be used to treat refractory joint complaints, but because of possible GI side effects including disease exacerbation, they should be used sparingly in individuals with IBD.

Osteoporosis and decreased bone mineral density (BMD) are frequent in children with IBD—up to 41% with CD and 25% with UC (Jose & Heyman, 2008). Osteoporosis and consequent increased fracture rates are increased in children and adolescents with IBD. Corticosteroids are associated with decreased BMD, but in a study of children a similar proportion of osteoporosis is reported in non–corticosteroid-treated (12%) and corticosteroid-treated (11%) individuals with IBD (Jose & Heyman). Decreased BMD can be caused by malabsorption of calcium and vitamin D, macronutrient and micronutrient deficiencies, decreased level of physical activity, estrogen deficiency in females, and—importantly—corticosteroid use (Dubinsky, 2008). In CD a major factor in decreased BMD is the inhibition of bone formation by cytokines (Griffiths & Buller, 2004). In UC, decreased bone density is most often associated with long-term corticosteroid use.

Dermatologic Manifestations

Dermatologic manifestations occur in up to 5% to 15% of individuals with IBD (Griffiths & Buller, 2004; Jose & Heyman, 2008). Erythema nodosum presents with tender, reddened nodules that commonly appear on the anterior aspect of the lower leg, although the lesions may be seen on the foot, back of the leg, or the arm. Erythema nodosum is seen more often with CD (8% to 15%) than with UC (4%). It usually occurs when the intestinal disease is active but does not indicate severity (Griffiths & Buller, 2004). Therapy involves treating the underlying bowel disease.

Pyoderma gangrenosum is a more serious dermatologic condition that may be found in 1% to 5% of individuals with UC and 1% to 2% of those with CD. It is usually seen in those with active pancolitis, but it can occur even when the disease is in remission. The lesions typically appear on the anterior aspect of the lower leg as erythematous pustules or nodules that spread rapidly to adjacent skin. They develop into burrowing ulcers with dark red or purple borders surrounding deep skin ulcerations with necrotic centers (Jose & Heyman, 2008; Powell & O'Kane, 2002). Lesions may develop even before bowel symptoms, during quiescent disease, or following colectomy (Jose & Heyman, 2008). Control of the intestinal disease can result in healing of these lesions, but topical or systemic therapy directed at the lesions themselves may also be necessary. Recurrence of pyoderma gangrenosum is common and arthritis develops in about 40% of individuals with IBD and pyoderma gangrenosum (Jose & Heyman, 2008; Powell & O'Kane, 2002).

Visual Changes

Ophthalmologic involvement related to IBD correlates with disease activity and is reported in 1.6% to 4.6% of individuals with UC and 3% to 6.3% of individuals with CD (Jose & Heyman, 2008). Episcleritis and uveitis are the two most common conditions, and iritis and conjunctivitis may develop. Episcleritis is characterized by painless hyperemia of the sclera and conjunctiva without loss of vision and rarely progresses if left untreated. Uveitis is usually symptomatic, causing pain or possibly decreased vision. Acute anterior uveitis is an ophthalmologic emergency. Systemic or topical steroids are essential to prevent progression to blindness (Jose & Heyman). Children treated with corticosteroids are also at increased risk for cataracts and elevated intraocular pressure (reported in 22% of children with IBD), although glaucoma has been reported in children and adolescents without corticosteroid exposure (Jose & Heyman).

Hepatobiliary Complications

A particularly troublesome extraintestinal manifestation of IBD is hepatobiliary involvement, including small bile duct and large bile duct inflammation, chronic active hepatitis, drug-induced hepatitis, granulomatous hepatitis; cirrhosis, bile duct (cholangio-) carcinoma, fatty liver, amyloidosis, hepatic abscess, and cholelithiasis (Jose & Heyman, 2008). However, the most common and potentially serious hepatobiliary complication is primary sclerosing cholangiitis (PSC) that involves both intrahepatic and extrahepatic bile ducts and occurs in 1.6% to 7.4% of individuals with UC and 1% with CD (Jose & Heyman). PSC should be suspected in children or adolescents with elevated liver enzyme

levels, especially gamma-glutamyl transpeptidase and/or alkaline phosphatase out of proportion to the aspartate aminotransferase and alanine aminotransferase. To date, no effective therapy has been found for PSC, and the only definitive long-term treatment is liver transplantation.

Hepatobiliary complications in pediatrics, such as pericholangiitis, cirrhosis, and PSC, may precede the onset of IBD, may develop during active disease, or may even evolve after surgical resection (Jose & Heyman, 2008). Transient elevation of liver enzyme levels is common in IBD and appears to be related to medications or disease activity. Physical examination should carefully monitor for signs of liver disease including hepatic enlargement and/or portal hypertension. Gallstones (found in 13% to 34% of individuals with IBD) are more common in individuals with CD compared with UC. Gallstones seem to be related to the malabsorption of bile salts with subsequent cholesterol precipitation and calculus formation in the biliary system (Jose & Heyman, 2008).

Renal Changes

Renal calculi may complicate the course of individuals with IBD as a result of calcium oxalate or uric acid precipitation. These have been reported in 1% to 2% of children with IBD—the highest incidence occurring in children in CD after small bowel resection or ileostomy possibly secondary to frequent episodes of dehydration (Jose & Heyman, 2008). Children with severe ileal disease or resection of the ileum are at risk for formation of calcium oxalate stones (Jose & Heyman). Sudden onset of severe abdominal, back, or flank pain in children or adolescents with IBD should lead to the investigation for stones. Management consists of analgesia, hydration, alkalinization of urine for uric-acid stones, lithotripsy, and surgery if necessary (Jose & Heyman).

Perianal and Perirectal Disease

Perianal and perirectal disease is common in children with CD but is not seen in UC. Perianal disease is reported in 25% to 30% of children with CD and includes fissures, skin tags, fistulas, and abscesses (Fish & Kugathasan, 2004). Fistulas often become infected or may form an abscess near the intestine. Complaints of pain, fullness, fever, or drainage from the perianal area may alert clinicians to active perianal disease or abscess. If the area around the anus and rectum becomes involved, providers should question children and/or parents about the passage of air or stool through the vagina or the urethra, because this may indicate a rectovaginal or rectourethral fistula. Metronidazole has been most useful in treating perianal disease, but other therapies (e.g., corticosteroids, 6-MP, TPN, or cyclosporine) also may be used. Infliximab and adalimumab have been effective for fistulizing CD unresponsive to conventional therapy. Abscesses may require drainage either through a catheter inserted by an interventional radiologist or surgically. In cases of refractory perianal disease, surgery including drainage and placement of a seton or more involved procedures may be necessary (Ponsky et al., 2007).

Fulminant Colitis or Toxic Megacolon

Fulminant colitis presents with grossly bloody diarrhea, fever, tachycardia, abdominal pain with distention, decreased bowel sounds, and abnormal laboratory findings. When these symptoms are accompanied by a markedly distended colon on radiographs, toxic megacolon should be suspected (Leichtner & Higuchi, 2004). Fulminant colitis and toxic megacolon are medical emergencies and many individuals eventually require a colectomy. Toxic megacolon is reported in up to 5% of children and adolescents with UC and less often in CD (Leichtner & Higuchi). The incidence of toxic megacolon has decreased in part because of avoidance of opiates and antispasmodics and tests such as barium enema or colonoscopy during periods of severe colitis.

Lactose Intolerance

During periods of active disease, some children with IBD may experience symptoms of lactose intolerance, including bloating, abdominal cramping, and diarrhea, related to the intake of dairy products (Heyman & Committee on Nutrition, 2006). For this reason, some health care providers recommend that children eliminate lactose from their diet at the time of diagnosis and recovery to minimize confusion about a child's response to therapy. A breath hydrogen test may be performed to definitively diagnose lactose intolerance if such a clarification is needed. Without a clear history of lactose intolerance, eliminating dairy products from the diet is seldom warranted as these foods are a major source of a child's daily caloric and calcium intake. A significant proportion of children with IBD eventually are able to tolerate some lactose in their diet. Lactase supplementation may be taken orally or added to many dairy products so that individuals can ingest dairy products without developing symptoms of lactose intolerance.

Anemia

Chronic malnutrition, malabsorption, the interference of sulfasalazine with absorption of folate, and chronic blood loss increase the risk for vitamin B_{12} deficiency and hypochromic microcytic or iron deficiency anemia in children with IBD. Secondary anemia has been reported in 5% of children with UC and 70% of those with CD (Jose & Heyman, 2008). Treatment of anemia depends on the underlying cause. Daily supplementation with folic acid is recommended for children receiving sulfasalazine. Iron supplementation is recommended for children with iron deficiency anemia. Symptomatic anemia, especially in children with severe colitis, requires transfusion. Regular CBC monitoring is recommended for all children with IBD.

Hypercoagulability

About 1% to 2% of individuals with UC and CD have associated hypercoagulable states manifested by thrombosis and blood tests revealing thrombocytosis, low prothrombin time, and low partial thromboplastin time. Thromboembolism and thrombosis are less frequently reported among children (Jose & Heyman, 2008). Peripheral vein thrombosis and pulmonary emboli are less often reported among children compared with adults (Jose & Heyman). Postoperative thromboembolic events must be considered in follow-up of these children and adolescents after surgical procedures.

Carcinoma

Colorectal cancer (CRC) and adenocarcinomas are serious and life-threatening complications of IBD. CRC accounts for 15% of all deaths in adults with IBD. IBD-associated CRC accounts for only approximately 1% to 2% of cases with CRC in the general population; however, the mortality is higher than sporadic CRC (Stucchi et al., 2006). A significantly greater risk for intestinal malignancies exists among children with IBD than among those who do not have IBD, especially in individuals with pancolitis beginning in childhood.

The risk of malignancy in UC increases with the extent and duration of the disease and with a younger age at the time of diagnosis (Diefenbach & Breuer, 2006; Griffiths & Buller, 2004). The risk of cancer begins to increase 10 to 15 years after diagnosis (Diefenbach & Breuer, 2006). Children in whom pancolitis develops before 14 years of age have a cumulative CRC incidence rate of 5% at 20 years and 40% at 35 years. Children in whom the disease develops between 15 and 39 years of age have a cumulative incidence rate of 5% at 20 years and 30% at 35 years. This gives an estimate of an 8% risk of dying of colon cancer 10 to 25 years after diagnosis of UC if colectomy is not performed to cure the disease. The risk of CRC in CD is not as high as in UC. PSC can significantly increase the risk for CRC (Stucchi et al., 2006). The incidence of adenocarcinoma of the colon with CD is 4 to 20 times that of the general population. CD of the small bowel increases the risk up to 50 to 100 times higher for the development of small bowel adenocarcinoma (Diefenbach & Breuer, 2006). Much like UC, the cumulative risk for developing small bowel adenocarcinomas increases significantly after 8 to 10 years of small bowel disease, even if quiescent (Stucchi et al., 2006). Other factors increasing the risk are early age of disease onset, male sex, location and extent of the disease, smoking, and presence of strictures or fistulas. Unfortunately, the prognosis for small bowel adenocarcinoma is poor because of the delay and difficulty in diagnosis and advanced stage of cancer.

Most pediatric gastroenterologists agree that surveillance colonoscopy should be performed on children with UC, beginning about 8 years after diagnosis. Annual or biannual colonoscopies are recommended when biopsy findings are negative for dysplasia. Colonoscopy is recommended every 6 months when biopsies show indeterminant dysplasia. Colectomy is recommended when a biopsy shows any sign of dysplasia (Stucchi et al., 2006). Dysplastic lesions and carcinomas may be difficult to detect in early stages, and although multiple biopsies during colonoscopy are recommended, lesions may be missed. Some gastroenterologists recommend prophylactic colectomy for individuals with long-standing UC, especially when diagnosed in childhood (Leichtner & Higuchi, 2004). The risk of developing a neoplasm in a pouch after IPAA surgery, while rare, supports a recommendation for performing pouchoscopy every 5 years (Leichtner & Higuchi, 2004; Stucchi et al., 2006).

Psychosocial Issues

Chronic disease alone places children and adolescents at risk for secondary psychiatric disorders. Studies comparing children and adolescents with IBD against healthy cohorts have found higher rates of psychological disturbance, including anxiety, depression, and problems in social functioning and self-esteem, but rates were generally similar to those of children with other chronic illnesses and only a subset have clinically significant problems (Mackner & Crandall, 2007; Perrin, Kuhlthau, Chughtai, et al., 2008).

Because of the relapsing and remitting course of IBD, lifestyle changes can occur unexpectedly as a result of disease exacerbation. Difficulty interacting with peers may result from school absenteeism, low self-esteem because of delayed growth and development (symptoms that can be embarrassing and limit social activities), and appearance-altering side effects from medications. Adolescents are particularly vulnerable because belonging to a particular social group and acceptance by peers in an important part of their identity (Mackner & Crandall, 2007). Mackner and Crandall (2007) found significantly impaired social functioning in 35% of those with disease diagnosed during adolescence compared with 5% of those diagnosed earlier in childhood.

Psychosocial factors such as family functioning and stress-coping strategies may be better predictors of behavioral/emotional functioning than illness factors or disease severity. Investigators are beginning to assess the QoL issues in childhood IBD with hopes of developing more effective early interventional strategies. Several questionnaires have been developed; the Impact Questionnaire to examine health-related quality of life (HRQoL) consists of "6 domains": bowel symptoms, systemic symptoms, social/functioning concerns, body image, test and treatment concerns, and emotional concerns (Perrin et al., 2008) and the Impact-II, which categorized IBD-related QoL into "4 domains" based on 33 items: general well-being and symptoms, emotional functioning, social interactions, and body image (Perrin et al.). In the Impact-II questionnaire, children with higher disease activity scores and other indicators of clinical activity had lower HRQoL (Perrin et al.).

Age and stages of psychosocial development also affect the ability of children with IBD to understand and participate in their own care and impact on adherence to the medical regimen prescribed by their pediatric gastroenterologist. Compliance rates for medications, especially during remission, are an ongoing problem. Adolescents have the lowest rate of adherence (50%) (Dubinsky, 2008). Family dysfunction and poor child coping strategies were associated with worse adherence (Dubinsky, 2008). This reinforces the need to address the psychological and psychosocial impact of IBD in the pediatric population and on their families. Support groups, the Internet, and camps specifically for children with IBD are additional resources for improved psychosocial functioning.

Prognosis

At this time, no prospective studies have been done to determine outcomes in pediatric IBD. The severity of presenting symptoms of IBD does not necessarily predict the course of the disease for a child, a frustrating aspect of IBD for both children and their parents. The spectrum of disease includes children and adolescents who remain in a sustained remission, those who have recurrent relapses and remission of disease, and those who have continuous active disease. Advances in medical therapy, especially the biologic agents, has improved QoL, reduced rate of hospitalizations and surgery, allowed fewer side effects from corticosteroids, and improved growth rates for a large proportion of children with UC and CD (Bousvaros et al., 2008b).

Most children with UC have a full, active life with good health despite having a chronic disease (Leichtner & Higuchi, 2004). Ten percent experience only their presenting episode, 25% have intermittent symptoms, 50% have chronic disease, and 20% have chronically active, incapacitating disease despite advances in medial therapy (Leichtner & Higuchi, 2004). As described above, UC can be "cured" by removing the colon, but this may not be the "true cure." Colectomy can result in resolution of symptoms and almost eliminate the risk of CRC, but it presents with its own risk and morbidities (Leichtner & Higuchi). The "true cure" will come from further study of the genetic basis of UC and its pathogenesis (Leichtner & Higuchi).

No known cure exists for CD and the course of the disease is unpredictable, characterized by recurrent exacerbation of symptoms (Diefenbach & Breuer, 2006). Freeman (2004) found the incidence of stricture (28.6%) and penetrating complications (46.4%) in children and the likelihood of surgery in CD remains high (56.3% within a mean time of 4.2 years) despite the more widespread use of immunosuppressive medications (Beattie et al., 2006; Gupta et al., 2007). Unfortunately, there is a high relapse rate after surgical intervention (Beattie et al., 2006).

Recently, intestinal mucosa healing has been proposed as the primary therapeutic objective in IBD, challenging previous views of clinical remission. This approach may modify the natural history of IBD and possibly decrease the chances of developing perforating disease (fistulas and abscesses) and/or fibrostenosis, especially in CD (Bousvaros et al., 2008a, b). Long-term use of biologic agents may lead to mucosal healing, although these medications are still being used with caution because of their high cost and uncertainty about safety. Biologic medications have had a substantial impact on the management of IBD, improving QoL, reducing hospitalizations and surgery, decreasing use and therefore side effects from corticosteroids, and improving growth rates (Bousvaros et al., 2008b). Emerging genetic factors may help predict individuals likely to have a more severe disease course and the development of safer therapies that individualize strategies and will be a critical part in the future management of pediatric IBD.

PRIMARY CARE MANAGEMENT

Health Care Maintenance
Growth and Development
Children with IBD should have growth parameters (height, weight, and BMI) measured and graphed on a National Center for Health Statistics chart at each primary care visit. For children with recently diagnosed IBD, a review of previous visit records to assess growth in the years before the diagnosis was made is useful. Such a review helps primary care providers assess any deceleration in growth rate. School health or athletic offices often may be of assistance in reconstructing the growth curve. Height and weight for age, BMI, and Tanner stage for pubertal development are growth parameters of particular importance. Once growth delay is identified as an actual or potential problem, bone age should be obtained to identify the child's remaining growth potential. Continued careful measurement and graphing of growth parameters are essential. Catch-up growth is considered adequate if children return to their pre-illness growth percentiles. Cognitive abilities are unimpaired in children with IBD, and development usually progresses normally, although psychosocial issues often surface in these individuals.

Diet
Diet and nutritional concerns for families of children and adolescents with IBD are extremely common. It is well known that diet can affect symptoms in IBD, but scientific evidence is lacking to suggest that diet is a major factor in the inflammatory process. However, close attention to the child's diet, once IBD is diagnosed, may help reduce symptoms. No single diet plan helps everyone with IBD; recommendations must be individualized depending on the type—CD or UC—and location of disease. Disease and/

or inflammation of the large intestine should allow for normal digestion and absorption in the small intestine. Disease of the small intestine can affect absorption of all nutrients, in particular carbohydrates, lipids, and micronutrients such as vitamin B_{12}, iron, and calcium. During periods of active disease, many children may feel more comfortable consuming a low-roughage diet. Narrowing of the small bowel or stricture formation may necessitate a low-residue diet and restriction of nuts, seeds, popcorn, and vegetables that are difficult to digest. The most important advice is to eat a well-balanced diet of proteins, calories, and nutrients. It should be stressed to the child's family that good nutrition is one of the ways the body restores itself to health. This is especially true with delayed growth when IBD is diagnosed before the onset of puberty.

Some individuals may feel more comfortable when they avoid certain foods and the child and family can be helped to identify such foods. Malabsorption, especially of carbohydrates, lactose, and fructose, may induce symptoms of diarrhea and gas. If lactose intolerance is suspected, a breath hydrogen breath test can be performed for a definitive diagnosis. Over-the-counter lactase in both pill form or lactase products (milk) are available. Practitioners must be aware that concerned parents, who feel able to attribute symptoms to multiple foods, may overly restrict the diet and make it much more difficult to achieve balanced nutritional goals. Such overrestriction may result in a diet that is unappealing to the child and too restrictive to provide enough calories for growth and development. Sometimes even "junk" food, which may be more appealing to children and adolescents, can have nutritious benefits when ingested in limited amounts (e.g., pizza, cheeseburgers, and milkshakes).

Many centers consider a nutritional assessment to be within the standard of care for children and adolescents with recently diagnosed IBD. The dietitian may assess a child's intake and nutritional status and, if necessary, counsel the child and family regarding augmentation of caloric and other nutrient intake. The dietitian may recommend oral iron for children and youths for iron deficiency from blood loss, vitamin B_{12} if they have undergone small bowel resection, vitamin D and calcium if they have evidence of bone disease, or a general multiple vitamin. Folic acid should be supplemented in individuals taking sulfasalazine. Calcium is the most common mineral deficiency seen in IBD, mostly as a result of the limited dietary intake of dairy products related to lactose intolerance or with long-term corticosteroid use. Calcium supplementation may be needed if requirements cannot be met by dietary means. Oral iron may be required more often in children and youths with UC than CD secondary to blood loss following inflammation and ulceration of the colon. If growth retardation associated with IBD is identified, nutritional supplementation with high-caloric formulas or an enriched diet is necessary; these are delivered orally or by nasogastric or gastrostomy tube. TPN administered through an intravenous catheter into a large blood vessel may be necessary when bowel rest is required or in severe disease. Consultation with a clinical nutritionist is beneficial for the family to help learn to increase calories in a palatable manner. With adequate calories, children or adolescents (i.e., before epiphyseal closure) may recover lost growth. As nutritional replenishment begins, children or youths with IBD may have greater caloric requirements than their unaffected peers. Recommendations for caloric intake range vary depending on age, nutritional status, growth rate, disease activity, and physical activity and may be more than 90 to 100 kcal/kg/day.

Safety

Children with IBD require no special restriction of activities. They should be encouraged to participate in all sports they enjoy. Vigorous activities (e.g., lacrosse or tackle football) should pose no problem for children in remission. Children with severe osteoporosis, however, should refrain from contact sports. Because (as in many populations with special needs) anxious families may tend to shelter their child from uncomfortable or tense situations, primary care providers can play an integral role in advocating for a normal lifestyle for these children.

Children and adolescents with IBD who plan to travel may need to make some special modifications. Consultation with a tropical medicine or travel clinic may be beneficial when travel abroad is planned. General considerations include the purity of the water supply, exposure to ova and parasites, and proper immunization.

Alcohol consumption by adolescents with IBD who are in remission is of the same concern as alcohol consumption by their unaffected peers. Alcohol ingestion may cause discomfort for some individuals with IBD. If so, these individuals should limit intake. Individuals taking metronidazole should be informed that alcohol intake can induce a disulfiram (Antabuse) type of reaction, primarily nausea and vomiting.

Children who are immunosuppressed should wear a medical identification/alert bracelet or use other easily identifiable means of communicating this fact to emergency medical personnel. Children who have received corticosteroids in the past year may need a stress dose of hydrocortisone at times of serious illness, accident, or surgery.

Immunizations

At diagnosis, children and adolescents should have a complete review of their immunization history to ensure immunizations are up to date and if not, they should be vaccinated before therapy is initiated. No change from the normal immunization schedule is necessary unless a child receives maintenance therapy of corticosteroids or other immunosuppressive agents (e.g., 6-MP, AZA, methotrexate, cyclosporine, and infliximab). These children should not receive live virus immunizations (measles, mumps, and rubella [MMR] or varicella) until the drugs have been tapered and they have not taken them for more than 3 months, but killed/attenuated vaccines can be safely administered even with immunocompromised children (Dubinsky, 2008). If this is not feasible or if exposure is of particular concern, a killed virus vaccine or condition-specific immunoglobulin may be given. Exposure to varicella infection in those who have not been vaccinated or had prior varicella infection and who are taking 6-MP or AZA warrants administration of varicella zoster immune globulin (VZIG) within 48 hours of exposure; the 6-MP or AZA then should be temporarily discontinued. Additionally, all children with IBD, particularly those who are immunosuppressed, should receive a yearly influenza vaccination.

Screening

Vision. Annual ophthalmic examinations are necessary to screen for ocular manifestations of IBD. Many individuals with ophthalmologic complications are asymptomatic, especially early in the disease course. In children or adolescents with iritis, examiners may note redness of the eye, eye pain, photophobia, or blurred vision. In uveitis, abnormal pupillary reaction may also be observed. Diagnosis of uveitis is made by slit-lamp examination. A reddened eye may be noted in episcleritis or conjunctivitis. Regardless of whether a child with IBD is receiving prolonged corticosteroid therapy, all affected individuals should be tested for glaucoma and cataracts; the recommended schedule is twice a year (Jose & Heyman, 2008). Any child with an abnormal ophthalmoscopic examination result or complaints of the previously mentioned symptoms should be referred to an ophthalmologist and back to the gastroenterology team for consideration of further treatment.

Hearing. Routine screening is recommended.

Dental. Children who are being treated with cyclosporine are at risk for gingival hyperplasia. Proper dental hygiene and the need for dental visits twice a year should be reinforced at each well-child visit.

Blood Pressure. Children who are taking cyclosporine or corticosteroids are at increased risk for hypertension. Their blood pressures should be measured and recorded at every visit. Evidence of hypertension should be reported to the gastroenterology team.

Hematocrit. Hemoglobin and hematocrit values should be measured yearly for children who are asymptomatic and have no history of anemia. A CBC count should be checked every 6 months or as needed for children with a history of anemia or those experiencing increased symptoms of their disease.

Urinalysis. No change in the usual protocol for screening is necessary unless the history indicates renal involvement or the child is experiencing symptoms indicative of any of the previously mentioned conditions.

Tuberculosis. Children receiving immunosuppressive therapy may not respond to testing for tuberculosis. Screening may be withheld until immunosuppressive drugs are discontinued. If exposure is suspected, a skin test control (e.g., *Candida* or histamine) may be placed along with the purified protein derivative of the tuberculosis tests to assess for anergy. Chest radiography may be necessary to screen for active disease. Tuberculosis screening and a chest x-ray must be done before treatment with infliximab because of the risk of reported disseminated tuberculosis.

Condition-Specific Screening

Even asymptomatic children and adolescents should be scheduled for regular follow-up by the gastroenterology team. At these visits the following condition-specific screening studies are typically obtained. Primary care practitioners must be aware that these studies should be routinely evaluated. In some circumstances, the primary care setting may be the most convenient or appropriate place to monitor these values.

Erythrocyte Sedimentation Rate and C-Reactive Protein Levels. An erythrocyte sedimentation rate (ESR) and/or C-reactive protein (CRP) levels should be measured yearly for asymptomatic children. CRP is sometimes favored over ESR since it is not affected by hematocrit or other serum proteins and may be a superior marker for intestinal inflammation (Leichtner & Higuchi, 2004). The ESR and CRP values may be used for some children with IBD as an index of disease activity. The ESR and CRP levels should be normal in children with inactive disease. A variation from baseline should be followed with close questioning about current disease activity and onset of new symptoms.

Fecal Occult Blood Test. For asymptomatic children, stool should be monitored yearly with a fecal occult blood reagent (e.g., Hemoccult, Beckman Coulter, Inc.) for the presence of occult blood. The results should usually be negative in children with inactive disease. Some children with IBD always have a trace of blood in their stool. Children whose stools are routinely normal but have a positive occult blood result should be assessed more carefully for indications of increased disease activity and anemia.

Chemistries. Children taking medications (including 5-ASA, AZA, 6-MP, methotrexate, tacrolimus, or cyclosporine) should have renal (i.e., BUN and creatinine levels) and liver enzyme studies (i.e., fractionated bilirubin, aspartate aminotransferase, alanine aminotransferase, gamma-glutamyl transpeptidase, and alkaline phosphatase values) monitored at least every 3 months throughout therapy. Liver enzymes studies and albumin levels should be assessed every year in otherwise asymptomatic children with IBD.

Lactose Intolerance. The diagnosis of lactose intolerance may be made empirically by eliminating lactose-containing products from the diet and monitoring for changes in symptoms such as abdominal cramping, distention, flatulence, and diarrhea. The diagnosis may also be made by the breath hydrogen test. Clinicians may also do a cursory screen for lactose intolerance by testing stool for reducing substances or testing the pH of the stool. An acidic pH (i.e., ≤6.0) could be indicative of lactose intolerance.

Osteoporosis and Decreased Bone Mineral Density. Individuals should undergo baseline bone densitometry scans with repeat examinations at 1- to 2-year intervals with long-term, high dose exposure to corticosteroids (Jose & Heyman, 2008). Bone density is measured using dual-energy x-ray absorptiometry (DEXA) scanning. Osteopenia is defined as a Z-score of −1.0 to −2.5, and osteoporosis is a Z-score lower than −2.5 (Jose & Heyman, 2008). Results should be interpreted using bone age or height age, not chronological age, which overestimates the extent of bone disease (Diefenbach & Breuer, 2006). Calcium and vitamin D supplementation should also be considered, especially if milk intake is limited.

Neurologic Examination. Children who are being treated with metronidazole should be assessed for peripheral neuropathy at each visit.

Endoscopy. Endoscopy may be performed during times of disease exacerbation, and routine colonoscopy should be performed in children with UC starting 8 to 10 years after diagnosis.

Common Illness Management
Differential Diagnosis

The symptoms of IBD and its associated problems vary. Symptoms of common childhood illnesses such as acute gastroenteritis or influenza-like illnesses may be difficult to differentiate from exacerbations of a child's underlying disease process. GI symptoms most likely concern or alarm the child, family, and primary care provider. Index of disease activity for some—but not all—children are the ESR or CRP, which may sometimes help to clarify a child's symptoms. Because these values are nonspecific indicators of systemic inflammation, and may not be specific indicators of IBD activity.

Intercurrent illnesses, such as a viral or bacterial gastroenteritis or another illness that must be treated with antibiotics, may contribute to flare-ups of a child's IBD. These illnesses may result from the alteration of the normal flora of the bowel (e.g., *C. difficile*) after antibiotic therapy.

Diarrhea. Children with IBD have bouts of gastroenteritis similar to those of their peers and family members. A child's physical examination and history should include an evaluation of any IBD-like symptoms, including the presence of any blood, pus, or mucus in the stool; cramping pain or urgency associated with bowel movements; weight loss or anorexia; and any symptoms that might be extraintestinal manifestations of the disease. A child's abdomen should be closely examined for any change. Stool cultures should always be obtained, because infections (e.g., with rotavirus, norovirus, *Yersinia*, *Campylobacter*, *Shigella*, and *C. difficile*) may mimic IBD. Children should be treated for any identified pathogen. Any child with prolonged symptoms, including bloody diarrhea (with no identified pathogen) or weight loss, should be referred to the gastroenterology team.

Abdominal Pain. Children with abdominal pain should be examined for any changes that might indicate a progression of the disease, fulminant colitis, or an obstruction. These children should be questioned about the similarity of their current pain to the pain experienced as a part of the IBD. Similarity to previous episodes, location of known disease, and history of accompanying symptoms that would indicate IBD rather than influenza or other acute conditions of the abdomen should guide practitioners. Many medications used to treat IBD may cause gastritis. Children often present with epigastric pain or reflux-like symptoms. A child who appears ill with acute pain should be immediately referred to the gastroenterology team; children with less acute symptoms should be monitored carefully with referral if the symptoms do not abate within 24 to 48 hours.

Vomiting. Vomiting in children with IBD, especially CD, could indicate an obstruction. The history and physical examination should elicit information about distention, associated pain and its relation to meals and the nature of the emesis (e.g., is it bilious?), and accompanying abdominal pain. As always, information about the child's bowel pattern and the nature of the stools should be gathered.

Skeletal Complaints. Children with IBD, especially those receiving corticosteroid therapy, are at increased risk for osteoporosis, aseptic necrosis of the hip or knee joints, and spinal fractures. In addition, children with IBD are more likely to have peripheral arthritis, servilities, and ankylosing spondylitis. Children with IBD who report back or hip pain require radiologic examination to adequately assess these symptoms. When children with IBD report joint pain, they should be questioned about the presence of erythema or swelling. Children with symptoms suggesting joint involvement should also be assessed for any increased disease activity.

Drug Interactions

Drugs used to treat IBD, as well as drugs used to treat other conditions in individuals with IBD, can cause a wide range of potentially serious interactions (Irving et al., 2007). Many drug interactions are of no clinical significance; an exhaustive review would be unwieldy, so only the most common and serious interactions are addressed, with particular attention to interactions that occur when both drugs are used concurrently in the treatment of individuals with IBD. Sulfasalazine decreases levels of folate, oral hypoglycemic agents, and digoxin when used concurrently (Irving et al.). Individuals receiving both 5-ASA and thiopurine-containing drugs may develop leukopenia (Irving et al.). Sulfasalazine potentiates the action of phenytoin (Dilantin), resulting in higher than expected blood values of this drug. Corticosteroid levels increase with oral contraceptives (especially prednisolone) and if taken with grapefruit juice (especially budesonide). Ciprofloxacin levels decrease when used concurrently with nutritional supplements and antacids. Metronidazole has a disulfiram (Antabuse)-type reaction when an individual ingests alcohol or alcohol-containing elixirs during drug therapy. Phenytoin and phenobarbital increase the elimination of metronidazole, but cimetidine decreases its clearance. Individuals taking lithium may experience elevations in lithium levels if they start taking metronidazole. Methotrexate levels increase with penicillin and tetracycline. Methotrexate and proton pump inhibitors when given concurrently can lead to myalgias. Cyclosporine levels increase with concurrent administration of antibiotics, antifungals, calcium channel blockers, oral contraceptives, oral hypoglycemic agents, and grapefruit juice (Irving et al.). Decreased cyclosporine levels can occur when given concurrently with antibiotics (rifampicin and trimethoprim), antiepileptic drugs (carbamazepine, phenytoin, and phenobarbital), red wine, vitamin E, and vitamin C (Irving et al.). Warfarin is affected by almost every drug used to treat IBD. Mesalazine, sulfasalazine, and thiopurines decrease the absorption of warfarin, whereas ciprofloxacin, metronidazole, and corticosteroids increase its absorption (Irving et al.). Nonsteroidal anti-inflammatory drugs should be avoided by most individuals with IBD because of the ulcerogenic effect and potential for GI bleeding.

Developmental Issues

Sleep Patterns

Children who are taking corticosteroids twice daily may feel agitated or euphoric at bedtime and may have difficulty sleeping. Dosage times may be shifted to alleviate this problem. Once the dose is decreased, a single dose may be given in the morning. Children experiencing a flare-up of disease or whose disease is under poor control may be troubled by the need to use the bathroom frequently during the night, which may make it difficult for them to feel well rested and refreshed in the morning.

Toileting

Because IBD is usually diagnosed in most children after they have accomplished toilet training, families of children with IBD do not typically face this issue. For children who are not toilet-trained, however, it is preferable to wait to start toilet training until the disease is in remission and the character of bowel movements is as close to normal as possible.

Incontinence is experienced by many individuals with IBD. Children who have frequent bowel movements accompanied by urgency often fear recurrence of this problem when they are in public. Children and families should be assisted in planning to prevent or handle such eventualities in a low-key way. In the context of an overview of a child's condition and its implications, the possibility of incontinence should be shared with the school nurse and classroom teachers, who can make plans to ensure that incidents will be handled with sensitivity and that the child may retain as much control and dignity as possible. Classroom teachers should be encouraged to move the child's seat closer to the door and to liberalize bathroom privileges so that he or she may inconspicuously leave the room. Primary care providers may suggest that an extra change of clothing be kept in the child's locker or the nurse's office. Reminders to use the bathroom before leaving home and at regular intervals may also help to reduce the occurrence of potentially embarrassing episodes.

Management styles vary among practitioners with respect to the use of antispasmodic agents for the relief of chronic diarrhea in children with mild IBD. Drugs such as loperamide (Imodium) should be used cautiously if needed in controlling symptoms during daytime activity.

Discipline

Behavioral expectations for children with IBD are similar to those of their unaffected peers. One area of concern may be the issue of compliance for children who are assuming responsibility for their treatment regimen. Children in whom IBD remains in remission may not perceive the need for their medications because they may essentially be asymptomatic and feeling well. The concept of remission and disease being present but not discernible is difficult for school-aged children or early adolescents to master. Because a large percentage of children with IBD are in early to middle adolescence, rebellion and testing are normal developmental issues. For adolescents with IBD, medications and treatment regimens can become a battleground for testing their independence. Primary care providers can help families identify ownership of responsibility for disease management. A particular risk facing children and adolescents with IBD is the abrupt discontinuation of steroid medications with its inherent hazards. In addition to a recurrence of IBD-related symptoms, children are at risk for adrenal crisis. Adolescents who are responsible for their own medication regimens, as well as their parents, should be educated about the significant risks associated with abruptly stopping steroid treatment.

Child Care

Parents of children with IBD should be encouraged to use the same guidelines for choosing child-care arrangements as for their well children. Because the onset of IBD commonly occurs later in childhood, the increased risk of diarrheal illness secondary to diaper-changing areas and daycare providers handling food often does not need to be addressed with these families. If a child becomes infected, the illness should be promptly treated and the child monitored for signs of exacerbation of the disease. The overriding philosophy, however, is not to unduly isolate a child from the normal activities of daily living.

Schooling

Children with CD and UC are as able to achieve in the classroom as their unaffected peers. Similar to many children with chronic conditions, children with IBD must juggle treatment schedules and cope with stigma, pain, fatigue, and, occasionally, frequent or prolonged school absences. Academic performance may ultimately reflect a child's struggle to overcome these hurdles (see Chapter 3).

The nature of the disease processes and treatment regimens often set children with IBD apart from their peers in significant ways, including the cushingoid facies of children receiving corticosteroid therapy, the need for embarrassing treatments such as the instillation of rectal medications and the use of nocturnal nasogastric feedings or restrictive diets. The isolation felt by children experiencing these treatments may cause them to limit participation in activities that enrich their school and extracurricular experiences. Alternatively, these children may choose not to comply with treatment regimens in an effort to "fit in." This behavior may establish a cycle of disease exacerbation and escalation of therapy that may concomitantly affect a child's academic achievement, reinforcing the child's sense of isolation. Sensitivity to these issues, creative problem solving, and anticipatory guidance by the primary care provider support the child and family in achieving as normal a lifestyle as possible. An issue often faced by individuals with IBD is the common misunderstanding by lay people and some in the medical community that IBD is a psychological disease. A primary role of health care providers is to educate school personnel and other significant adults in the child's life (e.g., club leaders, coaches, and daycare providers).

Sexuality

Adolescence is a time when concerns about body image, interpersonal relationships, and plans for the future are paramount. Therefore it is not unusual that adolescents or young adults with IBD are concerned about the possible effect of this diagnosis on their appeal as a sexual partner, their ability to perform sexually, and their fertility. The significant changes in appearance that adolescents with IBD must withstand often include late onset of puberty, weight gain, and acne—all of which contribute to their feelings of self-consciousness and stigmatization. Individuals with IBD may have stomas or perianal involvement, which can be disfiguring and may affect their feelings of sexual attractiveness or acceptability to another person. Positive feelings of self-worth and a sense of acceptance must be conveyed to adolescents with IBD. The option of joining a network of other adolescents with common concerns should be offered whenever possible. Formal organizations or casual social gatherings may provide opportunities for teens and families to obtain support and acceptance.

Sulfasalazine has been shown to cause infertility in men as a result of a decreased sperm count and dysmotility and sperm malformation. These effects are reversible, however, when men stop taking sulfasalazine for 3 months (*PDR*, 2008). No infertility is reported in men receiving the newer, oral 5-ASA preparations (*PDR,* 2008). Neither UC nor CD increases infertility in women with inactive disease. Some studies have indicated that women with CD have higher rates of infertility than control populations. It is believed that the most common cause of infertility in women with CD is the activity of the disease. Other factors include poor nutritional status, rectovaginal fistulas, and fear of becoming pregnant. A recent report suggests women who have had colectomies have more difficulty conceiving children compared with populations with no such surgery (Ording, Juul,

Berndtsson et al., 2002). Unfortunately, the reported estimates of both the relative risk of infertility after IPAA and the actual rate of infertility vary widely in the literature (Waljee et al., 2006). It is estimated that UC alone can cause up to a 15% increase in infertility. In a meta-analysis of 8 studies, Waljee et al. (2006) found a 50% increase risk of infertility after colectomy with a J-pouch. The outcome of pregnancy in women with IBD approximates that of the general population, but some researchers have found a somewhat higher incidence of prematurity in infants born to mothers with IBD than in the general population (Leichtner & Higuchi, 2004).

Methotrexate is a known teratogen and must be used with care in sexually active adolescents. The need for birth control should be addressed with any adolescent female who is taking this medication (Markowitz, 2008).

Pregnancy does not increase the likelihood of a relapse of either UC or of CD, but if UC is active at the time of conception, the course of disease activity may be worse during the pregnancy (Leichtner & Higuchi, 2004).

Transition to Adulthood

Individuals with IBD do not typically require a specialized environment or assistance with activities of daily living. The embarrassing nature of many of the required medical therapies and symptoms of active disease make private living facilities most desirable for many individuals with IBD. Practitioners may help individuals to secure such accommodations.

Specialized programs to transition adolescents with IBD to adult care are not readily available. Many primary care providers have an informal policy of caring for their adolescent clients with IBD until they have weathered most of the anticipated developmental crises of late adolescence. It is best to wait to make this transition until the individual's disease is quiescent. To facilitate this transition, the pediatric gastroenterologist should begin seeing affected adolescents without their parents in the examination room to build a relationship that promotes independence and self-reliance and resembles in part the relationship they will have with their internist-gastroenterologist (Baldassano, Ferry, Griffiths, et al., 2002; Dubinsky, 2008). The subject of transition should be talked about months or years before it will occur (see Chapter 4). The benefits of the transition should be highlighted each time. The young adult and their parent should be made aware of the need for a physician who not only has expertise in IBD, but in "adult"-type problems such as pregnancy, fertility, cancer surveillance, and the common health problems of adulthood (Baldassano et al., 2002). It is important to identify the internist-gastroenterologist who recognizes that the young adult in whom IBD was diagnosed in childhood may have a different set of expectations than the young adult with a recent diagnosis (Baldassano et al.). It is not unusual for the transition process to be more difficult for the parents than the child.

Family Concerns

Families of children with IBD, similar to families of children with other chronic conditions, may focus on the child's symptoms and treatment regimen. In the case of families dealing with IBD, however, this often means disclosing such private and potentially embarrassing issues as toileting and personal hygiene.

The invasion of privacy felt by the child may become a source of stress for the entire family. Common concerns shared by children with IBD include personal appearance, physical endurance, diet, and their ability to fit in when sharing a meal or snacks with friends and family. These issues are magnified as these children enter adolescence and seek increased independence from their families and become increasingly self-conscious and concerned about body image and function. Poor communication and distrust between parent and child about disease activity and compliance with treatment regimens may result. If these children can become relatively independent in disease management before this difficult time, they and their families may develop confidence and trust in one another, perhaps alleviating or avoiding some of these conflicts.

Summer camp programs are now available for children with IBD. The goals of these camp programs are to allow children to participate in normal camp activities surrounded by their peers dealing with similar childhood issues (Dubinsky, 2008). An added bonus of IBD camps is an increase in self-esteem, altered perceptions and attitudes toward illness, and the knowledge that they are not alone.

IBD may affect children of many ethnic and religious backgrounds at a wide range of ages and with varied clinical presentations and severity. When cultural or religious practices focus on food and special dietary practices, these children may feel conflicted if disease activity makes some foods difficult to tolerate. Other than during times of disease activity, it is not typically recommended that children limit their diet. Children should be encouraged to maintain a diet as unrestricted and palatable as possible to encourage adequate caloric and other nutrient intake to promote optimal growth and development. Health care team members' sensitivity about dietary issues relating to both everyday life and special celebrations or religious observances is important. Practitioners should work in partnership with the family and child to develop a flexible plan of care that incorporates individual cultural concerns, such as religious feasts or times of fasting.

Resources

Organizations

Crohn's and Colitis Foundation of America, Inc.
386 Park Ave. S., 17th Floor
New York, NY 10016-8804
(800) 932-2423; (212) 685-3440
Website: www.CCFA.org
Email: info@ccfa.org

The Crohn's and Colitis Foundation of America (CCFA) is an organization with many chapters across the country that support research and provide education and support for its members and for members of the community. Individuals with IBD and their families are encouraged to join and attend meetings and educational offerings. Many chapters have subcommittees that specifically deal with issues related to the needs of children with IBD and their families. The CCFA also publishes educational books, pamphlets, and newsletters written for the lay public. Professional memberships are available.

Summary of Primary Care Needs for the Child with Inflammatory Bowel Disease

HEALTH CARE MAINTENANCE

Growth and Development

- Growth failure is a common problem for children with IBD but is more commonly seen in CD than UC.
- Growth parameters are important to measure and chart at each primary care visit.
- Cognitive abilities are unimpaired by IBD.

Diet

- No special diet is recommended. Referral to a nutritionist at time of diagnosis is recommended. Some children may be lactose intolerant, particularly when disease is active. Some children during active disease may have less pain following a diet low in roughage. Adequate caloric intake is essential for growth.
- If growth retardation has occurred, supplemental diet preparations may be beneficial.

Safety

- No special safety recommendations are necessary for a child with inactive disease.
- Children with osteoporosis should not participate in contact sports.
- Individuals taking metronidazole should be cautioned about an Antabuse-type reaction to alcohol.
- Take caution with travel, especially to tropical areas. Ova, parasites, and purity of water should be concerns.
- Immunosuppressed children should carry medical identification.

Immunizations

- No change in the normal immunization protocol is indicated unless a child is taking maintenance doses of immunosuppressive agents; in this case, no live vaccines should be administered, but immune globulin may be used with exposures.
- Yearly influenza vaccine is recommended for children receiving immunosuppressants.

Screening

- *Vision.* Annual ophthalmic examination is necessary at each visit. Twice-yearly ophthalmologist visits are recommended for a child taking maintenance doses of corticosteroids.
- *Hearing.* Routine screening is recommended.
- *Dental.* Routine care is adequate, but children taking cyclosporine are at increased risk for gingival hyperplasia.
- *Blood pressure.* Routine screening is recommended; if a child is taking cyclosporine or corticosteroids, blood pressure should be measured at every visit.
- *Hematocrit.* Hematocrit and hemoglobin values should be obtained yearly if a child is asymptomatic and has no history of anemia; otherwise a CBC should be obtained every 6 months or as necessary.
- *Urinalysis.* Routine screening is recommended unless a child has a history of fistulas or abscesses.
- *Tuberculosis.* Routine screening is recommended; defer while on immunosuppressive drugs; required to initiating infliximab.

Condition-Specific Screening

- *Erythrocyte sedimentation rate.* Check annually or as needed if a flare-up of disease is suspected.
- *Fecal occult blood test.* Check stool yearly and with potential disease flare-ups.
- *Chemistries.* Liver function studies should be monitored every year for an otherwise asymptomatic child with IBD. A child taking Dipentum, Asacol, or Pentasa should have renal functions studies monitored at least every 4 months. For a child receiving cyclosporine, 6-MP, or AZA, renal and liver function studies should be monitored every 4 months. A child taking 6-MP should have amylase and lipase levels tested every 4 months.
- *Lactose intolerance.* Check as indicated.
- *Neurologic examination.* Children receiving metronidazole should be assessed for paresthesias at each routine visit.
- *Bone mineral density.* Screening in children with CD is recommended.
- *Surveillance endoscopy.* There are new recommendations for annual or biannual colonoscopies.

COMMON ILLNESS MANAGEMENT

Differential Diagnosis

- *Diarrhea.* Rule out flare-up of disease, obtain cultures.
- *Abdominal pain.* Rule out flare-up of disease, gastritis, fulminant colitis, and obstruction.
- *Vomiting.* Rule out flare-up of disease and gastritis; assess for obstruction.
- *Skeletal complaints.* Rule out arthritic manifestations of the disease (i.e., sacroiliitis, ankylosing spondylitis, peripheral arthritis), aseptic necrosis of the femoral head, vertebral compression fractures, and osteoporosis.

DEVELOPMENTAL ISSUES

Sleep Patterns

- Children with IBD generally have no special needs; children receiving an evening dose of corticosteroids may have some difficulty sleeping. These children may also have some nighttime stooling, which interrupts sleep.

Toileting

- In most children, IBD is diagnosed after toilet training has been accomplished. When toilet training is a concern, it may be suggested that toilet training be instituted when the disease activity is quiescent.
- For older children with active disease, occasional incontinence may be an issue.
- Antispasmodics may be used cautiously for daytime incontinence.

Discipline

- Standard developmental counseling is advised; monitor adherence to treatment regimen.
- Children and families should be educated on the hazards of discontinuing treatment.

Summary of Primary Care Needs for the Child with Inflammatory Bowel Disease—cont'd

Child Care
• Standard developmental counseling is advised.

Schooling
• Children with IBD are as able to achieve in the classroom as their unaffected peers.
• Frequent or prolonged absences may interfere with school performance.
• School personnel must be educated about special issues related to IBD; any misunderstandings about a psychological cause of IBD should be alleviated.

Sexuality
• Self-esteem and body image issues are important to adolescents with IBD.
• Adolescents may have late onset of puberty as a result of growth retardation.

• Sulfasalazine may cause infertility in men while they are taking the drug.
• Pregnancy outcomes are similar to those of the general population.

Transition to Adulthood
• Self-care responsibilities may be gradually assumed by adolescents. Specialized environments and assistance with activities of daily living are not typically required by young adults with IBD.
• The transition to a provider specializing in care of adults is best done during periods of quiescent disease.

FAMILY CONCERNS
Privacy issues regarding toileting are often difficult for children and families. Because IBD affects individuals of disparate backgrounds and varies in its clinical presentation and severity, care of a child with IBD should be individualized. The practitioner should be sensitive to the needs of children and families whose cultural or religious practices focus on food if dietary restrictions are indicated during periods of active disease.

REFERENCES

Ahmed, S.F., Wong, J.S.C., & McGrogan, P. (2007). Improving growth in children with inflammatory bowel disease. *Horm Res, 68*, 117-121.

Baldassano, R., Ferry, R., Griffiths, G., et al. (2002). Transition of the patient with inflammatory bowel disease from pediatric to adult care: Recommendations of the North American Society for Pediatric Gastroenterology, Hepatology and Nutrition. *J Pediatr Gastroenterol Nutr, 34*, 245-248.

Barrett, J.C., Hansoul, S., Nicolae, D.L., et al. (2008). Genome-wide association defines more than 30 distinct susceptibility loci for Crohn's disease. *Nat Genet, 40*: 955-962.

Beattie, R.M., Croft, N.M., Fell, J.M., et al. (2006). Inflammatory bowel disease. *Arch Dis Child, 91*, 426-432.

Boirivant, M., & Strober, W. (2007). The mechanism of action of probiotics. *Curr Opin Gastroenterol, 23*, 679-692.

Borrelli, O., Cordischi, L., Cirulli, M., et al. (2006). Polymeric versus corticosteroids in the treatment of active pediatric Crohn's disease: A randomized controlled open design. *Clin Gastroenterol Hepatol, 4*, 744-753.

Bousvaros, A., Sylvester, M., Kugathasan, S., et al. (2006). Challenges in pediatric inflammatory bowel disease. *Inflamm Bowel Dis, 12*, 885-912.

Bousvaros, A., Morley-Fletcher, M., Pensabene, L., et al. (2008a). Research and clinical challenges in paediatric inflammatory bowel disease. *Dig Liver Dis, 40*, 32-38,.

Bousvaros, A., Murray, K., & Leichtner, A. (2008b). *Clinical Manifestations of Crohn's Disease in Children and Adolescents.* Available at www.utdol.com/utd/content/topic.do?topickey=pedigast/12528&view)uptodate.com. Retrieved January 17, 2008.

Cuthbert, A.P., Fisher, S.A., Mirza, M.M., et al. (2002). The contribution of *NOD2* gene mutations to the risk and site of disease in inflammatory bowel disease. *Gastroenterology, 122*, 867-874.

Davis, M., Andres, J.M., Christopher, D., et al. (2007). Antibodies to *Escherichia coli* outer membrane porin C in the absence of anti-*Saccharomyces cerevisiae* antibodies and anti-neutrophil cytoplasmic antibodies are an unreliable marker of Crohn's disease and ulcerative colitis. *J Pediatr Gastroenterol Nutr, 45*, 409-413.

De Ridder, L., Benninga, M.A., Taminiau, J.A.J.M., et al. (2007). Infliximab use in children and adolescents with inflammatory bowel disease. *J Pediatr Gastroenterol Nutr, 45*, 3-14.

Diefenbach, K., & Breuer, C.K. (2006). Pediatric inflammatory bowel disease. *World J Gastroenterol, 12*, 3204-3212.

Dubinsky, M. (2008). Special issues in pediatric inflammatory bowel disease. *World J Gastroenterol, 14*, 413-420.

Ephgrave, K. (2007). Extra-intestinal manifestations of Crohn's disease. *Surg Clin North Am, 87*, 673-680.

Freeman, H.J. (2004). Comparison of longstanding pediatric-onset and adult-onset Crohn's disease. *J Pediatr Gastroenterol Nutr, 39*, 183-186.

Fish, D., & Kugathasan, S. (2004). Inflammatory bowel disease. *Adolesc Med Clin, 15*, 67-90.

Gerasimidis, K., McGrogan, P., Hassan, K., et al. (2008). Dietary modifications, nutritional supplements and alternative medicine in paediatric patients with inflammatory bowel disease. *Aliment Pharmacol Ther, 27*, 155-165.

Graham, T.O., & Kandil, H.M. (2002). Nutritional factors in inflammatory bowel disease. *Gastroenterol Clin, 31*, 203-219.

Griffiths, A.M., & Buller, H.B. (2004). Inflammatory bowel disease. In W.A. Walker, P.R. Durie, J.R., Hamilton, et al. (Eds.), *Pediatric Gastrointestinal Disease.* Hamilton, Ontario, Canada: BC Decker, 2004.

Griffiths, A.M., & Hugot, J.P. (2004). Inflammatory bowel disease; Crohn's disease. In W.A. Walker, P.R., Durie, J.R., Hamilton, et al.(Eds.), *Pediatric Gastrointestinal Disease. Hamilton,* Ontario, Canada: BC Decker, 2004.

Gupta, N., Bostrom, A., Kirschner, B., et al. (2007). Gender differences in presentation and course of disease in pediatric patients with Crohn's disease. *Pediatrics, 120*, e1418-e1425.

Gupta, N., Cohen, S.A., Bostrom A.G., et al. (2006). Risk factors for initial surgery in pediatric patients with Crohn's. *Gastroenterology, 130*, 1069-1077.

Hardin, D., Kemp, S., & Allen, D. (2007). Twenty years of recombinant human growth hormone in children: Relevance to pediatric care providers. *Clin Pediatr, 46*, 279-286.

Heuschkel, R., Afzal, N., Wuerth, A., et al. (2002). Complementary medicine use in children and young adults with inflammatory bowel disease. *Am J Gastroenterol, 97*, 382-388.

Heyman, M.B., & Committee on Nutrition. (2006). Lactose intolerance in infants, children and adolescents. *Pediatrics 118*, 1279-1286.

Heyman, M.B., Garnett, E.A., Wojcicki, J., et al. (2008). Growth hormone treatment for growth failure in pediatric patients with Crohns. *J Pediatr, 153*, 651-658.

Heyman, M.B., Kirschner, B.S., Gold, B.D., et al. (2005). Children with early-onset inflammatory bowel disease (IBD): Analysis of a pediatric IBD consortium registry. *J Pediatr, 146*, 35-40.

Higuchi, L., & Bousvaros, A. (2007). *Diagnosis of inflammatory bowel disease in children and adolescents, and epidemiology and etiology of inflammatory bowel disease in children and adolescents.* Available at www. utdol.com/utd/content/topic.do?topickey=pedigast/12528&view)uptodate.com. Retrieved December 19, 2007.

Hyams, J., & Markowitz, J.F. (2005). Can we alter the natural history of Crohn disease in children? *J Pediatr Gastroenterol Nutr, 40*, 262-272.

Hyams, J., Markowitz, J., Otley, A., et al. (2005). Evaluation of the pediatric Crohn disease activity index: A prospective multicenter experience. *J Pediatr Gastroenterol Nutr, 41*, 416-421.

Hyams, J., Markowitz, J., & Wyllie, R. (2000). Use of infliximab in the treatment of Crohn's disease in children and adolescents. *J Pediatr, 137*, 192-196.

Irving, P., Shanahan, F., & Rampton, D.S. (2007). Drug interactions in inflammatory bowel disease. *Am J Gastroenterol, 102*, 1-13.

Jani, N., & Regueiro, M.D. (2002). Medical therapy for ulcerative colitis. *Gastroenterol Clin North Am, 31*, 147-167.

Jose, F., & Heyman, M. (2008). Extraintestinal manifestation of inflammatory bowel disease. *J Pediatr Gastroenterol Nutr, 46*, 124-133.

Karp, S.M., & Koch, T.R. (2006). Nutrient supplements in inflammatory bowel disease. *Dis Month, 52*, 211-220.

Katz, J.A. (2004). Treatment of inflammatory bowel disease with corticosteroids. *Gastroenterol Clin North Am, 33*, 171-189.

Katz, S. (2002). Update in medical therapy of ulcerative colitis: A practical approach. *J Clin Gastroenterol, 34*, 397-407.

Kozuch, P., & Hanauer, S. (2008). Treatment of inflammatory bowel disease: A review of medical therapy. *World J Gastroenterol, 14*, 354-377.

Kugathasan, S., & Amre, D. (2006). Inflammatory bowel disease-environmental modification and genetic determinants. *Pediatric Clinics of North America, 53*, 727-749.

Kugathasan, S., Nebel, J., Skelton, J.A. et al. (2007). Body mass index in children with newly diagnosed inflammatory bowel disease: Observations from two multicenter North American inception cohorts. *J Pediatr, 151*, 523-527.

Langmead, L., & Rampton, D.S. (2006). Complementary and alternative therapies for inflammatory bowel diseases. *Aliment Pharmacol Ther, 23*, 341-349.

Leichtner, A.M., & Higuchi, L. (2004). Ulcerative colitis. In W.A. Walker, O. Goulet, R.E., Kleinman, et al. (Eds.), *Pediatric Gastrointestinal Disease*, Hamilton, Ontario, Canada: BC Decker.

Levine, A., Broide, E., Stein, M., et al. (2002). Evaluation of oral budesonide for treatment of mild and moderate exacerbations of Crohn's disease in children. *J Pediatr, 140*, 75-80.

MacDonald, A. (2006). Omega-3 fatty acids as adjunctive therapy in Crohn's disease. *Gastroenterol Nurs, 29*, 295-301.

Mack, D.R., Langton, C., Markowitz, J., et al. (2007). Laboratory values for children with newly diagnosed inflammatory bowel disease. *Pediatrics, 119*, 1113-1128.

Mackner, L.M., & Crandall, W.V. (2007). Psychological factors affecting pediatric inflammatory bowel disease. *Curr Opin Pediatr, 19*, 548-552.

Mamula, P., Mascarenhas, M.R., & Baldassano, R.N. (2002). Biological and novel therapies for inflammatory bowel disease in children. *Pediatr Gastroenterol Nutr, 49*, 1-25.

Markowitz, J. (2008). Current treatment of inflammatory bowel disease in children. *Dig Liver Dis, 40*, 16-21.

Markowitz, J.F., Grancher, K., Kohn, N., et al. (2000). A multicenter trial of 6-mercaptopurine and prednisone in children with newly diagnosed Crohn's disease. *Gastroenterology, 119*, 895-902.

Newby, E.A., Sawczenko, A., Thomas, A.G., et al. (2005). Interventions for growth failure in childhood Crohn's disease. *Cochrane Database of Systematic Reviews 3*. Art No: CD003873. DOI:10, 1002/14651858.CDOO3873.pub2.

Nieuwenhuis, E.E.S., & Escher, J.C. (2008). Early onset IBD: What's the difference? *Dig Liver Dis, 40*, 12-15.

Nikolaus, S., & Schreiber, S. (2007). Diagnostics of inflammatory bowel disease. *Gastroenterology. 133*, 1670-1689.

Ogura, Y., Bonen, D.K., Inohara, N., et al. (2000). A frame shift mutation in NOD2 associated with susceptibility to Crohn's disease. *Nature, 31*(411), 603-606.

Oliva-Hemker, M., & Fiocchi, C. (2002). Etiopathogenesis of inflammatory bowel disease: The importance of the pediatric perspective. *Inflamm Bowel Dis, 8*, 112-128.

Ording, O.K., Juul, S., Berndtsson, I., et al. (2002). Ulcerative colitis: Female fecundity before diagnosis, during disease and after surgery compared with a population sample. *Gastroenterology, 122*, 15-19.

Perrin, J.M., Kuhlthau, K., Chughtai, A., et al. (2008). Measuring quality of life in pediatric patients with inflammatory bowel disease: Psychometric and clinical characteristics. *J Pediatr Gastroenterol Nutr, 46*, 154-171.

Physicians' Desk Reference. (2008). Montvale, NJ: Medical Economics Data Production.

Podolsky, D.K. (2002). Inflammatory bowel disease. *N Engl J Med, 347*, 417-429.

Ponsky, T., Hindle, A., & Sandler, A. (2007). Inflammatory bowel disease in the pediatric patient. *Surg Clin North Am, 87*, 643-658.

Powell, F.C., & O'Kane, M. (2002). Management of pyoderma gangrenosum. *Dermatol Clin, 20*, 29-38.

Present, D.H. (2002). Serological tests are not helpful in managing inflammatory bowel disease. *Inflamm Bowel Dis, 3*, 227-228.

Razack, R., & Seidner, D.L. (2007). Nutrition in inflammatory bowel disease. *Curr Opin Gastroenterol, 23*, 400-405.

Reddy, J.G., & Loftus, E.V. (2006). Safety of infliximab and other biologic agents in the inflammatory bowel diseases. *Gastroenterol Clin North Am, 35*, 837-855.

Ruemmele, F.M., Roy, C.C., Levy, E., et al. (2000). Nutrition as primary therapy in pediatric Crohn's disease: Fact or fancy? *J Pediatr, 136*, 285-291.

Rufo, P.A., & Bousvaros, A. (2007). Challenges and progress in pediatric inflammatory bowel disease. *Curr Opin Gastroenterol, 23*, 406-412.

Sanborn, W.J., & Targan, S.R. (2002). Biologic therapy of inflammatory bowel disease. *Gastroenterology, 122*, 1592-1608.

Sands, B.E. (2006). New therapies for the treatment of inflammatory bowel disease. *Surg Clin North Am, 86*, 1045-1064.

Shen, B. (2007). Complications of IBD-related pouch surgery. *Gastroenterol Hepatol, 3*, 678-680.

Stucchi, A.F., Aarons, C.B., & Becker, J.M. (2006). Surgical approaches to cancer in patients who have inflammatory bowel disease. *Gastroenterol Clin North Am, 35*, 641-673.

Szajewska, H., Setty, M., Mrukowicz, J., et al. (2006). Probiotics in gastrointestinal disease in children: Hard and not-so-hard evidence of efficacy. *J Pediatr Gastroenterol Nutr, 42*, 454-475.

Tamboli, C.P. (2007). Current medical therapy for chronic inflammatory bowel diseases. *Surg Clin North Am, 87*, 697-725.

Targan, S.R., & Karp, L.C. (2007). Inflammatory bowel disease diagnosis, evaluation and classification: State-of-the art approach. *Curr Opin Gastroenterol, 23*, 390-394.

Turner, D., Otley, A.R., Mack, D., et al. (2007). Development, validation and evaluation of a pediatric ulcerative colitis activity index: A prospective multicenter study. *Gastroenterology, 133*, 423-432.

Waljee, A., Waljee, A., Morris, A.M., et al. (2006). Threefold increased risk of infertility: A meta-analysis of infertility after ileal pouch anal anastomosis in ulcerative colitis. *Gut, 55*, 1575-1580.

Xavier, R.J., & Podolsky, D.K. (2007). Unravelling the pathogenesis of inflammatory bowel disease. *Nature, 44*, 427-434.

Ziring, D.A., Wu, S.S., Mow, W.S., et al. (2007). Oral tacrolimus for steroid-dependent and steroid-resistant ulcerative colitis in children. *J Pediatr Gastroenterol Nutrition, 45*, 306-311.

Zocco, M.A., Zileri Dal Verme, L., Cremonini, F., et al. (2006). Efficacy of lactobacillus GG in maintaining remission of ulcerative colitis. *Aliment Pharmacol Ther, 23*, 1567-1574.

31 Juvenile Rheumatoid Arthritis

Karla B. Jones and Gloria C. Higgins

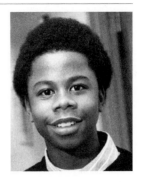

Etiology

Chronic arthritis in childhood represents a heterogeneous group of diseases, of which the two most common forms are juvenile rheumatoid arthritis (JRA) and juvenile spondyloarthropathy (JSpA). *Chronic arthritis* is defined as swelling within a joint or limitation in the range of movement with joint pain and tenderness that persists for at least 6 weeks and for which all other causes are excluded (Cassidy & Petty, 2005a).

Over the past three decades, international leaders in the field of pediatric rheumatology have debated the criteria for classification of childhood arthritis (Duffy, Colbert, Laxer, et al., 2005). The International League of Associations for Rheumatology (ILAR) classification criteria (Petty, Southwood, Manners, et al., 2004) using the juvenile idiopathic arthritis (JIA) terminology is increasingly being used on a worldwide basis. It has largely replaced the European League Against Rheumatism (EULAR) criteria for juvenile chronic arthritis (Table 31-1). In the United States, however, the American College of Rheumatology (ACR) criteria for JRA is still widely used in clinical practice and for billing purposes. Therefore, the specific conditions of JRA/JIA and JSpA are either referred to individually or in general as "chronic arthritis" for the purposes of clarity in this chapter. Moreover, the importance of recognizing JSpA in any discussion of chronic arthritis in children is emphasized because JSpA is frequently underdiagnosed or misdiagnosed (Burgos-Vargos, 2002).

The etiology of chronic arthritis in childhood is unknown. This condition is not a single disease entity but represents a heterogeneous group of phenotypes with several modes of onset (Cassidy & Petty, 2005a). Differences in onset and clinical course should be considered when researching causation and treatment. Current hypotheses focus on the roles of inflammatory and immune dysregulation, infection, psychological stress, trauma, and hormonal factors as potential contributing factors in a child with a genetic predisposition. Inflammation in JRA results from the interaction of different cell types (myeloid, lymphoid, and stromal) and the mediators they release (Sullivan, 2005). Recent research has shown that children with chronic arthritis have elevated levels of numerous cytokines, including tumor necrosis factor–alpha (TNF-α); macrophage inhibitory factor; interleukin (IL)-1, IL-6, IL-8; interferon-γ; and several chemokines (CCL-2, CCL-3, CCL-11, CXCL-9, CXCL-10), with different profiles among the different JRA onset types (deJager, Hoppenreijs, Wulffraat, et al., 2007; Saxena, Aggarwal & Misra, 2005). Epidemiologic studies have shown familial,

seasonal, geographic, and ethnic differences among the subtypes of chronic childhood arthritis, suggesting environmental and genetic factors (Kurahara, Grandinetti, Fujii, et al., 2007; Prahalad, Shear, Thompson, et al., 2002; Saurenmann, Rose, Tyrrell, et al., 2007).

Susceptibility to JRA is determined by a complex interaction of genetic and environmental factors. JRA does not tend to occur in multiple family members. When JRA is observed in more than one family member, it is most likely to be found in two siblings (Phelan & Thompson, 2006); however, sibling pairs with JRA are still rare (Moroldo, Chaudhari, Shear, et al., 2004). The observation that even identical twins do not have a high concordance for JRA suggests that other influences, such as environment and chance, are important. The division of JRA into different subtypes based on clinical characteristics has been reflected in differences in genetic associations among the subtypes. However, even within one subtype of JRA, it is clear that multiple genes are involved.

Human leukocyte antigen (HLA) molecules are encoded within the major histocompatibility complex (MHC) region on human chromosome 6. HLA proteins are responsible for antigen presentation to T cells. Some HLA molecules may be more effective in presenting certain antigens to autoreactive T cells (Prahalad, 2004). Certain subtypes of JRA are associated with certain HLA alleles (i.e., pauciarticular JRA with alleles of HLA-DR5). Association of JRA with groups of HLA antigens that tend to be inherited together (extended haplotype) also has been shown. In a genome-wide scan of 121 families with 247 affected children with JRA, differences in five other chromosome regions besides MHC had significant correlations with JRA (Thompson, Moraldo, Guyer, et al., 2004). There are many different genes within each of these chromosome regions. In addition to HLA genes, some of the other individual genes for polymorphisms that may be associated with JRA susceptibility include *CTLA4* (a regulator of T cell activation), macrophage migration inhibitory factor, and IL-6 (Phelan & Thompson, 2006).

In contrast to JRA, a high familial occurrence of JSpA exists among children, parents, and first-degree relatives. The genetic marker HLA-B27 is present in about 60% to 90% of children with JSpAs but is also present in about 8% of the general white population. The high prevalence of HLA-B27 in healthy individuals makes it an inappropriate screening test for JSpA. It is clear that, like JRA, spondyloarthropathies have a polygenic etiology (Breban, 2006). HLA-B27 is a family of at least 31 different alleles, some of which are strongly associated with spondyloarthropathies, whereas others are not (Khan, Mathieu, Sorrentino, et al., 2007). Further, certain HLA-B27 alleles tend to be inherited as part of an extended haplotype along with other HLA alleles that also influence disease susceptibility. Genes outside the MHC complex also appear to confer disease susceptibility (Breban,

The authors would like to acknowledge the work done by Gail R. McIlvain-Simpson, Patricia M. Reilly, Patricia A. Rettig, Stephanie L. Merhar and Randy Q. Cron on previous editions of this chapter.

TABLE 31-1

Comparison of Classifications of Chronic Arthritis in Children

ACR	EULAR	ILAR
Juvenile rheumatoid arthritis	Juvenile chronic arthritis	Juvenile idiopathic arthritis
Systemic	Systemic JCA	Systemic
Polyarticular	Polyarticular JCA	Polyarticular RF-negative
	Juvenile rheumatoid arthritis	Polyarticular RF-positive
Pauciarticular	Pauciarticular JCA	Oligoarticular Persistent Extended
	Juvenile psoriatic arthritis	Psoriatic arthritis
	Juvenile ankylosing spondylitis	
		Enthesitis-related arthritis
		Other arthritis

Data from Taketomo, C., Hodding, J.H., & Kraus, D.M. (2008). *Pediatric Dosage Handbook* (15th ed.). Hudson, OH: Lexi-Comp.
Key: *ACR,* American College of Rheumatology; *EULAR,* European League Against Rheumatism; *ILAR,* International League of Associations for Rheumatology; *RF,* rheumatoid factor.

2006; Khan et al., 2007). Despite a large body of research in recent years, there is no clear explanation of how HLA-B27 and other genes contribute to the pathogenesis of the spondyloarthropathies.

Incidence and Prevalence

The estimated incidence and prevalence of childhood chronic arthritis differ markedly across a range of studies, in part because of the discrepancies in classification criteria. A review of 34 epidemiology studies reported a prevalence range of 0.07 to 4.01 per 1000 children, and an incidence range of 0.0008 to 0.226 per 1000 children per year for chronic arthritis (Manners & Bower, 2002). The specific incidence of JRA based on ACR criteria has varied from 2 to 20 per 100,000 per year (Cassidy & Petty, 2005a). The prevalence of JRA based on ACR criteria ranges from 16 to 150 per 100,000 (Cassidy & Petty, 2005a). Based on the review by Manners and Bower (2002), the prevalence of enthesitis-related arthritis/JSpA would vary between 0.2 and 54 cases per 100,000 children. The incidence of JSpA may be higher than reported because of several factors, including differing nomenclature and criteria for diagnosis and classification, as well as a lack of clear boundaries between different arthropathies of childhood (Hofer, 2006).

Diagnostic Criteria

The diagnostic criteria for JRA are listed in Box 31-1. Misdiagnosis of JRA results when the following four key points are missed. (1) Arthralgia, or joint pain, alone is not sufficient to make the diagnosis, arthritis must be present. (2) The arthritis must persist for *at least* 6 weeks. (3) All other causes of chronic arthritis in children must be excluded. These causes include, but are not limited to, other pediatric rheumatic diseases such as JSpA, lupus, dermatomyositis, vasculitis, sarcoidosis, scleroderma, and periodic fever syndromes. In addition, nonrheumatic causes of arthritis must be ruled out, including metabolic, infectious, neoplastic, congenital, traumatic, and degenerative

BOX 31-1

Criteria for the Classification of Juvenile Rheumatoid Arthritis

1. Age at onset <16 years.
2. Arthritis (i.e., swelling or effusion, or presence of two or more of the following signs: limitation of range of motion, tenderness or pain on motion, and increased heat) in one or more joints.
3. Duration of disease >6 weeks.
4. Type of onset defined by type of disease in first 6 months:
   a. *Polyarthritis:* five or more inflamed joints.
   b. *Oligoarthritis:* fewer than five inflamed joints.
   c. *Systemic:* arthritis with characteristic fever.
5. Exclusion of other forms of juvenile arthritis.

From Cassidy, J.T., Petty, R.E., Lindsley, C.B., et. al. (Eds.). (2005). *Textbook of Pediatric Rheumatology* (5th ed.). Philadelphia: Elsevier Saunders.

causes. (4) There are no signs, symptoms, or results of laboratory investigations pathognomonic for JRA or JSpA. Children should be referred to a pediatric rheumatology center when the clinician suspects an underlying rheumatic, inflammatory, or autoimmune disorder.

Clinical Manifestations at Time of Diagnosis

A joint with arthritis exhibits one or more of the following signs of inflammation: swelling, warmth, redness, pain or tenderness, and/or reduced range of motion. Swelling results from an intra-articular effusion or hypertrophy (thickening) of the synovial membrane (Figure 31-1). Synovitis may develop insidiously and exist for months or years without causing detectable joint damage, or may damage cartilage, subchondral bone, or other joint structures in a relatively short time (Buchmann & Jaramillo, 2004; Cassidy & Petty, 2005a). Clinical features range from mild synovitis in one joint with no systemic symptoms to moderate or severe disease in many joints.

Clinical Manifestations at Time of Diagnosis

- Joint pain, swelling, stiffness, decreased mobility
- Limp, refusal to walk, or hip pain
- Unexplained rash or fever
- Prolonged or cyclical fevers
- Muscle weakness associated with rash
- Multisystem disease

Common clinical manifestations in addition to synovial inflammation include morning stiffness and stiffness after a period of inactivity. The duration of stiffness is a good indicator of disease activity (Cron & Finkel, 2002). Mild stiffness resolves within a few minutes of walking; however, severe stiffness may take several hours to dissipate.

Children with arthritis may not complain of pain, and the manner in which they do so depends on their age, disease status, and psychosocial measures, such as social support, stress, and locus of control (Schanberg, Anthony, Gil, et al., 2003; Thastum, Herlin, & Zachariae, 2005). Many children present with painless joint effusions (Weiss & Ilowite, 2007) and some may have joint contractures. However, because these children are able to maintain normal activity levels, the diagnosis is often delayed. Unfortunately, delay in diagnosis and treatment can have serious consequences for the child, including

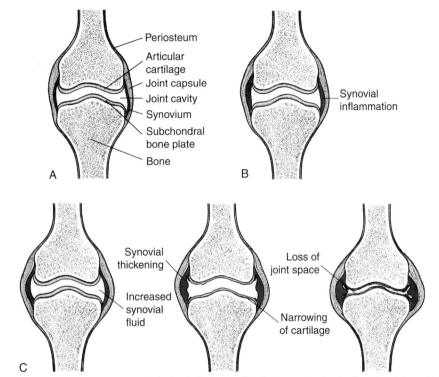

FIGURE 31-1 **A,** Normal diarthrodial joint. **B,** Early synovitis. **C,** Progressive destruction of an inflamed joint.

permanent leg length discrepancy (Iesaka, Kubiak, Bong, et al., 2006) and permanent vision loss if uveitis is present (Foster, 2003).

The history and physical examination are key to diagnosis of chronic inflammatory arthritis. Paradoxically, children whose chief complaint is musculoskeletal pain alone are highly unlikely to have chronic inflammatory arthritis. In a study of 414 children referred to a pediatric rheumatology service over a 2-year period, 111 children were referred for pain as an isolated complaint. Of these 111 children, only one child had a chronic inflammatory disease (McGhee, Burks, Scheckels, et al., 2002).

Another pitfall in the diagnosis of JRA is the erroneous belief that antinuclear antibody (ANA) and/or rheumatoid factor (RF) are sensitive and specific for diagnosis. At least 10% of healthy children have a positive ANA result, with a higher percentage in children who have relatives with autoimmune diseases. Therefore the rate of false-positive ANA results is too high for this test to be a good predictor of JRA. Rheumatoid factor is rarely positive in healthy children but is present in only a small proportion of children with JRA. Therefore the utility of RF as a screening tool is very limited. This test should generally be ordered for prognostic value after a diagnosis of inflammatory arthritis is made clinically (Table 31-2). The primary care provider must remember that childhood arthritis, except for polyarticular RF-positive JRA, is a totally different disease entity with different clinical and diagnostic parameters from the adult form of rheumatoid arthritis (RA).

Types of Onset

Manifestations at the time of onset and throughout the first 6 months of the disease determine classification into one of three major subtypes: pauciarticular, polyarticular, or systemic JRA (see Table 31-2). These subtypes are defined by the number of joints involved and extra-articular features. They are characterized by differences in patterns in severity of joint disease, immunogenetics, age at onset, and sex of the child (Cassidy & Petty, 2005a; Jarvis, 2002). JRA typically manifests exacerbations or "flares" followed by periods of improvement. Exacerbations may occur during episodes of acute illness or stress. The frequency and duration of flares are unpredictable but are easily recognized and should be rapidly treated. Children, especially those with systemic JRA, may also experience constitutional symptoms, such as fever, anorexia, weight loss, growth failure, and fatigue.

Pauciarticular JRA. Almost 60% of children with JRA have the mildest form, pauciarticular JRA, which involves four or fewer joints during the first 6 months of the disease. In this type of JRA, the peak age of onset is between 1 and 2 years of age, and the female:male ratio is 5:1. The most commonly affected joints are the knee, ankle, and elbow (Petty & Cassidy, 2005a). Often only one joint, typically the knee, is involved. A classic presentation of pauciarticular disease is a toddler with a limp, no complaints of pain, and a large knee effusion with a flexion contracture on examination. Physical findings may also include thigh and calf atrophy of the involved side and a leg length discrepancy. Uveitis is a major complication in this group, especially in those who are ANA positive, and it is imperative that the child see a pediatric ophthalmologist at onset and at designated periodic intervals (see Associated Problems). Children with pauciarticular onset may continue to have a pauciarticular course or a polyarticular course may develop any time after the first 6 months (Petty & Cassidy, 2005a).

Polyarticular JRA. Approximately 30% of children with JRA have five or more affected joints (polyarticular onset) during the

TABLE 31-2

Characteristics of Chronic Arthritis in Children by Type of Onset

Characteristic	Polyarthritis	Oligoarthritis (Pauciarticular Disease)	Systemic Disease
Percent of cases	30	60	10
Number of joints involved	≥5	≤4	Variable
Age at onset	Throughout childhood; peak at 1-3 yr	Early childhood; peak at 1-2 yr	Throughout childhood; no peak
Sex ratio (F/M)	3:1	5:1	1:1
Systemic involvement	Systemic disease generally mild; possible unremitting articular involvement	Systemic disease absent; major cause of morbidity is uveitis	Systemic disease often self-limited; arthritis chronic and destructive in 50% of individuals
Occurrence of chronic uveitis	5%	5%-15%	Rare
Frequency of seropositivity			
Rheumatoid factors	10% (increases with age)	Rare	Rare
Antinuclear antibodies	40%-50%	75%-85%*	10%
Prognosis	Guarded to moderately good	Excellent except for eyesight	Moderate to poor

From Cassidy J.T., Petty, R.E., Lindsley, C. B., et al. (Eds.). (2005). *Textbook of Pediatric Rheumatology* (5th ed.). Philadelphia: Elsevier.
*In girls with uveitis.

first 6 months of the disease. RF is rarely positive in JRA in general and is present in only approximately 10% of the children with this type of arthritis. Those in the small subgroup with polyarticular JRA and RF positivity are more likely to have early onset of erosive arthritis, rheumatoid nodules, and a chronic course persisting into adulthood (Jarvis, 2002; Petty & Cassidy, 2005b). Extra-articular manifestations can include fatigue, low-grade fevers, anemia, osteopenia, mild lymphadenopathy, and rheumatoid nodules. The greatest disability occurs with unremitting neck, jaw, and hip arthritis. Conversely, children with RF-negative arthritis, which is much more common, usually exhibit less aggressive joint destruction but have widespread large and small joint involvement (Oen, Malleson, Cabral, et al., 2003). Laboratory findings in polyarticular JRA include elevated or normal erythrocyte sedimentation rate (ESR), leukocyte count, and platelet count.

Systemic JRA. Systemic JRA (about 10% of all children with JRA) presents with severe systemic involvement that may precede the arthritis by weeks or months. The diagnostic hallmark of this type of arthritis is the fever pattern. The fevers are characterized by daily or twice-daily spiking temperatures higher than 102°F (38.8°C), with a rapid return to normal or below baseline. The fever usually occurs in the late afternoon or evening in conjunction with the classic systemic JRA rash. The rash consists of discrete, small (2 to 6 mm), evanescent (fleeting), salmon-pink, generally circumscribed macular lesions. This rash may become confluent, with larger lesions developing pale centers and pale peripheries. It is seen most commonly on the trunk, extremities, and over pressure areas, but the face, palms, and soles also may be involved. The rash is most prominent during fever spikes and may be visible only after the skin is rubbed or scratched. Stress or a hot bath may also induce the rash (Petty & Cassidy, 2005c). Arthritis may be absent at onset, but arthralgias or myalgias are usually present. Other systemic features include diffuse lymphadenopathy, hepatosplenomegaly, leukocytosis, thrombocytosis, progressive anemia, elevated ESR, elevated C-reactive protein, and increased serum ferritin (Behrens, Beukelman, Gallo, et al., 2008). Normochromic, normocytic anemia of chronic disease also may be present (White, 2003). Other laboratory abnormalities

BOX 31-2

Criteria for the Classification of Spondyloarthropathy

Inflammatory spinal pain
or
Synovitis
- Asymmetric *or*
- Predominantly in the lower limbs and one or more of the following:
  - Buttock pain alternating between right and left gluteal areas
  - Enthesopathy
  - Inflammatory bowel disease
  - Positive family history
  - Psoriasis
  - Sacroiliitis
  - Urethritis, cervicitis, or acute diarrhea within one month before arthritis

Reprinted from Dougados, M., Van Der Linden, S., Juhlin, R., et al. (1991). The European Spondyloarthropathy Study Group preliminary criteria for the classification of spondyloarthropathy. *Arthritis Rheum 34*(10), 1218-1227, with permission of the Wiley-Liss, Inc. a subsidiary of John Wiley & Sons, Inc.

may include elevated D-dimers, hypoalbuminemia, elevated transaminases, elevated aldolase levels, and hypergammaglobulinemia (Behrens et al., 2008; Laxer & Schneider, 2004). Once arthritis develops, joint involvement is usually polyarticular, involving the wrists, carpal bones, knees, ankles, tarsal bones, neck, and any or all other joints. Macrophage activation syndrome (MAS) can develop in children with systemic JRA; MAS is an uncommon but acute complication associated with morbidity and sometimes death (Kelly & Ramanan, 2007).

Juvenile Spondyloarthropathies. Four discrete entities comprise the chronic JSpAs (Box 31-2): seronegative enthesopathy and arthropathy (SEA) syndrome, juvenile ankylosing spondylitis, psoriatic arthritis, and arthritis associated with inflammatory bowel disease (IBD) (see Chapter 30). The JSpAs occur predominantly in males, except for psoriatic arthritis, which has a slightly higher percentage of females. Few studies related to the geographic and ethnic differences in the frequency of JSpAs exist, but a low incidence has been reported in African Americans and Japanese individuals (Cassidy & Petty, 2005b). JSpAs also are known for a more chronic waxing and waning disease course than JRA. A significant distinguishing feature of the JSpAs is the presence of enthesitis, which is absent in children with JRA. Enthesitis is inflammation at tendon and ligament insertion sites into bone. Most commonly these sites are found around the knees and feet (Cassidy & Petty, 2005b). The mechanism for enthesitis is thought to be similar to arthritis except that the inflammation does not occur within a defined joint capsule. Certain forms of reactive arthritis and Reiter syndrome are also considered in the category of SpAs but are not usually chronic and are not discussed in this chapter.

SEA syndrome. SEA (seronegative enthesopathy and arthropathy) syndrome is probably the most common form of JSpA. *Seronegative* refers to ANA-negative and RF-negative, and *arthropathy* refers to the fact that joint pain, not frank arthritis, is all that is required to make the initial diagnosis (Burgos-Vargos, 2002). SEA syndrome typically affects boys who are usually HLA-B27 positive, and there is often a family history of chronic lower back pain, psoriasis, or known SpAs. Enthesitis on examination and the pattern of involved joints are often clues to the diagnosis (Hofer, 2006). SEA syndrome is sometimes the precursor for other forms of JSpAs such as juvenile ankylosing spondylitis (JAS).

Juvenile ankylosing spondylitis. Because the criteria are so strict, true JAS is uncommon in childhood but does affect some older adolescent boys (Gensler & Davis, 2006). Ultimately axial skeleton involvement with sacroiliitis and lumbosacral spine arthritis develop in boys with JAS. This can be quite debilitating and is often best assessed clinically by the modified Schöber test, which measures lower back movement, and radiologically by magnetic resonance imaging (MRI) scan (Puhakka, Jurik, Egund, et al., 2003). True JAS often requires aggressive pharmacotherapy and physical therapy to maintain good range of motion and function of the pelvis, lower back, and lower extremities.

Psoriatic arthritis. Children with psoriasis and arthritis are said to have *juvenile psoriatic arthritis* (PsA). The diagnosis of PsA or probable PsA can be made even in the absence of psoriasis by the presence of arthritis and nail pits, dactylitis, or a strong family history for psoriasis (Stoll & Nigrovic, 2006). Two peaks of onset occur in juvenile PsA. The first occurs in young children who are more likely to be girls with dactylitis, small joint involvement, and ANA positivity. The second peak occurs in older children of either gender with enthesitis and axial joint disease. Uveitis is equally represented in both groups (Stoll, Zurakowski, Nigrovic et al 2006).

Arthritis associated with inflammatory bowel disease. Up to 30% of children with inflammatory bowel disease (IBD)—either Crohn's disease or ulcerative colitis (see Chapter 30)—develop chronic arthritis at some point during their illness. The onset of arthritis may occur before, concurrently with, or after the diagnosis of IBD. A recent study of adults with IBD revealed the prevalence of SpA and ankylosing spondylitis (AS) to be 45.7% and 9.9%, respectively (Turkcapar, Toruner, Soykan, et al., 2006). In a study of children referred to a pediatric gastroenterology clinic for suspected IBD, 24% met criteria for JSpA and all had diagnoses of IBD, indeterminate colitis, or lymphoid nodular hyperplasia (Conti, Borrelli, Anania, et al., 2005). There is an association with the inflammation of the bowels and inflammation of joints in the SpAs, and several immune-based hypotheses connecting the gut

and the joints have been proposed (Baeten, DeKeyser, Mielants, et al., 2002). The arthritis of IBD often begins peripherally but may eventually affect the axial skeleton. Moreover, the bowel disease may eventually become quiescent, but an aggressive form of axial arthritis not unlike that of JAS may develop later.

Treatment

Management of chronic arthritis in childhood is most successful with early diagnosis and institution of early aggressive treatment with targeted interventions. The cornerstones of treatment are antiinflammatory and disease-modifying medication, with newer, more effective treatments recently emerging. Interdisciplinary, family-centered treatment interventions incorporate the team approach and include the family and child, pediatric rheumatologist, advanced practice nurse, clinic nurse, primary care provider, physical therapist, occupational therapist, and social worker. Consultations with the ophthalmologist, orthopedist, psychologist, dietitian, orthodontist, interventional radiologist, and other pediatric specialists are sought as indicated.

Treatment

Goals of Treatment
- Induce disease remission
- Decrease systemic and joint inflammation
- Prevent disease complications and disability
- Promote maximal growth and development
- Promote psychosocial well-being of child and family

Treatment Plan
- Pharmacologic therapy
  - Nonsteroidal antiinflammatory drugs (NSAIDs)
  - Disease modifying antirheumatic drugs (DMARDs)
  - Corticosteroids
  - Biologic response modifiers
- Exercise and therapy: aerobic, range of motion, and stretching exercise program
- Physical therapy, occupational therapy, splints, orthotics, adaptive devices, and supportive footwear
- Nutritional counseling
- Social support
- Surgery

Key: *IV,* intravenous; *PO,* by mouth; *SQ,* subcutaneous.

Pharmacologic Therapy

Treatment of chronic arthritis in childhood has made great strides in the past half-century. At one time, aspirin was the only antiinflammatory medication used and many children with chronic arthritis eventually required wheelchairs or they were blinded by uveitis. The pace of development of new therapies has increased most dramatically in the past 10 years.

In general, JRA and the JSpAs are treated similarly. Specific pharmacologic agents used to treat JRA and the JSpAs are identified in Table 31-3. Nonsteroidal anti-inflammatory drugs (NSAIDs) remain one of the cornerstones of treatment for the childhood chronic arthritides (Weiss & Ilowite, 2007); naproxen is the most commonly used (Brunner, Kim, Ballinger, et al., 2001). There may be a trend among pediatric rheumatologists toward less frequent use of NSAIDs in

TABLE 31-3

Pharmacologic Therapy for Juvenile Rheumatoid Arthritis

Drug	Trade Name	Dosing	Side Effects	Laboratory Monitors
I. NONSTEROIDAL ANTIINFLAMMATORY DRUGS (NSAIDs)*				
Naproxen sodium[†]	Anaprox Naprosyn Aleve (OTC)	15 mg/kg/day bid	*For all NSAIDs:* abdominal pain, dizziness, drowsiness, fluid retention, gastric ulcers and bleeding, greater susceptibility to bruising or bleeding, heartburn, indigestion, lightheadedness, nausea, rash, reduction in kidney function, anemia, increase in liver enzymes, behavioral changes. *For naproxen and some others:* pseudoporphyria with sun exposure	CBC with differential, UA, BUN, creatinine, and LFTs initially, at 6 wk then every 3-6 mo.
Ibuprofen[†]	Advil (OTC) Motrin IB (OTC) Nuprin (OTC) Motrin (Rx)	30-40 mg/kg/day tid		
Indomethacin[†]	Indocin Indocin SR	1-2 mg/kg/day tid or qid 75 mg daily or bid	*For Indomethacin:* depression, severe headaches, "spaced-out" feeling	
Tolmetin sodium	Tolectin	30 mg/kg/day tid Maximum 1800 mg/day		
Nabumetone[‡]	Relafen	500 or 750 mg po bid		
Oxaprozin	Daypro	22-32 kg: 600 mg daily 32-54 kg: 900 mg daily > 55 kg: 1,200 mg daily		
Sulindac[‡]	Clinoril	2-6 mg/kg/day bid Maximum 400 mg/day		
Meloxicam[†]	Mobic	0.125 mg/kg/day		
COX-2 Inhibitor				
Celecoxib	Celebrex	≥ 10 kg to ≤25 kg: 50 mg bid > 25 kg: 100 mg bid	Same as traditional NSAIDs, but less likely to cause gastric ulcers, bleeding, and bruising *Cautions:* sensitivity to sulfonamides or allergies to aspirin or other NSAIDs	
II. DISEASE MODIFYING ANTIRHEUMATIC DRUGS (DMARDs)				
Methotrexate (MTX)	Rheumatrex Trexall	10-15 mg/m²/dose or 1 mg/kg/dose weekly Up to 40 mg subcutaneously or orally	Nausea, vomiting, mouth sores, increased liver enzymes, myelosuppression, hair loss *Cautions:* abnormal blood count, liver or lung disease, active infection or fever; NO alcohol; causes birth defects if taken during pregnancy	CBC with differential and LFTs every month ×6, then every 2 mo
Sulfasalazine	Azulfidine Azulfidine EN-Tabs	30-50 mg/kg/day bid Maximum 2 g/day	Stomach upset, diarrhea, dizziness, headache, light sensitivity, itching, rash, loss of appetite, nausea, vomiting, increased liver enzymes, lowered blood count *Cautions:* allergy to sulfa or aspirin; kidney, liver, or blood disease; avoid prolonged sun exposure; take with food; do not take with Maalox or Mylanta-type antacids	

From Taketomo, C., Hodding, J.H., & Kraus, D.M. (2006). *Pediatric Dosing Handbook* (13th ed.). Hudson, OH: Lexi-Comp.

*Pediatric dose of NSAIDs based on mg/kg should not exceed adult dose. Do not take NSAIDs with other OTC NSAIDs. Always take NSAIDs with food. Remind parents that NSAIDs are mainly to treat chronic inflammation and are to be continued as prescribed even if child does not complain of pain.

[†]Available as suspension.

[‡]Drugs not listed as mg/kg are actual adult doses; pediatric doses are estimated based on a 70-kg adult.

[§]Taken q AM or bid.

‖More effective and more likely to caused increased side effects when same total daily dose is divided throughout the day.

[¶]No FDA approved doses for children.

Key: *BP,* blood pressure; *BUN,* blood urea nitrogen; *CBC,* complete blood count; *LFTs,* liver function tests; *SQ,* subcutaneously; *TB,* tuberculosis; *UA,* urinalysis.

TABLE 31-3

Pharmacologic Therapy for Juvenile Rheumatoid Arthritis—cont'd

Drug	Trade Name	Dosing	Side Effects	Laboratory Monitors
III. CORTICOSTEROIDS				
Prednisolone§‖	Prelone† Pediapred† Orapred†	0.5-2 mg/kg/day varies with disease Used mostly for sJRA	Indigestion, weight gain, increased appetite, mood changes, insomnia *With chronic therapy:* Cushingoid features, weight gain, striae, osteoporosis, cataracts, glaucoma, elevated blood glucose, immunosuppression *Cautions:* active infection, hypertension, osteoporosis	CBC with differential, BP every month, yearly ocular examinations
Prednisone§‖	Deltasone Orasone			
IV. BIOLOGIC RESPONSE MODIFIERS				
Etanercept	Enbrel	0.8 mg/kg/wk as single SQ injection or divided twice weekly Maximum 50 mg per week	Possible redness, itching, or swelling at injection site for SQ; possible infusion reactions for IV Increased susceptibility to infections *Cautions:* hold drug if active infection, no live-virus vaccines *For TNF inhibitors:* rare lupus-like syndrome, neurologic syndromes, cytopenias	*For TNF inhibitors:* Obtain baseline TB skin test and chest x-ray to rule out TB.
Adalimumab	Humira	SQ every other wk. 15 to <30 kg: 20 mg ≥ 30 kg: 40 mg		
Infliximab	Remicade	IV infusion week 0, 2, 6; then every 4-8 wk¶		
Abatacept	Orencia	IV at 0, 2, 4 weeks, then every 4 wk < 75 kg: 10 mg/kg 75-100 kg: 750 mg > 100 kg: 1000 mg		

favor of intra-articular corticosteroids and early aggressive treatment (Cron, Sharma, & Sherry, 1999; Ravelli & Martini, 2007).

Intra-articular corticosteroids are the second most common form of treatment for pauciarticular JRA (Petty & Cassidy, 2005a); triamcinolone hexacetonide is considered the most effective (Eberhard, Sison, Gottlieb et al. 2004) because of its longer duration of action and excellent safety profile (Neidel, Boehnke, & Kuster, 2002). The most common use of intra-articular steroids is in pauciarticular JRA, although multiple joints may be injected with the child under sedation or general anesthesia. The use of real-time imaging, such as ultrasound, during injection is becoming more common (DeSmet, 2004).

Slow-acting antirheumatic drugs (SAARDs) or disease-modifying antirheumatic drugs (DMARDs) are more aggressive treatment than NSAIDs and may be used either initially or after NSAID failure. The most commonly used DMARD for SEA syndrome is sulfasalazine (Cron et al., 1999; Weiss & Ilowite, 2007). Methotrexate is the most common DMARD for all forms of JRA (Brunner et al., 2001; Cron et al., 1999) based on its high efficacy-to-side effect profile in children (Weiss & Ilowite, 2007) and is commonly used in combination with other agents. Methotrexate is also effective for uveitis resistant to topical steroids (Foeldvari & Wierk, 2005). Methotrexate may be given orally or subcutaneously; the latter is associated with better absorption and fewer gastrointestinal (GI) side effects (Weiss & Ilowite, 2007). DMARDs such as gold and D-penicillamine are rarely, if ever, used to treat chronic childhood arthritis (Weiss & Ilowite).

For the sickest children, particularly those with systemic-onset JRA, systemic glucocorticoids are often necessary to control disease activity. The steroids are usually given as daily oral doses and as weekly to monthly IV boluses. Unfortunately, systemic corticosteroids are

associated with many adverse effects, including striae, cushingoid features, hirsutism, weight gain, reduced growth velocity, diabetes, glaucoma, cataracts, and osteopenia (Laxer, 2005). More aggressive therapy may be necessary to limit steroid usage to the shortest possible duration. Immunosuppressive medications such as cyclosporine (Ruperto, Ravelli, Castell et al., 2006) and cytotoxic agents such as cyclophosphamide (Chen, Chen, Yeh et al., 2004) have been effective for some individuals. However, these medicines may be associated with significant short-term and long-term complications, such as opportunistic infections, infertility, mutagenesis, and oncogenesis.

The introduction of biologic response modifiers, which inhibit cytokines or cellular immune responses, has been revolutionary for treatment of JRA and JSpA. These medications generally have been used after failure of older, less expensive therapies, but earlier use is likely to become more common. A growing number of biologic medications are available for adults with RA. To date, three biologic medications have been approved for JRA (or JIA) in the United States—etanercept (Enbrel), adalimumab (Humira), and abatacept (Orencia). Etanercept and adalimumab, administered by subcutaneous injection, inhibit TNF-α, a potent pro-inflammatory cytokine. Etanercept was the first available biologic agent for JRA and has been shown to be safe and effective in the treatment of polyarticular JRA unresponsive to methotrexate (Lovell, Reiff, Ilowite et al., 2008a). Adalimumab recently received an FDA indication for treatment of JRA (Lovell, Ruperto, Goodman et al., 2008b). The other available TNF-α inhibitor approved for adults with RA, infliximab (Remicade, given intravenously) has been tested in children in controlled trials (Ruperto, Lovell, Cuttica et al., 2007) and has been used successfully in clinical practice for JRA (Ravelli & Martini, 2007). Abatacept, an inhibitor of lymphocyte activation by co-stimulatory blockade, is FDA approved for children 6 years and older with severe polyarticular JRA (Bristol-Myers Squibb, 2008; Ruperto et al., 2007). Anakinra (Kineret), an IL-1 receptor antagonist, has been useful in the treatment of systemic JRA in small, open, clinical trials (Pascual, Allantaz, Arce, et al., 2005; Lequerré, Quatier, Rosellini, et al., 2008) but is not FDA approved for use in children. Randomized, blinded, placebo-controlled trials are in progress for rilonacept (Arcalyst), a fusion protein of human IL-1 receptor extracellular domain with human IgG1 Fc domain, and of tocilizumab, a humanized monoclonal antibody against IL-6 receptor (Yokota, Imagawa, Mori, et al., 2008) for treatment of systemic JRA. Newer biologic response modifiers such as rituximab (Rituxan, a cytotoxic antibody against B lymphocytes) have also been used to treat JRA (Kuek, Hazleman, Gaston, et al., 2006) but also lack FDA approval for children.

Thalidomide has been explored as a therapy for steroid-dependent JRA with some success (Lehman, Schechter, Sundel, et al., 2004). Teratogenicity and neurotoxicity are some limiting factors for its use, although congeners with fewer side effects may be developed. Some very ill children with JRA in whom other treatments have failed have received stem cell transplantation (Brinkman, deKleer, ten Cate et al., 2007). Because the number of such children has been small, the long-term efficacy, side effects, and mortality rate of this treatment have not been determined.

Exercise and Therapy

Studies have shown that children and adolescents with JRA have impaired aerobic and anaerobic exercise capacity (Lelieveld, van Brussel, Takken et al., 2007; van Brussel, Lelieveld, van der Net, et al., 2007). Existing evidence does demonstrate that individualized conditioning programs, such as aerobic exercise and aquatic training, have both physical and psychological benefits. These programs have the potential to increase aerobic capacity, muscular strength, endurance, and stamina for daily activities without aggravating joint disease (Epps, Ginnelly, Utley, et al., 2005; Klepper, 2007; Singh-Grewal, Schneiderman-Walker, Wright, et al., 2007).

Physical and occupational therapy goals include the following: (1) increasing range of motion, endurance, strength, and conditioning; (2) teaching principles of joint protection and energy conservation; (3) using appropriate splints; (4) recommending modalities and assistive devices; and (5) improving performance of activities of daily living (Athreya & Lindsley, 2005; Cakmak & Bolukbas, 2005). Today, with early, advanced, aggressive pharmacotherapy, many children with arthritis may not require physical therapy or splints. Unfortunately, if treatment is delayed for a child with persistently swollen joints, the child may hold the joints in a position of comfort, usually flexion. This position contributes to a flexion contracture with decreased joint mobility, and causes joint malalignment. Such a child may require therapy and splinting to reduce residual limitations after the institution of medications.

Occupational therapists usually evaluate and fabricate splints for the upper extremities, whereas physical therapists construct splints for the lower extremities, including foot orthotics. Splints can be useful adjuncts to therapy to regain motion in an involved joint or to rest a joint experiencing a disease flare. Three categories of splints are used: resting splints, corrective splints, and functional splints (Cakmak & Bolukbas, 2005). Resting splints are used during active disease. Night resting splints place the wrist in a cock-up position (i.e., 20 degrees of wrist extension) and are the most common. Corrective splints include both serial casting and dynamic splints. Functional splints include supportive wrist splints

---

> **BOX 31-3**
>
> ## Children with Chronic Arthritis: Presurgical Considerations
>
> - Stop NSAID therapy 4 to 7 days before surgery (or at the surgeon's discretion) to prevent excessive bleeding.
> - With long-term steroid use, give stress dose of corticosteroids PO/IV to prevent adrenal insufficiency.
> - Consult pediatric anesthesiologist for airway considerations. With neck or TMJ disease, obtain cervical and TMJ imaging studies.
> - Give prophylactic antibiotics for total joint replacements or if child is taking corticosteroids.
> - Monitor a child's preoperative CBC and platelet count.

Key: *CBC*, complete blood count; *IV*, intravenously; *NSAID*, nonsteroidal antiinflammatory drug; *PO*, by mouth; *TMJ*, temporomandibular joint.

---

that can be worn during the day, ankle-foot orthoses, molded shoe inserts, and heel cups (Cakmak & Bolukbas).

Nutritional Counseling

Nutritional counseling is recommended particularly for children who are underweight, overweight, systemically ill, or receiving long-term steroid therapy. Nutritional education and dietary changes are necessary to minimize weight gain associated with long-term treatment with corticosteroids (see Primary Care Management).

Social Support

The chronicity and unpredictability of childhood arthritis and the necessary lifestyle changes lead to many situations in which psychological support is helpful. Counseling, support groups, and peer activities such as camps for children with chronic diseases are helpful adjuncts to care.

Surgery

Orthopedic surgery plays a very limited but important role in correcting joint deformities or replacing joints entirely (Cassidy & Petty, 2005a). Arthroscopy is rarely performed for synovial biopsy or synovectomy. Synovectomy may be beneficial in select cases for pain relief and to improve range of motion but does not alter the long-term outcome (Cassidy, 2005). For a child with functional impairment or secondary mechanical problems, soft tissue releases, osteotomies, posterior capsulotomy, and tendon lengthening may be performed (Iesaka et al., 2006). Children with micrognathia (small, receded jaw) may profit from a combined orthodontic and surgical approach to temporomandibular disease.

Total joint replacements are beneficial to those with marked disability and pain secondary to joint destruction (Kitsoulis, Siamopoulou, Beris, et al., 2006a). Total hip and knee replacements usually result in major improvements in functional ability (Kitsoulis, Stafilas, Siamopoulou, et al., 2006b; Palmer, Mulhall, Thompson, et al., 2005). As a child approaches adulthood and reaches bone maturity, reconstructive surgery plays a more vital role. Preoperative considerations for joint surgery and other surgical procedures are listed in Box 31-3.

Complementary and Alternative Therapies

Complementary and alternative medicine (CAM) is often used because of fear of side effects from conventional medications and the perception that the child's condition is not improving with such therapy (Feldman et al., 2004). Studies reveal that 33.9% to 92% of parents of children with rheumatic diseases report giving treatments, products, or therapies not prescribed by a physician (Feldman et al., 2004; Hagen et al., 2003; Rouster-Stevens et al, 2008). Commonly used products include vitamins, minerals, copper bracelets, herbal remedies, and fish oil; services are provided by chiropractors, homeopaths, manual healers, and other practitioners (Hagen et al.). Other interventions used include music, massage, spiritual healing and support groups (Rouster-Stevens et al.). Because parents are often reluctant to divulge their usage of CAM to the primary care provider, it is important to create an accepting environment where frustrations with conventional treatment can be aired and unproven remedies openly discussed. Primary care providers can help families differentiate between harmless and potentially harmful interventions and help them evaluate the claimed efficacy of unconventional remedies (Sibinga et al. 2004). Very few controlled clinical trials for alternative therapies have been done with children; therefore the risks and benefits are unknown (Hagen et al., 2003). Potential risks include interaction with prescribed medications, adverse side effects, and strain on the provider-client relationship (Kemper & O'Connor, 2004). Warn parents to be wary of any product that is labeled as a "cure" and to discuss any additional treatments with the rheumatology team.

Cognitive behavioral therapy may be used to reduce stress, pain, and psychological disability (Simon et al., 2002). Anecdotal reports from families reveal that some children benefit from massage, relaxation techniques, visual imagery, and exercise such as tai chi or yoga. A study of 13 children with JRA showed significant pain reduction after an 8-week program of cognitive behavioral therapy. The investigators taught the children progressive relaxation, meditative breathing, and guided imagery (Walco, Varni & Ilowite, 1992). Benefits include improved coping, pain control, and self-confidence. Moreover, the results were sustained 12 months after the intervention.

Anticipated Advances in Diagnosis and Treatment

JRA and JSpAs are complex disorders that are influenced by both genetic predisposition and environment. Abundant evidence indicates that both innate immunity (primitive inflammatory responses) and adaptive immunity (antigen presentation, recognition by specific receptors on T and B cells, and specific response) are involved (Malmström, Trollmo, & Klareskog, 2004). Most current therapies, including biologic response modifiers, are directed toward relatively late events in the pathogenesis of arthritis. Although cytokines are likely to remain targets of arthritis treatment for many years (McInnes & Liew, 2005), basic science progress in other areas such as receptor-mediated cell interaction, microenvironment, vascular biology, and gene regulation will allow development of treatments more tailored to early and critical events. It seems likely that in the future, complete remission of JRA off medications may be an attainable goal for many affected children.

Associated Problems of Juvenile Rheumatoid Arthritis and Treatment

Uveitis

Uveitis (i.e., iridocyclitis) is one of the most devastating complications associated with JRA and remains one of the major causes of visual impairment in children (Foster, 2003). Uveitis of JRA is a chronic, anterior nongranulomatous inflammation that primarily affects the iris and ciliary body (Petty & Cassidy, 2005a). Persistent uveitis can lead to multiple ocular complications, such as glaucoma, cataracts, band keratopathy, posterior synechiae, and loss of vision (Jarvis, 2002). Risk factors associated with developing uveitis include female gender, young age, ANA positivity, and pauciarticular onset (Heiligenhaus, Niewerth, Ganser, et al., 2007b). Uveitis is generally *asymptomatic;* therefore regular screening with a slit-lamp examination, preferably by a pediatric ophthalmologist, is required for early detection (see Table 31-4). When uveitis is symptomatic, the child may experience ocular pain and redness, change in vision, photophobia, and headache. The pattern of remissions and exacerbations of uveitis does not parallel articular disease (Kotaniemi, Savolainen, Karma et al., 2003).

Associated Problems of Juvenile Rheumatoid Arthritis and Treatment

- Uveitis
- Skeletal and growth abnormalities
  - Systemic growth delay
  - Local growth disturbances: overgrowth or undergrowth
    - Leg-length discrepancy
    - Shortened limb, brachydactyly
    - TMJ, micrognathia, mandibular undergrowth, dental malocclusion
  - Cervical spine fusion C2-C3
  - Atlantoaxial subluxation or instability
  - Scoliosis
  - Hip limitations, erosions, or protrusions
  - Joint contractures
  - Feet: valgus of hindfoot and/or hallux valgus
  - Gait disturbances
- Anemia of chronic disease
- Systemic JRA
  - Hepatosplenomegaly
  - Lymphadenopathy
  - Pericarditis
  - Pleuritis
  - Nutritional problems and/or protein-energy malnutrition

The estimated prevalence of uveitis in children with chronic arthritis differs greatly across a range of studies (Kotaniemi et al., 2003). Recent studies report a prevalence of 12% to 20.1% (Grassi, Corona, Casellato, et al., 2007; Heiligenhaus et al., 2007a, b). Early, aggressive treatment of the uveitis with topical corticosteroid drops with or without a mydriatic drug has been effective in preserving the vision of children without advanced disease (Petty & Cassidy, 2005a). Low-dose weekly methotrexate is considered the drug of choice for treating uveitis resistant to topical corticosteroids (Foeldvari & Wierk, 2005). Cataracts and glaucoma are associated with topical corticosteroid drops, and therefore oral or subcutaneous methotrexate is being used more frequently and earlier in the course of uveitis therapy (Heiligenhaus et al., 2007b). Over the past few years, infliximab and etanercept have been used effectively for treatment-resistant uveitis, although infliximab may be more effective than etanercept (Foeldvari, Nielsen, Kümmerle-Deschner, et al., 2007; Tynjälä, Lindahl, Pittonkanen, et al., 2007). Adalimumab has also recently been shown to treat uveitis effectively (Biester, Deuter, Haefner, et al., 2007).

Children with JSpA may develop a *symptomatic* iritis manifested by acute onset of eye pain, redness, and photophobia. The iritis is typically unilateral, recurrent, and frequently without residua (Heiligenhaus et al., 2007a, b). With acute iritis, ophthalmology evaluation and treatment are required only when the eye symptoms are present. Therefore the child with JSpA does not need more than routine eye screening.

Skeletal and Growth Abnormalities

Generalized or local growth disturbances develop in up to 30% of children with chronic arthritis (Cassidy & Petty, 2005a; White, 2003). Disease severity is a crucial factor in the association among skeletal abnormalities, bone mineralization, and impaired bone formation (Burnham & Leonard, 2004). Each subgroup of JRA affects growth differently. Children with systemic onset and those requiring long-term steroid therapy experience growth failure more than children with the other types of onset and therapy (Petty & Cassidy, 2005c). Factors contributing to short stature and growth abnormalities are largely a result of poor disease control, including undertreatment, side effects of corticosteroids, poor nutritional status, temporomandibular joint (TMJ) disease, vertebral fractures, and hip and knee contractures (Packham & Hall, 2002a).

Chronic hyperemia of inflammation in a joint may accelerate maturation of the epiphyseal plates, resulting in skeletal overgrowth of the affected extremity (Prieur, 2004). This process is characteristically seen in children with early-onset pauciarticular disease who have unilateral knee involvement, bony enlargement of the medial femoral condyle, and valgus deformity (Bowyer, Roettcher, Higgins et al., 2003; Skyttä, Savolainen, Kautiainen, et al., 2005). Eventually, limb shortening may result in chronic arthritis when premature fusion of the epiphyseal growth plates occurs in the affected extremity (Cassidy & Petty, 2005a).

TMJ involvement may lead to growth aberrations of the mandible and destruction of the condyle of the mandible, causing micrognathia, which has dental, nutritional, hygienic, speech, and cosmetic consequences. With destructive TMJ disease, combined orthodontic and reconstructive surgery may improve function, decrease pain, and improve appearance (Billiau, Hu, Verdonch et al., 2007) Thus early treatment with adequate therapy, including the use of intra-articular injections of the TMJ, is imperative to prevent complication (Arabshahi, DeWitt, Cahill, et al., 2005).

Characteristic abnormalities of the cervical spine in systemic or polyarticular disease include apophyseal joint space narrowing, irregularity and undergrowth of the vertebral bodies, fusion (especially at C2-C3), and atlantoaxial subluxation or instability leading to impingement on the spinal cord and brainstem (Cassidy & Petty, 2005a; Prieur, 2004). Stiffness and pain of the cervical spine with rapid loss of extension and rotation are common early findings in polyarticular JRA (Laiho, Savolainen, Kautiainen, et al., 2002). Children with chronic arthritis have structural scoliosis more often than unaffected children because of the postural curves associated with asymmetrical involvement of the lower limb joints causing pelvic tilting (Witt & Swann, 2004).

Hip pathology occurs in 30% to 50% of children with chronic arthritis. It is almost always bilateral and usually is associated with polyarticular arthritis. These children experience limitation of full flexion, abduction, and rotation (Prieur, 2004). Over time, anatomic changes in the hip as a result of persistent inflammation may include femoral head overgrowth, decreased development of the femoral neck, and acetabular modifications with erosions or protrusions (Spencer & Bernstein, 2002). A compensatory lumbar lordosis can occur with a hip contracture. Flexion contractures of the knees are common. Valgus of the knee with compensatory valgus deformity of the hindfoot and varus of the forefoot can develop in children with arthritis of the knee joint (Prieur, 2004). Subtalar joint involvement often results in a valgus deformity or, rarely, in a varus deformity.

Anemia of Chronic Disease

The anemia most often seen in JRA is a result of the anemia of chronic disease and is more severe in systemic JRA. Its pathogenesis is unclear, but its severity correlates with underlying disease activity and inflammation. The anemia of systemic JRA usually presents with low iron and transferrin levels, as well as with an elevated serum ferritin level that does not typically respond to iron supplementation (White, 2003). The anemia of chronic disease is normocytic and may be related to abnormal levels of IL-6 and hepcidin (Ganz, 2006). In children with poor nutrition or NSAID-induced GI blood loss, however, iron deficiency anemia may also develop, resulting in microcytosis and hypochromia (Ashorn, Verronen, Ruuska, et al., 2003).

Systemic Disease

Systemic JRA can include significant extra-articular manifestations, including hepatosplenomegaly, lymphadenopathy, pericarditis, pleuritis, or other serositis (Laxer & Schneider, 2004). Nutritional problems, in particular protein-energy malnutrition, are common in systemic JRA.

Prognosis

The prognosis for children with chronic arthritis depends on the disease type and course, symmetry of joint involvement, early hip joint involvement, duration of ESR elevation, and RF positivity (Adib, Silman, & Thomson, 2005). A recent study suggests that children with JSpA and JRA have a relatively favorable prognosis, with only half requiring rheumatology care in adulthood (Minden, Niewerth, Listing, et al., 2002). Different criteria for classification and remission, in addition to a lack of uniform methods to assess outcome, make a comparison of studies difficult (Adib et al., 2005; Cassidy & Petty, 2005a). About 60% of children with chronic arthritis reach adulthood with no active synovitis or functional limitation (Packham & Hall, 2002a). Before the use of biologic agents, more than 25% of those with polyarticular JRA and nearly half of the children with systemic JRA had functional limitations. After 5 years of follow-up, two thirds of children in those subsets had radiographically evident joint space damage (Bowyer et al., 2003). Future studies are expected to show a more favorable prognosis because of the current trend toward early, aggressive treatment and the availability of newer, targeted biologic agents.

Children with pauciarticular arthritis have a good prognosis for articular disease. In a long-term follow-up study 10 years after disease onset, 47% of children were in remission and 85% had no functional limitations (Oen, Malleson, Cabral, et al., 2002). One study of long-term outcome and prognosis of children with pauciarticular disease identified two to four affected joints, upper limb involvement, and high ESR as predictors for poor outcome (Guillaume, Prieur, Coste, et al., 2000). The prognosis with regard to uveitis is less favorable, however, ranging from remission without sequelae to severe visual loss (Sherry, Mellins, Sandborg, et al., 2004).

Children with a polyarticular course have a fair to poor prognosis for articular disease. Adolescents presenting with a positive RF level follow a course similar to those with adult-onset RA with development of persistent erosive joint disease (Oen et al., 2002). Children with systemic disease can have a monocyclic course with remission, a polycyclic course with exacerbations of systemic disease activity, or a course of persistent polyarticular arthritis without systemic features (Singh-Grewal, Schneider, Bayer, et al., 2006). A long-term follow-up study of individuals in this subset revealed that 75% had undergone joint replacement and 62.5% had Health Assessment Questionnaire scores in the severe disability range (Packham & Hall, 2002a). The prognosis for those with JSpAs is just as variable depending on onset type, course, and complications. Children with sacroiliitis, reduced spinal flexion, ankle and hip arthritis in the first 6 months, the presence of HLA-DRB1*08, and persistently elevated ESR are more likely to have unfavorable physical outcomes (Flatø, Hoffmann-Vold, Reiff, et, al., 2006).

PRIMARY CARE MANAGEMENT

Health Care Maintenance

Growth and Development

Linear growth may be retarded or delayed during periods of active disease, resulting in shorter stature in children with chronic arthritis than in healthy children (Packham & Hall, 2002a). Therefore monitoring of height and weight via the National Center for Health Statistics (NCHS) growth chart is important. Some children have growth abnormalities that persist into adulthood. Children with chronic arthritis often have osteopenia (Lien, Selvaag, Flatø, et al., 2005) and are recognized by the National Institutes of Health to be at risk for osteoporosis (National Institute of Arthritis and Musculoskeletal and Skin Diseases, 2005). Factors contributing to the development of low bone mineral density include longer duration of disease, higher number of active and mobility restricted joints, high ESRs, glucocorticoid use, and decreased weight-bearing activities (Celiker, Bal, Bakkaloğlu, et al., 2003). One study has shown that calcium supplementation in children with JRA results in a small but statistically significant increase in total body bone mineral density (Lovell, Glass, Ranz, et al., 2006). Therefore assessment and recommendation of adequate calcium and vitamin D intake by foods, milk, and/or supplementation is crucial. Children with arthritis have higher calcium needs than healthy children, and children receiving long-term steroid treatment have an even higher requirement (up to 1800 mg calcium per day). Excessive weight gain also may occur as a result of decreased activity, depression, poor nutrition, or corticosteroid usage.

Children with chronic arthritis generally do not have any cognitive or language delay; however they may have a delay in fine and gross motor skills. Fine motor skills are less likely to be delayed if the young child is provided with toys and activities that encourage hand manipulation. Limited mobility and decreased opportunities to actively interact with their peer group place the child at a risk for both motor and social delays. In these areas, the child's rheumatology team, occupational therapist, and physical therapist can be valuable resources for primary care providers (Athreya & Lindsley, 2005).

The acquisition of independence and self-care skills may be delayed in children with JRA. Certain skills, such as transition from a bottle to a cup or toilet training, should be postponed during periods of diagnosis or of active disease. Children with severe JRA often fall behind in acquiring hygiene, toileting, dressing, feeding, and handwriting skills. Regression in performance of these skills is common during acute illness and may be sustained during remissions as a result of lowered parental expectations and continued reinforcement of a child's dependent behaviors. Adaptive clothing (e.g., shoes with Velcro closures) and dressing aids can facilitate activities of daily living. Every office visit can be an opportunity for discussion about and promotion of independence in a child with arthritis. Educational materials are available for parents of children with arthritis regarding growth and development (see Resources). Moreover, developmentally appropriate functional assessment and quality of life (QoL) measures for children with arthritis exist. These include the following standard and validated tools: the Childhood Health Assessment Questionnaire (CHAQ), the Juvenile Arthritis Functional Assessment Scale (JAFAS) and Report (JAFAR), and the Juvenile Arthritis Self-Report Index (JASI) (Duffy, 2005).

Diet

Nutritional problems are common in JRA. Factors contributing to the occurrence of these problems include increased inflammatory activity (i.e., hypercatabolism in the systemic subgroup), anorexia, GI side effects of medication, physical limitations, depression, poor food choices, and limited movement of the TMJs (Cleary, Lancaster, Annan, et al., 2004). In addition, increased weight gain can occur with corticosteroid use as a result of increased appetite and fluid retention.

Alternative diets and dietary supplements have long been popular with people with rheumatic disease. The most common unconventional dietary remedies for arthritis are avoiding nightshade vegetables (e.g., potatoes and eggplant) and acidic foods (e.g., tomatoes), increasing dietary omega-3 fatty acids (found in fish), fasting, herbal remedies, and megavitamin therapy (Henderson, 2002). Although omega-3 fatty acids have been shown to cause improvement in adult RA (Goldberg & Katz, 2007), neither this nor any other specific dietary intervention has been proven to ameliorate the symptoms of arthritis in children. Given the current knowledge of childhood arthritis and diet, educating families about proper nutrition for a growing child with a chronic condition and evaluating potentially harmful dietary manipulations, especially those involving nutrient restrictions, are important responsibilities of the primary care provider. Nutritional education and referral to a dietitian may be indicated.

Safety

Education about medication safety is an important responsibility of the primary care provider. All medications must be kept in childproof containers out of reach of young children, which is especially important when older children assume responsibility for self-care. Because of their limited grip strength, special grippers may be used to open containers. Children taking long-term immunosuppressive drugs are encouraged to wear Medic-Alert bracelets or necklaces. Photosensitive skin reactions may occur with several JRA medications, including naproxen and other NSAIDs, methotrexate, sulfasalazine (Azulfidine), and hydroxychloroquine (Plaquenil). Therefore, hypoallergenic sunblock lotion with a minimum sun protection factor (SPF) of 45 should be used routinely on exposed skin.

TABLE 31-4

Ophthalmologic Screening Schedule

JRA Subtype at Onset	Arthritis Onset <6 yr of age			Arthritis Onset >6 yr of age	
	First 4 yr after onset, examine every:	Next 3 yr after onset, examine every:	After 7 yr from onset, examine every:	First 4 yr after onset, examine every:	After 4 yr from onset, examine every:
Pauci-ANA-positive	3 mo	6 mo	12 mo	6 mo	12 mo
Pauci-ANA-negative	6 mo	6 mo	12 mo	6 mo	12 mo
Poly-ANA-positive	3-4 mo	6 mo	12 mo	6 mo	12 mo
Poly-ANA-negative	6 mo	6 mo	12 mo	6 mo	12 mo
Systemic	12 mo	12 mo	12 mo	12 mo	12 mo

Adapted from Cassidy, J., Kivlin, J., Lindsley, C., et al. (2006). Ophthalmic examinations in children with juvenile rheumatoid arthritis, *Pediatrics, 117*,1843-1845.

Orthotic appliances are often recommended to prevent or correct deformities. Important safety issues related to splint wearing include care of the splint to maintain integrity, proper skin care, signs and symptoms of a poorly fitted splint (e.g., potential pressure points), and proper splint application. The splint should be adjusted to maintain correct function and ensure that the child has not outgrown it. Superficial heat and cold modalities are often recommended to relieve joint pain and stiffness. Determining the type of applications used by the family and reviewing safety precautions specific to each type of application are important.

Some children with JRA use adaptive equipment to minimize joint stress and increase independence. Adaptive equipment should be evaluated for the safety of all family members. Bath safety can be improved by the use of safety strips, rubber mats, wall grab bars, and tub chairs. As with all family members, a home fire safety plan should include a specific plan for the child with JRA.

Immunizations

Children with chronic arthritis in disease remission who are not taking immunosuppressive medications can receive all routine immunizations. If possible, children with arthritis should be immunized on schedule. Children whose immunocompetence is altered by antimetabolites such as methotrexate or by large doses of corticosteroids (≥2 mg/kg/day or ≥20 mg/day if weight is >10 kg, a dose usually reserved for children with severe systemic JRA) should not receive live vaccines for at least 3 months after discontinuation of these medications (AAP & Committee on Infectious Diseases, 2006). The polio vaccine is now administered as an inactivated virus (IPV). Live vaccinations (varicella, measles, mumps, rubella [MMR], rotavirus [RotaTeq]) may be administered to children with JRA whose only exposure to steroids are topically applied ophthalmic medication, intra-articular injections, or low-dose maintenance and/or physiologic doses (AAP & Committee on Infectious Diseases). It is not known whether the newer biologic agents pose a significant risk for receipt of live vaccines. At this time, children receiving these agents should avoid being immunized with live vaccines. All children with chronic arthritis should receive the current recommended influenza vaccine each year. Early concerns that influenza immunization may cause a disease flare seem to be unjustified (McCann, 2007). Overall, there has been widespread concern about the possibility of immunizations causing a flare of the underlying disease or immunologic disorder in chronic arthritis. Anecdotal experience views this as a potential problem, but scientific data to support this theory do not exist (Heijstek, Pileggi, Zonneveld-Huijssoon, et al., 2007; Kasapçopur, Çullu, Kamburoðlu-Goksel, et al., 2004). These concerns should not discourage primary care providers from immunizing children with chronic arthritis with inactivated vaccines.

Screening

Vision. A thorough funduscopic examination and visual acuity screening should be performed at each routine office visit. At the time of diagnosis, every child must be examined for uveitis by an ophthalmologist. Frequent ophthalmologic examinations are recommended for children at risk for uveitis, glaucoma, and cataracts. Young children with ANA-positive arthritis are at greatest risk for development of ocular inflammation. The Rheumatology and Ophthalmology Sections of the American Academy of Pediatrics (Cassidy, Kivlin, Lindsley, et al., 2006) have developed an ophthalmologic screening schedule (Table 31-4). More frequent follow-up is needed for children with active uveitis. Medications such as corticosteroids can cause glaucoma or cataracts. Children taking hydroxychloroquine (Plaquenil) should have a baseline and yearly ophthalmologic examination that includes visual field determinations.

Hearing. Routine office screening is recommended.

Dental. Dental visits should occur at least every 6 months and more frequently if malocclusions, crowded teeth, and dental caries occur as a result of TMJ disease. Orthodontic referrals are made as needed. Increased incidence of dental caries can occur in children with JRA, possibly because of poor oral hygiene secondary to TMJ or upper extremity limitations (Welbury, Thomason, Fitzgerald, et al., 2003). Malocclusions and crowded teeth occur as a result of micrognathia (Savioli, Silva, Ching, et al., 2004). Children with JRA should be checked for bleeding gums and poor dental hygiene. In these situations, consultation with the pediatric rheumatology team and the dentist is necessary. Orthodontic referrals are made as needed. Dental work for children in whom thrombocytopenia or leukopenia develop should be postponed until blood cell counts have returned to normal. Individuals with joint replacements should receive prophylactic antibiotics before dental work (see Chapter 21 for prescribing details).

Blood Pressure. Routine screening is recommended. Mild hypertension may occur in children taking NSAIDs. Steroid-induced hypertension can occur, although it is less frequent when lower doses are prescribed (Laxer, 2005).

Hematocrit. Hematologic testing is frequently ordered by the rheumatologist to screen for disease activity and medication toxicity so routine screening may not be required in the pediatric office.

Urinalysis. Routine urinalyses are generally checked at least every 6 months by the rheumatologist to screen for disease activity and medication toxicity.

Tuberculosis. Routine screening is recommended, especially before the initiation of TNF inhibitors.

Common Illness Management

Differential Diagnosis

Children with an established diagnosis of chronic arthritis will seek care for common childhood illnesses from the primary care provider. Several signs and symptoms of common illnesses must be differentiated from a potential arthritis flare or from arthritis treatment, side effects, or toxicity.

Differential Diagnosis

Chronic Arthritis versus Treatment Side Effects versus Other Illness
- *Fever:* rule out systemic JRA fever vs. infectious process.
- *Dermatologic symptoms:* rule out systemic JRA rash vs. infectious process vs. photosensitive skin reaction.
- *Otologic symptoms:* rule out referred TMJ pain vs. infectious process.
- *Respiratory symptoms:* rule out pleuritis vs. cricoarytenoid arthritis vs. infectious process.
- *Gastrointestinal symptoms:* rule out NSAID gastropathy vs. drug-induced GI bleeding vs. IBD associated with JSpA.
- *Renal symptoms:* rule out urinary tract infection vs. medication toxicity.

Fever. The fever of systemic JRA is easily differentiated from the fever of an infectious process because of the characteristic pattern with normal or below-normal temperature most of the day with once- or twice-daily high spikes. In addition, children with systemic JRA often appear toxic and have a pronounced classic rash during the febrile spikes but are relatively well when afebrile. A careful history and complete physical examination usually determine the source of the fever.

Dermatologic Symptoms. Primary care providers should be familiar with the classic rash associated with systemic JRA—a salmon-pink, evanescent, macular rash typically appearing on the trunk and extremities that coincides with fever spikes. Other types of rashes are rarely seen as part of the JRA condition and should be assessed and treated as for children without JRA.

Photosensitive skin reactions may occur with several medications used to treat JRA, including naproxen, methotrexate, sulfasalazine, and hydroxychloroquine. The most common rash is pseudoporphyria associated with naproxen (Naprosyn, Anaprox) and other NSAIDs (Schäd, Kraus, Haubitz, et al., 2007).

Otologic Symptoms. TMJ arthritis may cause referred pain to the ear, which should be considered when evaluating children for otitis media.

Respiratory Symptoms. Cricoarytenoid arthritis (i.e., laryngeal arthritis) can cause stridor, dyspnea, and cyanosis in JRA. Pleuritis and pericarditis can occur in systemic JRA. Very rarely, methotrexate therapy may lead to hypersensitivity pneumonitis (Laxer & Schneider, 2004).

Gastrointestinal Symptoms. GI symptoms commonly occur in children with JRA who take NSAIDs and/or glucocorticoids. Studies have shown that GI symptoms occur in 39% to 58% of children with JRA (Brunner, Johnson, Barron, et al., 2005; Weber, Brune, Ganser, et al., 2003). In one study, 45 children were

evaluated endoscopically for GI pathology. Of these children, 20 children (44%) had histologically mild chronic gastritis, and an additional 7 children (15.6%) had significant upper GI tract pathology (Ashorn et al., 2003). Although peptic ulcers are rare in children receiving NSAID treatment, they may present as chronic anemia secondary to occult blood loss. The classic peptic ulcer symptom of epigastric pain that improves with eating and worsens with an empty stomach is more common in adolescents and is virtually absent in young children. IBD should be ruled out in children experiencing major GI problems. A careful history and physical examination, as well as consultation with the pediatric rheumatologist as needed, will help the primary care provider to evaluate the differential diagnoses.

Renal. Urinary tract infection versus renal toxicity from medications must be considered with abnormal urinalysis results.

Drug Interactions

Potential interactions exist between medications commonly used to treat JRA and over-the-counter or prescription drugs used to manage common pediatric conditions. Major drug interactions of concern to primary care providers are identified in Box 31-4. Generally, providers should not discontinue a child's condition-specific medications without consulting the pediatric rheumatologist. Conditions warranting temporary cessation of arthritis medications may include the following: (1) exposure to chickenpox in unimmunized children; (2) significant bleeding of the nose, gums, or GI tract; and (3) significant emesis and dehydration as a result of infectious illness. On the other hand, children taking long-term corticosteroids may need increased steroid supplementation at times of significant illness. Communication with the rheumatology team is essential in these circumstances.

Developmental Issues

Sleep Patterns

Sleep abnormalities are common in children with JRA (Bloom, Owens, McGuinn, et al., 2002; Passarelli, Roizenblatt, Len, et al., 2006). They may also fatigue more readily during flares and require periods of rest during the day. Teaching a child to recognize body signals, set limits and priorities, pace activities, and plan ahead will help conserve energy. The severity and duration of morning stiffness increases with increased disease activity. Recommendations to alleviate morning stiffness include administration of medications 30 to 60 minutes before rising and stretching in a warm bath or shower before starting daily activities. In addition, the use of flannel sheets, thermal underwear, warmed clothing, and a sleeping bag may decrease morning stiffness.

Toileting

The acquisition of self-care skills may be delayed in children with JRA. Toilet training should be postponed during periods of active disease because a child may lack the motivation and physical capability to perform tasks necessary for successful toileting. Limitations in the upper and lower extremities may make it difficult for children to transfer on and off the toilet, manage toilet paper, and undress. Safety bars and elevated toilet seats are reliable assistive devices for children with lower extremity involvement. For children with upper extremity limitations, effective aids for wiping after toileting can be obtained from occupational therapists.

BOX 31-4
Drug Interactions

- Concurrent use of NSAIDs and glucocorticoids may increase risk of GI side effects.
- Antacids may alter the absorption rate of NSAIDs and glucocorticoids, resulting in subtherapeutic levels.
- Methotrexate concentrations are increased by NSAIDs, which is generally not a concern in weekly low-dose methotrexate therapy.
- Concomitant use of methotrexate and alcohol may increase the risk of GI and hepatic side effects.
- Sulfonamides may displace or be displaced by other highly protein-bound drugs (e.g., NSAIDs, methotrexate). Monitor children for increased effects (i.e., increased hepatotoxicity) of highly bound drugs when sulfonamides (e.g., trimethoprim/sulfamethoxazole [Bactrim]) are added.
- Estrogen-based oral contraceptives may decrease the clearance and increase the serum concentration and toxic effects of corticosteroids and cyclosporine.
- NSAIDs plus acetaminophen increases the risk of adverse hepatic side effects.
- NSAIDs displace anticoagulants from protein-binding sites.

Adaptive clothing and dressing aids can facilitate toileting. In severely affected children, bedpans, urinals, and commodes may also be required at night if pain and stiffness limit mobility.

Discipline

Parents of children with arthritis may have difficulty dealing with their guilt and concern over their child's condition. They may become overprotective and not handle behavioral issues as firmly as they would if the child was not "sick." In addition, overindulgence during periods of active disease alternating with normalization of discipline practices during remissions fosters inconsistent limit setting. The primary care provider can reinforce normalcy in childhood expectations, responsibilities, and chores, as well as appropriate behavioral expectations and discipline.

Child Care

Parents of children who are taking medications may have difficulty locating child-care providers who are willing to administer medications. For caregivers who accept this responsibility, parents can prepare a list that includes the name, dose, time, and method of administration, as well as the side effects of each medication. Caregivers need to understand that chronic arthritis is characterized by fluctuations in disease activity and symptoms. Therefore a child's functional capacity, energy level, and developmental progress may change on different days. Education about the child's abilities, limitations, disease, and treatments is likely to decrease anxiety among caregivers and promote appropriate interactions among caregivers, children, and families. Infants and young children with chronic arthritis may be eligible for special education services and related services under Public Laws 99-457 and 101-476 (see Chapter 3).

Schooling

Children with chronic arthritis can participate fully in school, physical education, and extracurricular activities with certain interventions and adaptations listed in Table 31-5. Many children have special needs that must be communicated to the school by verbal and written communication and addressed in an individualized educational plan (IEP) (see Chapter 3). Most pediatric

TABLE 31-5
Common School Problems for Students with Chronic Arthritis

Problem	Intervention Strategies
Difficulty climbing stairs/walking long distance	Elevator permit Schedule classes to decrease walking and climbing Two sets of books: keep one in appropriate class, other at home Wheelchair if needed Proper footwear: supportive sneakers
Inactivity, stiffness as a result of prolonged sitting	Move! Change position every 20 minutes Sit to the side or back of the room to allow for standing or walking without disturbing the class Ask to be assigned jobs that permit walking (pass/collect papers)
Difficulty carrying books/cafeteria tray	Accessible desk Rolling backpack for books Two sets of books Determine cafeteria assistance plan or pack lunch (helper, reserved seat, wheeled cart)
Handwriting problems (slow, messy, painful)	Use "fat" pen/pencil, crayons or pencil/pen grips Felt tip pen Stretch hands about every 10 minutes Tape recorder for note-taking Computer for reports Alternatives for timed tests (oral test, extra time, computer) Educate teacher; messy writing may be unavoidable at times
Difficulty with shoulder movement, dressing, putting on coat, boots, tying shoes	Loose-fitting clothing, without buttons or zippers Velcro closures Adaptive equipment from an occupational therapist Assistance may be needed for some things, especially on "stiff days"
Reaching locker, opening locker	Locker modification/alternative place for storage Two lockers Key for locker instead of combination
Raising hand	Devise alternative signaling method

---

rheumatology centers have a standard letter for school personnel that describes the condition and recommended adjustments. Educating school personnel about morning stiffness and variability of clinical manifestations is very important. Severe disease flares or surgery may necessitate temporary home instruction and should be planned for in a child's IEP. Primary care providers can periodically question children and parents about school-related problems such as fatigue, distractibility, limited mobility, absences, and medications. The provider may interface with the family, school staff, and pediatric rheumatology team to identify and remedy problems before, or when, they occur. The student can participate in school athletic programs with modifications as necessary. Swimming as a sport is strongly encouraged because it strengthens muscle groups around joints, provides good range of motion therapy, is less stressful on joints than weight-bearing activities of contact sports, and promotes aerobic fitness.

Sexuality

Sexual maturation may be delayed in adolescents with chronic arthritis, especially in those with systemic disease. Menarche occurs later in girls with JRA than in unaffected controls, particularly in those taking glucocorticoids (Rusconi, Corona, Grassi, et al., 2003). In one long-term follow-up study of 246 adults with JRA, the mean age of first sexual experience was later in adolescents with JRA (19.3 years) compared with the general population (17.0 years). However, more than one third (37.6%) of these individuals reported being sexually active before transfer to an adult rheumatologist (Packham & Hall, 2002b). Therefore contraceptive advice is important and should include discussion of interactions among arthritis medications and various oral contraceptives, as well as any potential effects of arthritis medications on fetal development.

Fertility is not impaired in women with JRA, but the rate of miscarriage and preterm birth is higher than in healthy controls (Packham & Hall, 2002b; Ostensen, Almberg, & Koksvik, 2000). At delivery, cesarean section may be necessary in some women because of poor hip abduction or a small pelvis (Packham & Hall, 2002b). Because of these factors, early referral to an obstetrician for women with JRA who are pregnant is very important.

Transition to Adulthood

Thoughtful planning for transition into adulthood is necessary and useful. The optimal goal of health care transition planning for the teenager with arthritis is to provide coordinated, uninterrupted care that addresses the developmental topics of this age period, including vocational, career, sexuality, independence, and financial issues (McDonagh, Shaw, & Southwood, 2006). Successful health care transition is influenced by a number of variables, including availability of adult rheumatologists, availability of staff time/resources to coordinate transition, delayed emotional maturity and learned dependency of some adolescents, fear of "moving on" to adult care, overprotectiveness of parents, health insurance restrictions, and/or lack of health insurance (Shaw, Southwood, McDonagh, et al., 2004). The primary care provider can promote the transition process for the teenager in many ways. The provider can help the family identify a local adult rheumatologist, encourage independence in self-care, address adolescent developmental issues, counsel parents and teens, refer to community programs as needed, and collaborate with the multidisciplinary team (Burns, Sadof, & Kamat, 2006). A coordinated transition program for adolescents with JRA resulted in improvement in adolescent health related QoL, adolescent and parent knowledge and satisfaction, and prevocational readiness (McDonagh, Southwood, Shaw, et al., 2007).

Family Concerns

Raising a child with chronic arthritis can be difficult. There are many misconceptions about arthritis. Families must repeatedly explain and educate others that arthritis is not just a problem to be quickly remedied by the multitudes of treatment offered on television advertisements and in magazines. Others often believe that arthritis is a condition that affects only the elderly and are often in disbelief when children discuss their arthritis. After hearing about the diagnosis of arthritis, well-meaning family and friends sometimes tend to overwhelm the family with information about the diagnosis and "cures" of which they have heard or read. Children with arthritis often appear healthy, which makes it difficult to explain their need for modifications at school and work. They have appropriate concerns about school attendance, sports participation, growth, and any limitations that make them feel different. Parents have concerns about long-term side effects of medications (e.g., fertility), whereas children are more concerned about the short-term effects (e.g., cushingoid facies with corticosteroids).

Children are asked to engage in several treatment regimens, such as medications, exercise, lifestyle changes, and added appointments to the primary care provider, rheumatologist, ophthalmologist, and other specialists. The child, adolescent, or parent may decide not to comply with the recommendations. Families and older children need to be made aware of the risk/benefit ratios of treatments and the consequences of poor adherence to treatment regimens. The primary care provider has the longest relationship with the family and can therefore encourage and support adherence, refer to social services (e.g., when finances or transportation interfere with treatment), and promote parental supervision and organization when necessary (Raphoff, 2002). Teaching problem-solving and decision-making skills, as well as using contracts, are helpful strategies to use with the adolescent.

A review of multiple studies has shown progressive improvement in outcomes and QoL for children with chronic arthritis. However, many children and adolescents with chronic arthritis have ongoing difficulties related to health status and social, educational, and vocational function (Duffy, 2005). Key family resources and programs are available through several organizations. Families of children with chronic arthritis are strongly encouraged to use these educational and support services.

Resources

American Juvenile Arthritis Organization (AJAO)
Arthritis Foundation
P.O. Box 7669
Atlanta, GA 30357-0669
(404) 872-7100 (×6277); (800)-283-7800
Website: www.arthritis.org

AJAO is a council of the Arthritis Foundation devoted to serving the special needs of children, teens, and young adults with childhood rheumatic diseases and their families by providing local, regional, and national family conferences; quarterly newsletters; and printed educational materials for children, parents, and health professionals. In addition, local chapters of the Arthritis Foundations may offer summer camps, pen pal clubs, and family support groups. Educational literature and information about these programs are available via the Arthritis Foundation website including (but not limited to):

- "Arthritis in Children," "When your Student Has Arthritis" (pamphlets)
- *Kids Get Arthritis Too* (newsletter)
- *Arthritis Today* (magazine)

Other Resources

National Institute of Arthritis and Musculoskeletal and Skin Diseases Information Clearinghouse, NIAMS/National Institutes of Health; www.nih.gov/niams/healthinfo.

The Pediatric Rheumatology International Trials Organization. Patient education information in several different languages is available; www.printo.it/pediatric-rheumatology.

American College of Rheumatology; www.rheumatology.org.

Information on rheumatic diseases and medications: www.rheumatology.org/public/factsheets/index.asp.

Validated Disease Activity and Quality of Life Questionnaires: www.rheumatology.org/sections/pediatric/tools.asp?aud=mem.

Transition Resources

Post-secondary education for individuals with disabilities:

The George Washington University
HEATH Resource Center
2134 G St., N.W.
Washington, DC 20052-0001
(202) 973-0904; Fax (202) 994-3365
Website: www.heath.gwu.edu/

National Center on Secondary Education and Transition
Institute on Community Integration
University of Minnesota
6 Pattee Hall, 150 Pillsbury Dr. SE
Minneapolis, MN 55455
(612) 624-2097; Fax (612) 624-9344
Website: www.ncset.org

Summary of Primary Care Needs for the Child with Juvenile Rheumatoid Arthritis

HEALTH CARE MAINTENANCE

Growth and Development

- Linear growth may be delayed during active systemic disease.
- Catch-up growth occurs with disease control or during remission.
- Increased calcium needs as children may be osteopenic.
- Corticosteroids may suppress growth at doses >0.15 mg/kg/day.
- Poor weight gain may be a result of systemic disease.
- Excessive weight gain may occur as a result of decreased activity, depression, poor nutrition, or corticosteroid usage.
- Gross motor delays and temporary regressions are not uncommon during periods of flares/active disease.
- Fine motor skills are less likely to be affected.
- Developmentally appropriate quality of life assessments are needed.

Diet

- Nutritional problems are common.
- Increased inflammatory activity, anorexia, GI side effects of medication, physical limitations, depression, corticosteroid usage, poor food choices, and limited movement of TMJ may contribute to nutritional problems.
- Daily vitamin should be added.
- "Arthritis diets" should be evaluated for nutritional adequacy, and families should be educated about proper nutrition for a growing child with a chronic disease.

Safety

- Childproof containers should be used for medications.
- Children taking immunosuppressive agents should wear a Medic-Alert bracelet or necklace.
- Sunblock should be used on exposed skin because of photosensitive skin reactions with some medications.
- Safety issues related to splint wear, heat and cold applications, and adaptive equipment should be reviewed.

Immunizations

- Children who are not taking immunosuppressive drugs or experiencing systemic disease symptoms should be routinely immunized.

- In the absence of neurologic symptoms, a child with classic, intermittent JRA fever can be immunized during febrile episodes.
- No live-virus vaccines (varicella, MMR, rotovirus) should be given to children receiving antimetabolites, large doses of corticosteroids, or biologic agents.
- All children with chronic arthritis should receive the current recommended influenza vaccine each year.

Screening

- *Vision:* A funduscopic examination and acuity screening should be performed at each visit. Children should be examined by an ophthalmologist for uveitis (see Table 31-4). Children taking topical or systemic steroids require close ophthalmologic follow-up.
- *Hearing:* Routine visits are recommended.
- *Dental:* Children with TMJ involvement and micrognathia should have frequent dental visits (at least every 6 months). Prophylactic antibiotics should be used for dental work in children with total joint replacements or those taking steroids.
- *Blood pressure:* Routine screening is recommended.
- *Hematocrit:* CBC, differential, ESR, C-reactive protein, platelet count, and liver function tests are routinely ordered by the rheumatologist to monitor disease activity, response to therapy, drug toxicity, and assess for anemia of chronic disease.
- *Urinalysis:* Urinalysis is routinely ordered by the rheumatologist to monitor disease-related factors
- *Tuberculosis:* Routine screening is recommended.

COMMON ILLNESS MANAGEMENT

Differential Diagnosis

- *Fever:* Classic, intermittent JRA fever should be differentiated from infectious process.
- *Dermatologic:* Rheumatoid rash should be ruled out in systemic JRA. Drug-related photosensitivity skin reactions should be ruled out.
- *Otologic:* TMJ arthritis with referred ear pain should be differentiated from otitis media.

Summary of Primary Care Needs for the Child with Juvenile Rheumatoid Arthritis—cont'd

- *Respiratory:* Colds and flu may cause arthritis flare-ups. Infectious process must be differentiated from pleuritis or cricoarytenoid arthritis.
- *Gastrointestinal:* Drug-related GI symptoms should be differentiated from a gastroenteritis infection. Drug-related gastropathy should also be differentiated from IBD associated with JspA.
- *Renal:* Urinary tract infection should be distinguished from medication toxicity.

DEVELOPMENTAL ISSUES

Sleep Patterns
- Fatigue associated with disease flares may necessitate rest periods during the day.
- Recommendations to promote comfort and sleep and to alleviate morning stiffness (e.g., use of electric blanket with timer and morning bath or shower) should be discussed with the family.

Toileting
- Training should be postponed during periods of active disease.
- Assistive devices may be needed with individuals with severe disease, joint deformities, and limited mobility.

Discipline
- Overprotection, overindulgence, and inconsistent limit setting should be identified. Reinforce the need for consistent expectations (e.g., daily chores). Discuss impact of chronic arthritis on age-specific developmental tasks so parents have a framework for decision making about discipline.

Child Care
- Caregivers need to be knowledgeable of medications, use of assistive devices, and applying splints.
- Parents should provide caregivers with information about the child's medications.
- Caregivers should be educated on the effect of JRA on a child's functional capacity, energy level, and developmental progress.
- Home-based, single-provider daycare setting rather than group child care is recommended for children taking steroids or immunosuppressants.

Schooling
- Individuals with Disabilities Education Improvement Act (IDEA) entitles most students with JRA to occupational therapy, physical therapy, adaptive physical education, and transportation between school, home, and facilities where services are provided (see Table 31-5).
- Most students with JRA can participate in modified school athletic programs "to their own tolerance level."
- Disease flares or surgery may necessitate home instructions for a brief period.
- Teaching families about their educational rights and how to advocate for their child in school is important.

Sexuality
- Puberty may be delayed in children with JRA.
- Discussion of puberty, sexual activity, appropriate contraception, and pregnancy is imperative with all adolescents.
- Medication modifications (i.e., methotrexate is an abortifacient and is teratogenic) must be made before planning a pregnancy.

Transition to Adulthood
- Adolescents can be referred to the state office of vocational rehabilitation for assistance with post-secondary educational opportunities.
- Primary care providers can assist the family with decisions regarding health care, psychosocial, vocational, financial, and family issues.
- Teenagers are advised to avoid drinking any alcohol. Alcohol significantly increases the risk of liver toxicity when taking methotrexate.

FAMILY CONCERNS
- Family frustration and concern over the lack of a cure and the unpredictability of the illness should be acknowledged.
- The impact of the illness on the child's ability to fully participate in school, sports, and social activities raises concerns for parents.
- Multiple treatment regimens and concern about side effects may lead to nonadherence.
- Referral for psychosocial and family issues may be necessary.

REFERENCES

Adib, N., Silman, A., & Thomson, W. (2005). Outcome following onset of juvenile idiopathic inflammatory arthritis: II. Predictors of outcome in juvenile arthritis. *Rheumatology, 44*(8), 1002-1007.

American Academy of Pediatrics & Committee on Infectious Diseases (2006). *2006 Red Book: Report of the Committee on Infectious Diseases.* (27th ed). Elk Grove, IL; American Academy of Pediatrics.

Arabshahi, B., Dewitt, E.M., Cahill, A.M., et al. (2005). Utility of corticosteroid injection for temporomandibular arthritis in children with juvenile idiopathic arthritis. *Arthritis Rheum, 52*(11), 3563-3569.

Ashorn, M., Verronen, P., Ruuska, T., et al. (2003). Upper endoscopic findings in children with active juvenile chronic arthritis. *Acta Paediatr, 92*(5), 558-561.

Athreya, B.H., & Lindsley, C. (2005). A general approach to management of rheumatic disease in children. In J.T. Cassidy, R.E. Petty, C.B. Lindsley, et al. (Eds.), *Textbook of Pediatric Rheumatology,* (5th ed.). Philadelphia: Elsevier.

Baeten, D., DeKeyser, F., Mielants, H., et al. (2002). Immune linkages between inflammatory bowel disease and spondyloarthropathies. *Curr Opin Rheumatol, 14*(4), 342-336.

Behrens, E.M., Beukelman, T., Gallo, L., et al. (2008). Evaluation of the presentation of systemic onset juvenile rheumatoid arthritis: Data from the Pennsylvania systemic onset juvenile arthritis registry (PASOJAR). *J Rheumatol, 35*(2), 343-348.

Biester, S., Deuter, C., Haefner, M.H., et al. (2007). Adalimumab in the therapy of uveitis in childhood. *Br J Ophthalmol, 91*(3), 274-276.

Billiau, A.D., Hu, Y., Verdonch, A., et al. (2007). Temporomandibular joint arthritis in juvenile idiopathic arthritis: Prevalence, clinical and radiologic signs, and relation to dentofacial morphology. *J Rheumatol, 34*(9), 1925-1933.

Bloom, B.J., Owens, J.A., McGuinn, M., et al. (2002). Sleep and its relationship to pain, dysfunction, and disease activity in juvenile rheumatoid arthritis. *J Rheumatol, 29*(1), 169-173.

Bowyer, S.L., Roettcher, P.A., Higgins, G.C., et al. (2003). Health status of patients with juvenile rheumatoid arthritis at 1 and 5 years. *J Rheumatol, 30*(2), 394-400.

Breban, M. (2006). Genetics of spondyloarthritis. *Best Pract Clin Rheumatol*, *20*(3), 593-599.

Brinkman, D.M., de Kleer, I.M., ten Cate, R., et al. (2007). Autologous stem cell transplantation in children with severe progressive systemic or polyarticular juvenile idiopathic arthritis: Long-term follow-up of a prospective clinical trial. *Arthritis Rheum*, *56*(7), 2410-2421.

Bristol-Myers Squibb News Release. (2008, April 8), *U.S. Food and Drug Administration approves ORENCIA (abatacept) for the treatment of moderate-to-severe polyarticular juvenile idiopathic arthritis (JIA) in patients six years and older.* Available at http://newsroom.bms.com/article_display.cfm?article_id=5249. Retrieved May 12, 2008.

Brunner, H.I., Kim, K.N., Ballinger, S.H., et al. (2001). Current medication choices in juvenile rheumatoid arthritis II—Update of a survey performed in 1993. *J Clin Rheumatol*, *7*(5), 283-285.

Brunner, H.I., Johnson, A.L., Barron, A.C., et al. (2005). Gastrointestinal symptoms and their association with health-related quality of life of children with juvenile rheumatoid arthritis: Validation of gastrointestinal symptom questionnaire. *J Clin Rheumatol*, *11*(4), 194-204.

Buchmann, R.F., & Jaramillo, D. (2004). Imaging of articular disorders in children. *Radiol Clin North Am*, *42*(1), 151-168.

Burgos-Vargos, R. (2002). Juvenile onset spondyloarthropathies: Therapeutic aspects. (extended report). *Ann Rheum Dis*, *61*(Suppl 3), iii33-iii39.

Burnham, J.M., & Leonard, M.B. (2004). Bone disease in pediatric rheumatologic disorders. *Curr Rheumatol Rep*, *6*(1). 79-78.

Burns, J.J., Sadof, M., & Kamat, D. (2006). The adolescent with a chronic illness. *Pediatr Ann*, *35*(3), 206-210. 214-216.

Cakmak, A., & Bolukbas, N. (2005). Juvenile rheumatoid arthritis: Physical therapy and rehabilitation. *South Med J*, *98*(2), 212-216.

Cassidy, J.T. (2005). Juvenile rheumatoid arthritis. E.D.Harris, R.C.Budd, M.C.Genovese, et al. (Eds.) *Kelley's Textbook of Rheumatology*, (7th ed.). Philadelphia: Elsevier Saunders.

Cassidy, J.T., Kivlin, J., Lindsley, C., et al. (2006). Ophthalmologic examinations in children with juvenile rheumatoid arthritis. *Pediatrics*, *117*(5), 1843-1845.

Cassidy, J.T., & Petty, R.E. (2005a). Chronic arthritis in childhood. In J.T. Cassidy, R.E. Petty, C.B. Lindsley, et al. (Eds.), *Textbook of Pediatric Rheumatology* (5th ed.). Philadelphia: Elsevier.

Cassidy, J.T., & Petty, R.E. (2005b). Juvenile ankylosing spondylitis. In J.T. Cassidy, R.E. Petty, C.B. Lindsley, et al. (Eds.), *Textbook of Pediatric Rheumatology* (5th ed.). Philadelphia: Elsevier.

Celiker, R., Bal, S., Bakkaloğlu, A., et al. (2003). Factors playing a role in the development of decreased bone mineral density in juvenile chronic arthritis. *Rheumatol Int*, *23*, 127-129.

Chen, C.Y., Chen, L.C., Yeh, K.W., et al. (2004). Sequential changes to clinical parameters and adhesion molecule following intravenous pulse cyclophosphamide and methylprednisolone treatment of refractory juvenile idiopathic arthritis. *Clin Exp Rheumatol*, *22*(2), 259-264.

Cleary, A.G., Lancaster, G.A., Annan, F., et al. (2004). Nutritional impairment in juvenile idiopathic arthritis. *Rheumatology*, *43*(12), 1569-1573.

Conti, F., Borrelli, O., Anania, C., et al (2005). Chronic intestinal inflammation and seronegative spondyloarthropathy in children. *Dig Liver Dis*, *37*(10), 761-767.

Cron, R.Q., & Finkel, T.H. (2002). Approach to child with joint pain. In S. West (Ed.) *Rheumatology Secrets*, (2nd ed.). Philadelphia: Hanley and Belfus.

Cron, R.Q., Sharma, S., & Sherry, D.D. (1999). Current treatment by United States and Canadian pediatric rheumatologists. *J Rheumatol*, *26*(9), 2036-2038.

deJager, W., Hoppenreijs, E.P., Wulffraat, N.M., et al. (2007). Blood and synovial fluid signatures in patients with juvenile idiopathic arthritis: A cross-sectional study. *Ann Rheum Dis*, *66*(5), 589-599.

DeSmet, A.A. (2004). Ultrasound-guided injections and aspirations of the extremities. *Semin Roentgenol*, *39*(1), 145-154.

Duffy, C.M. (2004). Measurement of health status, functional status, and quality of life in children with juvenile idiopathic arthritis: Clinical science for the pediatrician. *Pediatr Clin North Am*, *52*(2), 359-372.

Duffy, C.M., Colbert, R.A., Laxer, R.M., et al. (2005). Nomenclature and classification in chronic childhood arthritis: Time for a change? *Arthritis Rheum*, *52*(2), 382-385.

Eberhard, B.A., Sison, M.C., Gottlieb, B.S., et al. (2004). Comparison of the intraarticular effectiveness of triamcinolone hexacetonide and triamcinolone acetonide in treatment of juvenile rheumatoid arthritis. *J Rheumatol*, *31*(12), 2507-2512.

Epps, H., Ginnelly, L., Utley, M., et al. (2005). Is hydrotherapy cost-effective? A randomized controlled trial of combined hydrotherapy programmes compared with physiotherapy land techniques in children with juvenile idiopathic arthritis. *Health Technol Assess*, 1-59. iii-iv, ix-x *9*(39).

Feldman, D.E., Duffy, C., De Civita, M., et al. (2004). Factors associated with the use of complementary and alternative medicine in juvenile idiopathic arthritis. *Arthritis Rheum*, *51*(4), 527-532.

Flatø, B., Hoffmann-Vold, A.M., Reiff, A., et al. (2006). Long-term outcome and prognostic factors in enthesitis-related arthritis: A case-control study. *Arthritis Rheum*, *54*(11), 3573-3582.

Foeldvari, I., Nielsen, S., Kümmerle-Deschner, J., et al. (2007). Tumor necrosis factor–alpha blocker in treatment of juvenile idiopathic arthritis-associated uveitis refractory to second-line agents: Results of a multinational study. *J Rheumatol*, *34*(5), 1146-1150.

Foeldvari, I., & Wierk, A. (2005). Methotrexate is an effective treatment for chronic uveitis associated with juvenile idiopathic arthritis. *J Rheumatol*, *32*(2). 362-365.

Foster, C.S. (2003). Diagnosis and treatment of juvenile idiopathic arthritis-associated uveitis. *Curr Opin Ophthalmol*, *14*(6), 395-398.

Ganz, T. (2006). Molecular pathogenesis of anemia of chronic disease. *Pediatr Blood Cancer*, *46*(5), 554-557.

Gensler, L., & Davis, J.C. (2006). Recognition and treatment of juvenile-onset spondyloarthropathies. *Curr Opin Rheumatol*, *18*(5), 507-511.

Goldberg, R.J., & Katz, J. (2007). A meta-analysis of the analgesic effect of omega-3 polyunsaturated fatty acid supplementation for inflammatory joint pain. *Pain*, *129*(1-2), 210-223.

Grassi, A., Corona, F., Casellato, A., et al. (2007). Prevalence and outcome of juvenile idiopathic arthritis-associated uveitis and relation to articular disease. *J Rheumatol*, *34*(5), 1139-1145.

Guillaume, S., Prieur, A.M., Coste, J., et al. (2000). Long-term outcome and prognosis in oligoarticular-onset juvenile idiopathic arthritis. *Arthritis Rheum*, *43*(8), 1858-1865.

Hagen, L.E.M., Schneider, R., Stephens, D., et al. (2003). Use of complementary and alternative medicine by pediatric rheumatology patients. *Arthritis Rheum*, *49*(1), 3-6.

Heijstek, M.W., Pileggi, G.C., Zonneveld-Huijssoon, E., et al. (2007). Safety of measles, mumps and rubella vaccination in juvenile idiopathic arthritis. *Ann Rheum Dis*, *66*(10), 1384-1387.

Heiligenhaus, A., Mingels, A., Heinz, C., et al. (2007a). Methotrexate for uveitis associated with juvenile idiopathic arthritis: Value and requirement for additional anti-inflammatory medication. *Eur J Ophthalmol*, *17*(5), 743-748.

Heiligenhaus, A., Niewerth, M., Ganser, G., et al. (2007b). Prevalence and complications of uveitis in juvenile idiopathic arthritis in a population-based nation-wide study in Germany: Suggested modification of the current screening guidelines. *Rheumatology*, *46*(4), 1015-1019.

Henderson, C. (2002). The use of dietary supplements in rheumatic diseases: What evidence exists? *Biomechanics*, *4*(9), 1-10.

Hofer, M. (2006). Spondyloarthropathies in children—Are they different from those in adults? *Best Pract Res Clin Rheumatol*, *20*(2), 315-328.

Iesaka, K., Kubiak, E.N., Bong, M.R., et al. (2006). Orthopedic surgical management of hip and knee involvement in patients with juvenile rheumatoid arthritis. *Am J Orthopsychiatry*, *35*(2), 67-73.

Jarvis, J. (2002). Juvenile rheumatoid arthritis: A guide for pediatricians. *Pediatr Ann*, *31*(7), 437-446.

Kasapçopur, Ö., Çullu, F., Kamburoğlu-Goksel, A., et al. (2004). Hepatitis B vaccination in children with juvenile idiopathic arthritis. *Ann Rheum Dis*, *63*(9), 1128-1130.

Kelly, A., & Ramanan, A.V. (2007). Recognition and management of macrophage activation syndrome in juvenile arthritis. *Curr Opin Rheumatol*, *19*(5), 477-481.

Kemper, K.J., & O'Connor, K.G. (2004). Pediatricians' recommendations for complementary and alternative medical (CAM) therapies. *Ambul Pediatr*, *4*(6), 482-487.

Khan, M.A., Mathieu, A., Sorrentino, R., et al. (2007). The pathogenic role of HLA-B27 and its subtypes. *Autoimmun Rev*, *6*(3), 183-189.

Kitsoulis, P.B., Siamopoulou, A., Beris, A.E., et al. (2006a). Total hip and knee arthroplasty for juvenile rheumatoid arthritis. *Folia Med*, *48*(3-4), 42-49.

Kitsoulis, P.B., Stafilas, K.S., Siamopoulou, A., et al. (2006b). Total hip arthroplasty in children with juvenile chronic arthritis: Long-term results. *J Pediatr Orthopsychiatry*, *26*(1), 8-12.

Klepper, S.E. (2007). Making the case for exercise in children with juvenile idiopathic arthritis: What we know and where we go from here. *Arthritis Rheum*, *57*(6), 887-890.

Kotaniemi, K., Savolainen, A., Karma, A., et al. (2003). Recent advances in uveitis of juvenile idiopathic arthritis. *Surv Ophthalmol*, *48*(5), 489-502.

Kuek, A., Hazleman, B.L., Gaston, J.H., et al. (2006). Successful treatment of refractory polyarticular juvenile idiopathic arthritis with rituximab. *Rheumatology*, *45*(11), 1448-1449.

Kurahara, D.K., Grandinetti, A., Fujii, L.L., et al. (2007). Visiting consultant clinics to study prevalence rates of juvenile rheumatoid arthritis and childhood systemic lupus erythematosus across dispersed geographic areas. *J Rheumatol, 34*(2), 425-429.

Laiho, K., Savolainen, A., Kautiainen, H., et al. (2002). The cervical spine in juvenile chronic arthritis. *Spine J, 2*(2), 89-94.

Laxer, R. (2005). Pharmacology and drug therapy. In J.T. Cassidy, R.E. Petty, C.B. Lindsley, et al. (Eds.), *Textbook of Pediatric Rheumatology* (5th ed.). Philadelphia: Elsevier.

Laxer, R., & Schneider, R. (2004). Systemic-onset juvenile chronic arthritis. In D.A. Isenberg, P.J. Maddison, P. Woo, et al. (Eds.), *Oxford Textbook of Rheumatology* (3rd ed.). Oxford: Oxford University Press.

Lehman, T.J., Schechter, S.J., Sundel, R.P., et al. (2004). Thalidomide for severe systemic-onset juvenile rheumatoid arthritis: A multicenter study. *J Pediatr, 145*(6), 856-857.

Lelieveld, O.T., van Brussel, M., Takken, T., et al. (2007). Aerobic and anaerobic exercise capacity in adolescents with juvenile idiopathic arthritis. *Arthritis Rheum, 57*(6), 898-904.

Lequerré, T., Quatier, P., Rosellini, D., et al. (2008). Interleukin-1 receptor antagonist (anakinra) treatment in patients with systemic-onset juvenile idiopathic arthritis or adult onset Still disease: Preliminary experience in France. *Ann Rheum Dis, 67*(3), 302-308.

Lien, G., Selvaag, A.M., Flatø, B., et al. (2005). A two-year prospective controlled study of bone mass and bone turnover in children with early juvenile idiopathic arthritis. *Arthritis Rheum, 52*(3), 833-840.

Lovell, D.J., Glass, D., Ranz, J., et al. (2006). A randomized controlled trial of calcium supplementation to increase bone mineral density in children with juvenile rheumatoid arthritis. *Arthritis Rheum, 54*(7), 2235-2242.

Lovell, D.J., Reiff, A., Ilowite, N.T., et al. (2008a) Safety and efficacy of up to eight years of continuous etanercept therapy in patients with juvenile rheumatoid arthritis. *Arthritis Rheum, 58*(5), 1496-1504.

Lovell, D.J., Ruperto, N., Goodman, S., et al. (2008b). Adalimumab with or without methotrexate in juvenile rheumatoid arthritis. *N Engl J Med, 359*(8), 810-820.

Malmstrøm, V., Trollmo, C., Klareskog, L. (2004). The additive role of innate and adaptive immunity in the development of arthritis. *Am J Med Sci, 327*(4), 196-201.

Manners, P., & Bower, C. (2002). Worldwide prevalence of juvenile arthritis—Why does it vary so much? *J Rheumatol, 29*, 1520-1530.

McCann, L.J. (2007). Should children under treatment for juvenile idiopathic arthritis receive flu vaccination? *Arch Dis Child, 92*(4), 366-368.

McDonagh, J.E., Shaw, K.L., & Southwood, T.R. (2006). Growing up and moving on in rheumatology: Development and preliminary evaluation of a transitional care programme for a multicentre cohort of adolescents with juvenile idiopathic arthritis. *J Child Health Care, 10*(1), 22-42.

McDonagh, J.E., Southwood, T.R., Shaw, K.L., et al. (2007). The impact of a coordinated care programme on adolescents with juvenile idiopathic arthritis. *Rheumatology, 46*(1), 161-168.

McGhee, J.L., Burks, F.N., Sheckels, J.L., et al. (2002). Identifying children with chronic arthritis based on chief complaints: Absence of predictive value for musculoskeletal pain as an indicator of rheumatic disease in children. *Pediatrics, 110*(2), 354-359.

McInnes, I.B., & Liew, F.Y. (2005). Cytokine networks—Toward new therapies for rheumatoid arthritis. *Nat Clin Pract Rheumatol, 1*(1), 31-39.

Minden, K., Niewerth, M., Listing, J., et al. (2002). Health care provision in pediatric rheumatology in Germany—National rheumatologic database. *J Rheumatol, 29*(3), 622-628.

Moroldo, M.B., Chaudhari, M., Shear, E., et al. (2004). Juvenile rheumatoid arthritis affected sibpairs: Extent of clinical phenotype concordance. *Arthritis Rheum, 50*(6), 1928-1934.

National Institute of Arthritis and Musculoskeletal and Skin Diseases. (2005, March). *Juvenile osteoporosis.* Available at www.niams.nih.gov/Health_Info/Bone/Bone_Health/Juvenile/juvenile_osteoporosis.asp. Retrieved January 11, 2008.

Neidel, J., Boehnke, M., & Kuster, R.M. (2002). The efficacy and safety of intraarticular corticosteroid therapy for coxitis in juvenile rheumatoid arthritis. *Arthritis Rheumatol, 46*(6), 1620-1628.

Oen, K., Malleson, P.N., Cabral, D.A., et al. (2002). Disease course and outcome of JRA in a multicenter cohort. *J Rheumatol, 29*(9), 1989-1999.

Oen, K., Malleson, P.N., Cabral, D.A., et al. (2003). Radiologic outcome and its relationship to functional disability in juvenile rheumatoid arthritis. *J Rheumatol, 30*(4), 832-840.

Ostensen, M., Almberg, K., & Koksvik, H.S. (2000). Sex, reproduction, and gynecological disease in young adults with a history of juvenile chronic arthritis. *J Rheumatol, 27*(7), 1783-1787.

Packham, J.C., & Hall, M.A. (2002a). Long-term follow-up of 246 adults with juvenile idiopathic arthritis: Functional outcome. *Rheumatology, 41*(12), 1428-1435.

Packham, J.C., & Hall, M.A. (2002b). Long-term follow-up of 246 adults with juvenile idiopathic arthritis: social function, relationships and sexual activity. *Rheumatology, 41*(12), 1440-1443.

Palmer, D.H., Mulhall, K.J., Thompson, C.A., et al. (2005). Total knee arthroplasty in children with juvenile rheumatoid arthritis. *J Bone Joint Surg, 87*(7), 1510-1514.

Pascual, V., Allantaz, F., Arce, E., et al. (2005). Role of interleukin-1 (IL-1) in the pathogenesis of systemic juvenile idiopathic arthritis and clinical response to IL-1 blockade. *J Exp Med, 201*(9), 1479-1486.

Passarelli, C.M., Roizenblatt, S., Len, C.A., et al. (2006). A case-control sleep study in children with polyarticular juvenile rheumatoid arthritis. *J Rheumatol, 33*(4), 796-802.

Petty, R.E., & Cassidy, J.T. (2005a). Oligoarthritis. In J.T. Cassidy, R.E. Petty, C.B. Lindsley, et al. (Eds.), *Textbook of Pediatric Rheumatology* (5th ed.). Philadelphia: Elsevier Saunders.

Petty, R.E., & Cassidy, J.T. (2005b). Polyarthritis. In J.T. Cassidy, R.E. Petty, C.B. Lindsley, et al. (Eds.), *Textbook of Pediatric Rheumatology* (5th ed.). Philadelphia: Elsevier Saunders.

Petty, R.E., & Cassidy, J.T. (2005c). Systemic arthritis. In J.T. Cassidy, R.E. Petty, C.B. Lindsley, et al. (Eds.), *Textbook of Pediatric Rheumatology* (5th ed.). Philadelphia: Elsevier Saunders.

Petty, R.E., Southwood, T.R., Manners, P., et al. (2004). International League of Associations for Rheumatology Classification of Juvenile Idiopathic Arthritis: Second Revision, Edmonton, 2001. *J Rheumatol, 31*(2), 390-392.

Phelan, J.D., & Thompson, S.D. (2006). Genomic progress in pediatric arthritis: Recent work and future goals. *Curr Opin Rheumatol, 18*(5), 482-489.

Prahalad, S. (2004). Genetics of juvenile idiopathic arthritis: an update. *Curr Opin Rheumatol, 16*(5), 588-594.

Prahalad, S., Shear, E.S., Thompson, S.D., et al. (2002). Increased prevalence of familial autoimmunity in simplex and multiplex families with juvenile rheumatoid arthritis. *Arthritis Rheum, 46*(7), 1851-1856.

Prieur, A.F. (2004). Rheumatoid factor negative polyarthritis in children. In D.A. Isenberg, P.J. Maddison, P. Woo, et al. (Eds.), *Oxford Textbook of Rheumatology*, (3rd ed.). Oxford: Oxford University Press.

Puhakka, K.B., Jurik, A.G., Egund, N., et al. (2003). Imaging of sacroiliitis in early seronegative spondyloarthropathy. *Acta Radiol, 44*(2), 218-229.

Raphoff, M. (2002). Assessing and enhancing adherence to medical regimens for juvenile rheumatoid arthritis. *Pediatr Ann, 31*(6), 373-379.

Ravelli, A., & Martini, A. (2007) Juvenile idiopathic arthritis. *Lancet, 369*(9563), 767-778.

Rouster-Stevens, K., Nageswaran, S., Arcury, T., et al. (2008). How do parents of children with juvenile idiopathic arthritis (JIA) perceive their therapies? *BCM Complement Altern Med., 8*, 25. Published online June 2, 2008.

Ruperto, N., Lovell, D.J., Cuttica, R., et.al (2007). A randomized, placebo-controlled trial of infliximab plus methotrexate for treatment of polyarticular-course juvenile rheumatoid arthritis. *Arthritis Rheum, 56*(9), 3096-3106.

Ruperto, N., Ravelli, A., Castell, E., et al. (2006). Cyclosporine A in juvenile idiopathic arthritis. Results of the PRCSG/PRINTO phase IV post marketing surveillance study. *Clin Exp Rheumatol, 24*(5), 599-605.

Rusconi, R., Corona, F., Grassi, A., et al. (2003). Age at menarche in juvenile rheumatoid arthritis. *J Pediatr Endocrinol Metab, 16*(Suppl 2), 285-288.

Saurenmann, R.K., Rose, J.B., Tyrrell, P., et al. (2007). Epidemiology of juvenile idiopathic arthritis in a multiethnic cohort: Ethnicity as a risk factor. *Arthritis Rheum, 56*(6), 1974-1984.

Savioli, C., Silva, C.A., Ching, L.H., et al. (2004). Dental and facial characteristics of patients with juvenile idiopathic arthritis. *Rev Hosp Clin Fac Med Sao Paulo, 59*(3), 93-98.

Saxena, N., Aggarwal, A., & Misra, R. (2005). Elevated concentrations of monocyte derived cytokines in synovial fluid of children with enthesitis-related arthritis and polyarticular types of juvenile idiopathic arthritis. *J Rheumatol, 32*(7), 1349-1353.

Schäd, S.G., Kraus, A., Haubitz, I., et al. (2007). Early onset pauciarticular arthritis is the major risk factor for naproxen-induced pseudoporphyria in juvenile idiopathic arthritis. *Arthritis Res Ther, 9*(1), R10.

Schanberg, L., Anthony, K.K., Gil, K.M., et al. (2003). Daily pain and symptoms in children with polyarticular arthritis. *Arthritis Rheum, 48*(5), 1390-1397.

Shaw, K.L., Southwood, T.R., McDonagh, et al. (2004). Developing a programme of transitional care for adolescents with juvenile idiopathic arthritis: Results of a postal survey. *Rheumatology, 43*(2), 211-219.

Sherry, D.D., Mellins, E.D., Sandborg, C.I., et al. (2004). Juvenile idiopathic arthritis. In D.A. Isenberg, P.J. Maddison, P. Woo, et al. (Eds.), *Oxford Textbook of Rheumatology* (3rd ed.). Oxford: Oxford University Press.

Sibinga, E.M., Ottolini, M.C., Duggan, A.K., et al. (2004). Parent-pediatrician communication about complementary and alternative medicine use for children. *Clin Pediatr*, *43*(4), 367-373.

Simon, L., Lipman, A., Jacox, A., et al. (2002). *Guideline for the Management of Arthritis Pain in Osteoarthritis, Rheumatoid Arthritis, and Juvenile Chronic Arthritis, APS Clinical Practice Guidelines Series, No. 2.* Glenview, IL: American Pain Society.

Singh-Grewal, D., Schneider, R., Bayer, N., et al. (2006). Predictors of disease course and remission in systemic juvenile idiopathic arthritis. *Arthritis Rheum*, *54*(5), 1595-1601.

Singh-Grewal, D., Schneiderman-Walker, J., Wright, V., et al. (2007). The effects of vigorous exercise training on physical function in children with arthritis: A randomized, controlled, single-blinded trial. *Arthritis Rheum*, *57*(7), 1202-1210.

Skyttä, E., Savolainen, A., Kautiainen, H., et al. (2005). Stapling of knees with valgus deformity in children with juvenile chronic arthritis. *Clin Exp Rheumatol*, *23*(2), 270-272.

Spencer, C.H., & Bernstein, B.H. (2002). Hip disease in juvenile rheumatoid arthritis. *Curr Opin Rheumatol*, *14*(2), 536-541.

Stoll, M.L., & Nigrovic, P.A. (2006). Subpopulations within juvenile psoriatic arthritis: a review of the literature. *Clin Dev Immunol*, *13*(2-4), 377-380.

Stoll, M.L., Zurakowski, D., Nigrovic, L.E., et al. (2006). Patients with juvenile psoriatic arthritis comprise two distinct populations. *Arthritis Rheum*, *54*(11), 3564-3572.

Sullivan, K. (2005). Inflammation in juvenile idiopathic arthritis. *Pediatr Clin North Am*, *52*(2), 335-357.

Thastum, M., Herlin, T., & Zachariae, R. (2005). Relationship of pain-coping strategies and pain specific beliefs to pain experience in children with juvenile idiopathic arthritis. *Arthritis Rheum*, *53*(2), 178-184.

Thompson, S.D., Moraldo, M.D., Guyer, L., et al (2004). A genome-wide scan for juvenile rheumatoid arthritis in affected sibpair families provides evidence of linkage. *Arthritis Rheum*, *50*(9), 2920-2930.

Turkcapar, N., Toruner, M., Soykan, I., et al. (2006). The prevalence of extraintestinal manifestations and HLA associations in patients with inflammatory bowel disease. *Rheumatol Int*, *26*(7), 663-668.

Tynjälä, P., Lindahl, P., Pittonkanen, V., et al. (2007). Infliximab and etanercept in the treatment of chronic uveitis associated with refractory juvenile idiopathic arthritis. *Ann Rheum Dis*, *66*(4), 548-550.

van Brussel, M., Lelieveld, O.T., and van der Net, J., et al. (2007). Aerobic and anaerobic exercise capacity in children with juvenile idiopathic arthritis. *Arthritis Rheum*, *57*(6), 891-897.

Walco, G.A., Varni, J., & Ilowite, N.T. (1992). Cognitive-behavioral pain management in children with juvenile rheumatoid arthritis. *Pediatrics*, *89*(6), 1075-1089.

Weber, P., Brune, T., Ganser, G., et al. (2003). Gastrointestinal symptoms and permeability in patients with juvenile idiopathic arthritis. *Clin Exp Rheumatol*, *21*(5), 657-662.

Weiss, J.E., & Ilowite, N.T. (2007). Juvenile idiopathic arthritis. *Rheum Dis Clin North Am*, *33*(3), 441-470.

Welbury, R.R., Thomason, J.M., Fitzgerald, J.L., et al. (2003). Increased prevalence of dental caries and poor oral hygiene in juvenile idiopathic arthritis. *Rheumatology*, *42*(12), 1445-1451.

White, P. (2003). Clinical features of juvenile rheumatoid arthritis. In M.C. Hochberg, A.J. Silman, J.S. Smolen, et al. (Eds.), *Rheumatology*, (3rd ed.). London: Mosby.

Witt, J.D., & Swann, M. (2004) Surgery in children. In D.A. Isenberg, P.J. Maddison, P. Woo, et al. (Eds.), *Oxford Textbook of Rheumatology* (3rd ed.). Oxford: Oxford University Press.

Yokota, S., Imagawa, T., Mori, M., et al. (2008). Efficacy and safety of tocilizumab in patients with systemic-onset juvenile idiopathic arthritis: A randomized, double-blind, placebo-controlled, withdrawal phase III trial. *Lancet*, *371*(9617), 998-1006.

32 Kidney Disease, Chronic

Melanie S. Klein

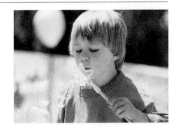

Etiology

Early recognition and management of renal failure is essential to minimize its potentially devastating consequences. Causes of chronic kidney disease (CKD) are varied and can be broadly categorized as (1) congenital, hereditary, or cystic diseases; (2) obstructive uropathy, glomerulonephritis; (3) secondary glomerulonephritis and vasculitis; (4) interstitial nephritis and pyelonephritis; (5) diabetes; (6) hypertension; and (7) malignancies. Children younger than 5 years of age most commonly present with congenital abnormalities, whereas older children are more likely to present with acquired diseases such as various forms of glomerulonephritis or inherited disorders (Vogt & Avner, 2007). Hypertensive nephrosclerosis and diabetic nephropathy, the most common causes of renal failure in adults, are rare in children.

In recent years, academic research has focused on the study of the genetic origin and expression of a variety of diseases. The goal of genetic research is to provide new opportunities for diagnosis, treatment, and ultimately prevention of certain medical conditions. This trend in molecular study has not eluded the renal community. In fact, research is increasingly being focused on determining the genetic basis for certain renal diseases in pediatric and adult patient populations. Examples of pediatric kidney diseases on which genetic research has been focused include but are not limited to the following: Wilm's tumor, focal segmental glomerulosclerosis (FSGS), Alport's syndrome, and polycystic kidney disease (PKD).

Wilm's tumor, a rapidly developing tumor of the kidney, usually affects children younger than 6 years and is now thought to be associated with the expression of the *WT1, WT2,* or *WT3* tumor suppressor genes (Khoury, 2005; Ghanemn, van Steenbruge, Nijman et al, 2005).

Focal segmental glomerulosclerosis, the most common cause of acquired CKD in children, is a major cause of idiopathic steroid–resistant nephritic syndrome and often progresses to end-stage kidney disease. It can also occur secondary to human immunodeficiency virus (HIV) disease and obesity. It is characterized by significant proteinuria, decreased serum albumin levels, elevated cholesterol and triglyceride levels, normal C3 and C4 complement levels, and edema. Approximately 20% of children with FSGS respond to prednisone treatment, but the disease is often progressive and leads to end-stage renal disease (ESRD) in most children. Individuals affected by FSGS display variable disease progression and responses to treatment. Genetic mutations have been identified within the nephrin gene, assisting researchers to identify specific gene mutations involved in the pathologic process (Vogt & Avner, 2007; Reidy & Kaskel, 2007).

Alport's syndrome is a genetic defect of glomerular basement membranes that results in hematuria and can lead to ESRD. High-frequency sensorineural deafness and ocular defects are also associated with Alport's syndrome. Because it is carried on the X chromosome, males have more severe disease than females, and although it usually progresses to ESRD in adulthood, it can occur during adolescence (Lau &Wyatt, 2005).

PKD is a genetic disorder that takes two major forms: autosomal dominant polycystic kidney disease (ADPKD) and autosomal recessive polycystic kidney disease (ARPKD). ADPKD is caused by a mutation in one of two genes, *PKD-1* and *PKD-2*. ARPKD, which occurs less frequently, is caused by mutations in a single gene: polycystic kidney and hepatic disease 1 *(PKHD-1).* Both forms can result in pediatric renal failure as a result of cyst formation; however, ADPKD typically occurs later in life, whereas ARPKD is typically diagnosed in infancy or in early childhood and approximately 50% of affected children who survive the neonatal period progress to ESRD within the first decade of life (Avner & Sweeney, 2006). The identification of a gene mutation in a patient with polycystic kidneys can identify which form of the disease is present. In addition, differentiating between ADPKD and ARPKD has important implications for genetic counseling of the affected families.

Active research involving the genetic link between these and other renal diseases is currently under way. The hopes are that this research will lead to new diagnostic, therapeutic, and preventative approaches to managing children with renal failure.

Incidence and Prevalence

In the most comprehensive collection of data available, the United States Renal Data System (USRDS, 2007) identified 104,927 newly diagnosed individuals with ESRD in the United States in 2005. Children up to 19 years of age beginning treatment for ESRD comprised 1.3% (i.e., 1325) of this total. Over the past decade, the number of new cases of pediatric ESRD (<19 years) has increased from a total of 1161 children in 1995 to 1325 children in 2005 and the incidence increases with age. Males have a higher incidence and prevalence of CKD than females in all age groups—but especially in the age group of children younger than 5 years because congenital renal disorders are more common in males. As of December 2005, point prevalence counts estimated 514,688 people of all ages with ESRD, with children up to 19 years of age representing 1.4% of the total (USRDS).

Diagnostic Criteria

Staging of Chronic Renal Failure

Assessment of the glomerular filtration rate (GFR) is the most important test for determining kidney function. GFR is a good indicator for CKD. In children, the Schwartz formula is used to determine GFR (expressed in mL/min/1.73 m²). This formula takes

---

BOX 32-1

Schwartz Formula for Calculating Creatinine Clearance

GFR (mL/min/1.73 m^2) = k (Height)/serum creatinine
- k = Constant
  - k = 0.33 in premature infants
  - k = 0.45 in term infants to 1-year-old
  - k = 0.55 in children to 13 years and adolescent females
  - k = 0.65 in adolescent males
- Height in cm
- Serum creatinine in mg/dL

---

into account the child's age and weight in addition to the serum creatinine level (Box 32-1).

CKD is a broadly used term and may be described in four stages. Stage 1 is asymptomatic and corresponds to a GFR of equal to or greater than 90 mL/min/1.73 m^2. Children in stage 2 have a GFR between 60 and 89 mL/min/1.73 m^2. The diagnosis of CKD is made when there is documented kidney damage or the GFR is <60 for 3 months. Stage 3 corresponds to a GFR of 30 to 59 mL/min/1.73 m^2; laboratory features of this stage include hyperkalemia, hyperphosphatemia, hypocalcemia, and anemia. Renal osteodystrophy (ROD) and rickets can also begin to appear. A severe decrease in GFR is noted in stage 4, which correlates with a GFR of 15 to 29 mL/min/1.73 m^2. Abnormalities noted in stage 4 often include metabolic acidosis, anemia, and reduction in appetite. Stage 5 disease is considered kidney failure and is associated with a GFR of <15 mL/min/1.73 m^2. Severe clinical, laboratory, and radiologic abnormalities can be seen and renal replacement therapy (RRT) by dialysis or transplantation is usually initiated (National Kidney Foundation [NKF], 2002; Kraut, 2007; Vogt & Avner, 2007).

Children with congenital disorders or whose renal disease begins in infancy are at greatest risk for significant growth failure and progression to ESRD. Children with congenital renal anomalies often also have abnormalities of other organ systems according to the period of embryonic development and gestational stage at which the problem occurred. Genetic counseling is recommended for future family planning.

Early detection of renal failure and the establishment of the exact cause of CKD is important for the following reasons: (1) timely surgical intervention, as early as in utero, is possible in some congenital obstructive disorders, minimizing the amount of renal damage acquired prenatally; (2) disorders may require different treatments and have varying prognoses; (3) genetic counseling and early diagnosis and treatment of similarly affected siblings should be initiated if a hereditary or metabolic disease is involved; and (4) the timing and donor selection for renal transplantation may be altered in diseases with a high incidence of recurrence in renal allografts. Unfortunately, it is not always possible to determine the cause, especially when a child is already experiencing CKD. A renal biopsy may be indicated for diagnosis and/or prognosis and treatment recommendations.

Clinical Manifestations at Time of Diagnosis

Symptoms at the time of diagnosis vary depending on the primary renal disease and the amount of residual renal function (RRF). Children with CKD may exhibit a few or many common signs and symptoms of renal failure.

Clinical Manifestations at Time of Diagnosis

- Fluid and electrolyte and acid-base abnormalities
  - Hyperkalemia
  - Fluid volume overload
  - Sodium imbalance
- Metabolic abnormalities
  - Alterations in calcium and phosphorus
  - Increased secretion of parathyroid hormone
- Hormone alteration
  - Decreased production of erythropoietin
  - Blood pressure may be elevated
- Uremia
  - Decreased energy, increased fatigue
  - In severe uremia: congestive heart failure, pericarditis, GI bleeding, and encephalopathy may occur
- Growth retardation

Fluid, Electrolyte, and Acid-Base Abnormalities

As renal function decreases, solute, fluid, and toxins accumulate in the blood (i.e., uremia). Alterations in calcium, phosphorus, and acid-base metabolism begin to develop. Impairment of bicarbonate resorption and decreased acid and ammonia excretion lead to metabolic acidosis. Hyperkalemia occurs as a result of excessive potassium intake, metabolic acidosis, and reduced renal excretion and—if untreated—can be fatal, causing peaked T waves, flattened P waves, and widened QRS complex; this scenario typically signals the onset of ventricular fibrillation and, potentially, cardiac arrest (Raja & Coletti, 2006). Hypokalemia, although less common, can result from the use of diuretics or be caused by tubular defects, such as renal tubular acidosis (Vogt & Avner, 2007).

Most children with CKD retain the ability to maintain sodium and water balance. Children with hypertension, edema, or heart failure may require a sodium-restricted diet and/or diuretic therapy to control symptoms of fluid overload. Infants and young children with congenital renal abnormalities (e.g., hypoplasia, dysplasia, and obstructive uropathy) can produce a "salt-wasting state" so severe that it impairs growth. In children with salt-losing nephropathy, serum sodium levels may remain within normal limits because of volume contraction, but often high-volume, low-caloric density feeding with sodium supplementation is needed to maintain a healthy sodium and fluid balance (Vogt & Avner, 2007).

Metabolic Abnormalities

Decreased kidney function results in the retention of phosphate wastes, which results in elevated serum phosphorus levels. Hyperphosphatemia causes calcium resorption from bone and increased stimulation by the parathyroid gland to secrete more parathyroid hormone (PTH) to enhance phosphate excretion and leads to calcium-phosphate deposition in the renal interstitium and blood vessels. Serum levels of 1,25-dihydroxycholecalciferol decrease as GFR worsens. Active vitamin D deficiency decreases intestinal calcium absorption and impairs the skeletal response to PTH, further promoting mild hypocalcemia. This circular mechanism ultimately results in secondary hyperparathyroidism. Vitamin D deficiency also promotes PTH secretion, causing additional bone resorption. Disturbance in the calcium-phosphorus-bone metabolism relationship causes ROD. In children, ROD resembles rickets. Bone deformities, bone pain, muscle weakness, slipped capital femoral epiphyses, and subperiosteal resorption of bone with widening of the metaphyses are commonly seen (Vogt & Avner, 2007). Of particular concern is the development of cardiovascular calcifications that result from hyperphosphatemia with an increased calcium-phosphorus product (Mitsnefes, 2008; Goodman, 2005; Vogt & Avner, 2007).

Hormone Alteration

At least 90% of all erythropoietin (EPO) is produced in the kidney; consequently, renal failure causes a deficiency in EPO. In utero, the liver is the primary source for EPO production. After birth, peritubular interstitial cells in the kidney assume this function. The decreased oxygen supply within those cells causes increased production of EPO. In kidney failure, the GFR is reduced, leading to decreased energy consumption and causing a relative excess of oxygen, thereby causing a decreased production of EPO (Koshy & Geary, 2008). EPO deficiency in addition to iron, vitamin B_{12}, and/or folic acid deficiencies, and a shorter life span of red blood cells (RBCs), result in anemia and its manifestations (Vogt & Avner, 2007). Excessive renin production, coupled with volume overload, may lead to hypertension in children with CKD (Vogt & Avner).

Uremia

The inability of the kidneys to rid the body of nitrogenous wastes leads to a syndrome called *uremia*. Uremia is defined as symptomatic renal failure associated with metabolic events and complications (Raja & Coletti, 2006). A child with CKD may initially exhibit a loss of normal energy and increased fatigue on exertion. Such fatigue often develops gradually and goes unnoticed. These children may prefer sedentary activities to active play. Physical examination may reveal a slightly listless, pale child whose hemoglobin is low. Blood pressure may be elevated or normal. Secondary amenorrhea is common in adolescent girls. Urine output may remain normal or decrease in volume but with decreased solute clearance.

As renal failure worsens, its manifestations become more pronounced. Children become more fatigued and uninterested in play, have a poor appetite, and are less capable of accomplishing schoolwork as their attention span diminishes and memory becomes erratic from toxin accumulation. Anemia worsens and calcium-phosphorus levels become increasingly unbalanced, accelerating the development of ROD. Symptoms of severe uremia can include congestive heart failure, pericarditis, uremic pleuritis, encephalopathy, and gastrointestinal (GI) bleeding (Raja & Coletti, 2006).

Growth Retardation

Growth retardation is a significant consequence of chronic renal failure (CRF) in children and is the symptom that occasionally leads to the diagnosis of renal disease. At the time of dialysis initiation, children with ESRD are, on average, approximately 1.6 standard deviations (SDs) below the mean height for their age and the deficit worsens to almost 2 SDs below the mean at 24 months after starting dialysis. Growth retardation is more pronounced in younger children and males with ESRD (North American Pediatric Renal Transplant Cooperative Study [NAPRTCS], 2007).

Treatment

Treatment goals include restoring and maintaining the child's health and improving growth and developmental level of function to the highest degree possible. As significant psychosocial, emotional, and financial stressors accompany chronic medical conditions, the child and family should be provided with psychological and emotional support from a specialized and multidisciplinary renal team. Treatment is based on the severity of the clinical manifestations of CKD. Approaches include conservative medical management and—eventually—RRT.

Treatment

Conservative Management
- Fluid, electrolyte, and blood pressure control
- Anemia management
- Metabolic control and calcium and phosphate homeostasis
- Managing growth retardation

Renal Replacement Therapy (RRT)
- Peritoneal dialysis (CAPD, CCPD, or NIPD)
- Hemodialysis
- Transplantation

Conservative Management

Fluid, Electrolyte, and Blood Pressure Control. Early recognition and management of biochemical imbalances may prevent adverse consequences. Fluid overload and hypertension may be controlled by limiting total fluid intake to total output volume plus insensible losses, restricting salt intake, and using diuretic and antihypertensive medications. The control of hypertension limits damage to the renal arterioles and slows the progression of CKD. Thiazide and loop diuretics help control the volume-dependent hypertension in CKD, although thiazides are effective only in children with a GFR >30% of normal. In stages 4 and 5, furosemide should be the preferred drug (Hadtstein & Schaefer, 2007). Although central alpha-agonists, beta blockers, peripheral vasodilators, calcium channel blockers, angiotensin-receptor blockers, and angiotensin-converting enzyme (ACE) inhibitors are groups of drugs available for CKD-associated hypertension, some of these drugs are not acceptable for use in young children. Hypertension must be controlled primarily by, or in consultation with, a pediatric nephrologist.

Hyperkalemia can be controlled through dietary restriction of high-potassium foods, use of bicarbonate for intracellular mobilization and acidosis prevention, and use of sodium polystyrene (Kayexalate, 1 g/kg/dose) to remove potassium from the body (Vogt & Avner, 2007). Metabolic acidosis may be controlled by use of alkalinizing medications (e.g., sodium citrate [Bicitra] or sodium bicarbonate tablets).

Anemia Management. Treatment is aimed at increasing RBC production and decreasing RBC loss. Administration of synthetic human recombinant erythropoietin (r-HuEPO, epoetin alfa, [Epogen, Procrit]; EPO, or darbepoetin alfa [Aranesp]) produced by recombinant DNA technology is the gold standard for treatment of anemia associated with CKD. Depending on the drug used, the current stage of renal failure, and desired hematocrit level, dosing can be given one to three times per week for EPO and one to four times per month for darbepoetin. The dose must be carefully titrated to prevent a rapid rise in hematocrit and possible hypertensive crisis (Vogt & Avner, 2007). As the desired erythropoiesis is achieved, iron stores become depleted. Iron supplementation (oral or intravenous) is usually required. The current goal of iron therapy is to maintain transferring saturation levels >20% and serum ferritin at >100 ng/mL (Koshy & Geary, 2008). With the advent of hormone replacement, blood transfusions are rarely recommended. Risks associated with transfusions are increased risk of acquiring viral or bacterial infections, hemolytic transfusion reactions, administrator error, and transfusion-related lung injury (Goodnough, 2005). If transfusions are required, filtered and washed leukocyte-poor RBC mass is usually preferred over whole blood. Oral therapy is often the initial route of iron supplementation, but a lack of therapeutic response secondary to decreased poor absorption, poor medication adherence, and GI side effects may warrant a change to intravenous iron supplementation. Transferrin saturation and ferritin levels should be monitored, along with RBC indices. Expected results include an increased slowing of disease progression, increased energy, decreased risk of hospitalization and mortality, and increased physical performance and school attendance (Koshy & Geary, 2008). Refer to the "Anemia" section of the NKF's Kidney Disease Outcome Quality Initiative (K/DOQI) Guidelines for further discussion (NKF, 2006b).

Metabolic Control and Calcium and Phosphate Homeostasis. Control of calcium and phosphate balance prevents ROD and secondary hyperparathyroidism. Dietary phosphate restrictions significantly limit a child's intake of dairy products. Medications used include phosphate binders to remove excess phosphate from the blood and vitamin D replacement therapy with calcitriol (Rocaltrol), paricalcitol (Zemplar), or doxercalciferol (Hectorol) (Vogt & Avner, 2007).

Managing Growth Retardation. Growth retardation is a significant consequence of CKD in children and is the symptom that occasionally leads to the diagnosis of renal disease. Factors associated with poor growth in CKD include inadequate nutrition, metabolic acidosis, and ROD (Mahan & Warady, 2006).

In addition to the aforementioned metabolic factors, children with CKD have increased circulating levels of growth hormone (GH), but a reduced response to GH and insulin-like growth factor, thought to be secondary to uremia. This resistance is thought to be important in the reduction of linear bone growth, leading to growth impairment. Also observed are abnormalities in the gonadotropic hormones, which likely contribute to the suboptimal pubertal growth and development that has been noted in pediatric CKD (Mahan & Warady, 2006).

Recombinant human growth hormone (rhGH) has been shown to safely and effectively improve growth in children with CKD, and long-term therapy with rhGH can result in catch-up growth and possibly lead to a final (adult) height within the normal range. Before rhGH therapy is started, optimal nutritional management and dialysis efficacy should be achieved, the PTH level should be normal or reduced if very high, and the baseline parameters should be established for funduscopic examinations, pubertal stage, biochemical assays, and hip and knee radiographs (Mahan & Warady, 2006).

Renal Replacement Therapy

As CKD progresses into stage 5, conservative management is no longer adequate and treatment with either dialysis or transplantation is typically required. As ESRD approaches, it is important to have ongoing discussions about the future and options for dialysis and transplantation with the child (if of suitable age) and parents. Family education regarding the different modalities of therapy should commence while the child's CKD is in stage 4. Touring the pediatric dialysis center and introducing the child and parent to one or more well-adjusted families with a child treated with dialysis or who has experienced a transplant are helpful ways to prepare children and families.

Indications for the timing of RRT are individualized, with consideration given to the following clinical and psychosocial factors: fluid status, electrolyte imbalances, growth failure, acidosis, or uremic symptoms, including nausea and vomiting, anorexia, and poor school performance (Vogt & Avner, 2007; White, Gowrishankar, Feber et al., 2006). Absolute indicators include uncontrollable hypertension, pulmonary edema, uremic encephalopathy and pericarditis, and refractory nausea and emesis (Greenbaum & Schaefer, 2004) (Box 32-2).

The many special needs of children help determine the modality of RRT selected. Because of the problems associated with small blood vessels for vascular access, hemodialysis (HD) in young children may not be practical. If a family is supportive and lives a long distance from the pediatric dialysis center, peritoneal dialysis (PD) may be preferred. Children older than 13 years are more likely to start HD than PD as their initial treatment modality (NAPRTCS, 2007). Transplantation is the overall preferred modality, however, because it offers the best chance of improvement in educational and psychological functioning (Fischbach, Edelfonti, Sröder et al., 2005). For children on transplant lists between 2003 and 2004, the median time/wait (in days) to first transplant from a cadaveric donor was 778 for children younger than 1 year of age, 360 for ages 1 to 5 years, 430 for ages 6 to 10 years, and 567 for ages 11 to 17 years (Organ Procurement and Transplantation Network [OTPN], 2008a). Children may have more live related kidney donors—especially parents—available to them, which may allow for preemptive transplant, foregoing the need for prolonged dialysis. Improved technology and more effective medications promote better survival (i.e., of both child and graft) with transplantation and offer the child and family greater potential to live a less restricted life. All treatment modalities have both positive and negative aspects. The child and family must understand that

---

BOX 32-2

Timing for Initiating Renal Replacement Therapy

RELATIVE INDICATORS
- Age of child
- GFR <10%
- Primary renal disease and comorbid conditions
- Failure to thrive
- Developmental delay
- Inability to function at school
- Inadequate electrolyte and metabolic control
- Poor nutritional status

ABSOLUTE INDICATORS
- Pulmonary edema
- Uncontrollable hypertension
- Pericarditis
- Uremic encephalopathy
- Refractory nausea and emesis

a kidney transplant is not a *cure* for CKD but is another treatment approach and can be successful only through carefully guided immunosuppression management with frequent clinical assessments (see Chapter 37).

Initiation of dialysis or transplantation is traumatic for the child and family, even with pre-ESRD counseling, but the stress is worse if the child is very ill. Denial is a strong coping mechanism, however, and is supported when a child feels "well" despite a significantly elevated creatinine level.

Peritoneal Dialysis. For children who need RRT, PD is the preferred choice over HD with the ultimate goals of renal transplantation and minimization of dialysis time (Cass & Nuchtern, 2004). Approximately 60% of children with ESRD who use dialysis are treated by PD (NAPRTCS, 2007).

PD uses the peritoneum as a filtering membrane to remove waste products and excess fluid from the vascular system. The peritoneal membrane surface area per kilogram of body weight is approximately twice as large in infants as in adults. Transport of solutes across the membrane is also more efficient in children than adults, requiring smaller, more frequent exchange cycles (Geary, 2004). Access to the peritoneal membrane is through a catheter placed in the child's abdomen. Two types of peritoneal dialysis catheters are used: those for acute dialysis and those for chronic dialysis. Acute peritoneal catheters are fairly rigid and are either straight or slightly curved. They are made to be placed at the bedside. Because of technical and infectious complications associated with acute catheters, chronic catheters are most frequently used. Chronic peritoneal catheters are created with either silicone or polyurethane and have one or two polyethylene terephthalate (Dacron) cuffs, which elicit an inflammatory response in the tissue to form granulation tissue. This tissue secures the catheter in place and prevents bacterial migration into the peritoneum. A sterile solution (dialysate) of electrolytes and glucose is instilled through the catheter into the peritoneal space. Dialysate volume is calculated at 600 to 1400 mL/m^2/cycle, depending on the time of day and the type of PD. Because the size of the peritoneal membrane correlates with the body surface area (BSA) of the child, volume calculations should be based on BSA rather than weight and should consider any residual renal function the child may have (Verrina & Perfumo, 2004). Waste particles are removed from the blood across the peritoneal membrane by diffusion, and excess water is removed by osmosis. Ultrafiltration is regulated by the amount of glucose in the dialysis solution in concentrations of 1.5%, 2.5%, and 4.25%. The amount of ultrafiltrate that can be removed depends on the glucose concentration of dialysis solution used and the transport characteristics of the peritoneal membrane, classified as high, high-average, low-average, or low. The amount and duration of cycles prescribed is individualized for each child according to her or his transport classification. In other words, a child who is a "high transporter" would benefit from short, frequent cycles and a "low transporter" from slower, fewer cycles with a last fill (fluid left in the abdomen for an entire day) or a mid-day exchange (an exchange done manually in the middle of the day) (Chadha & Warady, 2001).

Continuous ambulatory peritoneal dialysis (CAPD) is a manual dialysis regimen that delivers three to five dialysate bag exchanges daily into the peritoneum, with dwell times of 3 to 4 hours during the day and a long dwell overnight. CAPD affords greater freedom because no machine is required. Performing three to five exchanges during the day is time consuming, however, and inconvenient at work or school. Continuous cycling peritoneal dialysis (CCPD) uses a similar concept but uses an automated cycler; all exchanges can be performed at night while the child and parents sleep, so the daytime is free of exchanges. After the last cycle is completed, the peritoneum is then filled with dialysate that may or may not be exchanged at some point throughout the day. Nighttime intermittent peritoneal dialysis (NIPD) is similar to CCPD, except no dialysate is left in the peritoneum at the end of the treatment.

Meticulous care is crucial with CAPD, NIPD, and CCPD to prevent contamination and infection at the catheter exit site and within the peritoneum. Current data show that this infection, called *peritonitis,* occurs more frequently in CAPD than APD and infectious complications are the most common cause of death in children receiving long-term PD. Peritonitis episodes are highest in individuals up to 1 year of age and decrease in frequency with age (NAPRTCS, 2007; Auron, Simon, Andrews et al, 2007). The key features of peritonitis include abdominal pain, cloudy effluent with white blood cell (WBC) count >100/mm^3 and 50% neutrophils; and positive Gram stain or positive culture of microorganism(s) (Auron et al. 2007; Sharma & Blake, 2008). Data from NAPTRCS (2007) indicate that placement of double-cuffed catheters with a curved tunnel and downward exit site direction helps prevent peritonitis. Despite this, the most common type of pediatric catheter in use is a Tenckhoff (Tyco Healthcare Group, Mansfield, MA) single-cuffed peritoneal catheter that is curled with a straight tunnel and a lateral exit site orientation. Ideally, the catheter should not be used for 2 to 3 weeks after placement to allow healing and decrease the risk of complications such as leaking at the catheter site (Rönnholm & Holmberg, 2006).

Staphylococcus aureus infection is the most common cause of peritonitis (Rönnholm & Holmberg, 2006). Early use of intraperitoneal antibiotics for suspected peritonitis usually resolves the infection without catheter replacement. The most commonly used antibiotics are the cephalosporins and vancomycin; however, with the increase in vancomycin-resistant organisms, routine use of vancomycin is not recommended and careful selection of the appropriate antibiotic is essential. Although treatment courses vary from center to center, daily dosing of intraperitoneal antibiotics for 14 to 21 days, depending on the causative organism, is common (Sharma & Blake, 2008). Repeated or persistent peritonitis can result in catheter colonization and require catheter replacement. Multiple episodes of infection can also lead to the loss of membrane permeability by scarring, often requiring a change to HD. Other clinical problems associated with PD include hernia development, leaking, catheter exit site or tunnel infection, catheter migration, cuff extrusion, and catheter outflow obstruction by the omentum or other intraabdominal structures (NAPRTCS, 2007; Brandt & Brewer, 2004).

PD has many advantages over HD. Because PD is performed either continuously (as in CAPD) or over 8 to 10 hours every night (with CCPD or NIPD), better control of blood pressure and volume status can be maintained with fewer dietary restrictions, leading to better growth and development. Because PD is done in the home, caregivers must be taught to technically perform dialysis; however, it is a relatively simple procedure. Vascular access required for HD can be difficult to achieve and maintain in young children. Treating a child with home PD also offers educational and psychological advantages. Seventy-eight percent of children treated with PD attend school full-time and 9% attend part-time, compared with 53% and 28% of those children who use HD. It is a simple and safe procedure that can be performed at home without the psychological trauma associated with repeated fistula venipunctures. Perhaps the most attractive features of PD is that it interferes less with normal daily activities and offers more control to the child and family. A child who uses PD can attend school every day with little or no interruption, and family vacations are easier to arrange (Vogt & Avner, 2007; Cass & Nuchtern, 2004; NAPRTCS 2007). There is, however, a down side: A common reason for PD failure is family "burnout" from the repetitive daily regimen of PD. Providing respite care may provide a solution in some cases. Nonadherence is common, particularly in the adolescent population. The presence of an external catheter can affect body image. In children with excessive glucose absorption, obesity further complicates self-esteem issues. By preventing peritonitis and exit site infections, promoting good nutrition, and assisting with the psychosocial aspects of chronic peritoneal dialysis, PD can be considered a potential long-term therapy (Mendley, Fine, & Tejani, 2001; Holloway, 2001).

Hemodialysis. HD, which is usually performed three or four times per week, offers the advantage of more rapid correction of fluid, electrolyte, and metabolic abnormalities over PD. HD requires vascular access, dialyzer, and blood lines; an HD delivery system with a blood pump and many monitoring devices; heparin to prevent clotting; pediatric nephrologists; and the specialized skills of nurses, social workers, and nutritionists. As the blood passes through the filtering membrane, waste particles diffuse across the membrane from the blood while excess water is ultrafiltrated by negative pressure into the waste dialysate. The 3- to 5-hour process is constantly monitored for pressure changes, air detection or leaks, chemical imbalance, and temperature, in addition to the child's vital signs. Blood flow rates, medications, and fluid volumes are calculated based on the weight of the child (refer to the Hemodialysis Adequacy sections of the NKF's 2006 DOQI guidelines; NKF, 2006a). Complications associated with HD include anemia as a result of ESRD plus blood loss from frequent blood sampling or accidental clotting of the dialyzer system, access thrombosis, headache, nausea, vomiting, cramping, hypotension, and infections (Fischbach et al., 2005; Shroff, Wright, Ledermann et al., 2003). Children who weigh less than 10 kg are not as well suited for HD because they require very specialized and intensive nursing expertise (NKF, 2006a) and may require up to five or six HD sessions per week to achieve adequate fluid and hemodynamic balance.

Maintaining a patent and infection-free vascular access is the greatest challenge of HD. Internal or external vascular access is necessary to deliver blood to the extracorporeal dialysis circuit for solute and fluid removal (Figures 32-1 and 32-2). Currently access is categorized in two types: permanent and temporary. Permanent access is created surgically and includes the arteriovenous (AV) fistula, AV graft, and dual-lumen catheters with Dacron cuffs. A maturation time of at least 2 weeks for a graft or 6 weeks to 4 months for a fistula is required before the access can be used (Cass & Nuchtern, 2004). After this time, the fistula or graft is accessed through a special fistula-needle cannulation. A catheter can be accessed immediately after placement. An internal fistula is preferred for children because it lessens the risk of complications (Cass & Nuchtern, 2004). NAPRTCS data (2007) show 77.3% of children treated with HD receive their treatments through an external catheter, whereas only 12.5% have access through AV fistulas and 7.6% through AV grafts. Unfortunately, many small children have

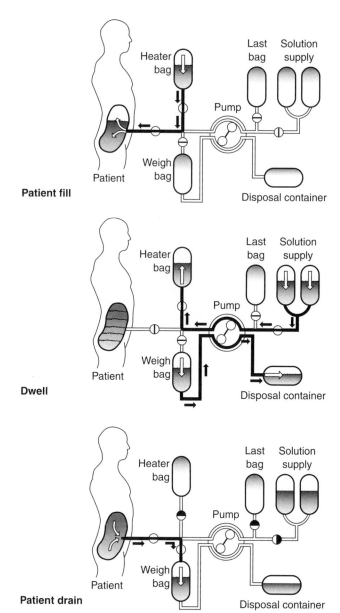

FIGURE 32-1 An example of a system used for cycler-assisted peritoneal dialysis. The solution is heated before use and weighed after use. The last bag of solution may have a different concentration to last throughout the day. From National Institutes of Health, National Institute of Diabetes and Digestive and Kidney Diseases. (April, 2001). *Treatment Methods for Kidney Failure: Peritoneal Dialysis.* Publication No. 01-4688. Reprinted with permission.

insufficient extremity blood flow to maintain a fistula or graft, and a central venous catheter may be the only option for dialysis access. Temporary access is accomplished through an indwelling central venous catheter that can be placed at the bedside through either the femoral or internal jugular veins and is used for emergent dialysis or in children who require dialysis for a short period. Failure of access, external or internal, is common secondary to infection; obstruction of the access device secondary to fibrin sheath formation around an external catheter; thrombosis, or vascular stenosis (Cass & Nuchtern, 2004). Access sites are at a premium and must be preserved because these children eventually require multiple vascular accesses. Potential problems warrant early assessment and

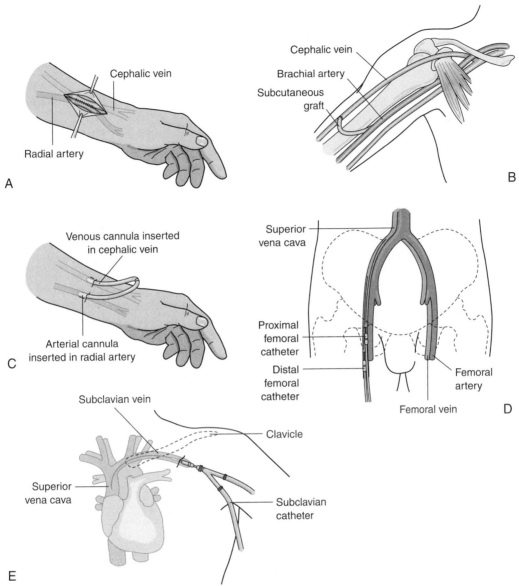

FIGURE 32-2 Frequently used methods for gaining vascular access for hemodialysis. **A,** Arteriovenous fistula; **B,** arteriovenous graft; **C,** external arteriovenous shunt; **D,** femoral vein catheterization; and **E,** subclavian vein catheterization. From Phipps, W.J., Sands, J.K., & Mack, J.F. (1999). *Medical-Surgical Nursing: Concepts and Clinical Practice* (6th ed.). St. Louis: Mosby. Reprinted with permission.

intervention. Preservation of potential access sites should begin at the time of CKD diagnosis. The nondominant arm should not be used for venipuncture. A single venipuncture or placement of an IV catheter at age 2 can render the vein useless at age 10, making it impossible to use for creation of an AVF (Cass & Nuchtern).

PD is technically easier to perform than HD in infants and small children. In many cases, however, PD may be medically contraindicated. Although morbidity and mortality are high, even very small infants can successfully undergo HD using specialized equipment and supplies adaptable to neonatal volume requirements (Geary, 2004). All medications and fluid volumes in pediatric HD are calculated based on a child's weight and medical condition. Pediatric HD should be performed in a pediatric dialysis center. If distance to a pediatric dialysis center is problematic, adolescents can receive dialysis in adult centers but risk the lack of comprehensive

assessment and therapies provided by a pediatric center. In such cases, the pediatric primary care provider's role becomes more important in ensuring continuity of care for a child with ESRD. Older children in very stable condition might be considered, on an individual basis, for home HD. HD takes time away from normal activities, such as school and play, and procedures and access care can be threatening to both the child and family. Child-life specialists and art and music therapists who provide emotional support and teach coping skills by instituting play, art, or musical therapy, as well as social workers who give emotional and financial family counseling are important members of the treatment team.

Transplantation. Renal transplantation is usually preferred for children with ESRD and, with careful planning, may be a primary therapy, bypassing the need for dialysis. Preemptive transplants account for 25% of primary transplants. Although children younger than 3 months have received transplants, that number has consistently decreased since 1996 and none were done in 2006. Live, related-donor sources accounted for 52% of all pediatric transplants reported in the NAPRTCS group since 1987; however, for transplants done in 2006, that percentage was significantly lower: 39% (NAPRTCS, 2007). Because transplantation is the preferred option and donor kidneys are scarce, eligible donors include live immediate family members; live, related donors outside the immediate family; as well as live, unrelated donors. Forty-nine confirmed transplants across ABO-compatible barriers have been done to date. This area of inquiry merits further study as the early data suggests that graft outcomes are satisfactory in those recipients whose anti-A titer history is low (1:4) (NAPRTCS). Adult kidneys may be transplanted into small children with intraabdominal placement; parents are the majority of live donors (80%) for pediatric recipients (NAPRTCS). Laparoscopic nephrectomy can allow live donors to return to work and regular activities sooner and may increase overall use of live donors. Aside from surgical techniques, careful medical management is the key to maintaining a successful kidney transplant (see Chapter 37). With a successful renal transplant, children have a better chance of achieving desired growth and development, attending school regularly, and leading a more normal life.

Complementary and Alternative Therapies

The most common complementary therapy used in renal diseases is the use of fish oil (omega-3 fatty acids) for treatment of IgA nephropathy. IgA nephropathy is one of the most common types of glomerulonephritis and can result in proteinuria, an elevated serum creatinine level, and/or hypertension (Dillon, 2001). It is thought that the omega-3 fatty acids have an antiinflammatory effect. Their effectiveness is highly debated because some studies have found that the use of fish oil reduces the risk of elevated creatinine levels and slows progression of renal disease, while other studies have found no beneficial effect (Hogg, Fitzgibbons, Atkins et al., 2006). Fish oil can prolong bleeding times, without the GI side effects of aspirin; inhibit intimal hyperplasia in autogenous vein grafts; decrease turbulence in the bloodstream, and decrease shear stress within the endothelial cells. These effects introduced the concept that use of fish oil may reduce the rate of graft thrombosis in individuals treated with HD (Schmitz, 2002).

Although no comprehensive studies have been completed, preliminary evidence suggests that a diet rich in phytoestrogens, such as soy protein and flaxseed, can slow the progression of renal disease. The mechanism of action is unknown, but the theory is that phytoestrogens may act as antioxidants, reduce proteinuria and hyperlipidemia, and stabilize the GFR (Velasquez, 2001).

Not all complementary therapies are considered beneficial and are potentially harmful to individuals with CKD. Drug-herb interactions are abundant and usually unknown to the individual seeking alternative therapy. Garlic, ginseng, and gingko biloba can potentiate the effects of anticoagulant such as aspirin and warfarin. St. John's wort affects the metabolism of antidepressants, digoxin, warfarin, and cyclosporin. In 2004, the Food and Drug Administration banned the sale of dietary supplements with ephedra as this herb had an unreasonable risk of injury, cardiovascular complications, and death. Noni juice, made from the fruit of the noni tree, has a concentration of potassium similar to that of orange and tomato juice and has been associated with hyperkalemia in individuals

with CKD (National Center for Complementary and Alternative Medicine [NCCAM, 2007/2008]; Bagnis, Deray, Baumelou, et al., 2004). Much study is needed in this area to provide safe, alternative choices for the treatment of the effects of CKD.

Anticipated Advances in Diagnosis and Management

Early Detection and Referral

The primary care provider's early detection of potential renal problems and referral of the child to a pediatric nephrologist often can prevent irreversible renal damage. Early and close monitoring of vesicoureteral reflux, including periodic urine cultures, voiding cystourethrograms to monitor degree and any improvement of reflux, and renal scans to detect scarring, sometimes can prevent permanent damage. Renal deterioration and failure may be prevented with antibiotic prophylaxis to prevent recurrent urinary tract infections (UTIs); however, with the continued concerns over drug-resistant bacteria, studies are investigating whether reflux in children can be managed safely without antibiotic prophylaxis (Bauer & Kogan, 2008). Surgical intervention is indicated in some children with severe reflux and recurrent UTIs, despite antibiotic prophylaxis. Posterior urethral valves and urethral atresia can cause severe hydronephrosis in utero and may be detected by a prenatal sonogram. Percutaneous placement of a stent, while in-utero, or open fetal surgery can be performed to decrease fetal hydronephrosis until surgical correction of valves can be accomplished, but the success rates of stent placement are only about 50% and carry high risks of shunt-related complications (Yiee & Wilcox, 2007).

Biomarkers such as GFR and proteinuria have been commonly used to help diagnose and manage CKD. Current research investigating new biomarkers, such as urinary protein excretion of very specific proteins, may better define diagnoses and types of kidney dysfunction (Lemley, 2007).

Significant technical advances in the treatment of infants and children with CKD have occurred over the past decade. More children are receiving dialysis or transplant for ESRD, surviving longer, and living with a higher quality of life. This longevity and improved quality can be credited to some of the following developments: use of r-HuEPO and GH in children with CKD via subcutaneous, intravenous, and intraperitoneal routes; greater compliance to kinetic modeling calculations, biochemical parameters, and clinical responses to individually tailor the adequacy of dialysis and improve efficiency; early and aggressive correction of electrolyte and metabolic imbalances; and prevention of associated consequences of ESRD.

Because children represent such a small percentage of the overall ESRD population, it is not cost effective for manufacturers to produce dialysis supplies geared to small children. Therefore pediatric supplies are very costly and in limited supply. Pediatric dialysis nurses must be creative and innovative to "rig" adult devices for use with children. PD innovations include various disconnect methods and design of smaller and simpler, computer-driven, suitcase-size portable PD cyclers that propose decreased risk of infection, promote easier PD exchanges, and improve quality of life. HD equipment now has computerization capabilities, allowing for more refined individualized treatment. A greater dependence on computerization will guide the future of education, communication, data collection and analysis, and research.

The Internet has made it possible for both professionals as well as lay individuals to access education, peer consulting, continuing education sites for licensure and certification updates, and discussion groups (see Resources later in the chapter). Nutritional information and recipes can be downloaded, and dialysis and transplant medications can be researched. Electronic journals related to nephrology are available for professionals and interested individuals.

Many new medications to treat problems associated with CKD—especially immunosuppressive therapy for transplantation—are being tested, approved, and released for use. Improved immunosuppression may reduce selected side effects of current medications and prolong graft survival.

Associated Problems of Chronic Kidney Disease and Treatment

Electrolyte Abnormalities

Electrolyte disturbances are probably the most common abnormalities found in renal failure. Hyperkalemia (i.e., potassium >5.5 mEq/L) is a frequent problem in CKD management, even after initiation of dialysis. Aggressive infant nutrition to improve brain growth and developmental potential may provide higher dietary potassium levels than desired. Infant formulas specifically designed for infants with renal failure can be treated with Kayexalate before use. Kayexalate leaches the potassium from the formula and replaces it with sodium. Children often find it difficult to adhere to a low-potassium diet. In children treated with dialysis, overall electrolyte control can be better established by PD or CCPD because of the continuous steady state of dialysis clearance as opposed to the intermittent clearance of HD.

Associated Problems of Chronic Kidney Disease and Treatment

- Electrolyte abnormalities
- Anemia
- Hypertension
- Cardiovascular disorders
- Neurologic complications
  - Aluminum toxicity
  - Uremic neuropathy
  - Encephalopathy
- Calcium and/or phosphrous disorders and renal osteodystrophy
- Dermatologic manifestations
- Gastrointestinal manifestations
- Intercurrent illness

Anemia

The primary cause of anemia in CKD is decreased RBC production as a result of decreased production and release of EPO and iron deficiency. Other contributing factors include shorter RBC life span because of retained inflammation, vitamin B_{12} and folate deficiencies, severe hyperparathyroidism, hemolysis, effects of cytotoxic or immunosuppressive medications, and blood loss associated with HD treatments and laboratory testing (Koshy & Geary, 2008). Treatment includes iron supplementation and administration of r-HuEPO. The goal of treatment is to maintain a hemoglobin level of 11 to 12 g/dL (NKF, 2007).

Hypertension

Hypertension is common in children with all stages of CKD and is one of the most common sequelae of pediatric CKD. More than 63% of children with stage 1 CKD have hypertension; that percentage increases as disease progresses to more than 80% of children with stage 4 or 5 CKD (Hadtstein & Schaefer, 2007).

Aside from treating the primary renal disease, proper control of hypertension is the most helpful task in slowing the progression of renal disease and reducing the risk of end-organ complications such as cardiovascular and ocular disease. Managing hypertension in children receiving dialysis includes nonpharmacologic interventions, such as exercise, reducing obesity, smoking cessation, restricting fluid and dietary salt, and ultrafiltrating excess fluid from the child through dialysis. Antihypertensive medications are used when nonpharmacologic methods are unsuccessful. ACE inhibitors and angiotensin II type I receptor blockers help to slow the rate of renal tissue injury by minimizing glomerular hyperfiltration, although renal function must be monitored closely because ACE inhibitors can quickly reduce function in some children; sexually active girls must use contraception (Hadtstein & Schaefer, 2007). Other classes of medications used include alpha- and beta-blockers, diuretics, and vasodilators.

Cardiovascular Disorders

Abnormal cardiac function associated with CKD can be attributed to hypertension, anemia, uremia, and vascular calcifications. Congestive heart failure can occur as a result of fluid overload, severe hypertension, or uremic myocardiopathy. The presence of anemia and AV shunting (from the vascular access) can increase cardiac workload and contribute to congestive heart failure. As with the general population, cardiovascular disease advances with age, but the risk for cardiovascular disease is significantly higher for individuals with ESRD than in the general population. Approximately 20% to 25% of deaths in individuals either undergoing dialysis or after transplantation are caused by cardiovascular disease (Mitsnefes, 2008). Heart murmurs are common in children with CKD as a result of anemia, hypertension, and volume overload. Electrocardiographic abnormalities are associated with left ventricular hypertrophy and hyperkalemia. Uremic pericarditis is a less common manifestation, seen with long-standing severe renal failure, and requires urgent dialysis given the high risk of intrapericardial hemorrhage and tamponade (Palevsky, 2005). Treatment of uremic pericarditis includes daily dialysis with ultrafiltration and surgical drainage of the pericardium.

Neurologic Complications

Neurologic manifestations are attributed to retention of uremic toxins. Multiple studies have noted neuropsychological abnormalities in children with CKD. Such abnormalities include general developmental delays, cerebral atrophy, poor school performance, memory deficits, and impairment of language development. Renal transplantation has been shown to improve some of these neurologic symptoms of CKD/ESRD; however, residual effects can be seen (Gipson, Wetherington, Duquette et al., 2007).

Aluminum Toxicity. A syndrome of progressive neurologic deterioration in children with CKD has been linked to aluminum toxicity, which caused speech disorders, seizures, dementia, and a slow EEG. By 1990, the avoidance of aluminum-based phosphate binders and improvements in dialysis water purification significantly decreased exposure to aluminum and its resultant neurotoxic manifestations (Gipson et al., 2007). Calcium-based phosphate binders are now used to control hyperphosphatemia; these binders are safer and more effective than their aluminum-based predecessors.

Uremic Neuropathy. Uremic neuropathy symmetrically affects the distal portions of the extremities, with the lower extremities more affected than the upper extremities. Signs of neuropathy caused by uremia include muscle weakness, a reduction in deep tendon reflexes, muscle wasting, and impaired vibration sense (Krishnan, 2007). Uremic neuropathy may be improved with adequate dialysis and relieved by successful transplantation.

Encephalopathy. Encephalopathy may be seen in advanced renal failure. Children may exhibit early symptoms, including headache, depression, fatigue, and listlessness. Hiccups, myoclonic twitching, memory loss, decreased attention span, drowsiness, impaired speech, and psychosis appear as deterioration in renal function progresses (Chan, Williams, & Roth, 2002; Wolfson & Maenza, 2002). Rapid reduction of urea from blood through highly efficient HD may cause cerebral edema, which results in the syndrome of dialysis disequilibrium. When a very high BUN level is present, the rate of urea clearance must be reduced until control of BUN is obtained. Mannitol can be given through the dialysis circuit to minimize the osmotic changes and treat seizures caused by this syndrome (Himmelfarb, Chuang, & Schulman, 2008).

Calcium and/or Phosphorus Disorders and Renal Osteodystrophy

Growth retardation and ROD are significant problems for children with ESRD. Loss of renal function results in the decreased ability of the kidneys to excrete phosphorus, resulting in hyperphosphatemia, which stimulates (PTH) production and suppresses vitamin D synthesis. This, in turn, inhibits the absorption of calcium, further stimulating the production of PTH and causing disturbances in skeletal metabolism, including high or low bone turnover lesions, osteomalacia, and osteoporosis, collectively known as *renal osteodystrophy* (Hamdy, 2007). Dietary phosphorus restriction in children with renal problems is difficult because it curtails intake of dairy products and meat. It is especially difficult to provide adequate nutrition to infants with CKD because of this restriction. Low-phosphorus formulas such as Similac PM 60/40 (Abbott Nutrition) for infants, dietary phosphorus restriction in older children, and use of non–aluminum-based phosphorus binders, such as calcium carbonate, calcium acetate, and sevelamer (Renagel), help to keep the serum concentration of phosphorus within the normal range in an attempt to prevent bony deformities and normalize growth velocity (Vogt & Avner, 2007).

Renal osteodystrophy (ROD) is a significant complication in growing children because of their open epiphyses and rapid bone mineralization. Clinical manifestations include varus and valgus deformities, fractures, rickets, muscle weakness, growth retardation, bone pain, extraskeletal calcifications in soft tissues and organs, and epiphyseal slipping of the femoral head. Development of ROD can be lessened by early and aggressive vitamin D therapy with calcitriol (Rocaltrol), paricalcitol (Zemplar), or doxercalciferol (Hectorol), as well as adequate metabolic control by diet, medication, and adequate dialysis (Vogt & Avner, 2007).

Dermatologic Manifestations

CKD-associated pruritus is a common complaint and its pathophysiologic mechanism is poorly understood. Symptoms can vary in severity from intermittent pruritus lasting a few minutes per day to symptoms that continue throughout the day; pruritus tends to be more severe at night (Patel, Freedman, & Yosipovich, 2007). As a child's course progresses toward ESRD, calcium and phosphorus imbalances can lead to metastatic calcifications of the skin (Robinson-Bostom & DiGiovanna, 2000).

Gastrointestinal Manifestations

Uremic symptoms of anorexia, nausea, vomiting, stomatitis, and halitosis improve with adequacy of dialysis and control of anemia. Many children gain weight after starting dialysis, and most who are well dialyzed and have normal hemoglobin and hematocrit levels have a good appetite and high energy level.

Intercurrent Illness

The development of intercurrent illnesses in children with CKD must be thoroughly assessed and appropriately managed to prevent further complications and promote optimal health. Infection, especially of the vascular access and peritoneum, is a frequent and common complication. Heart failure, pericarditis, pulmonary edema, and GI disease may occur with uremia. Children treated with immunosuppressive therapy, either because they have received a renal transplant or have conditions such as lupus or nephrotic syndrome, are much more susceptible to infections (Simon & Levin, 2001).

Prognosis

Although medical reasons often dictate the preferred treatment modality, infants and children can be treated by either PD or HD. With recent technical advances, small children can be more safely and effectively treated with HD conducted at pediatric dialysis centers. The use of newer medications may delay the onset of CKD in some diseases and more effectively treat problems children may encounter during HD and PD.

Advances in medical technology have resulted in the development of better antirejection management for renal transplant recipients with fewer adverse reactions or side effects. If a transplant is rejected, children must return to either PD or HD while waiting for another transplant. Unfortunately, many children develop high percentages of reactive antibodies to a large potential donor pool. Therefore the wait for a second or third transplant may be long.

Recent advances in equipment, expendable supplies technology, and medications have improved the potential quality of life for children receiving HD, PD, or for those who have received a transplant, allowing them to pursue a more normal lifestyle. The self-esteem of children affects their quality of life and prognosis of morbidity and mortality. Many factors may contribute to poor self-esteem in children with ESRD. Every effort should be made to provide interventions that enhance the self-esteem of children of all ages.

Although the long-term survival of children with ESRD has increased over the past 20 years, the mortality rate remains high. Cardiovascular disease accounts for 40% to 50% of all deaths, and infectious diseases account for approximately 20%. The overall mortality rate for children receiving long-term RRT is 30 times higher than expected for age, and the life expectancy for children receiving dialysis is 40 to 60 years less, and for transplant patients, about 20 to 25 years less than that of an age- and race-matched U.S. population (Groothoff, 2005; Mitsnefes, 2008).

Early recognition of CKD and its complications and aggressive treatment should help reduce morbidity and mortality in children with this condition.

PRIMARY CARE MANAGEMENT

Health Care Maintenance

Growth and Development

Incorporating developmental and behavioral assessments into primary health care evaluations can help identify deviations and promote early intervention. Children with renal disease may not have any clinical signs except stunted growth. Many children exhibit growth retardation at the time of referral to the pediatric nephrologist, but inadequate growth remains a problem for many individuals—including those undergoing dialysis. Except for infancy, the next greatest physical growth stage is during puberty. Children with CKD often have delayed linear growth and development of secondary sexual characteristics. Decreased estrogen and testosterone levels may occur.

Accurate growth measurements should be taken at the initial visit and at least every 3 to 4 months thereafter and plotted on appropriate growth charts for children older than 2 years. Measuring and monitoring of head circumference growth should be done every 3 to 4 months for all children between the ages of 2 and 3 years to assess neurologic potential. Children younger than 2 years should be assessed monthly for changes in growth (Secker, 2004). The weight-height index provides a measure of a child's weight relative to height and should be performed at each visit; a low index suggests malnutrition. At the onset of puberty, serial measurements using the Tanner scale should be done to monitor pubertal development. Children taking growth hormone should undergo Tanner staging every 3 to 4 months (Singh, Mulder, & Palmer, 2008).

Developmental assessment should be done with the onset of CKD and repeated at 2- to 9-month intervals, depending on a child's age and disease severity. Although the timing of milestones may be delayed, children with CKD have the same developmental needs as healthy children and must progress through the same developmental stages. To best help a child attain developmental milestones, the level of development attained must be assessed. Assessment tools (see Chapter 2) are useful in obtaining objective data. The effect of the disease process on the child's psychological status, school attendance, intellectual performance, and social development should be assessed every 6 to 9 months.

Diet

Although protein restriction may delay progression of CKD, it is not acceptable in children. In addition to growth and developmental delay in children, poor nutrition—especially with low serum albumin levels—is associated with increased morbidity and mortality. Nutritional problems are manifested long before ESRD is reached and continue after RRT is initiated. Evaluation and regular follow up with a registered dietician with renal experience is essential as part of a goal to achieve and maintain optimal growth and development in the child with CKD (Secker, 2004).

Children receiving PD experience a feeling of fullness soon after eating small amounts because of abdominal distention from the volume of peritoneal fluid. This sensation often leads to the active refusal of meals or oral feedings. Symptoms of gastroesophageal reflux are common and can further impair feedings. Protein and amino acids are constantly lost through the peritoneum because the pore size is easily permeable to albumin transfer. Children receiving PD have increased protein requirements (i.e., 2.3 to 3.0 g/kg in infants, 1.7 to 2.0 g/kg in toddlers and children, and approximately 1.5 g/kg in adolescents) (NKF, 2000).

Energy requirements are based on the recommended dietary allowance for children with increased physical activity and range from 98 to 108 kcal/kg in infants to 40 to 55 kcal/kg in adolescents (NKF, 2000). Glucose absorption from the dialysate in both HD and PD provides calories, occasionally resulting in obesity. Anemia control via r-HuEPO injections results in increased appetite and energy level and eventual weight gain, which helps reduce the incidence of malnutrition in children with CKD. Intradialytic parenteral nutrition is provided in some dialysis centers, but it is cost prohibitive and reserved for those children with severe malnutrition who cannot tolerate enteral feedings (Secker, 2004).

Parents of infants and small children soon become frustrated with unsuccessful efforts to get children to eat the recommended calories and protein. Children with renal failure are often poor eaters and more than 70% experience symptoms of gastroesophageal reflux. Supplemental tube feedings by orogastric, nasogastric, or gastrostomy tube or button may be instituted early in renal insufficiency as an important and useful therapy to ensure better nutritional intake with less stress to the family (Secker, 2004; NKF, 2000). Unpalatable additives of corn or safflower oil and glucose polymers (Polycose; Ross Nutrition) can easily be instilled by tube along with medications as needed to supplement a child's oral feedings. The formula calculation for supplemental feedings should be determined with the help of a nutritionist familiar with the special needs of children with renal failure. The current recommendation is to aggressively treat infants with caloric and protein intake above the recommended daily allowance (RDA) to help improve physical and cognitive growth.

Dietary restrictions change with ESRD modality. In HD, potassium and phosphorus generally govern the dietary prescription. Greater dietary freedom is possible with PD, and protein may be increased. The posttransplant diet also has restrictions of no added salt, low fat, and low cholesterol to prevent hypertension and obesity. Because eating is a social custom in our society and not solely for sustenance, pizza may be the favorite food of a child with CKD, making dietary restrictions difficult. Phosphorus restriction limits dairy products and most children are expected to drink milk. Fluid restriction depends on a child's urinary output volume and is calculated by intake volume allowed being equal to output plus 500 to 600 mL (insensible loss). The primary care provider should obtain the dietary management plan from the nephrology team to reinforce family education.

Safety

Although children with CKD should be encouraged to pursue normal childhood activities, some considerations and limitations must be kept in mind. Delay in cognitive and gross motor development may result in these children being academically and physically slower than classmates, as well as smaller in size. Children with CKD may become the brunt of jokes and unkind comments. In response to a challenge, these children may retaliate and attempt to accomplish something of which they are physically incapable, possibly injuring themselves and/or others in the process.

Some children require special occupational and physical therapy programs to enhance their physical ability and improve skills and stamina. Bike helmets and knee pads can be used to help prevent easy bruising. Children should be encouraged to wear a Medic-Alert bracelet or necklace to notify other health care providers of their CKD status, medication needs, and other possible complications.

Children taking immunosuppressive therapy are more at risk for infections and their injuries heal more slowly. Children with an HD internal vascular access (i.e., AV fistula or graft) must be taught to monitor the blood flow in their access several times per day and cautioned against allowing blood pressure measurement or venipuncture in their affected arm; they also should not wear restrictive clothing or accessories that can lead to venostasis and clotting. Children with indwelling central venous catheters should not be allowed to swim to prevent serious infection through the catheter (NKF, 2008). Swimming with PD catheters is controversial and may require special catheter and exit site care procedures.

ROD may predispose children to fractures or cause bone pain on exertion. Physical activity, however, should be encouraged to promote physical and mental health. Group aerobic exercise programs, camping, group games at picnics, and other fun outings are excellent ways to promote controlled exercise, encourage independence, and help raise self-esteem.

Immunizations

Routine immunizations should be given to children with CKD except for a few specific disease conditions and therapies. Immunosuppressive therapy is used not only with transplantation but also to treat some renal conditions, including glomerulonephritis, nephrotic syndrome, and lupus nephritis. Immunosuppression is generally an indication for withholding live-virus immunizations, including the measles-mumps-rubella (MMR) and varicella vaccine (AAP & Committee on Infectious Diseases, 2006). Immunizations should be withheld until a child is in remission and off corticosteroid therapy for at least 1 month (Orenstein & Pickering, 2007); exceptions are determined by weighing the risks versus the benefits on an individual basis for children who are steroid resistant or have frequent relapses. Disease-specific immunoglobulins may be given after known exposure. Varicella infection in children with a transplant is associated with significant morbidity and mortality. Reports of mortality caused by posttransplant varicella range from 5% to 25% (Smith & McDonald, 2006). Children without positive antibody titers should be immunized before transplant or immunosuppressive therapy if possible. The rates of seroconversion in children with renal failure are lower than in healthy children. However, immunizations are effective enough to warrant vaccination of this population before transplantation (Campbell & Herold, 2005). Children should continue to receive varicella zoster virus immunoglobulin (VZIG) within 96 hours after exposure to minimize adverse occurrences (Verma & Wade, 2006). Pneumococcal and inactivated influenza vaccines are recommended for children with CKD and active nephrotic syndrome because of their increased susceptibility to infections (AAP & Committee on Infectious Diseases, 2006).

Even though r-HuEPO has decreased the need for blood transfusions in children with ESRD, hepatitis B is still a risk. If a child has never been vaccinated or has received previous vaccination but has negative titers for hepatitis B antigen, the hepatitis vaccine series should be started as soon as possible so the series can be completed before possible transplant. Because the antibody response to the hepatitis B vaccine may be diminished with CKD, these children can be given higher doses of vaccine and immunized on an accelerated schedule with the first and second doses 4 weeks apart and the second and third doses 8 weeks apart (Campbell & Herold, 2005). Hepatitis B and C viral screening are also recommended in individuals receiving dialysis or awaiting transplantation (Tokars, Arduino, & Alter, 2001). As part of the transplant evaluation process, extensive immunologic screening is performed to determine exposure to a variety of infectious diseases including HIV.

Screening

Vision. A yearly eye examination by a pediatric ophthalmologist is recommended. The eyes should be examined for scleral calcification caused by hypercalcemia or uncontrolled hyperphosphatemia. The fundus should be examined for arterial narrowing, hemorrhages, exudates, and papilledema secondary to hypertension. Cataract assessment should be included for any child treated with steroid therapy.

Hearing. An annual assessment by an audiologist is recommended. High-frequency sensorineural deafness is characteristic of Alport's syndrome (Lau & Wyatt, 2005). Hearing loss can also result from use of ototoxic drugs (e.g., furosemide and gentamicin).

Dental. Routine dental care (every 6 months) and vigilant oral hygiene is recommended for children with CKD. Although is it not uncommon for physicians to prescribe antibiotic prophylaxis for children receiving immunosuppressive medications and those who have indwelling catheters, grafts, or fistulas for dialysis, data are insufficient to support this practice and the American Heart Association does not recommend antibiotic prophylaxis unless the child has a prior history of infective endocarditis (Wilson, Taubert, Gewitz, et al, 2007; Raja & Colleti, 2006).

Children with renal disease often have enamel defects. Poor nutritional intake may lead to poor mineralization of teeth. In an effort to improve nutrition, small children with CKD may be allowed to use a bottle for a longer time, resulting in deformities of the primary teeth. Use of oral iron for anemia may stain teeth; liquid preparations should be placed in the mouth past the teeth.

Drug-induced gingival hyperplasia may occur in children with CKD receiving drugs such as phenytoin (Dilantin) for seizures, calcium channel blockers (e.g., nifedipine [Procardia] or verapamil [Calan]) for hypertension, and cyclosporine (Neoral) for immunosuppression in transplant, lupus, and nephrotic syndrome treatment. Good dental and oral hygiene with mechanical stimulation by daily brushing and flossing, gingival massaging, and plaque control can contain the gum growth to within acceptable limits; however, gingivectomy treatment by surgical excision or laser has been used but has shown a relapse of enlargement within 1 year and leads to fibrotic scarring of the gingival tissue (Farge, Ranchin, & Cochat, 2006).

Blood Pressure. Three blood pressure measurements should be taken at each visit and at periodic intervals, depending on a child's clinical condition. Initiation and follow-up of antihypertensive therapy should be done in consultation with the pediatric nephrologist. "White coat hypertension" (i.e., higher blood pressure in clinics) can be reduced by use of automated monitoring devices.

Ambulatory blood pressure monitors are worn for 24 hours and can give better insight to the true daily overall blood pressure at rest and during activity and facilitate more ideal medical management (Hadtstein & Schaefer, 2007).

Hematocrit. Routine screening may be deferred if a recent complete blood count (CBC) is included with the other renal function tests. Anemia is a chronic problem that is usually monitored by the nephrology team.

Urinalysis. Routine screening is not necessary because of the frequent urinalysis done by the nephrology team. Some children with CKD have little to no urine output, so urinalysis is not indicated.

Tuberculosis. Yearly screening is recommended.

Condition-Specific Screening

Blood Work. The nephrology team regularly monitors the CBC, serum ferritin, iron, transferrin, folate, and reticulocyte counts to assess the anemia management. Serum electrolyte, BUN, creatinine, calcium, phosphorus, alkaline phosphatase, protein, albumin, cholesterol, and liver function tests help monitor renal function and treatment efficacy. Metabolic acidosis must be promptly identified and treated to prevent bone demineralization and growth retardation. PTH levels should be monitored every 3 to 6 months and correlated with radiologic findings for prevention and/or management of ROD. Fasting blood levels are best for monitoring cholesterol and triglycerides, which is difficult in small children or infants. Viral titers for varicella zoster virus, cytomegalovirus, herpes simplex virus, Epstein-Barr virus, hepatitis profile (i.e., hepatitis A virus, hepatitis C virus, hepatitis B virus [HBV], antibody to HBV), rubella, rubeola, and HIV should initially be monitored as a baseline, then before transplant, and periodically as determined by the pediatric nephrologist.

Cardiac Screening. A chest radiograph and baseline electrocardiogram and echocardiogram should initially be performed and then again at 6- to 12-month intervals to assess the cardiovascular status of children with CKD.

Radiologic Screening. Radiologic bone studies can show evidence of subperiosteal resorption of bone and widening of the metaphyses in children with ROD (Vogt & Avner, 2007). Examination of the hands and knees should initially be obtained and then again at 6-month intervals to assess for improvement or worsening of ROD and compare bone age with chronological age to determine growth potential. Bone density studies and bone biopsies are helpful but less commonly used methods of assessing bone mineralization in children. For children taking growth hormone, bone age films should be obtained yearly as treatment should be discontinued when the epiphyses close (Mahan & Warady, 2006).

Common Illness Management

Differential Diagnosis

Infections. Children with CKD may be at greater risk for routine infections and their sequelae because of a compromised immune system. Primary care providers should evaluate and manage routine pediatric problems (e.g., influenza, urinary tract or GI infections, and fever), consulting the pediatric nephrologist about a child's hydration status and residual renal function, as well as antibiotic selection and dose related to a child's renal disease and residual function. Temporary alterations in a child's dialysis program may be necessary during illness. If other common benign causes of fever have been ruled out, fever related to a dialysis access infection or peritonitis should be managed directly by the pediatric nephrologist.

Gastrointestinal Symptoms. Nausea and vomiting are common symptoms in childhood. Decreasing renal function must be ruled out in children with mild renal failure, especially in the absence of associated fever.

Headaches. Uncontrolled hypertension should be ruled out in children with CKD complaining of frequent headaches.

Drug Interactions

The most important factors to consider in pharmacokinetics are the extent to which the drug is excreted by the kidney, the degree of renal impairment, and the drug's interactions with various other medications needed in the ESRD treatment regimen.

Once the GFR drops below 50 mL/min/1.73 m², care must be taken to adjust the dosing of certain medications. Loading doses usually do not need to be adjusted and in subsequent dosing, the adjustment is usually made by either decreasing the dose, lengthening the interval between doses, or both (Munar & Singh, 2007).

Children with anemia and CKD receiving a calcium- (not aluminum)-based phosphate binder given with food or within 30 minutes after eating should wait at least 1 hour before taking oral iron because the two medications are antagonistic, compromising the desired effect (Lacy, Armstrong, Goldman et al., 2008). Depending on the specific medication, dosage calculations should be based on the weight, BSA, and/or pubertal stage—not the chronologic age—of a child with CKD. Medications that are removed by dialysis (i.e., vitamins, some antihypertensive medications, and aminoglycoside antibiotics) should be given after dialysis (i.e., at night with CAPD or in the morning with CCPD or NIPD). The pediatric nephrologist should be consulted for appropriate medication selection and dosage adjustment.

Children with CKD may need to take up to 40 pills daily, which requires much determination and perseverance for both the child and the parents. Transplant medications can total up to 6 or 7 different medications (and comprise 30 or 40 pills) and are critical to the life of the transplant; even one missed dose can cause a rejection episode. Avenues to promote therapeutic adherence must be explored with the child and family (Ringewald, Gidding, Crawford et al., 2001).

Developmental Issues

Sleep Patterns

Sleep disturbances are common in children receiving dialysis. Complaints included sleep-disordered breathing, restless leg syndrome/periodic leg movements, and excessive daytime sleepiness (Davis, Baron, O'Riordan, et al., 2005). Children of all ages should be encouraged to assume a normal sleep pattern at night. Most children can sleep undisturbed with nocturnal CCPD/NIPD treatment. An increased need for sleep and lethargy or depression may indicate increasing renal failure and should be reported to the pediatric nephrology team. Restlessness, insomnia, or cramps may indicate the need for more dialysis time or physical activity to promote rest.

Toileting

Children with CKD may be oliguric, anuric, or have normal urine output, as determined largely by the cause of the renal disorder. Congenital abnormalities, such as neuropathic bladder, posterior urethral valves, and vesicoureterorenal reflux cause malformations of the lower urinary tract and often require surgical intervention and creation of a urinary diversional system to preserve renal function or prepare for kidney transplantation (Adams, Mehls, & Wiesel, 2004). The adolescent with a urinary stoma and appliance may have difficulty emotionally accepting the diversional system and participating in peer activities. Families and children need instruction in care of the stoma and supportive care as indicated.

Even after corrective urologic surgery, some children may be unable to achieve urinary continence. Toilet training for urinary continence is often deferred until after transplant if a child is capable of urinary continence. Female children and their parents should be taught to wipe properly to prevent UTIs. Bowel training should be initiated when a toddler is developmentally ready.

Discipline

Many parents are hesitant to set limits with their child because of anxiety, guilt, or ambivalence about their child's diagnosis. Children with chronic conditions need discipline—the same as any other child. Many parents eventually realize that one of the best things they can do is treat their child like any other child. All children need to develop self-discipline, regardless of their health status. Parents need to foster development of that skill by setting limits and enforcing them by the use of "time-outs" for younger children or removing privileges from older children and granting them back as rewards as the child modifies the unacceptable behavior (Arthritis Foundation, 2008).

Children receiving HD can have difficulty accepting the painful procedure of venipuncture required for each treatment. For pain associated with procedures, management techniques (e.g., guided imagery, hypnosis, and progressive muscle relaxation) can be taught to children and their parents. Topical anesthetics (e.g., eutectic mixture of lidocaine and prilocaine [EMLA] cream) are commonly used in many pediatric dialysis centers. Involvement of child-life professionals to engage the child in play therapy helps children work through these difficult situations and lets parents or other caregivers know their unexpressed thoughts.

Children should be encouraged to participate in their care by performing achievable tasks and making decisions. Giving the child input on when and where to take their medications, including body sites for growth hormone or recombinant growth hormone injections, is acceptable. Once a schedule is agreed on, it is important stick to it. It can make it easier for the child to cope with unpleasant tasks when he or she knows when they are coming and will be completed.

Child Care

Children with CKD are not restricted from daycare. Because children receiving corticosteroid therapy are more susceptible to infections, home care or small-group child care is recommended. Daycare and preschool settings provide stimulation for learning and sharing with other children and may be a positive situation, especially if classes are small. When child care is used, the caregiver must be taught about the child's dietary restriction, medications, and any special treatment regimen. Specific instructions should be given in writing, with a telephone contact in case of questions. The nephrology team should encourage children receiving CAPD and their parents to arrange the dialysis schedule around the child-care hours whenever possible. If a child has a vascular access, those entrusted as caregivers must be given instructions on potential emergencies and actions to be taken.

Schooling

School-age children must be encouraged to attend school fulltime. CAPD exchanges should be scheduled around school activities with the least interference possible, or nocturnal CCPD/ NIPD might be preferable for school-age children. Changes in schedules to accommodate after-school activities can be discussed with the pediatric nephrology team. Pediatric HD centers should include a school teacher or tutor to help children with missed schoolwork. A dual school-home educational program may be established with both teachers communicating with each other for continuity of the child's learning. Children with renal disease may need a note to be allowed extra trips to the bathroom because of a small bladder capacity or infection, to perform intermittent catheterization, to drink more or less fluids, or receive assistance with ureterostomy or central venous catheter care. Some children need to be assigned to a school with a nurse in attendance daily, but this does not mean that the child needs to be in special education classes. The pediatric nephrology team may need to provide educational materials on specific CKD management and in-service presentations on a child's physical or emotional needs to school personnel, in addition to participating in a child's individualized educational plan (IEP) conference. Parents need to be informed about laws protecting their child's educational rights (see Chapter 3).

Poor school performance must be evaluated for contributing factors, including family disharmony. Cognitive deficits have been correlated with more advanced CKD and congenital etiologies (Gipson et al., 2007).

Adolescence can be a time of turbulence that is associated with transition, maturational crises, and adjustment (Holmbeck, 2002). Table 32-1 highlights some of the differences, problems, and interventions related to cognitive, physical, and psychosocial development in adolescents with ESRD.

Sexuality

The onset of puberty and the pubertal growth spurt is delayed by approximately 2 years in children with ESRD (Schaefer, 2007). Adolescent males with ESRD may show delayed development of genitalia, pubic hair, and testicular size and decreased sperm counts. A successful transplant usually returns hormonal function and fertility capability to normal. These are important issues in adolescent sexuality and preparation for adulthood, as well as for families of small children concerned about the ability of their child to have a normal life.

Adolescents with CKD must be counseled about birth control, sexually transmitted diseases, and acquired immunodeficiency syndrome (AIDS). Females with CKD and hypertension or coagulopathies should avoid estrogen-containing combined hormonal contraceptives because of the risk of thromboembolism (Gittes & Strickland, 2005).

Characteristics of Adolescents with ESRD by Developmental Domain

Expected Difference from Normal Development	Manifestations or Potential Problems	Prevention and Interventions
COGNITIVE ASPECTS		
Should move from concrete to abstract thinking at 12 to 15 years of age. May have excessive school absences for medical reasons and slower or accelerated learning, which must be individualized. Academic achievement is less affected with later onset of chronic renal failure (CRF). Renal failure (RF) affects acquisition of new skills, attention, and speed of processing data.	Advanced education requires greater ability to abstract, which is reflected in competency or scholastic testing and academic scores. Concrete thinkers lack the ability to apply general principles from one event to another. Academic delay may result in school disinterest and dropout. Hearing and/or vision problems may be CRF related. More difficulty in learning new skills. Attention and responses aided by good biochemical control and worsened by nonadherence.	Concrete thinkers need care plan that realizes immediate goals; abstract thinkers can work with long-range goals. Incorporate results from academic and/or neuropsychomotor skills testing to guide improvement. Encourage school attendance and participation in extracurricular activities. Encourage adherence to care plan. Encourage opportunities for responsible decision making, problem solving, and development of own beliefs and values. Help prepare for transition into adulthood.
PHYSICAL ASPECTS		
Linear growth retardation is affected by treatment modality and steroids. Decreased effect and/or production of growth and sex hormones. Delayed onset of puberty. *Girls:* 10.5 to 14 years of age, with menarche onset at about 13 years. *Boys:* 12 to 16.5 years; delay in development of secondary sexual characteristics and sexually active behavior. Nutritional needs vary with age: *Protein:* 0.8-1 g/kg needed *Calories:* 38-60 cal/kg needed Phosphorus restricted. Anemia present.	Short stature (i.e., 1-3 SD below norm). Does not follow height-weight curve pattern of puberty. Compares size to peers. *Girls:* Delay in breast enlargement, pubic hair, menarche. *Boys:* Delay in testes and/or scrotal growth, pubic hair, penile size and ability to erect and ejaculate, muscle mass increase, voice change to deeper pitch. May be underweight or overweight. May rebel at ESRD treatment regimen through dietary indiscretions, especially in peer groups. May be nonadherent with medications, especially those causing visible side effects. May develop ROD with rickets or fractures; hypocalcification by bone radiographs. Fatigue or shortness of breath from anemia.	Early diagnosis and RRT. Child and family education about normal growth and/or development and expected alterations. Encourage diet and medication adherence, physical activities and exercise, and physical independence. Consider use of growth hormone; teach self-administration. Encourage self-participation in care plan. Provide sexuality education at individual level of understanding. Encourage optimal nutrition to promote best growth potential. Encourage dietary adherence; work with dietitian to include as many favorite foods as possible. Consider meal pattern of school lunches, fast-food stops with peers. Focus on positive—not negative—nutrition. Encourage taking phosphate binders. Consider early use (pre-RRT) of epoetin alfa; teach self-administration; monitor.
PSYCHOSOCIAL ASPECTS		
Interruption of or inability to master adolescent developmental tasks; dependency vs. independency conflict; identity quest; body image dissatisfaction; peer group identity desired; future planning. Self-esteem influenced by actual and perceived image and peer response. Risk for lower self-esteem greater with negative body image, poor peer and family relationships, strong family dependence. Delayed psychosexual development.	Coping behaviors used include denial, regression, projection, displacement, anger, acting out, increased risk taking, being disruptive, resentment, being argumentative, challenging authority. Vacillates between child (compliant) and rebel (noncompliant). May sublimate poor academic performance with physical prowess. Fears peer rejection, loneliness, depression, and withdrawal despite strong need for friends and social support. May avoid sexual relationships and activity or experiment to prove sexual worth.	Promote achievement of developmental tasks; foster independence and autonomy. Allow controlled choices. Encourage activities that enhance positive self-esteem and self-worth. Encourage healthy group activities in community, school, church, camps, support groups. Evaluate self-concept through assessment tools. Encourage ventilation of feelings of sexuality and provide education for understanding. Assist in preparation for transition into adulthood.

From Taylor, J.H. (1994). *Enhancing development in the adolescent with ESRD.* Presentation at ANNA symposium, Dallas. Adapted with permission.

Transition to Adulthood

Children with CKD eventually become adults with CKD. The road to independence and career development begins before a child reaches adulthood. The consequences of childhood noncompliance with phosphate binders are evidenced by ROD in adult life. Individuals with short stature from growth retardation or bone disease may require assistive devices to drive. Hypertension, diabetes, and impaired vision may result in other long-term health problems. Individuals must be encouraged to eat a healthy diet and avoid drug, alcohol, and tobacco use. Chronic illness during childhood and adolescence can interfere with the natural maturation process.

Immaturity, together with an adolescent's sense of invincibility, learned dependency on parents and health care professionals, and rebellion or anger directed toward the illness or treatment can contribute to nonadherence to medications and treatment. The goal of transition is to provide coordinated, continuous health care (Bell, 2007). In addition, care plans that emphasize self care can help prepare teens for this stage. Most important, a successful transition is achieved through a positive mental attitude of overcoming adverse situations into successful lives. The American Association of Kidney Patients (AAKP) can supply dozens of adult role models (see Resources later in the chapter).

Family Concerns

A child's CKD affects the entire family. Parents may have to deal with the following: (1) feelings of shock and disbelief; (2) anger; (3) loss; (4) guilt at causing renal failure; (5) depression; (6) fatigue and burnout associated with constant care and appointments; (7) inadequacy at not being able to heal or fix the problem; (8) frustration with the medical establishment for no cure; (9) overprotection versus being too lenient; (10) marital stress; and (11) financial worries. Frequent trips to the dialysis center or clinic, daily or nightly PD treatments, and additional physical care interfere with family schedules, school, extracurricular activities, and outings.

Attention to family coping skills and dynamics and the behaviors of the child with CKD are important in identifying those children and families in need of extra support and counseling. Providing networking sessions is often helpful. Social support is important, particularly in adolescents when many physical, social and emotional changes occur. Child and family support can be provided by working in partnership with the child and family, strengthening positive informal social networks, and involving outside organizations to provide needed services (Pinkerton & Dolan, 2007). Families should be encouraged to continue normal activities (e.g., family outings, camps for children, and vacations) with previously arranged transient dialysis scheduling at a pediatric dialysis center if necessary.

A family's belief system must be considered. Religious practices may prohibit blood transfusions, even in life-threatening situations, or challenge that healing by faith alone is all that is needed. With children who are Jehovah's Witnesses, it may be advisable to start r-HuEPO administration early (before renal failure reaches end-stage), supplement iron stores with intravenous administration of iron, use of micro blood tubes for laboratory tests whenever possible, and use of cell-saver reinfusion during surgery (Remmers & Speer, 2006). An understanding of the family's background, religious and cultural beliefs and practices, dietary beliefs and practices associated with health care, and identification of the "primary leader" of the family (e.g., a great-grandmother) is valuable to health care professionals when effective interventions require altering a child or family's health care practices (Ritchie, Mapes, & Dailey, 1995).

Some renal diseases are linked to race and ethnicity. NAPRTCS data (2007) listed FSGS as the most common cause of renal failure in African American transplant patients, whereas aplastic/hypoplastic/dysplastic kidney disease and obstructive uropathy are the most common causes in white children.

Quality of life issues and the rights of parents versus rights of minor children are being discussed with no clear-cut answers (Levine, 2001). Some members of medical and legislative committees would argue that many children should not receive all ESRD services because of cost containment. Technologic advances in dialysis and transplant have improved the quality of life and increased life expectancy for thousands with ESRD while pacing the resources. Even the smallest, very ill infant might be treated with life-sustaining dialysis—but at a high cost. Extracorporeal membrane oxygenation with integrated hemofiltration is more widely performed today with positive results. Equipment, supplies, and professional expertise are more costly for infants with ESRD. Many of these infants have other congenital anomalies; morbidity and mortality are high in this early period. Some children will not become productive members of society, but others have demonstrated adequate growth and development with early and aggressive RRT and are attending regular school full-time and living fairly normal lives. Children with severe developmental or intellectual delays are being successfully treated with dialysis and transplantation, but they require considerable comprehensive and long-term care. Families need support as they make decisions about their child's care that will have emotional, ethical, and financial implications.

As of June 23, 2008, there were 839 children younger than age 17 listed on the United Network for Organ Sharing (UNOS) awaiting a kidney transplant (Organ Procurement and Transplantation Network, 2008b). Dialysis and/or transplant care is very expensive with American ESRD programs reaching a cost of $25.2 billion in 2002, up 11.5% from 2001, and is expected to reach $29 billion by 2010 (Warady & Chadha, 2007). On July 1, 1973, the Social Security Act was amended to provide Medicare benefits for persons younger than 65 years who were certified to have chronic kidney failure and require dialysis or transplantation (HR-1, Public Law 92-603). Because the Medicare payment process becomes quite complicated, families should be referred to the nephrology social worker for assistance in accessing available services. Additional financial assistance information is available through the National Kidney Foundation affiliates, the American Kidney Fund, and the American Association of Kidney Patients.

Resources

American Association of Kidney Patients (AAKP)
3505 E. Frontage Rd., Suite 315
Tampa, FL 33607
(800) 749-AAKP
Fax (813) 636-8122
Email: info@aakp.org

American Kidney Fund (AKF)
6110 Executive Blvd., Suite 1010
Rockville, MD 20852
(800) 638-8299
Email: helpline@kidneyfund.org
Website: www.kidneyfund.org
Free educational materials are available.

American Nephrology Nurses Association (ANNA)
East Holly Dr., Box 56
Pitman, NJ 08071-0056
(856) 256-2320
(888) 600-2662
Fax (856) 589-7463
Email: anna@ajj.com
Website: http://anna.inurse.com
Website: www.aakp.org

National Kidney Foundation (NKF)
30 East 33rd St.
New York, NY 10016
(800) 622-9010
Website: www.kidney.org
Contact the local chapter for educational assistance, summer camps, support groups, and financial information.

HCFA ESRD Networks

Divided into geographic regions, these networks are assigned to coordinate and review dialysis and transplant facilities to ensure the best possible care for individuals. Call the AAKP or NKF for the location of the network for your state.

Renal Physicians Association (RPA)

1700 Rockville Pike, Suite 220
Rockville, MD 20852
(301) 468-3515; Fax: (301) 468-3511
Email: rpa@renalmd.org
Website: www.renalmd.org

Other Online Resources

Medical Matrix: Service directory of patient education documents on the Internet, www.medmatrix.org.

PKD Foundation: Website for the research of polycystic kidney disease, www.pkdcure.org.

TransWeb: A site for transplant and organ donation information, www.transweb.org.

United Network for Organ Sharing (UNOS): www.unos.org.

United States Renal Data System (USRDS): www.usrds.org.

Summary of Primary Care Needs for the Child with Chronic Kidney Disease

HEALTH CARE MAINTENANCE

Growth and Development

- Despite advances in medical management, dialysis, and transplant, growth retardation is a major problem in children with CKD (most are ≥2 SDs below the mean height for their age).
- Accurate growth measurements should be taken at initial visit and every 3 to 4 months for children older than 2 years. Head circumference should be monitored every 3 to 4 months on all children between the ages of 2 and 3 years. Children younger than 2 years of age should be assessed monthly for changes in growth.
- Achievement of developmental milestones (all ages) is delayed; sexual maturation is delayed.
- Developmental assessment and Tanner staging should be monitored.
- Adolescent characteristics differ between early, middle, and late adolescence; areas of growth, cognition, identity, sexuality, emotionality, family, and peer relationships across the age span should be assessed.
- Ventilation of emotions; physical activity for emotional health, independence, and support groups should be encouraged.
- Aggressive nutrition, adequate dialysis efficiency, and growth hormone injections may improve growth.

Diet

- Protein and caloric needs in children with CKD are greater than the normal recommended daily allowance to enhance growth and development and offset losses (protein in PD). Glucose is absorbed in PD.
- Supplemental oral, nasogastric, or gastrostomy-tube feedings should be considered to improve nutrition.
- Dietary restrictions differ with change in ESRD modality.

Safety

- Children with CKD should be encouraged to live as normal and active lives as possible, with modifications as necessary. Occupational and physical therapy may improve skills and stamina.
- Medic-Alert bracelets are recommended.
- Immunosuppression and ROD increase risk of infection and fracture.

Immunizations

- Routine immunizations are recommended. Live-virus vaccines are prohibited in the immunosuppressed child.

- Influenza, pneumococcal, varicella, and hepatitis vaccines are recommended. Immunoglobulin is given after known exposure to virus (i.e., hepatitis, varicella-zoster).

Screening

- *Vision.* Routine annual examinations by a pediatric ophthalmologist are recommended to assess for calcification, arterial hemorrhages, and cataracts (if child is receiving steroid therapy), as well as vision testing.
- *Hearing.* Routine annual examinations are recommended; hearing should be monitored when a child is using ototoxic drugs.
- *Dental.* Routine dental care at 6-month intervals. Prophylactic antibiotics are not warranted except in a child with a previous history of infective endocarditis.
- Gingival hyperplasia, enamel defects, and poor mineralization should be monitored.
- *Blood pressure.* Blood pressure should be taken at all medical visits; frequency of measurement depends on blood pressure (BP) value. Correctly sized cuff should be used. Antihypertensive therapy should be managed by the pediatric nephrologist. Goal is normal BP.
- *Hematocrit.* Anemia is a chronic problem. CBC count is monitored by the pediatric nephrology team.
- *Urinalysis.* Routine screening is done by pediatric nephrology team if indicated.
- *Tuberculosis.* Yearly screening is done.

Condition-Specific Screening

- *Blood work.* CBC and RBC indices and folate studies, electrolytes, BUN, creatinine, calcium, phosphorus, alkaline phosphatase, albumin, ferritin, PTH, and iron are monitored regularly. Cholesterol, triglycerides, and viral titers periodically.
- *Cardiac screening.* Monitor chest x-ray, ECG, and echocardiogram every 6 to 12 months.
- *Radiologic screening.* Monitor bone radiographs for skeletal growth and ROD.

COMMON ILLNESS MANAGEMENT

Differential Diagnosis

- Routine pediatric care should be provided by a pediatric provider in collaboration with the pediatric nephrologist.

Continued

Summary of Primary Care Needs for the Child with Chronic Kidney Disease—cont'd

- Fever should always be assessed for etiology; fever related to a vascular access or PD catheter infection or peritonitis should be managed by the pediatric nephrologist. GI symptoms should be assessed for decreasing renal function.
- Headaches should be assessed for hypertension; BP should be controlled to normal.

Drug Interactions

- For all medications in CKD management, the route of excretion, degree of renal impairment, and interaction with other medications in CKD management should be known.
- Dosage of all medications should be calculated by weight—not age—of the child.
- Drugs excreted renally may require dosage adjustment.
- Calcium-based—not aluminum-based—phosphate binders should be used.
- Acetaminophen rather than aspirin or ibuprofen should be used for pain or fever.
- Absolute medication compliance is the key to a successful kidney transplant; many graft losses are because of noncompliance, especially in adolescents.
- Medication teaching should be related to child's developmental level.

DEVELOPMENTAL ISSUES

Sleep Patterns

- Increased fatigue and need for sleep may indicate decreasing renal failure.
- Restlessness, insomnia, or cramps may indicate need for increased dialysis time or more physical activity.

Toileting

- Children with CKD may have normal urine output, oliguria, or anuria. Urinary diversion may present greater difficulty for adolescents.
- Not all children can achieve urinary continence.
- Bowel training should begin when a child is developmentally ready.
- Proper wiping direction should be taught to female children and their parents.

Discipline

- Parents' own emotions may interfere with discipline of the child (e.g., overprotective or too lenient without discipline).
- Agree on a plan for medications or procedures and stick to it.
- Nonadherence with plan of care is a source of conflict.

- Children with CKD should learn self-discipline and begin taking responsibility for self-care as soon as possible.

Child Care

- The child care provider must be taught about diet, medications, special treatment regimen, and emergency measures.
- The dialysis schedule should be arranged around child-care hours.
- Children may be exposed to more infections in daycare.

School

- School attendance, when possible, should be encouraged or an alternative (home school, tutor, teacher in dialysis) provided.
- Teachers should be instructed about child's care plan and needs.
- Children may need additional school-based services to perform catheterizations, take medication, or deal with fatigue.
- An IEP should be established.
- Poor school performance should be evaluated for physical versus psychological factors contributing to cause.

Sexuality

- Delayed sexual development is common.
- Erectile dysfunction is common in males but may resolve with transplantation.
- Counseling on birth control, sexually transmitted diseases, HIV exposure should be provided.
- Responsibility toward transition into adulthood should be promoted.

Transition to Adulthood

- CKD makes independence difficult.
- Hypertension, diabetes, and impaired vision result in long-term health problems.
- Positive mental attitude is important.

FAMILY CONCERNS

- CKD affects the entire family; the goal is to strengthen the total family unit.
- Networking with the other families of children with CKD should be provided.
- Religious, ethnic, cultural, and racial factors affect adjustment to CKD and care.
- Ethical issues are closely related to economics and highly controversial.
- Health care team should practice patient advocacy.
- Cost containment has an effect on care.

REFERENCES

Adams, J., Mehls, O., & Wiesel, M. (2004). Pediatric renal transplantation and the dysfunctional bladder. *Transplant Intl, 17,* 596-602.

American Academy of Pediatrics & Committee on Infectious Diseases (2006). *Report of the Committee on Infectious Diseases.* 27th ed.. Elk Grove Village, IL: American Academy of Pediatrics.

Arthritis Foundation (2008). *Taking control. Helping children follow their medical treatment program: Guidelines for parents of children with rheumatic diseases.* Available at www.arthritis.org/ja-treatments-discipline.php. Retrieved June 28, 2008.

Auron, A., Simon, S., Andrews, W., et al. (2007). Prevention of peritonitis in children receiving peritoneal dialysis. *Pediatr Nephrol, 22,* 578-585.

Avner, E., & Sweeney, Jr., W. (2006). Renal cystic disease: New insights for the clinician. *Pediatr Clin North Am, 53,* 889-909.

Bagnis, C.I., Deray, G., Baumelou, A., et al. (2004). Herbs and the kidney. *Am J Kidney Dis, 44,* 1-11.

Bauer, R., & Kogan, B.A. (2008). New developments in the diagnosis and management of pediatric UTIs. *Urol Clin North Am, 35,* 47-58.

Bell, L. (2007). Adolescent dialysis patient transition to adult care: A cross-sectional survey. *Pediatr Nephrol, 22*(5), 720-726.

Brandt, M.L., & Brewer, E.D. (2004). Peritoneal dialysis in children. In B. Warady, F. Schaefer, R. Fine, et al. (Eds.), *Pediatric Dialysis*. Boston: Kluwer Academic.

Campbell, A.L., & Herold, B.C. (2005). Immunization of pediatric solid-organ transplantation candidates: Immunizations in transplant candidates. *Pediatr Transplant, 9*, 652-661.

Cass, D.L., and Nuchtern, J.G. (2004). Vascular access. In B. Warady, F. Schaefer, R.Fine, et al. (Eds.), *Pediatric Dialysis*, Boston: Kluwer Academic.

Chadha, V., & Warady, B.A. (2001). Adequacy of peritoneal dialysis in pediatric patients. In A.R. Nissenson, & R.N. Fine, (Eds.), *Dialysis Therapy*, (3rd ed.). Philadelphia: Hanley & Belfus.

Chan, J.C.M., Williams, D.M., & Roth, K.S. (2002). Kidney failure in children. *Pediatr Rev, 23*, 47-60.

Davis, I.D., Baron, J., O'Riordan, M.A., et al. (2005). Sleep disturbances in pediatric dialysis patients. *Pediatr Nephrol, 20*(1), 69-75.

Dillon, J.J. (2001). Treating IgA nephropathy. *J Am Soc Nephrol, 12*, 846-847.

Farge, P., Ranchin, B., & Cochat, P. (2006). Four-year follow-up of oral health surveillance in renal transplant children. *Pediatr Nephrol, 21*, 851-855.

Fischbach, M., Edelfonti, A., Scröder, C., et al. (2005). Hemodialysis in children: General practice guidelines. *Pediatr Nephrol, 20*, 1054-1066.

Geary, D.F. (2004). Initiation of maintenance renal replacement therapy in infancy. In B. Warady, F. Schaefer, R. Fine, et al. (Eds.), *Pediatric Dialysis*, Boston: Kluwer Academic.

Ghanemn, M.A., van Steenbruge, G.J., Nijman, R.J., et al. (2005). Prognostic markers in nephroblastoma (Wilms' tumor). *Urology, 65*, 1047-1054.

Gipson, D., Wetherington, C.E., Duquette, P.J., et al. (2007). The central nervous system in childhood chronic kidney disease. *Pediatr Nephrol, 22*, 1703-1710.

Gittes, E.B., & Strickland, J.L. (2005). Contraceptive choices for chronically ill adolescents. *Adolesc Med Clin, 16*, 635-644.

Goodman, W.G. (2005). Calcium and phosphorus metabolism in patients who have chronic kidney disease. *Med Clin North Am, 89*, 631-647.

Goodnough, L. (2005). Risks of blood transfusion. *Anesthesiol Clin North Am, 23*, 241-252.

Greenbaum, L., & Schaefer, F.S. (2004). The decision to initiate dialysis in children and adolescents. In B. Warady, F. Schaefer, R. Fine, et al. (Eds.), *Pediatric Dialysis*. Boston: Kluwer Academic.

Groothoff, J.W. (2005). Long-term outcomes of children with end-stage renal disease. *Pediatr Nephrol, 20*, 849-853.

Hadtstein, C., & Schaefer, F. (2007). Hypertension in children with chronic kidney disease: Pathophysiology and management. *Pediatr Nephrol, 23*, 363-371.

Hamdy, N.A.T. (2007). Calcium and bone metabolism pre- and post-kidney transplantation. *Endocrinol Metab Clin North Am, 36*, 923-935.

Himmelfarb, J., Chuang, P., & Schulman, G. (2008). Hemodialysis. In B.M. Brenner & S.A. Levine (Eds.), *Brenner & Rector's The Kidney*. Philadelphia: Saunders.

Hogg, R.J., Fitzgibbons, L., Atkins, C., et al. (2006). Efficacy of omega-3 fatty acids in children and adults with IgA nephropathy is dosage- and size-dependent. *Clin J Am Soc Nephrol, 1*, 1167-1172.

Holloway, M.S. (2001). Peritoneal dialysis orders in children. In A.R., Nissenson & R.N. Fine (Eds.), *Dialysis Therapy* (3rd ed.). Philadelphia: Hanley & Belfus.

Holmbeck, G.N. (2002). A developmental perspective on adolescent health and illness: An introduction to the special issues. *J Pediatr Psychol, 27*, 409-416.

Khoury, J.D. (2005). Nephroblastic neoplasms. *Clin Lab Med, 25*, 341-361.

Koshy, S., & Geary, D. (2008). Anemia in children with chronic kidney disease. *Pediatr Nephrol, 23*, 209-219.

Kraut, J. (2007). Chronic renal failure. In R. Rakel & E. Bope (Eds.), *Conn's Current Therapy 2007* (59th ed.). Philadelphia: Saunders.

Krishnan, A.V. (2007). Uremic neuropathy: Clinical features and new pathophysiological insights. *Muscle Nerve, 35*, 273-290.

Lacy, C.F., Armstrong, L.L., Goldman, M.P., et al. (2008). *Drug Information Handbook*. Hudson, OH: Lexi-Comp.

Lau, K., & Wyatt, R. (2005). Glomerulonephritis. *Adolesc Med Clin, 16*, 67-85.

Lemley, K. (2007). An introduction to biomarkers: Applications to chronic kidney disease. *Pediatr Nephrol, 22*, 1849-1859.

Levine, D.Z. (2001). Discontinuing immunosuppression in a child with a renal transplant: Are there limits to withdrawing life support? *Am J Kidney Dis, 38*, 901-915.

Mahan, J., & Warady, B. (2006). Assessment and treatment of short stature in pediatric patients with chronic kidney disease: A consensus statement. *Pediatr Nephrol, 21*, 917-930.

Mendley, S.R., Fine, R.N., & Tejani, A. (2001). Dialysis in infants and children. In J.T. Daugirdas, P.G. Blake, & T.S. Ing (Eds.), *Handbook of Dialysis* (3rd ed.). Philadelphia: Lippincott, Williams, & Wilkins.

Mitsnefes, M. (2008). Cardiovascular complications of pediatric chronic kidney disease. *Pediatr Nephrol, 23*(1), 27-39.

Munar, M.Y., & Singh, H. (2007). Drug dosing adjustments in patients with chronic kidney disease. *Am Fam Physician, 75*, 1487-1496.

National Center for Complementary and Alternative Medicine, National Institutes of Health (October 2007; updated June 2008). *Noni juice.* Available at http://nccam.nih.gov/health/noni/. Retrieved June 23, 2008.

National Kidney Foundation (NKF). (2000). *K/DOQI clinical practice guidelines for nutrition in chronic renal failure.* Available at www.kidney.org/professionals/kdoqi/guidelines_updates/doqi_nut.html. Retrieved June 23, 2008.

National Kidney Foundation (NKF). (2002). *K/DOQI clinical practice guidelines for chronic kidney disease.* Available at www.kidney.org/professionals/KDOQI/guidelines_ckd/p4_class_g1.htm. Retrieved June 23, 2008.

National Kidney Foundation (NKF). (2006a). *K/DOQI clinical practice guidelines and clinical practice recommendations (Hemodialysis adequacy).* Available at www.kidney.org/professionals/KDOQI/guideline_upHD_PD_VA/index.htm. Retrieved June 23, 2008.

National Kidney Foundation (NKF). (2006b). *K/DOQI clinical practice guidelines and clinical practice recommendations for anemia in chronic kidney disease.* Available at www.kidney.org/professionals/KDOQI/guidelines_anemia/index.htm. Retrieved June 23, 2008.

National Kidney Foundation (NKF). (2007). K/DOQI clinical practice guidelines and clinical practice recommendations for anemia in chronic kidney disease: 2007 update of target hemoglobin. *J Kidney Dis, 50*(3), 471-530.

National Kidney Foundation (NKF). (2008). *Hemodialysis catheters: How to keep yours working well.* Available at www.kidney.org/atoz/atozItem.cfm?id=166. Retrieved June 23, 2008.

North American Pediatric Renal Transplant Cooperative Study (NAPRTCS). (2007). *2007 Annual Report.* Available at https://web.emmes.com/study/ped/annlrept/annlrept2007.pdf. Retrieved June 23, 2008.

Orenstein, W.A. & Pickering, L.K. (2007). Immunization practices. In R. Kleigman, R. Behrman, H. Jenson, et al., (Eds.), *Nelson's Textbook of Pediatrics* (18th ed.). Philadelphia: Saunders.

Organ Procurement and Transplantation Network (OPTN). (2008a). *All Kaplan-Meier median waiting times for registrations listed: 1999–2004.* (Data report, as of June 20, 2008). Available at www.optn.org/latestData/step@.asp?; choose Category: Median Waiting Time; select Waiting Time by UNOS Status at Listing. Retrieved June 23, 2008.

Organ Procurement and Transplantation Network (OPTN). (2008b). *Waitlist: Organ by waiting time and age* (Data report as of June 20, 2008). Available at www.optn.org/latestData/step@.asp?; choose Category: Waiting List; select Organ by Waiting Time. Retrieved June 23, 2008.

Palevsky, P.M. (2005). Renal replacement therapy I: Indications and timing. *Crit Care Clin, 21*, 347-356.

Patel, T.S., Freedman, B.L., & Yosipovitch, G. (2007). An update on pruritus associated with CKD. *Am J Kidney Dis, 50*, 11-20.

Pinkerton, J., & Dolan, P. (2007). Family support, social, capital, resilience, and adolescent coping. *Child Family Soc Work, 12*, 219-228.

Raja, K., & Coletti, D. (2006). Management of the dental patient with renal disease. *Dent Clin North Am, 50*, 529-545.

Reidy, K., & Kaskel, F. (2007). Pathophysiology of focal segmental glomerulosclerosis. *Pediatr Nephrol, 22*, 350-354.

Remmers, P.A., & Speer, A.J. (2006). Clinical strategies in the medical care of Jehovah's Witnesses. *Am J Med, 119*, 1013-1018.

Richie, M.F., Mapes, D., & Dailey, F.D. (1995). Psychosocial aspects of renal failure and its treatment. In L.E. Lancaster. (Ed.), *Core Curriculum for Nephrology Nursing,* (3rd ed.). Pitman, NJ: Jannetti Publications.

Ringewald, J.M., Gidding, S.S., Crawford, S.E., et al. (2001). Nonadherence is associated with late rejection in pediatric heart transplant recipients. *J Pediatr, 139*, 75-78.

Robinson-Bostom, L., & DiGiovanna, J.J. (2000). Cutaneous manifestations of end-stage renal disease. *J Am Acad Dermatol, 43*, 975-986.

Rönnholm, K., & Holmberg, C. (2006). Peritoneal dialysis in infants. *Pediatr Nephrol, 21*, 751-756.

Schaefer, F. (2007). Growth and puberty. In R.N. Fine, S. Webber, D.Kelly, et al. (Eds.), *Pediatric Organ Transplantation*. Boston: Blackwell.

Schmitz, P.G. (2002). Prophylaxis of hemodialysis graft thrombosis with fish oil: Double-blind, randomized, prospective trial. *J Am Soc Nephrol, 13*, 184-190.

Secker, D. (2004). Achieving nutritional goals for children on dialysis. In B. Warady, F. Schaefer, R. Fine, et al. (Eds.), *Pediatric Dialysis*. Boston: Kluwer Academic.

Sharma, A., & Blake, P.G. (2008). Peritoneal dialysis. In B.M. Brenner, S.A. Levine (Eds.), *Brenner & Rector's The Kidney.* Philadelphia: Saunders.

Shroff, R., Wright, E., Ledermann, S., et al. (2003). Chronic hemodialysis in infants and children under 2 years of age. *Pediatr Nephrol, 18*, 378-383.

Simon, D.M., & Levin, S. (2001). Infectious complications of solid organ transplantation. *Infect Dis Clin North Am, 15*, 521-549.

Singh, A., Mulder, J., & Palmer, B. (2008). Endocrine aspects of kidney disease. In B.M., Brenner & S.A. Levine (Eds.), *Brenner & Rector's The Kidney* (8th ed.). Philadelphia: Saunders.

Smith, J.M., & McDonald, R.A. (2006). Emerging viral infections in transplantation. *Pediatr Transplant, 10*, 838-843.

Tokars, J.I., Arduino, M.J., & Alter, M.J. (2001). Infection control in hemodialysis units. *Infect Dis Clin North Am, 15*, 797-812.

*United States Renal Data System. (2007). *USRDS 2007 Annual data report: Atlas of chronic kidney disease and end-stage renal disease in the United States, The National Institutes of Health, National Institute of Diabetes and Digestive and Kidney Diseases.* Available at www.usrds.org/2007/ref/A_incidence_07.pdf. Retrieved June 25. 2008.

Velasquez, M.T. (2001). Dietary phytoestrogens: A possible role in renal disease protection. *Am J Kidney Dis, 37*, 1056-1068.

Verma, A., & Wade, J.J. (2006). Immunization issues before and after solid organ transplantation in children. *Pediatr Transplant, 10*, 536-548.

Verrina, E., & Perfumo, F. (2004). Technical aspects of the peritoneal dialysis procedure. In B. Warady, F. Schaefer, R. Fine, et al. (Eds.), *Pediatric Dialysis*, Boston: Kluwer Academic.

Vogt, B., & Avner, E. (2007). Renal failure. In R. Kleigman, R. Behrman, H. Jenson, et al. (Eds.), *Nelson's Textbook of Pediatrics* (18th ed.). Philadelphia: Saunders.

Warady, B., & Chadha, V. (2007). Chronic kidney disease in children: The global perspective. *Pediatr Nephrol, 22*(12), 1999-2009.

White, C.T., Gowrishankar, M., Feber, J., et al. (2006). Clinical practice guidelines for pediatric peritoneal dialysis. *Pediatr Nephrol, 21*(8), 1059-1066.

Wilson, W., Taubert, K.A., Gewitz, M., et al. (2007). Prevention of Infective Endocarditis: Guidelines from the American Heart Association: A guideline from the American Heart Association Rheumatic Fever, Endocarditis, and Kawasaki Disease Committee, Council on Cardiovascular Disease in the Young, and the Council on Clinical Cardiology, Council on Cardiovascular Surgery and Anesthesia, and the Quality of Care and Outcomes Research Interdisciplinary Working Group. *Circulation, 116*, 1736-1754. [Erratum in *Circulation* (2007), *16*(15), e376-e377.

Wolfson, A.B., & Maenza, R.L. (2002). Renal failure. In J.A. Marx, R.S. Hockberger & R.M.Walls (Eds.), *Rosen's Emergency Medicine: Concepts and Clinical Practice* (5th ed.). St. Louis: Mosby.

Yiee, J., & Wilcox, D. (2007). Management of fetal hydronephrosis. *Pediatr Nephrol, 23*(3), 347-353. Advance online publication. doi:10.1007/s00467-007-0542-y. Retrieved January 19, 2008.

*The data here have been supplied by the United States Renal Data System (USRDS). The interpretation and reporting of these data are the responsibility of the author(s) and in no way should be seen as an official policy or interpretation of the U.S. government.

33 Mood Disorders

June Andrews Horowitz and Carol Anne Marchetti

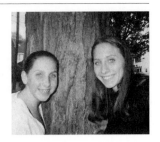

OOD disorders in children and adolescents are not a single clinical entity with a clearly determined etiology or predictable lifetime course. Rather, mood disorders include a range of mental health difficulties that feature depressed mood with or without mania and loss of pleasure or interest, and disorders characterized by mania in varying degrees with or without depression. All mood disorders in children and adolescents commonly manifest age-specific associated features. Even when diagnostic criteria for a mood disorder are met, a myriad of paths can lead to its development, continuation, and recurrence. Evidence supports both genetic and environmental contributions (Ryan, 2005). Moreover, research outcomes have indicated that children and adolescents who experience depression also frequently manifest a coexisting condition, most commonly an anxiety disorder (Sims, Nottelmann, Koretz, et al., 2007). When a bipolar disorder (BPD) is found, attention-deficit disorder, oppositional defiant disorder, anxiety disorders, conduct disorders, and substance use disorders are the most frequent coexisting conditions (Kowatch, Youngstrom, Danielyan, et al., 2005). Most important, determination of a mood disorder in children necessitates consideration of the severity and duration of symptoms, developmental factors, additional coexisting mental health and physical problems, and the degree of disability experienced (Turk, Graham, & Verhulst, 2007).

According to the *Diagnostic and Statistical Manual of Mental Disorders* (4th ed., text revision) *(DSM-IV-TR)* (American Psychiatric Association [APA], 2000), mood disorders encompass several diagnoses and their subtypes. Mood disorders are organized as depressive disorders (unipolar depression), BPDs, and two etiologically based diagnoses: mood disorder caused by a general medical condition and substance-induced mood disorder. The diagnoses falling under depressive disorders are distinguished from BPDs by a lack of any type of manic episode or features in the history. Conversely, BPDs do involve current or past manic episodes or manic features in the presentation. Table 33-1 summarizes the diagnostic categories that comprise the mood disorders according to *DSM-IV-TR.*

Etiology

The etiology of childhood mood disorders is multifaceted. Considerable evidence has accumulated to indicate that mood disorders are fundamentally the same when experienced by children, adolescents, and adults (Sadock & Sadock, 2007); nevertheless, developmental factors influence their onset, course, and prognosis. The research literature indicates that a variety of psychosocial and biologic factors contribute to development of a depressive disorder without a single causal pathway (Ryan, 2005). Even less is known

about the etiology of BPDs, although evidence suggests a strong genetic contribution (Turk et al., 2007). Further, it is likely that specific etiologic factors differ from child to child.

Psychosocial Factors

Models of depression have been developed from psychodynamic, interpersonal, cognitive, behavioral, and sociologic theoretical perspectives. No single model is adequate to (1) explain the variations across personal history, family and peer relationships, social environment, or other factors among youths who experience depression; or (2) explicate how some children with psychosocial risk factors for depression escape a mood disorder. However, several important psychosocial risks with empiric support include negative thinking, inadequate self-regulation, poor interpersonal relations, and family factors (Garber, 2006).

Negative Thinking. Cognitive theories of depression, developed in relation to adults (Beck, 1967; Seligman, 1975), focus on negative thinking as a cause of depressed mood. The *learned helplessness* model of depression first evolved from animal studies demonstrating that a lack of control over aversive events led to a state of helplessness (Seligman). In the revised model, cognitive attribution is the operative process. A negative attributional style in which a person takes responsibility for bad events and outcomes characterizes individuals prone to depression. Blaming oneself is an *internal attribution;* seeing the cause as unchanging is a *stable attribution;* and generalizing the cause to most situations is a *global attribution.* Such attributions create learned helplessness that can lead to hopelessness and ongoing depression (Abramson, Seligman, & Teasdale, 1978).

According to Beck's cognitive theory of depression (1967), biased and negative beliefs lead to faulty interpretations of life events. Problematic cognitive processing involves automatic thoughts about events based on selective attention to negative information, assumption of blame about events, exaggeration of negative outcomes, and minimization of positive aspects of events. Distortions in thinking—characterized as the *depressive cognitive triad* of thoughts about the self, the world, and the future—are thought to generate feelings of worthlessness and hopelessness that characterize depression. Rigid and enduring cognitive schemata guide information processing and do not yield to new information that could contradict negative self-perceptions.

Cognitive models of depressive disorders are useful templates for evaluation of distorted thinking and undergird cognitive therapy approaches to treatment. Clinicians who work with depressed youths validate the presence of negative interpretations of events, self-blame, and poor self-esteem. However, children and adolescents progress through developmental stages that are not

TABLE 33-1

Diagnostic *DSM-IV-TR* Categories for Mood Disorders

Diagnosis	Summary of Key Characteristics
Major depressive disorder	Presence of one or more major depressive episodes
Dysthymic disorder	Chronically depressed mood most days for at least 1 yr for children and adolescents; criteria not met for major depressive episode
Bipolar I disorder	Presence of one or more manic episodes or mixed episodes (i.e., manic *and* major depressive)
Bipolar II disorder	Presence of one or more major depressive episodes and one or more hypomanic episodes
Cyclothymic disorder	Chronic mood disturbance with alternating periods of hypomanic and depressive symptoms; criteria not met for major depressive episode or manic episode
Depressive disorder not otherwise specified	Disorders with depressive features that do not meet criteria for other disorders
Bipolar disorder not otherwise specified	Disorders with bipolar features that do not meet criteria for other disorders
Mood disorder caused by a general medical condition	Mood disturbance caused by direct psychological effects of a medical condition
Substance-induced mood disorder	Mood disturbance caused by direct physiologic effects of a substance

Data from American Psychiatric Association. (2000). *Diagnostic and Statistical Manual of Mental Disorders* (4th ed., Text Revision). Washington, DC: Author.

comparable to the adult cognitive processing on which this model is based (Mash & Wolfe, 2005). Therefore clinicians who are assessing a child for depression are cautioned to evaluate any cognitive distortions in relation to the child's developing sense of self.

Inadequate Self-Regulation. According to the self-control theory (Rehm, 1977), problems in self-monitoring, self-evaluation, and self-reinforcement contribute to development of depression. Children with inadequate self-regulation are likely to attend to negative events, establish excessively high standards for self-performance, furnish inadequate personal rewards, and use excessive self-punishment. Children with depression have shown self-regulation problems, although ongoing research is needed to provide more substantive evidence regarding etiologic mechanisms (Garber, 2006; Mash & Wolfe, 2005).

Poor Interpersonal Relations and Family Factors. Problematic peer relations have been associated with depression in children and adolescents. Negative interactive patterns, such as ongoing hurtful teasing and bullying, affect 15% to 25% of children and involve social exclusion, physical violence, threats, sexual and racial harassment, and public humiliation. Cyberbullying—electronic or online bullying—has escalated both the speed of delivering hurtful messages and pictures and the breadth of the audience. Youths who experience long-term teasing and bullying are at increased risk for detrimental psychological effects, including depression, anxiety, low self-esteem, social withdrawal, violent retaliation, and suicide (Bellenir, 2006; Health Resources and Services Administration, n.d.). Depressed youths also tend to exhibit aversive behaviors that produce annoyance and frustration in others (Mash & Wolfe, 2005)—exacerbating a cycle of rejection, withdrawal, social isolation, and ongoing depression.

The function of problematic family relations in development and continuation of childhood depressive disorders is yet to be explicated fully; however, direct and indirect family influences have been described (Avenevoli, Reis, & Merikangas, 2006). Family influences can include parental transmission of a genetic predisposition to a depressive disorder. When present, parental psychopathology has a negative effect on interactions within the family and interferes with the parent's ability to nurture, show affection, and support the child. Other family environmental factors, such as conflict, instability, substance abuse, and child maltreatment, may converge to increase the child's risk for development of a depressive disorder. Stress reaction models also have been proposed to explain how stressful life events, such as parental death, put children at risk for depression. In diathesis-stress models, individual vulnerability and the nature of the stressor interact to determine whether or not depression will result (Mash & Wolfe, 2005).

Biologic Factors

Contributions of psychophysiologic factors to childhood depressive disorders are being explored and are thought to underlie the expression of depressive symptoms. The ability of various antidepressant medications to alleviate depressive symptoms indicates that neurotransmitter systems contribute to development and maintenance of depression. In particular, deficits in the monoamine transmitters (norepinephrine, serotonin, and dopamine) and an excessive number of binding sites for these neurotransmitters are likely to be present in depressed individuals. Serotonin and norepinephrine are involved in functions of the limbic system regulating drives, emotions, and instincts. The monoamine hypothesis of depression is evolving to include the possibility that depression results from a deficiency in signal transmission from the monoamine neurotransmitter to its postsynaptic neuron, rather than from a deficiency in amounts of either the neurotransmitter or receptors (Preston, O'Neal, & Talaga, 2008).

Monoamine neurotransmitters and the neuroendocrine systems are related. The hypothalamic-pituitary-thyroid (HPT) axis and the hypothalamic-pituitary-adrenal (HPA) axis modulate reactions to stress and are associated with depression, particularly an excess activation of the HPA axis. Cortisol, a stress hormone related to depression, produces deleterious effects on the brain and arteries (Preston et al., 2008). Chronic stress may produce changes in monoamines in individuals who are prone to depression. Current research indicates that children and adolescents who experience depression may have increased sensitivity to stress rather than a chronic dysregulation (Mash & Wolfe, 2005). A cycle may be fueled by continued neuroendocrine activation related to stress that raises the risk for depression; chronic depressive symptoms may lead in turn to continued activation and repeated psychosocial stresses. Additional hormonal alterations, such as reduction in growth hormone (GH) secretion, may contribute to risk of depression in children and adolescents, and GH response may be a trait marker for at-risk children and adolescents. Whether these neurobiologic changes and dysregulations cause depression or result from depression is not definitively known (Stuart, 2005).

Even less is understood about the neurobiology of BPDs. Both structural and functional central nervous system (CNS) abnormalities are likely to be involved. The relatively positive response to pharmacotherapy and poor response to psychotherapy provide rather convincing evidence of biologic etiology for BPD (Preston et al., 2008). Nonetheless, no single biologic model is fully explanatory and further research is needed to increase understanding of the development and persistence of mood disorders among children and adults.

Known Genetic Etiology. Family studies support the existence of a moderate genetic link for depressive disorders (Avenevoli et al., 2006). Monozygotic twins are at higher risk for depressive disorders than are dizygotic twins. Major depressive disorder is 1.5 to 3 times more common among first-degree biologic relatives of individuals with this disorder (APA, 2000). Yet research has not identified specific genetic markers with high attributable risk for depression (Avenevoli et al.). Furthermore, environmental conditions likely influence gene expressivity.

Family, twin, and adoption studies provide empiric support for a genetic contribution to the etiology of BPD. Having one biologic parent with a BPD creates a 10% to 30% risk for the disorder. Odds increase to 75% when both parents have BPD. Among affected individuals, 90% have one or more biologic relatives with the disorder. Inheritance of BPD is likely multifactorial, and as many as 10 chromosomes may be involved. Nonetheless, because researchers have not identified a specific genetic marker and most individuals with BPD do not have an affected first-degree relative, practitioners are advised to continue to base their diagnoses on clinical history, presentation, and evaluation (Correll, Penzer, Lencz, et al., 2007). Moreover, as with depressive disorders, genetic and environmental factors are likely to interact, and multiple genes may have a modifying, causative, or protective role in development of BPDs.

Incidence and Prevalence

For children and adolescents, prevalence estimates for each of the diagnostic categories are less robust than for adults; however, evidence is accumulating that these disorders are serious problems for a significant number of youths, that they tend to persist and recur, and that prevalence increases with age. Preschool children rarely exhibit criteria for major depressive disorder. Overall prevalence for mood disorders is estimated as 1% to 2% for prepubertal children and 3% to 4% for adolescents within a 3- to 12-month time frame (Sims et al., 2007). Among youths hospitalized for psychiatric reasons, approximately 20% of school-age children and 40% of adolescents have major depressive disorders (Sadock & Sadock, 2007).

Childhood-onset dysthymic disorder (i.e., a disorder characterized by unremitting low-level depression) (see Table 33-1) is less common than major depressive disorder with rates from 0.6% to 1.7% (Mash & Wolfe, 2005) but may be as high as 5% to 8% among young adolescents (Sadock & Sadock, 2007). Because dysthymic disorder does not present with symptoms that meet criteria for major depressive disorder and may be more insidious or longstanding, many cases may remain unrecognized. More important, in many children and adolescents, a major depressive disorder occurs within 1 year of onset of dysthymic disorder (Sadock & Sadock).

BPD is less common than either major depressive disorder or dysthymic disorder. In pediatric populations, estimates have ranged from 0.04% to 1.2% (Sadock & Sadock, 2007). Rapid cycling of mood symptoms among children and adolescents may mask the presence of bipolar I disorder (i.e., mood disorder characterized by presence of mania with or without depression). Rapid mood cycling also may lead to higher estimates for the less severe diagnoses of bipolar II (i.e., depression with hypomania) and cyclothymic disorder (i.e., a disorder characterized by numerous periods of hypomanic symptoms) (see Table 33-1) (Mash & Wolfe, 2005); moreover, as many as 10% of adolescents may exhibit some variant of mania (Sadock & Sadock).

The recognition of pediatric BPD is increasing in psychiatric practice. Estimates of incidence are rising, and the average age of onset has fallen from the early 30s to late teens over the course of a single generation (Laraia, 2002). Diagnosis of BPD among children and adolescents has increased 40-fold from 1994–1995 to 2002–2003 (Moreno, Laje, Bianco, et al., 2007). Nevertheless, controversy continues among experts regarding appropriate diagnostic criteria for childhood- and adolescent-onset BPD.

Diagnostic Criteria

Before the 1980s, few researchers explored depression among children and adolescents, many clinicians debated its existence, and others considered depression to be part of normal development or a rare or transitory occurrence (Harrington, 2006; Scahill & Rains, 2005a). Childhood depressive disorders were not even included in the psychiatric diagnostic classification until publication of *DSM-III* (APA, 1980). Diagnostic criteria for mood disorders with onset in childhood and adolescence are set forth in the *DSM-IV-TR* (APA, 2000). Key characteristics for each of the conditions within the spectrum of mood disorders are listed in Table 33-1 and expanded in the following text.

Major Depressive Disorder

Major depressive disorder (Box 33-1), also referred to as *unipolar depression,* requires the presence of one or more major depressive episodes. According to the current *DSM-IV-TR* (APA, 2000), a depressive episode has common characteristics for adults as well as for children and adolescents. The essential feature of a major

---

BOX 33-1

Diagnostic Criteria for a Major Depressive Episode

- Five or more symptoms of either (a) depressed mood or (b) loss of interest or pleasure
  (a) Depressed mood most of the day, most days, and/or diminished interest
  or
  (b) Pleasure in all/most activities most of the day, most days
- Additional symptoms
  - Significant loss of weight when not dieting, or increase or decrease in appetite nearly every day (For children, failure to achieve expected weight gains is considered.)
  - Insomnia or excessive sleeping almost every day
  - Observable psychomotor agitation or retardation
  - Fatigue or reduced energy almost every day
  - Feeling worthless or excessively guilty (even if delusional) almost every day
  - Reduced ability to concentrate or think, or indecisiveness almost every day
  - Continuing thoughts of death or suicide without a plan, a plan to commit suicide, or a suicide attempt

Data from American Psychiatric Association. (2000). *Diagnostic and Statistical Manual of Mental Disorders* (4th ed., Text Revision). Washington, DC: Author.

depressive episode is a 2-week or longer period during which a person experiences depressed mood or loss of interest or pleasure (anhedonia) in most activities. In addition to one of these hallmarks, four or more of nine additional diagnostic criteria for a major depressive episode must be met, or an additional three if both depressed mood and anhedonia are present (for a total of at least five criteria). These criteria are found in Box 33-1. The presenting symptoms (1) must cause distress and functional impairment; (2) cannot meet criteria for a mixed episode (i.e., episode with mania); (3) cannot be caused by effects of a substance or medical condition; and (4) must not be better accounted for by the bereavement diagnosis (APA, 2000).

Dysthymic Disorder. Dysthymic disorder, also considered a unipolar depressive disorder, is characterized by a chronically depressed mood experienced most of the day, on more days than not, for at least 1 year for children and adolescents and for 2 years for adults (APA, 2000). The specifier "early onset" indicates occurrence before 21 years of age. As in major depressive disorder, mood may be more irritable or "cranky" than sad or "down." Two or more of the following symptoms are needed in addition to presence of depressed mood for a diagnosis of dysthymic disorder: "poor appetite or overeating, insomnia or hypersomnia, low energy or fatigue, low self-esteem, poor concentration or difficulty making decisions, and feelings of hopelessness" (APA, 2000, p. 377). Additional APA criteria specify conditions for diagnosis and factors for consideration in differential diagnosis by psychiatric clinicians.

Bipolar Disorders

In 2000, the National Institute of Mental Health (NIMH) convened a roundtable meeting to discuss controversial issues about BPD in children (NIMH, 2001). The participants reached consensus that clinicians could diagnose BPD in prepubertal children using *DSM* criteria. These experts identified two categories: (1) children who clearly meet *DSM-IV* criteria for a BPD; and (2) children who do not meet criteria but who may have BPD (i.e., although full diagnostic criteria are not met, these children experience severe impairment from symptoms of mood instability). For this latter group, the diagnosis of "BPD, not otherwise specified" may be used.

Mania, an abnormally and persistently expansive, elated, or irritable mood, is the hallmark of BPDs (APA, 2000). The subtypes of BPD are characterized by manic, mixed, and hypomanic episodes with and without depressive symptomatology (APA). Bipolar I disorder is characterized by one or more manic episodes with or without depression; bipolar II disorder is characterized by one or more major depressive episodes along with one or more hypomanic episodes.

To meet criteria for a manic episode, mania (i.e., abnormally and persistently expansive, elated, or irritable mood) must be present for at least 1 week. During the mood disturbance, three or more persistent and significant symptoms from the following list are required (four or more are required if mood is only irritable): grandiosity or exaggerated self-esteem; diminished need for sleep; excessive talkativeness or pressured speaking; racing thoughts or flight of ideas (i.e., rapid flow of thoughts); distractibility; psychomotor agitation or increased goal-driven behavior; and excessive activity involving pleasurable pursuits that are likely to result in problems. The mood disturbance must cause serious impairment in functioning (social, occupational, or academic),

require hospitalization to prevent harm to self or others, or include psychotic symptoms. Finally, manic symptoms are not attributable to substance use or a medical condition. Based on results of their study of children and adolescents who were evaluated for apparent BPD, Staton, Volness, and Beatty (2008) proposed that recurrent or chronic simultaneous occurrence of any two of the following symptoms of elation, grandiosity, or racing thoughts, and five of the *DSM-IV-TR* symptoms of mania will classify almost all children correctly.

A mixed episode consists of a period of at least 1 week during which criteria for both manic and major depressive episodes are met almost every day. Moods alternate rapidly across the spectrum of depression, irritability, and euphoria along with other symptoms of both types of episodes. A hypomanic episode consists of a period of 4 days or more during which elevated, expansive, or irritable mood is present. Other criteria for a manic episode are also met except that changes in functioning are less severe, hospitalization is not needed, and psychotic features are not present (APA, 2000).

Cyclothymic Disorder. A chronic mood disturbance with alternating periods of hypomanic and depressive symptoms characterizes cyclothymic disorder. Cyclothymic disorder is analogous to dysthymic disorder in depression. Hypomanic and depressive symptoms do not meet the threshold for severity, pervasiveness, or duration needed to meet criteria for a manic or major depressive episode, and hypomanic symptoms do not need to fulfill criteria for a full hypomanic episode. A diagnosis of cyclothymic disorder requires that children and adolescents exhibit symptoms for at least 1 year (the time frame for adults is 2 years' duration) and that no more than 2 months during this time are symptom free. Clinically significant distress and social or functional impairment also are required for a diagnosis. In addition, symptoms are not due to direct physiologic effects of a substance or general medical condition and cannot be better accounted for by schizoaffective disorder, or are not superimposed on schizophrenia, schizophreniform disorder, delusional disorder, or psychotic disorder not otherwise specified (APA, 2000).

Identifying Mood Disorders in Primary Care Settings

Primary care providers (PCPs) are expected to identify symptoms of a mood disorder among children and adolescents within the scope of their practices. Yet, limited time for routine health care visits, inadequate training, and scarcity of mental health services pose many challenges to early identification and appropriate treatment of these conditions. PCPs can use key clinical questions to first screen for common mental health problems among children and adolescents. Clinical questions should focus on how much a child or adolescent worries; experiences somatic complaints such as stomach aches and headaches; feels nervous, angry, irritable, depressed, sad, or afraid; or has thoughts of hurting or killing oneself (Melnyk, Brown, Jones, et al., 2003). Questions that address specific diagnostic criteria for mood disorders (see Table 33-1) are appropriate follow-up queries to positive responses during routine assessment.

A variety of mental health screening instruments can be useful in some pediatric primary care settings to aid in early identification of mental health problems. PCPs are cautioned that scores on screening instruments can never be substituted for expert clinical diagnostic evaluation. However, elevated scores on such screening instruments can provide baseline information to guide PCPs in making timely referrals, initiating treatment when indicated, and coordinating treatment with mental health providers. The *KySS (Keep Your Children/Yourself Safe and Secure) Guide to Child and Adolescent Mental Health Screening, Early Intervention and Health Promotion* (Melnyk & Moldenhauer, 2006) is a valuable resource for PCPs who seek to identify youths at risk for mental health problems. The instruments below are available for purchase and require varying levels of expertise to administer and score.

The K-SADS-PL instrument is a semi-structured diagnostic interview designed to assess psychopathology in youths (Kaufman, Birmaher, Brent, et al., 1996). The K-SADS-PL includes a screening interview that could be used by PCPs and is available online at www.wpic.pitt.edu/KSADS/ksads-pl.pdf. In addition, symptom measures for use in assessing children and adolescents include the Children's Depression Inventory (Kovacs, 2008), Reynolds Adolescent Depression Scale, 2nd ed. (Reynolds, 2008a), Reynolds Child Depression Scale (Reynolds, 2008b), the Mental Status Checklist—Children (Dougherty & Schinka, 2008a), and the Mental Status Checklist—Adolescent (Dougherty, Schinka, & PAR Staff, 2008b). Furthermore, although co-management by an experienced pediatric mental health clinician is optimal, guidelines are available for identification, assessment, management, and treatment of depression in primary care (Cheung, Zuckerbrot, Jensen, et al., 2007; Zuckerbrot, Cheung, Jensen, et al., 2007).

Clinical Manifestations at Time of Diagnosis

The signs and symptoms of mood disorders and other mental health problems are often more subtle than those of other common childhood ailments, yet the effects of psychiatric disorders can be pervasive and destructive. Early detection is essential.

Major Depressive Disorder

Descriptions such as feeling sad, gloomy, hopeless, down, blue, moody, grouchy, or depressed characterize mood. Apathetic or anxious mood may obscure the presence of an underlying depressed mood. Somatic complaints sometimes are the vehicle of expression for depression. To ascertain if the child or adolescent is feeling depressed, the clinician can question carefully and comment on nonverbal cues, for example, "You look like you might start to cry as you talk." Facial expression and body language also may infer depression. Children and adolescents often present with irritability and "cranky" mood, with angry outbursts over minor events and frustrations, rather than sadness (APA, 2000; Mash & Wolfe, 2005; Sadock & Sadock, 2007) (see Clinical Manifestations box).

Decreased interest or loss of pleasure also typifies a depressive episode. Family members may note reduced participation in activities and lack of enjoyment of formerly pleasurable activities. For children and adolescents, withdrawal from friends and activities, such as sports practice or school events, are cause for concern. Changes from previous behavior also characterize depression, including a drop in academic performance or conduct disturbances (APA, 2000; Mash & Wolfe).

Early Childhood Depression

Although research to validate clinical presentation of major depressive disorder for children and adolescents is limited, available data confirm that diagnostic criteria developed for adults apply within the context of a child's development. Luby, Heffelfinger, Mrakotsky and colleagues (2002) investigated the validity of developmentally modified *DSM-IV* criteria for preschool major depressive disorder. Preschool children with major depressive disorder displayed expected age-adjusted symptoms of depression based on diagnostic criteria, as well as neurovegetative signs, that is, "housekeeping functions," that include changes in sleep, appetite, and energy level (Sahler & Carr, 2007). Major depressive disorder symptoms differentiated these children from nonsymptomatic controls and controls with another psychiatric diagnosis. Anhedonia, or lack of pleasure in activities and play, could serve as a marker for major depressive disorder because only the depressed group exhibited this diagnostic sign. Death-related or suicidal themes in play also were present for 61% of the depressed group.

Clinical Manifestations at Time of Diagnosis

Mood	Somatic	Behavior	Loss of Pleasure or Interest	Cognitive
Irritable	Vague complaints without specific illness or injury	Drop in grades	Going through the motions	Poor concentration
Sad		Poor social, academic, or occupational functioning	Bored or apathetic attitude	Indecisiveness
Gloomy	Body or facial expressions of depressed mood		Not feeling satisfaction	Thoughts of death or suicide
Hopeless		Withdrawal or dropping out of activities or play	Lack of enjoyment in usual activities or play	Play themes of worthlessness, guilt, death, suicide, self-destruction
Down	Weight loss	Isolation from peers		
Blue	Decrease or increase in appetite	Frequent angry outbursts		Self-reproach
Moody		Temper tantrums (older child or adolescent)		Poor or exaggerated self-esteem
Grouchy	Failure to meet expected weight gains for age			
Depressed		Excessive goal-driven or pleasure-oriented activities		Slowed thoughts
Anxious	Insomnia or excessive sleeping			Distractibility
Apathetic		Flight of ideas or racing thoughts		Grandiosity
Angry	Diminished need for sleep			
Cranky	Pressured speech or excessive talkativeness			
Fatigue				
Feeling worthless	Low energy			
Guilty	Psychomotor retardation			
Abnormally expansive or elated	Psychomotor agitation			
Euphoric				

BOX 33-2

Proposed Adjustments to *DSM-IV-TR* Criteria for Depression in Preschoolers

Five (or more) of the following symptoms have been present *but not necessarily persistently** over a 2-week period and represent a change from previous functioning; at least one of the symptoms is either (1) depressed mood or (2) loss of interest or pleasure *in activities or play. If both (1) and (2) are present a total of only 4 symptoms is needed.*

1. "Depressed mood for a portion of the day for several days, as observed (or reported) in behavior. Note: may be irritable mood."
2. "Markedly diminished interest or pleasure in all, or almost all, activities or play for a portion of the day for several days (as indicated by either subjective account or observation made by others)."
3. "Feelings of worthlessness or excessive guilt (even if delusional) that may be evident in play themes."
4. "Diminished ability to think or concentrate, or indecisiveness, for several days (either by subjective account or as observed by others)."
5. "Recurrent thoughts of death (not just fear of dying), recurrent suicidal ideation without specific plan, or a suicide attempt or specific plan for committing suicide. Suicidal or self-destructive themes are persistently evident in play only" (p. 931).

Data from Luby, J.L., Heffelfinger, A.K., Mrakotsky, C., et al. (2002). Preschool major depressive disorder: Preliminary validation for developmentally modified *DSM-IV* criteria. *J Am Acad Child Adolesc Psychiatry, 41,* 928-937.
*Suggested changes in *DSM-IV-TR* diagnostic criteria are indicated in italics.

These data provide new evidence that preschool children manifest major depressive disorder with typical age-adjusted symptoms, including neurovegetative signs (Box 33-2).

Dysthymic Disorder

Compared with youths with major depressive disorder, children and adolescents with dysthymic disorder typically have fewer neurovegetative symptoms, such as sleep disturbance, agitation, or restless behavior; seldom exhibit anhedonia or social withdrawal; and are less likely to have thoughts of dying or somatic complaints (Mash & Wolfe, 2005). Moodiness, irritability, anger, sadness, poor self-esteem, and temper outbursts occur more prominently in dysthymic disorder than in major depressive disorder. Youths with dysthymic disorder may develop major depressive disorder. Clinicians may miss the presence of underlying dysthymia because the presentation of an acute major depressive episode is more florid. Overlapping diagnoses negatively affect long-term prognosis, therefore careful evaluation is merited.

Bipolar Disorders

A meta-analysis of seven studies (Kowatch et al., 2005) indicated that the most common symptoms among children and adolescents with BPD were increased energy, distractibility, and pressured speech. Irritability and grandiosity characterized four of five affected youths, and a majority also had elated mood, decreased need for sleep, or racing thoughts. About half of those affected experienced racing thoughts, and about a third manifested hypersexuality. Diagnosing mania in children, particularly young children, can be challenging because characteristic and developmentally normal behaviors of early childhood, such as magical thinking and rapid speech, can resemble the hallmark symptoms of BPD. Once again, this fact underscores the need for children to be evaluated by clinicians with expertise in child psychiatry.

BOX 33-3

Symptoms Associated with BPD that Are Rarely Associated with ADHD

1. Decreased sleep requirement
2. Prolonged (2-4 hours) episodes of intense rage
3. Hypersexuality
4. Morbid nightmares
5. Symptoms of psychosis (e.g., hallucinations, delusions, bizarre behavior)

Data from Preston, J. D., O'Neal, J. H., & Talaga, M. C. (2008). *Handbook of Clinical Psychopharmacology for Therapists* (5th ed.). Oakland, CA: New Harbinger Publications.

It is important for the PCP to recognize that any evidence of mania indicates the presence of a BPD rather than a depressive disorder. As discussed below, medications commonly used for depression can contribute to a triggering or escalation of mania. When any degree of mania is identified, the child should be referred to an experienced child psychiatric–mental health (PMH) clinician who is authorized to prescribe to ensure accurate diagnosis and appropriate treatment. Follow-up care by the PCP involves ongoing evaluation of symptoms and response to medication.

Furthermore, differential diagnosis of psychiatric conditions is challenging for clinicians, particularly distinguishing between attention-deficit/hyperactivity disorder (ADHD) and BPD (see Chapter 12 for a discussion of ADHD). Consideration of the criteria in Box 33-3 can assist in differentiating between these diagnoses.

Additionally, the following represent positive findings in the family history (i.e., blood relatives) that suggest a diagnosis of BPD rather than ADHD:

1. Suicide or attempted suicide
2. Severe substance abuse (alcohol and drugs)
3. Multiple marriages
4. Dramatic occupational instability (e.g., starting numerous businesses)
5. Hyperthymia (a state of chronic hypomania characterized by high energy, excessive productivity, gregariousness, impulsivity, and a decreased sleep requirement)

Treatment

Psychotherapy for Depressive Disorders

Children and adolescents typically respond well to psychotherapy for the treatment of depression provided by clinicians with expertise in child psychiatric practice and specialized psychotherapy training (Carr, 2008). Psychodynamic, cognitive-behavioral, and interpersonal therapy have demonstrated efficacy (Harrington, 2006; Ryan, 2005; Trowell, Joffe, Campbell, et al., 2007). Interventions such as psychoeducation and family therapy that directly involve parents and other family members in the treatment also may be helpful, particularly when a child is experiencing a crisis or loss, another family member is depressed, or family distress is evident. Family therapy also has been shown to be an effective treatment (Trowell et al.) and family support of treatment across modalities is critical to successful outcomes.

Psychotherapeutic approaches are classified according to their underlying theoretic concepts (i.e., interpersonal, psychodynamic, or cognitive-behavioral theories) but often are blended in practice. In addition, treatment may be adapted depending on the setting (i.e., inpatient or outpatient), and the approach to treatment (i.e., individual therapy, family therapy, or combination of psychotherapy and medication). Practice parameters are published in the *Journal of the American Academy of Child and Adolescent Psychiatry* and are available online at www.aacap.org/cs/root/member_information/practice_information/practice_parameters/practice_parameters.

Treatment

Depressive Disorders
- Psychotherapy
  - Interpersonal therapy
  - Psychodynamic therapy
  - Cognitive-behavioral therapy (CBT)
  - Adjunctive therapies
    - Child-centered
    - Family
    - Psychoeducational
- Psychopharmacologic therapy
  - Antidepressant medications
- Electroconvulsant therapy (ECT) (for severe depression only)

Bipolar Disorders
- Adjunctive psychoeducational therapy
- Psychopharmacologic therapy
  - Mood stabilizers
    - Lithium
    - Alternative mood stabilizers/anticonvulsants
  - Antipsychotics
  - Antihypertensives
  - Anxiolytic agent
- ECT (for acute mania only)

Interpersonal Therapy. Interpersonal therapy (IPT) has demonstrated efficacy as a treatment for depression, particularly when used to treat adolescents (Klomek & Mufson, 2006). IPT involves teaching strategies that help the child or adolescent relate to and connect with others, such as learning to describe one's thoughts and feelings. Ultimately such learning leads to the cultivation of empathy for and from others. The effects of depressive symptoms dissipate as the young person increases supportive interactions with family members and peers (Bostic & Prince, 2008). For younger children or those with cognitive or developmental challenges, play therapy in combination with family therapy is recommended to achieve these therapeutic goals.

Psychodynamic Psychotherapy. Psychodynamic therapy is based on the premise that a real or imagined loss leads to the development of depression. According to this model, a depressed child harbors aggressive impulses as a result of losses and directs these impulses inward. Thus the goal of psychodynamic psychotherapy for the treatment of depression is to help the child recognize the source of the aggressive impulses and work at integrating these impulses, and thereby improve self-esteem. The literature provides support for the effectiveness of psychodynamic therapy for treatment of youths with depression (Carr, 2008; Trowell et al., 2007). For young children, play therapy, with origins in this treatment framework, is the appropriate modality. For older children and adolescents, the treatment goal may be achieved through conversation or "talk therapy."

Cognitive-Behavioral Therapy. The literature provides substantive support for use of cognitive-behavioral therapy (CBT) as an effective treatment of depression in children and adolescents (Carr, 2008; Harrington, 2006; Ryan, 2005). The underlying principle of CBT is that emotional and behavioral difficulties stem from maladaptive thinking patterns, feelings, and behavioral responses. Thus CBT is based on the precept that a change in one's thoughts will lead to a change in both behavior and emotions. CBT is a problem-oriented therapy that targets cognitive distortions and also focuses on faulty attributions, poor self-esteem, and their behavioral manifestations. In practice, CBT comprises a combination of cognitive and behavioral therapeutic approaches that emphasize how children and adolescents may use thinking processes to reframe, restructure, and solve problems; complementary behavioral changes are encouraged (Sadock & Sadock, 2007).

Psychopharmacologic Therapy for Depression

Medication is frequently used in the management of pediatric and adolescent mood disorders (Table 33-2). In addition, pharmacotherapy for psychiatric disorders in children may enhance normal development or protect against brain damage. This damage results from the "kindling effect" of prolonged exposure to toxic levels of neurotransmitters (such as glutamate) or stress hormones (such as cortisol) (Preston et al., 2008, p. 226). Symptoms of mood disorder subtypes overlap and BPD can be more difficult to diagnose in younger children. Nevertheless, careful assessment and accurate diagnosis of this population are critical before developing a medication plan, as some antidepressants and stimulants can induce mania in youths with BPD and may be contraindicated. When stopping use of a medication or changing medications, weaning is advised with monitoring of discontinuation and depression symptoms.

Antidepressant Medications. Antidepressant medications work by inhibiting or potentiating the actions of neurotransmitters in the brain, particularly norepinephrine, serotonin, dopamine, and gamma-aminobutyric acid (GABA) (Jackson, 2006). The major classes of antidepressant medications include selective serotonin reuptake inhibitors (SSRIs) (e.g., fluoxetine, sertraline, paroxetine); atypical antidepressants (e.g., trazodone, bupropion); tricyclic antidepressants (TCAs) (e.g., imipramine, amitriptyline); and monoamine oxidase inhibitors (MAOIs) (e.g., phenelzine, tranylcypromine (Keltner, & Folks, 2005; Fava & Papakostas, 2008).

SSRIs are the newest class of antidepressants and the most widely used medications for treatment of depression in children and adolescents. SSRIs are the medication of choice primarily because of their favorable side effect profile. SSRIs act by potentiating the CNS action of serotonin and norepinephrine. Although SSRIs do not cause orthostatic hypotension or anticholinergic side effects, some of their side effects include restlessness, irritability, and insomnia (Fava & Papakostas, 2008).

Evidence supporting the effectiveness of SSRIs in treating child and adolescent depression is mixed. The Task Force Report of the American College of Neuropsychopharmacology (Mann, Emslie, Baldessarini, et al., 2006) indicated that in randomized controlled trials with depressed youths, only fluoxetine (Prozac) was clearly effective. Moreover, a systematic review and meta-analysis also indicated that only fluoxetine showed a moderately beneficial profile (Usala, Clavenna, Zuddas, et al., 2008). The authors found that "the combination of CBT and fluoxetine is significantly more effective

Text continued on p. 639

TABLE 33-2
Psychotropic Medications Used to Treat Childhood and Adolescent Mood Disorders

Medication	Typical Starting Dosage*	Typical Daily Dosage*	Side Effects	Use Guidelines and Efficacy (when data available)
SELECTIVE SEROTONIN REUPTAKE INHIBITORS (SSRIs)				Antidepressant medications approved for use in individuals over 12 yr; fluoxetine received FDA approval for treatment of depression and obsessive-compulsive disorder in children (January, 2003)
Citalopram (Celexa)	5 mg	5-40 mg	Gastrointestinal (GI): nausea, diarrhea, cramping, heartburn; Central nervous system (CNS): insomnia, agitation, restlessness, headache, tremor, insomnia, irritability; Genitourinary (GU): decreased libido	Similar to other SSRIs
Fluoxetine (Prozac)	5-10 mg	Children: 5-40 mg; Adolescents: 10-60 mg	Similar to other SSRIs; Most common: behavioral activation (e.g., motor restlessness, insomnia, disinhibition); Also reports of suicidal ideation and self-injurious behavior	Studied for treatment of depression in children and adolescents; support as first-line medication choice; strong evidence to date of efficacy as treatment of depression in children and adolescents.
Fluvoxamine (Luvox)	12.5-25 mg	50-200 mg	Similar to other SSRIs	FDA approved use (November, 2003) for children 8+ yr. Approved to treat obsessive-compulsive disorder in children
Sertraline (Zoloft)	12.5-25 mg	Children: 25-150 mg	Similar to other SSRIs	Studied for treatment of depression in children and adolescents; more evidence of efficacy needed for children but adequate support as first-line medication choice; modest evidence to date of efficacy as treatment of depression in adolescents; approved to treat obsessive-compulsive disorder in children
		Adolescents: 50-200 mg	One study of 33 children and adolescents demonstrated evidence of two cases of sertraline-induced mania	Evidence from adult studies shows that some individuals respond to low doses; hence clinicians should evaluate response before increasing dose
ATYPICAL/NOVEL ANTIDEPRESSANTS				
Bupropion (Wellbutrin)		Children: 50-200 mg; Adolescents: 100-250 mg	GI: nausea, vomiting, constipation; CNS: agitation, insomnia; Neurologic: tremors; Dermatologic: skin rashes; Low risk of seizures	Limited evidence of efficacy for treatment of attention-deficit/hyperactivity disorder (ADHD) in children and adolescents; more evidence needed
Trazodone (Desyrel)	Children 6-18 yr: 1.5-2 mg/kg/day in divided doses	Children 6-18 yr: 1.5-6 mg/kg/day	*Specific to trazodone:* GI: nausea, dyspepsia; CNS: orthostasis, sedation, restlessness; Cardiovascular: effects such as risk for atrial arrhythmia; GU: priapism	Not well studied in children and adolescents
Mirtazapine (Remeron)	Adults: 15-45 mg	Adults: 15-45 mg	*Specific to mirtazapine:* GI: increased appetite, weight gain; CNS: somnolence, dizziness	Not well studied in children and adolescents
Nefazodone (Serzone)	Adults: 200 mg	Adults: 150-600 mg	Hepatic: abnormal liver function tests (LFTs), "black box" risk warning; GI: nausea, dyspepsia, constipation, and varied symptoms	Not well studied in children and adolescents; *not recommended at this time for use with children and adolescents* because of risk of liver damage
Venlafaxine (Effexor)		75-150 mg in two or three divided doses with food; Adults: up to 375 mg	GI: dysphagia, eructation (belching), gastritis, stomach and mouth ulcerations, rectal hemorrhage, weight gain or loss	One study found drug to be no better than placebo in relieving depression in children

TRICYCLIC ANTIDEPRESSANTS (TCAs)

Drug	Dosage	Side Effects	Comments
		GI: weight gain CNS: tremor, agitation Cardiovascular: orthostatic hypotension, palpitations, hypertension, dizziness Anticholinergic: dry mouth, sweating, urinary retention and hesitance	Over 30 yr of use in children and adolescents; approved for use in individuals over 12 yr with depression; evidence for efficacy in treating children's depression is unconvincing Children can show tremendous variation in serum level at the same dosage of these drugs Before initiating treatment with TCA, an electrocardiogram (ECG) should be performed; ECG should be repeated with dosage adjustments, when maintenance dose is achieved, and semiannually during treatment Baseline assessment should include blood pressure, pulse, and a review of medical and family history (e.g., syncope, sudden death); children thought to be more sensitive to overdoses of TCAs than adults
Clomipramine (Anafranil, Apo-Clomipramine, Clopram, Novo-Clopamine, Placil) (also referred to as a serotonin reuptake inhibitor because of potential action)	25 mg/day, gradually increase divided dosages over first 2 wk to max of 200 mg/day Children 10+ yr: 25-200 mg/day Adolescents: 50-200 mg		Approved to treat obsessive-compulsive disorder in children
Desipramine (Norpramin, Pertofrane, Apo-Desipramine, Novo-Desipramine)	Children 6-12 yr: 1-3 mg/kg/day to a max of 5 mg/kg/day Children 12+ yr: 25-50 mg/day; may gradually increase to 250 mg/day	Children 6-12 yr: 1-5 mg/kg/day Children 12+ yr: 25-150 mg/day TCA most likely to alter electrical conduction through the heart; can also prolong the QT interval, which can increase risk of fatal ventricular tachycardia in susceptible individuals	
Nortriptyline (Allegron, Aventyl, Norventyl, Pamelor)	Children 6-12 yr: 10-20 mg/day in three or four divided doses Children 12+ yr: 30-50 mg/day in three or four divided doses, for a maximum of 150 mg/day		Modest evidence of efficacy in treating depression for adolescents

Data from Jackson, C. (Ed.). (2006). *Mosby's Pediatric Drug Consult (2006)*. St. Louis: Elsevier Mosby; Keltner, N.L., & Folks, D.G. (2005). *Psychotropic Drugs* (4th ed.). St. Louis: Mosby; Papolos, D., & Papolos, J. (2006). *The Bipolar Child: The Definitive and Reassuring Guide to Childhood's Most Misunderstood Disorder* (3rd ed.). New York: Broadway Books.; Preston, J.D., O'Neal, J.H., & Talaga, M.C. (2005). *Handbook of Clinical Psychopharmacology for Therapists* (4th ed.). Oakland, CA: New Harbinger Publications, Inc.; Sadock, B.J., & Sadock, V.A. (Eds.). (2007). *Kaplan & Sadock's Synopsis of Psychiatry: Behavioral Sciences/Clinical Psychiatry* (10th ed.). Philadelphia: Lippincott Williams & Wilkins; Scahill, L., & Rains, A. (2005a). Psychopharmacology for adolescents. In N.L. Keltner & D.G. Folks (Eds.), *Psychotropic Drugs* (4th ed.). St. Louis: Mosby; Scahill, L., & Rains, A. (2005b). Psychopharmacology for children. In N.L. Keltner & D.G. Folks (Eds.), *Psychotropic Drugs* (4th ed.). St. Louis: Mosby; Schatzberg, A.F., & Nemeroff, C.D. (2004). *The American Psychiatric Textbook of Psychopharmacology* (3rd ed.). Washington, D.C.: American Psychiatric Press; Takemoto, C.K., Hodding, J.H., & Kraus, D.M. (2008). *Pediatric Dosage Handbook* (15th ed.). Hudson, OH: Lexi-Comp.

*Dosages are indicated for children and adolescents when recommendations for each age-group are available. When not specified as child, adolescent, or adult dose, the dosages indicated are guidelines for use with children and adolescents. If child or adolescent dosage recommendations are not generally available, adult dosages are given. **Please note: Caution is recommended when prescribing and monitoring psychotropic medication use with children and adolescents;** many drugs require off-label use, demonstration of efficacy may be minimal, and dosages may not be clearly evidence based. Clinicians are advised to monitor changes in fda approvals, warnings, and new medications and uses.

Continued

TABLE 33-2

Psychotropic Medications Used to Treat Childhood and Adolescent Mood Disorders—cont'd

Medication	Typical Starting Dosage	Typical Daily Dosage	Side Effects	Use Guidelines and Efficacy (when data available)
MONOAMINE OXIDASE INHIBITORS (MAOIs)				
			GI: constipation, weight gain Cardiovascular: decreased heart rate, decreased vasoconstriction, hypotension, hypertensive crisis Anticholinergic: dry mouth, blurred vision, urinary hesitancy CNS: agitation, anxiety, restlessness, insomnia GU: anorgasmia or impotence Mood: euphoria, hypomania	Tyramine-containing foods (e.g., wine, aged cheese) should **not** be ingested by the person taking MAOIs
Phenelzine (Nardil) Tranylcypromine (Parnate)		Adults: 30-90 mg Adults: 20-60 mg		
MOOD STABILIZER				
Lithium	15-30 mg/kg body weight/day in three or four doses Adolescents: 300-600 mg increasing over 4-5 days to 1500-1800 mg	Adolescents: 600-1800 mg/day in divided doses	GI: weight gain, bloated feeling, diarrhea CNS: tremor, ataxia, cognitive slowing, sedation, sleeplessness, headaches, dyspepsia, dry mouth Cardiovascular: arrhythmia, conduction disturbances, hypotension GU: polyuria, polydipsia Dermatologic: hair loss, acne, rash	Several studies for prepubertal children to treat severe aggression; not approved for use in children <12 yr, although limited use reported; evidence to support safe and effective use in adolescents During first month, check serum level q wk and then monthly; thyroid q 4-6 mo, renal function q 6-12 mo; baseline ECG needed and repeated yearly Serum levels: therapeutic or normal level: 0.6-1.2 mEq/L; adverse reactions at 1.5 mEq/L; toxic reaction at 2.0-3.0 mEq/L; lethal reactions at >4 mEq/L Draw blood in AM 8-12 hr after last dose and before morning dose Maintenance of adequate hydration essential
ALTERNATIVE MOOD STABILIZERS/ANTICONVULSANTS				
Carbamazepine (Tegretol, Apo-Carbamazepine, Carbatrol, Epitol, Teril)	Adults: 200 mg twice daily	Children: 10 mg/kg/day (max 600 mg/day in three divided doses) Increase by 200 mg/day in adolescents Dose to reach serum level of 4-12 mcg/mL	Multiple side effects reported Specific side effects as noted by medication GI: nausea and vomiting, weight gain, GI upset CNS: sedation, poor coordination, dizziness, irritability, diplopia, tremors ECG, hemoglobin, hematocrit Dermatologic: skin reactions and rashes, transient hair loss, acne Hematologic: blood dyscrasias including agranulocytosis (most serious), leukopenia, aplastic anemia (rare), agranulocytosis, thrombocytopenia (dose related) Eyes, ears, nose, and throat (EENT): blurred vision Renal: hyponatremia Hepatic and pancreatic: hepatotoxicity and pancreatitis (rare)	Minimally studied in children, may be useful for aggression; laboratory work weekly to monitor plasma levels; after stabilization, monitor monthly; baseline or complete blood count (CBC) with differential, white blood count (WBC), platelet count, LFTs; after stabilization, CBC and LFTs q wk for 1 mo, monthly for 4 mo, q 3 mo thereafter; evaluate CBC for blood dyscrasias
Gabapentin (Neurontin)		Adults and children >12 yr: 900-1800 mg in three divided doses	Specific to gabapentin: GI: increased appetite, weight gain CNS: sedation, tremor, ataxia, incoordination	Open trials and case reports with adults indicate effectiveness for rapid cycling; may be more effective to treat bipolar II and in combination with another mood stabilizer; not used for children <12 yr

Drug	Dosage		Side effects	Comments
Lamotrigine (Lamictal)	Adolescents: 12.5-25 mg/day with slow increase by 12.5 mg q 7-10 days Adults: 25-50 mg/day	Adolescents: 75-100 mg/day may be effective, but up to 225 mg required Adults: 100-500 mg	Specific to lamotrigine: CNS: cognitive blunting ("spacing out") Cardiac: restlessness, dizziness, conduction changes Dermatologic: rash (particularly in combination with valproate, higher dosages, during first 8 wk of treatment, and in children), Stevens-Johnson syndrome in 1%-2% of children and 0.1% of adults (severe allergic and sometimes fatal reaction; stop use immediately and treat with corticosteroids)	Used only for children >16 yr; valproate doubles plasma levels of lamotrigine; sertraline increases plasma levels of lamotrigine; carbamazepine and phenobarbital lower plasma levels of lamotrigine; alcohol increases severity of lamotrigine's side effects
Tiagabine (Gabitril)	Start low and increase weekly until good response or until max dosage reached	32 mg max dose/day	CNS: dizziness, fatigue, unstable gait	FDA approved for treatment of convulsant disorders in adolescents; more evidence needed to show efficacy for bipolar treatment over other agents; may be helpful after other agents tried with limited effect Decreased levels of contraceptives
Topiramate (Topamax)	Adults: 25 mg/day	Adults: increase by 1-3 mg/kg/day q1-2 wk up to 5-9 mg/kg/day in two divided doses 200-600 mg/day	GI: weight loss, anorexia CNS: sedation, fatigue, dizziness GU: dysmenorrhea and menstrual disorder EENT: diplopia, vision abnormality Respiratory: upper respiratory infection (URI), pharyngitis, sinusitis Miscellaneous: leukopenia	
Valproate/valproic acid (Depakene, Depakote)	10-15 mg/kg/day in divided doses	May increase by 5-10 mg/kg/day q wk; not to exceed 60 mg/kg/day in two or three divided doses Children and adults: dosage to reach serum level of 50-100 mcg/mL	GI: nausea, vomiting, constipation, weight gain, toxic hepatitis, hepatic failure, pancreatitis CNS: sedation, drowsiness, dizziness, incoordination, tremors, headache, depression GU: polycystic ovaries (more likely when treatment started in teen years Hematologic: thrombocytopenia, leukopenia, lymphocytosis Dermatologic: transitory hair loss, skin eruptions Hepatic: hepatotoxicity (rare in children under 10 yr) Pancreatic: pancreatitis (potentially fatal and rare, usually associated with use of multiple anticonvulsants)	Approved for treatment of epilepsy in children and adults Minimal studies with adolescents conducted to date During first 1-2 mo, serum levels checked q 1-2 wk and liver function tests (LFTs) and CBC q mo and then q 6-12 mo; potential for development of polycystic ovaries raises question about risk benefit ratio for use in adolescent girls

ANTIPSYCHOTIC MEDICATIONS

| | | | Traditional neuroleptics/antipsychotics (e.g., chlorpromazine, haloperidol, thioridazine, thiothixene) have significant side effects including:
CNS: sedation
Cardiovascular: hypotension
Anticholinergic: dry mouth, constipation, blurred vision
Extrapyramidal side effects: dystonia, rigidity, akathisia; long-term use associated with tardive dyskinesia
Neuroleptic malignant syndrome (NMS; severe muscular rigidity, autonomic system instability, changing levels of consciousness) can be fatal; associated with high-potency drugs prescribed in high doses and with rapid increase in dosing; if NMS is suspected, treat symptoms and stop the drug | With traditional neuroleptics, consider risk and monitor signs of abnormal movements that may indicate tardive dyskinesia
Use lowest possible dose, and withdraw slowly, evaluate changes in symptom severity
Newer atypical antipsychotic drugs (e.g., risperidone, lonazapine, quetiapine, loxapine) generally better tolerated |

Continued

TABLE 33-2

Psychotropic Medications Used to Treat Childhood and Adolescent Mood Disorders—cont'd

Medication	Typical Starting Dosage	Typical Daily Dosage	Side Effects	Use Guidelines and Efficacy (when data available)
ANTIPSYCHOTIC MEDICATIONS—cont'd				
Aripiprazole (Abilify)	Adolescents 10-17: 2 mg/day	2-30 mg/day		High-potency antipsychotic; Abilify associated with a decrease in EPS, less sedating, and fewer metabolic side effects (e.g., less weight gain)[†]; Abilify can cause nausea and anxiety, particularly at the beginning of treatment[‡]; Abilify is unique in that it not only blocks but also adjusts dopamine levels and also affects serotonin
Haloperidol (Haldol, Apo-Haloperidol, Novoperidol, Peridol, Serenace)	Children: 0.25-0.5 mg/kg/day in two or three divided doses; Adults: 0.5-5 mg/day in two or three divided doses	Children: 1-3 mg/day; Adolescents/adults: 2-10 mg	Causes more extrapyramidal side effects than chlorpromazine or thioridazine but is less sedating	Most studied neuroleptic with children; effective for treatment of autism, schizophrenia, severe aggression, tics; studied in adolescents
Loxapine (Loxitane)	Adolescents: 10 mg bid	Adolescents: 60-100 mg		Studied in adolescents
Olanzapine (Zyprexa)	Children: 2 mg/day; Adolescents: 2-4 mg/day	5-20 mg/day	GI: increased appetite, weight gain	Limited data for use with children and adolescents
Quetiapine (Seroquel)		Adolescents: 100-400 mg		Limited data for use with children and adolescents
Risperidone (Risperdal)	Children and adolescents 10-17: 0.5 mg	1-3.5 mg, increased adverse effects >2.5 mg/day	Cardiovascular: higher incidence of cerebrovascular adverse events in elderly with dementia-related psychosis	Limited data to support use in children yet several studies to support use for behavioral dyscontrol; extensive evidence for use in adults; studied in adolescents
Thioridazine (Mellaril, Aldazine, Apo-Thioridazine)	Adolescents: 25-50 mg	Children: 0.5-3.0 mg/kg/day or 10-50 mg two or three times per day; Adolescents: 50-400 mg		
Thiothixene (Navane)	1-2 mg	Children: 5-40 mg; Adolescents: 8-40 mg		Approved to treat psychosis in children >12 yr; studied in adolescents; meager evidence for children <12 yr suggests less sedation than low-potency neuroleptics and fewer side effects than high-potency neuroleptics
Ziprasidone (Geodon)		40-160 mg/day	Extended QTc intervals seen in children	Low potency, less sedating, less weight gain associated with its use as compared to other neuroleptics; however, side effects can include: sedation, EPS, tardive dyskinesia, nausea, and anxiety (especially initially)
ANXIOLYTIC AGENT				
Buspirone (BuSpar, Buspirex, Bustab)	2.5-5 mg	Children: 10-20 mg; Adolescents: 60 mg max dose in three divided doses	CNS: fatigue, sleep disturbance, headache, restlessness, agitation, depression, anxiety, confusion; GI: abdominal discomfort, nausea	Minimally studied in children; improvement in anxiety and aggression; If there is no evidence of improvement after 6 wk, buspirone should be discontinued

[†]Medpage Today. (2008). Retrieved from www.medpagetody.com/Psychiatry/BipolarDisorder/tb/1987 on January 26, 2008.
[‡]Preston, J.D., O'Neal, J.H., & Talaga, M.C. (2008). Handbook of Clinical Psychopharmacology for Therapists (5th ed.), Oakland, CA: New Harbinger Publications.

than placebo, fluoxetine or CBT" (p. 70). Based on another systematic review of available literature, Ryan (2005) indicated that CBT and IPT have merit as treatments of depression among youths but cautions that trained clinicians are often scarce or unavailable in many locations. In addition, there is good evidence for the efficacy of fluoxetine in child depression and some evidence for citalopram and nefazodone, but little for other agents (Ryan).

The action of TCAs appears to be similar to that of the SSRIs, but TCAs are not the first choice of antidepressant medication for the treatment of depression in children because of their more troublesome side effect profile and because of evidence that they are ineffective (Mann et al., 2006; Stark, Sander, Hauser, et al., 2006). However, imipramine is an approved and frequently used treatment for enuresis, and clomipramine is approved to treat childhood obsessive-compulsive disorder. Most common side effects include anticholinergic reactions (e.g., dry mouth, dizziness), weight gain, and insomnia.

Although a few open studies have provided evidence of benefit of MAOIs in the treatment of both depression and ADHD in children, MAOI usage is not recommended among the pediatric population. Patients who are taking MAOIs must avoid ingesting foods that have monoamine agonist activity or foods containing tyramines, such as aged meats and cheeses, wine, and certain legumes. Combining MAOIs with the forbidden foods can result in a life-threatening hypertensive crisis. Because of this risk, clinicians tend to prescribe MAOIs to youths only in very unusual situations, such as incapacitating, recurrent depression that has been resistant to treatment with SSRIs, atypical antidepressants, and TCAs (Stark et al., 2006). [NOTE: Given that MAOIs are seldom used to treat children, discussion of these medications here is limited. Please refer to a drug reference manual for more information, such as *Essential Pharmacology: The Prescriber's Guide* (Stahl, 2006)].

Judging the effectiveness of a particular antidepressant in a particular child requires the evaluation of target symptoms that are being treated (such as anhedonia or neurovegetative signs) and also patience, as the full effect of the medication may not be felt for several weeks. In addition, many parents and clinicians are surprised that prepubertal children may require higher doses of psychotropic medications because of their faster metabolic processes. As a result, clinicians, parents, and young patients may falsely conclude that a medication is not efficacious when, in fact, the dosage has been insufficient (Preston et al., 2008).

Psychotherapy for Bipolar Disorders

Although there is no evidence that psychotherapy can help to treat the core symptoms of BPDs in children, adjunctive psychosocial therapies can address the functional impairments of affected individuals and families. Supportive therapy helps families to cope with the devastating social and emotional effects of the disorder and promotes adherence to medication regimens. Additionally, psychosocial interventions, such as establishing predictable routines and learning de-escalation strategies, can reduce the intensity and frequency of symptoms (Bostic & Prince, 2008).

Psychopharmacologic Therapy for Bipolar Disorders

The treatment of BPD in the pediatric population is evolving and is receiving greater attention in the psychiatric community, as evidenced by the roundtable meetings that have been convened by the American Academy of Child and Adolescent Psychiatry (AACAP) and the National Institute of Mental Health (NIMH) (Bostic, & Prince, 2008). In 2007 the AACAP issued practice parameters that address the assessment, diagnosis, treatment, and research regarding pediatric BPD (McClellan, Kowatch, Findling, et al., 2007). Given evidence of a biologic cause of this condition and the related functional and psychosocial problems, a sensible treatment strategy for moderate to severe cases combines psychopharmacology and psychotherapy. Medication is widely used to eliminate manic (or mixed) and depressive symptoms and to prevent recurrence (see Table 33-2 and Psychopharmacology Therapy section above).

Mood stabilizers, such as lithium and anticonvulsants, are the mainstays of treatment for BPDs (Jackson, 2006). Although lithium can treat both mania and depression, it requires careful monitoring and may not be effective or tolerated in all cases. Prescription of a combination of drugs within different classes frequently is necessary to treat the complex and varied symptoms of BPD. For example, a child may take a mood stabilizer to achieve some balance in mood, an antipsychotic medication to treat manic symptoms and severe behavioral disturbances, and an antidepressant to relieve depressive features of the illness. Without the protection of a mood stabilizer, use of antidepressants, and in many cases stimulants, can lead to increased anxiety, aggression, temper tantrums, cycling of mood, and induction of mania. Given limited research evidence and potential risks, careful administration of combined drug therapies to children and adolescents is warranted (Scahill & Rains, 2005a). These medications should be initiated and adjusted by an expert PMH clinician with prescribing authority. The PCP has a major role in monitoring effectiveness and side effects in collaboration with the PMH clinician, the youth, and parents.

Regulatory Aspects of Psychopharmacology

The research literature regarding pharmacologic treatment of childhood mood disorders is limited and many treatment recommendations are based on evidence from adult studies. Most antidepressant medications used in pediatrics are approved for individuals older than 12 years (Keltner & Folks, 2005; Scahill & Rains, 2005a, 2005b), yet clinicians frequently turn to medications even in younger children to reduce distressing symptoms and to prevent escalation of related functional and social problems.

Psychopharmacologic management of the majority of psychiatric childhood disorders involves the practice called *off-label prescribing* (Lakhan & Hagger-Johnson, 2007). In off-label use clinicians prescribe drugs for disorders other than those indicated in the U.S. Food and Drug Administration (FDA)–approved labeling for those products. Off-label prescribing is *not* a violation of federal law, and the FDA does not regulate such professional practice decisions. Moreover, lack of evidence to guide prescribing and dosing for children is not limited to psychopharmacologic agents, because medications from many classes have not been tested adequately in children (McEvoy, 2008). Without adequate research involving pediatric populations, labeling and marketing of medications require a disclaimer to indicate that safety and effectiveness have not been established for children.

Although psychopharmacologic treatment for children and adolescents is widespread and often effective, there is at least a perception of increased liability and risk concerning such practices (Lakhan & Hagger-Johnson, 2007). PCPs who prescribe medication, whether FDA-approved or off-label, without a psychiatric referral are practicing outside their area of specialization, particularly for children and adolescents with a major psychiatric disorder. The best practice for a PCP is always to consult with a pediatric psychiatrist or other pediatric mental health professional with prescribing expertise. Given the shortage of pediatric psychiatrists in poor and rural communities (Thomas & Holzer, 2006), this consultation may be challenging to set up. However, any time a PCP detects symptoms indicative of a moderate to severe mood disorder, suspects a BPD, or identifies suicidal ideation, intent, or a plan a psychiatric referral is essential. Subsequent medication management by PCPs is appropriate when collaborative practice with PMH colleagues is in place. Such collaboration is likely to reduce risk and produce the safest, most efficacious outcomes for treatment of mood disorders among children and adolescents (see Table 33-2).

Black Box Warning. On October 14, 2004, the FDA required pharmaceutical companies to place a "black box warning" on all antidepressant medications distributed in the United States, alerting clinicians, parents, and patients to exercise care and special concern when considering these particular medications. The FDA advisory cautions that these medications ". . . increase the risk of suicidal thinking and behavior (suicidality) in children and adolescents with major depressive disorder (MDD) and other psychiatric disorders" (APA and AACAP, 2005; FDA, 2004). The advisory also explains that suicidality has been found in a small proportion of children and adolescents in the early stages of taking antidepressant medication, and that there were no completed suicides among children taking antidepressants in the studies that led to this warning. Although the background research is not explained in the actual black box medication guide, the guide explains that "depression and other serious illnesses are the most important causes of suicidal thoughts and actions" and that the risk of suicidal thoughts and behaviors tends to occur early in treatment (www.fda.gov/cder/drug/antidepressants/antidepressants_MG_2007.pdf.) The FDA is considering a similar warning for children taking anticonvulsants, although in this case the risk seems to be greater in children with epilepsy than in children using anticonvulsants as mood stabilizers (FDA, 2008a). The association of suicide with mood disorders is further discussed below.

Although the FDA does not prohibit the use of antidepressants for children and adolescents, the agency recommends that clinicians and parents closely monitor children and adolescents who are taking antidepressants for worsening signs of depression or other unexpected changes in behavior, such as restlessness or elation. Although the APA and AACAP indicate that the frequency and nature of monitoring should be individualized to the needs of child and family, the FDA recommends that a child receiving antidepressants be seen by the prescribing clinician once a week for the first 4 weeks of treatment; every other week for the second month of treatment; and at the end of the twelfth week on medication (APA and AACAP, 2005).

Electroconvulsive Therapy

Older children and adolescents who have been resistant to alternate forms of treatment sometimes receive electroconvulsive therapy (ECT) for treatment of severe depression and acute mania. When rapid relief is required because of suicidal intent, risk for self-harm, or exhaustion, ECT may be an alternative treatment to consider. Specifically, when an adolescent does not respond to two

adequate courses of psychotropic medication treatment and severe symptoms persist, then ECT may be warranted (Findling, Feeney, Stansbrey, et al., 2004; Turk et al., 2007). Although ECT generally is safe and may be effective when administered correctly, many people expect that the treatment is painful and view it as barbaric and archaic. Because of these common misperceptions about ECT, extensive education is essential when this treatment option is proposed. Moreover, there is little documentation of how often ECT is actually used to treat children and adolescents. Further, it is important to note that the effectiveness of ECT in the treatment of refractory depression in children is unknown because of inadequate data (Young, 2007).

Complementary and Alternative Therapies

Complementary and alternative therapies for the treatment of many childhood disorders and ailments have been a topic of intense interest and research in the United States in recent years, and their use has been increasing over time (Smith & Mischoulon, 2008). A central tenet underpinning these treatment approaches is that people heal themselves and physicians, nurses, and others assist in the process. Cost containment and relative noninvasiveness also are attractive features of many of these therapies. However, evidence of treatment efficacy for children and adolescents is limited.

St. John's Wort. Many individuals use St. John's wort *(Hypericum perforatum)*, a whole plant product with antidepressant properties, to treat their depression. St. John's wort is licensed in Germany and used extensively throughout Europe for treatment of insomnia, anxiety, and depression, and it surpasses sales of fluoxetine by a wide margin. Action involves inhibition of uptake of serotonin, norepinephrine, and dopamine and inhibition of binding to GABA receptors. St. John's wort reduces serum levels of theophylline, digoxin, cyclosporine, tacrolimus, coumadin, antiretrovirals, amitryptyline, and oral contraceptives (Alpert, 2008). Its use is associated with increased photosensitivity and poses a theoretic risk for serotonergic crisis when taken with other agents that have similar action. St. John's wort is neither regulated nor approved as a depression treatment in the United States so dosage and composition are not standardized. However, St. John's wort may help to reduce mild depression (Keltner & Folks, 2005; Smith & Mischoulon, 2008). Ongoing placebo-controlled clinical trials and comparative studies with SSRIs are likely to yield data about efficacy for different types of depression, comparison with other antidepressants, and long-term maintenance (Keltner & Folks).

Light Therapy. Light therapy (phototherapy) is used for seasonal affective disorder, a depressive disorder associated with reduced sunlight exposure during autumn and winter. Treatment involves daily exposure to full-spectrum wavelengths (such as sunlight) from a high-intensity lamp. The pineal gland receives information about light exposure through nerve pathways. This gland secretes melatonin, a sleep-inducing hormone associated with depression of mood and mental agility. Melatonin secretion is highest during winter under conditions of reduced sunlight. Thus light therapy may help to reduce melatonin production and resultant effects on mood and associated features of depression (Sadock & Sadock, 2007). Reasonable evidence supports use of light therapy as a treatment for children and adolescents (Findling et al., 2004; Jom, Allen, O'Donnell, et al., 2006).

Exercise. Exercise has demonstrated positive effects on depression (Sadock & Sadock, 2007). Exercise produces physiologic and psychological benefits that include a reduced stress response and increased well-being. Athletes and others who regularly engage in physical activity attest to positive feelings (e.g., "runner's high") associated with release of endorphins triggered by exercise. Positive effects of exercise have long been recognized and encouraged as complementary treatment for depression, although additional research with children and adolescents is warranted.

Anticipated Advances in Diagnosis and Management

Most youths with mood disorders do not receive treatment, and even when referrals are made for mental health services, many families do not follow up to obtain care (Melnyk et al., 2003). Furthermore, mental health services for children are in short supply and inadequate in scope, coverage, and accessibility: "Primary care clinics have become the 'de facto' mental health clinics for teens with mental health problems such as depression; however, there is little guidance for primary care professionals who are faced with treating this population" (Cheung, Zuckerbrot, Jensen, et al., 2008, p. e101). Experts from family medicine, pediatrics, nursing, psychology, and child psychiatry support identification and management of adolescent depression in primary care settings with referral and co-management with mental health clinicians (Cheung et al., 2008). They also agree that, in some circumstances, ongoing monitoring, treatment with SSRIs, and psychotherapy can be initiated from primary care settings. However, PCPs often feel that they lack the training, time, and reimbursement potential for taking on this kind of mental health management.

A critically important goal for health care reform is the integration of mental health services into primary care, starting with the increased training in screening and management of common mental health conditions for PCPs, specifically pediatric nurse practitioners and pediatricians (Melnyk et al., 2003). PMH advanced practice nurses, as well as nurse practitioners dually certified in pediatrics and mental health, are ideal clinicians to function in an integrated care model, providing expert and flexible provision of services. Creation of consultation systems between pediatric and mental health clinicians could bridge the gap when a waiting list exists, when mental health services are not readily accessible, and when PCPs are responsible for monitoring responses to treatment provided by mental health specialists. Emerging technology could provide remote access for mental health consultation when access to expert services is limited.

Questions remain regarding whether SSRIs, psychotherapy, or a combined approach of an SSRI and psychotherapy (CBT or other modality) is the best first-line treatment approach. Although there are ethical, methodologic, and practical barriers to pediatric research, more randomized, controlled trials including children from diverse ethnic and socioeconomic backgrounds and with coexisting conditions and developmental delays are needed to test the efficacy and safety of medications and therapeutic modalities (Preston et al., 2008). Since 1998, the FDA has implemented a combination of regulations and financial incentives (i.e., patents) for drug companies that implement efficacy studies in children and adolescents. Hence, although a paucity of published research findings still exists concerning use of psychoactive medications with children

and adolescents, we can expect that this research database will increase significantly in the near future (Preston et al.).

Clinical investigators also are exploring less invasive treatment options. Examples of such methods for the treatment of mood disorders include light therapy and repeated transcranial magnetic stimulation (Findling et al., 2004; Jom et al., 2006).

Recent developments in the field of genetics may lead to a better understanding of the complex causes of mood disorders and better diagnosis and treatment of these conditions. But genetic advances also present challenges for researchers and clinicians, as youths affected by mood disorders, their families, and potential partners attempt to use this information to manage their conditions and make decisions about the future. Health care professionals will need preparation to address potential effects of new discoveries on family relationships (Smoller, Finn, & Gardner-Schuster, 2008).

Associated Problems of Mood Disorders and Treatment

Although research-based evidence about the interface between mood disorders and other illnesses is limited to date, it is logical to expect that youths with mood disorders are more prone to stress-related illnesses and accidents than their non affected peers. Children with mood disorders often exhibit hyperactivity and impulsivity that are associated with aggressive behavior. Furthermore, hyperactivity, impulsivity, and associated aggressive behavior put them at higher risk for falls and accidents, leading to self-injury and injury of others. Social, academic, and occupational problems commonly accompany mood disorders.

Associated Problems of Mood Disorders and Treatment

- Accidents
- Suicide
- Stress-related somatic complaints and problems
- Hyperactivity and impulsivity
- Injury to self or others
- Social, academic, and occupational difficulties
- Coexisting conditions
  - Anxiety disorders (highest)
  - Attention deficit and disruptive behavior disorders
  - Substance use disorders
  - Tourette syndrome

Accidents

Impulsive behavior associated with BPDs sometimes results in accidents. When children present with frequent accidents associated with making poor judgments or feeling frustrated, a covert BPD might be present. Further, a child, adolescent, or parent might describe a suicidal gesture as an accident because of denial or shame. When PCPs observe a pattern of injuries from accidents, assessing the child or adolescent for signs of depression, mania, or hypomania and suicidal ideation is appropriate; if one of these problems is suspected, referral for a mental health evaluation is needed. Children with a diagnosed mood disorder also require ongoing monitoring of self-injurious behavior during primary care visits.

Suicide

In the United States, suicide is the third leading cause of death among young people ages 15 to 24 years (Mann et al., 2006). A dramatic rise in suicide incidence also has occurred among younger children between the ages of 5 and 12 years; suicide rates among these youngsters have more than doubled in the past two decades. Incidence statistics tend to underreport suicide because many suicidal deaths are recorded as "accidents." Moreover, interpreting changing trends is a challenging endeavor. Shain (2007) reported that suicide rates for adolescents increased by 300% from 1950–1990, decreased from 1990–2003, and then increased after 2003. Shain hypothesized that the decrease in use of SSRIs in response to the FDA advisory warning may have had an unintended effect of increasing suicidal risk as a result of inadequate treatment of depression.

Although numerous factors, such as divorce or death of a parent, can prompt young people to attempt to take their own lives, depression and psychotic thinking clearly put youths at higher risk for suicide. Depression often leads to feelings of hopelessness and helplessness, and psychosis can result in a suicide attempt as a response to a hallucination. Suicidal thoughts, threats, or gestures always must be taken very seriously, and children with mood disorders are considered to be at high risk for self-harm. Evaluation includes assessment of the following factors that increase suicide risk (Brendel, Lagomasino, Perlis et al., 2008):

- Evidence of suicidal or homicidal thoughts, intent, or plan
- Availability of means for suicide and lethality of method
- Psychiatric history
- History of suicide attempts or threats
- Family history of suicide or psychiatric illness
- A tumultuous early home environment

Stress-Related Somatic Complaints and Problems

Children and adolescents commonly come for primary care visits because of somatic complaints, such as headaches, sleep disturbances, fatigue, and stomach aches. When a physical illness cannot fully explain somatic symptoms, emotional distress might be contributing to the problem. After ruling out possible illnesses or when such illnesses do not explain symptoms completely, exploring another source of the problem is warranted. In addition, when physical symptoms persist or occur in relation to stressful situations, a mental health problem might be present. Children sometimes express emotional distress and depressed feelings as physical symptoms. Depressive disorders in particular may present with fatigue and sleep disturbance.

Coexisting Conditions

Coexisting conditions and overlap of symptoms from other psychiatric disorders are common and tailored interventions may be required (Bostic & Prince, 2008). Fewer than one third of children and adolescents with a diagnosis of a depressive disorder are experiencing only depression (Stark et al., 2006). Anxiety disorders are the most frequently co-occurring conditions, followed by attention deficit and disruptive behavior disorders and substance-related disorders (Mash & Wolfe, 2005). In a study to differentiate ADHD from major depressive disorder, 16% of youths with ADHD also had major depressive disorder (Diler, Daviss, Lopez, et al., 2007).

Furthermore, the researchers discerned that mood/anhedonia symptoms and cognitive symptoms, including thoughts of suicide, distinguished between major depression and ADHD, but few neurovegetative symptoms did so.

BPD in children rarely occurs as a single diagnosis. Typically, a cluster of symptoms that suggest other disorders, such as ADHD, oppositional defiant and conduct disorders, substance abuse, or Tourette syndrome (see Chapter 41), accompanies BPDs. Among youths seen for evaluation of possible BPD, preexisting ADHD, disruptive behavior problems, substance abuse problems, anxiety disorders, and suicidal ideation are common (Mash & Wolfe, 2005).

Prognosis

Depressive disorders typically have a long-term course with periods of remission that vary across diagnoses and individuals. Major depressive disorder has a high rate of recurrence. At least 60% of individuals with a single episode experience another episode, and 5% to 10% subsequently have a manic episode. Partial remission rather than complete remission also increases the likelihood of additional episodes (APA, 2000). Most children and adolescents with a depressive disorder experience recovery. However, evidence indicates that recovery requires treatment over time (i.e., several months to years), the presence of coexisting mental health problems complicates recovery, and the severity at onset increases the likelihood of future episodes (Turk et al., 2007).

Dysthymic disorder is likely to have an insidious onset during childhood, adolescence, or early adulthood, with a chronic course. Major depressive disorder may be superimposed over a dysthymia. The spontaneous remission rate for dysthymic disorder may be as low as 10%; however, active treatment significantly improves outcomes (APA, 2000).

BPDs tend to have a chronic course. BPD recurs in 90% of individuals who have a single manic episode. The majority of affected persons experience remission of symptoms between episodes, 20% to 30% continue to experience mood instability and other ongoing mood symptoms, and up to 60% have interpersonal and occupational or school difficulties between acute episodes. The course of BPD characterized by hypomania rather than mania tends to be less severe, and most individuals return to a good functional level between episodes; however, about 15% of affected individuals continue to have interpersonal and occupational or school difficulties. Dysthymic disorder and cyclothymic disorder tend to have an early and insidious onset and follow a chronic course. When cyclothymic disorder is present, the risk for development of a more serious BPD is 15% to 50% (APA, 2000). Thus mood disorders have a high risk of recurrence of episodes, and many of these conditions have a chronic lifetime course.

When individuals experience recurrence of depression or mania, they also are at risk for self-harm. Repeated major depressive episodes contribute to hopelessness that can prompt suicidal ideation and actions. The cyclic nature of manic episodes, with or without alternating periods of depression, impairs judgment and therefore increases risk for self-harm through unintentional accidents, dangerous behaviors, and suicide attempts. Thus to evaluate the prognosis for any child or adolescent with a mood disorder, the long-term risk for self-harm merits ongoing consideration.

PRIMARY CARE MANAGEMENT

Health Care Maintenance
Growth and Development
Mood disorders are not associated with specific alterations in normal physical growth and development, and therefore regular age-appropriate screening is recommended. However, failure to achieve expected weight gains for children, weight loss without dieting, or increases or decreases in appetite constitute a criterion for a major depressive episode requiring additional evaluation when detected during any primary health care encounter. If undetected and untreated, underlying depression could thwart a child's normal growth over time. In addition, psychopharmacologic treatment may cause appetite and weight changes. TCAs, MAOIs, mood stabilizers, some antipsychotics, and possibly atypical/novel antidepressants (notably mirtazapine [Remeron]) frequently cause weight gain that may be distressing to children and adolescents and requires monitoring.

Interruptions in social development frequently result from or even contribute to the development and chronic course of mood disorders. Failure to reach academic standards for grades in school and poor social integration may threaten psychosocial development of affected youths. Thus evaluating information about functioning at home, in school, and in social settings is an important component of regular developmental monitoring.

Diet
Changes in eating patterns may occur with mood disorders. Decreased or increased appetite and changes in food preferences often develop as early signs of mood disorders. Hoarding and binge eating can be seen across these disorders. Excessive eating may be an attempt to fill a sense of emptiness or to self-soothe in depressive disorders. During mania, children and adolescents may become "too busy" to stop for a meal. Poor nutrition results from binge eating, filling up on junk food and sweets, or inadequate intake of calories and nutrients during mania. Nutritional planning and, in severe cases, a nutritional consultation are needed to ensure that affected children and adolescents maintain adequate dietary intake. Increased risk for development of a coexisting eating disorder requires careful monitoring throughout treatment and recovery phases. In addition, because psychotropic medications can cause changes in appetite and weight, dietary and weight monitoring and education about the side effects of medications are important clinical actions during primary care encounters.

Safety
Assessment of the potential for self-injury because of poor judgment and risky behavior also is needed when depression or a hypomanic or manic episode is suspected or evident. For example, adolescents who have driving violations, especially speeding, are at risk for self-injury and harming others. Risk behaviors necessitate careful monitoring and may require parental limitations on privileges and even hospitalization in extreme situations to ensure safety.

Safety considerations also accompany psychotropic medication use. Referral to psychiatric practitioners to initiate medication use and to provide periodic evaluation over the course of treatment is recommended as appropriate and safe primary care practice when treating mood disorders in children and adolescents. Risk of overdose, particularly with TCAs, antipsychotics, lithium, and antiepileptic drugs, and the potential for serious adverse reactions necessitate intensive education of affected youths and their parents at initiation of treatment and follow-up education at every health care visit. As mentioned previously, medication interactions with rarely used MAOIs pose significant risks. In addition, SSRIs, as well as antipsychotic and antiepileptic drugs, all interact with other medications metabolized through cytochrome P pathways (Preston et al., 2008).

Youths with mood disorders may attempt to self-medicate by using substances, including alcohol and street drugs. Substance use can mask mood disorder symptoms and places youths at risk for overdose, accidents, impulsive sexual activity, sexual assault, and fighting. Although assessment of substance use among older children and adolescents is an important component of primary care, ongoing evaluation is essential whenever a youth has a mood disorder.

Educating parents and affected youths about psychotropic drugs is an essential component of primary care. Clinicians share medication management with children and adolescents being treated and their families. Educational goals include understanding the medication's purpose, desired effects, dosage, and administration; related tests and monitoring; potential side effects and adverse effects; risk for overdose; possible interactions and dietary requirements; and anticipated time frame for treatment (Box 33-4).

Immunizations
Routine immunizations are recommended per latest CDC recommendations (CDC, 2009).

Screening
Vision. Routine screening for vision is recommended (Box 33-5). To ensure that symptoms of withdrawal, low self-esteem, distractibility, irritability, and impaired attention are not partially caused by impaired sight, conducting vision screening when assessing for a mood disorder is recommended.

Hearing. Routine screening for hearing is recommended. To ensure that symptoms of withdrawal, low self-esteem, distractibility, irritability, and impaired attention are not partially caused by impaired hearing, conducting hearing screening when assessing for a mood disorder is recommended.

Dental. Routine screening is recommended.

Blood Pressure. Routine screening is recommended. Blood pressure should be monitored regularly during the first several weeks of medication treatment if novel antidepressants, TCAs, MAOIs, or atypical antipsychotics are prescribed, and it should be monitored every few months thereafter. If MAOIs are in use, the risk of hypertensive crisis is serious if the required diet is not followed carefully or if drug interactions occur (Alpert, 2008; Keltner & Folks, 2005). In such instances, blood pressure screening or monitoring is ineffective because onset is rapid and requires immediate emergency treatment. Thus, in the rare instances in which MAOIs are used, education about the risks associated with diet and medications is essential.

Hematocrit. Routine screening is recommended unless the child is taking specific medications below.

Urinalysis. Routine screening is recommended.

Tuberculosis. Routine screening is recommended.

BOX 33-4

Parent Education for Specific Psychotropic Drugs

ANTIDEPRESSANTS

- Tricyclics can be fatal in overdose. Drug administration should be supervised, and the drug should be securely stored.
- Other medications, including antibiotics and over-the-counter agents, may interact with antidepressants. Hence, all medications should be reviewed with the primary clinician.
- The selective serotonin reuptake inhibitors (SSRIs) can cause motor restlessness, insomnia, and irritability.
- In OCD and depression, there may be a lag between initiation of treatment and clinical response.

ANTIPSYCHOTIC AGENTS

- Antipsychotic drugs are part of a comprehensive program to treat psychosis and may be added on in small doses to treatment regimes for other conditions.
- Traditional antipsychotic medications can cause dystonic reactions, especially early in treatment.
- Watch for muscle rigidity, inability to remain still, and new abnormal movements.
- Review the risk of tardive dyskinesia and withdrawal dyskinesia before treatment.

MOOD STABILIZERS/ANTICONVULSANTS

- Some medications require monitoring of serum levels (involves drawing blood samples).
- Lithium can cause serious and even fatal reactions if serum level is too high.
- With lithium, keep child well hydrated with adequate liquids (10-12 glasses of water per day) and extra care during exercise and hot weather.
- Topiramate (Topamax) can reduce effectiveness of oral contraceptives.
- Valproate (Depakote) is associated with polycystic ovary syndrome; use with caution in girls.
- Many side effects can occur with these medications: report changes to primary care practitioner (PCP) to evaluate.
- Some side effects may decrease over time.
- Contact PCP if serious side effects occur: vomiting, severe tremor, severe sedation, muscle weakness, and dizziness.
- Gastrointestinal effects and weight gain occur with many of the drugs: give with food, encourage healthy diet (decrease high-calorie foods and drinks) and moderate exercise.
- Sedation, blood changes, and skin problems occur with some drugs.
- Learn side effects for particular medication from PCP and follow instructions for follow-up health care visits, observe changes, know changes that are serious and require immediate action, and use measures to reduce effects as suggested by PCP.

From Scahill, L. & Rains, A. (2005b). Psychopharmacology for children. In N.L. Keltner & D.G. Folks (Eds.), *Psychotropic Drugs* (4th ed.). St. Louis: Mosby. Modified with permission.

BOX 33-5

Screening

VISION AND HEARING

- Determine if symptoms are related to vision or hearing deficits

SPEECH AND LANGUAGE

- Additional evaluation if treatment does not correct any abnormalities

BLOOD PRESSURE

- Baseline readings before starting medication treatment
- Monitor throughout treatment
- Alter dose or change medication if persistent elevation
- Stop medication immediately if extreme increase and seek emergency intervention

CARDIAC

- Baseline blood pressure, complete blood count (CBC), and electrocardiogram (ECG) before starting tricyclic antidepressants (TCAs) and atypical antipsychotics
- Repeat if dosage is changed or if PR interval ≥0.22 seconds, QRS ≥130% of baseline, pulse >140/90 mm Hg

DRUG TOXICITY SCREENING

- Monitor for safety-specific recommendations for each drug class

---

Condition-Specific Screening

Speech and Language. If psychomotor retardation is present when a depressive disorder is suspected, or if rapid speech flow is noted when a manic episode is suspected, additional speech and language evaluation may be indicated. However, if other symptoms of a mood disorder are present and meet diagnostic criteria, treatment for the appropriate mood disorder is implemented first. If speech and language do not normalize in relation to improvement of other symptoms, then additional evaluation of speech and language is needed.

Cardiac Function. Children taking TCAs and some antipsychotic medications are at risk for adverse cardiac effects, including tachycardia, prolonged QTc interval, arrhythmias, and orthostatic hypotension (Preston et al., 2008). Obtaining baseline blood pressure, complete blood count (CBC), and electrocardiogram (ECG) is recommended. If a dosage is changed, blood pressure, CBC, and ECG should be repeated. Lowering the dosage is warranted when the PR interval reaches 0.22 seconds or QRS reaches 130% of baseline on ECG, heart rate is greater than 140 beats/min, or blood pressure is higher than 140/90 mm Hg.

Drug Toxicity Screening. Medications used to treat mood disorders have various adverse effects. Screening and safety monitoring recommendations are provided for the most commonly prescribed medications and for selected drugs in practice with specific recommendations (Keltner & Folks, 2005; Preston et al., 2008; Scahill & Rains, 2005a, 2005b; Schatzberg & Nemeroff, 2004). (See Table 33-2 for additional medication information.)

TCAs. An ECG should be done at baseline, and regular blood pressure and pulse checks should be done; evaluate family history for cardiac disease. Repeat ECGs with each dosage increase; and every 3 months when the maintenance dose is reached.

MAOIs. Monitor diet and avoid contraindicated foods, medications, and substances.

Lithium. Laboratory work should be done weekly to monitor plasma levels; after stabilization, monitor monthly. Most individuals experience some toxic effects with levels over 1.5 mEq/L, and levels over 2.0 mEq/L are associated with life-threatening side effects. Baseline ECG should be recorded. Because lithium can cause alterations in kidney function, blood urea nitrogen (BUN) and creatinine levels should be checked every 4 to 6 months; because lithium can cause goiter or hypothyroidism, a thyroid-stimulating hormone test should be done every 4 to 6 months.

Carbamazepine (Tegretol). Laboratory tests should be performed weekly to monitor plasma levels; after stabilization, monitor monthly. Baseline ECG should be recorded. Baseline hemoglobin, hematocrit, CBC with differential, white blood cell (WBC) count, platelet count, and liver function tests (LFTs) should be done. Monitoring recommendations vary, but a conservative plan is as follows: CBC and LFTs weekly for 1 month, monthly for 4 months, and every 3 months thereafter. Evaluate CBC for blood dyscrasias, especially agranulocytosis and leukopenia (rare). Order tests if rash, lethargy, fever, weakness, malaise, vomiting, anorexia, increased urinary frequency, jaundice, easy bruising, bleeding, or mouth ulcers occur. Stop the drug if neutrophil count drops below 1000/mm³ or if hepatitis occurs.

Valproate/valproic acid (Depakote). Baseline and periodic CBC and LFTs should be obtained. Suggest scheduling laboratory tests as for carbamazepine (Tegretol).

Topiramate (Topamax). Baseline and periodic serum bicarbonate levels to assess for metabolic acidosis should be done (Stahl, 2006).

Antipsychotic Medications

Chlorpromazine (Thorazine). Baseline and periodic (e.g., every 3 to 6 months) CBC and LFTs should be done.

Atypical Antipsychotic Agents

Risperidone (Risperidal); quetiapine (Seroquel); aripiprazole (Abilify). Baseline weight, BMI, waist circumference, blood pressure, fasting plasma glucose, and fasting lipid profile should be obtained before starting treatment. Patients who are overweight (BMI >95th percentile for age) have high blood pressure (>95th percentile for age and height), prediabetes (fasting plasma glucose 100-126 mg/dL), diabetes (fasting plasma glucose ≥126 mg/dL), or dyslipidemia (increased total cholesterol, low-density lipoprotein cholesterol, and triglycerides; decreased high-density lipoprotein cholesterol) should be referred for nutritional counseling before starting treatment. BMI should continue to be monitored for 3 months, then on a quarterly basis. Blood pressure, fasting plasma glucose, and fasting lipids should be measured within 3 months of starting treatment and then annually, but earlier and more frequently in patients who are diabetic or for those who have gained more than 5% of their initial body weight (Medpage Today, 2008; Stahl, 2006).

Common Illness Management

Differential Diagnosis

Differential diagnosis is an important issue in relation to all mood disorders for children and adolescents. Considerable overlap in symptoms with several other psychiatric disorders requires evaluation of diagnostic *DSM-IV-TR* criteria across conditions. Several other disorders require evaluation including, but not limited to, anxiety disorders, ADHD, substance use disorders, and eating disorders. Common problems seen by PCPs that include weight loss, somatic complaints, fatigue, recurrent injuries, and school failure have overlapping presentations with mood disorders. A detailed and thorough history is often the best strategy to help the clinician create an accurate timeline of the onset of symptoms. The youth and the parent or other important person in the child's life may be of great assistance in providing these critical data.

Anxiety often accompanies other symptoms of depressive disorders among children and adolescents and tends to emerge as a coexisting condition as age and severity increase. Distractibility and inattention, characteristics of ADHD, overlap with symptoms of depressive disorders and BPDs. All other diagnostic criteria merit careful evaluation to differentiate these diagnoses.

Youths who experience depression or mania often use alcohol and drugs in an attempt to manage symptoms or because of their poor judgment. If criteria for any substance use disorder are met, co-occurring conditions exist and both disorders require active treatment. Moreover, safety risks result from illegal use of substances, interactions of substances with prescribed medications, and increased incidence of accidents. Therefore even if diagnostic criteria for a substance use disorder are not met, the reasons, pattern, and effects necessitate exploration, and strategies to promote and monitor abstinence are important components of care.

Differential Diagnosis

- Adjustment disorders
- Anxiety disorders
- Attention-deficit/hyperactivity disorder
- Eating disorders
- Recurrent injuries
- Somatic complaints
- Substance use disorders

Weight loss and reduced appetite that can occur in depressive disorders might appear like signs of anorexia nervosa; however, individuals with anorexia typically retain their desire for food even when restricting intake and mood changes can emerge as a secondary problem to the eating disorder. Binge eating, a component of bulimia nervosa, can occur with mania. Obtaining a detailed report for food intake from a single day, exploring perceptions of food and body characteristics, and evaluating other impulsive behaviors will assist the clinician to differentiate eating disorders from mood disorders (see also Chapter 25). Weight loss among children and adolescents with mood disorders requires careful investigation to detect a possible underlying illness (Becker, Mickley, Derenne et al., 2008).

Somatic complaints may be expressions of emotional distress but also may indicate another illness or problem. Fatigue is a common symptom of depression but is also associated with many physical illnesses. PCPs can evaluate such symptoms by asking the child about other signs related to the diagnosed mood disorder and about signs of other suspected illnesses. For example, a stomach ache might indicate emotional upset or a gastrointestinal disorder. Before attributing a somatic complaint to a mood disorder, investigation of a possible physical cause is needed. Recurrent injuries require thorough evaluation in addition to safety education and assessment of judgment and functioning. For example, frequent falling from athletic equipment on a playground might indicate self-injurious motivation, impulsiveness, or a physical problem such as a neurologic disorder. Poor school performance or failure could be caused by exacerbation of a mood disorder or by another problem, such as a learning or developmental disorder.

Drug Interactions and Adverse Drug Effects

Drug interactions can occur with concurrent use of two or more psychotropic agents or when a psychopharmacologic drug interacts with a medication used to treat a different problem. Youths being medicated for mood disorders are at risk for both types of drug interactions. Monitoring drug plasma levels is indicated when interactions have the potential to raise or lower levels to an extent that safety or efficacy is affected and when careful monitoring is indicated to judge safety and efficacy of dosage, such as with lithium use.

Antidepressants. SSRIs have a more benign profile than earlier TCA and MAOI antidepressants, including less risk from cumulative effects with concomitant CNS depressants such as alcohol, antihistamines, or anticholinergic drugs (Schatzberg & Nemeroff, 2004). However, significant drug interactions are associated with SSRIs. Fluoxetine (Prozac) and sertraline (Zoloft) are powerful inhibitors of the cytochrome P (CYP) 450 2D6 pathway, which could interfere with the analgesic actions of codeine and increase the plasma levels of some beta blockers and of atomoxetine (Strattera). Fluoxetine can increase the concentration of certain antipsychotics (e.g., thioridazine [Mellaril] or aripiprazole [Abilify]), which can cause dangerous cardiac arrhythmias. Grapefruit juice increases sertraline levels. Similarly, the clearance of diazepam (Valium) and trazodone (Desyrel) may be reduced, thus increasing plasma levels. CYP 3A4 inhibition may increase levels of alprazolam (Xanax), buspirone (BuSpar), and triazolam (Halcion) (Stahl, 2006).

Serotonin syndrome, a rare and potentially fatal adverse reaction to SSRIs, presents with heightened restlessness, confusion, and lethargy and may progress to myoclonus, hyperthermia, and rigor. Serotonin syndrome may result from overstimulation of the serotonergic centers. The risk for occurrence is greatest when a clinician changes medication from an SSRI to an MAOI; or when SSRIs are used in combination with substances taken to produce a high, such as dextromethorphan, amphetamines, or Ecstasy (methylenedioxy methamphetamine [MMDA]), or with triptans used to treat migraine headaches. Fortunately, MAOIs are seldom used for the treatment of depression because pharmacologic options with more favorable side effect profiles are available (Rusyniak & Sprague, 2005).

Changing from an SSRI to an MAOI requires that at least five half-lives elapse between the cessation of one medication and the initiation of the second; the long half-life of fluoxetine (Prozac) necessitates a 5-week washout period. A 2-week waiting period is recommended to change from an MAOI to an SSRI. SSRIs and antipsychotic medications may reduce metabolism and clearance of TCAs, causing a rise in TCA blood levels (Alpert, 2008; Scahill & Rains, 2005a, 2005b).In addition, albuterol should not be used in conjunction with TCAs or MAOIs due to their additive effects on the vascular system (Ogbru, 2008).

Mood Stabilizers. Drug treatment of mania also poses risks for adverse effects and interactions. Lithium has few clinically significant drug interactions; however, a risk of kidney damage exists. Lithium is cleared by the kidneys with an approximate half-life of 14 to 30 hours. Young people tend to have a faster lithium clearance rate than older adults. Changes in hydration, renal function, and sodium levels alter lithium serum levels; diuretics increase lithium levels by 30% to 50%. Agents that may produce interactions with lithium are diuretics, nonsteroidal antiinflammatory agents (e.g., ibuprofen, naproxen), neuroleptics, potassium, and antiarrhythmics (Perlis & Ostacher, 2008; Schatzberg & Nemeroff, 2004).

Anticonvulsants, used as mood stabilizers in BPD, have significant interactions with other medications cleared through the liver. Valproate (Depakote) is highly protein bound; therefore interactions, including valproate toxicity, may occur with other protein-bound medications, most notably aspirin. Valproate also weakly inhibits drug oxidation on several CYP pathways, resulting in increased serum concentrations of TCAs, phenobarbital, and phenytoin. Co-administration of microsomal enzyme-inducing drugs, such as carbamazepine (Tegretol), can decrease serum concentrations of valproate, and drugs that inhibit metabolism, such as fluoxetine (Prozac), can increase levels (Alpert, 2008; Schatzberg & Nemeroff, 2004; Stahl, 2006). Carbamazepine induces metabolism of other drugs by the liver and is highly protein bound. Thus this medication decreases plasma levels of many other medications, including TCAs, antipsychotics (particularly haloperidol), thyroid hormones, hormonal contraceptives, antiasthmatics (e.g., prednisone, methylprednisone, theophylline), warfarin, valproate, benzodiazepines, and neuroleptics. Drugs that inhibit carbamazepine metabolism, including erythromycin, calcium channel blockers (diltiazem, verapamil), danazol, isoniazid, valproate, and SSRIs, will increase serum levels. Other anticonvulsants, notably gabapentin and lamotrigine, have drug interactions: Gabapentin may interact with antacids and cimetidine; and lamotrigine may interact with carbamazepine, phenobarbital, phenytoin, primidone, and valproate. Topiramate (Topamax) may decrease phenytoin (Dilantin) and valproate levels. Also, carbamazepine, phenytoin, and valproate may increase the clearance of topiramate, possibly requiring higher doses. (Alpert, 2008; Schatzberg & Nemeroff, 2004; Stahl, 2006).

Currently, haloperidol (Haldol), risperidone (Risperdal), aripiprazole (Abilify) are the only antipsychotic medications that have been approved by the U.S. FDA for use in children and adolescents (U.S. FDA, 2008b; Correll, 2008); however, quetiapine (Seroquel) is also used as a mood stabilizer. Preliminary data indicate that children and adolescents are more prone to experience sedation and extrapyramidal side effects (e.g., dystonia, parkinsonian symptoms) from antipsychotic medications than are adults. Hyperprolactinemia and age-inappropriate weight gain with related metabolic abnormalities are also more prevalent among this population. Quetiapine can prolong the QTc interval and may interact with other QT interval prolongers, such as macrolide antibiotics. Aripiprazole is metabolized on the CYP 2D6 pathway and could interact with both fluoxetine and quetiapine. In summary, PCPs are urged to exercise caution and monitor medications and combination therapies closely.

Developmental Issues
Sleep Patterns

Sleep disturbances characterize mood disorders. Although sleep patterns among children and adolescents who experience mood disorders may not mirror the sleep of adults with depressive or BPDs (Mash & Wolfe, 2005), sleeping difficulties are common symptoms. Excessive sleeping, too little sleep, disrupted sleep, and poor quality of sleep all contribute to irritability, poor school performance, and fatigue or agitation. The depressed child may sleep more or have insomnia that may be related to a coexisting anxiety disorder or may be due to anxiety associated with the depression. The child with BPD may cycle from periods of very little sleep and hyperactivity to periods of utter exhaustion during which the child may want to sleep all day. A coexisting hyperactivity disorder could also profoundly affect sleep cycles. As previously mentioned, the sedating effects of many psychoactive medications must also be considered.

Changes in sleep patterns may be one of the early signs of an incipient mood episode. Eliciting an account of recent sleep patterns, including any changes from usual patterns, from parents and pediatric clients will assist PCPs to identify signs that might signify a mood disorder. Keeping a sleep diary can assist youths and their parents to track patterns and monitor response to treatment. Improvement is expected with treatment; in addition, implementing good sleep habits, including a regular bedtime, avoidance of caffeine in the evening, and relaxing routines before sleep, can assist in normalizing sleep patterns.

Toileting

Mood disorders generally are not associated with significant difficulties in toileting. In some instances, however, problems with bedwetting and soiling have been seen in children with BPD (Papolos & Papolos, 2006).

Discipline

Mood disorders can create tremendous interactive problems for children and adolescents in various environments, including the home, the classroom, and the playground. Parents and teachers may perceive depressed children who are frequently quiet and withdrawn as being uncooperative. Children with BPD are prone to aggressive behavior and outbursts that are disruptive; these behaviors might alienate them from the other children who fear for their own safety. All children and adolescents with mood disorders are prone to irritability that often translates into lack of cooperation and lack of respect. If adults treat symptoms as discipline problems without treating the underlying disorder, discipline will be ineffective and likely exacerbate the undesired behaviors. Consistent limit setting and clear explanations of behavioral contingencies are appropriate discipline strategies. Enforcing rules regarding safety also is essential for purposes of protection.

Child Care

Although no specific problems concerning child care are associated with mood disorders, children with these disorders can present a challenge to child-care providers. These children frequently have trouble relating to peers. Irritability makes them difficult to be around and tends to push others away. Children with BPD typically have periods of disruptive behavior that can cause safety problems and interfere with group activities. In addition, a lack of pleasure (anhedonia), a cardinal symptom of depressive disorders, limits engagement in usual social activities and even casual peer pastimes. Regular schedules and placement in small family settings or centers with high staff/child ratios and stable personnel are ideal. Once a diagnosis has been made, child-care personnel should be educated about the condition and management in the setting. These issues necessitate careful placement with consistent, caring caregivers for child care to be successful—not always an easy goal.

Schooling

Not surprisingly, children with mood disorders, particularly BPDs, frequently experience a great deal of difficulty in school. Successful school performance requires concentration, alertness, proper behavior, individual performance, teamwork, and an ability to consolidate information quickly. A downward slide in grades, difficulty managing school-related activities, and behavior problems in the classroom are indicators that students might be experiencing a mood disorder. Although such behavioral signs are associated with many health-related problems among youth too, often they fail to trigger evaluation for a mood disorder. Poor concentration, irritability, disorganization, lack of self-confidence, or grandiosity interferes with academic work. In addition, the factors discussed above

in relation to social problems also lead to difficulties in school, most notably withdrawal, bullying, and fighting.

Without timely evaluation and treatment, school-related problems can escalate and may lead to academic failure and even dropping out of school among adolescents. In severe cases, hospitalization and residential placement may be needed. In such instances, removal from school becomes necessary, and academic tutoring or schooling in a residential treatment setting must substitute for usual school attendance. Children with mood disorders often have trouble making transitions and may have coexisting conditions that make them easily distracted and inattentive. In addition, medications may have a sedating effect that makes it difficult for these children to stay awake (Papolos & Papolos, 2006).

Clearly, children with mood disorders often require special accommodations in school that are guaranteed by federal law (see Chapter 3). PCPs may help the child and family obtain educational services, negotiate modification of the educational program, or collaborate with the therapist. An individualized educational plan (IEP) may assist the student to function in the classroom. For example, a student may require adjustments in assignments, setting, or teaching modality to learn effectively. To create a viable plan, consultation is needed among learning specialists in the school system, teachers, the guidance counselor or school psychologist, and the PCP and psychiatric clinician involved in the student's care. The PCP appropriately provides information to involved school personnel, with parental consent and student assent, and monitors progress.

Sexuality

Depressive disorders may affect sexuality by reducing interest and performance ability among adolescents (APA, 2000). More important for young people, difficulty establishing close relationships may interfere with the development of healthy sexuality. In addition, BPDs are associated with poor judgment during manic episodes that could lead to impulsive sexual behavior and related risks for unwanted pregnancy and sexually transmitted diseases (STDs). PCPs are encouraged to discuss dating and sexual behavior and to provide early contraceptive education, and pregnancy and STD testing. Because medications to manage BPDs (i.e., carbamazepine, topiramate) can reduce the effectiveness of hormonal contraceptives, alternative or dual birth control methods (e.g., use of condoms with birth control pills, higher doses of oral contraceptives, or depot medroxyprogesterone) are recommended (Zieman, Hatcher, Cwiak et al., 2007). Condoms also provide some protection against STDs. Exploring risks associated with sexual behavior may assist older children and adolescents to make responsible choices. In addition, genetic counseling may be indicated, given available knowledge about genetic factors in etiology of mood disorders, particularly for BPDs.

If pregnancy occurs and is maintained, continuation of psychotropic medications requires careful evaluation by all involved providers, including obstetric and perinatal specialists and a PMH specialist in psychopharmacology. Because all psychotropic drugs diffuse across the placenta, the FDA has not approved any psychotropic medication for use during pregnancy. Psychotropics vary in teratogenic potential. Nonetheless, determining a plan involves evaluation of severity of mood disorder symptoms and risk of relapse versus risks of medication use. Thus a careful case-by-case analysis of risks versus benefits for the pregnant adolescent and fetus is needed to determine the best treatment plan (Wang, Nonacs, Viguera, et al., 2008). Clearly, these complex issues necessitate collaboration among PCPs, psychiatric providers, parents/guardians, and affected adolescents.

Transition to Adulthood

Symptoms associated with mood disorders typically interfere with the ability of affected children and adolescents to relate to peers, develop intimate relationships, and manage responsibilities—important goals in preparation for transition into adulthood. Although hypomanic symptoms initially may help affected youths to be popular and engage in a whirlwind of activities, as irritability and disorganization increase with mania, social engagement and functional ability decrease. Poor social relationships and impaired performance in school or work are hallmarks of mood disorders that directly interfere with a successful transition to adulthood. Separation from family is particularly difficult because a consistent and supportive home environment promotes recovery and helps to prevent relapse. Moreover, being sensitive to cultural practices and values is essential because the meaning of transition to adulthood varies. Effective transitions to college or work and moving away from home involve planning for continuation of treatment, including crisis management, and development of ways to maintain connection with family members, such as visits and contact by telephone and e-mail.

Adolescents with mood disorders may face trouble managing future responsibilities. If substance abuse also is present, difficulties multiply. Obtaining occupational preparation and holding a consistent job are challenging tasks. Functioning in the work world is necessary to receive health insurance, to obtain housing, and to manage other financial obligations. Failure to establish stable employment in adulthood leads to ongoing dependency on family or government programs with increased risk for homelessness and a course of chronic mental illness. PCPs play an important role in encouraging affected adolescents and their families to plan appropriately for education and occupational preparation, and to anticipate the need for ongoing or episodic treatment suitable to the young person's diagnosis and its severity.

Family Concerns

Mood disorders can also take a toll on the family as a whole. The "well" siblings may harbor feelings of resentment as the "ill" child gets special accommodations based on the condition. The child with BPD also may embarrass family members with angry public outbursts of rage (Papolos & Papolos, 2006). Coping with the vicissitudes of mood and behavior, especially for children with rapid-cycling BPDs, is a daily challenge for families (Box 33-6).

Families also face other worries. Stigma associated with mental illness may lead to shame and isolation. Concerns about possible genetic transmission can create feelings of guilt and anger, as well as anxiety about future generations. Parents often worry that symptoms will worsen over time and that their child will be unable to live independently or to fulfill their hopes for a productive and happy life.

Financial concerns often worry parents. Difficulty obtaining adequate health care coverage for psychiatric disorders, particularly when a long-term course develops, creates real financial burden and stress for families. Efforts at state and federal levels to pass and enforce legislation for mental health parity have improved coverage for pediatric care; however, adequacy of services, especially for pediatric chronic conditions, varies widely and remains a long-term concern.

BOX 33-6

The Rapid-Cycling Bipolar Child: A Day of Mood Swings

- *Mornings:* Difficult to arouse; resists getting up, dressed, and off to school; irritable with a tendency to snap and gripe or sullen and withdrawn.
- *Midday:* The darkness lifts, and the bipolar child enjoys a few clear hours, enabling the child to focus and take part in school.
- *Late afternoon:* The child becomes increasingly wild, wired, euphoric in a giddy and strained way; laughs too loudly and too long; play has a flailing and aggressive quality; temper tantrums when needs are not met.
- *Late evening:* Behavior can continue well into the night, accounting for the difficulty getting up in the morning.

TREATMENT

- Conventional psychopharmacology recommended for adults
- Stable schedules; no caffeine, drugs, or alcohol
- Individual therapy to help learn to balance the day and resolve crises that can trigger a mood change
- Family therapy so that parents and siblings can learn how to help

From Laraia, M.T. (2002). Bipolar disorder: Bipolar depression, rapid cycling, children, and pharmacology. *APNA News, 14,* 13. Reprinted with permission.

Resources

Organizations, support groups, and informational websites are available resources for families. The following is a list of resources and organizations as presented by Demitri and Janice Papolos in *The Bipolar Child: The Definitive and Reassuring Guide to Childhood's Most Misunderstood Disorder* (3rd. ed.) (2006).

Family Voices, Inc.
2340 Alamo SE, Suite 102
Albuquerque, NM 87106
(505) 867-2368; (888) 835-5669; Fax: (505) 872-4780
Email: kidshealth@familyvoices.org
Website: www.familyvoices.org

Lithium Information Center
c/o Madison Institute of Medicine
7617 Mineral Point Dr., Suite 300
Madison, WI 53717
(608) 827-2470; Fax: (608) 827-2479
Email: mim@miminc.org
Website: www.miminc.org/aboutlithinfoctr.asp

National Federation of Families for Children's Mental Health
9605 Medical Center Dr.
Rockville, MD 20850
(240) 403-1901 ; Fax: (240) 403-1909
Email: ffcmh@ffcmh.org
Website: www.ffcmh.org

Internet Resources

The Bipolar Child (Website for Demitri and Janice Papolos)
Website: www.bipolarchild.com

Pendulum Resources
Website: www.pendulum.org

Organizations

Child and Adolescent Bipolar Foundation
1000 Skokie Blvd., Suite 570

Wilmette, IL 60091
(847) 256-8525; Fax: (847) 920-9498
Website: www.bpkids.org
Depression and Bipolar Support Alliance
730 N. Franklin St., Suite 501
Chicago, IL 60654-7225
(800) 826-3632; Fax: (312) 642-7243
Website: www.dbsalliance.org/site/PageServer?pagename=home
Mental Health America
2000 N. Beauregard St., 6th Floor
Alexandria, VA 22311
(800) 969-6642; (703) 684-7722; Crisis Help Line:
   (800) 273-TALK; Fax: (703) 684-5698
Website: www.nmha.org

National Alliance for the Mentally Ill (NAMI)
Colonial Place Three
2107 Wilson Blvd., Suite 300
Arlington, VA 22201-3042
(703) 524-7600; (800) 950-NAMI (6264); Fax (703) 524-9094
Website: www.nami.org
National Alliance for Research on Schizophrenia and Depression
60 Cutter Mill Rd., Suite 404
Great Neck, NY 11021
(516) 829-0091; (800) 829-8289; Fax: (516) 487-6930
Website: www.narsad.org
E-mail info@arsad.org

Summary of Primary Care Needs for the Child or Adolescent with a Mood Disorder

HEALTH CARE MAINTENANCE

Growth and Development

- Failure to achieve expected weight gains, weight loss without dieting, and increases or decreases in appetite require additional evaluation.
- Psychopharmacotherapy may cause appetite and weight changes.
- Failure to reach academic standards and poor social integration may threaten psychosocial development of affected youth. Evaluate information about functioning at home, in school, and in social settings.

Diet

- Decreased or increased appetite, hoarding, binge eating, and changes in food preferences can occur.
- During mania, children and adolescents may become "too busy" to stop for a meal.
- Poor nutrition results from binge eating, filling up on junk food and sweets, or inadequate intake of calories and nutrients during mania.
- Increased risk for development of a coexisting eating disorder requires careful monitoring throughout treatment and recovery phases.
- Psychotropic medications can cause changes in appetite and weight. Monitor diet and weight, and educate about side effects of medications.

Use of monoamine oxidase inhibitors (MAOIs) requires a special diet that excludes foods high in tyramine and avoidance of foods and drug interactions that may cause hypertension, anticholinergic effects, or sympathomimetic effects. (Please refer to a drug reference book for more details.*)

Safety

- Suicidal thoughts, threats, or gestures always must be taken seriously, and children and adolescents with mood disorders are considered to be at high risk for self-harm.
- When a hypomanic or manic episode is suspected or evident, assess potential for self-injury because of poor judgment and risk-taking behavior.
- Risk of overdose, particularly with tricyclic antidepressants (TCAs), and potential for serious adverse reactions necessitate intensive education of affected youths and their parents at initiation of treatment and follow-up education at every health care visit.
- Medication and dietary interactions with use of MAOIs pose special risks.

Immunizations

- No changes in the routine schedule of immunizations are needed.

Screening

- *Vision.* Routine age-related screening for vision is recommended.
  - Ensure that symptoms of withdrawal, low self-esteem, distractibility, irritability, and impaired attention are not caused in part by impaired sight by conducting vision screening when assessing for a mood disorder.
- *Hearing.* Routine age-related screening for hearing is recommended.
  - Ensure that symptoms of withdrawal, low self-esteem, distractibility, irritability, and impaired attention are not caused in part by impaired hearing by conducting hearing screening when assessing for a mood disorder.
- *Dental.* Routine screening is recommended.
- *Blood Pressure.* Routine screening is recommended.
  - Baseline blood pressure assessment and regular monitoring should be done during the first several weeks of medication treatment if TCAs, MAOIs, or atypical antipsychotics are prescribed; monitoring should be every few months thereafter.
  - If MAOIs are in use, risk of hypertensive crisis is serious if the required diet is not followed carefully or if drug interactions occur. Education is essential to prevent this type of crisis.
- *Hematocrit.* Routine screening is recommended.
- *Urinalysis.* Routine screening is recommended.
- *Tuberculosis.* Routine screening is recommended.

Condition-Specific Screening

- *Speech and language.* If speech and language do not normalize after treatment is implemented, additional evaluation of speech and language is needed.
- *Cardiac function.* Children taking TCAs and antipsychotics are at risk for cardiac effects, including tachycardia, prolonged QTc interval, and orthostatic hypotension.
  - Obtaining baseline blood pressure, complete blood count (CBC), and electrocardiogram (ECG) is recommended.

---

*Jackson, C. (Ed.). (2006). *Mosby's Pediatric Drug Consult*. St. Louis: Elsevier Mosby.

Continued

Summary of Primary Care Needs for the Child or Adolescent with a Mood Disorder—cont'd

- If a dosage is changed, blood pressure, CBC, and ECG should be repeated.
- Lowering the dose is warranted when the PR interval reaches 0.22 seconds or QRS reaches 130% of baseline, heart rate is >140 beats/min, or blood pressure is >140/90 mm Hg.
- *Drug toxicity.* Monitor for safety and follow specific recommendations for each class of drugs.

COMMON ILLNESS MANAGEMENT

Differential Diagnosis

- Overlap in symptoms with several other psychiatric disorders and common childhood illnesses requires evaluation of diagnostic *DSM-IV-TR* criteria and an assessment of physical symptoms.
- The clinician must determine which symptoms are occurring in isolation and which appear to be associated with or caused by another physical or psychological ailment.
- A detailed and thorough history from youth and parent or other caregiver is often the best strategy to help the clinician create an accurate timeline of the onset of symptoms.
- The most common psychiatric disorders to be considered as differential diagnoses include: adjustment disorder, posttraumatic stress disorder (PTSD), anxiety disorders, attention-deficit/hyperactivity disorder (ADHD), eating disorders, and substance use disorders.
- Discerning between a symptom of a known mood disorder and a symptom that may represent another problem is difficult at times. To determine the most accurate diagnosis, careful observations are required, sometimes over an extended period. Routine common illness management with attention to potential drug interactions is needed.

Drug Interactions

- Combination therapy increases the risk for drug interactions.
- Changing from one class of drugs to another can produce interactions.
- Selective serotonin reuptake inhibitors (SSRIs) in combination with MAOIs, designer drugs of abuse, and other medications can produce a potentially lethal interaction: serotonin syndrome. Follow guidelines carefully if changing from MAOI to SSRI and vice versa.
- SSRIs, particularly fluoxetine, are inhibitors of their own metabolism and can inhibit metabolism of other medications on the same CYP pathway.
- Lithium is cleared by the kidneys with an approximate half-life of 14 to 30 hours.
- Young people tend to have a faster lithium clearance rate than older adults.
- Safe treatment requires regular monitoring of lithium serum levels.
- Toxic effects from lithium typically occur with serum levels >1.5 mEq/L, and levels >2.0 mEq/L are associated with life-threatening side effects.
- Changes in hydration, renal function, and sodium levels will alter lithium serum levels.
- Valproate is metabolized by the liver and is highly protein bound; therefore interactions may occur with other metabolized or protein-bound medications. Valproate's weak inhibition of drug oxidation results in increased serum concentrations of drugs that undergo oxidative metabolism.
- Co-administration of many other medications can decrease or increase serum concentrations of valproate, requiring careful evaluation of all medications administered. Valproate toxicity can result from co-administration with other protein-bound medications.
- Carbamazepine decreases plasma levels of many other medications, including TCAs, thyroid hormones, hormonal contraceptives, and neuroleptics.
- Drugs that inhibit carbamazepine metabolism, including erythromycin, calcium channel blockers diltiazem and verapamil, and SSRIs, will increase serum levels.
- Topiramate (Topamax) may decrease phenytoin (Dilantin) and valproate levels, as well as levels of combined hormonal contraceptives.
- Quetiapine can prolong the QTc interval and may interact with other QT interval prolongers, such as macrolide antibiotics.
- Aripiprazole is metabolized on CYP 2D6 pathway and could interact with both fluoxetine and quetiapine.

DEVELOPMENTAL ISSUES

Sleep Patterns

- Change in sleep patterns may be an early sign of a mood disorder. Excessive sleeping, too little sleep, disrupted sleep, and poor quality of sleep are common symptoms.
- Abnormal sleep contributes to irritability, poor school performance, and fatigue or agitation.
- In bipolar disorder, the affected youths may alternate between periods of very little sleep and hyperactivity to periods of utter exhaustion during which the child may want to sleep all day.
- Sedating effects of many medications must be considered when evaluating sleep.
- Eliciting an account of recent sleep patterns helps identify signs of a mood disorder.
- Keeping a sleep diary helps track patterns and monitor response to treatment.
- Implementing good sleep habits, including a regular bedtime, avoidance of caffeine in the evening, and relaxing routines before sleep, helps normalize sleep patterns.

Toileting

- Mood disorders generally are not associated with significant difficulties in toileting. Problems with bedwetting and soiling sometimes occur with bipolar disorder.

Discipline

- Parents and teachers may interpret withdrawal or irritability as a lack of cooperation or respect. Children with bipolar disorder are prone to aggressive behavior and disruptive and alienating outbursts.
- Consistent limits and clear explanations of behavioral contingencies are appropriate discipline strategies. Enforcing rules regarding safety also is essential for purposes of protection.

Summary of Primary Care Needs for the Child or Adolescent with a Mood Disorder—cont'd

Child Care

- Children frequently have trouble relating to peers. Irritability makes them difficult to be around and tends to push others away.
- Children with symptoms or diagnosis of a bipolar disorder typically have periods of disruptive behavior that can cause safety problems and interfere with group activities.
- A lack of pleasure or interest limits engagement in social activities.
- Regular schedules and placement in small family settings or centers with high staff/child ratios and stable personnel are ideal.

Schooling

- A downward slide in grades, difficulty managing school-related activities, and behavior problems in the classroom can indicate a mood disorder.
- Poor concentration, irritability, disorganization, lack of self-confidence or grandiosity, and withdrawal or fighting interfere with academic work.
- School-related problems can escalate and lead to academic failure and dropping out.
- In severe cases, hospitalization and residential placement may need to substitute for usual school attendance.
- Children often require special accommodations, and an Individualized Educational Plan (IEP) may assist affected students to function in the classroom.

Sexuality

- Interest and performance ability may lessen among adolescents.
- Difficulty establishing close relationships may interfere with development of healthy sexuality.

- Bipolar disorders are associated with poor judgment during manic episodes that could lead to promiscuous behavior and related risks for unwanted pregnancy and sexually transmitted diseases (STDs).

Transition to Adulthood

- Mood disorders interfere with being able to relate to peers, develop intimate relationships, and manage responsibilities.
- Appropriate adjunctive therapeutic approaches include social skills training, academic and occupational counseling, and education in life skills.

FAMILY CONCERNS

- Mood disorders take a toll on the family. "Well" siblings may harbor feelings of resentment as the "ill" child gets special accommodations based on the condition.
- The child with bipolar disorder also may embarrass family members with angry public outbursts of rage.
- Concerns about possible genetic transmission can create feelings of guilt and anger, and anxiety about future generations.
- Difficulty obtaining adequate health care coverage for long-term psychiatric conditions creates real financial burden and stress for families.
- National organizations, local support groups, and informational websites are available resources for families.

REFERENCES

Abramson, L.Y., Seligman, M.E., & Teasdale, J.D. (1978). Learned helplessness in humans: Critique and reformulation. *J Abnorm Psychol, 37*, 49-74.

Alpert, J.E. (2008). Drug-drug interactions in psychopharmacology. In T.A. Stern, J.F. Rosenbaum, M. Fava, et al. (Eds.), *Massachusetts General Hospital Comprehensive Clinical Psychiatry*. Philadelphia: Mosby Elsevier.

American Psychiatric Association (APA). (1980). *Diagnostic and Statistical Manual of Mental Disorders*. (3rd ed.). Washington, DC: Author.

American Psychiatric Association (APA). (2000). *Diagnostic and Statistical Manual of Mental Disorders: DSM-IV-TR* (4th ed., Text Revision). Washington, DC: Author.

American Psychiatric Association (APA) and American Academy of Child and Adolescent Psychiatry (AACAP). (2005). *The use of medication in treating childhood and adolescent depression: Information for physicians.* Available at http://parentsmedguide.org/physiciansmedguide.htm. Retrieved January 24, 2008.

Avenevoli, S., Reis, K., & Merikangas, R. (2006). Implications of high-risk family studies for prevention of depression. *Am J Prev Med, 31*, S126-S135.

Beck, A.T. (1967). *Depression: Clinical, Experimental, and Theoretical Aspects.*. Philadelphia: University of Pennsylvania Press.

Becker, A., Mickley, D.W., Derenne, J.L., et al. (2008). Eating disorders: Evaluation and management. In T.A. Stern, J.F. Rosenbaum, M. Fava, et al. (Eds.), *Massachusetts General Hospital Comprehensive Clinical Psychiatry*. Philadelphia: Mosby Elsevier.

Bellenir, K. (2006). *Mental Health Information for Teens: Health Tips About Mental Wellness and Mental Illness* (2nd ed.). Detroit: Omnigraphics.

Bostic, J.Q., & Prince, J.B. (2008). Child and adolescent psychiatric disorders. In T.A. Stern, J.F. Rosenbaum, M. Fava, et al. (Eds.), *Massachusetts General Hospital Comprehensive Clinical Psychiatry*. Philadelphia: Mosby Elsevier.

Brendel, R.W., Lagomasino, I.T., Perlis, R.H., et al. (2008). The suicidal patient. In T.A. Stern, J.F. Rosenbaum, M. Fava, et al. (Eds.), *Massachusetts General Hospital Comprehensive Clinical Psychiatry*. Philadelphia: Mosby Elsevier.

Carr, A. (2008). Depression in young people: Description, assessment and evidence-based treatment. *Dev Neurorehabil, 11*, 3-15.

Centers for Disease Control and Prevention (CDC). (2009). *Recommendations and guidelines: 2009 child and adolescent immunization schedules for persons aged 0-6 years, 7-18 years, and "catch-up schedule."* Available at www.cdc.gov/vaccines/recs/schedules/child-schedule.htm. Retrieved March 22, 2009.

Cheung, A.H., Zuckerbrot, R.A., Jensen, P.S., et al. (2007). Guidelines for adolescent depression in primary care (GLAD-PC): II. Treatment and ongoing management. *Pediatrics, 120*, e1313-1326.

Cheung, A.H., Zuckerbrot, R.A., Jensen, P.S., et al. (2008). Expert survey for the management of adolescent depression in primary care. *Pediatrics, 121*, e101-e107.

Correll, C.U. (2008). Antipsychotic use in children and adolescents: Minimizing adverse effects to maximize outcomes. *J Am Acad Child Adolesc Psychiatry, 47*(1), 9-20.

Correll, C.U., Penzer, J.B., Lencz, T., et al. (2007). Early identification and high-risk strategies for bipolar disorder. *Bipolar Disord, 9*, 324-338.

Diler, R.S., Daviss, W.B., Lopez, A., et al. (2007). Differentiating major depressive disorder in youths with attention deficit hyperactivity disorder. *J Affect Disord, 102*, 125-130.

Dougherty, E.H., & Schinka, J.A. (2008a). *Mental Status Checklist—Children.* Lutz, FL: Psychological Assessment Resources.

Dougherty, E.H., Schinka, J.A., & PAR Staff, et al. (2008b). *Mental Status Checklist—Adolescent.* Lutz, FL: Psychological Assessment Resources.

Fava, M., & Papakostas, G. (2008). Antidepressants. In T.A. Stern, J.F., Rosenbaum, M. Fava, et al. (Eds.), *Massachusetts General Hospital Comprehensive Clinical Psychiatry.* Philadelphia: Mosby Elsevier.

Findling, R.L., Feeney, N.C., Stansbrey, R.J., et al. (2004). Somatic treatment for depressive illnesses in children and adolescents. *Pediatr Clin North Am, 27,* 113-137.

Food and Drug Administration (FDA). (2008a). *Antiepileptic drugs* (January 31, 2008). Available at www.fda.gov/medwatch/safety/2008/safety08. htm#Antiepileptic. Retrieved September 7, 2008.

Food and Drug Administration. (2008b). *Clinical review: Aripiprazole.* Available at www.fda.gov/cder/foi/ped_review/2008/021436S017_Aripiprazole_Clinical_BPCA.pdf. Retrieved March 23, 2009.

Food and Drug Administration (FDA). (2004). FDA *Public Health Advisory: Suicidality in children and adolescents being treated with antidepressant medications* (October 15, 2004). Available at www.fda.gov/cder/drug/antidepressants/SSRIPHA200410.htm Retrieved February 8, 2009.

Garber, J. (2006). Depression in children and adolescents: Linking risk research and prevention. *Am J Prev Med, 31,* S104-S125.

Harrington, R. (2006). Affective disorders. In C. Gillberg, R. Harrington, & H.C. Steinhausen (Eds.), *A Clinician's Handbook of Child and Adolescent Psychiatry.* New York: Cambridge University Press.

Health Resources and Services Administration. (n.d.). *Stop bullying now!* Available at http://stopbullyingnow.hrsa.gov. Retrieved June 7, 2008.

Jackson, C. (Ed.) (2006). *Mosby's Pediatric Drug Consult (2006).* St. Louis: Elsevier Mosby.

Jom, A.F., Allen, N.B., O'Donnell, C.P., et al. (2006). Effectiveness of complementary and self-help treatments for depression in children and adolescents. *Med J Aust, 185,* 368-372.

Keltner, N.L., & Folks, D.G. (2005). *Psychotropic Drugs.* 4th ed. St. Louis: Mosby.

Kaufman, J., Birmaher, B., Brent, D. et al. (1996). Kiddie-SADS-present and lifetime Version (K-SADS-PL). Available at www.wpic.pitt.edu/KSADS/ksads-pl. Retrieved January 25, 2009.

Klomek, A.B., & Mufson, L. (2006). Interpersonal psychotherapy for depressed adolescents. *Child Adolesc Psychiatr Clin North Am, 15,* 959-975.

Kovacs, M. (2008). *Children's Depression Inventory.* Lutz, FL: Psychological Assessment Resources.

Kowatch, R.A., Youngstrom, E.A., Danielyan, A., et al. (2005). Review and meta-analysis of the phenomenology and clinical characteristics of mania in children and adolescents. *Bipolar Disord, 7,* 483-496.

Lakhan, S.E., & Hagger-Johnson, G.E. (2007). The impact of prescribed psychotropics on youth. *Clin Pract Epidemiol Ment Health, 3,* 21.

Laraia, M.T. (2002). Bipolar disorder: Bipolar depression, rapid cycling, children, and pharmacology. *APNA News, 14*(6), 12-13.

Luby, J.L., Heffelfinger, A.K., Mrakotsky, C., et al. (2002). Preschool major depressive disorder: Preliminary validation for developmentally modified *DSM-IV* criteria. *J Am Acad Child Adolesc Psychiatry, 41,* 928-937.

Mann, J.J., Emslie, G., Baldessarini, R.J., et al. (2006). Perspective: ACNP task force on SSRIs and suicidal behavior in youth. *Neuropsychopharmacology, 31,* 473-492.

Mash, E.J. & Wolfe, D.A. (Eds.). (2005). *Abnormal Child Psychiatry* (3rd ed, Belmont, CA: Thompson Wadsworth.

McClellan, J., Kowatch, R., Findling, R.L., et al. (2007). Practice parameters for the assessment and treatment of children and adolescents with bipolar disorder. *J Am Acad Child Adolesc Psychiatry, 46,* 107-125.

McEvoy, V. (2008, March 31). Pediatricians left guessing at drug doses. *Boston Globe,* March 31, 2008, C1, C3. Available at www.boston.com/news/health/articles/2008/03/31/pediatricians_left_guessing_at_drug_doses. Retrieved January 12, 2009.

Medpage Today (2008). *AACAP: Atypical antipsychotic scores at adult doses for children and adolescents.* Available at www.medpagetoday.com/Psychiatry/BipolarDisorder/tb/1987. Retrieved January 26, 2008.

Melnyk, B.M., Brown, H.E., Jones, D.C., et al. (2003). Improving the mental/psychosocial health of US children and adolescents: Outcomes and implementation strategies from the National KySS Summit. *J Pediatr Health Care, 17,* S1-S24.

Melnyk, B.M., & Moldenhauer, Z. (Eds.). (2006). *The KySS (Keep Your Children/Yourself Safe and Secure) Program Guide to Child and Adolescent Mental Health Screening, Early Intervention and Health Promotion (KySS).* Cherry Hill, NJ: National Association of Pediatric Nurse Practitioners.

Moreno, C., Laje, G., Bianco, C., et al. (2007). National trends in the outpatient diagnosis and treatment of bipolar disorders in youth. *Arch Gen Psychiatry, 64,* 1032-1039.

National Institute of Mental Health (NIMH) (2001). National Institute of Mental Health Roundtable on prepubertal bipolar disorder. *J Am Acad Child Adolesc Psychiatry, 40,* 871-878.

Ogbru, O (2008). Albuterol and ipratropium inhaler. Available at www.medicinenet.com/albuterol-inhaher_solution/article.htm. Retrieved January 25, 2009.

Papolos, D., & Papolos, J. (2006). *The Bipolar Child: The Definitive and Reassuring Guide to Childhood's Most Misunderstood Disorder* (3rd ed.). New York: Broadway Books.

Perlis, R.H., & Ostacher, M.J. (2008). Lithium and its role in psychiatry. In T.A. Stern, J.F. Rosenbaum, M. Fava, et al. (Eds.), *Massachusetts General Hospital Comprehensive Clinical Psychiatry,* Philadelphia: Mosby Elsevier.

Preston, J.D., O'Neal, J.H., & Talaga, M.C. (2008). *Handbook of Clinical Psychopharmacology for Therapists* (5th ed.). Oakland, CA: New Harbinger Publications.

Rehm, L.P. (1977). A self-control model of depression. *Behav Ther, 8,* 787-804.

Reynolds, W.M. (2008a). *Reynolds Adolescent Depression Scale* (2nd ed.). Lutz, FL: Psychological Assessment Resources.

Reynolds, W.M. (2008b). *Reynolds Child Depression Scale.* Lutz, FL: Psychological Assessment Resources.

Rusyniak, D.E., & Sprague, J.E. (2005). Toxin-induced hyperthermic syndromes. *Med Clin North Am, 89,* 1277-1296.

Ryan, N.D. (2005). Treatment of depression in children and adolescents. *Lancet, 366,* 933-940.

Sadock, B.J., & Sadock, V.A. (Eds.). (2007). *Kaplan & Sadock's Synopsis of Psychiatry: Behavioral Sciences/Clinical Psychiatry* (10th ed.). Philadelphia: Lippincott Williams & Wilkins.

Sahler, O.J.Z., & Carr, J.E. (2007). *The Behavioral Sciences and Health Care* (2nd ed.). Cambridge, MA: Hogrefe.

Scahill, L., & Rains, A. (2005a). Psychopharmacology for adolescents. In N.L. Keltner & D.G. Folks (Eds.), *Psychotropic Drugs* (4th ed.). St. Louis: Mosby.

Scahill, L., & Rains, A. (2005b). Psychopharmacology for children. In N.L. Keltner & D.G. Folks (Eds.), *Psychotropic Drugs* (4th ed.). St. Louis: Mosby.

Schatzberg, A.F., & Nemeroff, C.D. (2004). *The American Psychiatric Publishing Textbook of Psychopharmacology* (3rd ed.). Washington, DC: American Psychiatric Publications.

Seligman, M.E. (1975). *Helplessness: On Depression, Development, and Death* San Francisco: W.H. Freeman.

Shain, B.N. (2007). Suicide and suicide attempts in adolescents. *Pediatrics, 120,* 669-676.

Sims, B.E., Nottelmann, E., Koretz, D., et al. (2007). Prevention of depression in children and adolescents. *Am J Prev Med, 32,* 451-455.

Smith, F.A., & Mischoulon, D. (2008). Natural medications in psychiatry. In T.A. Stern, J.F. Rosenbaum, M. Fava, et al. (Eds.), *Massachusetts General Hospital Comprehensive Clinical Psychiatry.* Philadelphia: Mosby Elsevier.

Smoller, J.W., Finn, C.T., & Gardner-Schuster, E.E. (2008). Genetics. In T.A. Stern, J.F. Rosenbaum, M. Fava, et al. (Eds.), *Massachusetts General Hospital Comprehensive Clinical Psychiatry.* Philadelphia: Mosby Elsevier.

Stahl, S.M. (2006). *Essential Psychopharmacology: The Prescriber's Guide.* New York: Cambridge University Press.

Stark, K.D., Sander, J., Hauser, M., et al. (2006). Depressive disorders during childhood and adolescence. In E.J. Mash, & D.A. Wolfe, (Eds.) *Treatment of Childhood Disorders* (3rd ed.). New York: Guilford Press.

Staton, D., Volness, L.J., & Beatty, W.W. (2008). Diagnosis and classification of pediatric bipolar disorder. *J Affect Disord, 105,* 205-212.

Stuart, G.W. (2005). Emotional response and mood disorders. In G.W. Stuart, & M.T. Laraia (Eds.), *Principles and Practice of Psychiatric Nursing* (6th ed.). St. Louis: Elsevier Mosby.

Thomas, C.R., & Holzer, C.E. III (2006). The continuing shortage of child and adolescent psychiatrists. *J Am Acad Child Adolesc Psychiatry, 45,* 1023-1031.

Trowell, J., Joffe, I., Campbell, J., et al. (2007). Childhood depression: A place for psychotherapy. An outcome study comparing individual psychodynamic and family therapy. *Eur Child Adolesc Psychiatry, 16,* 157-167.

Turk, J., Graham, P., & Verhulst, F. (2007). *Child and Adolescent Psychiatry: A Developmental Approach* (4th ed.). New York: Oxford University Press.

Usala, T., Clavenna, A., Zuddas, A., et al. (2008). Randomised controlled trials of selective serotonin reuptake inhibitors in treating depression in children and adolescents: A systematic review and meta-analysis. *Eur Neuropsychopharmacol, 18,* 62-73.

Wang, B.C. Nonacs, R.M., Viguera, A.C., et al. (2008). Psychiatric illness during pregnancy and the postpartum period. In T.A. Stern, J.F. Rosenbaum, M. Fava, et al. (Eds.), *Massachusetts General Hospital Comprehensive Clinical Psychiatry*. Philadelphia: Mosby Elsevier.

Young, C. (Ed.). (2007). *BMJ Clinical Evidence Handbook* (Summer ed.). Tavistock Square, London: BMJ Publishing Group.

Zieman, M., Hatcher, R.A., Cwiak, C., et al. (2007). *A Pocket Guide to Managing Contraception*. Tiger, GA: Bridging the Gap Foundation.

Zuckerbrot, R.A., Cheung, A.H., Jensen, P.S., et al. (2007). Guidelines for adolescent depression in primary care (GLAD-PC): I. Identification, assessment, and initial management. *Pediatrics, 120*, e1299-e1312.

34 Muscular Dystrophy, Duchenne

Vanessa Battista

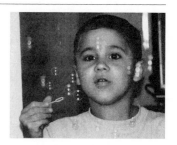

Etiology

Muscular dystrophy (MD) is a group of inherited diseases characterized by muscle tissue weakness and atrophy. There are nine different types of MD: Becker, congenital, Duchenne, distal, Emery-Dreifuss, facioscapulohumeral, limb-girdle, myotonic, and oculopharyngeal. Table 34-1 summarizes the inheritance pattern, age of onset, type of muscle affected, and rate of progression for each of the nine types of MD (Muscular Dystrophy Association [MDA], 2006). Although the focus of this chapter is on boys with DMD, much of the diagnostic processs, treatment, and primary care is similar across types of MD.

Duchenne muscular dystrophy (DMD), the most common form of muscular dystrophy in children, is named after a French neurologist who first described it in 1868 (Duchenne de Boulogne, 1973). DMD is primarily a disease of skeletal and heart muscle but can also affect cognition. DMD is X-linked and thus primarily affects boys, although female carriers can be affected (Darras, Menache, & Kunkel, 2003). DMD is a chronic, degenerative, and eventually fatal disorder, with children appearing normal at birth and deteriorating throughout childhood. Life expectancy in DMD is truncated. The majority die before age 30 (Hinton & Goldstein, 2007), although with supportive care some individuals live longer (Kohler, Clarenbach, Boni, et al., 2005).

DMD is caused by a mutation in the dystrophin gene at position Xp21 (Monaco, Neve, Colletti-Feener, et al., 1986). It is one of the largest genes in the human genome, with 79 exons (Stockley, Akber, Bulgin, et al., 2006), having a high proclivity for mutations. Approximately two thirds (70%) of boys with DMD have large deletions or duplications in the dystrophin gene and the other third (30%) have smaller insertion or deletion mutations, splice mutations, or other small point mutations (Aartsma-Rus, van Deutekom, Fokkema, et al., 2006). Deletions may occur at any point along the dystrophin gene, with most occurring in two "hot spots" within the gene (Mendell, Buzin, Feng, et al., 2001). These deletions or mutations disrupt essential functional domains of the dystrophin molecule, resulting in a truncated and unstable dystrophin protein with impaired function (Muntoni, Torelli, & Ferlini, 2003).

In muscles, dystrophin is part of a protein complex. Dystrophin-deficient muscle fibers are susceptible to contraction-induced tears that allow calcium influx and ultimately lead to muscle fiber necrosis (Eagle, Baudouin, Chandler, et al., 2002). Muscle fiber regeneration can only partially compensate so that fibers are progressively replaced by fat and connective tissue. The dystrophin protein is nearly absent in the muscles of boys with DMD (Hoffman & Wang, 1993) and partially absent in Becker muscular dystrophy (BMD), a milder form of muscular dystrophy. The gene also codes for protein products that localize to other tissue types, including the brain, and the absence of these products is associated with cognitive dysfunction (Felisari, Martinelli-Boneschi, Bardoni, et al., 2000).

Incidence and Prevalence

DMD is the most common genetically determined neuromuscular disease of childhood and shows no predilection for race or ethnic group. It occurs in 1 in 3500 live male births, with an incidence of approximately 2 per 10,000 males worldwide (National Human Genome Research Institute, 2007). An X-linked disease, there is a 50% chance that a male child will be affected with DMD and a 50% chance that a female child will be a carrier if the mother carries the defective gene (Darras et al., 2003). Although girls typically are asymptomatic, up to 8% of female carriers manifest mild proximal muscle weakness or cardiomyopathy (Williams, 2007).

Diagnostic Criteria

DMD is a well-characterized inherited disorder with a strong genotype-phenotype relationship (Kemper & Wake, 2007). Recent advances in molecular diagnoses have made it possible to identify precise mutations in up to 90% of individuals with a DMD phenotype (Griggs & Bushby, 2005), thus allowing for more accurate genetic diagnoses.

Laboratory Testing: Creatine Kinase

If DMD is suspected, elevated serum creatine kinase (CK) concentrations support the diagnosis and may be an initial indicator of the disease. Sometimes these concentrations are detected incidentally by the primary care provider (PCP). In DMD, CK will be greater than 10 times normal and can reach as high as 10,000 to 50,000 IU/L (Darras et al., 2003). CK is an enzyme concentrated in muscle and is released into the blood with muscle damage. Serum CK is highest at birth in those with DMD and then gradually declines as muscle mass decreases throughout the course of the disease (Williams, 2007). Alanine aminotransferase (ALT) and aspartate aminotransferase (AST) are also released from damaged muscle (Darras et al., 2003). This may inadvertently be considered a sign

The author expresses heartfelt gratitude to Petra Kaufmann, MD, MSc, Associate Director of the Pediatric Neuromuscular Center at the Columbia University Medical Center and Ritamarie John, Dr NP, MSN, CPNP-PC, Program Director for the Pediatric Nurse Practitioner Program at Columbia University School of Nursing for their thoughtful review of this chapter.

TABLE 34-1

Summary of Nine Types of Muscular Dystrophy

Type of Muscular Dystrophy	Inheritance Pattern	Age of Onset	Type of Muscle Affected	Rate of Progression
Becker muscular dystrophy (BMD)	X-linked recessive	Childhood to adulthood	Less severe form of DMD	Slower than DMD
Congenital muscular dystrophy (CMD)	Autosomal recessive or dominant or de novo	At or near birth	General muscle weakness	Mainly slow but varies with type
Duchenne muscular dystrophy (DMD)	X-linked recessive	Early childhood	General muscle weakness, proximal greater than distal	Ususaly slow
Distal muscular dystrophy (DD)	Autosomal dominant or recessive	Childhood to adulthood	Hands, forearms, calf	Slow
Emery-Dreifuss muscular dystrophy (EDMD)	X-linked recessive or autosomal dominant	Childhood to early adolescence (usually by age 10)	Shoulder, upper arm, calf	Slow; sudden death may occur due to cardiac problems
Facioscapulohumeral muscular dystrophy (FSH or FSHD)	Autosomal dominant or de novo	Adolescence to early adulthood (usually by age 20)	Eyes and mouth, shoulders, upper arms, and calf initially, then abdominal and hip	Slow, with periods of rapid deterioration
Limb-girdle muscular dystrophy (LGMD)	Autosomal dominant or recessive	Childhood to adulthood	Shoulder and pelvic girdles (limb) initially	Slow
Myotonic muscular dystrophy (MMD)	Autosomal dominant	Congenital form at birth, or adolescence to adulthood	Face, calf, forearms, hands, and neck initially; gastrointestinal, vision, cardiac, or respiratory complications later	Slow
Oculopharyngeal muscular dystrophy (OPMD)	Autosomal dominant or recessive	Adulthood (usually forties or fifties)	Eyelids and throat initially, facial and limb later	Slow

From Muscular Dystrophy Association. (2006). *Diseases in the MDA program, master list.* Available at www.mda.org/disease/40list.html. Retrieved June 15, 2008.

of liver disease. Therefore CK concentrations should be checked in boys with elevated ALT and AST and no other hepatic symptoms (Darras et al.).

Muscle Biopsy

Immunohistochemistry analysis of the biopsied muscle shows absence of dystrophin in DMD (Mendell et al., 2001). Currently, muscle biopsy is mainly used to distinguish between DMD and BMD, in young children without a family history of the disease and after genetic testing is negative. Because it is anxiety provoking and typically requires anesthesia in children, biopsy should be avoided whenever possible (Mendell et al.).

Electromyography

Electromyography (EMG) is the recording of muscle electrical activity at the time of needle insertion, at rest, and during muscle contraction (Biggar, 2006). EMG confirms the presence of a muscle disease and excludes neurogenic disease through the measurement of electrical activity in the muscle. However, it is nonspecific and rarely used in the diagnosis of DMD (Darras et al., 2003).

Newborn Screening, Testing, and Family Planning

Newborn screening has several potential benefits and risks in DMD. Benefits include identifying a cohort of children eligible for trials aimed at developing new therapies or assessing the effectiveness of early treatment; avoiding the potentially difficult and time-consuming process of establishing a diagnosis; enabling families to become knowledgeable and develop strategies for managing complex health care needs in advance; and informing future reproductive planning (Kemper & Wake, 2007). However, because

of the large number of possible mutations associated with DMD, molecular genetic screening is not feasible for newborn screening (Kemper & Wake).

Women with a familial history of DMD can undergo carrier testing to make informed reproductive choices. Pretest and posttest counseling is required and reproductive options may need to be discussed, including pregnancy with or without prenatal testing, preimplantation diagnosis, pregnancy by egg or sperm donation, parenting by adoption, or remaining childless (Pagon et al., 2001).

Clinical Manifestations at Time of Diagnosis

The first sign of DMD is slow acquisition of motor milestones; walking is often not achieved until 18 months of age. Around 2 to 3 years of age, boys with DMD may appear to be "somewhat clumsy," and by ages of 3 to 5, they often have difficulty keeping up with their peers on the playground (Hinton & Goldstein, 2007). Weakness progresses at different rates but is consistent in its pattern; proximal muscles weaken before distal, legs weaken before arms, and extensors weaken before flexors (McDonald, Abresch, Carter, et al., 1995). Initially, boys have difficulty running, jumping from a standing position, and climbing stairs; and they may experience frequent falls (Darras et al., 2003).

As weakness progresses, the Achilles tendons become contracted, causing boys to shift the weight onto the balls of their feet, a compensatory mechanism known as toe walking (Williams, 2007). Often this is associated with exaggerated lumbar lordosis. Muscles have a firm, "rubbery" consistency and calf muscles appear larger, known as calf pseudohypertrophy (Darras et al., 2003). When asked to get up from a sitting position on the floor, boys will typically get into a knee-elbow position, extend their elbows and

Clinical Manifestations at Time of Diagnosis

SLOW ACQUISITION OF MOTOR MILESTONES
- 18 months: Start walking
- Age 2 to 3 years: "Somewhat clumsy"
- Age 3 to 5 years: Difficulty keeping up with peers

CONSISTENT PATTERN OF WEAKNESS THAT VARIES IN RATE
- Proximal muscles weaken before distal muscles
- Legs weaken before arms
- Extensors weaken before flexors

PHYSICAL PRESENTATION
- Difficulty running, jumping from a standing position, climbing stairs
- Frequent falls
- Toe walking
- Calf pseudohypertrophy
- Positive Gowers' maneuver
- Lumbar lordosis

Treatment

Therapies
- Physical
- Occupational
- Recreational
- Aqua
- Speech

Adaptive Equipment
- Orthotic devices
- Customized mobility and seating

Surgery
- Achilles tendon release surgery
- Posterior spinal fusion
- Sedation and anesthesia precautions

Respiratory Devices
- Noninvasive positive-pressure ventilation (NIPPV)
- Mechanical insufflator-exsufflator (MIE)
- Suction Machine

Pharmacologic Therapy

Cardiac
- ACE inhibitors, beta-blockers, diuretics, digoxin to treat progressive abnormalities

Corticosteroid Therapy
- Increase strength, performance, pulmonary function, and progression of weakness
- Benefits vs. risks

knees, bring their hands and feet as close together as possible, and then raise their rears in the air and, using their arms as support, will "walk" their hands up their legs to get into a standing position; this movement is known as the Gowers' maneuver (Hinton & Goldstein, 2007). If the diagnosis of DMD is suspected by the PCP, simple tests can be preformed during physical examination to detect proximal weakness such as asking the child to run, jump, climb stairs, and get up from the floor (Bushby, Bourke, Bullock, et al., 2005).

Treatment

There is currently no cure for DMD, and the plan for disease management should be individualized. The goals of treatment for boys with DMD should be consistent with maintaining mobility, maximizing muscle strength performance and pulmonary function, and optimizing performance of activities of daily living. Treatment plans should be determined by boys' developmental and functional needs. Goals of care should be centered on a multidisciplinary approach including specialists from the following areas: clinical genetics, neurology, pulmonology, cardiology, nutrition, rehabilitation medicine, orthopedics, and neuropsychology (American Thoracic Society [ATS], 2004).

Therapies

Physical, Occupational, Recreational, and Aqua Therapies. Because of the progressive nature of DMD, it is important for rehabilitation specialists to proactively determine ways to maximize the independence and quality of life of boys with DMD (Liu, Mineo, Hanayama, et al., 2003). Physical therapy aims at maintaining range of motion and preserving muscle function while minimizing muscle damage. It also plays an important role in pain management (Bushby & Straub, 2005). Stretching and passive range-of-motion exercises are often recommended; however, there is little evidence to document the exact type of physiotherapy that is most advantageous (Bushby & Straub). Proper selection of adaptive equipment optimizes independent function, minimizes complications such as skin breakdown and musculoskeletal pain, and improves the quality of life for boys and their caregivers (Hinton & Goldstein, 2007).

Boys with DMD should be encouraged to participate in adapted activities that enhance quality of life and minimize muscle damage such as adapted sports, gardening (Liu et al., 2003), arts and crafts, chess, card games, and computer activities. Playing music, especially small wind instruments that can be held such as the clarinet, may improve their respiratory function. Aquatherapy is especially helpful as being in water may relieve pressure on the joints and make exercises easier to perform, allowing boys with DMD to move their extremities much farther and more often.

Speech Therapy. Early treatment of DMD typically includes speech therapy as children with DMD have significantly higher rates of speech and developmental delay (Hinton, Fee, & Batchelder, 2007). Early initiation of speech therapy helps improve the quality of life for young children with DMD (Hinton et al.).

Adaptive Equipment

Orthotic Devices. Orthotic devices and braces assist with walking and posture and should be prescribed to meet the evolving needs of boys with DMD. Most devices are lightweight and custom designed to fit inside a shoe and provide support by maintaining foot alignment while boys are standing or walking. Once wheelchair-dependent, boys may still wear braces to avoid contractures and maintain proper alignment of the extremity and foot. As boys grow and their needs for support progress, these devices will need to be modified to maintain proper function and fit. Most orthotic devices are recommended by a physical therapist, prescribed by the PCP or other specialist (e.g., neurologist), and fitted for by an orthotist.

The specific device recommended depends of the stage of the disease. During the initial stage of independent ambulation, intervention should be limited to the foot and ankle complex (Stevens, 2006) and usually includes the use of ankle-foot orthotics (AFOs) and knee-ankle-foot orthotics (KAFOs), starting with nighttime use (Leitch,

Raza, Biggar, et al., 2005). Most commonly, night splints are employed to stretch the Achilles tendon and reduce forefoot gait (Hinton & Goldstein, 2007); they may also slow the progression of weakness of equinovarus deformities (Stevens, 2006). AFOs and KAFOs should be properly fitted because boys will likely refuse to wear them if they are uncomfortable. Daily stretching exercises and proper bracing help prevent the development of contractures and will also provide extra stability (Do, 2002). Once ambulation ceases, orthotic intervention should focus on the spine and again on the foot and ankle because preservation of hip and knee joints is difficult (Stevens, 2006).

Customized Mobility and Seating. By ages 10 to 12, most boys with DMD are chronically fatigued and become fully wheelchair-dependent. Manual wheelchairs may be used initially, but as boys become increasingly dependent, a motorized wheelchair is needed (Hinton & Goldstein, 2007) and should be custom fitted for each child. Motorized chairs are controlled electronically, typically by a joystick that is located near the child's dominant hand; if muscle strength in the upper extremities becomes affected, adaptations can be made for other ways to control chair movement. Wait time for a custom-built chair can be lengthy, and the process should be started as soon as the need is anticipated and before the use of a chair becomes absolutely necessary. The PCP can assist in ordering the chair and with follow-up to ensure as timely delivery as possible.

Custom-made adaptive seating helps reduce lateral curvature (Liu et al., 2003). Pain and numbness caused by long hours of sitting are relieved with conventional flotation pads or cushions; anterior trunk support facilitates eating; and a semireclining chair is useful to make toileting easier. Adjustable seating systems are preferred anticipating disease progression, especially because health insurance does not usually permit frequent modifications or renewals (Liu et al.).

Surgery

Achilles Tendon Release Surgery. Although historically used in the 1970s (Spencer & Vignos, 1962), achilles tendon release surgery is sometimes still performed to assist in managing contractures. If done, it needs to be considered with caution in boys with DMD and combined with the use of KAFOs. It may extend the ambulatory period by approximately 2 years, although factors such as remaining strength, motivation, and residual walking ability also play a role (Stevens, 2006). If the boy is weak in ambulation with early evidence of distal muscle weakness and contractures, surgery may lead to overlengthening of the tendon and result in further weakness (Do, 2002).

Posterior Spinal Fusion. Posterior spinal fusion for scoliosis in DMD has been highly effective in stabilizing the spine and maintaining seating balance and comfort. It is also associated with a significant decrease in the rate of respiratory decline (Velasco, Colin, Zurakowski, et al., 2007). Corrective surgery that includes appropriate coverage for cardiac and respiratory complications may be a successful treatment modality (Bushby & Straub, 2005); however, it is not without risk. A systematic review of 402 studies involving scoliosis surgery in DMD concluded that without randomized controlled clinical trials specifically aimed to evaluate its effectiveness, no evidence-based recommendations could be made (Cheuk, Wong, Wraige, et al., 2007). New approaches to scoliosis surgery (i.e., growing rod insertion or Vertical Expandable Prosthetic Titanium Rib (VEPTR) insertion) hold promise but little outcome data is available and these procedures are available at only a few surgical centers. The uncertainty of benefits and potential risks should be discussed with families. Quality of life, functional status, respiratory function, and life expectancy should be considered (Cheuk et al.).

Sedation and Anesthesia Precautions. A consensus statement by the American College of Chest Physicians states that boys with DMD have an increased risk for complications when undergoing sedation or general anesthesia, which include potentially fatal reactions to inhaled anesthetics and certain muscle relaxants, upper airway obstruction, hypoventilation, atelectasis, congestive heart failure, cardiac dysrhythmias, respiratory failure, and difficulty weaning from mechanical ventilation (Birnkrant, Panitch, Benditt, et al., 2007). A plan, including a preoperative pulmonary and cardiac evaluation, should be tailored to meet the specific needs of the patient and the surgery. Anesthesiologists should avoid using depolarizing agents (Bushby & Straub, 2005). Respiratory complications can occur during the postoperative period (Bushby & Straub), and aggressive airway clearance and extubation to positive pressure ventilation should be used to help reduce the frequency and severity of these complications (Kaira & Amin, 2005). PCPs should refer to the American College of Chest Physicians Consensus Statement for specific guidelines when educating families regarding the risks associated with sedation and anesthesia in DMD (Birnkrant et al., 2007).

Respiratory Devices

Respiratory complications are common as DMD progresses. Devices that are prescribed to augment maximal insufflations, noninvasive ventilation, and assisted coughing should ideally be introduced in outpatient settings (Bach, 2004) before the onset of a respiratory emergency. A variety of nasal prongs and face masks are available, and a respiratory therapist can assist in finding one that fits comfortably. Ideally, a pulmologist should manage the respiratory complications of DMD, although in some instances the PCP may be involved and should be knowledgeable about commonly used devices. The settings of respiratory equipment should be monitored by a respiratory therapist who is knowledgeable in neuromuscular diseases and can educate families in the proper use of these devices.

Symptoms of respiratory weakness usually begin at nighttime and are initially supported with the nocturnal use of noninvasive positive-pressure ventilation (NIPPV), which allows for the entry of more air into the lungs. As weakness progresses, boys may use NIPPV increasingly during the day, especially when in stages of advanced disease or after scoliosis repair surgery (Kaira & Amin, 2005). A mechanical insufflator-exsufflator (MIE) can be used to deliver deep insufflations until lungs are fully expanded, followed immediately by deep exsufflations during which lungs are fully emptied and the chest wall retracted (Bach, 2004). A suction machine can also be used to aid in secretion and mucus removal. MIE is well tolerated in boys with DMD and provides short-term benefits by improving bicarbonate clearance and respiratory muscle performance (Fauroux, Guillemot, Aubertin, et al., 2008). This, in turn, may help prevent the onset of respiratory infections such as pneumonia. Ventilatory support by NIPPV may be a good option in advanced disease in terms of portability and ease of use (Kaira & Amin, 2005). In cases when contraindications to NIPPV exist or NIPPV is not successful, invasive mechanical ventilation via tracheostomy may be warranted (Kaira & Amin); however, this option should be discussed thoroughly before a decision is made.

Pharmacologic Therapy

Cardiac. Electrocardiograms and echocardiograms should be performed regularly to check for evidence of cardiomyopathy. If necessary, pharmacotherapies may be prescribed that improve heart contractility and reduce the heart's workload (American Academy of Pediatrics [AAP], 2005). Angiotensin-converting enzyme (ACE) inhibitors and beta-blockers are considered first-line heart failure therapy, along with the use of diuretics and occasionally digoxin (Markham, Spicer, & Cripe, 2005), to improve heart contractility and reduce the heart's workload (Hinton & Goldstein, 2007). Early treatment with an ACE inhibitor may delay the onset and progression of prominent left ventricle dysfunction in boys with DMD (Duboc, Meune, Lerebours, et al., 2005).

Corticosteroid Therapy. Practice parameters regarding corticosteroid treatment of DMD set forth by a subcommittee of the American Academy of Neurology suggest that daily corticosteroid treatment with prednisone (0.75 mg/kg/day) increases muscle strength, performance, and pulmonary function and significantly decreases the progression of weakness (Moxley, Ashwal, Pandya, et al., 2005). The general medical consensus is that daily corticosteroids should be offered to boys with DMD while they are still ambulating (Biggar, Harris, Eliasoph, et al., 2006). Both prednisone (0.75 mg/kg/day) and deflazacort (0.9 mg/kg/day) (Biggar et al., 2006) significantly slow disease process and functional loss in boys with DMD (Balaban, Matthews, Clayton, et al., 2005); however, deflazacort has not been given Food and Drug Administration (FDA) approval for use in the United States (Campbell & Jacob, 2003).

Steroid treatment is not without side effects. Boys with DMD on long-term corticosteroid therapy have a significantly decreased risk of scoliosis and an increase of 3 or more years of independent ambulation, yet they are also at an increased risk of vertebral and lower limb fractures (King, Ruttencutter, Nagaraja, et al., 2007). The PCP must monitor boys receiving steroid therapy carefully for weight gain; growth suppression; hypertension; cushingoid appearance; skin changes, such as acne, hirsutism, hyperpigmentation, skin thinning, and striae; altered behavior; osteoporosis leading to vertebral fracture; and cataracts (Balaban et al., 2005; Gedalia & Shetty, 2004). Many parents and health care providers believe that the benefits of corticosteroid treatment outweigh the adverse effects.

Complementary and Alternative Therapies

A growing number of families in Western countries are turning to alternative therapies such as massage, acupuncture, magnets, biofeedback and relaxation training, and hypnosis (Bushby & Straub, 2005), or alternative drug therapies such as nutritional supplements or Chinese traditional medications, despite the fact that research has resulted in disparate outcomes in DMD (Urtizberea, Fan, Vroom, et al., 2003). Families should be informed of the lack of existing research for alternative therapies in DMD and made aware of any known effects, potential hazards, or toxicities of Chinese traditional medicines that have been demonstrated in studies involving other conditions (Urtizberea et al.).

Anticipated Advances in Diagnosis and Management

Ongoing advances in preclinical research reveal promising therapeutic prospects, including novel strategies aimed at replacing the mutated gene (gene therapy), replacing affected cells (cell therapy), repairing the defective gene (exon skipping), and compensating for the absence of dystrophin (drug therapy) (Cossu & Sampaolesi, 2007). Strategies under development include growth-modulating agents that increase muscle regeneration and delay muscle fibrosis (Bogdanovich, Krag, Barton, et al., 2002); antiinflammatory or second-messenger signal-modulating agents that affect immune response (Balaban et al., 2005; Biggar et al., 2006); antisense oligonucleotides (AONs) with exon-skipping capacity (splice donor or acceptor sites during pre–messenger ribonucleic acid [pre-mRNA] splicing) (Aartsma-Rus et al., 2006; McClorey, Moulton, Iverson, et al., 2006); and agents targeted to suppress stop codon mutations (aminoglycosides and other pharmacologic agents) (Hamed, 2006). Given the recent advances within the field, effective therapy seems to be an achievable goal (Foster, Foster, & Dickson, 2006).

Progress in understanding the molecular basis of muscle regeneration and maintenance has also contributed new insights toward finding an effective treatment. Individuals with DMD have irregularities that stem from erroneous expression of genes regulated by *PGC-1α*, a gene that regulates the activity of several genes involved in muscle maintenance and regeneration (Russell, Feilchenfeldt, Schreiber, et al., 2003). Laboratory experiments with mice have shown that increasing the expression of this gene may be a useful treatment for DMD and may slow or even halt disease progression (Handschin, Choi, Chin, et al., 2007). Drug screens are currently being conducted to identify drugs that would simulate the expression of this gene (Cohn, van Erp, Habashi, et al., 2007). Other promising research has shown that inhibiting the activity of transforming growth factor–beta (TGF-β) may be beneficial by improving muscle regeneration (Cohn et al., 2007). Long-term administration (6 months or longer) of losartan, an antihypertensive drug, showed improved muscle structure and function in dystrophin-deficient mice, suggesting that although it may not reverse dystrophin deficiency, it may provide long-term benefits by allowing muscle regeneration to keep pace with muscle degeneration (Kuehn, 2007).

PTC124 is another promising approach, targeted for the 10% to 15% of cases of DMD that involve a nonsense mutation, which serves to prematurely stop translation of the dystrophin gene. This potential treatment would allow the ribosome to read through stop-codon and produce dystrophin, yet still obey normal signals to stop translation. Recent tests of the drug have shown that it can lead to the production of enough dystrophin to restore muscle function in laboratory experiments with mice that have a DMD-like disorder (Welch, Barton, Zhuo, et al., 2007). The advantage of this treatment is that it is a small molecule that can be easily swallowed in pill form and also that there is a large margin between an effective and toxic dose, allowing for the feasible delivery of a safe and effective dose. Clinical trials of PTC124 are currently underway, which will serve as a good test of the broader effectiveness of the drug (Kuehn, 2007).

A potential challenge in finding a cure is the fact that not all affected individuals have the same mutation and thus the same strategies may not be beneficial for everyone. Despite these challenges, it is reasonable to expect that the next decade will see great advances in the field of treatment for DMD (van Deutekom & van Ommen, 2003).

Associated Problems of Duchenne Muscular Dystrophy and Treatment

Secondary problems associated with DMD usually result from increasing muscle weakness as boys grow older and the disease progresses.

Associated Problems of Duchenne Muscular Dystropy and Treatment

- Pulmonary effects
  - Weakened cough
  - Respiratory insufficiency
  - Respiratory tract infections
  - Sleep-related disturbances
- Cardiac dysfunction
  - Cardiomyopathy
- Cognitive impairments
  - Lower than average IQ
  - Deficient immediate verbal memory skills
- Language impairments
- Motor impairment
  - Contractures and gait changes
  - Scoliosis
  - Osteoporosis and fractures
- Feeding and swallowing difficulties
- Obesity
  - Weight gain caused by limited movement or corticosteroid therapy
- Constipation
- Decubitus ulcers
- Psychosocial and behavioral issues
  - Distractibility and poor attention span
  - Low frustration threshold
  - Features of obsessive-compulsive behavior
  - Anxiety
  - Depression

Pulmonary Effects

Chest wall and diaphragmatic muscle weakness causes weakened cough and respiratory insufficiency in DMD (Bushby & Straub, 2005). Boys with DMD exhibit an inability to maintain normal respiratory function in conditions of stress, respiratory infection, general anesthesia, exercise, and sleep (Kaira & Amin, 2005). Significant problems arise with viral respiratory infections and the inability to adequately clear secretions; pneumonia frequently occurs (Kaira & Amin, 2005). Cough-assist devices should be prescribed, along with prompt antibiotic treatment for respiratory infection (Bushby & Straub, 2005).

Progressive muscle deterioration leads to pulmonary complications (Hinton & Goldstein, 2007). The forced vital capacity (FVC) declines by 5% to 10% per year and affected boys begin to lose the ability to cough effectively, increasing the risk for pneumonia (Biggar, 2006). A decreasing FVC is an indication of increasing respiratory insufficiency, which may lead to higher rates of chest infections or more insidious signs of respiratory failure such as

weight loss, loss of appetite and energy, increased waking, and general malaise (Bushby & Straub, 2005). Prevention and treatment of increasing respiratory insufficiency through the prophylaxis and treatment of chest infections with immunization, cough augmentation techniques, prompt treatment with antibiotics when necessary (Bushby & Straub, 2005), and close collaboration with an experienced respiratory therapist is warranted.

Cardiac Dysfunction

Approximately 9% of boys experience cardiac complications by ages 9 to 13; 67% are affected by age 16; and in time, all individuals with DMD will be affected (Hinton & Goldstein, 2007). Cardiac dysfunction may manifest as pronounced fatigue, altered duration and quality of sleep, unexplained weight loss or gain, changes in daily activities not related to weakness, chest pain, dizziness, palpations, syncope, abnormal cardiac rate or rhythm, tachypnea, diminished pulses, murmurs, hepatomegaly, edema, abdominal pain, or vomiting (Markham et al., 2005). Because most boys are wheelchair-dependent by the time cardiac changes develop, the typical cardiac symptoms such as exercise intolerance may not be manifested, making cardiac decompensation more difficult to diagnose (Biggar, 2006).

Cardiomyopathy is a major cause of mortality in individuals with DMD (Bushby & Straub, 2005). Cardiac evaluations should be performed biannually during early childhood and yearly starting at approximately 10 years of age; carriers of DMD should be made aware of the risk of developing cardiomyopathy and should have a complete cardiac evaluation at least every 5 years starting at 25 to 30 years of age (AAP, 2005). Because skeletal muscle and cardiac muscle may not be equally affected in DMD at any given time (Markham et al., 2005), it is possible that skeletal muscle may be well preserved but cardiomyopathy exists.

Cognitive Impairments

Many boys with DMD have nonprogressive cognitive impairment, but some have average or above average intelligence (Darras et al., 2003). The average intelligence quotient (IQ) of boys with DMD falls approximately 1 standard deviation (SD) lower than the population mean (Cotton, Voudouris, & Greenwood, 2005). Mildly reduced IQ with lower verbal than performance IQ and mildly affected visual attention and short-term memory processing may be present (Marini, Lorussoc, D'Angeloc, et al., 2007). Speech delay, developmental delay, and social problems also are all significantly more common (Hinton et al., 2007). Cognitive profiles may show selective deficits in verbal skills that improve over time and treating these as early as possible is beneficial (Hinton & Goldstein, 2007).

Language Impairments

Boys with DMD are at increased risk for a language delay and language difficulties. School-age boys with DMD have good receptive vocabularies (word comprehension) yet limited verbal immediate memory or working memory skills. Overall, boys have more difficulty following long verbal instructions and this can ultimately limit academic achievement (Hinton et al., 2007). It has been hypothesized that the lack of dystrophin characteristic of DMD produces effects on the maturation of the cerebellum, whose involvement has been suggested in verb and syntactic processing, although this is not entirely clear (Cyrulnika & Hinton, 2008).

Motor Impairment

Contractures and Gait Changes. During middle childhood, as boys with DMD lose skeletal muscle strength and endurance and painful multifocal contractures develop, pelvic muscles weaken and lumbar lordosis develops. Boys with DMD begin using a waddling, or "Trendelenburg" gait (Biggar, 2006). Waddling caused by weakness of the gluteus medius and maximus and subsequent inability to support a single leg stance and weakness of the quadriceps requires that forward motion be propagated by circumducting each leg and leaning forward toward the opposite side to maintain balance (Do, 2002). With disease progression, contractures of the hip flexors, knee flexors, and plantar flexors will develop (Stevens, 2006). Daily stretching exercises and proper bracing should be employed (Do, 2002).

Scoliosis. Progressive scoliosis usually develops in the second decade of life once boys lose the ability to walk. If left untreated, scoliotic curves in DMD generally progress to greater than 80 degrees (Velasco et al., 2007) producing pain, difficulty with positioning, and compromised respiratory status (Hinton & Goldstein, 2007). Boys with DMD may elect spinal fusion surgery, which is best performed either before or soon after a teen becomes wheelchair-dependent (Sengupta, Mehdian, McConnell, et al., 2001).

Osteoporosis and Fractures. Boys with DMD have low bone mineral density even before the loss of independent ambulation; long-term corticosteroid treatment further increases the risk for osteoporosis (Bushby et al., 2005). Appropriate monitoring and supportive treatment are indicated.

Feeding and Swallowing Difficulties

Feeding difficulties occur with DMD, particularly during the advanced stages of the disease. Boys should be sent to a speech and language pathologist (SLP), an occupational therapist, or a swallowing team for a clinical feeding and swallowing evaluation. A videofluoroscopy swallow study may detect any difficulties as food moves from the esophagus to the stomach, although this type of assessment may not be of additional benefit in DMD beyond eliciting a careful feeding history and observation of feeding difficulties (Aloysius, Born, Kinali, et al., 2008). The oral phase of swallowing is most significantly affected in DMD and in most boys the pharyngeal phase of swallowing is readily initiated but is weak with incomplete pharyngeal clearance leaving pharyngeal residue, which can trigger episodes of choking. Insufficient or effortful chewing combined with weak clearance may also predispose boys to choking episodes (Aloysius et al.).

Obesity

Obesity is common in boys with DMD, partially because of decreased physical activity that accompanies disease progression and partially from the side effects of corticosteroid therapy and inappropriate caloric intake (Bushby et al., 2005). Weight gain can occur over a range of prednisone dosages (0.3 to 1.5 mg/kg/day), but some of the weight gained is fat and some of it is muscle (Moxley et al., 2005). This elucidates one of the benefits of corticosteroid therapy but also poses a challenge for providers in defining "excessive weight gain" in boys with DMD (Moxley et al.).

Constipation

Constipation, worsened by a lack of mobility and dehydration, is a common problem. Constipation and bowel regularity should be evaluated continually, especially with disease progression and subsequent limited physical activity and decreasing ambulation. Constipation can be managed by the PCP or a nutritionist knowledgeable in neuromuscular disorders either nutritionally (Hinton & Goldstein, 2007) or, if necessary, pharmacologically, with senna, docusate, or polyethylene glycol (Bushby et al., 2005).

Decubitus Ulcers

Skin problems may arise when bony prominences rub against surfaces as a result of positioning in chairs or beds. Decubitus ulcers can occur quickly and vigilant skin management is necessary. Frequent repositioning, especially at nighttime, should be done to prophylactically prevent against the development of pressure sores, and bony prominences should be protected with soft coverings. Medical attention should be sought as soon as any skin breakdown is detected.

Psychosocial and Behavioral Issues

Psychological and behavioral problems have been reported for boys with DMD (Weidner, 2005). In younger boys with DMD, behavior problems may be a consequence of language delay. Notably, younger boys are more likely to have increased social problems such as immaturity and poor peer relationships (Hinton, Nereo, Fee, et al., 2006). Behavioral problems also may be a normal mechanism for coping with the disease and its challenges (Weidner, 2005). Behavioral problems may include distractibility, low frustration threshold, poor attention span, anxiety, features of obsessive-compulsive behavior, or depression (see Chapters 33 and 41) (Biggar, 2006). A range of behaviors can be associated with varying age, disease progression, intellectual level, and environmental background. Recommendations for specific treatment must be based on individual assessment (Hinton & Goldstein, 2007).

Many psychological adjustments also accompany DMD, such as facing separation and loss; experiencing and expressing emotions (including anger, guilt, sadness, loss of control, resentment of increased demands); and changing values, expectations, roles, and responsibilities. Older boys are more likely to experience adjustment difficulties (Reid & Renwick, 2001), including depression, social isolation, poor attention span, and anxiety, as the physical limitations of their disease further remove them from their peers (Weidner, 2005).

Prognosis

DMD is ultimately fatal. The majority of individuals with DMD do not live beyond the third decade of life (Kohler et al., 2005). Most affected individuals eventually succumb to respiratory complications or cardiopulmonary issues. Hospice services may be helpful in providing supportive and palliative care.

PRIMARY CARE MANAGEMENT

Health Care Maintenance

Growth and Development

Most boys with DMD initially experience normal growth and development, but the rate of growth likely will be altered as boys become increasingly limited in physical activity, after the initiation of corticosteroid therapy, and as muscle mass declines with disease progression. Twenty-four hour energy expenditure in boys with DMD is estimated to be approximately 25% lower than in unaffected children (Bach, 2004). This accounts for an increase in weight without a simultaneous increase in height (Moxley et al., 2005). PCPs should monitor growth parameters at every visit with the appropriate measurement devices and plotting of weight, length or height, head circumference, and body mass index (BMI) (when appropriate). In general, most boys can be started on a 1200 to 1500 kcal daily diet when corticosteroid therapy is initiated. In boys with advanced stage DMD, weight may be drastically reduced, and it has been reported that boys weigh 70 lb, on average, at the point when ventilatory assistance becomes necessary (Bach, 2004).

It is important that anthropomorphic measurements be assessed as accurately as possible, especially as the disease progresses. In the rare instance that an infant or small boy presents with DMD, weight should be measured using an electronic digital infant scale. From approximately ages 2 to 10 years, boys should stand on a scale to be weighed, if able to stand independently. For boys who are unable to stand independently but can easily be held by a caregiver, the caregiver's weight should be subtracted from the total. Starting at age 10 to 12 years, or when a boy with DMD becomes fully dependent on a wheelchair, he should be weighed in his chair by rolling onto the platform of a digital electronic scale. The first time this is done the boy should be weighed in his chair and then safely transferred onto a stationary chair while the wheelchair is weighed independently; the weight of the chair should then be subtracted from the total weight. The chair weight should be recorded in the boy's chart for future use. The provider should remove any excess baggage or cushions from the chair and should ask if any modifications have been made to the chair at every visit.

Length or height should be measured using the standing scale if the boy is able to stand up straight or lying down if the boy is small or unable to stand. If an accurate height is unable to be determined with the boy lying down, because of contractures or obesity, length should be assessed by measuring the length from joint to joint, starting at the boy's heel and ending at the crown of his head. Head circumference should be measured with the boy lying down, if possible. BMI measurements, although calculated, may be misleading when assessing obesity in DMD because they fail to incorporate perimuscular and intramuscular lipid infiltrations and thus do not accurately reflect whether excess weight is attributable to obesity or edema (Pessolano, Suarez, Monteiro, et al., 2003). Standard measurements of BMI, including skinfold thickness (ST), underestimate excessive body fat and should be used at the provider's discretion. Indices that incorporate the assessment of the compartmental distribution of fat and muscle (Pessolano et al.), such as bioelectrical impedance analysis (BIA) (Mok, Beghin, Gachon, et al., 2006), are preferable although not always available.

Initially, boys with DMD appear to be developing normally. At age 2 to 3, slight motor impairments are apparent and boys will be perceived as clumsy and have difficulty keeping up with their peers on the playground (Hinton & Goldstein, 2007). As muscles continue to weaken, boys will have difficulty walking and become wheelchair-dependent, eventually needing assistance with all activities that require the use of legs, arms, and trunk (Hinton & Goldstein). Boys should be encouraged to remain as active as possible while in their wheelchairs; for example, they should be encouraged to pursue activities with their hands such as playing a

small instrument, playing a wheelchair-accessible sport, or working with handheld toys or puzzles.

Diet

A decrease in energy expenditure should be considered when calculating the daily caloric needs of boys with DMD. An equation has been derived to guide providers in calculating the daily recommended caloric intake (Bach, 2004):

$$\text{Daily energy intake in kcal} = 2000 - \text{Age (year)} \times 50$$

Keep in mind that this equation is a guideline. For wheelchair-dependent, minimally active boys the following calculation, which takes into account the height of the child, may be more appropriate (Ekvall & Cerniglia, 2005):

$$9\text{-}11\,\text{kcal}/\text{Height (in cm)}$$

PCPs should use clinical judgment in determining caloric needs and reducing obesity, and should consult with a nutritionist when necessary. Caloric adjustments should be made for boys at the time when ventilatory support substitutes for inspiratory muscle function (Bach, 2004). Healthy food choices, portion control, and selecting low-sodium foods should also be part of nutritional planning, and adjustments should then be tailored to meet individual nutritional needs throughout the course of the disease.

If swallowing difficulties develop, recipes are available for texture-adapted meals that facilitate swallowing and minimize aspiration (Bach, 2004), and boys can also be put on a pureed-food diet. Liquids can be thickened using commercially prepared products such as "Thick It," and nutritional dietary formulations can be prescribed to supplement meals and increase caloric intake, if necessary. In extreme cases of dysphagia a percutaneous endoscopic gastrostomy (PEG) tube may be necessary to ensure safe feeding. The risks and benefits of this intervention should be discussed with the child, caregiver, and health care provider.

The risk for osteoporosis may be treated with intravenous biphosphonates under the guidance of an expert in bone metabolism (Bushby et al., 2005). There is insufficient evidence to warrant the use of oral biphosphonates prophylactically; however, many providers do recommend bone density loss prophylaxis through calcium and vitamin D supplementation (Bushby et al.). If the provider believes that calcium and vitamin D intake through diet and sunshine are inadequate, supplementation to reach a daily intake of 1000 mg of calcium and 400 units of vitamin D may be advised (Bushby et al.), but the effects of these interventions are not proven (Hinton & Goldstein, 2007).

Safety

Young boys with DMD initially may not be restricted in physical activity but should be adequately supervised and normal safety precautions should be taken. As muscle weakness progresses and gait changes ensue, boys with DMD may experience unexpected falls. Thus extra precautions should be taken regarding bath safety. Both the home and school environment should be kept safe and clear from objects on the floor and sharp edges and corners to safeguard against injurious falls. When a boy becomes wheelchair-dependent, the home and school environment should be made wheelchair accessible. An adapted car seat with additional neck support or a wheelchair-accessible vehicle will become necessary to ensure safety while traveling. The MDA often can arrange and cover the cost of a home evaluation to assess for accessibility, suggest adaptations to ensure safety, and help plan necessary modifications. When necessary, the PCP can complete forms to augment a move to accessible housing or an apartment building with an elevator. Home emergency plans should be made to accommodate a boy in a wheelchair, and local police and fire departments should be alerted to facilitate safety during an emergency.

Immunizations

Unless specifically contraindicated, immunizations for healthy children, as recommended by the AAP, should be given to children with chronic conditions (AAP, 2006), such as DMD. Intramuscular (IM) injections should be given in the locations normally recommended for age, using a needle long enough to reach the muscle, when possible. In boys with DMD with decreased muscle mass, IM injections should be given in the best available muscle, as per the AAP guidelines.

Boys with DMD have cardiorespiratory involvement and are at increased risk for complications of influenza, varicella, and pneumococcal infection. Annual immunization with inactivated influenza vaccine is recommended for boys with DMD who are 6 months and older, following the Centers for Disease Control and Prevention (CDC) guidelines (AAP, 2006). PCPs should also encourage all family members and household contacts to be immunized as well. Given the risk for pulmonary disease, boys should be immunized with heptavalent pneumococcal polysaccharide-protein conjugate vaccine (PPCV-7) before age 2 and boys ages 2 and older should receive 23-valent pneumococcal polysaccharide vaccine (PPCV-23) as recommended for age and immunization status (AAP, 2006).

For children receiving systemic corticosteroid therapy, empiric guidelines recommend that children receiving low or moderate doses (less than 2 mg/kg/day of prednisone or its equivalent, or less than 20 mg/day if weight is greater than 10 kg) can receive live-virus vaccines (AAP, 2006). The recommended dose of corticosteroid therapy for boys with DMD puts them in this category (prednisone: 0.75 mg/kg/day and deflazacort: 0.9 mg/kg/day) (Biggar et al., 2006). If the dose increases, live vaccines should be avoided (AAP, 2006).

Screening

Vision. Routine screening is recommended for boys with DMD. Boys on steroid therapy should be monitored annually by a pediatric ophthalmologist for early detection of cataracts or glaucoma (Moxley et al., 2005).

In addition to full-length dystrophin, two other shorter proteins are transcribed from the DMD gene *(Xp21)* and are expressed in the retina (Costa, Oliveira, Feitosa-Santana, et al., 2007). As compared with age-matched peers, 66% of boys with DMD have some red-green color defect. However, the vision changes are generally subclinical. In most instances boys accommodate for slightly impaired color vision and may not recognize the discrepancy until adulthood (Costa et al.). Color vision testing is only warranted if a boy complains of disturbances in color vision.

Hearing. Although hearing loss is not widely reported, cochlear hair cells express dystrophin. In animal models, decreased dystrophin may lead to a depletion of neurotransmitters, inducing a sensorineural hearing loss (Chen, Chen, Wang, et al., 2002). It is recommended that boys with DMD have routine auditory examinations (ATS, 2004) to ensure early detection of any hearing disability and subsequent adoption of appropriate protection against further noise-induced damage (Chen et al., 2002).

Dental. Early and routine screening is recommended. Adaptive equipment such as a built-up toothbrush may be necessary if a boy loses hand function with disease progression, and boys may need assistance with daily oral hygiene. Boys should be treated by a dentist who has experience with children with neuromuscular disorders, and the dental office should be wheelchair accessible with ample space for either a wheelchair or transfer to the dental chair, if necessary (Mielnik-Blaszczak & Malgorzata, 2007).

Blood Pressure. Blood pressure should be measured at every visit because of possible hypertension resulting from corticosteroid therapy (Seth & Aggarwal, 2004).

Hematocrit. Routine screening is recommended. A complete blood count (CBC) with differential and bicarbonate measurement by arterial or free-flowing blood gas is recommended annually for nonambulatory patients (ATS, 2004).

Urinalysis. Routine screening is recommended.

Tuberculosis. Routine screening is recommended, especially before steroid treatment is initiated (Reznik & Ozuah, 2006).

Condition-Specific Screening

See Table 34-2.

Pulmonary Function Testing. Pulmonary function testing (PFT) to measure forced vital capacity (FVC) should be part of the regular assessment of all boys with DMD (Bushby & Straub, 2005). Boys should be referred, at minimum, for an annual visit with a pulmonologist before confinement to a wheelchair; twice yearly after age 12, wheelchair-dependent, or when FVC falls below 80% predicted; and more frequently as indicated by disease progression (ATS, 2004).

Other Screenings. The following condition-specific screenings are recommended for boys with DMD.

Respiratory. (1) Annual chest radiograph if wheelchair-dependent; (2) oxyhemoglobin saturation by pulse oximetry; end-tidal carbon dioxide; spirometric measurements of FVC, forced expiratory volume in 1 second (FEV_1), and maximal midexpiratory flow rate; maximum inspiratory and expiratory pressures; and peak cough flow at every visit; (3) evaluation for obstructive sleep apnea, oropharyngeal aspiration, gastroesophageal reflux, and asthma, as indicated; and (4) pulmonary evaluation before any type of surgery (ATS, 2004).

Cardiac. (1) Noninvasive cardiac evaluation, including an echocardiogram and electrocardiogram, at the time of diagnosis and then every 2 years until age 10 and annually thereafter (Meune & Duboc, 2006); and (2) cardiac evaluation before any type of surgery (ATS, 2004).

The PCP should refer boys with DMD to specialists in the following areas depending on screening results and as the need arises: neurology, pulmonology, cardiology, ophthalmology, gastroenterology/nutrition, rehabilitation medicine, orthopedics/neurosurgery, and neuropsychology (ATS, 2004). Considering boys' specific needs, specialized management of DMD may be best handled in a multidisciplinary care setting if available. Care coordination between specialists may best be managed by the PCP (see Chapter 9). Figure 34-1 represents the specialists that should be involved in the management of DMD.

Common Illness Management

Differential Diagnosis

Respiratory Tract Infections. Boys with DMD are prone to respiratory tract infections, and the risks for infection should be considered in the office evaluation of febrile illness (Kaira & Amin, 2005). For any fever that persists for several days with or without accompanying symptoms of infection, the child with DMD should be seen by a PCP for routine management. Physical assessment and laboratory work should be done as routinely appropriate for the presentation of a child with fever.

TABLE 34-2
Summary of Disease-Specific Screening

Disease-Specific Screening	Recommended Frequency
Pulmonary function testing (PFT)	Every visit with PCP or pulmonologist*
Chest radiograph	Annual when wheelchair-dependent[a]
Oxyhemoglobin saturation (by pulse oximetry)	Every visit with pulmonologist
Cardiac evaluation	Biannual visit before age 10; annual after age 12*
Pulmonary evaluation	Annual visit before age 10; biannual visits after age 12, when wheelchair-dependent, or FVC ≤80% predicted*
Presurgical clearance	Clearance by pulmonologist and cardiologist before every procedure[a]

*American Thoracic Society. (2004). American Thoracic Society documents: Respiratory care of the patient with Duchenne muscular dystrophy, ATS consensus statement. *Am J Respir Crit Care Med, 170,* 456-465.

Boys with DMD with impaired cough are at increased risk for aspiration, atelectasis, and pneumonia (Kaira & Amin, 2005). These risks should be considered when a boy with DMD has symptoms of respiratory illness. Management with appropriate antibiotics, along with careful monitoring for the resolution of the infection, is necessary. A history of prolonged cough with respiratory infections or need for frequent antibiotics to treat chest congestion reflects an inability to clear respiratory secretions effectively and should be monitored carefully. Referral to a pulmonologist may be warranted.

There is a high probability of pneumonia occurring after an initial upper respiratory infection or other illness such as influenza in boys with advanced DMD. Pneumonia can also be caused by aspiration or gastroesophageal reflux and can lead to severe, life-threatening respiratory complications. The use of an MIE device that helps to clear secretions may be helpful. Precautions should be taken to avoid dehydration, and hospitalization may be an option for the purpose of close observation. The importance of monitoring carefully and contacting the pulmonologist if the condition worsens should be emphasized.

Pain Management. Pain can be exercise related, temperature modulated, and palpation induced. The back is the most common site for pain in DMD, followed by the leg, shoulder, and neck (Bushby & Straub, 2005). Pain can be caused by abnormal posture or gait; ligament sprains or falls resulting from joint instability caused by severe weakness; muscle cramping and contractures; possible nerve impingement; or pressure areas resulting from prolonged use of a wheelchair (Bushby & Straub). Therapeutic approaches to pain include physical therapy, occupational therapy, massage therapy, chiropractic care, nerve blocks, several analgesic

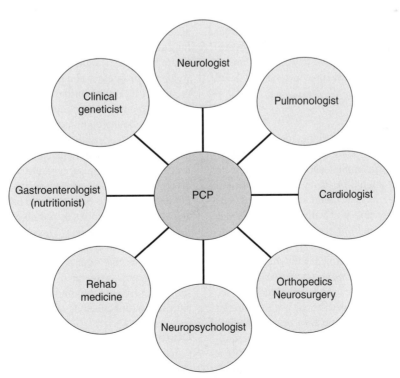

FIGURE 34-1 Specialists involved in multidisciplinary care.

Differential Diagnosis

- *Respiratory tract infections:* upper or lower respiratory tract infection (URI or LRI) vs. aspiration, atelectasis, or pneumonia caused by prolonged cough, chest congestion, or influenza complicated by respiratory muscle weakness
- *Pain management:* common injury-related pain from exercise, sprains, or falls vs. condition-related pain caused by abnormal posture or gait; injury secondary to instability due to severe weakness; muscle cramping and contractures; possible nerve impingement; or pressure areas resulting from prolonged use of wheelchair
- *Gastrointestinal problems:* common gastrointestinal (GI) illness vs. malfunction of smooth muscle lining in the GI tract or complications of chronic constipation due to immobility

---

drugs (most commonly nonsteroidal antiinflammatory drugs [NSAIDs], used with limited success), gabapentin, carbamazepine, muscle relaxants, and tricyclic antidepressants, as well as several alternative therapies (see earlier section) (Bushby & Straub). Pain management is an important aspect of care for the boy with DMD because it has an impact on mobility, school performance, recreational activities, and overall quality of life (Bushby & Straub). Pain is usually effectively managed by the PCP, but if it becomes severe or seemingly unmanageable, referral to a pain management team may be warranted.

Gastrointestinal Problems. Gastrointestinal (GI) symptoms in boys with DMD are thought to be caused by the malfunction of smooth muscle lining the GI tract (Bushby & Straub, 2005). Caregivers should carefully monitor the frequency and consistency of stools, straining efforts associated with bowel movements, and evidence of abdominal distention associated with constipation. Constipation can be managed by the PCP or a nutritionist knowledgeable in neuromuscular disorders either nutritionally or pharmacologically (or both). The development of complications of chronic constipation such as urinary tract infections and bowel impaction should be carefully assessed by the PCP, and referral to a gastroenterologist should be made if the provider suspects a GI complication.

Drug Interactions

Boys with DMD often receive corticosteroid therapy, as described on p.658. There are no specific pharmaceutical contraindications for corticosteroids; however, immunosuppression can occur with larger doses. Precautions should be taken when administering live virus vaccinations (see immunization section). The same precautions should be taken for any boy with DMD who has a concurrent immunosuppressive condition requiring the use of other immunosuppressive agents.

Cardiac medications are being prescribed with gaining popularity for boys with DMD (see cardiac section). Angiotensin-converting enzyme (ACE) inhibitors and beta-blockers are sometimes prescribed, along with the occasional use of diuretics and digoxin (Markham et al., 2005). The use of cardiac medications for boys with DMD should be monitored closely by a cardiologist and precautions should be taken for any possible interactions with other drugs, such as nonsteroidal antiinflammatory drugs (NSAIDs) (see Chapter 21).

Developmental Issues

Sleep Patterns

Boys with DMD have needs regarding healthy sleep patterns that increase as their mobility decreases. Necessary objects (e.g., commode, tissues, water, book, music, remote control, call bell) should be located in close proximity while arm function remains intact. Boys should be repositioned intermittently throughout the night to prevent the development of pressure sores and to maintain comfort, and the use of electric blankets should be considered in cold climates to avoid excess weight of heavy blankets.

Sleep-related disturbances (SRDs), namely obstructive sleep apnea (OSA) and hypoventilation (Kaira & Amin, 2005), increase with age in DMD. The conventional approaches to managing disease progression usually start by monitoring for SRDs. Custom-made intraoral appliances may be necessary to bring the mandible forward and open the airway in cases of OSA (Bach, 2004). Supportive treatment with nocturnal use of noninvasive positive-pressure ventilation (NIPPV) may be helpful (Bach). Boys with DMD respond very well to long-term use of NIPPV with improved longevity of at least 10 years and good quality of life, especially when combined with other treatment modalities (Eagle et al., 2002). Use of NIPPV is usually effective in treating SRD that is not complicated by scoliosis, obesity, or severe muscle weakness (Bach, 2004). SRD can be monitored best by polysomnogram, which involves monitoring electroencephalographic (EEG) and cardiorespiratory parameters during sleep (Kaira & Amin, 2005). However, this is not always available and can be burdensome to families. Instead, overnight pulse oximetry testing can be conducted in the home. Overnight sleep studies should be done as soon as boys show signs of OSA or when they become wheelchair dependent.

Toileting

Because signs of DMD usually manifest after the developmentally appropriate age for toilet training, boys generally are trained like all children. Boys should be encouraged to use the toilet for as long as possible and may require assistance as ambulation becomes limited. Transfers to the toilet may become increasingly difficult as weakness progresses and boys become wheelchair-dependent, and the use of a portable urinal or a commode may be necessary. Occupational and physical therapists should provide input regarding adaptive toileting equipment.

PCPs can work with families to develop toileting plans for both home and school that include designated individuals to assist with toileting and that are acceptable to both the child and the caregiver, being mindful that boys may be sensitive about this topic. For example, some boys prefer to have bowel movements at home and only use the toilet or portable urinal at school to urinate or for emergency situations. The use of a condom catheter or adult diapers should also be considered when it may not be possible to use an accessible bathroom, such as during travel, and to avoid embarrassment associated with accidents. Finally, consideration should be given to the timing of laxatives or other supplements to aid constipation when developing a plan for toileting.

Discipline

Caregivers and teachers may discipline boys with DMD differently than their siblings and peers and should be encouraged to remain consistent when disciplining all children using techniques that are appropriate for the child's developmental and cognitive ability. The need for more services aimed at psychological problems, peer support, and professional counseling merit attention in DMD (Chen, Chen, Jong, et al., 2002). Boys should be assessed by their PCPs in the same manner as other children for abuse and neglect, and any signs should be appropriately reported.

Child Care

Early in life boys with DMD can receive childcare in traditional settings. As boys' needs progress, the decision can be made to transition care to an early intervention program or an inclusive child care program tailored to meet the boys' individual functional and cognitive abilities.

Schooling

Boys with DMD face considerable academic obstacles, partly because of their physical disabilities and subsequent hardships associated with placement in the proper academic setting (Hinton & Goldstein, 2007). Some boys with DMD require early intervention (EI) services before age 3, but support likely will be needed by school entry. An individualized educational program (IEP) should be instituted as soon as feasible (see Chapter 3). Some boys also require special education (Hinton & Goldstein, 2007). It is essential that boys are challenged to work to their full potential; in some instances boys are placed erroneously in classrooms that are below their intellectual level of functioning based on their physical disabilities (Muscular Dystrophy Association [MDA], 2005).

Teachers must be made aware of the child's potential difficulties with keeping up with class work and homework; written language and writing tasks; paying attention and concentrating; and peer interactions. Appropriate accommodations must be made for special transportation; physical accessibility of the school and classroom; positioning and seating; adaptive physical education; medical care; curriculum modifications and tutoring, if necessary; and therapies that may interrupt the day (MDA, 2005). Some boys require a paraprofessional to help with personal needs or to assist them throughout the day. Transportation to and from school can also be an issue, and the PCP may be asked to complete paperwork for the board of education to authorize a more direct bus route, assistance getting on and off the school bus, or a bus equipped for wheelchairs.

School-age boys may participate in after-school programs provided through the school system or may be cared for by family members or private babysitters who are prepared to meet their needs. In adolescence, day programs are sometimes available for boys that promote socialization and life skills while still providing supervision so that parents can work.

Sexuality

By the time most boys reach the appropriate age for the development of intimate relationships, they are wheelchair-bound and dependent in activities of daily living. As a result, many young men are unable to function independently and may not experience intimate sexual relationships. Adolescents with DMD do, however, go through regular pubertal development and may have sexual desires, sometimes expressed through masturbation. This behavior should not be discouraged and should be handled appropriately as with any adolescent in this developmental stage. Adolescents with DMD should be educated regarding sexual development and healthy and safe sex practices, if appropriate. This may also be beneficial in fostering healthy self-esteem. Given the unlikelihood that those affected with DMD will become sexually active, it is rare for the condition to be passed down from affected males. However, sexual education should be initiated by the PCP when appropriate since some adolescents with DMD may have healthy sexual relationships.

Transition to Adulthood

As boys get older they are often faced with the challenge of combining their intellectual and physical capabilities to find skills that they are both capable of and enjoy doing. If possible, some adolescents will choose to enroll in vocational or college preparation programs. Some boys may also attend college, and special classroom and dorm room accommodations should be made. Educational support such as tutoring or specialized test circumstances should be provided during this time if needed, as adolescents may struggle with the increasing demands of education at this level. If boys succeed with vocational or educational training, specialized jobs may be acquired that are compatible with their intellectual and physical capabilities.

Recent advances in supportive care and therapeutic strategies aimed at slowing disease progression have led to increases of survival into adulthood (Kohler et al., 2005). In appropriate instances, and before age 18, the issue of guardianship should be addressed. Parents (or current legal guardians) may consider obtaining guardianship to ensure involvement in medical care and decision making in legal matters. Obtaining guardianship can be costly and involves a lengthy amount of paperwork but should be granted in court without difficulty for adolescents with DMD.

Changing needs regarding therapy, adaptive equipment, and assistance with activities of daily living should be assessed on a regular basis, and proper accommodations should be made for adolescents who are able to attend vocational programs or college and obtain employment. When it becomes too difficult to transfer older boys into cars, an accessible van may be necessary and special arrangements made to facilitate vacation and travel plans. PCPs may be asked to provide documentation to augment accessible travel, especially when traveling by airplane. In some instances, adolescents may be able to drive with the use of adaptive equipment and technology.

Individuals with DMD may be very social and well liked among their peers. Social status and positive self-esteem should be considered when transitioning to adulthood, and individual or group psychotherapy may be beneficial during this time. In some instances, individuals may choose to live independently. Men with DMD report feeling materially, socially, and symbolically marginalized by inaccessible environments, social arrangements that limit their involvement in community life, and negative social experiences as a result of their physical disabilities (Gibson, Young, Upshur, et al., 2007), whereas others anecdotally report living very full, independent lives requiring only some assistance.

Independence should be stressed and adolescents should have a role in decision making as much as possible, especially if and when life support is considered. The transition to adult medicine may also be necessary at this time and can be especially difficult as families become comfortable with pediatric providers who have cared for their children from a very young age (see Chapter 4). PCPs should facilitate conversations regarding the end of life if and when families and adolescents with DMD are ready.

Palliative care can begin as early as the time of diagnosis and should be provided by teams consisting of health care providers and family members to develop solutions as issues arise throughout the course of the disease (Weidner, 2005). As illness progresses, the level of psychosocial and emotional stress for the family living with DMD rises, providing the opportunity to develop a palliative care plan, tailored specifically to the family's individual needs and communication style. The plan usually includes treatment, stress management, respite services, anticipatory guidance, familial support at critical periods, and assistance in decision making, and may include hospice care and bereavement support (Weidner). The early introduction of a palliative care team allows a relationship of trust to develop, and serves as the foundation for the interventions necessary to meet the needs that arise during the care of a child with a chronic, life-threatening condition such as DMD (Weidner).

Family Concerns

The care of boys with DMD presents many complex issues and should be focused on the entire family, especially considering that more than one child is commonly affected within a family. Supportive care, based on palliative principles, should be provided throughout the course of the disease. The PCP should also provide suitable anticipatory guidance throughout the disease course and should facilitate decision making regarding end-of-life care. The PCP must be aware of psychosocial needs and should make referrals for individual, family, and genetic counseling as an essential early intervention for DMD.

A study conducted with families of children with DMD specifically explored the relationship between child-related factors of disability level and age at diagnosis and family-related factors of caregiver health, income and employment, family support, and family hardiness in relation to overall family functional ability. Results suggest that family-related factors of caregiver health and levels of hardiness and support have an impact on families' abilities to function effectively (Chen & Clark, 2007). Family function displayed a significant correlation with the child-related factor of age at diagnosis, but not with disability level, suggesting that parents of children who were diagnosed younger had more time to adapt to the diagnosis of DMD and to garner information about the disease and how to cope with its effects on the family. Health care providers should be sensitized to the array of stresses and losses experienced by the family and the boy affected with DMD as they experience physical, educational, social, and emotional changes.

Caring for boys with DMD can be overwhelming, and caregivers may understandably get frustrated and tired. In some instances, respite services may be available for families of boys with DMD. The setting should be accessible with adequate adaptations and caregivers who are prepared to meet the special needs associated with DMD. Families need support as they attempt to normalize family life, capitalize on personal strengths, and make use of a resource network (Chen et al., 2002). The PCP should provide families of boys with DMD with an array of resources from the time of diagnosis and throughout the progression of the disease. Some of these are summarized in the resources section.

Resources

American Occupational Therapy Association (AOTA)
(800) 668-8255
Website: www.aota.org

American Physical Therapy Association (APTA)
(703) 684-APTA
Website: www.apta.org

Americans with Disabilities Act (ADA)
(800) 949-4232

ADA Technical Assistance Program
Website: www.adata.org

Centers for Disease Control and Prevention (CDC)
U.S. Department of Health and Human Services
1600 Clifton Rd., N.E.
Atlanta, GA 30333
(800) 311-3435; (404) 639-3311; (404) 639-3543
Email: inquiry@cdc.gov
Website: www.cdc.gov

Muscular Dystrophy Association
3300 East Sunrise Dr.
Tucson, AZ 85718-3208
(520) 529-2000; (800) 344-4863; Fax: (520) 529-5300
Email: mda@mdausa.org
Website: www.mda.org

Muscular Dystrophy Family Foundation
3951 N. Meridian St., Suite 100
Indianapolis, IN 46208-4062
(317) 923-6333; (800) 544-1213; Fax: (317) 923-633
Email: mdff@mdff.org
Website: www.mdff.org

National Institute of Arthritis and Musculoskeletal and Skin Diseases (NIAMS)
National Institutes of Health, DHHS
31 Center Dr., Room 4C02 MSC 2350
Bethesda, MD 20892-2350
(301) 496-8190; (877) 22-NIAMS (226-4267)
Email: NIAMSinfo@mail.nih.gov
Website: www.niams.nih.gov

National Institute of Child Health and Human Development (NICHD)
National Institutes of Health, DHHS
31 Center Dr., Room 2A32 MSC 2425
Bethesda, MD 20892-2425
(301) 496-5133; Fax: (301) 496-7101
Website: www.nichd.nih.gov

Parent Project Muscular Dystrophy (PPMD)
1012 North University Blvd.
Middletown, OH 45042
(513) 424-0696; (800) 714-KIDS (5437); Fax: (513) 425-9907
Email: info@parentprojectmd.org
Website: www.parentprojectmd.org

SATH (Society for Accessible Travel and Hospitality)
Website: www.sath.org

Winners on Wheels (WOW)
Website: www.wowusa.com

Books for Younger Children

Dobbs, J. (2004). *Kids on Wheels*. Shanghai, China: No Limits Communications. Pamphlets for kids in wheelchairs.

Dwight, L. (1998). *We Can Do It!* Long Island City, NY: Star Bright Books.

Maguire, A. (2000). *Special People, Special Ways*. Arlington, TX: Future Horizons.

Mayer, M. (1993). *A Very Special Critter*. New York: Random House/Golden Books.

Thomas, P., & Harker, L. (2005). *Don't Call Me Special*. Hauppauge, NY: Barron's Educational Series.

Wenger, B., & Green, A. (2005). *Dewey Doo-It Helps Owlie Fly Again*. Irvine, CA: RandallFraser Publishing.

Books for Family Members and Siblings of Children with Special Needs

Blackburn, L. B. (1991). *I Know I Made It Happen: A Gentle Book About Feeling Guilty*. Omaha: Centering Corporation.

Farrell, M. (1995). *Marrying Malcolm Murgatroyd*. NY: Farrar, Strauss & Giroux.

Heegaard, M. (1988). *When Someone Very Special Dies: Children Can Learn to Cope with Grief*. Minneapolis: Woodland Press.

Heegaard, M. (1991). *When Someone Has a Very Serious Illness: Children Can Learn to Cope with Loss and Change*. Minneapolis: Woodland Press.

Meyer, D.J., & Gallagher, D. (2005). *The Sibling Slam Book: What It's Really Like to Have a Brother or Sister with Special Needs*. Bethesda, MD: Woodbine House.

Meyer, D.J., & Pillo, C. (1997). *Views from Our Shoes: Growing Up with a Brother or Sister with Special Needs*. Bethesda, MD: Woodbine House.

Moynihan, R. & Haig, R.D. (1989). *Whole Parent Whole Child: A Parents' Guide to Raising a Child with a Chronic Illness*. Wayzata, MN: DCI Publishing, Inc.

Siegel, I.M. (1989). *Muscular Dystrophy in Children: A Guide for Families*. New York: Demos Medical Publishing.

Summary of Primary Care Needs for the Child with Duchenne Muscular Dystrophy

HEALTH CARE MAINTENANCE

Growth and Development
- Close surveillance of growth is necessary, adapting measurement techniques is necessary as disease progresses.
- Monitor growth parameters at every visit with the appropriate measurement and plotting of weight, length or height, head circumference, and BMI.
- Monitor development and need for adaptive equipment.

Diet
- Encourage boys to remain as active as possible and to maintain a healthy weight by making healthy food choices.
- Closely monitor weight gain with decreasing mobility and exercise and corticosteroid use.
- Consider a decrease in energy expenditure when calculating daily caloric needs using an appropriate formula: Daily energy intake in kcal = 2000 − Age (in years) × 50, or 9 to 11 kcal/Height (in cm), and individualize plans as necessary.
- Consider calcium and vitamin D supplementation when on corticosteroid therapy.
- Diet modifications and adaptive equipment needed with disease progression.

Safety
- Instruct families in keeping both the home and school environment safe and clear from objects on the floor and sharp edges and corners.
- Assist in arranging a home evaluation to assess for accessibility.
- Suggest adaptations to ensure safety.
- Assist in relocation to accessible housing or an apartment building with an elevator, when necessary.
- Instruct families to notify local police and fire departments to facilitate safety during an emergency.

Immunizations
- Routine immunizations should be given on schedule.
- All family members should be immunized against influenza on an annual basis.
- Administer heptavalent pneumococcal polysaccharide-protein conjugate vaccine (PPCV-7) before age 2, and boys ages 2 and older should receive 23-valent pneumococcal polysaccharide vaccine (PPCV-23) as recommended for age and immunization status.
- Systemic corticosteroid therapy can cause immunosuppression. Empiric guidelines recommend that children receiving low or moderate doses (<2 mg/kg/day of prednisone or its equivalent, or <20 mg/day if weight is >10 kg) can receive live-virus vaccines; however, the AAP guidelines should be referred to if the dose increases, in which cases live vaccines should be avoided.

Screening
- *Vision*. Routine screening is recommended. Annual pediatric ophthalmologist referral is needed for boys on steroid therapy.
  - Mild color-blindness may be present.
- *Hearing*. Routine screening is recommended.
- *Dental*. Routine screening and early referral to a dentist is recommended.
- *Blood pressure*. Screen at every visit after start of corticosteroid treatment.
- *Hematocrit*. Routine screening for anemia. Annual complete blood count and arterial or free-flowing blood gas for nonambulatory patients is recommended.
- *Tuberculosis*. Routine screening for boys at increased risk and before the onset of steroid treatment.

Condition-Specific Screening
- Pulmonary function tests (PFTs); chest radiograph if wheelchair-dependent; oxyhemoglobin saturation by pulse oximetry; spirometic

Continued

Summary of Primary Care Needs for the Child with Duchenne Muscular Dystrophy—cont'd

measurements of FVC, FEV_1, and maximal midexpiratory flow rate; maximum inspiratory and expiratory pressures; peak cough flow; noninvasive cardiac evaluation; pulmonary and cardiac evaluations before any type of surgery; evaluation for obstructive sleep apnea, oropharyngeal aspiration, gastroesophageal reflux, and asthma as indicated and anthropomorphic measurements reflective of nutritional status are routinely assessed at multidisciplinary care settings.

COMMON ILLNESS MANAGEMENT

- *Respiratory tract infections.* Distinguish between common viral or bacterial illness vs. respiratory tract infection resulting from impaired respiratory muscle function and treat appropriately. Be aware of frequent upper or lower respiratory tract infections (URIs or LRIs) and assess for aspiration, atelectasis, or pneumonia caused by prolonged cough, chest congestion, or influenza complicated by respiratory muscle weakness.
- *Pain management.* Treat condition-related pain caused by abnormal posture or gait; injury secondary to instability due to severe weakness; muscle cramping and contractures; possible nerve impingement; or pressure areas resulting from prolonged use of wheelchair with proper analgesics.
- *Gastrointestinal problems.* Assess for complications due to malfunction of smooth muscle lining in the GI tract and refer to a gastroenterologist if necessary. Treat complications of chronic constipation resulting from immobility.

DEVELOPMENTAL ISSUES

Sleep Patterns

- Instruct in repositioning to prevent the development of pressure sores and to maintain comfort.
- Assess for early signs of sleep-related disturbances, namely obstructive sleep apnea (OSA) and hypoventilation, and order overnight sleep studies.
- Initiate the use of NIPPV when appropriate.

Toileting

- Encourage age-appropriate toilet training.
- Obtain input from occupational/physical therapists regarding adaptive equipment.
- Develop toileting plans for both home and school that include designated individuals to assist with toileting.

Discipline

- Encourage caregivers to remain consistent when disciplining all children using developmentally appropriate techniques.
- Routinely assess for and report any signs of abuse and neglect.

Child Care

- Child care can be provided in traditional or specialized settings.

Schooling

- Boys should be challenged to achieve their maximum potential in school and should be placed in an intellectually appropriate classroom setting.
- Early intervention (EI) services, an Individualized Educational Program (IEP), and special education may be required.
- Therapeutic interventions may be provided in school and frequent classroom interruptions should be weighed.
- Assist in obtaining classroom and transportation accommodations and personal aides or paraprofessionals, if required.
- Discuss vocational or college preparation programs with eligible adolescents.
- Assist in finding appropriate after-school programs and respite programs (that are accessible with adequate adaptations).

Sexuality

- Many adolescents will not experience intimate sexual relationships.
- Educate regarding sexual development and healthy and safe sex practices, when appropriate.

Transition to Adulthood

- Independence should be maintained as long as possible.
- Consider guardianship issues before age 18.
- Facilitate discussions regarding life-supportive therapies, end of life issues.
- Regularly assess for quality of life.

FAMILY CONCERNS

- Care presents many complex and evolving issues and should focus on the entire family.
- Provide anticipatory guidance.
- Advocate and provide support regarding separation and loss; experiencing and expressing emotions; and changing values, expectations, roles, and responsibilities.
- Be aware of psychosocial needs and refer for counseling services as needed.
- Initiate and participate in palliative care plans with familial input.

REFERENCES

Aartsma-Rus, A., van Deutekom, J.C.T., Fokkema, I.F., et al. (2006). Entries in the Leiden Duchenne muscular dystrophy database: An overview of mutation types and paradoxical cases that confirm the reading-frame rule. *Muscle Nerve, 34*, 135-144.

Aloysius, A., Born, P., Kinali, M., et al. (2008). Swallowing difficulties in Duchenne muscular dystrophy: Indications for feeding assessment and outcome of videofluoroscopic swallow studies. *Eur J Paediatr Neurol. 12*(3), 239-245.

American Academy of Pediatrics (AAP). (2005). Clinical report: Cardiovascular health supervision for individuals affected by Duchenne or Becker muscular dystrophy: Section on cardiology and cardiac surgery. *Pediatrics, 116*(6), 1569-1573.

American Academy of Pediatrics (AAP). (2006). *Red Book: 2006 Report of the Committee on Infectious Diseases* (27th ed.). Elk Grove Village, IL: Author.

American Thoracic Society (ATS). (2004). American Thoracic Society documents: Respiratory care of the patient with Duchenne muscular dystrophy, ATS consensus statement. *Am J Respir Crit Care Med, 170*, 456-465.

Bach, J.R. (2004). *Management of Patients with Neuromuscular Disease.* Philadelphia: Hanley & Belfus.

Balaban, B., Matthews, D., Clayton, G.H., et al. (2005). Corticosteroid treatment and functional improvement in Duchenne muscular dystrophy: Long-term effect. *Am J Phys Med Rehabil, 84*(11), 843-850.

Biggar, W.D. (2006). Duchenne muscular dystrophy. *Pediatr Rev, 22*(3), 83-88.

Biggar, W.D., Harris, V.A., Eliasoph, L., et al. (2006). Long-term benefits of deflazacort treatment for boys with Duchenne muscular dystrophy in their second decade. *Neuromusc Disord, 16*, 249-255.

Birnkrant, D.J., Panitch, H.B., Benditt, J.O., et al. (2007). American College of Chest Physicians consensus statement on the respiratory and related management of patients with Duchenne muscular dystrophy undergoing anesthesia or sedation. *Chest, 132*(6), 1976-1986.

Bogdanovich, S., Krag, T.O.B., Barton, E.R., et al. (2002). Functional improvements of dystrophic muscle by myostatin blockade. *Nature, 420*(6914), 418-421.

Bushby, K., Bourke, J., Bullock, R., et al. (2005). The multidisciplinary management of Duchenne muscular dystrophy. *Curr Pediatr, 15*, 292-300.

Bushby, K., & Straub, V. (2005). Nonmolecular treatment for muscular dystrophies. *Curr Opin Neurol, 18*, 511-518.

Campbell, C., & Jacob, P. (2003, September 8). Deflazacort for the treatment of Duchenne dystrophy: A systematic review. *Neurology, 3*(7), Article 10.1186. Available at www.biomedcentral.com/1471-2377/3/7. Retrieved April 23, 2007.

Chen, J.Y., Chen, S.S., Jong, Y.J., et al. (2002). A comparison of the stress and coping strategies between the parents of children with Duchenne muscular dystrophy and children with a fever. *Int Pediatr Nurs, 17*(5), 369-379.

Chen, J.Y., & Clark, M.J. (2007). Family function in families of children with Duchenne muscular dystrophy. *Fam Community Health, 30*(4), 296-304.

Chen, T.J., Chen, S.S., Wang, D.C., et al. (2002). Increased vulnerability of auditory system to noise exposure in *mdx* mice. *Laryngoscope, 112*, 520-525.

Cheuk, D.K.L., Wong, V., Wraige, E., et al. (2007). Surgery for scoliosis in Duchenne muscular dystrophy. *Cochrane Database of Systematic Reviews, 2007*(1). Retrieved December 15, 2007, from the Cochrane Library Database.

Cohn, R.D., van Erp, C., Habashi, J.P., et al. (2007). Angiotensin II type 1 receptor blockade attenuates TGF-beta-induced failure of muscle regeneration in multiple myopathic states. *Nat Med, 13*(2), 204-210.

Cossu, G., & Sampaolesi, M. (2007). New therapies for Duchenne muscular dystrophy: Challenges, prospects, and clinical trials. *Trends Molecular Med, 13*(12), 520-526.

Costa, M.F., Oliveira, A.G.F., Feitosa-Santana, C., et al. (2007). Red-green vision impairment in Duchenne muscular dystrophy. *Am J Hum Genet, 80*, 1064-1075.

Cotton, S.M., Voudouris, N.J., & Greenwood, K.M. (2005). Association between intellectual functioning and age in children and young adults with Duchenne muscular dystrophy: further results from a meta-analysis. *Developmental Medicine & Child Neurology, 47*(4), 257-265.

Cyrulnika, C.E. & Hinton, V.J. (2008). Duchenne muscular dystrophy: A cerebellar disorder? *Neuroscience & Biobehavioral Reviews, 32*(3), 486-496.

Darras, B.T., Menache, C.C., & Kunkel, L.M. (2003). Dystrinopathies. In H.R. Jones, Jr., D.C. De Vivo, & B.T. Darras (Eds.), *Neuromuscular Disorders of Infancy, Childhood, and Adolescence: A Clinician's Approach.* Philadelphia: Elsevier Science.

Do, T. (2002). Orthopedic management of the muscular dystrophies. *Curr Opin Pediatr, 14*, 50-53.

Duboc, D., Meune, C., Lerebours, G., et al. (2005). Effect of perindropril on the onset and progression of left ventricular dysfunction in Duchenne muscular dystrophy. *J Am Cardiol Assoc, 45*, 855-857.

Duchenne de Boulogne, G.B.A. (1973). Recherches sur la paralysie musculaire pseudohypertrophique, ou paralysie myo-sclerosique. (Studies on pseudohypertrophic muscular paralysis or myosclerotic paralysis.). In R.H. Wilkins, & I.A. Brody (Eds.), *Neurological Classics.* New York: Johnson Reprint.

Eagle, M., Baudouin, S.V., Chandler, C., et al. (2002). Survival in Duchenne muscular dystrophy: Improvements in life expectancy since 1967 and the impact of home nocturnal ventilation. *Neuromusc Disord, 12*(10), 926-927.

Ekvall, S.W., & Cerniglia, Jr., F. (2005). Myelomeningocele. In S.W. Ekvall & V.K. Ekvall (Eds.), *Pediatric Nutrition in Chronic Diseases and Developmental Disorders.* New York: Oxford University Press.

Fauroux, B., Guillemot, N., Aubertin, G., et al. (2008). Physiological benefits of mechanical insufflation-exsufflation in children with neuromuscular diseases. *Chest.* Available at http://chestjournal.org/cgi/content/abstract/chest.07-1615v1. Retrieved December 15, 2007.

Felisari, G., Martinelli-Boneschi, F., Bardoni, A., et al. (2000). Loss of Dp140 dystrophin isoform and intellectual impairment in Duchenne dystrophy. *Neurology, 55*, 559-564.

Foster, K., Foster, H., & Dickson, J.G. (2006). Gene therapy progress and prospects: Duchenne muscular dystrophy. *Gene Ther, 13*, 1677-1685.

Gedalia, A., & Shetty, A.K. (2004). Chronic steroid and immunosuppressant therapy in children. *Pediatr Rev, 25*(12), 425-434.

Gibson, B.E., Young, N.L., Upshur, R.E.G., et al. (2007). Men on the margin: A Bourdieusian examination of living into adulthood with muscular dystrophy. *Soc Sci Med, 65*(3), 505-517.

Griggs, R.C., & Bushby, K. (2005). Continued need for caution in the diagnosis of Duchenne muscular dystrophy. *Neurology, 64*, 1498-1499.

Hamed, S.A. (2006). Drug evaluation: PTC-124—a potential treatment of cystic fibrosis and Duchenne muscular dystrophy. *IDrugs, 9*(11), 783-789.

Handschin, C., Choi, C.S., Chin, S., et al. (2007). Abnormal glucose homeostasis in skeletal muscle-specific PGC-1alpha knockout mice reveals skeletal muscle-pancreatic beta cell crosstalk. *J Clin Invest, 117*(11), 3463-3474.

Hinton, V.J., Fee, R., & Batchelder, A. (2007, November). *Cognitive/Behavioral Diagnoses Associated with Duchenne Muscular Dystrophy* [abstract]. Abstract presented at the meeting of the American Public Health Association (APHA), Washington, DC.

Hinton, V.J., & Goldstein, E.M. (2007). Duchenne muscular dystrophy. In M.M.M. Mazzocco & J.L. Ross (Eds.), *Neurogenetic Developmental Disorders: Variation of Manifestation in Childhood.* Cumberland, RI: MIT Press.

Hinton, V.J., Nereo, N., Fee, R., et al. (2006). Social behavior problems in boys with Duchenne muscular dystrophy. *Dev Behav Pediatr, 27*(5), 1-7.

Hoffman, E.P., & Wang, J. (1993). Duchenne-Becker muscular dystrophy and the nondystrophic myotonias: Paradigms for loss of function and change of function of gene products. *Arch Neurol, 50*, 1227-1237.

Kaira, M., & Amin, R.S. (2005). Pulmonary management of the patient with muscular dystrophy. *Pediatr Ann, 34*(7), 531-535.

Kemper, A.R., & Wake, M.A. (2007). Duchenne muscular dystrophy: Issues in expanding newborn screening. *Curr Opin Pediatr, 19*(6), 700-704.

King, W.M., Ruttencutter, R., Nagaraja, H.N., et al. (2007). Orthopedic outcomes of long-term daily corticosteroid treatment in Duchenne muscular dystrophy. *Neurology, 68*, 1607-1613.

Kohler, M., Clarenbach, C., Boni, L., et al. (2005). Quality of life, physical disability, and respiratory impairment in Duchenne muscular dystrophy. *Am J Respir Crit Care Med, 172*(8), 1032-1036.

Kuehn, B.M. (2007). Studies point way to new therapeutic prospects for muscular dystrophy. *J Am Acad Med, 298*(12), 1385-1386.

Leitch, K.K., Raza, N., Biggar, D., et al. (2005). Should foot surgery be performed for children with Duchenne muscular dystrophy? *J Pediatr Orthop, 25*(1), 95-97.

Liu, M., Mineo, K., Hanayama, K., et al. (2003). Practical problems and management of seating through the clinical stages of Duchenne's muscular dystrophy. *Arch Phys Med Rehabil, 84*(6), 818-824.

Marini, A., Lorussoc, M.L., D'Angeloc, M.G., et al. (2007). Evaluation of narrative abilities in patients suffering from Duchenne muscular dystrophy. *Brain Lang, 102*(1), 1-12.

Markham, L.W., Spicer, R.L., & Cripe, L.H. (2005). The heart in muscular dystrophy. *Pediatr Ann, 34*(7), 531-535.

McClorey, G., Moulton, H.M., Iversen, P.L., et al. (2006). Antisense oligonucleotide-induced exon skipping restores dystrophin expression in vitro in a canine model of DMD. *Gene Ther, 13*(19), 1373-1381.

McDonald, C., Abresch, R., Carter, G., et al. (1995). Profiles of neuromuscular diseases: Duchenne muscular dystrophy. *Am J Phys Med Rehabil, 74*(5), 70-92.

Mendell, J.R., Buzin, C.H., Feng, J., et al. (2001). Diagnosis of Duchenne dystrophy by enhanced detection of small mutations. *Neurology, 57,* 645-650.

Meune, C., & Duboc, D. (2006). How should physicians manage patients with Duchenne muscular dystrophy when experts' recommendations are not unanimous? *Dev Med Child Neurol, 48*(10), 863-864.

Mielnik-Blaszczak, M., & Malgorzata, B. (2007). Duchenne muscular dystrophy—a dental healthcare program. *Special Care Dentist, 27*(1), 23-25.

Mok, E., Beghin, L., Gachon, P., et al. (2006). Estimating body composition in children with Duchenne muscular dystrophy: Comparison of bioelectrical impedance analysis and skinfold-thickness measurement. *Am J Clin Nutr, 83,* 65-69.

Monaco, A.P., Neve, R.L., Colletti-Feener, C., et al. (1986). Isolation of candidate cDNAs for portions of the Duchenne muscular dystrophy gene. *Nature, 323,* 646-650.

Moxley, R.T., Ashwal, S., Pandya, S., et al. (2005). Practice parameters: Corticosteroid treatment of Duchenne dystrophy. *Neurology, 64,* 13-20.

Muntoni, F., Torelli, S., & Ferlini, A. (2003). Dystrophin and mutations: One gene, several proteins, multiple phenotypes. *Lancet Neurology, 2,* 731-740.

Muscular Dystrophy Association. (MDA). (2005). *A Teacher's Guide to Neuromuscular Disease* (brochure). Tucson, AZ: Muscular Dystrophy Association.

Muscular Dystrophy Association. (MDA). (2006). *Diseases in the MDA program, master list.* Available at www.mda.org/disease/40list.html. Retrieved June 15, 2008.

National Human Genome Research Institute. (2007, October 11). *Learning about Duchenne muscular dystrophy.* Available at www.genome.gov/19518854. Retrieved December 24, 2007.

Pagon, R.A., Hanson, N.B., Neufeld-Kaiser, W., et al. (2001). Genetic consultation. *West J Med, 174*(6), 397-399.

Pessolano, F.A., Suarez, A.A., Monteiro, S.G., et al. (2003). Nutritional assessment of patients with neuromuscular diseases. *Am J Phys Med Rehabil, 82*(3), 182-185.

Reid, D.T., & Renwick, R.M. (2001). Relating familial stress to the psychosocial adjustment of adolescents with Duchenne muscular dystrophy. *Int J Rehabil Res, 24*(2), 83-93.

Reznik, M., & Ozuah, P.O. (2006). Tuberculin skin testing in children. *Emerg Infect Dis, 12*(5), 725-728.

Russell, A.P., Feilchenfeldt, J., Schreiber, S., et al. (2003). Endurance training in humans leads to fiber type-specific increases in levels of peroxisome proliferator-activated receptor-gamma coactivator-1 and peroxisome proliferator-activated receptor-alpha in skeletal muscle. *Diabetes, 52*(12), 2874-2881.

Sengupta, D.K., Mehdian, S.H., McConnell, J.R., et al. (2001). Pelvic or lumbar fixation for the surgical management of scoliosis in Duchenne muscular dystrophy. *Spine, 27,* 2072-2079.

Seth, A., & Aggarwal, A. (2004). Monitoring adverse reactions to steroid therapy in children. *Indian Pediatr, 41,* 349-357.

Spencer, G.E., & Vignos, P.J. (1962). Bracing for ambulation in childhood progressive muscular dystrophy. *J Bone Joint Surg Am, 44,* 234-242.

Stevens, P.M. (2006). Lower limb orthotic management of Duchenne muscular dystrophy: A literature review. *J Prosthet Orthotics, 18*(4), 111-119.

Stockley, T.L., Akber, S., Bulgin, N., et al. (2006). Strategy for comprehensive molecular testing for Duchenne and Becker muscular dystrophies. *Genetic Testing, 10*(4), 229-243.

Urtizberea, J.A., Fan, Q.S., Vroom, E., et al. (2003). Looking under every rock: Duchenne muscular dystrophy and traditional Chinese medicine. *Neuromusc Disord, 13*(9), 705-707.

van Deutekom, J.C.T., & van Ommen, G.J.B. (2003). Advances in Duchenne muscular dystrophy gene therapy. *Genetics, 4,* 774-783.

Velasco, M.V., Colin, A.A., Zurakowski, D., et al. (2007). Posterior spinal fusion for scoliosis in Duchenne muscular dystrophy diminishes the rate of respiratory decline. *Spine, 32*(4), 459-465.

Weidner, N. (2005). Developing an interdisciplinary palliative care plan for the patient with muscular dystrophy. *Pediatr Ann, 34*(7), 547-552.

Welch, E.M., Barton, E.R., Zhuo, J., et al. (2007). PTC124 targets genetic disorders caused by nonsense mutations. *Nature, 447*(7140), 87-91.

Williams, O. (2007). Diseases of muscle. In Brust, J.M.C. (Ed.), *Current Diagnosis and Treatment in Neurology.* New York: McGraw-Hill.

35 Myelodysplasia

Cynthia Colen Lazzaretti and Caroline Pearson

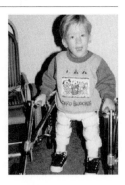

Etiology

Neural tube defects (NTDs) are malformations of the central nervous system (CNS) during embryonic development. The embryologic development of the CNS begins early in the third week of gestation with the formation of the primitive neural tube from the neural plate. The process of neurulation produces the functional nervous system (i.e., the future brain and spinal cord). Closure of the human neural tube begins in the midcervical region and proceeds simultaneously in the cranial and caudal directions (Lew & Kothbauer, 2007). If the neural tube fails to close, the process of neurulation is interrupted, which results in the imperfect formation of the brain and spinal cord at a focal point (Lew & Kothbauer). Anencephaly is the incomplete development of the forebrain, and is usually incompatible with life. Encephalocele, herniation of the brain and meninges through a defect in the skull, is the least common of the NTDs. *Spina bifida,* or *myelodysplasia,* is a collective term for malformations of the spinal cord and is the most common NTD. This defect can occur at any level of the spinal cord, although it more commonly affects the lumbar and sacral spine. The extent of nerve tissue and spinal cord involvement varies, with altered body function at and below the level of the defect (Table 35-1).

The neurologic deficits sustained by the fetus with an NTD are postulated to occur in stages, as a "two hit" hypothesis. In this theory, the first "hit" is the original defect in neurulation that creates the NTD and any associated myelodysplasia, and the second "hit" is the secondary trauma to the spinal cord as a result of its exposure to the intrauterine environment (Stiefel, Copp, & Meuli, 2007). This has led to investigations in fetal surgery for myelodysplasia to avoid this secondary injury and improve functional outcome (Hirose, Farmer, & Albanese, 2001).

The cause of NTDs is unknown, but there appears to be a combination of environmental and genetic factors. The genetic predisposition is through an autosomal recessive mechanism, with the risk of recurrent NTD-affected pregnancies increased to 10 times that found in the general population (Geisel, 2003). Abnormalities such as trisomies 9, 13, and 18 and Meckel-Gruber syndrome account for a small proportion of NTDs. Genetic studies have failed to identify any one gene in humans that can cause myelodysplasia (Padmanabhan, 2006).

Exposure to various teratogens, including valproic acid, carbamazepine, cytochalasin, calcium antagonists, and hyperthermia, has been implicated in NTDs (Padmanabhan, 2006). Maternal infections (e.g., rubella, cytomegalovirus [CMV], toxoplasmosis) and metabolic conditions (e.g., phenylketonuria, diabetes) are also capable of causing malformations of the CNS. Further study of the mechanisms of these teratogens may elucidate some of the genetic programs responsible for normal neurulation (Padmanabhan).

Incidence and Prevalence

NTDs occur in 1 in 1500 births, with an estimated 3000 pregnancies affected each year by an NTD, with some fetal demise through spontaneous or induced losses (Williams, Rasmussen, Flores, et al., 2005). The prevalence of NTDs varies by race/ethnicity, with the highest rates occurring among Hispanic women and the lowest among black and Asian women (Rader & Scheeman, 2006). The spina bifida rate per 100,000 live births declined 25% from 1995 to 2000 and 13% from 2000 to 2005 (Centers for Disease Control and Prevention [CDC], 2008b). The rate for 2005, 17.96 per 100,000 live births, was the lowest ever reported (CDC, 2007). The anencephaly rate declined 36% from 1991 to 1995 and was unchanged from 1995 to 2005 (CDC, 2008b). Reasons for the observed declining incidence include increasing use of prenatal screening in the form of alpha-fetoprotein (AFP) assay and ultrasonography, both of which are done early enough in the pregnancy to allow the parents the choice of terminating the pregnancy. The medical emphasis on folic acid supplementation, as detailed later, has also resulted in a significant reduction in NTDs.

There is an overall risk of birth defects with poor prenatal care and maternal nutritional deficiencies; in particular, maternal or fetal folate deficiency is associated with the occurrence of NTDs. Genetic defects that alter folic acid metabolism and absorption have also been implicated in NTDs (Geisel, 2003). Intervention studies in the 1980s and 1990s demonstrated a 50% to 70% reduction in NTDs with preconceptual folic acid intake (Williams et al., 2005).

In 1992 the U.S. Public Health Service published the recommendation that all women of childbearing age consume 0.4 mg (400 mcg) of folic acid daily to prevent NTDs (Spina Bifida Association of America [SBAA], 2008a). Women who have had a pregnancy with an NTD should consume 0.4 mg of folic acid every day when not planning to become pregnant, and they should consult their health care provider about following the August, 1991 U.S. Public Health Service guideline for consumption of 4 mg (4000 mcg) of synthetic folic acid daily beginning 1 month before they start trying to get pregnant and continuing through the first 3 months of pregnancy (SBAA, 2008a). Synthetic folic acid is approximately twice as absorbable as naturally occurring food folate because of the complex structure of folate (Hasenau & Covington, 2002). There is some evidence that adding vitamin B_{12} to folic acid may further decrease the incidence of NTDs (Ray, Wyatt, Thompson, et al., 2007).

A recently published report from the CDC shows that folic acid intake has increased over the past few years, and the rate of NTDs has declined by 26% (CDC, 2008a). However, among all women of childbearing age, those ages 18 to 24 years have the lowest reported daily use of folic acid supplements. Because women in this age-group account for nearly one third of all births in the United States, education about folic acid consumption should be targeted to this population.

Diagnostic Criteria

With routine antenatal ultrasonography, most cases of myelodysplasia are diagnosed in utero. An elevated maternal AFP may also indicate the presence of an NTD (Reece & Hobbins, 2006). It is important to note that a closed NTD may not alter the AFP levels. When AFP levels are elevated, amniocentesis is indicated. High-resolution ultrasound or fetal magnetic resonance imaging (MRI) is also helpful in documenting the lesion, its approximate level, and the presence or absence of hydrocephalus or other cerebral anomalies, such as a Chiari II malformation. The purpose of prenatal diagnosis is two-fold; first, it offers the parents the option to terminate the pregnancy, and second, if the parents choose to continue the pregnancy, prenatal diagnosis provides the family and health care team the opportunity to physically and emotionally prepare for the birth of the child. Genetic counseling should be offered at this time as well.

Further diagnostic tests in the postnatal period (e.g., ultrasonography, computed tomography [CT] scan, MRI) are necessary to determine other neurologic or systemic anomalies, such as hydromyelia, diastematomyelia (split cord malformation), hydronephrosis, and hip dysplasia. In preparation for surgery, a full cardiopulmonary assessment is critical to rule out any cardiac anomalies or airway problems.

Clinical Manifestations at Time of Diagnosis

NTDs can vary in severity, from the congenital malformation of vertebrae alone to extensive involvement of the spinal cord and surrounding structures of nerve, bone, muscle, and skin. Myelodysplasia is classified based on the pathophysiology of the lesion or defect (Figure 35-1).

TABLE 35-1

Functional Alterations in Myelodysplasia Related to Level of Lesion

Level of Lesion	Functional Implications
Thoracic	Flaccid paralysis of lower extremities
	Variable weakness in abdominal trunk musculature
	High thoracic level may have respiratory compromise
	Absence of bowel and bladder control
High lumbar	Voluntary hip flexion and adduction
	Flaccid paralysis of knees, ankles, and feet
	May walk with extensive braces and crutches
	Absence of bowel and bladder control
Midlumbar	Strong hip flexion and adduction
	Fair knee extension
	Flaccid paralysis of ankles and feet
	Absence of bowel and bladder control
Low lumbar	Strong hip flexion, extension and adduction, knee extension
	Weak ankle and toe mobility
	Absence of bowel and bladder control
Sacral	"Normal" function of lower extremities
	May have impaired bowel and bladder function

Clinical Manifestations at Time of Diagnosis

- Congenital malformation of vertebrae
  - Spina bifida
  - Meningocele
  - Myelomeningocele
- Cutaneous abnormalities above the vertebrae
  - Tufts of hair
  - Dimpling
  - Hemangiomas
  - Dermoid cysts
- Lower extremity weakness or atrophy
- Foot deformities
- Bowel and bladder disturbances

Spina bifida occulta (SBO) is the failed fusion of the vertebral arches that surround and protect the spinal cord and may involve a small portion of one vertebra or the complete absence of bone. SBO is often a benign, incidental finding, occurring in about 20% of individuals of North American descent (Sairyo, Goel, Vadapalli, et al., 2006). However, it may be associated with underlying spinal cord anomalies, such as myelomeningoceles, lipomyelomeningoceles, diastematomyelia (split spinal cord), and a tethered spinal cord (Lew & Kothbauer, 2007). Often there are cutaneous abnormalities such as tufts of hair, dimpling, hemangiomas, and

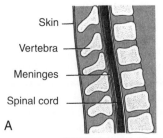
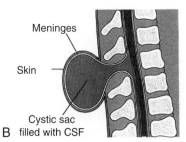
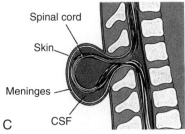

FIGURE 35-1 Diagram showing section through **A,** normal spine; **B,** meningocele; and **C,** myelomeningocele.

dermoid cysts located above the area of the defect. A child may be asymptomatic at birth or have leg weakness and atrophy, bowel and bladder disturbances, or foot deformities. If left untreated, a child may develop these symptoms later in life.

A meningocele is an NTD in which there is congenital absence of the vertebral arches and cystic dilation of the meninges through the defect (Lew & Kothbauer, 2007). At birth the infant has a protruding sac on the back at the level of the defect. This sac is filled with cerebrospinal fluid, and the overlying skin is usually normal. In a pure meningocele, there are no abnormalities of the spinal cord, and infants remain asymptomatic before and after the repair. It is difficult to know the true incidence of meningoceles because there is usually some involvement of the spinal cord or nerve roots at the area of the defect. However, it is believed to be less than one twentieth as frequent as myelomeningocele (McComb, 1999).

Myelomeningocele is the most severe form of an NTD in which there is cystic dilation of meninges and a dysfunctional spinal cord through an open defect. Like meningoceles, infants have a protruding sac at the level of the defect. However, the overlying muscle and skin are usually dysplastic. Associated problems include hydrocephalus, Chiari II malformation, musculoskeletal deformities, and a neurogenic bowel and bladder.

Treatment

Initial treatment for meningocele and myelomeningocele is early surgical closure of the defect to prevent infection and further damage of exposed neural tissue (Dias, 2005). Careful assessment of the infant before and during the surgical closure often aids in determination of the depth and extent of involvement. Large lesions may require a complex closure, using muscle flaps and allogeneic skin grafts (Danish, Samdani, Storm, et al., 2006). Hydrocephalus is often not apparent at birth but becomes evident in most children in the first week of life, after the spinal defect is repaired. Approximately 85% of children born with myelomeningocele will require early placement of an internal shunt system to control the hydrocephalus (Tulipan, Sutton, Bruner, et al., 2003). The incidence of shunting varies with the level of the spinal defect, with higher-level lesions causing more severe cases of hydrocephalus (Rintoul, Sutton, Hubbard, et al., 2002) (see Chapter 29).

Treatment

- Assess level of involvement
  - Ultrasonography
  - Computed tomography (CT) scan
  - Magnetic resonance imaging (MRI) scan
- Surgical closure of deformity
- Evaluation and treatment for hydrocephalus
- Comprehensive multidisciplinary team approach to care
- Rehabilitation
- Prevention

The multisystem involvement of this diagnosis requires a comprehensive multidisciplinary team approach to treatment. This team may include nurses, neurosurgeons, urologists, orthopedists, neurologists, pediatricians, physical therapists, occupational therapists, and social workers. It is very important that the primary care provider, the multidisciplinary team, and the community resources and program work collaboratively so that the child can attain optimum function. Long-term treatment focuses on habilitation, prevention of secondary conditions, and management of associated problems.

Anticipated Advances in Diagnosis and Management

Since 1998, in utero myelomeningocele repairs have been performed in the United States with mixed results. Early outcomes suggest a decreased need for ventriculoperitoneal shunting, consistent resolution of the Chiari II malformation, and neurologic improvement in leg function. However, there is an increased risk of obstetric complications, such as oligohydramnios, premature rupture of membranes, preterm labor and delivery, and fetal demise (Johnson, Sutton, Rintoul et al., 2003). The impact of prenatal surgery on bowel and bladder function remains unknown (Carr, 2007).

Further research is required to determine whether the risks of intrauterine surgery outweigh the potential benefits. In 2003, the National Institute of Child Health and Human Development (NICHD) initiated a multicenter, prospective, randomized controlled trial comparing long-term outcomes in fetuses undergoing in utero repair at 19 to 25 weeks gestation to those fetuses delivered by elective cesarean section near term with postnatal closure. The Management of Myelomeningocele Study (MOMS) is estimated to be complete in December 2011 (NICHD, 2007).

Current research in bladder management involves an artificial somatic-autonomic reflex pathway procedure for bladder control. This procedure involves an anastomosis between the ventral efferent (motor) roots of L5 and S3 (Xiao, 2005). This intervention treats the cause of neurogenic dysfunction and not the end result of the neuropathy, as with bladder reconstruction. The potential benefits could radically change the future of children with spina bifida, eliminating the consequences of bladder reconstruction and intermittent catheterization (Joseph, 2005).

Associated Problems of Myelodysplasia and Treatment

Arnold-Chiari II Malformation

Chiari II (Arnold-Chiari II) malformation is a serious, potentially life-threatening malformation that invariably occurs in 95% of children with myelodysplasia (Dias, 2005). The Chiari II malformation may be a clinically silent phenomenon or cause catastrophic events (e.g., cardiac or respiratory arrest). The malformation compresses and essentially stretches the posterior region of the cerebellum and brainstem downward through the foramen magnum into the cervical space (Figure 35-2). The brainstem houses the 12 cranial nerves, and pressure on this region results in cranial nerve dysfunction (Table 35-2). The exact pathogenesis of the malformation is not known. It is believed an abnormal pressure differential caused by an open spinal defect leads to a small posterior fossa and abnormal development and displacement of the brainstem and cerebellum (McLone & Dias, 2003).

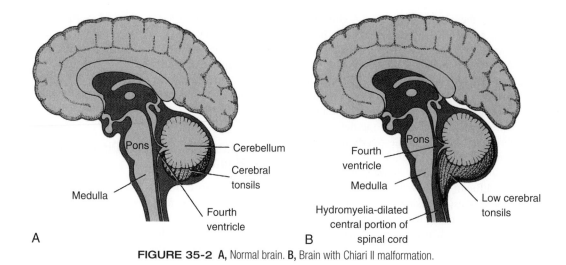

FIGURE 35-2 **A,** Normal brain. **B,** Brain with Chiari II malformation.

Associated Problems of Myelodysplasia and Treatment

- Arnold-Chiari II malformation
- Hydrocephalus
- Seizures
- Skin breakdown
- Cognitive deficit
- Learning issues
- Altered motor and sensory function
- Musculoskeletal deformities
- Urinary dysfunction
- Bowel dysfunction
- Visual problems
- Latex allergic reactions

TABLE 35-2

Implications of Cranial Nerve Dysfunction in Myelodysplasia

Cranial Nerve	Functional Implications
CN I: Olfactory	Sense of smell
CN II: Optic	Visual acuity, visual fields
CN III: Oculomotor	Raises eyelids; constricts pupils; moves eyes up, down, and medially
CN IV: Trochlear	Moves eyes down
CN V: Trigeminal	Sensory innervation to face, tongue; opens and closes jaw
CN VI: Abducens	Moves eyes laterally (out)
CN VII: Facial	Closes eyelids; motor and sensory for facial muscles; secretion of lacrimal and salivary glands
CN VIII: Acoustic	Hearing; equilibrium
CN IX: Glossopharyngeal	Gag, swallow; taste
CN X: Vagus	Muscles of larynx, pharynx, soft palate; parasympathetic innervation
CN XI: Spinal accessory	Shoulder shrug
CN XII: Hypoglossal	Moves tongue

Hydrocephalus

Hydrocephalus results from the Chiari II malformation and obstruction of the fourth ventricle. Infants with myelodysplasia and hydrocephalus can have increased head circumference and bulging fontanel, although they may appear asymptomatic until their spinal defect is repaired. Head ultrasounds are commonly used to monitor ventriculomegaly along with serial head circumference measurements. The decision to place a ventriculoperitoneal shunt is made based on the rate of increasing ventriculomegaly (see Chapter 29).

Seizures

Seizures occur in approximately 15% to 25% of children with myelodysplasia and are most likely related to cerebral anomalies, such as cortical heterotopias and polymicrogyria (McLone & Dias, 2003). The risk increases in those who have had CNS infections, multiple shunt failures, or a history of respiratory insufficiency or arrest (see Chapter 26).

Skin Breakdown

Newborns are at great risk for developing infection secondary to the altered skin integrity over the malformed spine, which is a possible complication until the lesion has completely healed. The risk of skin breakdown continues throughout a child's life span as a result of altered sensory function below the level of the lesion.

Urinary and fecal incontinence in conjunction with altered sensation greatly increases the risk of skin breakdown.

Cognitive Deficit

Most children with myelodysplasia and hydrocephalus have intelligence quotient (IQ) scores in the average to low average range, and IQ is influenced by the level of lesion, motor function level, and CNS complications. Cognitive skill patterns in myelodysplasia and hydrocephalus are dynamic and are affected by neurologic development, as well as associated medical conditions and procedures (Matson, Mahone, & Zabel, 2005). The precise nature of the neuropsychological deficits in hydrocephalus is not completely known; several factors (e.g., etiology, raised intracranial pressure, ventricular size, shunt treatment complications) have been shown to influence cognition. Complications, such as infections, trauma, intraventricular hemorrhage, and other brain abnormalities, are important determinants of the ultimate cognitive status, putting the child at a higher risk of cognitive impairment. A higher level of spinal lesion is a marker for more severe anomalous brain development, which, in turn, is associated with poorer neurobehavioral outcomes in a wide variety of domains that determine levels of independent functioning (Fletcher, Copeland, Frederick, et al., 2005).

Learning Issues

Children with myelodysplasia and hydrocephalus have a high rate of learning disabilities, particularly in math (Fletcher et al., 2005). In addition, attention problems are common and usually need to be treated, given the significant impact of such problems on functioning at home and school (Fletcher et al.) (see Chapter 12). Neuropsychological assessments should be conducted more frequently in children with myelodysplasia and hydrocephalus than in children with more "static" conditions, and testing may be requested in response to suspected cognitive symptoms of hydrocephalus. Serial use of standardized neuropsychological tests can help distinguish true cognitive changes related to hydrocephalus from academic "declines" experienced by these children during known periods of educational stress and increased self-organizational expectations (Matson et al., 2005).

Altered Motor and Sensory Function

Motor and sensory functions below the level of the lesion are invariably altered. This dysfunction may include paralysis, weakness, spasticity of lower extremities, and sensory loss. Altered motor and sensory function may also impair peristalsis, leading to constipation, impaction, and fecal incontinence. Education should start early so secondary complications of skin breakdown can be minimized. Further deterioration may occur as the child grows and increased tension is placed on the tethered spinal cord, causing changes in bladder, bowel, and motor function. This may indicate the need for further diagnostic studies and neurosurgical intervention.

Musculoskeletal Deformities

Musculoskeletal deformities related to myelomeningocele may include clubfeet, dislocated hips, contractures, and deformities caused by decreased activity and improper musculoskeletal alignment from altered embryonic development and muscle group imbalance. Spinal deformities (e.g., scoliosis, kyphosis, gibbus) are also common as the child grows, and management poses a challenge. Multiple medical comorbidities, such as insensate skin and chronic urinary tract infections (UTIs), make care of the child with spinal deformities difficult (Guille, Sarwark, Sherk, et al., 2006). Habilitation is essential to promoting optimum functional independence and requires close collaboration of the child's physical and occupational therapists, the family, and the myelodysplasia team. Orthotics and assistive devices such as walkers, crutches, wheelchairs, and adaptive equipment for activities of daily living are often needed and require close monitoring and adjustments for growth and to prevent skin irritation. Close monitoring of muscle strength is important in assessing early signs of spinal cord tethering as indicated by changes in motor function.

Urinary Dysfunction

Neurogenic bladder occurs in the majority of children with myelodysplasia and results in incontinence; however, all newborns with myelodysplasia have normal kidney function. The nerves that innervate the bladder are impaired, which can result in detrusor sphincter dyssynergy, incomplete emptying, high-pressure bladder, reflux, and incompetent sphincter. The goal of bladder management is to preserve kidney and bladder function and urinary continence.

Clean intermittent catheterization (CIC) is the most commonly used method to help achieve urinary continence. Ideally, CIC should be started at birth, but if not it should begin at the normal time for toilet training. If a child has been catheterized from birth every 3 to 4 hours, the concept of using the toilet for the procedure should be introduced at this time. The procedure is ideally taught to the parents and other individuals involved in the child's direct care. Instituting this procedure often causes varying emotions in parents related to the child's disabilities. Fear of injuring the child, difficulties with genital touching, and frustration with the mechanics of the procedure are common. Psychologic and emotional concerns must be addressed before parents can be expected to understand and comply with the recommendations.

If continence is not attained by catheterization alone, medications, such as anticholinergics and sympathomimetics, may be used in conjunction with catheterization to relax the bladder, thereby decreasing bladder pressure and the risk of reflux and increasing bladder capacity. Botulinum toxin type A (Botox) is being used to temporarily delay surgery for bladder augmentation and may be useful as a diagnostic tool (Altaweel, Jenack, Bilodequ, et al., 2006). The goal of Botox is to temporarily increase bladder capacity before surgically enlarging or augmenting the bladder. Continence may also successfully be achieved through use of surgical interventions (e.g., artificial urinary sphincter, bladder neck reconstruction, bladder augmentation, creation of continent stomas, and establishment of an artificial somatic-autonomic reflex pathway (Joseph, 2005; McAndrew & Malone, 2002).

Bowel Dysfunction

Neurogenic bowel occurs in the majority of children with myelodysplasia and results in incontinence because of impaired sensation and impaired sphincter control. Constipation is common as a result of decreased bowel motility. Bowel management in infancy to toddler age should focus on preventing constipation. Skin integrity is at risk because of incontinence, and good skin care habits are essential.

Visual Problems

Abnormalities of the cerebellum and brainstem, as well as pressure on the cranial nerves (CNs) that control eye movements (i.e., CN III [oculomotor], CN IV [trochlear], and CN VI [abducens]), may result in a dysconjugate gaze, esotropia, or nystagmus. There is an increased risk of refractive errors and amblyopia in children with myelodysplasia, and many require corrective lenses.

Latex Allergic Reactions

Research studies recently have shown that up to 73% of children and adolescents with myelodysplasia are sensitive to latex (Box 35-1) as measured by blood test or by a history of an allergic reaction (Levey, Demetrides, Hamilton, et al., 2007). Clinical manifestations involve urticaria, angioedema, rhinitis, conjunctivitis, asthma, and generalized anaphylactic reaction (Patriarca, Nucera, Pollastrini, et al., 2002). Serious systemic reactions usually occur after mucosal exposure to latex devices or during surgical

Latex Allergic Reactions

- *Irritant contact dermatitis:* Dry, itchy, irritated areas, usually on the hands, caused from using gloves—not a true allergy
- *Allergic contact dermatitis* (delayed hypersensitivity): May include symptoms such as watery eyes, eczematous skin eruptions, or dermatitis
- *Immediate allergic reaction:* Immediate hypersensitivity to exposure, which may include symptoms of rhinitis, conjunctivitis, wheezing, bronchospasm, facial swelling, tachycardia, laryngeal edema, and hypotension (NIOSH, 1997)

Centers for Disease Control and Prevention (CDC). (1997). *Preventing allergic reactions to natural rubber latex in the workplace.* Available at www.cdc.gov/niosh/latexalt.html. Retrieved April 17, 2008.

procedures, but may occur under a variety of other circumstances in daily life (Rendeli, Nucera, Ansili, et al., 2006). Latex avoidance from birth and at home is believed to be the cornerstone for the primary prevention of latex sensitization, that is, to prevent immunoglobulin E (IgE) antibodies in nonsensitized children (Nieto, Mazon, Pamies, et al., 2002). A list of common latex products in the home/community and hospital is available on the Spina Bifida Association of America website (SBAA, 2007).

Careful history should be elicited regarding signs and symptoms of latex allergy. Three types of reactions may occur (see Box 35-1). Type I reaction is an immediate hypersensitivity to exposure and may include such symptoms as rhinitis, conjunctivitis, wheezing, bronchospasm, facial swelling, tachycardia, laryngeal edema, and hypotension. Individuals with type I reaction to latex are at extreme risk for developing anaphylaxis and must be treated accordingly (see Chapter 10). Those who experience type IV are at lower risk for developing anaphylaxis, but constant sensitization may predispose them to anaphylaxis. Avoidance of latex products is extremely important in preventing allergic reactions. Refer individuals to an allergist if latex allergy is suspected.

Prognosis

Myelodysplasia is a chronic condition. The prognosis depends on the success of prophylactic and acute treatment for potential and actual complications that affect each body system. Improved ventricular shunt systems have helped to reduce complications of malfunction and infection (see Chapter 29). Implementation of aggressive urologic management with CIC starting in the newborn period and improved surgical options for bladder management have greatly reduced the incidence of renal damage and failure. Treatments and interventions will be necessary throughout the child's life span and are individualized to the child's needs and rendered when indicated by the clinical presentation, assessment, and evaluation. Life-threatening complications remain despite the vast improvement in treatment and management. If untreated or not treated quickly enough, shunt malfunction can lead to brainstem herniation and death. Those with symptomatic Chiari malformations necessitating tracheostomies and feeding tubes are at risk of aspiration and pulmonary compromise and arrest. Independent living and gainful employment are realistic goals and are directly affected by cognitive development; achievement of functional independence; good, consistent medical follow-up; and continued collaboration of the family, the child, community and school resources, and the medical team.

PRIMARY CARE MANAGEMENT

Health Care Maintenance
Growth and Development

The growth and development of a child with myelodysplasia are affected by the level of the defect, the motor and sensory impairment, and the presence of hydrocephalus. As with all children, monitoring growth by obtaining routine heights and weights during follow-up in a spina bifida clinic, as well as with their primary care provider, and plotting them on a standardized growth chart is crucial. Obtaining heights may be difficult, depending on the child's ability to stand. If necessary, the primary care provider should measure the full body length with the child supine or by using arm span. Because of shortening of the spine and muscle atrophy, these children often fall below the 10th percentile in height. Short stature and precocious puberty are commonly seen in children with myelodysplasia. Hydrocephalus and Chiari II malformations increase the risk of hypothalamopituitary dysfunction, such as central precocious puberty and growth hormone deficiency (Rotenstein & Bass, 2004). If suspected, these children should be referred to an endocrinologist.

Obesity is a common problem in children with myelodysplasia as a result of decreased levels of activity and can cause problems with skin breakdown and orthotic fitting. Obesity may also interfere with development of a positive self-image. Educating the family and child about healthy eating habits must begin early to establish healthy patterns (see Chapter 36).

Head circumference should be monitored closely by the primary care provider during infancy and early childhood. If there is progressive enlargement in head size, a referral to a neurosurgeon or a spina bifida clinic should be made (see Chapter 29).

Motor development may be affected and is directly related to the level of the lesion (see Table 35-1). The degree of weakness, paralysis, and decreased sensation varies. Early orthopedic and physical therapy assessment and intervention are extremely important to prevent contractures, minimize deformities, and monitor muscle strength and flexibility. Surgical intervention is often recommended and sometimes required to achieve proper muscle balance and body alignment for problems common to this population (e.g., dislocated hips, scoliosis, kyphosis, clubfeet) that would limit the child's potential. Monitoring for orthotics, adaptive equipment, and mobility needs is ongoing throughout the child's life.

Promoting upright positioning and independent mobility is essential for the child's overall growth and development. As the child grows and develops, other adaptive equipment (i.e., braces, wheelchairs) is used to increase mobility and independence. Each child's treatment program varies because of differences in motivation, both the child's and the family's, and access to and availability of resources.

The rate at which cognitive development and intellectual skills are acquired depends on a child's interaction with the environment, the severity of the defect, and the presence of hydrocephalus. Infants should be considered at risk for cognitive and developmental delays, and early intervention services should be implemented in infancy. As part of a developmental approach to assessment of children with myelodysplasia and hydrocephalus, baseline neuropsychological testing is critical in this process of detecting cognitive changes related to acute hydrocephalus (Matson et al., 2005). Language development is usually on track, although difficulties have been noted in the development of pragmatic communication and the construction of meaning (Fletcher, Barnes, & Dennis, 2002). In discussing the long-term outcomes of myelodysplasia with hydrocephalus with families, particular attention should be devoted to learning and attention difficulties, and to the probable explanation for these difficulties, which involves anomalous brain development associated with myelodysplasia and hydrocephalus (Fletcher et al., 2005). Close monitoring of hydrocephalus and the ventriculoperitoneal shunt is important.

Diet

Early nutritional assessment and guidance are essential parts of the care of children with myelodysplasia.

Infancy is an excellent time to guide and educate parents on nutritional needs. It is important to teach parents early about the dangers of overfeeding, especially in children who are less mobile and therefore have fewer caloric needs. Preventing obesity and avoiding the pattern of using food as a reward are primary goals in the nutritional management of children with myelodysplasia.

The child's diet should include plenty of fluids to lessen the chance of constipation and the incidence of UTIs. Dietary management is important in controlling the consistency of stools and in avoiding constipation. A diet high in fiber and low in constipating foods is usually recommended. Medications to soften stool or stimulate passage may be indicated. During infancy, problems related to a Chiari II malformation may cause feeding problems affecting growth. Compression on CN IX (glossopharyngeal), CN X (vagus), and CN XII (hypoglossal) can affect gag and swallowing and increase the risk of aspiration, resulting in symptoms of failure to thrive, pneumonia, and respiratory compromise. The spina bifida team or the pediatric neurosurgeon should be consulted. Children and adolescents may have increased difficulty with swallowing, gagging with different textures, and choking. MRI imaging and modified barium swallow may be indicated to definitively assess and diagnose. In children with severe Chiari II symptoms, a gastrostomy tube may be needed to prevent aspiration and malnutrition.

Children with known latex sensitivity or allergy should avoid plant products that contain the same allergy-producing proteins found in natural rubber latex because they may cause an allergic cross reaction. These include bananas, avocados, kiwis, plums, peaches, cherries, apricots, figs, papayas, tomatoes, potatoes, and chestnuts.

Safety

There are numerous safety issues specific to children with myelodysplasia. The congenital defect affects nerve function at and below the level of the defect on the spine, thus altering mobility and sensation of bone, muscle, and skin tissue below the level of the defect. This decreased sensation puts a child at greater risk for injuries such as burns, fractures, and skin breakdown. With proper body positioning, frequent position changes, and assurance that adaptive equipment fits properly and is used correctly, the risk of skin breakdown can be reduced. Tepid water should be used for bathing to prevent burns. The condition of the child's skin should be checked at least twice daily for redness and irritation. As soon as children are competent to assume this responsibility, they should be taught how to perform a thorough skin check.

The potential for limited cognitive ability and altered judgment exists in these children. An awareness of limitations is essential to help these children with issues such as independence, decision making, self-care, and sexuality. Instructions on the proper use of equipment for mobility (e.g., wheelchairs, braces, crutches) should be appropriate to the child's developmental and cognitive abilities.

Parents of children with seizures should be instructed on how to intervene safely and appropriately during a seizure (see Chapter 26).

Latex allergy can be life threatening; therefore the primary care provider must inform and educate the parents and individual of this potential sensitivity and the importance of avoiding contact with latex, observe for signs, document the allergy, and prescribe Epipen for home and school. Examples of products that may contain latex are surgical gloves, balloons, catheters, and bandages. (A list of such products and alternatives for use is available from the Spina Bifida Association of America [SBAA, 2007]). Individuals with latex sensitivity should carry an Epipen, a letter documenting the allergy, and nonlatex gloves, as well as wear a Medic-Alert bracelet indicating the allergy (SBAA, 2008b).

Immunizations

Routine immunizations are recommended. Alterations in the immunization schedule for children with seizures and hydrocephalus are addressed in Chapters 26 and 29. Parents should be informed of the risk of possible latex allergy reaction from immunization vials/syringes containing latex. A review of data in the Vaccine Adverse Event Reporting System (VAERS) reported the risk of allergic reactions in persons allergic to latex to be very low (Russell, Pool, Kelso, et al., 2004). Consideration should be given to not using multiple-dose vials containing latex when administering immunizations because they may increase the risk of exposure.

Screening

Vision. Because of the high incidence of visual and perceptual deficits, ocular palsies, and astigmatism in children with myelodysplsia, practitioners should assess for these conditions during routine screening. Referral to an ophthalmologist is recommended at 6 months of age for routine assessment and yearly thereafter, unless positive findings are noted earlier.

Hearing. Routine screening is recommended. Children with myelodysplasia who have shunts for hydrocephalus are often hypersensitive to loud noises. Awareness of this finding may alleviate parental concern. Use of aminoglycosides may cause hearing deficits, and hearing should be evaluated after treatment.

Dental. Routine screening is recommended. Dentists should be notified of the increased risk of latex allergy. Information should be given for safe, alternative nonlatex products. The neurosurgeon of children with hydrocephalus and shunts undergoing dental procedures should be consulted regarding the use of antibiotic prophylaxis. The American Academy of Pediatric Dentistry (AAPD) recommends antibiotic prophylaxis for children with ventriculoatrial (VA) shunts. In contrast, ventriculoperitoneal (VP) shunts do not involve any vascular structures and do not require antibiotic protection (AAPD, 2005).

Blood Pressure. Routine screening is recommended. Children with known renal problems such as urinary reflux or a history of hypertension should have more frequent assessment. Persistent

---

BOX 35-2

Condition-Specific Screening

- Complete blood count
- Serum creatinine
- Scoliosis
- Latex allergy

Differential Diagnosis

- Chiari II malformation
- Tethering of the spinal cord
- Hydrocephalus
- Urinary tract infections
- Fevers
- Gastrointestinal symptoms

---

elevated readings should be communicated to the child's urologist. In rare cases, persistent hypertension may be a sign of shunt malfunction.

Hematocrit. Routine screening is recommended.

Urinalysis. Baseline urinalysis and urine cultures are obtained in newborns. If a UTI is suspected, a urine culture and sensitivity should be obtained by catheterization (bag specimens have been noted to have a higher chance of contamination). A positive urine culture should be reported to the child's urologist.

Tuberculosis. Routine screening is recommended.

Condition-Specific Screening (Box 35-2)

Complete Blood Count. If an individual is receiving long-term antibiotic therapy (e.g., sulfonamides) for prevention of UTIs, complete blood counts should be done approximately every 6 months to monitor changes.

Serum Creatinine. Serum creatinine should be checked routinely in newborns as a baseline study for renal function and should be repeated if changes on renal ultrasound are noted.

Scoliosis. Screening for scoliosis in children with myelodysplasia should begin during the first year of life and continue throughout adolescence. Spine radiographs should be obtained yearly or as indicated.

Latex Allergy. All children with myelodysplasia should be treated as latex sensitive from birth. Skin testing and blood testing or in vitro testing is available. Standardized skin testing is not available in the United States, so the reliability and consistency of results vary. In vitro testing is intended for diagnosis of individuals with suspected latex allergy and not as a screening tool. These tests are very specific when the clinical symptoms are severe but less specific when symptoms are ambiguous.

Common Illness Management

Differential Diagnosis

Chiari II Malformation. Approximately 15% to 30% of children with myelodysplasia develop neurologic deterioration related to the Chiari II malformation (Dias, 2005). Symptoms may develop at any age but are most common during infancy. The infant's symptoms may include apnea, respiratory difficulties, stridor, and the classic barking cough of croup. Primary care providers must be cautious not to dismiss these findings as a simple upper respiratory infection but must consider the possibility that these symptoms result from pressure on the CN IX (glossopharyngeal), CN X (vagus), or CN XII (hypoglossal) nerves. A depressed or absent gag may be present, leading to possible aspiration pneumonia. Feeding difficulties, poor weight gain, and symptoms of failure to thrive may also be present. Older children often have headaches, neck pain, upper extremity weakness, spasticity, and progressive scoliosis.

Treatment focuses on symptomatic relief of the presenting problems (e.g., gastrostomy tube and tracheostomy may be placed for absent gag and cough). Clinical indications for a surgical decompression include severe brainstem dysfunction, cranial nerve dysfunction, and hydromyelia. It is very important to determine that the shunt is functioning and the intracranial pressure is normal before considering surgical intervention for the Chiari II malformation. Recent studies show a 50% to 80% recovery rate with early decompressive surgery (Dias, 2005).

Tethering of the Spinal Cord. Myelodysplasia is not a progressive condition; thus any signs of deterioration should be evaluated closely by the primary care provider and the specialists. Virtually all children with myelodysplasia have signs of spinal cord tethering on MRI as a result of the defect and subsequent surgical closure. It is estimated that 10% to 30% of children with myelodysplasia will, at some time, require surgery to untether the spinal cord (Hudgins & Gilreath, 2004). Signs and symptoms can include decreased muscle strength, worsening gait, pain, spasticity, changes in bowel and bladder function, and scoliosis. The decision to intervene surgically requires careful assessment of the symptoms, the impact on the child's function, and the results of diagnostic studies, such as urodynamic studies, spinal x-rays, and MRI. Early detection and release of the tethered cord can stabilize or reverse deterioration in most cases. However, the probability of neurologic morbidity increases with second or third tethered cord releases (Hudgins & Gilreath, 2004).

Hydrocephalus. Most individuals have an internal shunt system to treat hydrocephalus. The differential diagnosis of shunt malfunction and infection must be considered in the presence of lethargy, fever, visual changes, gastrointestinal distress, and headache (see Chapter 29).

Urinary Tract Infections. Urinary tract infections (UTIs) are common among children with myelodysplasia. Fever associated with UTIs may be mild or severe. Other symptoms may include abdominal pain, vomiting, cloudy, malodorous urine, and increased voiding. These symptoms should alert the primary care provider to obtain a urine specimen by catheterization for culture. Frequency and burning may be masked because of decreased sensation. A positive culture should be reported to the child's urologist, especially in cases with urinary reflux. Treatment of positive cultures may vary depending on the individual's urologist. Bacteriuria is found in many children with myelodysplasia, especially those who perform CIC, and is termed "asymptomatic bacteriuria." These children do not require antibiotic therapy or prophylactic suppression unless there is documented vesicoureteral reflux or symptoms such as fever, dysuria, or new-onset incontinence. In the absence of vesicoureteral reflux, there is little risk of renal scarring (Baskin & Kogan, 2005). Children with urinary reflux need continuous antibiotic coverage as recommended by their urologist.

Fevers. Fever is a symptom found in many common childhood illnesses. Causes of fever may include shunt infection and malfunction, UTI, skin breakdown, and cellulitis. Particular consideration must be given to the presence of a fever because it may lower the seizure threshold in these children.

Fever of unknown origin may be the result of an undetected fracture of an insensate extremity. Osteoporosis associated with paralysis, decreased weight bearing, and inactivity, especially after immobilization in a cast, may contribute to the occurrence of fractures. An undetected burn of insensate areas may also result in fever. Careful examination of the area for swelling, redness, or abrasions should be undertaken by the practitioner. Obtaining a complete history from the individual and the parents may assist in determining if there has been recent trauma.

Gastrointestinal Symptoms. Nausea, vomiting, and diarrhea are all common symptoms in children. In children with myelodysplasia, however, a heightened concern is necessary because nausea and vomiting may be symptoms of shunt malfunction. UTIs may also be the cause of gastrointestinal distress. Children who have had a bladder augmentation and also have referred pain to the shoulder should seek immediate medical attention because this could indicate a urinary leak into the peritoneum. A child with a neurogenic bowel may become impacted with stool, leading to gastrointestinal distress. The presence of diarrhea may be misleading because liquid stool passes around the impacted stool. A radiograph of the kidneys, ureters, and bladder (KUB) may help differentiate diarrhea from impaction.

In children with a high lesion, practitioners should consider the possibility of appendicitis as a cause of nausea, vomiting, or fever; the classic symptom of pain may be altered as a result of the decreased sensation.

Drug Interactions

Many children with myelodysplasia are on routine medication therapy. Potential interactions among these and other medications must be carefully considered when additional medications are prescribed. Commonly used drug categories are as follows:

1. Antibiotics are given for treatment of UTIs or prophylaxis, including amoxicillin (Amoxil), trimethoprim-sulfamethoxazole (TMP-SMX), and nitrofurantoin (Furadantin). If a child requires other antibiotic therapy for common childhood illness, such as ear infections, the antibiotic for the UTI is discontinued during the needed course of treatment. Bladder irrigations containing antibiotics are used much less frequently.
2. Anticholinergics, most commonly oxybutynin chloride (Ditropan) and tolterodine (Detrol), are used to assist in urinary continence and reduce high bladder pressure. Oxybutynin chloride can cause heat prostration in the presence of high environmental temperatures. Both Ditropan and Detrol are available in extended-release or long-acting forms that require administration only once per day The child must be able to swallow pills. Anticholinergics may delay absorption of other medications given concomitantly in these children (*Physicians' Desk Reference* [PDR], 2008).
3. Stool softeners, stimulants, and bulk formers aid in evacuation of stool. Many products are used for this purpose, and most are over-the-counter drugs. None of these should be administered in the presence of abdominal pain, nausea, vomiting, or diarrhea.

4. Anticonvulsants are given to control seizure activity and include phenobarbital, phenytoin sodium (Dilantin), and carbamazepine (Tegretol). Concomitant administration of carbamazepine with erythromycin may result in toxicity (*PDR,* 2008) (see Chapter 26).

Developmental Issues

Sleep Patterns

Individuals with Chiari II malformation may experience sleep apnea, increased stridor, and snoring with sleep. These children are at increased risk for sudden respiratory arrest. Sleep studies are helpful in determining the severity of the sleep disorder and the need for positive airway pressure, such as bilevel positive airway pressure BiPAP and continuous positive airway pressure (CPAP). Parents must also be able to perform cardiopulmonary resuscitation in the event of an arrest. Alteration in the child's normal sleep pattern (e.g., longer naps, increased frequency of naps) may indicate increased intracranial pressure from a shunt malfunction (see Chapter 29). In addition, sleep may be interrupted if a child needs to be repositioned during the night to prevent pressure sores and skin breakdown from developing.

Toileting

Bowel and bladder continence is essential in the development of positive self-esteem and optimum functioning. A child's physical abilities and psychological readiness for toileting should be assessed. Children who are unable to sit without adaptive devices or unable to master self-dressing skills need special consideration when toileting is introduced. A physical or occupational therapist should be consulted about the use of bars or adaptive seats. Special clothing or underwear may be helpful to make access to the perineum easier.

It is desirable for children to master self-care methods of toileting before entering school. Urinary and fecal incontinence can lead to difficulties socially, as well as to issues with skin care. Bowel management should be monitored from birth to avoid constipation and impaction. Aggressive management of constipation early on (birth to 3 years) results in greater success when training for bowel continence (Baskin & Kogan, 2005). At age 2 to 3 years the concept of toileting should be introduced to children. The goals of bowel management are to maintain soft, formed stools and develop a regular schedule of evacuation on the toilet every 1 to 2 days to avoid impaction or soiling between bowel movements. These goals can be accomplished by having the child sit on the toilet at regular times, taking advantage of the gastrocolic reflex by toileting after meals, and increasing abdominal pressure by blowing bubbles, tickling the child to make him or her laugh, or placing the child's legs on a stool to increase pressure by hip flexion.

Stool consistency is crucial to developing a good bowel program. Bulking agents (e.g., Benefiber) taken with increased fluids are a key factor in avoiding constipation and eventual impaction. Miralax is often used in conjunction with bulking agents to promote transit time. Children should assume responsibility for timed evacuation and good perineal care as physical and cognitive development allows.

The use of medicinal aids may also be necessary to control the consistency or to aid in evacuation. A number of agents are available, including stimulants, softeners, and lubricants. The antegrade continence enema (ACE) and more recently the laparoscopic ACE (LACE) are operative procedures being used frequently in children who have failed at aggressive bowel management programs. The ACE involves surgical placement of a continent stoma to the bowel that can be catheterized for the administration of enemas for predictable bowel movements. The ACE is flushed every day or every other day with water through a catheter that is inserted into the stoma. It is a simple procedure with the goal of the child being able to manage the procedure independently.

It is important to remember that the program of management varies from child to child. A sympathetic manner in working with a child helps to avoid feelings of guilt and blame for unavoidable accidents.

Self-catheterization is a realistic goal to accomplish for most children by early school age. An individualized approach accounting for the child's readiness is important in achieving this goal. Providing young children with an anatomically correct doll and catheter often helps them master the skill. In children with limited cognitive abilities and poor manual dexterity, adaptation, such as an abdominal continent stoma, should be considered in an effort to enable independence for the child. Noncompliance with self-catheterization may become an issue in adolescence when catheterization is used as a focus in the fight for independence.

Discipline

There can be a wide range of emotional responses to having a child with a chronic disability, requiring some degree of psychological adjustment (Trute & Heibert-Murphy, 2002). The feeling of the need to overprotect a child with a disability is not uncommon and can affect a child's independence and social adjustment. Children with such a complex long-term condition are at increased risk for experiencing psychosocial adjustment problems that may affect the parents' and family members' response to discipline. The need for discipline, direction, and encouragement of independence should be addressed early in a child's life (Lollar, 2001).

Child Care

Primary care providers should be familiar with early intervention programs and child-care placements available in the community because these programs for infants vary from state to state. Preschoolers are eligible for placement in public programs that meet their physical and educational needs. It is important that the daycare or educational setting be notified in advance about a prospective student so that the staff can be educated regarding the child's abilities and medical care needs and a smooth transition can be facilitated (see Chapter 3). The child's bladder and bowel program and procedures should be taught to the care provider, as well as education regarding medication administration. The care providers should be educated regarding signs and symptoms of shunt malfunction, UTI, and latex precautions.

Many children with myelodysplasia have adaptive equipment to aid in mobilization, maintain appropriate body alignment, prevent further deformity, and increase independence. Daycare providers should be aware of proper application and fit of the equipment. It is also important to communicate the child's actual motor and sensory capacity to prevent injury.

A list of emergency telephone numbers must accompany these children. If possible, primary care providers should be available to answer questions and concerns from child-care staff.

Schooling

Learning disabilities are common in children with myelodysplasia. Problems may occur in perceptual-motor skills, comprehension, attention, activity, memory, organization, sequencing, and reasoning. In addition, attention problems are common and usually need to be treated, given the significant impact of such problems on functioning at home and school (Fletcher et al., 2005). Concerns regarding learning disabilities and attention disorders should be addressed early in the educational process so the identified needs may be met and adaptations made to minimize educational problems and frustrations for the child, family, and educators. Neuropsychological testing in addition to psychological testing should be part of the educational planning. School performance can be further compromised by frequent absences as a result of illness or medical treatment.

Federal laws protect the rights of children with disabilities to access appropriate education (see Chapter 3). Individualized educational plans (IEPs) must be formulated to take care of each child's specific needs, including educational and physical requirements. The primary care provider, the child, and the family must actively collaborate with the school in this planning process. Each of the child's particular needs must be addressed in the IEP, including the necessity for catheterization; timed toileting; administration of medications; physical, occupational, and speech therapies; and individual counseling. These needs may require assistance from an aide.

School personnel should be aware of any adaptive equipment and its purpose and function and should involve the child's physical and occupational therapists in adapting the school environment for optimum functioning. Elevators may help a child to get to classes in a timely manner and minimize fatigue.

As children get older, they may choose to use a wheelchair for mobilization in school. This should be viewed as a means of increasing mobility and independence instead of decreasing independence. Ideally, the school should be free of structural barriers to enable the child to move freely and participate in all activities. Special provisions must be made for safe departure from the building in the event of an emergency, as well as transportation to and from home (i.e., wheelchair van or bus). Individuals with a known latex allergy will need assistance in identifying and avoiding latex in school. Common sources of latex in the school environment include art supplies, pencil erasers, and gym mats or floors. The school nurse or allergists are possible resources to assist in this process.

Both myelodysplasia and hydrocephalus affect quality of life because of the chronicity and multisystem impact of these conditions. Associated social disadvantages include decreased opportunity for peer relationships, prolonged dependency on parents, and decreased community acceptance (Kripalani, 2000). Children with myelodysplasia often have low self-concepts, low levels of general happiness, and high levels of anxiety. Awareness of these potential problems is helpful for those working with children with myelodysplasia. Emotional independence is the foundation that supports the successful development of physical independence. Appropriate referrals for further psychological intervention and support may be advised. Primary care providers should encourage these children to be involved in extracurricular activities such as clubs, scouting, and sporting activities to enhance peer relationships, self-esteem, and independence (Lollar, 2001).

Academic planning and career counseling must take into consideration an individual's physical as well as cognitive abilities. Education and vocational training should prepare individuals to be successful in employment, independent living, and social relationships (Johnson & Dorval, 2001).

Sexuality

The issues of sexuality and reproduction are major areas of concern for children with myelodysplasia and their parents. Information regarding sexual function, intimacy, and reproduction should be discussed early and continued throughout childhood and adolescence. The development of good self-esteem and peer relationships is important in developing satisfying intimate relationships. As with all children, sex education should begin at home with information also available through the educational system and further addressed by the spina bifida clinic team. If a primary care provider does not feel skilled in gynecologic care, the child should be referred to a sensitive specialist with experience examining individuals with disabilities.

Women with myelodysplasia are capable of normal fertility, but do have unique health care concerns and may be entering adulthood with little information as to what to expect. Likewise, their health care providers do not have the benefit of evidence-based research that comprehensively address issues these women face related to reproduction or aging (Jackson & Mott, 2007). Birth control methods must be carefully evaluated on an individual basis. The importance of folic acid supplementation must be discussed and reinforced. The high incidence of latex allergies in this population prohibits the use of latex condoms and diaphragms; however, nonlatex condoms are available, and information should be made available by the primary care provider and the spina bifida team. Because of increased risk for UTI with intercourse, women not taking routine antibiotics should take prophylactic antibiotics before and after intercourse.

Although individuals with myelodysplasia have normal sex drives, unless sensation exists in the bulbourethral, bulbocavernosus, and perineal muscles of both genders, orgasm is not likely (Cardenas, Topolski, White, et al., 2008). Women may benefit from the use of additional lubricating gels when attempting intercourse because vaginal lubrication in response to sexual arousal does not occur with lower spinal cord injury. Counseling regarding sexually transmitted diseases and pregnancy is essential, including the use of nonlatex condoms.

Pregnancy in women with myelodysplasia is complicated by physical deformity, the presence of ventriculoperitoneal shunts, previous abdominal surgery for urologic and bowel management, varying degrees of impaired renal function, and hypertension. Early prenatal care is important, especially for screening the fetus for NTDs. Results of a recent survey suggest that there are gaps in obstetricians' and gynecologists' knowledge of risk factors for conception, strategies for prenatal diagnosis, and prognosis for affected individuals (Shaer, Chescheir, & Schulkin, 2007). Genetic counseling should be offered and encouraged.

In men with myelodysplasia, the level of spinal lesion will predict their capacity for erection and ejaculation A thorough history regarding erections and ejaculations is important in determining potential sexual function. Fertility in men with myelodysplasia is less likely than in the general population because of inadequate erectile function, semen quality, and factors of socialization

(Baskin & Kogan, 2005). Erectile dysfunction and fertility treatments may be of great benefit for these individuals.

Transition to Adulthood

Transition planning is a process mandated by law that must begin by age 14 years (see Chapters 3 and 4). Amendments under the Individuals with Disabilities Education Improvement Act (2004) require that goals and objectives related to employment and postsecondary education, independent living, and community participation be included in IEPs no later than age 16 years.

A successful transition is possible if there is ample preparation, motivation on the part of the young adult and family, and involvement of the school and appropriate community resources. Decision-making skills that relate to community living are necessary to a successful transition and must begin early. Development of a social support system including peers is needed to prevent social isolation that can lead to depression and loneliness and an inability to access medical care (Johnson & Dorval, 2001).

The survival rate of individuals with myelodysplasia has increased dramatically over the past 25 years, and thus the issue of transition has become a primary focus for the continued care of persons with myelodysplasia. Coordinated care is of equal importance for adults, though, unfortunately, adult multidisciplinary clinics are very rare. Adults must learn to navigate the already complex medical system and piece together their care. The organization and planning required of them because of their complex medical condition and possible limited cognitive skills greatly affect the success of a smooth transition (Matson et al., 2005). This puts the adult at great risk for suboptimum care and follow-up. Primary health care should be provided by health professionals interested in and committed to working with this high-risk population. This necessary transition of care has been met with reluctance by many adult health care providers for a number of reasons, including lack of familiarity with the complex needs of individuals with myelodysplasia. Providers may perceive this population as having a negative economic effect on their practice. Access to health care insurance can be a challenge for individuals not on state-funded insurance. Many health insurances purchased for individuals have preexisting medical clauses, thus excluding coverage for spina bifida–related care.

Coordinated multidisciplinary care, education of health care providers and clients, costs, and promotion of client-directed care are issues that need to be addressed. A few adult programs have been developed in various parts of the United States. Further information can be obtained from the Spina Bifida Association of America (www.sbaa.org).

Family Concerns

Raising a child with myelodysplasia represents a considerable challenge to parents' psychological well-being (Vermaes, Janssens, Bosman, et al., 2005). Studies indicate that the extent to which myelodysplasia affects parents depends on the quality of parents' partner relationship, family climate, and support from informal social networks (Vermaes et al., 2005). Families of children with myelodysplasia experience long-term grief for the "loss of the normal child" at birth. This grief is expressed repeatedly as the child fails to achieve developmental milestones.

The risk for sudden death as a result of a shunt malfunction or complications related to the Chiari II malformation is a chronic and intense stress on the family system. This stress, in addition to the other complex needs of these children, often results in families overprotecting the child and treating him or her as a "perpetual child" (Johnson & Dorval, 2001). Families may be hesitant or fearful of allowing others to care for their child because of the child's special needs. Parents should be encouraged to treat their child as a member of the family, not the center of the family.

Resources

The multisystem involvement of this condition requires frequent hospitalizations, surgeries, outpatient services, and multidisciplinary care. These factors, in addition to items such as special equipment or medications that may be needed by these children, place a tremendous financial burden on parents. The health care system recognizes the many needs of children with myelodysplasia and their families and offers physical, emotional, spiritual, and social care. Nevertheless, no individual understands or feels the problems these children

and families face in their day-to-day lives as well as another child or family with the same disorder. Therefore support groups and opportunities available to provide this network of support within the community not only are necessary but also have proven to be a major factor in coping and adaptation for these families. The following are a few support systems available to families. Each region has its own community-based network or local chapter. It is important that the primary care provider be aware of available local resources.

Hydrocephalus Association
870 Market St., Suite 705
San Francisco, CA 94102
Website: www.hydroassco.org
Spina Bifida Association of America
4590 MacArthur Blvd. NW, Suite 250
Washington, DC 20007-4226
(202) 944-3285; (800) 621-3141
Website: www.sbaa.org

Summary of Primary Care Needs for the Child with Myelodysplasia

HEALTH CARE MAINTENANCE

Growth and Development
- Height may be measured in the supine position.
- Both precocious puberty and short stature are reported.
- Obesity is common in these children as a result of lack of motor activity.
- Head size may be enlarged if child is diagnosed with hydrocephalus; measure head circumference at each visit, until sutures are fused.
- Motor delays are common and depend on level of lesion. Surgical intervention for proper muscle balance may be necessary.
- Promoting upright positioning and independent mobility is a goal.
- Cognitive ability varies, and testing and early intervention are recommended.

Diet
- Caloric intake should be monitored to minimize potential for obesity.
- Caution parents about using food as a reward.
- Diet should include increased fluids to lessen chance of constipation and urinary tract infections.
- Regurgitation, vomiting, and difficulties with gag reflex need to be evaluated for increased intracranial pressure and Chiari II malformation.
- Children with latex allergies may have allergic reactions to some foods.

Safety
- Increased risk of injuries (i.e., burns, fractures, skin breakdown) may occur as a result of decreased sensation and mobility.
- Skin integrity should be checked twice daily.
- Cognitive deficit may alter judgment regarding safety and use of equipment.

- Proper body positioning, frequent position changes, and proper fit of adaptive equipment are recommended.
- Education on emergency care of seizures is recommended.
- Increased risk for latex allergy. Educate on common sources of latex to avoid. Medic-Alert bracelets identifying allergy are recommended. Epipens are necessary for severe reactions.

Immunizations
- Routine immunizations are recommended. Multidose vials may have latex tops and should be avoided.
- Immunizations are not contraindicated in children with seizures. Consultation with a pediatric neurologist is recommended for children with severe or poorly controlled seizures.

Screening
- *Vision.* These children have a high incidence of visual deficits such as ocular palsies, astigmatism, and visual-perceptual deficits. Children should be evaluated by an ophthalmologist at 6 months of age and yearly thereafter.
- *Hearing.* Routine screening is recommended. Children may have hypersensitivity to loud noises if they have shunts. If children are exposed to aminoglycosides or have a history of central nervous system (CNS) infection, hearing should be evaluated by an audiologist.
- *Dental.* Routine care is recommended. Latex precautions are required. Antibiotic prophylaxis is not needed in children with ventriculoperitoneal shunts for hydrocephalus but is recommended for children with ventriculoatrial shunts.
- *Hematocrit.* Routine screening is recommended.
- *Urinalysis.* Baseline urinalysis and cultures should be obtained in the newborn period.
  - Bladder catheterization is recommended for obtaining urine for cultures.
  - Positive cultures should be reported to urologist to determine treatment.

Summary of Primary Care Needs for the Child with Myelodysplasia—cont'd

- *Tuberculosis.* Routine screening is recommended.
- *Blood pressure.* Routine monitoring is recommended. Children with renal problems may develop hypertension and should have more frequent monitoring. In rare cases, persistent hypertension may be a sign of shunt malfunction.

Condition-Specific Screening

- *Blood tests.* Complete blood counts (CBCs) should be obtained frequently on children treated with sulfonamides for urinary tract infection (UTI) prevention. Serum creatinine should be done on newborns and then as indicated when changes appear on renal ultrasound (i.e., hydronephrosis).
- *Scoliosis.* Screening for scoliosis should be done yearly from birth through adolescence.
- *Latex allergies.* Latex precautions include monitoring for signs and symptoms and educating the child, family, and other care providers. Epipen is needed for severe reactions.

COMMON ILLNESS MANAGEMENT

Differential Diagnosis

- *Chiari II malformation.* Symptoms may include respiratory difficulties, stridor, croupy cough, absent gag reflex, or headache, or upper body weakness in older children. Refer to neurologist/neurosurgeon for evaluation.
- *Tethered cord.* Symptoms may include scoliosis, altered gait pattern, changes in muscle strength and tone, disturbance in urinary and bowel patterns, and back pain: rule out tethered cord.
- *Shunt malfunction.* See Chapter 29.
- *Fevers.* Rule out shunt or CNS infection, UTI, and fracture or injury of insensate area.
- *Gastrointestinal symptoms.* Rule out increased intracranial pressure with nausea and vomiting, UTI, fecal impaction, and appendicitis.

Drug Interactions

- No routine drug therapy exists, but children frequently take daily medications.
- Antibiotics are commonly given to prevent or treat UTI.
- Anticholinergics are given to assist in urinary continence training.
- Stool softeners and bulking agents are used to prevent constipation.
- Anticonvulsants are used if seizures are present (see Chapter 26).
- Evaluate for possible interactions on an individual basis.

DEVELOPMENTAL ISSUES

Sleep Patterns

- Apnea, increased stridor, and snoring may occur in children with symptomatic Chiari II malformation. Sleep studies may be indicated.
- Lethargy may indicate increased intracranial pressure.
- Children may need to be repositioned during the night to prevent skin irritation resulting in fatigue.

Toileting

- Aggressive bowel and bladder management should begin early to avoid delay in continence.
- Independence should be encouraged when developmentally and physically appropriate. Parents should be trained in cardiopulmonary resuscitation (CPR).
- Bulking agents and stool softeners may be used daily to prevent constipation.
- Bowel regimens will vary. Antegrade continence enemas (ACEs) are sometimes used.
- Intermittent catheterization is common, and compliance may be an issue during adolescence.

Discipline

- These children are at an increased risk of psychosocial adjustment problems.
- They have a need for discipline and encouragement toward independence.

Child Care

- Special medical care procedures must be taught to daycare personnel.
- Care providers must be educated regarding signs and symptoms of shunt malfunction, UTIs, and latex allergies and precautions.
- Early intervention programs are ideal for infants and toddlers.
- Daycare personnel must know how to use adaptive equipment and check for injury.
- Emergency contact information is necessary.

Schooling

- Learning disabilities and attention problems are common.
- Neuropsychological testing is recommended.
- Frequent school absences may occur because of illness or medical treatments.
- Federal laws protect children with disabilities. Special physical needs must be tended to during school hours.
- Special provisions may be necessary for adaptive equipment, wheelchairs, transportation, accessibility, and safety in emergencies.
- Latex items must be removed from the classrooms.
- Children may have adjustment problems because of low self-esteem and functional limitation. Participation in extracurricular activities may help with peer relationships.
- Families need assistance in individualized educational plan (IEP) hearings.

Sexuality

- Sexuality and reproductive health should be introduced early.
- Precocious puberty may occur.
- Sexual functioning may be altered because of sensory impairment.
- Women have normal fertility, so birth control is important when sexually active. Latex condoms and diaphragms must be avoided.
- Men may not be able to have erection or ejaculation depending on level of spinal lesion.
- Genetic counseling is recommended.

Continued

Summary of Primary Care Needs for the Child with Myelodysplasia—cont'd

- Early prenatal care is required because of possible complications related to urinary function, scoliosis, VP shunts, and lower body lack of sensation.

Transition to Adulthood

- Primary health care needs, independent living, vocational training, and socialization all must be addressed in transition planning (see Chapter 4).
- Social support systems are needed for independent living.

- Cognitive deficits and functional limitation must be evaluated for independent living.

FAMILY CONCERNS

- Parents suffer chronic grief for loss of "normal" child.
- Stress is related to frequent hospitalizations, surgeries, and need for multidisciplinary care.
- Caring for these children can be a financial burden on families.

REFERENCES

Altaweel, W., Jenack, R., Bilodequ, C., et al. (2006). Repeated intradetrusor botulinum toxin type A in children with neurogenic bladder due to myelomeningocele. *J Urol, 175*(3 pt 1), 1102-1105.

American Academy of Pediatric Dentistry (AAPD). (2005). *Clinical guideline on antibiotic prophylaxis for dental patients at risk for infection.* Available at www.guideline.gov. Retrieved .

Baskin, L., & Kogan, B. (2005). *Handbook of Pediatric Urology.* (2nd ed.). Philadelphia: Lippincott Williams & Wilkins.

Cardenas, D., Topolski, T., White, C., et al. (2008) Sexual functioning in adolescents and young adults with spina bifida [electronic version]. *Arch Phys Med Rehabil, 89*(1), 31-35.

Carr, M.C. (2007). Fetal myelomeningocele repair: Urologic aspects. *Curr Opin Urol, 17*(4), 257-262.

Centers for Disease Control and Prevention (CDC). (2007). *Trends in spina bifida and anencephalus in the United States: 1991-2005* [electronic version]. National Center for Health Statistics.

Centers for Disease Control and Prevention (CDC). (2008a). Use of supplements containing folic acid among women of childbearing age—United States, 2007 [electronic version]. *MMWR Morb Mortal Wkly Rep, 57*(01), 5-8.

Centers for Disease Control and Prevention (CDC). (2008b). Quickstats: Spina bifida and anencephaly rates—United States, 1991, 1995, 2000, and 2005 [electronic version]. *MMWR Morb Mortal Wkly Rep, 57*(01), 15.

Danish, S.F., Samdani, A.F., Storm, P.B., et al. (2006). Use of allogeneic skin graft for the closure of large meningomyeloceles: Technical case report [electronic version]. *Neurosurgery, 58*(4 Suppl 2), E376.

Dias, M.S. (2005). Neurosurgical management of myelomeningocele (spina bifida) [electronic version]. *Pediatr Rev, 26*(2), 50-60.

Fletcher, J.M., Barnes, M., & Dennis, M. (2002). Language development in children with spina bifida. *Semin Pediatr Neurol, 9*(3), 201-208.

Fletcher, J.M., Copeland, K., Frederick, J.A., et al. (2005). Spinal lesion level in spina bifida: A source of neural and cognitive heterogeneity. *J Neurosurg Pediatr, 102*, 268-279.

Food and Drug Administration (FDA). (2007). *Parent guide to immunizations.* Available at www.fda.gov. Retrieved. April 17, 2008.

Geisel, J. (2003). Folic acid and neural tube defects in pregnancy [electronic version]. *J Perinat Neonat Nurs, 17*(4), 268-279.

Guille, J., Sarwark, J., Sherk, H., et al. (2006). Congenital and developmental deformities of the spine in children with myelomeningocele. *J Am Acad Orthop Surg, 14*(5), 294-302.

Hasenau, S., & Covington, C. (2002). Neural tube defects prevention and folic acid. *MCN Am J Matern Child Nurs, 27*, 87-91.

Hirose, S., Farmer, D., & Albanese, C. (2001). Fetal surgery for myelomeningocele. *Curr Opin Obstet Gynecol, 13*, 215-222.

Hudgins, R.J., & Gilreath, C.L. (2004). Tethered spinal cord following repair of myelomeningocele. *Neurosurg Focus, 16*(2), 1-4.

Jackson, A.B., & Mott, P.K. (2007). Reproductive health care for women with spina bifida [electronic version]. *Scientific World Journal* (7), 1875-1883.

Johnson, C.P., & Dorval, J. (2001). *Transitions into Adolescence. Spina Bifida Association of America Fact Sheet.* Washington, DC: Spina Bifida Association of America.

Johnson, M.P., Sutton, L.N., Rintoul, N., et al. (2003). Fetal myelomeningocele repair: Short-term clinical outcomes. *Am J Obstet Gynecol, 189*(2), 482-487.

Joseph, D.B. (2005). Bladder rehabilitation in children with spina bifida: State-of-the-art [electronic version]. *J Urol, 173*(6), 1850-1851.

Kripalani, H.M. (2000). Quality of life in spina bifida: Importance of parental hope. *Arch Dis Child, 83*, 749-758.

Levey, E., Demetrides, S., Hamilton, R., et al. (2007). Current prevalence of latex sensitization in children with spina bifida with use of latex precautions [electronic version]. *Oral Presentation Cerebrospinal Fluid Research 2007, 4*(Suppl 1), S13.

Lew, S.M., & Kothbauer, K.F. (2007). Tethered cord syndrome: An updated review. [electronic version]. *Pediatr Neurosurg, 43*(3), 236-248.

Lollar, D. (2001). *Learning Among Children with Spina Bifida. Spina Bifida Association of America Fact Sheet.* Washington, DC: Spina Bifida Association of America.

Matson, M., Mahone, M., & Zabel, A. (2005). Serial neuropsychological assessment and evidence of shunt malfunction in spina bifida: A longitudinal case study [electronic version]. *Child Neuropsychol, 11*, 315-332.

McAndrew, H.F., & Malone, P.S. (2002). Continent catheterizable conduits: Which stoma, which conduit and which reservoir? *BJU Int, 89*, 86-89.

McLone, D.G., Dias, M.S. (2003). The Chiari II malformation: Cause and impact. *Childs Nerv Syst, 19*, 540-550.

National Institute of Child Health and Human Development (NICHHD). (2007). *Management of Myelomeningocele Study (MOMS)* [electronic version]. Available at www.ClinicalTrials.gov. Retrieved. April 17, 2008.

Nieto, A., Mazon, A., Pamies, R., et al. (2002). Efficacy of latex avoidance for primary prevention of latex sensitization in children with spina bifida. *J Pediatr, 140*(3), 370-372.

Padmanabhan, R. (2006). Etiology, pathogenesis and prevention of neural tube defects. *Congen Anomalies, 46*, 55-67.

Patriarca, G., Nucera, E., Pollastrini, E., et al. (2002). Sublingual desensitization: A new approach to latex allergy problem. *Anesth Analg, 95*, 956-960.

Physicians' Desk Reference (PDR). (2008). (ed. 62). Montvale, NJ: Medical Economics Co., Inc.

Rader, J.I., & Scheeman, B.O. (2006). Prevalence of neural tube defects, folate status, and folate fortification of enriched cereal-grain products in the United States [electronic version]. *Pediatrics, 117*(4), 1394-1399.

Ray, J.G., Wyatt, P.R., Thompson, M.D., et al. (2007). Vitamin B$_{12}$ and the risk of neural tube defects in a folic-acid–fortified population. *Epidemiology, 18*(3), 362-366.

Reece, E.A., Hobbins, J.C. (2006). *Clinical Obstetrics. The Fetus and Mother* (2nd ed.). Blackwell Publishing.

Rendeli, C., Nucera, E., Ansili, E., et al. (2006). Latex sensitization and allergy in children with myelomeningocele [electronic version]. *Childs Nerv Syst,* (22), 28-32.

Rintoul, N.E., Sutton, L.N., Hubbard, A.M., et al. (2002). A new look at myelomeningoceles: Functional level, vertebral level, shunting, and the implications for fetal intervention. *Pediatrics, 3*(109), 409-413.

Rotenstein, D., & Bass, A.N. (2004). Treatment to near adult stature of patients with myelomeningocele with recombinant human growth hormone [electronic version]. *J Pediatr Endocrinol Metab, 17*(9), 1195-1200.

Russell, M., Pool, V., Kelso, J., et al. (2004). Vaccination of persons allergic to latex: A review of safety data in the Vaccine Adverse Event Reporting System (VAERS) [electronic version]. *Vaccine, 23*(2004), 664-667.

Sairyo, K., Goel, V.K., Vadapalli, S., et al. (2006). Biomechanical comparison of lumbar spine with or without spina bifida occulta. A finite element analysis [electronic version]. *Spinal Cord, 44*, 440-444.

Shaer, C., Chescheir, H., & Schulkin, J. (2007). Myelomeningocele: A review of the epidemiology, genetics, risk factors for conception, prenatal diagnosis, and prognosis for affected individuals. *Obstet Gynecol Surv, 62*(7), 471-479.

Spina Bifida Association of America (SBAA). (2007). *Latex list.* Available at www.sbaa.org. Retrieved April 17, 2008.

Spina Bifida Association of America (SBAA). (2008a). *Folic acid.* Available at www.sbaa.org. Retrieved April 17, 2008.

Spina Bifida Association of America (SBAA). (2008b). *Latex allergy in spina bifida.* Available at: www.sbaa.org. Retrieved April 17, 2008.

Stiefel, D., Copp, A.J., & Meuli, M. (2007). Fetal spina bifida in a mouse model: Loss of neural function in utero. *J Neurosurg, 106*, 213-221.

Trute, B., & Heibert-Murphy, D. (2002). Family adjustment to childhood developmental disability: A measure of parent appraisal of family impacts. *J Pediatr Psychol, 27*(3), 271-280.

Tulipan, N., Sutton, L.N., Bruner, J.P., et al. (2003). The effect of intrauterine myelomeningocele repair on the incidence of shunt-dependent hydrocephalus. *Pediatr Neurosurg, 38*(1), 27-33.

Vermaes, I., Janssens, J., Bosman, A., et al. (2005). Parents' psychological adjustment in families of children with spina bifida: A meta-analysis [electronic version]. *BMC Pediatr, 5*, 32.

Williams, L.J., Rasmussen, S.A., Flores, A., et al. (2005). Decline in the prevalence of spina bifida and anencephaly by race/ethnicity: 1995-2002 [electronic version]. *Pediatrics, 116*(3), 580-586.

Xiao, C.G. (2005). Reinnervation for neurogenic bladder: Historic review and introduction of a somatic-autonomic reflex pathway procedure for patients with spina cord injury or spina bifida [electronic version]. *Eur Urol, 49*(1), 22-29.

36 Obesity

Mary Margaret Gottesman, Margaret A. Brady,
Bonnie Gance-Cleveland and Karen G. Duderstadt

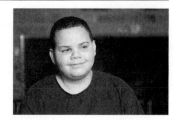

Etiology

Obesity is the result of an imbalance in energy intake from food compared to energy expenditure in physical activity. Multiple factors influence both the occurrence and extent of obesity in any individual (Anderson & Butcher, 2006). These factors include genetic inheritance, physical activity, the hormone leptin, the intrauterine environment, and the greater "obesogenic environment"—the built, economic, social, school, and cultural environment and the home and parenting behaviors that affect the child's lifestyle choices in food, activity, inactivity, and sleep (Koplan, Liverman, & Kroak, 2005).

Estimates of heritability vary widely from as little as 16% to as much as 85% for body mass index (BMI) and from 35% to 63% for body fat percentage (Yang, Kelly, & He, 2007). A longitudinal study including twins and families by the National Heart, Lung, and Blood Institute (NHLBI) suggested that heritability accounts for 40% to 80% of BMI levels (Borecki, Higgins, Schreiner, et al., 1998). In comparison, a longitudinal community-based study, the Framingham Heart Study, reports a 40% to 50% heritability estimate (McQueen, Bertram, Rimm, et al., 2003). According to many experts in the field of childhood obesity, having two obese parents increases the child's risk for overweight and obesity. The exact contribution of various genes to obesity is unclear. What is clear from numerous studies of fraternal and homozygous twins, adoption studies, and family studies is that heritability and its expression through ethnicity play an important role in the prevalence and severity of obesity (Allison, Kaprio, Korkeila, et al., 1996; Stunkard, Berkowitz, Schoeller, et al., 2004). In the United States, all ethnic minority groups are at higher risk for overweight. Among children, strong racial/ethnic differences in the prevalence of childhood obesity emerge early in life regardless of socioeconomic status (SES) (Freedman, Wang, Thornton, et al., 2008).

Interestingly, obesity caused by the influence of a single gene is extremely rare. At least 35 research studies implicate linkages between BMI and specific regions of chromosomes 2, 3, 6, 11, 13, and 20 with odds of over a thousand to one in favor of a true genetic linkage. Twenty-two genes have at least five studies each supporting their contribution to obesity via energy homeostasis, thermogenesis, adipogenesis, leptin, insulin levels, or a combination of these processes (Lagou, Scott, Manios, et al., 2008; Yang et al., 2007). Coregulation of function through gene-gene interaction and complex intracellular hormonal peptide signaling systems governing individual cell function also influence the risk for and severity of obesity. Consequently, obesity is as diverse in its root causes as are the individuals in whom it occurs.

Childhood obesity is a feature of several genetic conditions, including Down syndrome (see Chapter 24), as well as Prader-Willi, Bardet-Biedl, hereditary Cushing, Mehmo, and Alström syndromes. Children with isolated growth hormone deficiency, X-linked syndromic mental retardation, and Albright hereditary osteodystrophy also are at high risk for obesity (Barlow & Expert Committee, 2007).

Physical Activity

Although it is well known that genetic heritage interacts with diet in terms of the digestion and absorption of nutrients and the regulation of energy metabolism and cellular growth processes, there is less appreciation for the role of genetic influence on physical activity. Estimates of heritability for physical activity are between 29% and 62% (Beunen & Thomis, 2006; DeLaney, Bray, Harsha, et al., 2004). Genes influence physical performance through the programming of cellular maximal oxygen uptake and skeletal muscle metabolism. Individuals with high levels of oxygen uptake and skeletal muscle metabolism perform better in a wide variety of athletic skills requiring endurance. The positive rewards for excellence in athletic pursuits foster continued participation and weight maintenance, whereas poor performance in physical activities generally elicits negative feedback from peers and adults, discouraging continued engagement in physical activities (Faith, Leone, Ayers, et al., 2002; Gray, Janicke, Ingerski, et al. 2008). This is a lived reality for children and adolescents every day in schools, recreation centers, and sports clubs the world over. Funding for public school programs is often insufficient to support physical education and sports for the majority of students. Low-income families are less likely to be able to pay athletic fees and purchase the uniforms and equipment formerly provided by schools for participation, placing low-income children at greater risk for overweight through inactivity.

Whereas physical activity is the positive side of energy expenditure, relative physical inactivity during sedentary activities such as television viewing leads to energy conservation through low metabolic demand. Television viewing is the most researched aspect of sedentary behavior (Boynton-Jarrett, Thomas, Peterson, et al., 2003). More than 15 years of study have identified a consistent link between a sharp increase in risk for overweight and obesity for each additional hour of television viewing beyond 2 hours of viewing per day (Proctor, Moore, Gao, et al., 2003). A recent study finds, however, that the culprit in weight gain may be more the energy consumption (food intake) accompanying television viewing rather than the lack of activity (Epstein, Roemmich, Robinson, et al., 2008; Matheson, Killen, Wang, et al., 2004).

Leptin

Leptin, a hormone produced in fatty tissue, plays an important role in influencing the brain and behavior and is one of the most widely studied hormones influencing appetite and hunger (Paz-Filho, Ayala, Esposito, et al., 2008). Its level is in direct proportion to the amount of adipose tissue in the body. Leptin binds to the ventral medial nucleus of the hypothalamus, also known as the appetite center. It signals the brain about the body's level of energy storage and the need for food, inhibiting the production of neuropeptide Y and anandimide, both potent stimulants of feeding behavior (Lomenick, Clasey, & Anderson, 2008). Conversely, it promotes the production of the appetite suppressants alpha-melanocyte stimulating hormone (α-MSH) and peptide YY_{3-36} (PYY_{3-36}); during sleep, melatonin interacts with insulin to suppress appetite (Louis & Myers, 2007).

Intrauterine Factors

The intrauterine environment is one of the most potent in determining a child's risk for overweight and obesity (Gillman, Rifas-Shiman, Berkey, et al., 2003). Current research suggests that both large for gestational age and small for gestational age infants are at increased risk for later overweight and obesity (Oken & Gillman, 2003; Simmons, 2004). Mothers who are overweight before conception and those gaining an excessive amount of weight during pregnancy provide a glucose- and fatty acid–rich intrauterine environment that alters fetal insulin production and fuels excessive fetal growth (Kramer, Morin, Yang, et al., 2002). This nutrient-rich intrauterine environment appears to program the child's metabolism to demand excessive energy intake after birth (Rasmussen & Kjolhede, 2008).

Conversely, a nutrient-poor environment during pregnancy from maternal undernutrition, ill health, placental vasoconstriction caused by smoking, or placental malformation and dysfunction appears to trigger metabolic energy conservation after birth in small for gestational age infants (Oken & Gillman, 2003). Researchers posit that the metabolic programming of the nutrient-poor intrauterine environment triggers the function of a "thrifty gene." This gene leads the child's body to perceive even normal levels of nutrients as excessive and results in the storage of energy in fat for future episodes of nutrient deficit (Gluckman, Hanson, Beedle, et al., 2008).

Obesogenic Environment

The environment also has a significant impact on the rapidly increasing prevalence of childhood obesity. In nearly every part of the world the prevalence of obesity has increased, even in developing countries (Wang & Lobstein, 2006). Human intelligence and ingenuity have created an "obesogenic environment" that fosters a mismatch between energy consumption and energy expenditure (Bellisari, 2008).

The *availability of food* contributes to the incidence of obesity (Rose-Jacobs, Black, Casey, et al., 2008). Food scarcity is no longer the issue it once was for the vast majority of humans. Technology has allowed us to create low-cost, good-tasting, energy-dense foods (Bray, Nielsen, & Popkin, 2004). In addition, most humans living in industrialized, modern nations no longer engage in hard physical labor. Labor-saving devices are plentiful and inexpensive. Walking is no longer a major mode of transportation. Whereas human environments and lifestyles have changed dramatically in the

last century, our genetic makeup has not. The human body remains programmed for the conversion of excess energy intake into fat cells for the days of starvation and high energy demand that are no longer a reality.

The *built environment* also influences the rates of childhood obesity (Sallis & Glanz, 2006; Taylor, Floyd, Whitt-Glover, et al., 2007). The degree of neighborhood safety for outdoor play, the presence or absence of sidewalks for walking safely to school, bussing of students to school, and the presence and capacity of community parks and recreation centers all influence opportunities for energy expenditure through physical activity (Fitzgibbon & Stolley, 2004; Gómez, Johnson, Selva, et al., 2004). The presence or absence of lower-cost major grocery stores versus mom-and-pop stores influences the availability and affordability of high-nutrient, low-calorie food options such as fresh fruits and vegetables, fish, and lean meat. The presence and density of fast food restaurants also influences food choices and, hence, calorie intake (Block, Scribner, & DeSalvo, 2004).

The *economic* and *social environments* affect family lifestyles. For many children in the United States, family life has changed dramatically since the early twentieth century (Nicklas, Morales, Linares, et al., 2004). Greater numbers of single-parent families and families with both parents working outside the home mean there is less time available for shopping for and preparing meals, eating, and playing together as a family. Parents more frequently turn to eating outside the home or bringing in fast food for meals. Meals prepared at home are generally richer in calcium sources, as well as fruits and vegetables, and lower in fat and energy than meals eaten outside the home (Lindsay, Sussner, Kim, et al., 2006; Neumark-Sztainer, Eisenberg, Fulkerson, et al., 2008; Neumark-Sztainer, Wall, Story, et al., 2004). Recent data support a 40% increase in the likelihood of childhood overweight when the meals are not prepared at home and significantly greater risk for overweight when eating at fast food establishments, especially among white young adults (Larson, Neumark-Sztainer, Story, et al., 2008; Pereira, Kartashov, Ebbeling, et al., 2005).

Daycare and *school environments* also affect childhood obesity. Research has shown that there is a difference in weight gain and the quality and quantity of food intake between children cared for at home and those who are in child-care settings (Lumeng, Gannon, Appugliese, et al., 2005). In a large, national sample of infants 9 months of age and younger in child care, infants in child care experienced less breastfeeding, earlier introduction of solid foods, and greater weight gain than infants cared for at home by their mothers (Kim & Peterson, 2008; Monteiro & Victora, 2005; Owen, Whincup, Odoki, et al., 2002). Both formula feeding and the introduction of solid foods increase the risk for early excessive weight gain (Kramer, Guo, Platt et al., 2004). Breastfeeding and breast milk offer important protective benefits to infants, including a more favorable growth pattern that is not associated with later obesity (Hediger, Overpeck, Kuczmarski, et al., 2001). A larger national sample of nearly 16,000 kindergartners found that children who had been in family, friend, and neighborhood care settings and non-Latino children in Head Start were more likely to be obese than children who had not attended daycare before starting kindergarten (Maher, Li, Carter, et al., 2008). However, in contrast, Latino kindergartners who had been in nonparental child care were less likely to be obese. Recent data demonstrate that most excessive weight gain occurs before age 5 and is significantly predictive of weight at 9 years of age and future cardiometabolic risk, highlighting the critical role of early diet and physical activity patterns on adult health (Gardner, Hosking, Metcalf et al., 2009).

The school environment is second only to the child's home in influencing the child's quality of nutrition, activity level, and mental health (Andrews, Peterson, & Duncan, 2007). Most school districts lack standards for the educational preparation of food service directors, much less food service workers (Finkelstein, Hill, & Whitaker, 2008). Without adequate knowledge of good nutrition and quality food preparation practices, school breakfast and lunch programs are often higher in total fat and saturated fat content than recommended by the National School Lunch Program (NSLP) with only two thirds of schools offering two fruit and vegetable choices (Finkelstein et al., 2008; U.S. Department of Agriculture [USDA], 2005). Interestingly, the current NSLP guidelines do not require that school lunch programs serve fruit and vegetables, nor do they prohibit offering foods fried in fat.

With decreases in funding from property and sales taxes, schools have sought to make up the difference in funding levels by offering foods to students through partnerships with fast food restaurants and vending machine contracts (Kubik, Lytle, Hannan, et al., 2003). These strategies have allowed schools to maintain programming but have increased the availability to children during the school day of cheap, high-caloric foods and beverages rich in fats and sugar (Johnson-Taylor & Everhart, 2006).

Political policies such as "No Child Left Behind" also have had unintended negative consequences on the school resources devoted to nutrition and physical education, as well as the time allotted for recess. With the emphasis on passing achievement tests to progress in school and graduate, school boards and school officials have increased instructional time by sacrificing recess time, physical education, health classes, and other extracurricular activities. The decrement in physical education and recess opportunities coupled with the availability of energy-dense, nutrient-poor food service and vending machine choices has led to many schools becoming unhealthful, obesogenic environments for their students.

Culture influences the onset of obesity in multiple ways (Kumanyika, 2008). Ethnic foods and their traditional preparation are important ways group members preserve and celebrate their heritage. Culture determines the acceptable foods for its members and their most desirable preparation. Culture also dictates the acceptable types of physical activity for each gender, generally supporting sports participation for males more than females. Gene-environment interactions are an aspect of culture as well. For example, obesity rates are higher among Japanese and Mexican American immigrants to the United States compared with their counterparts who have not immigrated. Thus individuals at high risk genetically for obesity entering a highly obesogenic environment significantly increase their risk for becoming overweight and obese (Talmud & Stephens, 2004).

Incidence and Prevalence

Obesity is the most serious long-term health risk currently facing America's children (Katzmarzyk, Baur, Blair, et al., 2008). The World Health Organization (WHO) now recognizes obesity as one of the most important, worldwide, public health issues (WHO, 2003). The problem is most prominent among developed countries, and the United States has the highest prevalence of overweight children and adolescents in the world. In the last two decades, the percentage of overweight and obese school-age children and adolescents in the United States has more than tripled (Ogden, Carroll, Curtin, et al., 2006).

The National Health and Nutrition Examination Survey (NHANES) shows the prevalence of overweight among preschool-age children ages 2 to 5 years to be 14%, doubling between 1988 and 2004 (National Center for Health Statistics, 2007). A startling 31.9% of children and adolescents were overweight and 16.3% reached the obese level with a BMI at or above the 95th percentile for age (Ogden, Carroll, & Flegel, 2008). NHANES data showed that 11.3% of children and adolescents in the United States ages 2 through 19 years were severely obese with BMIs exceeding the 97th percentile for age and gender (Ogden et al., 2008). This segment of children and adolescents represents those at greatest risk for the cardiovascular and metabolic complications of obesity (Ford, Mokdad, & Ajani, 2004).

Most concerning in the current epidemic of overweight and obesity is the overrepresentation of children living in low-income families, particularly racially and ethnically diverse children (Grahm, 2005; Shrewsbury & Wardle, 2008). The obesity rate is 20% for non-Hispanic black children ages 2 to 19 years, and another 35.1% are overweight (Ogden et al., 2006). The rates for overweight and at risk for overweight in Mexican American children (ages 2 to 19 years) are 19.2% and 37%, respectively (Stovitz, Schwimmer, Martinez, et al., 2008). Prevalence rates for overweight Native American children, though varying greatly among tribes, have been estimated as high as 40% (Zephier, Hime, Story, et al., 2006). A national study of 3-year-olds examining racial and ethnic differences among urban, low-income families found that 35% of the study children were overweight, with Hispanic children twice as likely as black or white children to be overweight or obese (Kimbro, Brooks-Gunn, & McLanahan, 2007).

Diagnostic Criteria

Research has shown that both parents and providers often fail to recognize excessive weight gain, even when significant (Killion, Hughes, Wendt, et al., 2006; Mitchell, Wake, Canterford, et al., 2008: Shibli, Rubin, Akons, et al., 2008). Therefore it is important to obtain accurate growth measures, to calculate BMI for children 2 years of age and older. Because BMI values are not standardized for children less than 2 years of age and because younger children normally have greater amounts of adipose tissue, the AAP and the CDC recommend the use of weight-for-length to describe body fatness in infants and young toddlers (Kuczmarski, Ogden, Guo et al., 2002: Krebs, Himes, Jacobson et al., 2007). A weight-for-length value above the 95th percentile in this age-group defines overweight. Accurate plotting on standard growth charts is essential (available at www.cdc.gov/growth-charts).

BMI is a measure of body weight adjusted for height and defines overweight and obesity. BMI is calculated by dividing the individual's weight in kilograms by the square of height in meters. Although BMI does not measure body fat directly and fails to account for other factors affecting the risks of overweight such as fat distribution, muscle mass, genetics, and level of physical fitness, it is a clinically useful tool for assessing degree of body fatness and the recommended measure for identifying overweight and obesity for both children and adults by the World Health Organization, the Centers for Disease Control and Prevention (CDC), the National Association of Pediatric Nurse Practitioners (NAPNAP), the American Academy of Pediatrics (AAP), the National Heart Lung, and Blood Institute (NHLBI), the American Medical Association (AMA), and the American Heart Association (AHA) (AMA, 2007; Krebs et al., 2007; Kuczmarski et al., 2002; Lissau, Overpeck, Ruan, et al., 2004; NAPNAP, 2006; NHLBI, 2007; Poirier, Giles, Bray, et al., 2006).

BMI alone is insufficient for identifying the child's or adolescent's full degree of risk from excessive weight gain. It is important for the practitioner to interpret the child's risk within the context of the family health history, the child's growth pattern over time, and all relevant clinical information in assigning degree of risk in relation to BMI and body fat.

The AAP Expert Committee (Barlow & Expert Committee, 2007) defines overweight as having a BMI for age and gender between the 85th and 94th percentiles. The term "obese" applies to children and adolescents having a BMI between the 95th and 98th percentile for age and gender (Barlow & Expert Committee). The term "obesity" denotes markedly excessive body fat more accurately than the previously used term "overweight" and indicates the serious health risks associated with high adiposity, including significant risk for cardiovascular disease (Freedman, Khan, Mei, et al., 2002). For older adolescents, obesity is defined as a BMI of 30 kg/m^2, the adult obesity cutoff. NAPNAP, AHA, AAP, and AMA recommend at least annual determination of BMI for children and adolescents beginning at 2 years of age and every 3 to 6 months if the child meets the criteria for overweight or obesity. This valid and clinically acceptable tool has the added benefit of continuity with the recommended standard measurement for monitoring adult weight (Krebs et al., 2007).

The AAP and others also have recognized the need for an additional cut off point to identify the severely obese child and adolescent (AMA, 2007). Consequently, experts have agreed that a BMI at or above the 97th percentile for age and gender identifies those children and adolescents who are severely obese and who should receive priority for the most intensive level of intervention (Spear, Barlow, Ervin, et al., 2007).

Much attention has been focused recently on the value of the waist-to-hip ratio as a superior measure of risk for the comorbidities of overweight. However, data do not find that it is superior to BMI (Mei, Grummer-Strawn, Pietrobelli, et al., 2002). In addition, it is more difficult to obtain valid and reliable measurements of waist and hip size, as well as measurements of various types of skin-fold thickness. Therefore these measurements are not currently recommended for use in primary care (Krebs et al., 2007).

Clinical Manifestations at Time of Diagnosis

Common findings at the time of diagnosis include excessive truncal adipose tissue, although providers may not recognize early overweight simply through visual inspection. The severely obese child or adolescent may also have tachypnea on exertion, such as climbing onto the examination surface, and may be pale and sweaty even in a cool examination room. A waddling gait or limp during ambulation, bowed legs, or apparently painful feet may also mark the obese child's presentation. Pubertal females may have severe acne and fine hair over the face and parts of the body.

Clinical Manifestations at Time of Diagnosis

- Excessive truncal adipose tissue
- Signs and symptoms of associated problems
- Early development of secondary sexual characteristics
- Acanthosis nigricans

Adapted from Krebs, N.F., Himes, J.H., Jacobson, D., et al. (2007). Assessment of child and adolescent overweight and obesity. *Pediatrics, 120,* S193-S228.

Overweight and obese children require a thorough physical examination. This is necessary to identify the extent of their excessive weight gain, to identify all associated problems, and to plan treatment that addresses all of their health care needs (Krebs et al., 2007).

The development of secondary sexual characteristics before age 8 for white girls, before age 7 in black girls, and before age 9 in males signals early-onset puberty and is frequent among overweight and obese children. In girls it is a risk factor for polycystic ovary syndrome. Distinguishing between adipose tissue and the true glandular enlargement or thelarche in girls and gynecomastia in boys can be challenging. In girls, darkening of the areola and prominence of the nipple indicate the onset of true thelarche. Adipose tissue also may cause the examiner to falsely identify micropenis in boys. In boys, true micropenis and undescended testes along with truncal obesity suggest the possibility of Prader-Willi syndrome.

Acanthosis nigricans, a velvety, hyperpigmented plaque, occurs more often in darker-skinned and overweight children. It occurs most often in the axillae, groin, and body folds, over the dorsal neck surface, and over joint surfaces. Its presence has been thought to be a strong indication of hyperinsulinemia; however, recent data suggest it may not be a strong predictor of the presence of metabolic abnormalities (Krebs et al., 2007).

Treatment

Obesity affects almost every body system and contributes to the development of a variety of obesity-related medical conditions. In addition to referral to specialists for management of the complications of obesity, primary care providers work with the child and family to improve their nutrition and physical activity patterns to achieve a BMI at or below the 85th percentile for gender, age, and height (Golan & Crow, 2004; Spear et al., 2007). Primary prevention is the first treatment strategy.

Preventing Childhood Overweight: Establishing Energy Balance

Once established, obesity is difficult to reverse. In fact, other than surgical intervention for adolescents, there are no high-quality, evidence-based treatments with demonstrated long-term effectiveness for children (Summerbell, Ashton, Campbell, et al., 2003). Prevention of overweight and obesity remains the most important strategy for stemming the epidemic of childhood obesity.

Individuals achieve their best health when there is a daily balance between energy intake from food and energy expenditure in growth and activity (Fogelholm, 2008). Assessment of the family's history for risk factors for obesity and cardiovascular disease and individual and family patterns of nutrition, activity, and inactivity

Treatment

Prevention
- At least annual growth measurements
- At least annual body mass index (BMI) determination and plotting
- Explanation of growth to parents
- At least annual nutrition review and education
- At least annual physical activity review and education
- At least annual review of screen time and education

Recommended daily dietary intake
- Five or more servings of fruits and vegetables
- One 4-ounce serving of 100% fruit juice
- Two or three servings of fat-free or low-fat milk or equivalent dairy foods
- Six to eleven servings of grain, at least half from whole grain
- Two servings of lean meats, fish, or vegetable protein
- Water as supplemental beverage
- Fat-free or low-fat milk
- Avoid all sweetened beverages

- Avoid *trans* fats
- Emphasize monounsaturated and polyunsaturated fat sources
- Limit saturated fat intake

Recommended physical activity
- At least 60 minutes per day of moderate to vigorous physical activity to maintain weight
- At least 90 minutes per day of moderate to vigorous physical activity to lose weight
- No more than 2 hours per day of screen time

Staged Treatment for Obesity (see Table 36-3)
Pharmacologic Therapy
- Sibutramine
- Orlistat

Bariatric Surgery
Strengthening Parenting Skills and Family Motivation

Adapted from Barlow, S.E, & Expert Committee (2007). Expert Committee recommendations regarding the prevention, assessment, and treatment of child and adolescent overweight and obesity: Summary report. *Pediatrics, 120,* S164-S192; Gidding, S.S., Dennison, B.A., Birch, L.L., et al. (2005). Dietary recommendations for children and adolescents: A guide for practitioners: Consensus statement from the American Heart Association. *Circulation, 12,* 2061-2075.

provide the basis for interventions (Gidding, Dennison, Birch, et al., 2005). Prevention strategies focus on improving the quality and quantity of nutrient intake, ensuring effective levels of physical activity to balance energy intake, and limiting inactivity through education, lifestyle counseling, and motivational interventions by a team of health professionals (Sullivan, Beste, Cummings, et al., 2004). Assessments of the family's and child's or adolescent's readiness to change, as well as their treatment preferences, guide practitioners in supporting changes in these fundamental aspects of daily life (Prochaska & Sallis, 2004).

Recommended Dietary Intake

The U.S. Department of Agriculture (USDA) has set the standards for a high-quality diet for Americans 2 years of age and older (USDA, 2005) (Figure 36-1). The optimal daily diet is one rich in fruits, vegetables, and whole grain foods. The 2005 *Dietary Guidelines for Americans* recommend at least five servings each day of fruits and vegetables. Fruits and vegetables are high in micronutrients and fiber, but low in calories when fat and fat-containing products are not added. Because 100% fruit juice is rich in natural fructose sugars, the AAP recommends that juice be limited to no more than 4 ounces per day at any age (Spear et al., 2007). Sweetened beverages, including sweetened milk, soda, lemonade, sweetened iced tea, and coffee, as well as fruit juice drinks and juice-flavored drinks, should be limited because they contribute to overweight and obesity (Elliott, Keim, Stern, et al., 2002). Even small decrements in sugar and sweetened beverage intake have been shown to lower excessive weight gain (Rodearmel, Wyatt, Stroebele, et al., 2007).

Children need 6 to 11 servings of grain products daily, at least half of which should be from whole grain products. Children with higher levels of physical activity need more servings, and less active children need fewer servings. Whole grain products contain more vitamins and fiber than do nonenriched, refined grain products. The additional fiber in fruits, vegetables, and whole grain products creates greater feelings of satiety, thus limiting food and calorie intake. Fiber also removes fat from the digestive tract, limiting its absorption and promoting digestive function.

TABLE 36-1

Calories per Day by Gender, Age, and Level of Activity

Age in Years	Sedentary	Moderately Active	Active
MALE			
2-3	1000	1000-1400	1000-1400
4-8	1400	1400-1600	1600-2000
9-13	1800	1800-2200	2000-2600
14-18	2200	2400-2800	2800-3200
19-30	2600	2600-2800	3000
FEMALE			
2-3	1000	1000-1400	1000-1400
4-8	1200	1400-1600	1400-1800
9-13	1600	1600-2000	1800-2200
14-18	1800	2000	2400
19-30	2000	2000-2200	2400

Adapted from U.S. Department of Agriculture. (2005). *Dietary guidelines for healthy Americans.* Available at www.health.gov/DietaryGuidelines/dga2005/document/default. htm. Retrieved June 23, 2008.

The intake of fat deserves particular attention. Pediatric experts recommend a low-fat, but not fat-free, diet for children (Van Horn, Obarzanek, Barton, et al., 2003). Fat is a necessary part of the diet to meet the active, growing child's energy requirements. However, fats are energy rich (9 calories per gram) compared with carbohydrates and proteins (4 calories per gram). Fat intake should ideally be no more than 30% of daily calorie intake with less than 10% of fat from saturated fat sources, none from trans fat, and the remainder from polyunsaturated and monounsaturated fat sources. Healthier fat choices include canola, olive, and soy oils and soft margarines.

Protein is a critical element in the daily diet and is never stored in adipose tissue. Plant protein sources such as those from soy and legumes, as well as lean meats, are the preferred sources for protein at all ages.

Calcium sources are an important part of the diet for growing children who need to build the foundation of maximal bone density by the end of adolescence. Dairy foods are the richest, most

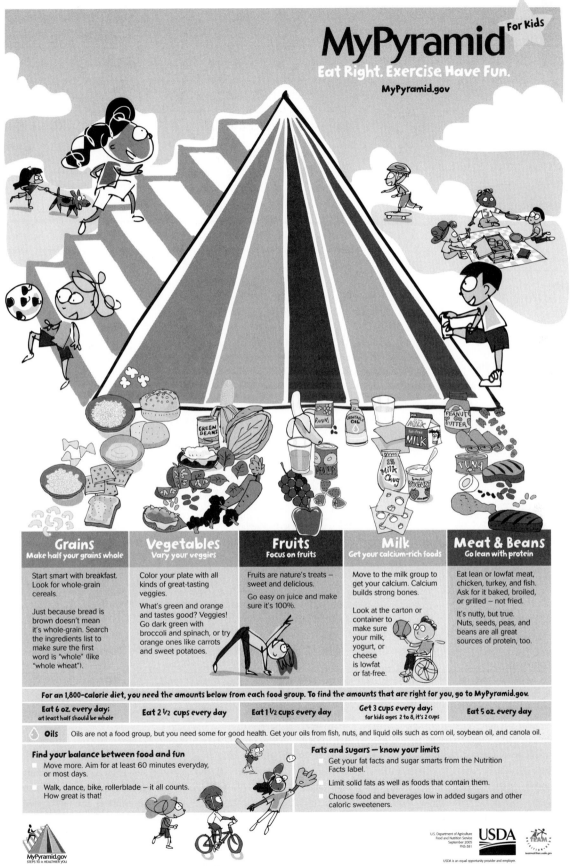

FIGURE 36-1 Children's Food Pyramid. From the U.S. Department of Agriculture Food and Nutrition Service. (2005). My Pyramid for kids. Available at http://teamnutrition.usda.gov/Resources/mpk_poster2.pdf. Retrieved October 16, 2008.

TABLE 36-2

Serving Sizes and Number of Servings for Age 1 to 6 Years and At Varying Calorie Intake Levels Irrespective of Age

Serving Size	No. of Servings		Serving Size	No. of Servings			
	1-3 Yr	4-6 Yr		1600 cal.	2000 cal.	2600 cal.	3100 cal.
GRAINS							
¼-½ slice bread 4 tbsp cooked cereal, rice, pasta ¼ cup dry cereal 1 or 2 crackers	6	6	1 slice bread 1 cup of ready-to-eat cereal ½ cup rice, pasta, or cereal	6	7-8	10-11	12-13
VEGETABLES							
1 tbsp of cooked vegetable	2-3	3-5	1 cup raw leafy ½ cup cooked or raw other vegetables ¾ cup vegetable juice	3-4	4-5	5-6	6
FRUITS							
½ piece fresh fruit ¼ cup fruit canned, cooked ¼ -½ cup juice	2-3	2	¾ cup fruit juice 1 medium fruit ¼ cup dried fruit ½ cup fresh, frozen, canned fruit	4	4-5	5-6	6
LOW-FAT OR FAT-FREE DAIRY FOODS							
>12 months old should have low-fat milk	2 500 mg calcium/day	2 800 mg calcium/day	1 cup milk 1 cup yogurt 1½ oz cheese	3 1200-1500 mg calcium/day 9- to 18-year-olds	3	3	3-4
MEAT, POULTRY, FISH, EGG							
	2	2	2-3 oz cooked meats, poultry, fish 1 egg	2	2	2	2-3
NUTS, SEEDS, LEGUMES							
a. 2 tbsp cooked beans or peas b. Only creamy peanut butter spread thinly on a cracker/bread c. Omit seeds and nuts	2	2	1 tbsp peanut butter ⅓ cup nuts 2 tbsp seeds ½ cup cooked dry beans or peas	3-4	4-5	1	1
FAT, OIL							
Moderate use until 2 years old (about 50% of total calories)		Sparingly	1 tsp soft margarine 1 tbsp low-fat mayonnaise, salad dressing, vegetable oil	2	2-3	3	4

Adapted from American Academy of Pediatrics. (2004). *Pediatric Nutrition Handbook* (5th ed.). Elk Grove Village, IL: AAP; Dietz, W.H., & Stern, L. (Eds.). (1999). *Guide to Your Child's Nutrition.* New York: Villard; U.S. Department of Agriculture. (2005). *Dietary Guidelines for Healthy Americans.* Available at www.health.gov/Dietaryguidelines/dga2005/document/default.htm. Retrieved June 23, 2008.

bioavailable source of calcium. Because of the energy density of milk fat, low-fat or nonfat dairy products are better choices than products with full milk fat content. Low-fat milk is now recommended at 12 months of age (Daniels et al., 2008). Nonfat products are best for those adolescents who have completed puberty and entered the phase of weight maintenance.

An important strategy in preserving a healthy weight is raising parent awareness of the average daily calorie needs for gender, age, and level of activity (Table 36-1), number of servings of each macronutrient group per day, and serving sizes appropriate to the child's age and activity level (Table 36-2). A serving is the age-appropriate amount of a food typically eaten at one sitting. A portion is the amount of a food type eaten at any one sitting. Thus one portion may contain two or more servings of a food group. Serving sizes vary with the age of the child; for example, a serving of cooked vegetables for a 9-month-old infant is one tablespoon, and it is one-half cup for a 7-year-old. Research shows that portion sizes have increased dramatically for many prepared foods (Smiciklas-Wright, Mitchell, Mickle, et al., 2003). Serving a larger portion of food results in greater food consumption by individuals 5 years of age and older (Diliberti, Bordi, Conklin, et al., 2004). Limiting portion sizes is an important strategy for limiting energy intake from food.

TABLE 36-3
Staged Approach to Obesity Treatment

Components	Implementation
STAGE 1: PREVENTION PLUS ≥5 servings of fruits and vegetables per day ≤2 hours of television per day No television in bedroom Decrease sugar-sweetened beverages Portion control Daily breakfast Decrease eating out Family meals At least 60 minutes of moderate to vigorous physical activity per day	Setting: primary care provider (PCP) office Personnel: PCP or staff Visits: Based on readiness to change and severity of condition Advance stage based on progress, medical condition, risks, length of time, and readiness to change
STAGE 2: STRUCTURED WEIGHT MANAGEMENT *In addition to above:* Balanced macronutrient diet Limit energy-dense foods High protein Self/parent monitoring Medical screening: laboratory tests Mental health referral for parenting skills, family conflict, motivation (as needed)	Setting: PCP office + registered dietitian (RD) Personnel: PCP + RD Visits: monthly tailored and based on readiness to change and severity of condition Advance to next stage based on progress, age, medical condition, risks, length of time, and readiness to change

STAGE 3: COMPREHENSIVE, MULTIDISCIPLINARY TREATMENT
Referral to community weight management center or specially trained staff in addition to all of above
More frequent visits (monthly) with assessment of measures
Multidisciplinary approach (dietitian, psychiatrist, physical therapist, medical doctor [MD], nurse practitioner [NP], physician's assistant [PA])
Behavioral modification training for parents
Strong parental involvement initially
Group sessions may be helpful
	Setting: PCP coordinates care
	Community weight management program:
	  Pediatric weight center
	  Commercial programs
	Personnel: Interdisciplinary team: behavior, RD, PCP
	Visits: weekly; include nutrition, exercise, and behavioral counseling
	Advance depending on response, age, health risk, and motivation

STAGE 4: TERTIARY CARE TREATMENT Pediatric weight management center	Multidisciplinary team Personnel: behavioral counselor, medical social worker (MSW), psychologist, RN, NP, RD, mental health care provider, exercise specialist, may involve surgeon Visits: according to protocol

Adapted from Spear, B.A., Barlow, S., Ervin, C., et al. (2007). Recommendations for treatment of child and adolescent overweight and obesity. *Pediatrics, 120,* S254-S288.

Recommended Physical Activity

Food consumption must be balanced with energy expenditure through physical activity and avoidance of sedentary behavior to achieve energy balance. Studies consistently link increased physical activity with decreased BMI in children and adolescents (Gidding, Barton, Dorgan, et al., 2006; Saris, Blair, van Baak, et al., 2003). In addition to the physiologic benefits of physical activity, moderate and intense levels of activity improve mood and attention (Berkey, Rockett, Gillman, et al., 2003; Dunn, Trivedi, Kampert, et al., 2005). Other studies indicate that regular moderate to vigorous physical activity reduces cardiovascular risk factors, whether or not the person loses weight (Meyer, Kundt, Lenschow, et al., 2006; McGavok, Sellers, & Dean, 2007; McMurray, Harrell, Creighton, et al., 2008). Current guidelines recommend that children and adolescents participate in 60 minutes or more of daily moderate- to vigorous-intensity physical activity (Ekelund, Yngve, Brage, et al., 2004; Spear et al., 2007). Children who are obese may need to start with shorter periods of moderate to vigorous physical activity with a gradual increase to recommended levels over time (Butte, Puyau, Adolph, et al., 2007).

When advising families and children who are obese, it is important to emphasize the following: activities should be chosen that are fun and use large muscle groups; the entire family should engage in activities together on as close to a daily basis as possible; negative comments on appearance or performance should be avoided; and increases in physical activity should be gradual, as should be decreases in television viewing time (Epstein, Paluch, Kilanowski, et al., 2004; Epstein, Paluch, Roemmich, et al., 2007; Salmon, Booth, Phongsavan, et al., 2007). A desirable workout pattern includes a 5- to 10-minute warm-up period, stretching, the workout, a cool-down period, and ending with more stretching. Highly recommended activities include water activities because adipose tissue increases buoyancy, making sustained activity easier. If good supervision is available, weight training is a good idea because overweight children have more muscle mass. Strength sports such as football, wrestling, and javelin, hammer, and discus throwing are all good choices.

Staged Treatment for Obesity

The Expert Committee recommendations (Barlow & Expert Committee, 2007) suggest a staged approach to treatment (Table 36-3). Although evidence supports the components of these stages, research has not established the effectiveness of this approach as a complete protocol for preventing and managing overweight and obesity (Barlow & Expert Committee).

Stage 1: Prevention Plus. The prevention plus stage is an appropriate place to start for all children and adolescents who are overweight or obese. The goal of this stage is for the child's BMI to move toward the 85th percentile. It may take 3 to 6 months for the recommended changes in this stage to produce a noticeable change in BMI. Advancement to stage 2 may be recommended if the child is not making adequate progress, the BMI has increased, comorbidities have developed or worsened, or the child and family indicate readiness for more aggressive management.

Stage 2: Structured Weight Management. The second stage of treatment focuses on the same behavioral changes as stage 1 (improving nutrition quality, increasing physical activity, and decreasing inactivity), as well as offering additional behavioral counseling. This stage requires staff with special training in behavior change and involves more frequent weight management visits, greater intervention structure, and close monitoring of progress toward behavior change goals. In stage 2 the nutrition plan includes education regarding a balanced-macronutrient diet, limitation of energy-dense foods, provision of structured daily meals and snacks, increased behavior monitoring to ensure meeting of recommendations, and positive reinforcement strategies. Regular meetings with a registered dietitian with pediatric obesity experience is desirable. Weight loss should not exceed 1 pound per month for children 2 to 11 years of age or 2 pounds per month for adolescents 12 years of age and older. Weight maintenance in youths who are continuing to grow in height is an indication of adequate progress. Monthly follow-up is recommended. Indications of failure to make progress at this stage are the same as for stage 1: an increase in BMI, appearance of new comorbidities or worsening of existing comorbidities, and child and family readiness for more intensive treatment.

Stage 3: Comprehensive, Multidisciplinary Intervention. The components of treatment at this stage include all of the strategies included in stages 1 and 2 with an increase in the intensity of behavior change strategies, more frequent weight management visits, and specialty referral as available. Negative energy balance is the goal at this stage. Structured behavioral modification to alter diet and physical activity, systematic evaluation of body measurements, dietary intake, and physical activity mark this stage. Weight loss goals remain the same as those outlined previously. Providers may also refer the individual to a commercial weight loss program that meets the criteria for safety and appropriateness for children and adolescents (Box 36-1).

Stage 4: Tertiary Care Intervention. Stage 4 treatment involves referral to a specialized pediatric obesity center. Youths with severe obesity who are unable to decrease their degree of adiposity and mitigate their health risks through lifestyle interventions and who meet the criteria receive this level of care. Criteria for this most intensive level of care include attempted weight loss at stage 3; the maturity to understand the possible risks associated with stage 4 interventions; and willingness to maintain physical activity, to follow a prescribed diet, and to participate in behavior modification. Treatment strategies may include meal replacement, a very-low-energy diet, pharmacotherapy, or bariatric surgery.

Pharmacologic Therapy

Weight loss medications must be used with caution in the care of children because of the absence of scientific evaluation of their effectiveness and the unknown, long-term effects of these

---

BOX 36-1

Criteria for Commercial Weight Loss Program for Youths

1. The program should be specifically designed for children and adolescents.
2. Behavior modification emphasizes cultural sensitivity, positive reinforcement, and sensitivity to body image issues; incorporates family; and requires frequent visits.
3. Nutrition and exercise components are conducted by trained professionals.
4. Cost of program is affordable to the family.
5. Culturally appropriate interventions are used.
6. Outcomes of intervention are monitored.
7. Attrition rate is low.
8. Evidence-based alternative and complementary methods are used and use of over-the-counter medications is avoided.

Adapted from Spear, B.A., Barlow, S., Ervin, C., et al. (2007). Recommendations for treatment of child and adolescent overweight and obesity. *Pediatrics, 120,* S254-S288.

---

substances on the growth and development of children. Few guidelines are available for the safe use of weight loss medications in the pediatric population, and lifestyle modification remains the preferred treatment (Daniels et al., 2008; Spear et al., 2007). Research suggests that youths with a BMI at or above the 97th percentile are at very high risk for biochemical abnormalities and severe adult obesity, leading some experts to elect more aggressive treatments such as pharmacotherapy with orlistat (Xenical, Allī) or sibutramine (Meridia), the only medications approved for use in children (McCrindle, Urbina, Dennison, et al., 2007).

Orlistat is a reversible lipase inhibitor that blocks the action of lipase, preventing the breakup and absorption of fat in the lumen of the stomach and intestine. Orlistat blocks absorption of about 25% of the fat in a meal, decreasing the absorption of triglycerides and cholesterol (Chanoine, Hampl, Jensen, et al., 2005). The unabsorbed fat is excreted in the stool. Side effects include abdominal cramping, flatus, and oily bowel movements. It is available over the counter. One 60 mg capsule is taken with every meal that contains fat or up to 1 hour after the meal, but no more than three times per day. Because it blocks fat absorption, it increases the risk for fat-soluble vitamin deficiencies. Vitamin supplements are recommended to decrease this risk.

Sibutramine is an appetite suppressant preventing the reuptake of serotonin, norepinephrine, and, to a lesser extent, dopamine. It is currently licensed for use in adolescents 16 years of age or older (Berkowitz, Fujioka, Daniels, et al., 2006). The usual dose is one 10 mg capsule once per day. After 1 month, it may be titrated upward to 15 mg if the medication is well tolerated but ineffective at 10 mg. Some children may only tolerate a low dose at 5 mg once per day. Among the most concerning side effects is vasoconstriction, leading to increased heart rate and blood pressure. Because vasoconstriction may persist even after significant weight loss, it is a poor choice for children with hypertension. Other common side effects include headache, dry mouth, constipation, and insomnia.

Pharmacotherapy alone has not been proven effective in the treatment of obesity (Berkowitz, Wadden, Tershakovec, et al., 2003). Medication in conjunction with a structured lifestyle modification results in an average weight loss of 5% to 10%, which plateaus after 4 to 6 months. Weight regain is common when medication is discontinued. Children and youth who may benefit from pharmacotherapy should not be managed in primary care; rather, they should be referred to a pediatric tertiary care center for evaluation and treatment.

Bariatric Surgery

Bariatric surgery is the treatment of last resort. Depending on the type of procedure, adolescents may expect to lose 50% to 70% of their excess weight. The AAP has established criteria for bariatric surgery based on data from adult studies (Inge, Krebs, Garcia, et al., 2004); these criteria include adolescents who are physically mature (determined by sexual maturity rating for girls 13 years of age or older and boys 15 years of age and older), have a BMI of 50 or more with significant comorbidities, have experienced failure of a formal, 6-month weight loss program, and are capable of adhering to the long-term lifestyle changes required after surgery. Most adolescent candidates for bariatric surgery also have significant psychological issues, especially mood disorders (Zeller, Roehrig, Modi, et al., 2006). Assessing psychological readiness is therefore difficult and is done most appropriately by an experienced mental health provider (Inge et al., 2004).

Fortunately, adolescents have fewer complications from surgery than do adults (Nadler, Young, Ren, et al., 2007). After the surgical procedure, careful, lifelong supervision is indicated to ensure optimal postoperative weight loss, and eventual weight maintenance (Apovian, Baker, Ludwig, et al., 2005). The long-term effects of this surgery on both the physical and psychological health of adolescents is unknown (Loux, Haricharan, Clements, et al., 2008). A large, prospective, multicenter trial to evaluate the effects of bariatric surgery on adolescents is underway (Inge, Zeller, Harmon, et al, 2007).

Strengthening Parenting Skills and Motivation

Studies of obesity treatment have demonstrated the importance of parents' participation in weight control (Golan, 2006; Lindsay et al., 2006). Parents serve as role models for healthy lifestyle choices for their children when they provide healthy foods within the home and monitor the eating and physical activity patterns of their children (Faith, Calamaro, Dolan, et al., 2004). Clinicians influence children's health behaviors by teaching and supporting parents in their important family leadership roles by providing age-appropriate anticipatory guidance (Barlow & Expert Committee, 2007).

Motivational interviewing (MI) is a technique for establishing a collaborative relationship with children and their families that reflects the value of partnership with families. Both NAPNAP's *Identifying and Preventing Overweight in Childhood: Clinical Practice Guidelines* (NAPNAP, 2006) and the *Expert Committee recommendations on the assessment, treatment, and prevention of child and adolescent overweight and obesity* (AMA, 2007) urge pediatric providers to learn and use MI techniques to create effective treatment partnerships with families. MI strategies recognize that making healthier lifestyle choices is really in the hands of the family and individual; providers cannot instill the motivation to change or make needed changes happen (Miller & Rollnick, 2002). The role of the provider is to support the family and individual in moving forward in readiness to change, increasing family and individual confidence in effectively making change, and facilitating development of workable plans to make changes and overcome barriers to change (Rollnick, Miller, & Butler, 2008).

Complementary and Alternative Therapies

There are no studies of complementary and alternative (CAM) therapies addressing the management of obesity in children. A recent study found that adults who were obese had a higher usage of traditional medical care and lower use of CAM therapies than adults of normal weight (Bertisch, Wee, & McCarthy, 2008). Nevertheless, studies show that obese adults use a variety of CAM therapies, particularly dietary changes and supplements to aid weight loss (Cerniak, 2008).

The safety and effectiveness of popular diets based on severe carbohydrate restriction have not been established for children, nor have protein-sparing, modified fast diets (Gibson, Peto, Warren, et al., 2006). Both pose a potential threat to children's growth and development. The majority of dietary change studies have focused on middle-aged adults, primarily women. In the short term, low-carbohydrate diets result in greater weight loss and better adherence than do low-fat diets. Low-carbohydrate, high-protein diets increase feelings of satiety and have similar weight loss percentages compared with low-fat, high-carbohydrate diets (Dansinger, Gleason, Griffith, et al., 2005; Gardner, Kiazand, Alhassan, et al., 2007). Differences in weight loss among various diet plans disappear after 1 year.

Acupuncture is the most studied CAM therapy for obesity in adults. However, small study sample sizes and weak study designs provide inadequate data on effectiveness (Cabioglu & Ergene, 2006). Likewise, there are no quality data to support the effectiveness of hypnotherapy in augmenting weight loss (Kirsch, 1996).

Both animal and human studies have demonstrated that tea extracts promote thermogenesis and increase energy expenditure, possibly aiding weight loss. There were no significant differences in weight loss between dieting adults using green, black, and oolong tea extracts and those not using them (Nagao, Hase, & Tokimitsu, 2007). Similar lack of effectiveness also marked the use of garcinia cambogia and citrus aurantium (bitter orange) (Haaz, Fontaine, Cutter et al., 2006; Heymsfield, Allison, Vasselli, et al., 1998; Mattes & Bormann, 2000).

Conjugated linoleic acid (CLA) in triglyceride form at 4 to 5 grams per day resulted in greater weight loss in a randomized, double-blinded, placebo-controlled trial in a small sample of adults (Gaullier, Halse, Høye, et al., 2005). CLA given as free fatty acids showed no effect on weight loss. Meta-analyses of chitosan, a polysaccharide that blocks fat absorption in animal studies, concluded that the studies examined were methodologically flawed and definite benefit and safety could not be determined (Pittler & Ernst, 2005).

Anticipated Advances in Diagnosis and Management

Effective prevention of childhood overweight remains elusive. Although the literature abounds with behavioral change theories and behavioral intervention study data, both are insufficient to guide practitioners in assisting families and children to select and implement healthier lifestyle choices. In addition, most health professionals receive little or no educational preparation in behavioral change strategies and advanced communication techniques.

In the short term, treatment will continue to focus on developing safe and effective drug therapies with low side-effect profiles for use with children (NHLBI, 2007). Surgeons will continue to improve gastric banding and gastric bypass surgical techniques, while generating the data needed to evaluate the long-term safety and effectiveness of these surgeries on weight loss and the reduction of cardiovascular risks in adulthood.

In the more distant future, genetic data for individuals will lead to prevention and intervention strategies tailored to the genetic makeup of the individual. A better understanding of gene-environment interactions will allow health professionals to further customize interventions to maximize child health.

Associated Problems of Childhood Obesity and Treatment

Cardiovascular Problems

A three-generation family genogram is helpful in identifying the extent of heritable risk (Zhu, Yan, Ge, et al., 2008). Beginning with the biologic grandparents, a detailed history for obesity and cardiovascular conditions should be obtained (Salbe, Weyer, Lindsay, et al., 2002). This should include overweight and obesity in all family members, diabetes mellitus, hypertension, stroke, hypercholesterolemia, atherosclerosis, sudden death of grandparent or parent under 55 years of age for men and under 65 years of age for women, and heart disease as evidenced by myocardial infarction, treated angina, coronary catheter intervention procedure, or coronary artery grafting procedure before age 55 (Krebs et al., 2007; Toschke, Beyerlein, & von Kries, 2005).

Hypertension is common among children who are overweight and obese, with 13% having an elevated systolic blood pressure and 9% having elevated diastolic blood pressure (Faulkner, Gidding, Portman, et al., 2008; Krebs et al., 2007). Treatment for hypertension should follow the NHLBI recommendations in addition to treatment to reduce BMI (NHLBI, 2004). Elevation at or above the 95th percentile but not 5 mm Hg higher than the 99th percentile during the follow-up visit indicates stage 1 hypertension and the need for a thorough evaluation for hypertension and a weight management plan appropriate to the child's BMI percentile. Finally, if the child's blood pressure is 5 mm Hg higher than the 99th percentile during three resting pressures 10 to 15 minutes apart, the child has stage 2 hypertension. Additional hypertension evaluation and treatment should begin immediately for the symptomatic child or within 1 week for the asymptomatic child.

Lipid profile abnormalities are one of the most common obesity-related comorbidities (Kwiterovich, 2008). Autopsies of young victims of motor vehicle accidents have shown that fatty plaque develops within the carotid artery medial intima even during the early preschool years. A fasting lipid profile should be obtained when the child's BMI is at or above the 85th percentile, even in the absence of other risk factors. Total cholesterol levels of less than 170 mg/dL are acceptable, levels of 170 to 199 mg/dL are in the borderline category, and levels of 200 mg/dL or greater are elevated (Daniels, Greer, & Committee on Nutrition, 2008). Low-density lipoprotein (LDL) levels of less than 110 mg/dL are acceptable, levels of 110 to 129 mg/dL are borderline, and levels of 130 mg/dL or greater are elevated. Children with lipid abnormalities and their families should be instructed on a reduced-fat, reduced-cholesterol diet. If the levels are highly elevated and do not respond to dietary changes, the child should be referred to a pediatric cardiologist or lipid specialist for assessment of the benefits and risks of medication to normalize serum lipids (Daniels, Greer, & Committee on Nutrition). Abnormal serum triglyceride levels (above 110 mg/dL) and low high-density lipoprotein (HDL) levels (40 mg/dL or lower) respond well to increased physical activity (Kavey, Allada, Daniels, et al., 2006). It is critical, then, that clinicians develop skill in forming effective partnerships with families and children to improve the level of physical activity. If this fails, pharmacotherapy with lipid-lowering statin drugs has proven safe and effective in children, reversing carotid intimal thickening (Reinehr, Wunsch, de Sousa, et al., 2008).

Endocrine Disorders

Type 2 diabetes mellitus is a significant complication of obesity seen predominantly after 10 years of age among adolescents (see Chapter 23). Features most predictive of type 2 diabetes include a slow onset that is often asymptomatic, obesity, a strong family history of type 2 diabetes, ethnic minority group membership, acanthosis nigricans, and the absence of autoimmune disorders (Jones, 2008; Libman & Arslanian, 2007). Unlike children with type 1 diabetes, children with type 2 diabetes are unlikely to have ketoacidosis (Rewers, Klingensmith, Davis, et al., 2008). Girls are at greater risk for type 2 diabetes; research shows that as young as 5 years of

---

Associated Problems of Obesity and Treatment

- Cardiovascular problems
  - Hypertension
  - Dyslipidemia
- Endocrine disorders
  - Type 2 diabetes mellitus
  - Polycystic ovary syndrome (POS)
  - Hypothyroidism
  - Primary Cushing syndrome
  - Metabolic syndrome
- Respiratory disorders
  - Asthma
  - Pulmonary edema
- Orthopedic disorders
  - Painful joints
  - Bony injury
  - Slipped capital femoral epiphysis (SCFE)
  - Tibia vara (Blount's disease)
- Gastrointestinal problems
  - Cholecystitis with and without gallstones
  - Nonalcoholic fatty liver disease (NAFLD)
  - Gastroesophageal reflux
  - Constipation
- Sleep disturbances
  - Disordered sleep
  - Obstructive sleep apnea
- Neurologic problems
  - Pseudotumor cerebri
- Psychological consequences
  - Low self-esteem
  - Depression
  - Suicidal ideation
  - Suicide

age, girls are more insulin resistant than boys (Murphy, Metcalf, Voss, et al., 2004; Syme, Abrahamowicz, Leonard, et al., 2008).

Children with these risk factors should be screened for this condition (Pinhas-Hamiel & Zeitler, 2007). Screening should start before puberty in high-risk children (Daniels et al., 2008) and be repeated every 2 years. A fasting glucose of 126 mg/dL or higher indicates diabetes and requires referral to a pediatric endocrinologist. Fasting glucose levels of 100 mg/dL or higher are considered prediabetes, indicating future risk for diabetes (Alberti, Zimmer, Shaw, et al, 2004; Saib, Hunt, Ford, et al., 2008).

Experts recommend aggressive management with weight loss, exercise, and, if necessary, metformin (Glucophage) or a sulfonylurea drug such as chlorpropamide (Diabinese) (Peterson, Silverstein, Kaufman, et al., 2007). The metformin dose for children and adolescents 10 to 16 years of age starts at 500 mg twice daily up to a maximum dose of 2000 mg per day (Turkowski, Lance, & Bonfiglio, 2008). The extended-release form of metformin has not been studied in children. Metformin is superior to sulfonylureas in that it is does not cause hypoglycemia because it does not raise serum insulin levels. However, the side effects of metformin are substantial and include nausea, vomiting, and diarrhea.

In contrast, sulfonylurea drugs act by increasing insulin secretion by the beta cells of the pancreas. They are taken orally 30 minutes before breakfast and their peak action is 60 minutes after the dose. They should not be used by children or adolescents with kidney, heart, or liver disease or individuals with allergy to sulfa drugs. Like metformin and similar drugs, common side effects include nausea, vomiting, diarrhea, and abdominal pain (Turkowski et al., 2008). They also increase sensitivity to sunlight, so it is important that those taking these drugs use sunscreen with a sun protection factor (SPF) of 30 or more when out in the sun.

The microvascular consequences of diabetes are accelerated in children with type 2 diabetes compared with type 1 diabetes. Careful monitoring of kidney function via testing for albumin spillage in the urine and for eye disease via twice-yearly ophthalmologic evaluation is critical (Matyka, 2008).

Polycystic ovary syndrome occurs more frequently in adolescents and young women who are obese. Infrequent menstrual cycles are the most common symptom (Jasik & Lustig, 2008). Facial acne and hirsutism are also common. Laboratory assessment may reveal insulin resistance, type 2 diabetes, or metabolic syndrome. Diagnosis is based on reproductive hormone laboratory tests (Blank, Helm, McCartney, et al., 2008). Monitoring by an endocrinologist, a gynecologist, or an adolescent specialist is indicated to protect fertility (Tfayli & Arslanian, 2008).

Metabolic syndrome is a multisystem abnormality associated with obesity and type 2 diabetes. Important clinical features predictive of insulin resistance include a positive family history of obesity and type 2 diabetes, being either small or large for gestational age at birth, or a history positive for maternal gestational diabetes (Gahagan & Silverstein, 2003; Maclaren, Gujral, Ten, et al., 2007). Clinical features found in childhood include acanthosis nigricans, premature adrenarche, obesity, and pseudoacromegaly (Shaw, 2007; Weiss, Dziura, Burgert, et al., 2004). During adolescence, the presence of tall stature, pseudoacromegaly, violaceous striae, skin tags, and amenorrhea should suggest the need for evaluation for metabolic syndrome.

Obesity places the child at significant risk for metabolic syndrome in adulthood (Sun, Liang, Huang, et al., 2008). In the adult population, the constellation of dyslipidemia, glucose intolerance, abdominal obesity, and hypertension define the diagnostic criteria for metabolic syndrome. In contrast, there is considerable disagreement among pediatric researchers and clinicians regarding the markers of metabolic syndrome in children and adolescents (Goodman, Daniels, Morrison, et al., 2004; Lottenburg, Glezer, & Turatti, 2007; Pietrobelli, Malavolti, Battistini, et al., 2008). The physiologic changes evolving during puberty (i.e., falling serum lipids and increased insulin resistance, and rapid growth in height with changing blood pressure) may be incorrectly diagnosed as metabolic syndrome (Huang, Nansel, Belsheim, et al., 2007); adolescents diagnosed with metabolic syndrome in the pubertal years often fail to meet the criteria for the diagnosis 2 to 3 years later (Goodman, Daniels, Meigs, et al., 2007; Nguyen, Srinivasan, Xu, et al., 2008).

Weiss and colleagues (2004) have proposed the following criteria for diagnosing metabolic syndrome in children and adolescents: BMI Z-score of 2.0 (97% for sex and age); triglyceride level above the 95th percentile; HDL-cholesterol (HDL-C) level below the 5th percentile; systolic and diastolic blood pressure for gender, age, and height above the 95th percentile; and impaired glucose tolerance with a 2-hour serum glucose level greater than 140 mg/dL but less than 200 mg/dL. Applying these criteria to a sample of 470 adolescents who were obese, 4.8% of white adolescents, 2.0% of black adolescents, and 5.6% of Hispanic adolescents who were obese received the diagnosis of metabolic syndrome. A higher BMI Z-score and the presence of glucose intolerance were most predictive of metabolic syndrome. High serum triglycerides and low HDL-C were the most common findings among all of the obese adolescents.

A recent study of 85 obese adolescents by Love-Osborne, Nadeau, Sheeder, and colleagues (2008) found that adding liver ultrasound examination and fasting glucose tolerance testing improved the diagnostic accuracy in their sample. Impaired glucose tolerance testing and fatty liver on ultrasound were significantly more common in adolescents with true metabolic syndrome. Because of the importance of insulin resistance and its sequelae, Maclaren and colleagues (2007) have proposed that metabolic syndrome be renamed insulin resistance syndrome (IRS) in children and adolescents. The contribution of underlying inflammatory processes are also under examination (Wärnberg & Marcos, 2008).

Hypothyroidism should be ruled out in cases of obesity with stunted linear growth, fatigue, and decline in academic performance (Libman, Sun, Foley, et al., 2008). Symptoms may include a goiter. Thyroid function tests are not indicated in youths with normal linear growth and the absence of symptoms other than obesity.

Primary Cushing syndrome is extremely rare and also involves stunted linear growth, moon facies, a buffalo hump across the shoulders, and violaceous striae (Nieman, Biller, Findling, et al., 2008). Referral to an endocrinologist is indicated if Cushing syndrome is suspected.

Respiratory Disorders

Wheezing and shortness of breath on exertion are common among overweight and obese children (Glazebrook, McPherson, MacDonald, et al., 2006). Although risk factors for both obesity and asthma overlap significantly, such as membership in a minority group and living in the inner city, some researchers also believe that obesity independently contributes to asthma (Taveras, Rifas-Shiman, Camargo, et al., 2008). Shibli and colleagues (2008) found that asthma and stridor were much more common among obese infants and toddlers, suggesting that airway narrowing and respiratory compromise begin as soon as obesity is present even in the youngest children. Although cross-sectional studies consistently demonstrate a link between higher rates of asthma and obesity in children from the preschool years through adolescence, the findings from prospective studies are inconsistent (Abramson, Wamboldt, Mansell, et al., 2008; Litonjua & Gold, 2008). It is not clear whether asthma and fear of provoking symptoms cause children to become inactive and, eventually, obese or whether obesity itself causes asthma to develop (Story, 2007). Fat does compress airways and contribute to their greater reactivity to temperature changes and other triggers.

There is a common underlying feature of inflammation in both obesity and asthma. In addition, a protein underlying insulin resistance has been identified in the lungs of obese mice, leading researchers to postulate a common genetic foundation for both conditions (Story, 2007). Children who have shortness of breath or exercise intolerance should receive pulmonary function testing to identify reversible airway obstruction and an appropriate asthma management plan (Taveras et al., 2008). Weight loss improves asthma symptoms in children as well. Because increased physical activity is helpful in controlling weight gain and facilitating weight loss, pediatric professionals should provide counseling on strategies to minimize asthma symptoms that interfere with physical activity.

Wheezing and coarse rales may also indicate pulmonary edema from the additional stress placed on the cardiovascular system. An elevated respiratory rate at rest and dyspnea in the prone position also suggest possible pulmonary edema. Pulmonary edema is more likely to occur among overweight children who were preterm infants and who have residual chronic lung disease. It is also more likely to happen among overweight children with special health care needs accompanied by limited mobility and impaired cardiac or respiratory function.

Orthopedic Disorders

The unique features of children's bones place children who are overweight or obese at greater risk for orthopedic disorders. Overweight and obese children experience more fractures and musculoskeletal discomfort than do children with normal weight (Taylor, Theim, Mirch, et al., 2006). Because of the greater porosity of their bones, children are more likely to suffer nondisplaced fractures such as buckle and greenstick fractures that are more difficult to identify. In addition, bone porosity increases the risk for fracture because the ligaments are stronger than the bones. Excessive weight places tremendous stress on growth plates, increasing the risk for displacement and deformity. Because pain and frequent injuries interfere with much-needed physical activity, early intervention, including physical therapy, may limit weight gain in these children.

Slipped capital femoral epiphysis (SCFE) can occur in children of any weight but is seen more frequently in obese children 9 to 16 years of age. Its presentation includes knee and hip pain, as well as a limp with walking. On physical assessment, there is limited range of motion of the hip, and diagnosis is made via frog-leg, lateral radiographic imaging of the hips. Treatment is immediate referral to orthopedic surgery for pinning of the femoral epiphysis.

Tibia vara (bowing of the lower extremity), or Blount's disease, also occurs more often in children who are obese than in children with normal weight. Diagnosis is made by anteroposterior radiographic views of the affected knee taken while the child is standing. Treatment is referral to an orthopedic surgeon.

Gastrointestinal Problems

Cholelithiasis or *gallstones* are more prevalent in children who are obese. Rapid weight loss increases the risk of developing this condition. Classic symptoms include intermittent episodes of intense, colicky pain in the right upper quadrant (RUQ) of the abdomen. However, milder pain and epigastric pain may be the initial symptoms. Physical examination reveals RUQ tenderness. Abdominal ultrasound evaluation reveals the presence of gallstones and cholecystitis.

Nonalcoholic fatty liver disease (NAFLD) is a condition consisting of steatosis, steatohepatitis, fibrosis, and cirrhosis resulting from a fatty liver. NAFLD causes no symptoms in most individuals (Riley, Bass, Rosenthal, et al., 2005). Some children have RUQ abdominal pain and demonstrate tenderness to palpation or mild hepatomegaly during abdominal palpation. Serum alanine aminotransferase (ALT) and aspartate aminotransferase (AST) levels may be elevated, and are good screening tests for the presence of this condition. ALT and AST levels twice the normal level should prompt referral to a hepatologist. Ultrasonography reveals changes consistent with NAFLD; however, it cannot determine the degree of inflammation or fibrosis. Liver biopsy is the standard method for diagnosis. Weight loss leads to improvement in the condition, and studies are in progress evaluating treatment with medications (Lavine & Schwimmer, 2004).

Gastroesophageal reflux and *constipation* increase in severity with obesity. Treatment for these conditions is the same as for children of normal weight; however, the clinician should be aware of the increased likelihood of the conditions with obesity and treat the overweight condition as well.

Sleep Disturbances

Sleep-disordered breathing is common among overweight and obese children (Verhulst, Aerts, Jacobs, et al., 2008) Parents report loud snoring, pauses in sleeping, restless sleep, and daytime sleepiness, (Chen, Beydoun, & Wang, 2008; Patel & Hu, 2008; Taveras et al., 2008). With every increase in BMI of 1 kg/m², the risk for obstructive sleep apnea (OSA) increases 12% (Gozal & Kheirandish-Gozal, 2009). These authors also found a six-fold increase in propensity for excessive daytime sleepiness among obese children compared to normal weight children with an equivalent severity of OSA. The exact cause of this phenomenon is not clear. Some researchers believe that both obesity and OSA are low grade inflammatory disorders that increase levels of inflammatory mediators associated with increased sleepiness or other compounds influencing sleepiness yet to be identified (Vgontzas, Bixler, & Chrousos). Sleep apnea disturbs sleep, resulting in poor attention, poor academic performance, and enuresis (Barlow & Expert Committee, 2007; Durmer & Dinges, 2005). Diagnosis is made through polysomnography. If severe, it may lead to right ventricular hypertrophy and pulmonary hypertension.

On physical examination, children frequently have enlarged tonsils. Removal of tonsils and adenoids may be indicated if weight loss does not improve the condition. Research on treatment is limited, but recent reports of successful treatment with nasal budesonide (Kheirandish-Gozal & Gozal, 2008) may offer some relief to children with mild sleep apnea. Continuous positive airway pressure (CPAP) and bilevel positive airway pressure (BiPAP) therapy may be required for sleep. BiPAP is especially helpful for children and adolescents with impaired respiratory function of the chest muscles, central hypoventilation in which the signals from the brain to the respiratory muscles are absent, or both.

Neurologic Disorders

Pseudotumor cerebri is a very rare condition, but there is an increased incidence in children who are obese (Marton, Feletti, Mazzucco, et al., 2008). Symptoms include severe headache with photophobia, diplopia, and blurred vision. Funduscopic examination reveals blurred optic disks and indicates the need for immediate referral to a pediatric neurologist. Untreated, the condition leads to loss of vision.

Psychological Consequences

Research consistently shows that overweight and obesity carry a negative stigma that often damages the self-esteem and social development of children (Puhl & Latner, 2007; Zeller, Reiter-Purtill, & Ramey, 2008). Children who are overweight experience an increased prevalence of psychiatric disorders (Buddeberg-Fischer, Klaghofer, Krug, et al., 2006; Lumeng, Gannon, Cabral, et al., 2003; Waring & Lapane, 2008). Depression is an important comorbidity experienced by children and youths who are overweight and may require treatment with medications, many of which increase the risk for overweight. Sexual and physical abuse may increase the risk of severe obesity. In addition, overweight children are often the recipients of bullying and teasing (Janssen, Craig, Boyce, et al., 2004; Sjöberg, Nilsson, & Leppert, 2005; Swallen, Reither, Haas, et al., 2005). Their overall quality of life may be significantly impaired, as indicated by findings that children who are obese and their parents rate their quality of life similar to that of children with cancer undergoing treatment and significantly worse than a normative population of children (Falkner, Neumark-Sztainer, Story, et al., 2001; Latner, Stunkard, & Wilson, 2005; Schwimmer, Burwinkle, & Varni, 2003). Regardless of ethnicity or gender, emotional distress often accompanies increasing weight, although distress has been found to be less severe among black as compared with white children and adolescents (Young-Hyman, Tanofsky-Kraff, Yanovski, et al., 2006). All children being treated for overweight or obesity should be evaluated for psychiatric disorders and depression and referred for counseling and treatment if indicated (Goldschmidt, Aspen, Linton, et al., 2008).

Most concerning is the link between suicide ideation and overweight (Eaton, Lowry, Brener, et al., 2005). Adolescents who perceive themselves as slightly overweight (85th to 94th percentile) or very overweight (95th percentile or greater) were significantly more likely to experience depression than those who thought their weight was appropriate. Teens who were overweight were also 2.5 times more likely to have suicide ideation than those teens who perceived their weight as normal (adjusted odds ratio for adolescents at 95th percentile or greater). How adolescents perceive their body weight may be more important than their actual weight in terms of increased likelihood of suicidal behavior. Regardless of body mass index (BMI), extreme perceptions of weight appear to be a significant risk factor for suicidal behavior (Mustillo, Worthman, Erkanli, et al., 2003).

Prognosis

Children and adolescents who are obese are more likely to become obese adults (Freedman, Khan, Serdula, et al., 2005). The higher the BMI is in childhood, the greater the probability the problem will persist into adulthood (Guo, Wu, Chumlea, et al., 2002). In girls with a BMI at or above the 95th percentile during childhood, the probabilities of being obese as an adult were 20% to 39.9% if the girl was 3 to 5 years of age, 40% to 59.9% if she was 6 to 11 years of age, and 60% or greater if she was 17 to 20 years of age at the time the BMI was recorded. For boys with a BMI at or above the 95th percentile during childhood, the risk of becoming an obese adult was less than 20% if the boy was 3 to 4 years of age, 20% to 39.9% if he was 5 to 11 years of age, and 60% or greater if he was 17 to 20 years of age at the time the BMI was recorded (Guo et al.).

BMI greater than the 85th percentile in childhood and adolescence correlates with adverse physical health, increased morbidities, decreased mental health, poor socioeconomic outcomes, and increased mortality rates (Janssen, Katzmarzyk, Srinivasan, et al., 2005; Viner & Cole, 2006). Studies suggest that children who are overweight and obese have an increased risk for heart disease, atherosclerosis, type 2 diabetes mellitus, colorectal cancer, gout, hip fracture, arthritis, and early death during their adult years (Barlow & Expert Committee, 2007; Lee, 2008).

The burden of obesity in the population, particularly high-risk and ethnically diverse populations, will exceed the capacity of the current health care delivery system to deliver treatment for obesity or for the associated conditions (Kumanyika & Obarzanek, 2003). Treatment of obesity cannot necessarily reverse the long-term health effects of overweight, particularly when it begins in childhood. This represents a significant challenge to health professionals and health care organizations to design strategies to identify children at risk for overweight and to implement programs for children and adolescents with sedentary lifestyles (Caballero, Clay, Davis, et al., 2003; Crawford, Gosliner, Anderson, et al., 2004; Kropski, Keckley, & Jensen, 2008). Prevention makes good economic sense as well for both public and private health care payers (Cawley & Liu, 2008; Skinner, Mayer, Flower, et al., 2008). Nearly 10% of all health care expenditures in the United States are for obesity-related health problems, with Medicare and Medicaid financing about half of these costs (Evans, Finkelstein, Kamerow, et al., 2005; Finkelstein, Fiebelkorn, & Wang, 2003).

PRIMARY CARE MANAGEMENT

Health Care Maintenance
Growth and Development

Primary prevention of childhood obesity is critical. Each well visit from birth through young adulthood offers the opportunity for primary care providers to measure and plot the individual's growth parameters, as well as interpret the child's growth for parents and child (Treuth, Butte, & Sorkin, 2003; Treuth, Butte, Adolph, et al., 2004). Parents are often unaware of their child being overweight, and over one third of parents of overweight children reported that they were never told that their child was overweight for the child's height and gender (Ogden & Tabak, 2006). Each health care maintenance visit is an opportunity for education regarding diet and exercise appropriate for the child's age and identification of excessive weight gain and additional concurrent risk factors (Danhauer, Oliveira, Myll, et al., 2004).

Growth measurements should be obtained and plotted, as well as calculating and plotting the BMI. Discussion of these values and their interpretation with older children, adolescents, and parents is an important strategy for enlisting and retaining family commitment to making healthier lifestyle choices. Changes in growth patterns also alert providers to the need to alter the plan of care to a higher stage of intensity with continued gains in weight and BMI, as well as providing the opportunity for positive reinforcement for effective efforts in weight maintenance or weight loss (Singh, Mulder, Twisk, et al., 2008).

A recent study showed that infants and toddlers who were obese based on a weight-for-length percentile equal to or greater than the 95th percentile often experienced developmental delays, especially gross motor delays, early in life (Shibli et al., 2008). This study and others suggests that decreased physical activity and overweight begin early in life and children who are overweight and obese are less likely to be physically active (Wittmeier, Mollard, & Kriellaars, 2008).

At all ages, decreases in physical activity are associated with increases in BMI and can lead to delay in physical skill development and peer socialization (McKenzie, Baquero, Crespo, at al., 2008; Trost, Sallis, Pate, et al., 2003). Limiting screen time, which includes video game use, television, and non-homework computer use, to no more than 2 hours per day and ensuring that the child has access to frequent periods for vigorous activity in a safe environment should start during the early years of development (Leatherdale & Wong, 2008; Teran-Garcia, Rankinen, & Bouchard, (2008).

Team sports and physical education classes are not only important opportunities for weight control, they are also opportunities for socialization with peers, fun, and skill building. Because overweight children are less likely to perform well in team sports and physical education classes, they are more likely to experience peer rejection and ridicule, as well as negative comments and attitudes from their parents, coaches, and teachers. Negative feedback has a powerful, damaging impact on the time spent in physical activity, exacerbating not only the extent and persistence of overweight, but also promoting problems in psychological and emotional well-being among obese children and adolescents (Lemeshow, Fisher, Goodman, et al., 2008).

Diet

Energy intake through healthful nutrition is one half of the equation for obtaining and maintaining best health at all ages. In general, amounts of food eaten are underestimated and amounts of physical activity are overestimated. Education on practical ways to balance nutrition and physical activity is a critical intervention at wellness visits. Education needs to be sufficiently detailed to be useful, conveyed in literacy-friendly ways, and tailored to the cultural preferences of the family (Finkelstein, French, Variyam, et al., 2004).

During infancy, education includes encouragement and knowledgeable support of breastfeeding, as well as education about the infant's changing hunger and satiation cues. Research suggests that exclusive breastfeeding confers a protective benefit against overweight, particularly for white children (Buyken, Karaolis-Danckert,

Remer, at al., 2008; Grummer-Strawn & Mei, 2004). Research also demonstrates that excessive early weight gain in the first 4 months of life significantly increases the risk for later child overweight (Hadler, Colugnati, & Sigulem, 2004). The weight gain patterns of breastfed infants demonstrate a slower rate of weight gain compared with that of bottle-fed infants during infancy (Stettler, Kumanyika, Katz, et al., 2003; Stettler, Tershakovec, Zemel, et al., 2000; Stettler, Zemel, Kumanyika, et al., 2002). The mechanism of this difference is not clear. Researchers have hypothesized that it is due to greater infant control of feeding initiation and intake during breastfeeding (Cope & Allison, 2008: Gluckman et al., 2008). In contrast, parents who formula feed their infants may be less in tune with the infant's hunger and satiation cues. Thus parents who are formula feeding their infant, even partially, need instruction in recognizing the feeding cues of their infant. Other key skills for infant feeding include use of a pacifier or rocking and holding versus feeding an infant whenever he or she cries, growth patterns and weight expectations, delaying solid foods until the second 6 months of life, and the value of play and tummy time in promoting infant activity (NAPNAP, 2006).

For toddlers and preschoolers, recommendations focus on providing only healthful choices in foods and beverages; offering a varied, low-fat diet rich in fruits, vegetables, and whole grains; and avoiding food battles by allowing the child to decide when and how much to eat (Atkin & Davies, 2000; Briefel, Reidy, Karwe, et al., 2004; Farrow & Blissett, 2008). For school-age children, anticipatory guidance focuses on understanding growth patterns during the prepubertal and pubertal years, supporting healthy choices in eating and physical activity, providing family meal times, limiting screen time, and ensuring adequate sleep. Adolescents benefit both physically and emotionally from family meals, support and encouragement for 60 minutes of daily moderate to vigorous physical activity, adequate nightly sleep, and limits on screen time (Franko, Affenito, Thompson, et al., 2008).

Feeding patterns also affect weight gain in infants and children (Kim & Peterson, 2008). Data support a relationship between excessive weight gain and skipping breakfast, frequent snacking (also termed "grazing") on energy-dense foods, eating while watching television, and eating outside the home (Dubois, Farmer, Girard, et al., 2008; Epstein, Paluch, Beecher, et al., 2008). Excessive parental control of access to food and eating also increase the risk for overweight and obesity by blunting the child's responsiveness to sensations of hunger and satiety and by increasing the desirability of energy-dense, forbidden foods (Birch, Fisher, & Davison, 2003; Spruijt-Metz, Lindquist, Birch, et al., 2002; Wake, Nicholson, Hardy, et al., 2007). When these forbidden foods become available, children tend to overeat them, fostering overweight. Serving large portions also leads to overeating among children 5 years of age and older.

In contrast, family mealtimes promote the intake of more nutritious foods, while also supporting positive mental health (Fulkerson, Neumark-Sztainer, Hannan, et al., 2008; Gable, Chang, & Krull, 2007). Therefore experts recommend that children eat breakfast daily, that children observe regular mealtimes and snack times with only healthful foods and beverages served in the home, that family mealtimes be a priority and occur as often as possible, and that portion sizes be reduced to reflect recommended serving sizes for age, gender, and activity level (Fisher, Rolls, & Birch, 2003).

Culturally mediated attitudes about foods and eating practices must be discussed before addressing any changes in feeding practices so that the parent and child feel that their concerns are heard by the clinician (Lumeng, 2008). Likewise, addressing parental and child behaviors around feeding practices and food choices is important. Eating in the absence of hunger and using food as a reward for good behavior or to relieve stress are learned behaviors.

Safety

Age-appropriate safety concerns should be addressed with parents. Parents of overweight young children experience significant difficulty in finding appropriate car seats to accommodate their child's large body size (Trifiletti, Shields, Bishai, et al., 2006). Infant and toddler car seats have weight restrictions for tested safety effectiveness and an overweight or obese child may surpass these weight limits.

Because many overweight and obese children are the victims of teasing and bullying, primary care providers should discuss with the parents, child, and adolescent safe ways to avoid and handle these unwelcome and hurtful situations. Parents should also be educated about the behavioral and affective signs of bullying and hurtful teasing their son or daughter may be reluctant to reveal. Clinicians should also partner with their local school districts to promote a safe and violence-free environment for all students at all ages.

Immunizations

Routine immunizations are recommended.

Screening

Vision. Routine screening is recommended except when children are diagnosed with type 2 diabetes. Children and adolescents with type 2 diabetes need a thorough ophthalmologic evaluation at diagnosis and annually thereafter (see Chapter 23). Children with pseudotumor cerebri also require annual eye examinations by a pediatric ophthalmologist and sooner if the child complains of severe headache, double vision, or blurred vision.

Hearing. Routine screening is recommended.

Dental. Routine screening is recommended. Children who are overweight and obese may have a higher incidence of dental caries because of their intake of foods high in sugar and frequent snacking behavior. Regular brushing of teeth and flossing should be encouraged, as well as regular dental visits and the appropriate use of fluoride.

Blood Pressure. Blood pressure elevation frequently accompanies overweight and obesity in children and adolescents because of the associated increase in blood volume servicing the adipose tissue. Blood pressure monitoring should occur at least annually and preferably at each health encounter. Care needs to be taken to ensure an accurate blood pressure measurement with a cuff that covers 80% of the upper right arm. Blood pressure measurements should be compared with standards for the child's gender, height, and age (NHLBI, 2004).

If the initial measurement is at or above the 90th percentile, the measurement should be retaken at least once during the visit. If it remains elevated, repeat measurements should be taken weekly for 3 weeks to determine the presence of hypertension. Weight loss through a low-fat diet and increase in vigorous physical activity is the first line of treatment. Families require monthly, intensive education and supervision to achieve weight loss goals and monitor

changes in blood pressure. If blood pressure remains elevated after 6 months of dietary and activity intervention, medication to control blood pressure should be added to ongoing efforts to achieve weight loss.

Hematocrit. Routine screening is recommended. The incidence of anemia has been reported to be higher in children who are obese (Ausk & Ioannou, 2008; Nead, Halterman, Kaczorowski, et al., 2004); therefore, if the diet history reflects low or marginal intake of foods rich in iron, the clinician should obtain a screening hematocrit/hemoglobin. Children being treated for extreme obesity with extremely low-calorie diets or bariatric surgery and those with high-risk conditions associated with obesity should have blood work done regularly by the tertiary treatment center. These children should be managed in conjunction with specialty care providers.

Urinalysis. Routine screening is recommended. However, in the presence of obesity and a positive family history for diabetes mellitus, urine screen for ketones and glucose should be obtained at least annually, particularly in children 10 years of age or older who are at greatest risk for the onset of type 2 diabetes mellitus. If the parent notes or the child complains of excessive thirst and frequent urination, a urinalysis should also be obtained. Constipation with concomitant urinary tract infections may also occur due to lack of physical activity and diets low in fiber. The risk for urinary tract infections also increases with the use of orlistat because the adolescent may not be able to control forceful diarrhea and the urinary meatus and urethra may become contaminated with bacteria from stool, especially in females.

Tuberculosis. Routine screening is recommended.

Condition-Specific Screening

Lipid Profile. Children who are overweight and obese are at increased risk for dyslipidemia, particularly if dyslipidemia and early cardiovascular disease (CVD) are in the child's family history. Recommendations from NHLBI released in 2009 include obtaining a non-fasting lipid profile and calculation of the non-HDL level for all children between 9 and 11 years of age. Because lipid values fluctuate during puberty, particularly after the child reaches a sexual maturity rating of 3, no routine screening is recommended between 12 and 18 years of age. Non-HDL is calculated by subtracting the high-density Lipoprotein (HDL) cholesterol value from the total cholesterol value. A non-HDL level greater than 145 mg/dL, or an HDL cholesterol value under 40 mg/dL indicates dyslipidemia.

If profiles are elevated, the provider should review the family history for risk factors, update the history, obtain a detailed assessment of the child's typical daily food intake with particular emphasis on sources of fat, and obtain a detailed assessment of the child's daily and weekly activity and inactivity patterns. A 6-month trial of a low fat diet, increase in physical activity and limitation of screen time to one hour or less per day should be initiated. A fasting lipid profile should then be obtained. If the lipid profile has normalized, maintain the dietary and lifestyle changes and reassess the child every 6-12 months. If the triglyceride level is 500 mg/dL or higher, a referral should be made to a pediatric preventive cardiologist. Research shows that early treatment with statin drugs is safe in older school-age children and adolescents, effectively reversing carotid intimal thickening caused by fatty plaque formation (de Jongh, Lilien, op't Roodt, et al., 2002; de Jongh, Ose, Szamosi, et al., 2002; McCrindle, Ose, & Marais, 2003).

Glucose and Insulin Testing. Fasting glucose or oral glucose tolerance test should be obtained in the presence of risk factors for type 2 diabetes and hyperinsulinemia. In addition to overweight and obesity, these include a positive family history for type 2 diabetes, the presence of acanthosis nigricans on physical examination, tachycardia and excessive sweating at rest, polydipsia, and polyuria. Testing should begin at 10 years of age and occur at least every 2 years or sooner with a change in symptoms or family history. Fasting insulin levels are not recommended at this time because there are no reliable pediatric reference standards.

Thyroid Function Tests. Enlargement of the thyroid gland in the presence of impaired linear growth and a BMI at or above the 97th percentile suggests possible hypothyroidism. Thyroid screening is not necessary if symptoms other than being overweight are not present. They are often done as part of the initial workup for obesity to reassure the family that hypothyroidism is not the cause of the child's increased weight.

Pulse Rate. The resting pulse rate is an important vital sign for the overweight and obese child. An increased pulse rate often reflects a lack of physical fitness, whereas a low pulse rate may suggest hypothyroidism.

Common Illness Management

Respiratory Disorders

Respiratory disorders pose a special challenge to children who are overweight and obese. Because of the frequent comorbidity of asthma, the common cold and other respiratory triggers may provoke exacerbations. It is critical that these children have a current and effective asthma plan, that they have adequate supplies of medications and administration equipment at home and at school, and that both parents and children are skilled and knowledgeable in their use. Adolescents taking sibutramine should avoid the use of most over-the-counter cough and cold medications that could lead to dangerous elevations of blood pressure or heart rate.

The overweight and obese child is at greater risk for skin breakdown and infections in the intertriginous skin areas. Common infections include candidal infections in skin folds of the neck, groin, and axillae, as well as the vagina in girls. Repeated candidal infections should prompt the primary care provider to evaluate the child for the onset of type 2 diabetes.

Staphylococcal skin infections, especially abscesses such as pilonidal cysts, are more common among overweight and obese children. These children often find it more difficult to maintain good skin hygiene. They also tend to perspire, experience more friction between skin surfaces, and have clothing that fits snugly, all of which contribute to skin breakdown and infection. Since community-acquired methicillin-resistant *Staphylococcus aureus* (MRSA) has increased in prevalence, it is important for the clinician to culture all abscesses and boils requiring drainage and identify children colonized with MRSA.

Drug Interactions

There are no standard drugs used in the management and treatment of obesity. If the individual child has type 2 diabetes (see Chapter 23) or asthma (see Chapter 11), the clinician should be aware of possible interactions with medications used to treat these associated problems. Children on medications for mood disorders (see Chapter 33) may have significant difficulty losing weight because

many of the psychotropic medications used to treat depression and anxiety cause weight gain. Excessive weight gain is also likely for children on atypical antipsychotic medications such as resperidone and anticonvulsants (see Chapter 33). When rapid weight gain, overweight, or obesity is a concern for these children, primary care providers should consult with the specialists managing the child's seizure, behavior, and mood disorders to consider the possibility of changing to alternative medications with a lower risk for excessive weight gain.

Differential Diagnosis

- *Respiratory disorders:* may trigger asthma exacerbation
- *Wheezing:* may indicate an asthma exacerbation or pulmonary edema
- Skin infections
  - Fungal
  - Bacterial

Serious drug interactions may occur between medications used to treat severely obese adolescents and other medications commonly used in this population. Allī should not be taken together with cyclosporine, an immune suppressant, because it alters its absorption and lowers serum levels. Allī can be taken 2 hours before or 2 hours after a dose of cyclosporine.

Sibutramine produces similar drug interactions to that of other serotonergic agents (Turkowski et al., 2008). Sibutramine should not be combined with a selective serotonin reuptake inhibitor (SSRI) or monoamine oxidase inhibitor (MAOI) drug. The combination of these drugs increases the risk for suicidal ideation and suicide, as well as death as a result of a serotonin storm. If the child is on an SSRI or MAOI, at least a 2-week drug-free period should precede the start of sibutramine. Conversely, drug therapy with an SSRI or MAOI should start only after sibutramine has been stopped for 2 weeks. Caution should be used in combining sibutramine with migraine treatment medications and opiates. In addition, children and adolescents should be cautioned to avoid using over-the-counter cough and cold medications containing decongestants that cause vasoconstriction, because these could add to the vasoconstriction and hypertensive effects of sibutramine.

Metformin's blood levels are increased by up to 40% when given with cimetidine (Tagamet) (Turkowski et al., 2008). Because gastrointestinal symptoms are common in overweight and obese children, clinicians should avoid this deadly combination and alert parents, children, and adolescents to avoid accepting prescriptions for this drug. Families and adolescents also should be warned about the possibility of lactic acidosis, which is fatal in 50% of the cases in which it occurs. Symptoms include weakness, dyspnea, cardiac arrhythmias, muscle spasms, feeling cold, and light-headedness. This is most likely to occur in individuals with impaired liver and kidney function and those with congestive heart failure.

Sulfonylurea antidiabetic agents cause severe hypoglycemia when taken with alcohol or oral miconazole (Turkowski et al., 2008). Children and adolescents should be instructed in recognizing the symptoms of hypoglycemia, including feeling hot, sweating, tachycardia, feelings of hunger, and light-headedness. They should always have a ready sugar source with them. Drugs that cause hyperglycemia, threatening diabetic control when used with sulfonylurea, include estrogen-containing contraceptives, antibiotics, antihypertensives, rifampin, MAOI drugs, dilantin, thiazide and phenothiazide diuretics, prednisone, and thyroid supplements.

Developmental Issues

Sleep Patterns

Data clearly indicate linkages among child obesity, increased risk for obstructive sleep apnea or disordered sleep, impaired attention, and impaired school performance (Muzumdar & Rao, 2006; Verhulst, et al., 2008). Children of all ages should be encouraged to receive adequate sleep. A recent study found a significant correlation between shorter sleep duration in school-age children and likelihood of being overweight (Patel & Hu, 2008). The authors hypothesize a biologic link between sleep duration and obesity, possibly involving levels of circulating leptin and ghrelin, both of which have been implicated in the regulation of appetite. Inadequate sleep may also interfere with the child's ability to participate in sufficient exercise for weight management. Importantly, exercise promotes high-quality sleep, which improves mood, memory, school performance, and behavior. Adequate sleep and exercise enhance the management of many conditions associated with obesity.

Toileting

As a consequence of low activity levels and diets low in fiber, overweight children are at risk for constipation and, with constipation, enuresis. As with all children, health professionals should inquire about the regularity of pain-free defecation and daytime or nighttime enuresis. Children and adolescents who are taking medications to block the absorption of fat have fatty, liquid stools that are difficult to control. These changes are often responsible for discontinuation of the medication.

Discipline

All children benefit from age-appropriate limit setting. In the context of childhood obesity, limit setting, supervision, and role modeling by parents for their children are critical in managing overweight and obesity.

For children of most ages, parents and child care providers are in charge of food selection, purchase, preparation, and the determination of eating times for family members. If unhealthful foods are not brought into the home or offered to children as a choice, children will eat more healthful diets. Serving only nutritious foods will also avoid the use of restrictive practices such as withholding preferred, calorie-dense foods from overweight children. This strategy enhances the desirability of low-nutrient, energy-dense foods and often results in the overeating of these foods when access is obtained.

A more helpful message is that there really are no bad foods, but there is a need to limit calorie intake to match calorie output in physical activity. When parents monitor their children's activity, encourage active play often each day, and limit television and other forms of screen time, their children have more discretionary calories to devote to highly palatable, energy-dense foods. It is also important to discuss the impact of food advertising on child food requests and preferences; less television viewing decreases the child's exposure to advertising.

Positive reinforcement is the best strategy to use in building good dietary and physical activity habits. The use of inexpensive nonfood reinforcements such as stickers and the award of "special time" with parents to do whatever the child prefers are effective ways to value the child's healthful food and activity choices. Because the use of food as a reward is potentially harmful, it is important to counsel parents in avoiding this behavior. This is a particular issue for low-income parents for whom the purchase of a candy bar as a reward is affordable whereas the purchase of a new book as a reward may not be affordable.

Parents of overweight and obese children often have heightened concerns about how best to address the need to make healthful changes in the family's diet and worry about the child perceiving them as behaving in a mean manner. Parents of younger children may be quelled by tantrums over demands for unhealthful foods and are often tempted to give in to their child because they feel helpless or too stressed to deal not only with dietary changes for the family but also the child's protests, which can be embarrassing in public. When counseling, the clinician needs to dispel the parents' perception that the child will view them as being mean when they refuse to purchase and prepare unhealthful foods or reduce the frequency of such food. It is setting a critically important example for lifelong good health for their child and sends a strong message of caring concern to the child. Although it is important to acknowledge the difficulty of taking on this challenge, it is also important to offer concrete help to the parent in developing specific strategies for implementing a healthier diet for the family and overcoming the barriers they anticipate.

Child Care

When an infant or young child is overweight, parents must pay close attention to the child-care arrangements. Top priorities include high-quality nutrition provided in appropriate feeding environments and many opportunities for safe, vigorous physical activity (Pate, Pfeiffer, Trost, et al., 2004). The child-care provider should avoid the use of food for distraction, comfort, or reward; offer only healthful foods in appropriate serving sizes on a predictable schedule; and be skillful in engaging the more sedentary child in active, physical play in at least 10-minute bouts throughout the day, both indoors and outdoors.

Research shows that even older toddlers and preschoolers demonstrate less interest in playing with overweight peers (Musher-Eizenman, Holub, Miller, et al., 2004). It is essential that child-care providers be watchful for any teasing or avoidance of play and social time with the overweight child and that they know how to handle these situations skillfully.

Schooling

Academic success is linked to long-term positive social and economic outcomes. Research data are emerging about the academic and the emotional and social consequences of childhood overweight. A longitudinal study by Gable, Britt-Rankin, and Krull (2008) involving a sample of 8000 children from kindergarten through third grade revealed that decreased academic achievement in reading and math was associated with childhood overweight. Furthermore, teacher ratings of children's academic ability and emotional well-being were lower for children who were overweight than for those children who were normal weight. Not surprisingly, overweight children also rated themselves lower in academic abilities and social and emotional well-being than did their normal-weight counterparts, and their self-reported assessments of their interpersonal skills were also lower.

Obese children often become the targets of bullying and frequently are the victims of taunting remarks about their weight (Eisenberg & Newmark-Sztainer, 2008; Janssen et al., 2004). Clinicians should inquire about whether or not the child has been the victim of bullying or teasing at each visit. If this has been a serious problem, with permission from the child and family, the primary care provider should call the school to discuss the problem and encourage immediate intervention to prevent further abuse.

When obese children can no longer participate or be successful in the physical activities that their peers are enjoying, social distancing may take place between the child who is overweight and his or her normal-weight peers. Overweight children are less likely to perform well in team sports and physical education classes. They may experience peer rejection and ridicule, as well as negative comments from peers, coaches, and teachers. This negative feedback can further discourage the child from participating in physical education and school sports, exacerbating not only the extent and persistence of overweight, but also social distancing from peers.

Schools are the natural environment for children. Primary care providers should attempt to influence community school programs to establish physical education programs to address the activity capabilities and needs of all children, including children who are overweight and obese.

Sexuality

Teens who are overweight often face additional challenges related to his or her developing concept of personal sexuality. In comparison with average-weight female teens, adolescent girls who are obese are less likely to date because of fewer dating opportunities available to them. In addition, both adolescent males and females report greater dissatisfaction with their dating status than do their normal-weight counterparts (Chen & Brown, 2005). Thus obesity may exert a negative influence on the teen's ability to develop intimate romantic relationships (Halpern, Udry, Campbell, et al., 1999; Pearce, Borgers, & Prinstein, 2002). Not surprisingly, a study of college students revealed that obesity stigmatization continues during young adulthood. Individuals who are obese are rated by college students as the least preferred sexual partners; males ranked women who were obese significantly lower as preferred sexual partners than females did for males who were obese (Chen & Brown, 2005). However, views of physical attractiveness are culture bound. Race and ethnicity have been associated with total body and weight esteem. Some ethnic groups prefer the more "robust or Mona Lisa" look for adolescent females and label that look as "sexy" and physically attractive (Komblau, Pearson, & Breitkopf, 2007).

In a study of 522 black adolescent females that controlled for BMI, researchers demonstrated a relationship between being dissatisfied with one's body image and never using condoms during sexual intercourse and being more likely to engage in unprotected vaginal sex (Wingood, DiClemente, Harrington, et al., 2002). For adolescent females in this study, BMI per se was not a risk factor for unintended pregnancy; rather, a negative body image was the greatest risk factor.

The selection of a contraceptive for an adolescent female who is obese should take into consideration some contraceptives' potential for added weight gain or decreased efficacy in overweight women. For instance, the Evra contraceptive patch is less effective in women weighing more than 90 kg, and medroxyprogesterone acetate (Depo-Provera) has the disadvantage of weight gain associated with its use (Gerlt & Starr, 2009).

Being overweight has been linked with earlier secondary sexual development in females compared with their peers who are not overweight (Cesario & Hughes, 2007). Changes in body image brought on by the emergence of early sexual maturation in girls can be a source of anxiety for these children and result in increased teasing. Similarly, pseudogynecomastia caused by excess adipose tissue rather than excess glandular tissue, is associated with obesity and often is viewed as an embarrassment for the overweight adolescent male. Teens with this problem are commonly self-conscious and reluctant to go without a heavy shirt to cover their chest.

Transition to Adulthood

Many of the principles on transition of the adolescent who is overweight or obese to adult services are similar to transitioning of all adolescents with chronic health conditions (see Chapter 4). The teen who is obese or at risk for overweight typically has chronic health care issues that are likely to continue and often worsen during adulthood as excessive weight gain continues. Finding an adult primary health care provider who is willing and able to work effectively with teens or young adults who are overweight is challenging. With age and advancing weight, coexisting physical health conditions such as increased cholesterol levels, hypertension, type 2 diabetes, orthopedic conditions that impair mobility, and a host of other problems may either emerge or become more severe, requiring more medical interventions and care by specialists (Morrison, Friedman, Wang, et al., 2007). The pediatric primary care provider should assist the family in selecting an adult primary care provider who enjoys working with young adults and has a reputation for effectively working with adults who are overweight.

Key to transition planning for adolescents who are overweight or obese is the provision of education about the need for a lifelong commitment to obtaining and maintaining an appropriate weight through healthy diet patterns and eating behaviors and daily physical activity (Menschik, Ahmed, Alexander, et al., 2008). During adolescence, the pediatric primary care provider should strive to establish an effective relationship with the adolescent that supports the teen's engagement in learning about the risks accompanying obesity and their crucial role in making the commitment to important lifestyle changes for the teen's best health. Both parents and the clinician should ensure the adolescent's knowledge of his or her own health history and family health history and health record. Adolescents should also be provided with and encouraged to keep and understand their health records, including growth charts, blood pressure readings, and diagnostic tests and results. Self-management, not restrictions or requirements of others, should be emphasized.

Developing a practice's directory of local community resources for youths and adults who are overweight, such as facilities for exercise with flexible payment plans and weight management programs such as Weight Watchers, is helpful in transitioning the adolescent to adult independent care. Recommending support groups such as Overeaters Anonymous (OA), which has both a youth and an adult program, may be beneficial and provides the message that self-management must be a lifelong strategy for weight control. OA has a brochure for children 10 years of age and under, *The Twelve Steps and Twelve Traditions of Overeaters Anonymous: A Kids View* (2008) (www.oa.org/pdf/A_Kids_View.pdf).

Family Concerns

Clinicians often view counseling of parents and children about the prevention and treatment of overweight and obesity as a challenging task. Parents and children who recognize the need for lifestyle change may also feel overwhelmed and unable to reverse unhealthful habits and behaviors that are part of their daily lives and routines.

The clinician must collaborate with parents and their child to develop an action plan that will provide them with a sense of empowerment. First, it must be determined if the parents recognize lifestyle factors that put their child at risk for being overweight and the potential long-term health risks. Some ethnic groups view a "chubby" baby as being ideal or healthy, and a thin baby or child as less healthy (Crawford, Story, Wang, et al., 2001; McArthur, Anguiano, & Gross, 2004). Families with multiple family members who are overweight may also not recognize the health risks, but attribute their size to family physical characteristics instead of lifestyle patterns (Wardle, Robb, Johnson, et al., 2004). The clinician may encounter major resistance from parents who do not believe that the BMI standards used to determine overweight are appropriate standards for their child (West, Raczynski, Phillips, et al., 2008).

Parents may be more motivated to seek healthier eating practices and to provide increased opportunities for physical activity for their child when they realize not only the health consequences but also the negative social consequences for the child of being overweight. Interestingly, parents and children often express more concerns about the visible signs of obesity, such as acanthosis nigricans and striae and want to know how they can "remove" these unsightly skin markings, than they do about the long-term health consequences.

Making significant changes in lifestyle is a complex process. Recognition that there is a problem requiring change is the first step in this process. At each and every health visit, primary care providers should offer support and encouragement for taking action, assist the family and child in exploring barriers to action, build confidence in taking action, and work with them on a concrete plan for action that works in their lives once they are ready to move forward.

Uncovering parental perceptions and concerns about what would be required to change to more healthful nutrition and physical activity facilitates the change process. Many parents and children believe a "radical starvation" diet will be imposed making them always feel hungry, or that the changes will mark them as "different" from other children.

Children who are obese may be just as resistant to counseling about physical activity and incorporating this into their lives as they may be to adopting more healthful food choices. Recommendations for increased physical activity are often thought to mean doing strenuous exercise they feel incapable of doing. It is important to discuss acceptable types of enjoyable physical activity that appeal to them and a gradual but planned increase in daily physical activity and decrease in screen time. The most successful solutions and choices come from the parents and children themselves.

Unfortunately, there are no easy solutions for preventing and treating overweight in today's society. The primary care provider's challenge is to skillfully support parents and children in building the confidence and competence to take effective action for the best health of all family members.

Resources

Parents

Baylor University's Nutritional Research Center

Offers calculators for child and adult BMI, Healthy Eating Calculator, Kids Energy Calculator, and a weblink to the popular Portion Distortion Quiz.

Website: www.bcm.edu/cnrc

CDC: Activity

Contains a wealth of information about understanding the need for daily physical activity and ways to ensure that you are expending enough calories each day safely. Includes many interactive features.

Website: www.cdc.gov/nccdphp/dnpa/physical/measuring

CDC: Fruits and Vegetables

Information on fruits and vegetables, recipes, and helpful ideas on increasing their consumption.

Website: www.fruitsandveggiesmorematters.gov

Child Development Institute

Provides excellent resources such as *Good Nutrition for Kids and Teens,* an informational fact sheet.

Website: www.childdevelopmentinfo.com/health_safety/nutrition.shtml

Children's Hospitals—Information Sites

Here is a list of some children's hospitals that provide websites with outstanding information for parents and their children about overweight, physical activity, and nutrition. Enter the website and search for health information/topic and overweight or obesity.

Arkansas Children's Hospital

Website: www.archildrens.org

Children's Hospital Boston

Website: www.childrenshospital.org

The Children's Hospital of Philadelphia

Website: www.chop.edu

Cincinnati Children's Hospital

Website: www.cincinnatichildrens.org

Seattle Children's Hospital

Website: www.seattlechildrens.org

Gerber Parents Resource Center

Has an excellent resource for parents titled *Start Healthy*™ Feeding Plan. The booklet discusses the what, when, and how to feed babies and toddlers. The information comes in both English and Spanish versions.

Website: www.gerber.com

KidsHealth

Parents site: Fact sheets and helpful suggestions for parents about this problem.

Website: www.kidshealth.org/Search01.jsp

Nutrition.gov

Great tips on shopping, meal planning, and recipes.

Website: www.nutrition.gov/nal_display/index.php?info_center=11&tax_level=1

Parents Action for Children

This website offers parents information (booklets and DVDs) in English and Spanish about raising healthy children.

Website: http://parentsaction.org

USDA Food and Nutrition Service

Site designed for parents and caregivers to provide information on healthy eating, being more physically active, and acting as a role model for children. A very useful resource is their *Eat Smart. Play Hard ™ Healthy Lifestyle.*

Website: www.fns.usda.gov/eatsmartplayhardhealthylifestyle/Default.htm

We Can

Terrific website with a great deal of information and interactive features about childhood overweight and prevention of obesity. Many practical tips and resources.

Website: www.nhlbi.nih.gov/health/public/heart/obesity/wecan/learn-it/index.htm

Zero to Three

Provides practical information for parents about health, nutrition, and physical activity.

Website: www.zerotothree.org/site/PageServer

School-Age Children

Connect for Kids

A healthy eating and active living website for parents and children. It uses technology to interest and educate school-age children about nutrition and physical activity.

Website: www.kidnetic.com

Connect for Kids' obesity resource advocacy site has information and activities for school-age children ages 9 and older. It provides physical activity and nutrition advice, activities, and links to other related sites.

Website: www.connectforkids.org/obesity_resource

Kids-Health

Fact sheets and helpful suggestions for children about this problem.

Website: www.kidshealth.org/Search01.jsp

MyPyramid

A site with recipes, information, and activities for children.

Website: www.mypyramid.gov/kids/index.html

Nutrition Explorations

Interactive and colorful way to learn about healthful eating. Recipes and activities are included.

Website: www.nutritionexplorations.org/kids/nutrition-main.asp

VERB: It's what you do

Information on being physically active. There are six games you can customize for yourself.

Website: www.verbnow.com

Adolescents

Connect for Kids

Obesity resource for teens. It provides physical activity and nutrition advice, activities, and links to other related sites.

Website: www.connectforkids.org/obesity_resource

Kids-Health

Fact sheets and helpful suggestions for teens about this problem.

Website: www.kidshealth.org/Search01.jsp

Clinicians

Access to Child and Teen BMI Calculator

Information about nutrition, physical activity, and obesity.

Website: www.cdc.gov/nccdphp/dnpa/obesity/childhood

Website: www.cdc.gov/nccdphp/dnpa/obesity

Action for Healthy Kids

A nonprofit organization dedication to addressing the epidemic of overweight, undernourished, and sedentary youth.

Website: www.actionforhealthykids.org

American Academy of Pediatrics (AAP) Overweight and Obesity Website

Contains family, community, and professional resources.

Website: www.aap.org/healthtopics/overweight.cfm

American School Food Service Association/School Nutrition Association

Lists many key articles and resources related to overweight in schoolchildren.

Website: www.schoolnutrition.org:8765/query.html?col=snasite&col=snafiles&qt=overweight%20in%20children&charset=iso-8859-1

Centers for Disease Control and Prevention (CDC): Healthy Youth: Health Topics Childhood Overweight

Information about prevalence, science-based strategies, policy guidance, and national, state, and local programs.

Website: www.cdc.gov/HealthyYouth/overweight

NAPNAP

The National Association of Pediatric Nurse Practitioner (NAP-NAP) developed clinical practice guidelines to assist clinicians in the prevention of overweight in children. Healthy Eating and Activity Together (HEAT™) can be ordered online. This clinical practice guideline is also available through the Agency for Healthcare Quality and Research (www.ahrq.gov). NAPNAP also has an informative brochure that is a nutritional guide for infants and children entitled *Starting Solids.*

Website: www.napnap.org

National Alliance for Nutrition and Activity (NANA)—Model School Wellness Policies

This website provides information about the model school wellness policies related to nutrition and physical activity for children in school settings. Model school wellness policies are identified.

Website: www.schoolwellnesspolicies.org

USDA Food and Nutrition Service

Lists of key studies about nutrition and overweight in children.

Website: http://65.216.150.153/texis/search?pr=FNS

This site also contains a wealth of information for parents and children of all ages regarding nutrition, including food pyramids. Search for "childhood overweight."

Website: www.usda.gov

U.S. Department of Health and Human Services (National Institute of Health) Weight-control Information Network (WIN)

Provides excellent resources (booklets) on the topic of overweight, physical activity and weight control for health professionals and the general public.

Website: http://win.niddk.nih.gov

Summary of Primary Care Needs for the Child with Obesity

HEALTH CARE MAINTENANCE
Growth and Development
- Regular measures of growth and their plotting are key to alerting the clinician and family about changes in the growth pattern presaging the onset or the worsening of overweight and obesity.
- Measure height and weight at each visit and plot them on the 2000 CDC growth charts.
- Calculate the BMI and plot it on the growth chart for all children 2 years of age and older.
- Plot weight-for-length for infants and toddlers ≤ 2 years of age.
- Review the growth chart with the parent, older child, and adolescent, explaining meaning.
- Alert parents, older children, and adolescents to excessive weight gain.
- Review daily nutrition, physical activity level, and amount of screen time when upward changes become evident across weight and BMI percentiles.

Diet
- Educate parents, older children, and adolescents about the need to balance energy intake from food with energy output in physical activity.
- Provide regular nutritional counseling at every well-child visit in literacy-friendly ways, adapting advice to the family's culture.
- Encourage and support new mothers to choose breastfeeding.
- Encourage cue-based feeding throughout infancy at home and in child care.
- Instruct parents to avoid using food as a reward, eating for comfort, and negative or coercive feeding practices that promote excessive weight gain.
- Set a regular schedule for meals, including daily breakfast, and snacks and provide only healthful foods.
- Allow the child to determine whether or not to eat and how much to eat if he or she is eating.
- Serve meals at the family table as often as possible.
- Serve a low-fat diet rich in fruits, vegetables, whole grains, sources of calcium, and lean meat, fish, or vegetable protein.

Safety
- Assist the family in securing a safety seat system for their vehicle that best protects the child because many seats have weight limits.
- Prepare the family and child with anticipatory guidance about best ways to handle bullying and teasing about the child's weight.
- Promote local school policies that ensure a violence-free environment for all children.

Immunizations
- Routine immunizations are recommended.

Screening
- *Vision.* Routine screening is recommended for children without type 2 diabetes.
  - Thorough ophthalmologic evaluation is recommended at least annually for children with type 2 diabetes, and more often with changes in vision.
- *Hearing.* Routine screening is recommended.

- *Dental.* Routine screening is recommended.
  - Caries may be more prevalent among overweight children with a high sugar intake.
- *Blood pressure.* Blood pressure should be obtained at least annually, preferably at every health visit.
  - Blood pressure should be compared to norms established by NHLBI for gender, age, and height for both diastolic and systolic pressure.
  - If the blood pressure is ≥ the 90th percentile, two more pressures should be obtained at 10- to 15-minute intervals during the visit. If the blood pressure remains elevated, the child should return weekly for 3 weeks for blood pressure measurement to establish the diagnosis of hypertension.
  - If the child receives the diagnosis of hypertension, offer counseling on weight loss, nutrition quality, and increased physical activity. Recheck the blood pressure in a month.
  - If 6 months of diet and activity therapy fail to result in weight loss and a drop in blood pressure below the 90th percentile, refer the child for specialist care.
- *Hematocrit.* Routine screening is recommended.
  - Screen more often if the nutrition history indicates a diet low in iron sources, the child is on a severely restricted diet, or the child has had bariatric surgery.
- *Urinalysis.* Routine screening is recommended.
  - For children 10 years of age or older who are obese with a positive family history of type 2 diabetes, annual urine screens for ketones and glucose are warranted.
  - More frequent urine screening is also appropriate for obese children with constipation, enuresis, or encopresis.
- *Tuberculosis.* Routine screening is recommended.

Condition-Specific Screening
- *Lipids.* Serum lipid screening is recommended for children who are overweight or obese with a positive family history of dyslipidemia, high cholesterol, early heart disease requiring a palliative procedure, or early death from heart disease, before age 55 in men and age 65 in women.
  - If the random screen reveals lipid abnormalities, a fasting serum lipid panel should be obtained.
  - If the fasting lipid panel reveals elevated triglycerides and LDL cholesterol or a low HDL cholesterol value, evaluate the child's diet and activity patterns. Instruct the family and child on needed changes, because weight loss and increased physical activity are often effective treatments for dyslipidemias.
  - If values remain elevated, refer to a lipid specialist for management.
- *Glucose and insulin testing.* Fasting serum glucose and glucose tolerance testing should be obtained for the child who is overweight or obese with a positive family history for type 2 diabetes, or if the child has acanthosis nigricans, tachycardia and excessive sweating at rest, or polydipsia and polyuria.
  - For the overweight or obese child with a negative family history for type 2 diabetes and in the absence of the signs and symptoms listed above, fasting glucose levels and oral glucose tolerance testing should begin at 10 years of age and be repeated every 2 years or sooner with a change in family history or the child's presentation.

Continued

Summary of Primary Care Needs for the Child with Obesity—cont'd

- Insulin levels are not established for children of varying ages and different genders; therefore insulin levels are not recommended at this time.
- *Thyroid function tests.* Routine thyroid tests are not recommended for children who are overweight and obese in the absence of signs and symptoms of hypothyroidism such as bradycardia, thyroid enlargement, impaired linear growth, and a BMI ≥ the 97th percentile.

COMMON ILLNESS MANAGEMENT

Differential Diagnosis

- *Respiratory disorders.* Viral infections of the upper respiratory tract may provoke asthma exacerbations. Primary care providers should annually update the overweight and obese asthmatic child's asthma care plan and assess child and parent knowledge and skill in the use of medications and delivery systems. Assure rescue inhalers are available at home and school and that they have not expired.
  - Overweight and obese children with asthma should receive the flu vaccine annually.
- *Skin rashes.* Children who are overweight and obese children are prone to both fungal and staphylococcal skin infections.
  - It is important to culture wound drainage to identify MRSA-positive skin infections to ensure effective treatment.

Drug Interactions

- *Orlistat* or *Allī* should not be taken within 2 hours of the immune suppressant cyclosporine because it alters the blood level of the immune suppressant.
- *Sibutramine* should not be combined with selective serotonin reuptake inhibitors (SSRIs) or monoamine oxidase inhibitor (MAOI) drugs because this may provoke suicidal ideation, suicide, or serotonin storm.
  - Over-the-counter cough and cold medications containing decongestants should be avoided when taking sibutramine because they may augment the vasoconstrictive and hypertensive effects of sibutramine.
  - Caution should also be used in prescribing migraine medications and opiates for children using sibutramine.
- *Metformin* serum levels are increased by 40% when cimetidine is taken concomitantly.
- Hyperglycemia occurs when *sulfonylurea drugs* are taken with estrogen-containing medications, antibiotics, antihypertensives, rifampin, MAOI drugs, dilantin, thiazide and phenothiazide diuretics, prednisone, and thyroid supplements.
- Hypoglycemia occurs when *sulfonylurea drugs* are taken with alcohol or oral miconazole.

DEVELOPMENTAL ISSUES

Sleep Patterns

- Many children and adolescents who are overweight have disordered sleep patterns, hypoventilation syndrome, and obstructive sleep apnea. Adequacy of sleep and the presence of symptoms such as snoring should be assessed for at each wellness visit. Referrals may be necessary for sleep studies or evaluation for tonsillectomy and adenoidectomy.
- Poor quality of sleep is associated with problems in memory and behavior. Sleep disorders should be considered with reports of school failure or behavior problems.

Toileting

- Constipation is more common among overweight and obese children who lack adequate levels of physical activity and fiber in the diet.
- Enuresis and encopresis, as well as bladder infections, are more common among children with constipation.
- Orlistat and Allī may cause uncontrollable diarrhea.

Discipline

- Parents of children who are overweight need detailed counseling on reasonable limits on food and beverage purchases and choices, as well as limiting the child's amount of screen time.
- Advise parents to monitor and support 60 minutes of daily active play and moderate to vigorous physical activity. Being active together as a family is important.
- Advise parents to avoid the use of food or sedentary time as rewards. Recommend family activities, stickers, or just special time with the parents as appropriate rewards.
- Help identify parents' concerns regarding needed family lifestyle changes and barriers to change.

Child Care

- Advise parents to carefully evaluate feeding and activity practices in child care and preschool settings, selecting providers who respect infant cues for feeding, offer only healthful food and snacks, and ensure regular active play throughout the day.
- In preschool, providers should be alert to recognizing and effectively dealing with teasing or exclusion of overweight peers from play groups.

Schooling

- Overweight and obese children are at increased risk for poor academic performance, possibly as a consequence of impaired sleep.
- Overweight and obese children are also frequently the victims of bullying and teasing that damages self-esteem. Children and parents need counseling and support to address these difficult situations.
- Many children who are overweight or obese are embarrassed to participate in physical education classes and sports. It is important to work with schools to include children of all levels of ability and skill in physical education and sports.

Sexuality

- Overweight and obese adolescents of both genders are less likely to view themselves as attractive and seldom have the social and dating experiences they desire to have.
- Effective contraception may be more difficult to achieve for females who are obese because some contraceptives are less effective in overweight females and many hormone-based options promote weight gain.
- Early pubarche is common, especially in girls. They require sensitive education and guidance about the care of their changing bodies and handling social pressures.
- Gynecomastia is a concerning and embarrassing problem for many obese males.

Transition to Adulthood

- Clinicians should assist the adolescent in finding an adult health care provider with expertise in the care of overweight and obese young adults.

Summary of Primary Care Needs for the Child with Obesity—cont'd

- Young adults need to be assisted in assuming responsibility for independent self-management of a healthful diet and physically active lifestyle, as well as the management of any comorbid conditions.
- Primary care providers need to develop a ready list of community resources to support healthful nutrition, cooking and shopping skills, and physical activity.

FAMILY CONCERNS

- A collaborative partnership with the family is the most effective way to approach significant lifestyle change to improve child health.
- Cultural barriers and family concerns must be explored and plans of care adapted to the concerns, needs, and preferences of each family and child.
- Families should be active partners in developing the plan of care for lifestyle change at home.

REFERENCES

Abramson, N.W., Wamboldt, F.S., Mansell, A.L., et al. (2008). Frequency and correlates of overweight status in adolescent asthma. *J Asthma, 45,* 135-139.

Alberti, G., Zimmer, P., Shaw, J., et al., for the Consensus Work Group. (2004). Type 2 diabetes in the young: The evolving epidemic. The International Diabetes Federation Consensus Workshop. *Diabetes Care, 27,* 1798-1811.

Allison, D.B., Kaprio, J., Korkeila, M., et al. (1996). The heritability of body mass index among an international sample of monozygotic twins reared apart. *Int J Obes Relat Metab Disord, 20,* 501-506.

American Medical Association (AMA). (2007). *Expert Committee recommendations on the assessment, treatment, and prevention of child and adolescent overweight and obesity.* Available at www.ama-ssn.org/ama1/pub/upload/mm/433/ped_obesity_recs.pdf. Retrieved June 25, 2008.

Anderson, P.M., & Butcher, K.F. (2006). Childhood obesity: Trends and potential causes. *Future Child, 16,* 19-45.

Andrews, J.A., Peterson, M.A., & Duncan, S.C. (2007). A cognitive-behavioral mechanism leading to adolescent obesity: Children's social images and physical activity. *Ann Behav Med, 34,* 287-294.

Apovian, C.M., Baker, C., Ludwig, D.S., et al. (2005). Best practice guidelines in pediatric/adolescent weight loss surgery. *Obesity Res, 13,* 274-282.

Atkin, L.M., & Davies, P.S. (2000). Diet composition and body composition in preschool children. *Am J Clin Nutr, 72,* 15-21.

Ausk, K.J., & Ioannou, G.N. (2008). Is obesity associated with anemia of chronic disease? A population-based study. *Obesity, 16*(10), 2356-2361.

Barlow, S.E., & Expert Committee (2007). Expert Committee recommendations regarding the prevention, assessment, and treatment of child and adolescent overweight and obesity: Summary report. *Pediatrics, 120,* S164-S192.

Bellisari, A. (2008). Evolutionary origins of obesity. *Obesity Rev, 9,* 165-180.

Berkey, C.S., Rockett, H.R.H., Gillman, M.W., et al. (2003). One-year changes in activity and in inactivity among 10- to 15-year-old boys and girls: Relationship to change in body mass index. *Pediatrics, 111,* 836-843.

Berkowitz, R.I., Fujioka, K., Daniels, S.R., et al. (2006). Effects of sibutramine treatment in obese adolescents: A randomized trial. *Ann Intern Med, 145,* 81-90.

Berkowitz, R.I., Wadden, T.A., Tershakovec, A.M., et al. (2003). Behavior therapy and sibutramine for the treatment of adolescent obesity: A randomized controlled trial. *J Am Med Assoc, 289,* 1805-1812.

Bertisch, S.M., Wee, C.C., & McCarthy, E.P. (2008). Use of complementary and alternative therapies by overweight and obese adults. *Obesity, 16,* 1610-1615.

Beunen, G., & Thomis, M. (2006). Gene driven power athletes? Genetic variation in muscular strength and power. *Br J Sports Med, 40,* 822-823.

Birch, L.L., Fisher, J.O., & Davison, K.K. (2003). Learning to overeat: Maternal use of restrictive feeding practices promotes girls' eating in the absence of hunger. *Am J Clin Nutr, 78,* 215-220.

Blank, S.K., Helm, K.D., McCartney, C.R., et al. (2008). Polycystic ovary syndrome in adolescence. *Ann N Y Acad Sci, 1135,* 76-84.

Block, J.P., Scribner, R.A., & DeSalvo, K.B. (2004). Fast food, race/ethnicity, and income: A geographic analysis. *Am J Prev Med, 27,* 211-217.

Borecki, I.B., Higgins, M., Schreiner, P.J., et al. (1998). Evidence for multiple determinants of the body mass index: the National Heart, Lung, and Blood Institute Family Heart Study. *Obesity Res, 6,* 107-114.

Boynton-Jarrett, R., Thomas, T.N., Peterson, K.E., et al. (2003). Impact of television viewing patterns on fruit and vegetable consumption among adolescents. *Pediatrics, 112*(6), 1321-1326.

Bray, G.A., Nielsen, S.J., & Popkin, B.M. (2004). Consumption of high-fructose corn syrup in beverages may play a role in the epidemic of obesity. *Am J Clin Nutr, 79,* 537-543.

Briefel, R.R., Reidy, K., Karwe, V., et al. (2004). Toddlers' transition to table foods: Impact on nutrient intakes and food patterns. *J Am Diet Assoc, 104,* S38-S44.

Buddeberg-Fischer, B., Klaghofer, R., Krug, L., et al. (2006). Physical and psychosocial outcome in morbidly obese patients with and without bariatric surgery: A 4 1/2-year follow-up. *Obesity Surg, 16,* 321-330.

Butte, N.F., Puyau, M.R., Adolph, A.L., et al. (2007). Physical activity in non-overweight and overweight Hispanic children and adolescents. *Med Sci Sports Exerc, 39,* 1257-1266.

Buyken, A.E., Karaolis-Danckert, N., Remer, T., et al. (2008). Effects of breast-feeding on trajectories of body fat and BMI throughout childhood. *Obesity, 16,* 389-395.

Caballero, B., Clay, T., Davis, S.M., et al. (2003). Pathways: A school-based, randomized controlled trial for the prevention of obesity in American Indian schoolchildren. *Am J Clin Nutr, 78,* 1030-1038.

Cabioglu, M.T., & Ergene, N. (2006). Changes in levels of serum insulin, C-peptide and glucose after electroacupuncture and diet therapy in obese women. *Am J Chin Med, 34,* 367-376.

Cawley, J., & Liu, F. (2008). Correlates of state legislative action to prevent childhood obesity. *Obesity, 16*(1), 162-167.

Cerniak, E.P. (2008). Potential applications for alternative medicine to treat obesity in an aging population. *Alternat Med Rev, 13,* 34-42.

Cesario, S.K., & Hughes, L.A. (2007). Precocious puberty: A comprehensive review of literature. *J Obstet Gynecol Neonat Nurs, 36,* 263-274.

Chanoine, J.P., Hampl, S., Jensen, C., et al. (2005). Effect of orlistat on weight and body composition in obese adolescents: A randomized controlled trial. *J Am Med Assoc, 293,* 2873-2883.

Chen, E.Y., & Brown, M. (2005). Obesity stigma in sexual relationships. *Obesity Res, 13,* 1393-1397.

Chen, X., Beydoun, M.A., & Wang, Y. (2008). Is sleep duration associated with childhood obesity? A systematic review and meta-analysis. *Obesity, 16,* 265-274.

Cope, M.B., & Allison, D.B. (2008). Critical review of the World Health Organization's (WHO) 2007 report on evidence of the long-term effects of breastfeeding: Systematic reviews and meta-analysis with respect to obesity. *Obesity Rev, 9.*

Crawford, P.B., Gosliner, W., Anderson, C., et al. (2004). Counseling Latina mothers of preschool children about weight issues: Suggestions for a new framework. *J Am Diet Assoc, 104,* 387-394.

Crawford, P.D., Story, M., Wang, M.C., et al. (2001). Ethnic issues in the epidemiology of childhood obesity. *Pediatr Clin North Am, 48,* 855-878.

Danhauer, S.C., Oliveira, B., Myll, J., et al. (2004). Successful dietary changes in a cardiovascular risk reduction intervention are differentially predicted by biopsychosocial characteristics. *Prev Med, 39,* 783-790.

Daniels, S.R., Greer, F.R., & Committee on Nutrition (2008). Lipid screening and cardiovascular health in childhood. *Pediatrics, 122,* 198-208.

Dansinger, M.L., Gleason, J.A., Griffith, J.L., et al. (2005). Comparison of the Atkins, Ornish, Weight Watchers, and Zone diets for weight loss and heart disease risk reduction: A randomized trial. *J Am Med Assoc, 293,* 43-53.

de Jongh, S., Lilien, M.R., op't Roodt, J., et al. (2002). Early statin therapy restores endothelial function in children with familial hypercholesterolemia. *J Am Coll Cardiol, 40*(12), 2122-2124.

de Jongh, S., Ose, L., Szamosi, T., et al. (2002). Efficacy and safety of statin therapy in children with familial hypercholesterolemia: A randomized, double-blind, placebo-controlled trial with simvastatin. *Circulation, 106,* 2231-2237.

DeLaney, J.P., Bray, G.A., Harsha, D.W., et al. (2004). Energy expenditure in African American and white boys and girls in a 2-y follow-up of the Baton Rouge children's study. *Am J Clin Nutr, 79,* 268-273.

Diliberti, N., Bordi, P.L., Conklin, M.T., et al. (2004). Increased portion size leads to increased energy intake in a restaurant meal. *Obesity Res, 12,* 562-568.

Dubois, L., Farmer, A., Girard, M., et al. (2008). Social factors and television use during meals and snacks is associated with higher BMI among pre-school children. *Public Health Nutr, 12,* 1-13.

Dunn, A.L., Trivedi, M.H., Kampert, J.B., et al. (2005). Exercise treatment for depression: Efficacy and dose response. *Am J Prev Med, 28,* 1-8.

Durmer, J.S., & Dinges, D.F. (2005). Neurocognitive consequences of sleep deprivation. *Semin Neurol, 25,* 117-129.

Eaton, D.K., Lowry, R., Brener, N.D., et al. (2005). Associations of body mass index and perceived weight with suicide ideation and suicide attempts among US high school students. *Arch Pediatr Adolesc Med, 159,* 513-519.

Eisenberg, M., & Neumark-Sztainer, D. (2008). Peer harassment and disordered eating. *Int J Adolesc Med Health, 20,* 155-164.

Ekelund, U., Yngve, A., Brage, S., et al. (2004). Body movement and physical activity energy expenditure in children and adolescents: How to adjust for differences in body size and age. *Am J Clin Nutr, 79,* 851-856.

Elliott, S.S., Keim, N.L., Stern, J.S., et al. (2002). Fructose, weight gain, and the insulin resistance syndrome. *Am J Clin Nutr, 76,* 911-922.

Epstein, L.H., Paluch, R.A., Beecher, M.D., et al. (2008). Increasing healthy eating vs. reducing high energy-dense foods to treat pediatric obesity. *Obesity, 16*(2), 318-326.

Epstein, L.H., Paluch, R.A., Kilanowski, C.K., et al. (2004). The effect of reinforcement or stimulus control to reduce sedentary behavior in the treatment of pediatric obesity. *Health Psychol, 23,* 371-380.

Epstein, L.H., Paluch, R.A., Roemmich, J.N., et al. (2007). Family-based obesity treatment, then and now: Twenty-five years of pediatric obesity treatment. *Health Psychol, 26,* 381-391.

Epstein, L.H., Roemmich, J.N., Robinson, J.L., et al. (2008). A randomized trial of the effects of reducing television viewing and computer use on body mass index in young children. *Arch Pediatr Adolesc Med, 162,* 239-245.

Evans, W.D., Finkelstein, E., Kamerow, D.B., et al. (2005). Public perceptions of childhood obesity. *Am J Prev Med, 28,* 26-32.

Faith, M.S., Calamaro, C., Dolan, M.S., et al. (2004). Mood disorders and obesity. *Curr Opin Psychiatry, 17*(1), 9-13.

Faith, M.S., Leone, M.A., Ayers, T.S., et al. (2002). Weight criticism during physical activity, coping skills, and reported physical activity in children. *Pediatrics, 110*(2), e23.

Falkner, N.H., Neumark-Sztainer, D., Story, M., et al. (2001). Social, educational, and psychological correlates of weight status in adolescents. *Obesity Res, 9,* 32-42.

Farrow, C.V., & Blissett, J. (2008). Controlling feeding practices: Cause or consequence of early child weight? *Pediatrics, 121,* e164-e169.

Faulkner, B., Gidding, S.S., Portman, R., et al. (2008). Blood pressure variability and classification of prehypertension and hypertension in adolescence. *Pediatrics, 122,* 238-242.

Finkelstein, D.M., Hill, E.L., & Whitaker, R.C. (2008). School food environments and policies in US public schools. *Pediatrics, 122,* e251-e259.

Finkelstein, E., Fiebelkorn, I.C., & Wang, G. (2003). National medical spending attributable to overweight and obesity: How much, and who's paying?. *Health Aff, 3,* 219-226.

Finkelstein, E., French, S., Variyam, J.N., et al. (2004). Pros and cons of proposed interventions to promote healthy eating. *Am J Prev Med, 27*(3S), 163-171.

Fisher, J.O., Rolls, B.J., & Birch, L.L. (2003). Children's bite size and intake of an entrée are greater with large portions than with age-appropriate or self-selected portions. *Am J Clin Nutr, 77,* 1164-1170.

Fitzgibbon, M.L., & Stolley, M.R. (2004). Environmental changes may be needed for prevention of overweight in minority children. *Pediatr Ann, 33*(1), 45-49.

Fogelholm, M. (2008). How physical activity can work? *Int J Pediatr Obesity, 3*(S1), 10-14.

Ford, E.S., Mokdad, A.H., & Ajani, U.A. (2004). Trends in risk factors for cardiovascular disease among children and adolescents in the United States. *Pediatrics, 114*(6), 1534-1544.

Franko, D.L., Affenito, S.G., Thompson, D., et al. (2008). What mediates the relationship between family meals and adolescent health issues? *Health Psychol, 27,* S109-S117.

Freedman, D.S., Khan, L.K., Mei, Z., et al. (2002). Relation of childhood height to obesity among adults: The Bogalusa Heart Study. *Pediatrics, 109,* e23-e29.

Freedman, D.S., Khan, L.K., Serdula, M.K., et al. (2005). The relation of childhood BMI to adult adiposity: The Bogalusa Heart Study. *Pediatrics, 115,* 22-27.

Freedman, D.S., Wang, J., Thornton, J.C., et al. (2008). Racial/ethnic differences in body fatness among children and adolescents. *Obesity, 16*(5), 1105-1111.

Fulkerson, J.A., Neumark-Sztainer, D., Hannan, P.J., et al. (2008). Family meal frequency and weight status among adolescents: Cross-sectional and 5-year longitudinal associations. *Obesity. 16,* 2529-2534.

Gable, S., Britt-Rankin, J., & Krull, J.L. (2008). *Ecological predictors and developmental outcomes of persistent childhood overweight.* United States Department of Agriculture. Contractor and Cooperator Report No, 42. June (2002).

Gable, S., Chang, Y., & Krull, J.L. (2007). Television watching and frequency of family meals are predictive of overweight onset and persistence in a national sample of school-aged children. *J Am Diet Assoc, 107,* 53-61.

Gahagan, S., & Silverstein, J. (2003). Prevention and treatment of type 2 diabetes mellitus in children, with special emphasis on American Indian and Alaska Native children. *Pediatrics, 112,* e328.

Gardner, C.D., Kiazand, A., Alhassan, S., et al. (2007). Comparison of the Atkins, Zone, Ornish, and LEARN diets for change in weight and related risk factors among overweight premenopausal women: The A to Z Weight Loss Study: A randomized trial. *J Am Med Assoc, 297,* 969-977.

Gardner, D.S.L., Hosking, J., Metcalf, B.S., Jeffery, A.N., Voss, L.D., & Wilkin, T.J. (2009). Contribution of early weight gain to childhood overweight and metabolic helth: A longitudinal study (EarlyBird 36). *Pediatrics, 123,* e67-e73.

Gaullier, J.M., Halse, J., Høye, K., et al. (2005). Supplementation with conjugated linoleic acid for 24 months is well tolerated by and reduces body fat mass in healthy, overweight humans. *J Nutr, 135,* 778-784.

Gerlt, T., & Starr, N.B. (2009). Gynecologic conditions. In C.E. Burns, A.M. Dunn, M.A. Brady, et al. (Eds.). *Pediatric Primary Care* (4th ed). St. Louis: Saunders Elsevier.

Gibson, L.J., Peto, J., Warren, J.M., et al. (2006). Lack of evidence on diets for obesity for children: A systematic review. *Int J Epidemiol, 35,* 1544-1552.

Gidding, S.S., Barton, B.A., Dorgan, J.A., et al. (2006). Higher self-reported physical activity is associated with lower systolic blood pressure: The Dietary Intervention Study in Childhood (DISC). *Pediatrics, 118,* 2388-2393.

Gidding, S.S., Dennison, B.A., Birch, L.L., et al. (2005). Dietary recommendations for children and adolescents: A guide for practitioners: Consensus statement from the American Heart Association. *Circulation, 112,* 2061-2075.

Gillman, M.W., Rifas-Shiman, S.L., Berkey, C.S., et al. (2003). Maternal gestational diabetes, birth weight, and adolescent obesity. *Pediatrics, 111,* e221.

Glazebrook, C., McPherson, A.C., MacDonald, I.A., et al. (2006). Asthma as a barrier to children's physical activity: Implications for body mass index and mental health. *Pediatrics, 118,* 2443-2449.

Gluckman, P.D., Hanson, M.A., Beedle, A.S., et al. (2008). Fetal and neonatal pathways to obesity. *Frontiers in Hormonal Research, 36,* 61-72.

Golan, M. (2006). Parents as agents of change in childhood obesity—from research to practice. *Int J Pediatr Obesity, 1*(2), 66-76.

Golan, M., & Crow, S. (2004). Parents are key players in the prevention and treatment of weight-related problems. *Nutr Rev, 62,* 39-50.

Goldschmidt, A.B., Aspen, V.P., Linton, M.M., et al. (2008). Disordered eating attitudes and behaviors in overweight youth. *Obesity, 16,* 257-264.

Gómez, J.G., Johnson, B.A., Selva, M., et al. (2004). Violent crime and outdoor physical activity among inner-city youth. *Prev Med, 39,* 876-881.

Goodman, E., Daniels, S.R., Meigs, J.B., et al. (2007). Instability in the diagnosis of metabolic syndrome in adolescents. *Circulation, 115,* 2316-2322.

Goodman, E., Daniels, S.R., Morrison, J.A., et al. (2004). Contrasting prevalence of and demographic disparities in the World Health Organization and National Cholesterol Education Program Adult Treatment Panel III definitions of metabolic syndrome among adolescents. *J Pediatr, 145,* 445-451.

Gozal, D., & Kheirandish-Gozal, L. (2009). Obesity and excessive daytime sleepiness in prepubertal children with obstructive sleep apnea. *Pediatrics, 123,* 13-18.

Grahm, E.A. (2005). Economic, racial, and cultural influences on the growth and maturation of children. *Pediatr Rev, 26,* 290-294.

Gray, W.N., Janicke, D.M., Ingerski, L.M., et al. (2008). The impact of peer victimization, parent distress and child depression on barrier formation and physical activity in overweight youth. *J Dev Behav Pediatr, 29*, 26-33.

Grummer-Strawn, L.M., & Mei, Z. (2004). Does breastfeeding protect against pediatric overweight? Anaylsis of longitudinal data from the Centers for Disease Control and Prevention pediatric nutrition surveillance system. *Pediatrics, 113*, e81-e86.

Guo, S.S., Wu, W., Chumlea, W.C., et al. (2002). Predicting overweight and obesity in adulthood from body mass index values in childhood and adolescence. *Am J Clin Nutr, 76*, 653-658.

Haaz, S., Fontaine, K.R., Cutter, G., et al. (2006). Citrus aurantium and synephrine alkaloids in the treatment of overweight and obesity: An update. *Obesity Rev, 7*, 79-88.

Hadler, M.C.M., Colugnati, F.A.B., & Sigulem, D.M. (2004). Risks of anemia in infants according to dietary iron density and weight gain rate. *Prev Med, 39*, 713-721.

Halpern, C.T., Udry, J.R., Campbell, B., et al. (1999). Effects of body fat on weight concerns, dating, and sexual activity: A longitudinal analysis of black and white adolescent girls. *Dev Psychol, 35*, 721-736.

Hediger, M.L., Overpeck, M.D., Kuczmarski, R.J., et al. (2001). Association between infant breastfeeding and overweight in young children. *J Am Med Assoc, 285*, 2453-2460.

Heymsfield, S.B., Allison, D.B., Vasselli, J.R., et al. (1998). Garcinia cambogia (hydroxycitric acid) as a potential antiobesity agent: A randomized controlled trial. *J Am Med Assoc, 280*, 1596-1600.

Huang, T.T., Nansel, T.R., Belsheim, A.R., et al. (2007). Sensitivity, specificity, and predictive values of pediatric metabolic syndrome components in relation to adult metabolic syndrome: The Princeton LRC follow-up study. *J Pediatr, 152*, 185-190.

Inge, T.H., Krebs, N.F., Garcia, V.F., et al. (2004). Bariatric surgery for severely overweight adolescents: Concerns and recommendations. *Pediatrics, 114*, 217-223.

Inge, T.H., Zeller, M., Harmon, C., et al. (2007). Teen-longitudinal assessment of bariatric surgery: Methodological features of the first prospective multi-center study of adolescent bariatric surgery. *J Pediatr Surg, 42*, 1969-1971.

Janssen, I., Craig, W.M., Boyce, W.F., et al. (2004). Association between overweight and obesity with bullying behaviors in school-aged children. *Pediatrics, 113*, 1187-1194.

Janssen, I., Katzmarzyk, P.T., Srinivasan, S.R., et al. (2005). Utility of childhood BMI in the prediction of adulthood disease: Comparison of national and international references. *Obesity Res, 13*, 1106-1115.

Jasik, C.B., & Lustig, R.H. (2008). Adolescent obesity and puberty: The "perfect storm." The menstrual cycle and adolescent health. *N Y Acad Sci, 1135*, 265-279.

Johnson-Taylor, W.L., & Everhart, J.E. (2006). Modifiable environmental and behavioral determinants of overweight among children and adolescents: Report of a workshop. *Obesity, 14*, 929-966.

Jones, K.L. (2008). Role of obesity in complicating and confusing the diagnosis and treatment of diabetes in children. *Pediatrics, 121*, 361-368.

Katzmarzyk, P.T., Baur, L.A., Blair, S.N., et al. (2008). International conference on physical activity and obesity in children: Summary statement and recommendations. *Int J Pediatr Obesity, 3*, 3-21.

Kavey, R.E.W., Allada, V., Daniels, S.R., et al. (2006). Cardiovascular risk reduction in high-risk pediatric patients: A scientific statement from the American Heart Association Expert Panel on Population and Prevention Science; the Councils on Cardiovascular Disease in the Young, Epidemiology and Prevention, Nutrition, Physical Activity and Metabolism, High Blood Pressure Research, Cardiovascular Nursing, and the Kidney in Heart Disease; and the Interdisciplinary Working Group on Quality of Care and Outcomes Research: Endorsed by the American Academy of Pediatrics. *Circulation, 114*, 2710-2738.

Kheirandish-Gozal, L., & Gozal, D. (2008). Intranasal budesonide treatment for children with mild obstructive sleep apnea syndrome. *Pediatrics, 122*, e149-e155.

Killion, L., Hughes, S.O., Wendt, J.C., et al. (2006). Minority mothers' perceptions of children's body size. *Int J Pediatr Obesity, 1*, 96-102.

Kim, J., & Peterson, K.K. (2008). Association of infant child care with infant feeding practice and weight gain among US infants. *Arch Pediatr Adolesc Med, 162*, 727-733.

Kimbro, R.T., Brooks-Gunn, J., & McLanahan, S. (2007). Racial and ethnic differences in overweight and obesity among 3-year-old children. *Am J Public Health, 97*, 298-305.

Kirsch, I. (1996). Hypnotic enhancement of cognitive-behavioral weight loss treatments: Another meta-reanalysis. *J Consult Clin Psychol, 64*(3), 517-519.

Komblau, I.S., Pearson, H.C., & Breitkopf, C.R. (2007). Demographic, behavioral, and physical correlates of body esteem among low-income female adolescents. *J Adolesc Health, 41*, 566-570.

Koplan, J.P., Liverman, C.T., & Kroak, V.I. (2005). *Preventing childhood obesity: Health in the balance.* Washington, DC: National Academies Press.

Kramer, M.S., Guo, T., Platt, R.W., et al. (2004). Feeding effects on growth during infancy. *J Pediatr., 145*, 600-605.

Kramer, M.S., Morin, I., Yang, H., et al. (2002). Why are babies getting bigger? Temporal trends in fetal growth and its determinants. *J Pediatr, 141*, 538-542.

Krebs, N.F., Himes, J.H., Jacobson, D., et al. (2007). Assessment of child and adolescent overweight and obesity. *Pediatrics, 120*, S193-S228.

Kropski, J.A., Keckley, P.H., & Jensen, G.L. (2008). School-based obesity prevention programs: An evidence-based review. *Obesity, 16*, 1009-1018.

Kubik, M.Y., Lytle, L.A., Hannan, P.J., et al. (2003). The association of the school food environment with dietary behaviors of young adolescents. *Am J Public Health, 93*, 1168-1173.

Kuczmarski, R.J., Ogden, C.L., Guo, S.S., et al. (2002). CDC growth charts for the United States: Methods and development. *Vital Health Stat, 11*, 1-190.

Kumanyika, S.K. (2008). Environmental influences on childhood obesity: Ethnic and cultural influences in context. *Physiol Behav, 22*(94), 61-70.

Kumanyika, S.K., & Obarzanek, E. (2003). Pathways to obesity prevention: Report of a National Institute of Health workshop. *Obesity Res, 11*, 1263-1274.

Kwiterovich, P.O. (2008). Primary and secondary disorders of lipid metabolism in pediatrics. *Pediatr Endocrinol Rev, 5*(Suppl 2), 727-738.

Lagou, V., Scott, R.A., Manios, Y., et al. (2008). Impact of peroxisome proliferator-activated receptors γ and δ on adiposity in toddlers and pre-schoolers in the GENESIS study. *Obesity, 16*, 913-918.

Larson, N.I., Neumark-Sztainer, D.R., Story, M.T., et al. (2008). Fast food intake: Longitudinal trends during the transition to young adulthood and correlates of intake. *J Adolesc Health, 43*, 79-86.

Latner, J.D., Stunkard, A.J., & Wilson, G.T. (2005). Stigmatized students: Age, sex, and ethnicity effects in the stigmatization of obesity. *Obesity Res, 13*, 1226-1231.

Lavine, J.E., & Schwimmer, J.B. (2004). Nonalcoholic fatty liver disease in the pediatric population. *Clin Liver Dis, 8*, 549-558.

Leatherdale, S.T., & Wong, S.L. (2008). Modifiable characteristics associated with sedentary behaviours among youth. *Int J Pediatr Obesity, 3*, 93-101.

Lee, J.M. (2008). Why young adults hold the key to assessing the obesity epidemic in children. *Arch Pediatr Adolesc Med, 162*, 682-687.

Lemeshow, A.R., Fisher, L., Goodman, E., et al. (2008). Subjective social status in the school and change in adiposity in female adolescents. *Arch Pediatr Adolesc Med, 162*, 23-28.

Libman, I.M., & Arslanian, S.A. (2007). Prevention and treatment of type 2 diabetes in youth. *Horm Res, 67*, 22-34.

Libman, I.M., Sun, K., Foley, T.P., et al. (2008). Thyroid autoimmunity in children with features of both type 1 and type 2 diabetes. *Pediatr Diabetes, 9* (pt 1), 266-271.

Lindsay, A.C., Sussner, K.M., Kim, J., et al. (2006). The role of parents in preventing childhood obesity. *Future Child, 16*, 169-186.

Lissau, I., Overpeck, M.D., Ruan, W.J., et al. (2004). Body mass index and overweight in adolescents in 13 European countries, Israel, and the United States. *Arch Pediatr Adolesc Med, 158*, 27-33.

Litonjua, A.A., & Gold, D.R. (2008). Asthma and obesity: Common early-life influences in the inception of disease. *J Allergy Clin Immunol, 121*, 1075-1084.

Lomenick, J.P., Clasey, J.L., & Anderson, J.W. (2008). Meal-related changes in ghrelin, peptide YY, and appetite in normal weight and overweight children. *Obesity, 16*(3), 547-552.

Lottenberg, S.A., Glezer, A., & Turatti, L.A. (2007). Metabolic syndrome: Identifying the risk factors. *J Pediatr, 83*(5 Suppl), S204-S208.

Louis, G.W., & Myers, M.G. Jr. (2007). The role of leptin in the regulation of neuroendocrine function and CNS development. *Rev Endocr Metab Disord, 8*, 85-94.

Loux, T.J., Haricharan, R.N., Clements, R.H., et al. (2008). Health-related quality of life before and after bariatric surgery in adolescents. *J Pediatr Surg, 43*, 1275-1279.

Love-Osborne, K.A., Nadeau, K.J., Sheeder, J., et al. (2008). Presence of the metabolic syndrome in obese adolescents predicts impaired glucose tolerance and nonalcoholic fatty liver disease. *J Adolesc Health, 42*, 543-548.

Lumeng, J.C. (2008). Mother knows best? Feeding styles and child obesity. *Contemp Pediatr, 25*, 32-48.

Lumeng, J.C., Gannon, K., Appugliese, D., et al. (2005). Preschool child care and risk of overweight in 6- to 12-year-old children. *Int J Obesity*, *29*, 60-66.

Lumeng, J.C., Gannon, K., Cabral, H.J., et al. (2003). Association between clinically meaningful behavior problems and overweight in children. *Pediatrics*, *112*, 1138-1145.

Maclaren, N.K., Gujral, S., Ten, S., et al. (2007). Childhood obesity and insulin resistance. *Cell Biochem Biophysiol*, *48*, 73-78.

Maher, E.J., Li, G., Carter, L., et al. (2008). Preschool child care participation and obesity at the start of kindergarten. *Pediatrics*, *122*, 322-330.

Marton, E., Feletti, A., Mazzucco, G.M., et al. (2008). Pseudotumor cerebri in pediatric age: Role of obesity in the management of neurological impairments. *Nutr Neurosci*, *1*, 25-31.

Matheson, D.M., Killen, J.D., Wang, Y., et al. (2004). Children's food consumption during television viewing. *Am J Clin Nutr*, *79*, 1088-1094.

Mattes, R.D., & Bormann, L. (2000). Effects of (-)-hydroxycitric acid on appetitive variables. *Physiol Behav*, *71*, 87-94.

Matyka, K.A. (2008). Type 2 diabetes in childhood: Epidemiological and clinical aspects. *Br Med Bull*, *86*, 59-75.

McArthur, L.H., Anguiano, R., & Gross, K.H. (2004). Are household factors putting immigrant Hispanic children at risk for becoming overweight: A community-based study in Eastern North Carolina. *J Community Health*, *29*, 387-404.

McCrindle, B.W., Ose, L., & Marais, A.D. (2003). Efficacy and safety of atorvastatin in children and adolescents with familial hypercholesterolemia or severe hyperlipidemia: A multicenter, randomized, placebo-controlled trial. *J Pediatr*, *143*, 74-80.

McCrindle, B.W., Urbina, E.M., Dennison, B.A., et al. (2007). Drug therapy of high-risk lipid abnormalities in children and adolescents: A scientific statement from the American Heart Association Atherosclerosis, Hypertension, and Obesity in Youth Committee, Council of Cardiovascular Disease in the Young, with the Council on Cardiovascular Nursing. *Circulation*, *115*, 1948-1967.

McGavok, J., Sellers, E., & Dean, H. (2007). Physical activity for the prevention and management of youth-onset type 2 diabetes mellitus: Focus on cardiovascular complications. *Diabetes Vasc Dis Res*, *4*, 305-310.

McKenzie, T.L., Baquero, B., Crespo, N.C., et al. (2008). Environmental correlates of physical activity in Mexican American children at home. *J Physical Activity Health*, *5*, 579-591.

McMurray, R.G., Harrell, J.S., Creighton, D., et al. (2008). Influence of physical activity on change in weight status as children become adolescents. *Int J Pediatr Obesity*, *3*, 69-77.

McQueen, M.B., Bertram, L., Rimm, E.B., et al. (2003). A QTL genome scan of the metabolic syndrome and its component traits. *BMC Genet*, *4* (Suppl 1), S96.

Mei, Z., Grummer-Strawn, L.M., Pietrobelli, A., et al. (2002). Validity of body mass index compared with other body-composition screening indexes for the assessment of body fatness in children and adolescents. *Am J Clin Nutr*, *75*, 978-985.

Menschik, D., Ahmed, S., Alexander, M.H., et al. (2008). Adolescent physical activities as predictors of young adult weight. *Arch Pediatr Adolesc Med*, *162*, 29-33.

Meyer, A.A., Kundt, G., Lenschow, U., et al. (2006). Improvement in early vascular changes and cardiovascular risk factors in obese children after a six month exercise program. *J Am Coll Cardiol*, *48*, 1865-1870.

Miller, W., & Rollnick, S. (2002). *Motivational Interviewing: Preparing People to Change* (2nd ed.). New York: Guilford Press.

Mitchell, R., Wake, M., Canterford, L., et al. (2008). Does maternal concern about children's weight affect children's body size perception at the age of 6.5? A community-based study. *Int J Obesity*, *32*, 1001-1007.

Monteiro, P.O.A., & Victora, C.G. (2005). Rapid growth in infancy and childhood and obesity in later life—a systematic review. *Obesity Rev*, *6*, 143-154.

Morrison, J.A., Friedman, L.A., Wang, P., et al. (2007). Metabolic syndrome in childhood predicts adult metabolic syndrome and type 2 diabetes mellitus 25-30 years later. *J Pediatr*, *152*, 201-206.

Murphy, M.J., Metcalf, B.S., Voss, L.D., et al. (2004). Girls at five are intrinsically more insulin resistant than boys: The programming hypotheses revisited—the Early Bird study. *Pediatrics*, *113*, 82-87.

Musher-Eizenman, D.R., Holub, S.C., Miller, A.B., et al. (2004). Body size stigmatization in preschool children: The role of control attributions. *J Pediatr Psychol*, *29*, 613-620.

Mustillo, S., Worthman, C., Erkanli, A., et al. (2003). Obesity and psychiatric disorder: Developmental trajectories. *Pediatrics*, *111*, 851-859.

Muzumdar, H., & Rao, M. (2006). Pulmonary dysfunction and sleep apnea in morbid obesity. *Pediatr Endocrinol Rev*, *3* (Suppl 4), 579-583.

Nadler, E.P., Young, H.A., Ren, C.J., et al. (2007). An update on 73 US obese pediatric patients treated with laparoscopic adjustable gastric banding: Comorbidity resolution and compliance data. *J Pediatr Surg*, *43*, 141-146.

Nagao, T., Hase, T., & Tokimitsu, I. (2007). A green tea extract high in catechins reduces body fat and cardiovascular risks in humans. *Obesity*, *15*, 1473-1483.

National Association of Pediatric Nurse Practitioners (NAPNAP) (2006). Early identification and prevention of childhood overweight. *J Pediatr Health Care*, *20*(2 Suppl), 3-63.

National Center for Health Statistics (NCHS). (2007). *Health, United States, 2007 with Chartbook on Trends in the Health of Americans*. Hyattsville, MD: National Center for Health Statistics.

National Heart, Lung, and Blood Institute. (2000). *The practical guide: Identification, evaluation, and treatment of overweight and obesity in adults*. Available at www.nhlbi.nih.gov/guidelines/obesity/practgde.htm. Retrieved August 1, 2008.

National Heart, Lung, and Blood Institute (NHLBI). (2004). *The fourth report on the diagnosis, evaluation, and treatment of high blood pressure in children and adolescents*. Available at: www.nhlbi.nih.gov/guidelines/hypertension/hbp_ped.htm. Retrieved August 1, 2008.

National Heart, Lung, and Blood Institute (NHLBI). (2007). *Working group report on future research directions in childhood obesity prevention and treatment*. Available at www.nhlbi.nih.gov/meetings/workshops/child-obesity/index.htm. Retrieved June 23, 2008.

Nead, K.G., Halterman, J.S., Kaczorowski, J.M., et al. (2004). Overweight children and adolescents: A risk group for iron deficiency. *Pediatrics*, *114*, 104-108.

Neumark-Sztainer, D., Eisenberg, M.E., Fulkerson, J.A., et al. (2008). Family meals and disordered eating in adolescents: Longitudinal findings from Project EAT. *Arch Pediatr Adolesc Med*, *162*, 17-22.

Neumark-Sztainer, D., Wall, M., Story, M., et al. (2004). Are family meal patterns associated with disordered eating behaviors among adolescents? *J Adolesc Health*, *35*, 350-359.

Nguyen, Q.M., Srinivasan, S.R., Xu, J.H., et al. (2008). Changes in risk variables of metabolic syndrome since childhood in prediabetic and type 2 diabetic subjects: The Bogalusa Heart Study. *Diabetes Care*, *31*, 2044-2049.

Nicklas, T.A., Morales, M., Linares, A., et al. (2004). Children's meal patterns have changed over a 21-year period: The Bogalusa Heart Study. *J Am Diet Assoc*, *104*, 753-761.

Nieman, L.K., Biller, B.M., Findling, J.W., et al. (2008). The diagnosis of Cushing's syndrome: An Endocrine Society clinical practice guideline. *J Clin Endocrinol Metab*, *93*, 1526-1540.

Ogden, C.L., Carroll, D., Curtin, L.R., et al. (2006). Prevalence of overweight and obesity in the United States, 1999-2004. *J Am Med Assoc*, *295*, 1549-1555.

Ogden, C.L., Carroll, M.D., & Flegal, K.M. (2008). High body mass index for age among U.S. children and adolescents, 2003-2006. *J Am Med Assoc*, *299*, 2401-2405.

Ogden, C.L., & Tabak, C.J. (2006). Children and teens told by doctors that they were overweight—United States, 1999–2002. *MMWR Morb Mortal Wkly Rep*, *54*, 848-849.

Oken, E., & Gillman, M.W. (2003). Fetal origins of obesity. *Obesity Res*, *11*, 496-506.

Owen, C.G., Whincup, P.H., Odoki, K., et al. (2002). Infant feeding and blood cholesterol: A study in adolescents and a systematic review. *Pediatrics*, *110*, 597-608.

Pate, R.R., Pfeiffer, K.A., Trost, S.G., et al. (2004). Physical activity among children attending preschools. *Pediatrics*, *114*, 1258-1263.

Patel, S.R., & Hu, F.B. (2008). Short sleep duration and weight gain: A systematic review. *Obesity*, *16*, 643-653.

Paz-Filho, G., Ayala, A., Esposito, K., et al. (2008). Effects of leptin on lipid metabolism. *Horm Metab Res*, *40*, 572-574.

Pearce, M.J., Borgers, J., & Prinstein, M.J. (2002). Adolescent obesity, overt and relational peer victimization, and romantic relationships. *Obesity Res*, *10*(5), 386-393.

Pereira, M.A., Kartashov, A.I., Ebbeling, C.B., et al. (2005). Fast-food habits, weight gain, and insulin resistance (the CARDIA study): 15-year prospective analysis. *Lancet*, *365*, 36-42.

Peterson, K., Silverstein, J.M., Kaufman, F., et al. (2007). Management of type 2 diabetes in youth: An update. *Am Fam Physician*, *76*, 658-666.

Pietrobelli, A., Malavolti, M., Battistini, N.C., et al. (2008). Metabolic syndrome: A child is not a small adult. *Int J Pediatr Obesity*, *3*(S1), 67-71.

Pinhas-Hamiel, O., & Zeitler, P. (2007). Clinical presentation and treatment of type 2 diabetes in children. *Pediatr Diabetes, 8*(Suppl 9), 16-27.

Pittler, M.H., & Ernst, E. (2005). Complementary therapies for reducing body weight: A systematic review. *Int J Obesity, 29*, 1030-1038.

Poirier, P., Giles, T.D., Bray, G.A., et al. (2006). Obesity and cardiovascular disease: Pathophysiology, evaluation, and effect of weight loss: An update of the 1997 American Heart Association scientific statement on obesity and heart disease from the Obesity Committee of the Council on Nutrition, Physical Activity, and Metabolism. *Circulation, 113*, 898-918.

Prochaska, J.J., & Sallis, J.F. (2004). A randomized controlled trial of single versus multiple health behavior change: Promoting physical activity and nutrition among adolescents. *Health Psychol, 23*, 314-318.

Proctor, M.H., Moore, L.L., Gao, D., et al. (2003). Television viewing and change in body fat from preschool to early adolescence: The Framingham children's study. *Int J Obesity, 27*, 827-833.

Puhl, R.M., & Latner, J.D. (2007). Stigma, obesity, and the health of the nation's children. *Psychol Bull, 133*, 557-850.

Rasmussen, K.M., & Kjolhede, C.L. (2008). Maternal obesity: A problem for both mother and child. *Obesity, 16*, 929-931.

Reinehr, T., Wunsch, R., de Sousa, G., et al. (2008). Relationship between metabolic syndrome definitions for children and adolescents and intima-media thickness. *Atherosclerosis, 199*, 193-200.

Rewers, A., Klingensmith, G., Davis, C., et al. (2008). Presence of diabetic ketoacidosis at diagnosis of diabetes mellitus in youth: The Search for Diabetes in Youth Study. *Pediatrics, 121*, e1258-1266.

Riley, M.R., Bass, N.M., Rosenthal, P., et al. (2005). Underdiagnosis of pediatric obesity and underscreening for fatty liver disease and metabolic syndrome by pediatricians and pediatric subspecialists. *J Pediatr, 147*, 839-842.

Rodearmel, S.J., Wyatt, H.R., Stroebele, N., et al. (2007). Small changes in dietary sugar and physical activity as an approach to preventing excessive weight gain: The America on the Move Family Study. *Pediatrics, 120*, e869-e879.

Rollnick, S., Miller, W.R., & Butler, C.C. (2008). *Motivational Interviewing in Health Care: Helping Patients Change Behavior*. New York: Guilford.

Rose-Jacobs, R., Black, M.M., Casey, P.H., et al. (2008). Household food insecurity: Associations with at-risk infant and toddler development. *Pediatrics, 121*, 65-72.

Saib, M.A., Hunt, L.P., Ford, A.L., et al. (2008). Elevated blood glucose concentrations during oral glucose tolerance test are associated with the presence of metabolic syndrome in childhood obesity. *Diabetic Med, 25*, 289-295.

Salbe, A.D., Weyer, C., Lindsay, R.S., et al. (2002). Assessing risk factors for obesity between childhood and adolescence: I. Birth weight, childhood adiposity, parental obesity, insulin, and leptin. *Pediatrics, 110*, 299-306.

Sallis, J.F., & Glanz, K. (2006). The role of built environments in physical activity, eating, and obesity in childhood. *Future of Children, 16*, 89-104.

Salmon, J., Booth, M.L., Phongsavan, P., et al. (2007). Promoting physical activity participation among children and adolescents. *Epidemiol Rev, 29*, 144-159.

Saris, W.H.M., Blair, S.N., van Baak, M.A., et al. (2003). How much physical activity is enough to prevent unhealthy weight gain? Outcome of the IASO 1st stock conference and consensus statement. *Obesity Rev, 4*, 101-114.

Schwimmer, J.B., Burwinkle, T.M., & Varni, J.W. (2003). Health-related quality of life of severely obese children and adolescents. *J Am Med Assoc, 289*, 1813-1819.

Shaw, J. (2007). Epidemiology of childhood type 2 diabetes and obesity. *Pediatr Diabetes, 8* (Suppl 9), 7-15.

Shibli, R., Rubin, L., Akons, H., et al. (2008). Morbidity of overweight (≥85th percentile) in the first 2 years of life. *Pediatrics, 122*, 267-272.

Shrewsbury, V., & Wardle, J. (2008). Socioeconomic status and adiposity in childhood: A systematic review of cross-sectional studies 1990-2005. *Obesity, 16*, 275-284.

Simmons, R. (2004). Fetal origins of adult disease: Concepts and controversies. *NeoReviews, 5*(12), e511.

Singh, A.S., Mulder, C., Twisk, J.W.R., et al. (2008). Tracking of childhood overweight into adulthood: A systematic review of the literature. *Obesity Rev, 9*, 474-488.

Sjöberg, R.L., Nilsson, K.W., & Leppert, J. (2005). Obesity, shame, and depression in school-aged children: A population-based study. *Pediatrics, 116*, e389-e392.

Skinner, A.C., Mayer, M.L., Flower, K., et al. (2008). Health status and health care expenditures in a nationally representative sample: How do overweight and healthy-weight children compare?. *Pediatrics, 121*, e269-e277.

Smiciklas-Wright, H., Mitchell, D.C., Mickle, S.J., et al. (2003). Foods commonly eaten in the United States, 1989-1991 and 1994-1996: Are portion sizes changing?. *J Am Diet Assoc, 103*, 41-47.

Spear, B.A., Barlow, S., Ervin, C., et al. (2007). Recommendations for treatment of child and adolescent overweight and obesity. *Pediatrics, 120*, S254-S288.

Spruijt-Metz, D., Lindquist, C.H., Birch, L.L., et al. (2002). Relation between mothers' child-feeding practices and children's adiposity. *Am J Clin Nutr, 75*, 581-586.

Stettler, N., Kumanyika, S.K., Katz, S.H., et al. (2003). Rapid weight gain during infancy and obesity in young adulthood in a cohort of African Americans. *Am J Clin Nutr, 77*, 1374-1378.

Stettler, N., Tershakovec, A.M., Zemel, B.S., et al. (2000). Early risk factors for increased adiposity: A cohort study of African American subjects followed from birth to young adulthood. *Am J Clin Nutr, 72*, 378-383.

Stettler, N., Zemel, B.S., Kumanyika, S.K., et al. (2002). Infant weight gain and childhood overweight status in a multicenter, cohort study. *Pediatrics, 109*, 194-199.

Story, R.E. (2007). Asthma and obesity in children. *Curr Opin Pediatr, 19*, 680-684.

Stovitz, S.D., Schwimmer, J.B., Martinez, H., et al. (2008). Pediatric obesity: The unique issues in Latino-American male youth. *Am J Prev Med, 34*, 153-160.

Stunkard, A.J., Berkowitz, R.I., Schoeller, D., et al. (2004). Predictors of body size in the first 2 y of life: A high-risk study of human obesity. *Int J Obesity Relat Metab Disord, 28*, 503-513.

Sullivan, C.S., Beste, J., Cummings, D.M., et al. (2004). Prevalence of hyperinsulinemia and clinical correlates in overweight children referred for lifestyle intervention. *J Am Med Assoc, 104*, 433-436.

Summerbell, C.D., Ashton, V., Campbell, K.J., et al. (2003). Interventions for treating obesity in children. *Cochrane Database of Systematic Reviews*(3), CD001872.

Sun, S.S., Liang, R., Huang, T.T., et al. (2008). Childhood obesity predicts adult metabolic syndrome: The Fels Longitudinal Study. *J Pediatr, 152*, 191-200.

Swallen, K.C., Reither, E.N., Haas, S.A., et al. (2005). Overweight, obesity, and health-related quality of life among adolescents: The National Longitudinal Study of Adolescent Health. *Pediatrics, 115*, 340-347.

Syme, C., Abrahamowicz, M., Leonard, G.T., et al. (2008). Intra-abdominal adiposity and individual components of the metabolic syndrome: Sex differences and underlying mechanisms. *Arch Pediatr Adolesc Med, 162*, 453-461.

Talmud, P.J., & Stephens, J.W. (2004). Lipoprotein lipase gene variants and the effect of environmental factors on cardiovascular disease risk. *Diabetes Obesity Metab, 6*, 1-7.

Taveras, E.M., Rifas-Shiman, S.L., Camargo, C.A., et al. (2008). Higher adiposity in infancy associated with recurrent wheeze in a prospective cohort of children. *J Allergy Clin Immunol, 121*, 1161-1166.

Taylor, E.D., Theim, K.R., Mirch, M.C., et al. (2006). Orthopedic complications of overweight in children and adolescents. *Pediatrics, 117*, 2167-2174.

Taylor, W.C., Floyd, M.F., Whitt-Glover, M.C., et al. (2007). Environmental justice: A framework for collaboration between the public health and parks and recreation fields to study disparities in physical activity. *J Phys Activity Health, 4*(Suppl 1), S50-S63.

Teran-Garcia, M., Rankinen, T., & Bouchard, C. (2008). Genes, exercise, growth and the sedentary, obese child. *J Appl Physiol, 105*, 988-1001.

Tfayli, H., & Arslanian, S. (2008). Menstrual health and the metabolic syndrome in adolescents. *Ann N Y Acad Sci, 1135*, 85-94.

Toschke, A.M., Beyerlein, A., & von Kries, R. (2005). Children at high risk for overweight: A classification and regression trees analysis. *Obesity Res, 13*, 1270-1274.

Treuth, M.S., Butte, N.F., Adolph, A.L., et al. (2004). A longitudinal study of fitness and activity in girls predisposed to obesity. *Med Sci Sports Exerc, 36*, 198-204.

Treuth, M.S., Butte, N.F., & Sorkin, J.D. (2003). Predictors of body fat gain in nonobese girls with a familial predisposition to obesity. *Am J Clin Nutr, 78*, 1212-1218.

Trifiletti, L.B., Shields, W., Bishai, D., et al. (2006). Tipping the scales: Obese children and child safety seats. *Pediatrics, 117*, 1197-1202.

Trost, S.G., Sallis, J.F., Pate, R.R., et al. (2003). Evaluating a model of parental influence on youth physical activity. *Am J Prev Med, 25*, 277-282.

Turkowski, B.B., Lance, B.R., & Bonfiglio, M.F. (2008). *Drug Information Handbook for Advanced Practice Nursing* (9th ed.). Hudson, OH: LexiComp.

U.S. Department of Agriculture (USDA). (2005). *Dietary guidelines for Americans.* Available at www.health.gov/DietaryGuidelines/dga2005/document/default.htm. Retrieved June 23, 2008.

Van Horn, L., Obarzanek, E., Barton, B.A., et al. (2003). A summary of the results of the dietary study in children (DISC): Lessons learned. *Prog Cardiovasc Nurs, 18*, 28-41.

Verhulst, S.L., Aerts, L., Jacobs, S., et al. (2008). Sleep disordered breathing, obesity, and airway inflammation in children and adolescents. *Chest, 134*, 1169-1175.

Vgontzas, A.N., Bixler, E.O., & Chrousos, G.P. (2006). Obesity related sleepiness and fatigue: The role of stress systems and cytokines. *Ann N Y Acad Sci, 1083*, 329-344.

Viner, R.M., & Cole, T.J. (2006). Who changes body mass between adolescence and adulthood? Factors predicting change in BMI between 16 year and 30 years in the 1970 British Birth Cohort. *Int J Obesity, 30*, 1368-1374.

Wake, M., Nicholson, J.M., Hardy, P., et al. (2007). Preschooler obesity and parenting styles of mothers and fathers: Australian national population study. *Pediatrics, 120*, e1520-1527.

Wang, Y., & Lobstein, T. (2006). Worldwide trends in childhood overweight and obesity. *Int J Pediatr Obesity, 1*, 11-25.

Wardle, J., Robb, K.A., Johnson, F., et al. (2004). Socioeconomic variation in attitudes to eating and weight in female adolescents. *Health Psychol, 23*, 275-282.

Waring, M.E., & Lapane, K.L. (2008). Overweight in children and adolescents in relation to attention-deficit/hyperactivity disorder: Results from a national sample. *Pediatrics, 122*, e1-e6.

Wärnberg, J., & Marcos, A. (2008). Low-grade inflammation and the metabolic syndrome in children and adolescents. *Curr Opin Lipidol, 19*, 11-15.

Weiss, R., Dziura, J., Burgert, T.S., et al. (2004). Obesity and the metabolic syndrome in children and adolescents. *N Engl J Med, 350*, 2362-2374.

West, D.S., Raczynski, J.M., Phillips, M.M., et al. (2008). Parental recognition of overweight in school-age children. *Obesity, 16*(3), 630-636.

Wingood, G.M., DiClemente, R.J., Harrington, K., et al. (2002). Body image and African American females' sexual health. *Journal of Women's Health and Gender-Based Medicine, 11*(5), 433-439.

Wittmeier, K.D.M., Mollard, R.C., & Kriellaars, D.J. (2008). Physical activity intensity and risk of overweight and adiposity in children. *Obesity, 16*(2), 415-420.

World Health Organization (WHO). (2003). *Process for a global strategy on diet, physical activity, and health.* Geneva, Switzerland: Author. Available at www.who.int/dietphysicalactivity/strategy/en/. Retrieved August 1, 2008

Yang, W., Kelly, T., & He, J. (2007). Genetic epidemiology of obesity. *Epidemiol Rev, 29*, 49-61.

Zeller, M.H., Reiter-Purtill, J., & Ramey, C. (2008). Negative peer perceptions of obese children in the classroom environment. *Obesity, 16*(4), 755-762.

Zeller, M.H., Roerhig, H.R., Modi, A.C., et al. (2006). Health-related quality of life and depressive symptoms in adolescents with extreme obesity presenting for bariatric surgery. *Pediatrics, 117*, 1155-1161.

Zephier, E., Hime, J.H., Story, M., et al. (2006). Increasing prevalences of overweight and obesity in Northern Plains American Indian children. *Arch Pediatr Adolesc Med, 160*, 34-39.

Zhu, H., Yan, W., Ge, D., et al. (2008). Relationships of cardiovascular phenotypes with healthy weight, at risk of overweight, and overweight in US youths. *Pediatrics, 121*(1), 115-122.

37 Organ Transplantation

Melanie S. Klein and Kathy Martin

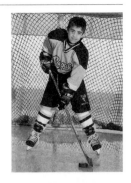

Etiology

Solid organ transplantation has evolved into an effective treatment for a variety of end-stage organ diseases. This complex surgical procedure is followed by a phase of intensive surgical and medical management leading to stable graft function with routine monitoring. The liver, kidney, and heart are the most commonly transplanted solid organs in the pediatric population. Intestine transplantation has recently become an accepted procedure for those children with volvulus, gastroschisis, necrotizing enterocolitis, pseudo-obstruction, intestinal atresia, or Hirschsprung's disease (Fryer, 2007). The Organ Procurement and Transplantation Network (OPTN) reported that 111 pediatric intestinal transplants were performed in the United States in 2007 (OPTN, 2009). Lung and heart-lung transplants are performed only when other treatments are not viable.

With increased success and survival following solid organ transplantation, the indications for transplantation of the kidney, liver, heart, and lung continue to increase (Table 37-1). The most common causes of renal failure resulting in end-stage renal disease (ESRD) requiring transplantation in children are obstructive uropathy, renal aplasia/hypoplasia/dysplasia, reflux nephropathy, focal segmental glomerulosclerosis, and chronic glomerulonephritis (North American Pediatric Renal Transplant Cooperative Study [NAPRTCS], 2007).

Liver transplantation is a treatment therapy for a variety of end-stage liver diseases (ESLDs) that can generally be categorized as progressive primary liver disease with anticipated hepatic failure, stable liver disease with a remarkable morbidity/mortality rate, hepatic-based metabolic disease, and acute liver failure. Biliary atresia, which is an obstructive biliary tract condition, accounts for at least 50% of the pediatric liver transplants performed (Tiao & Ryckman, 2006). A Kasai portoenterostomy may result in improved bile drainage if performed within an infant's first 120 days of life. Most of the children who have progressive liver disease after the procedure require transplantation within the first 2 years of life. Metabolic conditions that may require transplantation include Wilson's disease, alpha-1-antitrypsin deficiency, cystic fibrosis, and primary hyperoxaluria. The most common type of acute liver failure is viral hepatitis (Tiao & Ryckman).

Cardiomyopathy and congenital heart disease (CHD) (see Chapter 21) are the leading indications for heart transplantation in children, with more infant recipients having CHD and more adolescent recipients having a myopathy (Boucek, Aurora, Edwards, et al., 2007). Cystic fibrosis and pulmonary hypertension most commonly lead to end-stage lung disease requiring lung transplantation, with cystic fibrosis being the most frequent pretransplant diagnosis (Huddleston, 2006). Heart-lung transplantation is done very infrequently because of limited organ availability and advancements in lung transplants and surgery for congenital heart disease. The most common indication for heart-lung transplantation is CHD, which is associated with end-stage pulmonary vascular disease (Webber, McCurry, & Zeevi, 2006).

There are many renal conditions with genetic etiologies that can lead to chronic and end-stage renal disease (see Chapter 32). Genetic etiologies include Alport syndrome, focal segmental glomerulosclerosis (FSGS), Wilms' tumor, familial juvenile nephronophthisis, and polycystic kidney disease (PKD), either autosomal dominant (ADPKD) or autosomal recessive (ARPKD).

Though gene therapy is not available at this time, there is promise. Researchers are working to develop ways to not only identify the genes that cause inherited kidney and liver diseases but to treat conditions in transplanted organs (Isaka, 2006; Tiao & Ryckman, 2006). The hope is that this research will provide new technology to diagnose, treat, and even prevent renal and liver failure in children.

Several etiologies of liver disease requiring transplantation have a genetic predisposition. These include familial cholestasis, Alagille syndrome, Byler syndrome, Wilson's disease, and alpha-1-antitrypsin deficiency. In addition, some children with cystic fibrosis (see Chapter 22), an autosomal recessive disorder, may have secondary liver disease requiring transplantation.

Cardiomyopathy is a common indication for heart transplantation. The incidence of cardiomyopathy in children is not well documented. Etiology may be genetic, familial, or related to secondary causes such as infection, systemic disease, exposure to toxins, or malnutrition (Benson, 2004; Lee & Yeh, 2004). See Chapter 21 for additional discussion on the genetic etiology of cardiac conditions leading to transplantation.

Cystic fibrosis, an inherited disorder, is the most common indication for end-stage lung disease leading to lung transplantation (Huddleston, 2006). See Chapter 22 for additional discussion regarding the genetic etiology of cystic fibrosis.

Incidence and Prevalence

Transplantation provides an accepted treatment for a variety of end-stage organ conditions. As of January 25, 2008, the OPTN reported that nearly 100,000 adults and children were listed for solid organ transplantation at the end of 2005, with 2% of those candidates less than 18 years of age (OPTN, 2008a). In 2007, nearly 2000 children received a solid organ transplant. Of that group, 796 children younger than 18 years of age received renal transplants, 605 children received liver transplants, 60 received pancreas transplants, 4 received kidney/pancreas transplants, 52 received lung transplants, 3 received heart/lung transplants,

TABLE 37-1

Comparative Indications for Transplantation in Children by Organ*

Renal	Liver	Heart	Dual Transplants and Lung
Congenital Condition	**Cholestatic Disease**	**Cardiomyopathy**	**Heart and Liver**
Congenital nephrotic syndrome	Alagille syndrome	Dilated	Familial hypercholesterolemia with
Eagle-Barrett syndrome	Byler syndrome	Hypertrophic	ischemic cardiomyopathy
Renal dysplasia	Biliary atresia	Restrictive	Intrahepatic biliary atresia
Renal hypoplasia/aplasia	Familial cholestasis	**Congenital Heart Defects**	and dilated cardiomyopathy
Wilms' tumor	**Parenchymal Disease**	(select lesions)	**Liver and Kidney**
Obstructive uropathy	Budd-Chiari syndrome		Cystinosis
Reflux nephropathy	Congenital hepatic fibrosis		Oxalosis
Acquired Disease	Cystic fibrosis		**Heart and Lung**
Chronic pyelonephritis	Neonatal hepatitis		Congenital heart defects with elevated
Focal segmental glomerulosclerosis	Acute fulminant hepatic failure		pulmonary vascular resistance
Glomerulonephritis	Hepatitis B		**Lung**
Hemolytic-uremic syndrome	Hepatitis C		Cystic fibrosis
Henoch-Schönlein purpura	**Metabolic Disorders**		Primary pulmonary hypertension
IgA nephropathy	Alpha-1-antitrypsin deficiency		
Lupus nephritis	Glycogen storage disease, type IV		
Membranoproliferative	Tyrosinemia		
glomerulonephritis, types I and II	Wilson disease		
Renal infarct	**Hepatomas**		
Sickle cell nephropathy			
Hereditary Condition			
Alport syndrome			
Juvenile nephronophthisis			
Polycystic kidney disease			
Metabolic Disorders			
Cystinosis			
Oxalosis			

*This list includes the most common etiologies of end-stage organ failure; it is not all-inclusive.

111 received intestinal transplants, and 327 received heart transplants (OPTN, 2009).

Diagnostic Criteria

There are few published objective criteria for pediatric heart transplantation. Decreased exercise tolerance with peak oxygen consumption (VO_2) less than 10 mL/kg/min is an indication for heart transplant (Dipchand, 2004). In the absence of clear objective criteria, expected survival of less than 2 years and quality of life without transplant are important considerations (Webber, McCurry, & Zeevi, 2006).

Expected survival and quality of life are also key considerations for potential lung transplant recipients. Forced expiratory volume in 1 second (FEV_1) of less than 30% is the accepted threshold for lung transplantation assessment (Burch & Aurora, 2004).

Assessment of the glomerular filtration rate (GFR) is the most important test for determining kidney function. GFR is a good indicator for chronic kidney disease. In children, the Schwartz formula is used to determine GFR, which is expressed in mL/min/1.73 m². This formula takes into account the child's age and weight in addition to the serum creatinine level.

Chronic kidney disease (CKD) is a broadly used term and may be described in four stages. Stages 1 to 4 are defined by the progressive worsening of kidney function until stage 5 is reached. Stage 5 is considered kidney failure and is associated with a GFR of less than 15. Children in stage 5 manifest severe clinical, laboratory,

and radiologic abnormalities, and renal replacement therapy (RRT) by dialysis or transplantation is usually initiated (Kraut, 2007; National Kidney Foundation, 2002; Vogt & Avner, 2007).

In North America, pediatric end-stage liver disease (PELD) and the model of end-stage liver disease (MELD) were developed to accurately measure the severity of liver disease and to better predict the risk for dying or moving to an intensive care unit in the following 3 months. PELD takes into consideration the international normalized ratio (INR), total bilirubin, serum albumin, age less than 1 year, and height less than 2 standard deviations from the mean for age and gender; however, its accuracy is a subject of debate. The MELD score is based on bilirubin, INR, and serum creatinine and is used for adults and children greater than 11 years of age, because it has been recognized as more accurate than PELD in older children (Kerkar & Emre, 2007).

Clinical Manifestations at Time of Diagnosis

The symptoms and severity of illness of children with end-stage organ disease vary according to the specific condition and affected organ, as well as the length of illness, age of the child, and effectiveness of treatment.

Children with ESRD exhibit symptoms related to fluid and electrolyte imbalances, hypertension, fatigue, feeding intolerance, recurrent emesis, growth failure, edema, anemia, and rickets (Vogt & Avner, 2007). A complete discussion of the manifestations of chronic kidney disease is presented in Chapter 32.

Clinical Manifestations at Time of Diagnosis

RENAL	LIVER	HEART	LUNG
Anemia	Ascites	Arrhythmias	Exercise intolerance
Congestive heart failure	Coagulopathies	Cardiac murmurs	Growth retardation
Edema/hypervolemia	Encephalopathy	Congestive heart failure	Malnutrition
Elevated BUN and creatinine	Hepatomegaly	Growth retardation	Respiratory distress
Growth retardation	Hormone imbalance	Respiratory distress	
Hyperkalemia	Hyperammonemia	ST- and T-wave abnormalities	
Hyperlipidemia	Hypercholesterolemia	Tachypnea	
Hyperphosphatemia	Hypoalbuminemia		
Hypertension	Hypoglycemia		
Metabolic acidosis	Jaundice		
Pericarditis	Malnutrition		
Peripheral neuropathy	Portal hypertension		
Renal osteodystrophy	Splenomegaly		
Secondary hyperparathyroidism			

Key: *BUN*, blood urea nitrogen.

Children with liver disease may have an acute or chronic course of illness depending on the etiology and severity of the liver condition. Some children may remain stable for several years before transplantation with appropriate medical management, but others may have a moderate to rapid decline in hepatic function requiring emergent transplantation. Symptoms of liver dysfunction, such as those seen with biliary atresia, may include jaundice, hepatomegaly, splenomegaly, ascites, pruritus, xanthomas, and variceal bleeding. Hepatic enzymes, bilirubin, gamma-glutamyl transpeptidase phosphate (GGTP), and ammonia levels are elevated. Children who have had a Kasai portoenterostomy are also at risk for cholangitis. Other symptoms associated with liver failure may include delayed growth, malnutrition, rickets, osteomalacia with fractures, increased synthetic function, and encephalopathy.

Acute liver failure, by definition, progresses from jaundice to encephalopathy within 8 weeks from the onset of illness. Coagulopathies also occur within this time frame. With progression of hepatic dysfunction, cerebral edema increases causing intracranial hypertension, which can lead to irreversible neurologic damage, uncal herniation, and death (Fontana, 2006).

Complex CHD and cardiomyopathies requiring transplantation may have similar initial symptoms (see Chapter 21 for a review of CHD). Heart transplant candidates with CHD may have already undergone corrective or palliative surgery, which can make the transplant procedure more complicated (Alkhaldi, Chin, & Bernstein, 2006). Symptoms of cardiomyopathy vary depending on the child's age at onset of illness and the type of cardiomyopathy. The clinical manifestations of dilated cardiomyopathy include symptoms of congestive heart failure as a result of decreasing myocardial contractility. Other common clinical signs include an enlarged heart by chest radiography, nonspecific ST-T wave changes and sinus tachycardia on electrocardiography, and a gallop rhythm on auscultation. Nonspecific symptoms may include fever, vomiting, weight loss, or failure to thrive (Lee & Yeh, 2004).

Most children discovered to have hypertrophic cardiomyopathy do not have prominent cardiac symptoms because thickening of the left ventricular wall may remain stable or progress slowly. There is a positive family history in 30% to 60% of affected individuals (Benson, 2004). Children and young adults are at risk for episodes of syncope and sudden death during exercise when the left ventricular demand increases and obstruction to the outflow tract occurs. This diagnosis is sometimes first made on autopsy.

Lung transplant candidates have evidence of advanced chronic lung disease no longer alleviated by medical therapy, and poor quality of life. These children will generally have an FEV_1 less than 30%, poor tolerance on a 6- or 12-minute walk test demonstrated by poor arterial oxygen saturation, and declining nutritional status (Burch & Aurora, 2004). Decreased life expectancy and poorer quality of life most often accompany end-stage lung disease. However, quality of life occasionally does not mirror the child's clinical condition and must be assessed independently.

Treatment

Pretransplant Management

Conservative therapy of kidney disease consists of managing fluid, electrolyte, and metabolic imbalances, as well as hypertension and anemia (see Chapter 32). When conservative treatment for chronic kidney disease is no longer effective, ESRD care consists of hemodialysis, peritoneal dialysis, or renal transplantation (Vogt & Avner, 2007). Because of the deleterious effects of dialysis on children, preemptive renal transplantation, or transplantation before the initiation of dialysis, has become more common. As of 2000, nearly 25% of all renal transplants were preemptive (NAPRTCS, 2007). Because this goal is not always immediately attainable, such as in the cases of acute renal failure or chronic kidney disease with no available living donor, dialysis is often initiated. Transplantation is the treatment choice for children with ESRD to maximize survival, minimize the sequelae of uremia on growth and development, improve the overall quality of life for the child and family, and reduce the physiologic, psychological, and financial effects of end-stage disease.

Treatment

Pretransplant Management
Kidney
- Conservative therapy for kidney condition
- Dialysis

Liver
- Medical management to stabilize hepatic function
- Enteral supplementation
- Pharmacological treatment for symptoms
- Prevention of bleeding from esophageal and gastric varices

Cardiac
- Maximizing cardiac function and controlling symptoms of congestive heart failure
- Surgical intervention if necessary
- Control of arrhythmias
- Control of pulmonary hypertension
- ECMO for temporary bridge to transplantation

Evaluation for Transplantation
- Multidisciplinary evaluation
- Pretransplant surgical procedures
- Laboratory assessment

After Transplantation
- Immunosuppressive management
- Infection prophylaxis
- Graft evaluation

Children with chronic liver disease may be followed on an outpatient basis with medical management designed to optimize and stabilize hepatic function. To meet nutritional requirements, these children may require enteral supplementation, administration of fat-soluble vitamins, and/or total parental nutrition (TPN). Synthetic function of the liver, coagulation times, and ammonia levels, as well as electrolytes, fluid balance, and renal function, must be frequently monitored.

Medications may provide symptomatic relief to mitigate the effects of hepatic dysfunction. Ursodeoxycholic acid (UDCA, Ursodiol) may help decrease cholestasis. Pruritus may be lessened with single or combination therapy, including cholestyramine (Questran), phenobarbital, and antihistamines such as hydroxyzine (Atarax) (Bergasa, 2008). Rifampin (Rifadin) can be used in cases where other medications fail to control symptoms of itching. Its mechanism of action is unknown, but is thought to be related to a selective interaction of rifampin with the hepatobiliary transport of bilirubin (Silveira & Lindor, 2008). High ammonia levels may be improved by lactulose (Cephulac) (Han & Hyzy, 2006).

Recurrent cholangitis caused by biliary stasis and bacterial contamination in children who have had a Kasai procedure are common. Symptoms may include a fever of greater than 38°C (100.4°F), an elevated white blood cell count, and an increase in serum bilirubin concentration. Diagnosis is confirmed by positive blood cultures. Treatment includes an appropriately sensitive intravenous antibiotic followed by long-term prophylaxis with trimethoprim-sulfamethoxazole (Bactrim, Septra), metronidazole (Flagyl), or ciprofloxacin hydrochloride (Cipro).

Bleeding episodes from esophageal and gastric varices caused by portal hypertension can be temporized by sclerotherapy and band ligation (Heidelbaugh & Sherbondy, 2006). Sclerotherapy consists of the injection of a sclerosing agent into the varix with the goal of obliterating the targeted vessel. Band ligation involves the placement of small elastic bands that are endoscopically placed over a suctioned varix (Magno & Kalloo, 2008). In the event of massive bleeding refractory to sclerotherapy, transjugular intrahepatic portosystemic shunting (TIPS) may be required. Although this procedure may help stabilize a child during the waiting period, it is accompanied by a higher risk of hepatic encephalopathy (Heidelbaugh & Sherbondy, 2006).

Medical management of children with dilated cardiomyopathy consists of maximizing cardiac output and controlling symptoms of heart failure with digoxin, diuretics, and afterload reduction. Angiotensin-converting enzyme inhibitors (i.e., captopril [Capoten], enalapril [Vasotec]) for afterload reduction have been beneficial in optimizing cardiac function and decreasing the workload of the heart. Antiarrhythmics may be needed in some children. Anticoagulation therapy may help prevent thrombus formation in a dilated and poorly contracting heart (Lee & Yeh, 2004).

In contrast, medical management for hypertrophic cardiomyopathy consists of maintaining a normal preload and afterload while reducing ventricular contractility, usually accomplished with calcium channel blockers, as well as beta blockers, to decrease the septal muscle from obstructing the left ventricular outflow tract. Antiarrhythmics may be needed for ventricular arrhythmias but have not been shown to prevent sudden death. Surgical intervention can be attempted to remove muscle bundles in the left ventricular outflow tract to relieve obstruction. Surgical intervention is not recommended until medical management has failed because of the possibility of recurrent obstruction (Benson, 2004). The use of implanted cardioverter-defibrillator (ICD) devices in children waiting for heart transplant is controversial and does not have the same advantage as is observed in adults. Children with cardiomyopathy-related ischemia may have the greatest benefit from ICD implantation because they have the greatest risk of sudden death (Rhee, Canter, Basile, et al., 2007).

Children with CHD who develop ventricular dysfunction, lethal arrhythmias, and/or irreversible pulmonary hypertension are also managed medically until transplantation. Management is similar to dilated cardiomyopathy but may vary slightly depending on the type of CHD and previous operative or palliative procedures. Some children and adolescents with cyanotic heart defects may have additional management issues related to polycythemia, hypoxemia, and central nervous system (CNS) sequelae (see Chapter 21).

Mechanical circulatory support as a temporary bridge to heart transplantation has been traditionally provided with extracorporeal membrane oxygenation (ECMO) (Fiser, Yetman, Gunselman, et al, 2003). There are many limitations to this technology and it is a short-term (days to 2 or 3 weeks) therapy, which may not allow enough time for a suitable organ to become available for transplant. There has been encouraging development in ventricular assist devices (VADs) for pediatric patients. VADs for young children and infants are now available with the advantages of longer duration of circulatory support and the potential for patient mobility, including physical activity and even the return to normal daily activities (Arabia, Tsau, Smith, et al., 2006). VAD complications include infection and bleeding; however, the proportion of patients successfully bridged to transplant approaches 80% (Blume, Naftel, Bastardi, et al, 2006; Sharma, Webber, Morell, et al., 2006). Both VADs and ECMO are currently used in most large pediatric transplant centers depending on the circumstances of the patient.

As with other transplant candidates, optimization of their clinical condition is the primary aim for children before lung transplantation. This includes maximizing nutritional status, maintaining and improving physical endurance, and providing respiratory support (e.g., with supplemental oxygen) as necessary, and treating infections—especially in cystic fibrosis patients (Wise & Walsh, 2008).

Organ transplantation is an alternative to failed medical and surgical management of end-stage organ disease. A shortage of organ donors means that many children at the maximum limits of medical management may not survive until transplantation. Health care professionals, including transplant specialists and primary care practitioners, can play an important role by educating the public and dispelling myths about organ donation and organ transplantation.

Evaluation for Transplantation

Evaluation for organ transplantation requires a multidisciplinary approach that includes medical, surgical, nutritional, and psychosocial assessments with multiple diagnostic tests, laboratory data, radiologic testing, and consultant evaluations (Flattery & Dale, 2008). The evaluation process is organ specific and institution specific, but usually includes consultations by the transplant surgery staff; specialty medical services (e.g., nephrology, gastroenterology, anesthesiology, cardiology) and infectious disease specialists; nursing services with transplant coordinators, clinical nurse specialists, or nurse practitioners; psychosocial services through social work and psychiatry; nutritional therapists; behavioral medicine involving developmental and child life specialists; and physical and occupational therapists. Although not involved in direct care, financial counselors are also utilized to assist families with insurance and billing questions. Evaluations are usually scheduled on an outpatient basis in specialty clinics, with routine outpatient follow-up facilitated by the transplant coordinator during the waiting period. Children with more advanced disease, however, may be hospitalized during the evaluation and also require long-term hospitalization while waiting for transplantation.

Pretransplant surgical procedures may be necessary in some cases to provide corrective or palliative repairs to prepare or stabilize a child for transplantation. For example, infants with nephrotic syndrome or chronically infected urinary tracts may require a preemptive bilateral nephrectomy, followed by time to recover on dialysis, before proceeding to transplantation (Chavers, Najarian, & Humar, 2007).

Laboratory data commonly obtained for all children awaiting organ transplant include a complete blood count; a full chemistry profile to assess electrolytes, renal function, and nutritional status; and prothrombin and partial thromboplastin times. Serologic testing is also completed to diagnose previous infections with hepatitis A, B, and C, cytomegalovirus (CMV), Epstein-Barr virus (EBV), human immunodeficiency virus (HIV), herpes, and varicella-zoster virus. A child's immunization record is reviewed, and every attempt is made to administer delinquent vaccines if the child is well enough to tolerate a vaccination. Live vaccines, such as the measles, mumps, rubella (MMR) vaccine and varicella virus vaccine (Varivax), are not administered after transplantation because the child has an increased risk of acquiring the virus from a live vaccine when the immune system is suppressed (Diana, Posfay-Barbe, Belli, et al., 2007; Verma & Wade, 2006).

Blood typing to achieve ABO-matched organs is required for kidney, liver, lung, and most heart transplantations. In addition, human leukocyte antigen (HLA) matching is necessary in renal transplantation. Cytotoxic antibody crossmatch compatibility, percent panel reactive antibody (PRA), and HLA tissue typing are also completed. The transplant candidate with preexisting anti-HLA antibodies presents a significant challenge. The presence of anti-HLA antibodies increases the chance of antibody-mediated organ rejection (Dipchand, 2004). In the past several years, many strategies have been recommended to prevent and mitigate HLA sensitization. Some pretransplant strategies include limiting blood transfusions; immunosuppression with cyclophosphamide (Cytoxan), azathioprine (Imuran), and mycophenolate mofetil (CellCept); intravenous immune globulin (IVIG); and plasmapheresis (Shaddy & Fuller, 2005). The results of these interventions are variable and management protocols differ between transplant centers and organ groups.

Although most children with end-stage organ disease are suitable candidates for transplantation, there are some exclusion criteria. These criteria have decreased significantly over the past two decades because of innovations in care and advances in surgical techniques. Exclusion criteria vary by institution, but most centers agree that children with systemic sepsis, multisystem organ failure, and metastatic disease are not appropriate candidates. Individuals who are HIV positive, once considered an absolute contraindication to transplantation, are receiving transplants at some centers. Children with cystic fibrosis colonized with *Burkholderia cepacia* (genome 3) have a poorer posttransplant outcome and are not considered transplant candidates at many centers (Burch & Aurora, 2004). A history of medical nonadherence and poor social support may place the transplant recipient at increased risk for graft failure (Pearlman, 2002a). A referral to the local child and family services department may be necessary if a family is unable or unwilling to provide appropriate care to the child before or after transplant.

Following acceptance as a transplant candidate, a child is listed with the United Network for Organ Sharing (UNOS) according to organ-specific criteria. While waiting at home or in a community hospital for transplantation, the child is medically managed by the primary care provider, who must provide regular updates to the transplant center and inform the center of any deterioration or complications in the child's medical status. Because the primary care provider may also have developed a supportive relationship with the child and family during the diagnosis of the illness and pretransplant care, this caregiver may be best able to assess the child's and family's coping abilities, responses to stress, level of understanding, and adaptability. This assessment should be communicated to the transplant team to help build on the family's strengths as the family learns to cope with and adapt to the various stressors of the transplant process. The waiting period is variable, depending on the organ or organs needed, as well as the child's blood type, weight, and medical status. Waiting for a cadaveric organ may range from a few days to months and possibly years. It is a highly stressful time for family members as they hope for an organ before their child's condition deteriorates.

After Transplant

Immunosuppressive Management. Immunosuppressive regimens vary according to the organ transplanted and institution protocol, but the goals are similar: to maintain the lowest acceptable level of drug that maximizes stable and adequate functioning of the transplanted organ without drug toxicity. The most common posttransplant immunosuppressive medications used alone or in combination therapy to prevent rejection are cyclosporine (CSA, Neoral), tacrolimus (TAC/Prograf), prednisone, sirolimus (Rapamune), mycophenolate mofetil (MMF, Cellcept), and azathioprine (Imuran). Therapeutic levels and doses vary according to the organ transplanted, the length of time posttransplant, and the presence of infection or rejection.

Cyclosporine (CSA) has been the mainstay of solid organ transplantation since its introduction in the 1980s. Originally used in conjunction with steroids and azathioprine, this immunosuppressant revolutionized transplantation and resulted in dramatically improved survival rates. CSA inhibits the activity of calcineurin, which triggers transcription factors involved in interleukin-2 (IL-2) and other molecules critical for T cell activation (Chandraker, Iacomini, & Sayegh, 2007). Absorption of CSA is bile dependent because it is excreted and reabsorbed from bile through enterohepatic circulation. Consequently, therapeutic drug levels may be difficult to maintain in people receiving liver transplants, in other organ recipients with cholestasis due to hepatic dysfunction, and in people with external bile drainage. A microemulsion formulation of CSA absorbed independently of bile is available (Neoral) and is commonly used.

Although nephrotoxicity is the most significant side effect of CSA, it is dosage dependent and usually reversible. Acute nephrotoxicity may cause a sudden increase in the blood urea nitrogen (BUN) level and creatinine. Hyperkalemia, hyponatremia, metabolic acidosis, and hypomagnesemia may also occur. Chronic toxicity can result in nephropathy, which appears on biopsy as tubular changes, vascular changes, and/or interstitial fibrosis with tubular atrophy (MD Consult, 2008). Hypertension is common, especially when CSA is given in combination with high-dose corticosteroids, but is usually responsive to antihypertensive therapy with calcium channel blockers (e.g., nifedipine [Procardia], amlodipine [Norvasc], verapamil [Calan]) or beta-adrenergic blockers (e.g., atenolol [Tenormin], propranolol [Inderal], labetalol [Normodyne]). Calcium channel blockers, especially diltiazem (Cardizem), not only treat hypertension, but may also offer some protection against posttransplant coronary artery disease in heart recipients. Beta-adrenergic blockers may exacerbate chronotropic incompetence in children with heart transplants and are generally not used as first-line therapy. Angiotensin-converting enzyme (ACE) inhibitors should be avoided in people with marginal renal function or hyperkalemia. Although nephrotoxicity is a concern in all transplant recipients, it may be more critical in those with renal transplants because renal dysfunction may reflect not only CSA toxicity but also rejection and acute tubular necrosis.

CSA may cause gingival hyperplasia, hirsutism, gastrointestinal (GI) disorders, and an increased risk for infection and malignancy. Maintaining a low therapeutic CSA trough level may often decrease the risk or severity of these side effects.

Tacrolimus (Prograf, FK506) is a calcineurin inhibitor (CNI) that differs chemically from CSA, but has a similar mechanism of action. Approved for use in 1994, tacrolimus has been used as a primary immunosuppressant and as a treatment for steroid- or antibody-resistant rejection. Though studies have found similar efficacy between tacrolimus and CSA in terms of graft and patient survival, tacrolimus has been shown to further reduce the risk of acute rejection and has a more favorable side-effect profile (Gaston, 2006).

Individuals receiving tacrolimus-based immunosuppression have demonstrated lower rates of acute rejection than those on cyclosporine (Gaston, 2006). Tacrolimus has side effects similar to those of CSA, such as nephrotoxicity, but tacrolimus is associated with less hypertension, dyslipidemia, and cardiovascular disease than cyclosporine (Liu & Schiano, 2007). As with CSA, the severity of these side effects may be decreased or eliminated after transplantation as levels are decreased over time. Individuals on tacrolimus have higher rates of posttransplant diabetes mellitus (PTDM), particularly when used in conjunction with corticosteroids. Posttransplant lymphoproliferative disease (PTLD), particularly when associated with a primary EBV infection, has been associated with tacrolimus use (Liu & Schiano, 2007). Neurotoxicities, particularly hand tremors, are associated with CSA, but more so with tacrolimus use, though their severity can be improved with dose reductions. Other neurotoxic side effects include headaches, insomnia, and paresthesias (Hawbe, 2006). Hirsutism and gingival hyperplasia have not been reported with tacrolimus therapy.

Corticosteroids (Prednisone, Solumedrol) are also used for immunosuppressant effects and are part of the immunosuppressive regimen at most transplant centers, though studies are underway to develop steroid-sparing or steroid withdrawal regimens. The mechanism of action is not completely understood, but they are known to have broad antiinflammatory effects on cell-mediated immunity while leaving humoral immunity relatively intact (Smith & McDonald, 2005). The antiinflammatory effects of steroids may play a large role in protecting the transplanted organ. Depending on the dose and length of treatment, steroids produce a variety of mild to severe side effects. Stomach irritation, cushingoid facies, mood swings, acne, swelling and weight gain, hypertension, and insomnia are most commonly seen. Side effects of higher, long-term doses may include cataracts, glaucoma, hyperglycemia, delayed growth, osteoporosis, and muscle weakness.

Mycophenolate mofetil (MMF, Cellcept) was approved by the U.S. Food and Drug Administration (FDA) in 1995 for prevention of acute rejection in renal transplantation and has replaced azathioprine as part of the standard triple therapy. MMF is an antimetabolite agent that decreases the number of functional B and T lymphocytes and inhibits the response to human lymphocytes to antigen tolerance (Smith & McDonald, 2005). Its main side effects are GI distress and hematologic side effects such as anemia, leukopenia, and neutropenia.

Sirolimus (Rapamune), approved in 1999 for prevention of organ transplant rejection in patients older than 13 years of age, was originally found in soil samples from Easter Island and was developed into an immunosuppressant. Sirolimus inhibits the activation of the mammalian target of rapamycin (mTOR), which prevents the progression of the cell cycle, suppressing T lymphocyte activation and proliferation and antibody production. Sirolimus alone appears to cause less nephrotoxicity, neurotoxicity, and hypertension as compared with cyclosporine or tacrolimus (Paghdal & Schwartz, 2007); however, it does appear to potentiate the nephrotoxic effects of CSA and tacrolimus and so is useful in facilitation of CSA/tacrolimus-sparing regimens (Gaston, 2006). These regimens use lower doses of CSA and tacrolimus in the hopes of minimizing their nephrotoxic side effects. Side effects of sirolimus include hypercholesterolemia, nausea, and oral ulcers (Liu & Schiano, 2007).

In renal transplantation, triple combination therapy protocols are frequently employed, with nearly 60% of pediatric recipients on CSA/prednisone/MMF or tacrolimus/prednisone/MMF 1 year after transplant (NAPRTCS, 2007).

Studies are underway to determine the efficacy and safety of regimens that minimize, withdraw, or completely avoid corticosteroids or CNIs (Yang, 2006). The ability to wean and withdraw steroids from transplant recipients is beneficial for posttransplant health, as well as growth and development. With steroid withdrawal, side effects from long-term high-dose steroids (e.g., cushingoid facies, growth failure, osteoporosis, cataract formation, hypertension, diabetes, and an increased risk of infection) can be minimized or eliminated.

Infection Prophylaxis. Risk of opportunistic infections related to the use of immunosuppressive medications is a posttransplant concern. Prophylactic medications including antibiotics (trimethoprim-sulfamethoxazole), antivirals (acyclovir, ganciclovir), and antifungals (nystatin, Mycelex) are used to prevent infectious complications, particularly in the early posttransplant period (see section on infections on p. 724 for more detailed information).

Graft Evaluation. Once graft function has stabilized, most transplant centers prefer that pediatric transplant recipients return to the transplant center for an annual evaluation of the graft. Blood work and organ-specific testing are completed as indicated and may include an abdominal ultrasound, echocardiogram, chest x-ray, or renal flow scan. Biopsies of the transplanted organ are not routinely obtained unless there are clinically significant concerns. The evaluation is usually completed on an outpatient basis over 1 to 2 days, although a short-stay admission may be required following an invasive procedure such as a cardiac catheterization or biopsy.

Although follow-up varies by center, the majority of transplant centers prefer to manage the recipient's immunosuppressive therapy. The child's primary care provider will continue to see the child for routine childhood illnesses and examinations, with any fevers or illnesses reported to the transplant center as well. Although the child may have what appears to be a community virus, it is also important to assess the child for posttransplant viral infections, such as CMV or EBV. Laboratory results, obtained through a community health center or private practice, are sent to the transplant center for evaluation as well.

Complementary and Alternative Therapies

Because not much is known about herbal therapies and the effect of these therapies on the metabolism of medications, herbal remedies are not recommended in children awaiting transplant or with transplants. Additionally, herbal remedies are not regulated by the FDA. Limited information is available that reports interference with the absorption and/or metabolism of immunosuppressants and other medications. Any herbal or natural supplement that affects the activity of cytochrome P-450 3A4, a major drug-metabolizing enzyme, can affect the metabolism of calcineurin inhibitors, cyclosporine, and tacrolimus. It is thought that St. John's wort works in this way by inducing CYP3A4, which increases the metabolism of those medications, reducing the serum concentration of CSA or tacrolimus, and resulting in decreased immunosuppression, placing the child at risk for rejection and allograft loss (Filshie & Rubens, 2006). St. John's wort also interacts with medications such as digoxin, warfarin, and theophylline (Seeff, 2007). Other medication-herb interactions include ma-huang and ginseng, which interact with antihypertensives and increase blood pressure; aloe vera, which can decrease the effectiveness of diuretics; and echinacea, which stimulates the immune system, interfering with the effects of immunosuppressants (Mayo Foundation for Medical Education and Research, 2007). Additionally, herbs such as kava, ma huang (ephedra), and black cohosh have been associated with hepatic toxicity requiring transplantation (Seeff, 2007).

Anticipated Advances in Diagnosis and Management

Because the function of the liver is primarily metabolic, the challenge is to develop a device that could duplicate these complex chemical reactions. Currently, there are clinical trials evaluating different types of liver assist devices. The Molecular Absorbent and Recirculating System (MARS) is an extracorporeal system used for performing albumin dialysis. In this type of dialysis, blood circulates through a dialyzer filter that "cleans" the patient's albumin of protein-bound toxins. In a phase I trial, considerable decreases in ammonia and creatinine levels, intracranial pressure, and the severity of hepatic encephalopathy were noted. In addition to the MARS system, other liver assist devices are being studied. The HepatAssist Liver Support System uses a filter infused with porcine hepatocytes. This device was shown to lead to neurologic and hematologic improvements and has been successfully used as a bridge to liver transplantation (Barshes, Gay, Williams, et al., 2005).

Recipient and graft survival has improved significantly over the past three decades because of advances in immunosuppression, surgical techniques, organ preservation, and monitoring for infections, as well as a better understanding of postoperative management and intensive care medicine. New approaches to standard immunosuppressive protocols that result in optimum graft function with minimal side effects are being explored. Ongoing research is focused on immunosuppressive medications that more specifically inhibit the immune system and decrease the incidence of rejection, subsequently placing a child at less risk for long-term infection and nephrotoxicity. Steroid-free regimens, induction therapies, and weaning trials are innovative immunosuppressive protocols that are being investigated with the goal of inducing tolerance of the transplanted organ.

Approved for use in the late 1990s, daclizumab (Zenapax) and basiliximab (Simulect) are monoclonal antibodies used for the prophylaxis of acute organ rejection. They are chimeric antibodies, made of recombinant murine and human deoxyribonucleic acid (DNA), and work by directly inhibiting IL-2–expressing T lymphocytes (Baran, 2007). Daclizumab is administered before transplant and then every other week after transplant for a total of five doses, whereas basiliximab is given in two doses over a 5-day period, the first dose immediately before transplant and the second dose on postoperative day 4 (Lacy, Armstrong, Goldman, et al., 2008).

Induction therapy with antilymphocyte globulin (ATG, thymoglobulin) is being administered preoperatively or intraoperatively with the goals of decreasing rejection, delaying the first episode of rejection, or preventing or delaying the additional use of calcineurin inhibitors and their associated toxicities (Flynn, 2002). Induction therapy is becoming a more accepted treatment with promising early outcomes; however, the advantages of this type of immunosuppression must be balanced with the risk of infection and recurrent disease (Flynn).

Chimerism and Tolerance

Tolerance is an acquired modification that occurs within the host's immune system, leading to an indefinite survival of the allograft without the use of immunosuppressive medications (Weiss, Ng, & Madsen, 2006). Chimerism is a form of tolerance in which the donor and recipient's blood precursor cells live in coexistence and is quantified by measuring the relative numbers of neutrophils, monocytes, and lymphocytes of both donor and recipient origin in the bloodstream (Pierson, 2007). Though, until recently, scientific studies have only been performed in animal models, there is anecdotal evidence of tolerance achievement. Two patients with end-stage kidney disease and multiple myeloma were treated with simultaneous kidney and bone marrow transplants. In each case, the kidney and bone marrow were harvested from the same living donor. Over 5 years later, both patients continued to have normal allograft function off of all immunosuppression (Weiss et al., 2006).

Xenotransplantation

Cadaveric and living donor organ donations have been unable to meet the demands of the increasing numbers of individuals requiring organ transplantation for end-stage disease. Xenotransplantation is being studied as one option to supply the growing demand for organs, and in the past 20 years, research in this area has significantly increased (Sachs & Fishman, 2008). Xenotransplantation, the cross-species transplantation of organs, has been done experimentally since 1964 using nonhuman primates, sheep, and pigs (Weiss et al., 2006). Pig neural tissue has been implanted in some people with Parkinson's disease and the graft was maintained for many months on cyclosporine alone. Animal-to-human xenotransplantation has included a few experimental procedures. Pig and baboon livers were transplanted into individuals with fulminant hepatic failure, but none had long-term success (Makowka, Cramer, & Hoffman, 1993; Makowka, Wu, Hoffman, et al., 1994; Starzl, Fung, Tzakis, et al., 1993).

Although xenotransplantation would provide an increased source of organs, concern for transmitting infections from the animal source to the recipient and immunologic interactions between the recipient's immune system with the graft have deterred the progress of this strategy (Khalpey, Koch, & Platt, 2004). These concerns for cross-species, animal-derived pathogens have led to a self-imposed suspension of clinical applications of xenotransplantation by most clinicians (Sachs & Fishman, 2008).

ABO-Incompatible Heart Transplantation

Matching donor and recipient blood group has been a cornerstone of transplant management but often means an extended pretransplant waiting time until a blood group–matched donor is available (Boucek, 2001). The innovation of using incompatible blood group donors for infant heart transplant recipients has led to increased survival for this population (West, Pollock-Barziv, Dipchand, et al., 2001). The newborn immune system is immature and anti–blood group antibody (isohemagglutinins) is not yet developed, and this is postulated to allow acceptance of the incompatible blood group heart without rejection (Dipchand, 2004). There are no known differences in outcomes between infants who have received matched versus unmatched transplants. ABO-incompatible (ABOI) heart transplant recipients have specialized requirements regarding transfusion of blood products so that antibody against the recipient or donor blood group is not introduced (West et al., 2001). Primary care practitioners should be aware of these requirements if they have an ABOI transplant recipient in their care. In addition, the primary care practitioner may be involved in facilitating routine blood tests to monitor isohemagglutinin titers.

Living Donor Lung Transplantation

Living donor bilateral lobar transplantation has been performed for more than 10 years and involves the donation of a lower lobe from two separate living donors. This procedure addresses the issue of deceased donor shortages but is controversial because it places two donors at risk (Burch & Aurora, 2004; Webber, McCurry, & Zeevi, 2006). Living donor lung transplantation has similar outcomes to deceased donor lung transplants and is generally reserved for critically ill patients who cannot wait for a deceased donor transplant (Yamane, Date, Okazaki, et al., 2007). Whereas living lung donors may receive emotional benefits from their donation, they face similar potential complications to lung lobectomy for other indications, including pain, bleeding, infection, and other problems. Living lung donors can expect to have lung function within a normal range but have been shown to experience some decrease in exercise capacity (Prager, Wain, Roberts, et al., 2006).

Associated Problems of Solid Organ Transplantation and Treatment
Rejection

Rejection is an inflammatory response of the immune system in which the transplanted tissue is recognized as foreign. Acute cellular rejection most commonly occurs during the first 6 months after transplantation. This type of rejection is a T cell–mediated event and is usually reversible by increasing the level of immunosuppression. Chronic rejection develops over a longer period of time and is a combination of cellular and humoral immune responses. Increased immunosuppressive therapies may not resolve chronic rejection, and the graft may be lost.

Associated Problems

Rejection
- Acute: First 6 months after transplant
- Reversible
- Chronic: Slower process lasting months to years; leading cause of late graft loss

Infection
- Bacterial
- Viral
- Fungal
- Protozoan
- Symptoms of infection masked by immunosuppressive therapy
- Lymphoproliferative disorders

Renal dysfunction

Recurrent disease

Acute rejection is usually reversed if detected early and treated promptly. Acute rejection is a major cause of chronic allograft dysfunction, and multiple episodes of acute rejection can lead to poorer long-term outcomes (Gaston, 2006). Treatment varies by center and severity, but usually involves an increased level of baseline

TABLE 37-2

Clinical Signs of Organ Rejection

Liver	Kidney	Heart	Lung
Abdominal tenderness	Anorexia, oliguria, hypertension	Abdominal pain, vomiting	Decreased exercise tolerance
Acholic stools and bile-stained urine	Edema (particularly of lower extremities)	Cardiomegaly	Decrease in FEV$_1$ ≥ 0% from baseline
Ascites	Elevated BUN and creatinine	Elevated liver enzymes	
Fever (ALT, AST, GGTP), bilirubin, alkaline phosphatase	Fever	Fever (nonspecific)	
Jaundice	Lethargy, fatigue, malaise, irritability	Heart failure	
Lethargy, fatigue, malaise, irritability	Tenderness at the graft site	Hepatomegaly	
	Weight gain	Poor feeding and irritability (infants)	
		Sudden change in blood pressure	

Key: *ALT,* alanine aminotransferase; *AST,* aspartate aminotransferase; *BUN,* blood urea nitrogen; *FEV$_1$,* forced expiratory volume in 1 second; *GGTP,* gamma-glutamyl transpeptidase phosphate.

immunosuppression, increased corticosteroids, the addition of an adjunctive immunosuppressant such as azathioprine (Imuran), MMF, or sirolimus (Rapamune), and/or conversion of immunosuppression from CSA to tacrolimus. Muromonab-CD3 (OKT3), a monoclonal antibody, or antilymphocyte globulin or antithymocyte globulin (Thymoglobulin) may be used to treat rejection that is refractory to steroids and/or increased baseline immunosuppression (Kerkar & Emre, 2007; Tiao & Ryckman, 2006). Repeat biopsies may be performed to evaluate the effectiveness of treatment and determine changes in immunosuppression.

Symptoms of liver rejection include fever, elevated liver function tests, abdominal tenderness, irritability, and fatigue (Table 37-2). If left untreated, rejection may progress from mild to moderate symptoms to those of hepatic dysfunction: ascites, jaundice, acholic stools, bile-stained urine, pruritus, encephalopathy, decreased synthetic function, and renal dysfunction. A percutaneous liver biopsy may be performed to definitively diagnose rejection since elevated enzymes and fever may also be seen with infectious processes, biliary tract complications, or hepatic artery thrombosis. Chronic rejection occurs in 5% to 10% of children with liver transplants and is defined by the progressive disappearance of bile ducts with subsequent cholestasis and liver failure (i.e., vanishing bile duct syndrome) and may result in late graft loss (Jain, Mazariegos, Kashyap, et al., 2002; Tiao & Ryckman, 2006; Wallot, Mathot, Janssen, et al., 2002).

Advances in immunosuppressive therapy have significantly decreased the risk of both acute and chronic rejection. For children who received a renal transplant from 1987 to 1990, the probability of acute rejection was 54% for a living donor allograft and 69% for a deceased donor. In 2003 to 2005, those numbers decreased to 13% and 16%, respectively (NAPRTCS, 2007). Careful assessment is key because a low-grade fever and hypertension may be the only signs of early acute rejection. Other symptoms of rejection may include irritability, malaise, oliguria, increased BUN and creatinine levels, weight gain from fluid retention, swelling and tenderness at the graft site, edema of the lower extremities, and anorexia. Rejection is confirmed definitively through percutaneous renal biopsy and renal flow scan. Treatment varies based on center-specific immunosuppressive protocols and severity of rejection but usually involves an increased level of baseline immunosuppression, increased corticosteroids, and the possible addition of an adjunctive immunosuppressant. In children receiving cyclosporine, tacrolimus has been shown to be an effective rescue therapy (Burton & Rosen, 2006). Antibody therapy with antilymphocyte globulin (Thymoglobulin), daclizumab (Zenapax), or basiliximab may also

be used to reduce the immune response by temporarily blocking IL-2 receptors (Vester, Kranz, Testa, et al., 2001). Repeat biopsies may be performed to evaluate the effectiveness of treatment.

Acute and chronic rejection causes nearly half of all graft losses in renal transplantation (NAPRTCS, 2007). Chronic rejection is a slow process in which the transplant recipient progressively loses renal function, resulting in graft loss in 35% of all renal allograft failures (NAPRTCS, 2007).

Unlike acute rejection of the liver or kidney, children with heart transplants usually do not develop symptoms until rejection is severe. Most acute rejection is identified by echocardiogram or heart biopsy before the child is symptomatic. Severe rejection results in graft dysfunction that manifests as heart failure with tachycardia, tachypnea, arrhythmia, gallop rhythm, hepatomegaly, and cardiomegaly. Other symptoms may include shortness of breath, increased respiratory rate, edema and/or sudden weight gain, and changes in blood pressure. Nonspecific findings may include fever, irritability, and poor feeding, particularly in infants. Abdominal pain and vomiting secondary to decreased cardiac output and perfusion to the gastrointestinal tract may also be seen. Rejection is diagnosed through clinical assessment and echocardiography and confirmed by cardiac biopsy. Surveillance biopsies are performed more frequently in the early postoperative period and then less often as the risk of rejection decreases (Wise & Walsh, 2008).

Chronic rejection of the heart allograft is also known as transplant coronary artery vasculopathy (CAV). This is a progressive condition that usually occurs over many years resulting in graft loss. It is characterized by circumferential narrowing of the coronary artery and thickening of the intima and is detected by arteriography and dobutamine stress echocardiography. The risk of having CAV is less than 20% at 10 years after transplant; however, CAV is the most common cause of death at this point, accounting for greater than 30% of deaths at 10 years (Boucek et al., 2007). Retransplantation is the primary treatment for chronic rejection. Palliative treatment through stenting of discrete coronary artery lesions is of limited use because CAV tends to involve the entire length of the coronary artery and stenting will not improve disease in the small, distal vessels (Webber, McCurry, & Zeevi, 2006). Unfortunately, syncope or sudden death may be the first clinical sign of chronic rejection.

Acute rejection in the lung transplant recipient is most often identified by a decrease in lung function. Regular pulmonary function testing and home spirometry are used to identify changes in lung function. A decrease of 10% or more in FEV$_1$ is considered suspicious of rejection (Visner & Goldfarb, 2007). Transbronchial biopsy is used both as surveillance for rejection and follow-up to changes in pulmonary function (Webber, McCurry, & Zeevi, 2006).

Chronic rejection in lung transplantation is known as bronchiolitis obliterans syndrome (BOS) and manifests as progressive shortness of breath and decreased exercise tolerance with decreasing FEV_1 well below posttransplant baseline (White-Williams, Kugler, & Widmar, 2008). BOS is the most common cause of death in lung transplant recipients more than 2 years after transplant (Trulock, Christie, Edwards, et al., 2007), and nearly half of pediatric lung transplant recipients will have some evidence of BOS by 5 years after transplant (Webber, McCurry, & Zeevi, 2006).

Infection

The dilemma of transplantation is that an adequately suppressed immune system to prevent rejection must be balanced with one that is also competent in resisting infection. This delicate equilibrium can be easily disturbed when immunosuppression is increased to treat or avoid rejection. The common result is infection, which is a significant cause of morbidity and mortality following transplantation.

The period when the child is at highest risk for infections is within the first 6 months after transplant. During the early postoperative period, the first 30 days, infections related to surgical complications and donor- or recipient-derived infections are most common. These infections are usually the result of a preexisting chronic condition or infection, wound or line infections, pneumonia, urinary tract infections, and nosocomial infections (Fishman, 2007).

During months 1 to 6 after transplant, the most common infections are opportunistic infections such as *Pneumocystis jiroveci* (formerly *carinii*), polyoma virus, and adenovirus. CMV- and EBV-associated lymphoproliferative disorders are also seen during this time (Fishman, 2007).

Long-term infections are difficult to document because most transplant recipients are receiving care through primary settings where data on infections may not be accrued. At 6 months after transplant, those transplant recipients who have satisfactory graft function are on maintenance immunosuppression. Infections in this group are most commonly community acquired (e.g., pneumonia, CMV, and urinary tract infections) (Fishman, 2007).

Cytomegalovirus. CMV is a common viral infection following transplantation and is a significant source of morbidity and mortality in pediatric transplant recipients. CMV usually occurs within the first several months after transplant (Smith & McDonald, 2005). Children who are CMV-seronegative before transplant and receive a seropositive organ are at greater risk of developing primary disease. Additional risk factors include the intensity and duration of immunosuppression, particularly the use of antilymphocyte and antithymocyte therapies and acute rejection (Huprikar, 2007). CMV disease is manifested frequently as fever and neutropenia; however, other signs, including lymphadenopathy, hepatitis, thrombocytopenia, colitis, or chorioretinitis, can be seen as well (Fishman, 2007). Diagnosis is based on clinical presentation, viral cultures, serology (including newer assays such as PP65 tegument protein, a CMV antigenemia assay, and the polymerase chain reaction [PCR]), and histopathology (Fischer, 2006). Detecting antigenemia may result in earlier treatment and intervention before the development of clinical symptoms.

There are similarities in the prevention and treatment of CMV after transplant, but protocols are center specific. Ganciclovir (Cytovene) or valganciclovir (Valcyte) is widely used for the treatment of CMV disease due to its potent ability to inhibit viral DNA replication of the human herpes viruses. In pediatrics, intravenous (IV) ganciclovir is preferred because of the erratic absorption of the oral preparation. However, valganciclovir has been shown to have a greater bioavailability than oral ganciclovir and has a pharmacokinetic profile similar to IV ganciclovir (Huprikar, 2007). Hyperimmune anti-CMV-IgG, which contains antibodies against CMV, is also used in combination with ganciclovir to prevent or treat severe CMV disease and provides passive immunity to the child (Kerkar & Emre, 2007). The duration of antiviral therapy is based on the extent of CMV disease, the level of immunosuppression, presence of concurrent rejection or other infections, and institution protocols. Research into vaccines that would protect children from acquired CMV infection is underway (Schleiss, 2007).

Lymphoproliferative Disorders. EBV and associated posttransplant lymphoproliferative disorders (PTLDs) may range from a self-limiting mononucleosis to malignant monoclonal lymphoma. From 80% to 90% of all PTLDs are associated with EBV infections. EBV-negative lymphoproliferative disorders tend to occur later (longer than 1 year after transplant), tend to have a worse prognosis, and tend to have a poor response to therapy (Fishman, 2007; Loren & Tsai, 2005).

The incidence of PTLD is 2.6% to 9% in renal transplantation, 6.8% to 13% in liver transplantation, and 5% in cardiac transplantation. PTLD accounts for more than half of posttransplantation malignancies in pediatric transplant recipients, and has mortality rates as high as 60% (Al-Akash, Al Makadma, & Al Omari, 2005; Fishman, 2007; Webber, Naftel, Fricker, et al., 2006). Risk factors for EBV include young age, primary EBV infection after transplantation in EBV-seronegative recipients of EBV-seropositive organs, coexisting CMV infection, and exposure to antilymphocyte antiserum (Al-Akash et al., 2005; Fishman, 2007). Symptoms may include fever, malaise, tonsillitis, pharyngitis, abdominal-mass lesions, CNS disease, or GI disturbances (Fishman, 2007). Tumor-like infiltrates, as well as ulcerations of the GI tract with abdominal pain and bleeding, are seen in invasive disease.

Early diagnosis is vital to recovery and is based on clinical presentation, histopathology, laboratory studies, and radiographic findings. A biopsy is often performed on an accessible node, and a computed tomography (CT) scan is obtained to assess the chest and abdomen for enlarged nodes or disseminated disease. The EBV polymerase chain reaction (EBV-PCR) and EBV DNA quantification testing are sensitive tools that help monitor viral load and are used to track disease progression in transplant recipients (Kullberg-Lindh, Ascher, Saalman, et al., 2006).

Treatment and management of EBV and PTLD are controversial, although the reduction or discontinuation of immunosuppression with frequent monitoring of the EBV-PCR is generally accepted. Evaluation of graft function with biopsy is essential to monitor for rejection in the setting of reduced immunosuppression. Other treatments include the use of antiviral agents, chemotherapy, and anti-CD20 antibodies, such as rituximab, and irradiation (Al-Akash et al., 2005; Fishman, 2007).

***Pneumocystis jiroveci* (formerly *carinii*) Pneumonia.** Children who are immunosuppressed are at risk for *Pneumocystis jiroveci* (formerly *carinii*) pneumonia (PCP), a rare but serious infectious complication. Trimethoprim-sulfamethoxazole (TMP-SMX, Bactrim, Septra) is widely accepted as effective prophylaxis (Fonseca-Aten & Michaels, 2006). Most cases occur within 1 to 6 months after transplant. If a transplant recipient has fever and a lower respiratory tract infection and is not receiving prophylaxis, PCP should always be considered in the differential diagnosis—especially in the early posttransplant period.

Varicella-Zoster Virus. Varicella-zoster virus is a highly contagious childhood disease that can be potentially severe in the child who is immunocompromised (Dodd, Burger, Edwards, et al., 2001). Recommended therapy is administration of varicella-zoster immune globulin (VZIG) within 72 hours of exposure, as well as a reduction of immunosuppression to help prevent or decrease the severity of the illness. Approximately 50% of children treated with VZIG following direct exposure develop a mild form of the virus and are usually hospitalized to receive intravenous acyclovir until the lesions crust, followed by a course of oral acyclovir (Pearlman, 2002b). Successful management of varicella zoster infection with oral antiviral therapy alone has been described in heart transplant recipients who were otherwise well and off steroids (Dodd et al., 2001). Graft function should be monitored closely for rejection for several weeks in the setting of reduced baseline immunosuppression. Following an exposure to or outbreak of the disease, transplant recipients should be tested for immunity to varicella-zoster virus to determine whether precautions need to be taken with future exposures.

The varicella-zoster vaccine Varivax is routinely administered to immunocompetent children at 1 and 4 years of age. However, since this vaccine is a live virus, it is not recommended for use in the immunocompromised child. If the child awaiting transplant is at least 1 year old, the child is otherwise medically stable, and the transplant is not imminent, the vaccine should be administered before transplant (Verma & Wade, 2006).

Fungal Infections. Fungal infections usually occur during the early postoperative period. *Candida* causes the majority of posttransplant fungal infections, although *Aspergillus* can be seen more commonly in lung transplant recipients (Fonseca-Aten & Michaels, 2006). Fungal infections are usually opportunistic and manifest as noninvasive infections of the oropharynx, esophagus, or genitalia caused by high immunosuppressive levels. Noninvasive *Candida* appears as plaques on the oral mucosa or as a papular rash of the genitalia. Treatment with an oral "swish and swallow" solution of nystatin or topical nystatin ointment usually resolves a noninvasive infection. Invasive disease (fungemia) can develop related to surgical complications, steroid administration, broad-spectrum antibiotics, prolonged operative time, repeat laparotomies, retransplantation, and renal or respiratory compromise. Invasive disease causes fever, irritability, malaise, decreased appetite, or an erythematous central catheter site and is confirmed by blood, urine, throat, or wound cultures. Fungemia is treated with an intravenous antifungal agent with close monitoring of renal function (Cupples, Dumas-Hicks, & Burnapp, 2008).

Polyomavirus. Human polyomaviruses, composed of subgroups BKV, JCV, and SV40, are DNA viruses. BKV has been associated with polyomavirus-associated nephropathy (PVAN) and JCV with progressive multifocal leukoencephalopathy (Fishman, 2007). Serologic studies have shown 60% to 96% of adults with positive antibodies to BKV, and most children become seropositive

by age 10. From 2% to 8% of children with renal transplants are diagnosed with PVAN and this often precedes renal allograft dysfunction. Though not fully understood, transmission of BKV is thought to occur by oral-enteric or respiratory routes. Risk factors for PVAN include BKV-seropositive donors and BKV-negative recipients, age less than 5 years, reduced BKV-specific cellular immunity, and positive BKV viruria. Infection, typically asymptomatic in persons with an intact immune system, can cause hemorrhagic cystitis, interstitial nephritis, and ureteral stenosis in renal transplant recipients (Elidemir, Chang, Schecter, et al., 2007). Interstitial nephritis can mimic the symptoms of rejection, making the identification of BKV important when making treatment decisions. A renal biopsy is the current gold standard of diagnosis, though serum and urine assays using PCR are being used to assess response to therapy. Whereas intensified immunosuppression is used for rejection, a reduction of immunosuppression is appropriate for the treatment of BKV. There is limited anecdotal experience with the antiviral medications leflunomide and cidofovir and IVIG (Acott & Hirsch, 2007).

Renal Dysfunction

As patient and graft survival rates have increased, renal dysfunction and progression to chronic kidney disease has become an issue of concern. The incidence of renal dysfunction after pediatric heart transplant is 6% at 1 year and increases to 17% at 10 years (Lee, Christensen, Magee, et al., 2007). Pediatric liver transplant data are sparse; however, adult studies have shown that after liver transplantation, the glomerular filtration rate (GFR) falls to approximately 60% of the pretransplantation GFR within 6 weeks of surgery and as many as 10% of adult liver transplant recipients develop ESRD by 10 years (Campbell, Yagigi, Ryckman, et al., 2006; Liu & Schiano, 2007). One pediatric study noted that renal dysfunction was present in 32% at an average of 7 years after transplant (Campbell et al., 2006). Contributors to renal dysfunction include the use of calcineurin inhibitors, pretransplant renal disease, perioperative hemodynamic instability, hypertension, and diabetes (Liu & Schiano, 2007). Decreasing exposure to nephrotoxic medications and strict control and management of hypertension and proteinuria may have an impact in minimizing renal dysfunction (Campbell et al., 2006).

Recurrent Disease

In select causes of renal failure, there is a risk of posttransplant recurrence. Diseases such as hyperoxaluria and focal segmental glomerulosclerosis (FSGS) can both recur rapidly in the transplanted allograft. Recurrence rates of FSGS vary from 20% to 30%. Risk of graft failure secondary to recurrent FSGS is 25% (Trachtman, 2007; Vogt & Avner, 2007). Membranoproliferative glomerulonephritis (MPGN) can also recur, but the risk of recurrence is dependent on the specific type of MPGN. MPGN type II recurs in 90% of allografts, whereas type I only recurs in 25% (Vogt & Avner). Membranous nephropathy, immunoglobulin A (IgA) nephropathy, Henoch-Schönlein purpura, and hemolytic uremic syndrome are other renal diseases that may recur following transplantation.

There are particular liver diseases that can recur after transplant, as well. Viral infections such as hepatitis B or C, autoimmune diseases, hepatocellular carcinoma, and Budd-Chiari syndrome can all cause posttransplant allograft dysfunction (Burton & Rosen, 2006).

Prognosis

Pediatric transplantation has offered a second chance at life for thousands of children with end-stage organ disease. Although recipient and graft survival is high, long-term graft loss may be associated with late acute rejection, chronic rejection, recurrent disease, and nonadherence (NAPRTCS, 2007).

The first successful clinical trials in renal transplantation were conducted in 1962 at the University of Colorado (Starzl & Demetris, 1997). Before that series, a few isolated cases of renal transplantation between fraternal and identical twins were reported. Renal transplantation has evolved as the treatment choice for ESRD. Combined graft survival rates for living and cadaver kidney recipients have increased over time. The 1-year survival rates in the cohort group of children who received kidney transplant during 1987 to 1990 for cadaveric and living grafts were 75.2% and 89.4%, respectively, increasing in cohort group 2003 to 2006 to 95% and 97.5% (NAPRTCS, 2007).

Dr. Thomas Starzl pioneered pediatric liver transplantation, with the first surgery being performed in 1963 (Ahmed & Keefe, 2007). One-year survival was not achieved until 1967, and the survival rate was only 30% until the era of cyclosporine immunosuppression in the late 1970s to early 1980s. As of June 27, 2008, the OPTN reported a 90% survival rate at 1 year and an 84% survival rate at 3 years for children ages less than 1 year to 17 years who received a transplant between 1997 and 2004 (OPTN, 2008b).

In 2002, the model of end-stage liver disease (MELD) and pediatric end-stage liver disease (PELD) scoring system was introduced to more accurately predict who needs a liver transplant most urgently. The MELD is used for candidates over 12 years of age and the PELD is used for children age 11 and younger (UNOS, 2008). With the demand for donor livers far exceeding the supply, split-liver transplantation and living-related liver transplantation (LRLT) are being used as strategies to increase the donor pool. The split-liver procedure involves dividing the liver into two sections using various segments of the right or left lobe, depending on the size of the recipients. But due to technical difficulties and logistical obstacles, only a small number of large centers in North America routinely undertake split-liver transplantation. As results and outcomes improve, however, the use of partial-liver grafts probably will increase (Foster, Zimmerman, & Trotter, 2007). LRLT usually involves liver donation between a child with ESLD and an ABO-compatible donor, most commonly a biologic parent, but poses the ethical dilemma of placing a healthy donor at risk in order to save the life of a child. The evaluation for LRLT demands a full assessment of the risk-benefit ratio for the child, donor, and family.

Heart transplantation in humans was pioneered in the 1960s and pediatric transplants began in the 1980s (Dipchand, 2004; Wise & Walsh, 2008). There is now more than 25 years of pediatric heart transplant experience with continued improvements in patient and graft survival over time. Median survival (half-life) is the point at which 50% of recipients will be alive with a functioning transplant. The overall median survival for pediatric heart transplant recipients is 15.8 years for infants, 14.2 years for 1- to 10-year-olds, and 11.4 years for adolescents. Median survival for infant recipients who survive the first year after transplant cannot be computed, which reflects excellent outcomes. The expected half-life for 1- to 10-year-old recipients who survive the first year after transplant is 17.5 years and 15.2 years for adolescent recipients (Boucek et al., 2007).

Many children will require retransplantation at some point in the future. Although the number of reported retransplants is still low (35 in 2005), the number has doubled in the past 10 years (Boucek et al.).

Survival after lung transplant is not as robust as for most other organ groups. Survival at 1 year after lung transplant is 75% and 42% at 5 years (Webber, McCurry, & Zeevi, 2006). Children ages 6 to 10 years have the best outcomes, with 73% survival at 3 years. Adolescents have the worst outcomes, with 56% survival at 3 years (Horslen, Barr, Christensen, et al., 2007).

Although the use of parenteral nutrition (PN) has extended the lives of children with end-stage short gut syndrome, associated morbidities are common. These morbidities include PN-associated liver disease, venous access complications related to thrombosis and sepsis, and ultimately a lack of venous access (Fryer, 2007). The financial burden of daily TPN and associated care, as well as the psychosocial impact of a permanent indwelling line and connection to an infusion pump, are also stressors for these children and their families. Over the last 40 years, intestine transplantation has progressed from an experimental strategy to an accepted treatment for permanent intestinal failure. Graft and patient survival 5 years after transplantation is 38% and 54%, respectively, for isolated intestine and 44% and 47%, respectively, for a composite liver-intestine graft (Fryer).

PRIMARY CARE MANAGEMENT

Health Care Maintenance

Growth and Development

The goal of pediatric organ transplantation is for the child to achieve normal growth and development with an improved quality of life. Growth affects the emotional well-being of children and participation in the routine activities of childhood. Growth retardation is seen in all children with solid organ transplants, most likely from the effect of corticosteroid immunosuppression (Turkel & Pao, 2007). The primary care provider has an essential role in monitoring the child's long-term growth and development. Height, weight, and body mass index (BMI) should be routinely documented on standardized growth charts and evaluated (Peterson, Perens, Wetzel, et al., 2007).

Transplant candidates exhibit symptoms and effects of chronic disease such as anorexia, vomiting, malnutrition, anemia, and bone problems, which affect growth and development. Although transplantation may resolve some of these complications, immunosuppressive therapy with long-term and/or high-dose steroids also affects growth (Peterson et al., 2007). Aggressive nutritional support and minimization or discontinuation of steroids will contribute to growth. Increased or intensified nutritional support or growth hormone therapy may be required in some cases of growth retardation (Fuqua, 2006).

The average child awaiting renal transplant is nearly 2 standard deviations below the mean for height (NAPTRCS, 2007) at the time of transplantation. Growth after renal transplantation is affected by age at transplant, persistent hyperparathyroidism and renal osteodystrophy, graft function, and immunosuppressive medications (NAPTRCS, 2007; Sanchez, Kuizon, Goodman, et al., 2002). Of children transplanted before age 15 years, 70% remain below the third percentile for height as adults (Sanchez et al., 2002). Catch-up growth has been seen primarily in children who were under 6 years of age at the time of transplant, with children under 2 years of age showing the most improvement (NAPRTCS, 2007). Improvements in growth velocity have been seen with the use of growth hormone for children with chronic renal insufficiency, for children requiring dialysis, and for children with renal transplants (Mahan & Warady, 2006). The ability to wean or withdraw steroids may also affect growth and development.

Growth retardation in children with liver transplants is a result of malnutrition secondary to anorexia, vomiting, malabsorption, and inadequate oral intake (Mejia, Barshes, Halff, et al., 2007). The Studies of Pediatric Liver Transplantation (SPLIT), a cooperative research network of pediatric liver transplantation centers in the United States and Canada, reports that the pediatric liver transplant candidate is on average 1.4 standard deviations below the age- and gender-adjusted height level. Younger children (less than 5 years of age) have even greater height deficits, but also have the best catch-up growth within 24 months after transplant (SPLIT Research Group, 2001). Early liver transplantation in children with growth retardation has been found to restore growth potential, although age at time of transplant, gender, onset of puberty, and disease etiology also affected growth (Renz, de Roos, Rosenthal, et al., 2001).

Children with chronic conditions are more likely to have emotional, behavioral, and psychiatric symptoms than healthy children. The distribution of cause can be attributed to a variety of issues, including neurodevelopmental abnormalities; disruptions that occur in education because of illness, appointments, or hospitalizations; limited social experiences; and the physical effects of the chronic condition and its treatment (Turkel & Pao, 2007).

Cerebral atrophy has been seen in 12% to 23% of children with ESRD. Those at higher risk are children with congenital nephrotic syndrome, cystinosis, and Lowe's syndrome. Approximately 20% to 25% of young children with ESRD show general developmental delays. When compared with healthy siblings, children with ESRD were found to have lower intelligence quotients (IQs) and lower school achievement. Some studies have reported that successful renal transplantation in these children can help correct some of these deficits (Gipson, Wetherington, Duquette, et al., 2007).

Health-related quality of life for children after liver transplantation from the parents' perspective is lower than that of healthy children, but is similar to that of children with other chronic conditions (Bucuvalas, Britto, Krug, et al, 2003); however, perceptions of quality of life improve over time. The child's psychosocial functioning was predicted by the child's age at the time of transplant and maternal education (Bucuvalas, et al., 2003).

Many children with heart failure experience inadequate growth. Heart transplantation helps optimize linear growth and weight gain in this patient population. The majority of pediatric heart transplant recipients can achieve normal linear growth (Alkhaldi et al., 2006). Factors such as age at the time of transplant and length of steroid use after transplant can affect optimal growth. Observation of weight gain in the context of linear growth is important to ensure an appropriate BMI (Peterson et al., 2007). After heart transplantation most children return to school, participate in sports and age-appropriate activities, and are classified as a New York Heart Association Functional Class I with no activity restrictions (Webber, McCurry, & Zeevi, 2006). Behavior and cognitive function after heart and heart-lung transplantation has been measured in the

normal or low-normal range, with younger children exhibiting more developmental problems (Wray & Radley-Smith, 2005). Pretransplant diagnosis may also be a risk factor for psychological problems, with children with CHD having more difficulty (Wray & Radley-Smith, 2006). Although many children achieve good psychological outcomes after transplant, ongoing attention to this area of development is essential.

Information regarding growth and development after lung transplant is limited. Many children with cystic fibrosis are at risk for poor nutritional status and low BMI. There is emerging evidence that BMI improves after transplant, reflecting improved growth and nutrition (Dosanjh, 2002). Most children still surviving 3 years after their lung transplant have no activity limitations (Burch & Aurora, 2004).

Diet

Attention to nutritional management for children both before and after transplantation is crucial in achieving optimal wound healing, catch-up growth, and ultimately normal growth and development. After transplant, a child's diet is usually liberalized. Renal recipients may have mild to moderate sodium intake restrictions, and cardiac recipients are encouraged to maintain healthy eating habits, avoiding excessive intake of foods high in sodium and cholesterol. In addition, medication side effects may cause hyperkalemia, hypertension, hypomagnesemia, hypophosphatemia, hyperglycemia, or hyperlipidemia, necessitating a respective dietary restriction or supplement. Hyperlipidemia not controlled by diet and exercise, particularly in cardiac recipients, is often treated with lipid-lowering agents (Seipelt, Crawford, Rodgers, et al., 2004).

Some children may require enteral supplementation because of an inability to ingest adequate calories or meet fluid requirements after transplant. This can be related to taste changes secondary to oral medications or metabolic imbalances, gastroesophageal reflux, and abdominal fullness due to dwelling peritoneal dialysis solutions (National Kidney Foundation, 2000). Some transplant recipients may require tube feeding for a period of time after transplant purely to promote catch-up growth. Certain children have unique nutritional requirements, such as small bowel transplant recipients, who may continue with TPN and enteral tube feeding for several weeks or months after transplant. Most children can eventually be weaned from these therapies (Venick, Farmer, Saikali, et al., 2006). Children with cystic fibrosis after lung transplant continue to require nutritional management for elements of their disease process such as fat malabsorption, osteoporosis, and possibly diabetes, which are not changed with the transplant (Dosanjh, 2002).

Safety

As with all routine pediatric visits, counseling about safety issues (e.g., the proper use of car seats, seat belts, and bicycle helmets; child proofing the home) at a child's age and developmental level is necessary for all families with a child who has had an organ transplant. Because most children have good graft function and are prescribed maintenance doses of immunosuppression, good hand-washing techniques and avoidance of others with obvious infections are sound guidelines to decrease the risk of infection.

Activity. In children with a heart or heart-lung transplant, it is important to understand that the incisions in the heart sever the sympathetic and parasympathetic nerves, which ordinarily regulate the heart rate. This lack of neural connections is known as denervation. Without direct control of the CNS, the transplanted heart will beat faster in a resting state. This faster than normal rate is associated with normal cardiac function and the capability of sustaining vigorous physical activity. The transplanted heart depends on circulating adrenalin and related hormones produced by the adrenal gland, instead of a direct impulse from the brain, to change its rate. The transplanted heart may take up to 10 minutes before an increase in heart rate is seen in response to exercise, and up to 1 hour may pass after stopping exercise before a decrease in rate is seen (Hartley, Fisher, & Cupples, 2008). Another effect of denervation is that chest pain or angina pectoris cannot be perceived if coronary artery disease develops; however, some recipients may regrow these nerves and will experience the typical symptoms of coronary artery blockage if it develops. Consequently, coronary arteriograms and dobutamine stress echocardiograms are obtained to assess for evidence of vasculopathy.

Pediatric heart recipients are activity restricted for the first 6 to 8 weeks after surgery to allow the sternum to heal. Recipients should avoid bike riding, climbing, sit-ups, push-ups, roller skating, and contact sports and should also refrain from lifting, pushing, or pulling heavy objects during this period. After 8 weeks, all activities, as well as physical education class at school, may be resumed. Teens who are licensed drivers may also resume driving at 2 months after transplant. A physical therapist should instruct children on an exercise program before discharge from the hospital. This program consists of a 5-minute warm-up and cool-down period before and after peak physical activity. If a child shows signs of increased shortness of breath or fatigue, the cool-down period should begin. Physical education teachers should be informed of the heart recipient's additional exercise considerations.

Children who have received liver or kidney transplants are encouraged to resume previous activities, although there are some limitations in the early postoperative period. Push-ups or sit-ups, as well as activities that stretch or put pressure on the abdomen and incision, are to be avoided for 3 to 6 months. Recipients should avoid heavy lifting for at least 6 months. Although some centers discourage contact sports, most children can participate in age-appropriate activities as they develop greater endurance and fitness, such as soccer, softball, basketball, bicycling, skating, swimming, dancing, and gymnastics.

Some centers prefer that families notify the transplant center when they plan to travel for an extended period of time or to a foreign country. This notification is particularly important for children awaiting an organ transplant so that a means of communication is available in case an organ becomes available. Medication doses and schedules should always be maintained while a child is on vacation, and an adequate supply of medication should be taken with the child. Medications should be carried onto airplanes rather than being checked with luggage. Parents are encouraged to obtain Medic-Alert bracelets for their child to identify the child as a transplant recipient and provide the name and telephone number of the transplant center in case of an emergency. In addition, infectious disease precautions need to be taken with foreign travel to certain areas where immunizations may not be available for all children and adults.

Immunizations

Because of the inconsistent rates of serologic conversion of many vaccines after transplant, care should be taken to complete the schedule for routine immunizations before transplantation

whenever possible (Campbell & Herold, 2005). Children who have been previously immunized should have serologic testing for antibodies to vaccine-preventable diseases. Those children who are susceptible should be reimmunized (American Academy of Pediatrics [AAP] Committee on Infectious Diseases, 2006).

After transplant, primary care practitioners should follow the guidelines established for immunosuppressed children (AAP Committee on Infectious Diseases, 2006). Live-bacterial and live-virus vaccines are generally contraindicated in this population, and only inactivated vaccines (e.g., the inactivated polio and flu vaccines) should be administered. Unfortunately, no inactivated form of vaccination exists for measles, mumps, and rubella (MMR) or varicella. For those children who received the MMR or varicella vaccine before transplant, yearly serum titers should be drawn to verify immunity (AAP Committee on Infectious Diseases, 2006). Siblings of the transplant recipient should receive the MMR and varicella vaccines.

Children transplanted in infancy do not have the benefit of receiving MMR and varicella vaccines before transplant, and other chronically ill transplant candidates' vaccinations may be incomplete. Consequently, some transplant programs are investigating the administration of these live-virus vaccines after transplant with reasonable immunologic response and limited adverse events (Khan, Erlichman, & Rand, 2006). Despite these early successes, live-virus vaccines after transplant remain contraindicated by most transplant centers and should not be undertaken by the primary care practitioner.

Because children are more highly immunosuppressed in the early posttransplant period they may be unable to mount an immunologic response to vaccine, and no immunizations should be given during this time. The immunization schedule for children who are immunosuppressed should commence once the recipient is receiving maintenance immunosuppression. This time frame can vary by transplant center and organ group but is usually 3 to 12 months after transplant. If a child is receiving augmented immunosuppression to treat rejection, any scheduled immunizations should be postponed for at least 1 to 3 months.

The influenza vaccine should be administered annually to children with organ transplants who are 3 or more months after transplant. All family members living within the household should also receive the vaccine. Some transplant centers recommend respiratory syncytial virus (RSV) prophylaxis with palivizumab (Synagis) monthly to infant transplant recipients transplanted just before or during RSV season. There is no specific recommendation for RSV vaccine in immunocompromised children, but potential benefits in certain circumstances are acknowledged (AAP, 2003).

Hepatitis B is an infrequent but significant cause of decreased graft survival, morbidity, and mortality. Children awaiting transplant, particularly children with ESRD receiving dialysis, should be vaccinated against hepatitis B, if they did not already receive it, because it can be acquired through contact with blood products. Children whose hepatitis B vaccine is not up to date may receive it 3 to 12 months after transplantation following posttransplant guidelines. It is recommended that siblings, caretakers, and household contacts also be immunized.

Immunization policies vary by transplant center. The primary care provider should contact the transplant center for specific immunization guidelines for the child and family. Administration and maintenance of routine childhood vaccinations after transplant is one of the most important roles of the primary care provider with this patient population.

Screening

Vision. Routine screening is recommended. Because cataracts, glaucoma, and pseudotumor cerebri may be side effects of long-term steroid use, an annual ophthalmologic examination should be performed on children at risk for these conditions. CMV retinitis may occur as a result of a CMV infection and requires ophthalmologic follow-up until resolution. Children with no prior exposure to toxoplasmosis who receive organs from toxoplasmosis-positive donors require periodic ophthalmologic examinations. These children receive posttransplant prophylaxis with pyrimethamine (Daraprim) and folinic acid (Muñoz, Rodriguez, & Bouza, 2004).

Hearing. Routine screening is recommended. In addition, transplant recipients who received intravenous ototoxic medications (i.e., gentamicin, vancomycin) frequently before and after transplant are at risk for hearing deficits and should be referred to an audiologist for screening. Audiograms are recommended to determine the extent of hearing loss and to recommend interventions.

Dental. Biannual dental visits and good oral hygiene practices are recommended for children following organ transplantation. Gingival hyperplasia is commonly seen in children receiving cyclosporine or calcium channel blockers. Good dental and oral hygiene with mechanical stimulation by daily brushing and flossing, gingival massaging, and plaque control can contain the gum growth to within acceptable limits. Gingivectomy treatment by surgical excision or laser has been used, but has been shown to result in a relapse of enlargement within 1 year and lead to fibrotic scarring of the gingival tissue (Farge, Ranchin, & Cochat, 2006).

Antibiotic prophylaxis is no longer recommended for solid organ transplant recipients except for heart transplant recipients who have developed a cardiac valvulopathy or those recipients who have had a previous case of infective endocarditis (Wilson, Taubert, Gewitz, et al., 2007).

Blood Pressure. Because hypertension is a common side effect of some immunosuppressants, blood pressure measurement should be a part of all discharge teaching plans. If antihypertensive medications are prescribed, parents are instructed to measure the child's blood pressure before administering these medications. Administration guidelines, based on blood pressure parameters, should be clearly delineated for the child and family. Parents may be advised to maintain a record of blood pressure readings and administered antihypertensive medications so that the primary care provider and transplant team can monitor treatment and adjust medications. Antihypertensive medications are usually not required for the long term after transplant if the child is steroid free or if immunosuppressive levels are maintained at a low level.

A trend in nighttime hypertension in people with heart transplants has been noted. It is suspected that denervation of the transplanted heart plays a role in this as a result of decreased parasympathetic tone, which would normally contribute to lower blood pressure at night. Consequently, a single daytime blood pressure measurement may not accurately reflect the blood pressure profile, and occasional 24-hour blood pressure monitoring is recommended (O'Sullivan, Derrick, & Gray, 2005).

Hematocrit. The hematocrit is obtained with routine laboratory tests as recommended by the transplant center during the early postoperative period and through the primary care provider if the child is discharged from the transplant area. Laboratory tests are obtained frequently, up to weekly or twice weekly, during the first 3 months after the transplant and then with decreasing frequency over time. Children with renal transplants may develop anemia secondary to progressive renal dysfunction from recurrent disease or chronic rejection.

Urinalysis. Nephrotoxicity is a well-recognized complication of both tacrolimus and cyclosporine immunosuppressive therapy in all solid organ transplantation and can be detected in urine and blood specimens. The BUN and creatinine and the GFR are monitored to assess kidney function. Additionally, urine samples are obtained for urinalysis and culture in renal transplant recipients as a part of posttransplant management. Routine monitoring of the serum creatinine and total protein, as well as a urinalysis, is essential to screen for recurrent renal diseases, such as focal segmental glomerulosclerosis or membranoproliferative glomerulonephritis.

In children with liver and heart transplantation, urinalysis is obtained to monitor for nephrotoxicity resulting from immunosuppressive therapies. Otherwise, a urinalysis is obtained only if the child is symptomatic or as part of an evaluation of fever. Fever in the posttransplant period is usually diagnostic of rejection or infection. If rejection is ruled out, infection is likely, and cultures of urine, blood, stool, and sputum are obtained.

Tuberculosis. Some transplant centers may recommend a Mantoux-purified protein derivative (PPD) with an anergy panel in addition to chest radiography to evaluate a child for exposure to tuberculosis (TB) before transplantation. Though TB is rare in developed countries, individuals with solid-organ transplants have a 50- to 100-fold higher risk of infection than the general population. Treatment is with isoniazid, which can cause hepatotoxicity, so close monitoring of hepatic enzymes during treatment is warranted (Gasink & Blumberg, 2005).

Condition-Specific Screening

Posttransplant Blood Tests. Laboratory blood testing is usually obtained at weekly to biweekly clinic visits after discharge from the hospital. Laboratory tests vary depending on the organ transplanted, the length of time after transplant, current complications, and center-specific protocols. Leukopenia and neutropenia can be side effects of immunosuppressant or antiviral medications, and an adjustment of those medications may be required to avoid overimmunosuppression and decrease the risk of posttransplant infections. The most commonly obtained laboratory tests include a complete blood cell count with differential and a full chemistry profile, including glucose, BUN, creatinine, magnesium, phosphorus, bicarbonate, uric acid, aspartate aminotransferase (AST), alanine aminotransferase (ALT), gamma-glutamyl transpeptidase phosphate (GGTP), lactic dehydrogenase (LDH), creatine phosphokinase (CPK), cholesterol, and triglycerides.

Medication Levels. Trough levels of CSA, tacrolimus, or sirolimus are usually obtained with these routine tests. In addition, fasting lipids and glycated hemoglobin (HbA_{1c}) are done periodically to screen for hyperlipidemia and diabetes.

Maintenance Laboratory Testing. Laboratory testing decreases over time. By 6 months after transplant, the majority of children have stable graft function and require laboratory testing monthly. Long-term survivors commonly have laboratory testing completed every 2 to 3 months; however, laboratory tests may be required more frequently during episodes of infection or rejection as immunosuppressive mediations are adjusted. Children are followed closely until the episode of rejection or the infectious process resolves.

Common Illness Management

Differential Diagnosis

Fever. Children are more highly immunosuppressed for the first 3 to 6 months after transplantation and consequently are at greater risk for infection. As discussed previously, bacterial infections are most commonly seen in the early period related to the preexisting chronic condition, surgical complications, or nosocomial infections. Viruses and opportunistic infections are more common in the intermediate and late periods following transplantation. Fever, especially in the first 3 months after transplant, demands a thorough assessment. The differential diagnoses of rejection or infection must be investigated with each febrile episode, particularly in the early postoperative period. The primary care provider and the transplant specialist work cooperatively to evaluate and manage febrile episodes.

> *Differential Diagnosis*
>
> - *Fever:* Common childhood conditions vs. rejection
> - *Abdominal symptoms:* Common childhood conditions vs. obstruction in common bile duct, ulcers, small bowel obstruction, peritonitis, or rejection
> - *Vomiting and diarrhea:* May result in altered absorption of medications
> - *Metabolic abnormalities:* Hyperkalemia, hyperglycemia, and low CO_2 levels may be related to immunosuppressant medications

Abdominal Symptoms. Abdominal pain in children with liver transplants during the early postoperative period most commonly indicates a surgical complication, including a postoperative ileus, hepatic artery thrombosis, or portal vein thrombosis. Biliary complications may also cause abdominal pain and may occur in the early postoperative period, as well as weeks to months after transplant. Acute rejection of the liver may also cause abdominal pain.

Abdominal pain in renal transplant recipients, as well as tenderness in the kidney area, may be a symptom of a urinary tract infection (UTI), acute pyelonephritis, posttransplant lymphoproliferative disease, CMV infection, or rejection.

Although abdominal pain and vomiting in the child with a heart transplant may be a viral illness, this clinical presentation warrants an echocardiogram to evaluate for the possibility of rejection secondary to decreased cardiac output and decreased perfusion to the gastrointestinal tract.

As with the general pediatric population, the differential diagnoses of abdominal pain may also include intestinal obstruction, peptic ulcer disease, appendicitis, or viral or bacterial gastroenteritis. A definitive diagnosis is determined through clinical presentation, laboratory testing, and radiologic testing.

Vomiting and Diarrhea. Prolonged vomiting or diarrhea caused by a community-acquired virus may result in altered absorption of immunosuppressant medications leading to toxic or subtherapeutic blood levels that may place the child at risk. Parents should contact the transplant center if the child is unable to retain the immunosuppressive medication. The primary care provider will facilitate the transplant center's recommendations for immunosuppression and will supervise medical management of fluids and electrolytes. A protracted course of vomiting or diarrhea may result in hospitalization for intravenous administration of CSA or tacrolimus, fluid management, and any indicated workup for infection (Teets & Borisuk, 2004).

Metabolic Abnormalities. Children with stable graft function receiving maintenance immunosuppression usually do not experience metabolic abnormalities. Elevated levels of CSA and tacrolimus during the early postoperative period may result in hyperkalemia, hypophosphatemia, hypomagnesemia, or metabolic acidosis.

Drug Interactions

Cyclosporine (CSA) and tacrolimus (Prograf) are metabolized in the liver by the cytochrome P450 III system (Gaston, 2006). Metabolism of CSA or tacrolimus depends on liver function and other agents that induce or inhibit this enzyme system, subsequently affecting blood levels. Because primary care providers often prescribe medications for a variety of acute and chronic childhood illnesses, it is important that the family or health care provider contact the transplant center to discuss possible drug interactions. Drugs that interact with CSA or tacrolimus disrupt an otherwise stable level, which may result in drug-related neurotoxicities and nephrotoxicities (Table 37-3). Fluctuating levels may also increase the risk of infection or rejection.

Developmental Issues

Sleep Patterns

Sleep disturbances in children with end-stage organ disease are common and may be caused by the existing chronic condition, symptoms of organ deterioration (e.g., severe pruritus from liver disease), emotional distress, and the psychological effects of extended hospitalization. In addition, tacrolimus, CSA, and steroids are reported to cause insomnia. During periods of rejection when the child is treated with increased tacrolimus or CSA levels in addition to high-dose oral steroids or intravenous methylprednisolone, sleep patterns may be significantly altered and insomnia and irritability are common. Sleep is an important issue because there is evidence that childhood sleep disturbances are associated with behavioral, mood, and cognitive disturbances, as well as poor school performance and absenteeism (Davis, Baron, O'Riordan, et al., 2005).

Parents may find it helpful to maintain familiar home routines and rituals to the fullest extent possible while the child is hospitalized. Strategies to improve sleep include maintaining an organized sleep-wake cycle, avoiding late-afternoon napping, and minimizing evening television watching and caffeine intake (Davis et al., 2005). In some cases, professional counseling may help the child and family.

Toileting

Regression in toileting habits is expected in toddlers and preschoolage children during and after hospitalization. Care providers should be aware of this temporary regression and support children in regaining their toileting skills. Pediatric renal transplant recipients may have specific concerns and issues related to toileting and the establishment or reestablishment of urinary flow and continence.

TABLE 37-3

Drug Interactions with Cyclosporine, Tacrolimus, and Sirolimus

Drug	Cyclosporine (CSA) Increase	Cyclosporine (CSA) Decrease	Tacrolimus (Prograf) Increase	Tacrolimus (Prograf) Decrease	Sirolimus Increase	Sirolimus Decrease
CALCIUM CHANNEL BLOCKERS						
Diltiazem	X		X		X	
Nicardipine	X		X		X	
Nifedipine	X		X			
Verapamil	X		X		X	
Antifungals						
Fluconazole	X		X		X	
Itraconazole	X		X		X	
Ketoconazole	X		X		X	
Voriconazole			X		X	
ANTIBIOTICS						
Azithromycin	X					
Clarithromycin	X		X		X	
Doxycycline	X		X		X	
Erythromycin	X		X		X	
Nafcillin		X		X		X
Rifabutin		X		X		X
Rifampin		X		X		X
Telithromycin	X		X		X	
GASTROINTESTINAL AGENTS						
H$_2$ blockers	X					
Metoclopramide	X		X			
ANTICONVULSANTS						
Carbamazepine		X		X		X
Phenobarbital		X		X		X
Phenytoin		X		X		X
OTHERS						
Allopurinol	X					
Cimetidine	X		X			
Cyclosporine			X		X	
Danazol	X		X			
Estrogens	X					
Grapefruit juice	X		X			X
Methotrexate	X					
Progestins	X					
Propofol	X		X		X	
Protease inhibitors	X		X		X	
St. John's wort		X		X		X
Tacrolimus	X					

Data from Lacy, C.F., Armstrong, L.L., Goldman, M.P., et al. (Eds.). (2008). *Drug information handbook* (16th ed.). Hudson, OH: Lexi-Comp.

The initiation of urine flow for a child following renal transplantation is often a time of great excitement for the child and family. However, the child may have periods of incontinence while learning to recognize the body cues that signal the need to urinate and to control the urine flow.

Some heart and renal transplant recipients may require diuretic therapy, which may contribute to increased incontinence, consequently affecting toileting routines and new behaviors. When possible, diuretics should be administered early in the day to decrease nighttime incontinence, frequency of nightly urination, and sleep disruption. Incontinence and enuresis are common occurrences in the early posttransplant period, and parents should be counseled about the implications of the child's medical management on daily routines, as well as the need for emotional support for their child and consistency of home routines.

Discipline

A child's chronic condition affects the entire family, its system of functioning, and the roles within it. As a child with end-stage organ disease improves significantly after transplantation, former coping mechanisms used by the family, as well as parental roles and family dynamics, may no longer be successful. It is often difficult for families to make the transition from parenting a sick child to parenting a healthier one. Many parents continue to overprotect their child and now have the additional concerns of infection and rejection. Parents may have difficulty encouraging children to develop independence and peer relationships and are often reticent to integrate the child into school and community activities. In contrast, other parents may have trouble setting limits on inappropriate behavior and may overindulge the child.

The primary care provider plays an essential role in evaluating family dynamics and the parents' ability to appropriately discipline and nurture a child after transplantation. The caregiver can help parents achieve a balance between establishing age-appropriate and consistent limits and allowing the child some control in decision making. Encouraging independence helps promote confidence and positive self-esteem. Family counseling can be a highly effective method to help families cope with the ongoing stressors of the transplant process.

Child Care

Attendance at daycare centers is generally not recommended by most transplant centers for 1 to 3 months following transplantation because these children are usually more highly immunosuppressed during that time with a greater risk for infection. As immunosuppressive levels are decreased, routine social contact and participation in group activities and daycare programs may be resumed. Community-acquired viruses are usually tolerated well by children who are receiving lower-dose maintenance immunosuppression. However, parents should be informed by the primary care provider or daycare staff of any outbreaks of varicella or measles in the community or daycare center because these viruses could be potentially serious for the child with a transplant, particularly if the child was unable to be immunized before transplantation.

Schooling

Children are encouraged to return to school as soon as possible after transplantation to resume a normal routine, continue class work, and interact with peers. Although most children can return to the classroom within 3 months after transplantation, some children benefit from gradually increasing school attendance from a few hours daily to a full schedule as tolerated. Tutoring in the home, as provided by the school district, may be an ideal option when children have had an extended absence from school and are significantly behind in class content.

Parents are often hesitant to return their child to school because of concerns about exposure to infections, their perception of the child's fragility and increased demands on the child, and peer influences. Primary care providers should encourage the resumption of routine childhood activities and school while emphasizing the benefits of developmentally appropriate play, social interactions, and instruction. Teachers also have an important role in normalizing the child's school experience by accommodating medical absences and encouraging optimal academic performance. Children with chronic conditions leading to transplantation and children after transplantation may benefit from special education services, and an individualized education plan should be initiated (Well, Rodgers & Rubovits, 2006).

The child's medication schedule should be organized to accommodate the school day with minimal interruptions. Medications prescribed on a daily or twice-daily schedule are easily adaptable to the child's schedule. Frequent visits to the health office for medications or having a parent visit daily to administer medications is disruptive to the child's school routine and may emphasize the different needs of the child. Children may be particularly sensitive to these intrusions during adolescence.

Sexuality

The majority of children experience significant improvements in physical appearance following successful solid organ transplantation. Older school-age children and adolescents are very aware of these dramatically positive physical changes: increased energy and strength, a natural skin color following resolution of jaundice or cyanosis, a normal body shape in the absence of ascites or peripheral edema, increased growth and maturation, and the absence of appliances such as central venous lines, gastrostomy tubes, oxygen cannulas, or dialysis catheters. In addition, daily care routines, laboratory testing, clinic visits, and medical routines may be considerably minimized with stable graft function.

Recipients may also experience some negative effects to appearance and body image. The physical stigmata of immunosuppressive therapy with CSA and steroids include hirsutism, cushingoid facies, gingival hyperplasia, obesity, and short stature. Steroids may also intensify outbreaks of acne in adolescents and cause mood swings. Physical stigmata as a result of immunosuppressive therapy with tacrolimus are very rare, although a small percentage of children experience transient alopecia. Scarring from multiple surgeries, invasive lines and catheters, and other procedures is unavoidable. Parents and children are advised about skin care issues as they recuperate from surgery. Some adolescents are interested in minimizing scarring and any keloid formations and may benefit from a plastic surgery consultation. Professional counseling and support groups are also encouraged for this population because these children may be at risk for depression, nonadherence, or increased risk-taking behaviors.

Transplant education for adolescents should include information about puberty, sexual development, sexual activity/abstinence, birth control, and sexually transmitted diseases. Adolescents with chronic organ disease often experience delayed pubertal development. Following transplantation and stable graft function, there is often subsequent initiation or resumption of menses, progression of puberty, and return of libido (Sucato & Murray, 2004). Pretransplant and posttransplant counseling and education will help the adolescent prepare for and adapt to these sudden changes. Adolescent women should be referred to their primary care provider, teen clinic, or gynecology practitioner for birth control counseling and gynecologic examinations as indicated.

Sexual activity may resume at 6 to 8 weeks after transplantation. Sexually active adolescents can choose from any of the standard options for adolescent contraception, including hormonal contraception and emergency contraception after unprotected sex; however, estrogen- and progesterone-containing contraceptives interact with posttransplant immunosuppressive medications. They may increase levels of corticosteroids (prednisone), cyclosporine, tacrolimus, and sirolimus (Rapamune). Blood levels and signs of increased side effects should monitored (Sucato & Murray, 2004). Azathioprine can cause liver toxicity and mycophenolate mofetil can cause diarrhea, which may affect the absorption or metabolism of these contraceptive medications. Blood pressure control is important in these children because hypertension is a contraindication for estrogen- and progesterone-containing contraceptives. Bone density should be monitored in those adolescents who choose to use depot medroxyprogesterone acetate (Depo-Provera) (Sucato & Murray, 2004). The risks and benefits of contraception, side effects, and pregnancy must be considered before deciding on a method of contraception.

With increased long-term survival and a significantly improved physical status, pregnancy is now a more frequent occurrence for women with transplants. Successful pregnancies in recipients of solid organ transplants are possible but are not without certain risks and complications. Recommendations for planning a pregnancy may include discontinuation of teratogenic medications at least 3 months before suspending birth control, achievement of stable graft function with low levels of immunosuppression, and genetic counseling for recipients with an inherited etiology of organ disease. The pregnancy should be carefully monitored with close assessment of graft function and fetal development. In addition to routine prenatal care, the pregnant woman requires frequent monitoring to assess immunosuppressive levels and specific laboratory tests to evaluate for rejection caused by the physiologic changes of pregnancy. These women are at higher risk for spontaneous abortions, intrauterine growth retardation, preeclampsia, or worsening of preexisting hypertension. Premature deliveries and low birth weight in infants are also risks for women with transplants (Hawbe, 2006).

Transition to Adulthood

Adolescents with transplants struggle with the same issues of separation and developing independence and identity as their peers but within the context of adapting to the chronicity of transplantation (Kaufman, 2006). Because of a suppressed immune system, the transplant recipient has an increased risk of developing sexually transmitted diseases if safe sex practices are not followed. Drugs, alcohol, and cigarette smoking affect the transplanted organs and may possibly interfere with the metabolism of immunosuppressive medications. Tattoos and body piercings, which are popular among this age-group, also place transplant recipients at risk for infection. Deviation from prescribed medication and care routines is most often reported in adolescents can jeopardize the graft, resulting in rejection and ultimately graft loss and death (Simons & Blount, 2007). Providing support to the adolescent transplant recipient, engaging him or her in care decisions, and individualizing immunosuppression regimens and follow-up testing can help the adolescent incorporate necessary treatments into daily life activities.

Securing employment and obtaining insurance are significant concerns for the late adolescent entering college or the job force. An employer may be fearful of possible physical limitations and potential absences from work. Young adults eventually lose their parents' insurance coverage and must find health insurance through a private carrier or apply for medical assistance. Private insurance may be difficult to obtain because of a preexisting condition or employment issues. Although the expenses of transplantation decrease in the long term, an ongoing financial obligation remains for the recipient's lifetime. Medications, laboratory tests, and physical examinations are routinely required. Additional invasive testing and hospitalization may be necessary if the individual acquires an infection or has an episode of acute rejection. Transplant financial counselors and social workers from the transplant center offer counseling about insurance options, medication programs, and grants. Additionally, support groups and websites established by a variety of foundations, pharmaceutical companies, private individuals, and community groups provide information about the transplant process and resources.

Supporting adolescents during the transition to adulthood may be difficult for parents as they help their child achieve the developmental tasks of adolescence and as the adolescent assumes a greater responsibility for routine care. Individual and family counseling is recommended and encouraged. Consistent and routine communication with the transplant center may also help provide parents with strategies and advice in working through these complex issues within the context of transplantation. In addition, as the adolescent progresses chronologically and developmentally into adulthood, a gradual transition to an adult transplant center should be planned to better meet the needs of an adult transplant recipient.

Family Concerns

Transplantation is an exchange of end-stage organ disease for the chronic condition of transplantation. Although most families and recipients believe this is an acceptable trade-off, anxiety and apprehensions about the future may be ongoing. Long-term survival, the child's transition into adulthood, nonadherence with care, fear of rejection, late infections, possible retransplantation, and the child's future employment and quality of life are major concerns.

Medication nonadherence is a major cause of late rejection and other complications in solid organ transplantation. Because nonadherence is such a significant problem following transplantation, adherence to medication and care routines should be discussed with the child and family throughout the transplant process, from the pretransplant evaluation through chronic care follow-up. Between 5% to 50% of renal transplant recipients are reported to be noncompliant, with that rate increasing to as high as 64% in adolescents (Smith & McDonald, 2005). More than 60% of adolescent and young adult heart recipients acknowledged missing immunosuppression medication more than once per month (Stilley, Lawrence, Bender, et al., 2006). A small study of liver transplant recipients suggested that severe adverse outcomes of retransplantation and death were likely significantly associated with nonadherent behavior (Berquist, Berquist, Esquivel, et al., 2006). Medication is just one aspect of the posttransplant regimen. Follow-up testing, diet, exercise, and other lifestyle elements can be a challenge for the child and family to incorporate into their daily lives.

Nonadherence should always be considered in the differential diagnosis of rejection, particularly if the child is an adolescent and a long-term survivor. Risk factors for nonadherence include race, female gender, adolescent age, low socioeconomic status, cosmetic side effects of medications, distance from transplant center, and complexity and duration of medical regimen (Smith & McDonald, 2005). Maturity has been associated with better adherence among adolescent and young adult heart transplant recipients, with more mature individuals being more adherent (Stilley et al., 2006). The transplant team must work closely with the adolescent to ensure that the outcome and consequences of poor adherence to medical routines are understood. Repeated education about medications, rejection, infection, and chronic care requirements is essential and must be reinforced. Counseling with a psychologist or medical social worker may help the adolescent recognize the underlying causes of nonadherence and lead to changes to increase adherence. The transplant team should also make every effort to help by minimizing medication requirements and the number of daily dosages while working with the child to create a schedule that is supported by the child's daily routine, is easy to adhere to, and does not interfere with other activities. A system for routinely obtaining laboratory tests and communicating with the transplant coordinator is also imperative. In repeated cases of nonadherence, a contract may be helpful to delineate the responsibilities of the child and the transplant center, the adherence plan, and the consequences of breaking the contract. Ultimately, a referral to family services may be needed in some extreme cases.

The financial impact of transplantation may be another significant concern for families. The transplant surgery and initial hospitalization, possible repeat admissions, an array of medications, living expenses while at the transplant center, and ongoing expenses at home amass an enormous financial burden for many families. Financial support can come from third-party health insurance payers, community fundraising, state funding, or the family's own resources.

Ongoing communication, updated information, and emotional support from the transplant team and primary care providers will help families cope with the fears and uncertainty they may have about their child's future as they progress and adapt to life after transplantation.

Resources and Organizations

Alpha-1-Antitrypsin Disease
Website: www.alpha1.org
American Association of Kidney Patients (AAKP)
Website: www.aakp.org
American Heart Association (AHA)
Website: www.americanheart.org
American Liver Foundation
Website: www.liverfoundation.org
Astellas Pharma US, Inc.
Website: www.us.astella.com
Children's Liver Association for Support Services
Website: www.classkids.org
Children's Organ Transplant Association (COTA)
Website: www.cota.org
Donate Life America
Website: www.shareyourlife.org
Healthfinder Kids
Website: www.healthfinder.gov/kids
International Pediatric Transplant Association
Website: www.iptaonline.org
International Society for Heart and Lung Transplantation
Website: www.ishlt.org

International Transplant Nurses Society
Website: www.itns.org
The James Redford Institute for Transplant Awareness
Website: www.jrifilms.org
Minority Organ Tissue Transplant Education Program
Website: www.nationalmottep.org
MyHealthPassport
Website: www.sickkids.ca/good2go
National Foundation for Transplant
Website: www.transplants.org
National Kidney Foundation, Inc.
Website: www.kidney.org
National Transplant Assistance Fund and Catastrophic Injury Program
Website: www.transplantfund.org
North American Transplant Coordinators' Organization
Website: www.natco1.org
Novartis Pharmaceuticals
Website: www.pharma.us.novartis.com
Roche Pharmaceuticals
Website: www.rocheusa.com
Thomas Starzl Transplant Institute
Website: www.sti.upmc.edu
Transplant Health
Website: www.transplanthealth.com
Transplant Recipients' International Organization (TRIO)
Website: www.trioweb.org
Transplant Speakers International
Website: www.transplant-speakers.org
Transweb
Website: www.transweb.org
United Network for Organ Sharing (UNOS)
Website: www.unos.org
Wilson's Disease Association
Website: www.wilsonsdisease.org
Wyeth-Ayerst
Website: www.wyeth.com

Summary of Primary Care Needs for the Child with a Solid Organ Transplant

HEALTH CARE MAINTENANCE

Growth and Development

- Measure height and weight at each visit.
- Measure head circumference for children <3 years old at each visit.
- Linear growth may be compromised by long-term use of corticosteroids.
- Catch-up growth may be attained after transplantation.
- Growth hormone may be advised for children <1 year before renal transplantation and for children >1 year following renal transplantation.
- Improved physical development after transplantation has a positive effect on psychosocial development.
- Cognitive functioning should be monitored at regular intervals.
- Screening for depressive symptoms related to body image changes, side effects of medications, and adaptation to chronic condition may be advisable.

Diet

- A regular oral diet without restrictions is common following stable graft function, although renal recipients may have sodium restrictions.
- Enteral supplements may be needed to meet caloric requirements for catch-up growth and wound healing, particularly in younger children.
- Dietary restrictions are instituted when indicated for electrolyte imbalances or hyperglycemia.
- Children with heart transplant are on a heart-healthy diet.

Safety

- Good hand washing and avoidance of people with infection are recommended to decrease the risk of toxoplasmosis and other potential infections.
- Medic-Alert bracelets are recommended.

Summary of Primary Care Needs for the Child with a Solid Organ Transplant—cont'd

- The transplant center should be contacted before travel outside the United States or to report extended travel arrangements to give contact information.
- Activity and exercise are usually restricted for 6 to 8 weeks after transplant. Age-appropriate safety issues should be addressed as in the healthy pediatric population: seat belts, helmets, Mr. Yuk stickers, electrical outlet covers, and so on.

Immunizations

- All recommended immunizations should be administered at least 1 month before the transplant whenever possible.
- Interrupted immunization schedules can usually be resumed 3-6 months after transplantation.
- Live-virus vaccines are contraindicated in transplant recipients. Transplant recipients should receive inactivated vaccines when available.
- All routine childhood immunizations, including inactivated poliovirus (IPV); measles, mumps, rubella (MMR); and varicella vaccines, should be given to siblings and other close contacts.
- Transplant recipients and family members within the household should get the annual inactivated influenza vaccine.

Screening

- *Vision.* Routine screening is recommended. Pediatric transplant recipients receiving high-dose long-term steroid therapy are at risk for developing glaucoma and cataracts and may require more frequent examinations. Children with chronic CMV infection should be screened for infection-related retinitis.
- *Hearing.* Audiograms should be obtained to evaluate hearing loss in children who have received ototoxic drugs.
- *Dental.* Routine screening is recommended.
  - CSA may cause gingival hyperplasia. Antibiotic prophylaxis is indicated only for cardiac transplant recipients with valvular disease.
- *Blood pressure.* Blood pressure measurement should be obtained at each checkup.
  - If antihypertensive medications are prescribed, blood pressure should be checked and recorded before administration of each dose. A record of blood pressure results should be kept and assessed at each checkup. Further evaluation may be required for long-term hypertension.
- *Hematocrit.* Screening should be done per transplant center routine.
  - Anemia may occur as a result of renal dysfunction or recurrent disease.
- *Urinalysis.* Nephrotoxicity is a complication of cyclosporine and tacrolimus.
  - Additional screening is necessary in children with kidney transplants.
  - Immunosuppression may mask symptoms of urinary tract infection (UTI). Urinalysis should be obtained in children with fever and possible UTI.
- *Tuberculosis.* Screening with a PPD and anergy panel is recommended. Chest radiography is obtained if indicated. A lifetime course of isoniazid (INH) is recommended in patients with a positive PPD and chest films.

Condition-Specific Screening

- *Blood work.* Routine laboratory testing is obtained at regular intervals, usually weekly to monthly, depending on the time after transplant and any current episodes of infection or rejection.
- Tacrolimus, CSA, and/or sirolimus levels are also monitored regularly and adjusted as indicated per transplant center protocols.

COMMON ILLNESS MANAGEMENT

Differential Diagnosis

- *Fever.* The risk of bacterial, fungal, and viral infections is highest during the first 3 months after a transplant and whenever immunosuppression is maximized.
  - Immunosuppression may mask symptoms, so careful assessment of any fever is very important.
  - Normal childhood illnesses should be ruled out.
  - Fever may indicate organ rejection or infection.
- *Abdominal symptoms.* Abdominal pain should be investigated to rule out appendicitis or intestinal obstruction, ulcers, peritonitis, rejection, or posttransplant lymphoproliferative disorder (PTLD).
  - Abdominal pain in liver transplant recipients may be a sign of rejection or surgical complications.
  - Abdominal pain or vomiting may be a sign of rejection in heart transplant recipients.
  - Vomiting and diarrhea may lower therapeutic blood levels of immunosuppressant drugs.
- *Metabolic abnormalities.* Hyperkalemia can result from drug therapy.
  - Hyperglycemia may result from immunosuppressant medications.

Drug Interactions

- CSA and tacrolimus absorption is altered by phenytoin, phenobarbital, ketoconazole, fluconazole, erythromycin, diltiazem, and other drugs.
- When administered with anticonvulsants, higher doses of CSA may be needed to achieve a therapeutic range.
- Acetaminophen should be used instead of aspirin or ibuprofen.
- If the child is hypertensive, decongestants should be avoided.
- It is important for the primary care provider to contact the transplant center before prescribing any medication.

DEVELOPMENTAL ISSUES

Sleep Patterns

- End-stage organ disease, hospitalization, or drugs may alter sleep patterns.
- Familiar routines and rituals should be maintained when possible.

Continued

Summary of Primary Care Needs for the Child with a Solid Organ Transplant—cont'd

Toileting

- Regression in toddlers and preschoolers is to be expected.
- Children with renal transplantation may need to relearn body cues to achieve toilet training.
- Children taking diuretics may have difficulty with urinary continence and training.
- Emotional support is required as children learn skills.

Discipline

- Parental overprotectiveness is likely; parents may need help to promote independence in their children.
- Family counseling may be helpful.

Child Care

- Children may attend daycare by 3 months after surgery if immunosuppression requirements have been reduced.
- Precautions should be taken to limit exposure to communicable diseases.

Schooling

- Normal schooling should be resumed 1 to 3 months after transplantation.
- Additional academic help may be needed to attain grade level skills because of time lost.
- An Individualized Educational Program (IEP) should be initiated if school problems develop.

Sexuality

- The transplant experience may affect body image and self-esteem.
- Barrier methods of birth control are recommended.
- Childbearing is possible after transplantation.
- Physiologic strain on the maternal system must be monitored.
- Effects of immunosuppression on the fetus must be monitored.

Transition to Adulthood

- Many individuals have difficulty attaining independence.
- Body image and intimacy may be negatively affected.
- Concerns about employment and health insurance develop.
- Planning and preparation for eventual transition to adult primary and transplant care is important.

FAMILY CONCERNS

- Family concerns include the fear of rejection, search for a new organ, organ donor issues, and finances.
- Securing employment and continued health insurance may be difficult.
- Nonadherence with immunosuppressive therapy is a major problem that can result in graft loss. Counseling may be helpful.

REFERENCES

Acott, P., & Hirsch, H.H. (2007). BK virus infection, replication, and diseases in pediatric kidney transplantation. *Pediatr Nephrol, 22*, 1243-1250.

Ahmed, A., & Keefe, E. (2007). Current indications and contraindications for liver transplantation. *Clin Liver Dis, 11*, 227-247.

Al-Akash, S.I., Al Makadma, A.S., & Al Omari, M.G. (2005). Rapid response to rituximab in a pediatric liver transplant recipient with post-transplant lymphoproliferative disease and maintenance with sirolimus monotherapy. *Pediatr Transplant, 9*, 249-253.

Alkhaldi, A., Chin, C., & Bernstein, D. (2006). Pediatric cardiac transplantation. *Semin Pediatr Surg, 15*, 188-198.

American Academy of Pediatrics (AAP). (2003). Revised indications for the use of palivizumab and respiratory syncytial virus immune globulin intravenous for the prevention of respiratory syncytial virus infections. *Pediatrics, 112*, 1442-1446.

American Academy of Pediatrics (AAP) Committee on Infectious Diseases. (2006). Active and passive immunization. In L.K. Pickering (Ed.), *Red Book: 2006 Report of the Committee on Infectious Diseases* (27th ed.) Elk Grove Village, IL: American Academy of Pediatrics.

Arabia, F.A., Tsau, P.H., Smith, R.G., et al. (2006). Pediatric bridge to heart transplantation: Application of the Berlin Heart, Medos and Thoratec ventricular assist devices. *J Heart Lung Transplant, 25*, 16-21.

Baran, D.A. (2007). Induction therapy in cardiac transplantation: When and why? *Heart Failure Clin, 3*, 31-41.

Barshes, N., Gay, N., Williams, B., et al. (2005). Support for the acutely failing liver. *J Am Coll Surg, 201*, 458-476.

Benson, L.M. (2004). Hypertrophic cardiomyopathy. In R.M. Freedom, S.J. Yoo, H. Mikailian, et al. (Eds.), *The Natural History of Congenital Heart Disease*. New York: Blackwell Publishing.

Bergasa, N.V. (2008). Pruritus in primary biliary cirrhosis: Pathogenesis and therapy. *Clin Liver Dis, 12*, 385-406.

Berquist, R.K., Berquist, W.E., Esquivel, C.O., et al. (2006). Adolescent nonadherence: Prevalence and consequences in liver transplant recipients. *Pediatr Transplant, 3*, 304-310.

Blume, E.D., Naftel, D.C., Bastardi, H.J., et al. (2006). Outcomes of children bridged to heart transplantation with ventricular assist devices: A multiinstitutional study. *Circulation, 113*, 2313-2319.

Boucek, M.M. (2001). Breaching the barrier of ABO incompatibility in heart transplantation for infants. *N Engl J Med, 344*(11), 843-844.

Boucek, M.M., Aurora, P., Edwards, L.B., et al. (2007). Registry of the International Society of Heart and Lung Transplantation: Tenth official pediatric heart transplantation report—2007. *J Heart Lung Transplant, 26*, 796-807.

Bucuvalas, J.C., Britto, M., Krug, S., et al. (2003). Health-related quality of life in pediatric liver transplant recipients: A single-center study. *Liver Transpl, 9*, 62-71.

Burch, M., & Aurora, P. (2004). Current status of paediatric heart, lung and heart-lung transplantation. *Arch Dis Child, 89*, 386-389.

Burton, J.R., & Rosen, H.R. (2006). Diagnosis and management of allograft failure. *Clin Liver Dis, 10*, 407-435.

Campbell, A.L., & Herold, B.C. (2005). Immunization of pediatric solid-organ transplantation candidates: Immunizations in transplant candidates. *Pediatr Transplant, 9*, 652-661.

Campbell, K., Yagigi, N., Ryckman, F.C., et al. (2006). High prevalence of renal dysfunction in long-term survivors after pediatric liver transplantation. *J Pediatr, 148*, 475-480.

Chandraker, A., Iacomini, J.J., & Sayegh, M.H. (2007). Transplantation immunobiology. In B. Brenner & S. Levine (Eds.), *Brenner and Rector's the Kidney* (8th ed.). Saunders: Philadelphia.

Chavers, B., Najarian, J.S., & Humar, A. (2007). Kidney transplantation in infants and small children. *Pediatr Transplant, 11*, 702-708.

Cupples, S.A., Dumas-Hicks, D.H., & Burnapp, L. (2008). Transplant complications: infectious diseases. In L. Ohler & S. Cupples (Eds.), *Core Curriculum for Transplant Nurses*. St. Louis: Mosby Elsevier.

Davis, I.D., Baron, J., O'Riordan, M.A., et al. (2005). Sleep disturbances in pediatric dialysis patients. *Pediatr Nephrol, 20*, 69-75.

Diana, A., Posfay-Barbe, K.M., Belli, C., et al. (2007). Vaccine-induced immunity in children after orthotopic liver transplantation: A 12-yr review of the Swiss national reference center. *Pediatr Transplant, 11*, 31-37.

Dipchand, A.I. (2004). Heart transplantation. In R.M. Freedom, S.J. Yoo, H. Mikailian, et al. (Eds.), *The Natural History of Congenital Heart Disease*. New York: Blackwell Publishing.

Dodd, D.A., Burger, J., Edwards, K.M, et al. (2001). Varicella in a pediatric heart transplant population on nonsteroid maintenance immunosuppression. *Pediatrics, 108*, 80(5), E80. Available at www.pediatrics.org/cgi/content/full/108/5/e80. Retrieved January 6, 2008.

Dosanjh, A. (2002). A review of nutritional problems and the cystic fibrosis lung transplant patient. *Pediatr Transplant, 6*, 388-391.

Elidemir, O., Chang, I., Schecter, M., et al. (2007). BK virus-associated hemorrhagic cystitis in a pediatric lung transplant patient. *Pediatr Transplant, 11*, 807-810.

Farge, P., Ranchin, B., & Cochat, P. (2006). Four year follow-up of oral health surveillance in renal transplant children. *Pediatr Nephrol, 21*(6), 851-855.

Filshie, J., & Rubens, C. (2006). Complementary and alternative medicine. *Anesthesiol Clin North Am, 24*, 81-111.

Fischer, S.A. (2006). Infections complicating solid organ transplantation. *Surg Clin North Am, 86*(5), 1127-1145.

Fiser, W.B., Yetman, A.T., Gunselman, R.J., et al. (2003). Pediatric arteriovenous extracorporeal membrane oxygenation (ECMO) as a bridge to cardiac transplantation. *J Heart Lung Transplant, 22*, 770-777.

Fishman, J.A. (2007). Infection in solid organ transplant recipients. *N Engl J Med, 357*, 2601-2614.

Flattery, M.P., & Dale, C. (2008). Solid organ transplantation: The evaluation process. In L. Ohler & S. Cupples (Eds.), *Core Curriculum for Transplant Nurses*. St. Louis: Mosby Elsevier.

Flynn, B. (2002). Liver transplantation. In S. Cupples & L. Ohler (Eds.), *Transplantation Nursing Secrets*. Philadelphia: Hanley & Belfus.

Fonseca-Aten, M., & Michaels, M.G. (2006). Infections in pediatric solid organ transplant recipients. *Semin Pediatr Surg, 15*, 153-161.

Fontana, R. (2006) Acute liver failure. In M. Feldman, L.S. Friedman, & L.J. Brandt (Eds.), *Sleisenger and Fordtran's Gastrointestinal and Liver Disease Pathophysiology/Diagnosis/Management* (8th ed.). Philadelphia: Saunders.

Foster, R., Zimmerman, M., & Trotter, J.F. (2007). Expanding donor options: Marginal, living, and split donors. *Clin Liver Dis, 11*, 417-429.

Fryer, J. (2007). Intestinal transplantation: Current status. *Gastroenterol Clin North Am, 36*, 145-159.

Fuqua, J.S. (2006). Growth after organ transplantation. *Semin Pediatr Surg, 15*, 162-169.

Gasink, L.B., & Blumberg, E.A. (2005). Bacterial and mycobacterial pneumonia in transplant recipients. *Clin Chest Med, 26*, 647-659.

Gaston, R.S. (2006). Current and evolving immunosuppressive regimens in kidney transplantation. *Am J Kidney Dis, 47*, S3-S21.

Gipson, D., Wetherington, C.E., Duquette, P.J., et al. (2007). The central nervous system in childhood chronic kidney disease. *Pediatr Nephrol, 22*, 1703-1710.

Han, M.K., & Hyzy, R. (2006). Advances in critical care management of hepatic failure and insufficiency. *Crit Care Med, 34*(9), S225-S231.

Hartley, C., Fisher, G., & Cupples, S.A. (2008). Heart transplantation. In L. Ohler & S. Cupples (Eds.), *Core Curriculum for Transplant Nurses*. St. Louis: Mosby Elsevier.

Hawbe, V.Q. (2006). Posttransplantation quality of life: More than graft function. *Am J Kidney Dis, 47*, S98-S110.

Heidelbaugh, J.J., & Sherbondy, M. (2006). Cirrhosis and chronic liver failure: Part II. Complications and treatment. *Am Fam Physician, 74*, 767-776.

Horslen, S., Barr, M.L., Christensen, L.L., et al. (2007). Pediatric transplantation in the United States, 1996-2005. *Am J Transplant, 7*(pt 2), 1339-1358.

Huddleston, C.B. (2006). Pediatric lung transplantation. *Semin Pediatr Surg, 15*, 199-207.

Huprikar, S. (2007). Update in infections in liver transplantation recipients. *Clin Liver Dis, 11*, 337-354.

Isaka, Y. (2006). Gene therapy targeting kidney diseases: Routes and vehicles. *Clin Exp Nephrol, 10*(4), 229-235.

Jain, A., Mazariegos, G., Kashyap, R., et al. (2002). Pediatric liver transplantation: A single center experience spanning 20 years. *Transplantation, 73*, 941-947.

Kaufman, M. (2006). Role of adolescent development in the transition process. *Prog Transplant, 16*(4), 286-290.

Kerkar, N., & Emre, S. (2007). Issues unique to pediatric liver transplantation. *Clin Liver Dis, 11*, 323-335.

Khalpey, Z., Koch, C., & Platt, J. (2004). Xenograft transplantation. *Anesthesiol Clin North Am, 22*, 871-885.

Khan, S., Erlichman, J., & Rand, E.B. (2006). Live virus immunization after orthotopic liver transplantation. *Pediatr Transplant, 10*, 78-82.

Kraut, J. (2007). Chronic renal failure. In R. Rakel & E. Bope (Eds.), *Conn's Current Therapy 2007* (59th ed.). Philadelphia: Saunders.

Kullberg-Lindh, C., Ascher, H., Saalman, R., et al. (2006). Epstein-Barr viremia levels after pediatric liver transplantation as measured by real-time polymerase chain reaction. *Pediatr Transplant, 10*, 83-89.

Lacy, C.F., Armstrong, L.L., Goldman, M.P., et al. (Eds). (2008). *Drug Information Handbook*. (16th ed.). Hudson, OH: Lexi-Comp Inc.

Lee, C.K., Christensen, L.I., Magee, J.C., et al. (2007). Pre-transplant risk factors for chronic renal dysfunction after pediatric heart transplantation: A 10-year national cohort study. *J Heart Lung Transplant, 26*, 458-465.

Lee, K.J., & Yeh, T. (2004). Dilated cardiomyopathy. In R.M. Freedom, S.J. Yoo, H. Mikailian, et al. (Eds.), *The Natural History of Congenital Heart Disease*. New York: Blackwell Publishing.

Liu, L., & Schiano, T.D. (2007). Long-term care of the liver transplantation recipient. *Clin Liver Dis, 11*, 397-416.

Loren, A.W., & Tsai, D.E. (2005). Post-transplant lymphoproliferative disorder. *Clin Chest Med, 26*, 631-645.

Magno, P., & Kalloo, A.N. (2008). Endoscopic therapy for esophageal variceal hemorrhage. In J.L. Cameron (Ed.), *Current Surgical Therapy* (9th ed.). Philadelphia: Mosby.

Mahan, J.D., & Warady, B.A. (2006). Assessment and treatment of short stature in pediatric patients with chronic kidney disease: A consensus statement. *Pediatr Nephrol, 21*, 917-930.

Makowka, L., Cramer, D., & Hoffman, A. (1993). Pig liver xenografts as a temporary bridge for human allografting. *Xenotransplantation, 1*, 27-29.

Makowka, L., Wu, G.D., Hoffman, A., et al. (1994). Immunohistopathologic lesions associated with the rejection of pig to human liver xenograft. *Transplant Proc, 26*, 1074-1075.

Mayo Foundation for Medical Education and Research. (2007). *Herbal supplements: How they can interfere with surgery* (patient information). Available at www.mayoclinic.com/health/herbal-supplements/SA00040. Retrieved June 9, 2008.

MD Consult. (2008). *Cyclosporine* (drug monograph). Available at www.mdconsult.com/das/pharm/body/86921135-3/668905080/full/158. Retrieved January 4, 2008.

Mejia, A., Barshes, N., Halff, G., et al. (2007). Use of split-liver allografts does not impair pediatric recipient growth. *Liver Transplant, 13*, 145-148.

Muñoz, P., Rodriguez, C., & Bouza, E. (2004). Heart transplant patients. In J. Cohen & W. Powderly (Eds.), *Infectious Diseases* (2nd ed.). Edinburgh: Mosby.

National Kidney Foundation. (NKF) (2000). *K/DOQI clinical practice guidelines for nutrition in chronic renal failure*. Available at www.kidney.org/professionals/kdoqi/guidelines_updates/doqi_nut.html. Retrieved June 27, 2008.

National Kidney Foundation (NKF). (2002). *K/DOQI clinical practice guidelines for chronic kidney disease*. Available at www.kidney.org/professionals/KDOQI/guidelines_ckd/p4_class_g1.htm. Retrieved June 23, 2008.

North American Pediatric Renal Transplant Cooperative Study (NAPRTCS). (2007). *2007 annual report*. Available at https://web.emmes.com/study/ped/annlrept/annlrept2007.pdf. Retrieved January 25, 2008.

Organ Procurement and Transplantation Network (OPTN). (2008a). *Waitlist: Organ by waiting time and age* (Data report as of June 20, 2008). Available at www.optn.org/latestData/rptData.asp. Retrieved June 23, 2008.

Organ Procurement and Transplantation Network (OPTN). (2008b). *Liver Kaplan-Meier patient survival rates for transplants performed 1997-2004* (Data report as of June 20, 2008). Available at www.optn.org/latestData/rptData.asp. Retrieved June 27, 2008.

Organ Procurement and Transplantation Network (OPTN). (2009). *Transplants in the U.S. by recipient age* (Data report as of January 9, 2009). Available at www.optn.org/latestData/rptData.asp. Retrieved January 22, 2009.

O'Sullivan, J.J., Derrick, G., & Gray, J. (2005). Blood pressure after cardiac transplantation in childhood. *J Heart Lung Transplant, 24*, 891-895.

Paghdal, K., & Schwartz, R.A. (2007). Sirolimus (rapamycin): From the soil of Easter Island to a bright future. *J Am Acad Dermatol, 57*, 1046-1050.

Pearlman, L. (2002a). Pediatric solid organ transplantation. In S. Cupples & L. Ohler (Eds.), *Transplantation Nursing Secrets*. Philadelphia: Hanley & Belfus.

Pearlman, L. (2002b). Posttransplant viral syndromes. *Prog Transplant, 12*, 116-124.

Peterson, R.E., Perens, G.S., Wetzel, G.T., et al. (2007). Growth and weight gain of prepubertal children after cardiac transplantation. *Pediatric Transplantation*. Available at www.iptaonline.org. Retrieved January 5, 2008.

Pierson, R.N. (2007). Tolerance in heart transplantation: The Holy Grail, or an attainable goal? *Heart Failure Clin, 3*, 17-29.

Prager, L.M., Wain, J.C., Roberts, D.H., et al. (2006). Medical and psychologic outcome of living lobar lung transplant donors. *J Heart Lung Transplant, 25*(10), 1206-1212.

Renz, J.F., de Roos, M., Rosenthal, P., et al. (2001). Posttransplantation growth in pediatric liver recipients. *Liver Transplant, 7*, 1040-1055.

Rhee, E.K., Canter, C.E., Basile, S., et al. (2007). Sudden death prior to pediatric heart transplantation: Would implantable defibrillators improve outcome? *J Heart Lung Transplant, 26*, 447-452.

Sachs, D.H., & Fishman, J.A. (2008). Xenotransplantation. In B.M. Brenner (Ed.), *Brenner & Rector's the Kidney*. Philadelphia: Saunders.

Sanchez, C.P., Kuizon, B.D., Goodman, W.G., et al. (2002). Growth hormone and the skeleton in pediatric renal allograft recipients. *Pediatr Nephrol, 17*, 322-328.

Schleiss, M.R. (2007). Prospects for development and potential impact of a vaccine against congenital cytomegalovirus (CMV) infection. *J Pediatr, 151*, 564-570.

Seeff, L. (2007). Herbal hepatotoxicity. *Clin Liver Dis, 11*, 577-596.

Seipelt, I.M., Crawford, S.E., Rodgers, S., et al. (2004). Hypercholesterolemia is common after pediatric heart transplantation: Initial experience with pravastatin. *J Heart Lung Transplant, 23*, 317-322.

Shaddy, R.E., & Fuller, T.C. (2005). The sensitized pediatric heart transplant candidate: Causes, consequences, and treatment options. *Pediatr Transplant, 9*, 208-214.

Sharma, M.S., Webber, S.A., Morell, V.O., et al. (2006). Ventricular assist device support in children and adolescents as a bridge to heart transplantation. *Ann Thorac Surg, 82*, 926-932.

Silveira, M.G., & Lindor, K.D. (2008). Treatment of primary biliary cirrhosis: Therapy with choleretic and immunosuppressive agents. *Clin Liver Dis, 12*, 425-443.

Simons, L.E., & Blount, R.L. (2007). Identifying barriers to medication adherence in adolescent transplant recipients. *J Pediatr Psychol, 32*, 831-844.

Smith, J.M., & McDonald, R.A. (2005). Renal transplantation in adolescents. *Adolesc Med Clin, 16*, 201-214.

SPLIT Research Group. (2001). Studies of pediatric liver transplantation (SPLIT). *Transplantation, 72*(3), 463-476.

Starzl, T., & Demetris, A. (1997). History of renal transplantation. In R. Shapiro, R. Simmons, & T. Starzl (Eds.), *Renal Transplantation*. Stamford, CT: Appleton & Lange.

Starzl, T.E., Fung, J., Tzakis, A., et al. (1993). Baboon-to-human liver transplantation. *Lancet, 341*(8837), 65-71.

Stilley, C.S., Lawrence, K., Bender, A., et al. (2006). Maturity and adherence in adolescent and young adult heart recipients. *Pediatr Transplant, 10*, 323-330.

Sucato, G.S., & Murray, P.J. (2004). Gynecologic health care for the adolescent solid organ transplant recipient. *Pediatr Transplant, 9*, 346-356.

Teets, J.M., & Borisuk, M.J. (2004). Pediatric thoracic organ transplant: Challenges in primary care. *Pediatr Nurs, 30*, 23-30.

Tiao, G., & Ryckman, F.C. (2006). Pediatric liver transplantation. *Clin Liver Dis, 10*, 169-197.

Trachtman, H. (2007). Educational feature on focal segmental glomerulosclerosis (FSGS): An introduction. *Pediatr Nephrol, 22*, 26-27.

Trulock, E.P., Christie, J.D., Edwards, L.B., et al. (2007). Registry of the International Society for Heart and Lung Transplantation: Twenty-fourth official adult lung and heart-lung transplantation report—2007. *J Heart Lung Transplant, 26*, 782-795.

Turkel, S., & Pao, M. (2007). Late consequences of chronic pediatric illness. *Psychiatr Clin North Am, 30*, 819-835.

United Network for Organ Sharing (UNOS). (2008). *About the MELD/PELD calculator.* Available at www.unos.org/resources/MeldPeldCalculator. asp?index=97. Retrieved June 27, 2008.

Venick, R.S., Farmer, D.G., Saikali, D., et al. (2006). Nutritional outcomes following pediatric intestinal transplantation. *Transplant Proc, 38*, 1718-1719.

Verma, A., & Wade, J.J. (2006). Immunization issues before and after solid organ transplantation in children. *Pediatr Transplant, 10*, 535-548.

Vester, U., Kranz, B., Testa, G., et al. (2001). Efficacy and tolerability of interleukin-2 receptor blockade with basiliximab in pediatric renal transplant recipients. *Pediatr Transplant, 5*, 297-301.

Visner, G.A., & Goldfarb, S.B. (2007). Posttransplant monitoring of pediatric lung transplant recipients. *Curr Opin Pediatr, 19*, 321-326.

Vogt, B.A., & Avner, E.D. (2007). Renal failure. In R.E. Behrman, R.M. Kliegman, B.L. Stanton, et al. (Eds.), *Nelson Textbook of Pediatrics* (18th ed.). Philadelphia: Saunders.

Wallot, M.A., Mathot, M., Janssen, M., et al. (2002). Long-term survival and late graft loss in pediatric liver transplantation recipients: A 15-year single center experience. *Liver Transplant, 8*, 615-622.

Webber, S.A., McCurry, K., & Zeevi, A. (2006). Heart and lung transplantation in children. *Lancet, 368*, 53-69.

Webber, S.A., Naftel, D.C., Fricker, F.J., et al. (2006). Pediatric Heart Transplant Study Lymphoproliferative disorders after paediatric heart transplantation: A multi-institutional study. *Lancet, 367*, 233-239.

Weiss, M., Ng, C., & Madsen, J. (2006). Tolerance, xenotransplantation: Future therapies. *Surg Clin North Am, 86*, 1277-1296.

Well, C.M., Rodgers, S., & Rubovits, S. (2006). School re-entry of the pediatric heart transplant recipient. *Pediatr Transplant, 10*, 928-933.

West, L.J., Pollock-Barziv, S.M., Dipchand, A.I., et al. (2001). ABO-incompatible heart transplantation in infants. *N Engl J Med, 344*, 793-800.

White-Williams, C., Kugler, C., & Widmar, B. (2008). Lung and heart-lung transplantation. In L. Ohler & S. Cupples (Eds.), *Core Curriculum for Transplant Nurses*. St. Louis: Mosby Elsevier.

Wilson, W., Taubert, K.A., Gewitz, M., et al. (2007). Prevention of infective endocarditis: Guidelines from the American Heart Association: A guideline from the American Heart Association Rheumatic Fever, Endocarditis, and Kawasaki Disease Committee; American Heart Association Council on Cardiovascular Disease in the Young; American Heart Association Council on Clinical Cardiology; American Heart Association Council on Cardiovascular Surgery and Anesthesia; Quality of Care and Outcomes Research Interdisciplinary Working Group. *Circulation, 116*, 1736-1754.

Wise, B.V., & Walsh, G. (2008). Pediatric solid organ transplantation. In L. Ohler & S. Cupples (Eds.), *Core Curriculum for Transplant Nurses*. St. Louis: Mosby Elsevier.

Wray, J., & Radley-Smith, R. (2005). Beyond the first year after pediatric heart or heart-lung transplantation: Changes in cognitive function and behavior. *Pediatr Transplant, 9*, 170-177.

Wray, J., & Radley-Smith, R. (2006). Longitudinal assessment of psychological functioning in children after heart or heart-lung transplantation. *J Heart Lung Transplant, 25*, 345-352.

Yamane, M., Date, H., Okazaki, M., et al. (2007). Long-term improvement in pulmonary function after living donor lobar lung transplantation. *J Heart Lung Transplant, 26*, 687-692.

Yang, H. (2006). Maintenance immunosuppression regimens: Conversion, minimization, withdrawal, and avoidance. *Am J Kidney Dis, 47*, S37-S51.

38 Phenylketonuria

Alana L. Clements

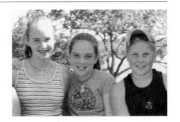

Etiology

Phenylketonuria (PKU) is an autosomal recessive biochemical genetic disorder that results in elevated plasma phenylalanine (Phe) levels. High levels of phenylalanine are toxic to the developing nervous system, and untreated individuals experience mental retardation and other complications, including microcephaly, seizures, and behavioral and psychiatric problems. PKU is caused by a mutation of the phenylalanine hydroxylase (PAH) gene on chromosome 12 and exposure to dietary phenylalanine, an essential amino acid found in most protein foods. Absence or deficiency of PAH halts the conversion of Phe to tyrosine (Tyr) and results in hyperphenylalaninemia (HPA).

More than 500 mutations (allelic variations) in the human PAH gene have been described and compiled in the PAH mutation database (www.pahdb.mcgill.ca). Mutations result from a variety of mechanisms, including insertions, deletions, missense and nonsense mutations, and deoxyribonucleic acid (DNA) splicing defects; missense mutations in PAH are the most commonly seen. Mutations change the DNA code for PAH, which is believed to have a deleterious effect on enzyme function secondary to misfolding and resultant enzyme instability (Scriver, 2007). All individuals inherit two PAH alleles—one from each parent—at the PAH locus. PKU is an autosomal recessive disorder; therefore an individual with one normal allele and one mutant allele will produce adequate functional PAH and will be an asymptomatic carrier of the disease.

Most cases of PKU result from allelic heterogeneity, whereby a different mutation is inherited from each parent, making the affected individual a compound heterozygote. Significant variations in specific PAH mutations are seen in different geographic areas and ethnic populations. Figure 38-1 depicts a family pedigree in which the affected child has inherited one allele for mild HPA and one allele for classic PKU.

The degree of hyperphenylalaninemia in an affected child cannot be accurately predicted from genotype information at the current time. Correlation of genotype with biochemical and metabolic phenotype has been established for some of the common genotypes and this information is available in the PAH mutation database (www.pahdb.mcgill.ca), but allelic heterogeneity complicates the analysis. Identifying genotype-phenotype correlations is currently a major area of interest because some new treatments for HPA may be, at least in part, genotype based (Scriver, 2007). There are many

challenges in this body of research related to the number of known mutations and the probable influence of modifier genes and environmental factors. For example, variations in transport of Phe into the brain may explain the existence of siblings with the same genotype at the PAH locus who exhibit different clinical phenotypes and the existence of the rare individuals with PKU who experience no neurologic damage (National Institutes of Health [NIH], 2000).

The metabolic pathway for Phe is predominantly in the liver. Phe not used for new protein synthesis is converted to Tyr for use in the biosynthesis of protein, melanin, thyroxine, and the catecholamines. Loss of PAH activity in PKU results in an increase in the serum concentration of Phe relative to that of Tyr and subsequently causes an accumulation of Phe metabolites such as phenylpyruvic acid, phenylacetic acid, and others. A high level of Phe inhibits the transport of large neutral amino acids into the brain, disrupting the synthesis of essential substances such as myelin, neurotransmitters, and other proteins. These deficiencies all contribute to the neuropathology of PKU, although the exact mechanisms of neurologic damage remain poorly understood and remain an important area of research (Anderson, Wood, Francis, et al., 2004, 2007; Channon, German, Cassina, et al., 2004; VanZutphen, Packman, Sporri, et al., 2007).

The Phe hydroxylation system is a complex biochemical reaction that requires the presence of oxygen, active site-bound Fe^{2+}, and the co-factor tetrahydrobiopterin (BH_4; see discussion later in this chapter). A deficiency in any enzyme involved in the synthesis or regeneration of BH_4 will result in HPA. BH_4 disorders, found in approximately 1% to 2% of individuals with HPA, are phenotypically and genotypically distinct from PKU, require different modes of therapy, and have a different prognosis. Testing for BH_4 disorders should be done in all newborns with HPA and in any child with microcephaly, mental retardation, seizure disorders, developmental delays, disturbances of tone and posture, hyperreflexia, movement disorders, hyperpyrexia, or other unexplained neurologic findings (Acosta & Yanicelli, 2001).

Offspring of women with PKU, who generally do not have PKU themselves, may be exposed to toxic levels of Phe in utero and experience the effects of maternal PKU (MPKU) syndrome (Clarke, 2003). MPKU syndrome is becoming an increasing cause for concern because large numbers of healthy young women with PKU are now reaching childbearing age. There are approximately 4000 women of reproductive age in the United States with PKU who are at high risk for giving birth to infants with MPKU syndrome if they fail to restrict dietary phenylalanine before and throughout pregnancy (Centers for Disease Control and Prevention [CDC], 2002). Despite the recommendation that all individuals with PKU follow

The authors gratefully acknowledge the contribution of Kathleen Schmidt Yule, the author of this chapter in previous editions.

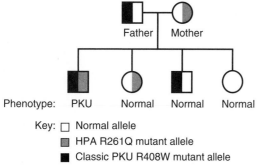

FIGURE 38-1 Hypothetical family pedigree showing segregation of mutant PKU and mutant HPA alleles with haplotype.

a Phe-restricted diet for life, nonadherence during adolescence is common. The success of dietary therapy in arresting the neurologic deficits caused by PKU has resulted in an increasing number of mentally retarded offspring with maternal PKU syndrome; the possibility exists that in one generation the incidence of PKU-related mental deficient could return to the level it was before newborn screening and treatment were available.

Incidence and Prevalence

In the United Sates, the incidence of PKU is 1 in 13,500 to 1 in 19,000; the incidence of non-PKU HPA is estimated to be 1 in 48,000 (NIH, 2000). There are no gender differences, although there is significant racial and ethnic variability, with an increased incidence in certain European white and Native American populations, and a decreased incidence in blacks, Hispanics, and Asians (Hardelid, Cortina-Borja, Munro, et al., 2008; NIH, 2000). For autosomal recessive disorders, carrier (heterozygote) frequency is calculated from PKU incidence (Nussbaum, McInnes, & Willard, 2001), and consequently the incidence of carrier frequency for PKU also varies among populations. For a population with a PKU incidence of 1 in 10,000, the carrier frequency is calculated to be 2%; that is, 1 in 50 people in that population possesses one copy of the mutated PKU gene. The nonuniform distribution of cases of PKU and its major alleles may be explained by migration, genetic drift, recurrent mutation, and intragenic recombination over the past 100,000 years (Scriver, Levy, & Donlon, 2008, updated).

The incidence of PKU is calculated from data collected through mandated newborn screening programs. An NIH consensus development panel on PKU (NIH, 2000) reviewed the Council of Regional Networks for Genetic Services National Newborn Screening Report (Newborn Screening Committee, 1999) and found several factors that confound incidence estimates of PKU: states do not uniformly report the number of infants born, the number of infants screened, the gender or race of the infant, or data about non-PKU HPA. In addition, there are variations in the blood phenylalanine levels considered diagnostic of PKU and HPA. For example, most states or provinces define classic PKU as blood Phe above 20 mg/dL, compared with four states that use 10 mg/dL as the cutoff value. Such discrepancies alter estimates of PKU incidence and lead to state-to-state differences in referrals for follow-up testing and treatment.

Diagnostic Criteria

Individuals with HPA caused by deficient PAH are historically classified as having classic PKU if their Phe levels are consistently greater than 1200 μmol/L (20 mg/dL),[*] mild PKU (sometimes referred to as variant PKU) for Phe levels between 600 μmol/L (10 mg/dL) and 1200 μmol/L (20 mg/dL), or mild HPA for Phe levels below 600 μmol/L (10 mg/dL) (Weglage, Pietsch, Feldmann, et al., 2001). There is variation in this terminology, however, and in some settings the term "non-PKU hyperphenylalaninemia" is used to refer to all individuals whose Phe levels are greater than 120 μmol/L (2 mg/dL) but less than 1200 μmol/L (20 mg/dL).

Screening of newborn infants for PKU is conducted in all U.S. states, Puerto Rico, the Virgin Islands, Guam, all provinces in Canada, and many other countries. Guthrie's method of detecting elevated Phe in a blood spot on a piece of filter paper became widely used in the 1960s. Applications of the method have changed over the years and have included the Guthrie Bacterial Inhibition Assay, automated fluorometric analysis, and high-performance liquid chromatography. In recent years, many states have begun to use tandem mass spectrometry (TMS or MS/MS) to screen newborn blood spots. TMS allows detection of elevated Phe and a large number of other metabolic disorders simultaneously, and it has been shown to reduce the incidence of false-positive results. Nevertheless, the cost, technical complexity, and need for sophisticated interpretation of the results obtained by TMS demand cautious adoption of the technology (NIH, 2000; Rinaldo, Tortorelli, & Matern, 2004).

Screening refers to efforts to distinguish persons who probably do have a condition from those who do not. Newborns with positive newborn screening tests for PKU may or may not actually have PKU; further testing is always required to make a diagnosis of PKU. Fewer than 30% to 50% of infants identified through newborn screening will ultimately be diagnosed with PKU or HPA (Wilcox & Cederbaum, 2002). An infant with a positive screening test should be referred to a metabolic specialty center for a diagnostic workup as soon as possible. This evaluation will reveal false-positive results or confirm the diagnosis of hyperphenylalaninemia, allowing treatment to be initiated immediately. Blood levels of Phe and tyrosine will be checked on all babies with a positive newborn screen for PKU to make this distinction. Parents of a newborn with a positive screening test are notified in various ways, depending on the policy of the regional screening laboratory. Dietary treatment of the child with PKU should ideally begin no later than 7 to 10 days after birth, and therefore it is imperative that every effort be made to avoid delays in the diagnostic process (NIH, 2000).

Although 98% to 99% of cases of hyperphenylalaninemia result from PAH deficiency, it is essential to rule out defects in the biopterin synthase group of enzymes, dihydropterin reductase (DHPR) deficiency, or PAH with decreased affinity for BH_4, because these require different therapies. Pterin metabolites in the urine and DHPR in the blood will be evaluated in all babies with hyperphenylalanemia (Acosta & Yannicelli, 2001; American College of Medical Genetics, 2006; Walter, Lee, & Burgard, 2006;

---

[*]To convert Phe from μmol/L to mg/dL, multiply μmol/L by 0.0165. To convert Phe from mg/dL to μmol/L, multiply mg/dL by 60.53.

Wilcox & Cederbaum, 2002). It is important to be cognizant of the finding that false-positive newborn screening results are not benign and have long-term effects on parental stress, as well as objective indices such as number of hospital visits during the first year of life; special attention should be paid to these families to ensure that they understand what testing was done, as well as the negative outcome (Gurian, Kinnamon, Henry, et al., 2006; Waisbren, Albers, Amato, et al., 2003).

DNA analysis to determine the specific PKU mutation may be suggested by the PKU specialty center. Direct DNA analysis of the PAH gene can be performed to determine the specific mutation present in a child with HPA. Currently, this information is not required for routine diagnostic or therapeutic decisions, but it may be useful for genetic counseling. For fetal diagnosis in families with a known history of HPA, the mode of testing depends on whether or not the mutations of the original proband are known. If the mutant alleles are known, chorionic villus sampling (CVS) or amniocentesis can be used to identify the carrier status of the fetus. If the mutant alleles are not known, identification of polymorphisms in the PAH gene is usually necessary. All individuals have identifiable normal variations in the DNA surrounding the PAH locus on chromosome 12 called restriction fragment length polymorphisms (RFLPs). Because specific RFLPs segregate with the PKU mutation on the PAH gene, they act as markers for PKU and are called PKU haplotypes (haps). Analysis of the parental haplotypes in association with the PAH mutation enables prenatal genetic counseling (Scriver, Levy, & Donlon, 2008, updated).

Despite screening efforts, some cases of PKU and HPA are diagnosed late or undiagnosed. False-negative screening results may occur if the blood is collected before the infant is 24 hours old. Early discharge of newborns from the hospital necessitates a second test, although there is a lack of uniformity in state policies related to repeat testing. Others at risk for a missed diagnosis of PKU include premature infants who are transferred to neonatal intensive care units shortly after birth, those whose parents refuse the screening test, or those born outside of a health care institution or who immigrate to the United States at a young age. Primary care providers should be alert to the possibility of PKU in any of these situations or when the child has unexplained signs and symptoms associated with untreated PKU. In addition, maternal PKU syndrome should be suspected in a child with unexplained microcephaly, cardiac defects, or other dysmorphology or developmental delay, because some women have asymptomatic forms of PKU or HPA.

Clinical Manifestations at Time of Diagnosis

Untreated Phenylketonuria

For more than 40 years, newborn screening has been successful in the prevention of clinical manifestations in children with PKU in the United States. Nevertheless, there remain a number of persons who experience the consequences of misdiagnosis, late diagnosis, or lack of metabolic control. Infants with PKU generally appear normal at birth, but they may have feeding difficulties, vomiting, and irritability soon after birth. Approximately one third of infants with untreated PKU demonstrate lack of increase in head circumference and infantile spasms with hypsarrhythmia or other abnormalities on electroencephalogram (EEG) after the

Clinical Manifestations at Time of Diagnosis

CLINICAL MANIFESTATIONS OF UNTREATED PHENYLKETONURIA
- Normal appearance at birth
- Fair pigmentation
- Irritability
- Neonatal vomiting
- Infantile spasms
- Generalized epilepsy
- Microcephaly
- Atopic dermatitis
- Mousy odor of urine and sweat
- Fine, rapid, irregular tremor
- Parkinson's-like movements
- Bony changes with altered growth patterns
- Delayed motor skills
- Delayed intellectual skills
- Delayed speech and language skills

CLINICAL MANIFESTATIONS OF MATERNAL PHENYLKETONURIA
- Fetal mental retardation
- Microcephaly
- Intrauterine and postnatal growth delay
- Congenital birth defects
  - Cardiac defects
  - Gastrointestinal defects
  - Other

first few months of life (Nyhan, Barshop, & Ozand, 2005; Walter et al., 2006). Infantile spasms (West syndrome) often occur as the first clinical sign of untreated PKU (Zhongshu, Weiming, Yukio, et al., 2001).

As the infant gets older, there are noticeable developmental delays and an unpleasant "mousy" or "musty" odor of the body or urine from the excretion of phenylacetic acid, a metabolite of the accumulated Phe. Mental retardation is generally severe, with a drop in developmental quotient to 50 points by 1 year of age and to 30 points by 3 years of age (Koch & Wenz, 1987). Neurologic features may include seizures (25%), EEG abnormalities (50%), tremors, tics, abnormalities of gait and posturing, and hypertonicity with hyperactive deep tendon reflexes (Rezvani, 2000). Excitability, autism, schizophrenia-like behaviors, and self-destructiveness have also been described in untreated individuals with PKU (Walter et al., 2006).

Children with untreated PKU have lighter skin, eyes, and hair than their unaffected siblings because of impaired melanin synthesis in the absence of sufficient levels of tyrosine. In children of ethnic backgrounds where black hair is expected, this feature will be expressed as hair that is brown or even reddish. Other physical manifestations of untreated PKU include eczema (20% to 40%), prominent maxilla with widely spaced teeth, enamel hypoplasia, and growth retardation that is more evident in boys (Nyhan et al., 2005; Rezvani, 2000; Walter et al., 2006).

Maternal Phenylketonuria Syndrome

Children of women with PKU are obligatory heterozygotes who can only have PKU if their father is a carrier; thus the vast majority do not have PKU. The greatest risk to these infants is prenatal exposure to high levels of Phe in the mother's blood. Until the 1980s

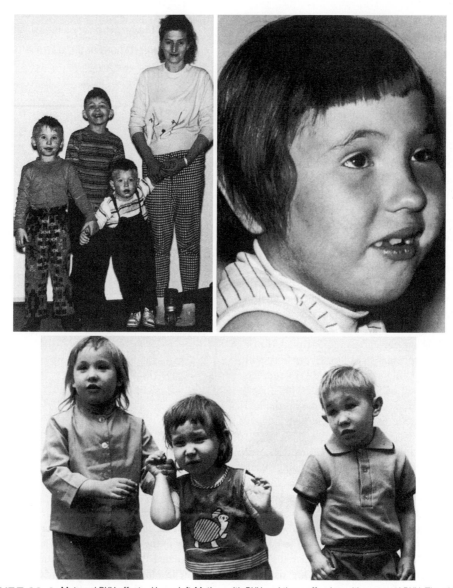

FIGURE 38-2 Maternal PKU effects. *Upper left,* Mother with PKU and three offspring with maternal PKU. The children do not have PKU. *Upper right,* Girl with maternal PKU. *Lower,* Three children of PKU mother. In addition to the relative microcephaly, note the subtle similarity in the facies, including the poorly defined philtrum. From Jones, K.L. (1997). *Smith's Recognizable Patterns of Human Malformation* (5th ed.). Philadelphia: Saunders. Courtesy of Dr. Witheld Zaleski, University of Saskatoon, Department of Pediatrics, Saskatoon, Saskatchewan. Reprinted with permission.

it was common to discontinue the diet in middle childhood, and presently lack of adherence to the recommended diet remains problematic. Return to diet once it has been discontinued is very difficult, even for women planning a pregnancy, and many pregnant women with PKU do not achieve dietary control before conception (CDC, 2002; Gambol, 2007).

Infants born to women with PKU who do not adhere to a low-Phe diet before and during pregnancy have a high incidence of mental retardation (93%), microcephaly (72%), and heart defects (14%) (Levy, Guldberg, Guttler, et al., 2001; Rouse, Azen, Koch, et al., 1997; Rouse, Matalon, Koch, et al., 2000). Other features of maternal PKU syndrome include intrauterine and postnatal growth delay and dysmorphic facial features that resemble fetal alcohol syndrome (Figure 38-2). There is also a higher incidence of other

birth defects in infants with maternal PKU syndrome, including dysgenesis of the corpus callosum (Nissenkorn, Michelson, Ben-Zeev, et al., 2001), tracheoesophageal fistula (Koch, Hanley, Levy, et al., 2003), bowel malrotation, bladder exstrophy, orofacial clefting, and eye abnormalities such as coloboma and cataracts (Walter et al., 2006).

In a pregnant woman with PKU, a transplacental gradient that favors the fetus results in a fetal/maternal ratio of Phe of about 1.5, although that ratio may be as high as 2.9 (Scriver, Levy, & Donlon, 2008, updated); thus studies of MPKU rely on maternal Phe levels, and these may not be valid indicators of the fetal level. Many studies document a dose-dependent teratogenic effect of maternal Phe on a developing fetus, which is more pronounced in the early weeks of pregnancy. Rouse and colleagues (1997) determined that at maternal Phe levels of 900 µmol/L (15 mg/dL), 85% of infants had microcephaly, 51% had postnatal growth retardation, and 26% had intrauterine growth retardation, compared with 6%, 4%, and 0%, respectively, if the maternal Phe level was less than 360 µmol/L (6 mg/dL). Levy and colleagues (2001) found that a basal maternal Phe level above 900 µmol/L (15 mg/dL) may be the threshold for congenital heart disease in the fetus and that a level above 1800 µmol/L (30 mg/dL) poses a significant risk of congenital heart disease. Phe levels of 2 to 6 mg/dL have been shown to pose relatively low risk of fetal anomalies and developmental disabilities, and this is the goal advised for most women (Koch et al., 2003). Review of the maternal PKU registry in the United Kingdom confirmed that initiating dietary restriction before conception significantly improved outcomes (Lee, Ridout, Walter, et al., 2005).

Treatment

Dietary modification is the primary treatment for PKU and for prevention of maternal PKU syndrome. It is well established that a Phe-restricted diet can prevent the severe neurologic consequences associated with untreated PKU. However, metabolic control in PKU may be difficult to achieve in practice; it requires frequent monitoring of blood Phe levels, maintaining a highly restrictive diet, careful monitoring of food intake, frequent visits to a PKU clinic, and supplementation with formula that many persons find unpalatable.

Treatment

- Phe-restricted diet to maintain levels
  - For children ≤12 years and for women before and throughout pregnancy: 120 µmol/L (2 mg/dL) to 360 µmol/L (6 mg/dL)
  - >12 years: 120 µmol/L (2 mg/dL) to 900 µmol/L (15 mg/dL), although an upper limit of 600 µmol/L (10 mg/dL) strongly encouraged
- Supplement tyrosine and other nutrients as needed
- Kuvan trial may be considered

The NIH consensus statement (NIH, 2000) on the management of PKU recommends that treatment of the neonate with PKU be initiated as soon as possible but no later than 7 to 10 days after birth. Blood Phe levels should be maintained between 120 µmol/L (2 mg/dL) and 360 µmol/L (6 mg/dL) until age 12 years. After age 12 years, Phe levels should be between 120 µmol/L (2 mg/dL) and 900 µmol/L (15 mg/dL), although 600 µmol/L (10 mg/dL) as an upper limit is strongly encouraged. For women of childbearing age, a Phe level between 120 µmol/L (2 mg/dL) and 360 µmol/L (6 mg/dL) should be achieved at least 3 months before conception and maintained throughout the pregnancy. Individuals with mild HPA whose Phe levels remain below 360 µmol/L (6 mg/dL) may remain on a natural protein diet.

The diet for PKU is far more involved than simple restriction of Phe. Since all naturally occurring food proteins contain (on average) 5% Phe and must be avoided, supplements are required to ensure adequate nutrient intake for optimum growth and development. The PKU treatment center team, which continually monitors the child's Phe tolerance, prescribes the diet. An individual's Phe and other nutrient requirements depend on many factors, including

PAH activity, age, growth rate, adequacy of energy and protein intake, and state of health. The precise tolerance for Phe varies, but for most individuals with PKU it is between 200 and 500 mg/day. Phe tolerance may change over time, so careful and continuous monitoring of individuals whose Phe intake is restricted is necessary to avoid both elevations and deficiencies of Phe. Long-term deficiencies of Phe from excessive restriction are also associated with adverse outcomes, including poor growth and development and, in some cases when treatment for PKU was first initiated, death (Acosta & Yanicelli, 2001; Scriver, Levy, & Donlon, 2008, updated; Seashore, 2008).

In the neonate, breast milk supplemented with Phe-free formula is recommended. If the infant is formula fed, one of the commercially available Phe-free elemental medical foods (EMFs) should be used in conjunction with the standard baby formula being used by the family. These products are modified protein hydrolysates in which Phe is removed, or they are mixtures of free amino acids that do not contain Phe. EMFs provide the essential amino acids in suitable proportions for the given age of the individual. As the infant begins to eat solid foods, the Phe content must be calculated and the amount of EMF adjusted to ensure that all nutrients are ingested in proper amounts and the desired blood Phe level is maintained. Parents invariably require the assistance of a nutritionist to accomplish these goals.

There is much controversy over the need for supplementation of certain nutrients for individuals on Phe-restricted diets. Tyrosine deficiency is a consequence of inadequate Phe metabolism in PKU, and it has been postulated that low Tyr levels may be responsible for learning difficulties in well-treated individuals with PKU. EMFs are enriched with Tyr, and clinicians often prescribe additional Tyr supplements. However, tyrosine supplementation in PKU has not been found to improve neuropsychological function in studies, and this is thought to be related to nonsustained plasma Tyr elevations after ingestion of the supplement with inadequate levels reaching the brain (Kalsner, Rohr, Strauss, et al., 2001). The potential dangers of fluctuating Tyr levels have prompted some researchers to recommend against additional supplementation and advocate reduction of the Tyr content in EMFs and the development of slow-release Tyr dietary compounds (Van Spronsen, van Rijn, Bekhof, et al., 2001).

Long-chain polyunsaturated fatty acids, including docosahexanoic acid (DHA) and arachidonic acid (AA), may be reduced in the blood of individuals treated for PKU, and blood lipid monitoring with supplementation of DHA and AA in deficient individuals is recommended (Moseley, Koch, & Moser, 2002). There is also evidence that supplementation with omega-3 long-chain polyunsaturated fatty acids from fish oil improves visual evoked potentials and motor function in children with treated PKU (Beblo, Reinhardt, Demmelmair, et al., 2007; Beblo, Reinhardt, Muntau, et al., 2001). Other dietary components commonly monitored and supplemented in individuals with PKU include vitamin B_{12}, folic acid, calcium, zinc, iron, phosphate, and selenium (NIH, 2000; Van Bakel, Printzen, Wermuth, et al., 2000).

Children with late-diagnosed PKU should also be placed on the Phe-restricted diet no matter how late they are identified. Improvements in behavior and neurologic status have been seen in individuals with severe retardation who had untreated PKU (Baumeister & Baumeister, 1998; Fitzgerald, Morgan, Keene, et al., 2000). In a study of 57 people with a late diagnosis with a mean intelligence quotient (IQ) of 44 at the time of diagnosis, institution of the Phe-restricted diet improved their mean IQ to 73 (Koch, Moseley, Ning, et al., 1999). In addition, return to diet for adults with PKU who have discontinued it has been shown to improve a variety of conditions, including brain magnetic resonance imaging (MRI) changes, agoraphobia, panic attacks, and recurrent headaches (Koch et al., 1999). Another study revealed that 60% of individuals reported an improved quality of life after resumption or initiation of the diet, though only 47% of those in this research group maintained dietary compliance (Gassió, Campistol, Vilaseca, et al., 2003).

In late 2007, the U.S. Food and Drug Administration (FDA) approved a new medication that is expected to be an important adjuvant to dietary treatment in some individuals with PKU (Pollack, 2007). Tetrahydrobiopterin (BH_4) is a co-factor in the phenylalanine hydoxylase system and has been shown to reduce Phe levels by 20% to 30% or greater in up to 50% of individuals with hyperphenylalaninemia. BioMarin Pharmaceuticals has developed and is now marketing BH_4 as Kuvan. It had originally been postulated that it would be possible to predetermine a person's response to BH_4 based on genotype-phenotype correlation, but the research is inconsistent and therefore the current recommendation is for all persons with PKU ages 8 and above who are interested to have a trial with Kuvan to determine their responder status (Zurfluh, Zschocke, Lindner, et al., 2008). Dosing range is 5 to 20 mg/kg/day, and different clinics will be using different algorithms to start children and adults on Kuvan and determine the appropriate dosage (Levy, Burton, Cederbaum, et al., 2007). Definition of "responders" also varies, but most providers would expect a responder to achieve a 20% to 30% decrease in plasma Phe level with the appropriate dose of Kuvan and no dietary change. This could allow for significant liberalization of the diet in these individuals. Of note, utilization of Kuvan may be limited by the prohibitive cost, which can be up to $200,000 per year for large adults, though people who are insured should have at least part of this cost covered (Pollack, 2007).

Effects of long-term use of BH_4 are currently unknown, but at least one European study has attempted long-term treatment with no significant ill effects (Trefz, Scheible, Frauendienst-Egger, et al., 2005). This same team has used BH_4 without dietary treatment in a small group of infants with mild PKU diagnosed on newborn screening. They have thus far witnessed no significant side effects and normal somatic and psychomotor development in this limited study. They note that further studies are necessary before offering medication alone as a clinical treatment for all infants with mild PKU.

Complementary and Alternative Therapies
Complementary therapies for PKU must be administered in conjunction with conventional dietary treatment. A person with PKU should not take dietary supplements or herbal remedies without the approval of the metabolic practitioner, because many of these contain high amounts of protein or aspartame. However, affected children and their families may derive significant benefit from relaxation training, spirituality, imagery, and therapies involving art, music, and touch. PKU, like any chronic condition requiring constant care and vigilance, places enormous stress on all involved. Online and local support groups and E-mail mailing lists for families with PKU may provide practical information and act as a resource for relevant complementary therapy programs.

Anticipated Advances in Diagnosis and Management

Although diet therapy is an effective treatment for PKU, some individuals have difficulty adhering to the strict regimen and experience poor outcomes as a result. Potential alternative treatments that are being investigated include somatic enzyme substitution or replacement and gene therapy, though little progress has been made on the latter. One promising therapy involves oral administration of recombinant phenylalanine ammonia lyase (PAL), an enzyme that degrades phenylalanine in the intestinal tract into *trans*-cinnamic acid that can be broken down in the liver of people with PAH deficiency. Animal studies and limited human studies suggest that PAL has the potential to make the PKU diet less restrictive for humans. The utility and feasibility of enzyme replacement using PAH continue to be evaluated, though less progress has been made. The challenge for all of these types of treatments is finding a formulation that has sufficient bioavailability, minimal side effects, and consistent effectiveness (Kim, Erlandsen, Surendran, et al., 2004).

Although liver transplants are unlikely to become standard therapy for a condition treatable by diet therapy, Phe tolerance was restored to a 10-year-old boy with PKU who received a liver transplant for concurrent active cirrhosis (Scriver, Levy, & Donlon, 2008, updated). Hepatocyte transplantation is under consideration for PKU; in this scenario, the person's own liver cells are removed, the normal PAH gene is inserted into the cells, and the cells are then reinserted into the person. Techniques for insertion of the PAH gene into skin, lymphocytes, or other human cells may eventually be able to restore normal Phe metabolism in people with PKU, but at the present time there are many obstacles to overcome in the field of gene therapy; some animal studies have been promising, but gene therapy for humans with metabolic disorders likely continues to be a long way off (Harding, Gillingham, Daghighi, et al., 2006; Scriver, Levy, & Donlon, 2008, updated; Spirito, Meneguzzi, Danos, et al., 2001).

Research on foods and supplements also shows promise for improving the lives of those affected by PKU. Glycomacropeptide (GMP) is a whey protein and the only known protein free of Phe; researchers have been able to successfully create foods out of GMP that were met with positive reviews by people with PKU who tried them. GMP foods may become commercially available in the future and may prove to be a useful adjunct to the current low-protein food options (Etzel, 2002; Lim, van Calcar, Nelson, et al., 2007; Ney, Hull, van Calcar, et al., 2008).

There is some evidence that large neutral amino acids (LNAAs) lower the brain Phe level by competing with phenylalanine for transport across the blood-brain barrier (Pietz, Kreis, Rupp et al., 1999). Brain Phe levels may now be measured using magnetic resonance spectroscopy (MRS), a specialized type of MRI (Giewska, Cyryowski, Jowiak, et al., 2001). Recent studies in Australia indicate that LNAAs are unlikely to be of benefit to individuals who are compliant with the consumption of their EMF and diet, but may improve functioning and decrease plasma Phe in people who are unable to maintain good control. Further studies are needed to refine our understanding of the utility of LNAAs (Giovannini, Verduci, Salvatici, et al., 2007; Schindeler, Ghosh-Jerath, Thompson, et al., 2007).

Regular blood Phe monitoring is an important aspect of care in PKU. Home monitoring devices are being developed (Andrade, 2002), and the possibility of a noninvasive monitoring device is being investigated (Miller, 2002). Such technologies would give the individual greater autonomy and potentially improve Phe control (Bilginsoy, Waitzman, Leonard, et al., 2005). Researchers are also working to create a test to monitor Phe levels through urine samples that could also potentially improve compliance with testing frequency (Langenbeck, Baum, Mench-Hoinowski, et al., 2005).

Associated Problems of Phenylketonuria and Treatment

Although dietary treatment has largely eliminated the severe problems associated with untreated PKU, questions remain about subtle abnormalities people with PKU may have with neurologic function, cognitive development, behavioral adjustment, school achievement, and physical health (NIH, 2000). Unfortunately, it is difficult to determine precisely what factors account for impairments; high Phe levels are presumed to cause the pathophysiologic changes in body systems, but low tyrosine levels, low fatty acid levels, or imbalances in other substances may also play a role. However, it is generally agreed, based on all the available evidence, that early and consistent Phe control is associated with better outcomes in all domains.

Associated Problems of Phenylketonuria and Treatment

- Consistent dietary treatment eliminates severe problems
- Neurologic changes
- Cognitive deficits
  - Poorer performance on intelligence quotient (IQ) tests
  - Cognitive difficulties related to planning, problem solving, and self-regulation
- Behavioral manifestations
  - Tendency toward depression, anxiety, phobias
  - Attention-deficit/hyperactivity disorder
- Dermatitis
- Decreased bone mineral density

Neurologic Manifestations

Abnormal findings in cerebral white matter on MRI have been observed in some individuals with PKU, likely related to a myelin defect secondary to elevated Phe and decreased Tyr. The clinical significance of white matter abnormalities remains unclear, and the severity of signs and symptoms may not consistently reflect the degree of visualized abnormality; people with more extensive white matter abnormalities, particularly those extending into frontal and subcortical regions, appear to have the most significant impairments in executive functioning and cognition. Reversal of cerebral white matter change has been observed when Phe restriction is resumed (Anderson et al., 2007). Some researchers believe that there are individual differences in the brain's vulnerability to Phe and that this vulnerability varies throughout the life span. Evidence suggests that maintaining Phe levels below 600 μmol/L minimizes cerebral white matter changes (Weglage et al., 2001). Abnormal visual and auditory evoked potentials have been identified in some individuals with treated PKU. Other signs of impaired nerve conduction found in some individuals who relax their dietary Phe restriction include hyperactive tendon reflexes, intention tremor, and abnormal EEG findings (NIH, 2000; Walter et al., 2006; Welsh & Pennington, 2000).

Cognitive Deficits

Dietary discontinuation before age 8 is associated with poorer performance on IQ tests; adults and adolescents on relaxed diets have stable IQ scores but may have poorer performance on measures of attention and speed of processing. Adults whose diet has been consistently maintained continue to show subtle deficits compared with unaffected controls in tasks of executive function, memory, and learning. However, these deficits were not consistent across all tasks performed in the study—in some, the adults with PKU performed as well as control subjects—and the researchers posited that perhaps these deficits actually represent slowed information processing (Channon et al., 2004). The variation in severity of disease and metabolic control at different ages makes it difficult to generalize these studies to an individual. However, it is clear that adolescence is the stage at which many children begin to discontinue their diet, and an increase in deficits of executive functioning corresponding with an increase in Phe have been found in multiple studies (VanZutphen et al., 2007).

The NIH Consensus Panel (NIH, 2000) also reviewed 37 studies reporting outcomes that involved school achievement, behavioral adjustment, or cognitive functions other than IQ tests. Poorer performance among persons with PKU was found in 29 of these studies, with the most prominent findings being diminished school achievement and greater difficulty on achievement tests. Cognitive difficulties reported included executive functions (planning, problem solving, self-regulation) and attention. The panel noted that many of these studies were limited by small sample sizes and inconsistent use of comparison groups but concluded that levels of Phe show moderate relationships to performance on measures of cognitive function and the presence of behavioral difficulties.

Evaluation of the relationship between various Phe levels and cognitive functioning remains an active area of research. Weglage and colleagues (2001) reported normal intellectual and educational outcomes in 31 adolescent subjects with mild HPA (persistent Phe levels between 360 and 600 μmol/L) when compared with unaffected controls. Griffiths, Demellweek, Fay, and colleagues (2000) found that verbal intelligence in the primary school years tends to normalize if blood Phe is maintained below 360 μmol/L in infancy, but spatial intelligence may remain poor. Huijbregts, de Sonneville, Licht, and colleagues (2002) found that people with PKU with Phe levels above 360 μmol/L exhibited lower speed of information processing, less ability to inhibit task-induced cognitive interference, less consistent performance, and a stronger decrease in performance level over time compared with control subjects. A recent large-scale literature review and meta-analysis confirmed that IQ and executive function are inversely influenced when diet is discontinued and thus Phe increased during childhood (Waisbren, Noel, Fahrbach, et al., 2007). Some of these neuropsychological changes can be mitigated by close adherence to the diet, and it is crucial to discuss these research findings with all families, but particularly those whose children are in poor control.

Behavioral Manifestations

Both anecdotal evidence and scientific evidence support the conclusion that certain neuropsychiatric and psychological deficits are more frequent in persons with PKU and that these may sometimes be relieved by a return to a strict diet. Anxiety, depression, anorexia, and agoraphobia may be associated with high blood Phe levels that decrease dopamine and serotonin in the brain. A link between PKU and autism (see Chapter 13) has also been noted, especially in late-treated individuals (NIH, 2000). Smith and Knowles (2000) reviewed 34 studies related to behavioral problems in people with treated PKU and found evidence that affected individuals are more prone to depression, anxiety, phobic tendencies, and isolation from peers; the authors suggested that these findings are related to a combination of the stress of maintaining the diet and the degree of neurobiologic impairment.

Attention-deficit/hyperactivity disorder (ADHD; see Chapter 12) may be more common in children with early-treated PKU than in the general population (Antshel, 2001; Welsh & Pennington, 2000). One study of 38 children with PKU found that 26% were using a stimulant to control symptoms of ADHD, compared with a matched control group and the population norm, in which 6.5% and 5% of children, respectively, were using stimulants; the plasma Phe of the children receiving stimulants was significantly higher than those not reporting problems with attention (Arnold, Vladutiu, Orlowski, et al., 2004). One explanation for some of the attention deficits noted in children with early-treated PKU was posited by Banich, Passarotti, White, and colleagues (2000), who found that interhemispheric interaction is compromised in the brains of these children as compared with normal controls.

Dermatitis

Scaling eczematous dermatitis is more prevalent in children with PKU, presumably because of the toxic effects of Phe and its metabolites. Skin and muscle indurations resembling scleroderma have been reported, especially on the arms and buttocks of young children with PKU. These skin manifestations have been noted to improve with better dietary control (NIH, 2000; Nyhan et al., 2005).

Decreased Bone Mineral Density

Decreased total bone mineral density and spine bone mineral density may occur in prepubertal children and adults with treated PKU; these changes are associated with an increased incidence of fractures (Modan-Moses, Vered, Schwartz, et al., 2007). Whether this is caused by a nutrient deficiency in the diet or a pathophysiology inherent in the disease remains unclear. Poor linear growth has also been seen in some children with PKU, and there is still debate as to whether or not this correlates with protein deficiency (Dobbelaere, Michaud, Debrabander, et al., 2003; Nyhan et al., 2005).

Prognosis

Individuals treated early for PKU may be expected to grow and develop normally. The lifelong outcome for children with well-treated PKU is yet to be observed, since the oldest treated individuals are currently in their forties. Several factors affect the prognosis for PKU, including age at time of diagnosis and Phe restriction, degree of metabolic control, and the specific mutation responsible. Adherence to the treatment regimen, a primary predictor of overall health in PKU, is undoubtedly affected by psychosocial factors.

PRIMARY CARE MANAGEMENT

Health Care Maintenance
Growth and Development

Growth is essentially normal for children with early-treated PKU on a controlled, Phe-restricted diet. Careful monitoring of height, weight, and head circumference on growth charts, as well as body mass index, is an especially important aspect of primary care of a child with PKU because efforts to limit Phe may result in inadequate protein or calorie intake. Head circumference, weight, and length should be measured at scheduled monthly intervals for the first year, then every 3 months until after the prepubertal growth spurt, and then every 6 months throughout adolescence to monitor adequacy of diet.

Cognitive deficits and learning difficulties may be present even in children with good dietary management (see section on Schooling). Development should be monitored in primary care in conjunction with the specialty provider. Referral to the PKU treatment center or neurology for psychological testing and developmental assessment is recommended. Young children with evidence of delay should be referred to early intervention programs (e.g., Birth to Three).

Diet

The goals of diet therapy are to maintain blood Phe levels in the safe range and provide adequate amounts of all other nutrients to support growth and prevent protein catabolism. The requirements for the PKU diet vary among individuals and throughout their lifetimes, and Phe levels must be monitored on a regular basis.

Consultation with a professional nutritionist experienced with PKU is an essential part of care. Dietary management of PKU is simple in theory but very difficult in reality. Parents are often overwhelmed to learn that their child has PKU, yet they must begin to make modifications immediately. Most parents have never heard of PKU at the time their newborn is diagnosed, so they have numerous concerns about the implications of having a genetic condition in the family, the child's prognosis, and the details of the treatment. It takes time for parents to adjust to the diagnosis and to the knowledge that this is a condition that will require lifelong attention and management.

Although the decision to breastfeed is a personal one, clinicians should inform women of the particular advantages of human breast milk for a newborn with PKU. Mature human breast milk has a mean Phe content of 48 mg/dL, which is lower than the mean Phe content of cow's milk (164 mg/dL) and common infant formulas such as Isomil (88 mg/dL) and Similac (59 mg/dL) (Acosta & Yanicelli, 2001). Formula-fed infants generally accept one of the commercially available Phe-free infant formulas. Since some Phe is essential in the diet, infants are also given a prescribed amount of a Phe-containing formula. Table 38-1 gives the recommended daily nutrient intakes for persons with PKU; these values provide general guidelines but cannot be a substitute for monitoring of Phe levels and nutritional indices. Frequent diet adjustments are necessary throughout life but especially in periods of rapid growth. PKU treatment centers have knowledgeable nutritionists to assist families.

TABLE 38-1

Recommended Daily Nutrient Intakes (Ranges) for Infants, Children, and Adults with Phenylketonuria

	Nutrient				
	Phe	Tyr	Protein	Energy	Fluid
Age	mg/kg	mg/kg	g/kg	kcal/kg	mL/kg
INFANTS					
0-3 mo	25-70	300-350	3.50-3.00	120 (95-145)	160-135
3-6 mo	20-45	300-350	3.50-3.00	120 (95-145)	160-130
6-9 mo	15-35	250-300	3.00-2.50	110 (80-135)	145-125
9-12 mo	10-35	250-300	3.00-2.50	105 (80-135)	135-120
	mg/day	g/day	g/day	kcal/day	mL/day
GIRLS AND BOYS					
1-4 yr	200-400	1.72-3.00	>30	1300 (900-1800)	900-1800
4-7 yr	210-450	2.25-3.50	>35	1700 (1300-2300)	1300-2300
7-11 yr	220-500	2.55-4.00	>40	2400 (1650-3300)	1650-3300
WOMEN					
11-15 yr	250-750	3.45-5.00	>50	2200 (1500-3000)	1500-3000
15-19 yr	230-700	3.45-5.00	>55	2100 (1200-3000)	1200-3000
>19 yr	220-700	3.75-5.00	>60	2100 (1400-2500)	2100-2500
MEN					
11-15 yr	225-900	3.38-5.50	>55	2700 (2000-3700)	2000-3700
15-19 yr	295-1100	4.42-6.50	>65	2800 (2100-3900)	2100-3900
>19 yr	290-1200	4.35-6.50	>70	2900 (2000-3300)	2000-3300

From Acosta, P.B., & Yannicelli, S. (Eds.). (2001). *The Ross Metabolic Formula System: Nutrition Support Protocols* (4th ed.). Columbus, OH: Ross Products Division/Abbott Laboratories. Reprinted with permission.

Solid foods should be introduced to infants with PKU as they would be for any infant, but parents must monitor and adjust the child's Phe intake. In general, protein foods are high in Phe, so foods to avoid include cheese, eggs, meat, milk, poultry, nuts, dried beans and peas, most breads, seeds, and peanut butter. Foods that are low in protein include fruits, fats, vegetables, sweets, and some cereals. Special low-protein breads, pasta, and cereal should be encouraged, because they will become an important part of the lifelong diet. Such products are commercially available, although many families prefer to prepare their own.

One common method for calculating Phe intake involves the use of exchanges, where one exchange is equal to 15 mg of Phe. Other practitioners prefer to instruct parents to calculate milligrams of Phe and to maintain a daily intake that will keep their blood level in the desired range. Some clinics recommend the use of a gram scale or use standard scoops and household measures.

Detailed lists of the Phe content in foods are available from the U.S. Department of Agriculture (USDA) Nutrient Database at www.nal.usda.gov/fnic/cgi-bin/nut_search.pl, medical food companies, the nutritionist at the metabolic clinic, or the National PKU News website at www.pkunews.org. Parents may be asked to weigh or measure and record all the food the child eats for 3 days before the clinic visit and blood test. This diet record allows the nutritionist to calculate necessary adjustments.

All persons with PKU require some Phe-free EMF to maintain proper nutrition. A typical individual requires three servings of EMF per day, and these generally accompany regular meals. In any case, optimal growth and Phe homeostasis are best maintained by distributing the protein intake throughout the day. The EMF products look and taste very different from milk, and many individuals find them unpalatable. EMF ingestion is critical for the health of the child with PKU because it contains both supplemental Phe-free protein and vitamins and minerals the children might lack secondary to the restricted diet, therefore parents and significant others need to be very careful not to communicate any distaste for the product. Most children readily accept the EMF if it is started early and if the family has a positive attitude about it. The use of straws and "sippy cups" often facilitates EMF ingestion. Some children prefer to have flavorings added to the formula, such as Tang, Kool-Aid mixes, chocolate syrup, concentrated fruit juice, or flavor packets available from the EMF company. The nutritionist must approve such flavorings, and great care must be taken to avoid any product containing aspartame, which is converted to Phe in the gastrointestinal tract. Older children may choose to take their EMF in the form of a capsule or bar. Scientific Hospital Supplies (www.shsna.com) makes Phe-free protein capsules that replace formula; however, more than 100 capsules per day may be required. Many states require that insurance companies or state agencies provide formula and/or low-protein foods for individuals with PKU (www.pkunews.org).

Parents should follow the instructions supplied by the manufacturer when preparing EMF products. The amount of powder to be ingested should be carefully measured, although the volume of liquid to be used may be adjusted according to individual preferences. Some children prefer a more concentrated mixture so they have to drink less. It is important that all the powder is ingested, and this may necessitate further dilution of any remaining "sludge" in the bottom of the container. Most people prefer to mix a 24-hour supply of the EMF and store it in the refrigerator for use the following day. These products should not be heated beyond 130.1°F (54.5°C) to avoid a chemical reaction that alters their protein structure. The shelf life of EMF products is limited, and parents should note the expiration date on the can.

Many children exhibit feeding problems at some point in their development, and children with PKU are no different. However, parents may be more concerned about such problems when they know that their child's health depends on adherence to a strict diet. Parents may be reassured that 1 or 2 days of poor intake will not harm the child, nor will occasional nonsustained elevations in Phe. As with any child, parents should not force feed. It is often useful to offer smaller portions; the child can always ask for more but may feel overwhelmed by large helpings. The EMF should be served first. Giving the child some choice in selection of foods and having large amounts of "free" foods available also are useful strategies. In an older child, extra protein-free foods may be necessary to meet calorie and energy requirements. These should be monitored carefully, however, because they often contain large amounts of sugar and fat and may lead to obesity if used in excess.

There are anecdotal reports of increased incidence of eating disorders in children with PKU. The idea of a young child being on a "diet" may cause confusion or abnormal perceptions about the meaning of food. As one young adult with PKU so aptly put it, "My main advice for parents of children with PKU is to try not to make PKU a big deal or a central issue in the child's life. What you eat is not even remotely close to being the most important aspect of life" (Beck, 1999).

Because diet for life is the primary treatment for PKU, it is important to initiate self-management at an early age. The child must be taught to make low-Phe food choices and to understand the importance of doing so. At the same time, great care must be taken not to make the child feel stigmatized by "different" eating habits. Overemphasizing the restrictions may instill undue fear or guilt in a young child. Establishing a balance between a healthy Phe-restricted diet and making the child feel normal takes a tremendous amount of effort and sensitivity on the part of parents and caregivers.

Safety

The only safety concerns particular to PKU are related to nutritional imbalances. Overrestriction resulting in long-term Phe deficiency may lead to aminoaciduria, hypoproteinemia, bone changes, decreased growth, anemia, mental retardation, and hair loss (Acosta & Yannicelli, 2001). Ingestion of Phe that exceeds the individual's tolerance leads to the complications associated with hyperphenylalaninemia. Occasional ingestion of a high-Phe substance such as aspartame is less deleterious than chronic lapses of the restricted diet. Teaching the child and significant others about the importance of a Phe-restricted diet is the best prevention against this hazard.

Immunizations

Routine immunizations are recommended.

Screening

Vision. Routine screening is recommended.

Hearing. Routine screening is recommended.

Dental. The diet for PKU includes a high proportion of carbohydrates to meet the daily requirement for calories. Dietary sugars are known to increase the risk for dental caries, although one study found no greater incidence in tooth decay in children with PKU (Lucas, Contreras, Loukissa, et al., 2001). To promote dental health, parents should be cautioned not to put the baby to bed with a bottle. Wean the infant to a cup as early as 6 months of age; offer foods such as fruits in place of more retentive forms of refined sugars, as well as liquid forms of carbohydrate that promote oral clearance. Fluoride supplementation is recommended if it is not added to the local water supply. Oral hygiene and dentist visits should be implemented soon after the teeth erupt. Children with PKU who were diagnosed late may require specialized dental care if they have enamel hypoplasia or abnormal tooth spacing.

Blood Pressure. Routine screening is recommended.

Hematocrit. Children on protein-restricted semisynthetic diets are at risk for inadequate intake of iron and other trace elements, though EMFs are supplemented with vitamins and minerals that children on restricted diets often lack. Hematocrit monitoring and related tests are part of the biochemical nutritional assessment done at the metabolic clinic. Primary care practitioners should communicate with the metabolic practitioner to determine the need for additional tests.

Urinalysis. Routine screening is recommended.

Tuberculosis. Routine screening is recommended.

Condition-Specific Screening (Box 38-1)

Blood Phe Monitoring. Plasma Phe and Tyr levels are evaluated twice weekly in newborns with PKU until concentrations are stabilized and approximate dietary Phe and Tyr requirements are known. Blood Phe is evaluated weekly until age 1 year, twice monthly until age 12 years, monthly after age 12 years, and twice weekly for pregnant women (NIH, 2000). Parents may be taught to collect the capillary blood samples on filter paper at home and return them to the metabolic clinic or other laboratory. The PKU treatment center team evaluates these results, and dietary adjustments are made as needed.

Nutritional Indices Monitoring. Nutrient intake is evaluated for Phe, Tyr, protein, and energy intake by the nutritionist on the PKU treatment team. Protein status is evaluated by plasma transthyretin, albumin, or prealbumin levels every 3 months in infants and every 6 months in children and adolescents. The metabolic treatment team also monitors for insufficient intake of iron, folate, vitamin B_{12}, and other nutrients (Acosta & Yannicelli, 2001).

BOX 38-1

Condition-Specific Screening

Newborn with positive screening test
- Quantitative tests for Phe and Tyr
- Pterin metabolites in urine
- Dihydropterin reductase (DHPR) in blood

Blood Phe monitoring
- Twice weekly with Tyr levels until stable
- Weekly until age 1 year
- Twice monthly until age 12 years
- Monthly after age 12 years
- Weekly or twice weekly in pregnant women

Nutritional indices monitoring
- Plasma transthyretin, albumin, or prealbumin every 3 months in infants, every 6 months in children and adolescents
- Iron, folate, vitamin B_{12} levels per nutritionist

Common Illness Management
Differential Diagnosis

Well-nourished children with PKU respond to infection and trauma in the same way as any child. Children with chronically elevated Phe levels may exhibit the associated signs and symptoms of PKU, including eczematous skin lesions, musty body odor, and cognitive and neurologic sequelae.

Management during Illness and Surgery. Minor uncomplicated surgery with general anesthesia does not cause a major alteration in the blood Phe level. Febrile illness and trauma are normally accompanied by protein catabolism, which may result in elevation of plasma Phe concentrations. These elevations are generally transient and do not require additional Phe monitoring. Supportive measures should be undertaken to limit protein catabolism; liberal volumes of fruit juices, liquid gelatin, caffeine-free soft drinks, or electrolyte formulas (e.g., Pedialyte) without aspartame should be allowed. Polycose powder or liquid or a Phe-free additive recommended by the medical food company may be mixed with the fluids. Acetaminophen, ibuprofen, antibiotics, or other medications may be recommended or prescribed as for any child, but the Phe content of these substances must be taken into consideration. EMFs are reinstituted as soon as possible, initially at half strength. If parenteral amino acid solutions are indicated for any reason, involvement of a specialist familiar with PKU is essential (Acosta & Yannicelli, 2001).

Drug Interactions

Aspartame. Aspartame (L-aspartyl-L-phenylalanine methyl ester [APM]) is contraindicated in individuals with PKU because it is converted to phenylalanine in the gastrointestinal tract. Currently marketed under the brand names NutraSweet, Equal, or Canderel, aspartame must be identified on the label of all products with the statement "Phenylketonurics: Contains phenylalanine." This popular artificial sweetener is used in numerous foods, chewing gums, drinks, and liquid medicines. A quart of aspartame-sweetened fruit drink contains 280 mg of Phe, more than one half the daily allowance for a child with PKU (Scriver, Levy, & Donlon, 2008, updated).

Parents should be cautioned about aspartame in over-the-counter medications or vitamins or any product labeled "sugar free." The exact amount of Phe in medications must be calculated as part of a child's daily Phe intake. A variety of resources are available for information about the Phe content of medications, including the manufacturer, the product information, a pharmacist, and the *Physicians' Desk Reference* (PDR). The National PKU News Website has a frequently updated list of the Phe content of over-the-counter and prescription medications (http://www.pkunews.org/diet/asptable.htm); a few of the common ones are listed in Table 38-2.

Developmental Issues
Sleep Patterns

There are no particular sleep disturbances associated with PKU. Routine counseling about establishing and maintaining healthy sleep habits is recommended. Children who have behaviors consistent with ADHD may have an increase in sleep problems.

Toileting

Children with PKU achieve bowel and bladder control at the same age as children without PKU. If Phe levels are chronically elevated, the child may be more prone to eczematous skin lesions

TABLE 38-2
Phe Content of Selected Medications*

Product	Phe content
Amoxicillin 250 mg chew tabs (WarnerChilcott)	2 mg/tablet
Augmentin 200 mg/5 mL suspension	7 mg/5 mL
Benadryl Allergy chewables	4.2 mg/tablet
Children's Advil chewable tablets 50 mg chewable grape flavor	2.1 mg/tablet
Dramamine chewable tablets	1.5 mg/tablet
Flintstones Complete chewable tablets	2 mg/tablet
Pedialyte freezer pops	16 mg/pop
Triaminic softchews cough and sore throat	28.1 mg/tablet

*NOTE: This information was taken from www.pkunews.org/diet/asptable.htm, updated September 2007. It is provided only as an example and must be confirmed with the manufacturer, because formulations change frequently.

that are associated with an increased risk for diaper rash. There is a characteristic musty smell to urine containing Phe metabolites, but this does not occur in children with well-treated PKU.

Discipline

Parenting strategies for the child with PKU are the same as for any child. Positive reinforcement of good behavior is always more effective than negative reinforcement of undesirable behavior. Limit setting and consistent expectations are essential, even if the parent has ambivalent feelings because the child has a chronic condition.

Food is an important social factor in any child's life, and how it is managed from the very beginning by parents can determine the success of the therapy. A major pitfall in disciplining children with PKU is to use food as a reward system and the need for blood tests as punishment. It is critical to establish healthy habits when the child is very young, because the child must begin to make the right food choices independently once school age is reached.

Child Care

All individuals in the child's home environment should be knowledgeable about the Phe-restricted diet and the preparation of the EMF products. Grandparents and other caregivers play an essential role in supporting the diet and should be included in educational sessions at the metabolic clinic or in primary care. Everyone who spends time with the child must support the parents' efforts to provide the diet and resist the temptation to "treat" the child to ice cream or other restricted foods. Most daycare providers will feed the child whatever the parents send but will need to be educated about the importance of dietary restrictions and the potential hazards of sharing protein foods with other children at daycare. Parents devise creative ways to make their child feel "normal," such as preparing low-Phe "look-alike" treats to take to birthday parties or other activities that involve food. As the child's primary advocates, parents find themselves teaching others in the community about PKU on a constant basis.

Schooling

Children with PKU are likely to progress in school just like other children. Although there is some evidence of an increased risk for ADHD or mild cognitive dysfunction, most experts agree that these may be minimized with good control of Phe. If a child needs to be evaluated for an individualized educational program (IEP), the primary care or metabolic care provider may be involved in reviewing the plan or communicating information about the child. Children with PKU may undergo psychological testing at the PKU treatment center, including developmental assessments, language development tests, intelligence tests, and tests of executive functioning or attention. Ideally, testing is initiated at 6 months of age, continued every 6 months until 2 years of age, and done at annual or 3-year intervals thereafter. For optimal performance, it is important that the child's blood Phe level be in maintenance range on the day of testing.

School personnel may have little or no knowledge of or experience with PKU. It is often necessary for the professionals at the metabolic clinic or the primary care practice or the parents to educate teachers, cafeteria personnel, and school administrators about the child's special needs. The school nurse may be enlisted to assist with these efforts. A useful publication, "A Teacher's Guide to PKU," is available through the Texas Department of Health at www.dshs.state.tx.us/newborn/teachpku.shtm. This booklet explains PKU and gives teachers specific guidelines related to dietary restrictions.

Because diet is the primary aspect of life affected by PKU, cafeteria personnel can be of great help in preventing the child from feeling different. Many parents report that their children have positive experiences with school meals thanks to the willingness of the personnel to provide detailed information about weekly cafeteria menus, to heat meals sent from home, to weigh portions, or to give the child specially prepared items. Open and frequent communication between the family and the school is essential.

Sexuality

Sexual development and curiosity are no different for children with PKU than for any other child. Females with PKU must be educated from an early age about strict Phe control before and throughout pregnancy. The best approach to prevention of maternal PKU is to foster adherence to diet at all times. Numerous educational materials are available for parents and adolescents related to sexuality and PKU. These may be obtained from the metabolic center or through some of the resources available to families online. Discussions of contraception and the implications of being a woman with PKU should be individualized and approached with sensitivity. PKU peer support groups, online chat rooms, and written materials and videos designed specifically for adolescents with PKU are available.

Transition to Adulthood

All adolescents face the challenges of peer pressure, desire for independence from authority figures, and social and emotional change. Adolescents with conditions such as PKU or diabetes need much support to adhere to a restricted diet and to take their medical foods. Despite clinic recommendations to adhere to the diet for life, studies have shown that adolescents often discontinue the diet (NIH, 2000). Pediatric metabolic clinics may not routinely follow individuals with PKU after age 18 years. It is not unusual for persons in this age-group to abandon routine medical care for a variety of reasons. Every effort must be made to ensure that individuals with PKU receive continuing primary care and metabolic follow-up given the recent compelling evidence of the benefits of lifelong

therapy and the need to prevent the growing problem of maternal PKU syndrome.

Before the 1980s, most adults with PKU relaxed or discontinued Phe restriction. Consequently, many adults with PKU are currently attempting to reinstitute the diet. This has proved to be very difficult, and individuals may benefit from the guidance of professionals who can promote adherence, primary care providers, family counseling, and peer support mechanisms. Previously untreated adults with PKU may show improvement in behavior, neurologic status, and IQ (Koch et al., 1999) after institution of a low-Phe diet, and specific protocols are available (Acosta & Yannicelli, 1997; Dolan, Koch, Bekins, et al., 2000).

The transition is helped if children start assisting in calculating their daily intake and mixing their formula at an early age. It is also important for adolescents to be reminded that high levels of Phe can be found in all types of food and drink, including alcohol, and all of these must be considered in planning their daily intake.

Special Concerns of Women of Childbearing Age

Contact with a metabolic clinic is often lost in adulthood, so primary care practitioners have an essential role in the prevention of MPKU syndrome. Women of childbearing age must prevent pregnancy or maintain Phe levels between 120 µmol/L (2 mg/dL) and 360 µmol/L (6 mg/dL) before conception to prevent birth defects in the fetus and potential developmental and behavioral disabilities in their offspring. Practitioners who care for adolescents and women with PKU or HPA should reinforce this at every opportunity and counsel women of childbearing age with PKU or HPA to have their blood levels checked and to achieve metabolic control of Phe before becoming pregnant. However, practitioners should also be prepared to give guidance regarding the significant barriers to good metabolic control. Returning to control after going off diet can be very difficult. Also, obtaining insurance coverage for EMF can be a challenge, and the cost of formula and low-protein foods can be prohibitive for some people. Many obstetric providers are unfamiliar with the management of PKU, so ensuring that women with PKU who are of childbearing age continue to be followed by a metabolic provider familiar with PKU is of the utmost importance. Ideally, a practitioner familiar with PKU or one who is in close association with such an expert will provide prenatal care.

Pregnancy in women with PKU is a medical challenge. Phe must be restricted, but adequate tyrosine, vitamins, and other nutrients must be supplied. Special EMF products and detailed guidelines for nutrition management are available (Acosta & Yannicelli, 2001). Currently, BH$_4$ is not being used during pregnancy in women with PKU. Biomarin has created a pregnancy registry, and it is hoped that more will be understood about the benefits and risks of using BH$_4$ during pregnancy in the future.

Several factors affect a woman's adherence to a Phe-restricted diet in pregnancy, including age, socioeconomic status, and social support. Women with higher intellectual levels are more likely to follow dietary guidelines; thus women with late-diagnosed or inadequately treated PKU are at greater risk for having affected offspring. In one study, young age and economic factors were the two most significant barriers to good control before and during pregnancy (Brown, Fernhoff, Waisbren, et al., 2002). Strategies that have improved dietary adherence in pregnant women include the use of specially trained resource mothers and maternal PKU camps. Internet-based and other methods for tracking and communicating with women at risk are currently being developed. The researchers and providers involved in the maternal phenylketonuria project continue to investigate strategies to prevent MPKU (Clarke, 2003).

Phenylketonuria in Men

Although much emphasis had been placed on adherence to diet in women with PKU owing to the grave effects of Phe on the fetus, young men should also be counseled about the importance of diet for life and supported in this endeavor by their primary care practitioner. The benefits of Phe level maintenance include decreased depression, agitation, and aggressiveness and improved attention span, concentration, and skin condition. Men with PKU and their partners may also wish to have genetic counseling to discuss the risks of having a child with PKU before conceiving.

Family Concerns

Families often have a difficult time adjusting to the frequent clinic visits, blood draws, and rigid diet control required to care for a child with PKU. As with any new diagnosis of a chronic condition, each family will react differently and some may have more difficulty during this time than others. Cultural practices have an impact on the family's acceptance and management of PKU. Beliefs about disease causality, customs related to parenting, and dietary preferences are just some of the factors a practitioner must consider in order to provide comprehensive care.

Successful treatment of a child with PKU requires the support and commitment of everyone involved with the child. More than one individual in the home should be knowledgeable about the Phe-restricted diet, preparation of EMF products, and obtaining blood samples. It is not necessary or advisable for the entire family to adopt the eating habits of the child with PKU, although children in vegetarian families may have less difficulty adhering to the protein-restricted PKU diet. The focus of mealtime discussions should be on topics other than the food.

Raising a child with PKU can be very expensive. The financial burden of PKU is variable, owing to inconsistent policies on the part of third-party payers, Medicare/Medicaid, and other entities regarding funding for medical and supportive care, formula, and low-protein foods. A list of state laws and policies related to reimbursement for formula and foods is posted on the National PKU News website (www.pkunews.org), and the regional metabolic center should also be able to provide this information. Although most states require coverage for infant formula, many do not cover the cost of foods. The primary care provider may need to intercede on behalf of the parents in negotiating coverage of the expenses of EMF, low-protein medical foods, and blood Phe monitoring.

The diagnosis of PKU has implications for blood relatives of the affected child. Parents with a child with PKU are obligate carriers of the disorder and face a 25% recurrence risk in subsequent pregnancies. Other children in the family, grandparents, and the child's aunts and uncles may also be carriers. A metabolic specialist, a genetic counselor, or a specially trained nurse, social worker, psychologist, or other provider can provide genetic counseling. Carrier testing is available for families whose mutations are known, although some individuals prefer not to know, because there is some psychological burden associated with knowledge of one's own or one's family member's genetic information. Parents with a child with PKU may choose to prevent another affected pregnancy through contraception, prenatal diagnosis with pregnancy termination, or preimplantation genetic diagnosis. Factors shown to have the greatest impact on reproductive decisions of parents with a child with a metabolic disorder include stress, worry about the child's future, difficulty meeting the child's needs, and lower functional level of the child (Read, 2002).

Resources

Numerous supports are available for families with PKU. The metabolic clinic will provide information and referrals, but parents increasingly use the World Wide Web as a resource. This has led to a change in health care, whereby consumers come to clinicians with questions about information they have gathered. Many levels of information are available to consumers on the Internet, from full-text articles in leading medical journals to informal discussions in chat rooms. Providers have a responsibility to assist individuals to evaluate such resources. PKU is a rare disease, and parents quickly become informed consumers who educate others about their child's condition. Two organizations provide comprehensive guides to current information and resources.

National PKU News

This nonprofit organization is dedicated to providing accurate and up-to-date information to families and professionals. The website (www.pkunews.org) provides direct information and links to a wide variety of resources related to PKU. The organization also publishes a newsletter three times per year. Membership in the organization, subscriptions to the newsletter, and additional information may be obtained by contacting the following or through the website:

National PKU News
6869 Woodlawn Ave. NE, #116
Seattle, WA 98115-5469
(206) 525-8140
Website: pkunews.org

The following are some items of interest on the PKU News website:

- Articles about all aspects of PKU, including personal stories written by parents and teens
- Diet information, including low-protein food companies, lists of Phe content in foods and medicines, order forms for PKU cookbooks, screening and treatment guidelines, and practical information about dietary adherence for all age-groups
- Information about legislation to cover PKU costs
- Summaries of current research related to PKU
- Information about support groups, PKU treatment centers, meetings, camps, and other events
- A comprehensive list of audiovisual and written materials about PKU; includes materials appropriate for professionals, parents, and siblings
- Instructions for joining the PKU E-mail mailing list

There are more than 1000 subscribers to this mailing list from more than 20 countries. Its purpose is to provide a vehicle for communication among families of children with PKU, young adults with PKU, and professionals treating PKU. This busy mailing list supports a wide range of comments and inquiries about cooking tips, low-protein recipes, issues related to diet management, low-protein food sources, and information about other support groups. It is not intended to be a source of medical information or advice, although professionals occasionally respond to questions.

Children's PKU Network

This national nonprofit organization aims to address the special needs and concerns of children and families with PKU. The website (www.pkunetwork.org) provides information and links to multiple resources. Materials may also be obtained by contacting the following:

Children's PKU Network
3970 Via De La Valle, Ste. 120
Del Mar, CA 92014
(800) 377-6677(toll-free); (858) 509-0767
Fax: (858) 509-0768
Email: pkunetwork@aol.com

Some items of interest on the Children's PKU Network website include the following:

- General information about the disorder
- Information about how to obtain free "Express Packs" that contain booklets, videos, and other materials about PKU; available both for families of a newborn with PKU and women with PKU of childbearing age who are contemplating pregnancy and are at risk for having a fetus with maternal PKU syndrome

- Crisis intervention programs
- Scholarship information
- Research clearinghouse
- Information about food scales
- Links to other organizations that might provide useful information or assistance
- A comprehensive list of low-protein food companies and links to other PKU-related publications and resources

Other Web Sites

Texas Department of Health

A Teacher's Guide to PKU, a booklet that explains PKU and gives teachers specific guidelines related to dietary restrictions.
Website: www.dshs.state.tx.us/newborn/teachpku/shtm

University of Washington

A Babysitters' Guide to PKU, a booklet that explains the basic principles of PKU and the special diet that must be followed.
Website: depts.washington.edu/pku/pdfs/babysitter.pdf

USDA Nutrient Database

Detailed lists of Phe content in foods.
Website: www.nal.usda.gov/fnic/cgi-bin/nut_search.pl

PAHdb: Phenylalanine Hydroxylase Locus Knowledgebase

An online database of the mutations in the human PAH gene.
Website: www.pahdb.mcgill.ca

U.S. National Library of Medicine

A website sponsored by the U.S. National Library of Medicine that provides a brief review of many genetic conditions, including PKU, and is especially useful for families awaiting the follow-up results of a positive newborn screen.
Website: www.ghr.nlm.nih.gov/condition=phenylketonuria

Summary of Primary Care Needs for the Child with Phenylketonuria

HEALTH CARE MAINTENANCE

Growth and Development

- Growth should be normal on a Phe-restricted diet.
- Careful monitoring of growth charts is necessary to ensure adequate nutrient intake and to avoid obesity from high-carbohydrate, high-fat foods.
- Development should be monitored with psychological and behavioral testing.

Diet

- Breastfeeding is recommended for infants.
- Involvement of a professional nutritionist is essential.
- Phe-restricted diet is for life.
- Dietary modifications are dictated by blood Phe and Tyr levels.
- Self-management of Phe-restricted diet should be initiated early in childhood.
- Elemental medical food (EMF) products should be prepared as prescribed and taken with meals.
- Avoid overemphasis on the diet as the central issue in the child's life.

Safety

- Only individuals with a diagnosis of PKU should ingest EMF products as prescribed.
- Occasional high Phe levels are unlikely to be detrimental.

Immunizations

- Routine immunizations are recommended.

Screening

- *Vision.* Routine screening is recommended.
- *Hearing.* Routine screening is recommended.
- *Dental.* Early evaluation is recommended because of the high-carbohydrate diet.
- *Blood pressure.* Routine screening is recommended.
- *Hematocrit.* Hematocrit is part of the nutritional assessment at metabolic clinic; routine screening is not usually required.
- *Urinalysis.* Routine screening is recommended.
- *Tuberculosis.* Routine screening is recommended.

Condition-Specific Screening

- Blood Phe monitoring
- Nutritional indices monitoring

COMMON ILLNESS MANAGEMENT

- Catabolic state related to common childhood illness should be prevented with adequate hydration and caloric intake. Transient Phe increases during periods of illness are expected. Analgesics, antipyretics, and antibiotics should be used as for any child, but formulations with the lowest Phe content should be sought.

Summary of Primary Care Needs for the Child with Phenylketonuria—cont'd

Drug Interactions

- Aspartame ingestion is contraindicated.
- Check Phe content of all medications.

DEVELOPMENTAL ISSUES

Sleep Patterns

- Routine counseling is recommended.

Toileting

- Routine counseling is recommended.

Discipline

- Expectations are normal based on age and developmental level.
- Avoid use of food as a reward system and blood tests as punishment.

Child Care

- All care providers must be aware of dietary modifications.

Schooling

- Children with good Phe control generally progress normally.
- Developmental testing should be done as indicated and educational support given as needed.
- School personnel must be made aware of child's dietary restrictions.
- School cafeteria personnel should be aware of child's dietary restrictions and instructed on preparation of Phe-restricted meals.

Sexuality

- Young women with PKU should be educated about the risks of maternal PKU syndrome and the need to adhere to Phe-restricted diet before conception and throughout pregnancy.

Transition to Adulthood

- All individuals should remain on a Phe-restricted diet for life. There are no special considerations related to alcohol consumption, although types of alcohol have varying amounts of Phe and adolescents should be reminded that this must be included in their calculations of daily Phe intake.
- Participation in PKU support groups and professional counseling as needed are recommended for adults with PKU and their families. Some metabolic clinics have special programs that help transition adolescents from pediatric to adult care. Other clinics provide metabolic care throughout the life span and are equipped to handle the changing issues and concerns that arise as children with PKU transition to self-management.

FAMILY CONCERNS

- Many barriers exist that prevent persons with PKU from adhering to the diet, including complexity and inconvenience, poor palatability and cost of the foods, and psychosocial factors.
- Multiple supports are available and should be promoted by the practitioner.
- Genetic counseling for all family members is advisable.

REFERENCES

Acosta, P.B., & Yannicelli, S. (1997). *Ross Metabolic Formula System: Nutrition Support Protocol for Previously Untreated Adults with Phenylketonuria.* Columbus, OH: Ross Products Division/Abbott Laboratories.

Acosta, P.B., & Yannicelli, S. (Eds.). (2001). *Ross Metabolic Formula System: Nutrition Support Protocols* (4th ed.). Columbus, OH: Ross Products Division/Abbott Laboratories.

American College of Medical Genetics. (2006). *Newborn screening ACT sheet [increased phenylalanine] phenylketonuria (PKU).* Available at www.acmg.net/resources/policies/ACT/ACT-sheet_Phenylalanine_5-2-06_ljo.pdf. Retrieved December 4, 2007.

Anderson, P.J., Wood, S.J., Francis, D.E., et al. (2004). Neuropsychological functioning in children with early-treated phenylketonuria: Impact of white matter abnormalities. *Dev Med Child Neurol, 46*(4), 230-238.

Anderson, P.J., Wood, S.J., Francis, D.E., et al. (2007). Are neuropsychological impairments in children with early-treated phenylketonuria (PKU) related to white matter abnormalities or elevated phenylalanine levels? *Dev Neuropsychol, 32*(2), 645-668.

Andrade, J.D. (2002). ChemChip project at the University of Utah. *National PKU News, 14*(1), 1.

Antshel, K. (2001). ADHD and PKU. *National PKU News, 13*(2), 3.

Arnold, G.L., Vladutiu, C.J., Orlowski, C.C., et al. (2004). Prevalence of stimulant use for attentional dysfunction in children with phenylketonuria. *J Inherit Metab Dis, 27*(2), 137-143.

Banich, M.T., Passarotti, A.M., White, D.A., et al. (2000). Interhemispheric interaction during childhood. II. Children with early-treated phenylketonuria. *Dev Neuropsychol, 18*(1), 53-71.

Baumeister, A., & Baumeister, A. (1998). Dietary treatment of destructive behavior associated with hyperphenylalaninemia. *Clin Neuropharmacol, 21*(1), 18-27.

Beblo, S., Reinhardt, H., Demmelmair, H., et al. (2007). Effect of fish oil supplementation on fatty acid status, coordination, and fine motor skills in children with phenylketonuria. *J Pediatr, 150*(5), 479-484.

Beblo, S., Reinhardt, H., Muntau, A.C., et al. (2001). Fish oil supplementation improves visual evoked potentials in children with phenylketonuria. *Neurology, 57*(8), 1488-1491.

Beck, T. (1999). My life with PKU. *National PKU News, 10*(3), 11-12. Available at www.astro.sunysb.edu/tracy/mystory.html. Retrieved January 16, 2009.

Bilginsoy, C., Waitzman, N., Leonard, C.O., et al. (2005). Living with phenylketonuria: Perspectives of patients and their families. *J Inherit Metab Dis, 28*(5), 639-649.

Brown, A.S., Fernhoff, P.M., Waisbren, S.E., et al. (2002). Barriers to successful dietary control among pregnant women with phenylketonuria. *Genet Med, 4*(2), 84-89.

Centers for Disease Control and Prevention (CDC). (2002). Barriers to dietary control among pregnant women with phenylketonuria—United States, 1998-2000. *MMWR Morb Mortal Wkly Rep, 51*, 117-120.

Channon, S., German, E., Cassina, C., et al. (2004). Executive functioning, memory, and learning in phenylketonuria. *Neuropsychology, 18*(4), 613-620.

Clarke, J.T. (2003). The maternal phenylketonuria project: A summary of progress and challenges for the future. *Pediatrics, 112*(6 pt 2), 1584-1587.

Dobbelaere, D., Michaud, L., Debrabander, A., et al. (2003). Evaluation of nutritional status and pathophysiology of growth retardation in patients with phenylketonuria. *J Inherit Metab Dis, 26*(1), 1-11.

Dolan, B.E., Koch, R., Bekins, C., et al. (2000). *Diet intervention guidelines for adults with untreated PKU*. Available at www.pkunews.org/adults/guide.htm. Retrieved February 12, 2008.

Etzel, M.R. (2002). Glycomacropeptide (GMP) update. *National PKU News*, *14*(1), 2.

Fitzgerald, B., Morgan, J., Keene, N., et al. (2000). An investigation into diet treatment for adults with previously untreated phenylketonuria and severe intellectual disability. *J Intellect Disabil Res*, *44*(pt 1), 53-59.

Gambol, P.J. (2007). Maternal phenylketonuria syndrome and case management implications. *J Pediatr Nurs*, *22*(2), 129-138.

Gassió, R., Campistol, J., Vilaseca, M.A., et al. (2003). Do adult patients with phenylketonuria improve their quality of life after introduction/resumption of a phenylalanine-restricted diet? *Acta Paediatr*, *92*(12), 1474-1478.

Giewska, M., Cyryowski, L., Jowiak, I., et al. (2001). A diet with large neutral amino acids supplementation as a combined treatment for difficult to control or late diagnosed patients with PKU—preliminary data. *J Inherit Metab Dis*, *24*(Suppl 1), 22. (abstract).

Giovannini, M., Verduci, E., Salvatici, E., et al. (2007). Phenylketonuria: Dietary and therapeutic challenges. *J Inherit Metab Dis*, *30*(2), 145-152.

Griffiths, P.Y., Demellweek, C., Fay, N., et al. (2000). Wechsler subscale IQ and subtest profile in early treated phenylketonuria. *Arch Dis Child*, *82*(3), 209-215.

Gurian, E.A., Kinnamon, D.D., Henry, J.J., et al. (2006). Expanded newborn screening for biochemical disorders: The effect of a false-positive result. *Pediatrics*, *117*(6), 1915-1921.

Hardelid, P., Cortina-Borja, M., Munro, A., et al. (2008). The birth prevalence of PKU in populations of European, South Asian and Sub-Saharan African ancestry living in South East England. *Ann Hum Genet*, *72*, 65-71.

Harding, C.O., Gillingham, M.B., Daghighi, E., et al. (2006). 219. Persistent correction of hyperphenylalaninemia following liver-directed, rAAV2/8-mediated gene therapy for murine phenylketonuria (PKU). *Mol Ther*, *13*(S84), S84.

Huijbregts, S.C., de Sonneville, L.M., Licht, R., et al. (2002). Sustained attention and inhibition of cognitive interference in treated phenylketonuria: Associations with concurrent and lifetime phenylalanine concentrations. *Neuropsychologica*, *40*(1), 7-15.

Kalsner, L.R., Rohr, F.J., Strauss, K.A., et al. (2001). Tyrosine supplementation in phenylketonuria: Diurnal blood tyrosine levels and presumptive brain influx of tyrosine and other large neutral amino acids. *J Pediatr*, *139*(3), 421-427.

Kim, W., Erlandsen, H., Surendran, S., et al. (2004). Trends in enzyme therapy for phenylketonuria. *Mol Ther*, *10*(2), 220-224.

Koch, R., Hanley, W., Levy, H., et al. (2003). The maternal phenylketonuria international study: 1984-2002. *Pediatrics*, *112*(6), 1523-1529.

Koch, R., Moseley, K., Ning, J., et al. (1999). Long-term beneficial effects of the phenylalanine restricted diet in late diagnosed individuals with phenylketonuria. *Mol Genet Metab*, *67*(2), 148-155.

Koch, R., & Wenz, E. (1987). Phenylketonuria. *Ann Rev Nutr*, *7*, 117-135.

Langenbeck, U., Baum, F., Mench-Hoinowski, A., et al. (2005). Predicting the phenylalanine blood concentration from urine analyses. An approach to noninvasive monitoring of patients with phenylketonuria. *J Inherit Metab Dis*, *28*(6), 855-861.

Lee, P., Ridout, D., Walter, J., et al. (2005). Maternal phenylketonuria: Report from the United Kingdom registry 1978-97. *BMJ*, *90*(2), 143.

Levy, H., Burton, B., Cederbaum, S., et al. (2007). Recommendations for evaluation of responsiveness to tetrahydrobiopterin (BH4) in phenylketonuria and its use in treatment. *Mol Genet Metab*, *92*(4), 287-291.

Levy, H.L., Guldberg, P., Guttler, F., et al. (2001). Congenital heart disease in maternal phenylketonuria: Report from the Maternal PKU Collaborative Study. *Pediatr Res*, *49*(5), 636-642.

Lim, K., van Calcar, S.C., Nelson, K.L., et al. (2007). Acceptable low-phenylalanine foods and beverages can be made with glycomacropeptide from cheese whey for individuals with PKU. *Mol Genet Metab*, *92*(1-2), 176-178.

Lucas, V.S., Contreras, A., Loukissa, M., et al. (2001). Dental disease and caries related oral microflora in children with phenylketonuria. *ASDC J Dent Child*, *68*(4), 263-267.

Miller, D. (2002). Acoint works on non-invasive phenylalanine monitoring device. *National PKU News*, *14*(1), 1-2.

Modan-Moses, D., Vered, I., Schwartz, G., et al. (2007). Peak bone mass in patients with phenylketonuria. *J Inherit Metab Dis*, *30*(2), 202-208.

Moseley, K., Koch, R., & Moser, A.B. (2002). Lipid status and long-chain polyunsaturated fatty acid concentrations in adults and adolescents with phenylketonuria on phenylalanine-restricted diets. *J Inherit Metab Dis*, *25*(1), 56-64.

National Institutes of Health. (2000). Phenylketonuria (PKU): Screening and management. *NIH Consensus Statement*, *17*(3). Available at:www.nichd.nih.gov/publications/pubs/pku/index.htm. Retrieved December 4, 2007.

Newborn Screening Committee (1999). *The Council of Regional Networks for Genetics Services (CORN). National Newborn Screening Report—1994*. Atlanta: CORN.

Ney, D.M., Hull, A.K., van Calcar, S.C., et al. (2008). Dietary glycomacropeptide supports growth and reduces the concentrations of phenylalanine in plasma and brain in a murine model of phenylketonuria. *J Nutr*, *138*(2), 316.

Nissenkorn, A., Michelson, M., Ben-Zeev, B., et al. (2001). Inborn errors of metabolism: A cause of abnormal brain development. *Neurology*, *56*(10), 1265-1272.

Nussbaum, R., McInnes, R., & Willard, H. (2001). *Thompson and Thompson Genetics in Medicine* (6th ed.). Philadelphia: Saunders.

Nyhan, W.L., Barshop, B.A., & Ozand, P.T. (2005). *Atlas of Metabolic Diseases* (2nd ed.). London: Hodder Arnold.

Pietz, J., Kreis, R., Rupp, A., et al. (1999). Large neutral amino acids block phenylalanine transport into brain tissue in patients with phenylketonuria. *J Clin Invest*, *103*(8), 1169-1178.

Pollack, A. (2007, December 14). Agency approves drug to treat genetic disorder that can lead to retardation [electronic version]. *New York Times*. Available at http://www.nytimes.com/2007/12/14/health/14genetic.html?scp=2&sq=KUVAN&st=cse. Retrieved January 16, 2009.

Read, C.Y. (2002). Reproductive decisions of parents of children with metabolic disorders. *Clin Genet*, *61*, 268-276.

Rezvani, I. (2000). Defects in metabolism of amino acids: Phenylalanine. In R.E. Behrman, R.M. Kliegman, & H.B. Jenson (Eds.), *Nelson Textbook of Pediatrics* (16th ed.). Philadelphia: Saunders.

Rinaldo, P., Tortorelli, S., Matern, D. (2004). Recent developments and new applications of tandem mass spectrometry in newborn screening. *Curr Opin Pediatr*, *16*(4), 427-433.

Rouse, B., Azen, C., Koch, R., et al. (1997). Maternal phenylketonuria collaborative study (MPKUCS) offspring: Facial anomalies, malformations, and early neurological sequelae. *Am J Med Genet*, *69*, 89-95.

Rouse, B., Matalon, R., Koch, R. et al. (2000). Maternal phenylketonuria syndrome: Congenital heart defects, microcephaly, and developmental outcomes. *J Pediatr*, *136*(1), 57-61.

Schindeler, S., Ghosh-Jerath, S., Thompson, S., et al. (2007). The effects of large neutral amino acid supplements in PKU: An MRS and neuropsychological study. *Mol Genet Metab*, *91*(1), 48-54.

Scriver, C.R. (2007). The PAH gene, phenylketonuria, and a paradigm shift. *Hum Mutat*, *28*(9), 831-845.

Scriver, C.R., Levy, H., Donlon, J. (2008; updated). *Hyperphenylalaninemia: Phenylalanine hydroxylase deficiency*. Available at www.ommbid.com/OMMBID/the_online_metabolic_and_molecular_bases_of_inherited_disease/b/abstract/part8/ch77. Retrieved February 3, 2009.

Seashore, M.R. (2008, May 22). *Personal communication*.

Smith, I., & Knowles, J. (2000). Behaviour in early treated phenylketonuria: A systematic review. *Eur J Pediatr*, *159*(Suppl 2), S89-S93.

Spirito, F., Meneguzzi, G., Danos, O., et al. (2001). Cutaneous gene transfer and therapy: The present and future. *J Gene Med*, *3*(1), 21-31.

Trefz, F.K., Scheible, D., Frauendienst-Egger, G., et al. (2005). Long-term treatment of patients with mild and classical phenylketonuria by tetrahydrobiopterin. *Mol Genet Metab*, *86*(Suppl 1), S75-S80.

Van Bakel, M.M., Printzen, G., Wermuth, B., et al. (2000). Antioxidant and thyroid hormone status in selenium-deficient phenylketonuric and hyperphenylalaninemic patients. *Am J Clin Nutr*, *72*(4), 976-981.

Van Spronsen, F.J., van Rijn, M., Bekhof, J., et al. (2001). Phenylketonuria: Tyrosine supplementation in phenylalanine-restricted diets. *Am J Clin Nutr*, *73*(2), 153-157.

VanZutphen, K.H., Packman, W., Sporri, L., et al. (2007). Executive functioning in children and adolescents with phenylketonuria. *Clin Genet*, *72*(1), 13-18.

Waisbren, S.E., Albers, S., Amato, S., et al. (2003). Effect of expanded newborn screening for biochemical genetic disorders on child outcomes and parental stress. *J Am Med Assoc*, *290*(19), 2564-2572.

Waisbren, S.E., Noel, K., Fahrbach, K., et al. (2007). Phenylalanine blood levels and clinical outcomes in phenylketonuria: A systematic literature wreview and meta-analysis. *Mol Genet Metab*, *92*(1-2), 63-70.

Walter, J., Lee, P., & Burgard, P. (2006). Hyperphenylalinemias. In J.Fernandes, J.M. Saudubray, G. Van den Berghe et al. (Eds.), *Inborn Metabolic Disease: Diagnosis and Treatment*, (4th ed.). New York: Springer.

Weglage, J., Pietsch, M., Feldmann, R., et al. (2001). Normal clinical outcome in untreated subjects with mild hyperphenylalaninemia. *Pediatr Res*, *49*(4), 532-536.

Welsh, M.C., & Pennington, B.F. (2000). Phenylketonuria. In K.O. Yeats, D. Ris, & H.G. Taylor (Eds.), *Pediatric Neuropsychology: Research, Theory, and Practice.* New York: Guilford Press.

Wilcox, W.R., and Cederbaum, S.D. (2002). Amino acid metabolism. In J.M. Connor, R. Pyeritz, B. Korf, (Eds.) (2002). *Emery and Rimoin's Principles and Practice of Medical Genetics*, (4th ed.). Philadelphia: Saunders.

Zhongshu, Z., Weiming, Y., Yukio, F., et al. (2001). Clinical analysis of West syndrome associated with phenylketonuria. *Brain Dev*, *23*(7), 552-557.

Zurfluh, M.R., Zschocke, J., Lindner, M., et al. (2008). Molecular genetics of tetrahydrobiopterin-responsive phenylalanine hydroxylase deficiency. *Hum Mutat*, *29*(1), 167-175.

39 Prematurity

Michelle M. Kelly

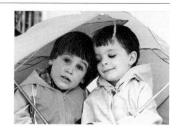

Etiology

The March of Dimes (MOD) estimates that the number of preterm births, as a percentage of all live births, rose to a staggering 12.5% in 2004 (Martin, Hamilton, Sutton, et al., 2006), and recent published data show a further increase to 12.7% in 2005 (National Vital Statistics System, 2005). This is an overall increase of more than 30% since 1981 (Institute of Medicine [IOM], 2007). The condition of premature infants and the philosophies that dictate their care underwent major changes from the late 1970s through the mid-1990s (Buchh, Graham, Harris, et al., 2007). New technologies, mechanical ventilators, antenatal steroids, and surfactant changed the fate of infants born too early. Since the late 1990s, however, outcome data have become relatively stable (Buchh et al.).

To understand prematurity one must first understand the terminology used to classify infants born too early and too small. Preterm is used to describe infants born before the completion of 37 weeks of gestation. To describe the degree of prematurity we label infants from 34 to 37 weeks of gestation as late preterm, those born from 32 to 34 weeks of gestation as moderately preterm, and those born before 32 weeks of gestation as very preterm.

Prematurity can also be described in terms of birth weight, recognizing that for these infants, size matters. Low birth weight (LBW) infants are those born weighing less than 2500 grams (5 lb, 8 oz). Very low birth weight (VLBW) infants weigh less than 1500 grams at birth (3 lb, 5 oz), and extremely low birth weight (ELBW) infants weight less than 1000 grams (2 lb, 3 oz). This terminology is important to understand when discussing outcomes and prognosis for these infants. Table 39-1 defines other important neonatal terminology put forth by the American Academy of Pediatrics (AAP) (2004).

For as many as 50% of all premature births, there is no identifiable etiology (March of Dimes [MOD], 2007). Risk factors of prematurity include a combination of medical, social, and environmental factors: stress, poverty, domestic violence, smoking, drug abuse, poor nutrition, inadequate prenatal care, lower levels of education, intrauterine infections, uteroplacental insufficiency, incompetent cervix, and multiple gestations (Giarratano, 2006) (Box 39-1). Other clinical features have been identified in mothers who deliver preterm: black (African American race), a low body mass index (BMI) (less than 19.8 kg/m²), a large interpregnancy weight loss (greater than 5 kg/m²), contractions late in the second trimester, smoking, cervical shortening, and short interpregnancy interval (less than 18 months) (Spong, 2007). A history of prior preterm birth, a family history of preterm births, and a history of preterm premature rupture of membranes (pPROM) are also identified risk factors for preterm birth (Giarratano, 2006; Reedy, 2007).

Incidence and Prevalence

The rate of preterm birth for infants less than 32 weeks of gestation has remained relatively constant since the 1980s. Births between 32 and 36 weeks of gestation make up a significant portion of the overall increase in premature births in the United States (Reedy, 2007). Although assistive reproduction has increased the number of multiple-gestation births, this does not fully explain the increase in premature births (MOD, 2007). Black women experience significantly higher rates of prematurity (17.8% in 2003) than other races (IOM, 2007). Asian and Pacific Islander women have the lowest rate at 10.5% with Hispanic, white and American Indian women falling between.

Preterm birth has surpassed congenital anomalies as the primary cause of perinatal morbidity and mortality (Reedy, 2007). Preterm birth cost American society $26 billion in 2005, or $51,600 per infant born prematurely; $33,200 for medical care, $3800 for maternal delivery, $1200 for early intervention services, $2200 for special education, and a staggering $11,200 in lost household and labor market productivity (IOM, 2007). Respiratory distress syndrome (RDS) and LBW are the second and third most expensive hospital diagnoses, respectively, for all ages in the United States (Reedy, 2007). After hospital discharge, premature infants continue to require more care than term infants. Wade and colleagues report that preterm infants receive an average of 20 office visits during the first year of life well beyond the average of 12 office visits received by term infants and more prescriptions than term infants, primarily for respiratory medications and antibiotics (Wade, et al., 2009). Their study excluded the sickest of premature infants, those discharged on mechanical ventilation or with VP shunts.

Diagnostic Criteria

The assignment of gestational age is most accurately based on a calculation using the first day of the mother's last menstrual period (LMP). In absence of this data point, ultrasound dating during the first half of pregnancy may be used. Because of significant weight and size variation, ultrasound dating later in pregnancy is less accurate. When neither accurate LMP data nor early ultrasound data are available, physical and neurologic findings during the first few hours of life can be used to provide a rough estimate of gestational age (AAP & American College of Obstetricians and Gynecologists [ACOG], 2002; Ballard, Khoury, Wedig, et al., 1991; Dubowitz, Dubowitz, & Goldberg, 1970).

TABLE 39-1
Neonatal Terminology

Expression	Definition
Appropriate for gestational age	Birth weight between 10%-90% for age
Chronologic age	Time elapsed since birth
Corrected age	Chronologic age minus the number of weeks born before 40 weeks
Extremely low birth weight	Birth weight <1000 grams
Gestational age	Time elapsed between first day of last menstrual period and day of delivery
Large for gestational age	Birth weight >90% for age
Late preterm	Born between 34-37 weeks of gestation
Low birth weight	Birth weight <2500 grams
Moderately preterm	Born between 32-35 weeks of gestation
Postmenstrual age	Gestational age plus chronologic age
Preterm	Born less than 37 weeks of gestation
Small for gestational age	Birth weight <10% for age
Very low birth weight	Birth weight <1500 grams
Very preterm	Delivered at less than 32 weeks of gestation

Adapted from American Academy of Pediatrics (2004). Policy statement: Age terminology during the perinatal period. *Pediatrics, 114,* 1362-1364; Engle, W.A., Tomashek, K.M., Wallman, C., & Committee on Fetus and Newborn. (2007). Clinical report: "Late-preterm" infants: A population at risk. *Pediatrics, 120,* 1390-1401. DOI: 10.1542/peds.2007-2952.

BOX 39-1
Risk Factors for Prematurity

RISK FACTORS
- Prior preterm delivery
- Family history of preterm births
- Uteroplacental insufficiency
- Incompetent cervix/cervical shortening
- Uterine anomalies
- Multiple gestation
- Assistive reproductive technology
- Preterm premature rupture of membranes
- Polyhydramnios
- Chorioamnionitis
- Contractions late in the second trimester
- Short interpregnancy interval (<18 months)
- Low BMI (<19.8 kg/m²)
- Large interpregnancy weight loss (>5 kg/m²)
- Stress

- Poverty/lower level of education
- Drug abuse/smoking
- Poor nutrition
- Inadequate prenatal care
- Black (African American) race

FETAL INDICATIONS FOR PRETERM DELIVERY
- Intrauterine demise of identical twin
- Low biophysical profile
- Hydrops fetalis
- Intrauterine growth restriction

MATERNAL INDICATIONS FOR PRETERM DELIVERY
- Severe preeclampsia
- Chorioamnionitis
- Placenta previa/abruption
- Uncontrolled diabetes
- Cardiovascular compromise

Clinical Manifestations at Time of Diagnosis

The infant who is delivered moderately or extremely premature will appear distressed, appear smaller, and have less ability to achieve the transition from intrauterine to extrauterine life. Respiratory distress, poor skin integrity, hypothermia, hypoglycemia, and a lack of subcutaneous fat characterize the premature newborn. The late preterm infant may appear to be of good weight and may begin to transition appropriately, but will fail to maintain this stability.

Clinical Manifestations at Time of Diagnosis

- Neuromuscular and physical maturity indicators developed by Ballard et al.*
- Low birth weight
- Distressed transition to extrauterine life
- Poor skin turgor, decreased subcutaneous fat
- Hypothermia
- Difficulty feeding, hypoglycemia

*Ballard, J.L., Khoury, J.C., Wedig, K., et al. (1991). New Ballard score, expanded to include extremely premature infants. *J Pediatr,* 119, 417-423.

Treatment
Prevention

Effective methods for prevention of prematurity and for prolonging pregnancy are elusive, as is the ability to predict which mother/fetal dyad will deliver prematurely. Fetal fibronectin and transvaginal ultrasound measurements of cervical length are two assessments made by the obstetric provider to predict preterm delivery (Reedy, 2007). Fetal fibronectin, a biochemical marker that is abnormal in the cervicovaginal mucus after 22 weeks, is more likely to be positive in those delivering preterm. A positive fetal fibronectin result equates to an increased risk of spontaneous preterm delivery from 3% to 10% whereas a negative fetal fibronectin result suggests that there is a less than 1 in 100 chance that delivery will occur in the subsequent 7 to 10 days (Reedy). Some obstetric providers use this test to assist in determining the need for tocolysis. However, as many as 90% of one study group with a negative fetal fibronectin result went on to deliver prematurely, making it a significantly insensitive test (Spong, 2007).

Currently, the use of 17-alpha-hydroxyprogesterone during pregnancy is believed to be useful in prolonging the pregnancy of a woman with a history of previous preterm birth (Spong, 2007). For women who have had a previous preterm delivery, this medication provides hope that subsequent pregnancies might be prolonged to at least 35 weeks. Maternal bed rest, at home or in hospital, is commonly prescribed to mothers with preterm labor; however, there is little evidence to either support or refute its efficacy in prolonging pregnancy. Prophylactic tocolytics are of no benefit, although tocolysis in the presence of preterm labor may prolong pregnancy to allow administration of maternal corticosteroids (Spong).

Treatment of the Fetus

Some treatments are aimed not at stopping the preterm delivery, but improving the clinical condition of the fetus at delivery. Antenatal corticosteroids will accelerate fetal lung maturation; decrease the incidence and severity of RDS; and decrease the incidence of some associated morbidities, including bronchopulmonary dysplasia (BPD), intraventricular hemorrhage (IVH), and necrotizing enterocolitis (NEC) for infants born before 32 weeks of gestation (ACOG, 1998; National Institutes of Health, 2000) (see Associated Problems of Prematurity box). The use of maternal corticosteroids (two 12 mg doses of betamethasone given 24 hours apart) is currently recommended for use in women between 24 and 34 weeks of gestation with clinical indications of possible preterm delivery (Spong, 2007). It is most effective when administered within 1 to 2 weeks of delivery. Current research underscores the importance of steroid administration even for the threatened, moderately preterm delivery. The EPIPAGE (Etudes Epidemiologique sue les Petits Ages Gestationnels) study group showed that as many as 28% of infants born at 33 weeks of gestation required mechanical ventilation (Marret, Ancel, Marpeau, et al., 2007).

When feasible for the mother/fetal dyad, they should be transferred to a center with expertise in management of preterm labor, high-risk deliveries, and care of high-risk newborns. This proactive transfer will improve infant outcomes and allow the mother and infant to be in the same location after delivery. Regardless of delivery site, there should be at least one person whose primary responsibility is the neonate and who is capable of initiating resuscitation. Either that person or someone else who is immediately available should have the skills required to perform a complete resuscitation (AAP & ACOG, 2002).

Treatment

- Prevention
  - Adequate prenatal care
  - 17-alpha-hydroxyprogesterone for women with previous preterm delivery
- Treatment in utero
- Antenatal corticosteroids
- Delivery in a facility equipped for high-risk deliveries
- Treatment of complications of prematurity
  - Treatments are aimed at supporting the immature body systems of the infant (see Associated Problems of Prematurity box)

Complementary and Alternative Therapies

The MOD advocates improved public awareness of the signs of preterm labor so that actions may be taken to prolong pregnancy at least long enough for maternal corticosteroid administration. High levels of chronic stress, catastrophic events, and negative psychosocial events may increase the risk of preterm delivery (IOM, 2007). The link between stress and premature labor is not well understood; however, stress-mediated hormones may play a role. The MOD advocates healthy stress-relieving interventions, including healthy diet, adequate amounts of sleep, yoga for pregnancy, meditation, and relaxation techniques, and avoiding alcohol, drugs, and cigarettes (MOD, 2006). Herbal preparations and folk medicines are poorly regulated; their compositions may vary by manufacturer and supplier. In high doses, some herbal preparations (e.g., angelica, juniper, mugwort, nutmeg, pennyroyal raspberry tea, saffron, sage) can act as an abortifacient (Bright, 2002; Fetrow & Avila, 1999).

The use of "Kangaroo Care," or skin-to-skin contact during the neonatal intensive care unit (NICU) stay, even for the most vulnerable infant is becoming a more mainstream treatment. Infants who are held in skin-to-skin contact experience extended periods of sleep, increased weight gain, improved respiratory status, and more stable oxygen saturations (Smith, 2007). Mothers experience increased breast milk production during skin-to-skin contact with their infants, and both parents report improved bonding with their infant (Smith).

Parents must be asked about home remedies, cultural practices, and alternative medicines used with their preterm infant. Primary care providers must be open to exploring the therapeutic potential of complementary and alternative therapies with the safety of the infant as their principal concern. Many therapies may not demonstrate scientific efficacy, but may not be harmful. Others, however, may interfere with treatment plans, may be harmful, or may simply be a financial burden that outweighs its benefit.

Anticipated Advances in Diagnosis and Management

The MOD and other research bodies are continually striving to discover a marker or a combination of markers that will identify the pregnancy at risk for preterm delivery and effective strategies for prolonging pregnancy to as close to term as feasible for both the mother and the fetus. In addition, the IOM (2007) recommends future research into improved medical treatments for both infants and mothers; the causes of racial, ethnic, and socioeconomic disparity among prematurity birth rates; and an understanding of the social impact of prematurity on public programs and services.

Research is ongoing to identify the efficacy of treatments such as cervical cerclage and omega-3 fatty acids. Development of effective therapies for the treatment of inflammatory diseases of pregnancy (i.e., pPROM, chorioamnionitis, maternal-fetal infections) is critical. Currently, these conditions increase the risk of white matter injury and subsequent development of cerebral palsy (CP) through a proinflammatory cytokine cascade (Marret et al., 2007) (see Chapter 18).

Infection and neonatal sepsis complicate the care of infants and have a negative impact on morbidity and mortality rates for premature infants. The development of a screening mechanism for infection that is highly sensitive, with excellent positive and negative predictive values, will improve the care of mothers and infants (Ng & Lam, 2007). This test should require a minimal amount of blood; should be quick, simple, and automated; and ultimately should be able to differentiate among fungal, bacterial, and viral infections (Ng & Lam, 2007). Studies into chemokines, cytokines, cell surface markers, acute-phase reactants, and protein markers hold significant promise for identification of infection (Ng & Lam, 2007).

Research into feeding and nutrition needs of infants continues, particularly the extremely premature and the late preterm infant. Breast milk feeding should be the ultimate goal for infant nutrition, and research into improving the caloric quality of breast milk is underway. Commercially available formulas will continue to evolve. Products aimed specifically at the ELBW infant with gastroesophageal reflux are needed.

A further imperative is challenging the belief that delivery at 34 weeks of gestation produces an infant that is "early but okay" (Reedy, 2007). Moderately preterm infants equate to 25% of all NICU admissions (Kirby, Greenspan, Kornhauser, et al., 2007). Increases in preterm birth rates have been greatest among infants 32 to 36 weeks of gestational age. Late preterm and moderately preterm infants display signs of immature physiologic function (Engle, Tomashek, Wallman, et al., 2007; Kirby et al., 2007). Research indicates that these infants are indeed vulnerable. Although they may have significantly lower mortality rates than very premature infants, they cannot be seen as "almost term" or any other label that negates the realities of their immature physiology.

Associated Problems of Prematurity and Treatment

The comorbidities of prematurity have variable expression. Physiologically immature body systems cannot be forced into accelerated development, so the ramifications depend on the organ system

---

> *Associated Problems* of Prematurity and Treatment
>
> - Apnea
> - Chronic lung disease
> - Patent ductus arteriosus
> - Sepsis
> - Intraventricular hemorrhage (IVH)/periventricular leukomalacia (PVL)
> - Retinopathy of prematurity
> - Anemia
> - Nutrition
> - Gastroesophageal reflux
> - Necrotizing enterocolitis

---

affected. Nosocomial infections and risks inherent to the required lifesaving therapies further complicate the infant's young life.

Apnea

Apnea of prematurity is defined as sudden cessation of breathing that lasts for at least 20 seconds or is accompanied by bradycardia and oxygen desaturation in an infant less than 37 weeks of gestational age. Apnea can be categorized by its etiology: central apnea occurs as a result of immature respiratory control mechanisms; obstructive apnea occurs due to the collapsibility of the chest wall and diaphragm; mixed apnea results when components of both types coexist. Apnea of prematurity and newborn periodic breathing patterns are consequences of an immature respiratory control system (Stokowski, 2005). Apnea of prematurity is believed to resolve by 37 weeks of postconceptual age (PCA), but may persist to 43 to 44 weeks PCA, particularly in children born at less than 28 weeks of gestation. This prolonged incidence of apnea/bradycardia events in the extremely premature infant may indicate that the central nervous system develops slower in these infants (Stokowski). During the NICU stay, methylxanthines are the primary choice of pharmacologic treatment for apnea of prematurity (Ambalavanan & Whyte, 2003). Caffeine is preferred over theophylline owing to its lower toxicity and slower elimination rate (Stokowski, 2005). The timing between resolution of apneic events and NICU discharge varies among institutions, generally 3 to 7 days for the otherwise stable infant (Stokowski). Most NICUs prefer to discontinue methylxanthines at least 1 week or more before hospital discharge.

Chronic Lung Disease

In the 1960s, neonatal lung injury and its radiographic findings were classified as bronchopulmonary dysplasia (BPD) by Norway, Rosan, and Porter (1967). The terms BPD and chronic lung disease (CLD) of prematurity are often used interchangeably in medical literature. The American Thoracic Society (2003) defines BPD for infants born less than 32 weeks of gestation as the need for supplemental oxygen at 28 days of life. For infants born greater than 32 weeks of gestation, it is defined as the need for supplemental oxygen at 36 weeks of corrected age.

The progression and treatments of BPD have undergone many changes during the last 40 years. Ventilation strategies, the routine use of antenatal steroids, and exogenous surfactant therapy have increased the viability of very premature infants. Physiologic conditions including surfactant deficiency, pneumonia, sepsis, meconium aspiration, pulmonary hypoplasia, persistent pulmonary hypertension, and congenital anomalies predispose the premature infant to the development of CLD (American Thoracic Society, 2003). Chronic lung disease complicates all other aspects of care, increases the financial and social burden of the family, and is a predictor for cognitive, motor, and academic delays (O'Shea, Nageswaran, Hiatt, et al., 2007). For infants with CLD, supplemental oxygen after hospital discharge improves growth, decreases pulmonary hypertension, and decreases right ventricular workload. Use of diuretics, bronchodilators, and corticosteroids is controversial; therefore benefits should be balanced with potential adverse effects.

Patent Ductus Arteriosus

The ductus arteriosus is a fetal shunt that connects the pulmonary artery with the descending aorta and facilitates blood return to the placenta. The term infant will experience functional closure of the ductus arteriosus during the first 24 to 96 hours of life (DiMenna, Laabs, McCloskey, et al., 2006). However, this functional closure may be delayed in preterm infants because of an altered response to oxygen, greater sensitivity to circulating prostaglandins, increased blood flow through the duct, increased pulmonary vascular resistance, and the size of the lumen of the ductus (DiMenna et al., 2006). Persistent ductal patency occurs in approximately 50% of LBW infants and 80% of ELBW infants, resulting in increased pulmonary blood flow and volume overload in the left ventricle (DiMenna et al.). Most preterm infants with PDA will have clinical symptomatology including a systolic murmur, bounding peripheral pulses, and pulmonary venous congestion by the third postnatal day.

Prostaglandin synthesis inhibitors and fluid restriction have been shown to be effective for PDA closure in the first 3 to 4 weeks of life (DiMenna et al., 2006). Indomethacin and ibuprofen lysine are two prostaglandin synthesis inhibitors. Indomethacin has been used for PDA treatment for decades. Recently, however, the use of ibuprofen lysine has been favored because it results in less thrombocytopenia and compromised urinary output. Surgical ligation may be indicated when the infant is refractory to medications or the infant is not a candidate for medical treatments.

Sepsis

Infection is the cause of death in 50% of newborn fatalities occurring on the first day of life (Wright Lott, 2006). Over half of all NICU admissions will be treated at least once for sepsis during their hospital course (Adams-Chapman & Stoll, 2006). Infants who have had an infection during the neonatal period are more likely to have comorbidities associated with adverse outcomes, such as severe IVH, periventricular leukomalacia (PVL), BPD, exposure to postnatal steroids, and impaired head growth (Adams-Chapman & Stoll).

Prevention of infection is a critical goal in the care of the preterm infant; however, immunologic limitations, physiologic stress, inadequate nutrition, and nosocomial exposures in the NICU constantly challenge this goal. The preterm infant born before 32 weeks of gestation receives a limited quantity of the maternal antibody immunoglobulin G (IgG) that normally crosses the placenta in greater quantities late in the third trimester. In addition, the preterm infant has limited ability to generate IgG, which, coupled with deficiencies in complement, neutrophil, and phagocytic function, places the preterm infant at greater risk for sepsis.

The most common bacteria in the newborn are gram-positive cocci, particularly group B beta-hemolytic streptococci (GBS) (Wright Lott, 2006); however, there has also been a resurgence of gram-negative bacteria (Adams-Chapman & Stoll, 2006).

Early-onset suspected sepsis should be treated with an ampicillin and an aminoglycoside, typically gentamicin, because the combination will provide coverage for *Streptococcus* species, *Escherichia coli,* and *Listeria* (Wright Lott, 2006). After the initial newborn period, the potential pathogens increase to include *Staphylococcus aureus, Staphylococcus epidermidis, Pseudomonas,* or *Bacteroides fragilis,* requiring different medication combinations (Wright Lott).

Intraventricular Hemorrhage/Periventricular Leukomalacia

Most intraventricular hemorrhages (IVHs) occur within the first 2 days of life, with some occurring up to day 7 (Papile, 2002). The gestational age at birth is inversely related to the occurrence of IVH; the younger the infant at birth, the more likely to develop an IVH (Papile). The classification used for IVH, described by Papile, Burstein, Burstein, and colleagues in 1978, includes the following: grade I, germinal matrix hemorrhage; grade II, intraventricular hemorrhage; grade III, intraventricular hemorrhage with dilation of the ventricle; and grade IV, intraventricular hemorrhage with extension of bleeding into the brain parenchyma. Treatment for most IVHs is supportive; however, if hydrocephalus develops, treatment aimed at minimizing brain injury is crucial (see Chapter 29).

The American Academy of Neurology and the Practice Committee of the Child Neurology Society recommend routine cranial ultrasounds during the first 7 to 14 days of life on all infants born less than 30 weeks of gestation and then repeated between 36 to 40 weeks of postmenstrual age (Ment, Bada, Barnes, et al., 2002). Serial monthly ultrasounds, or magnetic resonance imaging (MRI) before discharge, may be performed to identify the development of periventricular leukomalacia (PVL).

PVL may be seen with grades III or IV hemorrhage and may be the result of a multifactoral process of cytoxic injury, vascular compromise, and hypoxic ischemic events. From 3% to 4% of infants born weighing less than 1500 grams are diagnosed with PVL (Adams-Chapman & Stoll, 2006). The presence of PVL and higher-grade IVH equates to significant risk factors for neurodevelopmental impairment.

Retinopathy of Prematurity

Retinopathy of prematurity (ROP) is a process of incomplete vascularization of the retina and the arresting of normal retinal development due to preterm birth. If untreated, this condition can lead to visual impairment and blindness (Early Treatment for Retinopathy of Prematurity Cooperative Group, 2005). ROP develops in phases and is classified by stages. Phase I occurs as the normal vascularization is interrupted by the relatively hyperoxic extrauterine life, and results in vascular injury and retinal avascularity. The second phase of abnormal neovascularization is a response to the increased demands of the developing retina and the relative hypoxia experienced from the vascular injury. Retinal examinations must be performed by an ophthalmologist who is experienced and confident with examinations of the preterm infant (AAP Section on Ophthalmology, 2006). The most recent recommendations for screening include all infants with birth weights less than 1500 grams, infants less than 30 weeks of gestation, select infants between 1500 and 2000 grams, and those greater than 30 weeks of gestation with unstable clinical course or those determined by the neonatologist to be at increased risk (AAP Section on Ophthalmology, 2006). Follow-up examinations should continue, with frequency determined by

the ophthalmologist until full vascularization is complete (AAP Section on Ophthalmology).

Anemia

At birth, the relative increase in oxygen content and the increase in oxygen delivery to the tissues results in a decrease of erythropoietin (EPO) production and suppression of erythropoiesis. The subsequent physiologic anemia of infancy results in the full-term infant's hemoglobin falling to 11 g/dL by 8 to 12 weeks of age. In the preterm infant this response occurs more rapidly and with a more significant decrease in hemoglobin. This situation is further aggravated by reduced iron stores, blood loss through repeat blood draws, and the infant's short erythrocyte survival time. Transfusions of red blood cells are necessary in 80% of all VLBW infants and 95% of all ELBW infants (Aher & Ohlsson, 2006).

Because no single, specific definition for anemia exists in this population, the hemoglobin level or hematocrit value must be assessed in light of an infant's age and clinical condition. Tachycardia, tachypnea, apnea, poor growth, feeding difficulties, increased oxygen requirement, and acidosis are nonspecific symptoms of anemia. In the preterm infant, comorbidities including CLD, RDS, LBW, congenital heart disease, and problematic apnea may worsen the physiologic symptoms.

Blood transfusions in the preterm infant come with all of the risks of transfusion as in the full-term infant (hemolytic transfusion reactions, transfusion-acquired infections) and some specific risks inherent in the premature population. Blood transfusion in the preterm infant may increase the risk of retinopathy of prematurity and necrotizing enterocolitis. Donor exposure can be limited in preterm infants if blood bank policies are in place to provide repeat transfusions from the same unit of blood.

In preterm infants at risk for repeat transfusion, recombinant human erythropoietin may be used because physiologic erythropoietin levels are anticipated to be low for a prolonged period. Treatment with recombinant human erythropoietin has been shown to reduce the rate of transfusion by one per infant (Aher & Ohlsson, 2006). Although this may not appear to be a significant reduction, it may prevent exposure to a new donor. An adverse effect of recombinant human erythropoietin is neutropenia, but this will resolve with discontinuation of medication (Young & Mangum, 2007).

Nutrition

Parenteral Nutrition. Parenteral nutrition consisting of carbohydrates, lipids, amino acids, electrolytes, and other micronutrients is a lifesaving source of nutrition for premature infants. Nutrition for premature infants must balance caloric intake with the demands of comorbid conditions, immature metabolic and gastrointestinal systems, and risks of immunologic insufficiency (Heiman & Schanler, 2007). Parenteral nutrition is not the ideal nutritional source, but it provides the infant with a means of receiving nutrition when enteral nutrition is either not yet tolerated, or not an option because of other clinical conditions. Complications of parenteral nutrition are mechanical, metabolic, or infectious in nature. Mechanical and infectious complications are related to the intravenous delivery catheter, central or peripheral, as a source of infection, infiltrate, or other mechanical malfunction. Metabolic complications include cholestasis (defined as direct bilirubin greater than 2 mg/dL in an infant receiving parenteral nutrition for over 2 weeks), hyperglycemia or hypoglycemia, abnormal mineral or electrolyte levels, and elevated triglycerides.

Enteral Feeding. The ultimate nutritional goal for any infant is tolerance of enteral feedings that supply adequate volume and calories for sustained growth. Small-volume trophic feeds increase production of gastric hormones, including gastrin and motilin, and support gut maturation and should be started as early in the NICU course as able. These feeds of 10 to 20 mL/kg/day are ideally started with human breast milk. Infants exposed to early trophic feeds show higher energy intake and weight gain, tolerate feedings sooner, require less supplemental oxygen, experience less sepsis, and are discharged sooner (Panigrahi, 2006). Early attainment of full enteral feedings is crucial to adequate growth and bone mineralization during the postnatal period. Poor nutrition and inadequate intakes of calcium and phosphorus place the preterm infant at risk of fractures and rickets. Early feedings are typically delivered via nasogastric or orogastric tube. Some infants are thought to be mature enough to begin nutritive sucking with adequate respiratory control as early as 32 weeks of gestation; however, in most infants this develops between 34 and 36 weeks of gestation (Thomas, 2007).

Once enteral feedings, oral or by gavage, are established, volume is increased to a minimum of 150 mL/kg/day. If weight gain lags, the volume or caloric density of the feedings may need to be manipulated to promote adequate weight gain. With formula-fed infants, using commercially available formulas at 24, 27, or 30 kcal/oz may provide the additional calories. For breast milk–fed infants the selective feeding of hind milk may provide the infant milk with a two- to three-fold increase in fat content (Heiman & Schanler, 2007). This can be obtained by pumping the foremilk and hind milk in separate containers. The mother does this by interrupting pumping after a few minutes of free-flowing milk and changing the collection bottles (Hurst, 2007). For the infant who is nursing, the mother may initiate pumping, and then place the infant to the breast.

There is decreased protein content of more mature breast milk as compared with the milk expressed during the first month of lactation. The mature breast milk may be unable to provide the rapidly growing infant all that it requires. Premature infants fed unfortified breast milk may have abnormal laboratory markers of nutrition (Heiman & Schanler, 2007). Fortified human milk for infants less than 1500 grams at birth promotes short-term improvement in weight gain, length, head circumference, and bone mineral content. Donor-banked breast milk must be pasteurized, and this will alter its nutritional and immunologic properties (Heiman & Schanler).

The AAP's 2005 recommendations reinforce the immunologic and neurodevelopmental benefits of human milk for all infants, especially the preterm infant. Vohr, Poindexter, Dusick, and colleagues (2007) evaluated ELBW infants at 18 and 30 months after discharge who received breast milk during the NICU stay; they found improved Bayley behavior scores for emotional regulation, motor quality, and total behavior scores. Of note, 77% of the infants evaluated at 30 months stopped receiving breast milk after NICU discharge, highlighting the value of breast milk exposure early in the infant's life (Vohr et al., 2007). When educating mothers at risk for delivering prematurely, it is important to highlight these benefits of breast milk. Most mothers, even those who had little or no intention of breastfeeding, can be persuaded to pump their breasts while their fragile infant is in the NICU. They feel comforted by the research that even if they are unable to continue to breastfeed after discharge, they have positively affected their infant's future and potentially improved the infant's outcome.

Gastroesophageal Reflux

Gastroesophageal reflux (GER) refers to the retrograde passage of gastric contents from the stomach into the esophagus and is caused by decreased lower esophageal sphincter (LES) tone. The incidence of GER is significantly increased in premature or neurologically impaired infants (Hibbs & Lorch, 2006). Approximately 3% to 10% of preterm infants are diagnosed with GER. Frequent GER may produce esophageal mucosa injury, esophagitis with dysmotility, poor feeding, irritability, and crying (Jadcherla, 2002). Although some infants experience aspiration, cyanosis, and vomiting in relation to GER, research does not support a causal relationship between GER and apnea (Poets, 2004). However, infants with CLD account for up to 70% of neonatal cases of GER (Jadcherla, 2002).

Despite traditional practices, head-of-bed elevation has no effect on either the incidence or the symptoms of GER in infants younger than 2 years of age (Craig, Hanlon-Dearman, Sinclair, et al., 2004). Thickened feeds may be helpful in reducing symptoms; however, all research into infants with GER is confounded by the reality that most GER will improve as the infant ages (Craig et al., 2004). Thickened feeds may be difficult for the preterm infant to consume because of the extra energy required to suck the thickened liquid from the nipple. Commercial formulas with rice proteins marketed for treatment of reflux may be easier for the infant to bottle feed and may improve GER symptoms. Currently, however, these formulas are only available in 20 kcal/oz standard formula varieties. Gastric acid suppressors and more recently proton pump inhibitors are medications being utilized for the management of symptoms of GER in children. Consultation with a gastroenterologist is beneficial for infants showing poor weight gain, poor feeding, or discomfort.

Necrotizing Enterocolitis

Although many conditions have been implicated as causative agents for necrotizing enterocolitis (NEC), the only clear predisposing condition for NEC is prematurity. NEC is a gastrointestinal emergency that may develop insidiously over days or acutely as a life-threatening event. Nonspecific symptoms include abdominal distention, feeding intolerance, gastric residuals, guaiac-positive stools, bilious vomiting, and lethargy. Untreated, NEC may rapidly progress to respiratory failure, acidosis, decreased perfusion, shock, and disseminated intravascular coagulation (DIC) (Panigrahi, 2006). Early and aggressive treatment includes antibiotics, bowel rest, serial radiographic studies to evaluate the bowel, and supportive therapies for DIC and shock. Pneumatosis intestinalis and portal vein gas are pathopneumonic signs of NEC. Perforation of the bowel may lead to bowel necrosis and the need for surgical resection. Peritoneal drainage has emerged as a nonsurgical treatment option for those infants too small or too unstable for surgical resection of the damaged bowel (Panigrahi, 2006). If surgery is performed, preservation of the ileocecal valve is a positive outcome predictor. Periods of bowel rest and feeding intolerance expose the infant to complications of prolonged intravenous access and parenteral nutrition.

Caution must be exercised when restarting feeds in these infants. Strictures may develop in infants with or without surgical intervention. Sequelae related to strictures, short bowel syndrome, abscess formation, cholestasis, and NEC recurrence complicate their nutritional care. Infants who underwent surgery for NEC are more likely to measure below the 10th percentile for weight, length, and head circumference at 18 and 22 months of age than those who were managed medically (Ehrenkranz, Dusick, Vohr, et al., 2006). This discrepancy is probably related to the severity of illness and continued effects of gastrointestinal complications. Research into the use of nutritional probiotics and amino acid supplementation as protective measures for the premature gut is ongoing (Panigrahi, 2006).

Prognosis

Survival data from the MOD reveals that at 36 weeks of gestation survival is the same as term infants. Infants 32 to 35 weeks of gestation have a 98% survival rate, infants 28 to 31 weeks of gestation have a 90% to 95% survival rate, infants 27 weeks of gestation have an 87% survival rate, and infants 26 weeks of gestation have an 80% survival rate (MOD, 2007). Survival drops off significantly at younger gestational ages with many neonatologists using 23 weeks as the edge of viability. These statistics relate to survival, and do not describe the associated morbidities experienced by these children.

Predictors for outcome cannot focus on gestational age or birth weigh alone. Social factors, medical comorbidities, and access to early intervention services all play a role. Infants with neonatal infections experience a higher likelihood of CP, lower mental developmental index (MDI) scores, lower psychomotor and developmental index scores, visual impairments, and impaired growth (Adams-Chapman & Stoll, 2006). Marlow, Hennessy, Bracewell, and colleagues (2007) found that former extremely premature infants who were participating in mainstream education at 6 years of age performed 1 standard deviation below their peers in the same school setting in visuospatial, perceptuomotor, attention-executive, and gross motor function. The EPIPAGE study group, evaluating 30 to 34 weeks of gestation infants at 5 years of age, found that 25% of these infants had cognitive impairment such that special education was warranted (Marret et al., 2007).

ELBW infants have periods of malnutrition that may result in a decreased number of brain cells and behavior, learning, and memory deficits (Ehrenkrantz et al., 2006). However, infants with higher rates of weight gain showed remarkably lower incidence of CP, improved neurologic mental and psychomotor development, and lower rehospitalization rates (Ehrenkrantz et al.).

The late preterm infant may be admitted to the regular nursery and cared for by the primary care provider from birth. In some institutions, the baby may be admitted to the NICU, but there is tremendous pressure to discharge this infant with its mother after 2 to 4 days. A 2007 clinical report by the AAP labels the late preterm infant as a population at risk. Neonatal mortality rate, death between 0 and 27 days of life, is four to six times higher in this group than in full-term infants, and immature body systems place them at risk for central apnea, cold stress, hypoglycemia, jaundice/hyperbilirubinemia, and feeding difficulties (Engle et al., 2007). These infants are susceptible to CP, speech delays, neurodevelopmental handicaps, and behavioral abnormalities and have a higher hospital readmission rate than other infants born more preterm (Engle et al.).

PRIMARY CARE MANAGEMENT

Health Care Maintenance

Growth

As a standard of care, premature infants are discharged from the NICU when they are physically mature. This state is typically achieved when the infant is breathing without respiratory support, feeding orally (either by breast or bottle), maintaining adequate temperature, and doing all of these activities while showing a sustained pattern of growth. Growth can and will be limited by the infant's endurance and coordination with oral feeds. Feedings that last more than 30 minutes may tire the infant and expend more calories than the baby is able to consume (Ritchie, 2002). Weight gain trends should be well established before discharge from the NICU. Growth charts from the NICU should be part of the discharge summary and be incorporated into the medical chart in the primary care practice. Measurements for length, weight, and head circumference should be plotted according to corrected age.

Weight gain of at least 20 to 30 g per day is desirable (Verma, Sridhar, & Spitzer, 2003). Growth targets for premature infants are listed in Table 39-2. VLBW infants may display increased weight gain for length in the initial postdischarge period; however, this is not an indication for restriction of oral intake (Carlson, 2005). Despite improvement in nutritional products, premature infants lag behind their peers in future growth. Based on the National Center for Health Statistics/Centers for Disease Control and Prevention (NCHS/CDC) 2000 growth curves, 20% to 30% of ELBW infants will plot below the 10th percentile at 30 months of age (Greer, 2007; Kuczmarski, Ogden, Guo, et al., 2002). Suboptimal early catch-up growth and plotting below the 10th percentile at 2 years of age is a predictor of small size at 5 and 8 years of age (Marshall, 2003; Thureen & Hay, 2005). Long-term follow-up of VLBW infants suggests that at 14 years of age, they remain smaller for height, weight, and head circumference than their peers (Greer, 2007). Comorbidities such as BPD may have a negative impact on infant growth; ideally, additional protein, not lipids or carbohydrates, should be added to supply the extra calories needed for optional growth (Thureen & Hay, 2005). The rapid growth expected for premature infants during the first year of life requires higher intakes of calcium and phosphorus than term infants (Greer, 2007). A nutritionist familiar with the needs of medically complex premature infants should be consulted if growth is difficult to attain.

TABLE 39-2

Growth Rates of Preterm Infants through 18 Months of Age

Age (Months)	Weight (g/day)	Length (cm/month)	Head Circumference (cm/month)
1	26-40	3-4.5	1.6-2.5
4	15-25	2.3-3.6	0.8-1.4
8	12-17	1-2	0.3-0.8
12	9-12	0.8-1.5	0.2-0.4
18	4-10	0.7-1.3	0.1-0.4

Data from Verma, R.P., Sridhar, S., & Spitzer, A.R. (2003). Continuing care of NICU graduates. *Clin Pediatr, 42,* 299-315.

Development

It is not possible to predict with certainty which child born prematurely will develop disability. Infants with PVL are at risk for developmental delay; however, a normal cranial ultrasound does not preclude disability (Donohue & Graham, 2007). Characteristics of prematurity and LBW alone are poor predictors of CP. Recent research looking at means of predicting CP found that the combination of a normal cranial MRI and normal Neurobehavioral Assessment of the Preterm Infant (NAPI) performed at 36 weeks of postmenstrual age had a negative predictive value of 97% (Donohue & Graham, 2007). Most parents could be reassured that their infant may not develop CP if both of those tests were negative at 36 weeks of postmenstrual age. No test or combination of tests had a positive predictive value of over 50%. ELBW infants have a 10% to 30% rate of CP whereas VLBW infants have a CP rate of 2 per 1000, which is twice the rate found in the general population (Donohue & Graham).

Developmental screening is imperative for all children, but it has special implications in the premature infant (AAP Council on Children with Disabilities: Section on Developmental Behavioral Pediatrics, 2006). Global developmental screening and achievement of developmental milestones should occur at routine intervals and at any time concern is raised by the caregivers or the health care provider (AAP Joint Committee on Hearing, 2007). Parental reports of developmental concern have a high correlation to actual delays and should be addressed promptly. A standardized developmental screening tool (see Chapter 2) should be used, and the use of a developmental growth chart is advocated (AAP Council on Children with Disabilities, 2006). Multiple screening tools are listed in the AAP's Algorithm for Developmental Surveillance and Screening. This algorithm also details the process, requirements, and recommendations of developmental screening by the primary care provider. Once a potential delay is identified on a routine screening, referral for medical and developmental evaluation should take place as quickly as possible (AAP Council on Children with Disabilities). It is important for primary care providers to develop relationships with local programs, services, and resources for early intervention services, as well as local medical specialists who provide developmental evaluations.

Diet

Nutrition in the preterm infant after hospital discharge continues to be a challenge; 90% of infants are less than the 10th percentile of reference fetal weights at hospital discharge (Greer, 2007). While in the NICU, the parents are taught to be hyperfocused on good weight gain, because it is a marker of homeostasis and a criterion for discharge. Some preterm infants will meet all parameters of discharge except the ability to orally feed the volume of milk or formula necessary for sustained growth.

Parents may be taught to place and maintain a nasogastric tube for administration of gavage feedings. Small research studies and anecdotal parental reports appear to support this practice. Strum (2005) studied a small sample of infants discharged on home gavage feedings and found a 10- to 12-day shorter hospital length of stay, positive parental reports, and no hospital readmissions related to the feedings. Gastrostomy tubes may be indicated for preterm infants who fail to improve their oral intake after discharge, or for whom the severity of other underlying conditions makes attainment of oral feedings unlikely.

During the first outpatient visit, caregivers should be questioned regarding the frequency and duration of feedings, how breast milk is stored, how formula is prepared, and the infant's general ability to feed. NICU discharge instructions should be reviewed. Typical instructions may include feedings every 3 hours with one 5-hour period of sleep. Caregiver discharge education regarding premature infant feeding cues should be reinforced, particularly looking for alertness and rooting. Crying is a late sign of hunger in the premature infant. Intake volumes of preterm infants able to feed ad libitum may vary from 200 to 350 mL/kg/day (Greer, 2007).

Breast milk has been shown to improve the health and cognition of premature infants and to have a protective effect for up to 2 years (Vohr et al., 2007). Premature infants fed unfortified breast milk are at risk for osteopenia and may benefit from fortification (AAP Section on Breastfeeding, 2005; Carlson, 2005). Human milk–fed premature infants should be monitored carefully for growth and weight gain. Laboratory evaluations of serum phosphorus and alkaline phosphatase should also be followed. NICU discharge summaries should include the most recent laboratory values and highlight values that may indicate nutritional deficiencies. If serum phosphorus is less than 4.5 mg/dL or alkaline phosphatase is elevated greater than 1000 IU/mL, supplementation may be indicted (Greer, 2007). Infants fed unfortified breast milk must receive supplemental iron (2 to 4 mg/kg/day). Changes to the vitamin D intake recommendations were made in 2008. Current recommendations for vitamin D supplementation are that breast fed and partially breastfed infants should receive 400 IU/day of vitamin D beginning within the first few days of life (AAP Committee on Nutrition, 2008). Test weighing, in which the fully clothed infant is weighed, then breastfed, then weighed again, is a useful tool for mothers who are breastfeeding their premature infant at home (Hurst, 2007). One gram of weight gain following the feeding equates to one milliliter of milk intake (Hurst, 2007). Precise scales can typically be rented from providers of breast pumps. Provision of an objective measure of intake can reassure parents and health care providers of the amount of milk transferred by the infant, or provide evidence to support the need for complementary feedings. Often the preterm infant receiving breast milk is discharged from the NICU taking only a few feedings at the breast per day. This may be due to the child's need for complementary feedings, the desire to provide the infant with breast milk pumped and frozen earlier in lactation, the child's skill at breastfeeding, the mother's intention to continue some bottle feedings after hospital discharge, or the mother's ability to be at the hospital. The primary care provider and the mother should collaborate to achieve a feeding plan that will provide the nutrition the infant needs to sustain growth and encourage a positive feeding experience for the family.

Heiman and Schanler (2007) recommend a "triple approach" to feeding the premature infant. They advocate breastfeeding, supplemental feedings, and pumping. Infants at risk of poor growth should be breastfed, but should also receive complementary feedings of enriched discharge formula (Heiman & Schanler). Close follow-up of growth and biochemical markers of nutrition is crucial. Lactation support for the family after hospital discharge is critically important to ensure continuation of breast milk feedings. Herbal supplements are not recommended by the MOD because of the lack of research regarding their safety. Caution should be used with other supplements aimed at increasing milk supply or treating common ailments.

Enriched transitional formulas have higher calcium, phosphorus, protein, fat, and calories than term formulas (Greer, 2007). The formula-fed infant may be fed transitional formulas safely for up to 12 months (Carlson, 2005). Enriched transitional formulas may also be used in conjunction with breast milk feedings to increase the calories, protein, and minerals received by the infant. Use of these formulas may mean that supplemental vitamins and iron are not needed (Greer, 2007). Multivitamins and iron are indicated for the premature infant fed term formula (Greer).

There are no official postdischarge recommendations for nutrition of the preterm infant because of the paucity of research and lack of conclusive studies regarding these special infants. It appears prudent to optimize nutritional intake during the first year of life when catch-up growth is indicated. Research by Ehrenkranz and colleagues (2006) provides evidence of improved outcomes at 18 and 22 months of age in infants who displayed higher rates of growth during the NICU admission. Concern exists, however, regarding premature infants being at elevated risk of developing metabolic syndrome or cardiovascular disease from "preprogramming" caused by the rapid weight gain necessary for catch-up growth. Current science cannot prove or disprove this claim. It is possible that actual adolescent or adult weight and cardiovascular health status may be found to be more predictive variables.

Water and juices lack nutritional value and should not be offered to preterm infants less than 6 months of age (AAP Section on Breastfeeding, 2005). Additional foods, as recommended for the term infant, should be offered when the preterm infant demonstrates adequate head control, interest in feeding, and a decrease in tongue thrust. This typically occurs between 4 and 8 months of corrected age. Premature infants may develop feeding problems later in childhood. These issues may initially have a physiologic basis (i.e., GER, fatigue related to respiratory disease), but later manifest as a learned behavioral response (Thoyre, 2007). Children with a history of GER symptoms as an infant have a 20% incidence of feeding issues characterized as food refusal, being upset during meals, or prolonged mealtimes at 1 year of age, despite full resolution of the GER symptoms. For premature infants, poor oral motor functioning at discharge is a risk factor for needing feeding support services, but as many as 40% of infants with normal oral motor functioning at discharge had at least one feeding problem at 6 months of age (Thoyre). Comorbidities associated with prematurity accentuate the likelihood of feeding problems later in childhood. Feeding difficulties, if present, are a source of extreme stress in the family of a premature child. Every attempt should be made to refer them to speech and feeding specialists familiar with premature infants to facilitate the development of a pleasurable feeding experience for the child and the family.

Safety

Home monitoring is prescribed with significant geographic and practice-based variability. The AAP recommends home monitors for any infant discharged on mechanical ventilation, infants with complex medical needs, or those who are at increased risk of recurrent episodes of apnea, bradycardia, and hypoxemia after discharge. Families should understand that there is no proven relationship between apnea of prematurity and sudden infant death syndrome (SIDS) (AAP Committee on the Fetus and Newborn, 2003). Home monitoring is not aimed at preventing SIDS, rather at early detection of prolonged apneic events (Stokowski, 2005).

Whereas some parents view the home monitor as reassuring, other families perceive it as cumbersome and stress producing. Home monitoring may limit daycare and baby-sitting choices for the family, adding further stress to the family dynamics.

Discharge teaching for parents and all caregivers of an infant on home monitoring include observation of the infant, stimulation of the infant, cardiopulmonary resuscitation, and operation of the monitor. The AAP further recommends that for infants discharged on monitors, the monitor should be discontinued at 43 weeks of postconceptual age or at cessation of extreme events, whichever occurs last (AAP Committee on the Fetus and Newborn, 2003). The mechanism for discontinuing the monitor varies significantly, with practices ranging from invasive studies before discontinuation, monitor downloads, or merely the parental preference to stop as the deciding factor.

Before hospital discharge, all infants less than 37 weeks of gestation should have a "period of observation" in a car safety seat to monitor for apnea, bradycardia, and desaturation (AAP, 1999). Despite this recommendation, 20% of this age-group is not tested, and great variability exists in the actual definition of the car seat challenge (Williams & Martin, 2003). In 2007, the stability of infant car safety seat challenge results was looked at in consecutive 90-minute tests separated by 12 to 36 hours; 86% had consistent results and all of the infants with inconsistent results were less than 3 days of age (DeGrazia, 2007). This evaluation highlights the instability of the respiratory control centers of late preterm infants during the first days of transition to extrauterine life. Infants in another study were found to be as likely to have apnea and bradycardia events in either a car safety seat or a car bed, suggesting that it is the restraint rather than the device that contributes to the events (Salhab, Khattak, Tyson, et al., 2007).

The National Center for Safe Transportation of Children with Special Needs (n.d.) sets forth some recommendations for car safety seat selection for premature and LBW infants (www.preventinjury.org/SNTmedCond.asp). A smaller, infant-only seat, with a distance from the lowest set of harness slots to the bottom of the seat that is short enough so that the harness is at or below the infant's shoulders, is preferred. The distance from the crotch strap to the back of the seat should be short enough so that the infant's bottom is held back against the seat and does not slide forward. Rolls may be placed laterally to center the infant in the seat; however, items should not be placed under or behind the infant (Figure 39-1). These recommendations, as well as those from the AAP's 2007 Car Safety Seat Guide, are summarized in Box 39-2. It is important to remember that as these children get older they may still be smaller than their peers and should use booster seats until they meet the recommended weight and height for adult seat belts.

Travel with a preterm infant poses some challenges. Feedings require frequent stops, and an adult should ride in the back seat with the infant. For the infant home on oxygen and monitoring, traveling may be even more difficult. Monitoring equipment should have battery backup for at least twice as long as the trip. All equipment should be secured to prevent them from becoming projectiles in an accident. Air travel is best avoided until the infant has developed mature respiratory control and is off supplemental oxygen.

Anticipatory guidance for other safety issues should be based on developmental age and ability as for term infants.

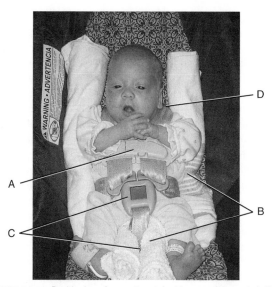

FIGURE 39-1 Positioning of premature infant in car safety seat. *A*, Retainer clip positioned on infant's chest. *B*, Blanket rolls on both sides of trunk and between crotch strap and infant. *C*, Distance from lowest set of harness slots to the bottom of the seat should allow the harness to be at or below infant's shoulders. *D*, Distance from crotch strap to the back of the seat should be such that the infant's bottom is held back against the seat.

BOX 39-2

Premature Infant Specific Recommendations for Travel

1. Before hospital discharge the infant should be observed for a period of time to assess the infant's respiratory stability in the semiupright position of a car seat.
2. Choose a safety seat with smaller dimensions. Use rolls or side supports to center the infant in the seat. Avoid use of items behind the infant.
3. Use a car safety seat without a shield or tray harness.
4. Be sure that monitors and other equipment have a battery power for at least twice the duration of the trip.
5. Secure monitors or other equipment because they may become projectiles during an accident.
6. Car beds may be indicated for infants unstable in a semiupright position.
7. When possible, an adult should ride in the back seat with the infant.
8. Locate car safety seat inspection centers at www.seatcheck.org.

Adapted from National Center for Safe Transportation of Children with Special Needs. (n.d.). Considerations for restraint selection. Available at: www.preventinjury.org/SNTmedCond.asp. Retrieved January 4, 2008; NHTSA website: www.boosterseat.gov.

Immunizations

The premature infant is particularly at risk for missing immunizations. One of the most effective and successful feats of modern medicine is the prevention of infectious diseases through active immunization with vaccines (Meissner, Anderson, & Pickering, 2004). Historically, concerns arose when premature infants showed increased incidence of apnea and bradycardia following the whole-cell pertussis vaccine. Preimmunization apnea, severity of illness at birth, young chronologic age, and lower weight are potential predictions for postimmunization apnea (Klein, Massolo, Greene, et al., 2008). The AAP recommends

that all preterm and LBW infants receive recommended vaccines, at full doses, at the same chronologic age as their fullterm peers regardless of gestational age and birth weight (Saari & Committee on Infectious Diseases, 2003). All 2-month immunizations may be given simultaneously in preterm and LBW infants (Saari & Committee on Infectious Diseases, 2003). In practice, if the infant is still hospitalized when receiving the 2-month immunizations, these may be spread out over a few days. Combination vaccines are appropriate for use in premature infants, but those containing hepatitis B components should be delayed until the baby is 6 weeks and over 2000 grams (Gad & Shah, 2007). With twins and higher multiples, sibling immunizations should be coordinated whenever possible. Immunizations provided during the infant's NICU stay should be clearly documented on the infant's discharge summary.

If a mother's hepatitis B status is unknown, the preterm infant born less than 2000 grams should receive a dose of hepatitis B vaccine and hepatitis B immune globulin (HBIG) within 12 hours of birth. For the infant less than 2000 grams, this dose does not count in the regular series and should be repeated according to the immunization schedule. The HBIG may be delayed if the infant is over 2000 grams for up to 7 days pending the mother's HbSAg testing (Saari & Committee on Infectious Diseases, 2003).

Protective immunity is of paramount importance to premature infants. Family and caregivers should be vaccinated yearly for influenza. Caregivers should receive boosters for diseases that may have waning efficacy; most cases of pertussis occurring in children less than 12 months of age can be attributed to waning immunity of the adult and adolescent caregivers of these children. Parents and caregivers of preterm infants may benefit from a Tdap booster rather than a Td booster (Gad & Shah, 2007).

Respiratory syncytial virus (RSV) poses a special threat to the premature infant. RSV enters the body through the nose, mouth, and eyes, infecting the respiratory mucosa. The virus produces various respiratory symptoms from nasal congestion, cough, wheezing, nasal flaring, retractions, apnea, and cyanosis (Austin, 2007). The virus can survive on hands for 30 minutes and on countertops, toys, and other surfaces for several hours. Palivizumab (Synagis) is recommended as prophylactic treatment for RSV among high-risk infants. In the United States, at-risk infants should receive palivizumab monthly from October-November through March-April according to the AAP guidelines (AAP, 2003). For infants discharged during these months, the series may begin before NICU discharge. Follow-up injections may be given by a home care nurse or at the primary care office (Austin, 2007). These injections do not significantly reduce RSV-related mortality rate, are expensive, and must be given monthly. Palivizumab does appear to reduce the severity of the disease in the preterm infant as evidenced by decreased hospital admissions. Indications for palivizumab therapy are listed in Box 39-3. Infants born less than 32 weeks of gestation and those less than 35 weeks of gestation with two risk factors are potential candidates for palivizumab. Of note, smoking in the home has been excluded as a risk factor for RSV. The AAP in the 2006 policy statement regarding bronchiolitis strongly recommends that infants not be exposed to passive smoking and states that the family has the ability to eliminate this risk factor completely by not smoking (AAP Subcommittee on Diagnosis and Management of Bronchiolitis, 2006).

BOX 39-3

Palivizumab Indications for the Prevention of Respiratory Syncytial Virus (RSV)

- Infants <24 months of age with CLD requiring treatment within 6 months of anticipated start of RSV season
- Infants <24 months of age with hemodynamically significant cyanotic or acyanotic congenital heart disease
- Infants <6 months of age at start of RSV season, born <32 weeks of gestation
- Infants <12 months of age at the start of RSV season, born <28 weeks of gestation
- Infants <6 months of age at the start of RSV season, born 32-35 weeks of gestation, *and* who have two or more of the following risk factors: daycare, school-age siblings, exposure to environmental pollutants, congenital abnormalities of the airway, and severe neuromuscular disease

Data from American Academy of Pediatrics. (2003). Policy statement: Revised indications for the use of palivizumab and respiratory syncytial virus immune globulin intravenous for the prevention of respiratory syncytial virus infection. *Pediatrics, 112*, 1442-1446.

Screening

Vision. Premature infants at risk for vision loss due to ROP must have clearly defined follow-up plans before NICU discharge. Primary care practitioners must not only verify that these appointments are being kept, but that these infants have ongoing ophthalmologic evaluations. Nurse practitioners should follow recommendations for screening for strabismus, amblyopia, and other vision deficits. Preterm infants, with or without ROP, are at risk of developing strabismus, cataracts, amblyopia, and glaucoma (AAP Section on Ophthalmology, 2006). The long-term complications of ROP continue to evolve as generations of infants with ROP survive into adulthood.

Hearing. NICU graduates make up half of the infants with abnormal hearing screens. Risk factors specific to the premature population include NICU admission for over 5 days, assisted ventilation, hyperbilirubinemia approaching exchange levels, receipt of ototoxic medications (including loop diuretics), and extracorporeal membrane oxygenation (ECMO) (AAP Joint Committee on Hearing, 2007). All term and preterm infants should have automated auditory brainstem response (ABR) screening before hospital discharge. If the infant fails screening in either ear, referral should be made to an audiologist with expertise with infants with hearing loss for rescreening and for comprehensive evaluation for both ears. Infants who have passed their ABR but who have identified risk factors for hearing loss should have a full diagnostic evaluation at any time concern is raised by the family or health care provider and by 24 to 30 months of age (AAP Joint Committee on Hearing, 2007).

Once hearing loss is confirmed, the infant should be immediately referred to early intervention services so that services can be in place before 6 months of age. Of children with confirmed hearing loss, 30% to 40% experience other developmental delays or disabilities (AAP Joint Committee on Hearing, 2007). Additional referrals should include pediatric otolaryngology and pediatric ophthalmology, as well as the option of genetic evaluation.

Dental. Prolonged orotracheal intubation affects the growing palate and may contribute to high arched palates, deep palatal grooves, and impaired future dentition. Nasal and mask continuous positive airway pressure devices may lead to nasal septum and upper lip or gum line deformities. Dental eruption may be delayed in premature infants and may be further delayed with poor growth or nutrition. Fluoride supplements should follow term infant recommendations. Referral to a pediatric dentist should occur as with any term infant, or earlier if there is concern regarding dentition.

Blood Pressure. Preterm infants may be at risk for developing hypertension, possibly related to complications from umbilical artery catheters or other facets of prematurity. Unlike full-term children who should have blood pressure screenings starting at age 3, premature infants should have blood pressure measurements at all routine well examinations. Hypertension screening should be done several times in the first year of life and then routinely in childhood. If concern regarding hypertension is identified before NICU discharge, blood pressure screenings may be provided by the NICU. If blood pressure equipment of the appropriate size is not available to the primary care provider, the NICU may facilitate these screenings. Hypertension is defined as repeated blood pressure measurements that are greater than the 95th percentile for age, gender, and weight, and childhood hypertension is a risk factor for hypertension in adulthood (National High Blood Pressure Education Program Working Group on High Blood Pressure in Children and Adolescents, 2004). Pediatric cardiac evaluations including echocardiogram are indicated if hypertension is identified.

Hematocrit. Understanding of the natural course of anemia of infancy is important. Whereas the physiologic nadir of hemoglobin in term infants occurs around 8 weeks, the preterm infant may experience this nadir at 5 weeks. The need for hematocrit screening should be determined based on the infant's history and current health status. Birth weight, nutritional support, use of exogenous erythropoietin, iron intake, and last hematocrit will help determine the frequency of screening. Although hematocrit levels below 25% are not typically well tolerated, transfusion should only be undertaken when the infant is experiencing ill effects from anemia, not at an arbitrary hematocrit level.

Urinalysis. Routine screening is recommended.

Tuberculosis. Routine screening is recommended.

Condition-Specific Screening

Inguinal hernias are more common in the premature infant. Surgical management of these conditions is not similar to the term infant; however, some consideration must be given to timing of surgical intervention. It is preferred to delay outpatient surgeries until the infant is 52 weeks of postconceptual age. Referral to a pediatric surgeon is appropriate at the time of identification of the hernia.

Common Illness Management
Differential Diagnosis

Respiratory Infections. Respiratory infections are a frequent cause of hospital readmission for the preterm infant. The risk of acquiring lower respiratory infection is correlated to the infant's age, with the highest morbidity in the first year of life and decreasing thereafter.

Bronchiolitis is a process of acute inflammation, edema, bronchospasm, and necrosis of epithelial cells lining the small airway of the lungs (AAP Subcommittee on Diagnosis and Management of Bronchiolitis, 2006). Clinical symptoms include rhinorrhea, cough, wheezing, tachypnea, increased respiratory effort, grunting, nasal flaring, and retractions. RSV is the most common etiology. Bronchiolitis is problematic for any infant, but for the premature infant, with or without underlying respiratory disease, bronchiolitis can be severe.

The 2006 AAP practice guidelines advocate diagnosis made based on clinical symptoms and history, avoiding the use of invasive laboratory testing (AAP Subcommittee on Diagnosis and Management of Bronchiolitis, 2006). Treatment recommendations are supportive, with current research failing to support the use of bronchodilators and corticosteroids. Inhaled bronchodilators may be used only if clinical symptoms improve after administration; however, sustained effects are unlikely. Antibacterials are indicated to treat a coexisting bacterial infection. Supplemental oxygen should be administered if pulse oximetry is below 90%. Intravenous fluids are indicated for those infants unable to maintain adequate hydration with oral intake. Good hand washing and the use of alcohol-based rubs by caretakers are advocated and imperative to help prevent the spread of respiratory and other illnesses (AAP Subcommittee on Diagnosis and Management of Bronchiolitis, 2006).

Differential Diagnosis

- Respiratory infections
  - Increased susceptibility to respiratory infections, especially RSV
  - Give RSV prophylaxis and flu vaccine during season
- Other viral infections
  - Herpes simplex virus types 1 and 2
- Bacterial infections
  - Nonspecific symptoms require early investigation and identification of bacterial group B streptococcus, *Chlamydia*, *Staphylococcus aureus*, and *Escherichia coli*

Other Viral Illnesses. The incubation period for perinatal exposure to herpes simplex virus (HSV) is variable, ranging from 2 days to 6 weeks. It is important to keep HSV in the differential, even with a negative family history, because the vast majority of cases occur in infants whose mother has no clinical symptoms and no history of HSV. Signs can include lethargy, poor feeding, respiratory distress, herpetic lesions, and seizures. Parents should be advised to avoid exposing the infant to individuals with any illness, including cold sores, fever blisters, and any vesicular lesions. If suspected, surface cultures should be obtained and acyclovir treatment should be instituted.

Bacterial Infections. Organisms such as *Chlamydia*, GBS, *Staphylococcus aureus*, *Streptococcus pneumoniae*, *Haemophilus influenzae* type b (Hib), or *Escherichia coli* may colonize in an infant during birth or hospitalization and place the infant at significant risk. Preterm infants with sudden temperature instability should be evaluated for sepsis. This evaluation is similar to the workup for a full-term infant; however, there should be a higher degree of suspicion with these vulnerable infants. Signs of infection may be subtle at first in the infant (e.g., change in oral intake or bowel patterns, pallor, lethargy, irritability, or respiratory distress). For the medically fragile premature infant, the parent may report a change in baseline status. These concerns should be taken seriously. Empiric antibiotic therapy should be begun after obtaining cultures. Any infant with obtundation, cyanosis,

respiratory compromise, seizures, or apnea should be considered a medical emergency and immediate hospitalization is imperative.

Developmental Issues

Sleep Patterns

The sleep patterns of preterm infants may differ from those of full-term infants. Nutritional needs may require frequent nighttime feedings for months after discharge. Some infants may be hypersensitive to lights and noise, whereas others may have become accustomed to the noise of the NICU and find it difficult to settle in the relatively quiet home environment. Parents should be instructed on the importance of the "back to sleep" positioning for prevention of sudden infant death syndrome (SIDS) (AAP Task Force on SIDS, 2005). Home apnea monitors are not aimed at preventing SIDS; however, some parents develop a false sense of security regarding sleep positioning. At times infants are placed prone in the NICU, and parents may imitate this positioning at home. Nurse practitioners should reinforce the need for supine positioning during sleep, while encouraging prone positioning or tummy time while awake to prevent positional plagiocephaly from occurring. Other recommendations include a separate crib in the parents' room, a firm sleeping surface, removing loose bedding and soft objects from the crib, offering pacifiers, and avoiding overheating (AAP Task Force on SIDS, 2005). The practice of co-bedding, either with the infant in bed with the parents or multiples sharing a crib for sleep, is not recommended.

Toileting

Toileting should begin when the child shows signs of readiness, as with any healthy child. Gross and fine motor delays may hamper independent toileting and should be taken into consideration.

Discipline

Parents may feel unwilling to discipline their child and continue to see the child as vulnerable. The premature infant can be irritable and a difficult child to console. Altered bonding and vulnerable child issues may lead to behavioral issues not related to prematurity or developmental disability. Parents should be encouraged to use discipline as they would with any other child based on appropriate developmental expectations. Parent education should include cautions about shaken baby syndrome and other forms of intentional or unintentional child abuse.

Child Care

Increased exposure to respiratory, gastrointestinal, and other infectious diseases occurs with children attending daycare. Preterm infants are especially vulnerable to these diseases and should be protected as much as possible. A single child-care provider in the child's home is ideal (Austin, 2007). When that is not feasible, smaller day centers with designated infant caregivers are preferable over large, multicaregiver daycare centers. Regardless of the site, the parents must be diligent in educating other caregivers regarding the special needs of their preterm infant.

Schooling

Premature infants with developmental issues should be referred to early intervention programs. These programs can be continued until the child is 3 years old, when school-based services should take over. The primary health care provider, as well as the early intervention support persons, can help identify school readiness and the appropriate timing for transition of services. Socialization and other supports from the classroom environment are important for the child with potential for behavioral or learning difficulties. Families of preterm infants who have adopted a vulnerable child mentality may benefit from the separation imposed by a daily school routine (see Chapter 3).

Sexuality

Men and women who were born preterm do not face reproductive issues other than those that may be inherent in any medical or developmental sequelae of their prematurity. However, premature birth and family history of premature birth have been shown to be risk factors for premature birth. This information should be communicated with families and with the children as they approach sexual maturity.

Transition to Adulthood

Transition to adolescence and adulthood may be more difficult for children and families with children born preterm. Although children who were premature infants have positive views of their own health status (Zwicker & Harris, 2008), their medical and developmental comorbidities may complicate their transition to adulthood. This may be a source of contention within the family. Parents may perceive the preterm adolescent's health and development as negatively affecting the adolescent's quality of life whereas the adolescent does not (Zwicker & Harris, 2008).

Developmental and behavioral problems may be exaggerated during the turbulence of adolescence. If growth has been suboptimal, these children may face a stigma of being smaller than their peers. As with all children with chronic conditions, the quest for independence in adolescence can be hampered by their medical status and their family's belief that they are vulnerable. Parental overprotection can lead to rebellion and low self-esteem. During adolescence, concerns about physical appearance are paramount, and cosmetic deformities may cause significant anguish. Efforts to limit the teen's angst over scars or deformities should be made; cosmetic repair may be helpful in some cases.

As more and more ELBW infants and extremely premature infants are surviving into adolescence and adulthood, adult health care providers will need to be more familiar with these comorbidities. Adult survivors of retinopathy of prematurity pose specific challenges for adult retinal specialists.

Strong, open communication between parents and adolescents is ideal and may facilitate a less difficult transition to adulthood. In some cases, professional support may be beneficial.

Family Concerns

Families of preterm infants have multiple issues to work through. If preterm delivery is threatened or if the mother has a difficult pregnancy, the families are in constant fear of what will happen to the baby. Once the baby is born, there is the constant struggle with guilt over "not having done enough" to prolong the pregnancy. During the NICU stay, parents live in constant fear that the infant will die; if the infant survives, parents may worry about the future—will their child be able to go to school, play sports, drive a car, and become a productive adult? Grief over the loss of what was imagined to be the ideal pregnancy and birth of a child can be overwhelming. Financial concerns may become a tremendous stressor for the family as well. The health care provider must try to promote a balance that will permit the child to realize his or her full potential.

Mothers of preterm infants experience intense emotional distress and fatigue from the care requirements of the infant. They may exhibit symptoms of depression, especially during the first 6 months after birth (Shandor Miles, Holditch-Davis, Schwartz, et al., 2007). These 6 months typically consist of the NICU stay and the early months after hospital discharge. Caregivers with this level of emotional distress will have difficulty bonding with their infant and may have difficulty facing the needs of their preterm infant at home. Pediatric providers will have the opportunity to have more contact with the family at this point than the mother's medical team, and should have information regarding local counseling providers. Extended family can also provide support and respite care to the parents. Davis, Sweeney, Turnage-Carrier, and colleagues (2004) found that preterm infants evaluated at school age, who had two involved caregivers, regardless of marital state, are more likely to perform at grade level. This underscores the importance of family and community support for the child and the parents of a child with chronic health needs.

Resources
Support Organizations
March of Dimes
Supports education and research to decrease birth defects.
(888) MODIMES (663-4637)
Spanish-speaking number: (800) 925-1855
Website: www.marchofdimes.com

National Center for the Safe Transportation of Children with Special Needs
Provides information regarding preventing injury in automobiles
(800) 620-0143
Website: www.preventinjury.org

National Organization of Mothers of Twins Club, Inc.
National organization to support parents of twins or higher multiple births.
(800) 243-2276
Website: www.nomotc.org

Zero to Three
Parent and professional resource center for early childhood development.
(202) 638-1144
Website: www.zerotothree.org

Online Resources
Nemours/KidsHealth.Org
Online resource for parents, health professionals, and children.
Website: www.kidshealth.org

NICHD
Information on preterm birth and labor.
Website: www.nichd.nih.gov/health/topics/preterm_labor_and_birth.cfm

NLM
Information on prematurity.
Website: www.nlm.nih.gov/medlineplus/prematurebabies.html

Summary of Primary Care Needs for the Premature Infant

HEALTH CARE MAINTENANCE

Growth and Development

- Use corrected age to plot height, weight, and head circumference.
- All preterm infants are at risk for developmental delays.
- Use corrected age and a standardized developmental screening tool.
- Referrals to early intervention should occur as soon as delay is suspected.

Diet

- Nasogastric tube feedings may be indicated after discharge if all other criteria for discharge are met.
- Breastfeeding is recommended.
- Fortification of breast milk may be indicated if growth or laboratory values indicate the need.
- Multivitamins and iron supplementation are indicated for infants fed standard formula or unfortified breast milk. New recommendations for vitamin D should be followed.
- Enriched transitional formula may be used for up to 1 year after hospital discharge.
- Introduction of additional foods should be delayed until the infant shows signs of readiness. Juice and water are not appropriate until after 6 months of corrected age.

Safety

- Home monitoring is not aimed at preventing SIDS, but may be indicated as a tool to alert caregivers to prolonged apneic events.
- Infant-only car seats with smaller dimensions are recommended for preterm infants.
- Air travel should be delayed until the infant tolerates lower environmental oxygen concentrations.
- Anticipatory guidance is based on developmental age.

Immunizations

- Immunizations should be administered at the same chronologic ages recommended by the AAP for term infants
- Preterm infants after 6 months of age and their caretakers should receive the influenza vaccine yearly.
- Family/caregivers of preterm infants should receive pertussis boosters.
- RSV prophylaxis should be administered to at-risk infants according to AAP guidelines.

Screening

- *Vision.* Assessment of fixation, alignment, and funduscopic examination is recommended. Ophthalmologic follow-up is necessary for infants with ROP and yearly for all preterm infants.
- *Hearing.* Screening is recommended for all infants before hospital discharge.
- Referral to audiology and otolaryngology is recommended if hearing loss is suspected.
- *Dental.* Prolonged intubation affects palate and dentition.
- Tooth eruptions may be delayed, and teeth may be abnormally shaped or discolored.
- Routine fluoride supplementation is recommended after 6 months of corrected age.

- *Blood pressure.* Hypertension screenings should be done at 1, 2, 6, 12, and 24 months of age, and then routinely in childhood.
- Children with consistently elevated blood pressures should be evaluated for etiology.
- *Hematocrit.* Hematocrit values should be evaluated routinely based on history, nutritional status, and symptoms. Transfusions for low hemoglobin should be given only if infant is symptomatic.
- *Urinalysis.* Routine screening is recommended.
- *Tuberculosis.* Routine screening is recommended.

COMMON ILLNESS MANAGEMENT

Differential Diagnosis

- Risk of infection—particularly respiratory infection and bronchiolitis—is increased.
- RSV, HSV, *Chlamydia,* group B streptococcus, *S. aureus,* and *E. coli* must all be considered possible pathogens. Risk for *Streptococcus pneumoniae* and *Haemophilus influenzae* type b infections must be evaluated.

DEVELOPMENTAL ISSUES

Sleep Patterns

- Children may have disorganized sleep patterns.
- Premature infants with poor growth should be woken for feedings every 3-4 hours.
- Families should follow the "back to sleep" program while allowing time in the prone position when awake.
- Home monitors do not prevent SIDS.
- Co-bedding of multiples or with parents is discouraged.

Toileting

- Toileting readiness is based on developmental age.
- Gross motor delays may impede toilet training.

Discipline

- Children should be assessed for vulnerable child syndrome.
- Limits should be set as with any other child.
- The incidence of child abuse is higher than with other children.

Child Care

- Home care or small daycare programs are preferred over large daycare centers to limit infectious exposures.
- All caregivers should be comfortable with the special needs of the premature child.

Schooling

- Early intervention services may be continued until the child is transitioned to school-based services.
- Education services are crucial for the child with potential for developmental delays.

Sexuality

- Adolescents who were born preterm should have normal pubertal sexual development.
- There is an increased incidence of preterm delivery with a family history of preterm delivery.

Continued

Summary of Primary Care Needs for the Premature Infant—cont'd

Transition to Adulthood

- Preexisting developmental or behavior problems may become more exaggerated.
- Adolescents born preterm report a self-perception of a good quality of life.
- Concerns regarding medical consequences of prematurity, cosmetic deformities, parental overprotection, and communication should be addressed.

FAMILY CONCERNS

- Family concerns include guilt, grief, financial considerations, concerns about developmental outcomes, and attachment issues as a result of prolonged hospitalization.
- Symptoms of depression and intense emotional distress can affect parent-infant bonding and developmental outcomes.

REFERENCES

Adams-Chapman, I., & Stoll, B.J. (2006). Neonatal infection and long-term neurodevelopmental outcome in the preterm infant. *Curr Opin Infect Dis, 19,* 290-297.

Aher, S., & Ohlsson, A. (2006). Late erythropoietin for preventing RBC transfusion in preterm and or LBW infants. *Cochrane Database of Systematic Reviews, 3,* CD004868.

Ambalavanan, N., & Whyte, R.K. (2003). The mismatch between evidence and practice: Common therapies in search of evidence. *Clin Perinatol, 30,* 305-331.

American Academy of Pediatrics (AAP). (1999). Safe transportation of newborns at hospital discharge. *Pediatrics, 104,* 986-987.

American Academy of Pediatrics (AAP). (2003). Policy statement: Revised indications for the use of palivizumab and respiratory syncytial virus immune globulin intravenous for the prevention of respiratory syncytial virus infection. *Pediatrics, 112,* 1442-1446.

American Academy of Pediatrics (AAP). (2004). Policy statement: Age terminology during the perinatal period. *Pediatrics, 114,* 1362-1364.

American Academy of Pediatrics (AAP) & American College of Obstetricians and Gynecologists. (2002). *Guidelines for Perinatal care.* Washington, DC: Author.

American Academy of Pediatrics (AAP). Committee on the Fetus and Newborn. (2003). Perinatal care at the threshold of viability. *Pediatrics, 110,* 1024-1027.

American Academy of Pediatrics (AAP). Council on Children with Disabilities: Section on Developmental Behavioral Pediatrics Bright Futures Steering Committee and Medical Home Initiatives for Children with Special Needs Project Advisory Committee. (2006). Policy statement: Identifying infants and young children with developmental disorders in the medical home: An algorithm for developmental surveillance and screening. *Pediatrics, 118,* 405-420. DOI: 10.1542/peds.2006-1231.

American Academy of Pediatrics (AAP), Committee on Nutrition (2008). Clinical Report: Prevention of rickets and vitamin D deficiency in infant, children and adolescents. *Pediatrics, 122*(5), 1142-1152.

American Academy of Pediatrics (AAP) Joint Committee on Hearing. (2007). Policy statement: Principles and guidelines for early hearing detection and intervention programs. *Pediatrics, 120,* 898-921.

American Academy of Pediatrics (AAP) Section on Breastfeeding. (2005). Policy statement: Breastfeeding and the use of human milk. *Pediatrics, 115,* 496-506.

American Academy of Pediatrics (AAP) Section on Ophthalmology, American Academy of Ophthalmology American Association for Pediatrics Ophthalmology and Strabismus. (2006). Screening examination of premature infants for retinopathy of prematurity (ROP). *Pediatrics, 117,* 572-576. Errata in DOI: 10.1542/peds.2006-2162.

American Academy of Pediatrics (AAP) Subcommittee on Diagnosis and Management of Bronchiolitis. (2006). Clinical practice guidelines: Diagnosis and management of bronchiolitis. *Pediatrics, 118,* 1774-1793.

American Academy of Pediatrics (AAP) Task Force on Sudden Infant Death Syndrome. (2005). Policy Statement: The changing concept of sudden infant death syndrome: Diagnostic coding shifts, controversies regarding the sleep environment, and new variables to consider in reducing risk. *Pediatrics, 116,* 1245-1255.

American College of Obstetricians and Gynecologists (ACOG). (1998). *Antenatal Corticosteroid Therapy for Fetal Maturation. ACOG Committee Opinion.* Washington, DC: Author.

American Thoracic Society Documents. (2003). Statement on the care of the child with chronic lung disease of infancy and childhood. *Am J Respir Crit Care Med, 168,* 356-396.

Austin, J. (2007). Preventing respiratory syncytial virus in homebound premature infants. *Home Health Nurse, 25,* 429-432.

Ballard, J.L., Khoury, J.C., Wedig, K., et al. (1991). New Ballard score, expanded to include extremely premature infants. *J Pediatr, 119,* 417-423.

Bright, M.A. (2002). *Holistic health and healing.* Philadelphia: F.A. Davis.

Buchh, B., Graham, N., Harris, B., et al. (2007). Neonatology has always been a bargain—even when we weren't very good at it! *Acta Paediatr,* 659-663. DOI: 10.1111/j.1651-2227.2007.00247.x.

Carlson, S.E. (2005). Feeding after discharge: Growth, development and long-term effects. In R.C. Tsang, R.Uauy, B. Koletzko, et al. (Eds.), *Nutrition of the Preterm Infant: Scientific Basis and Practical Guidelines* (2nd ed.). Cincinnati, OH: Digital Educational Publishing.

Craig, W.R., Hanlon-Dearman, A, Sinclair, C., et al. (2004). Metoclopramide, thickened feedings, and positioning for gastroesophageal reflux in children under two years. *Cochrane Database of Systematic Reviews.3,* DOI: 10.1002/14651858.CD003502.pub2

Davis, D.W., Sweeney, J.K., Turnage-Carrier, C.S., et al. (2004). Early intervention beyond the newborn period. In C. Kenner & J.M. McGrath (Eds.), *Developmental Care of Newborns and Infants: A Guide for Health Professionals.* St. Louis: Mosby.

DeGrazia, M. (2007). Stability of the infant car seat challenge and risk factors for oxygen desaturation events. *J Obstet Gynecol Neonat Nurs, 36,* 300-307.

DiMenna, L., Laabs, C., McCloskey, L., et al. (2006). Management of the neonate with patent ductus arteriosus. *J Perinat Neonat Nurs, 20*(4), 333-340.

Donohue, P.K., & Graham, E.M. (2007). Earlier markers for cerebral palsy and clinical research in premature infants. *J Perinatol, 27,* 259-261.

Dubowitz, L.M., Dubowitz, V., & Goldberg, C. (1970). Clinical assessment of gestational age in the newborn. *J Pediatr, 77,* 1-10.

Early Treatment for Retinopathy of Prematurity Cooperative Group. (2005). The incidence and course of retinopathy of prematurity: Findings from the Early Treatment for Retinopathy of Prematurity Study. *Pediatrics, 116*(1). Available at www.pediatrics.org/cgi/content/full/116/1/15. Retrieved August 1, 2005.

Ehrenkranz, R.A., Dusick, A.M., Vohr, B.R., et al., for the NICHD Neonatal Research Network. (2006). Growth outcomes in the neonatal intensive care unit influences neurodevelopmental and growth outcomes of extremely low birth weight infants. *Pediatrics, 117,* 1253-1261.

Engle, W.A., Tomashek, K.M., Wallman, C., & the Committee on Fetus and Newborn (2007). Clinical report: "Late-preterm" infants: A population at risk. *Pediatrics, 120,* 1390-1401. DOI: 10.1542/peds.2007-2952.

Fetrow, C.W., & Avila, J.R. (1999). *Professional Handbook of Complementary and Alternative Medicines.* Springhouse, PA: Springhouse.

Gad, A., & Shah, S. (2007). Special immunization considerations of the preterm infant. *J Pediatr Health Care, 21,* 385-391.

Giarratano, G. (2006). Genetic influences of preterm birth. *MCN Am J Matern Child Nurs, 31*(3), 169-175.

Greer, F.R. (2007). Post-discharge nutrition: What does the evidence support? *Semin Perinatol, 31,* 89-95.

Heiman, H., & Schanler, R. (2007). Enteral nutrition for premature infants: The role of human milk. *Semin Fetal Neonat Med, 12,* 26-34.

Hibbs, A.M., & Lorch, S.A. (2006). Metoclopramide for the treatment of gastroesophageal reflux disease in infants. *Pediatrics, 118,* 746-752. DOI: 10.1542/peds.2005-2006.

Hurst, N.M. (2007). The 3 M's of breast-feeding the preterm infant. *J Perinat Neonat Nurs, 21,* 234-239.

Institute of Medicine (IOM). (2007). Preterm birth: Causes, consequences and prevention Committee on Understanding Premature Birth and Assuring Healthy Outcomes. Behrman, R.E., & Butler, A.S. (Eds). Washington, DC: The National Academies Press.

Jadcherla, S.R. (2002). Recent advances in neonatal gastroenterology: Gastroesophageal reflux in the neonate. *Clin Perinatol, 29*(1). Available at www.mdconsult.com. Retrieved January 27, 2005.

Kirby, S., Greenspan, J.S., Kornhauser, M., et al. (2007). Clinical outcomes and cost of the moderately preterm infant. *Adv Neonat Care, 7*(2), 80-87.

Klein, N.P., Massolo, M.L., Greene, J., et al. & Vaccine Safety Database. (2008). Risk factors for developing apnea after immunization in the neonatal intensive care unit. *Pediatrics, 121*, 463-469. DOI: 10.1542/peds.2007-1462.

Kuczmarski, R.J., Ogden, C.L., Guo, S.S., et al. (2002). 2000 growth charts for the United States: Methods and development, National Center for Health Statistics. *Vital Health Statistics, 11*(246). Available at www.cdc.gov/nchs/data/series_11/sr11_246.pdf. Retrieved March 30, 2009.

March of Dimes (MOD). (2006, November). *Stress and prematurity.* Available at www.marchofdimes.com/printableArticles/14332_23759.asp. Retrieved September 21, 2007.

March of Dimes (MOD). (2007, February). *Quick reference fact sheets: Preterm birth.* Available at www.marchofdimes.com/printableArticles/14332_1157.asp. Retrieved September 21, 2007.

Marlow, N., Hennessy, E.M., Bracewell, M.A., et al., & EPICure Study Group. (2007). Motor and executive function at 6 years of age after extremely preterm birth. *Pediatrics, 120*, 793-804. DOI: 10.1542/peds.2007-0440.

Marret, S., Ancel, P.Y., Marpeau, L., et al. (2007). Neonatal and 5 year outcomes after birth at 30-34 weeks gestation. *Obstet Gynecol, 110*(1), 72-80.

Marshall, D.D. (2003). Review article: Primary care follow-up of the neonatal intensive care unit graduate. *Clin Fam Practice, 5*(2). Available at: www.mdconsult.com. Retrieved January 27, 2005.

Martin, J.A., Hamilton, B.E., Sutton, P.D., et al. (2006). Births: Final data for 2004. *National Vital Statistics Report, 55*(1), Hyattsville, MD: National Center for Health Statistics. Available at www.wonder.cdc.gov/wonder/sci_data/natal/detail/type_txt/natal04/births04.pdf.

Meissner, H.C., Anderson, L.J., & Pickering, L.K. (2004). Commentary: Annual variation in respiratory syncytial virus season and decisions regarding immunoprophylaxis with palivizumab. *Pediatrics, 114*(4), 1082-1084.

Ment, L.R., Bada, H.S., Barnes, P., et al. (2002). Practice parameters: Neuroimaging of the neonate: Report of the quality standards subcommittee of the American Academy of Neurology and the practice committee of the Child Neurology Society. *Am Acad Neurol, 58*, 1726-1738.

National Center for Safe Transportation of Children with Special Needs. (n.d.). *Considerations for restraint selection.* Available at www.preventinjury.org/SNTmedCond.asp. Retrieved January 4, 2008.

National High Blood Pressure Education Program Working Group on High Blood Pressure in Children and Adolescents (2004). The fourth report on the diagnosis, evaluation and treatment of high blood pressure in children and adolescents. *Pediatrics, 114*, 555-576.

National Institutes of Health (NIH) (2000). Antenatal corticosteroids revisited: Repeat courses. *NIH Consensus Statement, 17*(1), 1-10.

National Vital Statistics System. (2005). Births: Preliminary data for 2005. Available at: www.cdc.gov.nchs/products/pubs/pubd/hestats/prelimbirths05/prelimbirths05.htm. Retrieved September 21, 2007.

Ng, P.C., & Lam, H.S. (2007). Diagnostic markers for neonatal sepsis. *Curr Opin Pediatr, 18*, 125-131.

Norway, W.H., Rosan, R.C., & Porter, D.Y. (1967). Pulmonary disease following respiratory therapy of hyaline-membrane disease: Bronchopulmonary dysplasia. *N Engl J Med, 276*(7), 357-368.

O'Shea, T.M., Nageswaran, S., Hiatt, D.C., et al. (2007). Follow-up care for infants with chronic lung disease: A randomized comparison of community- and center-based models. *Pediatrics*, e947-e957. DOI: 10.1542/peds.2006-1717.

Panigrahi, P. (2006). Necrotizing enterocolitis: A practical guide to its prevention and management. *Pediatr Drugs, 8*(3), 151-165.

Papile, L. (2002). Intracranial hemorrhage. In A.A. Fanaroff & R.J. Martin (Eds.), *Neonatal-Perinatal Medicine* (7th ed.). St. Louis: Mosby.

Papile, L., Burstein, J., Burstein, R., et al. (1978). Incidence and evolution of subependymal and intraventricular hemorrhages: A study of infants with birth weights less than 1500 grams. *Pediatrics, 92*(4), 529-534.

Poets, C.F. (2004). Gastroesophageal reflux: A critical review of its role in preterm infants. *Pediatrics, 113*(2), e128-e132.

Reedy, N.J. (2007). Born too soon: The continuing challenge of preterm labor and birth in the United States. *J Midwife Womens Health, 52*(3), 281-290.

Ritchie, S.K. (2002). Primary care of the premature infant discharged from the neonatal intensive care unit. *MCN Am J Matern Child Nurs, 27*(2), 76-84.

Saari, T., & Committee on Infectious Diseases. (2003). Clinical report: Immunization in special circumstances: Preterm and low birth weight infants. *Pediatrics, 112*, 193-198.

Salhab, W., Khattak, A., Tyson, J., et al. (2007). Car seat or car bed for VLBW infants at discharge home. *J Pediatr, 150*, 224-228. DOI: 10.1016/j.peds/2006.10.10.068.

Shandor Miles, M., Holditch-Davis, D., Schwartz, T.A., et al. (2007). Depressive symptoms in mothers of prematurely born infants. *J Dev Behav Pediatr, 28*, 36-44.

Smith, K. (2007). Sleep and Kangaroo Care: Clinical practice in newborn intensive care unit: Where the baby sleeps... *J Perinat Neonat Nurs, 21*(2), 151-157.

Spong, C.Y. (2007). Prediction and prevention of recurrent spontaneous preterm birth. *Obstet Gynecol, 110*(2 pt 1), 405-415.

Stokowski, L.A. (2005). A primer on apnea of prematurity. *Adv Neonat Care, 5*(3), 155-170.

Strum, L.D. (2005). Implementation and evaluation of a home gavage program for preterm infants. *Neonat Network, 24*(4), 21-25.

Thomas, J.A. (2007). Guidelines for bottle feeding your premature baby. *Adv Neonat Care, 7*, 311-318.

Thoyre, S. (2007). Feeding outcomes of extremely premature infants after neonatal care. *J Obstet Gynecol Neonat Nurs, 36*, 366-376.

Thureen, P.J., & Hay, W.W. (2005). Conditions requiring special nutritional management. In R.C. Tsang, R. Uauy, B. Koletzko, et al. (Eds.), *Nutrition of the preterm infant: Scientific basis and practical guidelines* (2nd ed.). Cincinnati, OH: Digital Educational Publishing.

Verma, R.P., Sridhar, S., & Spitzer, A.R. (2003). Continuing care of NICU graduates. *Clin Pediatr, 42*, 299-315.

Vohr, B.R., Poindexter, B.B., Dusick, A.M., et al., & National Institute of Child Health and Human Development National Research Network. (2007). Persistent beneficial effects of breast milk ingested in the neonatal intensive care unit of outcomes of extremely low birth weight infants at 30 months of age. *Pediatrics, 120*, e953-e959. v DOI: 10.1542/peds.2006-3227.

Wade, K.C., Lorch, S.A., Bakewell,-Sachs, S., Medoff-Cooper, B., Silber, J.H., & Escobar, G.J. (2009). Pediatric care for preterm infants after NICU discharge: high number of office visits and prescription medications. *Journal of Perinatology, 28*, 696-701.

Williams, L.E., & Martin, J.E. (2003). Car seat challenges: Where are we in implementation of these programs? *J Perinat Neonat Nurs, 17*(2), 158-163.

Wright Lott, J. (2006). State of the science: Neonatal bacterial infection in the early 21st century. *J Perinat Neonat Nurs, 20*(1), 62-70.

Young, T.E., & Mangum, B. (Eds.) (2007). *Neofax: A Manual of Drugs Used in Neonatal Care,* (20th ed.,). Montavale, NJ: Thomson Healthcare.

Zwicker, J.G., & Harris, S.R. (2008). Quality of life of formerly preterm and VLBW infants from preschool age to adulthood: A systematic review. *Pediatrics, 121*, e366-e376. DOI: 10.1542/peds.2007-0169.

40 Sickle Cell Disease

Robin H. Pitts and Elizabeth O. Record

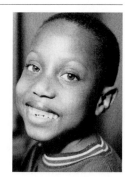

Etiology

Sickle cell disease (SCD) is a term used to describe several inherited, sickling hemoglobinopathy syndromes, including sickle–beta thalassemia (Hb Sβ° thal or Hb Sβ^{+} thal), sickle-C disease (Hb SC), and—most commonly—sickle cell anemia (Hb SS). Adult hemoglobin contains two pairs of polypeptide chains, alpha (α) and beta (β). Each of these hemoglobinopathy syndromes involves the mutated sickle hemoglobin (Hb S), which differs from normal hemoglobin (Hb A) by the substitution of a single amino acid, valine, for glutamic acid at the sixth position of the beta-globin chain (Driscoll, 2007).

SCD is a complex, chronic inflammatory condition characterized by hemolysis and vasoocclusion. Red blood cells (RBCs) that contain normal hemoglobin are pliable, biconcave discs with a life span of approximately 120 days. When deoxygenated, RBCs containing predominantly Hb S polymerize and form microtubules (i.e., rods) that distort the shape of the cell, characteristically to a crescent or sickle shape (Driscoll, 2007). In this form the cell is rigid and friable, causing vasoocclusion in the small vessels of the circulatory system. Hypoxia and acidosis, which may be caused by fever, infection, dehydration, or other factors, are known to induce this change in shape (Figure 40-1). Many times, however, the RBC changes shape without apparent provocation. To a limited degree, this change in shape is reversible, though not indefinitely. These cells eventually become irreversibly sickled cells (ISCs) with a life span of approximately 10 to 20 days. The fragility and shortened life span of these RBCs lead to chronic anemia, which serves as a stimulus for the bone marrow to create new RBCs, resulting in an elevated reticulocyte count. These stress reticulocytes have adhesion molecules that are expressed on their surfaces, contributing to adhesion onto the vascular endothelium. This sets in motion a cycle of abnormal adhesion–inflammation–increased adhesion that is continually occurring (Redding-Lallinger & Knoll, 2006). The vasoocclusion and hemolysis described previously are the hallmarks of sickle cell disease contributing to the complications that can occur in multiple organs of the body.

Fetal hemoglobin (Hb F) predominates from 10 weeks after conception through the remainder of gestation and normally begins to decline at 34 weeks. Hb F makes up 60% to 80% of the total hemoglobin at birth and declines to normal adult levels (1% to 2%) by 6 to 9 months of age (Frenette & Atweh, 2007). The remaining 20% to 40% of hemoglobin found at birth has the adult electrophoresis forms, Hb A and Hb A$_2$ or Hb S, if found to be affected. Hb F does not sickle, so it is unusual to find clinical manifestations of

the condition with significant amounts of Hb F. Because of this phenomenon, manifestations of SCD may not be clinically apparent until 4 to 6 months of age or later.

SCD has an autosomal recessive inheritance pattern. Both parents must carry some type of abnormal hemoglobin (i.e., one or both of them must carry sickle hemoglobin) for the condition to be manifested in their child. Carriers of SCD are described as having sickle cell trait (Hb AS). When two individuals, each of whom has sickle cell trait, elect to have a child, there is a 25% chance that they will have a child with sickle cell anemia (Hb SS). These individuals also have a 50% chance of having a child with sickle cell trait (Hb AS) and a 25% chance of having a child with entirely normal hemoglobin (Hb AA) with each pregnancy (Figure 40-2). Fifty states, the District of Columbia, the Virgin Islands, and Puerto Rico are now performing routine newborn screening for hemoglobinopathies, but screening is only available on request in six of these states (National Newborn Screening and Genetics Resource Center, 2008). Newborn screening identifies approximately 2000 infants per year with sickle cell hemoglobinopathies (Lane & Buchanan, 2002). Most screening programs use isoelectric focusing (IEF) of an elute from paper impregnated with blood that is used to screen for phenylketonuria, hypothyroidism, and other disorders, although some states rely on high-performance liquid chromatography (HPLC) or cellulose acetate electrophoresis. Most programs require a second test to verify accuracy of the diagnosis.

Incidence and Prevalence

SCD is one of the most common genetic conditions and is most often seen in individuals of African descent but is also found in other ethnic groups, including those from the Caribbean, Mediterranean, Arabian Peninsula, and India. In the United States, 1 in 12 black individuals (African Americans) is a carrier of the sickle cell gene, and 1 in 600 actually manifests the condition. In the United States, 70,000 people have sickle cell disease with 1000 babies being born with the condition annually (Centers for Disease Control and Prevention [CDC], 2008b).

Diagnostic Criteria

Prenatal diagnosis is available to couples known to be carriers of hemoglobinopathies. Diagnosis may be accomplished via chorionic villi sampling during the first trimester or amniocentesis during the

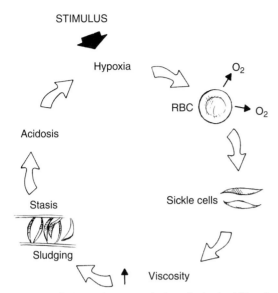

FIGURE 40-1 Cycle causing vasoocclusive episodes in sickle cell anemia. From Hockenberry, M., & Coody, D. (Eds.). (1986). *Pediatric Oncology and Hematology: Perspectives on Care.* St. Louis: Mosby.

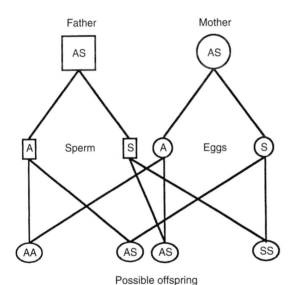

Possible offspring

FIGURE 40-2 Genetics of sickle cell anemia. Both parents possess one gene for normal hemoglobin *(A)* and one for sickle hemoglobin *(S)*. With each pregnancy, there is a 25% statistical chance that the child will have normal hemoglobin *(AA)* and a 25% chance that the child will have sickle cell anemia *(SS)*; 50% of the children will have the sickle cell trait *(AS)*. From Miller, D., & Miller, D. (author) and Baehner, R. (Ed.), (1990). *Blood Diseases of Infancy and Childhood* (6th ed.). St. Louis: Mosby.

second trimester. The method depends on the risks and benefits of the techniques involved; both are adequate to determine the diagnosis. To be beneficial, screening, follow-up, and diagnosis of SCD must be followed with prompt referral to knowledgeable providers of comprehensive care (National Institutes of Health [NIH], Division of Blood Diseases and Resources, 2002).

The sickle "prep," or solubility testing, is often used to screen infants and children for SCD. This test is inexpensive and rapidly performed but is not very specific. A sickle prep result will be positive for sickle cell trait, sickle cell anemia, and other sickle hemoglobinopathies but will not distinguish one from another (Kaye & Committee on Genetics, 2006). The definitive diagnosis of SCD is determined by performing a complete blood count (CBC), peripheral blood smear, and—most important—a quantitative hemoglobin electrophoresis. Measurement of hematologic indices is vitally important in the differential diagnoses of thalassemia syndromes and hemoglobinopathies. It is occasionally helpful to perform hematologic studies on a child's parents to confirm a diagnosis.

Clinical Manifestations at Time of Diagnosis

As a result of current newborn screening programs for hemoglobinopathies, infants are now identified before the onset of acute symptoms (Table 40-1). The anemia from which sickle cell anemia derives its name is broadly characterized as an uncompensated hemolytic anemia, in which a markedly shortened overall RBC survival (i.e., an increased rate of RBC destruction) is insufficiently balanced by the increase in production (i.e., erythropoiesis) to maintain normal levels of total RBC and hemoglobin.

Clinical Manifestations at Time of Diagnosis

NEONATES
- Normal birth weight
- No evidence of hemolytic anemia
- Hemoglobin electrophoresis shows no evidence of Hb A production
- Neonatal jaundice (when present) related to ABO hemolytic disease of the newborn, not to SCD

INFANTS AND TODDLERS
- Development of anemia
- Colic-like symptoms, often associated with feeding difficulties
- Generalized episodes of bone or abdomen pain preceded by acute, febrile infection
- Hand-foot syndrome associated with heat, pain, swelling, erythema
- Splenic hypofunction marked by presence of Howell-Jolly bodies in the blood smear
- Autosplenectomy preceded by splenomegaly in 73% of infants, followed by decrease in size
- Splenomegaly noted frequently during febrile episodes

EARLY CHILDHOOD
- Generalized vasoocclusive crisis (VOC) of bone or abdomen that may or may not be preceded by acute, febrile infection; seemingly triggered by emotional stress or abrupt weather changes
- Usually nonpalpable spleen but sometimes retained in Hb SC disease
- Males may develop priapism
- Biliary colic caused by stasis and gallstones
- Development of cerebral vasculopathy with cerebral infarction

LATE CHILDHOOD
- Gallstones with or without symptoms
- Delayed pubescence
- Females may have increased incidence of VOC with menses, presumably caused by hormonal changes
- Males may develop priapism
- Early signs of sickle retinopathy
- Early signs of sickle nephropathy

TABLE 40-1

Differential Diagnosis of Common Hemoglobinopathies

Clinical Severity	Hemoglobin (g/dL)	Hematocrit (%)	Mean Corpuscular Volume (MCV) (μ^3)	% of Reticulocytes	RBC Morphology*	Solubility Test	Electrophoresis (%)	Distribution of Hbg F
SS Moderate-severe	7.5 (6-11)	22 (18-30)	>80	11 (5-20)	Many ISCs, target cells, nucleated RBCs, normochromic H-J bodies	Positive	>90s <10F <3.6A_2	Uneven
SC Mild-moderate	10 (10-15)	30 (26-40)	75-95	3 (5-10)	Many target cells, aniso-poikilocytosis	Positive	50S 50C <5	Uneven
S/B° THAL Moderate-severe	8.1 (6-10)	25 (20-36)	<80	8 (5-20)	Marked hypochromia, microcytosis and target cells, variable ISCs	Positive	>80 S <20 F >3.5 A_2	Uneven
S/B + THAL Mild-moderate	11 (9-12)	32 (25-40)	<75	3 (5-10)	Mild microcytosis, hypochromia, rare ISCs	Positive	55-75S 15-30A <20F >3.5 A_2	Uneven
S/HP FH† Asymptomatic	14 (12-14)	40 (32-48)	<80	1.5 (1-2)	No ISCs, occasional target cells, and mild hypochromia	Positive	<70 S >30 F <2.5 A_2	Even
AS Asymptomatic	Normal	Normal	Normal	Normal	Normal	Positive	38-45 S 60-55 A 1-3 A_2	Uneven

From Charche, S., Lubin, B., & Reid, C. (1995). *Management and Therapy of Sickle Cell Disease*. NIH Publication No. 95-2117. Washington, DC: U.S. Government Printing Office.
*ICSs, Irreversibly sickled cells.
†*S/HPFH*, Sickle hereditary persistence of fetal hemoglobin.

The "Natural History of Sickle Cell Disease," a hallmark study by Powars (1975), indicated that in the first two decades of life, sickle cell anemia is marked by periods of clinical quiescence and relative physical well-being, interspersed with episodes of acute illness. This classic study supports that these illnesses are treatable by state-of-the-art medical care and are often preventable. The expression of untreated sickle cell anemia is often characterized by septicemia or meningitis (or both) during infancy, followed by cerebral vasculopathy with cerebral infarction during early childhood. Splenic hypofunction is present in nearly 30% of infants with sickle cell anemia by their first birthday and in 90% by age 6 years, accounting for the high risk of sepsis by polysaccharide-encapsulated organisms (Driscoll, 2007).

> **Treatment**
> - Supportive symptomatic care
>   - Aggressive treatment of fever and infection
>   - Maintenance of optimal hydration
>   - Maintenance of body temperature
>   - Penicillin prophylaxis
>   - Pneumococcal immunization
> - Drug therapy with hydroxyurea
> - Selective use of transfusions
> - Hematopoietic stem cell transplant in selected individuals

Treatment

Supportive Symptomatic Care

There is no cure for SCD short of bone marrow transplantation (BMT) (see Chapter 15). Despite the thorough understanding that exists among researchers and clinicians about the inheritance, diagnosis, and pathophysiology of SCD, treatment is essentially supportive and symptomatic. This therapy is aimed at aggressive treatment of infection and maintenance of optimal hydration and body temperature to prevent hypoxia and acidosis. Standard care includes bed rest, hydration, transfusions, analgesics, penicillin prophylaxis, and close follow-up and monitoring with a medical team specializing in sickle cell care. Treatment has moved from care during specific crises to the prevention of sickling episodes.

Drug Therapy with Hydroxyurea

One current method induces production of Hb F with hydroxyurea (HU) (NIH, 2002). HU, an S-phase cytotoxic drug, has been used to treat neoplastic diseases for many years (Driscoll, 2007). This is the first U.S. Food and Drug Administration (FDA)–approved medication for use in adults with SCD. For individuals with SCD, it increases production of Hb F through mechanisms that remain unclear. Expression of Hb F, in combination with the native Hb S, forms a diluted pool of RBCs with Hb F and Hb S. This combination reduces both the polymerization of the cells and the rate of hemolysis. Other observers note that HU decreases production of platelets and white blood cells (WBCs) and increases RBC survival time (Puffer, Schatz, & Roberts, 2007). Additionally, HU decreases cellular adhesion to the endothelium and increases microvascular perfusion (Puffer et al., 2007). Researchers recognize the complex interplay of sickle erythrocytes, leukocytes, vascular endothelium, platelets, plasma clotting factors, and certain mediators of inflammation in producing tissue ischemia and end-organ damage. Clinical trials aimed at modulating the effect of these various players are currently being studied (Frenette & Atweh, 2007).

Pediatric trials of HU therapy report significant improvement in Hb F production, mean corpuscular volume (MCV), and a mild to moderate increase in hemoglobin, which in turn reduces the number of sickle cell crises (Hankins, Ware, Rogers, et al., 2005). Growth failure in children with SCD has long been identified, probably secondary to their hypermetabolic state. Treatment with HU decreases the resting energy expenditure, thus improving the hypermetabolic state with better growth parameters than expected (Hankins et al., 2005). Children with greater than three hospitalizations a year for vasoocclusive crisis (VOC), priapism, or acute chest syndrome are potential candidates for this therapy (Zumberg, Reddy, Boyette, et al., 2005). They are generally started on 15 mg/kg of HU per day, with doses escalating by 5 mg/kg every 8 weeks if no signs or symptoms of toxicity are noted. The maximum dose is usually 30 mg/kg/day or maximum tolerated dose as determined by the health care team (NIH, 2002).

Administration of HU should be managed in a research-oriented practice because there is a theoretic risk of leukemia and a greater rate of deoxyribonucleic acid (DNA) mutations based on in vitro studies (Driscoll, 2007). Clinical observations have not detected an increased rate of cancer in people with sickle cell treated with HU (Hankins et al., 2005). The potential side effects of hydroxyurea (HU), such as myelosuppression of blood cells, particularly the WBCs and platelets, mandate strict monitoring of blood counts. However, the benefits of HU appear to far outweigh the risks as evidenced by the Multicenter Study of Hydroxyurea (MSH) (Steinberg, Barton, Castro, et al., 2003) follow-up observational study of 233 people over a 9-year period. This study demonstrated that HU reduced death rates by as much as 40% and reduced pain crisis, acute chest syndrome, and morbidity by almost half. The Hydroxyurea Safety and Organ Toxicity (HUSOFT) (Ware, Eggleston, Redding-Lallinger, et al., 2002) study indicated that HU therapy given to infants with SCD over a period of 2 years was safe, resulted in improved hematologic parameters, and potentially preserved splenic function. Many centers using HU with children require an informed consent before trial because of lack of FDA approval for this use in pediatrics. HU has the potential of reducing the incidence of both hemolytic and vasoocclusive manifestations of the condition; however, it is not an option for treatment of these complications in the acute setting.

Selective Use of Transfusions

A hallmark study done within the Cooperative Study of Sickle Cell Disease (CSSCD), Stroke Prevention in Sickle Cell Anemia (STOP I), looked at genetic markers, laboratory and radiographic indicators, and clinical findings that were predictive of stroke in this population (Adams, McKie, Hsu, et al., 1998). Over 2000 children, between ages 2 and 16, with Hb SS and Hb S$\beta°$thal were screened by transcranial Doppler (TCD) ultrasound. This noninvasive technique reliably demonstrates cerebral flow abnormalities. In particular, TCD demonstrates that high velocities (i.e., 200 cm/sec) in either the distal intracerebral or middle cerebral arteries are associated with an increased risk of subsequent stroke.

In the STOP I study, those identified with abnormal velocities were randomized to receive either monthly transfusions or no transfusion at all. The risk of stroke, about 10% in SCD, was reduced by 90% in those children treated with transfusions (Adams, 2000). This dramatic finding caused early termination of the study and a recommendation by the National Heart, Lung, and Blood Institute (NHLBI) that all children with Hb SS and Hb S$\beta°$thal be screened with TCD (Adams et al., 1998).

STOP II, using the population identified with abnormal TCD findings, studied the length of time that transfusion therapy is needed to normalize and retain normalization of the TCD findings (Adams & Brambilla, 2005). It also sought to determine if transfusions may be stopped after some period of time when risk of stroke has diminished (NIH, 2002). The study by Adams and Brambilla (2005) found that there is a significant risk of reverting to an abnormal TCD velocity or experiencing an overt stroke if transfusions are discontinued.

Children identified with high velocities are offered scheduled transfusions as a means of preventing stroke and its subsequent consequences. Further studies have indicated that those children with abnormal TCD should also be screened with magnetic resonance imaging (MRI) and magnetic resonance angiography (MRA) (Abboud, Cure, Granger, et al., 2004). Silent infarcts are seen on MRI in a substantial minority of children with SCD, even those with normal neurologic function. The combination of abnormal TCD and silent infarct on MRI further increases the risk of stroke or recurrent silent infarcts (Wang, 2007). These children should be aggressively treated with scheduled transfusion therapy.

In 1995, the CSSCD group completed another hallmark study evaluating preoperative transfusion needs of children with SCD (Koshy, Weiner, Miller, et al., 1995). It is well known that general anesthesia places an individual with SCD at increased risk for stroke, acute chest syndrome, and painful vasoocclusive crisis (Kokoska, West, Carney, et al., 2004). Standard protocol has been to transfuse individuals to a hemoglobin value of 11 g/dL with an Hb S level of 30% before surgery. In the Preoperative Transfusion Study, individuals were transfused to a preoperative level of 10 g/dL with an Hb S level of 60% (Koshy et al., 1995). Results suggest that stable individuals with Hb SS who are undergoing major elective surgery can safely be transfused to the lower level of 10 g/dL. Transfusion with limited phenotypic units of packed red blood cells (PRBCs) would most likely eliminate the alloimmunization observed from E, K, C, and Fy^a RBC phenotypes. There are currently no definitive data available that contraindicate preoperative transfusion in SCD.

Chronic transfusion (either for stroke, abnormal TCD findings, or other diagnostic state) induces iron overload. Chelation therapy to manage this complication must be addressed at the initiation of transfusions and again when the child shows evidence of iron overload (Wang, 2007). An alternative approach is transfusion by erythrocytapheresis (Nuss, Cole, Orsini, et al., 2008). In this method, sickled cells are selectively removed and replaced with normal red cells via a rapid, continuous-flow system that is similar to the production of pheresed units of platelets. Because normal erythrocytes are exchanged for sickled erythrocytes, the net gain of iron is greatly reduced or eliminated. Although this costly approach has merit, its application continues to be limited to a few sickle cell centers in the United States (Wang, 2007).

In the past, chelation treatment (removal of iron overload) has been very time intensive and compliance has often been very difficult to maintain. Traditional therapy included overnight infusion of deferoxamine (Desferal) multiple nights per week. An oral chelation agent, deferasirox (Exjade), was approved by the FDA in November 2005 (Lindsey & Olin, 2007). Extra iron binds to the drug, which then facilitates its removal from the body's circulation. The iron is primarily excreted in the feces. Exjade should be taken on an empty stomach at least 30 minutes before food, preferably at the same time every day. Occasional auditory and ocular disturbances have been reported with Exjade; therefore hearing and vision screening and follow-up are recommended while this medication is in use.

Hematopoietic Stem Cell Transplant

From a preventive point of view, providing genetic counseling for those individuals with sickle cell trait, prenatal diagnosis for pregnant women who are at risk for delivering a child with SCD, and education for parents of children newly diagnosed is the standard of care. As awareness has grown regarding the benefits of umbilical cord blood salvage, large-scale banking has begun in Europe and the United States (Kotz, 2007). The Sibling Cord Blood Donor Program (www.chori.org/Services/Sibling_Donor_Cord_Blood_Program/indexcord.html) in Oakland, California, currently offers free storage of cord blood for families considering the option of cord blood transplant.

Currently, hematopoietic stem cell transplant (HSCT) is the only intervention that can cure sickle cell disease. This approach is limited because only 24% of individuals have a human leukocyte antigen (HLA)–matched donor sibling. The National Marrow Donor Program is attempting to expand its minority representation with extensive recruitment. A total of less than 400 transplants are reported in the Center for International Blood and Marrow Transplant Research database despite having 70,000 persons afflicted with SCD in the United States (Shenoy, 2007). Eighty-eight percent of transplants are from HLA-matched sibling donors and 84% are younger than 16 years of age at transplant; graft rejection occurred in 9% (Shenoy, 2007). Overall survival after HSCT is 93%. Eighty-five percent of those surviving are sickle cell free (Bhatia & Walters, 2008).

Researchers are investigating the use of umbilical cord blood, unrelated donor cord blood, and mismatched related donors as alternative avenues for seeking donors (Reed & Vichinsky, 2001). Hematopoietic mixed chimerism, whereby a mix of donor cells and host cells remains after transplant, may be effective in ameliorating or eliminating the symptoms of SCD. Although this technique is not curative, mixed chimerism may be a suitable endpoint for stem cell therapies primarily because it prevents intravascular hemolysis (Wu, Gladwin, Tisdale, et al., 2007). In general, children selected for transplant demonstrate a morbid course of disease but not to the extent of irreversible organ damage, which would reduce chances for success; eligibility criteria are listed in Box 40-1.

Another consideration that limits this treatment approach is the morbidity associated with BMT, including risks for death, organ impairment, curtailed sexual function, and impaired motor and psychological function (see Chapter 15). Toxicity associated with transplant has been lessened by reducing the intensity of the pretransplant conditioning regimen (Locatelli, 2006). Other considerations include disturbance of family systems, cost-benefit ratios, the rights of siblings, and therapeutic adherence (Conboy, O'Brien, & Lowther, 2006). BMT options must be decisions shared by the health care workers and the family; differences in cultural background between the two, however, may impede the ability to negotiate informed consent (Conboy et al., 2006). Additionally, psychological screening and counseling of children and their families before and after transplant is critical for optimum psychosocial support (Vrijmoet-Wiersma & Koopman, 2006).

Complementary and Alternative Therapies

Researchers and those affected by SCD have long pondered why the severity of vasoocclusive crisis (VOC) seems to be more virulent in modern countries as compared with the disease evidenced by native Africans. Incidental reports of a native African yam that exhibits modulating powers to reduce the pain suffered by those afflicted with VOC have been anecdotally noted. Some community organizations thus suggest ingestion of yams as a preventive effort

---

BOX 40-1

Sickle Cell Disease: Eligibility for Pediatric Transplant

INCLUSIONS
- Children <16 years of age with sickle cell disease (Hb SS, Hb S, Hb Sβ° thalassemia)
- One or more of the following complications
  - Stroke or central nervous system event lasting longer than 24 hours
  - Impaired neuropsychological function and abnormal cerebral MRI
  - Recurrent acute chest syndrome or stage I or II sickle lung disease
  - Recurrent vasoocclusive painful episodes, or recurrent priapism
  - Sickle nephropathy (glomerular filtration rate [GFR]—30% to 50% of predicted normal)
  - Osteonecrosis of multiple joints
- Other considerations
  - RBC alloimmunization (≥2 antibodies) on chronic transfusion
  - Increased cerebral arterial velocity by transcranial Doppler

EXCLUSIONS
- Children older than 16 years of age
- HLA-nonidentical donor
- One or more of the following conditions
  - Lanzky performance score <70%
  - Acute hepatitis or biopsy evidence of cirrhosis
  - Renal impairment with GFR <30% of predictive normal
  - Stage III or IV of sickle lung disease

From European School of Haematology. (2006). *Handbook on disorders of iron homeostasis, erythrocytes and erythropoiesis.* Available at www.ironcurriculum.esh.org/activity/189103 chapter 13.pdf. Retrieved May 15, 2008.

despite lack of scientific studies. Part of the confusion regarding its effectiveness is confounded by the steep infant mortality rate experienced by African populations either from SCD, human immunodeficiency virus (HIV), or other infectious agents. Increased publicity surrounding "Noni" juice, a derivative of native herbs, as a preventive agent for VOC has recently been noted. This intervention is popular with families coming from Caribbean countries. As with African yams, no scientific studies have been recorded.

Massage, acupuncture, prayer, and relaxation techniques are effective as complementary therapies for pain associated with SCD. Most often these interventions are used in conjunction with pharmacologic agents. Inadequate insurance coverage of these interventions is a recurring barrier for many families (Yoon & Black, 2006). Nonpharmacologic forms of pain relief are useful adjuncts to pharmacologic therapy. Self-hypnosis, biofeedback, and distraction are particularly helpful, but must be taught to the child before a pain episode.

Anticipated Advances in Diagnosis and Management

Many other new treatment alternatives are being studied. These include, but are not limited to, butyric acid, clotrimazole, and nitric oxide. One of the main focuses of current research is related to the effects of SCD, inflammation, and cellular adhesion on the vascular endothelium (Telen, 2007).

Agents able to promote antisickling are also a very important part of current research. Butyrate is a short-chain fatty acid that has been shown to stimulate fetal hemoglobin production. Intermittent intravenous infusions effectively sustained Hb F response in some people, thus decreasing the amount of cells likely to sickle (Frenette & Atweh, 2007). Decitabine is another agent that has been found to increase Hb F and total hemoglobin when administered subcutaneously. Further studies are indicated (Saunthararajah, Hillery, Lavelle, et al., 2003).

Clinical trials are also looking into compounds to decrease sickle cell dehydration. Hydration of the red blood cell inhibits sickling and keeps overall hemoglobin concentration lower. Clotrimazole is routinely used to treat fungal infections but has been noted to prevent the loss of water from a RBC, and has shown in human pilot studies to increase RBC potassium content and slightly improve hemoglobin levels (Telen, 2007).

Nitric oxide plays a significant role in regulating vascular tone, cellular adhesion, and platelet aggregation (Weiner, Hibberd, Betit, et al., 2003). A trial of inhaled nitric oxide in children with VOC noted efficacy in pain control versus placebo use. Vasoactive drugs are key in advancing the treatment of painful episodes in children with SCD (Mack & Kato, 2006).

Gene therapy is a promising therapy in SCD that is being studied in many ways (Frenette & Atweh, 2007). It is being investigated as a means to inactivate the sickle gene, to increase expression of the gene for Hb F, or to introduce genes whose products can inhibit the polymerization of Hb S.

Associated Problems of Sickle Cell Disease and Treatment

Associated problems are primarily caused by the following: (1) vasoocclusion, a blockage of small blood vessels secondary to the clumping of sickled RBCs and increased adhesion of other circulating cells that causes tissue ischemia; and (2) hemolytic anemia and the resulting chronic hemolysis. The consequences of this vasoocclusion and chronic hemolysis lead to a state of chronic vasculopathy affecting nearly every organ in the body (Figure 40-3).

> **Associated Problems of Sickle Cell Disease and Treatment**
>
> - Functional asplenia
> - Acute splenic sequestration
> - Neurologic problems
> - Vasoocclusive crisis
> - Acute chest syndrome
> - Transient red cell aplasia
> - Hemolysis
> - Renal problems
> - Priapism
> - Skeletal changes
> - Ophthalmologic changes
> - Audiologic problems
> - Leg ulcers
> - Preparation for anesthesia, contrast medium
> - Cardiac problems
> - Hepatobiliary problems
> - Transfusion complications
>   - Formation of antibodies
>   - Iron overload
>   - Blood-borne pathogens

Functional Asplenia

Splenic function is normal at birth in infants with SCD, but by 6 months of age a state of splenic dysfunction develops, most likely as a result of massive infarction. By 1 year of age, approximately 30% of children with SCD have functional asplenia; 90% have functional asplenia by age 6 (Driscoll, 2007). Palpation of the spleen on physical examination is not an indication of splenic function. A palpable spleen in older children is thought to be the result of fibrosis and is almost exclusively found in individuals with Hb SC disease. The presence of Howell-Jolly bodies (e.g., "pocked cells") on blood smear confirms the condition of functional asplenia.

Splenic malfunction and failure to make specific immunoglobulin G (IgG) antibodies to polysaccharide antigens contribute to unusual susceptibility to infection. Without adequate splenic function, children with SCD are at high risk for infection from organisms such as *Streptococcus pneumoniae, Haemophilus influenzae,* and *Neisseria meningitides* (Driscoll, 2007). The advent of pneumococcal and *Haemophilus* influenza immunizations has significantly reduced this risk (Halasa, Shankar, Talbot, et al., 2007). Less common causes of bacteremia include other streptococci, *Escherichia coli, Staphylococcus aureus,* and gram-negative bacteria such as *Klebsiella* species, *Salmonella* species, and *Pseudomonas aeruginosa.* Other organisms associated with frequent infections in sickle cell anemia include *Mycoplasma* and *Chlamydia pneumoniae.* These organisms are often responsible for symptoms of pneumonia or acute chest syndrome, and human parvovirus B19 is often responsible for aplastic crisis in children with SCD (Wilson, Krishnamurti, & Kamat, 2003). Furthermore, those children chronically transfused have iron overload and become more susceptible to organisms such as *Yersinia enterocolitica,* as well as other

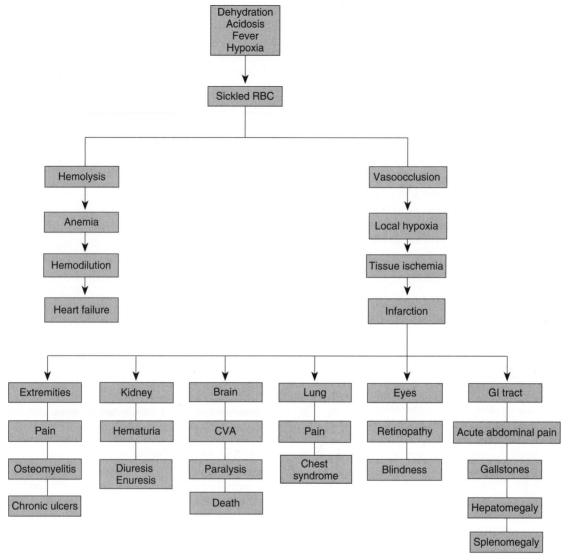

FIGURE 40-3 Tissue effects of sickle cell anemia. From Hockenberry, M., & Wilson, D. (2006). *Nursing Care of Infants and Children* (8th ed.). St. Louis: Mosby.

blood-borne pathogens seen in other transfused populations (Leclercq, Martin, Vergnes, et al., 2005).

Intervention should be threefold: (1) aggressive management of infectious episodes; (2) timely immunization (including HiB and pneumococcal vaccines [i.e., Prevnar and Pneumovax]); and (3) antibiotic prophylaxis. Because current pneumococcal vaccines do not cover all pathogenic strains, antibiotic prophylaxis is the standard of care for all young children with SCD and should be started at the time of diagnosis—preferably by 2 months of age (American Academy of Pediatrics Committee on Infectious Diseases [AAP], 2006). The usual doses for penicillin V or G are 125 mg twice daily for children under 3 years of age and 250 mg twice daily for those over 3 years of age. For children who are not adherent with oral antibiotic therapy at home, 1.2 million units of long-acting penicillin may be given intramuscularly every 3 weeks (AAP, 2006). If an individual is allergic to penicillin, erythromycin (20 mg/kg) may be substituted.

Some experts have recommended amoxicillin (20 mg/kg/day) or trimethoprim-sulfamethoxazole (4 mg/kg/day trimethoprim [TMP] to 20 mg/kg/day sulfamethoxazole [SMX]) for children under 5 years of age (AAP, 2006). As with other children taking antibiotics, the potential for fungal infections, gastrointestinal upset, and allergy exists.

The number of cases of penicillin-resistant invasive pneumococcal infections and the presence of nasopharyngeal carriage for those on penicillin prophylaxis may indicate that penicillin is no longer as effective at preventing invasive pneumococcal infections. The age at which prophylaxis should be discontinued is often an empirical decision (AAP, 2006). The landmark report of the Prophylactic Penicillin Study II established guidelines for discontinuing prophylaxis at 5 years of age (Falletta, Woods, Verter, et al., 1995). These guidelines continue to be standard of care and include the following: (1) children receiving regular medical attention; (2) those with no history of prior severe pneumococcal infection; and (3) those without surgical splenectomy. Consistent with these guidelines, all children having surgical splenectomies or a history of pneumococcal sepsis must continue penicillin prophylaxis indefinitely. Parents must be counseled to always seek immediate medical assistance with all febrile episodes.

Acute Splenic Sequestration Complication

In acute splenic sequestration complication (ASSC), blood flow into the spleen is adequate, but the vascular outflow system from the spleen to the systemic circulation is occluded. This occlusion results in a large collection of blood pooling in the spleen, causing significant enlargement. The systemic circulation may then be deprived of its needed blood volume, causing shock and cardiovascular collapse. The acute illness is associated with a hemoglobin level 2 g/dL or more below the child's baseline value with an acutely enlarged spleen (Lane & Buchanan, 2002). Children with Hb SS are susceptible to this at an early age (i.e., at under 5 years). Those with other variants of the disease may continue to be at risk until their teenage years because they maintain splenic circulation longer than children with Hb SS. Parents can be taught to palpate and measure their child's spleen using a simple measuring device such as a calibrated tongue blade (Figure 40-4). Knowledge of the child's steady state spleen size is essential in determining appropriate diagnosis and treatment during an acute event.

Management of ASSC necessitates hospitalization with immediate therapy, including transfusion. If shock is present, systemic circulation must be supported with fluids. Once adequate circulation is reestablished, however, the volume of fluid previously sequestered in the spleen is returned to the circulation, and circulatory overload must be avoided. In children with life-threatening episodes, splenectomy is recommended or else these children are placed on a chronic transfusion program (NIH, 2002). It is optimal to splenectomize a child after age 2 years. In contrast to the acute episodes, some children develop chronic, massive splenomegaly. Splenectomy is indicated in these children when pressure or pain from the enlarged spleen is evident or accompanied by thrombocytopenia, neutropenia, or severe anemia.

Neurologic Problems

The vasculature of the brain is subject to vasoocclusive episodes in children with SCD. The estimated age of the first cerebrovascular accident (CVA) differs significantly for children with Hb SS and Hb SC. The chances of a child with Hb SS having a first overt stroke by age 10 years is estimated at 11%, and the incidence of silent infarcts is approximately 17% in this same population (Wang, 2007). The estimated risk for a child with Hb SC is 3% (Wang). The risk factors are varied and continue to be identified. These factors include children with more severe anemia, low steady state hemoglobin levels, recent history of acute chest syndrome (ACS), elevated systolic blood pressure, low circulating oxygen levels, and asthma (Wang).

A transient ischemic attack (TIA) occurs when a blood vessel is partially occluded by a small embolus or vessel spasm. The manifestations may be focal and last less than 24 hours without residual deficit. A study by Miller, Macklin, Pegelow, and colleagues (2001) concluded that TIA was not an identified risk factor for stroke after accounting for the presence of silent infarcts. However, the general recommendation is that all children with recurrent TIAs receive the appropriate therapy for stroke prevention (i.e., chronic transfusion therapy).

When the affected vessel is completely occluded by thrombus or embolus—with or without narrowing of the vessel lining—a CVA occurs. Intracranial hemorrhage is a rare but usually fatal complication that occurs when blood vessel walls are thinned by intravascular sickling and then dilate and rupture. Computed tomography (CT), MRI, and MRA can show infarcts and areas of hemorrhage. MRI provides better detail of ischemia and can also show the patchy white matter abnormal signals that are present in individuals with SCD—both with and without neurologic deficits—and are thought to be due to disease in penetrating arterioles. MRA may show large vessel occlusive disease or aneurysms. It also allows detection of Moya-moya disease, a severe form of cerebral artery stenosis that can occur in Hb SS (Dobson, Holden, Nietert, et al., 2002). Symptoms include hemiparesis, aphasia, visual disturbances, seizures, and altered sensation, alertness, and mentation. Unless the diagnosis is in doubt, the MRI should be deferred until treatment is initiated (NIH, 2002).

Children and adolescents who have experienced an initial stroke have a 60% to 80% incidence of secondary stroke if no intervention is implemented after the first stroke insult (Wang, 2007). Initial treatment consists of an exchange transfusion and hydration.

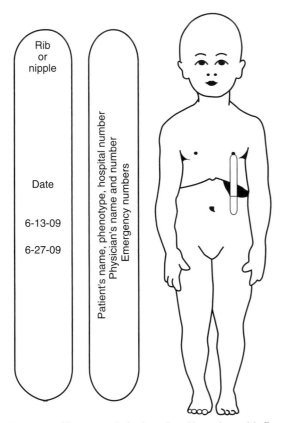

FIGURE 40-4 Measurement of spleen size with a spleen stick. From Eckman, J., & Platt, A. (1991). *Problem Oriented Management of Sickle Syndromes.* Atlanta: NIH Sickle Cell Center.

Hyperthermia increases cerebral metabolism and therefore should be treated. Hypotension is treated to prevent further ischemia. Admission to an intensive care unit (ICU) facilitates the treatment and observation that these children require. Chronic transfusion (every 3 to 4 weeks) therapy is the standard of care to prevent recurrent stroke.

Studies have implicated sickle cell disease itself and the impact of silent infarcts in children with SCD with decreased neurocognitive development (Schatz, 2004; Schatz, Brown, Pascual, et al., 2001). School-age children with SCD who do not show silent infarcts on MRI nevertheless show declining intelligence quotient (IQ) scores in verbal and math achievement scores with increasing age (Wang, Enos, Gallagher, et al., 2001). Eighty percent of children with SCD and stroke will have a cognitive deficit (King, White, McKinstry, et al., 2007). Assessment of neurocognitive development is warranted at an early age with ongoing evaluation of cerebral vessels by TCD for primary stroke prevention with children with Hb SS or Hb Sβthal.

Vasoocclusive Crisis

Painful, vasoocclusive episodes are the most common cause of emergency department visits and hospital admissions for individuals with SCD. Vasoocclusion is a physiologic process, but the resultant pain is a complex biopsychosocial event. Physiologic factors combined with social considerations (e.g., developmental stage, pain history, and family and child coping skills) contribute to the expression of vasoocclusion (Stinson & Naser, 2003). Each child exhibits an individualized pattern of duration, frequency, severity, and location of vasoocclusive crises. The hallmark of these crises is their unpredictability. A few children state that they are always in pain, but a small minority of children and adolescents with SCD account for more than 30% of hospital admissions for pain (Ellison & Shaw, 2007). There are two major kinds of assessment: rapid assessment of the acute episode to focus on pain intensity, prompt treatment, and relief, and comprehensive assessment of chronic pain induced by boney changes (NIH, 2002).

Precipitation of painful episodes in SCD has been related to numerous factors, including weather changes (i.e., warm to cold), stress, and menstrual cycles in females. The frequency of painful episodes is indirectly related to the Hb F level, and numerous painful crises are a prognostic sign for further complications as a result of sickling.

VOCs typically affect the lower back, femur, hips, and knees, although any area in the body or organ is subject to sickling episodes (Ellison & Shaw, 2007). In infants, the metatarsals and metacarpals can be involved resulting in dactylitis, a painful swelling of the hands and feet (Ellison & Shaw, 2007). In long bones, infarcts are most common in the shaft and are usually confined to the medulla. Muscular infarcts occasionally occur with secondary hemorrhage and myonecrosis and are clearly seen on CT and MRI scans. Abdominal pain is often referred pain from other sites and could also be mesenteric in origin. In adolescents, pain involving the vertebral bodies is often manifested.

The optimal treatment for VOCs is multimodal and includes treating any antecedent causes, improving circulation, and providing analgesia (Ballas, 2005). Treatment of antecedent causes includes correcting fever, hypoxia, and acidosis, as well as treating infection and dehydration (Ballas, 2005). History taking includes effective treatments at home, usual drugs, dosages, and side effects

during acute pain, and medications and timing since the onset of acute pain. Primary care providers must be aware that an extraneous illness possibly precipitated a painful episode and the child has two independent problems.

Hydration is an important part of improving circulation to the affected area. Children may be hydrated orally or intravenously with an electrolyte solution. Options for oral hydration include juice, bouillon, water, milk, sports drinks, Pedialyte, and Infalyte. Fluids given intravenously may include a normal saline bolus with care being taken not to tax the cardiovascular system with too large or rapid of a bolus.

Maintenance fluids of 5% dextrose with 0.25% normal saline, adjusted for serum chemistry results (NIH, 2002), should follow. The rate of fluids given should be approximately 1 to 1.5 times the maintenance volume. Circulation to infarcted areas may also be improved by the local application of heat (e.g., heating pad, warm bath, or whirlpool). Once comfort has been established, passive range of motion and massage may be initiated. These children should be encouraged to be as active as possible.

Severe pain should be considered a medical emergency that prompts timely and aggressive management. Analgesia may take several forms, including nonpharmacologic agents, nonsteroidal antiinflammatory drugs (NSAIDs), and oral or parenteral narcotics. Multimodal therapy, which includes several of these approaches, is more effective than single agents because each agent increases analgesia (Ballas, 2005). NSAIDs act on peripheral inflammatory pain receptors, and narcotics act centrally. This combination therapy may also contravene the "ceiling effect" that occurs with nonsteroidal drugs and acetaminophen, as well as have a significant narcotic-sparing effect. The dose given should begin at a standard therapeutic dose or a dose known to be therapeutic for a given child and then adjusted as needed. Placebos are never appropriate because they erode the trusting relationship between the health care provider and child.

Many narcotics have very brief half-lives, and care must be taken to administer them often enough for analgesic effect. For example, when a medication with a 12-hour half-life is used, dosing should be approximately every 2 hours to maintain consistent pain relief (Ellison & Shaw, 2007). Early in the course of a vasoocclusive episode, the vascular occlusion is constant—not intermittent. Therefore, early in the course of a painful episode, as-needed (i.e., prn) dosing is inappropriate; scheduled doses of narcotics should be given over the first 24 hours after admission for VOC. Later in the course, collateral circulation may develop or the occlusion may have decreased, improving vascular circulation to the infarcted area. It is preferable to control a child's pain early in the course of the illness and maintain control by frequent reassessment.

It is inappropriate to administer intramuscular injections to children for pain relief because an injection alone can be quite painful unless it is for a single dose and a longer half-life is desired (e.g., for outpatient management) or if intravenous (IV) access has not been obtained. Intrathecal catheters have been suggested as a route for analgesic administration for children who are hospitalized with severe, intractable pain but should not be considered before an adequate trial of maximal doses of systemic opioid and adjuvant medications are given. Patient-controlled analgesia (PCA) is also recommended if institutions are familiar with its use in children.

Because all pain episodes cannot be prevented, children and their families should be taught to manage mild pain and recognize symptoms that suggest serious problems. For mild pain, nonnarcotic medicines including acetaminophen, aspirin (provided there is no concurrent viral process or other contraindication), ibuprofen, and ketorolac are appropriate and may be given at the standard recommended dosages. Caution should be exercised with the use of NSAIDs in children with renal or liver complications. Optimal management requires adequate education of the child, family, and health care providers.

When children become significantly uncomfortable, they experience anxiety and, consequently, a heightened perception of pain. They may ultimately develop dysfunctional illness behavior as a result of inadequately treated pain. It is important for the child, family, and health care providers to have realistically attainable goals related to pain control. The goal of pain management should be prompt pain relief to a functional level. Relief could be defined as a pain intensity reduction of at least 50% to 60% from the upper end of the pain scale. The alleviation of pain provided by narcotics must be balanced against known side effects such as pruritus, nausea, constipation, and respiratory depression. Hospitalized children are routinely started on stool softeners and laxatives at the onset of opioid therapy and given standing orders for antihistamines for pruritus and antinausea medications. Side effects, such as respiratory depression, should be closely monitored by scheduled visual observations and pulse oximetry.

Several classic studies have documented the low prevalence of drug addiction within this population (Morrison, 1991; Pegelow, 1992). Despite these studies, health care providers continue to believe that drug addiction is a major problem among people with SCD, which is unfortunate because this misperception can interfere with the provision of adequate health care. Tolerance and physical dependence are expected pharmacologic consequences of long-term opioid use and should not be confused with addiction (NIH, 2002).

Acute Chest Syndrome

Acute chest syndrome (ACS) ranks second as a cause for hospitalization and is responsible for 25% of all deaths from SCD. ACS is an illness characterized by a new infiltrate on chest x-ray accompanied by pain, leukocytosis, hypoxia, cough, or fever (Walters, Nienhuis, & Vichinsky, 2002). ACS is a life-threatening complication that results from infection, pulmonary fat embolism, or pulmonary infarction (Lane & Buchanan, 2002). ACS can also be induced by respiratory depression caused by narcotics or general anesthesia. Twenty-five percent of individuals with SCD who undergo major surgery are shown to develop postoperative ACS (Walters et al., 2002).

Fever, cough, and tachypnea are often the only abnormal findings in children. ACS may be difficult to differentiate from and may be concurrent with pneumonia. Physical examination usually reveals tachypnea, but there may also be evidence of pulmonary consolidation, pleural effusion, a new pulmonary infiltrate, or pleural friction rub. Thirty-five percent of individuals with ACS will have a normal lung examination (Walters et al., 2002). Chest radiographic studies may be normal for the first few days, especially if a child is dehydrated.

ACS is often a fulminant process and may rapidly progress to pulmonary failure and death. Admission to the ICU may be necessary for close monitoring. Pulse oximetry and vital signs should be followed closely, and supplemental oxygen and further respiratory support should be provided as needed. All children should be encouraged to use scheduled incentive spirometry to fully aerate their lungs. Early transfusion may be necessary to prevent progressive problems because hypoxia will induce further sickling; partial or complete exchange transfusion may be needed (NIH, 2002). Pulmonary consultation is recommended to optimize early and aggressive treatment.

ACS is the most common cause of death in children with SCD. Pulmonary pressures increase during an episode of severe ACS resulting in pulmonary hypertension (pHTN) (Mekontso, Leon, Habibi, et al., 2008). pHTN is detected by echocardiogram (Ambrusko, Gunawardena, Sakara, et al., 2006), is associated with accelerated mortality rate, and is present in about 30% of adults with Hg SS. The prevalence in children with SCD is largely unknown. A recent study indicated that in children with SCD, a history of sepsis, ACS, or obstructive lung disease was a factor associated with pHTN (Michlitsch, Gardner, Vichinsky, et al., 2008). In a recent cohort study, 30% of children with SCD who were 10 years of age or older were found to have pHTN (Pashankar, Carbonella, Bazzy-Assad, et al., 2008). Recent recommendations at many comprehensive sickle cell centers include obtaining an echocardiogram annually after age 10 (Nelson, Adade, McDonough, et al., 2007). Frequent episodes of ACS and painful events are associated with shorter life spans (NIH, 2002). A study by Quinn, Shull, Ahmad, and colleagues (2007) showed that an episode of ACS in the first 3 years of life predicts recurrent ACS throughout childhood. Since ACS may be difficult to differentiate from pneumonia, primary care providers should empirically use antibiotics directed against *S. pneumoniae, H. influenzae, S. aureus,* and other pathogens commonly seen in community-acquired pneumonia.

Transient Red Cell Aplasia (formerly Aplastic Crisis)

Periodically, the bone marrow does not respond to a fall in hemoglobin and hematocrit values caused by the rapid turnover of RBCs. The hemoglobin and hematocrit values drop, and there is a lack of compensatory rise in the reticulocyte count that usually happens during or following a viral infection. Symptoms may include fever, more severe anemia than usual, headache, fatigue, and dyspnea, and the child may have signs of respiratory involvement or gastrointestinal involvement. Human parvovirus B19 has been implicated in 70% to 100% of episodes of transient red cell aplasia (TRCA) (NIH, 2002). Children being cared for during and shortly after a viral illness should be observed for unusual pallor or prolonged lethargy. Therapy includes slow transfusion to a hemoglobin level slightly above the baseline hemoglobin level. Recovery is indicated by a return of reticulocytosis.

Hemolysis

Hemolysis in SCD is usually of only moderate severity. The symptoms of anemia (e.g., pallor, fatigue, dyspnea) are not the hallmarks of this disorder. Hemolysis is generally associated with clinical observations of scleral icterus, tea-colored urine, and elevated bilirubin and urobilinogen levels. One long-term consequence of hemolysis is the high prevalence of gallstones in children with SCD. Pigmented gallstones develop in approximately 30% of children with SCD by age 18 (Wilson et al., 2003). Increased hemolysis may be triggered by bacterial infections, poisons, or glucose-6-phosphate dehydrogenase (G6PD) deficiency. Hemolysis accompanied by a brisk reticulocytosis requires no treatment.

Renal Problems

The environment within the renal medulla is characterized by low oxygen tension, acidosis, and hypertonicity. Therefore intravascular sickling occurs more rapidly in the kidney than in any other organ. Persistent proteinuria, beginning early in life, is the hallmark of sickle nephropathy that occurs in all forms of SCD, and is associated with severity of disease (Fitzhugh, Wigfall, & Ware, 2005). This intravascular sickling leaves the kidney with a relative inability to concentrate urine (i.e., hyposthenuria) or adequately acidify urine, which is an early sign of end-stage renal disease. The relative inability to concentrate urine often leads to enuresis or nocturia and also results in a relative inability to excrete potassium and uric acid.

Renal failure as a result of progressive sickle cell nephropathy affects 4% to 20% of adults with SCD (McKie, Hanevold, Hernandez, et al., 2007). Early detection of proteinuria may indicate the need for therapy to prevent chronic, progressive renal insufficiency (Fitzhugh et al., 2005). Several studies have shown that the presence of microalbuminuria precedes proteinuria and serves as an early marker for glomerular injury in SCD (Fitzhugh et al., 2005; McKie et al., 2007). The use of enalapril has been shown to reduce urinary protein excretion and normalize serum albumin. Combination therapy with hydroxyurea (HU) has been shown to further normalize the urine protein/creatinine ratio (Fitzhugh et al., 2005).

Gross hematuria may occur in children with SCD or sickle trait. Blood loss is usually minimal, resolving within 1 to 3 days with bed rest and hydration, and does not require transfusion. As with all individuals with gross hematuria, diagnoses of glomerulonephritis, tumor, renal stones, urinary tract infection, and bleeding disorders must be excluded. When other diagnoses have been eliminated, hematuria is often attributed to areas of ischemia or necrosis caused by sickled cells. Renal papillary necrosis, renal infarction, and perinephric hematoma (secondary to infarction) are all reported.

Priapism

Males with sickle cell anemia are subject to episodes of priapism. Priapism occurs when an accumulation of sickled cells obstructs the venous drainage of the corpora cavernosa of the penis, causing a prolonged and exquisitely painful erection of the penis. Priapism is not associated with sexual desire or excitement (Wilson et al., 2003). In addition, micturition is often difficult, and urinary retention may occur. If left untreated, irreversible fibrosis and impotency may occur. MRI is useful in demonstrating corporal destruction with development of intracorporeal fibrosis and hemosiderin deposition.

The mean age at manifestation is 12 years and by age 20, approximately 89% of all males with SCD will have experienced one or more episodes of priapism (Wilson et al., 2003). The following two general patterns of priapism are described:

1. Stuttering (recurrent) attacks lasting less than 3 hours that may precede a severe episode
2. Severe attacks lasting longer than 3 hours that may lead to impotence

At the onset, the child should be counseled to urinate (a full bladder aggravates priapism), drink extra fluids, and use oral analgesics (Maples & Hageman, 2004). Treatment of severe episodes also begins with conservative measures and after 3 hours includes progression to hospitalization, hydration, transfusions, pain management, and urologic consultation. Application of ice is inappropriate because it promotes vasoconstriction. Surgical intervention is considered if there is no detumescence after 4 to 6 hours of conservative treatment (NIH, 2002). Surgical measures aim to reestablish adequate venous outflow and circulation of the corporal body via aspiration and—if not successful—placement of a shunt (Wilson et al., 2003).

Prophylactic regimens include the addition of vasodilatory drugs including hydralazine and pseudoephedrine, alpha agonists and beta agonists, and chronic transfusion programs (Wilson et al., 2003). Despite intervention, impotence is a frequent complication of priapism. Research is currently looking into new pharmacologic agents, as well as improved surgical interventions, to address this troublesome complication (Maples & Hageman, 2004).

Skeletal Changes

SCD involves both hematologic and osseous abnormalities because it affects the two major functions of bone tissue: hematopoiesis and osteogenesis. Skeletal changes, such as dactylitis, which was previously discussed, occur as a result of expansion of the bone marrow and recurrent infarction in children with SCD. Back pain is common in older children and is recognized on radiographs by "fish-mouthed" vertebrae, which have decreased vertical height and increased width (Mulligan, 2004).

Sudden infarction causes acute symptoms of pain and must be differentiated from those of bacterial origin. Osteomyelitis is the second most common infection in children with SCD with *Salmonella* osteomyelitis occurring several hundred times more often in SCD as compared with the general pediatric population. It also accounts for 70% of bone infections in children with SCD (Wong, Skamoto, & Johnson, 2001). Common sites include the long bones and vertebral bones. Common symptoms consist of pain, warmth, and swelling, as well as limitation of motion to the affected area.

The pathophysiology of bone "erosions" in sickle cell anemia results from necrosis produced by repeated microinfarction. Repeated infarction may lead to avascular necrosis. This pathology most commonly involves the head of the femur but may also occur in the head of the humerus or fibula. Treatment includes physical therapy (PT) and judicious use of local heat and analgesics for pain relief (Shannon & Trousdale, 2004). A recent study evaluating PT alone compared with PT and surgical core decompression concluded that PT alone was as effective as core decompression and PT at improving hip function (Neumayr, Aguilar, Earles, et al., 2006). Both of these procedures are seen as temporary measures to forestall an eventual total hip replacement. There have been no prospective, randomized studies to assess safety or efficacy of these measures (NIH, 2002).

Ophthalmologic Changes

Ophthalmologic complications are a direct result of the vasoocclusive process within the eye. Because early stages of eye disease do not result in visual symptoms, they may go undiagnosed unless an eye examination is performed by an ophthalmologist. Most screenings begin at age 8 or 9, when the child is able to cooperate, although most defects occur during the second decade of life (Lane & Buchanan, 2002). These complications include nonproliferative retinopathy, proliferative retinopathy, and elevated intraocular pressure in the presence of hyphema. Nonproliferative retinopathy may not affect visual acuity. Proliferative sickle retinopathy can cause vitreous hemorrhage and subsequent retinal detachment and blindness. The occurrence of proliferative sickle retinopathy depends on an individual's age and type of hemoglobinopathy, and is progressive. Studies have confirmed that the risk of proliferative retinopathy is higher in Hb SC disease than it is in Hb SS disease (Downes, Hambleton, Chuang, et al., 2005). Individuals with sickle hemoglobinopathies who sustain blunt trauma and subsequent hyphema to the eye may quickly develop increased intraocular pressure, which is an ophthalmologic emergency (NIH, 2002).

Audiologic Problems

Vasoocclusive episodes within the circulation of the inner ear and the administration of ototoxic drugs may cause sensorineural hearing loss. This loss may be unilateral or bilateral but is generally manifested as a high-frequency deficit. A classic study by Gentry and Dancer (1997) showed a 12% failure rate in hearing as compared with a 1.6% rate in normal controls. As expected with hearing loss, speech screening should be implemented. Their findings showed that 10% of children with SCD had either an articulation disorder or a fluency disorder at a rate higher than expected.

Leg Ulcers

Leg ulcers are experienced by 25% to 75% of older children and adults with SCD, and are painful, indolent, and disfiguring (Trent & Kirsner, 2004). There is an increased risk in tropical regions, in males, and in those with a low hematocrit. Hb F appears to be protective (Kato, McGowan, Machado, et al., 2006). Trauma is believed to be a common cause of leg ulcers in SCD. Anemia, thrombocytosis, and venous incompetence are also thought to be contributing factors. Sickle cell ulcers classically appear as round, punched-out ulcers with raised margins, deep bases, and necrotic slough and can produce significant pain and limit movement (Trent & Kirsner, 2004). Those individuals with a history of ulcers have close to a 25% higher risk of developing future ulcerations (Trent & Kirsner). Early, prompt treatment includes bed rest, elevation, and wound care with antibiotics for cellulitic areas, but skin grafting and transfusion therapy may also be needed. The specific type of wound care is controversial and should be directed by a competent plastic surgeon.

Preparation for Anesthesia or Contrast Medium (Surgery or Radiologic Studies)

General anesthesia and hyperosmolar contrast medium are both known to induce sickling (Kokoska et al., 2004). If an operative or diagnostic procedure using these agents is anticipated, most hematologists suggest that children with SCD receive transfusion to a hemoglobin level of 10 g/dL. Children with Hb SC usually carry this hemoglobin value at baseline and most likely would not require a transfusion. Unusually high-risk children are the exception to this rule. All children undergoing tonsillectomies and adenoidectomies should be transfused, because these surgeries appear to be more serious for the child with SCD as a result of associated blood loss, fluid loss, and inability to orally hydrate (NIH, 2002). Additional measures such as warming the operating room, warming the IV fluids, or placing the child on a warming blanket during surgery are warranted (Kokoska et al., 2004). Aggressive hydration with intravenous fluids at 1 to 1½ times the maintenance rate given 8 to 24 hours before surgery is recommended.

Cardiac Problems

Over time the cardiovascular system accommodates to chronic anemia with increased cardiac output (Castro, Hoque, & Brown, 2003). This chronic volume overload causes cardiac enlargement. Although dilation and hypertrophy often occur, systolic and diastolic performance of the left ventricle in the resting state are usually preserved (NIH, 2002). Cardiac enlargement is often apparent on chest radiograph, the precordium is hyperactive, and a low-grade systolic ejection murmur may be heard in the second and third left intercostal spaces on examination. Cardiomegaly is an adaptation to anemia and alone should not be considered pathologic. Children with sickle cell anemia are subject to the same medical conditions as other children; therefore findings suggestive of congenital, rheumatic, or underlying heart disease should be investigated. In such cases, an echocardiogram and cardiac consultation are recommended. Machado, Kyle, Martyr, and colleagues (2007) report increased pulmonary pressures during exercise that may contribute to morbidity and mortality risk in individuals with SCD.

Hepatobiliary Problems

Biochemical and radiologic hepatic abnormalities are common in individuals with SCD. The ongoing elevated rate of RBC hemolysis generates an increase in serum bilirubin (Friedman, 2007). Likewise, elevations of the serum alkaline phosphatase and lactic dehydrogenase levels as a result of bone metabolism and hemolysis are often seen. Elevation in the serum alkaline phosphatase is common, particularly during pain crises. Children who have right upper quadrant pain, increased jaundice, and fever need careful evaluation and management (Box 40-2). Crisis pain involving the liver is often indistinguishable from acute cholecystitis. Transfused children are at risk for viral hepatitis and hepatic hemosiderosis, which can result in hepatic injury and fibrosis (Traina, Jorge, Yamanaka, et al., 2007).

Gallstones of bile or calcium bilirubinate are a common finding and easily seen via ultrasound. These gallstones are found in 14% to 30% of children with SCD and are most common in individuals with Hb SS (NIH, 2002). Ultrasonography indicates the onset of cholelithiasis as early as 2 to 4 years of age with increasing symptoms as the child gets older (Wilson et al., 2003).

Surgeons should be aware of the finding that concomitant common bile duct (CBD) stones have been reported in individuals with SCD and cholelithiasis. Both laparoscopic and open cholecystectomies are approved for individuals with SCD given that appropriate preoperative preparation is addressed (Friedman, 2007).

BOX 40-2

Common Sources of Abdominal Pain in Sickle Cell Anemia

- Gallstones
- Enlarged spleen/splenic sequestration
- Vasoocclusive crisis
- Hepatitis
- Biliary sludge
- Small bowel necrosis
- Pancreatic sickling
- Cirrhosis of various causes
- Intrahepatic cholestasis

A hepatic crisis (sometimes known as right upper quadrant [RUQ] syndrome or acute sickle hepatic crisis) may be indistinguishable from acute cholecystitis. RBC sequestration in the liver causes hepatocellular dysfunction, which decreases bilirubin excretion. This syndrome is most often self-limited and resolves within 2 weeks with IV fluid hydration and analgesia, but hepatic failure resulting from massive sickling has also been reported (Friedman, 2007).

Transfusion Complications

Individuals with SCD may need transfusions emergently, episodically, or chronically. Performing RBC phenotyping before transfusion avoids the problems associated with the development of RBC antibodies. Children requiring RBC transfusions should be given phenotypically matched units. Several centers have been successful in recruiting minority donors for extended matching for RBC antigens. This matching has markedly decreased the occurrence of alloimmunization and should be the standard for children needing chronic transfusions. The complications of transfusions include possible exposure to blood-borne infectious agents, formation of alloantibodies, and iron overload resulting from chronic or multiple transfusions. Individuals with iron overload experience progressive organ dysfunction, leading to iron-induced cardiac damage and death. Iron load is measured by serum ferritin levels and more specifically by liver biopsy.

Prognosis

In a classic study done over 30 years ago (Powars, 1975), a group of adults and children were longitudinally followed to determine the natural history of SCD. The disease effects in the adults tended to be chronic and organ related and the problems in the children were acute and often infectious. The predicted overall survival in one large cohort of individuals with Hb SS and Hb Sβ°thal at age 18 years was found to be 86%. A study by Reed and Vichinsky (2001) indicated that the overall mortality rate (at least in some regions of the United States) has decreased to less than 2% by age 10. The average longevity in persons with Hb SS genotype is 42 years for men and 48 years for women, whereas men and women with Hb SC genotype live to age 60 and 68 years, respectively (Ashley-Koch, Yang, & Olney, 2000).

Sickle cell disease is characterized by a highly variable phenotype within each genotype leading to varying severity of disease among the population. The CSSCD identified the following factors as predictors of adverse outcomes: lower hemoglobin level, lower Hg F level, increased pain rate, and an increased steady state WBC count (Miller, Sleeper, Pegelow, et al., 2000). This striking variability between genotypes provides another example of the variable presentation of symptoms and complications that must be considered by the primary care provider. Sickle thalassemia is reported to have lower rates of complications and mortality in children who inherit this genetic variant. The beta-globin gene cluster haplotypes further affect the severity of the disorder (Powars et al., 1994).

This information on genotypes assumes urgency in prenatal diagnosis and in making decisions about potentially life-threatening procedures (e.g., BMT). In the former case, the decision to continue a pregnancy can rest on the perceived future clinical course of a child. Factors determining the extremely variable clinical course include the following: (1) genetic factors (e.g., a thalassemia,

β-globin gene haplotypes, heterocellular hereditary persistence of Hb F, and high total hemoglobin); and (2) adherence to suggested clinical guidelines (e.g., penicillin prophylaxis, pneumococcal vaccinations, adequate hydration, and early recognition of life-threatening complications) (Chui & Dover, 2001).

The incidence of invasive pneumococcal disease has decreased by 68% since the advent of the pneumococcal conjugate vaccine (Prevnar) (Adamkiewicz, Silk, Howgate, et al., 2008). Adherence with prophylactic penicillin administration is critical in early years. Davis, Schoendorf, Gergen, and associates (1997) also reported that the survival of children with SCD improved significantly since 1968, but that a substantial number of deaths continue to occur outside the hospital. This finding raises concerns about whether care for acute illness is promptly sought and readily accessible. Improving parental knowledge (Logan, Radcliffe, & Smith-Whitley, 2002) about SCD has proven to correlate with increased use of appropriate and timely medical intervention. As early intervention decreases or eliminates deaths from sepsis, ACS, and splenic sequestration, the primary issue will be chronic organ damage, notably renal, neurologic, and pulmonary changes.

PRIMARY CARE MANAGEMENT

Health Care Maintenance

Growth and Development

When matched with controls of similar socioeconomic status, children with SCD have comparable physical parameters at birth, including weight, length, and head circumference, as well as similar 1- and 5-minute Apgar scores. Classic studies done by Modebe and Ifenu (1993) and Platt (1994) show that—starting at approximately 6 months of age and being clearly defined by the preschool years— those children with Hb SS and Hb Sβ° thal demonstrate a pattern of physical growth that is divergent from that of their unaffected peers. These children are shorter, weigh less, and have a smaller percentage of body fat and delayed bone age. Their muscle mass and head circumference, however, are comparable with those of their unaffected peers. Weight is affected more than height, and males are affected more than females. Later studies concur that physical delays in growth and development are common (Lawrence & Ryan, 2000; Silva & Viana, 2002). Pubertal changes are also delayed for both boys and girls. Normal height is often achieved by adulthood, but weight remains lower than that of controls. Neurodevelopment and skeletal maturation are also delayed (Hogan, Kirkham, Prengler, et al., 2006).

These changes are coincident with the usual physiologic waning of Hb F levels. It has also been noted that the growth of children who, for unknown reasons, persist in producing Hb F is usually not as delayed as that of other children with SCD. Children receiving chronic transfusions, however, maintain age-appropriate growth parameters, which suggests that hemolytic anemia plays a major role in the growth delay in children with sickle cell anemia.

As with standard well-child care, physical growth parameters should be measured and plotted on standardized growth charts every 3 to 4 months (Lane & Buchanan, 2002). The pattern of growth of an individual child, however, is more important than comparison with unaffected children.

Psychosocial researchers have studied the learning abilities, coping skills, anxieties, and self-concepts of unaffected children and those with SCD. Most studies conclude that children with SCD are well adjusted but vulnerable to experiencing impaired academic achievement often with other neuropsychological deficits (Berkelhammer, Williamson, Sanford, et al., 2007). Rates of mental illness in children and adolescents with SCD are no different than with other children from similar backgrounds but without SCD.

Beyond the expected significant psychosocial and intellectual deficits experienced by children with a history of stroke, researchers are now focusing on the incidence of subclinical deficits resulting from cerebral microvascular occlusion that are not apparent on routine neurologic examinations. Seventeen percent of children with SCD show evidence of silent infarct before age 14 years (Wang, 2007). In addition, there is also a 14-fold increase in the risk of clinical infarct if there is evidence of silent infarct (Miller et al., 2001). DeBaun, Schatz, Siegel, and associates (1998) have explored various neurocognitive tests to determine instruments sensitive and specific for identifying children with silent cerebral infarcts. Selected test results indicate impairment with fine and visual motor tasks, as well as with short-term memory skills. One recent meta-analysis concluded that children with SCD that show no silent stroke on MRI have on average a 4.3-point lower IQ score than their matched peers or siblings (Schatz, Finke, Kellet, et al., 2002).

Standardized tools such as the Denver Developmental Screening Test II are helpful when screening for developmental delay (Schatz, McClellan, Puffer, et al., 2008). Children found to be at developmental risk should be referred for a more thorough developmental assessment and connected with developmental services such as Birth to Three..The involvement of a consistent caregiver and the caregiver's rapport with a consistent health care provider are invaluable tools for monitoring developmental progress in children with SCD.

Diet

A child's diet should be well balanced with a generous amount of fluid. Diet during illness or disease exacerbation may include whatever nutritive dense solid foods children desire with oral fluids at one and a half times their usual fluid intake. Maintenance of daily fluid intake is essential in maintaining homeostasis in children with SCD. A fluid sheet, outlining times to increase fluids and amounts of oral fluids to be given, provides a handy reference to parents (Box 40-3).

Because of increased metabolic demands, children with SCD have a relative deficiency of energy, protein, and several micronutrients, so the recommended daily allowances for the normal population may not be applicable. Limited metabolic studies

---

| BOX 40-3 |

Sickle Cell Fluid Requirements

A child needs more fluids when:
1. He or she has a fever.
2. He or she has pain.
3. It's hot outside.
4. He or she is very active.
5. He or she is traveling.

Amount of fluids a child with sickle cell needs each day:
For every 5 lb of weight, child should have 1 cup (8 oz) of fluid.

From AFLAC Children's Cancer and Blood Disorders Service, Children's Healthcare of Atlanta, Atlanta, GA.

---

support the hypothesis that chronic hemolysis leads to a state of high protein turnover and increased metabolic requirements. One controlled study measuring energy expenditure in postpubertal males cited reduced physical activity as the compensatory mechanism for low energy intake that is inadequate to meet their higher metabolic demands, which led to a suboptimal nutritional state (Malinauskas, Sawchak, Koh, et al., 2001). Although reduced physical activity may allow the energy balance to be maintained in the short term, a persistent energy deficit leads to growth retardation.

Pica, the compulsive ingestion of certain nonfood items or nonnutritive substances, is an unusual behavior that has been classically associated with iron deficiency and lead poisoning. There appears to be an unusually high incidence of pica in children with SCD, especially those with low hemoglobin levels and high reticulocyte counts (Ivascu, Sarnaik, McCrae, et al., 2001). Pica can also be an emotional response to the stressors associated with chronic or recurrent pain (Lemanek, Brown, Armstrong, et al., 2002).

Folic acid therapy is recommended for all children with SCD (NIH, 2002). Supplemental iron therapy should not be prescribed unless a child is documented to have reduced iron stores as measured by serum iron, serum ferritin, and iron binding capacity.

Safety

Most children with sickle cell anemia regularly take oral medicines (e.g., folic acid, antibiotics, and narcotics) at home. Ingestion of narcotics beyond the prescribed amount can lead to lethargy and respiratory depression or death. All medicines should be safely stored. Adolescents should be cautioned about driving a car or using machinery while taking narcotics and be counseled that alcohol may potentiate the depressant effects of narcotics. Alcohol should also be avoided because it can cause dehydration and subsequent sickling. Smoking is strongly discouraged because it leads to vasoconstriction and concomitant problems. Parents should be cautioned about allowing exposure to reptiles as pets because of the risk of salmonella exposure (Lane & Buchanan, 2002).

Guidance regarding the importance of supplementing routine hydration in hot temperatures and with viral illnesses is essential. Recreational activities that involve prolonged exposure to cold, prolonged exertion, or exposure to high altitudes (i.e., greater than 10,000 feet) in an unpressurized aircraft should be avoided. Sports injuries should not be treated with ice because this can cause localized sickling. An awareness of each child's baseline spleen size is an important aspect of safety education when the child with sickle cell is engaging in physical activity.

Adolescents with SCD often demonstrate the same limit-testing and risk-taking behaviors as their unaffected peers. Parents must balance their child's need for safety with their child's need to become self-sufficient. An information card or Medic-Alert bracelet is often helpful in emergency situations.

Immunizations

The conventional schedule may be used for diphtheria-pertussis-tetanus (DaPT) vaccine, inactivated poliomyelitis vaccine (IPV), measles-mumps-rubella (MMR) vaccine, varicella vaccine, hepatitis A and B, *Haemophilus* type B (HiB) vaccines, pneumococcal conjugate vaccine (Prevnar), and meningococcal vaccines (CDC, 2008a). One dose of Pneumovax immunization against pneumococcal sepsis should be given at age 2 and again at age 5 years

TABLE 40-2

Recommended Schedule of Pneumococcal Immunizations in Previously Unvaccinated Children with Sickle Cell Disease

Product Type	Age at First Dose	Primary Series	Additional Doses
PPV23 (Pneumovax)	≥24 mo	1 dose at least 6-8 wk after last PCV7 dose	1 dose, 3-5 yr after first PPV23 dose

From Centers for Disease Control and Prevention. (2008). *Recommendations and guidelines: 2008 child and adolescent immunization schedules for persons aged 0-6 years, 7-18 years and "catch-up schedule."* Available at www.cdc.gov/vaccines/recs/acip. Retrieved January 16, 2008.

(Table 40-2). A booster dose after age 10 is also recommended (CDC, 2008a). It is important to emphasize that even with vigilant immunization and antibiotic prophylaxis, episodes of pneumococcal septicemia have occurred. Pneumovax may be given concurrently with the DaPT, IPV, MMR, influenza, and hepatitis B and HiB vaccines.

Children with hemoglobinopathies are identified as being at risk for influenza-related complications. Children with SCD are also known to be at high risk for bacterial infection, which could occur associated with concurrent viral infection. Therefore it is recommended that all children with SCD receive influenza vaccine on an annual basis (AAP, 2006).

Screening

Vision. During their first decade of life, children with SCD require routine screening. After age 10, they need an annual retinal examination by an ophthalmologist to screen for sickle retinopathy and possible intervention, especially for children with Hb SC (Lane & Buchanan, 2002). If a child sustains any eye trauma, referral to an ophthalmologist for evaluation of increased intraocular pressure or retinal detachment is necessary.

Hearing. Routine audiologic evaluations are recommended to screen for hearing loss related to vasoocclusion or hyperviscosity in the inner ear. Any abnormal findings on routine school screenings should be followed up on immediately. Sensorineural hearing loss has been occasionally described in this population.

Dental. Routine screening is recommended. Children with implanted venous devices should receive prophylactic doses of amoxicillin before invasive procedures, including aggressive oral hygiene (AAP, 2006).

Blood Pressure. Blood pressure should be measured at every visit. The risk for occlusive stroke increases with rises in systolic, but not diastolic, pressure. Children with high blood pressure values relative to this population (e.g., systolic pressures of 120 to 139 or diastolic pressures of 70 to 89 mm Hg) should be evaluated for renal dysfunction and pHTN (Gordeuk, Sachder, Taylor, et al., 2008).

Hematocrit. Routine hematocrit screening is not necessary because of regular CBC monitoring, which should be done every 4 to 6 months at a sickle cell treatment center (see later discussion).

Urinalysis. Urinalysis, with blood urea nitrogen (BUN) and creatinine, is performed at least yearly (see later discussion).

Tuberculosis. Routine screening is recommended.

Condition-Specific Screening

Pulse Oximetry. Readings should be obtained at every visit, noting changes from baseline. Because children with sickle cell disease are susceptible to infections that may progress to ACS, a baseline reading is invaluable in determining divergence from baseline.

Sleep Apnea. Notation of snoring and a history of restless sleep should be obtained at each visit, noting episodes of daytime sleepiness. Enlarged tonsils or adenoids may be the culprit in inducing episodes of sleep apnea, and if found on sleep study, is an indication for surgical removal. Oxygen desaturation occurs during these episodes and is a trigger for sickling events.

Hematologic Screening. CBC with differential and reticulocyte counts are obtained every 4 to 6 months (every 3 to 4 months for Hb SS and Hb $S\beta°$ thalassemia, and every 6 to 12 months for Hb SC and Hb $S\beta^+$ thalassemia). These screenings are useful in establishing baseline data and ascertaining bone marrow function. Determining the RBC phenotype of a well child who has not had a transfusion can expedite any future transfusions. Quantitative hemoglobin electrophoresis is obtained at 1 year of age to determine presence of fetal hemoglobin. Some comprehensive sickle cell centers test children during this time to correlate Hb F levels with clinical severity.

Renal Function Testing. A urinalysis should be performed and BUN and creatinine levels checked annually to monitor renal function. An inability to concentrate or acidify urine may be evident in the urinalysis and is commonly seen in children with SCD. Urobilinogen, a by-product of bilirubin metabolism, is also a frequent finding. Hematuria may be a manifestation of renal dysfunction secondary to SCD or other unrelated pathologic conditions. These children should be referred to a nephrologist for further evaluation and treatment if the hematuria is severe or casts are present in the urine. Proteinuria is the most common and early clinical manifestation of glomerular injury to the kidney. Follow-up requires a urine culture and sensitivity, and—if negative—a 24-hour collection of urine for protein quantitation. An elevation requires referral to a nephrologist.

Lead Poisoning. Determining free erythrocyte protoporphyrin (FEP) levels when screening children who may be at high risk for lead intoxication is not valid for children with SCD (Vichinsky, Kleman, Embury et al.,1981). Obtaining a serum lead level may be the most appropriate test to facilitate a diagnosis of lead poisoning.

Scoliosis. Scoliosis screenings should be done through late adolescence because of the delayed growth spurts of children with SCD.

Cardiac Function. Electrocardiography (ECG) and echocardiography (ECHO) may be performed every 1 to 2 years after age 5 to evaluate the impact of chronic anemia on ventricular function. Efforts should be made to establish whether symptoms of chest pain, dyspnea, or decreased exercise tolerance have occurred, and significant symptoms should be evaluated with exercise testing. Functional murmurs are frequently heard in these children because of chronic anemia, and parents should be counseled as to their compensatory mechanism.

Liver Function. Yearly liver function studies are helpful to evaluate RBC metabolism and liver function. Bilirubin is often elevated as a consequence of hemolysis, as well as liver disease. Bilirubin levels rise gradually until the third decade of life. Scleral icterus and tea-colored urine are indicative of bilirubin produced by the chronic hemolysis and are frequently seen. Alkaline phosphatase levels fall after periods of rapid growth in adolescence and reach lower levels in females than in males. Children on chronic transfusion programs should be screened yearly for HIV and hepatitis C.

Common Illness Management
Differential Diagnosis

Fever. As a result of functional asplenia, bacterial infection is a significant cause of morbidity and mortality in children with SCD. The incidence of bacteremia in children with SCD is highest among those under 2 years of age and declines from age 2 to 6 years. The most common pathogen in children under 6 years of age is *Streptococcus pneumoniae*. Antibiotic resistance to *S. pneumoniae* has been reported (AAP, 2006). Some children with SCD have cultured *S. pneumoniae* from the tonsillar beds despite appropriate doses of prophylactic penicillin. Caregivers must be alert to these exceptions and closely monitor antibiotic effectiveness and compliance with penicillin prophylaxis. Before the advent of Prevnar, the course of *S. pneumoniae* sepsis had been fulminant, with mortality rates reaching 24% to 50% (Poehling, Talbot, Griffin, et al., 2006).

Differential Diagnosis

- Fever
- Urinary tract infections
- Orthopedic symptoms
- Acute gastroenteritis
- Abdominal pain
- Anemia
- Respiratory distress
- Neurologic changes

Escherichia coli bacteremia is often associated with urinary tract infection and *Salmonella* species bacteremia with osteomyelitis. Capillary blockage by sickle cells may cause gut infarction, which—combined with defective function of the liver and spleen—allows for invasion by *Salmonella* species. This invasion, combined with expanded bone marrow and poor blood flow, provides an ischemic focus for *Salmonella* species localization.

Fever is a common finding during VOC, as well as during infectious episodes. There is no test or diagnostic tool to differentiate fever of an infectious origin from fever that results from inflammation secondary to infarction. Primary care providers must be aware of the fact that children may have two independent problems (e.g., infection and vasoocclusion), both of which require aggressive treatment and management. Some health care workers measure C-reactive protein (CRP), which might indicate an inflammatory reaction.

Any child having a temperature elevation (at or above 102.2°F [39°C]) should be given appropriate antibiotic coverage and treated as an outpatient, provided that a probable source of temperature elevation can be identified and the child is stable, can tolerate extra oral fluid, and looks well clinically. Careful follow-up at clinic visits in 24 and 48 hours with assurance of parental compliance is necessary for outpatient management.

BOX 40-4

Criteria for Admission and Inpatient Management

One or more of the following accompanied by a change in clinical status:

- "Seriously ill appearance"
- Hypotension
- Severe abdominal pain
- Poor perfusion
- Temperature >39°C (102.2°F)
- Hemoglobin <5 g/dL and clinical change from baseline
- Leukocyte count >30,000/mm^3 or <5000/mm^3
- Platelet count <100,000/mm^3 and clinical change from baseline
- Pain crisis that is unrelieved in 48 hours with home pain management
- Dehydration by examination or history
- Pulmonary infiltrate
- Prior history of sepsis
- No telephone or immediate access to the hospital
- Poor or no track record with previous prescriptions or appointments
- No prior training on monitoring for early signs of complications

Adapted from Platt, O. (1997). The febrile child with sickle cell disease: A pediatrician's quandary. *J Pediatr, 130,* 693-694.

Current treatment consists of prompt assessment of the child, followed by blood and urine cultures and administration of ceftriaxone or cefotaxime to all children. These cephalosporins have a half-life of 8 to 9 hours (Taketomo, Hodding, & Kraus, 2007), and effective bactericidal levels persist for 24 hours after a single dose. They are the ideal antibacterial agents for most of the bacterial pathogens likely to be associated with septic episodes in SCD, including *S. pneumoniae, Haemophilus* species, and *Salmonella* species. Children who appear toxic, have an extremely high fever and/or an unreliable caretaker, or to whom close outpatient follow-up is not possible should be hospitalized (Box 40-4).

All children with SCD should be considered at risk for fatal sepsis regardless of whether they are on penicillin prophylaxis and have received pneumococcal vaccinations. An aggressive search for the cause of the fever should include a CBC, blood culture, urinalysis, urine culture, chest radiograph, and possibly sinus radiographs if symptoms are suggestive of infection. Lumbar puncture should be performed if meningitis is suspected. Clinicians are increasingly aware of the development of penicillin-resistant organisms, which contribute to the difficulty of treating the child with a fever. Bacterial meningitis, suspected or proven to be caused by *S. pneumoniae,* should be treated with combination therapy of vancomycin and cefotaxime or ceftriaxone on all children at least 1 month of age. Based on culture and sensitivity results, penicillin or ceftriaxone should be continued and vancomycin discontinued if not needed. Rifampin is used if found to be sensitive to the identified organism (AAP, 2006).

Even common infections such as otitis media or sinusitis may precipitate a vasoocclusive crisis if fluid intake is reduced and dehydration and acidosis result. During periods of illness, a child must be assessed frequently for early signs of crisis. Maintaining fluid intake and controlling fever are critical.

Urinary Tract Infections. Asymptomatic bacteriuria, symptomatic urinary tract infection, and pyelonephritis occur much more commonly in individuals with SCD than in the general population. A child with a urinary tract infection or pyelonephritis should have a blood culture obtained because bacteremia is present more frequently in those children with SCD and a urinary tract infection.

Appropriate antibiotic therapy should be instituted and adequate follow-up, including a repeat culture, arranged. Further diagnostic studies (e.g., renal ultrasound or voiding cystourethrogram) should be done to exclude treatable conditions in children with pyelonephritis or recurrent urinary tract infection.

Orthopedic Symptoms. Areas of bone infarction may be easily confused with osteomyelitis or rheumatologic disorders. It is important to differentiate areas of infarction from areas of infection because children with SCD have an increased incidence of osteomyelitis. With both pathologic processes, a child may have an elevated WBC count, fever, and equivocal radiographic findings. Osteomyelitis, however, is more often associated with an increased number of immature granulocytes, bacteremia, and a purulent joint aspirate. Bone scans may be useful in differentiating osteomyelitis from areas of bone infarction. Bone marrow scans have also been used to further discriminate areas of infection from those of infarction, especially when a bone scan is equivocal. Opinions on the use of bone marrow scans are somewhat divergent, however, and largely depend on the level of expertise available at a given facility.

Acute Gastroenteritis. Vomiting and diarrhea must be carefully evaluated and managed in children with SCD because these children lack the ability to concentrate urine to compensate for decreased fluid intake or excess losses. Significant dehydration may quickly occur and lead to metabolic acidosis and increased sickling. If a child's oral fluid intake is less than that needed to maintain hydration, the child must receive IV hydration.

Abdominal Pain. Episodes of infarction of the abdominal organs (e.g., liver, spleen, abdominal lymph nodes) occur and may be quite painful. These abdominal crises should be differentiated from problems that would require surgical intervention (e.g., appendicitis, cholecystitis).

Abdominal pain and cramps found commonly in young children are possibly related to mesenteric ischemia. Normal bowel sounds with lack of ileus support nonsurgical management with adequate pain control. The duration may last days to weeks, with fluctuations in the severity of the pain. Abdominal pain triggered by constipation is a common complaint and may be treated with a combination of stool softeners and laxatives. Use of narcotics to treat VOC increases the risk of constipation, and bowel prophylaxis should be concurrent with pain management efforts.

Paralytic ileus is common during acute abdominal pain, making diagnosis problematic. Right upper quadrant pain creates further complications because intrahepatic sickling mimics cholecystitis. Neither ultrasound nor laboratory values aid in defining the process. Leukocytosis of 30,000 can be seen with both infarction and infection. Most children find that their sickle cell pain has a unique quality or character and they can often report whether their pain is typical of vasoocclusive pain. Deviation from a characteristic pattern (i.e., lower abdominal pain with persistent local tenderness) with symptoms lasting several hours suggests a surgical problem.

Anemia. Virtually all children with SCD are anemic at baseline. A child with SCD may periodically have acute lethargy and pallor. CBC and reticulocyte count should be obtained. If these reveal a significant drop in the hemoglobin and hematocrit levels, a child is probably experiencing an aplastic crisis or splenic sequestration. A fall in the hemoglobin and hematocrit values is usually a stimulus to the bone marrow, which then produces new RBCs in the form of reticulocytes. If the reticulocyte count is low

in the presence of low hemoglobin and hematocrit levels, a child is experiencing an aplastic crisis. If a child has an enlarged spleen, pallor, lethargy, and an associated drop in hemoglobin, he or she is likely to be experiencing splenic sequestration. Regardless of exact diagnosis, the child will require immediate hospitalization with close observation and transfusion.

Respiratory Distress. Increased respiratory rate and effort, chest pain, fever, rales, and dullness to percussion may indicate pneumonia or ACS. Infiltrates on chest radiograph may reflect either process. With ACS the chest radiograph may be clear in the first few days, but a pleural effusion is often seen. These children should receive antibiotics, hydration, analgesics, and oxygen as needed. Transfusion or partial exchange transfusion may be indicated, depending on the degree of respiratory distress. ACS is a medical emergency and necessitates hospitalization.

Neurologic Changes. A child who has a seizure, hemiparesis, blurred or double vision, or changes in speech, gait, or level of consciousness should have expedient neurologic and radiologic evaluation for the presence of stroke. These neurologic changes are a medical emergency and require exchange transfusion as soon as possible.

Drug Interactions

Antihistamines and barbiturates given concurrently with narcotics may cause respiratory depression, hypoxia, and further sickling. Diuretics and some bronchodilators, which have a diuretic effect, may cause dehydration and sickling and should be used with caution in children with SCD. Children receiving narcotics for pain control should be given stool softeners and cautioned about the use of alcohol or other sedatives.

Developmental Issues
Sleep Patterns

Because of chronic anemia, some children with SCD may fatigue more easily than their unaffected peers and may desire extra sleep. Parents often report that their child with SCD naps after coming home from school—a routine that can be encouraged. Snoring, in combination with daytime sleepiness, is an indication for a sleep study to determine if obstruction from enlarged tonsils or adenoids exists, particularly if pulse oximetry readings are below 90%.

Toileting

Toilet training should be initiated using the conventional guidelines to assess readiness for training. Bowel training usually progresses without difficulty. Bladder training progresses along normal developmental patterns in toddlers with SCD. Older children, however, may have difficulty concentrating urine and thus produce a large volume of dilute urine. This symptom is usually not seen until the second decade. Nevertheless, all children may need the opportunity to go to the toilet every 2 to 3 hours during the day. Primary enuresis often occurs in young children and commonly continues into the teenage years. It is especially troublesome when a child requires extra fluids during a VOC. Some children who previously achieved nighttime continence may develop secondary enuresis as subtle insults to the kidney occur. A pattern of enuresis typically emerges as a child begins having more "wet" than "dry" nights. This pattern may reflect the gradual loss of the kidneys' ability to concentrate urine. Daytime continence is unaffected by these renal changes.

Routine counseling regarding enuresis should be offered. Young children may initially use diapers. By the time a child reaches preschool or school age, however, the use of diapers often adversely affects the child's self-esteem and sense of mastery. Many families choose to wake the child once or twice during the night to urinate, but severe restriction of fluids is not wise because hydration needs must be met. Avoidance of caffeine ingestion during the evening hours may help prevent enuresis. Careful questioning by the primary care provider may point to a subclinical infectious process that can be treated. Parents need to be counseled regarding the physiology behind sickle cell enuresis in an effort to plan appropriate intervention aimed at preventing the loss of their child's self-esteem.

Discipline

Expectations for the behavior of children with SCD should vary little from those held for their unaffected siblings or peers. These expectations should be as clear and consistent as possible. Likewise, parents should strive to make discipline fair and consistent. Many parents are fearful of disciplining or setting limits for their child with SCD, especially because emotional stress is thought to possibly precipitate a VOC. Primary care providers can point out to parents that a lack of or inconsistency in setting limits may be more stressful to a child than consistently set limits. Parents should also be encouraged to note which behaviors their child consistently demonstrates when in pain (e.g., a certain pitch to his or her cry, a change in activity level, or changes in appetite) to help them discriminate episodes of pain from other behavior.

Child Care

Children with SCD can participate in normal daycare centers, although small group or home-centered daycare may be preferable because it provides less exposure to infections. Caregivers must be informed of a child's need for extra fluids and frequent need to void. They may also need to administer medications during daycare hours and must be instructed in this regard. Caregivers must be able to contact a parent or quickly seek medical care for the child in the event of fever, painful VOC, respiratory distress, or symptoms of stroke, all of which may be life threatening. It is commonly accepted that children attending daycare centers are at higher risk for acquiring community-based resistant infections, so health care workers must take this into consideration when prescribing antibiotic coverage.

Schooling

Parents are encouraged to meet with school officials before the beginning of each school year to allow them to communicate about the usual symptoms their child has relative to SCD. A plan should be developed for absences, makeup work, intermittent home-bound study (if necessary), and transfer of assignments from school to the home. These children are frequently eligible for special education services (see Chapter 3).

Many primary care providers play an active role in educating school officials about the needs of children with SCD. Some visit schools and give presentations, and others provide written materials (see Resources at the end of this chapter). The need for adequate hydration, frequent bathroom breaks, rest, physical education, and appropriate dress are all subjects for discussion by the health care team. School officials, in turn, can provide information about learning abilities and behavior. This open exchange of information helps ensure a successful school year for the student. Knowing whom to call when parents cannot be reached reduces anxiety on the part of school staff.

As previously discussed, some children with SCD and silent infarcts have declining IQs with increasing age. Recent research supports the need for early evaluation of *all* children with SCD because of their high risk for cognitive impairment (Thompson & Gustafson, 2002). Children with SCD should be referred for eligibility for special education services. Repeated testing to identify impairments affecting education may be necessary because of the possible progression of symptoms, especially from recurrent TIAs or small strokes (see Chapter 3). Children with splenomegaly should be cautioned about the risks for injury with contact sports. Modified physical education classes should be offered to keep these children engaged in group activities, which are important to their overall adjustment and well-being. Finally, school personnel should be counseled about the needs of children affected with chronic orthopedic problems (e.g., osteomyelitis or avascular necrosis of the femoral head). These children may need additional time to get to classes, or may need to obtain an elevator key during times of bone healing and or physical discomfort with ambulation.

Sexuality

Children with SCD progress through the Tanner stages in an orderly and consistent manner but usually experience puberty several years later than their unaffected peers, which can have significant adverse effects on their self-concepts. Once sexual maturation has occurred, fertility and contraception are important issues that must be addressed by primary care providers. For men, impotence is often a problem after a major episode of priapism. For female adolescents, menarche is often delayed by 2 to 2½ years, but fertility is normal. Decisions about contraception must take into account the attitudes, lifestyle, and maturity of the adolescent, as well as the hematologic ramifications of the method chosen. During pregnancy, close hematology follow-up is recommended for women with SCD.

Various contraceptive choices are available to adolescents with SCD, including all barrier forms of contraception (e.g., condoms for men, and foam and diaphragms for women). Women may also use oral contraceptives, preferably those brands containing low levels of estrogen.

Progesterone-only pills are useful because progestins stabilize the red cell membrane. Medroxyprogesterone (Depo-Provera) has also been used in this population and is often the method of preference (American College of Obstetricians and Gynecologists [ACOG], 2000). Adolescents with SCD should receive careful, repeated genetic counseling before puberty and during adolescence. They need to understand the pattern of transmission of SCD and the availability of testing for partners before conceiving a child.

Transition to Adulthood

Early vocational counseling should be offered to children and adolescents with SCD. Consideration should be directed toward the child's or adolescent's interests and intellectual abilities. Work in a climate-controlled environment is preferred over rigorous, outdoor work, which might trigger a crisis. SCD excludes a person from military service, so technical and academic training is encouraged. Many community-based sickle cell organizations offer scholarships for skilled and academic work. The Sickle Cell Disease Association of America, Inc. can direct families to local resources.

Families should be counseled about the progressive organ damage that develops as a child ages. Continuity of care by a knowledgeable primary care provider will afford the best quality of life and should be encouraged.

Insurance companies may deem individuals with SCD uninsurable. Local chapters of the Sickle Cell Foundation can provide counseling to such persons about options and resources.

Family Concerns

The families of children with SCD experience the same psychological ramifications as other families of children with chronic conditions, often in the context of limited resources. These families bear the additional burden of knowing that this disease is genetically transmitted. This knowledge can prompt feelings of overwhelming guilt and responsibility. Exacerbations of the condition often occur without provocation, prompting feelings of helplessness. Many manifestations of the condition are not objectively visible or measurable; therefore children with SCD can appear to be well when they are potentially extremely ill. Many parents are fearful that the therapeutic effects of narcotics and blood transfusions will be outweighed by their potentially deleterious effects.

Genetic counseling should be offered to the parents of a child with SCD at the time of the child's diagnosis and when subsequent pregnancies are contemplated. In addition to the black (African American) population, permeations of sickle hemoglobinopathies are found in Hispanics, Central Americans, Greeks, Arabs, Asians, and Caribbean natives. Each of these individuals brings his or her own view of health, coping, and wellness. Primary care providers must be mindful of the differences within and between cultures. Emphasis should focus on the different strengths families bring with them. For example, extended family support is a dominant feature in the black (African American) community and should play a role during crisis episodes.

Researchers show that black (African American) families prefer to use their family members as sources of support instead of using formal support groups. Among many minorities, close friends are considered kin and fulfill some functions of extended family members (Yoon & Black, 2006). When working with minority families, primary care providers need to explore and understand the effects of ethnicity on the family's daily life. Such understanding seeks out cultural practices (e.g., male and female roles and black [African American] language, communication styles, and family rituals). Instructions should be delivered to the head of the household. In contrast to the matriarchal leadership found in many black (African American) households, Muslim families center their decision making on the father or male head of the household. Strong church affiliations are often in place and offer consolation and hope leading to greater acceptance and improved quality of life.

Individuals espousing the Jehovah's Witness faith will deny blood transfusions to their children, placing extra stress on the primary care provider. Sensitive, open communication and vigilant intensive care management may prevent the need for transfusions and thereby support the religious beliefs of the family. In all instances, members of a particular ethnic or minority group should be consulted when actions or choices conflict with those of the medical care team.

Resources

Birth to Three
Website: www.birthto3.org
NIH Management and of Sickle Cell Disease (4th ed.).
Website: www.nhlbi.nih.gov/health/prof/blood/sickle/index.htm
Parent Handbook (Part I)
Website: www.vahealth.org/sicklecell/docs/Parents_Handbook_
    Sickle_Cell_Disease_Part_I.PDF.
Sickle Cell Disease Association of America (SCDAA)
Website: www.sicklecelldisease.org
Sickle Cell Disease: Information for School Personnel
Website: www.state.nj.us/health/fhs/sicklecell/index.shtml
Sickle Cell Information Center
Website: www.scinfo.org

Summary of Primary Care Needs for the Child with Sickle Cell Disease

HEALTH CARE MAINTENANCE

Growth and Development

- Children with SCD tend to weigh less and be shorter than their peers. Weight is affected more than height, and males are affected more than females. Weight and height should be checked and plotted every 3 to 4 months.
- Puberty is delayed for both sexes with Hb SS.
- Developmental impairment varies. Cerebral microvascular occlusion or stroke outcome can have an impact on intellectual and motor development. Refer for neurologic testing if screening results or clinical assessment warrants.

Diet

- Diet should be well balanced with a generous amount of fluid; fluid intake should be increased during a febrile illness, times of increased activity, environmental heat, dehydration, traveling, or while experiencing vasoocclusive crisis.
- Increased metabolic demands require additional protein, micronutrients, and food for energy.
- Pica is more common in children with sickle cell disease.
- Folic acid supplements are encouraged.

Safety

- Ingestion of narcotics beyond prescribed amount can lead to respiratory depression.
- Alcohol may cause dehydration and potentiate narcotics.
- Narcotics may impair judgment while driving or safe use of machinery.
- Smoking leads to vasoconstriction and is strongly discouraged
- Recreational activities that involve prolonged exposure to cold, prolonged exertion, or exposure to high altitudes should be avoided.

Summary of Primary Care Needs for the Child with Sickle Cell Disease—cont'd

Dehydration should be avoided. Ice should NEVER be used to treat injuries.
- A Medic-Alert bracelet is recommended.

Immunizations

- Routine standard immunizations are recommended.
- The pneumococcal vaccine should be given at 24 months, with a single booster given at 5 years with another booster given 5 years after the second immunization. Prevnar should be given as scheduled.
- An annual influenza vaccine is strongly recommended.
- Hepatitis A vaccination should be a part of each child's routine immunization schedule.

Screening

- *Vision.* Routine screening is recommended. At 10 years of age annual retinal examinations are recommended to rule out sickle retinopathy. If a child sustains eye trauma he or she must be referred to an ophthalmologist to rule out increased intraocular pressure or retinal detachment.
- *Hearing.* Routine audiologic examination is recommended. More frequent evaluation is warranted if clinical status indicates.
- *Dental.* Routine screening is recommended, as well as antibiotic prophylaxis prior to invasive procedures.
- *Blood pressure.* Blood pressure should be measured each visit. An increase in systolic pressure increases risk of stroke. Children with high blood pressures should be evaluated for renal dysfunction.
- *Hematocrit.* Routine hematocrit screening is deferred because of condition-specific screening.
- *Urinalysis.* Routine urinalysis is deferred because of condition-specific screening.
- *Tuberculosis.* Routine screening is recommended.

Condition-Specific Screening

- *Pulsoximetry.* Reading should be obtained at each visit and compared to baseline.
- *Sleep apnea.* Screen for snoring, restlessness, or daytime sleepiness, or enlarged tonsils or adenoids; these may induce sleep apnea and subsequent oxygen desaturation.
- *Hematologic screening.* A CBC with differential, platelet count, reticulocyte count, and RBC smear should be checked every 3 to 6 months.
- *Renal function screening.* BUN and creatinine levels should be checked routinely and a urinalysis done yearly. A child should be referred to a urologist if severe hematuria is noted or casts are found in urine.
- *Lead poisoning.* Lead screening using the EP level is unreliable; the serum lead level must be determined.
- *Scoliosis.* Screening should be extended to the late teens because of delayed puberty.
- *Cardiac function.* Both ECG and ECHO are recommended every 1 to 2 years after age 10 if clinically warranted.
- *Liver function.* Serum liver function tests should be done yearly. The gallbladder should be assessed via ultrasound if the child becomes symptomatic.
  - Transfused children should be routinely screened for HIV and hepatitis C.

COMMON ILLNESS MANAGEMENT

Differential Diagnosis

- *Fever.* A child with a temperature above 101.2°F (38.3°C) must be evaluated immediately, cultures taken, and ceftriaxone administered IM or IV. Outpatient management may be considered if the source of the fever can be identified, appropriate antibiotics are given, and reliable follow-up and reassessment as needed is ensured.
  - The child's age, past history, clinical condition, laboratory values, adherence with therapy, and ability to obtain follow-up care determine whether or not the child should receive inpatient care.
- *Urinary tract infections.* Asymptomatic bacteriuria, urinary tract infections, and pyelonephritis are more common with SCD.
  - Blood cultures should be done to rule out bacteremia if a urinary tract infection is diagnosed.
  - Treatment must cover cultured organisms, and follow-up is essential.
- *Orthopedic symptoms.* It is difficult to differentiate bone infarction from osteomyelitis or rheumatologic disorders. MRI studies are used to identify bone marrow infarction.
- *Acute gastroenteritis.* Significant dehydration may occur quickly and lead to acidosis and sickling. If oral intake is inadequate, IV hydration is needed.
- *Abdominal pain.* Abdominal pain crises may be differentiated from surgical problems by evaluating fever, hematologic changes, peristalsis, and response to symptomatic, supportive therapy.
- *Anemia.* Hemoglobin and hematocrit levels significantly lower than baseline may reflect aplastic crisis, hyperhemolytic crisis, or splenic sequestration. Splenic sequestration and aplasia may be life-threatening conditions.
- *Respiratory distress.* It is important that individuals are evaluated for ACS, which may be fulminant and require exchange transfusion.
- *Neurologic changes.* Neurologic changes may indicate stroke. Rapid, thorough evaluation is critical. Exchange transfusion should be performed as quickly as possible if stroke occurs.

Drug Interactions

- Antihistamines, alcohol, and barbiturates may potentiate sedation with narcotics.
- Diuretics and bronchodilators (which may have diuretic effects) may cause dehydration and sickling.
- Stool softeners are useful while on narcotics.

DEVELOPMENTAL ISSUES

Sleep Patterns

- Routine care is recommended. Clinical assessment of obstructive sleep apnea requires thorough evaluation.

Toileting

- Enuresis is often a long-term issue because of the large volume of dilute urine in this population.
- Nocturia may persist.

Discipline

- Expectations should be consistent, fair, and similar to those of unaffected peers and siblings.

Continued

Summary of Primary Care Needs for the Child with Sickle Cell Disease—cont'd

Child Care

- Caregivers must be mindful of fluid requirements, the importance of maintaining normal body temperature, and the critical importance of notifying parents of fever, signs of vasoocclusive crisis, or respiratory distress, and they must be able to administer medicines.

Schooling

- These children may have frequent, unpredictable absences.
- While at school, they need access to fluids and liberal bathroom privileges.
- They may participate in mainstream physical education as tolerated.
- Evaluation for special education services is warranted if the child is having difficulty with learning.

Sexuality

- Puberty may be delayed.
- Women usually have normal fertility patterns and may use all forms of birth control.

- Increased monitoring by a hematologist may be warranted during pregnancy.
- Men must be aware of the risk of impotency after multiple episodes of priapism.
- Genetic counseling is important.

Transition to Adulthood

- Early vocational counseling is recommended.
- Insurance problems may be encountered.

FAMILY CONCERNS

- Because SCD is genetically transmitted, there is a need for genetic counseling, as well as ongoing support to process feelings of guilt and responsibility.
- Support for cultural beliefs and family structure are important components of long-term care.

REFERENCES

Abboud, M., Cure, J., Granger, S., et al. (2004). Magnetic resonance angiography in children with sickle cell disease and abnormal transcranial Doppler ultrasonography findings enrolled in the STOP study. *Blood, 103*(7), 2822-2826.

Adamkiewicz, T., Silk, B., Howgate, J., et al. (2008). Effectiveness of the 7-valent pneumococcal conjugate vaccine in children with sickle cell disease. *Pediatrics, 121*(3), 562-569.

Adams, R. (2000). Lessons from the Stroke Prevention Trial in Sickle Cell Anemia (STOP) study. *J Child Neurol, 15*(5), 344-349.

Adams, R., & Brambilla, D. (2005). Discontinuing prophylactic transfusions used to prevent stroke in sickle cell disease. *N Engl J Med, 353*(26), 2769-2778.

Adams, R., McKie, V., & Hsu, L., et al. (1998). Prevention of a first stroke by transfusion in children with sickle cell anemia and abnormal results on transcranial Doppler ultrasonography. *N Engl J Med, 339*(1), 5-11.

Ambrusko, S., Gunawardena, S., Sakara, A., et al. (2006). Elevation of tricuspid regurgitant jet velocity, a marker for pulmonary hypertension in children with sickle cell disease. *Pediatr Blood Cancer, 47*(7), 907-913.

American Academy of Pediatrics (AAP). Committee on Infectious Diseases (L.K. Pickering, Ed.). (2006). *Red Book: 2006 Report of the Committee on Infectious Diseases* (27th ed.). Elk Grove Village, IL: American Academy of Pediatrics.

American College of Obstetricians and Gynecologists. (ACOG). (2000, July). The use of hormonal contraception in women with coexisting medical conditions. *Intl J Gynaecol Obstet, 18*, 93-106.

Ashley-Koch, A., Yang, Q., & Olney, R. (2000). Sickle hemoglobin (Hb S) allele and sickle cell disease: A huge review. *Am J Genet, 151*(9), 839-845.

Ballas, S. (2005). Pain management of sickle cell disease. *Hematol Oncol Clin North Am, 19*(5), 785-802.

Berkelhammer, L., Williamson, A., Sanford, S., et al. (2007). Neurocognitive sequelae of pediatric sickle cell disease: A review of the literature. *Child Neuropsychol, 13*, 120-131.

Bhatia, M., & Walters, M. (2008). Hematopoietic cell transplantation for thalassemia and sickle cell disease: Past, present and future. *Bone Marrow Transplant, 41*, 109-117.

Castro, O., Hoque, M., & Brown, B. (2003). Pulmonary hypertension in sickle cell disease: Cardiac catheterization results and survival. *Blood, 101*(4), 1257-1261.

Centers for Disease Control and Prevention (CDC). (2008a). *Recommendations and guidelines: 2008 child and adolescent immunization schedules for persons aged 0-6 years, 7-18 years and "catch-up schedule."* Available at www.cdc.gov/vaccines/recs/acip. Retrieved January 12, 2008.

Centers for Disease Control and Prevention. (2008b). *National Center on Birth Defects and Developmental Disabilities. Healthcare professionals*: Data and statistics. Available at www.cdc.gov/ncbddd/sicklecell/hcp_data.htm. Retrieved January 12, 2008.

Chui, D., & Dover, G. (2001). Sickle cell disease: No longer a single gene disorder. *Curr Opin Pediatr, 13*, 23-37.

Conboy, M., O'Brien, N., & Lowther, C. (2006). Evaluating preadmission preparation for pediatric stem cell transplant in the home environment: The parent's perspective. *Bone Marrow Transplant ACOG Practice Bulletin, 37*(Suppl 1). s282.

Davis, H., Schoendorf, K., Gergen, P., et al. (1997). National trends in the mortality of children with sickle cell disease, 1968-1992. *Am J Public Health, 87*(8), 1317-1322.

DeBaun, M., Schatz, J., Siegel, M., et al. (1998). Cognitive screening examinations for silent cerebral infarcts in sickle cell disease. *Neurology, 50*(6), 1678-1682.

Dobson, S., Holden, K., Nietert, P., et al. (2002). Moya-moya syndrome in childhood sickle cell disease: A predictive factor for recurrent cerebrovascular events. *Blood, 99*(9), 3144-3150.

Downes, S., Hambleton, I., Chuang, E., et al. (2005). Incidence and natural history of proliferative sickle cell retinopathy: Observations from a cohort study. *Ophthalmology, 112*(11), 1869-1875.

Driscoll, M. (2007). Sickle cell disease. *Pediatr Rev, 28*(7), 259-268.

Ellison, A., & Shaw, K. (2007). Management of vasoocclusive pain events in sickle cell disease. *Pediatr Emerg Care, 23*(11), 832-841.

Falletta, J., Woods, G., Verter, J., et al. (1995). Discontinuing penicillin prophylaxis in children with sickle cell anemia. *J Pediatr, 127*, 685-960.

Fitzhugh, C., Wigfall, D., & Ware, R. (2005). Enalapril and hydroxyurea therapy for children with sickle nephropathy. *Pediatr Blood Cancer, 45*(7), 982-985.

Frenette, P., & Atweh, G. (2007). Sickle cell disease: Old discoveries, new concepts, and future promises. *J Clin Invest, 117*(4), 850-858.

Friedman, L. (2007). Liver transplantation for sickle cell hepatopathy. *Liver Transplant, 13*(4), 483-485.

Gentry, B., & Dancer, J. (1997). Failure rates of young patients with sickle cell disease on a hearing screening test. *Percept Mot Skills, 84*, 434.

Gordeuk, V., Sachder, V., Taylor, J., et al. (2008). Relative systemic hypertension in patients with sickle cell disease is associated with risk of pulmonary hypertension and renal insufficiency. *Am J Hematol, 83*(1), 15-28.

Halasa, N., Shankar, S., Talbot, T., et al. (2007). Incidence of invasive pneumococcal disease among individuals with sickle cell disease before and after the introduction of the pneumococcal conjugate vaccine. *Clin Infect Dis*, *44*(11), 1428-1433.

Hankins, J., Ware, R., Rogers, Z., et al. (2005). Long-term hydroxyurea therapy for infants with sickle cell anemia: The HUSOFT extension study. *Blood*, *106*(7), 2269-2275.

Hogan, A., Kirkham, F., Prengler, M., et al. (2006). An exploratory study of physiological correlates of neurodevelopmental delay in infants with sickle cell anaemia. *Br J Haematol*, *132*(1), 99-107.

Ivascu, N., Sarnaik, S., McCrae, J., et al. (2001). Characterization of pica prevalence among patients with sickle cell disease. *Arch Pediatr Adolesc Med*, *155*(11), 1243-1247.

Kato, G., McGowan, V., Machado, R., et al. (2006). Lactate dehydrogenase as a biomarker of hemolysis-associated nitric oxide resistance, priapism, leg ulceration, pulmonary hypertension, and death in patients with sickle cell disease. *Blood*, *107*(6), 2279-2285.

Kaye, C., & Committee on Genetics. (2006). Newborn screening fact sheets: Sickle cell disease and other hemoglobinopathies. *Pediatrics*, *118*(3), 934-963.

King, A., White, D., McKinstry, R., et al. (2007). A pilot randomized education rehabilitation trial is feasible in sickle cell and strokes. *Neurology*, *68*(23), 2008-2011.

Kokoska, E., West, K., Carney, D., et al. (2004). Risk factors for acute chest syndrome in children with sickle cell disease undergoing abdominal surgery. *J Pediatr Surg*, *39*(6), 848-850.

Koshy, M., Weiner, S., Miller, S., et al. (1995). Surgery and anesthesia in sickle cell disease. Cooperative study of sickle cell diseases. *Blood*, *86*(10), 3676-3684.

Kotz, D. (2007). The gift of a cure. *U.S. News and World Report*, *142*(18), 59-60.

Lane, P., & Buchanan, G. (2002). Health supervision of children with sickle cell disease. *Pediatrics*, *109*(3), 526-534.

Lawrence, P., & Ryan, K. (2000). Sickle cell disease in children. *Adv Nurse Pract*, *9*(5), 48-57.

Leclercq, A., Martin, L., Vergnes, M., et al. (2005). Fatal *Yersinia enterocolitica* biotype 4 serovar 0:3 sepsis after red blood cell transfusion. *Transfusion*, *45*(5), 814-818.

Lemanek, K., Brown, R., Armstrong, F., et al. (2002). Dysfunctional eating patterns and symptoms of pica in children and adolescents with sickle cell disease. *Clin Pediatr*, *41*(7), 493-500.

Lindsey, W., & Olin, B. (2007). Deferasirox for transfusion-related iron overload: A clinical review. *Clin Ther*, *29*(10), 2154-2166.

Locatelli, F. (2006). Reduced-intensity regimen in allogenic hematopoietic stem cell transplantation for hemoglobinopathies. *Hematology Am Soc Hematol Educ Program*, *2006*, 398-401.

Logan, D., Radcliffe, J., & Smith-Whitley, K. (2002). Parent factors and adolescent sickle cell disease: Associations with patterns of health service use. *J Pediatr Psychol*, *27*(5), 475-484.

Machado, R., Kyle, A., Martyr, S., et al. (2007). Severity of pulmonary hypertension during vaso-occlusive pain crisis and exercise in patients with sickle cell disease. *Br J Haematol*, *136*(2), 319-325.

Mack, A., Kato, G. (2006). Sickle cell disease and nitric oxide: A paradigm shift?. *Int J Biochem Cell Biol*, *38*(8), 1237-1243.

Malinauskas, B., Sawchak, D., Koh, B., et al. (2001). Energy expenditure and intake in children with sickle cell disease during acute illness. *Clin Nutr*, *20*(2), 131-138.

Maples, B., & Hageman, T. (2004). Treatment of priapism in pediatric patients with sickle cell disease. *Am J Health System Pharm*, *61*, 355-363.

McKie, K., Hanevold, C., Hernandez, C., et al. (2007). Prevalence, prevention and treatment of microalbuminuria and proteinuria in children with sickle cell disease. *J Pediatr Hematol Oncol*, *29*(3), 140-144.

Mekontso, D., Leon, R., Habibi, A., et al. (2008). Pulmonary hypertension and cor pulmonale during severe acute chest syndrome in sickle cell disease. *Am J Respir Crit Care Med*, *177*(6), 646-653.

Michlitsch, J., Gardner, J., Vichinsky, E., et al. (2008). Clinical differences between children and adults with pulmonary hypertension and sickle cell disease. *Br J Haematol*, *140*(1), 104-112.

Miller, D., & Baehner, R. (Eds.). (1990). *Blood Diseases of Infancy and Childhood* (6th ed.). St. Louis: Mosby.

Miller, S., Macklin, E., Pegelow, C., et al. (2001). Silent infarction as a risk factor for overt stroke in children with sickle cell anemia: A report from the Cooperative Study of Sickle Cell Disease. *J Pediatr*, *139*, 385-390.

Miller, S., Sleeper, L., Pegelow, C., et al. (2000). Predictors of adverse outcomes in children with sickle cell disease. *N Engl J Med*, *342*, 83-89.

Modebe, O., & Ifenu, S. (1993). Growth retardation in homozygous sickle cell disease: Role of caloric intake and possible gender related differences. *Am J Hematol*, *44*(3), 149-154.

Morrison, R. (1991). Update on sickle cell disease: Incidence and choice of opioid in pain management. *Pediatr Nurs*, *17*(503), 76-77.

Mulligan, M. (2004). Regarding "fish" or "fish mouth" vertebrae. *Am J Roentgenol*, *182*(6), 1600.

National Institutes of Health (NIH), Division of Blood Diseases and Resources (2002). *The Management of Sickle Cell Disease*. (4th ed.). NIH Publication No. 02-2117 Washington, DC: U.S. Government Printing Office.

National Newborn Screening and Genetics Resource Center. (2008). National newborn screening status report 5/2/08. Available at www. genes-r-us.uthscsa.edu. Retrieved June 16, 2008.

Nelson, S., Adade, B., McDonough, E., et al. (2007). High prevalence of pulmonary hypertension in children with sickle cell disease. *J Pediatr Hematol Oncol*, *29*(5), 334-337.

Neumayr, D., Aguilar, C., Earles, A., et al. (2006). National Osteonecrosis Trial in Sickle Cell Anemia Study Group. Physical therapy alone compared with core decompression and physical therapy for femoral head osteonecrosis in sickle cell disease. Results of a multicenter study at a mean of three years after treatment. *J Bone Joint Surg Am*, *88*(12), 2573-2582.

Nuss, R., Cole, L., Orsini, E., et al. (2008). Pinch-off syndrome in patients with sickle cell disease receiving erythrocytapheresis. *Pediatr Blood Cancer*, *50*(2), 354-356.

Pashankar, F., Carbonella, J., Bazzy-Assad, A., et al. (2008). Prevalence and risk factors of elevated pulmonary artery pressure in children with sickle cell disease. *Pediatrics*, *121*(4), 777-782.

Pegelow, C. (1992). Survey of pain management therapy provided for children with sickle cell disease. *Clin Pediatr*, *31*, 211-214.

Platt, O. (1994). Mortality in sickle cell disease. *N Engl J Med*, *330*, 1639-1644.

Poehling, K., Talbot, T., Griffin, M., et al. (2006). Invasive pneumococcal disease among infants before and after the introduction of pneumococcal conjugate vaccine. *J Am Med Assoc*, *295*(14), 1668-1674.

Powars, D. (1975). Natural history of sickle cell disease—the first 10 years. *Semin Hematol*, *12*, 267-281.

Powars, D., Meiselman, H., Fisher, T., et al. (1994). Beta-S gene cluster haplotypes modulate hematologic and hemorrheologic expression in sickle cell anemia: Use in predicting clinical severity. *Am J Pediatr Hematol Oncol*, *16*(1), 55-61.

Puffer, E., Schatz, J., & Roberts, C. (2007). The association of oral hydroxyurea therapy with improved cognitive functioning in sickle cell disease. *Child Neuropsychol*, *13*(2), 142-154.

Quinn, C., Shull, E., Ahmad, N., et al. (2007). Prognostic significance of early vaso-occlusive complications in children with sickle cell anemia. *Blood*, *109*(1), 40-45.

Redding-Lallinger, R., & Knoll, C. (2006). Sickle cell disease—pathophysiology and treatment. *Curr Probl Pediatr Adolesc Health Care*, *36*(10), 346-376.

Reed, W., and Vichinsky, E. (2001). Transfusion therapy: A coming-of-age treatment for patients with sickle cell disease. *J Pediatr Hematol Oncol*, *23*(4), 197-201.

Saunthararajah, Y., Hillery, C., Lavelle, D., et al. (2003). Effects of 5-aza-2′-deoxycytidine on fetal hemoglobin levels, red cell adhesion, and hematopoietic differentiation in patients with sickle cell disease. *Blood*, *102*(2), 3865-3870.

Schatz, J. (2004). Brief report: Academic attainment in children with sickle cell disease. *J Pediatr Psychol*, *29*(8), 627-633.

Schatz, J., Brown, R., Pascual, J., et al. (2001). Poor school and cognitive functioning with silent cerebral infarcts and sickle cell disease. *Neurology*, *56*(8), 1109-1111.

Schatz, J., Finke, R., Kellet, J., et al. (2002). Cognitive functioning in children with sickle cell disease: A meta analysis. *J Pediatr Psychol*, *27*(8), 739-748.

Schatz, J., McClellan, C., Puffer, E., et al. (2008). Neurodevelopmental screening in toddlers and early preschoolers with sickle cell disease. *J Child Neurol*, *23*(1), 44-50.

Shannon, B., & Trousdale, R. (2004). Femoral osteotomies for avascular necrosis of the femoral head. *Clin Orthop Relat Res*, *418*, 34-40.

Shenoy, S. (2007). Has stem cell transplantation come of age in the treatment of sickle cell disease? *Bone Marrow Transplant*, *40*(9), 813-821.

Silva, C., & Viana, M. (2002). Growth deficits in children with sickle cell disease. *Arch Med Res*, *33*(3), 308-312.

Steinberg, M., Barton, F., Castro, O., et al. (2003). Effect of hydroxyurea on mortality and morbidity in adult sickle cell anemia: Risks and benefits up to 9 years of treatment. *J Am Med Assoc*, *298*(13), 1645-1651.

Stinson, J., & Naser, B. (2003). Pain management in children with sickle cell disease. *Pediatr Drugs*, *5*(4), 229-241.

Taketomo, C., Hodding, J., & Kraus, D. (2007). *Lexi-Comp's Pediatric Dosage Handbook* (14th ed.). Hudson, OH: Lexi-Comp.

Telen, M. (2007). Role of adhesion molecules and vascular endothelium in the pathogenesis of sickle cell disease. *Hematology Am Soc Hematol Educ Program*, *2007*, 84-90.

Thompson, R., & Gustafson, K. (2002). Neurocognitive development of young children with sickle cell disease through 3 years of age. *J Pediatr Psychol*, *27*(3), 235-244.

Traina, F., Jorge, S., Yamanaka, A., et al. (2007). Chronic liver abnormalities in sickle cell disease: A clinicopathological study in 70 living patients. *Acta Haematol*, *118*, 129-135.

Trent, J., & Kirsner, R. (2004). Leg ulcers in sickle cell disease. *Adv Skin Wound Care*, *17*(8), 410-416.

Vichinsky, E., Kleman, K., Embury, S., et al. (1981). The diagnosis of iron deficiency anemia in sickle cell disease. *Blood*, *58*(5), 963-968.

Vrijmoet-Wiersma, C., & Koopman, H. (2006). Psychological screening of children and their parents before haematopoietic stem cell transplantation: Results and implications for clinical practice. *Bone Marrow Transplant*, *37*(1). s263.

Walters, M., Nienhuis, A., & Vichinsky, E. (2002). Novel therapeutic approaches in sickle cell disease. *Hematology Am Soc Hematol Educ Program*, *2002*, 10-30.

Wang, W. (2007). Central nervous system complications of sickle cell disease in children: An overview. *Child Neuropsychol*, *13*(2), 103-119.

Wang, W., Enos, L., Gallagher, D., et al. (2001). Neuropsychologic performance in school age children with sickle cell disease: A report from the Cooperative Study of Sickle Cell Disease. *J Pediatr*, *139*(3), 391-397.

Ware, R., Eggleston, B., Redding-Lallinger, R., et al. (2002). Predictors of fetal hemoglobin response in children with sickle cell anemia receiving hydroxyurea therapy. *Blood*, *99*(1), 10-14.

Weiner, D., Hibberd, P., Betit, P., et al. (2003). Preliminary assessment of inhaled nitric oxide for acute vaso-occlusive crisis in pediatric patients with sickle cell disease. *J Am Med Assoc*, *289*(9), 1136-1142.

Wilson, R., Krishnamurti, L., & Kamat, D. (2003). Management of sickle cell disease in primary care. *Clin Pediatr*, *42*(9), 753-761.

Wong, A., Skamoto, K., & Johnson, E. (2001). Differentiating osteomyelitis from bone infarction in sickle cell disease. *Pediatr Emerg Care*, *17*(1), 60-63.

Wu, C., Gladwin, M., Tisdale, J., et al. (2007). Mixed haematopoietic chimerism for sickle cell disease prevents intravascular haemolysis. *Br J Haematol*, *139*(3), 504-507.

Yoon, S., & Black, S. (2006). Comprehensive, integrative management of pain for patients with sickle cell disease. *J Altern Complement Med*, *12*(10), 995-1001.

Zumberg, M., Reddy, S., Boyette, R., et al. (2005). Hydroxyurea therapy for sickle cell disease in community-based practices: A survey of Florida and North Carolina hematologists/oncologists. *Am J Hematol*, *79*(2), 107-113.

41 Tourette Syndrome and Obsessive-Compulsive Disorder

Naomi A. Schapiro

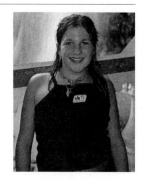

Etiology

Tourette syndrome (TS) is a neurobiologic condition characterized by vocal and motor tics that change over time and wax and wane in severity. Tics can be defined as "sudden, repetitive, stereotyped motor movements or phonic productions that involve discrete muscle groups" (Leckman, Bloch, King, et al., 2006, p. 1). Obsessive-compulsive disorder (OCD) is a neuropsychiatric condition characterized by recurrent and persistent thoughts that are experienced by the individual as intrusive, inappropriate, and distressing and by repetitive behaviors or mental acts that are aimed at preventing or reducing the distress (American Psychiatric Association [APA], 2000). Whereas OCD is usually classified by the APA as an anxiety disorder and TS as a movement disorder, there are several reasons for including the two conditions in the same chapter: recent studies have indicated that the same areas of the brain are involved in both conditions; genetic and family studies have linked the two conditions; and a disproportionate number of children have both diagnoses, suggesting a common or related origin.

As conditions that straddle the boundaries between voluntary and involuntary (Cohen & Leckman, 1999), TS and OCD have been claimed by both neurology and psychiatry. When the neurologist Gilles de la Tourette (1857–1904) first described nine individuals exhibiting the unusual movements and sounds of the syndrome that bears his name, he also described their compulsions (Lajonchere, Nortz, & Finger, 1996). The French psychologist and neurologist Pierre M.F. Janet (1859–1947) described OCD as a form of "psycholepsy," with neuronal discharges that were like tics of the mind (Rapoport, 1989), and reported success with behavioral treatments (Jenike, Baer, & Minichiello, 1998). Freud, who studied at the same Paris hospital as de la Tourette and Janet, believed in the relationship between neurologic factors and unconscious mental processes (Cohen & Leckman, 1999). Freud described tics in detail in his treatment of Frau Emmy von N (Cohen & Leckman) and attributed obsessions to overly strict toilet training in his famous Rat Man case, in which the individual was reportedly cured of obsessions by psychoanalysis (Freud, 1909/1973).

Until recently both TS and OCD were thought to have psychiatric origins (Coffey & Park, 1997; Rapoport, 1989). Noting haloperidol's efficacy in reducing tic severity, researchers began to explore the role of dopamine receptors and the limbic system in TS (Coffey & Park, 1997). It is currently thought that there is an underlying defect in TS of either excess dopamine or hypersensitivity of presynaptic or postsynaptic dopamine receptors (Leary, Reimschisel, & Singer, 2007). Research began to implicate the serotonin system in OCD after clinicians noted that OCD was refractory to traditional psychotherapy, but responded to particular serotonin reuptake inhibitors (Rapoport, 1989).

Studies suggest that basal ganglia dysfunction may be involved in TS (Mink, 2006) and OCD (Friedlander & Desrocher, 2006). Leckman and Cohen (1999) have postulated that specific cortico-striato-thalamo-cortical (CSTC) circuits convey cortical information throughout the basal ganglia and modulate systems that control different aspects of psychomotor behavior (Box 41-1 and Figure 41-1). Some of the circuits that convey information from the cortex throughout the basal ganglia are selectively disinhibited in both TS and OCD (Cohen & Leckman, 1999; Leary et al., 2007). In this conceptual model TS is seen as a disorder in which individuals are unable to inhibit premonitory sensory urges, leading to the emergence of motor and phonic behavior. In OCD, individuals are unable to inhibit specific innate worries, leading to the emergence of intense obsessions and compulsions. Current research does not dispute this model, but still has not clarified whether the primary neuroanatomic lesion is in the frontal cortex, the striatum, the thalamus, or the midbrain (Leary et al.).

Genetic Etiology

Genetic studies of TS are complicated by the lack of anatomic or physiologic markers, inconsistent diagnostic criteria, and the relative rarity of the syndrome (Keen-Kim & Freimer, 2006). Based on extended family studies, many researchers associate TS, chronic tics, OCD, and obsessive-compulsive symptoms as a spectrum of expression of the same underlying genetic disorder (Peterson, Pine, Cohen, et al., 2001). Earlier studies suggested an autosomal dominant model with sex-specific penetrance, accounting for the higher incidence of TS among boys (Alsobrook & Pauls, 1997). Current international research strategies, which include analysis of affected sibling pairs and complete genome screens of multigenerational families, indicate a complex and nonmendelian inheritance model, and the probability that more than one gene is involved (Tourette Syndrome Association International Consortium for Genetics, 2007).

Genetic studies of OCD encounter similar problems of symptom heterogeneity and decisions about inclusion or exclusion of coexisting conditions, such as mood or anxiety disorders (Miguel, Leckman, Rauch, et al., 2005). Studies of multigenerational families with multiple affected relatives have suggested several regions that may harbor a gene or genes for OCD (Grados & Wilcox, 2007). Candidate gene studies have implicated a gene for the glutamate transporter *SLC1A1* that may be involved in the inheritance of some OCD subtypes (Arnold, Sicard, Burroughs, et al., 2006).

Infectious or Autoimmune Influences

Swedo, Leonard, Mittleman, and colleagues (1997) coined the term Pediatric Autoimmune Neuropsychiatric Disorders Associated with Streptococcus (PANDAS) to describe a hypothesized subset of children with explosive onset of TS and OCD symptoms related to streptococcal infection. Sydenham chorea (SC), which involves abnormal movements, OCD-like symptoms, and emotional lability, is thought to be caused by a reaction between antibodies to group A beta-hemolytic Streptococcus and antigenic determinants in the basal ganglia, and researchers are looking at the overlap of symptom clusters of TS, OCD, and SC and the possibility of an immunologic cause for all three conditions (da Rocha, Correa, & Teixeira, 2008; Pavone, Parano, Rizzo, et al., 2006).

BOX 41-1

Brain Structures Thought to be Involved in Tourette Syndrome and Obsessive-Compulsive Disorder

- *Cerebral cortex:* Layer of gray matter that covers the surface of each cerebral hemisphere, consists primarily of six-layered neocortex containing functional modules: primary, sensory, and motor areas; unimodal association areas; multimodal association areas; and limbic areas.
- *Thalamus:* Acts as the gateway to cerebral cortex; relaying all sensory pathways, as well as circuits used by the cerebellum, basal ganglia, and limbic system.
- *Basal ganglia:* Group of subcortical nuclei that modulate output of the frontal cortex. Damage to the basal ganglia can cause disturbances of movement, alterations in muscle tone, and disturbances of cognition and motivation.
- *Striatum* (caudate nucleus, putamen, and ventral striatum): Major point of entry into basal ganglia circuitry, receiving inputs from cortical areas and projecting inhibitory outputs.

Incidence and Prevalence

A study of 11-year-old Swedish schoolchildren revealed an incidence of TS of 1.1% among boys and 0.5% among girls (Kadesjo & Gillberg, 2000). Other population studies of TS found rates ranging from 0.05% to 0.6% (Khalifa & von Knorring, 2005; Peterson et al., 2001). In contrast, as many as 10% to 20% of all school-age children have transient motor, and less commonly vocal, tics lasting less than 1 year (Peterson et al., 2001). A school-based study in the United States found that 22.3% of preschool children, 7.8% of school-age children, and 3.4% of adolescents in regular education classes had tics, as rated by their teachers (Gadow, Nolan, Sprafkin, et al., 2002). The relatively high prevalence of transient tic disorder might surprise primary care providers because the tics often resolve before the family seeks medical attention (Leckman, Bloch, King, et al., 2006). In up to 6% of school-age children, symptoms of either motor or vocal tics, but not both, persist for more than 1 year (Leckman, Bloch, King, et al., 2006).

In the population-based longitudinal study by Peterson and colleagues (2001), the point prevalence of OCD ranged from 1.8% to 5.5%. International community studies have found prevalence for OCD of between 2% and 4% of the population (Geller, 2006). Since adult onset is documented in some cases of OCD, and the prevalences of OCD in adult and pediatric studies are similar, Geller speculates that some cases of OCD in children remit before adulthood. Fireman, Koran, Leventhal, and colleagues (2001) found that the 1-year prevalence for pediatric cases of OCD treated in a large health maintenance organization (HMO) was only 0.13%, with the implication that many cases of symptomatically significant OCD are unrecognized and untreated.

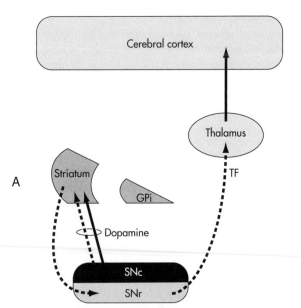
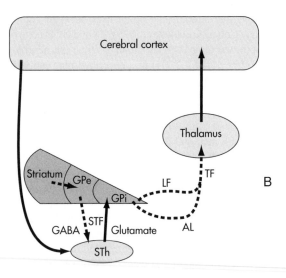

FIGURE 41-1 Two additional ganglia circuits of importance. Excitatory connections are in *solid line,* inhibitory connections are in *dotted line.* **A,** The substantia nigra is interconnected with the striatum. The pigmented, compact part of the substantia nigra *(SNc)* projects to the striatum, exciting some striatal neurons and inhibiting others; the striatum projects to the reticular part of the substantia nigra *(SNr),* which, like globus pallida interna *(GPi),* projects to the thalamus via the thalamic fasciculus *(TF).* **B,** The subthalamic nucleus receives inputs from the cerebral cortex and also is interconnected with the globus pallidus. (As described further in the text, this allows a substantial degree of subthalamic control over pallidal output.) Abbreviations for fiber bundles: *AL,* ansa lenticularis; *GPe,* globus pallida externa; *LF,* lenticular fasciculus; *STF,* subthalamic fasciculus; *TF,* thalamic fasciculus. A basal ganglia loop involving the centromedian and parafascicular nuclei of the thalamus is also prominent anatomically, but was omitted from these schematic diagrams because its functional significance is unclear. From Nolte, J. (2002). *The Human Brain: An Introduction to Its Functional Anatomy* (5th ed.). St Louis: Mosby.

TABLE 41-1
Tics and Tic Disorders

	Onset	Description	Prevalence	Diagnostic Criteria	Associations
Transient tics, history of	Usually 3-10 yr (before age 21)	Motor tics, rarely vocal tics	8%-20% of all children, boys > girls	Duration <12 mo	Possible family TS or tic disorders
Chronic tics, history of	Usually 3-10 yr (before age 21)	Simple and complex motor tics *or* vocal tics (rare); occasionally persist to adulthood	3%-6% of school-age children; boys > girls	Duration >12 mo	Possible family TS or tic disorders Possible ADHD, OCD, other behavioral or normal development
Tourette syndrome	Usually 3-10 yr (before age 21)	Simple and complex vocal and motor tics	0.05%-0.60%; boys > girls	Duration of vocal and motor tics >12 mo; bouts of tics; waxes and wanes; onset before 18-21 yr	Possible family history of TS or tic disorders Possible ADHD, OCD, other behavioral or normal development

Adapted from Schapiro, N.A. (2002). Dude, you don't have Tourette's. *Pediatr Nurs, 22,* 243-253. Reprinted with permission. Data from American Psychiatric Association. (2000). *Diagnostic and Statistical Manual of Mental and Psychiatric Disorders* (4th ed., Text Revision). Washington, DC: Author; Kadesjo, B., & Gillberg, C. (2000). Tourette's disorder: Epidemiology and comorbidity in primary school children. *J Am Acad Child Adolesc Psychiatry, 39,* 548-555; Khalifa, N., & von Knorring, A.L. (2005). Tourette syndrome and other tic disorders in a total population of children: Clinical assessment and background. *Acta Paediatr, 94,* 1608-1614; Leckman, J.F., Bloch, M.H., King, R.A., et al. (2006). Phenomenology of tics and natural history of tic disorders. *Adv Neurol, 99,* 1-16

Key: *ADHD,* attention-deficit/hyperactivity disorder; *OCD,* obsessive-compulsive disorder, *TS,* Tourette syndrome.

Obsessive-compulsive behaviors or OCD has been found in 20% to 60% of children in referral clinics with TS (Hounie, do Rosario-Campos, Diniz, et al., 2006; Kadesjo & Gillberg, 2000). Conversely, up to 10% of referred children with OCD have TS and 30% have tics (Hounie et al., 2006).

Diagnostic Criteria
Tourette Syndrome

TS is part of a spectrum of tic disorders, including transient tic disorder and chronic tic disorder (Table 41-1). Tics are exaggerations and repetitions of normal movements, in contrast with the movements of other disorders, such as myoclonus, chorea, or dystonias (Jankovic & Mejia, 2006). Although there are no clearly established guidelines to differentiate between tics and other movement disorders, the following characteristics would make a tic presentation "questionable": absence of current or historical facial tics, movements that do not wax and wane or change in location on the body, onset after age 18 with no prior history of tics, and presence of complex tics (see later discussion) with no history of simple tics (Woods, Piacentini, & Himle, 2007, p. 23).

Primary tics such as those in TS have no identifiable cause or may be genetic in origin. Conditions that could cause secondary tics or similar movements include Huntington disease, neuroacanthocytosis, head trauma, brain lesions in the basal ganglia, encephalitis, and some medications (Jankovic & Mejia, 2006). There is an increased incidence of tics in children with pervasive developmental disorder, although tics can sometimes be confused with the stereotypic movements common to children with autism (Canitano & Vivanti, 2007).

If symptoms of either motor or vocal tics, but not both, persist for more than 1 year, the child would be considered to have a chronic tic disorder (Leckman, Bloch, King, et al., 2006). Children with both vocal and motor tics that persist for more than 1 year generally fulfill the criteria for Tourette syndrome (APA, 2000). Diagnosis is based on history and observation, with no specific diagnostic tests available (Gilbert, 2006; Singer, 2005). See

BOX 41-2
Diagnostic Criteria for 307.23 Tourette's Disorder

A. Both multiple motor and one or more vocal tics have been present at some time during the illness, although not necessarily concurrently. (A *tic* is a sudden, rapid, recurrent, nonrhythmic, stereotyped motor movement or vocalization.)

B. The tics occur many times a day (usually in bouts) nearly every day or intermittently throughout a period of more than 1 year, and during this period there was never a tic-free period of more than 3 consecutive months.

C. The onset is before age 18 years.

D. The disturbance is not due to the direct physiological effects of a substance (e.g., stimulants) or a general medical condition (e.g., Huntington's disease or postviral encephalitis).

From American Psychiatric Association. (2000). *Diagnostic and Statistical Manual of Mental and Psychiatric Disorders* (4th ed., Text Revision). Washington, DC: Author. Reprinted with permission.

Box 41-2 for the *Diagnostic and Statistical Manual of Mental and Psychiatric Disorders,* 4th edition, Text Revision *(DSM-IV-TR)* criteria for TS.

Health care providers should keep in mind that most children with TS are able to suppress tics during an office visit (Gilbert, 2006), making it necessary for the provider to ask the child and caretakers about the tics and associated symptom severity and their impact on daily life. In specialty practice and research, tic symptoms are measured by self-report, interviews such as the Yale Global Tic Severity Scale, or direct observational methods, such as tic counts from videotapes (Leckman, Riddle, Hardin, et al., 1989; Woods et al., 2007).

Obsessive-Compulsive Disorder

The *DSM-IV-TR* (APA, 2000) defines obsessive-compulsive disorder (OCD) as obsessions or compulsions that are recognized by the individual as excessive or unreasonable, cause marked distress, interfere with normal functioning and/or take more than 1 hour a day, and are not restricted to symptoms of another disorder (e.g., food in eating disorder). Younger children frequently lack insight into the unreasonableness of their obsessions or compulsions, and

Diagnostic Criteria for 300.3 Obsessive-Compulsive Disorder

A. Either obsessions or compulsions:

Obsessions as defined by 1, 2, 3, and 4:

1. Recurrent and persistent thoughts, impulses, or images that are experienced, at some time during the disturbance, as intrusive and inappropriate and that cause marked anxiety or distress

2. The thoughts, impulses, or images are not simply excessive worries about real-life problems

3. The person attempts to ignore or suppress such thoughts, impulses, or images, or to neutralize them with some other thought or action

4. The person recognizes that the obsessional thoughts, impulses, or images are a product of his or her own mind (not imposed from without as in thought insertion)

Compulsions as defined by 1 and 2:

1. Repetitive behaviors (e.g., hand washing, ordering, checking) or mental acts (e.g., praying, counting, repeating words silently) that the person feels driven to perform in response to an obsession, or according to rules that must be applied rigidly

2. The behaviors or mental acts are aimed at preventing or reducing distress or preventing some dreaded event or situation; however, these behaviors or mental acts either are not connected in a realistic way with what they are designed to neutralize or prevent or are clearly excessive

B. At some point during the course of the disorder, the person has recognized that the obsessions or compulsions are excessive or unreasonable. Note: This does not apply to children.

C. The obsessions or compulsions cause marked distress, are time consuming (take >1 hour a day), or significantly interfere with the person's normal routine, occupational (or academic) functioning, or usual social activities or relationships.

D. If another Axis I disorder is present, the content of the obsessions or compulsions is not restricted to it (e.g., preoccupation with food in the presence of an eating disorder; hair pulling in the presence of trichotillomania; concern with appearance in the presence of body dysmorphic disorder; preoccupation with drugs in the presence of a substance use disorder; preoccupation with having a serious illness in the presence of hypochondriasis; preoccupation with sexual urges or fantasies in the presence of a paraphilia; or guilty ruminations in the presence of major depressive disorder).

E. The disturbance is not due to the direct physiological effects of a substance (e.g., a drug of abuse, a medication) or a general medical condition.

Specify if:

With poor insight: if, for most of the time during the current episode, the person does not recognize that the obsessions and compulsions are excessive or unreasonable

From American Psychiatric Association. (2000). *Diagnostic and Statistical Manual of Mental and Psychiatric Disorders* (4th ed., Text Revision). Washington, DC: Author. Reprinted with permission.

---

this insight is not required for the diagnosis of OCD in children (APA, 2000). Box 41-3 lists the *DSM-IV-TR* criteria for OCD.

In primary care, the provider can ask the child and caretakers about any unusual habits and their impact on daily functioning. Although they are not used for diagnosis, the current gold standards for measuring the level of functional impairment in specialty care and research are the Yale-Brown Obsessive Compulsive Scale (Y-BOCS) (Goodman, Price, Rasmussen, et al., 1989a and b) and the Children's Yale-Brown Obsessive Compulsive Scale (CY-BOCS) (Scahill, Riddle, McSwiggin-Hardin, et al., 1997). Geller, Doyle, Shaw, and colleagues (2006) found that eight items from the Child Behavior Checklist had good sensitivity, specificity, and negative and positive predictive values for OCD, which

might lead to a quicker screening tool for primary care providers. Ivarsson and Larsson (2008) found that just two questions, about obsessions and compulsions, performed as well as a longer screen for OCD.

PANDAS

Criteria for PANDAS include presence of either OCD and/or a tic disorder, age of onset between 3 and 11 years, episodic course of symptom severity, and association with group A beta-hemolytic streptococcal infection (Pavone, Parano, Rizzo et al., 2006). These criteria have been controversial, because both TS and OCD have an episodic course, and childhood infection with *Streptococcus* is common, yet epidemiologic studies have not yielded a consistent association between streptococcal infection and tics or OCD (Singer & Williams, 2006). In the clinical arena, deciding that any particular child with tics and OCD symptoms fits PANDAS criteria is difficult, given the high prevalence of both active streptococcal infections and strep carrier states in school-age children, and the lack of specific biologic markers that would distinguish PANDAS from a typical immune reaction to a streptococcal infection (King, 2006). Autoantibodies against the basal ganglia have been found in the peripheral blood of individuals with tics and/or OCD, but the ability of these antibodies to stimulate tic or OC symptoms in animal studies has been inconsistent (Hoekstra & Minderaa, 2005). Researchers have identified a serologic marker, the D18/B17 lymphocyte antigen, which is more commonly found in individuals with rheumatic fever, SC, childhood-onset OCD, and TS (Bottas & Richter, 2002), but these studies have not been replicated (Hoekstra & Minderaa).

Clinical Manifestations at Time of Diagnosis

Tourette Syndrome

Motor and Vocal Tics. Tics are commonly classified as simple or complex. Shoulder shrugging, neck twitching, and facial movements are examples of simple motor tics. Touching objects, skipping, and squatting in a rhythmic sequence (such as every four steps) are examples of complex motor tics. Simple vocal tics include sniffing, barking, coughing, yelling, and hiccupping. Complex vocal tics include repeating parts of words or phrases, talking to oneself, assuming different intonations, and uttering obscenities (Leckman, Bloch, King, et al., 2006; Singer, 2005).

Most children first develop tics in the head, neck, or upper extremities. In children who are eventually diagnosed with TS, many report that eye blinking was their initial tic, followed by other head and facial tics (Leckman, Bloch, Scahill, et al., 2006). Others report vocal tics such as throat clearing and sniffing to be an early symptom of TS (Gilbert, 2006) and less commonly of transient tic disorder (Leckman, Bloch, Scahill, et al., 2006). Once established, tics often occur in discrete bouts over the course of a day, with intertic intervals of 0.5 to 1 second, and intervals between bouts of tics lasting from minutes to several hours over the course of a day. These bouts may occur in a fractal pattern when plotted out on timelines, that is, a geometric pattern repeated at ever smaller scales to enable computer models to predict seemingly irregular events. It is possible that the well-known waxing and waning pattern of tics in TS may be a magnification of this shorter pattern (Leckman, Bloch, King, et al., 2006).

Clinical Manifestations at Time of Diagnosis

TOURETTE SYNDROME
- Tics wax and wane, come and go, irregular patterns
- Simple motor tics
  - Blinking
  - Jerking
  - Shoulder shrugging
  - Neck twitching
- Complex motor tics
  - Skipping
  - Touching
  - Squatting in rhythmic sequence
- Vocal tics
  - Coughing, throat-clearing
  - Sniffing
  - Barking
- Rare: coprolalia and copropraxia

OBSESSIVE-COMPULSIVE DISORDER
- Obsessions (typical categories)
  - Contamination
  - Catastrophic harm (especially to parent)
  - Aggressive or sexual urges
  - Scrupulosity (religious themes)
  - Symmetry urges, having objects arranged "just so" or to be "just so"
- Compulsions (examples)
  - Washing
  - Checking
  - Repeating
  - Touching
  - Counting
  - Ordering, arranging
  - Hoarding
  - Praying

Up to 90% of older children and adults with TS report some premonitory sensations related to their tics, whereas children younger than 10 are more likely to view their tics as completely involuntary (Leckman, Bloch, King, et al., 2006). Although many children are able to suppress their tics for some time, the urge to tic remains, and the tics must eventually be "released." Some children are able to remain relatively tic-free during school hours, only to engage in bouts of tics for several hours at home. Others report that tics are quiescent while they are engaged in an absorbing mental or physical task (Gilbert, 2006). Stress can exacerbate tics, but they can also increase when a child is in a relaxed state, such as watching television, and can be present during sleep (Gilbert, 2006; Singer, 2005).

Coprolalia and Copropraxia. Coprolalia (the involuntary uttering of obscenities, profanities, and racial slurs) and copropraxia (involuntary obscene gestures) tend to appear 4 to 7 years after the onset of tics, peaking during adolescence and greatly diminishing in adulthood. Although coprolalia is almost synonymous with TS in the popular media, it is a relatively rare phenomenon. The percentage of children with TS who exhibit these symptoms ranges from 8% in one study of a general pediatric practice, to 60% of children in a referred tertiary care practice. There is a high male-to-female ratio, ranging from 4.4:1 for coprolalia to 20:1 for copropraxia (Singer, 1997). These particular complex tics can jeopardize a child's safety, ability to stay in school, and ability to socialize (Leckman, Bloch, Scahill, et al., 2006).

Obsessive-Compulsive Behavior and Obsessive-Compulsive Disorder

Obsessions typically cluster in contamination themes, harm to self or others, aggressive or sexual themes, scrupulosity or religiosity, forbidden thoughts, or symmetry urges. Children and adolescents tend to have higher rates than adults of aggressive/harm obsessions, including fears of a catastrophic family event, such as the death of a parent. Adolescents tend to have higher rates of religious obsessions than either younger children or adults (Geller, 2006). Typical compulsions involve washing, checking, repeating, touching, counting, ordering and arranging, hoarding, or praying. Compulsions may involve either physical activities or mental rituals that are used to decrease anxiety associated with obsessions (APA, 2000). Hoarding is a more common compulsion in children and adolescents than in adults (Geller, 2006), and may be related to a subtype of OCD that includes higher instances of magical thinking, less insight, more symmetry and arranging, and higher rates of anxiety and somatic symptoms (Storch, Lack, Merlo, et al., 2007). Children with TS and OCD tend to have compulsions related to symmetry, completion, and perceptions of things being "just right" (Leckman, Bloch, Scahill, et al., 2006, p. 646).

Onset of OCD is usually gradual, but may be sudden or explosive. A majority of children with OCD will have multiple obsessions and compulsions over time, but some younger children have compulsions only (Geller, 2006). OCD symptoms tend to wax and wane, but persist over time in many children with the condition, although the specific obsessions and rituals may change. In some instances, parents are intimately involved in the rituals, typically offering the child repeated reassurance or helping the child avoid feared objects or situations (Chansky, 2000; Storch, Geffken, Merlo, et al., 2007). Other children and adolescents go to great lengths to hide their symptoms from others, including their parents and health care providers, for fear of being perceived as "crazy." An older child might be relatively secretive about hoarding, mental rituals, and bedtime rituals, for example. In comparing parent and child reports of OCD in a geographically and ethnically diverse study, researchers found that of 35 identified cases of OCD, only 4 were identified by parent report and 32 by child report, with one overlapping case (Rapoport, Inoff-Germain, Weissman, et al., 2000).

Treatment

Behavioral Treatments for Tics

Behavioral therapies rely on the child's awareness of premonitory urges to tic, present in most older children, adolescents, and adults, and attempt to change the behavioral response to this urge in order to reduce tics (Himle, Woods, Piacentini, et al., 2006). Habit reversal training consists of increasing awareness of the tic mechanisms, situations in which the tic is likely to occur and earliest signs of occurrences, and then developing a competing and incompatible physical response to the tic. In a review of both open and randomized controlled trials of children and adults using habit reversal therapy, Himle and colleagues (2006) found significant reductions in tics when compared with supportive psychotherapy and waiting list controls. Larger trials are currently underway. Exposure and response prevention (cognitive behavioral therapy) has also been found to be effective in adults (Verdellen, Keijsers, Cath, et al., 2004), and at least one study shows effect sizes of tic reduction to

---

BOX 41-4

Cognitive Behavioral Therapy (CBT)

1. Psychoeducation
   Framing OCD in a neurobehavioral model for parents and children, with analogies to medical illnesses
2. Cognitive training
   Teaching the child tactics for resisting OCD, such as "bossing back" the OCD symptom
3. Mapping OCD
   Detailing the child's specific obsessions and compulsions, particularly identifying the "transition zone" where the child is already able, at times, to win the battle against OCD
4. Graded exposure and response prevention (E/RP)
   Either imagined or actual exposures, in which the child is exposed to the feared object, action, or thought without performing the ritual

Data from March, J.S., & Mulle, K. (1998). *OCD in Children and Adolescents: A Cognitive Behavioral Treatment Manual.* New York: Guilford Press.

---

be larger than habit reversal training. Although behavioral therapies appear to be well tolerated, there is some concern that support for behavioral research might undo many years of public education by the Tourette syndrome community, emphasizing the involuntary nature of tics. Indeed, for many cases where tics are not bothersome, dangerous, or painful for the child, the best approach might simply be to allow the child to tic (Schapiro, 2002; Swain, Scahill, Lombroso, et al., 2007). However, behavioral research has received strong support from adults with TS who have often developed their own behavioral approach to tic suppression (Himle et al., 2006).

Cognitive Behavioral Therapy for OCD

Cognitive behavioral therapy (CBT) has become the cornerstone of treatment for OCD (March & Mulle, 1998) (Box 41-4). March and Mulle generally recommend a treatment plan of between 13 and 20 weekly sessions. A recent meta-analysis of randomized controlled pediatric trials involving either CBT or medication showed that CBT was more effective than control (wait list or placebo therapy) and that the effect sizes for CBT were larger than effect sizes for medication (Watson & Rees, 2008). In a review of 17 studies involving a variety of CBT configurations, individualized CBT was found to be "probably efficacious" and group and family CBT were found to be "possibly efficacious" (Barrett, Farrell, Pina, et al., 2008, p. 149) given limitations of study designs. A comparison of CBT and sertraline for treatment of OCD found CBT to be equally effective for children with and without tics (March, Franklin, Leonard, et al., 2007). Even early adolescents, who may not show the insight of older teens and adults, have shown improvement in group CBT with family involvement (Martin & Thienemann, 2005). Children as young as 5 to 8 years have been treated in modified CBT that addresses their cognitive and emotional development, as well as their greater dependence on parents, by including family members more directly in the groups (Freeman, Garcia, Coyne, et al., 2008).

Parental involvement and parent-child teamwork are crucial to the success of treatment, both in initiating the therapy and in helping with the child's "homework" between therapy sessions (Chansky, 2000; March & Benton, 2007). Working together with the therapist, the child helps pick the target ritual for extinction. If the target ritual is hand washing, for example, the parent must agree to limit the length of time the child spends washing, to the point

of escorting the child out of the bathroom (Chansky, 2000; March & Benton, 2007). If the ritual involves checking (e.g., for bugs in the bed, for the parent's forgiveness, or for locking the door), the parent must agree to limit the number of times the child is reassured. The parent reminds the child that OCD is playing tricks and trying to control the child. Although such limits may seem cruel in the face of a crying, anxious child, they are necessary in order to reinforce the message that the child can avoid the ritual without catastrophic consequences (Chansky, 2000).

If the child or adolescent with TS and/or OCD is seeing a therapist, the primary care provider should obtain written permission from the parent to communicate with the therapist and assent from the older child and adolescent, particularly if confidential issues might be involved.

Pharmacologic Therapy for Tics

Experts in TS care recommend starting medication (Table 41-2) for any associated conditions that may be present and cause impairment, such as OCD (see p. 801) or attention-deficit/hyperactivity disorder (ADHD) (p. 802 and Chapter 12), before beginning medication to reduce tics (Gilbert, 2006; Swain et al., 2007).

Pimozide (Orap) and haloperidol (Haldol), dopamine receptor antagonists, are approved by the U.S. Food and Drug Administration (FDA) to treat tics in children and adolescents (Kenney, Kuo, & Jimenez-Shahed, 2008), have a long history of use in TS, and have shown efficacy in randomized, placebo-controlled trials (Swain et al., 2007). Potential side effects of these medications, along with other neuroleptics, are extrapyramidal effects, tardive dyskinesia, cognitive dulling, sedation, and weight gain (Swain et al., 2007). In addition, haloperidol has been linked to QTc segment prolongation and cardiac arrhythmias (FDA, 2007). Atypical neuroleptics, such as risperidone (Risperdal) or olanzapine (Zyprexa), are sometimes used for explosive behavior and tics, and may have fewer side effects than older neuroleptics; however, they have been associated with greater weight gain. Aripiprazole (Abilify) has been used in adults with severe coprolalia (Ben Djebara, Worbe, Schupbach, et al., 2008). A rare but serious and potentially fatal adverse effect of any dopamine blocker is neuroleptic malignant syndrome, consisting of hyperthermia, muscular rigidity, myoglobinemia, and altered mental status. Neuroleptic malignant syndrome can occur even at low doses and tends to occur early in treatment (Rusyniak & Sprague, 2006).

The alpha-adrenergic receptor agonists clonidine (Catapres) and guanfacine (Tenex) have been used to treat tics and impulsivity in ADHD, with modest effects on motor tics and less effect on vocal tics (Kenney et al., 2008). Guanfacine causes less sedation and hypotension than clonidine. Because the medications have fewer adverse effects than neuroleptics, they are often tried first, even though they will help only a portion of children and adolescents with TS. Their primary use is in hypertension, and they can cause hypotension in some children, as well as irritability, insomnia, headache, dry mouth, and depression (Kenney et al., 2008; Swain et al., 2007).

Botulinum toxin blocks the release of acetylcholine at the neuromuscular junction and results in a temporary reduction in muscle activity that may last from weeks to months. It has been used sparingly to reduce severe tics in discrete muscle areas, such as the neck (Aguirregomozcorta, Pagonabarraga, Diaz-Manera, et al., 2008; Swain et al., 2007).

TABLE 41-2

Medications Used in the Treatment of Tourette Syndrome and Obsessive-Compulsive Disorder

Medication Class	Specific Examples	Uses	Notes	Side Effects	Interactions
Alpha-adrenergic receptor agonists	Clonidine, guanfacine	Tics, inattention, impulsiveness, hyperactivity	Effects mild, but often tried first; must be tapered off	Sedation, headaches, dry mouth, irritability	Additive sedation with antihistamines, opiates, alcohol
Neuroleptics	Haloperidol, pimozide, risperidone, aripiprazole, ziprasidone, olanzapine	Tics; risperidone, zisprasidone, aripiprazole used for rages, add-on to SSRIs for refractory OCD	Beneficial effects on tics noted for >30 yr	Sedation, weight gain, cognitive dulling, increased QT interval (pimozide), blood dyscrasias, neuroleptic	Macrolide antibiotics, grapefruit increased QT interval, tardive dyskinesia, additive sedation with other CNS depressants, fluoxetine ↑ levels of risperidone, aripiprazole, ziprasidone
SSRIs	Fluoxetine, fluvoxamine, sertraline	OCD, co-occurring depression	Dosage for OCD higher than antidepressant dosages	GI disturbance, sexual dysfunction, dry mouth, sweating, rare suicidal ideation (black box warning)	Additive effects with CNS depressants, may alter metabolism of phenobarbital, desipramine, codeine, central serotonin syndrome combined with dextromethorphan, triptans, Ecstasy, MAOIs, CYP 2D6, CYP 3A3/4 inhibitors, depending on medication
Tricyclic antidepressants	Imipramine, desipramine, nortryptyline, clomipramine	Clomipramine for OCD	Do not worsen tics, may be beneficial with coexisting depression, anxiety	Dry mouth, sweating, fatigue, dizziness, weight gain, tachycardia, increased QT interval, rare suicidal ideation (black box warning)	Difficult to monitor (same dose produces varying serum levels), hazardous in overdose, increased levels when combined with SSRIs
Stimulants	Dexedrine, methylphenidate	ADHD	May be effective alone or combined with alpha-adrenergic agonist, neuroleptic; may worsen tics in some children	Headache, anxiety, weight loss, possible increase in tics in some children	Increased cardiac effects with tricyclics, beta blockers

Data from Arnsten, A.F., Scahill, L., & Findling, R.L. (2007). Alpha-2 adrenergic receptor agonists for the treatment of attention-deficit/hyperactivity disorder: Emerging concepts from new data. *J Child Adolesc Psychopharmacol, 17*(4), 393-406; Harrison, J.N., Schneider, B., & Walkup, J.T. (2007). Medical management of Tourette syndrome and co-occurring conditions. In D.W. Woods, J.C. Piacentini, & J.T. Walkup (Eds.), *Treating Tourette Syndrome and Tic Disorders*. New York: Guilford Press; Taketomo, C.K., Hodding, J.H., & Kraus, D.M. (2008). *Pediatric Dosage Handbook: 2008-2009* (15th ed.). Hudson, OH: Lexi-Comp.

Key: *ADHD*, attention-deficit/hyperactivity disorder; *CNS*, central nervous system; *GI*, gastrointestinal; *MAOI*, monoamine oxidase inhibitor; *OCD*, obsessive-compulsive disorder; *SSRI*, selective serotonin reuptake inhibitor.

Pharmacologic Therapy for Obsessions and Compulsions

The first medication to show significant effect for OCD was clomipramine (Anafranil), a tricyclic serotonin reuptake inhibitor (Rapoport, 1989). Since then selective serotonin reuptake inhibitors (SSRIs) have largely supplanted clomipramine, due to a greater safety profile, particularly in overdose (Birmaher, Brent, Bernet, et al., 2007) and diminished side effects (Blier, Habib, & Flament, 2006; Goodman, Storch, Geffken, et al., 2006). Children taking clomipramine can gain a significant amount of weight, and can be at risk for cardiac arrhythmias and seizures. However, some medication trials have shown that clomipramine may be more effective than SSRIs (Geller, Biederman, Stewart, et al., 2003) (see Table 41-2).

Currently, clomipramine, fluoxetine (Prozac), sertraline (Zoloft), and fluvoxamine (Luvox) are FDA-approved to treat pediatric OCD (FDA, 2004). In a meta-analysis of pediatric drug trials for OCD, paroxetine (Paxil), fluoxetine, sertraline, and fluvoxamine were found to have comparable efficacy (Geller et al., 2003). In a randomized placebo-controlled trial comparing sertraline with CBT, either CBT alone (or with placebo) or sertraline and CBT were effective for most children, with the combination of CBT and sertraline showing the greatest benefit (March et al., 2007). Some children with OCD and tics showed less benefit from medication, but were just as likely to benefit from CBT and the combination of CBT and medication. Doses used in OCD are generally higher than doses used in depression, and medication effects may not be evident until 10 to 12 weeks after initiation (Goodman et al., 2006). Treatment benefits with medication do not seem to be maintained once medication is stopped, in contrast with CBT.

There are no long-term safety studies of SSRIs in children (Hetrick, Merry, McKenzie, et al., 2007). Although relatively well tolerated, adverse effects may include behavioral activation and akathisia, as well as mania in those with previously undetected bipolar disorder (BPD) (see Chapter 33) (Murphy, Segarra, Storch, et al., 2008). Some children experience nausea and stomach pain, particularly if the medication is started at a higher dose or increased rapidly. About 30% to 40% of adults report sexual dysfunction while taking SSRIs, and though the incidence appears to be lower in youths, there may be reluctance to discuss this issue by both youths and providers, leading to underreporting (Murphy et al., 2008). Younger children, less than age 7, may have a higher incidence of adverse effects (Zuckerman, Vaughan, Whitney, et al., 2007). A concern about growth retardation with long-term SSRI use has emerged with the publication of four case studies of children with TS or OCD and previously identified growth issues. The children showed abnormalities of growth hormone, which resolved when the SSRIs were discontinued in three of the cases (Weintrob, Cohen, Klipper-Aurbach, et al., 2002).

In 2004, the FDA issued a black box warning for all children and adolescents under age 18 taking antidepressant medication for any reason (FDA, 2004), citing a risk of increased suicidal ideation but no increase in completed suicides, early in treatment, in pediatric drug trials (see Chapter 33 for a more complete discussion). Although SSRIs have shown relatively greater efficacy for pediatric OCD when compared with pediatric depression, providers should remain alert and monitor children closely for physical, behavioral, and psychological adverse effects when these medications are initiated in children with OCD (Goodman et al., 2006).

Pharmacologic Therapy for Attention-Deficit/Hyperactivity Disorder with Tourette Syndrome or Obsessive-Compulsive Disorder

It had been thought that the stimulants used to treat ADHD (see Chapter 12) could exacerbate or even cause tics to appear, but this effect may have been coincidental: ADHD often surfaces before tics in children with both TS and ADHD, and tics themselves tend to wax and wane (Swain et al., 2007). In 2002, a study comparing children with TS and ADHD taking methylphenidate, methylphenidate and clonidine, and no medication found that children on no medication had more tics than the two treatment groups (Tourette Syndrome Study Group, 2002). Although there were some methodologic problems with the study (Gilbert, 2006), the results supported judicious use of stimulant medications for children with both tic disorders and TS, and follow-up studies have shown that most children with TS tolerate stimulants well (Erenberg, 2005; Gadow, Sverd, Nolan, et al., 2007). Alpha-adrenergic receptor agonists such as clonidine seem to decrease impulsivity but not inattention (Arnsten, Scahill, & Findling, 2007; Tourette Syndrome Study Group, 2002). Some children will benefit from medication for both OCD and ADHD (Goodman et al., 2006), although stimulants may increase obsessions and anxiety (Geller, 2006) and stimulants may decrease the metabolism of clomipramine.

To Medicate or Not to Medicate?

Because of the relative risk of side effects to modest benefit, most TS experts recommend trying behavioral and environmental measures before using medication, especially for tics, and to consider using medication for OCD or ADHD first if these are impairing function, beginning with one medication at a time (Harrison, Schneider, & Walkup, 2007). Packer (1997) and Ginsburg and Kingery (2007) emphasize the importance of distinguishing between symptoms that bother the child, and symptoms that bother the parent and siblings. For example, a parent who is unusually sensitive to environmental noise may be bothered by vocal tics that do not disturb the child (Packer, 1997). Providing parents, teachers, and classmates with information about tics and TS may be all that is needed for younger children. For children in middle school, whose tics are at their peak at the same time that their classmates

are least tolerant, a course of medication for tic suppression may be indicated, particularly for children with loud vocal tics (Gilbert, 2006).

The *Expert Consensus Treatment Guidelines for Obsessive Compulsive Disorder* (March, Frances, Carpenter, et al., 1997) recommends CBT first for younger children and milder symptoms of OCD. CBT plus serotonin reuptake inhibitors are recommended for moderate symptoms in children and adolescents; for severe OCD, the individual may need to begin medication alone before being able to engage in therapy. These recommendations have been reinforced in recent literature (Bjorgvinsson, Hart, & Heffelfinger, 2007; Flament, Geller, Irak, et al., 2007; Keeley, Storch, Dhungana, et al., 2007), with the added caveat that there seems to be a subset of individuals who do not respond to either CBT or serotonin reuptake inhibitors.

If needed, the goal of medication should be to use the lowest dose possible to bring the target symptom down to acceptable levels and to enhance the child's development. The doses of SSRIs used in OCD are often higher than those used in depression, and children with OCD may require treatment for a longer time than those with depression before benefits are seen (Blier et al., 2006). Many psychoactive medications have become household words, and children can have relatively sophisticated, if not necessarily accurate, understandings of their uses and reputations. When discussing the possibility of medication with a child and family, it is important to take into account their previous experiences with similar medications in other family members, and the differing concerns and opinions that parents, children, and their siblings may have (Rappaport & Chubinsky, 2000). The recommended medication regimens for target symptoms of TS, OCD, and ADHD are continually evolving, so it is important for the provider to ascertain how, when, and where the family has acquired knowledge about the medications, and for the provider to supply current information (Schapiro, 2002).

Complementary and Alternative Therapies

Confronted with limited efficacy and adverse effects for medications to reduce tics and control behavioral manifestations of both TS and OCD, many children and families turn to complementary and alternative treatments for these conditions (Kurlan, 2006). In one survey of families of children with TS, over 80% used some vitamins or supplements, most commonly calcium and magnesium, and a significant percentage had tried allergy treatment, homeopathy, or dietary changes (Mantel, Meyers, Tran, et al., 2004). There are some case reports of acupuncture being used for TS internationally (Wu, Li, & Kang, 1996), with more recent updates published in Chinese. The National Center for Complementary and Alternative Medicine (n.d.) does not list any current or recently completed trials for TS. In a 6-week randomized controlled trial, German researchers found a decrease in motor and vocal tics in adults treated with delta-9-tetrahydrocannabinol, an active ingredient in marijuana (Müller-Vahl, 2003).

Latitudes, a journal that promotes alternatives to medication for a variety of neurologic disorders, reports that controlling allergies and diet can help alleviate symptoms of TS, ADHD, and OCD (Association for Comprehensive NeuroTherapy, n.d.). A recent book published by the website's moderator (Rogers, 2005) encourages parents to look at the elimination of a variety of potential tic triggers, including cell phones, environmental toxins, food additives, allergies, and Candida, as well as the addition of a variety of supplements. The general difficulties of evaluating the efficacy of any particular treatment for tics are discussed below. In addition, the editors of *Latitudes* note that most parents are trying several modalities at once (e.g., amino acids and vitamins), making it more difficult to disentangle the effect of any one treatment. In an attempt to clarify community experience with food and tics, Müller-Vahl, Buddensiek, Geomelas, and colleagues (2008) surveyed German adults with TS and found that they associated caffeine, colas, black tea, refined sugar, and preservatives with increased tics, and no foods were noted to specifically decrease tics.

In an extensive review of alternative medical approaches and dietary supplements, Waltz (2000) found that many could be generally beneficial, but none were yet known to specifically diminish OCD symptoms. A more recent review recommended St. John's wort for OCD (Lakhan & Vieira, 2008); however, the studies cited were actually of adults with major depression. A randomized controlled trial of 60 adults with OCD found that St. John's wort was no more effective than placebo (Kobak, Taylor, Bystritsky, et al., 2005).

Anticipated Advances in Diagnosis and Management

The difficulties involved in making a clinical or laboratory diagnosis of PANDAS have been discussed previously; early studies of plasma exchange and immune globulin were promising but invasive (Perlmutter, Leitman, Garvey, et al., 1999) and evidence for the effectiveness of antibiotic treatment has been inconsistent (Garvey, Perlmutter, Allen, et al., 1999; Snider, Lougee, Slattery, et al., 2005). Despite the state of current research, children in community clinics are more likely to receive both a diagnosis of and antibiotic treatment for PANDAS than children in specialty clinics (Gabbay, Coffey, Babb, et al., 2008), attesting to continuing interest in this phenomenon among primary care clinicians. Research into PANDAS and other potential immune abnormalities, such as levels of CD19-positive B cells, in individuals with TS and OCD is ongoing (da Rocha et al., 2008; Hoekstra & Minderaa, 2005).

The working structural model for OCD, based on functional magnetic resonance imaging (fMRI) and the positive effects of serotonin reuptake inhibitors, has involved the orbitofrontal cortex and the striatum, but recently whole brain imaging has implicated other pathways in the frontal and parietal regions (Menzies, Chamberlain, Laird, et al., 2008). Some researchers are investigating the possible patterns of brain activation during obsessions and compulsions that involve harm avoidance as compared with those that involve feelings of incompleteness (Olatunji, Wilhelm, & Deckersbach, 2008). Medication research for OCD involves adding small doses of atypical neuroleptics, such as risperidone, to SSRIs (Goodman et al., 2006). Additional interest is focused on glutamate blockers, such as the medication riluzole used in amyotrophic lateral sclerosis, because OCD is thought to involve an excess of glutamate (Blier et al., 2006).

Newer atypical antipsychotic (dopamine-blocking) medications, such as aripiprazole (Abilify) and ziprasidone (Geodon), are being tried in clinical practice, with limited research data available. A number of other medications are under investigation for control of tics, including antiseizure medications (topiramate), dopamine agonists (pergolide), and calcium channel blockers (donepezil)

(Swain et al., 2007). Initial studies showing benefits for nicotine or mecylamine augmentation of neuroleptics were not replicated in randomized controlled trials (Swain et al., 2007). These studies highlight some of the problems in investigating medications for TS: the symptoms wax and wane, and any improvement may be spontaneous, rather than a medication effect; because tics vary by location, intensity, suppressibility, discomfort, and social impairment, they are difficult to quantify; and there are inherent reliability issues with any established tic rating scale (Gilbert, 2006; Swain et al., 2007).

Some centers have tried transcranial magnetic stimulation in adults with TS, and a few adults with intractable tics have undergone thalamic stimulation, or had electrodes placed in thalamic nuclei. These procedures are highly experimental (Swain et al., 2007).

Research about etiology and treatments for both TS and OCD is quite dynamic, with new findings appearing monthly. Primary care providers who are working with children who have TS and/or OCD are encouraged to check frequently for updated information.

Associated Problems of Tourette Syndrome and Obsessive-Compulsive Disorder and Treatment
Tourette Syndrome and Attention-Deficit/Hyperactivity Disorder

In ADHD, children exhibit developmentally inappropriate levels of inattention, impulsivity, and/or overactivity (APA, 2000) (see also Chapter 12). In a review of over 6000 individuals with TS from an international database, 55% were diagnosed with ADHD by their submitting physician (Freeman, 2007), including 55% of male children and 36% of female children in the database. Studies have shown that children with TS plus ADHD exhibit more internalizing and externalizing symptoms, poorer social adaptation, more difficulty sustaining attention, poorer scores on tests of verbal and performance intelligence, and more severe TS symptoms than children with TS alone (Gaze, Kepley, & Walkup, 2006; Spencer, Biederman, Harding, et al., 1998).

Obsessive-Compulsive Disorder and Attention-Deficit/Hyperactivity Disorder

Up to 53% of boys and 24% of girls with OCD also have ADHD (Geller, 2006). Out of concern that apparent symptoms of ADHD, such as inattention, might be due to unreported intrusive thoughts or compulsions, a study team compared children from a psychopharmacology clinic who fulfilled *DSM-IV* criteria for ADHD and

---

Associated Problems of Tourette Syndrome and Obsessive-Compulsive Disorder and Treatment

- ADHD
- Rage attacks
- Self-injurious behavior
- Body dysmorphic disorder and eating disorders
- Other psychiatric conditions (anxiety, bipolar)

Data from Gaze, C., Kepley, H.O., & Walkup, J.T. (2006). Co-occurring psychiatric disorders in children and adolescents with Tourette syndrome. *J Child Neurol, 21*(8), 657-664; Mathews, C.A., Waller, J., Glidden, D., et al. (2004). Self injurious behaviour in Tourette syndrome: Correlates with impulsivity and impulse control. *J Neurol Neurosurg Psychiatry, 75*(8), 1149-1155.

for ADHD plus OCD (Geller, Biederman, Faraone, et al., 2004; Geller, Biederman, Faraone, et al., 2002). There were no significant differences in core ADHD symptoms, scores on the Child Behavior Checklist, or functional academic impairment between the two groups, suggesting that the ADHD diagnosis represented an additional condition, rather than a variation of OCD presentation. In addition, the onset of ADHD preceded the onset of OCD symptoms in most subjects. The authors note that the presence of untreated ADHD might limit the ability of a child with OCD to focus on cognitive behavioral treatment.

Rage Attacks

Sudden, explosive outbursts of behavior are reported by 25% to 70% of children with TS who are referred to specialty clinics, depending on the site (Budman, Rockmore, Stokes, et al., 2003). These outbursts are described as stereotypic, with abrupt onset or unpredictable and primitive displays of aggression that are grossly out of proportion to provoking stimuli, and that threaten serious self-harm, property destruction, or injury to others. Outbursts are frequently directed at the child's mother, usually accompanied by autonomic activation, and appear impulsive and poorly modulated, rather than intentional goal-directed expressions of anger or manipulation. Children are typically described as showing empathy between attacks, with immediate remorse after the attack's resolution (Budman, Bruun, Park, et al., 2000; Budman et al., 2003). The relationship of rage attacks to tic severity and coexisting conditions, such as ADHD or OCD, is unclear and controversial (Swain et al., 2007). Parents have rated this symptom to be the least common and most distressing of all TS symptoms (Dooley, Brna, & Gordon, 1999). Children who have rage attacks are at risk for deterioration in home or school functioning (Budman et al., 2000; Dooley, 2006).

Self-Injurious Behavior

In the database of over 6000 individuals in the TS International Database Consortium, 14.3% of individuals had self-injurious behavior (SIB), as reported by their physicians (Freeman, 2007). However, older studies, some using client self-report, found prevalence ranging from 17% to 53% (Robertson & Orth, 2006). SIB ranges from picking at scabs and self-cutting, to touching hot stoves, poking oneself with sharp objects, headbanging, and eye injuries. Jankovic (1997) describes the behavior as straddling the line between a compulsion and a complex tic. Mathews, Waller, Glidden, and colleagues (2004) suggest that milder forms of SIB may be related to obsessions and compulsions, whereas more serious SIB may be more related to impulsivity, including rages. Although SIB may not involve a well-organized plan to inflict self-injury, individuals have been known to injure themselves significantly and to require hospitalization (Cheung, Shahed, & Jankovic, 2007).

Trichotillomania (recurrent pulling out of one's own hair) is more common in individuals with OCD (Franklin, Tolin, & Diefenbach, 2008) but may be more connected to other habit disorders (Lochner, Seedat, du Toit, et al., 2005). Individuals commonly report a trancelike state and positive reinforcement from the behavior that is different from the described experience of either a complex tic or a compulsion. Although individuals with OCD generally report more impairment than those with trichotillomania, OCD is also more amenable to treatment.

Body Dysmorphic Disorder and Eating Disorders

There are some similarities in age of onset, symptoms, and response to SSRIs between individuals with OCD and those with body dysmorphic disorder (BDD) (McKay, Gosselini, & Gupta, 2008), which is a preoccupation with a defect in appearance (APA, 2000). The joint preoccupation with symmetry and the feeling that something isn't "just right" are striking (see Chapter 25). In addition there are greater incidences of BDD in individuals and families with OCD (and vice versa) than would be expected to occur by chance (Phillips, 2000). However, there are also some phenomenologic differences: checking in OCD is done to decrease anxiety, whereas appearance checking in BDD often increases anxiety. In addition, individuals with OCD are usually aware of, and distressed by, the irrational nature of their obsessions and compulsions, whereas individuals with BDD generally do not display that kind of insight (McKay, Gosselini, & Gupta, 2008).

In a large genetics study of eating disorders, 41% of participants also had OCD, with no significant differences between those with anorexia nervosa and those with bulimia (Kaye, Bulik, Thornton, et al., 2004). Cumella, Kally, and Wall (2007) found that hospitalized women with eating disorders who also had OCD had more severe disease but similar treatment outcomes to women who did not have OCD if both conditions were treated simultaneously. Hospitalized adolescents with eating disorders in another study had only a 16.8% prevalence of OCD, still higher than the population at large (Salbach-Andrae, Lenz, Simmendinger, et al., 2008).

Other Psychiatric Conditions

Coffey, Biederman, Smoller, and associates (2000) found greater incidences of non-OCD anxiety disorders, particularly separation anxiety, as well as bipolar disorder, in children with severe TS. In a more recent study, over 90% of children with mild or moderate TS qualified for some coexisting psychiatric diagnosis (including ADHD and OCD) (Robertson, 2006). According to Coffey and associates (2000), the presence of a mood disorder was a better predictor of psychiatric hospitalization than merely the presence of ADHD or OCD. Gaze and colleagues (2006) caution that rates of coexisting conditions are lower in community samples, and that the demoralization associated with coping with multiple conditions (such as TS, OCD, and ADHD) may sometimes be confused with clinical depression.

A number of studies have found equally high rates of associated psychiatric conditions in children with OCD referred to treatment clinics (Geller, 2006). These included mood disorders, anxiety, disruptive behavior, developmental disorders, and enuresis. In one study of 120 children and adolescents with OCD, 35% had bipolar disorder, which was associated with earlier onset, more hoarding symptoms, and lower response to treatment (Masi, Perugi, Millepiedi, et al., 2007).

There have been some anecdotal accounts of repetitive hallucinations, particularly auditory hallucinations, in nonpsychotic children with TS who have other coexisting psychiatric conditions (Bruun & Budman, 1999; Schreier, 1999). Though the literature on nonpsychotic pediatric hallucinations is scant, a more recent study of children with auditory hallucinations showed an association with anxiety disorders (Best & Mertin, 2007). Because children may not spontaneously disclose this symptom, some clinicians recommend asking all children with TS about the presence of hallucinations (Bruun & Budman, 1999).

Prognosis

In a cross-sectional study of 36 children with TS who were contacted 7 years after diagnosis, Leckman, Zhang, Vitale, and associates (1998) found that tics began at a mean of 5.6 years of age, followed by progressive worsening and peaking at age 10. Whereas 22% of the sample had tics that were severe enough to jeopardize or prevent their functioning in school at the peak of symptoms, the tics steadily declined during adolescence, with 50% of the individuals virtually tic-free by age 18. Most of the remaining 18-year-olds experienced minimal to mild symptoms, whereas only 10% reported moderate or marked tics. A 2-year case-control longitudinal study of 41 children and adolescents with TS found that psychosocial stress was associated with increased levels of depression and obsessive-compulsive symptoms but not tic severity, whereas depression predicted increased tic severity (Lin, Katsovich, Ghebremichael, et al., 2007). Bloch, Peterson, Scahill, and colleagues (2006) surveyed adults with TS and found that worst-ever OCD symptoms peaked 2 years later than worst-ever tic symptoms, and that one third of participants still reported having OCD symptoms. For a small number of individuals with TS, tics and self injurious behavior associated with tics are severe enough to require hospitalization, with sequelae ranging from fractures to vision loss, burns, and suicidal ideation or attempts (Cheung et al., 2007).

Tic disorders are overrepresented in adults with ADHD, but the presence of tics does not affect the severity of ADHD; nor does the presence of ADHD affect the course of the tic disorder, which is generally diminished in adulthood (Spencer, Biederman, Faraone, et al., 2001). OCD, in contrast, has a variable course that tends to persist through adulthood, although Geller (2006) questions the validity of older studies, given current improvements in treatment. A meta-analysis of follow-up studies with a total of 521 pooled participants found that OCD persisted in 41% of those diagnosed as children, with 61% having OCD symptoms (Stewart, Geller, Jenike, et al., 2004).

Children with TS and OCD can be expected to attain normal developmental milestones and to achieve a normal life span. The lay literature notes that some professional athletes, artists, musicians, actors, professors, and health care professionals have TS and/or OCD (Shady, Jewers, Furer, et al., 2007).

PRIMARY CARE MANAGEMENT

Health Care Maintenance
Growth and Development

Children with both TS and OCD are generally thought to achieve normal growth and developmental milestones unless the child has additional conditions, such as pervasive developmental disorder or psychosis. One article has raised the concern about growth issues in children on long-term SSRIs (Weintrob et al., 2002), but there were only four children in the study, who had previously identified growth problems. Some medications used for TS or OCD may stimulate appetite, especially neuroleptics (such as haloperidol, pimozide, or risperidone) or alpha-adrenergic agonists (such as clonidine), and some serotonin reuptake inhibitors or SSRIs are associated with weight gain.

Although there are some cases of very early onset OCD, most children develop symptoms after age 7 (Geller, 2006). Parents and some providers may be concerned with distinguishing between developmentally normal rituals and obsessions of early childhood, and the rituals and obsessions associated with OCD, particularly in families with a history of tics or OCD among first-degree relatives. Normal childhood rituals bear some similarities to OCD-related rituals: needing things to be "just so," having lucky numbers, and having bedtime rituals. However, in children who are unaffected by OCD, the normal developmental rituals seem to aid in mastering anxiety and enhancing the child's socialization, whereas in OCD the rituals are distressing, isolating, and hinder daily life (Leonard, Goldberger, Rapoport, et al., 1990). In addition, whereas ritualized behavior starts to fade in children by age 7 or 8, OCD symptoms often start to increase at this age.

Some parents of young children who were later diagnosed with TS or OCD noted that their children had more separation anxiety than peers or siblings, more aggressive reactions to peers, more inflexibility, and more trouble with self-regulation (Shady et al., 2007).

Diet

Abrupt changes in dietary preferences may be a part of normal development or responses to contamination fears or other obsessions. In addition, there is an association of OCD with eating disorders (Salbach-Andrae et al., 2008) and individuals with both OCD and eating disorders go to great lengths to hide their preoccupations (Merlo, Storch, Murphy, et al., 2005; Waltz, 2000). A detailed discussion of food aversion and eating disorders is beyond the scope of this chapter (see Chapter 25); however, the growth and body mass index (BMI) charts of children with TS and/or OCD should be carefully maintained. Any failure to make or maintain expected gains in height and weight, failure to progress through puberty, or secondary amenorrhea in the absence of pregnancy should prompt a more careful history, examination, and referral to the appropriate specialists. If the child is already seeing a psychotherapist, close communication between the primary care provider and the therapist is essential.

In looking for alternatives to allopathic medications, parents sometimes try elimination diets or restrict the intake of foods thought to trigger tics or obsessive-compulsive symptoms. In these situations, it is important to work with the family to ensure adequate caloric and nutritional intake.

Safety

Some children with TS feel compelled to touch hot stoves, stand at the edge of precipices, or go through intersections with their eyes closed, risking injury at an age when they would be expected to "know better" (Mathews et al., 2004; Robertson & Orth, 2006). Self-injurious behavior is associated with both TS and OCD (Cheung et al., 2007; Shoval, Zalsman, Sher, et al., 2006). Some individuals with TS may have suicidal thoughts related to complex tics and compulsions (Cheung et al., 2007), and suicidal ideation is increased in both OCD and mood disorders (Shoval et al., 2006) (see Chapter 33). Although parents may not be able to prevent all risky or self-injurious behaviors in older children and adolescents, they should be alert to the possibility of such behaviors, and seek guidance from professionals with expertise in TS and OCD if they occur.

The treatment of self-injurious behaviors can be difficult, depending on whether the behavior is actually a complex tic or a compulsion (Jankovic, 1997). Medications that are intended to control tics can actually make compulsions worse, and medications for OCD do not usually diminish tics (Goodman et al., 2006). CBT can be quite helpful for compulsions, but the effect on tics is more modest (Barrett et al., 2008; Verdellen et al., 2004).

Adolescents with TS, like other adolescents with chronic conditions, may be more likely than their nonaffected peers to engage in risky behavior (Sawyer, Drew, Yeo, et al., 2007), but there is a paucity of research literature that describes their experiences. Adolescents with TS rate their overall quality of life as lower than adolescents without chronic conditions (Storch, Merlo, Lack, et al., 2007) and there may be additional risks for youths associated specifically with TS. Anecdotal accounts by adults with TS note that tobacco, alcohol, and marijuana use temporarily alleviates a variety of symptoms (Handler, 2004; Wilensky, 1999). The short-term benefits of cannabinoids are confirmed by emerging research in Germany (Müller-Vahl, 2003). For adolescents with TS and OCD whose tics, obsessions, and hyperactivity are not declining, symptom relief may be a compelling motivation for experimentation (Harrison et al., 2007; Schapiro, 2002).

Immunizations

Children with TS and OCD should be vaccinated following the schedule recommended by the American Academy of Pediatrics (AAP) (AAP Committee on Infectious Diseases, 2006; CDC, 2008).

Screenings

Vision. Routine screening is recommended.

Hearing. Routine screening is recommended.

Dental. Routine screening is recommended. Some children will note that their tics are set off by the vibrations in dental equipment and may need to have their teeth cleaned by hand.

Blood Pressure. Routine screening is recommended. Children taking medications such as clonidine, guanfacine, or stimulants should be routinely monitored and have additional screenings when medication is initiated and dosages are changed.

Hematocrit. Routine screening is recommended. Clozapine, an atypical neuroleptic, is associated with blood dyscrasias, and it would be prudent to monitor the complete blood count more frequently of children taking atypical neuroleptics.

Urinalysis. Routine screening is recommended.

Tuberculosis. Routine screening is recommended.

Condition-Specific Screening

Additional monitoring is advised with selected medications. An electrocardiogram is recommended before beginning or increasing doses of tricyclic antidepressants and pimozide, as well as periodic blood tests (depending on the medication) to measure drug levels, blood counts, or liver function tests.

Self-Injurious Behavior (SIB). The primary care provider should be particularly vigilant in examining the skin, hair, nails, and scalp of children with TS and OCD for signs of SIB.

Common Illness Management

Differential Diagnosis

Some children with undiagnosed tic disorders have sniffing and coughing tics (Leckman, Bloch, King, et al., 2006) that may be misdiagnosed as symptoms of an upper respiratory infection (URI) or allergy. Other children with TS notice an increase of symptoms

during fevers, viral illnesses, and allergy flare-ups (Swain et al., 2007). OCD and tic symptoms may begin or flare up explosively after a streptococcal infection (see PANDAS section earlier in this chapter). At this point, diagnosis and treatment of PANDAS remain experimental, and prophylactic antibiotics are not recommended (King, 2006).

When a child with OCD complains of typical childhood symptoms, such as headaches and stomachaches, it is hard for parents and providers to discern the cause: is the child obsessed with illness? Is there a serotonin imbalance implicated in headaches or stomachaches? Is the child constipated as a side effect of medication? Or is there is a serious health problem? After listening carefully to the child, parents may need to consult with the child's therapist and primary care provider.

Changes in skin condition and musculoskeletal complaints may be due to bruising from tics, holding unusual positions as part of a tic, or self-injurious behavior.

Drug Interactions

Erythromycin and other macrolide antibiotics can interact with medications such as pimozide or aripiprazole (dopamine blockers) to prolong the QT interval (Taketomo, Hodding, & Kraus, 2008). Dextromethorphan, a cough suppressant commonly found in over-the-counter medications and sometimes taken in high doses by adolescents for its psychoactive properties, may interact with fluoxetine to cause increased sedation, hallucinations, muscle dystonia, and hyperthermia, known as central serotonin syndrome. Ecstasy and related club or designer drugs, as well as triptans prescribed for migraines, may also cause central serotonin syndrome in interaction with SSRIs (Rusyniak & Sprague, 2006). SSRIs, dopamine blockers, and other psychoactive medications are metabolized through cytochrome P (CYP) pathways, and can each enhance or inhibit the metabolism on the same pathway of other medications the child might be taking. In addition, some children may have intrinsically

---

Differential Diagnosis

- Sniffing, coughing, throat clearing
    - Allergy
    - Upper respiratory infection
    - Vocal tics
- Pharyngitis
    - Streptococcal infection (observe for increase in tics or OCD)
    - Vocal tics (cough, throat clearing)
- Headache
    - Medication side effect (e.g., clonidine)
    - Somatic preoccupation or obsession
- Abdominal pain
    - Muscle tics (abdominal muscles)
    - Constipation related to toileting issues (OCD)
    - Constipation related to medication side effects
    - Somatic preoccupation or obsession
- Skin-mucosa changes
    - Bruising from tics
    - Self-injurious behavior
    - Nail biting
    - Trichotillomania
- Musculoskeletal complaints
    - Tics (muscle tightness, holding unusual positions)
    - Injury incurred during tic

slow or quicker metabolism along particular pathways (Lynch & Price, 2007). Fluoxetine and other CYP 2D6 pathway inhibitors can interact with codeine to prevent its breakdown to the active metabolite, thereby diminishing its analgesic properties (Taketomo et al., 2008). These examples should alert the provider to keep an accurate list of current medications and updated information about drug-drug interactions, and to ensure that parents and adolescents are aware of them as well.

Given the plethora of vitamins, supplements, and complementary and alternative medications available and evidence that many families of children with TS and OCD are using them (Mantel et al., 2004), providers should engage in an open dialog with the child and family about possible drug interactions with any alternative treatments. St. John's wort, dimethylglycine, and trimethylglycine, for example, can interact with SSRIs (Waltz, 2000).

Developmental Issues

Sleep Patterns

Children with TS can have difficulty falling or staying asleep if tics increase as they relax, or the bedclothes do not "feel right." Warm baths or massage can often temporarily diminish the tics, and some children benefit from having a soft mattress pad. Children with OCD, as noted previously, tend to have rituals they feel compelled to perform before bedtime, which can often delay sleep for several hours. If the child does not involve the parent in these rituals, the parent may not be aware of them. As with other rituals, bedtime rituals may be diminished with therapy and/or medication.

Toileting

Most children with TS and OCD are not diagnosed until school age, when toilet training is no longer an issue. However, Waltz (2000) notes that children who are later diagnosed with OCD may have had difficulties with toilet training, and often have obsessions and rituals related to toileting. There may be an increased incidence of encopresis and enuresis related to OCD symptoms (e.g., wetting or soiling connected to avoiding public bathrooms). As with other OCD symptoms, either CBT or medication or both combined may help.

Discipline

The typical cycle of relative suppressibility and release of tics in TS can lead to confusion and misguided attempts on the part of parents and teachers to use discipline or conditioning to stop the tics (Ginsburg & Kingery, 2007; Kenney et al., 2008). Part of the family's adjustment to a diagnosis of TS involves learning to understand, reinterpret, and accept their child's unusual behavior—often the very habits they have spent some time and energy encouraging the child to suppress (Leckman, Bloch, Scahill et al., 2006). When children with OCD begin treatment, there can be flare-ups of rituals. Parents will have to work with the child and therapist to decide which rituals to limit and which to ignore (Chansky, 2000; March & Benton, 2007).

Questions regarding the appropriateness of behavior, fairness to siblings, and consequences for behavior that is only partially under the child's control are complex, and families often benefit from support groups or other contact with parents of children with TS or OCD (Marsh, 2007; Schapiro, 2002). Structured training classes for parents of children with TS and OCD may be available in some

regions (Ginsburg & Kingery, 2007; Scahill, Sukhodolsky, Bearss, et al., 2006). Greene (2005) recommends a "basket" system for prioritizing behaviors of explosive children, including children with TS or OCD, with Basket A containing the behaviors needed to maintain safe child and family functioning, Basket B containing behaviors around which there is some room to teach the child negotiation skills, and Basket C containing behaviors the parent is willing to ignore for the time being (such as maintaining a clean room). Even with essential behaviors, parents may have to modify the way they customarily give commands and monitor adherence, in order to break cycles of coercive parent-child interactions (Ginsburg & Kingery, 2007).

In addition to developing an increased flexibility for acceptable behavior standards, parents may have to adjust their systems of consequences and rewards, as well. Most children respond well to positive reinforcement, and children with OCD in particular may need rewards because the acceptable behavior may provoke anxiety rather than being "its own reward" (Waltz, 2000). According to Greene (2005), timeouts are not helpful for children who would like to behave well, but lack the neurologic capability to work through frustrating situations without a meltdown. He recommends instead that parents help children avoid meltdowns by essentially acting as their surrogate frontal lobe: modeling and teaching them flexibility, verbal skills, and the ability to shift gears. For children who are engaging in explosive behavior, a safe place to regroup is important (Waltz, 2000).

Child Care

The combination of structure and flexibility is important for children with TS and OCD. Although children may not be formally diagnosed during the preschool years, they may have increased problems with adaptability and peer relationships, and child-care providers can provide important information to parents who have concerns about their child's intellectual and social development.

Schooling

According to Packer (2005), children with TS are more likely to need additional educational support than children without TS, but are not often referred for such support. Even though tics are not directly connected to learning disabilities, they may interfere with school functioning: arm tics may interfere with handwritten work and eye tics or head movements may interfere with reading (Gilbert, 2006). The tics and the effort to suppress them may internally distract the child enough to limit the ability to concentrate in the classroom, and fatigue and irritability increase as the day progresses (Kepley & Conners, 2007; Swain et al., 2007).

Children with TS can have dysgraphia and visual-motor integration problems, affecting all handwritten work and tasks that involve copying from the blackboard or from a test booklet to an answer sheet. Deficits in written expressive language are common, even in children who have no difficulty with reading or oral expression (Burd, 2007). Children with TS and ADHD will benefit from the same educational interventions as children without tic disorders who have ADHD (Kepley & Conners, 2007) (see Chapter 12).

Silent rituals associated with OCD, such as counting the number of times a letter occurs in reading, or avoiding the number 3 in math problems, can slow the child down considerably, without being apparent to either teachers or parents (Carter, Fredine, Findley, et al., 1999). Conversely, the child's rituals may be disruptive to the class, sometimes leading to the inaccurate labeling of compulsions as symptoms of oppositional defiant disorder (Carter et al., 1999). Children may get stuck on one task, may have rewriting compulsions, or may have difficulty making choices. Other children may be able to minimize their OCD symptoms at school, leaving teachers perplexed as to why assignments cannot be completed at home (Sabuncuoglu & Berkem, 2006). Individualizing a plan is key, as well as creating alliances with teachers and school personnel whenever possible. Their observations may be invaluable in tracking response to medication and behavioral treatment.

There are two levels of educational support available for children with TS or OCD attending public schools: written plans to provide access to educational programs/protection from discrimination (Section 504), and special education services (Burd, 2007). All children with TS and OCD can qualify for Section 504 protection, which might include preferential seating, parent input into teacher selection, allowing a child to stop an activity if "stuck," permission to leave the classroom to release tics, extra time on tests, and homework modification (Carter et al., 1999; Schapiro, 2002), with only a letter of diagnosis as documentation. Evaluations for services under the Individuals with Disabilities Education Improvement Act are more complex (see Chapter 3), but a parent can request an evaluation for an individualized educational program (IEP) in writing.

Children with TS often have particular talents in music, sports, the arts, or academic subjects. Some authors suggest that the involvement of children with TS in gifted programs, competitive sports, and drama could aid in school and social success (Shady et al., 2007). For adolescents, time spent practicing or in competition may be protective, providing increased time under adult supervision, as well as positive peer interactions (Schapiro, 2002).

Children with TS acknowledge more behavioral difficulties and dysphoric moods than children without TS, which increase with symptom severity (Storch et al., 2007). Studies tend to show more difficulties with peer relations for all children with TS (Woods, Marcks, & Flessner, 2007). Carter, O'Donnell, Schultz, and colleagues (2000) found that children with TS and without ADHD were similar in social adjustment to unaffected children, with the exception of school difficulties, but that ADHD status, obsessional symptoms, and family functioning were all related to social adaptation.

Children with OCD frequently have difficulty initiating and maintaining friendships. Preoccupation with obsessions often leaves little time or energy for friends. In addition, the desire to hide their obsessions and rituals from peers may lead to social isolation, and bullying by peers is associated with more severe symptoms, depressive symptoms, isolation, and behavioral difficulties at home (Storch, Ledley, Lewin, et al., 2006). Children with OCD may benefit from socialization groups, in which social skills are explicitly taught, and from structured activities, such as religious or community youth groups or sports. Other children may find it easier to socialize with just one child, for short periods (Waltz, 2000).

Sexuality

Unless affected by other conditions, physical sexual development and progression through puberty in children with TS and/or OCD are normal. However, the psychosocial aspects of sexuality in children with TS and OCD can be affected in several ways. In some individuals with TS, tics can be set off by touch or may increase during sexual activity. Adolescents with OCD may avoid any touch, including holding hands and kissing, because of contamination fears (Waltz, 2000). Sexual obsessions are common in OCD (Mula, Cavanna, Critchley, et al., 2008), including unwanted sexual thoughts, invasive thoughts that disrupt romantic or sexual activity, and obsessions or fears around being homosexual in teens who do not have same-sex attractions (Waltz, 2000). In addition, the medications used for TS and OCD, most notably SSRIs, have some effect on libido and sexual functioning (Murphy et al., 2008), which may be distressing for adolescents and may affect adherence to medications.

Adolescents with TS and OCD may not feel comfortable discussing sexuality with their parents, and may be reluctant to raise the issue to a health care provider, reinforcing the primary care provider's responsibility to discuss sexuality with all adolescents (Monasterio, Hwang, & Shafer, 2007). In the urge to prevent teen pregnancy and sexually transmitted diseases, it is important for providers to avoid reducing sexuality to intercourse and reproduction. Sexuality involves how one feels about one's own body, about touch and caring—difficult issues for any teen and even more so for teens with tics and/or compulsions.

Transition to Adulthood

Virtually all colleges receive some form of federal assistance and are required by law to provide services for students with disabilities. Although services vary from school to school, families who have struggled with public school systems for accommodations for their child with TS or OCD may find college disability services surprisingly easy to access. Parents should ensure that the adolescent with either an IEP or a 504 Plan has a reevaluation at the school within 3 years of entering college, in order to facilitate the transition (see Chapters 3 and 4). Parents can help students contact college disability services, and can help their adolescent prepare and submit documentation of any past services, but the responsibility for using college disability services rests with the young adult.

Most adolescents with TS find that their tics have dramatically decreased by adulthood (Leckman, Bloch, King, et al., 2006). Adults with ongoing motor and vocal tics, but without associated conditions, have few problems with mood, sleep, anger management, or self-injurious behavior (Freeman et al., 2000). However, these individuals may experience discrimination in education or employment, and older surveys of adults with TS have found higher rates of unemployment than in the general population (Woods, Marcks, & Flessner, 2007).

A few careers, including the military and some areas of law enforcement, may not be available to youths who have a history of any psychiatric illness or medication, including some of the medications used to treat TS and OCD (Waltz, 2000). Young adults with severe OCD or other associated psychiatric conditions may have limited options for employment, education, housing, and health care. Parents and the adolescent may benefit from hiring a case manager or working with their school's vocational rehabilitation services team to address transition to adulthood and independent living issues (Waltz, 2000).

It is important to remember that adults who are participants in current outcome studies often received a diagnosis of TS relatively late in life, may have been heavily medicated, and may not have encountered a receptive school system; adults with OCD may not have received effective treatment as a child or adolescent. It may be, with early diagnosis and effective care, that future adult outcomes will be much improved.

Family Concerns

The stress of parenting a child with TS was diminished for Taiwanese mothers receiving appropriate social support (Lee, Chen, Wang, et al., 2007). The child's adjustment after a diagnosis of TS may be related to parenting style (Cohen, Sade, Benarroch, et al., 2008), and to family functioning in general (Carter et al., 2000). These findings suggest that the child, as well as their parents, could benefit from the parents receiving emotional support after their child has been diagnosed with TS.

Parents and siblings of children with OCD experience stress in accommodating the child's rituals, and siblings may feel ashamed of the child's bizarre behavior at school. Chansky (2000) encourages parents to explain OCD as a medical condition to the child's siblings, and to validate the feelings of unfairness or possible embarrassment at their sibling's outbursts. Family meetings with the child's therapist to work out fair house rules may be helpful. Neuropsychiatric conditions have historically been associated with stigma, and are difficult for family members to explain to friends, relatives, and school personnel. Parents may not be used to the role of advocate for their child, and may not even be sure whether to disclose the diagnosis of TS or OCD. Families can benefit from sympathetic guidance by their primary providers as well as referral to the appropriate organizations and resources.

Resources

The resource section lists books and videos about TS and OCD that may help the child and families understand and cope with their unique circumstances.

Organizations
Tourette Syndrome Association, Inc. (TSA)
42-40 Bell Blvd., Suite 205
Bayside, NY 11361
(718) 224-2999
Website: www.tsa-usa.org
Obsessive-Compulsive Foundation, Inc. (OCF)
P.O. Box 961029
Boston, MA 02196
(617) 973-5801
Website: www.ocfoundation.org

Books for Adults and Older Adolescents
Chansky, T.E. (2000). *Freeing Your Child from Obsessive-Compulsive Disorder: A Powerful, Practical Program for Parents of Children and Adolescents.* New York: Crown Publishers.
Greene, R.W. (2005). *The Explosive Child: A New Approach for Understanding and Parenting Easily Frustrated, Chronically Inflexible Children.* New York: Harper Collins.

Handler, L. (2004). *Twitch and Shout: A Touretter's Tale.* Minneapolis: University of Minnesota Press.
March, J.S., & Benton, C.S. (2007). *Talking Back to OCD: The Program that Helps Kids and Teens Say "No Way"—and Parents Say "Way to Go."* New York: Guilford Press.
Marsh, T.L. (Ed.). (2007). *Children with Tourette Syndrome: A Parents' Guide* (2nd ed.). Bethesda, MD: Woodbine House.
Rapoport, J.L. (1989). *The Boy Who Couldn't Stop Washing: The Experience and Treatment of Obsessive-Compulsive Disorder.* New York: E.P. Dutton.
Traig, J. (2004). *Devil in the Details: Scenes from an Obsessive Girlhood.* New York: Little, Brown.
Waltz, M. (2000). *Obsessive-Compulsive Disorder: Help for Children and Adolescents.* Sebastopol, CA: O'Reilly & Associates.
Waltz, M. (2001). *Tourette's Syndrome: Finding Answers and Getting Help.* Sebastopol, CA: O'Reilly & Associates.
Wilensky, A.S. (1999). *Passing for Normal: A Memoir of Compulsion.* New York: Broadway Books.

Books for Children
Byalick, M. (2002). *Quit It.* New York: Delacorte Press.
Chowdhury, U., & Robertson, M. (2006). *Why Do You Do That? A Book about Tourette Syndrome for Children and Young People.* London: Jessica Kingsley Publishers.
Hesser, T.S. (1998). *Kissing Doorknobs.* New York: Delacorte Press.
Huebner, D. (2007). *What To Do When Your Brain Gets Stuck: A Kid's Guide to Overcoming OCD.* Washington, DC: Magination Press.
Peters, Dylan. (2007). *Tic Talk: Living with Tourette Syndrome. A 9 Year-Old Boy's Story in His Own Words.* Chandler, AZ: Little Five Store.
Wagner, A.P. (2004). *Up and Down the Worry Hill: A Children's Book about Obsessive-Compulsive Disorder and Its Treatment* (2nd ed.). Lighthouse Press.

Internet Resources
National Center for Complementary and Alternative Medicine
Website: http://nccam.nih.gov
Obsessive Compulsive Foundation
Website: www.ocfoundation.org
Obsessive-Compulsive Foundation Teen/Young Adult Site
Website: www.ocfoundation.org/organizedchaos
Overcoming OCD: A Guide for College Students
Website: www.ocdchicago.org/index.php/ocd-guides/overcoming-ocd
Tourette Syndrome Association
Website: www.tsa-usa.org
Tourette Syndrome Plus, Leslie Packer PhD
Website: www.tourettesyndrome.net

Summary of Primary Care Needs for the Child with Tourette Syndrome or Obsessive-Compulsive Disorder

HEALTH CARE MAINTENANCE
Growth and Development
- Growth is generally normal, although there are some recent concerns about growth of children on long-term medication, such as SSRIs.
- If growth slows or weight falls in older child/adolescent, consider eating disorder.
- Development generally normal.
- Rituals with OCD associated with isolation and distress, increase when normal childhood rituals are starting to diminish.
- Some parents report decreased flexibility and increased difficulties with regulation, even before emergence of specific symptoms.

Diet
- Abrupt changes in dietary preference may be due to obsessions/compulsions, especially around contamination.
- Increased risk of eating disorders in children with OCD.
- Parents may restrict intake in an attempt to eliminate triggers from foods or food additives.

Safety
- Excessive risk taking sometimes associated with complex tic behavior.
- Self-injurious behavior in both TS and OCD.
- Adolescents may self-medicate with alcohol and/or recreational drugs for symptom relief.

Immunizations
- Children with TS and OCD should be vaccinated following the schedule recommended by the American Academy of Pediatrics (2006).

Screening
- *Vision.* Routine screening is recommended.
- *Hearing.* Routine screening is recommended.
- *Dental.* Routine screening is recommended. Clean teeth by hand if tics set off by vibrations.
- *Blood pressure.* Routine screening is recommended. Children taking certain medications may need more frequent screening.
- *Hematocrit.* Routine screening is recommended. Additional frequency if taking atypical neuroleptics
- *Urinalysis.* Routine screening is recommended.
- *Tuberculosis.* Routine screening is recommended.

Condition-Specific Screening
- ECG if taking pimozide, other atypical neuroleptics, tricyclic antidepressants. More frequent monitoring of blood, liver function for some atypical neuroleptic medications,
- Careful observation for signs of self-injurious behavior.

COMMON ILLNESS MANAGEMENT
Differential Diagnosis
- Sniffing, coughing, throat clearing: allergy, upper respiratory infection, vocal tics.
- *Pharyngitis.* Streptococcal infection (observe for-tics or OCD), vocal tics (cough, throat clearing).
- *Headache.* Medication side effect (e.g., clonidine), somatic preoccupation or obsession
- *Abdominal pain.* Muscle tics (abdominal muscles), constipation related to toileting issues (OCD), or medication side effect, somatic preoccupation or obsession
- *Skin-mucosa changes.* Bruising from tics, self-injurious behavior, nail biting, trichotillomania
- *Musculoskeletal complaints.* Tics (muscle tightness, holding unusual positions), injury incurred during tic

Drug Interactions
- Pimozide and aripiprazole interact with macrolide antibiotics to prolong the QT interval.
- Dextromethorphan and club drugs such as Ecstasy interact with fluoxetine to increase the risk of central serotonin syndrome.
- SSRIs reduce the effectiveness of codeine for analgesia.
- St. John's wort and other supplements interact with SSRIs.

DEVELOPMENTAL ISSUES
Sleep Patterns
- Tics can increase as children relax, making falling asleep more difficult.
- Bedtime rituals can delay sleep for several hours; parents may not be aware of extent of rituals.

Toileting
- Some obsessions and rituals are related to toileting.
- Some medications increase constipation. Avoidance of public toilets may lead to constipation and encopresis.

Discipline
- It may be difficult to distinguish between tics and more voluntary behaviors.
- Flexibility needed to accept unusual behavior may be difficult for parents.
- Children with OCD may need rewards for avoiding rituals.
- Timeouts may not be effective for children with rage attacks.

Child Care
- A combination of structure and flexibility is needed.
- Daycare providers can give valuable feedback about socialization skills.

Schooling
- Tics and obsessions can interfere with concentration and written work.
- TS is associated with dysgraphia, visual-motor integration problems, and written expressive language.
- OCD may not be apparent to teachers, or child may disrupt class.
- All children are eligible for Section 504 accommodations, some for IEPs.
- Peer relations may be impaired.

Sexuality
- Tics may increase with touch or during sexual activity.
- Adolescents may avoid touch due to contamination fears.

Summary of Primary Care Needs for the Child with Tourette Syndrome or Obsessive-Compulsive Disorder—cont'd

- Sexual obsessions may interfere with relationships.
- SSRIs may decrease sexual desire and function.

Transition to Adulthood

- Tics often diminish significantly in adulthood.
- Individuals with TS and without other conditions have few behavioral problems, but may experience educational, employment, and housing discrimination.

- Severe OCD may limit educational, work, and independent living options.

FAMILY CONCERNS

- Decisions about disclosure of TS and OCD can be difficult.
- Siblings may feel that child's behavior is embarrassing, and families may need professional help to work out fair house rules.

REFERENCES

Aguirregomozcorta, M., Pagonabarraga, J., Diaz-Manera, J., et al. (2008). Efficacy of botulinum toxin in severe Tourette syndrome with dystonic tics involving the neck. *Parkinsonism Relat Disord, 14,* 443-445.

Alsobrook, J.P. II, & Pauls, D.L. (1997). The genetics of Tourette syndrome. *Neurol Clin, 15,* 381-393.

American Academy of Pediatrics (AAP) Committee on Infectious Diseases (2006). *Red book: 2006 report of the Committee on Infectious Diseases.* (27th ed.). Elk Grove Village, IL: American Academy of Pediatrics.

American Psychiatric Association (APA). (2000). *Diagnostic and Statistical Manual of Mental and Psychiatric Disorders.* (4th ed., Text Revision). Washington, DC: Author.

Arnold, P.D., Sicard, T., Burroughs, E., et al. (2006). Glutamate transporter gene *SLC1A1* associated with obsessive-compulsive disorder. *Arch Gen Psychiatry, 63,* 769-776.

Arnsten, A.F., Scahill, L., & Findling, R.L. (2007). Alpha-2 adrenergic receptor agonists for the treatment of attention-deficit/hyperactivity disorder: Emerging concepts from new data. *J Child Adolesc Psychopharmacol, 17*(4), 393-406.

Association for Comprehensive NeuroTherapy. (n.d.). Available at www.latitudes.org/index.html. Retrieved July 23, 2008.

Barrett, P.M., Farrell, L., Pina, A.A., et al. (2008). Evidence-based psychosocial treatments for child and adolescent obsessive-compulsive disorder. *J Clin Child Adolesc Psychol, 37,* 131-155.

Ben Djebara, M., Worbe, Y., Schupbach, M., et al. (2008). Aripiprazole: A treatment for severe coprolalia in "refractory" Gilles de la Tourette syndrome. *Mov Disord, 23,* 438-440.

Best, N.T., & Mertin, P. (2007). Correlates of auditory hallucinations in nonpsychotic children. *Clin Child Psychol Psychiatry, 12,* 611-623.

Birmaher, B., Brent, D., Bernet, W., et al. (2007). Practice parameter for the assessment and treatment of children and adolescents with depressive disorders. *J Am Acad Child Adolesc Psychiatry, 46,* 1503-1526.

Bjorgvinsson, T., Hart, J., & Heffelfinger, S. (2007). Obsessive-compulsive disorder: Update on assessment and treatment. *J Psychiatr Pract, 13,* 362-372.

Blier, P., Habib, R., & Flament, M.F. (2006). Pharmacotherapies in the management of obsessive-compulsive disorder. *Can J Psychiatry, 51,* 417-430.

Bloch, M.H., Peterson, B.S., Scahill, L., et al. (2006). Adulthood outcome of tic and obsessive-compulsive symptom severity in children with Tourette syndrome. *Arch Pediatr Adolesc Med, 160,* 65-69.

Bottas, A., & Richter, M.A. (2002). Pediatric autoimmune neuropsychiatric disorders associated with streptococcal infections (PANDAS). *Pediatr Infect Dis J, 21,* 67-71.

Bruun, R.D., & Budman, C.L. (1999). Hallucinations in nonpsychotic children. *J Am Acad Child Adolesc Psychiatry, 38,* 1328-1329.

Budman, C.L., Bruun, R.D., Park, K.S., et al. (2000). Explosive outbursts in children with Tourette's disorder. *J Am Acad Child Adolesc Psychiatry, 39,* 1270-1276.

Budman, C.L., Rockmore, L., Stokes, J., et al. (2003). Clinical phenomenology of episodic rage in children with Tourette syndrome. *J Psychosom Res, 55,* 59-65.

Burd, L. (2007). Educational needs of children with Tourette syndrome. In T.L. Marsh (Ed.), *Children with Tourette Syndrome: A Parents' Guide* (2nd ed.). Bethesda, MD: Woodbine House.

Canitano, R., & Vivanti, G. (2007). Tics and Tourette syndrome in autism spectrum disorders. *Autism, 11,* 19-28.

Carter, A.S., Fredine, N.J., Findley, D., et al. (1999). Recommendations for teachers. In J.F. Leckman & D.J. Cohen (Eds.), *Tourette's Syndrome—Tics, Obsessions, Compulsions: Developmental Psychopathology and Clinical Care.* New York: John Wiley & Sons.

Carter, A.S., O'Donnell, D.A., Schultz, R.T., et al. (2000). Social and emotional adjustment in children affected with Gilles de la Tourette's syndrome: Associations with ADHD and family functioning. Attention deficit hyperactivity disorder. *J Child Psychol Psychiatry, 41,* 215-223.

Centers for Disease Control and Prevention (CDC). (2008). *Epidemiology and Prevention of Vaccine-Preventable Diseases* (10th ed.). Washington, DC: Public Health Foundation. Available at www.cdc.gov/vaccines/pubs/pinkbook/default.htm. Retrieved March 25, 2009.

Chansky, T.E. (2000). *Freeing Your Child from Obsessive-Compulsive Disorder: A Powerful, Practical Program for Parents of Children and Adolescents.* New York: Crown Publishers.

Cheung, M.Y., Shahed, J., & Jankovic, J. (2007). Malignant Tourette syndrome. *Mov Disord, 22,* 1743-1750.

Coffey, B.J., Biederman, J., Smoller, J.W., et al. (2000). Anxiety disorders and tic severity in juveniles with Tourette's disorder. *J Am Acad Child Adolesc Psychiatry, 39,* 562-568.

Coffey, B.J., & Park, K.S. (1997). Behavioral and emotional aspects of Tourette syndrome. *Neurol Clin, 15,* 277-289.

Cohen, D.J., & Leckman, J.F. (1999). Introduction: The self under siege. In J.F. Leckman & D.J. Cohen (Eds.), *Tourette's Syndrome: Tics, Obsessions, Compulsions.* New York: John Wiley & Sons.

Cohen, E., Sade, M., Benarroch, F., et al. (2008). Locus of control, perceived parenting style, and symptoms of anxiety and depression in children with Tourette's syndrome. *Eur Child Adolesc Psychiatry, 17,* 299-305.

Cumella, E.J., Kally, Z., & Wall, A.D. (2007). Treatment responses of inpatient eating disorder women with and without co-occurring obsessive-compulsive disorder. *Eat Disord, 15,* 111-124.

da Rocha, F.F., Correa, H., & Teixeira, A.L. (2008). Obsessive-compulsive disorder and immunology: A review. *Prog Neuropsychopharmacol Biol Psychiatry, 32,* 1139-1146.

Dooley, J.M. (2006). Tic disorders in childhood. *Semin Pediatr Neurol, 13,* 231-242.

Dooley, J.M., Brna, P.M., & Gordon, K.E. (1999). Parent perceptions of symptom severity in Tourette's syndrome. *Arch Dis Child, 81,* 440-441.

Erenberg, G. (2005). The relationship between Tourette syndrome, attention deficit hyperactivity disorder, and stimulant medication: A critical review. *Semin Pediatr Neurol, 12,* 217-221.

Fireman, B., Koran, L.M., Leventhal, J.L., et al. (2001). The prevalence of clinically recognized obsessive-compulsive disorder in a large health maintenance organization. *Am J Psychiatry, 158,* 1904-1910.

Flament, M.F., Geller, D., Irak, M., et al. (2007). Specificities of treatment in pediatric obsessive-compulsive disorder. *CNS Spectr, 12*(2 Suppl 3), 43-58.

Food and Drug Administration (FDA). (2004, October 15). *FDA Public Health Advisory: Suicidality in children and adolescents being treated with antidepressant medications.* Available at www.fda.gov/cder/drug/antidepressants/SSRIPHA200410.htm. Retrieved July 22, 2008.

Food and Drug Administration (FDA). (2007, September 17). *Medwatch Safety Alert: Haloperidol.* Available at www.fda.gov/medwatch/safety/2007/safety07.htm#Haloperidol. Retrieved July 21, 2008.

Franklin, M.E., Tolin, D.F., & Diefenbach, G.J. (2008). Trichotillomania. In J.S. Abramowitz, D. McKay, & S. Taylor (Eds.), *Obsessive-Compulsive Disorder: Subtypes and Spectrum Conditions.* New York: Elsevier.

Freeman, J.B., Garcia, A.M., Coyne, L., et al. (2008). Early childhood OCD: Preliminary findings from a family-based cognitive-behavioral approach. *J Am Acad Child Adolesc Psychiatry, 47,* 593-602.

Freeman, R.D. (2007). Tic disorders and ADHD: Answers from a world-wide clinical dataset on Tourette syndrome. *Eur Child Adolesc Psychiatry, 16*(Suppl 1), 15-23.

Freeman, R.D., Fast, D.K., Burd, L., et al. (2000). An international perspective on Tourette syndrome: Selected findings from 3500 individuals in 22 countries. *Dev Med Child Neurol, 43,* 436-437.

Freud, S.F. (1909/1973). *Three Case Histories (P. Reiff, Trans.).* New York: Macmillan.

Friedlander, L., & Desrocher, M. (2006). Neuroimaging studies of obsessive-compulsive disorder in adults and children. *Clin Psychol Rev, 26,* 32-49.

Gabbay, V., Coffey, B.J., Babb, J.S., et al. (2008). Pediatric autoimmune neuropsychiatric disorders associated with streptococcus: Comparison of diagnosis and treatment in the community and at a specialty clinic. *Pediatrics, 122,* 273-278.

Gadow, K.D., Nolan, E.E., Sprafkin, J., et al. (2002). Tics and psychiatric comorbidity in children and adolescents. *Dev Med Child Neurol, 44,* 330-338.

Gadow, K.D., Sverd, J., Nolan, E.E., et al. (2007). Immediate-release methylphenidate for ADHD in children with comorbid chronic multiple tic disorder. *J Am Acad Child Adolesc Psychiatry, 46,* 840-848.

Garvey, M.A., Perlmutter, S.J., Allen, A.J., et al. (1999). A pilot study of penicillin prophylaxis for neuropsychiatric exacerbations triggered by streptococcal infections. *Biol Psychiatry, 45,* 1564-1571.

Gaze, C., Kepley, H.O., & Walkup, J.T. (2006). Co-occurring psychiatric disorders in children and adolescents with Tourette syndrome. *J Child Neurol, 21*(8), 657-664.

Geller, D.A. (2006). Obsessive-compulsive and spectrum disorders in children and adolescents. *Psychiatr Clin North Am, 29,* 353-370.

Geller, D.A., Biederman, J., Faraone, S., et al. (2002). Attention-deficit/hyperactivity disorder in children and adolescents with obsessive-compulsive disorder: Fact or artifact?. *J Am Acad Child Adolesc Psychiatry, 41,* 52-58.

Geller, D.A., Biederman, J., Faraone, S., et al. (2004). Re-examining comorbidity of obsessive compulsive and attention-deficit hyperactivity disorder using an empirically derived taxonomy. *Eur Child Adolesc Psychiatry, 13,* 83-91.

Geller, D.A., Biederman, J., Stewart, S.E., et al. (2003). Which SSRI? A meta-analysis of pharmacotherapy trials in pediatric obsessive-compulsive disorder. *Am J Psychiatry, 160,* 1919-1928.

Geller, D.A., Doyle, R., Shaw, D., et al. (2006). A quick and reliable screening measure for OCD in youth: Reliability and validity of the obsessive compulsive scale of the Child Behavior Checklist. *Compr Psychiatry, 47,* 234-240.

Gilbert, D. (2006). Treatment of children and adolescents with tics and Tourette syndrome. *J Child Neurol, 21,* 690-700.

Ginsburg, G.S., & Kingery, J.N. (2007). Management of familial issues in persons with Tourette syndrome. In D.W. Woods, J.C. Piacentini, & J.T. Walkup, (Eds.), *Treating Tourette Syndrome and Tic Disorders.* New York: Guilford Press.

Goodman, W.K., Price, L.H., Rasmussen, S.A., et al. (1989a). The Yale-Brown Obsessive Compulsive Scale. I. Development, use, and reliability. *Arch Gen Psychiatry, 46,* 1006-1011.

Goodman, W.K., Price, L.H., Rasmussen, S.A., et al. (1989b). The Yale-Brown Obsessive Compulsive Scale. II. Validity. *Arch Gen Psychiatry, 46,* 1012-1016.

Goodman, W.K., Storch, E.A., Geffken, G.R., et al. (2006). Obsessive-compulsive disorder in Tourette syndrome. *J Child Neurol, 21,* 704-714.

Grados, M., & Wilcox, H.C. (2007). Genetics of obsessive-compulsive disorder: A research update. *Expert Rev Neurother, 7,* 967-980.

Greene, R.W. (2005). *The Explosive Child: A New Approach for Understanding and Parenting Easily Frustrated, Chronically Inflexible Children.* New York: Harper Collins.

Handler, L. (2004). *Twitch and Shout: A Touretter's Tale.* Minneapolis: University of Minnesota Press.

Harrison, J.N., Schneider, B., & Walkup, J.T. (2007). Medical management of Tourette syndrome and co-occurring conditions. In D.W. Woods, J.C. Piacentini, & J.T. Walkup (Eds.) *Treating Tourette Syndrome and Tic Disorders.* New York: Guilford Press.

Hetrick, S., Merry, S., McKenzie, J., et al. (2007). Selective serotonin reuptake inhibitors (SSRIs) for depressive disorders in children and adolescents. *Cochrane Database Syst Rev*(3), CD004851.

Himle, M.B., Woods, D.W., Piacentini, J.C., et al. (2006). Brief review of habit reversal training for Tourette syndrome. *J Child Neurol, 21,* 719-725.

Hoekstra, P.J., & Minderaa, R.B. (2005). Tic disorders and obsessive-compulsive disorder: Is autoimmunity involved? *Int Rev Psychiatry, 17,* 497-502.

Hounie, A.G., do Rosario-Campos, M.C., Diniz, J.B., et al. (2006). Obsessive-compulsive disorder in Tourette syndrome. *Adv Neurol, 99,* 22-38.

Ivarsson, T., & Larsson, B. (2008). The obsessive-compulsive symptom (OCS) scale of the child behavior checklist: A comparison between Swedish children with obsessive-compulsive disorder from a specialized unit, regular outpatients and a school sample. *J Anxiety Disord, 22*(7), 1172-1179.

Jankovic, J. (1997). Tourette syndrome. Phenomenology and classification of tics. *Neurol Clin, 15,* 267-275.

Jankovic, J., & Mejia, N.I. (2006). Tics associated with other disorders. *Adv Neurol, 99,* 61-68.

Jenike, M.A., Baer, L., & Minichiello, W.E. (1998). An overview of obsessive-compulsive disorder. In M.A. Jenike & W.E. Minichiello (Eds.), *Obsessive-Compulsive Disorders: Practical Management* (3rd ed.). St. Louis: Mosby.

Kadesjo, B., & Gillberg, C. (2000). Tourette's disorder: Epidemiology and co-morbidity in primary school children. *J Am Acad Child Adolesc Psychiatry, 39,* 548-555.

Kaye, W.H., Bulik, C.M., Thornton, L., et al. (2004). Comorbidity of anxiety disorders with anorexia and bulimia nervosa. *Am J Psychiatry, 161,* 2215-2221.

Keeley, M.L., Storch, E.A., Dhungana, P., et al. (2007). Pediatric obsessive-compulsive disorder: A guide to assessment and treatment. *Issues Ment Health Nurs, 28,* 555-574.

Keen-Kim, D., & Freimer, N.B. (2006). Genetics and epidemiology of Tourette syndrome. *J Child Neurol, 21,* 665-671.

Kenney, C., Kuo, S.H., & Jimenez-Shahed, J. (2008). Tourette's syndrome. *Am Fam Physician, 77,* 651-658.

Kepley, H.O., & Conners, S. (2007). Management of learning and school difficulties in children with Tourette syndrome. In D.W. Woods, J.C. Piacentini, & J.T. Walkup, (Eds.), *Treating Tourette Syndrome and Tic Disorders.* New York: Guilford Press.

Khalifa, N., & von Knorring, A.L. (2005). Tourette syndrome and other tic disorders in a total population of children: Clinical assessment and background. *Acta Paediatr, 94,* 1608-1614.

King, R.A. (2006). PANDAS: To treat or not to treat? *Adv Neurol, 99,* 179-183.

Kobak, K.A., Taylor, L.V., Bystritsky, A., et al. (2005). St John's wort versus placebo in obsessive-compulsive disorder: Results from a double-blind study. *Int Clin Psychopharmacol, 20,* 299-304.

Kurlan, R. (2006). Future and alternative therapies in Tourette syndrome. *Adv Neurol, 99,* 248-253.

Lajonchere, C., Nortz, M., & Finger, S. (1996). Gilles de la Tourette and the discovery of Tourette syndrome. Includes a translation of his 1884 article. *Arch Neurol, 53,* 567-574.

Lakhan, S.E., & Vieira, K.F. (2008). Nutritional therapies for mental disorders. *Nutr J, 7,* 2.

Leary, J., Reimschisel, T., & Singer, H.S. (2007). Genetic and neurobiological bases for Tourette syndrome. In D.W. Woods, J.C. Piacentini, & J.T. Walkup (Eds.), *Treating Tourette Syndrome and Tic Disorders.* New York: Guilford Press.

Leckman, J.F., Bloch, M.H., King, R.A., et al. (2006). Phenomenology of tics and natural history of tic disorders. *Adv Neurol, 99,* 1-16.

Leckman, J.F., Bloch, M.H., Scahill, L., et al. (2006). Tourette syndrome: The self under siege. *J Child Neurol, 21,* 642-649.

Leckman, J.F., & Cohen, D.J. (1999). Evolving models of pathogenesis. In J.F. Leckman, & D.J. Cohen (Eds.), *Tourette's Syndrome—Tics, Obsessions, Compulsions: Developmental Psychopathology and Clinical Care.* New York: Wiley & Sons.

Leckman, J.F., Riddle, M.A., Hardin, M.T., et al. (1989). The Yale Global Tic Severity Scale: Initial testing of a clinician-rated scale of tic severity. *J Am Acad Child Adolesc Psychiatry, 28,* 566-573.

Leckman, J.F., Zhang, H., Vitale, A., et al. (1998). Course of tic severity in Tourette syndrome: The first two decades. *Pediatrics, 102*(1 pt 1), 14-19.

Lee, M.Y., Chen, Y.C., Wang, H.S., et al. (2007). Parenting stress and related factors in parents of children with Tourette syndrome. *J Nurs Res, 15,* 165-174.

Leonard, H.L., Goldberger, E.L., Rapoport, J.L., et al. (1990). Childhood rituals: Normal development or obsessive-compulsive symptoms? *J Am Acad Child Adolesc Psychiatry, 29,* 17-23.

Lin, H., Katsovich, L., Ghebremichael, M., et al. (2007). Psychosocial stress predicts future symptom severities in children and adolescents with Tourette syndrome and/or obsessive-compulsive disorder. *J Child Psychol Psychiatry*, *48*, 157-166.

Lochner, C., Seedat, S., du Toit, P.L., et al. (2005). Obsessive-compulsive disorder and trichotillomania: A phenomenological comparison. *BMC Psychiatry*, *5*, 2. Available at www.biomedcentral.com/1471-244X/5/2. Retrieved on July 31, 2008.

Lynch, T., & Price, A. (2007). The effect of cytochrome P450 metabolism on drug response, interactions, and adverse effects. *Am Fam Phys*, *76*, 391-396.

Mantel, B.J., Meyers, A., Tran, Q.Y., et al. (2004). Nutritional supplements and complementary/alternative medicine in Tourette syndrome. *J Child Adolesc Psychopharmacol*, *14*, 582-589.

March, J., & Benton, C.S. (2007). *Talking Back to OCD: The Program that Helps Kids and Teens Say "No Way"—and Parents Say "Way to Go."* New York: Guilford Press.

March, J., Frances, A., Carpenter, D., et al. (1997). Treatment of obsessive-compulsive disorder. The Expert Consensus Panel for obsessive-compulsive disorder. *J Clin Psychiatry*, *58*(Suppl 4), 2-72.

March, J., Franklin, M.E., Leonard, H., et al. (2007). Tics moderate treatment outcome with sertraline but not cognitive-behavior therapy in pediatric obsessive-compulsive disorder. *Biol Psychiatry*, *61*, 344-347.

March, J., & Mulle, K. (1998). *OCD in Children and Adolescents: A Cognitive-Behavioral Treatment Manual*. New York: Guilford Press.

Marsh, T.L. (2007). Adjusting to your child's diagnosis. In T.L.Marsh (Ed.), *Children with Tourette Syndrome: A Parents' Guide* (2nd ed.). Bethesda, MD: Woodbine House.

Martin, J.L., & Thienemann, M. (2005). Group cognitive-behavior therapy with family involvement for middle-school-age children with obsessive-compulsive disorder: A pilot study. *Child Psychiatry Hum Dev*, *36*, 113-127.

Masi, G., Perugi, G., Millepiedi, S., et al. (2007). Bipolar co-morbidity in pediatric obsessive-compulsive disorder: Clinical and treatment implications. *J Child Adolesc Psychopharmacol*, *17*, 475-486.

Mathews, C.A., Waller, J., Glidden, D., et al. (2004). Self-injurious behaviour in Tourette syndrome: Correlates with impulsivity and impulse control. *J Neurol Neurosurg Psychiatry*, *75*(8), 1149-1155.

McKay, D., Gosselini, J.T., & Gupta, S. (2008). Body dysmorphic disorder. In J.S. Abramowitz, D. McKay, & S. Taylor (Eds.), *Obsessive-Compulsive Disorder: Subtypes and Spectrum Conditions*. New York: Elsevier.

Menzies, L., Chamberlain, S.R., Laird, A.R., et al. (2008). Integrating evidence from neuroimaging and neuropsychological studies of obsessive-compulsive disorder: The orbitofronto-striatal model revisited. *Neurosci Biobehav Rev*, *32*, 525-549.

Merlo, L.J., Storch, E.A., Murphy, T.K., et al. (2005). Assessment of pediatric obsessive-compulsive disorder: A critical review of current methodology. *Child Psychiatry Hum Dev*, *36*, 195-214.

Miguel, E.C., Leckman, J.F., Rauch, S., et al. (2005). Obsessive-compulsive disorder phenotypes: Implications for genetic studies. *Mol Psychiatry*, *10*, 258-275.

Mink, J.W. (2006). Neurobiology of basal ganglia and Tourette syndrome: Basal ganglia circuits and thalamocortical outputs. *Adv Neurol*, *99*, 89-98.

Monasterio, E., Hwang, L.Y., & Shafer, M.A. (2007). Adolescent sexual health. *Curr Probl Pediatr Adolesc Health Care*, *37*, 302-325.

Mula, M., Cavanna, A.E., Critchley, H., et al. (2008). Phenomenology of obsessive compulsive disorder in patients with temporal lobe epilepsy or Tourette syndrome. *J Neuropsychiatry Clin Neurosci*, *20*, 223-226.

Müller-Vahl, K.R. (2003). Cannabinoids reduce symptoms of Tourette's syndrome. *Expert Opin Pharmacother*, *4*, 1717-1725.

Müller-Vahl, K.R., Buddensiek, N., Geomelas, M., et al. (2008). The influence of different food and drink on tics in Tourette syndrome. *Acta Paediatr*, *97*, 442-446.

Murphy, T.K., Segarra, A., Storch, E.A., et al. (2008). SSRI adverse events: How to monitor and manage. *Int Rev Psychiatry*, *20*, 203-208.

National Center for Complementary and Alternative Medicine. (n.d.). Available at http://nccam.nih.gov/research. Retrieved July 23, 2008.

Olatunji, B.O., Wilhelm, S., & Deckersbach, T. (2008). Tic-related obsessive compulsive disorder. In J.S. Abramowitz, D. McKay, & S. Taylor (Eds.), *Obsessive-Compulsive Disorder: Subtypes and Spectrum Conditions*. New York: Elsevier.

Packer, L.E. (1997). Social and educational resources for patients with Tourette syndrome. *Neurol Clin*, *15*, 457-473.

Packer, L.E. (2005). Tic-related school problems: Impact on functioning, accommodations, and interventions. *Behav Modif*, *29*, 876-899.

Pavone, P., Parano, E., Rizzo, R., et al. (2006). Autoimmune neuropsychiatric disorders associated with streptococcal infection: Sydenham chorea, PANDAS, and PANDAS variants. *J Child Neurol*, *21*, 727-736.

Perlmutter, S.J., Leitman, S.F., Garvey, M.A., et al. (1999). Therapeutic plasma exchange and intravenous immunoglobulin for obsessive-compulsive disorder and tic disorders in childhood. *Lancet*, *354*(9185), 1153-1158.

Peterson, B.S., Pine, D.S., Cohen, P., et al. (2001). Prospective, longitudinal study of tic, obsessive-compulsive, and attention-deficit/hyperactivity disorders in an epidemiological sample. *J Am Acad Child Adolesc Psychiatry*, *40*, 685-695.

Phillips, K.A. (2000). Connection between obsessive-compulsive disorder and body dysmorphic disorder. In W.K. Goodman, M.V. Rudorfer, & J.D. Maser (Eds.) *Obsessive-Compulsive Disorder: Contemporary Issues in Treatment*. Mahwah, NJ: Lawrence Erlbaum.

Rapoport, J.L. (1989). *The Boy Who Couldn't Stop Washing: The Experience and Treatment of Obsessive-Compulsive Disorder*. New York: E.P. Dutton.

Rapoport, J.L., Inoff-Germain, G., Weissman, M.M., et al. (2000). Childhood obsessive-compulsive disorder in the NIMH MECA study: Parent versus child identification of cases. Methods for the Epidemiology of Child and Adolescent Mental Disorders. *J Anxiety Disord*, *14*, 535-548.

Rappaport, N., & Chubinsky, P. (2000). The meaning of psychotropic medications for children, adolescents, and their families. *J Am Acad Child Adolesc Psychiatry*, *39*, 1198-1200.

Robertson, M.M. (2006). Mood disorders and Gilles de la Tourette's syndrome: An update on prevalence, etiology, comorbidity, clinical associations, and implications. *J Psychosom Res*, *61*, 349-358.

Robertson, M.M., & Orth, M. (2006). Behavioral and affective disorders in Tourette syndrome. *Adv Neurol*, *99*, 39-60.

Rogers, S.J. (2005). *Tics and Tourette's: Breakthrough Discoveries in Natural Treatments*. Royal Palm Beach, FL: Association for Comprehensive Neuro-Therapy.

Rusyniak, D.E., & Sprague, J.E. (2006). Hyperthermic syndromes induced by toxins. *Clin Lab Med*, *26*, 165-184. ix.

Sabuncuoglu, O., & Berkem, M. (2006). The presentation of childhood obsessive-compulsive disorder across home and school settings: A preliminary report. *School Psychol Int*, *27*, 248-256.

Salbach-Andrae, H., Lenz, K., Simmendinger, N., et al. (2008). Psychiatric comorbidities among female adolescents with anorexia nervosa. *Child Psychiatry Hum Dev*, *39*, 261-272.

Sawyer, S.M., Drew, S., Yeo, M.S., et al. (2007). Adolescents with a chronic condition: Challenges living, challenges treating. *Lancet*, *369*(9571), 1481-1489.

Scahill, L., Riddle, M.A., McSwiggin-Hardin, M., et al. (1997). Children's Yale-Brown Obsessive Compulsive Scale: Reliability and validity. *J Am Acad Child Adolesc Psychiatry*, *36*, 844-852.

Scahill, L., Sukhodolsky, D.G., Bearss, K., et al. (2006). Randomized trial of parent management training in children with tic disorders and disruptive behavior. *J Child Neurol*, *21*, 650-656.

Schapiro, N.A. (2002). "Dude, you don't have Tourette's": Tourette's syndrome, beyond the tics. *Pediatr Nurs*, *28*, 243-246, 249-253.

Schreier, H.A. (1999). Hallucinations in nonpsychotic children: More common than we think? *J Am Acad Child Adolesc Psychiatry*, *38*, 623-625.

Shady, G.A., Jewers, R., Furer, P., et al. (2007). Your child's development. In T.L. Marsh (Ed.), *Children with Tourette Syndrome: A Parents' Guide* (2nd ed.). Bethesda, MD: Woodbine House.

Shoval, G., Zalsman, G., Sher, L., et al. (2006). Clinical characteristics of inpatient adolescents with severe obsessive-compulsive disorder. *Depress Anxiety*, *23*, 62-70.

Singer, C. (1997). Tourette syndrome. Coprolalia and other coprophenomena. *Neurol Clin*, *15*, 299-308.

Singer, H.S. (2005). Tourette's syndrome: From behaviour to biology. *Lancet Neurol*, *4*, 149-159.

Singer, H.S., & Williams, P.N. (2006). Autoimmunity and pediatric movement disorders. *Adv Neurol*, *99*, 166-178.

Snider, L.A., Lougee, L., Slattery, M., et al. (2005). Antibiotic prophylaxis with azithromycin or penicillin for childhood-onset neuropsychiatric disorders. *Biol Psychiatry*, *57*, 788-792.

Spencer, T., Biederman, J., Harding, M., et al. (1998). Disentangling the overlap between Tourette's disorder and ADHD. *J Child Psychol Psychiatry*, *39*, 1037-1044.

Spencer, T.J., Biederman, J., Faraone, S., et al. (2001). Impact of tic disorders on ADHD outcome across the life cycle: Findings from a large group of adults with and without ADHD.. *Am J Psychiatry*, *158*, 611-617.

Stewart, S.E., Geller, D.A., Jenike, M., et al. (2004). Long-term outcome of pediatric obsessive-compulsive disorder: A meta-analysis and qualitative review of the literature. *Acta Psychiatr Scand, 110,* 4-13.

Storch, E.A., Geffken, G.R., Merlo, L.J., et al. (2007). Family accommodation in pediatric obsessive-compulsive disorder. *J Clin Child Adolesc Psychol, 36,* 207-216.

Storch, E.A., Lack, C.W., Merlo, L.J., et al. (2007). Clinical features of children and adolescents with obsessive-compulsive disorder and hoarding symptoms. *Compr Psychiatry, 48,* 313-318.

Storch, E.A., Ledley, D.R., Lewin, A.B., et al. (2006). Peer victimization in children with obsessive-compulsive disorder: Relations with symptoms of psychopathology. *J Clin Child Adolesc Psychol, 35,* 446-455.

Storch, E.A., Merlo, L.J., Lack, C., et al. (2007). Quality of life in youth with Tourette's syndrome and chronic tic disorder. *J Clin Child Adolesc Psychol, 36,* 217-227.

Swain, J.E., Scahill, L., Lombroso, P.J., et al. (2007). Tourette syndrome and tic disorders: A decade of progress. *J Am Acad Child Adolesc Psychiatry, 46,* 947-968.

Swedo, S.E., Leonard, H.L., Mittleman, B.B., et al. (1997). Identification of children with pediatric autoimmune neuropsychiatric disorders associated with streptococcal infections by a marker associated with rheumatic fever. *Am J Psychiatry, 154,* 110-112.

Taketomo, C.K., Hodding, J.H., & Kraus, D.M. (2008). *Pediatric Dosage Handbook: 2008-2009.* (15th ed.) Hudson, OH: Lexi-Comp.

Tourette Syndrome Association International Consortium for Genetics. (2007). Genome scan for Tourette disorder in affected-sibling-pair and multigenerational families. *Am J Hum Genet, 80,* 265-272.

Tourette Syndrome Study Group. (2002). Treatment of ADHD in children with tics: A randomized controlled trial. *Neurology, 58,* 527-536.

Verdellen, C.W., Keijsers, G.P., Cath, D.C., et al. (2004). Exposure with response prevention versus habit reversal in Tourette's syndrome: A controlled study. *Behav Res Ther, 42,* 501-511.

Waltz, M. (2000). *Obsessive-Compulsive Disorder: Help for Children and Adolescents.* Sebastopol, CA: O'Reilly & Associates.

Watson, H.J., & Rees, C.S. (2008). Meta-analysis of randomized, controlled treatment trials for pediatric obsessive-compulsive disorder. *J Child Psychol Psychiatry, 49,* 489-498.

Weintrob, N., Cohen, D., Klipper-Aurbach, Y., et al. (2002). Decreased growth during therapy with selective serotonin reuptake inhibitors. *Arch Pediatr Adolesc Med, 156,* 696-701.

Wilensky, A.S. (1999). *Passing for Normal: A Memoir of Compulsion.* New York: Broadway Books.

Woods, D.W., Marcks, B.A., & Flessner, C.A. (2007). Management of social and occupational difficulties in persons with Tourette syndrome. In D.W. Woods, J.C. Piacentini, & J.T. Walkup, (Eds.), *Treating Tourette Syndrome and Tic Disorders.* New York: Guilford Press.

Woods, D.W., Piacentini, J.C., & Himle, M.B. (2007). Assessment of tic disorders. In D.W. Woods, J.C. Piacentini, & J.T. Walkup (Eds.), *Treating Tourette Syndrome and Tic Disorders.* New York: Guilford Press.

Wu, L., Li, H., & Kang, L. (1996). 156 cases of Gilles de la Tourette's syndrome treated by acupuncture. *J Tradit Chin Med, 16,* 211-213.

Zuckerman, M.L., Vaughan, B.L., Whitney, J., et al. (2007). Tolerability of selective serotonin reuptake inhibitors in thirty-nine children under age seven: A retrospective chart review. *J Child Adolesc Psychopharmacol, 17,* 165-174.

42 Traumatic Brain Injury

Ann Milanese and Ann M. Riley

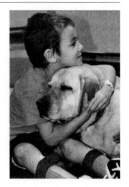

Etiology

Traumatic brain injury (TBI) is the most common cause of acquired disability and death in childhood (Schneier, Shields, Grim-Hostetler, et al., 2006). TBI is defined as a severe brain insult resulting from an external force, which may produce a reduced or altered state of consciousness. The Centers for Disease Control and Prevention (CDC) has called it "the silent epidemic" because of its high incidence and the often externally invisible presentation hallmarked by cognitive disability (Langlois, Rutland-Brown, & Thomas, 2005).

TBI is a diverse condition. There may be both primary and secondary injuries to the brain, and these injuries produce an array of complications, ranging from obvious physical disability to less visible but nonetheless incapacitating neuropsychological impairment (Giza, 2006). Although brain damage itself is believed to be irreversible (Marik, Varon, & Trask, 2002), aggressive acute management of TBI and intensive pediatric rehabilitation have greatly improved outcomes by minimizing associated complications, inducing therapeutic compensation, and preventing long-term impairments associated with poor cognitive and psychological adjustment.

Primary injury to the brain occurs from a direct traumatic force at the moment of impact and can be either focal or diffuse. Focal injuries are most commonly associated with a direct blow to the head. Examples of primary focal brain injuries include hematomas—epidural, subdural, and intracerebral. Diffuse injuries are the result of inertial forces causing microtrauma to nerves and blood vessels. The most common example is diffuse axonal injury, the result of violent motion of the brain inside the skull, as is experienced in a motor vehicle accident (Park & Hyun, 2004). Primary injury induces an acute response from the brain, in which a cascade of biochemical physiologic events can cause both direct neuronal damage and secondary brain injury (Marik et al., 2002).

Secondary injuries are generally understood as the resulting hypoxemia, acidosis, and chemical or metabolic response to cellular injury. The secondary injury cascade results in poor perfusion of the brain from systemic hypotension, intracranial hypertension, cerebral edema, or cerebral hemorrhage. There may be hypoxemia, seizures, hypercapnia, or infection. These secondary conditions significantly increase morbidity and mortality rates for children with TBI. It is these secondary responses, and the resulting injury to the brain, that are most amenable to medical and pharmacologic intervention, and thus can affect outcome. Although the damage from secondary complications is more diffuse in children than adults, it is also more likely to resolve during recovery and rehabilitation (Cronin, 2001).

There is no genetic predisposition to head injury itself. Certain behavioral conditions such as attention-deficit/hyperactivity disorder (ADHD) or mood disturbances constitute behavioral risk factors for TBI (Bloom, Levin, & Ewing-Cobbs, 2001) (see Chapters 12 and 33). These conditions may have a genetic component and are a frequent premorbid element of the pattern of risk-taking behaviors noted in children with TBI.

Children who are congenitally predisposed to bleeding disorders such as hemophilia (see Chapter 14) are more likely to sustain intracranial hemorrhagic complications from even mild head injuries.

Physical Mechanisms of Injury

The physical mechanisms of TBI are a result of direct injury, such as a penetrating object, or forces of deceleration, acceleration, coup-contrecoup, or rotational trauma (Figure 42-1). Deceleration occurs when the head strikes an immovable object; acceleration forces occur when a moving object strikes the head. A coup injury occurs when the brain strikes the cranium on the side of impact, and a contrecoup injury occurs when the brain rebounds and strikes the cranium on the contralateral side. Contrecoup injuries are considered more severe, and the size of the impact area affects the injury severity. The smaller the area of impact, the greater the severity of the injury, as a result of the concentration of force in a smaller area. Rotational trauma is characterized by a twisting of the brain during deceleration or acceleration. This can occur in combination with coup-contrecoup injuries, resulting in shearing of the tissues (Haider, 2006), or as a complication of inflicted trauma—from shaking—to children under age 2 (American Academy of Pediatrics [AAP] Committee on Child Abuse and Neglect, 2001).

Incidence and Prevalence

The reported annual rate of TBI in the United States is approximately 200 per 100,000 children (Langlois et al., 2005). At least 29,000 children experience permanent neurologic symptoms and another 7000 are fatally injured from head injuries each year. The two pediatric age-groups at highest risk for moderate to severe TBI are 0- to 4-year-olds and 15- to 19-year-olds, respectively (Langlois et al., 2005).

Data from a sample year period suggest an estimated 50,658 hospitalizations for TBI among children under 17 years of age in the United States, with a cost of more than $1 billion (Schneier et al., 2006). Hospital-related data and costs do not account for the large number of children who sustain concussions or mild TBIs and who

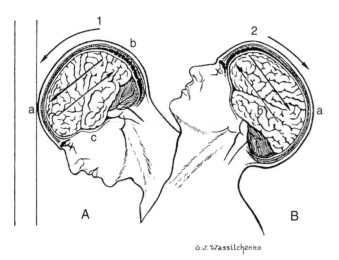

G.J. Wassilchenko

FIGURE 42-1 Coup and contrecoup head injury following blunt trauma. **A,** Coup injury: impact against object. Site of impact and direct trauma to brain *(a)*. Shearing of subdural veins *(b)*. Trauma to base of brain *(c)*. **B,** Contrecoup injury: impact within skull. Site of impact from brain hitting opposite side of skull *(a)*. Shearing forces through brain *(b)*. These injuries occur in one continuous motion—the head strikes the wall (coup), then rebounds (contrecoup). From Rudy, E. (1984). *Advanced Neurological and Neurosurgical Nursing.* St. Louis: Mosby. Reprinted with permission.

are not hospitalized, because the majority—75% to 90%—of head injuries are considered minor, requiring no acute intervention, but resulting in possible long-term risk and impairment (McAllister, 2005). Thus the actual rate of all TBIs in children remains unknown. The CDC estimates that there are 475,000 TBIs in children age 14 and under each year, with more in the 15- to 19-year-old age-group. An estimated 2.5 million to 6.5 million individuals of all ages are living with lasting effects of TBI (Langlois, Rutland-Brown, & Thomas, 2004).

Risk factors for TBI in children include age and sex, socioeconomic factors, and time of year. Males are more often affected than females, as high as 2:1 during adolescence. There is an increased incidence in low socioeconomic classes, and increased incidence in spring and summer (Alexander & Moore, 2001). Peak occurrence is during evenings, nights, weekends, and holidays when children are outside playing, swimming, riding bicycles, traveling in cars, or victims of gunshot wounds. A prior TBI within 6 to 12 months is a significant risk factor for a second TBI (Swaine, Tremblay, Platt, et al., 2007).

Head injuries in children commonly result from falls, child abuse, and bicycle and motor vehicle accidents. Child abuse is the main cause of head injury in children younger than 2 years of age (Keenan, Runyan, Marshall, et al., 2003). In 2- to 4-year-olds, falls are the main cause of head injury. In older children, bicycle, vehicle, and recreational accidents are the main cause of head injury. Of TBIs in children, 14% are moderate or severe, and 5% are fatal (Gualtieri, 2002; Langlois et al., 2004).

Although sports and recreation-related injuries (peak ages 5 to 24 years) account for 3% of hospitalized persons with TBI, approximately 90% of sports-related TBIs are mild traumatic brain injuries (MTBIs) and may go undetected or unreported (McCrea, 2008). Sports related concussions are typically the result of low-velocity impact causing confusion and disorientation but not loss

of consciousness (Meehan & Bachur, 2009). This leads to an underestimate of the actual incidence rate of MTBI. Collective epidemiologic indicators that review hospital-based studies, as well as estimates of those who do not seek hospital care, suggest a true incidence rate of approximately 500 per 100,000 population (Bazarian, 2005) instead of the 200 per 100,000 figure noted previously.

The most important aspect of TBI epidemiology is primary prevention. In 2006, the CDC made extensive efforts to educate parents, coaches, and medical care providers through the "Heads Up" program. The CDC's principal recommendations include the following: (1) use a seat belt or child safety seat for every car ride; (2) never drink or use drugs and then drive; (3) use appropriate sports helmets and protective equipment; and (4) "childproof" all living and playground areas (CDC, 2006).

Diagnostic Criteria
Head Injury Classification

Severity. Head injuries are classified by severity of response (mild, moderate, severe) during the immediate postinjury period. The Glasgow Coma Scale (GCS) was published in 1974 (Teasdale & Jennett, 1981). It remains the most reliable indicator of injury severity and short-term deterioration or improvement (Table 42-1). Mild head injuries, or concussions, are typically associated with GCS scores of 13 to 15. Moderate head injuries are typically associated with GCS scores of 9 to 12 (Table 42-2). Severe head injuries are associated with GCS scores of 8 or less and have significant potential long-term morbidity or mortality risks (Kraus, 2005). Because of the GCS's limitations for use in infants and preverbal children, individuals with a preinjury deficit (e.g., hemiparesis, cognitive deficit), or individuals who are intubated, a Children's Coma Scale (CCS) or Modified Glasgow Coma Scale was developed (Box 42-1) (Ghajar & Hariri, 1992). However, it is not used as commonly as the GCS.

Open or Closed. Open head injuries are the result of penetrating wounds to the skull such as falling onto sharp objects or gunshot wounds. In penetrating brain injuries, skull fragments tear the duramater. Open wounds are most commonly associated with focal brain pathology (Murdoch & Theodoros, 2001). Closed head injuries are the result of nonpenetrating wounds and can result in cerebral concussion, contusion, or hematoma.

Focal or Diffuse. Focal vascular lacerations or contusions occur when brain damage is localized to one area because of an expanding mass. Diffuse injuries occur when brain damage is widespread as a result of generalized brain edema or ischemia, systemic hypoxia, or hypotension. Children's brain injuries are most commonly diffuse closed-head injuries.

Types of Cranial Injury

Skull Fracture. Skull fractures are included in this discussion because they are a predictor for intracranial injury. Skull fractures occur when external forces exceed the skull's tolerance (Roth & Farls, 2000). Skull fractures may or may not result in bony displacement or swelling. The incidence of skull fracture is higher in children than in adults, especially in children younger than 2 years who have thinner cranial bones (Weiner & Weinberg, 2000). When fractures do occur, about 60% to 70% involve the parietal bone and are most often linear (Schutzman &

TABLE 42-1
Glasgow Coma Scale

		Child >2 Years Old or Adult			Child <2 Years Old or Developmentally Delayed	
Best eye-opening response	Spontaneously		4	Spontaneously		4
	To verbal command		3	Verbal command		3
	To pain		2	To pain		2
	No response		1	No response		1
Best verbal response	Oriented, converses		5	Coos, babbles		5
	Disoriented, converses		4	Irritable cry		4
	Inappropriate words		3	Cries to pain		3
	Incomprehensible sounds		2	Moans to pain		2
	No response		1	None		1
Best motor response To verbal command	Obeys		6	Spontaneous		6
To painful stimulus	Localizes pain		5	Withdraws—touch		5
	Flexion-withdrawal		4	Withdraws to pain		4
	Flexion-decorticate		3	Abnormal flexion		3
	Extension-decerebrate		2	Abnormal extension		2
	No response		1	None		1
Total			(3-15)			(3-15)

From Chipps, E.M., Clanin, N.J., & Campbell, V.G. (1992). *Neurologic Disorders.* St. Louis: Mosby; Hazinski, M.F. (1992). Neurologic disorders. In Hazinski, M.F. (Ed.), *Nursing Care of the Critically Ill Child.* St. Louis: Mosby. Adapted with permission.

TABLE 42-2
Severity of Head Injury

Mild	Moderate	Severe
Asymptomatic *or*	>10 min posttraumatic unconsciousness *or*	Respiratory distress *or*
Minimal loss of consciousness with rapid clearing of mental status *or*	Posttraumatic seizures *or*	Circulatory instability *or*
Headache *or*	Focal neurologic deficits *or*	Altered mental status (unresponsiveness, coma) *or*
Vomiting *or*	Retrograde amnesia lasting >30 min *or*	Marked irritability *or*
Irritability GCS 13-15	Evidence of depressed skull fracture, basilar skull fracture, or CSF leak *or*	Signs of increased intracranial pressure GCS ≤8
	Severe headache *or*	
	Persistent vomiting *or*	
	Irritability GCS 9-12	

From Fox, J. (1997). *Primary Healthcare of Children.* St. Louis: Mosby; Berman, S. (1997). *Pediatric Decision Making.* St. Louis: Mosby. Adapted with permissions.
Key: *CSF,* cerebrospinal fluid; *GCS,* Glasgow Coma Scale score.

BOX 42-1
Children's Coma Scale

Maximum score = 11
Minimum score = 3
Motor response (maximum score = 4)
  4 Flexes and extends
  3 Withdraws from painful stimulus
  2 Hypertonic
  1 Flaccid
Verbal response (maximum score = 3)
  3 Cries
  2 Spontaneous respirations
  1 Apneic
Ocular response (maximum score = 4)
  4 Pursuit
  3 Extraocular muscles (EOMs) intact, reactive pupils
  2 Fixed pupils or EOMs impaired
  1 Fixed pupil and EOMs paralyzed

From Ghajar, J., & Hariri, R. (1992). Management of pediatric head injury. *Pediatr Clin North Am, 39,* 1093-1125.

Greenes, 2001). Most linear fractures are associated with overlying hematomas or soft tissue swelling, and they typically heal without complications. Linear fractures can result from low velocity and blunt or compression trauma (Roth & Farls, 2000). They do not play a significant role in most brain injuries; however, in cases of mild head injury, the presence of a fracture increases the risk of intracranial injury four-fold (Evans & Wilberger, 1999).

Less common skull fractures include depressed and basilar fractures (Marik et al., 2002; Schutzman & Greenes, 2001). Depressed skull fractures occur in the presence of greater force velocity and blunt or compression trauma and can cause tissue damage or hemorrhage. Because of this, depressed skull fractures can be neurosurgical emergencies (Roth & Farls, 2000). Basilar fractures should be monitored more closely than linear fractures because of risk for cerebrospinal fluid leakage, infection, and cranial nerve palsies (Evans & Wilberger,1999).

Types of Intracranial Injury

Concussion or Mild Traumatic Brain Injury. The term *concussion* can be used interchangeably with the term *mild TBI* (MTBI). This is a transient alteration in mental status following head trauma (Schutzman & Greenes, 2001). In its 2003 report to Congress, the CDC recommended an "operational definition" of MTBI. MTBI includes any period of confusion, disorientation, or impaired consciousness; any period of memory disruption around the time of injury; or any observable neurologic changes, including irritability, seizures, or loss of consciousness less than 30 minutes (CDC, 2003). The intention in better defining MTBI was to encourage identification of MTBI to better quantitate the extent of the problem and better monitor outcomes.

Rapid acceleration/deceleration injuries or sudden blows to the head can cause concussions. A typical presentation (90% of cases) involves brief or no loss of consciousness and is often associated with sports-related injuries (McCrea, 2008; Meehan & Bachur, 2009). There may be anterograde and/or retrograde posttraumatic amnesia. Retrograde amnesia may predict more serious injury. The symptoms are usually reversible, but in some instances there may be subtle residual neurologic impairment (Collins, Iverson, & Lovell, 2003). The disturbance in brain function associated with MTBI is thought to be more related to disruption of brain metabolism than to specific structural brain damage (Giza & Hovda,

2001). Over the long term, some people experience a postconcussion syndrome, which includes changes in concentration, behavior, and personality (McAllister, 2005).

Contusion and Laceration. Cerebral contusions are the result of the brain moving within the skull, causing bruises along the surface of the brain. Cerebral contusions can occur at the site of impact (coup) and/or opposite the side of impact (contrecoup). Contusions are the most frequently seen lesions in older children following a head injury. Common locations for contusions include the frontal, occipital, and parietal areas.

Lacerations involve tearing of the cortical surface with damage to the surrounding tissues. Lacerations may also occur with contusions and are due to a penetrating head injury or depressed skull fracture (Roth & Farls, 2000).

Cerebral Hemorrhage. Cerebral hemorrhage, or hematoma, results in a mass lesion effect that causes elevated intracranial pressure (Figure 42-2). Among individuals with TBI, approximately 3% develop epidural hematoma (Hartl & Ghajar, 2005). These rare hematomas occur between the dura and the skull and are often arterial. Subdural hematomas occur in 30% of children with severe head injury (Marik et al., 2002). Blood collects between the dura and arachnoid meninges layer. Subdural hematomas are classified as acute (occurred in the past 48 hours), subacute (occurred in the past 2 to 14 days), and chronic (occurred more than 14 days ago). Intracerebral hemorrhage produces mass lesions primarily in the frontal and temporal lobes. These hemorrhages occur mainly in the presence of moderate and severe head injuries such as significant blows to the head or depressed skull fractures (Marik et al., 2002). Surgical evacuation of an intracerebral hemorrhage is necessary when medical therapies fail to decrease intracranial pressure.

Diffuse Axonal Injury. Diffuse axonal injury (DAI) is a term used to describe diffuse degeneration of white matter, global neurologic dysfunction, and diffuse cerebral swelling occurring at the time of impact. DAI results from axonal and microvascular shearing, which causes swelling, degeneration, and disconnection of axons (Marik et al., 2002).

Cerebral Edema. Cerebral edema, either focal or generalized, is the result of an increase in brain volume from intracellular or extracellular fluid. Peak occurrence for cerebral edema usually is up to 72 hours after a neurologic insult. It gradually resolves over a 2- to 3-week period. Cerebral edema may be caused by either the initial injury to the neuronal tissue or secondarily in response to the biochemical cellular injury cascade, hypoxia, hypercarbia, or cerebral ischemia. Because it increases brain volume, it causes the other intracranial components—blood and cerebrospinal fluid (CSF)—to be forced out of the relatively closed space of the cranium. Left untreated or poorly controlled, cerebral edema can have a devastating effect, resulting in intracranial hypertension and impaired cerebral perfusion. These can lead to neuronal tissue hypoxia, ischemia, cerebral herniation, and death (Jha, 2003).

Diagnostic Imaging. In 1999, the American Academy of Pediatrics (AAP), in collaboration with the American Academy of Family Physicians (AAFP), published a practice parameter for evaluating and managing minor closed head injury (AAP & AAFP, 1999). They commented on relative risk for intracranial injury and devised an algorithm for appropriate diagnostic imaging studies to clarify severity and to guide acute intervention.

Children considered at *high risk* of having intracranial injury are those who are difficult to arouse and have an abnormal neurologic examination, signs or symptoms of a skull fracture, irritability, progressively worsening vomiting, or a bulging fontanel. Children with any of these signs or symptoms should undergo a computed tomography (CT) scan. CT will accurately indicate the need for urgent neurosurgical interventions, such as evacuation of epidural or subdural hematoma.

Children considered at *moderate risk* of having an intracranial injury are those with four or fewer episodes of vomiting, loss of consciousness of less than 1 minute duration, reports of lethargy or irritability, skull fracture present more than 24 hours, behavior reportedly not at baseline, history of a fall onto a hard surface, a scalp hematoma, or history of unwitnessed trauma. They should receive a CT scan at the discretion of the health care provider. Children in the moderate-risk group who do not receive a CT scan should be observed in a medical facility for up to 6 hours for the development of neurologic symptoms.

Children considered at *low risk* of having intracranial injury are those who have fallen less than 3 feet and have a normal neurologic examination at least 2 hours after injury (AAP Committee on Child Abuse and Neglect, 2001). In low-risk children a CT scan is typically not warranted (Schutzman & Greenes, 2001). The exception is children younger than 2 years of age; they have a higher risk of intracranial injury even with minor mechanisms of injury (Schutzman & Greenes, 2001).

Clinical Manifestations at Time of Diagnosis

Clinical manifestations at the time of diagnosis vary, depending on the primary brain injury and the extent and involvement of secondary responses. Children with head injuries have varying degrees of alertness and responsiveness. Their presentation is influenced by the degree of increased intracranial pressure and by other

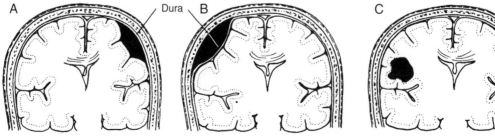

FIGURE 42-2 Different types of hematomas. **A,** Subdural. **B,** Epidural. **C,** Intracerebral. From Thelan, L.A., et al. (1994). *Critical Care Nursing: Diagnosis and Management* (2nd ed.). St. Louis: Mosby. Reprinted with permission.

metabolic factors. If the extent of secondary responses progresses, clinical symptoms may worsen in the hours after an injury.

Clinical Manifestations at Time of Diagnosis

- Varying degrees of alertness and responsiveness determined by degree of intracranial pressure (see Table 42-2)
- Loss of consciousness
- Headache
- Seizures
- Vomiting
- Hemiparesis
- Fixed dilated pupils
- Brain stem herniation

MANIFESTATION OF MTBI
- Asymptomatic
- Confusion
- Loss of consciousness for <1 minute
- Headache
- Vomiting
- Lethargy

A child with an epidural hematoma can exhibit fluctuating clinical manifestations with immediate loss of consciousness, followed by a lucid period of wakefulness, followed by rapid deterioration in neurologic status. Other symptoms and signs may include headache, seizure, vomiting, hemiparesis, and fixed and dilated pupils. Prompt identification and surgical management of a hematoma favors a positive outcome. Clinical manifestations of a subdural hematoma can range from headache and fatigue to seizures, papilledema, and hemiparesis.

Clinical manifestations of intracranial hemorrhage are headache, deteriorating level of consciousness, dilated pupil on the side of the hemorrhage, and hemiplegia on the opposite side of the hemorrhage.

Cerebral edema can cause increased intracranial pressure. Signs and symptoms of increased intracranial pressure include irritability, lethargy, nausea and vomiting, headache, photophobia, pupillary changes, abnormal reflexes, seizures, widening pulse pressure, bradycardia, and apnea. If this persists unchecked, cerebral herniation can ensue (Schutzman & Greenes, 2001). Clinical manifestations of herniation are changes in level of consciousness, abnormal respiratory patterns, loss of protective reflexes (e.g., gag or corneal), changes in blood pressure and pulse pressure with bradycardia, pupillary dysfunction, papilledema, changes in motor function or posturing, nausea and projectile vomiting, a positive Babinski's sign, and visual disturbances (Adelson & Kochanek, 2001).

Concussion or Mild Traumatic Brain Injury

Accurate identification of minor head trauma in children younger than 2 years can be challenging. A child may be initially asymptomatic despite having an intracranial injury. Therefore ongoing vigilance is essential when monitoring for behavioral and neurologic changes following an injury.

The AAP and AAFP (1999) algorithm (Figure 42-3) includes an approach to minor closed head injury in children older than 2, within the first 24 hours of the injury. Children with minor closed head trauma are defined as those with normal mental status at initial examination with no abnormal or focal findings on neurologic examination and have no physical evidence of a skull fracture. The parameter also considers those children who may have experienced temporary loss of consciousness (less than 1 minute), had a seizure or vomited, or exhibited postinjury headache or lethargy.

For a child with *mild closed head injury with no loss of consciousness,* an initial evaluation should include a thorough history, physical, and neurologic examination. Observation by a medical professional or by a competent, well-informed parent is sufficient, with the goal of recognizing worsening symptoms and seeking appropriate medical subspecialty assistance. Fewer than 1 in 5000 people with mild closed head injury with no loss of consciousness have intracranial injuries that require medical or neurosurgical interventions (AAP & AAFP, 1999). CT and magnetic resonance imaging (MRI) scans are not necessary because they provide only marginal benefits of early detection of intracranial injury. However, if imaging is desired, cranial CT is the preferred technique.

For a child *with mild closed head injury with loss of consciousness (less than 1 minute),* an initial evaluation should include a thorough history, physical, and neurologic examination. Although observation is sufficient, a cranial CT scan may be ordered at the discretion of the health care provider. Because children with signs and symptoms such as headache, vomiting, or lethargy are more likely to have intracranial injury, a cranial CT or MRI is the preferred brain imaging study.

Treatment
Mild Traumatic Brain Injury

Because most brain injuries are minor and observation is the most common treatment, instructions should be given to guardians/parents/caretakers describing postinjury signs and symptoms that may require medical attention After mild traumatic brain injury, or concussion, children should be observed for several weeks for symptoms suggestive of postconcussion syndrome (PCS). These symptoms can include dizziness, headache, irritability, poor concentration, sleep or appetite disturbance, or behavioral changes. PCS can persist for up to 1 year after injury (Roth & Farls, 2000).

Treatment

- Prehospital ("in the field") stabilization and evaluation
- Early treatment determined by severity of TBI
- Control hypoxia, increased cerebral CO_2, and brain edema
- Surgical intervention, if needed, for bleeding, trauma, or cerebral edema
- Coma recovery follows predictable patterns with variable time sequence
- Rehabilitation program and family involvement are keys to long-term recovery

---

Although children have generally good outcomes after MTBIs, repeated sports-related minor head injury is often associated with long-term cognitive and behavioral sequelae (McCrea, 2008). The CDC endorses a program of on-field concussion assessment and return-to-play guidelines (Box 42-2) (Lovell, Collins, & Bradley, 2004). Children who experience persistent MTBI symptoms should not return to competitive play or to recreational sports until the symptoms have completely abated (Meehan & Bachur,

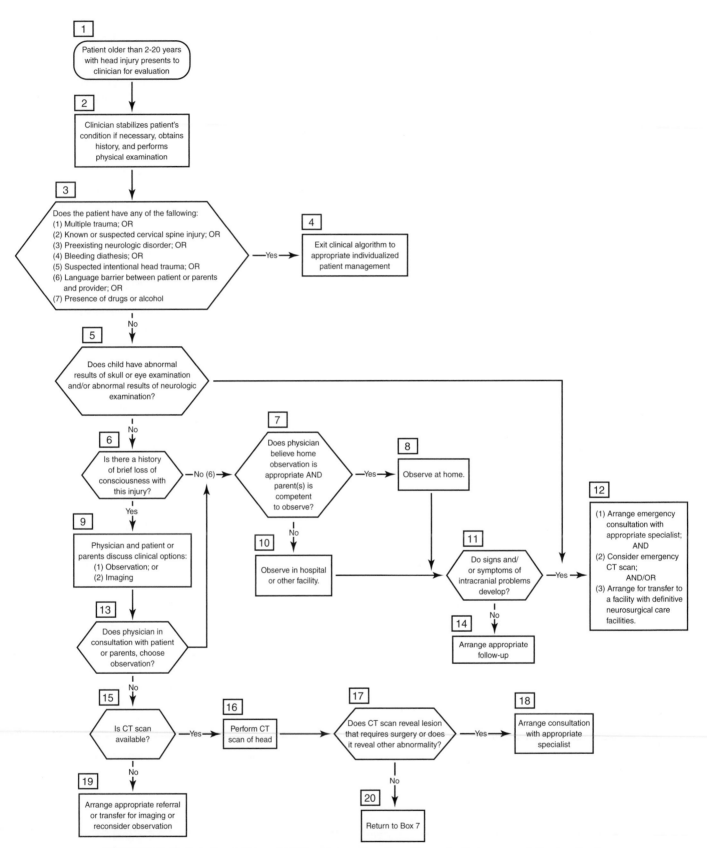

FIGURE 42-3 Evaluation and triage of mild head trauma. From Committee on Quality Improvement, American Academy of Pediatrics and Commission on Clinical Policies and Research, American Academy of Family Physicians. (1999). The management of minor closed head injury in children. *Pediatrics, 106*(6), 1407-1415.

Summary of Recommendations for Return to Sports Activity after Concussion

GRADE 1 CONCUSSION

Definition. Transient confusion, no loss of consciousness, and duration of post-traumatic amnesia between <5 and 30 minutes.

Management. Return to sports activity same day only if all symptoms resolve within 15 minutes; if a second grade 1 concussion occurs, no sports activity until asymptomatic for 1 week.

GRADE 2 CONCUSSION

- *Definition.* Transient confusion, loss of consciousness between 0 and 5 minutes, and a duration of posttraumatic amnesia >15-30 minutes but <24 hours.
- *Management.* No sports activity until asymptomatic for 1 full week; if a grade 2 concussion occurs on the same day as a grade 1 concussion, no sports activity until asymptomatic for 2 weeks.

GRADE 3 CONCUSSION

Definition. Concussion involving loss of consciousness >5 minutes, posttraumatic amnesia >24 hours.

Management. No sports activity until asymptomatic for 2 weeks.

For a second Grade 3 concussion: No sports activity until asymptomatic for 1 month.

If an intracranial pathology is detected on CT or MRI, no sports activity for remainder of season and the athlete should be discouraged from future return to contact sports.

Data from Lovell, M.R., Collins, M.W., & Bradley, J. (2004). Return to play following sports related concussion. *Clin Sports Med, 23*(3), 421-441.

BOX 42-3

Return to Play Progression for Competitive Contact Sports after Mild Traumatic Brain Injury

1. No activity until symptoms resolve
2. Light aerobic exercise (e.g., walking, stationary bicycle)
3. Sport-specific exercise (e.g., skating in hockey, running in soccer)
4. Noncontact training drills
5. Full-contact training after medical clearance
6. Full-contact game play

From McCrory, P., Johnston, K., Meeuwisse, W., et al. (2004). Summary and agreement statement of the second International Conference on Concussion in Sport, Prague 2004. *Br J Sports Med 2005,* 39(4), 196-204.

2009). Once postconcussive symptoms have resolved, there can be a graded return to play. The Concussion in Sport Group (McCrory, Johnston, Meeuwisse et al., 2004) proposes a gradual increase in intensity of athletic activity (Box 42-3). Neuropsychological testing is increasingly viewed as a necessary component in evaluating athletes who have had a concussion (Meehan & Bachur, 2009).

As part of the "Heads Up" initiative, the CDC has published an Acute Concussion Evaluation Form (ACE) (Figure 42-4); this is an evidence-based protocol to structure observations for suspected MTBI (CDC, 2006). It can also be administered serially, to track the resolution of symptoms over time.

Severe Traumatic Brain Injury

The goal of treatment of severe TBI is to stabilize the effects of the primary injury and prevent secondary injuries caused by hypoxia, hypercarbia, acidosis, free radicals, cerebral edema, seizures, infection, and aspiration, and to surgically treat correctable

intracranial lesions. Initial treatment at the scene of an accident begins with cervical stabilization and support of the airway, breathing, and circulation (Marik et al., 2002; Schutzman & Greenes, 2001). Successful medical management "in the field" is an important predictor of outcome.

Children who have sustained a severe TBI are best managed at a trauma center with neurologic and neurosurgical services and high-level pediatric intensive care. To minimize secondary injuries, treatment includes intubation, ventilation, fluid resuscitation, diuretics, and blood pressure monitoring (Marik et al., 2002). Adequate cerebral perfusion pressure at a minimum of 70 mm Hg is recommended to maximize perfusion and to avoid cerebral ischemia. Intracranial pressure monitoring is recommended in those with a GCS score of 8 or less. Intraventricular catheters have become the standard when treating severe head injuries and have been attributed to improved outcomes (Marik et al., 2002).

Management of severe brain injury can be divided into acute medical stabilization and intensive acute rehabilitation phases. These phases may flow together as children stabilize and become more tolerant of the stimulation and demands of the acute rehabilitation phase of care. The goals of treatment in children with TBI are to minimize complications and disability and to maximize the ability to function independently. An important goal within the acute inpatient rehabilitation setting is to plan the child's transition to the next level of care in the community, including outpatient medical care and therapies, and return to school.

Rehabilitation and Long-Term Management

Rehabilitation can hasten and maximize restoration of lost functions, promote adaptation to disabilities, and aid in age-appropriate independence and reintegration into family and school life. Rehabilitation can enhance the quality of life for both children with TBI and their families.

Most children with brain injuries undergo some spontaneous recovery in the first 6 months after injury. Deficits remaining after this period typically are more permanent (Goka, 2000). The GCS helps predict rehabilitation outcomes on the basis of four categories: mild, moderate, severe, and vegetative state (Table 42-3). There remains debate as to whether rehabilitation optimizes functional outcomes or quickens the time to reach the functional plateau (Cronin, 2001).

There is a broad range of possible symptoms after TBI. These include muscle movement and tone abnormalities with associated orthopedic problems, seizures, visual deficits, cognitive and behavioral deficits, and sleep disorders. Management of these symptoms requires an interdisciplinary approach to develop and implement an individualized treatment plan (National Institutes of Health [NIH] Consensus Development Panel on Rehabilitation, 1999).

A specialist in pediatric rehabilitation should direct the rehabilitation team. Rehabilitation reestablishes learning through repetitive and progressive stimulation. Daily repetition is thought to "reprogram" the brain, taking advantage of "experience dependent plasticity" (Giza, 2006), as well as helping a child to learn new ways of accomplishing old skills. Physical and occupational therapists attend to optimizing range of motion, strength, posture, and mobility. They use a number of modalities, including passive range of motion, strengthening exercises, limb splinting and bracing, and proper support and positioning. These approaches prevent physical deformities (e.g., joint contractures) that can result from prolonged

ACUTE CONCUSSION EVALUATION (ACE)
PHYSICIAN/CLINICIAN OFFICE VERSION
Gerard Gioia, PhD[1] & Micky Collins, PhD[2]
[1]Children's National Medical Center
[2]University of Pittsburgh Medical Center

Patient Name:_____
DOB: _____ Age:_____
Date:_____ ID/MR#_____

A. Injury Characteristics   Date/Time of Injury_____   Reporter: __Patient __Parent __Spouse __Other_____

1. Injury Description _____

_____

1a. Is there evidence of a forcible blow to the head (direct or indirect)?   __Yes __No __Unknown
1b. Is there evidence of intracranial injury or skull fracture?   __Yes __No __Unknown
1c. Location of Impact: __Frontal __Lft Temporal __Rt Temporal __Lft Parietal __Rt Parietal __Occipital __Neck __Indirect Force
2. Cause: __MVC __Pedestrian-MVC __Fall __Assault __Sports (specify)_____Other_____
3. Amnesia Before (Retrograde) Are there any events just BEFORE the injury that you/ person has no memory of (even brief)? __ Yes __No Duration
4. Amnesia After (Anterograde) Are there any events just AFTER the injury that you/ person has no memory of (even brief)? __ Yes __No Duration
5. Loss of Consciousness: Did you/ person lose consciousness?   __ Yes __No Duration
6. EARLY SIGNS: __Appears dazed or stunned __Is confused about events __Answers questions slowly __Repeats Questions __Forgetful (recent info)
7. Seizures: Were seizures observed? No__ Yes___ Detail_____

B. Symptom Check List*   Since the injury, has the person experienced <u>any</u> of these symptoms any <u>more than usual</u> today or in the past day?
Indicate presence of each symptom (0=No, 1=Yes).   *Lovell & Collins, 1998 JHTR*

PHYSICAL (10)			COGNITIVE (4)			SLEEP (4)			
Headache	0	1	Feeling mentally foggy	0	1	Drowsiness	0	1	
Nausea	0	1	Feeling slowed down	0	1	Sleeping less than usual	0	1	N/A
Vomiting	0	1	Difficulty concentrating	0	1	Sleeping more than usual	0	1	N/A
Balance problems	0	1	Difficulty remembering	0	1	Trouble falling asleep	0	1	N/A
Dizziness	0	1	**COGNITIVE Total (0-4)** ___			**SLEEP Total (0-4)** ___			
Visual problems	0	1	**EMOTIONAL (4)**						
Fatigue	0	1	Irritability	0	1				
Sensitivity to light	0	1	Sadness	0	1				
Sensitivity to noise	0	1	More emotional	0	1				
Numbness/Tingling	0	1	Nervousness	0	1				
PHYSICAL Total (0-10) ___			**EMOTIONAL Total (0-4)** ___						

(Add Physical, Cognitive, Emotion, Sleep totals)
Total Symptom Score (0-22) ___

Exertion: Do these symptoms <u>worsen</u> with:
Physical Activity __Yes __No __N/A
Cognitive Activity __Yes __No __N/A

Overall Rating: How <u>different</u> is the person acting compared to his/her usual self? (circle)

Normal 0 1 2 3 4 5 6 Very Different

C. Risk Factors for Protracted Recovery (check all that apply)

Concussion History? Y ___ N___	√	Headache History? Y ___ N___	√	Developmental History	√	Psychiatric History
Previous # 1 2 3 4 5 6+		Prior treatment for headache		Learning disabilities		Anxiety
Longest symptom duration Days__ Weeks__ Months__ Years__		History of migraine headache __ Personal __ Family_____		Attention-Deficit/ Hyperactivity Disorder		Depression
						Sleep disorder
If multiple concussions, less force caused reinjury? Yes__ No__				Other developmental disorder_____		Other psychiatric disorder _____

List other comorbid medical disorders or medication usage (e.g., hypothyroid, seizures)_____

D. RED FLAGS for acute emergency management: Refer to the emergency department with <u>sudden onset</u> of any of the following:

* Headaches that worsen	* Looks very drowsy/ can't be awakened	* Can't recognize people or places	* Neck pain
* Seizures	* Repeated vomiting	* Increasing confusion or irritability	* Unusual behavioral change
* Focal neurologic signs	* Slurred speech	* Weakness or numbness in arms/legs	* Change in state of consciousness

---

E. Diagnosis (ICD): __Concussion w/o LOC 850.0 __Concussion w/ LOC 850.1 __Concussion (Unspecified) 850.9 __Other (854) _____
__No diagnosis

F. Follow-Up Action Plan   Complete *ACE Care Plan* and provide copy to patient/family.
___ No Follow-Up Needed
___ Physician/Clinician Office Monitoring: Date of next follow-up _____
___ Referral:
  ___ Neuropsychological Testing
  ___ Physician: Neurosurgery____ Neurology____ Sports Medicine____ Physiatrist____ Psychiatrist____ Other_____
  ___ Emergency Department

ACE Completed by:_____   MD RN NP PhD ATC   © Copyright G. Gioia & M. Collins, 2006

This form is part of the "Heads Up: Brain Injury in Your Practice" tool kit developed by the Centers for Disease Control and Prevention (CDC).

FIGURE 42-4 Acute concussion evaluation (ACE). Courtesy of Gerard Gioia, Children's National Medical Center; Micky Collins, University of Pittsburgh Medical Center.

A concussion (or mild traumatic brain injury (MTBI)) is a complex pathophysiologic process affecting the brain, induced by traumatic biomechanical forces secondary to direct or indirect forces to the head. Disturbance of brain function is related to neurometabolic dysfunction, rather than structural injury, and is typically associated with normal structural neuroimaging findings (i.e., CT scan, MRI). Concussion may or may not involve a loss of consciousness (LOC). Concussion results in a constellation of physical, cognitive, emotional, and sleep-related symptoms. Symptoms may last from several minutes to days, weeks, months or even longer in some cases.

ACE Instructions

The ACE is intended to provide an evidence-based clinical protocol to conduct an initial evaluation and diagnosis of patients (both children and adults) with known or suspected MTBI. The research evidence documenting the importance of these components in the evaluation of an MTBI is provided in the reference list.

A. Injury Characteristics:

1. Obtain **description of the injury** – how injury occurred, type of force, location on the head or body (if force transmitted to head). Different biomechanics of injury may result in differential symptom patterns (e.g., occipital blow may result in visual changes, balance difficulties).

2. Indicate the **cause of injury**. Greater forces associated with the trauma are likely to result in more severe presentation of symptoms.

3/4. **Amnesia:** Amnesia is defined as the failure to form new memories. Determine whether amnesia has occurred and attempt to determine length of time of memory dysfunction – before (retrograde) and after (anterograde) injury. Even seconds to minutes of memory loss can be predictive of outcome. Recent research has indicated that amnesia may be up to 4-10 times more predictive of symptoms and cognitive deficits following concussion than is LOC (less than 1 minute).

5. **Loss of consciousness (LOC)** – If occurs, determine length of LOC.

6. **Early signs.** If present, ask the individuals who know the patient (parent, spouse, friend, etc) about specific signs of the concussion that may have been observed. These signs are typically observed early after the injury.

7. Inquire whether **seizures** were observed or not.

B. Symptom Checklist:

1. Ask patient (and/or parent, if child) to report presence of the four categories of symptoms since injury. It is important to assess all listed symptoms as different parts of the brain control different functions. One or all symptoms may be present depending upon mechanisms of injury. Record "1" for Yes or "0" for No for their presence or absence, respectively.

2. For all symptoms, indicate presence of symptoms as experienced within the past 24 hours. Since symptoms can be present premorbidly/at baseline (e.g., inattention, headaches, sleep, sadness), it is important to assess change from their usual presentation.

3. **Scoring**: Sum total number of symptoms present per area, and sum all four areas into Total Symptom Score (score range 0-22). (Note: most sleep symptoms are only applicable after a night has passed since the injury. Drowsiness may be present on the day of injury.) If symptoms are new and present, there is no lower limit symptom score. Any score > 0 indicates positive symptom history.

4. **Exertion:** Inquire whether any symptoms worsen with physical (e.g., running, climbing stairs, bike riding) and/or cognitive (e.g., academic studies, multi-tasking at work, reading or other tasks requiring focused concentration) exertion. Clinicians should be aware that symptoms will typically worsen or re-emerge with exertion, indicating incomplete recovery. Over-exertion may protract recovery.

5. **Overall Rating:** Determine how different the person is acting from their usual self. Circle "0" (Normal) to "6" (Very Different).

C. Risk Factors for Protracted Recovery: Assess the following risk factors as possible complicating factors in the recovery process.

1. **Concussion history:** Assess the number and date(s) of prior concussions, the duration of symptoms for each injury, and whether less biomechanical force resulted in re-injury. Research indicates that cognitive and symptom effects of concussion may be cumulative, especially if there is minimal duration of time between injuries and less biomechanical force results in subsequent concussion (which may indicate incomplete recovery from initial trauma).

2. **Headache history:** Assess personal and/or family history of diagnosis/treatment for headaches. Research indicates headache (migraine in particular) can result in protracted recovery from concussion.

3. **Developmental history:** Assess history of learning disabilities, Attention-Deficit/Hyperactivity Disorder or other developmental disorders. Research indicates that there is the possibility of a longer period of recovery with these conditions.

4. **Psychiatric history:** Assess for history of depression/mood disorder, anxiety, and/or sleep disorder.

D. Red Flags: The patient should be carefully observed over the first 24-48 hours for these serious signs. Red flags are to be assessed as possible signs of deteriorating neurological functioning. Any positive report should prompt strong consideration of referral for emergency medical evaluation (e.g. CT Scan to rule out intracranial bleed or other structural pathology).

E. Diagnosis: The following ICD diagnostic codes may be applicable.

850.0 (Concussion, with no loss of consciousness) – Positive injury description with evidence of forcible direct/indirect blow to the head (A1a); plus evidence of active symptoms (B) of any type and number related to the trauma (Total Symptom Score >0); no evidence of LOC (A5), skull fracture or intracranial injury (A1b).

850.1 (Concussion, with brief loss of consciousness < 1 hour) – Positive injury description with evidence of forcible direct/indirect blow to the head (A1a); plus evidence of active symptoms (B) of any type and number related to the trauma (Total Symptom Score >0); positive evidence of LOC (A5), skull fracture or intracranial injury (A1b).

850.9 (Concussion, unspecified) – Positive injury description with evidence of forcible direct/indirect blow to the head (A1a); plus evidence of active symptoms (B) of any type and number related to the trauma (Total Symptom Score >0); unclear/unknown injury details; unclear evidence of LOC (A5), no skull fracture or intracranial injury.

Other Diagnoses – If the patient presents with a positive injury description and associated symptoms, but additional evidence of intracranial injury (A 1b) such as from neuroimaging, a moderate TBI and the diagnostic category of 854 (Intracranial injury) should be considered.

F. Follow-Up Action Plan: Develop a follow-up plan of action for symptomatic patients. The physician/clinician may decide to (1) monitor the patient in the office or (2) refer them to a specialist. Serial evaluation of the concussion is critical as symptoms may resolve, worsen, or ebb and flow depending upon many factors (e.g., cognitive/physical exertion, comorbidities). Referral to a specialist can be particularly valuable to help manage certain aspects of the patient's condition. (Physician/Clinician should also complete the ACE Care Plan included in this tool kit.)

1. **Physician/Clinician serial monitoring** – Particularly appropriate if number and severity of symptoms are steadily decreasing over time and/or fully resolve within 3-5 days. If steady reduction is not evident, referral to a specialist is warranted.

2. **Referral to a specialist** – Appropriate if symptom reduction is not evident in 3-5 days, or sooner if symptom profile is concerning in type/severity.
   - Neuropsychological Testing can provide valuable information to help assess a patient's brain function and impairment and assist with treatment planning, such as return to play decisions.
   - Physician Evaluation is particularly relevant for medical evaluation and management of concussion. It is also critical for evaluating and managing focal neurologic, sensory, vestibular, and motor concerns. It may be useful for medication management (e.g., headaches, sleep disturbance, depression) if post-concussive problems persist.

FIGURE 42-4, cont'd Acute concussion evaluation (ACE).

TABLE 42-3
Glasgow Coma Scale: Outcomes

Category and Score	Description
Vegetative state (<5)	A persistent state of impaired consciousness.
Severe (5-8)	Child is conscious but requires 24-hour care and supervision because of cognitive, behavioral, or physical disabilities. Slow response time and difficulties with short-term memory predominate.
Moderate (9-12)	Child is expected to achieve eventual independence in activities of daily living and home and community activities with persistent disability. Children in this group may have memory impairments, hemiparesis, dysphagia, ataxia, and other neuromotor problems.
Mild (13-15)	Good recovery is expected. Child is able to reintegrate into normal social life. There may be mild persisting sequelae.

From Winkler, P. (1995). Head injury. In D. Umphred (Ed.), *Neurological Rehabilitation* (3rd ed.). St. Louis: Mosby. Adapted with permission.

immobilization and the effects of unbalanced muscle tone on a joint. Speech pathologists address feeding, communication, and some cognitive areas; early in the course, they ensure readiness and safety for oral feeding. As children move to higher levels of cognitive function, speech pathologists work closely with the psychology and educational staff to identify and address orientation and memory weaknesses that may affect recovery. The team's nurses, psychologists, psychiatrists, social workers, and child life/recreation therapists guide the challenging emotional, social, and behavioral aspects of a child's recovery. The parents and family are essential members of the rehabilitation team. They contribute prior knowledge of the child's behavioral style and capabilities, as well as understanding the culture and community to which the child will return.

The primary care provider (PCP) must be incorporated into the rehabilitation process. The PCP should be updated on the child's medical conditions and functional capabilities, the team of subspecialists providing services, and the types of therapy and equipment necessary after hospital discharge. Together, the PCP and the rehabilitation staff evaluate the community resources and services and activate the supports necessary for the child and family on returning home.

The process of recovery does not stop when a child is discharged from an inpatient unit. The decision to discharge a child from an inpatient rehabilitation program should be considered when reasonable safety has been achieved and when the child can tolerate a transition to a less intense and more community-based level of care. There is strong evidence that training family members to provide cognitive and motor therapy at home brings about more powerful improvements in cognitive and motor scores, compared with clinician-delivered therapy alone (Braga, Da Paz, & Ylvisaker, 2005). Ongoing medical, emotional, physical, and educational support for the child and family is essential, especially as the child moves forward and encounters the continuing developmental challenges common to all children.

A child with a brain injury may experience long-term motor impairments. The site of brain injury determines the type and extent of motor impairment. There may be ataxia, tremor, spasticity, and rigidity, which increase the risk of scoliosis and joint contractures. There is currently no effective medical or surgical intervention for ataxia. Propranolol may help reduce tremors. Attempts to control spasticity and rigidity should begin with oral medications including baclofen, dantrolene, and diazepam. A nerve blocker, such as botulinum toxin A, can be effective in reducing spasticity. Each nerve block can last for several months, but effects wear off and a child may require repeated injections. Intensive physical therapy or serial casting may improve function following botulinum toxin A injections. Surgical intervention may be warranted if attempts with oral medication, injections, and casting have not been satisfactory. Implantation of an intrathecal baclofen pump may be effective in relieving symptoms (Rawlins, 2004). Unfortunately, though these interventions may help reduce symptoms, they do not offer a cure. Careful monitoring and use of a variety of specialized treatment modalities should be considered. Collaboration with a physiatrist and orthopedist is usually indicated. Proper equipment and ongoing physical therapy are essential. Long-term physical management is crucial to support optimal function, mobility, and independence. Assistive devices (e.g., wheelchairs, walkers) and braces need to be assessed for safety and fit, especially as a child grows and gains weight.

Complementary and Alternative Therapies

Interventions such as music and art therapy, therapeutic recreation, acupuncture, and other alternative approaches are commonly used and seem intuitively positive; however, their efficacy has not been substantiated (NIH, 1999).

Anticipated Advances in Diagnosis and Management

Sports-related mild TBI is a challenging aspect of pediatrics practice. It has been historically difficult to achieve consensus on terminology, appropriate acute evaluation, and return-to-play standards. Additional research is needed around both prevention and neuropsychological outcomes of mild concussion and sports-related TBI. Current studies suggest that repeated mild concussions associated with sports injuries increase the risk for negative sequelae, including headaches, depression, and neurocognitive symptoms, the most common of which is memory loss (Bazarian, 2005). A few studies have considered MTBI outcomes by gender. The results suggest that females experience a higher rate of poor outcome, including persistent symptoms, depression, and a higher rate of PCS (Bazarian, 2005). This warrants additional consideration as to whether females are more vulnerable to the effects of MTBI or whether there are varying injury-related factors for females.

Current research interest in the acute management of children with head injuries involves preventing or treating secondary responses and secondary injuries. One promising theory holds that calcium influx is a major perpetrator of cellular damage. There have been attempts to decrease this type of brain damage after TBI with free radical scavengers, aminosteroids, calcium antagonists, glutamate antagonists, ion channel blockers, and adenosine agonists; however, these have not yet been proven to be clinically advantageous (Park, Bell, & Baker, 2008).

Some recent studies of people with severe TBI involve lowering body temperature to 89.6° to 91.4°F (32° to 33°C) for 24 hours within 8 hours of the trauma; preliminary results support decreased mortality risk and better neurologic outcomes (McIntyre, Fergusson, Hebert, et al., 2003).

Stem cell research offers promising theoretic possibilities for repairing or "rewiring" damaged areas of the brain. Current research is primarily on animal models. There is a suggestion that transplanted embryonic stem cells may improve functional outcomes; however, there are concerns about increased potential for brain tumors following stem cell transplantation (Riess, Molcanyi, Bentz, et al., 2007).

Associated Problems of Traumatic Brain Injury and Treatment

Associated Problems of Mild Traumatic Brain Injury

Mild traumatic brain injury can cause a range of problems from the more common post-concussive syndrome, to the rare but serious second impact syndrome. Although recovery from MTBI associated with sports-related injuries varies, instability changes in neuropsychological test scores and postural stability usually resolve in 7 to 10 days (Meehan & Bachur, 2009). After a first concussion, children and athletes have an increased risk of sustaining an additional concussive injury in the following week to ten days although the reasons for this increased risk are not clear (Meehan & Bachur).

Associated Problems of Traumatic Brain Injury and Treatment

Associated Problems of Mild Traumatic Brain Injury
- Postconcussion syndrome
- Confusion, disorientation
- Difficulty with school work
- Balance and coordination problems
- Second impact syndrome

Associated Problems of Moderate or Severe Traumatic Brain Injury
- Neurologic dysfunction
  - Posttraumatic hydrocephalus
  - Posttraumatic seizures
  - Abnormal motor and sensory function
- Impaired respiratory function
- Endocrine dysfunction
- Altered cognitive and neuropsychological functions
- Speech/communication deficits
- Psychiatric and psychosocial deficits

Additional Associated Problems

Postconcussion Syndrome. PCS can occur days to weeks after an initial mild head injury and can persist for up to a year after injury (McCrea, 2008). The most common symptoms include headaches, irritability, anxiety, behavioral disturbances, dizziness, fatigue, impaired concentration, forgetfulness, blurred vision, nausea, sleep disturbances, and noise sensitivity; management is symptomatic. Athletes who have had concussions should not return to play if they are still experiencing any of these symptoms. An objective assessment tool, such as the ACE (CDC, 2006) (see Figure 42-4), can be serially administered to help in documenting the persistence or resolution of postconcussion symptoms.

Second Impact Syndrome. Second impact syndrome (SIS) is an uncommon but catastrophic event following a relatively mild head trauma, usually during sports, sustained after an initial unresolved concussion. SIS is characterized by acute brain swelling and neurologic collapse. It is believed to be caused by impaired cerebral autoregulation. The acute swelling can be sudden, irreversible, and fatal (McCrory & Bercovic, 1998). Athletes at risk are those whose initial postconcussion symptoms, such as headache, visual changes, and difficulty with thinking and memory, have not completely resolved. Thus, following a head injury, athletes should not return to play until they have been examined and deemed to be free of postconcussion symptoms.

Associated Problems of Moderate or Severe Traumatic Brain Injury

Neurologic Dysfunction

Posttraumatic hydrocephalus. Posttraumatic hydrocephalus occurs in a small number of individuals after brain injury, most commonly in those who have suffered a subarachnoid hemorrhage. This may occur weeks or months after head injury. In children with severe head injury, cerebral ventriculomegaly may be due to cerebral atrophy, rather than true hydrocephalus. If a diagnosis of hydrocephalus is made, treatment may consist of placement of a valve-regulating shunt. Surgical management via a shunt relieves acute symptoms of increased intracranial pressure (see Chapter 29).

Posttraumatic seizures. The incidence of posttraumatic seizures in children is about 10% (Pellock, Dodson, & Bourgeois, 2001). Posttraumatic seizures are classified as early (i.e., occurring within 7 days of injury) or late (i.e., occurring 7 days after injury). Prophylactic administration of anticonvulsants during the first week reduces the incidence of early seizures. However, extended use of anticonvulsants does not reduce the incidence of late seizures. Thus anticonvulsants may be given prophylactically for 1 week to 1 month and then discontinued unless chronic seizures develop (Young, Okada, Sokolove, et al., 2004). The onset of late seizures varies greatly, from soon after the initial injury to 2 years following the injury (see Chapter 26). Chronic seizures are usually well controlled with anticonvulsant medications.

Abnormal Motor and Sensory Function. Common motor disabilities for children following severe head injury include spasticity, movement problems (i.e., ataxia), contractures, paralysis, and speech impairments. The incidence and severity increase with severity of injury and if prolonged coma follows the injury. Although 5% to 30% of children with TBI manifest some motor control problems, many experience improvements for up to 7 years after injury (Beaulieu, 2002). Occupational and physical therapies provided at regular intervals maximize balance, coordination, and strength. They can retrain individuals in assisted, and ultimately independent, ambulation and other functional activities leading to developmentally appropriate self-care and leisure pursuits. Adaptive equipment (crutches, walkers, wheelchairs, lifts, and mechanical seats) may be used as needed. Surgical and pharmacologic interventions are available to address motor problems (Cronin, 2001). There is also a risk of audiologic problems and visual deficits.

Impaired Respiratory Function. Impairments in respiratory function can follow TBI. Damage to the brain's respiratory centers may affect the ability to breathe independently, necessitating tracheostomy or mechanical ventilation; these may be temporary or permanent interventions. Neurologic impairments can affect posture by causing scoliosis or kyphosis. These can interfere with normal lung capacity.

Endocrine Dysfunction. After severe head injury children may experience hyperphagia, hypothyroidism, precocious puberty, amenorrhea, or growth failure (Alexander & Moore, 2001). There may be signs of antidiuretic dysfunction such as (1) diabetes insipidus, which manifests as hypernatremia, polydipsia, and polyuria, or (2) syndrome of inappropriate secretion of antidiuretic hormone (SIADH), which manifests as hyponatremia and decreased urinary output. These conditions usually resolve after the acute posttraumatic phase, but may become a lifelong issue for some children. An endocrinologist should evaluate any child with signs of endocrine dysfunction.

Precocious puberty may occur in association with head trauma as a result of potential disruption of the normal hypothalamus and pituitary function. Premature sexual characteristics can include isolated breast, axillary, or pubic hair development. If these are present, the child should be referred to a pediatric endocrinologist for more in-depth management.

Altered Cognitive and Neuropsychological Function. Alterations in cognitive ability and neuropsychological function are common and critically important areas of postinjury dysfunction. Deficits may occur in memory, word retrieval, naming, verbal organization, comprehension of verbal information, comprehension of verbal abstractions, verbal learning, and effective conversation. Difficulties in attention and concentration, poor judgment, and impulsivity may persist. For those children with prior problems in these areas, such as children with ADHD, these deficits may become more severe. There may also be perceptual impairment, poor motor planning, tactile sensory dysfunction, and spatial disorientation (Cronin, 2001). Neuropsychological testing can identify deficits. Special education designation is often helpful in providing essential school-based support.

Severe head injury may affect major milestone attainment or cause milestone regression. Developmental progress should be monitored, and, if needed, referrals to community services should be made for physical therapy, occupational therapy, and speech therapy, as well as special education.

Speech/Communication Deficits. Impairments in expressive and receptive language are common in children with TBI. Notable are deficits in memory, word retrieval, labeling, and verbal organization. Gains in motor function bring about improvement in motor speech. Language ability is primarily a cognitive (neuropsychological) function and may lag despite aggressive therapy by speech and language specialists (Cronin, 2001).

Psychiatric and Psychosocial Deficits. There is a risk for psychological sequelae after significant pediatric TBI (Wade, Taylor, Yeates, et al., 2006). Emotional or behavioral difficulties that predate the brain injury may be exacerbated and exaggerated, or new behavioral symptoms may occur. The most common pattern of psychiatric disorder among children who have sustained a severe TBI results from injury to the frontal lobes, which causes affective (mood) instability, aggression, impaired social judgment, and occasionally apathy or paranoia (Schwartz, Taylor, Drotar, et al., 2003). This used to be called "organic personality syndrome" (Max, Koele, & Smith, 1998) but more commonly resembles severe symptoms of ADHD. The most frequent symptoms seen

---

BOX 42-4

Additional Problems of Traumatic Brain Injury and Treatment

- Focal neurologic deficits
- Neurogenic pulmonary edema
- Pneumonia
- Gastrointestinal hemorrhage
- Cardiac dysrhythmias
- Disseminated intravascular coagulation
- Pulmonary emboli
- Heterotopic ossification
- Increased muscle tone
- Joint contractures
- Aspiration
- Hypertension
- Disturbances of respiratory control
- Hypopituitarism
- Impaired nutritional status
- Bladder incontinence
- Bowel incontinence
- Hyperphagia

Adapted from Chipps, E.M., Clanin, N.J., & Campbell, V.G. (1992). *Neurologic Disorders.* St. Louis: Mosby.

---

after severe TBI are anxiety, obsessive-compulsive disorders, and phobia symptoms (Vasa, Gerring, Grados, et al., 2002).

There is extensive risk for psychological and social dysfunction, which can exert a long-term negative impact on quality of life for children with TBI. This is related to difficulties in executive neurologic functioning in key areas, including adaptation to transitions and delaying gratification (Levin & Hanten, 2005).

Additional Problems Associated with Traumatic Brain Injury

A variety of other associated problems or complications can occur after TBI and are listed in Box 42-4. Primary care providers must recognize these as potential complications when providing care to children with a history of significant head injury.

Prognosis

There is an overall 95% survival rate for children who sustain TBI. Of the children who sustain a severe head injury, this decreases to 65% (Langlois et al., 2005). The best predictor of good neurologic outcome is maintenance of cerebral perfusion pressure greater than or equal to 50 mm Hg (Hackbarth, Rzeszutko, Sturm, et al., 2002). Risk factors for poorer outcomes include focal lesions in addition to a diffuse injury (Weiner & Weinberg, 2000), significant associated injuries, and related problems of hypoxia and hypotension. Important negative prognostic indicators include increased length of coma, deterioration in GCS scores in the first 24 hours, increasing age (up to 14), lower postresuscitation GCS scores, longer duration of posttraumatic amnesia (Salorio, Slomine, Grados, et al., 2005), pathologic neurologic reflexes, posttraumatic seizures, CT scan mass findings, and lack of availability of rehabilitation services.

Most children who become comatose as a result of a TBI eventually regain consciousness. Overall they fare better than adults in similar clinical states; that is, severity of injury and coma characteristics (Shewmon, 2000). The reasons for better neurologic outcomes in the pediatric population have not been completely elucidated, but could include the resilient properties of the immature brain (Beaulieu, 2002) or differences in the nature of injury for younger versus older children (i.e., falls vs. vehicular accidents). The duration of a coma (i.e., the length of time from its onset until the display of meaningful response to external stimuli) is directly proportional to severity of neurologic impairment (Alexander & Moore, 2001). A coma lasting less than 6 hours is rarely associated with severe neuropsychological problems; a coma lasting more than 7 days is generally associated with a decline in cognitive function.

The emerging MTBI literature casts doubt on the older view that mild head injuries were not associated with long-term sequelae and lost productivity (McCrea, 2008). This is particularly true of sports-related mild head injuries.

PRIMARY CARE MANAGEMENT

Health Care Maintenance

Growth and Development

Because of the risk of altered nutritional intake, weight and height should be measured and plotted on a growth chart at each health visit. Increasing head circumference in children under 24 months of age might indicate hydrocephalus; however, this is not a reliable indicator of hydrocephalus after the fontanels are closed.

Precocious puberty may occur in association with head trauma as a result of potential disruption of the hypothalamus and pituitary function. Premature sexual characteristics can include isolated breast, axillary, or pubic hair development. Referral to pediatric endocrinology is recommended for more in-depth management.

Severe head injury may affect major milestone attainment or cause regression. Therefore, developmental progress should be monitored and community services obtained for physical therapy, occupational therapy, and speech therapy as needed and available.

The pediatric literature supports positive long-term outcomes for the majority of children with mild brain injuries. However, for children who are early in their recovery course and for children at the more severe end of the MTBI spectrum (i.e., those who require hospital admission), as well as for children with moderate or severe brain injuries, there is a directly proportionate increase in cognitive and behavioral difficulties (Thompson & Irby, 2003). Thus it is important to maintain watchful observation around school and social functioning. The Conners Rating Scales (Conners, 1990) are examples of commonly employed and useful instruments to allow for parent and teacher rating of a child's functioning across settings—home, school, and community. These can enhance and objectify narrative descriptions of a child's adjustment after a TBI. Early referral to educational and mental health resources can help address problems associated with school and social failure.

Diet

After severe TBI children may experience swallowing difficulties because of oral-motor incoordination, dysphagia, or as the result of posture and upper extremity limitations. These can lead to aspiration or poor weight gain (Alexander & Moore, 2001). Placement of a gastrostomy tube, with fundoplication if there is significant gastroesophageal reflux, may be considered for long-term nutritional management. Placing an immobile child in a side-lying position during and after meals can minimize the potential for aspiration or gastroesophageal reflux. Immobility may lead to increased bone calcium loss as a result of inadequate weight bearing (Sholas, Tann, & Gaebler-Spira, 2005). It is also important to monitor for excess weight gain that may occur as a result of physical inactivity, poor awareness of satiety, or impulsive overeating. A child's ability to feed is often an area of focus for a family because of the emotional, social, and cultural values surrounding feeding and nutrition. Referrals to a gastroenterologist, nutritionist, or psychotherapist may be helpful. A registered dietitian can help guide fluid balance, appropriate caloric intake, and adequate nutrition for growth. The PCP can help a family to balance oral and nonoral feedings to simultaneously support nutritional and emotional goals.

Safety

As with all pediatric visits, counseling about safety practices and injury prevention for the child's age and developmental level is appropriate. Although it is impossible to prevent all minor head injuries, it is important to discuss preventing repeat head trauma. It is important to reinforce the use of appropriate motor vehicle passenger seat restraints; the use of helmets appropriate for recreational or competitive sports; and childproofing the home, the school, and community playgrounds.

Children with moderate to severe TBI are at an increased risk for future injury caused by neuropsychological and neurobehavioral deficits resulting in overactivity, poor judgment, impulsivity, aggression, and perceptual deficits similar to children with ADHD (see Chapter 12). In addition to direct supervision and school-based supports, there are psychopharmacologic options to improve day-to-day functioning. (Silver, Arciniegas, & Yudofsky, 2005). Stimulants, such as methylphenidate and dextroamphetamine, enhance selective attention and processing speed. Alpha agonists, such as clonidine and guanfacine, can assist with organization for sleep or for daytime cognitive functioning. Atypical antipsychotic agents, such as risperidone, can be helpful in cases of behavioral aggression. As with all psychotropic medications, the children need to be monitored both for target symptom abatement and for medication-specific side effects (Silver et al., 2005). Parents may need help in determining safe and appropriate adolescent responsibilities and activities, including driving.

The PCP must educate families, children, and school personnel regarding second impact syndrome, a rare but potentially serious complication. Children should not return to sports that pose a risk of a second brain injury until there is full resolution of neurologic and neuropsychological symptoms associated with the initial injury.

Immunizations

Routine immunizations are recommended. Immunizations can be given when the child's neurologic situation is stabilized. The risk of contracting preventable diseases and the risk of the immunization side effects should be discussed with the family. For children under 5 years of age, supplemental pneumococcal vaccines (PPV23) should be considered if the respiratory status is significantly compromised (AAP, 2006). Postimmunization fever management with antipyretics is recommended. Children with a known seizure history may be more susceptible to febrile seizures following the administration of diphtheria, tetanus, and acellular pertussis (DTaP) (AAP, 2006).

Screening

Vision. Vision can be adversely affected after a TBI. Children may experience symptoms of double vision, movement of fixed objects such as walls, eyestrain, visual fatigue, and loss of peripheral vision (Padula & Argyris, 2001). If visual deficits are suspected, a referral to a pediatric ophthalmologist should be made. Yearly screening for vision problems is recommended, even if deficits are not determined in the immediate postinjury period.

Hearing. Hearing can be adversely affected after TBI, and the most common sequelae are tinnitus, vestibular dysfunction, intolerance to loud/sudden noises, and sensorineural hearing impairment (Jury & Flynn, 2001). A referral to an audiologist should be made if there is a suggestion of hearing deficit. Routine periodic hearing screening is recommended even if deficits are not determined immediately.

Dental. Routine dental care is recommended. Children with head injuries may have fractured or missing teeth secondary to facial trauma and a pediatric orthodontist referral would be necessary. Anticonvulsant drugs may cause gingival hyperplasia.

Blood Pressure. Routine screening is recommended. Persistently elevated blood pressure should be carefully evaluated, particularly in the presence of an intracranial shunt (see Chapter 29).

Hematocrit. Routine screening is recommended.

Urinalysis. Routine screening is recommended. Low urine specific gravity may be an indicator of diabetes insipidus and high specific gravity may suggest SIADH.

Tuberculosis. Routine screening is recommended. If prophylactic medications are needed, evaluate potential drug interactions if the child is taking other medications.

Condition-Specific Screening

Posttraumatic Seizures. Family members and care providers should be knowledgeable about seizure precautions and seizure first aid (see Chapter 26). For children on anticonvulsant medication, periodic blood testing is necessary to determine medication blood levels and to test for hematologic side effects and liver dysfunction. These tests should be ordered in consultation with the child's neurologist (see Chapter 26).

Movement and Postural Problems. A motor evaluation, including assessment for scoliosis, contractures, weakness, and spasticity, should be conducted soon after discharge and annually, especially during periods of rapid height growth. Equipment and subspecialty evaluation might be indicated.

Skin Integrity. For those children who may have impaired mobility, sensation, nutrition, or cognitive status, frequent skin checks should be incorporated into daily care and should be included in visits to the PCP. It is essential to monitor for pressure areas, intertriginous infection, and skin breakdown. Appropriate equipment and proper fit and maintenance of equipment should also be ensured. This includes equipment used for mobility, as well as items such as gastrostomy tubes, tracheostomies, and urine and stool drainage systems.

> ### Differential Diagnosis
>
> - *Alterations in cognition or level of consciousness:* Know child's current baseline neurologic status.
> - *Fever* may increase potential for seizures in children with post-TBI seizures.
> - *Nausea and vomiting* may indicate shunt malfunction in children with posttraumatic hydrocephalus. Prolonged or severe vomiting may require aggressive rehydration in children with poor nutritional intake or limited oral-motor skills.
> - *Respiratory infections* pose risk of pneumonia and aspiration in the compromised child.
> - *Headaches* are common after TBI. Headache diaries may help determine frequency, intensity, and effectiveness of mild analgesics.

Alterations in Cognition or Level of Consciousness. Knowledge of the child's baseline neurologic status and behavior is the key to accurate assessment. A significant change or deterioration in cognitive function should be viewed as pathologic, and assessed further. Trauma, infections, tumors, and metabolic imbalances may cause alterations in arousal or cognition. Their onset may be sudden, subacute over a period of several days, or gradual over several weeks to months.

Fevers. Fevers are a common occurrence in the presence of viral and bacterial illnesses. Routine fever management is appropriate. In children with a history of seizures, the risk of seizures may increase during a febrile illness (see Chapter 26).

Nausea and Vomiting. Routine management of nausea and vomiting is advised. However, persistent vomiting or development of lethargy should be evaluated urgently in the child with an intracranial shunt (see Chapter 29).

Respiratory Infections. Children with severe neurologic or motor deficits are more prone to complications such as pneumonia or chronic aspiration. They require early and frequent assessment of respiratory function during periods of acute illness.

Headaches. Posttraumatic headaches can be concerning to the family. A headache diary can be valuable in recording onset, frequency, and associated symptoms. Symptom management with mild analgesics is usually adequate. If the headaches persist in frequency, further evaluation is recommended and a more specific medication may be warranted.

Drug Interactions

After a TBI a child may receive a variety of medications, including antiepileptics, stimulants for behavior, headache prophylaxis, and muscle relaxants for spasticity. In the event that additional medications such as antibiotics are necessary, it is important to consider potential drug interactions. There are a number of sources for this information, ranging from the pharmacist to the *Physicians' Desk Reference* (PDR) to online resources such as Epocrates (www.epocrates.com).

Common Illness Management
Differential Diagnosis

Like any other child, children with TBI are susceptible to common childhood illnesses; however, the management of these illnesses may differ depending on individual factors.

Developmental Issues
Sleep Patterns

Alterations in sleep patterns can be a challenge after TBI. Neurophysiologic sleep disruption can be compounded by posttraumatic stress disorder (PTSD). Transient insomnia should be treated symptomatically with short-term antihistamines (for their sedative effect), antidepressants, or other sleep aids such as melatonin or trazodone. Long-acting hypnotics are contraindicated because of potential impairment in daytime functioning. If PTSD is suspected, mental health referral is indicated for cognitive behavioral therapy, psychotherapy, and possible medications (Gerring, Slomine, Vasa, et al., 2002).

Good "sleep hygiene" is strongly recommended. This includes a regular bedtime routine that promotes an evening wind-down and a sleep period of at least 8 hours. Activities that can enhance sleep patterns include regular daily exercise, a soothing evening bath or shower to increase relaxation, and adjusting the timing of medication doses to promote sleep. Caffeine (in coffee, tea, or soft drinks), especially in the evening, late-evening exercise, and napping during the day should be avoided to encourage nighttime sleeping. Games and videos with violent or overstimulating content are also undesirable.

Toileting

Bowel and bladder continence may be disrupted after injury. These can generally be managed in conjunction with the rehabilitation team. Frequent toileting, or "trip training," can help reregulate bowel and bladder control. The first goal is bowel and bladder control during the waking hours, with subsequent targeting of nighttime continence. Fluid intake should be limited 2 hours before bedtime. If behavioral strategies are unsuccessful, consider the possibility of kidney disease, damage to the sacral nerves, or deficits in urine concentrating ability.

The child who is immobile is prone to constipation and can benefit from anticipatory guidance regarding its prevention and management. These children may require the use of natural or medicated stool softeners, glycerin suppositories, or additional fluid intake for assisted elimination. It is most helpful to establish a predictable pattern for bowel elimination, such as a warm drink and "sitting period" after the evening meal.

Discipline

Behavior and personality alterations should be anticipated following brain injury. Although it may be difficult to determine how TBI contributes to a child's behavior, the effects from brain injury should always be included in the differential diagnosis. Behavioral changes commonly seen after brain injury are anger, apathy, anxiety, depression, disinhibition, emotional lability, impaired judgment, and impulsivity (Alexander & Moore, 2001).

Parents and primary caretakers should be encouraged to be consistent with discipline and to reinforce normal household rules. Parents may have difficulty reinstating previous behavioral expectations after a catastrophic illness or injury. They may require support and encouragement around this area of "perceived vulnerability." Persistent behavioral difficulties at home, altered family and peer relationships, disruption in the school setting, or issues in the use of leisure time can generalize into other settings such as school and the community and can interrupt learning and socialization.

More extreme difficulties with behavior and discipline may respond to behavioral therapy techniques. Clear, simple expectations, explained at an appropriate cognitive level, need to take into account possible weaknesses in short-term memory and impulse control. It is important for care providers to be consistent in their style of discipline and behavior management. As with any behavioral intervention, avoid giving mixed or imprecise descriptions of desired behavior. The parents, care providers, and other family members should model desirable behavior. Pharmacologic management with stimulants or other psychotropic medications may be considered (see Chapter 12). These medications are best used in conjunction with behavioral therapy.

Child Care

Mildly disabled children may be appropriately cared for in a day-care or home care setting. For children in a daycare or preschool setting, an individualized health plan (IHP) can be useful in communicating medical information with early childhood educators.

Severely disabled children who are technology dependent may require assisted nursing care in the home or other "natural" settings. Federal funds from Title XX of the Social Security Act, also known as the Social Services Block Grant (SSBG), are available for respite services, homemaker services, and foster home care.

Schooling

Children who experience a TBI before age 3 years are eligible for early intervention services under the Birth to Three Service, which is mandated in the Individuals with Disabilities Education Improvement Act (IDEA) of 2004 (see Chapter 3). Early intervention programs are helpful in determining age-appropriate and developmentally enhancing activities. Other aspects of intervention include parent support, education, and training to create an environment that fosters the child's ability to work independently. IDEA also mandates preschool services, which include appropriate therapies for children with TBI if the resulting impairments affect the child's ability to learn.

The return to school represents a critical phase in recovery for all children with a head injury. Successful school reentry is determined by intellect and cognitive ability, social skills, and peer relationships. Home-based academic tutoring or part-time attendance may initially support the transition to a school program, especially if there is limited endurance or proneness to fatigue.

The child with TBI must be supported in the transition to school. Recommended transition services are (1) establishing communication among all persons caring for the child; (2) initiating an evaluation process, which may include neuropsychological testing; (3) integrating information in an interdisciplinary forum; (4) adapting education programs based on neuropsychological test results to meet the child's needs; (5) preparing the child for transitions; and (6) providing ongoing monitoring for possible late-developing problems (Cronin, 2001).

Depending on the depth and breadth of persistent deficits, children with TBI can receive services in regular classes or special education classes. They may be eligible for speech-language therapy, occupational or physical therapies, special services for hearing or visual impairments, behavior management, and counseling as components of an individualized educational program (IEP) (see Chapter 3).

Sexuality

Individuals who have sustained a head injury may have altered inhibition or may make socially inappropriate sexualized comments and gestures. These need to be addressed in the broader context of appropriate social behavior. Impairment in motor and sensory function or impaired communication may alter sexual functioning. Social isolation can diminish self-esteem and may contribute to inappropriate sexual behaviors. The onset of precocious puberty may further complicate sexuality.

Concerns about sexuality expressed by the child or adolescent, family, and significant others should be addressed directly and calmly. Weaknesses in impulse control and short-term memory may necessitate repeated conversation about these issues, as well as requiring emphasis from more than one individual in the child's life, such as the parents, teachers, counselor, pastor, or peer coach.

Transition to Adulthood

Traumatic brain injury may have a major effect on the subsequent education, vocational development, independent living skills, and future productivity of affected individuals. Supported living programs, supervised housing, shared services, or foster care should be evaluated with respect to the level of assistance provided for activities of daily living. Supervised work experiences may be necessary to develop appropriate skills and work habits to succeed in gainful employment and contribute to the community. Health care insurance coverage and financial assistance programs should also be addressed as adolescents enter adulthood (see Chapters 8 and 9).

Family Concerns

The stress of TBI can exert negative effects on the parents' mental health and can undermine parent-child and family relationships. Parents confront fears about immediate survival, current condition, and long-term needs. While caring for a child with TBI, parents may feel guilty about the incident that caused the TBI and their need to focus time and attention on the injured child, feeling neglectful of the child's siblings (Youngblut, 2000). Siblings can experience emotional disturbances, school problems, and aggression. Siblings may feel guilty, after initially experiencing a sense of relief that the injury happened to their brother or sister and not to them. It is helpful for parents, family members, and care providers to become actively involved in the day-to-day care of the injured child; this will reduce their sense of helplessness and build confidence (Wade et al., 2006). TBI support groups for parents and for siblings can offer reassurance and creative ideas to enhance coping.

Significant financial issues, change in employment because of care responsibilities, and conflict related to the parents' return to work may arise, adding to a family's stress. There may be anger if one parent was present at the time of the injury, such as driving the car in an accident. Beyond this, there may be disability or death of a parent as a result of the accident. One out of four of all occupant deaths among children ages 0 to 14 years involve a drinking driver. More than two thirds of these fatally injured children were riding with a drinking driver (Schults, 2004). Long-term family support and counseling can be extremely helpful. Families who seek support and work to cope with the situation may experience less stress and family dysfunction over time (Wade, Taylor, Yeates et al., 2001).

Caregivers of children with the most severe sequela and the greatest number of unmet needs report the most significant family burden (Aitken, McCarthy, Slomine, et al (2009). Primary care providers are in a key position to help locate comprehensive care services that are congruent with the child and family's cultural background. Primary care providers can facilitate the family's coping with the injury and help in setting attainable goals for recovery (Wade et al., 2001). Anticipatory guidance should incorporate the length of time that symptoms may occur and the importance of routine follow-up, especially during the first 12 months after injury (Youngblut, 2000).

Caring for a child with a head injury is a complex task because of the physical, cognitive, and psychosocial concerns that must be addressed. The following is a list of additional resources.

Resources

General Resources

American Speech, Language, Hearing Association
2200 Research Blvd.
Rockville, MD 20850-3289
(800) 638-8255
Website: www.asha.org

Brain Injury Association
1608 Spring Hill Rd., Suite 110
Vienna, VA 22182
(800) 444-6443 (Family Helpline)
Website: www.biausa.org

Centers for Disease Control and Prevention
National Center for Injury Prevention and Control
Heads Up: Brain Injury in Your Practice. Free Toolkit
Mailstop F41
4770 Buford Hwy. NE
Atlanta, GA 30341-3724
(800) CDC-INFO (232-4636)
Website: www.cdc.gov/ncipc/tbi

Family Caregiver Alliance
180 Montgomery St., Suite 1100
San Francisco, CA 94104
(415) 434-3388 or (800) 445-8106
Website: www.caregiver.org

Resources for Professionals

American Congress of Rehabilitative Medicine
6801 Lake Plaza Dr., Suite B-205
Indianapolis, IN 46220
(317) 915-2250
Website: www.acrm.org

Association of Rehabilitation Nurses
4700 W. Lake Ave.
Glenview, IL 60025-1485
(800) 229-7530
Website: www.rehabnurse.org

Summary of Primary Care Needs for the Child with a Traumatic Brain Injury

HEALTH CARE MAINTENANCE

Growth and Development

- Height and weight should be measured and plotted on growth charts for all children. Head circumference should be monitored at each visit until the fontanels are closed, at approximately 2 years of age.
- Monitor for pubertal development and for signs of precocious puberty and short stature.
- Screen and assess developmental, cognitive, and motor skills regularly. Monitor therapy intervention programs.
- Evaluate school and social functioning.

Diet

- Eating and feeding problems can contribute to poor growth patterns.
- Decreased physical activity and immobility may lead to excessive weight gain. Tailor intake to meet the child's nutritional needs.
- Decreased physical activity and immobility may contribute to loss of bone calcium and osteopenia. Monitor dietary calcium intake and encourage weight bearing in physical therapy and recreational activities.
- Monitor protective reflexes (i.e., gag) to minimize risk of aspiration.
- Occupational therapy or speech therapy can assist with safe and optimal feeding programs.

Safety

- Increased risk of falls is present as a result of instability, poor coordination, potential seizures, and delays in motor skill acquisition.
- Provide anticipatory guidance on general safety precautions.
- Review emergency seizure procedures.
- Evaluate desirability of participating in risk-taking sports and activities. Ensure the use of proper protective equipment.
- Evaluate adolescent's cognition, attention, and neuromuscular status. Counsel on driving or use of motorized vehicles.

Immunizations

- Routine immunizations are recommended
- Children with posttraumatic seizures may be at increased seizure risk.
- Fever prophylaxis with acetaminophen or ibuprofen, not aspirin, is recommended.

Screening

- *Vision.* Complete postinjury evaluation during the recovery period, with correction of minor deficits. Yearly screening is recommended.
- *Hearing.* Complete postinjury evaluation for hearing and vestibular deficits during the recovery period. Refer for correction of minor deficits.
- *Dental.* Routine screening.
  - Evaluate for possible dental trauma after a head injury.
  - More frequent evaluations may be necessary for children on seizure medications.
- *Blood pressure.* Monitor blood pressure with each visit.
- *Hematocrit.* Routine screening is recommended.
- *Urinalysis.* Routine screening is recommended, including specific gravity for diabetes insipidus and SIADH.
- *Tuberculosis.* Routine screening is recommended. If prophylactic medications are needed, evaluate potential drug interactions in children receiving other medications.

Condition-Specific Screening

- *Posttraumatic seizure therapy.* Monitor complete blood count (CBC) and chemistry panels along with anticonvulsant levels for the first 6 months after injury and periodically thereafter.
- *Movement and postural problems.* Assess for scoliosis, contractures, weakness, and spasticity, especially during growth spurts.
  - Ensure access to appropriate assistive devices.
- *Skin integrity.* Examine skin for pressure areas, breakdown, and signs of superficial infection.

COMMON ILLNESS MANAGEMENT

Differential Diagnosis

- A thorough knowledge of baseline neurologic status and behavior is key in assessing significance of deviations.
- Risk of seizures is increased with acute illness and fever.
- Consider the potential for increased intracranial pressure in the presence of an intracranial shunt with signs of nausea and vomiting.
- Evaluation of headaches requires careful history, neurologic examination, and symptom management.

Drug Interactions

- Potential drug interactions can occur if the child is taking epileptic drugs, stimulants for behavior, headache prophylaxis, and/or muscle relaxants for spasticity. Careful monitoring is required.

DEVELOPMENTAL ISSUES

Sleep Patterns

- Disruption in sleep patterns may be evident. A structured behavioral approach may be helpful. "Sleep hygiene" is recommended.

Toileting

- Bowel and bladder continence may be delayed in younger children or disrupted in older children who previously had voluntary control. A progressive training program with positive reinforcement will help reestablish control as cognition improves.
- Monitor for and manage chronic constipation.

Discipline

- Anticipate alterations in behavior and personality and institute early support and guidance. Recommend standard developmentally appropriate discipline with reinforcement of usual household rules.
- Manage persistent difficulties with behavior modification and discipline. Evaluation by a behavior specialist may be warranted.
- Anxiety, depression, and emotional lability may require mental health referral.

Child Care

- Assistance in identifying and accessing community respite care services for children with severe TBI is a priority area.

Schooling

- "Birth to Three" referral for assessment and intervention is recommended.
- Cognitive changes may persist from weeks to many months following head trauma.

Continued

Summary of Primary Care Needs for the Child with a Traumatic Brain Injury—cont'd

- Fully assess learning needs and individualize approaches as soon as feasible after the injury.
- Children with significant TBI sequelae are eligible for special education. Families may require assistance with the individualized educational program (IEP) process.
- If formal neuropsychological and school performance testing is needed, the local school district must provide it.

Sexuality

- Monitor for precocious or delayed puberty. Refer to endocrinologist if these are present.
- Impairment in communication, motor, and sensory function or impaired behavioral self-regulation may alter sexual functioning. Anticipatory guidance in counseling is advised.

Transition to Adulthood

- TBI can have a major effect on the future education, vocational development, and independent living skills of the affected adolescent. School guidance and vocational counseling are essential.
- Establish working relationships with local adult PCPs and subspecialists.

FAMILY CONCERNS

- Severe stresses on the family unit arise following a head injury. Support groups or family counseling for parents and siblings may be helpful.
- Comprehensive care that is congruent with and respectful toward the child's and family's cultural background is a key element for successful coping.

REFERENCES

Adelson, P.D., & Kochanek, P.M. (2001). Head injury in children. *J Child Neurol, 13*(1), 2-15.

Aitken, M.E., McCarthy, M.L., Slomine, B.S., et al. (2009). Family burden after traumatic brain injury in children. *Pediatrics, 123*, 199-206.

Alexander, J., & Moore, D. (2001). Primary care for children with brain injury. *N C Med J, 62*, 344-348.

American Academy of Pediatrics (AAP) & American Academy of Family Physicians. (1999). The management of minor closed head injury in children. *Pediatrics, 104*(6), 1407-1415.

American Academy of Pediatrics (AAP). Committee on Child Abuse and Neglect. (2001). Shaken baby syndrome: Rotational cranial injuries—technical report. *Pediatrics, 108*(1), 206-210.

American Academy of Pediatrics (APP). (2006). *Red Book Report of the Committee on Infectious Diseases.* Elk Grove Village, IL: Author.

Bazarian, J.J. (2005). Mild traumatic brain injury in the United States, 1998-2000. *Brain Inj, 19*(2), 85-90.

Beaulieu, C.L. (2002). Rehabilitation and outcome following pediatric traumatic brain injury. *Surg Clin North Am, 82*(2), 393-408.

Bloom, D.R., Levin, H., & Ewing-Cobbs, L. (2001). Lifetime and novel psychiatric disorders after pediatric traumatic brain injury. *J Am Acad Child Adolesc Psychiatry, 40*(5), 572-579.

Braga, L.W., Da Paz, A.C., & Ylvisaker, M. (2005). Direct clinician delivered versus indirect family supported rehabilitation of children with traumatic brain injury. *Brain Inj, 19*(8), 819-831.

Centers for Disease Control and Prevention (CDC). (2003). *Report to Congress on mild traumatic brain injury in the United States.* Available at www.cdc.gov/ncipc/tbi/mtbi/report.htm. Retrieved January 21, 2009.

Centers for Disease Control and Prevention (CDC). (2006). *Heads up: Brain injury in your practice.* Available at www.cdc.gov/ncipc/tbi/physicians_tool_kit.htm. Retrieved January 21, 2009.

Collins, M.W., Iverson, G.L., & Lovell, M.R. (2003). On field predictors of neuropsychological and symptom deficit following sports related concussion. *Clin J Sports Med, 13*(4), 222-229.

Conners, C.K. (1990). *Conners' Rating Scales, Revised (CRS-R).* Los Angeles: Western Psychological Services.

Cronin, A.F. (2001). Traumatic brain injury in children: Issues in community function. *Am J Occup Ther, 55*(4), 377-384.

Evans, R., & Wilberger, J.E. (1999). Traumatic disorders. In C. Goetz & E. Pappert (Eds.), *Textbook of Clinical Neurology.* Philadelphia: Saunders.

Gerring, J., Slomine, B., & Vasa, R., et al. (2002). Clinical predictors of post-traumatic stress disorder after closed head injury in children. *J Am Acad Child Adolesc Psychiatry, 41*(2), 157-165.

Ghajar, J., & Hariri, R. (1992). Management of pediatric head injury. *Pediatr Clin North Am, 39*, 1093-1125.

Giza, C. (2006). Lasting effects of pediatric traumatic brain injury. *Indian J Neurotrauma, 3*(1), 19-26.

Giza, C., & Hovda, D. (2001). The neurometabolic cascade of concussion. *J Athletic Training, 36*(3), 228-235.

Goka, R.S. (2000). Mild traumatic brain injury: Treatment paradigms. In G. Jay, (Ed.), *Minor Traumatic Brain Injury Handbook.* Boca Raton, FL: CRC Press.

Gualtieri, C.T. (2002). Brain injury and mental retardation. In *Psychopharmacology and Neuropsychiatry.* Philadelphia: Lippincott Williams & Wilkins.

Hackbarth, R.M., Rzeszutko, K.M., Sturm, G., et al. (2002). Survival and functional outcome in pediatric traumatic brain injury: A retrospective review and analysis of predictive factors. *Crit Care Med, 30*(7), 1630-1635.

Haider, A. (2006). Mechanism of injury predicts outcome in traumatic brain injury. *J Surg Res, 130*(2), 328.

Hartl, R., & Ghajar, J. (2005). Neurosurgical interventions. In J.M. Silver, T.W. McAllister, & S.C. Yudofsky (Eds.), *Textbook of Traumatic Brain Injury.* Washington, DC: American Psychiatric Publishing.

Jha, S.K. (2003). Cerebral edema and its management. *Med J Armed Forces India, 59*, 326-331.

Jury, M.A., & Flynn, M.C. (2001). Auditory and vestibular sequelae to traumatic brain injury: A pilot study. *N Z Med J, 114*(1134), 286-288.

Keenan, H.T., Runyan, D.K., Marshall, S.W., et al. (2003). A population-based study of inflicted traumatic brain injury in young children. *J Am Med Assoc, 290*(5), 621-626.

Kraus, J.F. (2005). Epidemiology. In J.M. Silver, T.W. McAllister, & S.C. Yudofsky (Eds.), *Textbook of Traumatic Brain Injury.* Washington, DC: American Psychiatric Publishing.

Langlois, J.A., Rutland-Brown, W., & Thomas, K.E. (2004). *Traumatic Brain Injury in the United States: Emergency Department Visits, Hospitalizations, and Deaths. Atlanta: Centers for Disease Control and Prevention, National Center for Injury Prevention and Control.*

Langlois, J.A., Rutland-Brown, W., & Thomas, K.E. (2005). The incidence of traumatic brain injury among children in the United States: Differences by race. *J Head Trauma Rehabil, 20*(3), 229-238.

Levin, H.S., & Hanten, G.H. (2005). Executive functions after traumatic brain injury in children. *Pediatr Neurol, 33*(2), 79-93.

Lovell, M.R., Collins, M.W., & Bradley, J. (2004). Return to play following sports related concussion. *Clin Sports Med, 23*(3), 421-441.

Marik, P.E., Varon, J., & Trask, T. (2002). Management of head trauma. *Chest, 122*(2), 699-711.

Max, J.B., Koele, S.L., & Smith, W.L. (1998). Psychiatric disorders in children and adolescents after severe traumatic brain injury: A controlled study. *J Am Acad Child Adolesc Psychiatry, 37*(8), 832-840.

McAllister, T.W. (2005). Mild brain injury and the postconcussion syndrome. In J.M. Silver, T.W. McAllister, & S.C. Yudofsky (Eds.), *Textbook of Traumatic Brain Injury.* Washington, DC: American Psychiatric Publishing.

McCrea, M.A. (2008). *Mild Traumatic Brain Injury and Postconcussion Syndrome: The New Evidence Base for Diagnosis and Treatment.* New York: Oxford University Press.

McCrory, P., Johnston, K., Meeuwisse, W., et al. (2004). Summary and agreement statement of the second International Conference on Concussion in Sport, Prague 2004. *Br J Sports Med 2005, 39*(4), 196-204.

McCrory, R., & Bercovic, S.F. (1998). Second impact syndrome. *Neurology, 50*, 677-683.

McIntyre, L.A., Fergusson, D.A., Hebert, P.C., et al. (2003). Prolonged therapeutic hypothermia after traumatic brain injury in adults: A systematic review. *J Am Med Assoc, 289*(22), 2992-2999.

Meehan, W.P., & Bachur, R.G. (2009). Sport-Related Concussion. *Pediatrics, 123*, 114-123.

Murdoch, B.E., & Theodoros, D.G. (2001). Introduction Epidemiology, neuropathophysiology, and medical aspects of traumatic brain injury. In B.E. Murdoch & D.G. Theodoros (Eds.), *Traumatic Brain Injury*: San Diego CA: Singular Publishing Group.

National Institutes of Health (NIH) Consensus Development Panel on Rehabilitation of Persons with Traumatic Brain Injury. (1999). Rehabilitation of persons with traumatic brain injury. *J Am Med Assoc, 282*(10), 974-983.

Padula, W.V., & Argyris, S. (2001). *Post-Traumatic Vision Syndrome: Part 1.* Neuro-optometric. Rehabilitation Association International, Inc.

Park, C.O., & Hyun, K.H. (2004). Apoptic change in response to magnesium therapy after moderate diffuse axonal injury in rats. *Yonsei Med J, 45*(5), 908-916.

Park, E., Bell, J.D., & Baker, A.J. (2008). Traumatic brain injury: Can the consequences be stopped?. *Can Med Assoc J, 178*(9), 1163-1170.

Pellock, J.M., Dodson, W.E., Bourgeois, B.F.(Eds.) (2001). *Pediatric Epilepsy Diagnosis and Therapy*, New York: Demos.

Rawlins, P.K. (2004). Intrathecal baclofen therapy over ten years. *J Neurosci Nurs, 16*(4), 322-327.

Riess, P., Molcanyi, M., Bentz, K., et al. (2007). Embryonic stem cell transplantation after experimental traumatic brain injury dramatically improves neurological outcome, but may cause tumors. *J Neurotrauma, 24*(1), 216-225.

Roth, P., & Farls, K. (2000). Pathophysiology of traumatic brain injury. *Crit Care Nurs Q, 23*(3), 14-25.

Salorio, C., Slomine, B., Grados, M., et al. (2005). Neuroanatomic correlates of CVLT-C performance following pediatric traumatic brain injury. *J Int Neuropsychol Soc, 11*(6), 686-696.

Schneier, A.J., Shields, B.J., Grim-Hostetler, S., et al. (2006). Incidence of pediatric traumatic brain injury and associated hospital resource utilization in the United States. *Pediatrics, 118*(2), 483-492.

Schults, R.A. (2004). Child passenger deaths involving drinking drivers. *MMWR Morb Mortal Wkly Rep, 53*(4), 77-80.

Schutzman, S.A., & Greenes, D.S. (2001). Evaluation and management of children younger than two years of age with apparently minor head trauma: Proposed guidelines. *Pediatrics, 107*(5), 983-993.

Schwartz, L., Taylor, H.G., Drotar, D., et al. (2003). Long-term behavior problems following pediatric traumatic brain injury: Prevalence, predictors, and correlates. *J Pediatr Psychol, 28*(4), 251-263.

Shewmon, D.A. (2000). Coma prognosis in children. *J Clin Neurophysiol, 17*(5), 467-472.

Sholas, M.G., Tann, B., & Gaebler-Spira, D. (2005). Oral bisphosphonates to treat disuse osteopenia in children with disabilities: A case series. *J Pediatr Orthop, 25*(3), 326-331.

Silver, J.M., Arciniegas, D.B., & Yudofsky, S.C. (2005). Psychopharmacology. In J.M. Silver, T.W. McAllister, & S.C. Yudofsky (Eds.), *Textbook of Traumatic Brain Injury.* Washington, DC: American Psychiatric Publishing.

Swaine, B.R., Tremblay, C., Platt, R.W., et al. (2007). Previous head injury is a risk factor for subsequent head injury in children. *Pediatrics, 119*, 749-758.

Teasdale, G., & Jennett, B.J. (1981). *Management of Head Injuries.* Philadelphia: F.A. Davis.

Thompson, M., & Irby, J. (2003). Recovery from mild head injury in pediatric populations. *Semin Pediatr Neurol, 10*(2), 130-139.

Vasa, R.A., Gerring, J., Grados, M., et al. (2002). Anxiety after severe pediatric closed head injury. *J Am Acad Child Adolesc Psychiatry, 41*(2), 148-157.

Wade, S.L., Taylor, G.H., Yeates, K.O., et al. (2001). The relationship of caregiver coping to family outcomes during the initial year following pediatric traumatic injury. *J Consult Clin Psychol, 69*(3), 406-415.

Wade, S.L., Taylor, G.H., Yeates, K.O., et al. (2006). Long-term parental and family adaptation following pediatric brain injury. *J Pediatr Psychol, 31*(10), 1072-1083.

Weiner, H.L., & Weinberg, J.S. (2000). Head injury in the pediatric age group. In P.R. Cooper & J. Golfinos (Eds.), *Head Injury.* New York: McGraw-Hill.

Young, K.D., Okada, P.J., & Sokolove, P.E., et al. (2004). A randomized, double-blinded, placebo-controlled trial of phenytoin for the prevention of early posttraumatic seizures in children with moderate to severe blunt head injury. *Ann Emerg Med, 43*(4), 435-446.

Youngblut, J.M. (2000). Effects of pediatric head trauma for children, parents, and families. *Crit Care Nurs Clin North Am, 12*(2), 228-235.

Index

A

AACAP. *See* American Academy of Child and Adolescent Psychiatry
AAKP. *See* American Association of Kidney Patients
AAP. *See* American Academy of Pediatrics
Abdominal pain
  with bleeding, 256
  in celiac disease, 321
  in IBD, 581
  in sickle cell disease, 783b, 788
Abilify. *See* Aripiprazole
ABO-incompatible heart transplantation, 722
Absence epilepsy
  childhood, 492
  juvenile, 492
Absence seizures, 490
  atypical, 490
Absenteeism, 53
Absolute neutrophil count, calculation of, 297b
Academic performance
  factors of, 53–54
  in terminal illness, 56–57
Access
  health care, in adults, 67–68
  hemodialysis, 613f
  implanted venous, device, 246
  vascular, problems, 296, 296b
Accidents, with bipolar disorder, 641
Accommodation plan, 43, 44, 504
Acculturation, biculturalism and, 92–93
ACE. *See* Acute Concussion Evaluation
Acid-base abnormality, 608
Acquired immunodeficiency disease (AIDS)
  associated problems with, 532–534
  camps for, 549
  CDC cases by, 528t
  complementary and alternative therapies for, 532
  diagnostic criteria for, 529
  National groups for, 541
  National Pediatric, Network, 541–543
  opportunistic infections in, 533
  perinatal, number of, 529t
  prognosis of, 534
  pulmonary disease in, 533–534
  Ryan White HIV/AIDS program, 127
ACTH. *See* Adrenocorticotropic hormone
Activity
  body mass index and, 700
  calories by, 690t
  in CHD, 399f
  in diabetes mellitus, 432
  after heart transplantation, 728

Activity *(Continued)*
  in obesity, 686
  after organ transplantation, 727–728
  of plasma renin, 376
  in schools, 35–36
  sports
    after concussion, 821b
    after traumatic brain injury, 821b
Acupuncture
  for obesity, 695
  for sickle cell disease, 777
Acute adrenal insufficiency, 376b
  differential diagnosis of, 377
Acute bleeding disorders, 248
Acute chest syndrome, with sickle cell disease, 781
Acute Concussion Evaluation (ACE), 822–823f
Acute graft-vs.-host disease, 269–270
Acute infectious conjunctivitis, differential diagnosis of, 160
Acute splenic sequestration complication, 779
Acute viral rhinitis, differential diagnosis of, 160
Acyanotic heart defects, 387f
Adaptive equipment, for muscular dystrophy, Duchenne, 656–657
Addiction
  Paul Wellstone and Pete Domenici Mental Health Parity and Addiction Equity Act of 2008, 120
  to stimulant medication, 205–206
Adenoidectomy, 353
Adenoid-type facies, in allergic rhinitis, 149f
ADHD. *See* Attention-deficit/hyperactivity disorder
Adolescence
  ADHD in, 201
  attitudes of, 64–65
  autonomy in, 64
  chronic conditions in, 25
  cognitive ability in, 64
  death rates in, 5t
  decision making during, 107–108
  developmental tasks during, 61–65
  early, 63t
  glucocorticoids in, 379
  kidney disease in, 621t
  mental health issues in, 67
  mineralocorticoids in, 379–380
  obesity resources in, 706
  problem solving in, 64
  relationships in, 64–65
  self-competence in, 64
  sexual development in, 65
  substance abuse in, 67
  successful, 64

Adolescent Self-Management and Independence Scale (AMIS), 67
Adrenalectomy, in CAH, 373
Adrenal insufficiency, acute, 376b
  differential diagnosis of, 377
Adrenals
  glucocorticoid production by, 364
  steroid pathways of, 365f
Adrenal suppression, corticotropin-releasing hormone antagonists for, 373
Adrenocorticotropic hormone (ACTH)
  for epilepsy, 495–497t
  stimulation test, 367
Adrenomedullary dysfunction/epinephrine deficiency, 369
Adulthood transition
  in ADHD, 213–214
  allergies with, 162
  in asthma, 190
  in autism, 236
  in bleeding disorders, 258
  in CAH, 379–380
  in cancer, 307
  in celiac disease, 322
  in cerebral palsy, 340
  in CHD, 400
  in cleft palate, 359
  to community living, 70–71
  in cystic fibrosis, 422
  decision making process in, 109
  in diabetes mellitus, 441–442
  in Down syndrome, 464–465
  in eating disorders, 475
  in epilepsy, 508–509
  in fragile X syndrome, 523–524
  after HSCT, 280
  in hydrocephalus, 558
  in IBD, 583
  in JRA, 601
  in kidney disease, 621
  legislation for, 61t
  in mood disorders, 648
  in muscular dystrophy, 665–666
  in myelodysplasia, 681
  in obesity, 704
  after organ transplantation, 733
  outcome data for, 60, 61t
  in phenylketonuria, 750
  after prematurity, 768
  in seizures, 508–509
  in sickle cell disease, 789–790
  after traumatic brain injury, 824
  in TS/OCD, 808–809
  unsuccessful, 60

Note: Page numbers followed by b, f, and t indicate boxes, figures and tables, respectively.

834